Gynecologic and Obstetric Surgery

GYNECOLOGIC AND OBSTETRIC SURGERY

EDITED BY

David H. Nichols, MD

Visiting Professor of Obstetrics, Gynecology, and Reproductive Biology
Harvard Medical School, Boston, Massachusetts

Past Professor and Chairman of Obstetrics and Gynecology
Brown University School of Medicine, Providence, Rhode Island

Chief of Pelvic Surgery
Vincent Memorial Gynecologic Service
Massachusetts General Hospital, Boston, Massachusetts

WITH 66 CONTRIBUTORS

with 1150 illustrations

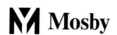 Mosby

St. Louis Baltimore Boston Chicago London Philadelphia Sydney Toronto

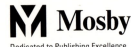

Mosby

Dedicated to Publishing Excellence

Senior Editor: Stephanie Manning
Developmental Editor: Barbara S. Menczer
Project Manager: Linda Clarke
Production Editor: Arofan Gregory
Cover Design: Susan Lane

Printed in the United States of America

Mosby–Year Book, Inc.
11830 Westline Industrial Drive
St. Louis, Missouri 63146

Library of Congress Cataloging in Publication Data

Gynecologic and obstetric surgery / edited by David H. Nichols; with
    66 contributors.
        p.   cm.
    Includes bibliographical references and index.
    ISBN 0-8016-6245-1
    1. Generative organs, Female—Surgery.   2. Obstetrics—Surgery.
I. Nichols, David H., 1925-   .
    [DNLM: 1. Delivery.   2. Genital Diseases, Female—surgery.
    3. Genitalia, Female—surgery.   4. Pregnancy Complications—surgery.
    5. Urinary Tract—surgery.   WP 660 G99557 1993]
RG104.G93   1993
618.0459—dc20
DNLM/DLC
for Library of Congress   92-48463
                                                               CIP

93 94 95 96 97 CL/MY 9 8 7 6 5 4 3 2 1

CONTRIBUTORS

Lejla V. Adamyan, M.D.
Head of Operative Gynecology Department
All-Union Scientific-Research Center
    for Maternal and Child Health Care
Moscow, Russia

Joseph F. Amaral, M.D.
Assistant Professor of Surgery
Brown University School of Medicine
Rhode Island Hospital
Providence, Rhode Island

Professeur Pierre Arnould
Université Claude Bernard
Service de Gynecologie-Obstetrique
Hospital Edouarde Herriot
Lyon, France

Michael S. Baggish, M.D.
Professor of Obstetrics and Gynecology
University of Illinois School of Medicine;
    Chairman
Department of Obstetrics and Gynecology
Ravenswood Hospital Medical Center
Chicago, Illinois

Hugh R.K. Barber, M.D.
Professor of Clinical Obstetrics-Gynecology
Cornell University Medical College;
Director
Department of Obstetrics and Gynecology
Lenox Hill Hospital
New York, New York

David L. Barclay, M.D.
Clinical Professor of Obsetrics and Gynecology
University of Arkansas for Medical Sciences
Little Rock, Arkansas

Douglas Brown, Ph.D.
Ethics Research and Curriculum Consultant
Department of Obstetrics and Gynecology
Louisiana State University Medical Center
New Orleans, Louisiana

Erich Burghardt, M.D.
Professor and Chairman
Department of Obstetrics and Gynecology
University of Graz
Graz, Austria

†**Luigi Carenza,** M.D.
Professor and Chairman
Department of Obstetrics and Gynecology
University of Rome
Rome, Italy

Marshall W. Carpenter, M.D.
Associate Professor of Obstetrics and Gynecology
Brown University;
Director of Maternal-Fetal Medicine
Women and Infants Hospital of Rhode Island
Providence, Rhode Island

Donald R. Coustan, M.D.
Professor and Chairman of Obstetrics and Gynecology
Brown University;
Obstetrician and Gynecologist-in-Chief
Women and Infants Hospital of Rhode Island;
Surgeon-in-Chief
Rhode Island Hospital
Providence, Rhode Island

Professeur Daniel Dargent
Université Claude Bernard
Service de Gynecologie-Obstetrique
Hopital Edouard Herriot
Lyon, France

Professor Sir John Dewhurst
Emeritus Professor of Obstetrics and Gynecology
University of London
Institute of Obstetrics and Gynecology
Queen Charlotte's Maternity Hospital
Harefield, Middlesex, England

William J. Dignam, M.D.
Professor
Department of Obstetrics and Gynecology
University of California, Los Angeles School of Medicine
Los Angeles, California

Raphael Durfee, M.D.
Retired Professor of Reproductive Medicine
University of California School of Medicine
San Diego, California

Thomas E. Elkins, M.D.
Professor and Chair
Department of Obstetrics and Gynecology
Louisiana State University Medical Center
New Orleans, Louisiana

†Deceased.

Sebastian Faro, M.D., Ph.D.

Professor
Department of Obstetrics and Gynecology
Baylor College of Medicine
Houston, Texas

Augusto G. Ferrari, M.D.

Professor
Milano, Italy

Celso-Ramón García, M.D.

William Shippen, Jr. Emeritus Professor of Obstetrics and Gynecology
Department of Obstetrics and Gynecology
University of Pennsylvania Medical Center
Philadelphia, Pennsylvania

Frank Girardi, M.D.

Department of Obstetrics and Gynecology
University of Graz
Graz, Austria

Robert M. Goldwyn, M.D.

Clinical Professor of Surgery
Harvard Medical School;
Head
Division of Plastic Surgery
Beth Israel Hospital
Boston, Massachusetts

A. Gerson Greenburg, M.D., Ph.D.

Professor of Surgery
Chairman (acting)
Department of Surgery
Brown University;
Chief of Surgery
The Miriam Hospital
Providence, Rhode Island

Reginald Hamlin, M.D.

Addis Ababa Fistula Hospital
Addis Ababa, Ethiopia

Charles B. Hammond, M.D.

E.C. Hamblen Professor and Chairman
Department of Obstetrics and Gynecology
Duke University Medical Center
Durham, North Carolina

Ronald E. Hempling, M.D.

Associate Program Director
Department of Gynecologic Oncology
Roswell Park Cancer Institute
Buffalo, New York

Jaroslav F. Hulka, M.D.

Professor
Department of Reproductive Endocrinology
University of North Carolina School of Medicine
Chapel Hill, North Carolina

Robert B. Hunt, M.D.

Clinical Instructor
Department of Obstetrics and Gynecology
Harvard Medical School
Boston, Massachusetts

W. Glenn Hurt, M.D.

Professor
Department of Obstetrics and Gynecology
Medical College of Virginia School of Medicine
Virginia Commonwealth University
Richmond, Virginia

Neil D. Jackson, M.D.

Department of Gynecology
Massachusetts General Hospital
Boston, Massachusetts

Jacqueline C. Johnson, M.D.

Gynecologic Oncology Fellow
Georgetown University
Washington, DC;
Department of Obstetrics and Gynecology
Lennox Hill Hospital
New York, New York

Charles M. Jones III, M.D.

Assistant Professor
Department of Obstetrics and Gynecology
Medical College of Virginia School of Medicine
Virginia Commonwealth University
Richmond, Virginia

Raymond A. Lee, M.D.

Professor of Obstetrics and Gynecology
Chair, Division of Gynecologic Surgery
Mayo Medical School
Rochester, Minnesota

John L. Lewis, Jr., M.D.

Chief, Gynecology Service
Memorial Sloan-Kettering Cancer Center
New York, New York

Ankica Lukic, M.D.

Assistant of Obstetrics and Gynecology
University of Rome "La Sapienza"
Rome, Italy

L. Russell Malinak, M.D.

Professor
Department of Obstetrics and Gynecology
Baylor College of Medicine
Houston, Texas

Charles M. March, M.D.

Professor
Department of Obstetrics and Gynecology
University of Southern California School of Medicine
Los Angeles, California

Douglas J. Marchant, M.D.

Professor
Department of Obstetrics and Gynecology
Brown University School of Medicine
Providence, Rhode Island

Dan C. Martin, M.D.

Reproductive Surgeon
Baptist Memorial Hospital;
Clinical Associate Professor
Department of Obstetrics and Gynecology
University of Tennessee, Memphis
Memphis, Tennessee

John J. Mikuta, M.D.

Franklin Payne Professor and Director
Division of Gynecologic Oncology
Department of Obstetrics and Gynecology
University of Pennsylvania Medical Center
Philadelphia, Pennsylvania

George W. Mitchell, Jr., M.D.

Professor
Department of Obstetrics and Gynecology
The University of Texas Health Science Center at San Antonio
San Antonio, Texas

Colonel Kunio Miyazawa, M.D.

Professor
Department of Obstetrics and Gynecology
Uniformed Services University of the Health Sciences
F. Edward Hebert School of Medicine
Bethesda, Maryland

George W. Morley, M.D.

Associate Chairman and
Norman F. Miller Professor
Gynecologic Oncology
Department of Obstetrics and Gynecology
University of Michigan Medical School
Ann Arbor, Michigan

John D. Nash, M.D.

Chairman
Department of Obstetrics and Gynecology
National Naval Medical Center;
Assistant Professor
Uniformed Services
University of the Health Sciences
Bethesda, Maryland

Beth E. Nelson, M.D.

Professor and Director of Gynecologic Oncology
Department of Obstetrics and Gynecology
University of Massachusetts Medical Center
Worcester, Massachusetts

James H. Nelson, Jr., M.D.

Professor and Director
Department of Gynecologic Oncology
New York Medical College
Westchester County Medical Center
Valhalla, New York

Catherine Nicholson, M.D.

Addis Ababa Fistula Hospital
Addis Ababa, Ethiopia

Flavia Nobili, M.D.

Assistant of Obstetrics and Gynecology
University of Rome "La Sapienza"
Rome, Italy

John R. Oliver, M.D.

Clinical Instructor
Department of Obstetrics and Gynecology
University of Southern California
Los Angeles, California

Robert C. Park, M.D.

Department of Obstetrics and Gynecology
Walter Reed Army Medical Center
Washington, DC

Richard H. Paul, M.D.

Department of Obstetrics and Gynecology
Women's Hospital
Los Angeles, California

Samantha M. Pfeifer, M.D.

Research Fellow in Reproductive Endocrinology and Infertility
University of Pennsylvania Medical Center
Philadelphia, Pennsylvania

M. Steven Piver, M.D.

Chief
Department of Gynecologic Oncology
Roswell Park Cancer Institute
Clinical Professor
Division of Gynecologic Oncology
State University of New York at Buffalo
Buffalo, New York

Warren C. Plauché, M.D.

Professor and Associate Dean for Clinical Affairs
Department of Obstetrics and Gynecology
Louisiana State University School of Medicine
New Orleans, Louisiana

Gunther Reiffenstuhl, M.D.

Professor
Department of Obstetrics and Gynecology
Baden, Austria
Former Director University Clinic
Munster, Westfalen, Germany
Salzburg, Austria

A. Cullen Richardson, M.D.

Assistant Professor
Department of Obstetrics and Gynecology
Emory University School of Medicine
Atlanta, Georgia

Daniel K. Roberts, M.D., Ph.D.

Professor and Chairman
Department of Obstetrics and Gynecology;
Professor
Department of Pathology
University of Kansas School of Medicine, Wichita;
Chief, Obstetrics/Gynecology Service
HCA/Wesley Medical Center
Wichita, Kansas

Stephen C. Rubin, M.D.

Gynecology Service
Memorial Sloan-Kettering Cancer Center
New York, New York

Devereux N. Saller, Jr., M.D.

Assistant Professor of Obstetrics and Gynecology
University of Rochester
Rochester, New York

Peter E. Schwartz, M.D.

Professor
Director, Gynecologic Services
Department of Obstetrics and Gynecology
Yale University
New Haven, Connecticut

Seymour I. Schwartz, M.D.

Professor and Chairman
Department of Surgery
University of Rochester School of Medicine
Rochester, New York

Sumner A. Slavin, M.D.

Assistant Clinical Professor of Surgery
Harvard Medical School;
Associate in Plastic and Reconstructive Surgery
Beth Israel Hospital
Boston, Massachusetts

John T. Soper, M.D.

Associate Professor
Division of Gynecologic Oncology
Department of Obstetrics and Gynecology
Duke University Medical Center
Durham, North Carolina

Phillip G. Stubblefield, M.D.

Professor
Department of Obstetrics and Gynecology
University of Vermont College of Medicine
Chief of Obstetrics and Gynecology
Maine Medical Center
Portland, Maine

Richard Turner-Warwick, M.D.

Senior Surgeon
The Middlesex Hospital;
Senior Urological Surgeon
St. Peter's Hospitals Group;
Senior Lecturer
The London University Institute of Urology
London, England

James M. Wheeler, M.D.

Assistant Professor
Department of Obstetrics and Gynecology
Baylor College of Medicine
Houston, Texas

Robert Zacharin, M.D.

Consultant Gynecologist
Alfred Hospital;
Consultant to the Royal Australian Navy
Melbourne, Victoria, Australia

PREFACE

"A little learning is a dang'rous thing;
Drink deep, or taste not the Pierian spring:
There shallow draughts intoxicate the brain,
And drinking largely sobers us again."

ALEXANDER POPE

Knowing how to perform surgery is important, but knowing *when, what,* and *why* to perform it is even more important.

Gynecologic surgeons must master fundamental technical skills and develop sound decision-making ability in order to select and implement appropriate surgical solutions to problems encountered in obstetrics and gynecology—the health care of women. This text addresses these needs as a compendium of currently recognized indications and techniques for both transabdominal and transvaginal surgical procedures.

There are numerous surgical publications available to the professional practitioner; however, long, all-inclusive reference works, atlases of operations, and presentations of personal opinion are less than satisfactory as textbooks for gynecologic surgery. Responding to the need for a text designed to promote clinical effectiveness in gynecologic surgery, I have focused this work on (1) surgical principles and techniques (some of relatively recent vintage that the reader may not have learned during residency), and (2) decision-making skill, the ability to choose the most appropriate among several surgical alternatives (the operation that best fits the needs of a particular patient).

All the operations described in this book are currently recommended and performed. I believe that the gynecologic surgeon's familiarity with these procedures will provide a framework for the day-to-day practice of gynecologic surgery and will stimulate the development of solutions to most of the troublesome surgical problems that arise both in the operating room and in clinical practice.

Pelvic disease and genital anomalies are truly international in distribution and patient disability—just as are the solutions to these problems. I believe that the observations and experiences of one national group of surgeons may be exportable and transferable to the surgeons of other nations whose subjects have the same disability and problems. Therefore among the contributors to this book are several providing an international perspective.

I share most of the gynecologic surgical views of the late Thomas Ball, author of *Gynecologic Surgery and Urology,* with whom I participated long ago in a lively correspondence and discussion of basic concepts and treatment options. Mosby has given a gracious and affirmative response to my request for reproduction of many of Ball's original drawings and plates. Chapter 72 was originally written by Thomas Ball, while he was an Associate Clinical Professor of Obstetrics and Gynecology at the University of California School of Medicine at Los Angeles. I have used his work as the basis for the chapter that appears here. These views, discussed over 30 years ago, are still relevant and timely, as are those of countless gynecologic surgeons throughout the world, reflecting upon the eternity and catholicism of these significant problems of women of all lands and places—past, present, and future. As we observe the sustained increase in life span over the past 90 years, the importance of quality of life as the redeeming feature of longevity becomes self-evident. When significant but surgically correctable urogynecologic problems exist that detract from this quality of life, their solution becomes the responsibility of the gynecologic surgeon. The solutions are dynamic in their identity, and the options for treatment are evolutionary. Many of the various available options for solutions are what this book is all about.

Well into an era of vastly increasing cost for hospitalization and surgery, it is necessary that, in order for appropriate surgical care to remain affordable, the right operation must be chosen for the right patient and expertly performed the first time. Reoperation is costly in time, suffering, risk, and money. Delivery of care correctly the first time can help keep our care affordable by the public and thus cost-effective.

This book, therefore, blends present practice with the proven lessons of the past and the surgical dreams of the future. It is in this context presented as one "state-of-the-art compendium" that covers perspectives for surgeons at all levels of training and experience.

ACKNOWLEDGMENTS

Assembling and phrasing my chapters for this manuscript would have been impossible without the patient and skilled editorial assistance of Gail Martin, the friendly pressures of Barbara Menczer, and the confident perspective of Elaine Steinborn. Mosby editor Stephanie Manning, who conveyed the initial invitation to do this book, has been patient beyond all understanding.

Some of the international chapters were submitted in their native language, and the translation skills of fellow physicians Samuel Levin, Joseph DeMartino, and Nicole Chavest were of timely and inestimable help.

Lori Vaskalis was recruited to execute much of the original artwork and taught me the simplistic beauty of transcontinental communication by fax for the preliminary sketches. John LaRiviere, near at hand, gave his assignments his undivided attention. Some of the previously published drawings of Daisy Stillwell, Melford Diedrick, and Allison Boiselle are gratefully reproduced.

Finally, I have drawn heavily upon my professional contacts with fellow surgeons the world over, as well as the study of their texts and of those of our predecessors. Although they are too numerous to mention, I wish to convey my grateful acknowledgment of their contributions.

David H. Nichols, M.D.

To
Lorraine
the best of the best

CONTENTS

PART V

SURGERY OF THE UPPER GENITAL TRACT

PART VI

**OPERATIONS FOR RESTORATION
OF FERTILITY**

COLOR PLATES

Part I

THE BASIS OF GYNECOLOGIC SURGERY

Chapter 1

HISTORY OF GYNECOLOGIC SURGERY

Raphael Durfee

The evolution of gynecologic surgery, as with other surgery, cannot succeed without the development of hemostasis, surgical anesthesia, and asepsis plus antisepsis. These depend on advances in (1) instruments, sutures, ligatures, and bandaging; (2) wound treatment; (3) the art of examination; (4) knowledge of human anatomy; (5) use of drugs; (6) awareness of physiologic principles; and (7) ability to pass such knowledge along through formal instruction. Operations on the human female pelvis deal with a highly vascular area, which can lead to extensive blood loss, and an area exquisitely sensitive to pain and especially vulnerable to infection. These factors had to be addressed to allow the successful development of gynecologic surgery.

This chapter explores the origins of current gynecologic surgical procedures. A list of suggested readings is included as a resource for readers who wish additional information.

SURGICAL MILESTONES

Initial medical care was heavily influenced by magic, astrology, religion, mythology, and the supernatural. These elements were separated from medicine only after many centuries. Yet the earliest accounts of manipulation of the human body, the most complicated of which we know as surgery, began with and have always included procedures associated with complicated childbirth.

The practice of surgery in the ancient world was characterized by practical responses to the situations found by observation of the patient. Although some medical knowledge was noted in early documents (Fig. 1-1), such as the Sushruta, most was passed along by word of mouth or by tradition.

Seventeenth century

Improvements in surgery, specifically gynecologic surgery, were stimulated by the Renaissance. The first major additions in terms of procedures and instruments were developed in the seventeenth century. For example, Trautmann, in 1600, performed the first successful cesarean operation, without anesthesia or asepsis. de Castro used a silk or horsehair suture dipped in aqua sublimati to ligate a hypertrophied clitoris; in addition, he excised a prolapsed uterus by daily increased tension on a ligature.

van Roonhuyze, the outstanding gynecologic surgeon of the seventeenth century, wrote the first text on gynecologic surgery, performed cesarean sections, described vaginal atresia and obstruction, reported a case of ruptured uterus, repaired vesicovaginal fistulae, extirpated totally prolapsed uteri, opened an obstructed urethra, and performed plastic surgery on a deformed urethra. He revived the method of wound drainage that was used by Greek surgeons and is considered by some to be the father of surgical gynecology.

Eighteenth century

Although this period did not see extensive advances in gynecologic surgical practice, some developments are of note, as listed here:

1. Excision of ovarian cysts found in extensive hernias was proposed.
2. Increased numbers of perineal lacerations were repaired successfully.
3. Abdominal tumefactions that contained abdominal pregnancies were opened and the contents were removed.
4. Intrapelvic abscesses were incised and drained, primarily through the vagina.

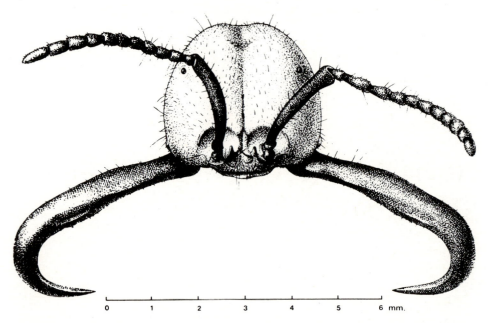

0 1 2 3 4 5 6 mm.

Fig. 1-1. The ant—the first surgical wound clip. (From the *Sushruta,* in Topoff HR: The social behaviour of army ants, *Scientific American,* Nov., 1972, Scientific American Inc., New York.)

Advances were also made in instrumentation.

The specific identification of gynecologic abnormalities was the foremost contribution of the eighteenth century. All kinds of uterine abnormalities, from congenital to positional to prolapses to cancer and benign tumors, were described. Vaginal relaxations without any terms attached were considered; variations of ectopic pregnancy were recognized and categorized. Urinary incontinence was differentially diagnosed, which revealed that there were causes other than vesicovaginal fistula.

Nineteenth century

The 1800s ushered in the explosive growth in the practice of surgery in gynecology. Although this was not as profound as the advances made in the twentieth century, much of the basis for modern gynecologic surgery was established at this time. Surgical methods evolved with some carryover from the 1700s, which included solutions to the three obstructions to operative therapy, specifically, problems of hemostasis, relief of pain, and antisepsis and asepsis.

Before the nineteenth century, gynecologic surgery was limited to the external genitalia, cervix and vagina, perineal lacerations, vesicovaginal fistula, ovariotomy on occasion, hysterectomy (although this was extremely hazardous), laparotomy (rarely), and incision and drainage of pelvic abscess. These were often beyond the limit of many surgeons, and failures were numerous.

In the early 1800s, interest was high in the etiology of uterine infection, malposition, and vaginal discharges. The first text of the era was devoted entirely to gynecologic surgery; it was fairly complete and well illustrated. The terms *anteflexion* and *retroflexion* were proposed.

In the nineteenth century, hemostasis was addressed, and many clamps and methods were devised for individual vessel ligation. Yet it remained for 20th century surgeons to perfect instruments and procedures for their use.

Twentieth century

The first 40 to 50 years of the 1900s were absorbed in the surgical treatment of many gynecologic problems and disease. Laparotomy had become just barely reasonable as had both vaginal and abdominal hysterectomy.

Knowledge of fallopian tube disease, endometriosis, and pelvic pain problems led to specific operations to treat some of the more common of these. The invention of the Bovie cautery in 1928 led to its use in the treatment of endometriosis and pelvic inflammatory disease. Improvements in surgical techniques were universal, with new instruments, improved sutures, self-retaining retractors, better surgeon's gloves, the use of sterile caps, and improved masks with sterile gowns and shoe covers and scrub clothes, all in the early 1900s, greatly reduced wound infection.

The establishment of residency programs and a well-developed examination in obstetrics and gynecology changed the capability of the surgeon immensely and created a true specialty. Bolstered by the American Board in the 1930s, gynecology became divorced from general surgery. By 1945, at least 75 to 100 procedures were generally used to treat the female pelvic organs.

The antibiotic era enlarged the scope of gynecologic surgery. The availability of blood from established blood banks further increased the amount and kind of gynecologic surgery that was attempted. Methods for sterilization were developed, and, in the 1950s, a simple, safe, and effective procedure for suction removal of uterine contents was introduced in England.

The many new diagnostic instruments and techniques opened up another entire area of surgical treatment. Laparoscopy, which followed culdoscopy in the middle 1900s, permitted a wide variety of operations in the pelvis, from new methods of tubal ligation to lysis of adhesions, treatment of pelvic inflammatory disease and endometriosis, excision of benign ovarian pathology, and several other procedures, even myomectomy. Posterior colpotomy and culdoscopy allowed the introduction of simple invasive pelvic operations. All of these were greatly enhanced, if not replaced, by laparoscopically-guided surgery. A final contribution was the innovation of laser surgery, which, combined with laparoscopy and hysteroscopy, has revolutionized much of gynecologic surgery.

Microsurgery was introduced into gynecology in the mid-1970s and has developed into a major area of expertise in gynecologic surgery. Residual tubal disease, pelvic adhesions, ectopic pregnancy, endometriosis, and many other pelvic problems are managed by combinations of the new methods. In vitro fertilization (IVF) and gamete intrafallopian transfer (GIFT) were made possible by ultrasonography (US). As an ancillary procedure, US facilitates all of these manipulations and has extended into even more exotic areas in the management of infertility difficulties, intrauterine fetal surgery, uterine excision, and ovarian transplantation, which is really in its infancy. Other methods of surgery in the female pelvis seem crude and bulky by comparison with microsurgery.

Progress has been made in the treatment of gynecologic cancer by surgical methods, but not at the same pace as the remainder of gynecology, primarily because of the characteristics of the disease. This is especially true in ovarian malignancy.

SPECIFIC AREAS
Diagnosis

Hysterosalpingography. The 1895 discovery of x-rays was quickly followed by discovery of many of their uses. For example, liquid bismuth was injected through the cervical canal to find a possible ectopic pregnancy, and collargol injection was used to diagnose uterine tumors as well as tubal patency. A delayed film was used to verify patency of the tube, and this technique combined with peritoneography came to be termed *hysterosalpingography* (HSG). Water-soluble Hypaque is used for hysterosalpingography, but a modified Lipiodol still has value in some cases for diagnosis and treatment of tubal obstruction. The technique has been improved with better cannulas, water-soluble injection media, local anesthesia for the cervix, relaxation premedication, possible use of antiprostaglandins, use of the fluoroscopic monitor together with a magnifier, cinematography, spot and delayed films, and image intensification. Combination with US increases the potential for this medium.

Cystoscopy. In 1805, Bozzini tried to visualize the interior of the urethra with a double catheter and candlelight; he was reprimanded by the Medical Society of Vienna, but this proved to be the origin of endoscopy. With improvements, the method was used to identify polyps in the uterine cavity in 1869. Nitze put a light and an endoscope together and made the first truly functional cystoscope that could be used for endoscopy in parts of the body other than the bladder. With the invention of the air cystoscope, gynecologic urology was born.

The Brown-Buerger water cystoscope has been the workhorse for the urologist and gynecologist. The use of CO_2 and placement of the patient in a lithotomy rather than the awkward knee-chest position were added in the 1970s. The visualization of the bladder through the clear, weightless medium was superb, but of even greater importance was the observation of the urethrovesical junction and the action of the bladder neck with passage of urine in normal and abnormal states. Voiding cystograms illustrated the passage of urine with absolute clarity. As a result, various forms of urinary incontinence can be identified and classified, even if the etiology is still in question, as is the act of the release of urine and the maintenence of continence.

Hysteroscopy. From its first use in 1880 until as recently as 1980, hysteroscopy has been regarded as everything from limited to dangerous. Serious visualization problems occurred, some related to insufficient dilation of the endometrial cavity and some to inadequate lighting. Difficulties with blood loss were also common.

The fiberoptic light introduced in the 1950s was a great improvement, but there was still the problem of blood. An ingenious balloon hysteroscope unfortunately pressed on the endometrium, causing blood to obstruct the view through the balloon wall and preventing any manipulation through the instrument. In 1968, use of a glass-fiber hysteroscope allowed visualization of a fetus, the inner surface of the uterine wall in pregnancy, the onset of labor, and the inner surface and lumen of the fallopian tube. Concentrated dextran, which is still in use today, was introduced in 1971, as was use of a cervical cap and CO_2. A colpohysteroscope, developed in 1979, revolutionized the applications of diagnostic hysteroscopy.

Culdoscopy. As early as 1898, posterior colpotomy incisions were used for the treatment of intrapelvic diseases. Endoscopic observation of the pelvic cavity originated in 1935, using the principle of negative intraabdominal pressure and the knee-chest position. The negative pressure distended the abdominal cavity for observation through the cul-de-sac attained by a posterior colpotomy incision, with a straight endoscope. Culdocentesis had been used for hundreds of years, and proximity of the posterior vaginal wall to the pouch of Douglas was a natural avenue for endoscopy. By 1942, this was pronounced a success and in 1944 the term *culdoscopy* was established. Photography was accomplished by 1953. However, because of the unwieldy position, difficulties with anesthesia, and somewhat limited observational capability, culdoscopy gave way to peritoneoscopy.

Laparoscopy. Laparoscopy, which is a much better term for the process of intraabdominal observation with distention, has eventually eliminated culdoscopy. As early as 1900, a cystoscope was inserted through a paracentesis wound. An abdominal endoscopy was performed with the patient in Trendelenburg's position, the first time a female pelvis underwent laparoscopy. Laparoscopy was used successfully for the diagnosis of ectopic pregnancy, for coagulation of fallopian tubes, for aspiration of ovarian and paraovarian cysts, for lysis of pelvic adhesions, and for identification of ruptured and unruptured ectopic pregnancies.

Despite the potential diagnostic and therapeutic impact, laparoscopy fell into disfavor for a few years. But Palmer, in 1947, published several cases of laparoscopy. The first atlas on laparoscopy was published in 1968, and the American Association of Gynecologic Laparoscopists was founded in 1972. Public courses of instruction were given, and the procedure became popular once again. Combined hysteroscopy and laparoscopy have proven invaluable in many cases; but, more importantly, the extent to which endoscopic surgery has expanded in the past 15 years is amazing. The impact of these procedures on the specialty of obstetrics and gynecology cannot be estimated, and the future possibilities remain limitless.

Ultrasonography. The use of ultrasound as a diagnostic medium developed as a spin-off from the studies of sonar (underwater sound) by the U.S. military in World War II, especially through the investigative committee for antisubmarine detection. It was first applied to the brain, and, in 1961, the first fetal head biparietal measurements were made. In the late 1900s ultrasound was used in combination with surgery. Vaginal ultrasound is better for the adnexal areas.

Papanicolaou vaginocervical smear and colposcopy. In 1943, Papanicolaou and Traut published a procedure that was to be one of the most important in contemporary times: the diagnosis of uterine cancer by the vaginal smear. This has been the most widespread, reliable, and inexpensive cancer screening device ever conceived. Refinements have been made in the manner of collection of material for the smears and to some extent in differential cytologic stains. The validity of the test is based on research establishing the fundamentals of cytology.

Invention of an optical instrument that permitted high magnification of the surface of the uterine cervix allowed development of a process named *colposcopy.* Earlier described cervical atypia had motivated production of this magnification instrument. The method was very popular in Europe. One of the difficulties with colposcopy was the confusion in terminology regarding the tissues observed.

Biopsy. Methods for cervical biopsy and uterine curettage of the endometrial cavity were not readily used until the 1900s. The use of cone biopsy, aside from abortion or for retained products of conception, was limited until the endocrine influence on uterine and cervical tissues came to be understood. Since then, not only has endometrial biopsy developed into a most valuable modality in the diagnosis of malignancy but it is also used to establish dates for endometrial response to hormones in the menstrual cycle. Defects in either tissue response or the nature and quantity of hormone secretion can also be determined. The development of suction curettage increased the degree to which intrauterine samples could be taken in an office situation and the small curettes first used have been refined. Gross biopsy of the cervix has improved with the creation of specialized instruments for the purpose.

Cone biopsy of the cervix became an integral part of the diagnosis of early or premalignant change (see discussion of conization on p. 15).

Ureteroscopy and tubaloscopy. Both of these procedures are products of the expertise of the late 1980s and early 1990s. The highly refined visualization instruments of contemporary times have led to exploration of both the ureter and the fallopian tube lumens to an extensive degree. Internal tubal pathology can be visualized to such an extent that decisions as to therapy are possible.

Instruments

Vaginal speculum. The design of the vaginal speculum has varied dramatically over the centuries. Among the earliest was a complicated speculum that consisted of four blades that tapered inward and were attached to a ring. The blades had four rods attached to them and, with outside pressure, they opened inside the vagina.

The laser. Development of the laser was based on the quantum theory of Planck (1900) and Bohr's description of the energy system in the hydrogen atom (1913). The development of the gaseous laser had particular application in medicine, with the CO_2 and YAG lasers proving the most useful in gynecology. Colposcopy is essential for use of the laser for the cervix. Laparoscopy combined with the laser allows the delivery of treatment in several kinds of pelvic disease. It is widely used for vulvar as well cervical disease and has been used in the treatment of VAIN in the vagina.

Laser photoradiation treatment for various cancers of the genital tract has been used since 1982. The more promising areas of laser surgery are infertility and debilitating pelvic disease (endometriosis). The following are some of the operations that use the laser that have been of great benefit:

1. In mid-segment tubal obstruction for anastomosis
2. In proximal and distal tubal occlusion
3. Lysis of adhesions
4. Endometriosis ablation
5. Myomectomy and plastic operations of the uterus
6. Laser combined with microsurgery
7. Hysteroscopic laser total ablation of the endometrium
8. Laser resection of Asherman's adhesions
9. Laser resection of intrauterine septa

These were all introduced in the 1980s. Clearly the future holds incredible possibilities for the application of lasers in gynecology.

Hemostasis

The control of blood loss is one of the most important factors in the development of gynecologic surgery because of the intense vascularity of the female pelvic area. Yet it took many years to produce the simple process of ligation of a blood vessel, even though ancient people developed remarkable capability with the bandage and showed surprising inventiveness with the creation of surgical instruments. The concept of the tourniquet was established but not applied for hemostasis. Manual compression and pressure with tight wrapping with pliable materials was the extent of hemostasis in early times, but it is probable that other materials were applied to a wound that bled.

Greco-Roman medicine, which included the Alexandrian school, was advanced for its time, and used ligation to accomplish hemostasis (Fig. 1-2). Hot iron cautery or boiling oil were also used to control blood loss.

The origin of the hemostatic forceps may well have been described by Erasistratus, who stated that a lead forceps used for dental purposes was in the temple of the oracle at Delphi. A much finer and smaller forceps was greatly needed. The Roman tenaculum was revived and soon was generally used to pull up a vessel for ligation; it was modified to become a ligature carrier. A dissection forceps was developed out of similar necessity, and a device for holding it closed was added. In about 1829, surgeons began twisting the cut ends of vessels with a square-beaked forceps with two nuts and a bar that moved.

For the remainder of the 1800s, surgeons followed the principle for forci-pressure and clamps. Another contribution to the application of ligature was, of course, the use of sterilized, chromacized catgut by Lister.

Hemostasis in the modern sense began with Pare and his invention of the clamp known as the "bec de corbin" (Fig. 1-3) or "raven's beak." In the years that followed, variations were invented such as a "crane's bill forceps" with long pincers. Many devices were created to manage the stump of the ovarian pedicle after ovariotomy; one example is Cintrat's constrictor (Fig. 1-4). The further pursuit of a compression forceps brought about crude instruments for constriction of the blood vessels, such as the use of two wooden pieces tied with cord.

The development of the hemostatic clamp was enhanced in the United States by Halsted with the introduction of a fine-nosed, small instrument and clear emphasis on the techniques of arterial ligation, both free and within tissue.

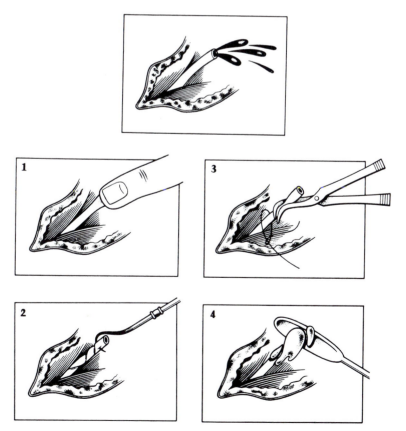

Fig. 1-2. Hemostasis methods by Galen. (From Majno G: *The healing hand*, Cambridge, Mass, 1975, Harvard University Press.)

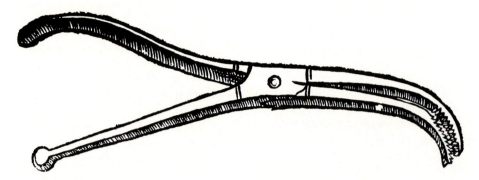

Fig. 1-3. Hemostatic clamp "bec de corbin." (From Pare A: *The collected works of Ambrose Pare,* Pound Ridge, New York, 1968, Milford House [Translated by T Johnson].)

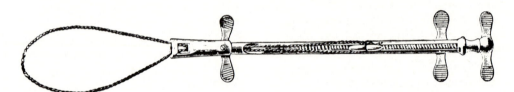

Fig. 1-4. Pedicle constrictor by Cintrat. (From Doyen E: *Surgical therapeutics and operative technique,* vol 1, New York, 1917, William Wood [Translated by H Spencer-Browne].)

Cautery

There are many illustrations of the various kinds of cautery instruments used throughout surgical history. One thing they all shared was unimaginable pain.

In the early 1900s, Cushing devised a silver clip for vessel occlusion, which was modified to steel and presently tantalum or tellurium for this purpose. Together with Bovie, Cushing developed the "sparking" device that used controlled electricity. Since 1928, the Bovie machine, with modifications, has been the instrument of choice for cautery in gynecologic surgery, especially pelvic surgery. Despite the efficiency of the Bovie machine, broad areas of constant discharge of blood have required the added control of various substances, including treated cottons and substances such as Gel-Foam. More recently, other substances have been created to produce local hemostasis without forming adhesions.

Blood replacement

Early in the twentieth century, Nuttal established the identification of different kinds of blood by a precipitin test, Landsteiner described the blood groups, and blood transfusions were made practical. This discovery has been greatly improved with the discovery of the Rh factor and many more tests of blood.

Position

The physical placement of a woman in a position to allow the approach to her external and internal genitalia for surgery or examination is essential. Records of early Hindu medicine illustrated a basic position for this purpose. There are also illustrations in the records of ancient Greece indicating both the wide lithotomy position for removal of a bladder stone and fixation of a woman to a ladder with inversion of her body for succussion to reduce pelvic organ prolapse.

The lithotomy position was adapted in numerous ways in the 1800s (Fig. 1-5). One of the problems with lithotomy was the uncomfortable manner of support for the legs when an assistant was unavailable. Several ingenious devices were created to meet this need, ranging from complicated mechanical apparatus to simple bands mounted on a steel vertical bar. Other positions were developed for gynecology—Sim's, extended lithotomy, knee-chest, low lithotomy, Trendelenberg, and supine.

Anesthesia

The ancient recorded instances of the use of anesthetic agents are few. In Greece about 1000 years BC, "nepenthe" was used to anesthetize patients for surgery, and Helen of Troy used a form of opium dissolved in wine to produce insensibility. In India, a drug named "samohini," presumably a narcotic herb or a combination of herbs, was used to put a patient to sleep; another drug named "samojani," apparently a stimulant, was used to awaken the patient. Mention has also been made of the use of henbane and hashish for anesthesia and another drug to reverse their action. In China (225 BC), wine loaded with hashish was used for pain relief during surgery.

"Sweet vitriol" (later named ether) was apparently dis-

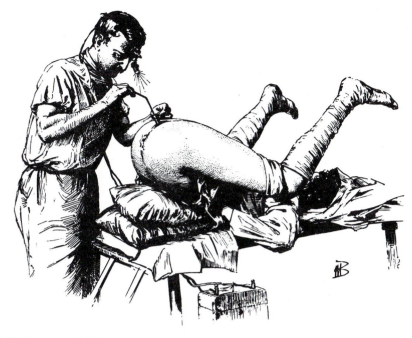

Fig. 1-5. Exaggerated lithotomy for air cystoscopy. (From Kelly H: *Operative gynecology,* vol 1, New York, 1902, D. Appleton.)

covered in Spain, but it was Paracelsus in 1540 who described the potential for insensibility of the mixture (sulfuric acid and alcohol); it was not named for almost 200 years. Paracelsus also described the value of a mixture of opium and alcohol known as "laudanum."

Anesthesia in the 1600s was attempted by the use of cold and compression. Mesmer introduced a form of hypnosis to produce lack of sensibility to pain. Oxygen and nitrous oxide were discovered in the late 1700s, and experiments were done with the inhalation of nitrous oxide ("laughing gas") that produced a loss of cerebral control, a concept that led to the development of inhalation anesthesia.

Morphine was extracted from opium in 1806; ether was inhaled to allay painful stimuli; and chloroform was discovered in 1831. During the mid-eighteenth century in the United States, various uses of ether and nitrous oxide were demonstrated, with a public presentation of surgery under ether anesthesia at the Massachusetts General Hospital. Also at this time, ether and chloroform were used to ease the pain of childbirth, which was promoted by Simpson in England. Morphine was introduced as a preanesthetic medication, and cyclopropane was suggested for anesthesia. Corning used cocaine for epidural anesthesia, which led to the use of spinal anesthesia. In 1899, Tuffier developed "twilight sleep" for management of the pain of labor, which often proved lethal for the child.

Caudal anesthesia was promoted in the early twentieth century. Continuous caudal anesthesia was introduced in 1942, and, with the development of continuous epidural anesthesia, pain control in labor could be extended to ce-

sarean section. The intravenous use of pentothal was further developed in the early 1900s and became almost routine when its safety was ensured by the development of intratracheal intubation. Nitrous oxide and cyclopropane have been made practical, and many newer agents have been used successfully for pain relief.

Asepsis

Based on the improvements in the microscope, the discoveries and theories of Pasteur, the development of the etiology of postpartum sepsis (streptococci), and the support of this theory, Lister in 1869 introduced the concept of sterility needed for all aspects of surgery, which included the patient's skin.

The introduction of sterile gloves by Halsted in the late nineteenth century facilitated the prevention of infection during surgery. This was followed by the use of the surgical mask, which prevents contamination of a surgical wound by personnel in the surgical suite. The evolution of the surgical uniform soon followed, with caps, shoe covers, scrub suits, gowns and tight-fitting gloves. This completed the improvement in prevention of outside contamination of surgical wounds.

The steam autoclave eliminated another potential area for bacterial contamination with surgery by high temperature sterilization of all materials to come into contact with the patient. Elaborate skin preparation, including removal of body hair the night before surgery, was simplified by the use of iodine preparations, which are highly effective skin cleaners. Body hair is frequently not removed at all or only in minimal amounts at the present time.

The surgeon's scrub techniques, also once long and arduous with soaps and dips with bacteriostatic solutions, have been reduced by the use of modern chemicals; studies have indicated a proper, easier method for satisfactory, virtually bacteria-free hands and fingernails. However, none of this compares with the cataclysmic advent of the antibiotic era, which began in the 1920s and 1930s and crystallized in the 1940s with the sulfa drugs, penicillins, mycotics, and others. These medications, properly used, have revolutionized all surgery and especially gynecologic surgery. Although the vagina, by its structure and location, has never been bacteria free, the use of antibiotic drugs has greatly reduced the threat of sepsis. Prophylactic antibiotics, although still a controversial subject, have probably reduced morbidity by a high degree, as demonstrated in many studies of vaginal hysterectomy or suspected uterine or tubal infections. Postoperative antibiotics used as indicated have been even more effective in the management of wounds and infections.

Disorders
Fallopian tube disease

Ectopic pregnancy. Extrauterine pregnancy was known in ancient times, with accounts of abdominal pregnancy found for at least 1000 years. In addition, the contents of spontaneous drainage from abdominal abscesses usually from near the umbilicus, very commonly contained decomposed fetal elements. Almost all ectopic pregnancies were found at the time of anatomic dissection, which was when the first lithopedion was described, or at a postmortem autopsy, which is when tubal ectopics were recognized.

In the mid-1800s, laparotomy was suggested for ectopic pregnancy; however, this was disregarded in favor of exotic methods for destruction of the tubal fetus, which ranged from poisons, to hormones, to electricity. In 1883, a successful exploratory laparotomy and adnexectomy were performed. Once the surgery had been established for ruptured ectopic pregnancy, lives were saved by this procedure.

The development of a reliable pregnancy test improved the management of early ectopic pregnancy cases. Although the early urine test took too long to assist in cases of severe internal hemorrhage, it was helpful in nonemergent situations. With later developments, the rapidity and reliability of early pregnancy tests have not only saved lives, but fallopian tubal tissues as well. Contemporary tests are read in minutes and can be performed anywhere.

The etiology and management of extrauterine gestation were reassessed in 1976. Several reports have noted the success of laparoscopic diagnosis and management for early unruptured tubal ectopics. Early diagnosis and conservative treatment have reduced mortality from this problem to nearly nothing except in Third World countries.

Pelvic inflammatory disease. Inflammation and severe pelvic infections have been recognized for several hundred years and were attributed ordinarily to cellulitis of the uterus. Tubal involvement was always secondary and was rarely diagnosed by pelvic examination. Hunter in 1775 was the first to recognize chronic tubal infections. Various other reports appeared, but it was neither recognized nor accepted as involving the pelvis primarily; rather the uterus was always considered the primary infected organ.

Pelvic abscesses that pointed into the vagina had been incised and drained since before the Middle Ages, a practice continuing until the early 1800s (Fig. 1-6). The concept of conservative preservation of the ovaries with tubal excision and salpingostomies with the idea of preserving fertility found support.

In the United States, the first laparotomy for salpingitis was done in 1887 with excision of just one tube; a bilateral adnexectomy and hysterectomy were also done at the same time. This radical procedure came to be accepted by several surgeons in both the United States and Europe.

Hot cautery was also used for hemostasis. From 1886 until 1890, several different surgeons in both the United States and Europe treated pyosalpingitis and hydrosalpingitis with surgery and drainage.

Partial adnexal removal proved ineffective, and severe bilateral disease was treated by supravaginal hysterectomy. Conservative cures were lengthy, and frequently recurrence of the infection ultimately resulted in a "pelvic clean-out." This was widespread and severely debilitated the patient. Antibiotics revolutionized the treatment of pelvic inflammatory disease and allowed for much more conservative surgery. Techniques improved in tuboplasty and reached a high level with the introduction of microtubal surgery.

Much of the severe, irreversible adnexal disease is no longer seen except in Third World countries. The role of pelvic and tubal infection in the etiology of tubal ectopic pregnancy became well recognized in the twentieth century, and therapeutic surgery for pelvic inflammatory disease was performed with this in mind.

Pelvic organ prolapse. This gynecologic problem is one of the oldest on record, even earlier than vesicovaginal fistula, which has been demonstrated in an Egyptian mummy. Uterine prolapse, including inversion, was treated in several ways, ranging from pleasant medications to entice the uterus back into the abdominal cavity, to odorous ones to drive it up into place, to one method in which the woman was inverted and shaken severely. Hundreds of combinations of materials have been placed in the vagina and the woman's legs tied together sometimes for long periods of time. Probably the first pessary was one half of a sun-dried pomegranate. Ancient medical documents are filled with prescriptions of all kinds for treatment of pelvic organ prolapse.

By the time of the Renaissance, diagnoses of genital prolapse were made with greater accuracy and the specifics of the insertion of pessaries were demonstrated. Very little progress was made until the 1800s when interest in the

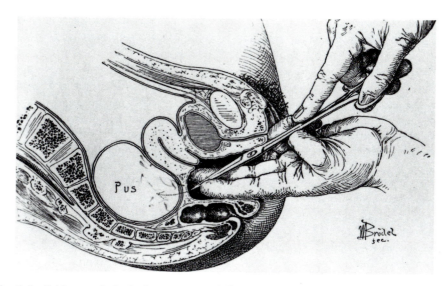

Fig. 1-6. Culdocentesis for both treatment and diagnosis. (From Kelly H: *Operative gynecology,* vol 2, New York, 1902, D. Appleton.)

subject was high; differentiation of the kind of prolapse was made and congenital prolapse, even in children, was identified.

Surgical procedures began to be developed in the 1800s; one of the first was a vaginal constriction operation. Later mucosal denudation and bringing of the round ligaments up through the inguinal canal were used. The term for procedures associated with vaginal mucosa was *elytrorrhaphy*. The vaginal walls were burned with cautery and caustic chemicals and even purposely infected to produce dense scars to cure the prolapse. The vulva and labia were attacked in the 1840s and 1850s. Forms of infibulation and several methods of suture of the labia that included apposition were used. The use of cautery and permanent silver sutures together with all of the above were eventually abandoned, but not until after some women were terribly tortured.

In the middle 1800s, there was a return to cervical amputation and destruction by pressure to produce a heavy cicatrix at the vaginal apex. Perineoplastic surgery was also advocated. Sims in 1866 described a cystocele and inadvertently performed an anterior vaginal repair that resembled the technique used in modern times. In 1877, Le Fort introduced his vaginal occlusion operation, which has survived to contemporary times. There were many complicated combined operations in the late 1800s.

Hadra in 1884 introduced the idea that obstetric injury to the pelvic structures was the probable etiology of pelvic organ prolapse. A combined multiple procedure was created, with amputation of the cervix and imbrication of the uterine ligaments into the vaginal apex with silver wires. The operation was modified by Fothergill in 1908 and came to be known as the "Manchester operation"; it was

very popular in England but not in the United States. Kelly suggested anterior and posterior repairs; his suburethral Lembert style stitch tightened the urethrovesical junction and has proved to be the best method for the restoration of urinary continence in cases of symptomatic cystocele. Almost all vaginal repairs use some form of the Kelly suture.

The first vaginal hysterectomy for the treatment of prolapse was done in 1861, the first suprapubic suspension of the vagina in 1890. Abdominal hysterectomy has been used for prolapse, and the broad and cardinal ligaments have been shortened and imbricated into the cervical stump.

Vaginal prolapse proved to be difficult to correct. Uterine inversion was seriously considered but rejected because of the mortality associated with it. Several methods for both manual and instrument reduction of the inversion were suggested, some of which were very strange. Vaginal surgery with reversion to cervix amputation in chronic cases was used, as was an abdominal operation.

Surgery for pelvic organ prolapse increased in the twentieth century. Operations were done simply because the tissues hung down into or out of the vagina, or because the prolapsed tissues produced severe symptoms of pain and pressure. Also, some were associated with urinary incontinence with or without difficult defecation. Much of the surgery was associated with vaginal hysterectomy for prolapse with asymptomatic anterior and posterior vaginal relaxation. In these cases, a token anterior and posterior vaginal repair was recommended without extensive dissection.

Overcorrection of the posterior vagina and perineum resulted in criticism of posterior vaginal repairs. Recently there have been careful corrections of this error. Prophylactic procedures for the prevention of recurrence of uterine or vaginal prolapse have also been done.

Enterocele and massive vaginal prolapse. Enterocele, which is the true pelvic hernia, was adequately described in the 1800s. As early as 1912, surgery was suggested for the correction of enterocele together with other vaginal wall relaxations. An abdominal procedure was developed for elevation of the rectum, which works equally well for obliteration of cul-de-sac hernias in women. Although transvaginal colpopexy was first reported in 1892, it lay forgotten until rediscovered in 1951 by an operation that obliterated the cul-de-sac and repaired the hernia. Before the 1950s, enterocele repairs were usually done vaginally. In general, these followed the basic surgical principles of herniorrhaphy anywhere. By the mid-1960s, postoperative vaginal prolapse was sometimes treated by colpocleisis and vaginectomy. The Le Fort operations were used frequently for these problems, but had been modified so that much more vaginal mucosa was removed than in the initial procedure. Prophylactic imbrication of the sacrouterine ligaments at the time of hysterectomy was suggested to prevent formation of an enterocele, and fascia lata strips were used to correct enterocele or the prolapsed vagina. Other recent surgeries include an abdominal surgery for vaginal and uterine prolapse; a composite vaginal vault suspension with fascia lata; pulsion enterocele and use of a levator muscle plication with vaginal vault fixation for repair of vaginal prolapse or enterocele; and uterosacral ligament and cardinal ligament suspension of the vagina. A unique, simple vaginal suspension by use of specially placed nonabsorbable suture through the vaginal apex and the sacrospinous ligament has been especially effective. Variations of these techniques have been implemented over the past 10 to 15 years with the addition of Dacron tape supports for the relaxed pelvic organs and the continued use of Marlex mesh slings and replacement of destroyed support in the pelvis.

Endometriosis. Endometriosis probably was first described by Rokitansky in 1861 when he referred to a complicated term for an adenomatous cystosarcoma of uterine tissue origin in the ovary. Russell described endometriosis as aberrant portions of the müllerian duct found in an ovary. Sampson in 1921 described endometriosis and its possible etiology in a landmark article. Aside from adhesions and carcinoma in the pelvis, this was a fairly common but not recognized disease.

The use of hysterectomy for endometriosis has allowed ovarian preservation, but this has been a point of contention for several years. Description of the anatomy of the pelvic autonomic nerves identified the proper tissue to be removed with presacral neurectomy, a procedure designed to relieve pain in the pelvis, including that caused by endometriosis. Several studies of endometriosis have observed the effect of suppressive hormones on the disease (1950 to 1962). Numerous definitive surgical procedures have been proposed for the treatment of pelvic endometriosis. In contemporary times, combined hormone therapy,

laser, and microsurgery have continued the therapeutic approach to this apparently increased disease.
Fistula
Vesicovaginal fistula. This entity has been one of the worst nonlethal occurrences in gynecology. It has often been difficult to diagnose and always difficult to treat. Van Roonhuyse was one of the few in the past who was successful with surgery for this problem. In the 1700s, very little could be done; Desault in 1799 provided the prevalent views of the time for management of the fistula: the use of a lint, a wax vaginal pessary, and an inlying bladder catheter.

In 1834, Gosset enunciated the basic principles of the surgical treatment of vesicovaginal fistula. With the patient in the knee-chest position, the fistula edges were freshened, interrupted sutures of gilded wire were twisted closed, a catheter was left in the bladder, and the patient remained in a prone position postoperatively. This combination was forgotten until Sims.

It remained, however, for Sims to provide the procedure of choice for many years. Sims placed his patient in the lateral prone position that carries his name, used silver sutures with lead bars and perforated shot, and was eminently successful. One of his followers, Emmet, had done more than 300 cases of both vesical and rectal vaginal fistulae by 1868 and achieved a very high success rate; Emmet is considered the first great vaginal plastic surgeon in the United States. In the late third of the nineteenth century, many modifications and additions were made, among them a repair of the fistula from the vesical side by Trendelenburg. Other improvements occurred in the twentieth century.

Rectovaginal fistula. Rectovaginal fistula was another entity known for a long time without acceptable treatment. Some of the surgery for this problem was associated with the information gained from the difficulties with repair of the totally ruptured perineum. These fistulae were categorized as due to obstetric trauma, syphilis, malignancy, or congenital disorder.

Over most of the eighteenth century, the concept was to consider the area a complete perineal rupture that included the fistula, and treat the entire area. A series of many operations were created for repair of the ruptured perineum. A form of dedoublement was used for this repair; such wide dissection allowed for the excellent apposition of tissues and also encouraged movement of the rectum, which disturbed the continuity of the fistula. When the fistula was high up in the vagina, the tissues were separated and the rectal side was sutured first with some displacement; then the vagina was closed so that the original tract was disrupted. Lembert sutures were placed in the fistulous orifice of the rectal wall, after a transverse incision, and then the vagina and perineum were closed by dedoublement. An autoplastic movable flap was created, and silver wire was frequently used for these procedures.

About 1880, a flap of vaginal mucosa was created to

cover the defect. This was improved in the early 1900s and, in modified form, is still used in modern practice.

Contemporary suture material has eliminated silver wire and encourages the process of repair due to reduced local tissue irritation.

Malignancy. In 1595, Schenck reported several rare lesions, including a large tumor that forced the vagina open and was successfully excised; a large ovarian tumor in an amenorrheic young girl; several congenital anomalies, among them a bicornuate uterus; and a tumor of the ovary filled with hair, wax, pus, and fluid. These are the first clear descriptions of ovarian carcinoma and dermoid cyst. Schenck used the term *molea aquea,* which probably was a hydatid mole; a mole described by de Vega in 1564 weighed 12 lb. Schenck described both fleshy mola and fibroids and the calcified variety.

Surgical treatment of gynecologic carcinoma was not a very successful enterprise until the twentieth century. Vulvar and clitoral disease was known to ancient surgeons, and the amputation or excision attempted was a miserable failure. Innumerable benign measures were made to cope with carcinoma, also to no avail. Amputation of prolapsed carcinomatous tissue has been done from time to time throughout the course of history. Many of these tissues were literally burned away with red iron cautery in a fashion similar to the treatment of breast tumors. Ovarian cancer was relieved by both vaginal and abdominal drainage with obvious failure.

Treatment of cervical malignancy was attempted more than other gynecologic cancers, perhaps partially because of its accessibility and the many variations of observable growth. Clark in 1812 first described an unusual change in the cervix that he called a cauliflower excrescence because of its appearance. Clarke introduced the term *carcinoma uteri* in 1821. It was not until Virchow in 1850 that the cellular nature of these cancers was recognized. By 1870, galvanocautery had been used for amputation because its use reduced blood loss immeasurably.

Vaginal hysterectomy was introduced for removal of a malignant uterus, and abdominal hysterectomy was also tried in an effort to cure the disease. These operations fostered the development of both types of uterine extirpation but did not affect the cancer. By 1888, the use of abdominal hysterectomy for both cervical and endometrial carcinoma had advanced considerably; at that time, Pawlik passed a catheter into the left ureter before a vaginal hysterectomy, providing some protection against ureteral trauma with the surgery. Catheterization of the ureters was not used again until 1892. Halsted's radical breast surgery in 1895 encouraged a more radical approach to the surgical treatment of both kinds of uterine cancer. Clark in 1895 performed a wide dissection abdominal hysterectomy and ligated the uterine arteries next to the internal iliac. He then dissected the ureter free and ligated the broad and cardinal ligaments as far lateral as possible; he did not remove the pelvic lymph nodes. Rumpf, however, actually

dissected the pelvic nodes in a live patient in 1895.

Kelly had used a straight tube cystoscope with the patient in the knee-chest position and passed catheters into both ureters before these extensive hysterectomies. Wertheim in 1900 performed a logical and meticulous radical hysterectomy for cervix cancer.

Endometrial carcinoma was recognized and accurately described in 1813, with fundal sarcoma identified in 1845. Virchow described carcinosarcoma of the fundus, and coexistent squamous and adenocarcinoma were identified by Kaumann in 1894. Vaginal hysterectomy had been done for endometrial carcinoma but most surgeons were more comfortable with abdominal hysterectomy, and some preferred to leave the adnexa intact.

Salpingitis isthmica nodosa was diagnosed by Chiari in 1887, who suspected possible malignancy and found an inflammatory lesion instead. In 1896, Cullen identified uterine adenomyosis; at one time this was thought to be carcinoma.

Ovarian pathology had been known for many years. Hodgkin in 1829 was the first to describe papillomatous ovarian growths. Virchow in 1848 developed some organization of ovarian pathology, but an entirely appropriate system has never been developed. Waldeyer in 1870 and Olshausen in 1877 established the histogenesis of ovarian tumors. Various benign and malignant ovarian tumors were described in the 1800s from papillary cystomata, the germ cell origin tumors, fibromas, hemorrhagic cysts, and corpus luteum cysts to sclerocystic ovaries. The management of these tumors is described in the sections on ovarian surgery.

Vulvar and vaginal carcinomas, although identified and locally treated by excision or cautery much earlier, were more adequately managed in the twentieth century. Wide local excision of the clitoris was popular for malignant and benign disease; in the early 1900s, a true radical vulvectomy was done for carcinoma of the clitoris, which established the possibility of this operation for all kinds of vulvar cancer, including carcinoma of Bartholin's gland. Lymph gland excision with this operation was also introduced.

Gynecologic pathology as divulged by persons such as Novak, who may well be the first gynecologic pathologist, led to specific surgical approaches to all gynecologic malignancy. Diagnosis was enhanced by the screening Pap smear, tissue biopsy, increased cytologic knowledge, and colposcopy.

Myomata uteri. Uterine tumors have been described under the term *mola* since the establishment of Greek medicine. Galen referred to a solid uterine tumor as a "scleroma." For the next several centuries, solid uterine tumors were confused with all other pelvic masses. Salius in the 1500s called it "uterine stone." It was not until postmortem autopsy became possible that any true knowledge of these tumors was obtained. Hunter in the late 1700s wrote a treatise of fibroids that defined their nature; they were then variously called "fleshy tubercles" or "tubercular tumors." Vogel in 1843 established the characteristic tissues microscopically. Uterine carcinoma was substantially separated from myomas in the early 1800s; by 1862, Klob identified malignant changes in a fibroid.

The treatment, as noted in 1868, involved slough, absorption, excision, ecrasement (crushing), enucleation, and "gastrotomy" (laparotomy). Other techniques included morcellation, hot iron cautery, incision of the capsule and removal of the fibroid by finger dissection, and electrolysis. In 1861, an extensive removal of a myoma, including morcellation, was accomplished per vaginum. Atlee in the United States did a myomectomy in 1843 and classified fibroids as extrauterine, intrauterine, and intramural.

Because laparotomy was so lethal, vaginal myomectomy became popular. By 1901, hundreds of cases were reported. Cervical myomectomy was first done in the late 1800s. Myomectomy in a pregnant woman was done in 1874.

As the techniques for hysterectomy improved in the early 1900s, the indications for the operation for myomata increased. Mayo in 1911 advocated hysterectomy or myomectomy for uterine fibroids; he followed Kelly and Cullen who in 1907 had produced a classic book on myomata uteri. Bonney in England (1948) introduced the use of a flap of tissue to cover any large areas that were left after removal of an extensive amount of tissue; this was known as the Bonney hood.

Since 1976, hysterectomy and myomectomy have been advocated to treat myomas. Meigs delineated the syndrome bearing his name and suggested that in some cases a myoma could stimulate a similar production of fluid. Malignant changes in myomas were noted over the next few years.

Myomectomy in infertility was reported in 1975; this stimulated several other reports of similar conditions and successes. Symptoms of large myomas included stress incontinence. Tomographic studies of these tumors were done in 1981, and the endocrine relationships of these tumors with the pituitary and ovary were postulated. The analogue of GnRh was investigated as a tool to shrink myomas.

Hysteroscopic removal of submucous myomas was introduced in 1983 and has become very popular. The procedure has been combined with the use of a resectoscope or with the adaptation of the laser to ablation of the tumor. This has made the procedure much easier for the patient with a minimal hospital stay and no painful incisions. The laser has been used with the laparoscope for pedunculated myomas and in some reports of subserosal and intramural tumors as well. An excellent mastery of intraabdominal laser surgery through the laparoscope is required. These operations use a video component, which allows the surgeon to exercise technique on a broad screen instead of being limited to visualization through the long tube of a laparoscope. Hemostasis can be a problem with these procedures, but management improves constantly.

PROCEDURES
Surgery of the vagina

The conditions of the vagina for which primary surgery is indicated include benign tumors, cysts, malignancy, endometriosis, and local abscesses in the vaginal wall. Other surgical conditions that engage the vagina are in association with adjacent organs and pelvic relaxation, congenital anomalies, and posttraumatic residual problems.

Benign tumors of the vagina have been managed by sharp and blunt dissection and excision; many are removed by Bovie cautery or, more recently, the laser. Retention cysts in old vaginal lacerations or incisions are removed by local excision.

Vaginal malignancy has been treated by surgery almost exclusively in the twentieth century and only under very strict protocols. Olshausen in 1895 introduced a procedure for extirpation of the vagina for primary malignancy, and a few total vaginectomies were performed in the early 1900s. By the middle 1900s, the treatment of choice was irradiation, but it has been suggested that low-placed cancers could be treated much the same as carcinoma of the vulva. Total vaginectomy with pelvic exenteration has been performed since the invention of the Bricker ileal loop bladder. Total vaginectomy for severe adenosis has been suggested since the importance of eradicating this potentially premalignant lesion, particularly in diethylstilbestrol (DES)-exposed young women, was realized. Total vaginectomy with radical hysterectomy has been done for clear cell adenocarcinoma with success. Partial vaginectomy for confined carcinoma in situ of the vagina has been recommended in contemporary times.

Metastatic malignant lesions, most commonly from endometrial carcinoma, have been managed by combined vaginectomy and radical hysterectomy with or without lymphadenectomy, but several oncologists favor irradiation for such lesions. Other metastatic lesions such as melanoma, choriocarcinoma, or breast carcinoma are usually managed conservatively unless radical surgery is thought to be the best therapeutic method. Endometriosis of the vagina is probably best treated by wide excision, especially if it is in or near the adjacent bladder or rectum. Use of the laser in the past 10 years has been helpful in the treatment of vaginal endometriosis. Local abscesses are incised and drained with added antibiotic therapy.

Surgery of the cervix

The cervix is the most abused organ in the female genital tract. From the earliest of times, some form of treatment of cervical disease has been used. Removal of growths of the cervix was done, and many applications of various medications were common. Leeches were used in the genital tract for treatment of cervical disease. Archigenes treated cervical carcinoma by surgery; there is a question as to the use of hysterectomy for that purpose, but this was probably amputation of the cancerous cervix; blood loss was probably controlled by cautery.

Soranus identified the cervix even more accurately than his predecessors; it may be that many reported prolapsed uteri were primarily the cervix. Polybos, Hippocrates' son, clearly described the cervix in the first written text of gynecology ever recorded. Galen stated that midwives examined the cervix for diagnostic purposes, spoke of cervical "erosion," and quoted Celsus on the use of gold or silver dilators to dilate the cervix and also to hold the vagina open after surgery.

Aetios described cervical stenosis, laceration, ulcer (erosion), and spongy tents to dilate the cervix; ligated polyps with waxed silk thread; and stated that cervical carcinoma was incurable.

Cophon from Salerno described the cervix and its orifice; it was open in intercourse and closed in pregnancy. He identified it as a site for sexual pleasure, and he was the originator of the term "seven-celled uterus." Lanfranchi, the father of French surgery, described the dilation of a hard cervix with sounds made of lead; in some cases, it was necessary to incise as well as dilate. The first accurate delineation of the cervical canal was by Eustachio. Fallopio detailed a description of the cervix and stated that it should never be included as part of the vagina.

In the eighteenth century, there was another expansion of interest in anatomy. Verheyen properly used the term *fundus,* wrote of a fundal-cervical sphincter, and identified the cervical mucosa. Bianchi and Naboth both described the rugae of the cervical canal; the latter identified the occlusion cysts that carry his name.

This was an era of preoccupation with cervical and uterine polyps. Literally hundreds of complicated instruments were created for polyp removal. They were excised, crushed, cauterized, and ligated. There were no authenticated hysterectomies for cervical carcinoma, but amputations were done, obviously without a cure. It is of interest that there is no mention of hemostasis in any of these reports.

The instruments used in cervical surgery carried exotic names: ecraseur, uterotomist, uteroceps, hysterotomist, and hysterotome. Despite a myriad of vaginal speculae invented at this time, cervical amputation was barbaric; the cervix was exposed by use of a speculum, it was grasped with a double-toothed Museaux vulsellum, the speculum was then removed, and by slow and heavy traction the cervix was pulled down external to the vulva! Twenty minutes to half an hour was common for this task. Many women died from hemorrhage. Amputation fortunately did not persist and yielded instead to an even more potentially hazardous operation known as vaginal hysterectomy.

The mid-nineteenth century was marked by an explosion in gynecologic surgery. Baker-Brown wrote the first definitive book on gynecologic surgery in 1854; in it, only cervical stenosis, polyps, and cancer were considered. Many new instruments were devised to facilitate removal of the cervix especially for cancer, but these were still bloody and without adequate hemostasis. de L'Isere invented very complicated devices to amputate or crush the cervix.

Cautery amputation began to be used for conditions other than cancer, for example, prolapse. Sims was the first to cover the cervical stump with mucous membrane. Lisfranc pulled the cervix down to the vulva for amputation by use of Muzeux forceps. The operation lost favor but once more was brought back with the performance of excision of cone-shaped tissue in the late 1800s, probably the precursor of the cone biopsy.

In 1950, a proposal was made for a plastic procedure to treat the incompetent cervix by a surgical reduction of the widespread internal cervical os by local excision and application of sutures. In 1952, a cervical ligation was done with a strip of fascia lata to reinforce a damaged or congenitally abnormal cervix that could not hold a pregnancy past the fifth month. A strip of exocervix was denuded for about 1 cm and closed with catgut.

In 1965, Benson and Durfee introduced the idea of abdominal cervical cerclage in pregnancy when the vaginal procedure was not possible. Several other modifications of cerclage followed the original. One was very simple and effective, employing a heavy suture in and out of the tissue. One advantage of this was that it could be cut and removed when the patient was ready for labor. Different kinds of foreign material have been used for cerclage: nylon, horsehair, heavy silk ("Wurm procedure"), and Mersilene. Glass or plastic ring pessaries have also been used to hold the cervix closed, but it is difficult to keep them at the proper level. An inflatable silicone cuff has been applied to the internal cervical os, and Smith-Hodge pessaries have also been used with some success.

Several modifications of cerclage have been introduced in the past 10 to 20 years, none of which is much of an improvement over the original operation.

Cervix conization

The first to suggest a circular excision of the central cervix was Lisfranc in 1815, but not until Emmet in 1874 was this recognized as an important procedure. Hyams in 1928 suggested electroconization; Ayre devised a special knife for the purpose of a cone biopsy (1948); and Sturmdorf in 1961 devised a method for covering the raw surface, which has stood the test of time.

There have been several attempts to improve the occlusion of the defect in the cervix which remains after conization, but none of them has been entirely successful. A modification of the original Sturmdorf procedure is still widely used.

Recently, cylindrical conization by the laser has been used extensively. Bellina and Baggish have emphasized how important it is that the careful exact technique of laser tissue removal be done to preserve a usable specimen for the pathologist. Those areas that remain apparently epithelialize readily, eliminating the problem of a proper mucosal cover.

Since approximately 1988 Townsend and others have used another method for conization, which employs a high-frequency electrical loop for incision of a portion of the external cervix for examination that has many advantages. As of 1992, this method has several advocates, but the skill and agility of the operator are still the most important point because it is very easy to overheat the tissue sample. LEEP, as it is called, has an excellent therapeutic application in superficial cervical lesions.

Surgery of the ovaries

The East Indians performed laparotomies and bilateral ovarian extirpation for "control of lust"; this operation is claimed to have been done for the Lydian kings to control "oversexed" women. Other historians have stated that the operation was done for hypersexuality even many years later.

Ovarian excision was apparently practiced in the 1500s, but there are no details. Australian natives also removed ovaries.

Houston (1701) performed a partial ovarian cystectomy and evacuated a great deal of material through a 4-inch incision, which had been enlarged a little at a time. When the cyst had been entirely emptied, the base of it was sutured to the abdominal wall. Hunter advocated removal of an ovarian cyst but did not actually do it. Pott removed an ovary that was in a hernial sac in 1756. Ovarian cysts were tapped through the vagina in 1760 and 1777; a cyst that obstructed the pelvis in a woman in labor was drained through the vagina in 1815; in the same year, a cyst was drained through the rectum.

Theden recorded the first ovariectomy in 1771, but this went largely unnoticed. Theden outlined the use of an inguinal incision, exposure of the cyst, puncture, evacuation, delivery of the sac, and ligation of the pedicle; this was a definitely proper method for the operation. McDowell, who has been called the "father of abdominal surgery," created a landmark in surgery in 1809 by a successful extirpation of an ovarian cyst without anesthesia; he sutured the ovarian pedicle to the abdominal incision for drainage. In 1821, Smith did an ovariotomy, without knowing of McDowell's technique. He sutured the pedicle and dropped it into the abdomen. All bleeding points as well as the pedicle were sutured with leather sutures. Clearly he was ahead of his time as to the details of the technique. Eight years later, Rogers ligated the pedicle vessels separately and tied each with animal suture.

Simpson created the term *ovariotomy* in 1844, and the operation became fairly common in the United States and Europe.

Wells was the great ovariotomist of England. He performed many operations with a high success rate due not only to meticulous technique but also to a high regard for cleanliness. He invented a clamp for the ovarian pedicle, then created a forci-pressure clamp for arteries. Tait, another great English gynecologic surgeon, devised many methods for ovarian surgery and performed many gynecologic operations, including the first laparotomy for ectopic pregnancy (1837).

For the remainder of the century, the only additions to the procedure were to leave the ligated ovarian pedicle in the abdominal cavity and eventually use the peritoneum to cover it.

Wedge resection for polycystic ovarian disease was common for about 40 years in the 1900s but has lost favor in view of endocrine management of the problem. Excision of endometriomas expanded with increased knowledge of that disease. Ovarian suspension has waxed and waned over the years, with very clear indications only in modern times. Ovarian transplantation into the uterine wall in certain cases of infertility was popular in the middle years but complications have almost eliminated the procedure.

Surgery can be a cure for stage Ia grade I ovarian carcinoma, but the diagnosis must be certain. Preservation of the contralateral ovary in these cases has become very controversial; in general, it may be limited to young women who desire to maintain fertility and even then in only very carefully selected cases with clear recognition of the risks. Many surgeons believe that the diagnosis must be of a well-differentiated mucinous malignancy to justify taking the chance. Bilateral ovarian excision with hysterectomy is the most accepted treatment today.

Omentectomy in the obvious absence of metastases in ovarian carcinoma is also a contentious subject and may be a matter of judgment. Until the latter part of the 1900s, lymph node dissection either for excision or for a diagnostic sample was usually not performed, but since the use of magnetic resonance imaging (MRI) and computed tomography (CT) scans, positive nodes are more common than formerly believed; therefore, node dissection is now included in surgery for ovarian carcinoma. Peritoneal cell samples are mandatory at the start of any laparatomy for ovarian carcinoma or even suspected disease. Since 1950, the second-look operation has become common but is still controversial; the recent use of laparoscopy instead of a second-look operation is not reliable nor successful.

Operations to debulk massive amounts of tumor have evolved over the past 50 years and are still a part of the surgical approach.

The application of a special catheter into the peritoneal cavity to implement improved direct dosage of chemotherapeutic agents has been another recent innovation. Bilateral ovarian excision was highly recommended for several years for breast carcinoma, but this is no longer generally performed. It is still generally accepted to do ovarian removal in all but very early cases of endometrial carcinoma.

Placement of the ovary in an accessible location for harvest of ova for IVF or GIFT programs has been common since 1975. Ovarian transplants, both autogenous or donor, have not realized accountability. Microsurgical lysis of adhesions with or without the laser has greatly improved ovarian reclamation.

Surgical treatment of vulvar disease

Surgery for diseases of the vulva is derived from ancient medicine. The procedure of amputating a hypertrophied clitoris is found in medical literature over the past 2000 years. Excision of external growth and pedunculated tumors and incision and drainage of abscesses are among the few gynecologic operations performed for over 1000 years.

Specific extensive removal of vulvar tissue was first accomplished by Basset for clitoral carcinoma in 1912. Taussig in 1929 introduced the importance of recognizing lymphatic metastases and lymphadenectomy. Conservative surgery for vulvar disease involved local excision and inguinal gland resection for melanoma unless the disease was extensive and deeply invasive. Pringle was among the first to discuss surgery for melanoma (1908). Conservative excision of superficial, confined, microinvasive carcinoma has been a method of choice.

The "skinning vulvectomy" was used for carcinoma precursors and for extensive symptomatic benign diseases. Simple vulvectomy has been the method of choice for several lesions, including carcinoma in situ, for the past 35 years. A modified simple vulvectomy has been used for intractable irritation and itch, as has intraepithelial injection with alcohol.

Extensive radical vulvectomy with inguinal gland resection and deep iliac lymph gland resection has also been used. Exenteration procedures that included the vulva and the vagina have been performed.

Combined irradiation and surgery has had mixed results. In extensive malignant vulvar or Bartholin gland involvement, wide radical vulvectomy with exenteration has been suggested.

Transsexual surgery with successful conversion of otherwise normal males to females was of interest in the 1960s. In the early 1950s, a team composed of a urologist, a gynecologist, and a plastic surgeon and directed by a psychiatric expert in transsexualism performed these conversion operations. Acceptable, functional external female genitalia and vagina were produced in genetic males with the otherwise unsolvable problem of confused sex identification. The knowledge gained from these procedures has helped immeasurably with plastic operations required because of burns or trauma in contemporary gynecology.

Plastic surgery

Uterine reunification. Plastic surgery of the uterus consists of the correction of intrauterine adhesions or synechiae, especially repair of the cavity that remains after myomectomy and the congenital anomalies. Although Fritsch first described uterine cavity adhesions in 1894, Asherman between 1948 and 1957 established the entire syndrome, which generally carries his name.

Hysteroscopic lysis of intracavitary adhesions is now accepted as the method of choice for management and treatment of this problem.

Excision of a rudimentary horn of the uterus and surgical correction of similar anomalies were done if indicated; on occasion, abdominal hysterectomy was performed. Rudimentary horns have been fused or unified by some excision followed by sutures. Diagnosis of a true bicornuate uterus may be made and a classification of the variants together with the septate uterus is very valuable in the selection of treatment. In 1907, a unification operation for a double and true and partial bicornuate uterus was introduced and proved very effective; it was later moderately modified and proved to be not as applicable to the septate uterus. Wedge excision and plastic repair of various types of septate uteri were also introduced; these operations became the standard for plastic uterine reunification.

Creation of a neovagina. Preliminary work was done in the 1880s to construct a neovagina. The advent of antibiotics, increased information about the use of skin grafts and intravaginal molds, and the apparent success with the use of bowel transplantation permitted an unusual number of procedures to be invented. Frank in 1940 proposed a method for creation of a neovagina that used dilators of increased size and length to invert the external tissue between the rectum and the urethra into a vaginal "pit." In 1977, Broadbent used a modification of this method, and Ingram in 1981 proposed the ingenious idea of using a bicycle seat with vertical dilators of various sizes placed so that the patient's weight when she sat on it would cause the desired penetration of the tissues of the area.

The surgical methods have frequently been very complicated, especially those using bowel transplantation. Skin flaps from the thighs and labia have been turned into a potential vaginal space. In 1895, Abbe did a procedure with an obturator and a skin graft that was highly successful; it was redescribed by McIndoe in 1938 and is one of the preferred methods in contemporary gynecology. Among the many variations is the stimulation of tissue growth over a mold. A vulvovaginal pouch that functioned externally as a vagina suitable for intercourse was especially useful in exenteration cases.

Hysterectomy

Hysterectomy, which was the proper term for any uterine extirpation, was introduced by Tillaux in 1879 and is the accepted designation.

Vaginal hysterectomy to the nineteenth century. Surgical procedures on the cervix preceded the evolution of vaginal hysterectomy, which was not performed until after a long period of experimentation with various medical therapies and many operations. These included amputations for all possible problems, among them carcinoma.

Vaginal hysterectomy for malignancy was first done in 1813. Recamier in 1829 performed a successful vaginal hysterectomy but injured the bladder. He was the first to consider the possibility of injury to the ureter in performance of the operation and to realize the importance of systematic ligation of the vessels and attention to a secure ligation of the ligaments of the uterus; in fact, vaginal hysterectomy has been named "Recamier's operation." Recamier held the severed uterine ligaments with his left hand and passed a curved needle mounted on a handle threaded with a strong suture to secure the tissues.

An improved method that included anesthesia, hemostasis, and antisepsis was developed and probably was the first operation for vaginal extirpation of a myomatous uterus. It also promoted the use of vaginal hysterectomy for benign conditions.

From the late 1890s to the early 1900s there was a division in the approach to pelvic operations. The vaginal and abdominal surgeons almost never used the alternative method, but, with time, most surgeons used both.

Schauta in 1890 performed a radical vaginal hysterectomy for cervical carcinoma and continued the procedure as late as 1909 in direct competition with the abdominal operation of Wertheim. Schauta incorporated the deep perineal incision introduced by Schuchardt in 1894. In that same year, Richelot in Paris published a text on vaginal hysterectomy and outlined nine benign indications for the operation. Benign conditions were now included more and more as indications for vaginal extirpation of the uterus.

The clamp operation was promoted by Hunter in New York in 1889; he left as many as 14 pairs of clamps attached to vessels and ligaments (Fig. 1-7).

Vaginal hysterectomy in the twentieth century. By the turn of the century, vaginal hysterectomy had begun to be an acceptable surgical procedure. Vaginal techniques were extremely varied and included the use of clamps alone, step-by-step ligation of small amounts of tissue and all vessels, use of braided Chinese silk or catgut, and use of cautery in place of a scalpel. There were as many variations in closure of the operative area as there were in the extirpation of the uterus and adnexa. By 1903, Pryor introduced clamps with detachable handles, which were removed at the completion of the operation and provided more postoperative comfort for the patient. Kennedy and Price reportedly did thousands of vaginal hysterectomies by the clamp method in the years from 1918 to 1927. By 1909, Schauta had perfected his radical vaginal hysterectomy.

Heany in 1934 introduced a technique for vaginal hysterectomy that has endured the passage of time and is the basic technical method for the operations (Fig. 1-8). Lash in 1941 proposed a method for reduction of uterine size that removed the myometrium and left a shell of uterine tissue, which could easily be removed. In 1942, Heaney secured the details of Lash's operation and indicated vaginal repair at the same time. The clear practical aspects of his technique cannot be denied.

Throughout the late 1940s, most of the 1950s, and then through the 1960s, there were many reports by many well-respected gynecologic surgeons in the United States.

In 1952, Ricci and Thom clearly identified the differ-

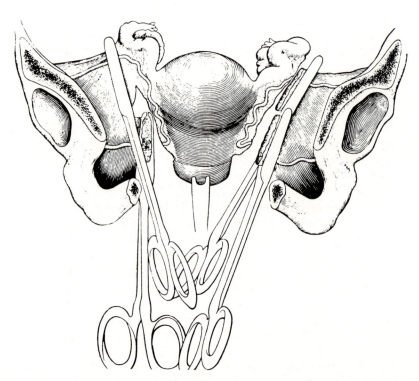

Fig. 1-7. Hysterectomy by clamp method, no ligatures or sutures. (From Pozzi S: *A treatise on gynecology,* vol 2, London, 1893, New Sydenham Society.)

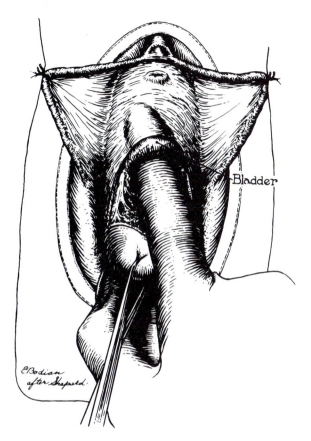

Fig. 1-8. Vaginal hysterectomy—start of dissection. (From Mattingly R, Thompson J: *Operative gynecology,* ed 6, Philadelphia, 1985, JB Lippincott.)

ence between total prolapse of the pelvic organs and a simulated condition of persistent hypertrophy and elongation of the cervix.

In 1953, Tauber presented his "stump stitch." Allen led in the use of vaginal hysterectomy, using preoperative curettage and an immediate posterior colpotomy to explore the pelvis, both of which prevented many serious mistakes. There were many modifications in the procedure and several reports of complications. The use of drains in the operative area was considered, and the concept of preoperative and postoperative antibiotics, which still has not been resolved, was introduced.

In 1957, McCall popularized the important contribution of imbrication of the sacrouterine ligaments and obliteration of the cul-de-sac after uterine removal, which prevented the development of postoperative enterocele.

In 1958, Werner and Sederl wrote on abdominal surgery by the vaginal route.

In 1959, Mitra presented his radical vaginal hysterectomy for cervical carcinoma combined with an extraperitoneal lymph gland dissection.

In 1962, Hofmeister and Wolfgram did an extensive study on the anatomic variance in the relationship of the

ureter in the cardinal ligament to the clamps and sutures of hysterectomy.

In the mid-1970s, recommendation was made for routine placement of a T-tube in the operative area for 24 hours, suggesting that there is some degree of accumulation of bloody fluid under the flaps and tissues that is invariably a source of infection. Suction drainage of the same areas had been suggested 10 years before. There has been considerable opposition to drains after this operation. About the same time, obesity was noted as an indication for the vaginal operation instead of the abdominal approach, because there is a much lower morbidity with the former.

Today, by use of the advances over the past 25 years, detailed techniques of vaginal hysterectomy have been developed by many operators. Injection with saline or hemostatic medications before the initial incisions in the vaginal mucosa have reduced operative blood loss. The newer synthetic suture materials have greatly improved the postoperative recovery, which, when combined with preoperative and postoperative prophylactic antibiotics, have made this almost an outpatient procedure. In the 1990s, vaginal hysterectomy combined with laparoscopic dissection of the uterine ligaments, with the exception of the cardinal ligaments and uterine arteries, has broadened the indications for vaginal hysterectomy.

Abdominal hysterectomy. Abdominal hysterectomy was derived from laparotomy and, to some degree, from vaginal hysterectomy. It was based on Guterblat's combined vaginal and abdominal operation (1813), which was followed by Delpech in 1830 and others who used the combined approach.

The early history of this operation is divided by the evolution of its use in benign versus malignant disease.

Abdominal hysterectomy for benign disease. The first abdominal hysterectomies for benign disease (myomata) followed the experience of Lizars (1825), Atlee (1849), and others, all of whom had begun a laparotomy for ovarian cysts and found large multiple myomata that caused them to abandon the procedure. Clay (1843) and Heath (1845) performed uterine amputation at the level of the internal cervical os for myomas; Clay removed the adnexa bilaterally with the uterus and thus carried out the first so-called panhysterectomy.

Schroder in 1878 introduced intraperitoneal management of the cervical stump (Fig. 1-9). An important step in this procedure was destruction of the mucous portion of the cervical canal with either Paquelin's cautery or strong carbolic acid; the cervical stump was then carefully sutured with silk and catgut sutures so as to close it securely.

Bardenhauer in 1881 performed a total abdominal hysterectomy and left the ligament ligatures to drain into the vagina. This report included an account of a broad transverse abdominal incision that extended nearly from one anterior superior spine to the other, which preceded all other transverse incisions that transected the rectus muscles.

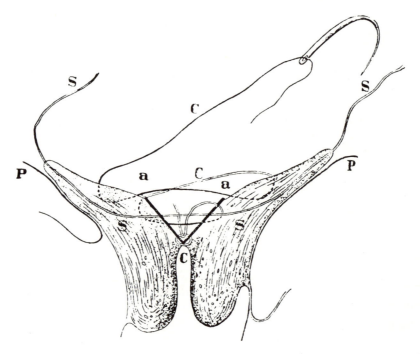

Fig. 1-9. Cervical stump closure at abdominal hysterectomy by Schroeder. (From Pozzi S: *A treatise on gynecology,* vol 1, London, 1896, New Sydenham Society.)

Although hysterectomy for carcinoma may have been questionably acceptable, the use of total hysterectomy for benign disease was even more questionable.

In an effort to improve the mortality rate, Fritsch in 1886 curetted a carcinoma and packed the uterus with iodoform gauze, using a permanganate wash in other situations. Freund in 1888 did a hysterectomy for myomata, used iodoform gauze, placed drains as indicated, and advocated bilateral excision of the ovaries when the operation was not considered possible. Martin in 1889 suggested oil-soaked sponges for protection of the intestines, used a temporary elastic ligature, freed the cervix through the vagina, and removed the uterus abdominally. Clifford used an ecraseur for supravaginal operations in 1889. Chrobak in 1891 shelled the uterus out of the serosa and amputated it very low into the cervix, leaving just a ring of tissue, and sutured the serosa to it. He was very successful with this operation.

Abdominal hysterectomy for malignancy. Apparently, the first total hysterectomy for carcinoma of the cervix was performed by Jones in the United States in 1867. In 1878, Freund reported a total hysterectomy for cervical carcinoma; his outline of the technique was remarkably progressive in that the procedure was highly disciplined with attention to the details of hemostasis and asepsis. Schroeder in 1879 did a total hysterectomy and vaginectomy for carcinoma.

Freund's later operations for uterine fundal carcinoma were done as a combined procedure with the cervix freed vaginally and the uterus and cervix then removed abdominally. In 1880, Rydygier revived the combined operation,

freed the cervix through the vagina, placed the patient in Trendelenburg's position, and used a midline incision. In cases where the rectus muscles were rigid, he transected them at the insertion on the pubis (clearly a predecessor to the Cherney incision). Crede excised part of the abdominal wall in such cases; when more space was needed, he packed the intestines and, on occasion, eventrated them onto the abdominal wall and kept them warm and wet. In 1889, Martin did a supravaginal hysterectomy first and then removed the cervix through the vagina. As of 1886, the mortality associated with abdominal hysterectomy for carcinoma was more than 67% from the procedure alone.

Abdominal hysterectomy in the twentieth century. The 1900s were the new era not only for hysterectomy for carcinoma, with the Wertheim procedure, but also for the onset of gynecologic surgery at its finest. Wertheim recorded his technique for radical hysterectomy with pelvic lymph node dissection in 1900. This was a classic example of the kind of perfection of technique that came to distinguish gynecologic surgery toward the middle and end of the century.

Abdominal hysterectomy came to be used more frequently for benign diseases in the early 1900s, with indications in myomata, endometriosis and adenomyosis, persistent uterine blood loss, pelvic inflammatory disease, and several less common problems (Fig. 1-10). Worrall in Australia devised the first intrafascial abdominal hysterectomy in 1914, and Masson at the Mayo Clinic in 1927 reported on a similar operation. Richardson in 1929 standardized the technique for hysterectomy on which almost all other such operations are based (Fig. 1-11); he further

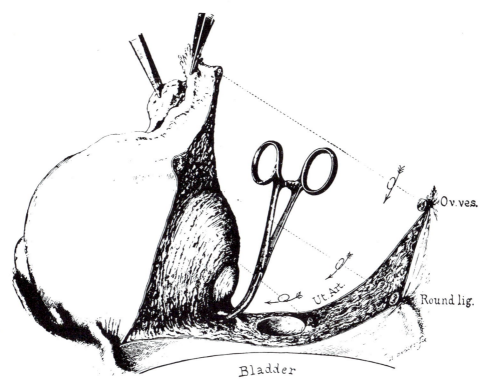

Fig. 1-10. Continuous abdominal supracervical hysterectomy by Kelly. (From Kelly H: *Operative gynecology,* vol 2, New York, 1902, D. Appleton.)

described a form of "intrafascial" dissection technique that employed a T-shaped incision in the pericervical fascia, facilitating its identification. The Mayo operation, patterned somewhat on Richardson, became a popular procedure by 1947 but was an extrafascial operation, as most hysterectomies are now.

In the 1940s, Meigs perfected the radical hysterectomy in the United States. By 1948, Brunschwig published details of his extensive exenteration with radical hysterectomy for cervical cancer; this was involved and consisted of removal of the pelvic organs, which included both bladder and rectum with the vagina and internal genitalia, with extensive lymph node dissection and the creation of abdominal stomas for both urine and fecal streams. His eventration of the intestines is a reminder of the work done in the 1800s.

Hysterectomy remained more or less static, with great improvements in mortality and morbidity due for the most part to the judicious application of antibiotic medications. The advent of the surgical clip was the newest innovation in hysterectomy in several decades. The use of clips for intestinal anastomosis was introduced by the Russians and used extensively in the United States but saw only limited application in hysterectomy. In 1968, staples were used to close the vagina in abdominal hysterectomy, supposedly isolating the vagina from the surgical field before the uterus and cervix were removed. By 1977, problems were noted with the metal staples in the apex of the vagina,

namely, severe dyspareunia. Absorbable ligature clips were introduced and applied to vaginal closure with much greater success.

The first to perform a hysterectomy with cesarean section was Storer in Boston in 1876. He was literally forced to do this operation because of hemorrhage after delivery of the child caused by the presence of myomata. This was a supravaginal operation. Unfortunately, the patient died about 3 days postoperatively.

In the past 2 or 3 years, there has been increased interest in the laparoscopically assisted hysterectomy; this is composed of a dissection of the round, broad, uteroovarian, and sometimes uterosacral ligaments through a laparoscope, in the 1990s with the use of clips. Once this has been accomplished, the cervix is dissected through the vagina, the cardinal ligaments are secured, the uterine vessels are also ligated vaginally, and the total hysterectomy is completed from below. This is an interesting exercise; the overall advantages, if any, are still to be realized.

Surgery for vesicourinary incontinence

Identification and classification of various urination situations were correlated with proper terminology before 1980. Enhorning established the urethral closure pressure profile in 1981.

Cystometry, electromyography, and microtransducers were introduced; simultaneous measurement of intravesical and intraurethral pressures was made possible. This work

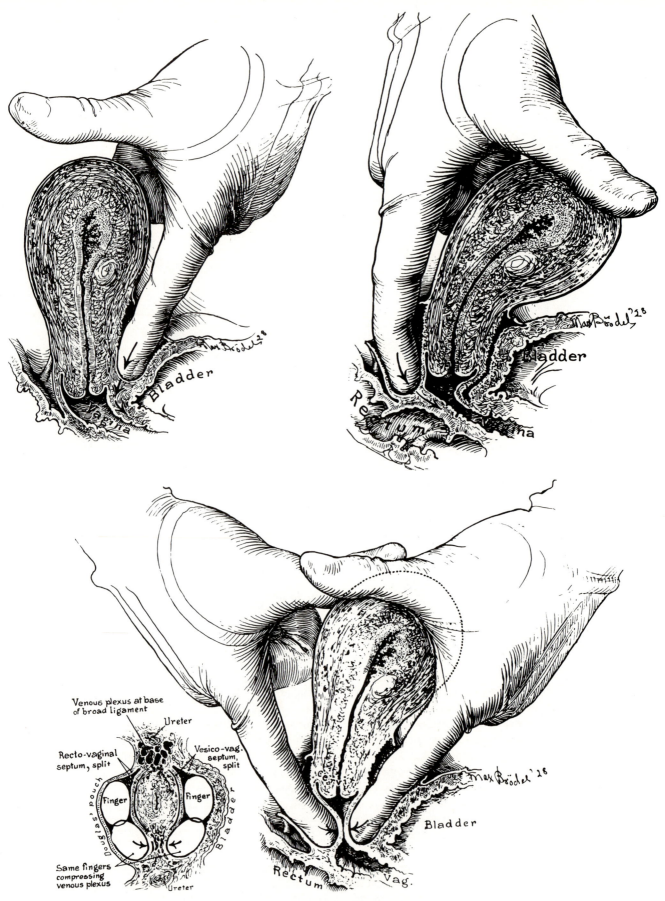

Venous plexus at base
of broad ligament

Ureter

Recto-vaginal
septum, split

Vesico-vag.
septum,
split

Douglas' pouch

Finger

Finger

Bladder

Same fingers
compressing
venous plexus

Ureter

Rectum

Vag.

Bladder

Rectum

Vagina

Bladder

Fig. 1-11. The Richardson abdominal hysterectomy. (From Richardson EH: *A simplified abdominal panhysterectomy*, Chicago, 1929, Surgical Publishers of Chicago.)

helped establish a postresidency fellowship in gynecologic urology.

Robertson in the 1970s devised a straight urethroscope based, in part, on the previous Kelly air cystoscope, which used CO_2 for bladder distention and provided a direct internal observation of the bladder neck and urethrovesical junction at all phases of the urination process; it also provided direct observation of the urethra throughout its entire length. It serves as a cystoscope as well and is used for urethrocystometrogram studies. The patient is in the lithotomy position, which preserves the normal anatomic relationships.

Diagnostic procedures were evaluated, and three important areas were noted: (1) the value of the Q-tip test; (2) the importance of the history with a description of urination in the patient's own words; and (3) the physical examination designed specifically to identify neurologic, muscular, and anatomic defects in incontinence cases. The Bonney stress test with upward movement of the vaginal wall was used to determine if anatomic replacement would solve the problem of stress urinary loss. Other studies included the use of posterior downward pull on the perineum with a Sims speculum or the posterior blade of Graves, the levator test, cystometry, urethral pressure profiles, electromyelography, uroflowmetry, radiographic studies such as urination video cystograms, and the use of direct cystoscopy.

In 1907, George R. White of Savanah described transvaginal reattachment of the anterior vaginal fornix to the arcus tendineus as a treatment for cystocele. This concept is not unlike the transabdominal paravaginal fixation operation. Kelly first illustrated his suture in 1911, and it is still the basis for most vaginal repairs of cystocele and urinary incontinence due to stress. Kennedy added an important procedure to these repairs in suggesting reinforcement of the integrity of the posterior length of the urethra. The invention of the polyglycolic suture material has improved anterior vaginal repairs if for no other reason than the elimination of much of the scar tissues. In the last 12 years, various authors have reported greater than 90% success with the basic Kelly-Kennedy vaginal repair in the treatment of urinary stress incontinence, but these results are not universal.

Furniss was the first in the 1900s to attempt suprapubic suspension of the vagina and urethra. The Marshal-Marchetti-Krantz (MMK) suprapubic elevation of the anterior vaginal wall, and with it the urethra (after some modification), has been highly successful since 1949. Burch in 1968 attached the suspension sutures to Cooper's ligament, also with success; however, even if popular because it is relatively easier, it is not anatomically correct. Various modifications of these procedures have been developed. Durfee simplified the MMK operation and facilitated suprapubic cystocele obliteration by the placement of vaginal suspension sutures in the undersurface of the cartilaginous central portion of the symphysis as well as one bilat-

erally to the condensed connective tissue of the obturator orifices.

Suspension of the urethrovesical region by a supportive "strap" of strong permanent tissue was another approach to the problem. Goebell demonstrated a "sling" operation using strips of abdominal rectus muscle fascia, which he brought down under the urethrovesical area and used to elevate the tissues anteriorly in 1910; this was modified later by Stoeckel and Frangenheim. Williams and TeLinde used a narrow synthetic strap for this purpose in 1962 but had to abandon it because of trauma to the undersurface to the bladder and urethra. A high percentage of these operations are unsatisfactory because of obstruction due to excessive scar formation.

Transplantation of other tissues under the relaxed anterior vaginal wall was attempted in 1918 by Taussig, who used tissues from the levator ani muscles. Other muscles used were the gracilis, the pyramidalis, the bulbocavernosis, and the pubococcygeus.

Procedures in which artificial materials have been used include the epiurethral suprapubic vaginal suspension by Sexton, who used both an artificial tape and a tendon from the forearm as a sling to suspend the vagina by inducing the perivaginal tissues to raise the anterior vaginal wall to the conjoined tendon bilaterally. Moir suggested a 1-inch-wide Mersilene gauze hammock for support of this area. A fibrin bean implantation was performed in 1975. The Politano procedure consists of endoscopic injection of Teflon under the mucosa of the bladder neck.

Surgical management of detrusor dysfunction was first approached by Ingelman-Sundberg in 1959 when he transsected the infravesical nerves. The key to success in this treatment lies in identifying those patients who will profit from the operations.

Several other exotic procedures have persisted, and there are many pharmaceutical approaches to these problems. The proper surgical procedure accurately and carefully done in cases where the problem has been definitely diagnosed has provided relief for many women.

TUBAL STERILIZATION AND ALTERNATIVE METHODS

Tubal sterilization and tubal ligation were first suggested by Blundell in 1823. Ovarian castration may have been practiced by ancient peoples for sterilization as well as for nymphomania, but this is unsubstantiated. Lungren in 1880 ligated the tubes for the first time. Porro performed a cesarean hysterectomy with the secondary intention of sterilization in 1876; Thomas in 1885 suggested tubal ligation as opposed to Porro's operation. Several surgeons performed the operation over the next 200 years. Duhrssen used a double ligature and was the first to perform tubal ligation by colpotomy. Fehrer and Buettner divided the tubes between two sutures in 1897, and Fritsch in 1897 suggested that at least 1 cm of tubal tissue be removed. Ruhl in 1898 cut the tube 5 cm from the uterus and sutured the ends to a vaginal incision. The tubes were removed at the cornua by Rose in 1898, and the cornual area was sutured closed. Intrauterine cauterization of the tubes was done with the use of silver nitrate and galvano-cautery. Uchida's procedure is the most effective.

Laparoscopy in the 1950s led to unipolar electrocoagulation tubal ligation, the Hulka spring clip, the Yoon plastic Falope ring, and bipolar cautery. Laparoscopy is the most popular method of sterilization in the nonpregnant or recently pregnant woman, although minilaparotomy immediately postpartum has many advocates. Pomeroy ligation with use of a large plain catgut double tie at cesarean section is very satisfactory.

SUGGESTED READINGS

Baas J: *Outlines of the history of medicine,* 2 vols, Huntington, New York, 1971, R Krieger (Translated by H Handerson).

Baggish M: *Basic and advanced laser surgery in gynecology,* Norwalk, Conn, 1985, Appleton Century Crofts.

Baker-Brown I: *Surgical diseases of women,* ed 2, London, 1861, John W Davies.

Benson R: *Current obstetric and gynecologic diagnosis and treatment,* Los Altos, Calif, 1978, Lange Medical Publications.

Bhisgratna K: *Sushruta samhita,* ed. 2, Varanasi, India, 1963, Chowkhamba Sanskrit Series Office.

Breasted J: *The Edwin Smith surgical papyrus,* Chicago, 1930, University of Chicago Press.

Bonney V: *Gynecological surgery,* ed 3, London, 1974, Balliere and Tindall.

Bucknell T, Ellis H: *Wound healing for surgeons,* London, 1984, Balliere and Tindall.

Channing W: *A treatise on etherization in childbirth,* London, 1848, W Ticknor and Co; (special edition, Birmingham, Alabama, 1990, Gryphon editions).

Cullen T: *Adenomyomata uteri,* New York, 1890, D Appleton and Co.

Cullen T: *Cancer of the uterus,* New York, 1900, D Appleton and Co.

Cushing H, Bovie W: Electro-surgery as an aid to removal of intracranial tumors, *Surg Gynecol Obstet* 47(6):751; 1928.

DeLancey J. Starr R: Histology of the connection between the vagina and levator ani muscles, *J Reprod Med* 35(8):765, 1990.

Dionis P: *Cours d'operations de chirugie,* ed 4, Paris, 1750, Chez D'Houry.

Doderlein ASG, Kronig B: *Operative gynakologie,* ed 5, Leipzig, 1924, Georg Thieme.

Doyen C: *Surgical therapeutics and operative technique,* New York, 1917, William Wood and Co. (Translated by H Spencer-Browne.)

Durfee R: Anterior vaginal suspension operation, *Am J Obstet Gynecol* 78(3):628, 1959.

Emge L, Durfee R: *Pelvic organ prolapse, 4000 years of treatment, Clin Obstet Gynecol* 4:997, 1961.

Engelmann G: The early history of vaginal hysterectomy, *Am Gynecol Obstet J* 31:521, 1895.

Garrison F: *An introduction to the history of medicine,* ed 4, Philadelphia, 1929, WB Saunders.

Gomel V: *Microsurgery in female infertility,* Boston, 1983, Little Brown.

Gomel V: *Laparoscopy and hysteroscopy in gynecologic practice,* Chicago, 1986, Year Book Medical Publishers.

Gray L: *Vaginal hysterectomy,* ed 3, Springfield, 1983, Charles Thomas.

Halban J, Seitz L: *Biologie und Pathologie des Weibes,* Berlin, 1924, Urban and Schwarzenberg.

Halsted W: *Surgical Papers,* Baltimore, 1924, Johns Hopkins Press.

Harvey S: *History of hemostasis,* New York, 1929, Paul Hoeber.

Hughes A: *A history of cytology,* London, 1959, Abelard Schuman.

Hunt R: *Atlas of female infertility surgery,* Chicago, 1985, Year Book Medical Publishers.

Hunt R, Seigler A: *Hysterosalpingography: techniques and interpretation,* Chicago, 1988, Year Book Medical Publishers.

Jones H, Rock J: *Reparative and constructive surgery of the female generative tract,* Baltimore, 1983, Williams and Wilkins.

Kelly H: *Operative gynecology,* ed 2, New York, 1900, Appleton and Company.

Kelly H, Noble CP: *Operative gynecology,* ed 3, New York, 1911, Appleton and Company.

Kelly H, Cullen T: *Myomata of the uterus,* Philadelphia, 1909, WB Saunders.

Keys T: *The history of surgical anesthesia,* ed 2, Boston, 1950, Milford House.

Leonardo R: *The history of surgery,* New York, 1943, Froben.

Leonardo T: *The history of gynecology,* New York, 1944, Froben.

Lister J: *Collected papers,* Oxford, 1909, Claredon Press.

Maino G: *The healing hand,* Cambridge, 1975, Harvard University Press.

Malgaigne J: *Surgery and Ambrose Pare,* Norman, Oklahoma, 1965, University of Oklahoma Press (Translated by W Hamby).

Malpas P: *Genital prolapse and allied conditions,* New York, 1955, Grune & Stratton.

Mann M: *American system of gynecology,* Philadelphia, 1888, Lea Brothers.

Marshall V, Marchetti A, Krantz K: Supra-pubic urethral vesical suspension, *Surg Gynecol Obstet* 78(3):628, 1959.

Martius N: *Die Gynekologischen Operationen,* Stuttgart, 1954, Georg Thieme.

Mattingly R, Thompson J: *TeLinde's operative gynecology,* ed 6, Philadelphia, 1985, JB Lippincott.

McDowell E: Three cases of expiration of diseases ovaria, *The Eclectic Repertory and Analytical Review* 7:242, 1817.

McKay W: *The history of ancient gynecology,* New York, 1901, Wiliam Wood.

Meigs J: *Surgical treatment of carcinoma of the cervix,* New York, 1954, Grune & Stratton.

Milne J: *Surgical instruments in Greek and Roman times,* Oxford, 1907, Clarendon Press.

Mukhopadhyaya G: *The surgical instruments of the Hindus,* Calcutta, 1913, Calcutta University.

Neuwirth R: *Hysteroscopy,* Philadelphia, 1975, WB Saunders.

Nichols D: *Clinical problems, injuries and complications of gynecologic surgery,* ed 2, Baltimore, 1988, Willams and Wilkins.

Nichols D, Randall C: *Vaginal surgery,* ed 3, Baltimore, 1989, Williams and Wilkins.

Novak E: *Gynecological and obstetrical pathology,* Baltimore, 1945, Williams and Wilkins.

Pare A: *The collected works of Ambrose Pare,* New York, 1968, Milford House (Translated by T Johnson from the first English edition, 1634).

Parsons L, Ulfelder H: *An atlas of pelvic operations,* New York, 1968, WB Saunders.

Patton G, Kistner R: *Atlas of infertility surgery,* ed 2, Boston, 1985, Little Brown.

Peham H, Amreich J: *Operative gynecology,* Philadelphia, 1934, JB Lippincott (Translated by L Ferguson). Phillips J: *Endoscopy in gynecology,* Downey, Calif, 1978, AAGL.

Ploss H, Bartels M, Bartels P: In Dingwell E, editor: *Woman,* St Louis, 1938, CV Mosby Co.

Pozzi SA: *Treatise on gynecology,* London, 1898, New Sydenham Society.

Preuss J: *Biblical and Talmudic medicine,* New York, 1978, Sanhedrin Press (Translated by F. Rosner).

Reich W, Nechtow M: *Pitfalls in gynecologic diagnosis and surgery,* New York, 1962, McGraw Hill.

Reiffenstuhl G, Platzer W: *Atlas of vaginal surgery,* Philadelphia, 1974, WB Saunders (Translated by E Friedman and J Friedman).

Ricci J: *One hundred years of gynecology,* Philadelphia, 1945, Blakiston.

Ricci J: *The development of gynecological surgery and instruments,* Philadelphia, 1949, Blakiston.

Ricci J: *The geneology of gynecology,* Philadelphia, 1950, Blakiston.

Ricci J: *The cystocele in America,* Philadelphia, 1950, Blakiston.

Richardson E: A simplified technique for abdominal panhysterectomy, *Surg Gynecol Obstet* 48:248, 1929.

Scultetus J: *Armamantarium surgicum,* 1655, Ulm edition (photocopy by Sautter K, 1919, Editions Medicina Rara Ltd; original by Agathon Presse, Baiersbraun, W Germany).

Sims J. On the treatment of vesico-vaginal fistulas, *Am J Med Sci* 23:59, 1852.

Thomas T: *A practical treatise on the diseases of women,* ed 4, Philadel-phia, 1874, Henry Lea.

Timor-Tritsch I, Rottem S: *Trans-vaginal ultra sound,* New York, 1988, Elesevier.

Ulin A, Gollub S: *Surgical bleeding,* New York, 1966, McGraw-Hill.

Wertheim E: Zur frage der radikal operation beim uterus krebs, *Arch Gynak* 61:627, 1900.

White GR: *An anatomical operation for the cure of cystocele,* JAMA 53:1707, 1909.

Chapter 2

PRACTICAL PELVIC ANATOMY FOR THE GYNECOLOGIC SURGEON

Gunther Reiffenstuhl

PELVIC CONNECTIVE TISSUE PLANES AND SPACES

An exact knowledge of the anatomy of the firm pelvic connective tissue is necessary for the gynecologic surgeon to find the appropriate blood vessels running within these tissues, thus saving the patient's blood during surgery. A precise knowledge of the location of the loose connective tissue is also significant because this tissue fills the spaces and potential spaces between the pelvic organs and the firm connective tissue ligaments that have to be exposed.

The term *pelvic connective tissue* is intended to include the entire system of connective tissue that surrounds the pelvic organs and extends into the subperitoneal area. This is bounded cranially by the pelvic peritoneum, caudally by the muscular pelvic floor, anteriorly by the symphysis, posteriorly by the sacrum, and laterally by the obturator and piriform muscles.

Operating in the correct layer—one of the most important prerequisites for successful vaginal and pelvic surgery—is only possible if the surgeon has exact knowledge of the anatomy of the connective tissue matrix and of the spaces filled with parenchyma (the so-called paraspaces) and enters them correctly.

This chapter uses the nomenclature of Amreich,[76] which is very practical, especially for the gynecologic surgeon.

Connective tissue matrix (firm pelvic connective tissue)

The vessels of the female pelvis always go in a precise direction from the pelvic wall through the extraperitoneal tissue to the uterus, vagina, bladder, rectum, and in the opposite direction from the pelvic organs to the pelvic wall. Because of the concentration of the connective tissue

surrounding the vessels, the columns extend in different directions. This connective tissue matrix was thought to be a fixation device of the pelvic viscera; but, after detailed study by Amreich, it became evident that it functions primarily as a device for conveying blood and lymphatic vessels and for organ embedding. The following subsections of the connective tissue matrix are differentiated based on their position and course (Fig. 2-1).

Horizontal connective tissue matrix

The horizontal connective tissue matrix extends from the symphysis beginning with the pubovesical ligament, mainly on the side of the vagina, in a horizontal direction sacrally up to the ischial spine and curves in accordance with the angle between the vagina and uterus into a frontal plate (frontal connective tissue matrix). The horizontal connective tissue matrix sends the vaginal and cervical column in a medial direction and finally forms the fascia for the vagina and cervix. Laterally, the horizontal part of the connective tissue matrix originates in the tendinous arch of the endopelvic fascia. This is a concentration of the levator fascia, which runs just below the tendinous arch of the levator ani muscle. The horizontal portion of this connective tissue matrix begins as a narrow insertion to the rear surface of the symphysis and broadens gradually in a posterior direction against the frontal connective tissue matrix, so that from above, it has the shape of a horizontal triangle with its point facing forward.

Frontal connective tissue matrix

The frontal connective tissue matrix is a continuation of the horizontal connective tissue matrix as it curves upward

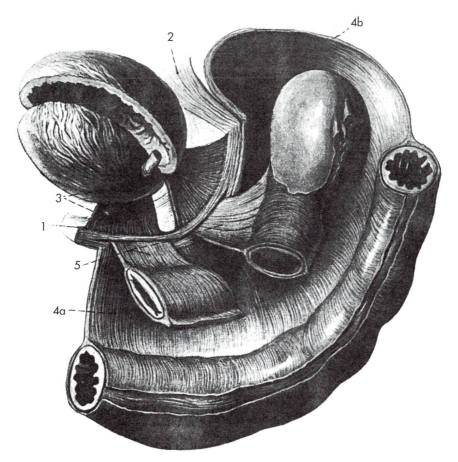

Fig. 2-1. Model of the pelvic connective tissue matrix (firm connective tissue). *1*, Horizontal connective tissue matrix; *2*, frontal connective tissue matrix (also called *ligamentum cardinale Mackenrodt*); *3*, bladder pillar (ligamentum vesicouterinum)—*a*, ascending, *b*, sagittal; *4*, rectal pillar (ligamentum rectouterinum)—*a*, descending, *b*, sagittal; *5*, vaginal-cervical column. (From Von Peham H, Amreich JA: *Gynaekologische Operationslehre*, Berlin, 1930, S Karger.)

at the large ischial foramen and rises to the point of separation of the uterine artery from the internal iliac artery. In a sagittal section, the entire connective tissue matrix has the shape of a sled runner whose point extends in a sacral direction. The horizontal part of the sled runner rests on the levator fascia; the curved part comes up in a cranial direction to a frontal plate. The frontal connective tissue matrix, also called the cardinal ligament of Mackenrodt, slowly decreases in mass in the caudocranial direction so that on sagittal section it assumes the shape of a wedge. It runs almost transversely from the uterus to the pelvic wall and, therefore, is often called the "lateral parametrium." The firm connective tissue of Mackenrodt's ligament in medial direction joins with the uterine vessels into the edge of the uterus, whereas in a lateral direction it continues upward along the pelvic sidewall into the firm connective tissue of the hypogastric vessels.

The frontal section of the connective tissue matrix can be anatomically described easily because all vessels of the urogenital tract are united within it and its lateral end is attached firmly to the pelvic wall. This fixation is especially tight because all the vessels of the pelvic viscera run

through it as they are being passed on by it to the larger vessels of the pelvic wall or they originate there.

The pelvic floor is mainly formed anatomically by the levator ani muscle and investing fascia, and in front by the urogenital diaphragm. The levator leaves a hiatus penetrated by the pelvic hollow organs (urethra, vagina, rectum). In the levator hiatus, the urethra (urinary bladder), vagina, and rectum are located one upon another, but then follow a curve of almost 90 degrees, typical for the genital tract, and are then located one behind another. The connective tissue matrix also follows this curve.

Ascending and sagittal bladder pillars

Three layers separate from the horizontal connective tissue matrix: (1) a connective tissue sheet ascending to the bladder (ascending bladder pillar), (2) a connective tissue sheet going in a caudal direction to the rectum (descending rectal pillar), and (3) a connective tissue sheet going in a medial direction to the vagina (horizontal vaginal column). But the frontal connective tissue matrix also passes the same three layers on to the pelvic organs, but these sheets have a different course because the pelvic organs are located behind one another. The bladder pillar branches off from the ventral surface of Mackenrodt's ligament and goes sagitally forward to the bladder (sagittal bladder pillar). Because of its importance as a vessel-conducting cord, this sagittal section of the bladder pillar also has its own name—"vesicouterine ligament." The name is not quite correct because the cord, as one might conclude from the name, does not go from the bladder to the side of the uterus, but instead from the bladder to the anterior surface of the frontal connective tissue matrix. The second layer originating from Mackenrodt's ligament runs from the posterior surface of this ligament in a sacral direction to the rectum (sagittal rectal pillar). This pillar is also called the rectouterine ligament, but, like the vesicouterine ligament, it contains an error in designation because it does not run from the rectum to the side of the uterus, but instead to the posterior surface of the frontal connective tissue matrix. The third layer originating from Mackenrodt's ligament runs as a frontal cervical column to the uterine neck. It contains the uterine vessels and forms the shell for the cervix.

Rectal pillar

The part of the rectal column going in a sacral direction (sagittal rectal column, uterosacral ligament) originates at the posterior surface of Mackenrodt's ligament and runs along the pelvic wall to the rectum. At its rear end, near the side wall of the rectum, the rectal pillar splits into an anterior layer that surrounds the rectum as fascia and into a posterior layer that attaches to the lateral mass of the sacrum at the level of S2-S4.

The part of the rectal pillar that runs from the posterior surface of Mackenrodt's ligament in a caudal direction (descending rectal column) is located next to the pelvic wall.

Vaginal cervical column

The connective tissue matrix in its entire expansion splits off lamellae in a medial direction to provide the fascial envelope for the pelvic organs (vaginal cervical fascia).

To expose the ureter vaginally, a knowledge of the connective tissue matrix and the subperitoneal hollow spaces filled with loose connective tissue is an absolute prerequisite.

Loose connective tissue

Between the firm columns of the connective tissue matrix on the one hand and the pelvic organs and the pelvic wall on the other hand, a series of actual or potential spaces is formed that are filled with loose connective tissue. If this loose connective tissue is removed or if it is pushed aside with the dissection scissors, the artificial or potential spaces form. The formation of the spaces exposes the firm connective tissue columns in which the blood vessels are contained (Fig. 2-2).

Prevesical space (of Retzius)

Laterally, the prevesical space borders on the lateral umbilical ligament. It may be demonstrated by bluntly separating the bladder from the rear surface of the symphysis in a downward direction using finger dissection. The space is filled with fat and loose connective tissue. Its visualization is important mainly during operations concerned with restoration of urinary continence.

Paravesical spaces

The paravesical spaces border laterally on the fascia of the obturator and the levator ani muscles, medially on the bladder and the bladder pillar, and in back the space runs up to Mackenrodt's ligament.

A paravesical space can be opened up from above by boring a hole with the closed scissors from the lateral parametrium laterally from the lateral umbilical ligament. Because the paravesical space is filled with fragile connective tissue and fat, it can be bluntly exposed easily all the way to the pelvic floor.

Vesicocervical and vesicovaginal spaces

Laterally, these spaces border on the ascending and sagittal bladder pillars, frontally on the urinary bladder, and behind on the cervix and vagina, respectively. The roof of these spaces is formed by the peritoneum (plica vesicouterina). These two spaces are separated because the rear flap of the bladder fascia is fixed to the front wall of the vagina and cervix by a small number of stronger connective tissue cords (supravaginal septum).

The vesicocervical and vesicovaginal spaces can be opened from above by transversely splitting the vesicouterine peritoneum in the midline, pushing the urinary bladder off the anterior wall of the cervix, and again in the midline by sharp dissection with the scissors, cutting through the supravaginal septum. In this way, the vesicocervical space is united with the vesicovaginal space. Then with a dissecting swab in the midline, the bladder can be bluntly pushed from the vagina. Bluntly pushing the urinary bladder away from the midline is not easy; also, it is not safe because this is where vessel-containing ascending and sagittal bladder pillars are located. (In the cranial parts of the bladder pillars, the outlet veins of the vesical plexus run to Mackenrodt's ligament to empty into the uterine veins, or to get directly into the veins of the pelvic wall.) The superior vesical artery also runs between these veins of the vesical plexus; it originates from the uterine artery and uses the bladder pillar (vesicouterine ligament) as passage to the bladder.

The ureter runs in the lowest part of the sagittal bladder pillar (the lateral wall of the vesicocervicovaginal space) in a kind of channel. If one works exactly on the midline when exposing the vesicocervical and vesicovaginal space, there is no danger of bleeding or of ureteral injury and the urinary bladder can be pushed off bluntly.

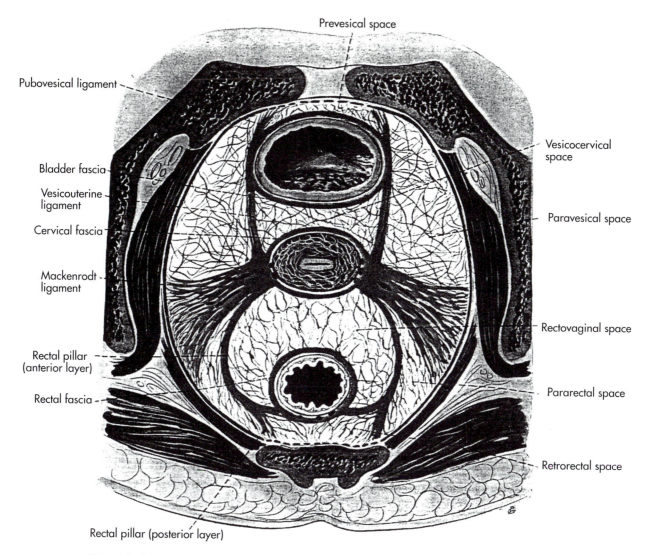

Prevesical space

Pubovesical ligament

Bladder fascia

Vesicouterine ligament

Cervical fascia

Mackenrodt ligament

Rectal pillar (anterior layer)

Rectal fascia

Rectal pillar (posterior layer)

Vesicocervical space

Paravesical space

Rectovaginal space

Pararectal space

Retrorectal space

Fig. 2-2. Schematic sectional drawing of the pelvis shows the firm connective tissue and the paraspaces (Amreich). The bladder, cervix, and rectum are surrounded by a connective tissue covering. The Mackenrodt ligament extends from the lateral cervix to the lateral abdominal pelvic wall. The vesicouterine ligament originating from the anterior edge of the Mackenrodt ligament leads to the covering of the bladder on the posterior side. The sagittal rectum column spreads both to the connective tissue of the rectum and the sacral vertebrae closely nestled against the back of the Mackenrodt ligament and lateral pelvic wall. Between the firm connective tissue bundles there is loose connective tissue (paraspaces). (From Von Peham H, Amreich JA: *Gynaekologische Operationslehre,* Berlin, 1930, S Karger.)

Rectovaginal space

Posteriorly the rectovaginal space borders on the rectum, anteriorly by the vagina, and laterally by the rectal pillars. (The sagittal rectal pillars are also called rear parametrium or rectouterine ligaments.) There is a thin layer of peritoneal fusion fascia (of Denonvilliers) fused to the undersurface of the posterior vaginal wall and extending from the most caudal portion of the cul-de-sac of Douglas to the most cranial portion of the perineal body. The roof of the rectovaginal space is formed by the peritoneum of the cul-de-sac of Douglas; caudally the vaginal fascia

and rectal fascia come more closely together just above the pelvic floor.

The rectovaginal space, which contains loose connective tissue, can be exposed by transversely cutting the peritoneum at the lowest point of the cul-de-sac of Douglas, and then bluntly separating the rectum from the vagina in the midline.

Pararectal space

The pararectal space medially borders on the rectal pillar and laterally borders on the large blood vessels of the pelvic wall or the levator and piriform muscles. Anteriorly it borders on Mackenrodt's ligament and posteriorly on the lateral parts of the sacrum. The roof is formed by the peritoneum. The caudal part of this space (e.g., during a Wertheim radical hysterectomy) is entered by penetrating with a finger around the curve of the connective tissue matrix. Here one has to stick closely to the sacrospinal ligament if one wants to separate the connective tissue matrix from the pelvic floor in the area of its knee. If the finger goes a little higher, in the area of the ischial foramen, it hits the appendage of Mackenrodt's ligament and may injure the genital veins.

After completely opening up the caudal sections of the pararectal space, one's finger arrives in the already exposed paravesical space and can reach into the front surface of Mackenrodt's ligament around the bend of the connective tissue matrix. In this way, the vessel-carrying ligament of Mackenrodt is exposed as a completely isolated condensation, which is important during a radical abdominal operation for carcinoma. After exposing the pararectal and paravesical spaces, the isolated Mackenrodt ligaments with their vessels can be ligated easily.

The pararectal space can be opened if, after separating the infundibulopelvic ligament, one splits the rear sheet of the broad ligament downward to the ureter and pushes the latter with its connective tissue layer aside.

Retrorectal space

Posteriorly the retrorectal space borders on the sacrum, anteriorly on the rectal fascia, and laterally at the height of S2-S4 on the rectal pillars, which also represent the separating wall of the pararectal spaces. Cranially, the retrorectal space changes into the retroperitoneal space, whereas in a caudal direction the space ends at the levator. The retrorectal space may be exposed by bluntly separating the rectum from the sacrum.

ARTERIES, VEINS, AND NERVES OF THE INTERNAL GENITALIA
Arteries of the internal genitalia (Fig. 2-3)

The main nutritional artery of the uterus is the uterine artery. In almost every patient it branches together with the residual umbilical artery from the internal iliac artery; rarely, it may originate directly from the hypogastric artery about 1 to 1.5 cm below the linea terminalis. The uterine artery has to be exposed when joining the so-called ovarian fascia at the lateral pelvic wall. The uterine artery then makes a medial turn and follows Mackenrodt's ligament

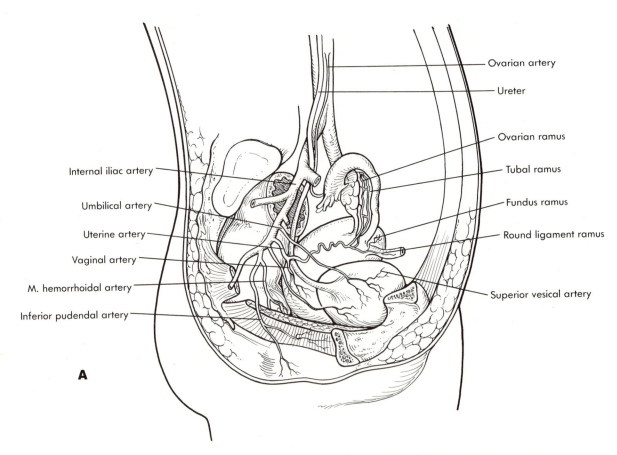

Fig. 2-3. Arteries of the internal female genitalia. **A,** Sagittal view of the right side of the pelvic arteries is shown. Notice the origin of the right ovarian artery from the aorta, which divides into an ovarian ramus and tubal ramus, and at the sides of the uterus anastomoses with uterine artery is shown, with ramus to the fundus and round ligament.

on its upper edge further medially. Inside this lateral parametrium, the uterine artery crosses the ureter. The crossing is located near the cervix about 1.5 to 2 cm lateral to the uterus. At the ureteral crossing, a small ramus uretericus branches from the uterine artery crossing cranially and caudally along the ureter. The uterine artery sends off the vaginal artery either before or after crossing the ureter. Approximately 0.5 cm lateral to the uterus, the uterine artery turns upward crossing onto the lateral margin of the uterus and sending off the rami uterini to the front and back of the uterus anastomosing to the opposite side. At the angle of the fallopian tube, the uterine artery finally branches into its four terminal arteries. The *fundus ramus,* penetrating into the muscle tissue of the uterine fundus, and the *round ligament ramus* are the weakest of the four branches leading underneath the fallopian tube to the round ligament, accompanying the round ligament to the inguinal canal and finally anastamosing to a branch of the inferior epigastric artery. The *tubal ramus* leads into the mesosalpinx and sends small branches to the fallopian tube until it reaches the infundibulopelvic ligament where it anastamoses with the ovarian artery. The *ovarian ramus,*

originating from the uterine artery below the ovarian proprium ligament, sends numerous branches to the ovary and continues into the ovarian artery, which originally had perfused the ovary alone. Branching almost immediately after the crossing of the uterine artery and the ureter, the cervical vaginal artery feeds the uterine cervix and the vagina.

The second largest artery in the internal genital area is the ovarian artery. Originating from the aorta below the renal arteries, it runs on the psoas muscle downward and crosses the ureter at the entrance of the small pelvis and reaches the ovary inside the infundibulopelvic ligament. A strong collateral branch connects the ovarian artery to the ovarian ramus and the tubal ramus of the uterine artery. The third artery concerned with perfusion of the internal genitals is the medial hemorrhoidal artery, which usually originates from the pudendal artery. It divides within Mackenrodt's ligament into a smaller branch, reaching the rectum through the descending rectum pillar and a stronger anterior branch extending into the horizontal connective tissue and the vaginal pillar to the vagina.

In the most caudal part of the vesicouterine ligament, the inferior vesical artery is surrounded by the draining

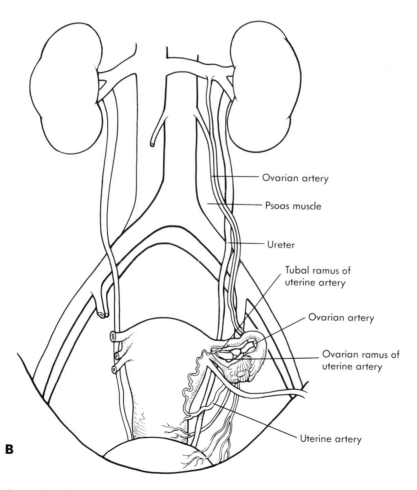

B

Fig. 2-3, cont'd. The right ureter is shown, coursing over the common iliac artery en route to the bladder. The common iliac artery divides into an internal and external branch, as shown, and the significant branches of the internal iliac are: the umbilical, the uterine, the vaginal artery, the middle hemorrhoidal artery, and the inferior pudendal artery as shown in **A**. Frontal view is shown in **B**. Note the ovarian artery and ureter coursing over the surface of the psoas muscle.

veins of the vaginal plexus. This artery is a direct branch of the internal iliac artery in the area of Mackenrodt's ligament. It uses the vesicouterine ligament to approach the bladder and vagina. Only the proximal part of the umbilical artery, being the main branch of the internal iliac in fetal life, is preserved. The distal part became the lateral umbilical ligament. The proximal part of the umbilical arteries and the superior vesical artery often consist of two branches parting on the upper edge of the sagittal pillar of the bladder (vesicouterine ligament). Similar to the inferior vesical artery, these two branches provide the bladder and the neighboring ureter with blood. The gynecologic surgeon must have detailed knowledge of the ureteral segments near the bladder because damaging any artery in the operative field may cause insufficient blood supply and perfusion followed by necrosis.

Veins of the internal genitalia (Fig. 2-4)

The veins go with parietal branches of the pelvic arteries and are, in their pelvic segments, often designed twice. The veins of the internal genitalia include the superior and inferior gluteal veins, and the ileolumbar, laterosacral, and obturator veins. The visceral branches of the veins are the internal pudendal vein (corresponding to the internal pudendal artery), which drains the deep vein of the clitoris; the posterior labial veins; and the inferior rectal veins. Entering the pelvis, the internal pudendal veins join the inferior gluteal veins. The vein plexus of the bladder, which drains the caudal segments of the bladder, flows into the internal iliac vein. The rectal vein branches surrounding the caudal segments of the rectum can drain either into the superior hemorrhoidal vein, which leads to the caudal vein, or into the medial hemorrhoidal vein, which flows into the internal iliac vein. The uterine and vaginal vein plexus are located between the posterior rectal vein plexus and the anterior vesical vein plexus. Combined, these are called the uterovaginal plexus. The uterovaginal plexus lies lateral to the vagina and the uterus, and it flows into the internal iliac veins. The vein draining the fundus of the uterus mainly uses the ovarian veins leading to the inferior vena cava. The venous drainage of the vagina is performed by the uterovaginal plexus situated in the walls of the paraspaces and flows into the internal iliac veins. All these vein plexus communicate with each other. The internal il-

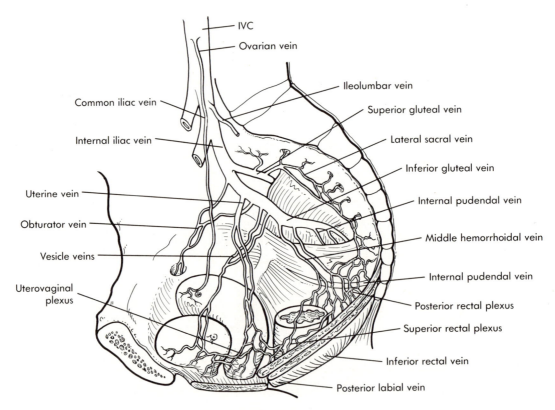

Fig. 2-4. The pelvic veins. A sagittal section shows the principle veins of the right side. Notice the uterovaginal plexes, the superior and inferior plexes, the middle hemorrhoidal veins, and internal pudendal vein and inferior gluteal vein. Together with the vesical veins, obturator veins, and uterine vein, they join the lateral and superior gluteal veins to form the internal iliac vein. The latter in company with the external iliac vein becomes the common iliac vein which proceeds directly to the vena cava. The right ovarian vein is shown.

iac vein combines with the external iliac vein, coming from the side to form the common iliac vein. The two common iliac veins join the inferior vena cava on the right side of the aorta.

The uterine and vaginal veins pass directly from Mackenrodt's ligament to the veins of the pelvic wall causing the extraordinarily firm attachment of Mackenrodt's ligament to the pelvic wall. Occasionally, the right obturator vein flows directly into the external iliac vein, and, in that case, the uterine, vaginal, and vesical veins are drained by the obturator vein. This newly created, strong vein is called the medial iliac vein.[29]

A perfect collated circulation of the venous backflow from the genitals is generally present because of the numerous venous connections and drainage into various drainage systems. Even if the hypogastric vein has been ligated, there is still enough drainage of the bladder coming from the genital into the caudal vein and the medial and superior hemorrhoidal veins. In addition, because the obturator iliac ramus is a communicating vessel between internal and external genitals, blood may flow into the external iliac vein. If the hypogastric vein is being ligated, only the drainage of the uterine, vaginal, vesical, and internal pudendal veins into the hypogastric vein is closed.

Special innervation of the internal genitalia

The celiac ganglion situated near the celiac artery is supposed to be the origin for the genital nerves. This ganglion receives parasympathetic branches from the pneumogastric (phrenic) and vagus nerves and sympathetic branches from the splanchnic nerves. The celiac ganglion is the origin for a number of nerve fibers covering the aorta (aortic plexus). The aortic plexus also receives fibers from the renal and the upper mesenteric ganglion. A bit below the renal arteries are the generally bilateral genital ganglia and the lower mesenteric ganglia (Fig. 2-5). The plexus of the prevertebral sympathetic nervous system reaches the size of about 1 cm in front of the fifth lumbar vertebrae in the branch of the aorta and can be seen, at least in thin persons, through the peritoneum of the posterior abdominal wall. In front of the sacral promontory, the plexus branches into the bilateral hypogastric plexus. This plexus borders the rectum very closely on both lateral faces and follows inside the rectal column to the posterior face of Mackenrodt's ligament. The largest ganglion located in that area is called Frankenhäuser's ganglion (Fig. 2-6). This ganglion receives parasympathetic branches from S2 to S4 (pelvic nerves) where the sensitive branches of the uterus also can be found. Frankenhäuser's ganglion is the origin of the nerve fibers of the uterus and vagina.

The fallopian tubes and ovaries are innervated by the "spermatic" plexus. The origin of this plexus is the superior part of the aortic plexus. It accompanies the ovarian artery downward and reaches the adnexa inside the infundibulopelvic ligament. In summary, nerves innervating the uterus, vagina, bladder, and rectum come from the sympathetic part from the lumbosacral bundle and the parasympathetic parts from the sacral plexus.

ARTERIES, VEINS, AND NERVES OF THE EXTERNAL GENITALIA
Urogenital and anal region

The internal pudendal artery and vein and the pudendal nerve after passing the minor ischiatic fossa are located in the pudendal (Alcock) canal inside of the internal obturator fascia (Fig. 2-7). The inferior rectal vein and artery (hemorrhoidal or anal vein and artery) branch here, and the inferior rectal nerves reach the anus through the fat tissues of the ischiorectal fossa.

Arteries. The internal pudendal artery branches into the perineal and clitoral artery at the posterior edge of the urogenital diaphragm. The perineal artery passes the perineum in the superficial perineal space of the urogenital region and finally forms the posterior labial rami, which supply the major and minor labia with blood. The clitoral artery, which is a continuation of the internal pudendal artery, sends out the vestibular artery at the region of the posterior edge of the urogenital diaphragm penetrating into the bulbus vestibuli. The clitoral artery is embedded in the urogenital diaphragm tissue. The two terminal branches of the clitoral artery are the profundus and dorsal clitoral artery. The profundus artery penetrates into the crurals of the clitoris coming from the diaphragm. The dorsal clitoral artery leads to the dorsum of the clitoris leaving the diaphragm closely underneath the symphysis. Clitoral erection is caused by the terminal branches of the internal pudendal artery (dorsal clitoral artery and vestibular artery); in an amputation of the clitoris, both dorsal and clitoral arteries need to be ligated for hemostasis. Although bleeding coming from the corpora cavernosa may easily be stopped by compression, it is more exact to suture the corpora.

Veins. The main vein is the internal pudendal vein, which does not drain the whole volume of the area. Another pond flows underneath the symphysis toward the vesicopudendal plexus. The dorsal superficial clitoral vein drains the corpus of the clitoris and the glands. The internal pudendal vein receives blood coming from the bulbus vestibuli in the bulbovestibular vein where the profundus clitoral vein also contributes. In addition, the internal pudendal vein drains the dorsal part of the labia through the posterior labial veins. The internal pudendal vein crosses along the posterior edge of the urogenital triangle and goes into the pudendal canal to the minor ischiadic foramen. Passing the infrapiriform foramen, it enters the small pelvis and flows into the internal iliac vein. The perineal veins do not have venous valves; therefore, if the tension of the pelvic floor muscles decreases, the venous blood flow will be obstructed. Chronic venous stasis causes the developing of varices including the area of the draining hemorrhoidal veins. Reconstruction of the pelvic floor muscles causes increasing tension in the pelvic floor and stops chronic venous stasis. The blood congestion of the

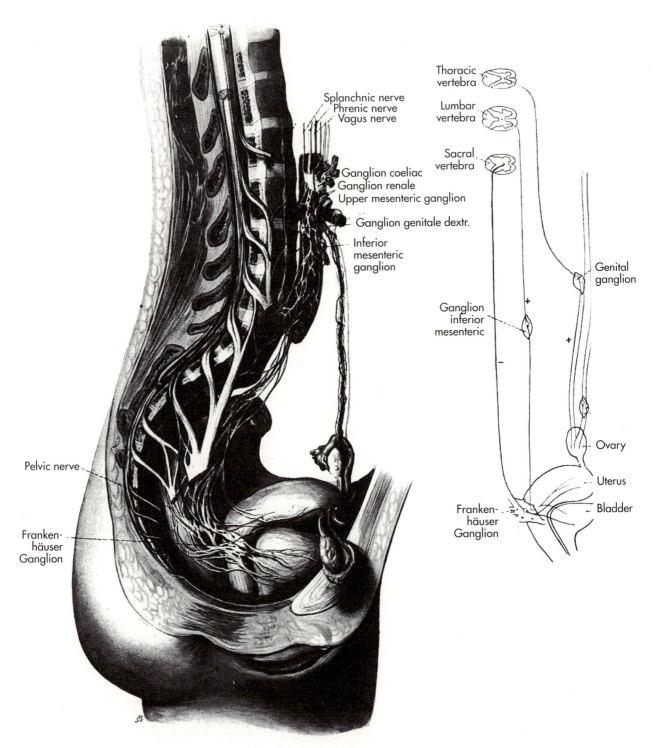

Fig. 2-5. Semischematic illustration of the genital innervation. (From Von Peham H, Amreich JA: *Gynaekologische Operationslehre*, Berlin, 1930, S Karger.)

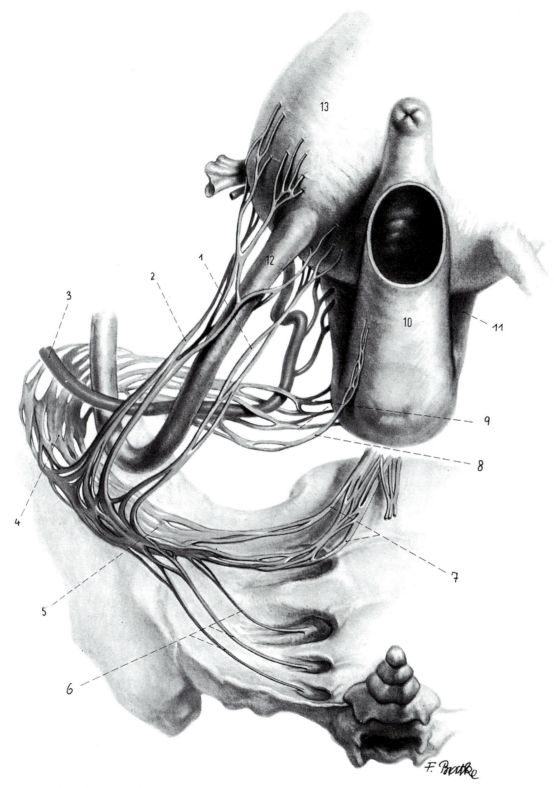

Fig. 2-6. Innervation of uterus, bladder and vagina, viewed from the perineum. *1*, Inferior vesical nerves; *2*, superior vesical nerves; *3*, uterine artery; *4*, uterine plexus (uterovaginal); *5*, plexus pelvinus (pelvic ganglion, inferior hypogastric plexus); *6*, pelvic nerves (parasympathetic); *7*, superior hypogastric plexus (sympathetic); *8*, vaginal ramus; *9*, uterine nerves; *10*, vagina; *11*, uterus; *12*, ureter; *13*, urinary bladder. (From Reiffenstuhl G, Platzer W: *Die Vaginalen Operationen. Chirurg Anatomie u Operationslehre*, Berlin, 1974, Urban-Schwarzenberg.)

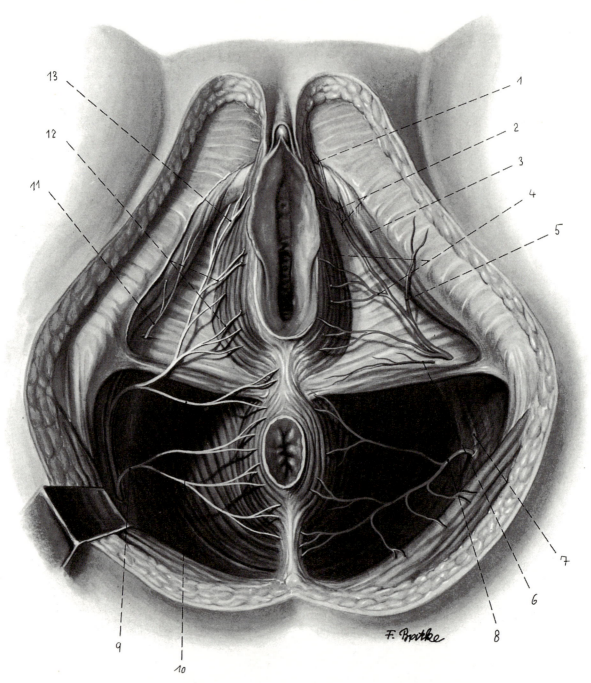

Fig. 2-7. The arteries and nerves of the pelvic floor as seen from below, demonstrating the branching of the internal pudendal artery and of the pudendal nerve. *1*, Dorsal clitoral artery; *2*, deep clitorial artery; *3*, ischiocavernosus muscle; *4*, bulbocavernosus muscle and the artery of the vestibular bulb; *5*, posterior labial artery; *6*, perineal artery; *7*, internal pudendal artery in Alcock's canal; *8*, inferior rectal artery; *9*, anal nerve; *10*, perineal nerve; *11*, branch innervating the ischiocavernosus muscle; *12*, posterior labial nerves; *13*, dorsal clitoral nerve. (From Reiffenstuhl G, Platzer W: *Die Vaginalen Operationen. Chirurg Anatomie u Operationslehre.* Berlin, 1974, Urban-Schwarzenberg.)

erectile phases (clitoris and bulbocavernosus body) probably is a secondary phenomenon.[38] Most of this blood comes from the arterial side.

Nerves. The pudendal nerve is thought to be the main nerve of the urogenital region. It passes the pudendal canal sending inferior rectal nerves (anal nerves) to innervate the external sphincter muscle of the anus and the anal skin area. At the posterior edge of the urogenital diaphragm, the pudendal nerve finally branches into the perineal and clitoral nerves. The perineal nerves terminate in the urogenital diaphragm into the posterior labial nerves, which innervate the dorsal part of the labia. Some of its fibers innervate the transverse superficial perineal muscle and the muscles of the swelling body. The clitoral nerve supplies the dorsum of the clitoris, the muscle of the urethra, and the deep transverse perineal muscle. These nerves are all branches of the pudendal nerve. The anococcygeal nerves also participate in the innervation of the urogenital and anal skin, originating from the coccygeal nerve and penetrating the pelvic diaphragm near the coccyx. They innervate the area around the coccyx toward the anus. The skin around the ischial tuberosity is innervated by perineal rami that originate from the posterior femoral nerve.

Perineal region

Arteries. The main vessel is the internal pudendal artery. The lateral and anterior segments of the labia are perfused by the anterior labial rami, which originate from the external pudendal and, therefore, from the femoral artery.

Veins. The deep veins have been discussed previously. On the dorsum of the clitoris, there is a superficial vein. This subcutaneous dorsal vein of the clitoris connects to the deep vessels of the clitoris but also to the subcutaneous veins of the pubic mons. More important are the anterior labial veins flowing into the external pudendal veins and finally being drained by the femoral veins.

Nerves. The pudendal nerve is the most important nerve for this region. Its posterior/labial nerves innervate the dorsal segment of the labia, and the dorsal/clitoral nerve covers the area of the clitoris. The anterior labial nerves, which are branches of the ilioinguinal nerve, reach the pubic mons, the ventral part of the major labia, and the clitoral prepuce.

The genital rami of the genital/femoral nerves participate in the neural supply of the major labia reaching the area accompanying the teres uteri ligament.

LYMPHATIC SYSTEM OF THE FEMALE GENITALS
Pelvic lymph nodes

The pelvic lymph nodes are mostly concentrated around the large arteries and veins. This means that the blood vessels of the pelvis are entwined by lymphatic nerves and vessels. It is of more use to discuss the lymphatics in certain groups based on their location near the arteries, although there is no other system in the body as well connected and transitional as the lymphatic system of the pelvis (Fig. 2-8).

Aortic lymph nodes. The nodes are located anteriorly, laterally, and superiorly to the aorta (Fig. 2-8, *A*).

Lateral common iliac lymph nodes. The nodes are located on the lateral face of the common iliac artery. The superficial lymph nodes can be seen easily at the lateral phase of the common iliac artery (Fig. 2-8, *B*). The deep lymph nodes of this group are attached to the posterior face of the common iliac vessels and, therefore, are hidden (Fig. 2-8, *C*). They can be exposed by following the lateral margins of the common iliac artery into the depths lying between the posterior face of the vessels and the psoas muscle.

Medial common iliac lymph nodes. The nodes are located on the medial face of the common iliac artery (Fig. 2-8, *D*).

Lateral external iliac lymph nodes. These nodes are located on the lateral edges of the external iliac artery. The superficial (Fig. 2-8, *E*) and deep lymph nodes (Fig. 2-8, *F*) are found caudal to the common iliac lymph nodes. These lymph nodes are not often exposed but can be found on the posterior surface of the external iliac vessels between the vessels and the psoas muscle.

Interiliac lymph nodes. All lymph nodes are located on the pelvic wall in the obturator fossa, which is limited by the medial face of the external iliac artery, by the lateral face of the internal iliac artery, and by the superior face of the obturator artery (Fig. 2-8, *G*). They can be divided into three groups: hypogastric lymph nodes located in the hypogastric angle (Fig. 2-8, *H*), obturator lymph nodes located along the obturator vessels and the obturator nerve (Fig. 2-8, *I*), and medial external iliac lymph nodes located on the medial face of the external iliac artery (Fig. 2-8, *J*). Usually the interiliac lymph nodes form a bunch surrounded by plenty of fat tissue. Starting distally at the femoral annulus extending cranially to the hypogastric angle, the lymph node packet caudally borders the obturator artery. The group of lymph nodes surrounding the femoral annulus at the place where the external iliac vessels meet the pelvic vessels mostly consist of three lymph nodes called annuli femoralis lymph nodes (Fig. 2-8, *K*). In this group, the lateral lymph node corresponds to the most distal lateral external iliac lymph node. The middle one is located on the external iliac vessels, and the medial one corresponds to the most distal obturator lymph node, known as Rosenmüller's node.

Superior gluteal lymph nodes. These are located at the branch of the internal iliac artery and the cranial gluteal artery situated on the medial phase of the cranial gluteal artery (Fig. 2-8, *L*).

Inferior gluteal lymph nodes. These are located on the branch of and along the inferior gluteal and internal pudendal artery, caudal to the obturator artery (Fig. 2-8, *M*). At the lateral insertion of Mackenrodt's ligament, they lie on the internal obturator muscle and the piriform muscle, on the sacral pelvis plexus. These lymph nodes can be found along the pelvic wall down to the lateral part of the infrapiriform foramen where the pudendal artery leaves the pelvis. This area corresponds to the region around the spine of the ischiatic bone. These lymph nodes are found on the pelvic wall partly anterior and partly posterior to the blood vessels.

Subaortic lymph nodes (promontoric). These are located in the aortic bifurcation on the fifth lumbar vertebra and the promontory (Fig. 2-8, *N*).

Sacral lymph nodes. These are located on the anterior face of the sacral bone in the basin of the medial and lateral sacral arteries (Fig. 2-8, *O*).

Cranial rectal lymph nodes. These are located at the posterior wall of the rectum in the basin of the cranial rectal artery.

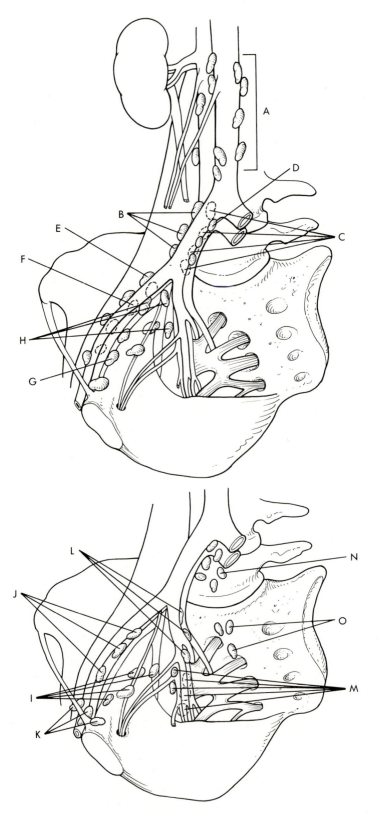

Fig. 2-8. The pelvic lymph nodes. *A*, Aortic lymph nodes; *B*, lateral common iliac lymph nodes (superficial); *C*, lateral common iliac lymph nodes (deep); *D*, medial common iliac lymph nodes; *E*, lateral external iliac lymph nodes (superficial); *F*, lateral external iliac lymph nodes (deep); *G*, interiliac lymph nodes; *H*, hypogastric lymph nodes; *I*, obturator lymph nodes; *J*, medial external iliac lymph nodes; *K*, femoral ring lymph nodes; *L*, superior gluteal lymph nodes; *M*, inferior gluteal lymph nodes; *N*, subaortic (promontorial) lymph nodes; *O*, sacral lymph nodes. (Adapted and redrawn from Reiffenstuhl G: *Das Lymphsystem d weiblichen Genitale*. Vienna, 1957, Urban-Schwarzenberg.)

The lymphatic drainage of the uterus and vagina can be traced by following the blood vessels of these organs to the lymphatic nodes on the pelvic wall.

Draining lymphatics of the cervix uteri. Figure 2-9 shows schematically the lymphatics leaving the cervix uteri. All groups of lymph nodes from number 1 to 10 are the station of the drainage of the cervix uteri. The actual extension of the lymphatics connecting the cervix uteri and the pelvic lymph nodes is shown in Figs. 2-10 to 2-14.

Draining lymphatics of the corpus uteri and the vagina. Figures 2-15 and 2-16 show schematics of the lymphatics originating at the corpus uteri and the vagina. Numbers 1, 5, 6, 8, and 9 are strongly marked because they belong to the lymph node stages mainly frequented by the lymphatics of the corpus uteri and vagina.

Lymphatic cord of Poirier-Seelig

At the lateral edge of the uterus there is a lymphatic cord first described by Poirier and confirmed by Seelig (Fig. 2-17). This lymphatic cord connects the uterine lymph vessels to the vaginal lymph vessels and even the ovarian and fallopian tube lymph vessels. This anatomic situation allows the carcinoma of the portio, above all cervical carcinoma, to metastasize cranially into the myometrium of the corpus uteri. The carcinoma cells may use the meridionally running anastamosis. For that reason, the cervical carcinoma cells may infiltrate the muscles of the corpus uteri with numerous cords of carcinoma and isolated fields or clusters right up to the uterine fundus. Because of the metastases spreading from the meridional to the radial lymph vessels and by retrograde cell transport,

Text continued on p. 49.

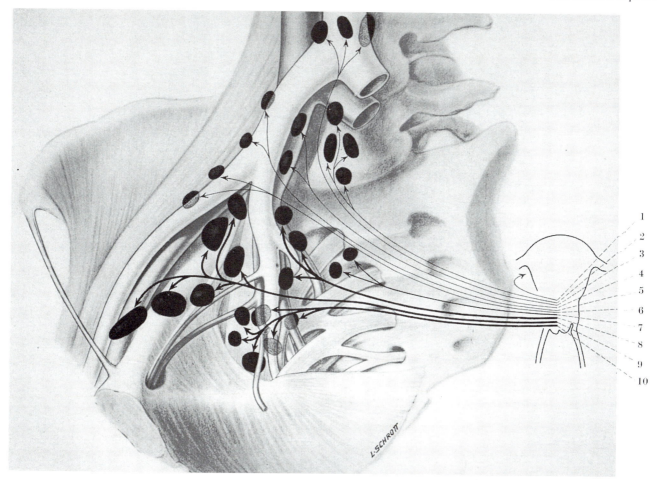

Fig. 2-9. Schematic illustration of the regional stages of the lymph nodes of the cervix. Channels 8, 9 and 10 are strongly marked because they feed main lymphatics of the cervix. Nevertheless, it has to be taken into consideration that in cases of carcinoma of the cervix, tumor cells easily could be spread directly to the pelvic lymph nodes by lymphatics number 1 to 7. Remember that the inferior gluteal lymph node being near to the ischiatic spine might be totally or partly hidden because of there localization behind the bigger vessels. Therefore, in Wertheim's radical procedure and modified procedures, it is technically very difficult if not relatively impossible to remove these lymph nodes (exemption Brunschwig's exenteration, discussed later on). These facts explain the occurrence of so-called "ischial spinous recurrence" in cancer of the cervix, which is not a real recurrence but more likely a primary of metastasis to lymph nodes. To (1) rectal, (2) subaortic (promontorial), (3) aortic, (4) medial common iliac, (5) lateral common iliac, (6) lateral external iliac, (7) sacral, (8) superior gluteal, (9) interiliac and (10) inferior gluteal lymph nodes. (From Reiffenstuhl G: *Das Lymphsystem d weiblichen Genitale,* Vienna, 1957, Urban-Schwarzenberg.)

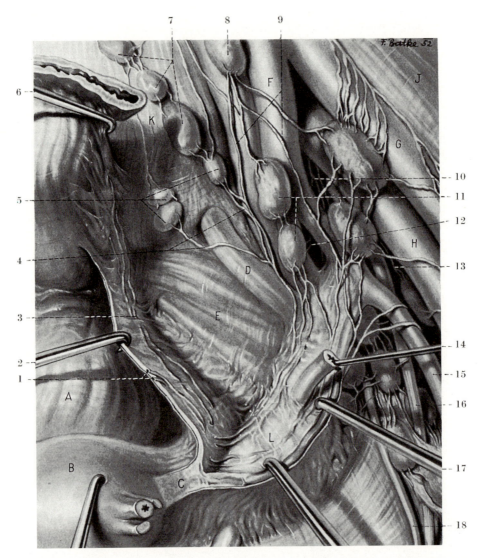

Fig. 2-10. Lymphatic drainage of the cervix to the pelvic wall and rectum. The recto-uterine ligaments (sagittal/rectal pillar or column) is drawn medially by a small retractor *(2)*. The lymphatics of the cervix *(3)* inside the sagittal/rectal pillar reach the posterior face of the rectum flowing into the superior rectal lymph nodes (not seen). The lymphatics marked with *(1)* extend cranially to the ureter sheet. Originating from the superior gluteal lymph nodes *(11)* efferent vessels lead to the medial common iliac lymph nodes *(8)*. Notice that cervical lymphatics *(4)* reach the sacral lymph nodes *(5)* located on the anterior sacrum without any interruption. These lymph nodes are likewise regional lymph node stage of the cervix. *A,* Rectum; *B,* uterus (intestinal surface); *C,* Mackenrodt's ligament (medial portion); *D,* first sacral nerve; *E,* piriform muscle; *F,* internal and *G,* external iliac arteries; *H,* external iliac vein; *J,* psoas muscle; *K,* promontory; *L,* Mackenrodt's ligament (posterior surface); *1,* cervical lymph vessels; *2,* recto-uterine ligament; *3* and *4,* cervical lymph vessels; *5,* sacral lymph nodes; *6,* rectum; *7,* subaortic (promontorial) and *8,* medial common iliac lymph nodes; *9,* cervical lymph vessels; *10,* efferent vessels; *11,* superior gluteal lymph nodes; *12* and *13,* efferent vessels; *14,* ureter; *15,* lateral umbilical ligament; *16,* obturator nerve; *17,* uterine and *18,* obturator arteries. (From Reiffenstuhl G: *Das Lymphsystem d weiblichen Genitale,* Vienna, 1957, Urban-Schwarzenberg.)

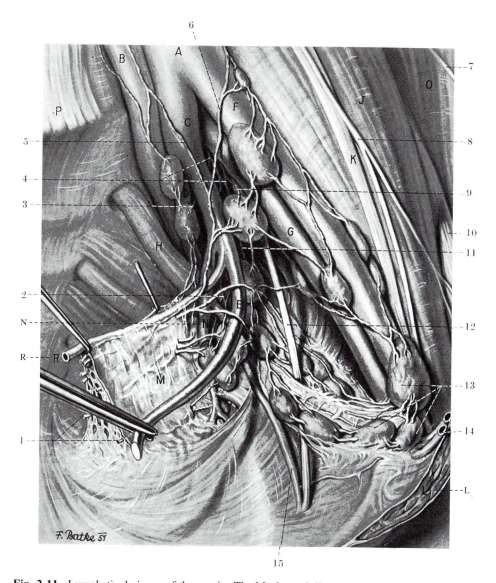

Fig. 2-11. Lymphatic drainage of the cervix. The Mackenrodt ligament was divided from the ureter. The superior border of the ligament is the uterine artery followed by several lymphatics flowing into the hypogastric and obturator lymph nodes. Efferent vessels of the cervix *(6)* pass the hypogastric lymph nodes and reach (without any interruption) the nodes of the lateral face of the external iliac artery. Further lymphatic vessels of the cervix pulled out by a small retractor follow at first the uterine artery and then join the superior gluteal lymph nodes surrounding the artery of the same name *(D)*. Other lymphatic drainages of the cervix flow into the inferior gluteal and the hypogastric lymph nodes located caudally to the obturator artery and partly covered by the lateral umbilical ligament. Notice the deep draining vessels *(2, 11* and *4)* coming from the inferior gluteal and the hypogastric lymph nodes, crossing underneath the big vessels of the pelvic wall to empty into the profound common iliac lymph nodes situated at the posterior face of the common iliac vessels *(A, B)* (see also Fig. 2-13). *A,* Common iliac artery; *B,* common iliac vein; *C,* internal iliac artery; *D,* superior gluteal artery; *E,* lateral umbilical ligament; *F,* external iliac artery; *G,* external iliac vein; *H,* first sacral nerve; *J,* psoas major and *K,* psoas minor muscles (tendon); *L,* internal oblique and transversus abdominis muscles; *M,* Mackenrodt's ligament; *N,* inferior gluteal-internal pudendal artery; *O,* iliac muscle; *P,* promontory; *R,* uterine artery; *1,* cervical lymph vessels; *2 to 4,* efferent vessels; *5 to 6,* cervical lymph vessel; *7,* lateral femoral cutaneous nerve; *8,* genitofemoral nerve; *9,* deep lateral external lymph node; *10,* femoral nerve; *11,* efferent vessel; *12,* obturator nerve; *13,* femoral ring lymph nodes; *14,* inferior epigastric vessel; *15,* obturator artery. (From Reiffenstuhl G: *Das Lymphsystem d weiblichen Genitale,* Vienna, 1957, Urban-Schwarzenberg.)

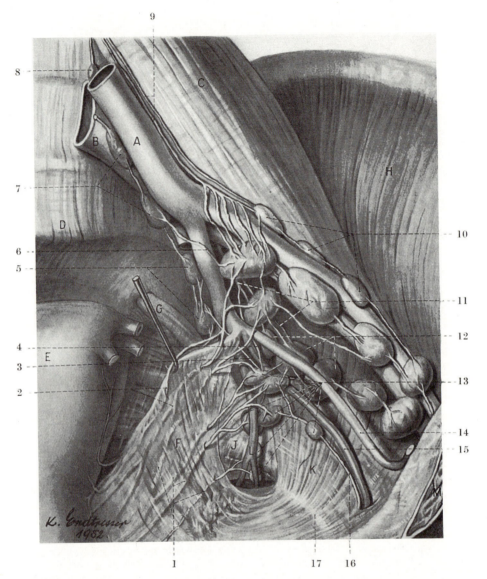

Fig. 2-12. Lymphatic vessels of the cervix *(1)* to the inferior gluteal lymph nodes. They go mainly to the pelvic wall in the basal segments of the lateral parametrium and then empty into the inferior gluteal lymph nodes *(13)* predominate. These nodes extend along the inferior gluteal-internal pudendal artery down as far to the infrapiriform foramen and, in part, lie behind the parietal blood vessels and are hidden by them. *A,* Common iliac artery; *B,* common iliac vein; *C,* psoas muscle; *D,* promontory; *E,* uterus; *F,* Mackenrodt's ligament; *G,* 1st sacral nerve; *H,* iliac muscle; *J,* sacral plexus; *K,* internal obturator muscle; *L,* internal pudendal-inferior gluteal artery; *M,* internal oblique and transverse abdominal muscles; *1* and *2,* cervical lymph vessels; *3* and *4,* efferent vessels; *5,* superior gluteal lymph nodes; *6,* efferent vessel; *7,* medial common iliac and *8,* deep lateral common iliac lymph nodes; *9,* lymphatic vessels; *10,* lateral external iliac lymph nodes; *11,* efferent vessels; *12,* interiliac (obturator) and *13,* inferior gluteal lymph nodes; *14,* lateral umbilical ligament; *15,* obturator artery; *16,* lymphatic vessel; *17,* tendinous arch of the levator ani muscle. (From Reiffenstuhl G: *Das Lymphsystem d weiblichen Genitale,* Vienna, 1957, Urban-Schwarzenberg.)

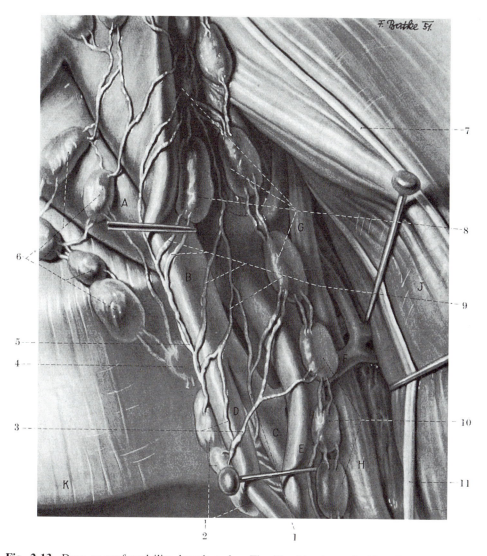

Fig. 2-13. Deep or profound iliac lymph nodes. The iliac blood vessels *(B to E)* were divided from the psoas muscle and pulled towards medial. The obturator nerve *(11)* and the psoas muscle *(J)* are forced laterally by two needles. In the deep recess the fourth lumbar nerve *(G)*, the lumbosacral trunk *(H)*, and the iliolumbal artery *(F)* are exposed. They are accompanied by the deep lateral common iliac lymph nodes *(8)* and the deep lateral external iliac lymph nodes *(10)*. The anatomical location of these lymph nodes is behind the parietal blood vessels and normally hidden by those vessels. When extirpating the deep external and common iliac lymph nodes, the iliolumbal artery *(F)* has to be exposed carefully to avoid damage. A, Left common iliac vein; *B*, left common iliac artery (posterior aspect); *C*, internal iliac artery (posterior aspect); *D*, external iliac artery (posterior aspect); *E*, external iliac vein (posterior aspect); *F*, iliolumbal artery; *G*, half of fourth lumbar nerve; *H*, lumbosacral trunk; *J*, psoas muscle; *K*, promontory; *1*, efferent vessels; *2*, lateral external iliac lymph nodes; *3*, efferent vessels; *4*, medial common iliac lymph node; *5*, lymph vessels; *6*, subaortic (promontorial) lymph nodes; *7*, genitofemoral nerve; *8*, deep lateral common iliac lymph nodes; *9*, efferent vessels; *10*, deep lateral external iliac lymph nodes; *11*, obturator nerve. (From Reiffenstuhl G: *Das Lymphsystem d weiblichen Genitale*, Vienna, 1957, Urban-Schwarzenberg.)

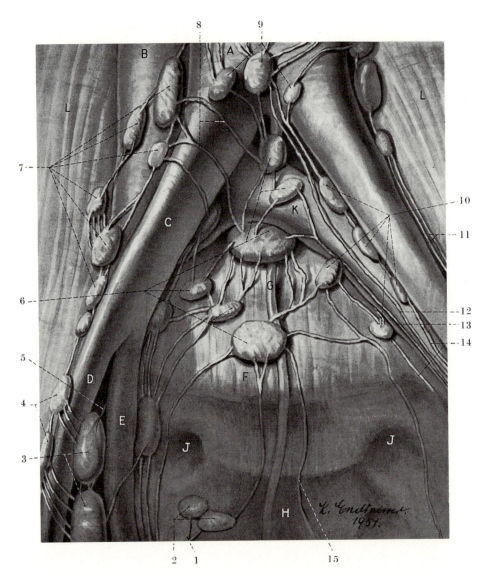

Fig. 2-14. Inflow and outflow of the subaortic (promontory) lymph nodes *(6)* which lie on the promontory *(F)* and in the aortic bifurcation angle and are interconnected by numerous lymph vessels so that the picture of a lymphatic plexus is created on the promontory. They are also regional lymph nodes of the cervix of the uterus because they are supplied by lymph vessels *(13)* coming from the cervix and being intermitted for the first time here. Other lymphatics of the cervix *(12)* pass the subaortic lymph nodes without emptying into them and first being interrupted by the aortic lymph nodes *(9)*. In conclusion, even the aortic lymph nodes are also a regional lymph node station of the lymphatic drainage of the cervix. Notice further the deep lymphatic vessels *(5)* starting from the hypogastric lymph nodes, undercrossing the internal iliac artery running upward and performing a connection to the deep common iliac lymph nodes. These are located behind the blood vessels of the same names and are not visible here. (Compare with Figs. 2-10, 2-11, and 2-13.) *A,* Aorta; *B,* inferior vena cava; *C,* right common iliac artery; *D,* external iliac artery; *E,* internal iliac artery; *F,* promontory; *G,* medial sacral artery; *H,* sacrum; *J,* first sacral foramen; *K,* left common iliac vein; *L,* psoas muscle; *1,* cervical lymph vessels; *2,* sacral; *3,* interiliac and *4,* lateral external iliac lymph nodes; *5,* efferent vessels; *6,* subaortic (promontorial) and *7,* lateral common iliac lymph nodes; *8,* efferent vessels; *9,* aortic and *10,* medial common iliac lymph nodes; *11,* lymph vessels; *12 to 15,* cervical lymph vessels. (From Reiffenstuhl G: *Das Lymphsystem d weiblichen Genitale,* Vienna, 1957, Urban-Schwarzenberg.)

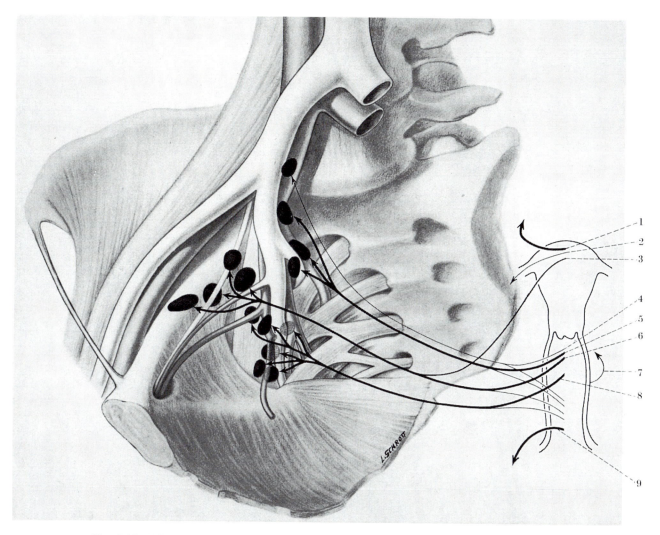

Fig. 2-15. Schematic illustration of the regional lymph nodes staging of the vagina and the corpus of the uterus. Lymphatic vessels number 1, 5, 6, 8 and 9 are strongly marked because they are emptying into the regional lymph node groups, mostly draining from the uterus, fundus, and vagina. Notice in comparison to Fig. 2-9 the partly hidden location of the inferior gluteal lymph node (gray) reached by vessel number 8. To *(1)* aorta, *(2)* inguinal, *(3)* interiliac, *(4)* medial common iliac, *(5)* superior gluteal, *(6)* interiliac, *(7)* rectal, *(8)* inferior gluteal, and *(9)* inguinal lymph nodes. (From Reiffenstuhl G: *Das Lymphsystem d weiblichen Genitale,* Vienna, 1957, Urban-Schwarzenberg.)

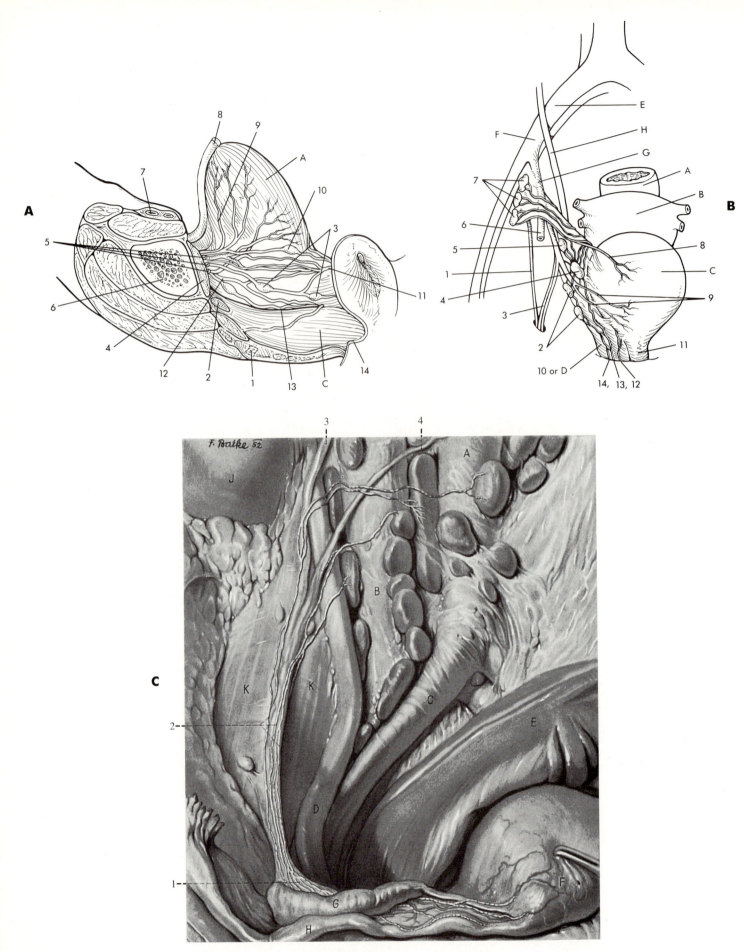

Fig. 2-16. For legend see opposite page.

Fig. 2-16. A, Lymphatic drainage of vagina, urethra and bladder. Vaginal lymph vessels *(13)* follow the vaginal artery upward to the lymph nodes of the pelvic wall. The course is interrupted by small paravaginal or juxtavaginal lymph nodes *(3)*. Other vaginal lymphatics *(15)* extend to the posterior face of the rectum *(C)* flowing into the rectal (anorectal) lymph nodes (therefore lymph node metastasis on the back side of the rectum from carcinoma of the vagina is possible). The draining lymph vessels of the intrapelvic segment of the urethra *(11)* sometimes are interrupted by an anterior vesical lymph node *(10)* and later proceed to the pelvic wall accompanied by the efferent lymphatic vessels of the bladder *(A)*. A, Urinary bladder; B, vagina; C, rectum; D, labium pudendi; *1,* sacral os; *2,* ischiatic nerve; *3,* juxtavaginal lymph nodes; *4,* internal obturator muscle; *5,* obturator nerve, artery and vein; *6,* os; *7,* femoral artery and vein; *8,* lateral umbilical ligament; *9,* lymph vessels of the urinary bladder; *10,* anterior vesical lymph node; *11,* urethral lymph vessels; *12,* vaginal artery; *13,* vaginal lymph vessels; *14,* anus; *15,* vaginal lymph vessel. **B,** Lymphatic drainage of the superior half of the vagina. The fatty-lymphnodal tissue of the obturator fossa were taken down the pelvic wall and clipped in a medial direction. Several vaginal lymph vessels *(12)* go upward to the draining lymph vessels of the cervix and turn along the superior vesical artery *(8)* emptying then all into the hypogastric lymph nodes *(7)*. Other vaginal lymph vessels *(13)* flow into a obturator lymph node *(4)* which has been medially exposed. From there, lymphatic connections go to a superior gluteal lymph node *(5)*. Notice further the course of the draining vaginal lymph vessels *(14)* flowing into an inferior gluteal lymph node *(2)*. A, Rectum; B, uterus (vesical surface); C, urinary bladder; D, vagina; E, common iliac artery; F, external iliac artery; G, internal iliac artery; H, ureter; *1,* obturator nerve; *2,* inferior gluteal lymph nodes; *3,* obturator artery; *4,* interiliac (obturator) lymph node; *5,* superior gluteal lymph node; *6,* lateral umbilical ligament; *7,* hypogastric lymph nodes; *8,* superior vesical artery; *9,* inferior vesical veins; *10,* vagina; *11,* urethra; *12* to *14,* vaginal lymph vessels. **C,** Lymphatic drainage of the fallopian tube, ovary and fundus of the uterus. Lymphatic vessels originating at the tube go either directly to the subovarian lymphatic plexus *(1)* or flow first into the lymph vessels draining the uterine fundus *(F)*. The lymphatics of the fundus follow the ovarian proprium ligament and mesosalpinx until reaching the subovarian plexus which mainly drains the ovary area. From that place the lymphatic vessels *(2)* extend along the ovarian blood vessels cranially, leaves the blood vessels near the lower kidney edge *(J)*, turns medially across the ureter *(D)* and flow into the upper aortic lymph nodes. A, Aorta; B, inferior vena cava; C, right common iliac artery; D, ureter; E, sigmoid; F, uterine fundus; G, right ovary; H, right fallopian tube; J, right kidney; K, psoas muscle; *1,* subovarian plexus; *2,* lymph vessels; *3,* ovarian vein; *4,* ovarian artery. (Adapted and redrawn from Reiffenstuhl G: *Das Lymphsystem d weiblichen Genitale,* Vienna, 1957, Urban-Schwarzenberg.)

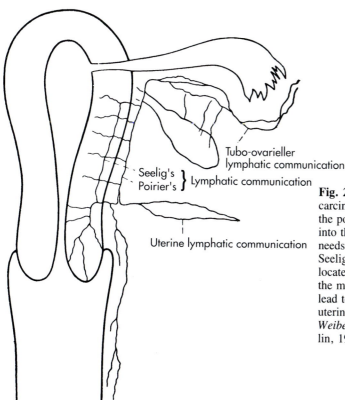

Tubo-ovarieller lymphatic communication

Seelig's
Poirier's } Lymphatic communication

Uterine lymphatic communication

Fig. 2-17. Lymphatic cord of Poirier. Possible metastasis of cervical carcinoma into the uterine corpus. Advanced cases of cancer in both the portio vaginalis and primarily the cervix can metastasize upwards into the myometrium of the uterine corpus. For such dissemination it needs anastomoses of the mucosal and myometrial lymphatics of Seelig which radiate to the meridionally coursing Poirier lymphatics, located along the border of the uterus. In this way they can intersperse the musculature of the uterine corpus with cancerous areas and also lead to development of metastatic colonies in the mucosa of the uterine corpus. (From Amreich IA: *Biologie und Pathologie des Weibes, Hdb d Frauenheilk u Gebtsch.* In Seitz-Amreich: *Bd. IV,* Berlin, 1955, Urban-Schwarzenberg.)

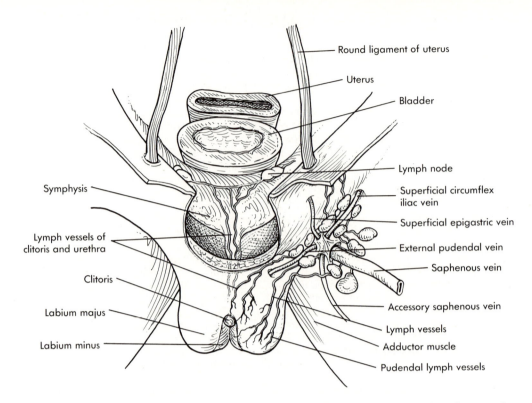

Fig. 2-18. Lymph drainage. (Adapted and redrawn from Reiffenstuhl G: *Das Lymphsystem d weiblichen Genitale,* Vienna, 1957, Urban-Schwarzenberg.)

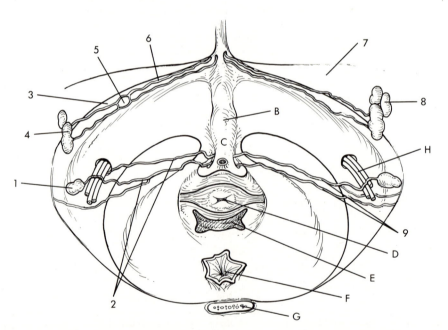

Fig. 2-19. Entrance of the extrapelvic lymph vessels into the pelvis and their course to the intrapelvic lymph nodes. View into the small pelvis from above. On the upper edge of the symphysis several lymph vessels (6) enter the pelvic cavity medially between the insertion of the rectus abdominal muscle (A). Then following the superior ramus of the pubic bone (3) they may reach on both sides the femoral ring lymph nodes (4, 8). Other lymph vessels (2) reach the pelvis together with the dorsal vein of the clitoris (C) following the inferior surface of the symphysis, then turn laterally and reach an obturator lymph node (1) on the left hand side whereas on the right hand side, they (9) empty finally into the hypogastric lymph nodes. In this manner, efferent lymphatic channels of the external genitals have reached lymph nodes of the pelvic wall as their regional stations. A, Rectus abdominis muscle; B, symphysis (posterior aspect); C, dorsal clitoridic vein; D, urethra; E, vagina; F, rectum; G, sacrum; H, obturator nerve, artery and vein; 1, obturator lymph node; 2, lymph vessels; 3, superior ramus of the pubic bone; 4, femoral ring lymph nodes; 5, lymph node; 6, lymph vessels; 7, inguinal ligament; 8, femoral ring lymph nodes; 9, lymph vessels. (Adapted and redrawn from Reiffenstuhl G: *Das Lymphsystem d weiblichen Genitale,* Vienna, 1957, Urban-Schwarzenberg.)

cervical cancer might cause isolated islands of tumor inside the mucous membrane of the corpus uteri. Even in the more cranially situated internal genitals, the fallopian tubes and ovaries, there might be an invasion by cells from the carcinoma of the cervix. These results are more likely to appear with corpus uteri carcinoma than with uterine cervical carcinoma.

Cervical cancer usually spreads into the vagina by continual growth and local infiltration of a superficial cancer cell population destroying the vaginal epithelium. In rare cases, metastatic disease carries carcinoma cells of the cervix in the lymph vessels of the cord of Poirier downward to the vagina by reversing the lymphatic flow direction. Small carcinoma cell aggregations infiltrate the rectal/vaginal septum, inside the paravaginal connective tissue.

Draining lymph vessels of bladder and urethra. The course of the lymphatics between bladder and lymph nodes of the pelvic wall is illustrated in Fig. 2-16, *A*. The lymphatics of the extrapelvic segment of the urethra are shown in Figs. 2-16, *B* and 2-16, *C*.

Draining lymph vessels of the labia and clitoris. The courses of the lymph vessels from the labia and clitoris to the inguinal lymph nodes, and also to the pelvic lymph nodes, are illustrated in Figs. 2-18 and 2-19.

LYMPHADENECTOMY

Every operation on a carcinoma should fulfill the following three demands:

1. If possible, the cancerous organ must be removed in total.
2. The surrounding tissue must be resected as much as possible.
3. The regional lymph nodes must be extirpated or resected.

It is probably impossible to remove all lymph nodes of the cervix uteri in a surgical procedure. The usual lymph node resection will always be incomplete because in procedures after Wertheim-Meigs, Latzko, or Okabajashi, the inferior gluteal lymph nodes are not removed. Radical extirpation of these lymph nodes would be complete only with resection of the gluteal pudendal vessels, which technically is not possible. Resection of these vessels of the pelvic wall fails because the veins accompanying the gluteal pudendal artery are very wide, have a thin wall, and are transformed into a cavernous system, having numerous anastomoses and buried in the fascia of the pelvic wall. Many people have tried to modify and extend the Wertheim procedure, but most procedures have not been successful in removing the gluteal lymph nodes. But Brunschwig's radical method of pelvic exenteration has been successful even in very advanced cases. To remove the inferior gluteal lymph nodes, the hypogastric artery must be ligated near its branch from the common iliac artery. Then the gluteal pudendal arteries are exposed and each is ligated. The hypogastric vein that lies underneath needs to be ligated with all its branches and then removed together

with the surrounding lymphatic and fatty tissue. After that, the sciatic nerve and its roots are totally exposed on each side. It is commonly felt that Brunschwig's procedure is too extended and dangerous as a palliative operation for carcinoma of the cervix or the uterus.

Inguinal lymph nodes

The inguinal lymph nodes are divided into superficial and deep lymph node groups. The superficial lymph nodes can be divided into a horizontal tract (parallel to the groin and vertical tract) along the great saphenous vein. The deep inguinal lymph nodes lie directly on the iliopsoas muscle and are covered by the superficial layer of the fascia lata. The fascia lata of the thigh is divided into two layers: the superficial one has a very small, oval opening—lamina cribriformis fossae ovalis—and goes medially into the ductus muscles fascia. The deep layer covers the psoas and pectinate muscles on the medial side and also the ductus muscle group. The superficial and deep inguinal lymph nodes are connected by anastamoses. The draining vessels of the vertical tract mainly go through the lateral group of the horizontal tract of the inguinal lymph nodes.

The draining vessels of the horizontal tract of the inguinal lymph nodes can be divided into three groups:

1. Numerous efferent vessels of the lateral inguinal lymph nodes pass the lateral side of the femoral artery and reach the pelvis by passing the lacuna of vessels (Fig. 2-20). On the lateral and the dorsal side of the external iliac artery, they turn upward and reach the lateral external iliac lymph nodes. From there, the lymph fluid flows through the common iliac and aortic lymph nodes. Sometimes there are interesting variations in the lymph vessels' directions. There are lymphatics moving from the lateral inguinal lymph nodes through the most lateral part of the lacuna of vessels along the intralacunal ligament into the pelvic cavity, which empty either into the distal external iliac lymph nodes and start going upward or turn without any intermission by the distal external iliac lymph nodes directly to the iliac or psoas muscle inside the iliac fossae and then flow cranially to the common iliac lymph nodes. In this way, there are lymphatic anastomoses of the lateral inguinal or distal external iliac lymph nodes into the common iliac lymph nodes.
2. Numerous efferent vessels of the inguinal lymph nodes pass with the femoral vein (and also femoral artery) central. They flow into the lymph nodes of the femoral ring (see Fig. 2-8, *K*) and mainly reach the medial external iliac nodes (see Fig. 2-8, *J*). The most medially situated lymph node of the group around the femoral ring is called Rosenmüller's lymph node. Its anterior part touches the femoral vein medially inside the lacuna of vessels and extends, depending on its size, over the horizontal ramus of the pubic bone. Rosenmüller's lymph node may not be developed but is then replaced

by a bunch of narrow lymph vessels. These flow from the lateral pelvic wall toward and into the external medial iliac lymph node. Starting from the external medial iliac lymph nodes, lymph vessels may lead to the obturator (Fig. 2-9, *I*), hypogastric (Fig. 2-8, *H*), and to the external iliac lymph nodes at the external iliac artery (Fig. 2-8, *J*).

3. After injection of contrast into the medial superficial inguinal lymph nodes, many efferent vessels leaving these lymph nodes and turning medially to the femoral

vein on the iliopsoas and pectineal muscles fascia later on the lacunar ligament upward, enter the pelvis through the most medial part of the vessel. Later they turn around the horizontal ramus of the pubic bone crossing underneath the pubic branches of the inferior epigastric artery and vein. They do not flow into the femoral ring lymph nodes—as expected for most of them—but pass Rosenmüller's lymph node medially and empty into the obturator and the inferior gluteal lymph nodes. The most caudal vessel of those lymphat-

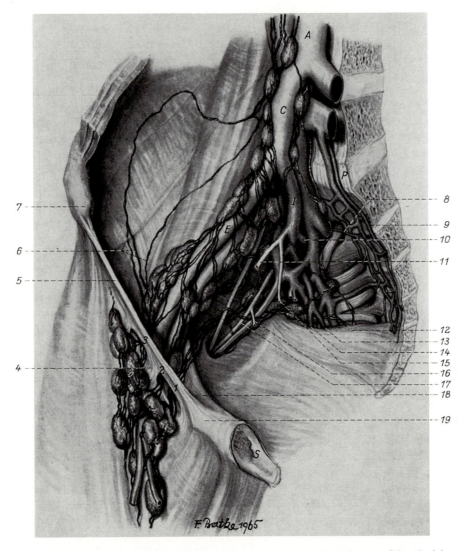

Fig. 2-20. Three groups of draining lymph vessels from the horizontal tract of inguinal lymph nodes to the pelvic lymph nodes. *3*, Lateral pathway to the lateral external iliac lymph nodes and the common iliac lymph nodes; *2*, median or midline pathway to the medial external iliac lymph nodes and the hypogastric lymph nodes; *F*, medial pathway to the obturator and inferior gluteal lymph nodes; *4*, connective tissue of the blood vessel canal and fascia (interlacunar ligament); *5*, inguinal ligament; *6*, bypasses from the inguinal respectively external iliac to the common iliac lymph nodes; *7*, anterior/superior iliac spine; *8*, lateral/sacral artery; *9*, medial sacral artery; *10*, superior gluteal artery; *11*, lateral umbilical ligament; *12*, lymph vessels to the gluteal region; *13*, inferior gluteal artery; *14*, inferior pudendal artery; *15*, uterine artery; *16*, inferior vesical artery; *17*, obturator artery; *18*, superior ramus of the pubic bone; *19*, tuberosity of the pubic bone. *A*, Aorta; *C*, common iliac artery; *E*, external iliac artery; *I*, internal iliac artery; *P*, promontory; *S*, symphysis. (From Reiffenstuhl G: *Das Lymphknoenproblem beim Carcinoma colli uteri und die Lymphirrdiatio pelvis. Direkte Bestrahlung des Beckenlymphsystems mit Isotopen*, Vienna, 1967, Urban-Schwarzenberg.)

ics drain performs anastamosis with the lymph vessel entering the pelvis by the obturator foramen. The lymphatic fluid flows further from the obturator lymph nodes and the inferior gluteal lymph nodes to the hypogastric, the superior gluteal, and sacral lymph nodes. The inferior gluteal lymph nodes also receive fluid from the gluteal region by lymphatics entering the pelvis through the infrapiriform foramen.

URETER

The ureter plays an important part in gynecologic operations. Its topographical relation to the organs and structures within the pelvis and on the pelvic wall is especially important. Finding it and sometimes exposing it are absolute prerequisites for its protection.

The ureter enters the small pelvis in front of or slightly medial to the sacral iliac junction; both sides are the same distance from the midline. To the outside convex arc, both ureters run along the small pelvic wall caudally to the back side of Mackenrodt's ligament. While performing this arc, they are more distant from each other than when entering the pelvis. The relation to the big vessels is not always constant. The ureter crosses either the common iliac artery or the external iliac artery. This is not caused by a different location of the ureter but by a different length of the common iliac artery.

After crossing the blood vessel, the right ureter lies either medially or medially and in front of the internal iliac artery and reaches the ovarian fossa. The ovarian fossa is a depression of the peritoneum between the internal and external iliac arteries. On the left side, the ureter mostly goes along the common iliac artery, then crosses in a sharp angle at the beginning of the internal iliac artery and reaches the ovarian fossa in front of the internal iliac artery. The ureter is covered in the described course by the parietal peritoneum to which it is fixed by the connective tissue surrounding itself. In some women the ureter produces a fold that can be followed from the entrance of the pelvis onto Mackenrodt's ligament. Laterally from the ureter there are the branches of the internal iliac vessels, the obturator artery, and the obturator vein and also the beginning of the lateral umbilical ligament. Above the pelvic floor, the ureter turns medially and ventrally into Mackenrodt's ligament. It stays at the back side of the ligament, then penetrates into the parametrium connective tissue. It passes the cervix of the uterus laterally in a small distance while going medially and ventrally. Of course, this very important location of the ureter near the cervix varies with the position of the uterus, which mostly is not strictly median or which is not strictly in midline. The distance of the right and left ureter to the cervix may, therefore, vary, which urges the surgeon to keep very close to the uterus to avoid damage of the ureter. Inside the parametrium, the ureter is located very close to the vessels. The uterine artery runs caudal lying lateral and somewhat medial to the ureter. Near the uterus, the uterine artery crosses over the ureter. The uterine and vaginal veins surround the ureter,

crossing and running below and above it, and finally lying lateral to the ureter and making their way to the internal iliac vein (Fig. 2-21).

In the middle of these vessels, the ureter, including its sheath, lies inside a canal running right through the parametrial connective tissue. The ureteral sheath is loosely connected to the wall of this canal, and it is not difficult to expose the ureter and its sheath if operating in the correct layer. The last segment of the ureter extends from the crossing with the uterine artery ventrally through its orifice into the bladder. At this location also the ureter lies in a preformed canal, which means it is not fixed to anything surrounding it. The ureter approaches the vaginal wall lateral to the uterine portio and then runs on top of the ventral vaginal wall. But, again, its only connection to the vaginal wall is by loose connective tissue. Cranially, the ureter comes very close to the floor of the vesicouterine cavity so that a fold is formed as soon as the ureter is forced backward.

The blood supply of the part of the pelvis dealing with the ureter is provided by different arteries, and there is always a certain range of individual variation. A branch of the ovarian artery might reach the ureter, and branches of the common and internal iliac, the iliolumbal and the superior gluteal and medial rectal arteries might belong to the feeding blood vessels. The ureteral segment near the bladder is supplied by a branch of the uterine artery that leaves the uterine artery and crosses near the ureter (Figs. 2-22 and 2-23). This branch is usually divided into an ascendent and descendent ramus; the descendent one anastamoses with branches of the superior and inferior vesical arteries that supply the ureter while ascending. Further on, a branch out of the vaginal artery very often leads into this net. Because of the rich blood supply, it is possible to ligate one of the branches in radical procedures. But the blood supply and the adventitial tissue of the ureter may not be destroyed or damaged. The venous drainage of the ureter is performed by the vesical vein plexus to the uterine plexus and indirectly to the ovarian and internal iliac vein.

For finding and sometimes exposing the ureter in the connective tissue matrix (Fig. 2-24), the pelvic ureter begins at the terminal on both sides at the sacroiliac articulation. The pelvic ureter first traverses the rectum pillar, then Mackenrodt's ligament, and finally the bladder pillar to reach forward to the bladder. Therefore, it is also subdivided in the small pelvis into three sections: (1) pars posterior in the rectouterine ligament; (2) pars intermedia in Mackenrodt's ligament; and (3) pars anterior in the vesicouterine ligament.

Clinical remarks

The 15-cm segment of the ureter inside the pelvis consists of a descending part describing a laterally convex turn and of an ascending urethrovesical (or juxtavesical) part beginning at the so-called knee of the ureter. The ascending juxtavesical segment changes its course if the inner

Text continued on p. 56.

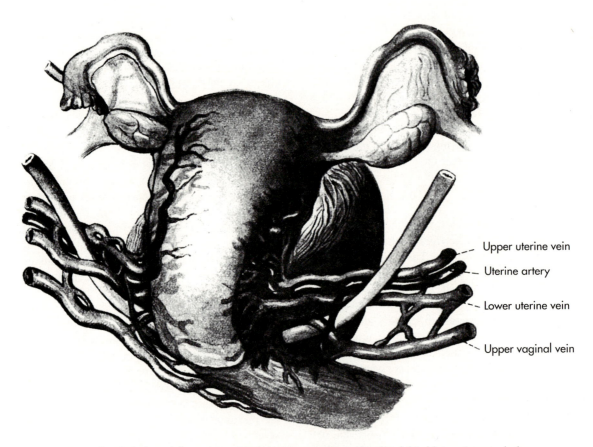

Upper uterine vein

Uterine artery

Lower uterine vein

Upper vaginal vein

Fig. 2-21. Relation of the ureter to its venous surroundings. On the right side, ureter runs in between lower uterine vein and upper vaginal vein, ventrally up to the bladder; on the left side, the ureter runs between uterine artery and the inferior uterine vein. (From Von Peham H, Amreich JA: *Gynaekologische Operationslehre,* Berlin, 1930, S. Karger.)

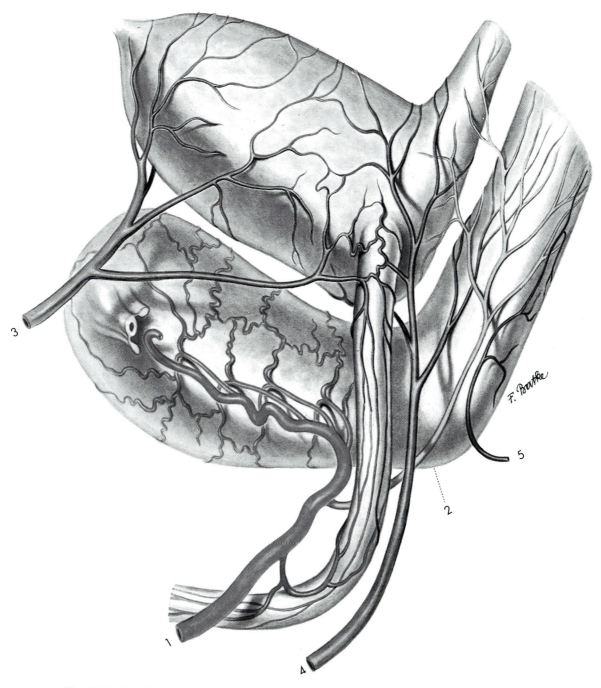

Fig. 2-22. Blood supply of the portion of the ureter near the bladder of the uterus in this area, of the more central parts of the urethra and of the vagina, as seen from the side. *1,* Uterine artery; *2,* vaginal artery; *3,* superior vesical artery; *4,* inferior vesical artery; *5,* branch of the inferior rectal artery. (From Reiffenstuhl G, Platzer W: *Die Vaginalen Operationen. Chirurg Anatomie u Operationslehre,* Berlin, 1974, Urban-Schwarzenberg.)

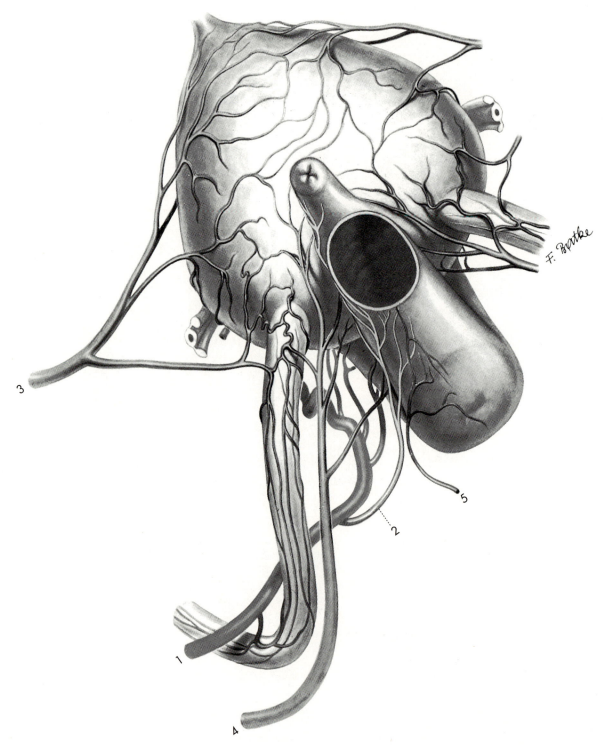

Fig. 2-23. Anteroinferior view of ureteral, uterine and urethral blood supply. *1* to *5*, see Fig. 2-22. (From Reiffenstuhl G, Platzer W: *Die Vaginalen Operationen. Chirurg Anatomie u Operationslehre*, Berlin, 1974, Urban-Schwarzenberg.)

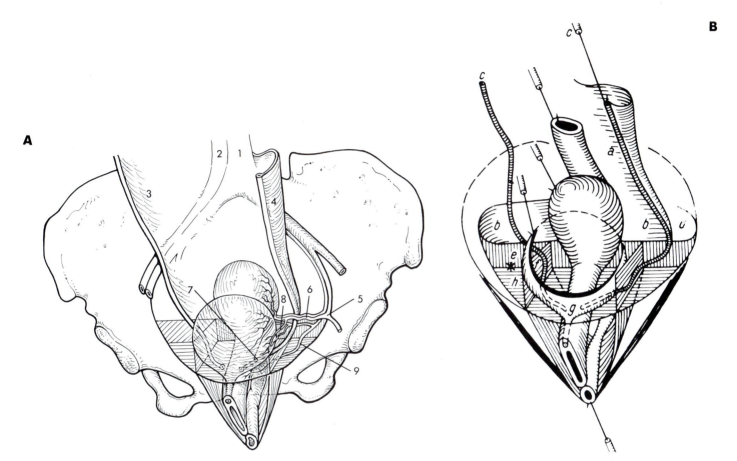

Fig. 2-24. A, Schematic representation of the pelvic connective tissue according to Amreich. Relative position of the ureter to the blood vessels. On the right, the ureter and its associated ureteral leaf *(3)* are left in place; on the left, the ureter and its leaf *(4)* are folded medially. In the course of the ureter in the pelvis, one differentiates posterior, intermediate, and anterior parts. The intermediate part of the ureter utilizes the middle portion of Mackenrodt's ligament in its course and is crossed there by the uterine artery *(5)*, which runs along the upper edge of the ligament and, as a rule, by one of its accompanying veins *(6)* as well. The anterior part *(7)* of the ureter follows a somewhat ascending course that tends toward the medial in the bladder pillar. The efferent veins of the vesical plexus and the superior vesical artery *(8)* lie cranially to the ureter; the vaginal veins *(9)* lie caudal to it. *1,* Aorta; *2,* inferior vena cava, *3,* ureteral leaf (anterior aspect); *4,* ureteral leaf (posterior aspect); *5,* uterine artery; *6,* uterine veins; *7,* ureter (anterior part); *8,* superior vesical artery and vein; and *9,* vaginal vein. **B,** Course of the ureter in the pelvic connective tissue. On the right side, the ureter *(c)* lies in place against the pelvic wall; on the left, with its leaf (the ureteral leaf *[a]* is an upward continuation of the sagittal rectal pillar *[b]*). It is detached from the pelvic wall and folded medially. Thereby a portion of an artificially produced cavity—the pararectal space *(d) (upper level)*—comes into view. The medial boundary of the space is formed by the rectal pillar *(b)*, now standing truly sagitally, with its ureteral leaf. The lateral boundary is formed by the pelvic wall. The ureter first runs in the ureteral leaf and the sagittal rectal pillar *(b)* and then utilizes the middle portion of Mackenrodt's ligament *(e)* and runs forward in the sagittal portion of the bladder pillar *(f)* until it reaches the bladder *(g)*. The paravesical space *(*)* is bounded medially by the bladder pillar *(f)*, laterally by the pelvic wall, dorsally by Mackenrodt's ligament *(e)*, caudally by the horizontal connective tissue foundation *(h)*, and cranially by the umbilical ligamental layers (a delicate leaf of connective tissue not shown here). *a,* Ureteral leaf; *b,* sagittal rectal pillar; *c,* ureter; *d,* pararectal space; *e,* Mackenrodt's ligament; *f,* sagittal bladder pillar; *g,* urinary bladder; *h,* horizontal connective tissue foundation; and *(*),* paravesical space. (From Reiffenstuhl G: *The lymphatics of the female genital organs,* Philadelphia, 1964, JB Lippincott.)

genitalia change position (Fig. 2-25). In a person suffering from cystocele, for example, the ureter approaches the bladder only at the lateral edge; whereas in a cystocele of a higher grade or in a prolapse it approaches the bladder laterally and from above (Fig. 2-26).

What happens to the course of the ureters in a woman having radical vaginal hysterectomy when the uterus is being pulled downward with the portio and vaginal cuff?

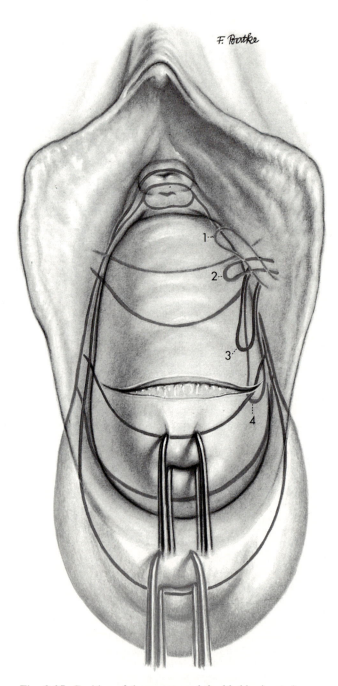

Fig. 2-25. Position of the ureters and the bladder in uterine prolapse. The ascending ureter in its normal original state *(1)* becomes almost horizontal *(2)* when the bladder sinks anteriorly. In more extensive cases with moderate *(3)* or severe *(4)* descensus uteri, the ureter descends vertically. (From Reiffenstuhl G, Platzer W: *Die Vaginalen Operationen. Chirurg Anatomie u Operationslehre,* Berlin, 1974, Urban-Schwarzenberg.)

The uterine vessels, the vessels feeding and surrounding the ureter, and the ureter itself (by the uterine artery at the crossing) are also being pulled downward together with the uterus. The pelvic knee of the ureter is transformed into a more or less sharp angular loop. After cutting the uterine vessels and dividing the vessels from the uterus, the ureter fits back into its former position. Then a radical excision of the paraspaces or parametrial spaces is possible without danger to the ureter. A second important point of the fixation of the ureter by a vascular framework appearing in exposure of the ureter for modified vaginal radical uterus extirpation is as follows: usually the surgeon looks for the ureter inside the vesicouterine ligament. But if the surgeon did not find the correct layer between vesical and vaginal fascia in the beginning of the operation when loosening the bladder, the operative field is almost always too close to the vagina and cervix. When the vesicouterine ligament is cut, the ureter does not become visible but remains covered by connective tissue (vaginal and cervical fascia). In such a case, the surgeon needs to dissect along the uterine vessels cranially until the vessels are reached; the ureter is fixed and can always be found there.

Damage to the ureter is more likely with abdominal than vaginal hysterectomy. In the vaginal procedure, lifting up the bladder after dissecting the supravaginal septum (the condensed connective tissue dividing the vesicovagi-

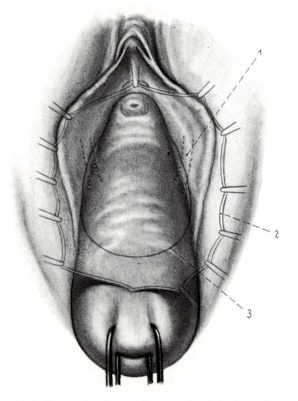

Fig. 2-26. Schematic view of the operative field in prolapse of the bladder and the vagina, showing section of the ureter near the bladder, the cut-edge of the vaginal wall and the operative margins diagrammatically. *1,* Ureteral course near the bladder; *2,* separated vaginal wall; *3,* edge of operative field. (From Reiffenstuhl G, Platzer W: *Die Vaginalen Operationen. Chirurg Anatomie u Operationslehre,* Berlin, 1974, Urban-Schwarzenberg.)

nal space from the vesicocervical space), the ureter is being stretched and, therefore, withdraws from the cervix, which it approaches in usual anatomic situation at about 1.5 cm (Fig. 2-27). In addition, the ureter can be forced laterally out of the operation field by the surgeon's finger forcing the bladder column laterally (Fig. 2-28). This procedure removes the knee of the ureter another 2 cm away from the cervix. In comparison to this in an abdominal procedure, the ureter is dissectable after exposure of the bladder, which has to be performed strictly in the midline

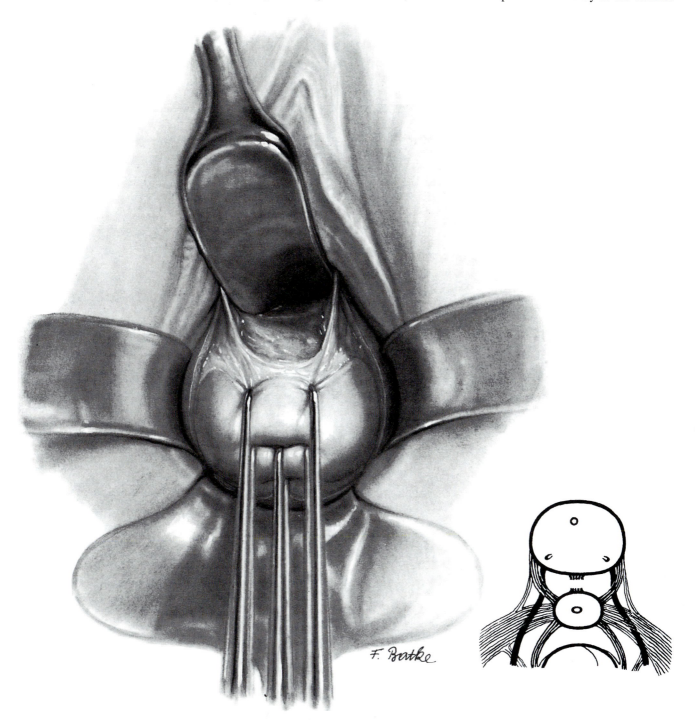

Fig. 2-27. Vaginal hysterectomy. Separating the lower pole of the bladder. The supravaginal septum is divided and the vesicocervical space is opened. The lower bladder pole is separated upward to the peritoneal reflection, being advanced with a spatula inserted in the vesicocervical space. Laterally, the bladder pillars (ligamentum vesicouterina), coursing from the bladder to the cervix, are stretched. Medial to the bladder pillars at the edge of the cervix are seen the uterine arteries. The diagram shows the anatomic relationships more clearly. (From Reiffenstuhl G, Platzer W: *Die Vaginalen Operationen. Chirurg Anatomie u Operationslehre,* Berlin, 1974, Urban-Schwarzenberg.)

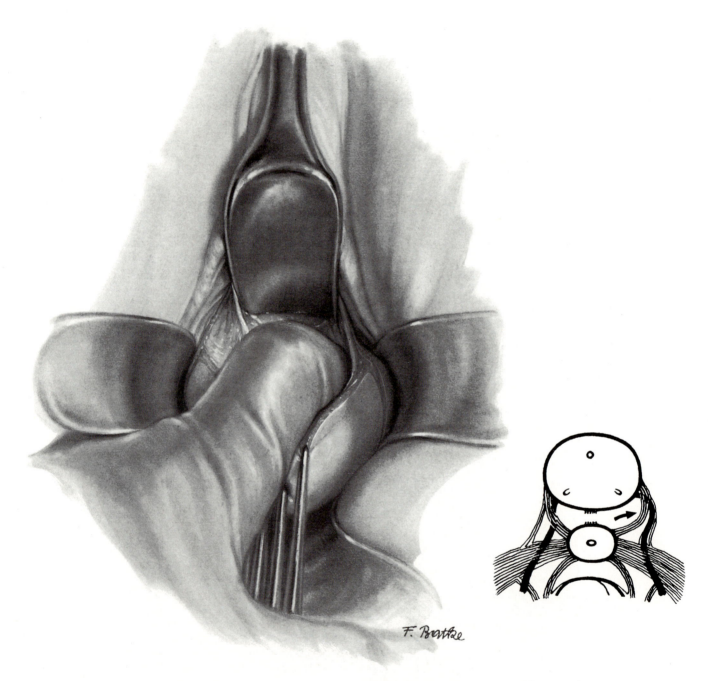

Fig. 2-28. Vaginal hysterectomy. Advancing the bladder. The bladder is held up with an anterior spatula inserted in the vesicocervical space. The surgeon pushes the fibers of the left bladder pillar laterally with his left index finger, thereby displacing the ureter, which courses in the bladder pillar, out of the operative field. This is shown in the schema. (From Reiffenstuhl G, Platzer W: *Die Vaginalen Operationen. Chirg Anatomie u Operationslehre,* Berlin, 1974, Urban-Schwarzenberg.)

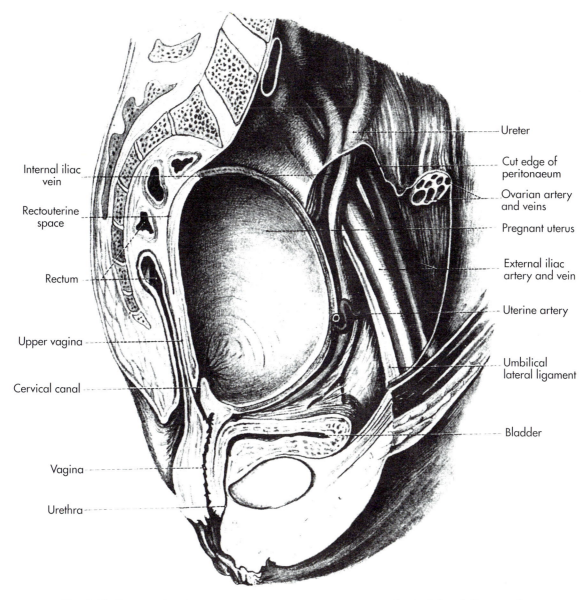

Internal iliac vein

Rectouterine space

Rectum

Upper vagina

Cervical canal

Vagina

Urethra

Ureter

Cut edge of peritonaeum

Ovarian artery and veins

Pregnant uterus

External iliac artery and vein

Uterine artery

Umbilical lateral ligament

Bladder

Fig. 2-29. Topography of the ureter in pregnant women. (From Tandler J, Halban J: *Topography of the female ureter,* Vienna, 1901.)

to avoid damage to blood vessels in the bladder column, and after forcing the bladder column laterally, best done with the smooth swab. The ureter, which crosses inside the bladder column, can be removed from the cervix at a 1- to 2-cm distance by forcing the bladder column laterally. Then it is no longer dangerous for the ureter to be clamped with the parametrial clamp. Also, it is not necessary to clamp the parametrium extended deep down to the upper part of the vagina because a later clamp—after opening the ventral fornix of the vagina—placed in the lateral vaginal fornix also clamps the rest of the parametrium. If this interaction is being followed and the most caudal clamp is not placed too far caudally, there is nothing to worry about. Possible ureteral damage is the most dangerous part of an abdominal hysterectomy.

In pregnant women, the relationships between ureter and uterus change (Fig. 2-29). The ureter is attached very closely to the lower uterus from the linea terminalis to the orifice into the bladder because the uterus fills out almost

all of the pelvis. Because of that, there is no distance between cervix and uterus in pregnant women.

Liberation of the ureter

The topography of the pelvic ureter might be considerably changed after serious inflammations in the area of the inner genitalia. Frequently, the liberation of the ureter has to be performed before excising a tumor of the adnexa or big myoma. The easiest place to find a ureter according to the pelvic anatomy is at the base of the infundibulopelvic ligament. For this procedure, the adnexa is lifted up with a ring forceps and the peritoneum is lifted up from the pelvic wall by forceps and cut close caudally to the ovarian vessels (Fig. 2-30).

A smooth, closed scissors is introduced into the peritoneal gap and the peritoneum is pulled away from the abdominal wall. The peritoneal cut can be enlarged caudally without damaging the blood vessels of the pelvic wall (Fig. 2-31).

In the depth of the peritoneal gap, the ureter can be found medially. In this area, the ureter has a close relationship to the peritoneum and is easily palpated by picking up the ureter between the second and third finger. In very difficult cases, as with adhesions and concretions, the ureter can be recognized by its peristaltic waves. A further

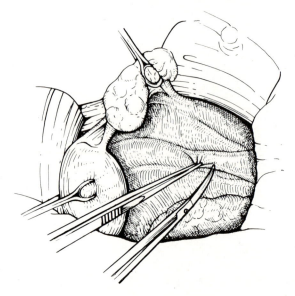

Fig. 2-30. Dissection of liberation of the ureter. Incision of the peritoneum of the pelvic wall. The adnexa is being lifted up by a forceps; the pelvic peritoneum is being pulled away from the pelvic wall by a forceps. The surgeon incises close and caudally to the ovarian vessels by using a smooth scissors. (From Reiffenstuhl G: *Dringliche gynakologische u gebh Operationen Chirurg. Operationslehre Breitner-Kraus-Zuckschwerdt, Bd VI,* Berlin, 1977, Urban-Schwarzenberg.)

liberation of the ureter until it enters the lateral parametrium should be done with closed scissors (Fig. 2-32). The ureter can be forced caudally quite easily.

In serious change caused by inflammation of the adnexa, the ureter might be fixed onto the tumor and has to be dissected very closely. Caution must be exercised so the ureteral adventitia is not damaged.

PELVIC FLOOR—PERINEAL REGION

The borders of the perineal region are the angle of symphysis, the inferior rami of the pubic bone, the ascendent ramus of the ischiatic bone, the lower edge of the sacrum, and the coccyx (Fig. 2-33). The pelvic floor is formed by two layers of muscle and connective tissue. The pelvic and urogenital diaphragms are shown in Fig. 2-34. Each is an incomplete seal of the pelvis, but this deficiency is met by shifting the two layers against each other.

Pelvic diaphragm

The muscular part of the pelvic diaphragm consists of the levator ani and coccygeal muscle and has the form of a funnel. The levator ani muscle originates at the pubic bone on the dorsal side of the pubic bone and at the transverse perineal ligament. It inserts at the tendineus ring of the obturator fascia to the ischial spine, then along the sacrospinous ligament to the coccyx (Fig. 2-33). The levator ani muscle can be divided into three parts corresponding to its course. The puborectal muscle is shown in Fig. 2-33, *d.* The fibers forming the so-called levator pillars or columns may be the most important part of the levator muscle in the gynecologist's opinion. These strong parts of the muscle cross caudally and dorsally along the sides of the ure-

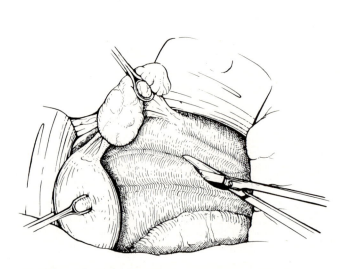

Fig. 2-31. Liberation of the ureter. Enlargement of the peritoneal gap. After pulling away the peritoneum from the pelvic wall by closed scissors, the peritoneal cut is being enlarged in caudal direction. (From Reiffenstuhl G: *Dringliche gynakologische u gebh Operationen Chirurg Operationslehre Breitner-Kraus-Zuckschwerdt, Bd VI,* Berlin, 1977, Urban-Schwarzenberg.)

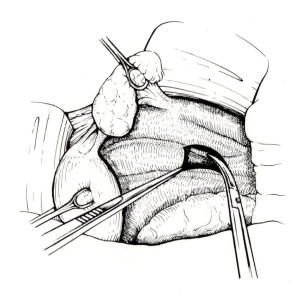

Fig. 2-32. Dissection of the ureter, liberation of the ureter. The pelvic peritoneum is incised; in the depth of the peritoneal gap, the ureter can be seen. With the closed scissors, it is being dissected further caudally. (From Reiffenstuhl G: *Dringliche gynakologische u gebh Operationen Chirurg Operationslehre Breitner-Kraus-Zuckschwerdt, Bd VI,* Berlin, 1977, Urban-Schwarzenberg.)

thra, vagina, and rectum performing a strong connection with the connective tissue of these organs. Certain fibers of the levator muscle cover the lateral and dorsal parts of the rectum and, after surrounding the rectum and coming around to the front joining the internal sphincter ani muscle, they support the rectum by performing a muscle loop. Certain parts of the puborectal muscle are called prerectal fibers (Fig. 2-33, c) because of their cross of the ventral wall of the rectum. Together with the perineal wedge (Fig. 2-34), they divide the levator opening, the so-called hiatus urogenitalis, from the anal hiatus. (The function of the prerectal fibers and the perineal wedge of the levator ani muscle is discussed below.)

Starting from the levator column of pillars, smooth and striated fibers of the muscle join the perineal wedge forming a loop around the vagina. The so-called levator vaginal muscle contractions of the levator columns stretch their ar-

cuate course, and reduce the genital hiatus and the diameter of the vagina. This process can be palpated in women by introducing a finger into the vagina and having the patient press as for defecation. If the levator columns drift apart, a descensus of the pelvic organs cannot be avoided. In the procedure of construction of an artificial perineum, the puborectal muscles may be considered very carefully because a combining of the left and right puborectal muscle guarantees a secure support of the pelvic organs.

The remaining fibers can be described as pubococcygeal and iliococcygeal (Fig. 2-33, f) muscle. They reach out to the top of the coccygeus passing the rectal coccygeal aponeurosis. The iliococcygeal muscle is a little weaker than the pubococcygeal muscle. The iliococcygeus originates at the fascia of the internal obturator muscle on the tendinous arc of the levator muscle and inserts at the coccyx and the lower parts of the sacrum. The pelvic diaphragm is com-

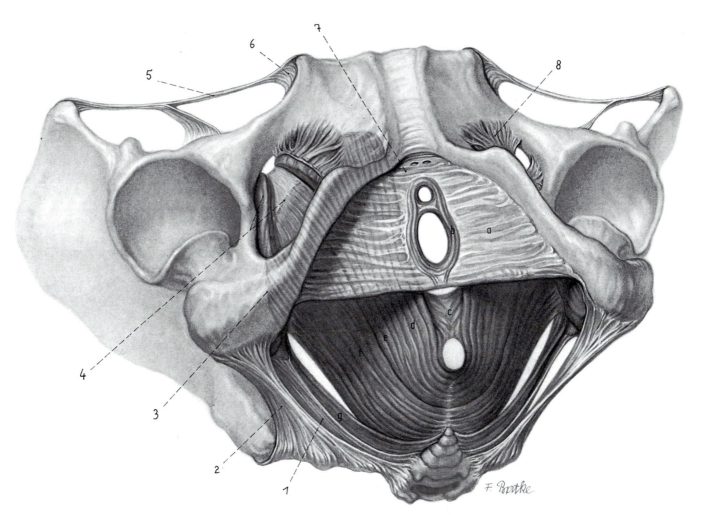

Fig. 2-33. Representation of the ligaments of the pelvis and of the urogenital and pelvic diaphragms. *1*, Sacrospinous ligament; *2*, sacrotuberous ligament; *3*, arcus tendineus of the obturator fascia (levator ani muscle); *4*, obturator internus muscle (cross section) and the arcus tendineus fasciae obturatoriae; *5*, inguinal ligament, arcus iliopectineus; *6*, lacunar ligament; *7*, transverse perineal ligament; *8*, obturator membrane; *a*, deep transverse perineal muscle; *b*, urethrovaginal muscle; *c*, prerectal fibers; *d*, puborectal muscle; *e*, pubococcygeus muscle; *f*, iliococcygeus muscle; *g*, coccygeus muscle. (From Reiffenstuhl G, Platzer W: *Die Vaginalen Operationen. Chirurg Anatomie u Operationslehre*, Berlin, 1974, Urban-Schwarzenberg.)

pleted dorsally by the coccygeal muscle (Fig. 2-33, g). The coccygeal muscle extends from ischiatic spine to the coccygeal and sacral bone. The sacrospinous ligament courses within the coccygeal muscle as its aponeurosis. Usually the pelvic diaphragm is innervated by a long branch of the sacral plexus (sacral nerve #4). The anatomic situation of the pelvic diaphragm is limited by the orifice of the rectum (anus).

The different parts of the levator muscle are combined and then have the name levator sheet. Berglas and Rubin studied the levator sheet in living women. In women, the levator sheet is a horizontal sheet with an opening near the symphysis (levator hiatus). Urethra, rectum, and vagina pass through this aperture. The levator plate is formed by

fusion of the pubococcygeal muscle posterior to the rectum. The vagina creates an especially weak point in the pelvic floor, and in this area a high incidence of hernias as cystoceles, rectoceles, and prolapse can be found. The levator ani muscle antagonizes the muscles of the abdominal wall. This muscle is responsible not only for support of the content of pelvis and abdomen, but also for maintenance and compensation of the intraabdominal pressure. Whenever one of the two components (muscle systems) is weakened or inactive for a certain period of time (e.g., by very narrow and strong corsetry), the opposite component compensates by not contracting for a longer period of time. A genital prolapse may be the result.

As soon as the vesicourethral fixation is dislocated out

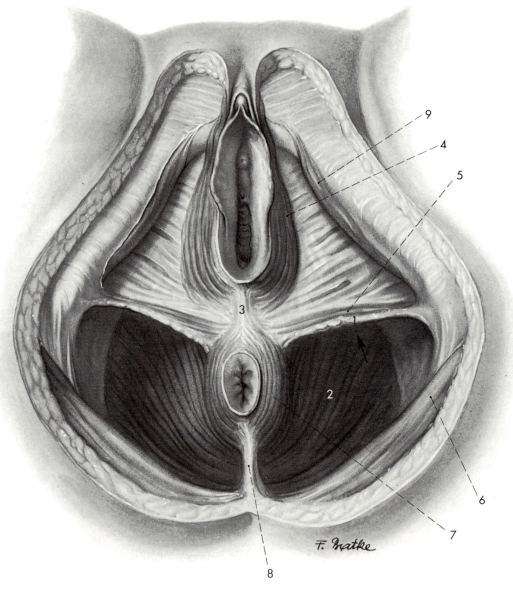

Fig. 2-34. Pelvic floor as seen from below with the urogenital diaphragm and the pelvic diaphragm in situ. *1*, Ischiorectal fossa *(arrow); 2*, levator ani muscle; *3*, perineum; *4*, bulbocavernosus muscle; *5*, superficial transverse perineal muscle; *6*, edge of the gluteus maximus muscle; *7*, external anal sphincter muscle; *8*, anococcygeal ligament; *9*, ischiocavernosus muscle. (From Reiffenstuhl G, Platzer W: *Die Vaginalen Operationen. Chirurg Anatomie u Operationslehre.* Berlin, 1974, Urban-Schwarzenberg.)

of the pelvic cavity, a descensus of the vagina and an incontinence of the bladder may result.

Urogenital diaphragm

The urogenital diaphragm extends inside the pubic angle and protects the wide levator aperture. There are openings for the vagina, urethra, and the dorsal clitoral vein (Fig. 2-35).

The urogenital diaphragm consists of the deep transverse muscle of the perineum (Fig. 2-33), which ends in the perineal wedge (Centrum tendineum).

The deep transverse muscle of the perineum originates from the ischiatic or pubic bone and, being invaded by connective tissue, crosses to the urogenital hiatus. The deep transverse muscle of the perineum encircles the urogenital hiatus in a way that a urogenital sphincter (urethral vaginal muscle) results. Frontally, the muscle fibers join the transverse perineal ligament (urethral ligament; Fig. 2-33, 7), which forms the ventral part of the urogenital diaphragm together with the arcuate pubic ligament. The free dorsal edge of the diaphragm is supported by the superficial transverse muscle of the perineum (Fig. 2-34, 5), which originates from the ischiatic tuberosity and inserts into the perineal wedge. The bulbocavernous and the ischiocavernous muscles (Fig. 2-34, 4 and 9) lie directly on the urogenital diaphragm. The two bulbocavernous muscles surround the vaginal aperture like a ring and can close this aperture by contraction. The bulbi vestibuli are above the urogenital diaphragm as are the major vestibular glands, the so-called Bartholin's glands (Fig. 2-35). The ducts perforate the urogenital diaphragm and course ventrally around the vaginal aperture to the orifice into the urogenital sinus near the hymen. In inflammatory disease of the vagina, these glands are very likely to be involved by forming an intraglandular abscess above the urogenital diaphragm. The pudendal nerve innervates the urogenital diaphragm. The vaginal, urethral, and urogenital diaphragm are grown together firmly. This is the reason for easy prolapse of the pelvic organs, vagina, bladder and uterus in case of damage of the pelvic floor.

PERINEUM

The knowledge of the anatomic structures of the perineum are important in colpoperineoplasty, episiotomy, and rupture of the perineum. The area between the anus and the vaginal orifice is of great importance in women. This region is called the perineum, which is about 2.5 cm in size. The rectovaginal septum meets the pelvic floor and enlarges concerning its muscle strength (Fig. 2-38). Fibers of many muscles join the rectovaginal septum and form a mass of muscle and connective tissue building up the central tendon of the perineum. Therefore, the central tendon is created by the connection of a lot of connective tissue and muscle fibers. The following structures belong to the central tendon of the perineum (Fig. 2-36): bulbocavernous muscle (originating bilaterally from the perineal wedge); superficial and deep transverse perineal muscle; prerectal fibers of the levator ani muscle; fibers of the rectal wall; superficial part of the external sphincter ani muscles. Also, the medial muscle fibers of the urethro-vaginal muscle (Fig. 2-36) join the central tendon of the perineum. Some smooth muscle bundles called rectovaginal muscles (Fig. 2-36) extending from the rectum to the vagina help to construct the perineal wedge. Smooth muscle fibers of the rectococcygeal muscle connecting to the levator fascia containing smooth muscles and the urogenital diaphragm help form the perineal wedge. A massive firm connective tissue wedge containing numerous muscle fibers is created.

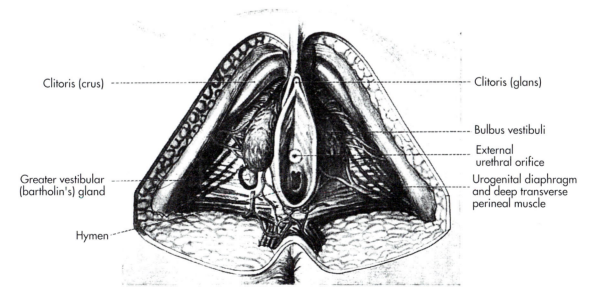

Clitoris (crus)

Greater vestibular (bartholin's) gland

Hymen

Clitoris (glans)

Bulbus vestibuli

External urethral orifice

Urogenital diaphragm and deep transverse perineal muscle

Fig. 2-35. The female urogenital diaphragm seen from below. Also illustrated are the swelling bodies or cavernosus bodies. On the right side the urogenital diaphragm is cut to show the major vestibular gland. (From Hafferl A: *Lehrbuch der Topographischen Anatomie,* Berlin, 1957, Springer-Verlag.)

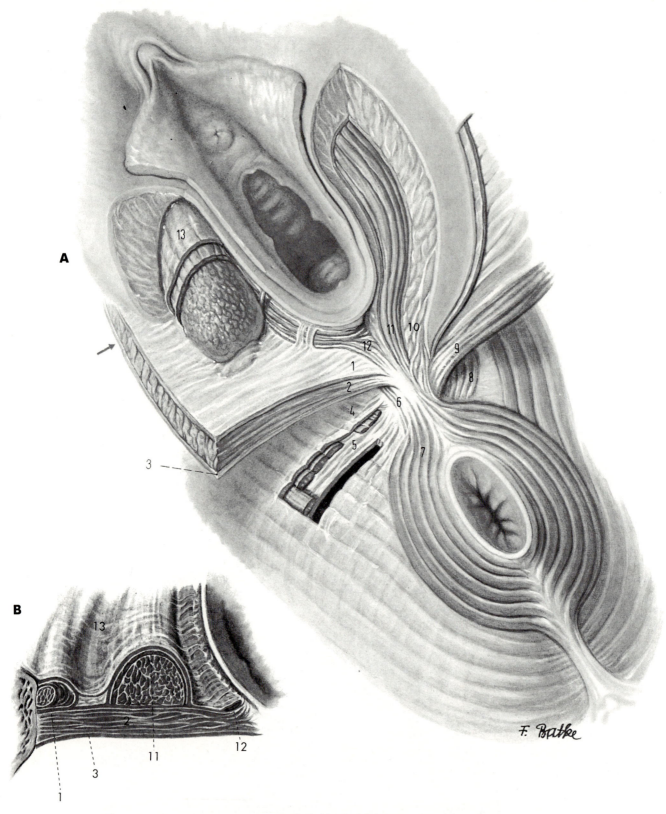

Fig. 2-36. A, Architecture of the perineum: diagonally striated musculature; smooth muscle, connective tissue, adipose tissue. *1,* Inferior urogenital fascia; *2,* deep transverse perineal muscle; *3,* superior urogenital fascia; *4,* inferior fascia of the pelvic diaphragm with smooth muscle fibers; *5,* superior fascia of the pelvic diaphragm with smooth muscle fibers; *6,* rectovaginal muscle; *7,* external anal sphincter muscle; *8,* prerectal fibers of the levator ani muscle; *9,* superficial transverse perineal muscle; *10,* deep transverse perineal muscle; *11,* bulbocavernosus muscle; *12,* urethrovaginal muscle; *13,* perineal muscle (superficial); *14,* ischocavernosus muscle. **B,** Section through the urogenital diaphragm (compare arrow in Fig. 2-36, **A**). (From Reiffenstuhl G, Platzer W: *Die Vaginalen Operationen. Chirurg Anatomie u Operationslehre.* Berlin, 1974, Urban-Schwarzenberg.)

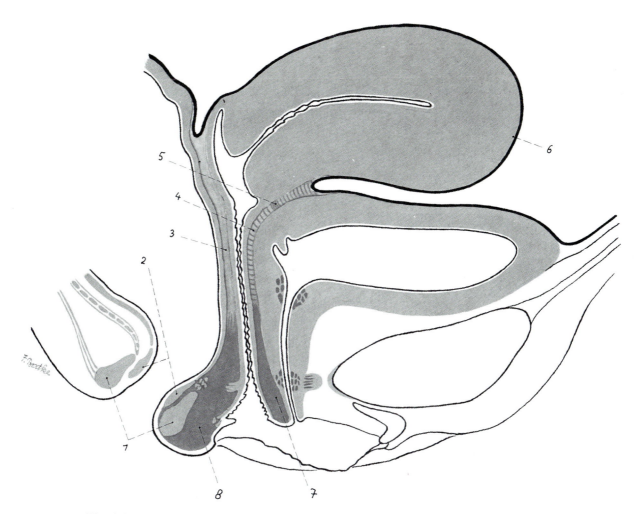

Fig. 2-37. Midline diagrammatic section of the perivaginal connective tissue. *1,* External anal sphincter muscle; *2,* internal sphincter; *3,* loose areolar connective tissue between vaginal and rectal fascias in the rectovaginal space; *4,* loose areolar connective tissue between vaginal and vesical or urethral fascias in the vesicovaginal or urethrovaginal space; *5,* supravaginal septum; *6,* peritoneum; *7,* dense connective tissue completely occupying the urethrovaginal space; *8,* dense fibrous tissue filling the rectovaginal space. (From Reiffenstuhl G, Platzer W: *Die Vaginalen Operationen. Chirurg Anatomie u Operationslehre,* Berlin, 1974, Urban-Schwarzenberg.)

Also called the perineal wedge or perineal body, it is the base for the perineum. The back of the wedge faces caudally; the other side facing cranially is formed by the rectovaginal septum (Figs. 2-37 and 2-38). The central tendon is an important part of the pelvic floor because just above it are the fornix of the vagina and the uterus. These structures have to be carried by the perineal body. An insufficiency of the perineal wedge might cause a descensus of the pelvic organs and a beginning of a prolapse (Fig. 2-39).

During delivery, the vagina is enlarged and the perineum is stretched extensively. In a very sudden increase in tension, the elasticity of the tissue might not be adequate so that ruptures of the central tendon of the perineum occur. Such ruptures of the perineum might extend cranially along the rectovaginal septum and cause a dissection of the vaginal wall from the rectal wall. They might even affect the anal sphincter muscle and the wall of

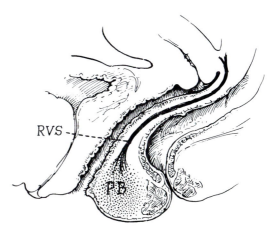

Fig. 2-38. Sagittal section shows the relationship between the rectovaginal septum *(RVS)* as it blends with the superior border of the perineal body *(PB).* (From Nichols DH, Randall CL: *Vaginal surgery,* ed 3, Baltimore, 1989, Williams & Wilkins.)

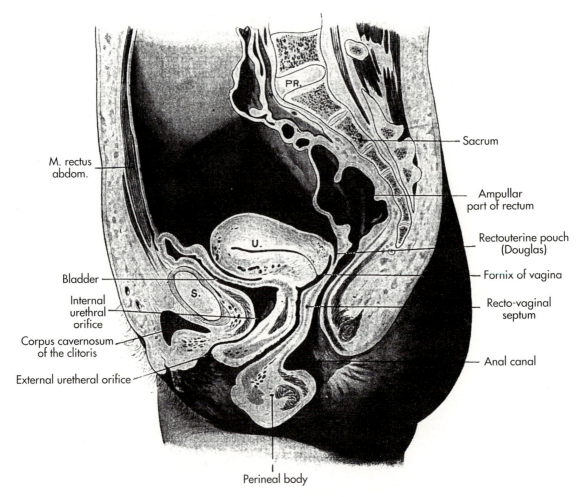

M. rectus
abdom.

Sacrum

Ampullar
part of rectum

Rectouterine pouch
(Douglas)

Fornix of vagina

Bladder

Internal
urethral
orifice

Recto-vaginal
septum

Corpus cavernosum
of the clitoris

Anal canal

External uretheral orifice

Perineal body

Fig. 2-39. Median cut through the pelvis of a 21-year-old woman. The perineal body carried the inner genitals. Its base is a strong area, from above the rectovaginal septum joins it. (From Corning HK: *Lehrbuch der Topograph Anatomie,* Wiesbaden, 1914, JF Bergmann.)

the rectum. The clinical importance of the perineal body and wedge is not only dividing the urogenital tract from gut but also the maintenance of the normal topography of the lower pelvic organs. This topic is discussed in Chapters 22 and 29.

FUNCTIONAL AND CLINICAL IMPORTANCE OF PELVIC FLOOR AND PELVIC CONNECTIVE TISSUE

The perineal muscles carry and fix the perineum. These muscles are firmly connected to the perineal body. They approach the central tendon of the perineum from the peripheral symmetric points and hold the perineal body in its place. They also protect it from the changing intraabdominal pressures so that it cannot form a prolapse. In this way, the perineal muscles are fixed by the central tendon and vice versa (Fig. 2-36). The wall of the lowest part of the vagina and the ventral wall of the anal part of muscles are also connected very closely to the central tendon. This part of the wall might form a prolapse only when their connections with the perineal body are destroyed. The

perineal body is damaged if the muscular or fascial connections are destroyed. Eventually, a prolapse might happen, without any previous trauma, if all parts of the perineum are weak or if the perineal body shrinks because of age. The urogenital diaphragm helps fix the lower vagina because the vagina and urethra are firmly grown together with the urogenital diaphragm. The central tendon of the perineum not only supports the topographical location of the lower genitalia, but the elastic perineal wedge also causes a turn of the perineal (anal) part of the rectum dorsally against the sacral part of the rectum. The turn of the dorsal rectal wall is about 2 cm ventrally from the coccyx (Fig. 2-40). This dorsal turn of the lower rectum, accompanied by the vagina (Richter), protects the lowest part of rectum and vagina from the intraabdominal pressure (Fig. 2-40).

The reason for this phenomenon is that the distal rectum and the lower vagina lie caudally to the levator sheet and the coccyx. The portio and the upper part of the vagina, however, usually lie near the sacral bone because of the perineal turn of the vagina.

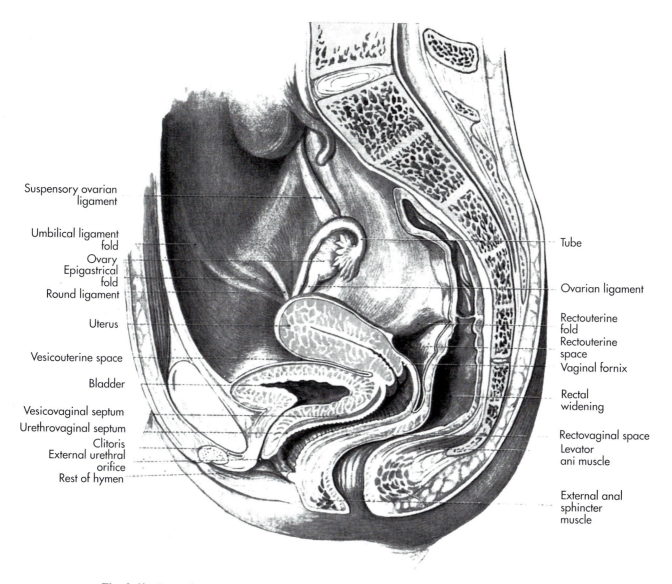

Suspensory ovarian
ligament

Umbilical ligament
fold
Ovary
Epigastrical
fold
Round ligament

Uterus

Vesicouterine space

Bladder

Vesicovaginal septum
Urethrovaginal septum
Clitoris
External urethral
orifice
Rest of hymen

Tube

Ovarian ligament

Rectouterine
fold
Rectouterine
space
Vaginal fornix

Rectal
widening

Rectovaginal space
Levator
ani muscle

External anal
sphincter
muscle

Fig. 2-40. Turn of the perineal part of rectum against the sacral part of the rectum which is also performed by the vagina. (From Hafferl A: *Lehrbuch der Topographischen Anatomie,* Berlin, 1957, Springer-Verlag.)

The proximal part of the vagina in a standing woman has a horizontal course. This phenomenon can be shown with casts of the vagina and lateral radiographs (Richter). The upper part of the vaginal portio and uterus lie, according to these situations, far away from the levator aperture. The closeness of the portio and uterus and the upper vagina to the sacrum is effected mainly by the cardinal ligament. These are very strong connective tissue bundles approaching the cervix and the upper vagina as Mackenrodt's ligament. The connective tissue of the pelvis is analogous to the shrouds of a sailboat holding the masts in correct position (Richter). In this way, the proximal vagina and the uterus with the portio are kept a distance away from the levator hiatus. This is of great importance for the following reason: once the uterus passes the gap of the levator muscle, all the inner genitals are pressed outside with a high power of intraabdominal pressure so that neither the connective tissue nor another tissue is able to control it or antagonize it. The inner genitals are kept in their position by the strong cardinal ligament, which holds the position of the portio and the cranial vagina near the sacral bone.

The vagina is kept in its position by two systems, one from above (cardinal ligament, parametrium) and one from below (levator muscle). Either one or both suspensory mechanisms might be destroyed in case of a genital prolapse. Tissue damage might be unilateral, and it is important to figure out which side is changed. Zacharin, Milley, and Nichols were able to demonstrate that the urethra is fixed not only at the back side of the pubic bone by the pubourethral ligament but also by the fascia of the urogenital diaphragm, similar to the vagina, and by the pubococcygeal muscle[77] (Fig. 2-41).

The pubourethral ligament contains smooth muscle fibers, contractive elements, controlled by the autonomic nervous system. If the urethra is hypermobile, this should be repaired by surgical procedure by suspension, by sup-

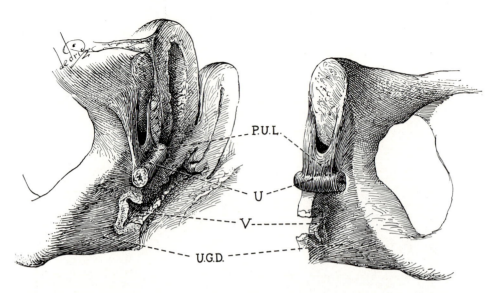

Fig. 2-41. Sagittal view shows the relationship between the pubourethral ligament *(PUL)* and urogenital diaphragm *(UGD)* in the human female. The urethra *(U)* and vagina *(V)* are shown in their relationship to the urogenital diaphragm. Note the bladder sketched into the drawing at the left. (From Milley PS, Nichols DH: The relationship between pubourethral ligaments and urogenital diaphragm in the human female, *Anat Rec* 170:281-284, 1971; reproduced with permission of the Wistar Institute Press.)

port, or by both. According to Nichols, different anatomic systems are responsible for support of the birth canal to various extents. These systems might be destroyed either isolated or in any combination, but in reconstructive surgery they must individually be taken into consideration.

Pelvic bones. The osseous pelvis is the fixation point for the muscular connective tissue. Congenital abnormalities, fractures, ruptures, or previous surgery might change the structures of bone and joints. This must be kept in mind when thinking of a repair operation.

Pelvic connective tissue. Fibrotic changes of the pelvic connective tissue might prevent a descensus. The connective tissue might be shortened by chronic inflammation, endometriosis, previous radiation, previous surgery, or chronic tension. The round ligament extending from the uterine fundus to the inguinal canal as an arc does not have any significant meaning in supporting the uterus.[19] But it is responsible to some degree for the anteversion of the uterus (in a low grade). Its most important function is the fixation of the uterus during childbirth. The cardinal ligament (Mackenrodt's) keeps the cervix and the proximal part of the vagina above the levator muscles in their position supported by the uterosacral ligaments. Tension on these ligaments might initiate dense fibrotic changes of the tissue (Fig. 2-42).

Every increase of abdominal tension normally is antagonized by the levator ani muscle. In this case, the pillars of the levator muscle contract, the hiatal diameter decreases but remains big enough to have a normal and especially an atrophic senile uterus pass through as soon as this

uterus happens to lie above the hiatus. The weight of the abdominal organs, which is normally neutralized by the atmospheric pressure and in the expiration even overcompensated by the suction of the lungs, gains importance as soon as the proximal vagina and the uterus are no longer kept in their place near the sacrum by the cardinal ligament. If the connection of the rectovaginal septum and the perineal body is damaged at the perineal wedge or the perineal body is shortened cranial-caudally without development of scars, a rectocele is very likely to be found.

A rectocele might also be called a hernia of the rectovaginal septum or the perineal body. The beginning of a rectocele can be found at the perineal curve. But very often the rectovaginal septum is pulled off the central tendon of the perineum at the borderline, the perineal body stays intact, so the curve is a little more cranially located than usual. Situations like these are caused by a high tension in the rectovaginal septum during delivery. The perineal body pulls off on the place of the rupture, and increased scar tissue develops. But even without any trauma during delivery such rectoceles are found, related to a deep Douglas pouch, which, according to Joachimovits,[27] can be looked on as an infantile stigma.

The aim of colpoperineoplasty is the reconstruction of a wedge of a body like the perineal body and approaching the two levator pillars or columns in the dorsal part of the hiatus. By sewing together a muscle bundle of these two muscles, a kind of a new central tendon may be constructed because the sewn muscles are transformed into scar tissue.

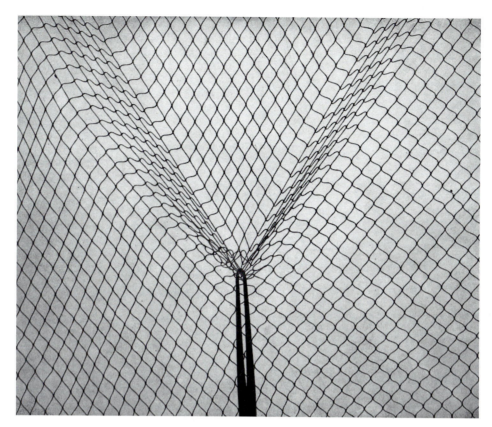

Fig. 2-42. The effect of traction on the connective tissue fibers of the cardinal and uterosacral ligaments is demonstrated. A forceps has been applied to the center of a piece of plastic net, and traction has been applied, demonstrating the distortion of the pelvic tissues resulting from traction on the cervix. Condensation and obliteration of intra-areolar spaces account for "ligaments" apparent at operation, reinforced by blood vessels, lymphatics, and nerves and their sheaths, both of which enter and exit along the lateral margin of the upper vagina. (From Nichols DH, Milley PS: *Clinical anatomy of the vulva, vagina, lower pelvis and perineum.* In Sciarra J, editor: *Gynecology and obstetrics,* Philadelphia, 1992, JB Lippincott.)

Prerectal fibers

The most medial muscle bundles of the levator muscle are called prerectal fibers (Fig. 2-33, *c*). These muscle fibers originate from the cranial ramus of the pubic bone and insert laterally on the craniodorsal perineal body.

Muscle contraction of these fibers pulls the perineal body and the connected parts of the rectovaginal septum into a cranial ventral direction. This can be interpreted as an additional protection from prolapse and descensus during increased intraabdominal pressure.

Elasticity of the central tendon

During delivery when the baby's head approaches deeper and the enlargement of the vagina begins, the central tendon, being the most elastic part of the perineum, is stretched in longitudinally. The rectovaginal septum is also stretched. The dilatation of the perineum would be almost impossible without the extreme elasticity of the central tendon. The size of the perineum is normally 2 to 3 cm; this can be enlarged to 10 to 15 cm during a delivery.

As the baby's skull reaches the pelvic floor, the perineal body is curved and more flattened. At the maximum dilatation, the perineal body lies on top of the levator muscle comparable to a cap on a head. The laboring patient continues to push the child's head, but the elasticity of the perineal body resists the pressure for a long time. Finally, when the central tendon is stretched as much as possible, the elastic resistance weakens. (This can be observed clinically; the child's head does not slip back in between the contraction of labor as quickly as it did before.) Further progress and delivery of the head do not happen unless the soft parts have been stretched and the vulva has been enlarged again and again.

The elastic tension of the central tendon is of great importance in other ways. The deep transverse perineal muscle and the external sphincter ani muscle insert at the tendineal body (Fig. 2-36, *2, 7*). This connection pulls the dorsal edge of the urogenital diaphragm in the midline toward the anus. This pulling causes an elastic tension all over the urogenital diaphragm, which may be controlled in different ways. This variable tone in the diaphragm, which is perforated by the urethra and on which the neck of the bladder rests, is a subsidiary mechanism to prevent urinary incontinence.

Smooth muscles in this area keep the tone but allow an extension of the tissue until the limits of its elasticity. If this is the case, smooth muscle fibers behave like concentrated connective tissue and help keep the internal genitalia in their position.

Striated muscles react very quickly and maintain both tone and balance, but they are not able to perform rhythmic contractions. The contracted muscles remain in a constant length, and balance and tone are maintained as a subsidiary tissue.

Elastic tissue consists of an irregular net, which antagonizes tension similar to an elastic band. In old age, the elasticity is decreased, which may cause the typical complication of descensus of vagina or uterus in elderly women.

Lost or decreased elasticity of the central tendon may be caused (1) by badly healed damages and their scars, (2) by shrinking of the connective tissue and loss of the elastic fibers in old age, or (3) by induration and shrinkage of the perineum in kraurosis vulvae or dyspareunia in the climacterium.[27]

Hernia of the vaginal stump

In a prolapse of the proximal part of the vagina, the paracolpic fixation is not sufficient. Normally even after vaginal or abdominal hysterectomy, the paracolpic suspensory keeps the proximal vagina in its place above the levator plate near the sacrum and far away from the hiatus of the levator muscle.

As long as the insufficiency of the paracolpic suspensory apparatus does not pass a certain grade, it can be repaired by a posterior vaginoplasty. A procedure including sewing of the levator muscles to reduce the genital hiatus, which means an extension of the levator plate causing a reduced diameter of the vagina, is the most proper operation in such a case.

In the case of a real vaginal prolapse, this procedure is not the right decision and will not have the same result. The levator muscles, as the only suspensory mechanism of the female genitals, (Halban and Tandler) cannot be upheld any longer (Richter). The large number of different procedures for treatment of a vaginal hernia in literature (see Richter, Nichols, Randall, Geburtsh) implies that neither vagina nor abdominal nor abdominovaginal operations has shown consistently good and satisfactory results. Several decades ago Amreich described a new method that was little used and finally forgotten. Later, Sederl, Richter, and Nichols, as disciples of Amreich and others, rediscovered the method, the vaginal sacrospinous fixation.

REFERENCES AND SUGGESTED READINGS

1. Averette HE Jr, Viamonte MI, Ferguson JH: Lymphangioadenography as a guide to lymphadenectomy, *Obstet Gynecol* 21:682, 1963.
2. Brunschwig A: Die Technik der Lymphadenektomie im Becken in Verbindung mit der radikalen Hysterektomie als Behandlung des Collumcarcinoms, *Presse Med* 724-726, 1955.
3. Collette JM: Envahissements ganglionnaires inguino-ilio-pelviens par lymphographie, *Acta radiol*, Stockholm 49:154, 1958.
4. Corning HK: *Lehrbuch der Topograph Anatomie*, Wiesbaden, 1913, JF Bergmann.
5. Dargent M, Guillemin G: The treatment of operable cancer of the cervix by the combination of radiation and surgery, *Cancer*, Philadelphia 8:53, 1955.
6. Dolan PA, Huges RR: Lymphography in genital cancer, *Surg Gynecol Obstet* 118:1286, 1964.
7. Frankenhauser: *Die Nerven der Gebarmutter*, Jena, 1867, W. Braumüller.
8. Fuchs WA: *Lymphographie u. Tumordiagnostik*, Heidelberg, 1965, Springer.
9. Fuchs WA, Böök-Hederström G: Inguinal and pelvic lymphography: a preliminary report, *Acta Radiol*, Stockholm 56:340, 1961.
10. Gerteis W: Die Lymphographie beim Genitalcarcinom der Frau, *Arch Gynäkol* 200:109, 1964.
11. Gitsch E: *Radioisotope in Geburtsh Gynäkol*, Berlin, 1977, Walter de Gruyter.
12. Gitsch E: Personal communication, 1990.
13. Gitsch E, Janisch H, Leodolter S: *Neue Erkenntnisse zum Problem einer radioaktiven Markierung der tiefen Lymphabflußgebiete des Beckens.* In Pabst, editor: *Nuklearmedizin*, Stuttgart, 1974, Schattauer, 370-373.
14. Gitsch E, Janisch H, Leodolter S: Zur Problematik der endolymphatischen P32 Applikation bei der Radioisotopen-Radikaloperation des Kollumkarzinoms vom Typ II, *Gynäkol Rundsch* 14:210, 1974.
15. Gitsch E, Janisch H, Tulzer H: Die Radikaloperation des Carcinoma colli uteri mit Radioisotopen vom Typ I, *Z Geburtsh Gynäkol* 175:253, 1971.
16. Gitsch E, Janisch H, Tulzer H: Die Isotopen-Radikaloperation des Kollumkarzinoms vom Typ II, *Schweiz Z Gynäkol Geburtsh* 3:121, 1972.
17. Gitsch E, Janisch H, Tulzer H: Progress in the radioisotope surgery of the cervical carcinoma, *Europ J Gynaecol Oncol* I:1, 1980.
18. Gulland GL: The development of lymphatic glands, *J Pathol* 2:447-485, 1894.
19. Hafferl A: *Lehrbuch der Topographischen Anatomie*, Berlin, 1957, Springer.
20. Heinen G: Personal communication, 1965.
21. Hellmann T: Studien über das lymphoide Gewebe: Die Bedeutung der Sekundärfollikel, *Beitr Path Anat* 68:333, 1921.
22. Hellmann T: *Lymphgefäß, Lymphknötchen und Lymphknoten.* In Möllendorf V: *Hdb d mikr Anat d Menschen, Bd VI*, Berlin, 1930, Springer.
23. Hillemanns HG: Die Reaktion des reg. Lymphknoten auf die therapeutische Ra-Rö-Bestrahlung beim Collumcarcinom, *Z Geburtsh Gynäkol* 149:156, 1957.
24. Hohenfellner R, Janisch H, Ludvik W: Die Lymphographie bei malignen Erkrankungen des Urogenitalsystems, *Geburtsh Frauenheilk* 25:298, 1965.
25. Janisch H: Zur Frage der Lymphgefäß und Lymphknotenregeneration nach Wertheimscher Radikaloperation: eine lymphographische Studie, *Geburtsh Frauenheilk* 28:646, 1968.
26. Janisch H, Leodolter S: On radioactive labelling of the lymph drainage regions of the pelvis, *Lymphology* 9:5, 1976.

27. Joachimovits R: *Das Beckenausgangsgebiet und Perineum des Weibes: eine anatomische und klinische Studie,* Wien, 1969, Wilhelm Maudrich.

28. Kinmonth JB: Lymphangiography in man, *Clin Sci* 11:13, 1952.

29. Kownatzki: *Die Venen des weiblichen Beckens,* Wiesbaden, 1907, JF Bergmann.

30. Latzko W, Schiffmann J: Klinisches und Anatomisches zur Radikaloperation des Gebärmutterkrebses, *Zbl Gynäkol* 43:689-705, 1919.

31. Meigs JV: *Surgical treatment of cancer of the cervix,* New York, 1954, Grune & Stratton.

32. Meigs JV, Sturgis SH: *Progress in gynecology, Vol I,* New York, 1950, Grune & Stratton.

33. Milley PS, Nichols DH: A correlative investigation of the human rectovaginal septum, *Anat Rec* 163:443, 1969.

34. Milley PS, Nichols DH: The relationship between the pubourethral ligaments and the urogenital diaphragm in the human female, *Anat Rec* 170:281, 1971.

35. Mitra S: Extraperitoneal lymphadenectomy and radical vaginal hysterectomy for cancer of the cervix (Mitra technique), *Amer J Obstet Gynecol* 78:191, 1959.

36. Nathanson IT: Extraperitoneal iliac lymphadenectomy in the treatment of cancer of the cervix. In Meigs JV, Sturgis SH, editors: *Progress in Gynecology, vol I,* New York, 1950, Grune & Stratton.

37. Navratil E: The Schauta-Amreich operation with and without lymphadenectomy. In Meigs JV, Sturgis SH, editors: *Progress in gynecology, vol IV,* New York, 1963, Grune & Stratton.

38. Nichols DH: International perspectives on vaginal surgery. In *Clinical Obstetrics and Gynecology,* New York, 1982, Harper & Row.

39. Nichols DH, Randall CL: *Vaginal surgery,* ed 3, Baltimore, 1989, William & Wilkins.

40. Noda: Mitteilung am Weltkrongreβ Gebh, *Gynäkol,* Berlin, 1985.

41. Okabayashi H: Radical abdominal hysterectomy for cancer of the cervix uteri, *Surg Gynecol Obstet* 33:335, 1921.

42. Pernkopf E: *Topographische Anatomie des Menschen: Lehrbuch und Atlas,* Berlin, 1941, Urban & Schwarzenberg.

43. Poppi A: L'apparato linfogliandolare nella puberta, *Riv Clin Pediat* 34:429, 1936.

44. Reiffenstuhl G: *Anwendung von radioaktiven Isotopen beim Collum-Carcinom der Frau auf Grund neuer anatomischer Kenntnisse,* Wien, 1955, Akademie der Wissenschaften.

45. Reiffenstuhl G: *Lymphsystem der Gebärmutter und Scheide.* In Seitz, Amreich: *Biologie und Pathologie des Weibes: Hdb d Frauenheilk u Gebh,* Bd IV, Berlin, 1955, Urban & Schwarzenberg.

46. Reiffenstuhl G: Die Beckenlymphknoten eines Falles von Mycloma plasmocellulare, *Z f Gynäkol* 78:75, 1956.

47. Reiffenstuhl G: Zur Frage der Nomenklatur der Beckenlymphknoten, *Wiener Klin Wschr* 68.247, 1956.

48. Reiffenstuhl G: Über Involution und Neubildung von Lymphknoten, *Arch f Gynäkol* 187:375-387, 1956.

49. Reiffenstuhl G: *Das Lymphsystem d weiblichen Genitale,* Berlin, 1957, Urban & Schwarzenberg.

50. Reiffenstuhl G: Vergleichende klinisch-anatomische Untersuchungen des Lymphsystems vom Neugeborenen und von Erwachsenen, *Geburtsh Frauenheilk* 18:1180, 1958.

51. Reiffenstuhl G: Zum Lymphknotenproblem des Carcinoma colli uteri: Häufugkeitsbefall der Lymphknoten und Radikalisierung der Lymphonodektomie, *Wiener Med Wschr* 109:294, 1959.

52. Reiffenstuhl G: *Das Lymphgefäβsystem des Affen.* In Hofer, Schultz, Starck: *Handbuch der Primatenkunde,* Bd III/2, Basel, 1960, S. Karger.

53. Reiffenstuhl G: *Lymphatic system of the ureter, bladder and urethra.* In Youssef AF: *Gynecological urology,* Springfield, IL, 1960, Charles C Thomas.

54. Reiffenstuhl G: Analyse von 60 Lymphonodektonomien bei der Wertheim'schen Radikalop Berichte III, *Weltkongreβ Gynäkol u Gebh,* 1961.

55. Reiffenstuhl G: Über das Vorkommen von Lymphcysten nach der Lymphonodektomie, *Wiener Med Wschr* 112:539, 1962.

56. Reiffenstuhl G: Über die Lokalisation der lymphogenen Aussaaten des Carcinoma colli uteri, *Wiener Med Wschr* 112:751, 1962.

57. Reiffenstuhl G: *The lymphatics of the female genital organs,* Philadelphia, 1964, JB Lippincott.

58. Reiffenstuhl G: The prognostic value of lymphography in carcinoma of the uterine cervix. In Rüttimann A: *Progress in lymphology,* Stuttgart, 1966, Georg Thieme.

59. Reiffenstuhl G: *Das Lymphknotenproblem beim Carcinoma colli uteri und die Lymphirradiatio pelvis: Direkte Bestrahlung des Beckenlymphsystems mit Isotopen,* Berlin, 1967, Urban & Schwarzenberg.

60. Reiffenstuhl G: Der prognostische Wert der Lymphographie beim Kollumkarzinom, *Geburtsh Frauenheilk* 27:590, 1967.

61. Reiffenstuhl G: Lymphknotenmetastasen beim Kollumkarzinom und ihre Behandlungsmöglichkeiten, *Z f Gynäkol* 90:966, 1967.

62. Reiffenstuhl G: *Dringliche gynäkologische u gebh Operationen.* In Breitner, Kraus, Zuckschwerdt: *Chirurg Operationslehre, Bd VI,* Berlin, 1977, Urban & Schwarzenberg.

63. Reiffenstuhl G: The clinical significance of the connective tissue planes and spaces, *Clin Obstet Gynecol* 25:4, 1982.

64. Reiffenstuhl G: Die vaginale Radikaloperation nach Schauter-Amreich zur Behandlung des Collumkarzinoms, *Arch Gynecol Obstet* 242:1, 1987.

65. Reiffenstuhl G, Platzer W: *Die Vaginalen Operationen: Chirurg Anatomie u Operationslehre,* Berlin, 1974, Urban & Schwarzenberg.

66. Reiffenstuhl G, Platzer W: *Atlas of vaginal surgery: surgical anatomy and technique,* Philadelphia, 1975, WB Saunders.

67. Richter K: Lebendige Anatomie der Vagina, *Geburtsh Frauenheilk* 26:1213, 1966.

68. Richter K: Die physiologische Topographie des weiblichen Genitale in moderner Sicht, *Z f Gynäkol* 34:1258, 1967.

69. Richter K: Die operative Behandlung des prolabierten Scheidengrundes nach Uterusextirpationen: ein Beitrag zur Vaginaefixatio sacrotuberalis nach Amreich, *Geburtsh Frauenheilk* 27:941-954, 1967.

70. Ruttimann A, del Buono MS, Cocchi U: Neue Fortschritte in der Lymphographie, *Schweiz Med Wschr* 91:1460, 1961.

71. Sederl J: Zur Operation des Prolapses der blindendigenden Scheide, *Geburtsh Frauenheilk* 18:824, 1958

72. Seelig A: *Ausbreitungswege des Gebärmutterkrebses,* Straβburg, 1894, Preisschrift.

73. Seelig A: Pathologisch Anatomische Untersuchungen über die Ausbreitungswege des Uteruscarcinoms im Bereiche des Genitaltractus, *Virchow's Arch* 140:80, 1895.

74. Tandler J, Halban H: *Topographie des weiblichen Ureters,* Wien, 1901, W. Braumüller.

75. Uhlenhuth E: *Problems in the anatomy of the pelvis,* Philadelphia, 1953, JB Lippincott.

76. von Peham H, Amreich JA: *Gynäkologische operationslehre,* Berlin, 1930, S Karger.

77. Wertheim E: *Die erweiterte abdominale Radikaloperation bei Ca colli uteri,* Berlin, 1911, Urban & Schwarzenberg.

78. Zacharin RF: The suspensory mechanism of the female urethra, *J Anat* 91:423, 1963.

Chapter 3

THE DYNAMICS OF PELVIC SUPPORT

Augusto G. Ferrari

Genital prolapse and urinary incontinence are the most important clinical manifestations that may result from (or co-exist with) functional anatomic deficit of the structures that form the so-called pelvic support mechanism.

To understand the pathogenic mechanism, some important considerations relative to the suspensory and support structures of the pelvic organs must be defined. When changing from a supine to a standing position, the abdominal pressure is elevated by a few centimeters of water (with small oscillations synchronous with the diaphragmatic movements). In a resting condition, even in the standing position, the structures that close the pathway from the pelvis normally are under very little pressure. Walking, running, many forms of work or sports activity, efforts that involve the Valsalva maneuver, coughing, laughing, sneezing, and so forth can cause an increase in abdominal pressure that for brief periods of time may reach and surpass 100 cm H_2O. In these situations, the pelvic support system is under strain.

The containment of the genital organs within the pelvis depends on the integrity of at least three systems: muscular, fascial, and neurologic. The pelvic organs—bladder, genital organs, and anal/rectal canal—literally are suspended to the bony pelvis by a connective tissue apparatus extending between the peritoneum and the pelvic upper aponeurosis formed by the so-called endopelvic fascia. The pelvic supports are attached to an intact suspensory apparatus that lies on the fascia of the pelvic muscles, which is the structure that directly supports gravitational weight. It is formed by the internal upper aponeurosis of the levator ani, which fuses at the level of the arcus tendineus with the fascia of the obturator internus, posteriorly with the presacral fascia, and anteriorly with the transversalis abdominal fascia. This fascial structure is continuous with very rich visceral connective fascial structures, in particular the perivaginal fascia. Underneath the pelvic upper aponeurosis, a complex muscular apparatus formed by the muscle of the pelvic diaphragm and the urogenital diaphragm form the dynamic support system. This is mediated by a tonic and phasic reflex activity through muscle fibers of type I and type II (fast twitch and slow twitch). This muscular apparatus has important functions integrated by the central nervous system. When there is an increase in abdominal pressure induced by changes in position or by physical activity, this muscular apparatus modulates its tonic activity. When there is a sudden increase in abdominal pressure like that induced by a strong episode of coughing, there is a corresponding series of rapid phasic muscular fiber contractions enhanced for short periods by contractions of fast twitch fibers.

During the filling phase of the bladder, there is an increase of activity detected by electromyogram (EMG), whereas during micturition phase, there is functional silence on EMG, an expression of muscular relaxation. The integration at the level of the central nervous system allows us to contract these muscles voluntarily in the face of voluntary interruption of micturition, in the initial phase of delay of the stimulus to micturition or defecation, and in numerous other circumstances. This muscular-fascial system of support dynamically antagonizes the expulsive forces gravitating on pelvic egress, protecting the overlying static suspensory apparatus, and intervening directly in the mechanism that guarantees containment and continence of the viscera. Prolapse and stress urinary incontinence are expressions, therefore, of a multifactorial pathology that can be related to traumatic or dystrophic factors that compromise the dynamic and static structures of pelvic support.

THE SUSPENSORY SYSTEMS

The pelvic viscera maintain reciprocal anatomic relations and connections with the bony pelvis by way of a suspensory system formed by a framework of connective tissue extending between the peritoneum and the levator upper aponeurosis named "endopelvic fascia." In this structure, we recognize "spaces" of loose areolar connective tissue (e.g., the paravesical spaces, pararectal spaces, vesicouterine space). The potential spaces are separated from one another by condensation of connective tissue containing within these septi the course of visceral hypogastric vessels and are called in surgical and anatomic terms the "pillars" that form the true suspensory system. These pillars originate posteriorly and laterally from the presacral and pelvic fascia, course medially and forward, fusing with the perivisceral connective tissue of the rectum, vagina, and bladder, terminating in the retropubic area. We recognize in the "pillars" pseudoligamentous structures, among which are the uterosacral and cardinal ligaments that constitute the posterior and lateral attachment systems to the region of the uterine isthmus and cervix, and also the pubovesical ligaments and vesicouterine ligaments that are the anterior segment of this suspensory system. This connective tissue architecture can be compared to a double arch. The ends of the points of attachment are the posterior lateral pelvic wall and the retropubic region. The base is wider posteriorly, and the two arches converge, suspending the vagina in its supradiaphragmatic segment included between the pelvic upper aponeurosis and the uterine isthmus region. The uterosacral ligaments are the most cranial and most consistent of this unique structure.

The vagina is fixed laterally in such a way that the anterior and posterior walls touch each other. That is due to lateral tension, whereas the posterior suspension determines the vaginal pelvic angle, which is acute posteriorly. This conformation of the vagina is important because it guarantees (1) the occlusive mechanism of the pouch of Douglas during increases of abdominal pressure; (2) the proper projection of the cervical isthmus region onto the fibrous center of the perineum, which is necessary to allow an adequate support of the uterus during body movement and expulsive efforts; and (3) the support of the cervical trigonal areas in both static and dynamic situations. When considering the pathogenesis of stress urinary incontinence, the anterior suspensory system of the vesical neck and urethra is often found to be very important. The system, not yet well-defined in its anatomic and functional details, forms suspensory structures to the pubic arch (pubourethral "ligaments"), to the anterior vaginal wall, and to the so-called levator vaginal attachments to the arcus tendineus and also the internal upper aponeurosis of the puborectalis muscles. Even in this area, there is a precise anatomic functional integration between suspensory connective tissue structures and musculofascial support structures formed by the puborectal muscles and the urogenital

diaphragm. Continence in the resting condition is ensured by the following factors:

1. The normal detrusor distention reflex (detrusor compliance)
2. The thickness of the urethral epithelium and its relation to age and endocrine stimulation
3. The presence and size of the subepithelial venous complex
4. The abundant elastic tissue present in all urethral layers
5. The urethral smooth muscle, which is still a source of contradiction and discussion not only as to its anatomic independence and functional independence of the detrusor muscle but also relative to a macral and microscopic description and to its innervation
6. The tone of the striated muscle of the external sphincter and of the muscles of the urogenital and pelvic diaphragms

In resting condition, all of these factors normally determine that the urethral pressure be higher than the vesical pressure. This condition is called the urethral closing pressure profile. During episodes of coughing and sudden increase of abdominal pressure, two accessory mechanisms increase this closing pressure to guarantee a positive differential pressure. With this mechanism aided by contraction of the striated pelvic muscles, this increased pressure occurs at the point of transition from the proximal two thirds to the distal third of the urethra. The second accessory mechanism is closure under stress, which refers to the passive increase of urethral closing pressure due to the transmission of abdominal pressure both on the bladder and on the external wall of the supradiaphragmatic urethra. The conditions present in order for these accessory mechanisms to be effective are (1) normal reflex activity of the striated muscles; (2) normal development and function of the striated muscle; (3) usual anatomic relations between the urethra, pelvic diaphragm, and urogenital diaphragm; and (4) the closure of the vesical neck during stress. If during stress the bladder neck becomes patent and there is disruption of the vesical closure, urine penetrates in the proximal urethra and the patient maintains continence only if the underlying muscular tone together with the intrinsic urethral pressure guarantees a positive differential ratio. If this is not present, a loss of urine synchronous with the stress but without participation of the detrusor occurs. For the patient to remain continent, the bladder neck must remain perfectly closed during stress. Patency of the neck and the proximal urethra during stress are necessary conditions for stress urinary incontinence to occur. The integrity of the suspensory structures at the level of the cervical or trigonal regions is essential for the maintenance of closure of the bladder neck under stress.

Some important questions of static and dynamic function and support remain to be clarified. Why is the presence of stress incontinence not necessarily related to urogenital prolapse? Why do we observe frequent episodes of severe stress incontinence in the absence of prolapse, or an absence of stress incontinence in the presence of a severe cystourethrocele? One hypothesis is that the maintenance of normal closure of the bladder neck is related, not so much to the integrity of the pubourethral ligaments, as to the integrity of the anatomic interorgan relationship between the cervical trigonal region and the vaginal wall (i.e., the collective integrity of the suspensory connective tissue structures of the urethra, trigone, and vagina). It is important that the dislocation under stress of the vaginal wall does not cause a disruption of the trigonal baseplate. Thus, various individual or combined lesions of the relations between urethra, trigone, and vagina can explain the presence of stress incontinence even in the absence of an evident cystourethrocele, whereas the integrity and preservation of the anatomic unity among organs of the system, the bladder neck, trigone, and vagina guarantee closure even in the presence of an obvious dislocation (cystourethrocele). Analysis of the cystographic radiologic images while the patient is applying stress substantiate this hypothesis: The radiologic integrity of the baseplate is coincident with continence even in the presence of considerable dislocation and large cystocele. On the contrary, the radiologic disruption of the baseplate does not always cause urinary stress incontinence because the accessory mechanisms related to the muscles of the pelvic floor may still guarantee continence in certain critical conditions.

DYNAMIC SUPPORT STRUCTURES

The musculature that forms the pelvic floor is divided into muscles of the urogenital diaphragm and those of the pelvic diaphragm. Except for the ischiocavernosus muscles, the other muscles that form the pelvic floor insert peripherally to osseous and ligamentous structures of the pelvic girdle. Inferiorly in the midline, they insert to the anococcygeal raphe posteriorly and to the fibrous center of the perineum anteriorly. Two of three perineal superficial muscles (bulbocavernosus and superficial transverse of the perineum) converge on the fibrous center of the perineum and the transverse deep muscle of the perineum and its superficial and deep upper aponeurosis and the anterior and medial bundles of the puborectal muscles with its upper aponeurosis. Therefore, one can understand how the fibrous center of the perineum is an important dynamic center of support for the vaginal wall, the cervical trigonal region, and the uterus. Loss of its anatomic integrity can be an important predisposition in the disruption of those delicate anatomic functional balances that protect from vaginal prolapse and from stress incontinence. Special attention should be given to the surgical reconstruction of defects of this structure in the operations both for uterovaginal prolapse and for stress incontinence.

The pelvic diaphragm is formed essentially by the levator ani muscles. A few anatomic considerations about its structure have important functional implications. Contrary to the classic view that defines the puborectal muscle as an

integral part of the levator, recent studies show that the puborectalis should be considered as an entity by itself not only because of its histologic characteristics and orientation of the muscle fibers but also because of its characteristic function. The puborectal muscles, therefore, form a true muscular arch surrounding the pelvic viscera that, when contracting, performs a double sphincteric containment and indirect containment action through the accentuation of the urethrovesical, vaginopelvic, and anorectal angles. The levator ani is characterized by a fusion posterior to the rectum called the levator plate (Fig. 3-1) and by an anterior part called the suspensory sling that fuses and fixes medially to the perivisceral connective tissues of the rectum, vagina, and urethra. The levator plate occupies a more or less horizontal orientation in the pelvis centrally fusing with a rectococcygeal raphe posteriorly, but with an anterior hiatus circumscribed by bundles of connective tissue that are fixed to the intrahiatal organs by connective tissue forming the so-called hiatal ligament. From a functional point of view, this anatomic interpretation is extremely important because whereas the puborectal muscle is active during the containment phase, the levator plate and the so-called suspensory sling act as an accessory opening mechanism in the evacuation phase. In summary, the main puborectal muscle bundle that is part of the dynamic system of support fulfills four main functions: (1) it guarantees opposing the vector of abdominal thrust to the suspension system, protecting it from dangerous and recurrent pressures; (2) it elevates the fibrous center of the perineum to make it coincide with the cervical and isthmic region of the uterus during sudden increases of abdominal pressure, helping to prevent prolapse of the uterus; (3) it accentuates the urethrovesical, and anorectal relationships in the mechanism of continence; and (4) it accentuates the vaginal-pelvic angle, preventing enterocele.

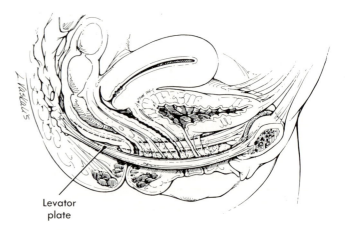

Levator plate

Fig. 3-1. A sagittal section of the pelvis demonstrates the almost horizontal upper vagina and rectum lying upon and parallel to the levator plate. The latter is formed by fusion of the pubococcygei muscles posterior to the rectum. The anterior limit of the point of fusion is the margin of the genital hiatus, immediately posterior to the rectum. It is the normal position of this levator plate that accounts for the anal rectal angle, which is shown.

PATHOGENESIS OF UROGENITAL PROLAPSE

Loss of the correct projection of the cervical isthmic region on the fibrous perineal center (generally secondary to a deficit of the uterosacral suspensory structures) represents the first episode of the uterine descensus through the genital hiatus. A forward displacement of the uterus with widening of the vaginal pelvic angle promotes uterine prolapse or often associated enterocele. Clinical confirmation of this is found in the frequent observation of subsequent enterocele and vaginal vault prolapse in patients who have undergone hysteropexy through ventral fixation. Anterior fixation of the uterus exposes the pouch of Douglas to the expulsive forces that, over time, promote the formation of large enterocele. Even the anterior colposuspension performed according to Burch, ignoring the normal uterine suspensory mechanism, can promote uterine prolapse of severe degree often in a short time. Defects of the perineal center are a cause of possible anterior prolapse (cystourethrocele) as well as the insufficience of the paravaginal connective suspensory tissues and anterior septae and posterior septae are causes of segmentary prolapse of the vaginal walls (cystourethrocele and rectocele). In the pathogenesis of urogenital prolapse, an important role is played by the musculofascial structures described. The lack of a valid support to the static suspensory structures exposes the internal pelvic organs to a sinking effect.

Biopsies of the puborectal muscles performed in the course of operations for prolapse have demonstrated surprisingly that with predictable dystrophic type lesions of the muscles, there are also structural changes of neurogenic origin. These observations substantiate the hypothesis that repeated pelvic floor stress is a cause of peripheral lesions of muscular innervation, with subsequent neurogenic myopathy and dynamic insufficiency. EMG studies performed in patients with prolapse when compared to controlled cases have confirmed, in numerous cases, the presence of tracing supportive of neurogenic myopathy. Also the studies of sacral potential, especially in the cases with stress incontinence, have demonstrated prolonged latency in the reflex response to stimuli. Whatever the initial damage, dystrophy or lesion of the suspensory structures, inefficiency of the musculofascial support systems, or primary or secondary deficit of pelvic muscle innervation, the end result is an evolving prolapse of various degree and severity in which deficits of the suspensory structures and support structures coexist because these structures are anatomically and functionally complementary.

Multiple factors have been incriminated in the pathogenesis of prolapse. Among these factors are traumatic episodes due to childbearing, multiparity, dystocia, and macrosomia. Separations and lacerations of upper aponeurotic muscular structures, partial tears of the musculature and its insertion, and lacerations of connective tissue suspension structures by hematomas may be the basis for precocious descensus or can form the basis for a prolapse developing later in life. No less important are dystrophic factors, including congenital insufficiency or acquired involution, or menopausal or senile atrophy of the musculofascial structures and ligamentous structures. In menopause, a progressive loss of elasticity of connective tissue occurs. More specifically, there is a decrease in organization of the subepithelial elastic lamina of the vagina with both degenerative changes and fragmentation. These alterations can, at times, predispose to prolapse in the nullipara. The studies of Zacharin have documented the existence of racial differences (more sturdiness of the pelvic floor in the Chinese women). Other studies emphasize the predisposition to prolapse in women who have certain pathologies as are included in the "joint instability syndrome" (hip dislocation, osteoartrosis, chondrocalcinosis, and so forth). In other cases, deficit of pelvic muscle innervation and altered neuroendocrine balances (spina bifida, endocrine obesity) are mentioned as primary causes. Chronic medical diseases and all the conditions that may be accompanied by repeated and prolonged increase in abdominal pressure (chronic constipation, chronic lung disease, obesity, and so forth) must be remembered. Many of these factors may coexist and synergistically determine prolapse. One also must remember the effects of iatrogenic factors, in particular gynecologic surgical procedures directed to suspension of the anterior vaginal wall and those procedures that are able to change the normal anatomic, topographic relationships or vaginal axis.

RELATIONS BETWEEN URINARY INCONTINENCE AND PROLAPSE

The clinical observation of an association between pathology of micturition and alteration in normal pelvic anatomy is frequent. However, the coexistence of incontinence in prolapse must not be considered on a basis of a simple and direct dependence; in fact, stress incontinence in prolapse implies lesions and functional alterations separate from the suspensory apparatus and support apparatus described and in a clinical situation must be evaluated separately. For example, stress urinary incontinence (1) may be present in the absence of prolapse; (2) may be absent in the presence of prolapse (when an incomplete chronic retention of urine may occur as in some cases of very large cystoceles and in many cases of total uterovaginal prolapse); (3) can accompany vaginal prolapse as an expression of the deterioration of both the suspensory and support system; (4) can be exacerbated by the development of genital prolapse; (5) can be aggravated by procedures for the correction of prolapse (urethrocystopexy, colpoplastic, and so forth); and (6) can be masked by the presence of prolapse. This last possibility (also called latent incontinence) is not always easy to document and occurs when a very large cystocele or rectocele or uterine prolapse does not allow the opening of the bladder neck, compressing it under stress versus the pubic arch.

BIBLIOGRAPHY

Al-Rawi ZS: Joint hypermobility in women with genital prolapse, *Lancet* 26:1439, 1982.

Berglas B, Rubin IC: Study of the supportive structures of the uterus by levator myography, *Surg Gynec Obstet* 97:677, 1953.

Bethoux A, Scali P, Blondon J: Physiopathologie et anatomie pathologique des prolapsus vaginaux, *Rev Prat* 21:1863, 1971.

Blaivus JG: Diagnostic evaluation of urinary incontinence, *Urology* 36:10, 1990.

Burch JC: Cooper's ligament urethrovesical suspension for stress incontinence, *Am J Obstet Gynecol* 100:764, 1968.

Campbell RM: The anatomy and histology of the sacrouterine ligaments, *Am J Obstet Gynecol* 59:1, 1950.

Candiani GB, Ferrari A: *Isterectomia vaginale,* Milano, 1986, Masson.

Candiani GB, Ferrari A: *Le disarmonie statico dinamiche nell' ambito pelvico. La Clinica Ostetrica e Ginecologica,* Milano, 1991, Masson.

Constantinou CE, Govan DE: Spatial distribution and timing of transmitted and reflexly generated urethral pressures in healthy women, *J Urol* 127:964, 1982.

Dickinson VA: Maintenance of anal continence: a review of pevic floor physiology, *Gut* 19:1163, 1978.

Gilpin SA et al: The pathogenesis of genitourinary prolapse and stress incontinence of urine. A histological and histochemical study, *Br J Obstet Gynaecol* 96:15, 1989.

Gosling F: The structure of the bladder and urethra, *Urology* 87:124, 1979.

Green TH: *Total prolapse of the vagina.* In Hafez ESE, Evans TN, editors: *The human vagina,* 1978, Biomedical Press.

Herzog AR, Fultz MM: Epidemology of urinary incontinence: prevalence, incidence and correlates in community populations, *Urology* 36:2, 1990.

Huisman AB: Morfologie van der vrouwelijke urethra, thesis, Groningen, Netherlands, 1979,

Hutch JA: A new theory of the anatomy of the internal urinary sphincter and the physiology of micturition. The base plate, *J Urol* 96:182, 1966.

Hutch JA: *Anatomy and physiology of the trigone, bladder, and urethra,* New York, 1972, Appleton.

Kamina P: *Anatomia ginecologica ed ostetrica,* Roma, 1975, Marrapese.

Milley PS, Nichols DH: The relationship between the pubourethral ligaments and the urogenital diaphram in the human female, *Anat Rec* 170:281, 1971.

Netter FH: Atlante di anatomia fisiopatologica e clinica. vol 3 Apparto riproduttivo. 1982, Ciba-Geigy II.

Nichols DH, Milley PS, Randall CL: Significance of restoration of normal vaginal depth and axis, *Obstet Gynecol* 36:251, 1970.

Nichols DH: Clinical pelvic anatomy, the types of genital prolapse and the choice of operation for repair, *R I Med J* 65:112, 1982.

Nichols DH, Randall CL: *Vaginal surgery,* ed 3, Baltimore, 1989, Williams & Wilkins.

Parks AG: Anorectal incontinence, *Proc R Soc Med* 68:21, 1975.

Platze WL: *Functional anatomy of the human vagina,* In Hafez ESE, Evans TN: *The human vagina,* 1978, Biomedical Press.

Richardson DA, Ostergard DR: The effect of uterovaginal prolapse on urethrovesical pressure dynamics, *Am J Obstet Gynecol* 146:901, 1982.

Richter K: Gynakologische Anatomie des Kleinen Beckens, *Synak Rdsch* 19(suppl 1):13, 1979.

Richter K: Massive eversion of the vagina: pathogenesis, diagnosis, and therapy of the true prolapse of the vaginal stump, *Clin Obstet Gynecol* 25:297, 1982.

Scali P: *Les prolapsus vaginaux et l'incontinence urinaire chez la femme,* Paris, 1980, Masson.

Shafik A: Pelvic double- sphincter control complex. Theory of pelvic organ continence with clinical application, *Urology* 6:611, 1984.

Smith ARB, Hosker GL, Warrell DW: The role of pudendal nerve damage in the aetiology of genuine stress incontinence in women, *Br J Obstet Gynaecol* 96:29, 1989.

Smith ARB, Hosker GL, Warrell DW: The role of partial denervation of the pelvic floor in the aetiology of genitournary prolapse and stress incontinence of urine. A neurophysiological study, *Br J Obstet Gynaecol* 96:24, 1989.

Wein AJ, Barret DM: *Voiding. Function and dysfunction,* St. Louis, 1988, Mosby–Year Book.

Wilson PM: Understanding the pelvic floor, *S Afr Med J* 7:1150, 1973.

Wilson PD, et al: Posterior pubo-urethral ligaments in normal and genuine stress incontinence women, *J Urol* 130:802, 1983.

Zacharin RF: "A chinese anatomy". The pelvic supporting tissues of the Chinese and occidental female compared and contrasted, *Aust N Z F J Obstet Gynaecol* 17:1, 1977.

Zacharin RF: Pulsion enterocele: review of functional anatomy of the pelvic floor, *Obstet Gynecol* 55:135, 1980.

Zacharin RF: *Pelvic floor anatomy and the surgery of pulsion enterocoele,* New York, 1985, Springer-Verlag.

Chapter 4

THE PHYSIOLOGIC STRESS OF SURGERY

Joseph F. Amaral
A. Gerson Greenburg

The "stress of surgery" is often invoked as a reason for a complication or a stormy perioperative course. Just what is "surgical stress"? In its simplest form, surgical intervention is a controlled traumatic injury, the goal of which is to correct an existing pathologic entity. This injury produces numerous alterations in homeostasis that lead to the activation of a series of physiologic reflexes aimed at restoring homeostasis. Both the alterations in homeostasis and the physiologic reflexes and responses may be viewed as surgical stress.

In the absence of major injury, sepsis, or starvation, alterations in homeostasis are usually small; the response is directed at fine tuning and integrating the physiologic functioning of the organism, and the overall stress is low. In the presence of major injury, sepsis, or starvation, alterations in homeostasis are multiple and intensified; the reflexes are directed at an integrated attempt to restore cardiovascular stability, preserve oxygen delivery, mobilize energy substrates, mobilize the supply of critical substrates, and minimize pain.[41] The stress is considerably greater with a major injury than with minor injury and, at a minimum, proportional to the degree of injury. However, the inability of a host to respond appropriately to stressors, as might occur in people with concurrent illnesses, may result in an overall surgical stress much greater than that anticipated. For example, the inability to respond to a drop in effective circulating volume results in further alterations in homeostasis as tissue perfusion and oxygen delivery are impaired.

Stressors represent alterations in homeostasis. They function as stimuli to a physiologic reflex response that makes up the neuroendocrine and metabolic responses to injury. Primary stimuli to the neuroendocrine reflexes include (1) changes in effective circulating volume; (2) changes in the concentrations of oxygen, carbon dioxide, or hydrogen ions of tissue or blood; (3) pain; (4) emotional stimuli such as fear and anxiety; (5) alterations in substrate availability; (6) changes in core or ambient temperature; and (7) sepsis (Fig. 4-1).[41]

All these stimuli must be perceived by specialized receptors that transduce the stimulus into electrical activity and transmit it to the brain. For example, a patient paraplegic from spinal cord transection at T4, undergoing a gastrectomy in the absence of a diminished circulatory volume fails to release adrenocorticotropic hormone (ACTH) in response to the operation but is capable of producing corticosteroids in response to intravenously administered ACTH.[35,48] The denervation prevents the afferent impulses from reaching the brain. Similarly, patients undergoing hip replacement under spinal anesthesia do not demonstrate an increase in vasopressin secretion during the procedure when compared with patients undergoing the same procedure under general anesthesia (Fig. 4-2).[18] However, as the effect of the spinal anesthetic wears off, the response is the same in both groups. This implies that postoperative pain and its perception are major stimuli to the neuroendocrine system.

RESPONSES TO SURGICAL STRESS
The baroreceptor reflex

Virtually all injuries are characterized by the loss of effective circulating volume.[41] This may result from the direct loss of blood, as in hemorrhage; from the loss or sequestration of plasma volume, as in dehydration and third-space losses; or from the inability of the body fluids to circulate, as in cardiac failure, pulmonary embolism, or tension pneumothorax. The loss of effective circulating volume is sensed by the high-pressure baroreceptors in the

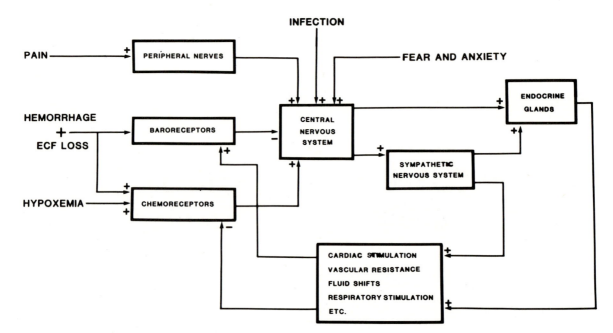

Fig. 4-1. Overview of the neuroendocrine reflexes induced by shock and injury. There are at least seven stimuli consequent to injury that elicit neuroendocrine reflexes. These include hypovolemia; pain; changes in Po_2, Pco_2, pH; infection; emotional arousal; changes in substrate availability; and changes in temperature. The most common of these are hypovolemia and pain. (From Gann DS, Amaral JF: *Endocrine and metabolic responses to injury.* In Schwartz SI, Shires GT, Spencer FC, editors: *Principles of surgery,* 1989, McGraw-Hill.)

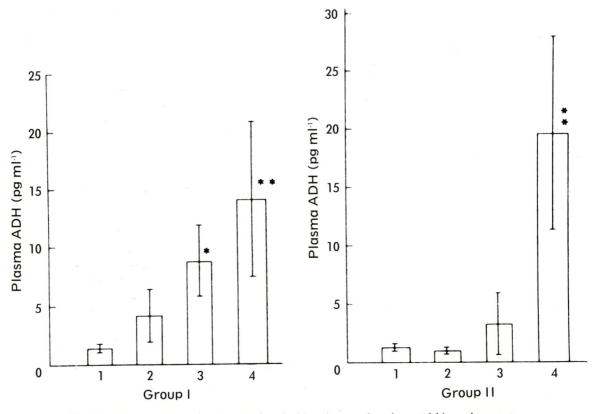

Fig. 4-2. Plasma vasopressin concentrations in 14 patients undergoing total hip replacement under general anesthesia (7 patients in group 1) or epidural anesthesia (7 patients in group II). Patients who underwent surgery under general anesthesia developed a progressive increase in plasma vasopressin, whereas those under epidural anesthesia demonstrated an increase only 4 hours after surgery and presumably as the anesthetic wore off. (From Bonnet F et al: *Br J Anesth* 54:29, 1982.)

aorta, carotid arteries, and renal arteries, which are sensitive to the arterial pressure and its rate of change, and by the low-pressure stretch receptors in the atria, which are sensitive to the atrial volume and its rate of change.[43,53] The total circulating volume and the effective circulating volume are not necessarily the same, because the total circulating volume is effective only to the extent that it is sensed by these receptors. For example, a patient with a tension pneumothorax or cardiac tamponade may have a total circulating volume greater than normal but be hypotensive because of an ineffective circulating volume caused by obstruction to cardiac outflow and filling. Similarly, even though the total circulating volume may be increased in congestive heart failure, the effective circulating volume as sensed by high- and low-pressure receptors is decreased.

The afferent signals from high-pressure baroreceptors and from low-pressure stretch receptors tonically inhibit the release of many hormones and the activities of the central and autonomic nervous systems (Fig. 4-3).[41] A decrease in effective circulating volume produces a decrease in baroreceptor and stretch receptor activity. This leads to

a release of the tonic inhibition of the neuroendocrine system, which results in the secretion of ACTH, vasopressin, renin, growth hormone, beta-endorphin, and catecholamines. These neuroendocrine effectors bring about further changes, including stimulation of cortisol secretion by the adrenal gland in response to ACTH; stimulation of the conversion of angiotensinogen to angiotensin in the vascular space by renin; stimulation of aldosterone secretion by the adrenal gland in response to ACTH and angiotensin II; stimulation of glucagon secretion by the pancreas in response to epinephrine; and inhibition of insulin secretion by the pancreas in response to epinephrine. The decrease in baroreceptor and in stretch receptor discharge also stimulates the vascular component of the sympathetic nervous system, leading to peripheral vasoconstriction, and to an increase in cardiac sympathetic nervous system activity and a decrease in cardiac parasympathetic nervous system activity that lead to an increase in heart rate and cardiac contractility. These mechanisms work in concert to preserve hemodynamic integrity and oxygen delivery—desirable homeostatic mechanisms.

The neuroendocrine and autonomic responses initiated

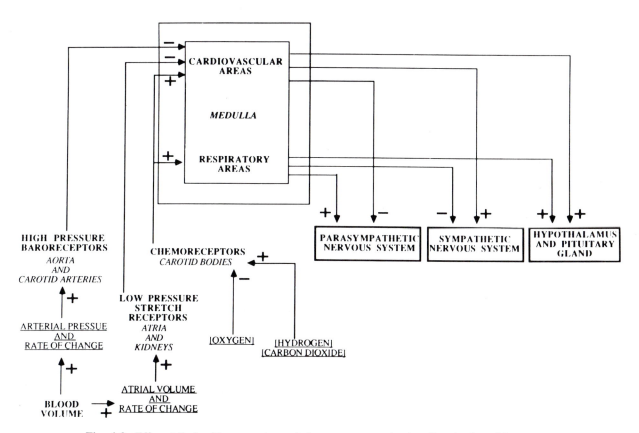

Fig. 4-3. Efferent limb of baroreceptor and chemoreceptor activation. Inactivation of baroreceptors or activation of chemoreceptors results in the stimulation of the hypothalamus and of the vascular component of the sympathetic nervous system. However, in contrast to the inactivation of baroreceptors, activation of chemoreceptors produces a decrease in cardiac sympathetic nervous system activity and an increase in parasympathetic activity. (From Gann DS and Amaral JF: *Endocrine and metabolic responses to injury.* In Schwartz SI, Shires GT, Spencer FC, editors: *Principles of surgery,* 1989, McGraw-Hill.)

by a decrease in effective circulating volume are proportional to the magnitude of the decrease. Therefore, the neuroendocrine response to a 20% hemorrhage is greater than that observed after a 10% hemorrhage.[13] However, many of the neuroendocrine and cardiovascular responses have maximal responses that are achieved usually when the effective circulating volume has been decreased by 30% to 40%. Further decreases in the effective circulating volume cannot be compensated for, and hypotension and decreased oxygen delivery ensue.

The chemoreceptor reflex

Changes in the concentration of oxygen, hydrogen ions, and carbon dioxide in the blood initiate cardiovascular, pulmonary, and neuroendocrine responses through the activation of peripheral chemoreceptors. These receptors, which are located in the carotid and the aortic bodies, are not activated under normal circumstances. However, decreases in the concentration of oxygen or, to a lesser extent, increases in the concentrations of hydrogen ions or carbon dioxide are sensed by these receptors and lead to activation of neuroendocrine reflexes.[41]

Activation of chemoreceptors stimulates the hypothalamus and the vascular component of the sympathetic nervous system (Fig. 4-3). In this regard, it is similar to the inactivation of baroreceptors and stretch receptors. The activation of chemoreceptors, in contrast to the inactivation of baroreceptors and stretch receptors, also produces a decrease in cardiac sympathetic nervous system activity and an increase in parasympathetic nervous system activity, leading to a decrease in heart rate and cardiac contractility.[54] In addition, chemoreceptor activation stimulates the respiratory center, leading to an increase in respiratory rate.

Pain and emotion

Pain and emotional arousal are characteristic of any injury and activate the neuroendocrine system. Pain, acting through projections of peripheral nociceptive fibers to the central nervous system (CNS), results in the stimulation of the thalamus and the hypothalamus.[41] Emotional arousal is produced by the perception or threat of injury and, through the limbic areas of the brain, invokes an emotional response of anger, fear, or anxiety. These emotional changes stimulate the neuroendocrine reflexes through projections from the limbic system to hypothalamic and lower brain stem nuclei. As a result, both pain and emotional arousal produce an increase in the secretion of vasopressin, ACTH, endogenous opiates, catecholamines, cortisol, and aldosterone and produce changes in the activity of the autonomic nervous system.

Substrate alterations

Changes in the plasma glucose concentration are the primary substrate alterations that activate neuroendocrine reflexes. The plasma glucose concentration is sensed by receptors in the hypothalamus (ventromedial nucleus) and the pancreas. A decrease in the plasma glucose concentra-

tion stimulates the release of catecholamines, growth hormone, cortisol, ACTH, beta-endorphin, and vasopressin through central pathways (hypothalamus and autonomic nervous system) and stimulates the release of glucagon both by central (autonomic nervous system) and by peripheral pathways (direct pancreatic activation).[10] In addition, the secretion of insulin is inhibited by central pathways (autonomic nervous system) and by the pancreas.

Temperature

Changes in the core temperature of the body are sensed in the preoptic area of the hypothalamus and lead to alterations in the secretion of many hormones, including ACTH, vasopressin, cortisol, epinephrine, growth hormone, catecholamines, aldosterone, and thyroxine.[49,73] The core temperature may change as a result of alterations in ambient temperature; the loss of the normal thermal insulating barrier (burns); inadequate blood flow (hypovolemia) or substrate supply (starvation); or inadequate peripheral vasoconstriction or vasodilation (sepsis).

Changes in the ambient temperature stimulate neuroendocrine reflexes, either directly or through changes in the core temperature. Similarly, infection may stimulate the neuroendocrine system directly through the action of endotoxin, or indirectly through secondary changes in blood volume, oxygen concentration, substrate concentrations, and pain, or through monokines released from inflammatory cells such as tumor necrosis factor and interleukin-1.

A surgical procedure evokes many of these stimuli during the operative and postoperative periods. To the extent that the stimuli can be minimized, so too will the overall stress of the procedure. To a large degree, this is the responsibility of anesthetic and perioperative management. These stimuli rarely occur singly. As a result of the similar pathways through which sensory inputs enter the CNS, integration of afferent signals can occur in the CNS with modulation of efferent signals, the response from the CNS. Consequently, the neuroendocrine response to a given stimulus is not an all-or-none phenomenon, nor is it always the same. The response depends, to a large extent, on the intensity and the duration of the stimulus; the presence of simultaneous and sequential stimuli that are qualitatively the same or different; the status of the receptor at the time of stimulation; and the time of day during which the stimulus occurs.

The dependence of the response to a stimulus on the intensity and duration of the stimulus, as well as the importance of CNS integration, is well described for cardiopulmonary reflexes and adrenomedullary secretion of catecholamines. Despite the potent activation of the sympathetic nervous system by small nonhypotensive hemorrhages, adrenomedullary secretion of catecholamines occurs only when hypotension develops. Because nonhypotensive hemorrhages have little, if any, effect on arterial baroreceptors, this finding suggests that inactivation of cardiac stretch receptors alone is not sufficient for the activation of catecholamine release. Similarly, activation of chemoreceptors alone or inactivation of baroreceptors in isolation produces potent sympathetic nervous system activity but little adrenal catecholamine secretion. However, adrenal catecholamine secretion does occur during hypotensive hemorrhages in which both receptors are activated, suggesting that high-pressure baroreceptors and low-pressure volume receptors both must be inactivated for adrenomedullary stimulation to occur.[41]

In addition to intensity and duration, the rate at which a stimulus is presented is also an important parameter in the modulation of efferent signals elicited by the stimulus. For example, Bereiter, Zaid, and Gann[13] demonstrated that the serum epinephrine concentration in the cat after hemor-

rhage is a function of the rate and the magnitude of the hemorrhage (Fig. 4-4). Whereas small hemorrhages, equivalent to 10% to 20% of the blood volume, elicited the same increase in serum epinephrine concentrations independent of the rate of hemorrhage, large hemorrhages, equivalent to 30% of the blood volume, elicited a greater response when they were performed rapidly (10%/min) rather than slowly (2%/min). Similar findings have also been reported for aldosterone, renin, and vasopressin.[24] Thus, the neuroendocrine response of an injured person with a loss of 30% blood volume in 1 hour may be considerably different from the response seen in a patient who loses 30% blood volume over 1 day.

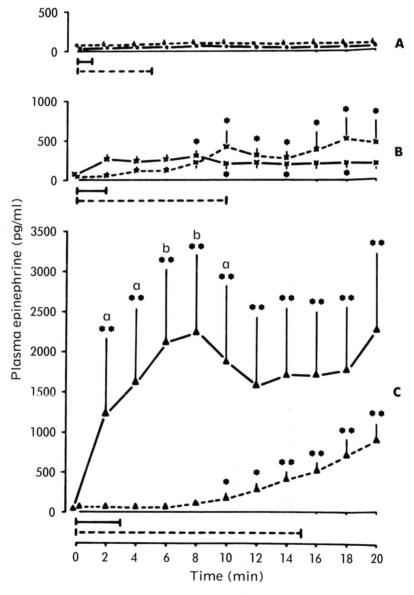

Fig. 4-4. Plasma epinephrine concentrations in response to graded blood loss in the cat at rapid and slow rates of hemorrhage. **A,** 10% hemorrhage, rapid rate = ●___● (n = 6), slow rate = ●-----● (n = 7). **B,** 20% hemorrhage, rapid rate = x___x (n = 11), slow rate = x-----x (n = 7). **C,** 30% hemorrhage, rapid rate = Δ___Δ (n = 8), slow rate = Δ-----Δ (n = 8). The horizontal bars under each figure represent the period of blood removal for each hemorrhage magnitude. *$p<0.05$, **$p<0.01$ vs control group. a. $p<0.05$; b. $p<0.01$ vs slow rate of hemorrhage. (From Bereiter DA et al: *Am J Physiol* 1986.)

The responsiveness of receptors in the transduction of the stimulus into neural activity is variable. For example, central osmoreceptors located in the hypothalamus, near the third ventricle, change their setpoint in response to other neural inputs.[15] Alterations of plasma osmolality and of effective circulating volume are potent stimuli to the secretion of vasopressin. Input from receptors monitoring these parameters interact in the CNS such that a change in the setpoint of the osmoreceptor occurs when the secretion of vasopressin is altered by neural input from baroreceptors. As a result, changes in the effective circulating volume do not eliminate the influence of the osmoregulatory system.[15,75] Instead, the change in the setpoint of the osmoreceptor makes it more or less sensitive to a given osmotic stimulus. Clinically, this situation is observed in the hypervolemic, hyponatremic patient who, despite an increased effective circulating volume, produces vasopressin in response to the low plasma osmolality. This is classically seen in the cirrhotic patient.

The sensitivity of some receptors, such as those of the adrenal cortex, changes as a function of the time of day. For example, despite a similar response of ACTH to hemorrhage when it occurs in the morning or in the evening, the secretory response of cortisol to ACTH is significantly greater in the evening.[37] The latter finding may have particular significance for patients undergoing emergency surgery, which is more likely to occur at night than during the day. Its importance in recovery from surgery, however, remains unknown. Nonetheless, it is important to recognize that a particular stimulus of the same magnitude, rate, and duration may have less of an effect under certain circumstances than under others.

The stimuli accompanying an operative procedure rarely occur singly. Upon injury or illness, the person is likely to perceive multiple stimuli simultaneously. Thus, the neuroendocrine response to injury is the summation of all the stimuli the person perceives and processes, and it is often different from the response to any single stimulus given alone. For example, Bereiter, Plotsky, and Gann[12] demonstrated that the secretion of ACTH was greater to hemorrhage and noxious stimulation than to hemorrhage or noxious stimulation alone (Fig. 4-5), and Overman and Wang[67] reported that, although a 40% hemorrhage alone produced 50% mortality, a 30% hemorrhage produced a similar mortality when combined with sciatic nerve stimulation.

In addition to multiple stimuli occurring simultaneously, it is not uncommon for multiple stimuli to occur sequentially. For example, a patient with an ectopic pregnancy may first experience pain from distention and rupture of the fallopian tube, then hypovolemia from a hemorrhage, and finally hypothermia as the hypotension progresses. According to classic endocrine feedback mechanisms, one might expect that the elevation of serum cortisol resulting from one set of stimuli would inhibit the release of ACTH by the second set. Under most circumstances, this is not true and the response is unchanged or

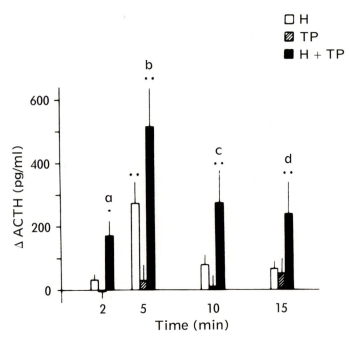

Fig. 4-5. Potentiation of the ACTH response to hemorrhage by nerve stimulation. H = hemorrhage, TP = tooth pulp, * = $p < 0.05$ vs baseline, ** = $p < 0.01$ vs baseline. (Letters above each sample time point denote intragroup individual comparisons: a = $p < 0.05$ H+TP vs TP, b = $p < 0.01$ H+TP vs TP or H, c = $p < 0.05$ H+TP vs H, d = $p < 0.05$ H+TP vs TP or H.) At all time points, the response of ACTH to hemorrhage and tooth pulp stimulation was greater than the response to either hemorrhage or tooth pulp stimulation alone. (From Bereiter DS et al: *Endocrinology* 113:1439, 1983.)

may actually be greater than the initial response (potentiation). The physiologic facilitation and potentiation have been demonstrated for cortisol and catecholamines in response to sequential hemorrhages of the same magnitude and to sequential operations (Fig. 4-6).[42,56,57] Potentiation of the adrenocortical response has also been shown when surgery has been performed 2 hours before an hypoxic stimulus but not 24 hours before.[71] Thus, the neuroendocrine response to injury, shock, and sepsis may modify the response to subsequent surgery, and the response to a second injury, such as surgery, may be considerably different from what it would have been had it occurred first.

Finally, the response to the stimuli consequent to injury may be modified by a variety of factors present in the person before injury, such as (1) ethanol and other recreational drugs, (2) concurrent medications, (3) drug withdrawal, (4) preexisting illness, and (5) old age. Among these modifiers, age is a particularly important one because the relative and absolute numbers of elderly persons in western industrialized society continue to increase. In the United States, approximately 11.3% of the population was older than age 65 in 1980.[83] This represents a 276% increase from the 4.1% observed in 1900 and a 140% increase from the 8.1% observed in 1950. By 2030, it is projected that 18% of the U.S. population will be over age 65.[83]

Because the aging population is at equal or greater risk for the development of medical problems requiring surgical intervention, surgeons are frequently called on to intervene in this group of patients. This decision is often confused by the aging process, such that elderly people are not offered surgical alternatives, particularly if the surgery is elective. Indeed, most studies comparing surgical intervention in elderly and nonelderly people note an increased morbidity and mortality in the elderly group.[4] This increase appears to be independent of the operative procedure. In part, old age alone may represent a risk for surgical intervention. This would not be surprising given the widespread impairment in physiologic function that is a consequence of senescence. However, recent studies strongly suggest that the risk of surgery in elderly patients is conferred by associated illnesses rather than old age itself.[19,46,70,74] That is, elderly people are not at an increased risk if they have no chronic illnesses.

Unfortunately, elderly people are likely to have associated illnesses. Del Guercio and Cohn[29] found only 13.5% of their population over age 65 to be "normal" by physiologic assessment. Foremost among the illnesses and aberrations present in elderly patients are malnutrition, cardiac disease, pulmonary dysfunction, renal impairment, and dementia. The greatest operative risk in any patient, young or old, is cardiac disease, whereas in elderly patients, dementia appears to confer the highest operative risk.[4,45]

Despite the increased risk conferred by associated illnesses and the decline in physiologic function with age, it appears as if virtually all types of surgical procedures can be performed in the elderly with morbidity and mortality similar to that observed in nonelderly patients if attention is paid to identifying the risk factors present in each individual patient; if aggressive measures are taken to correct these abnormalities when possible; and if lesser procedures are performed when severe deficits are present that cannot be corrected.

Rankin and Johnson[72] noted, ". . . some persons 50 years of age seem older than others of 70. However, due credit must be given these people, for without steadiness of fiber, they would never have reached the age of 70 years." Clearly, physiologic age is more important than chronologic age. Unfortunately, there are no objective scales to determine physiologic age with reference to chronologic age that predict risk. The Dripp's American Surgical Association and American Society of Anesthesiologists (ASA) physical status scale does allow for the identification of high-risk groups of patients based on simple subjective clinical criteria.[33,69] Using these criteria, patients in groups III and IV can be identified as high-risk patients. Marx, Mateo, and Orkin noted a 0 and 5% mortality in ASA groups I and II, respectively, whereas the mortality in groups III and IV was 25% and 45%, respectively, in patients over 70 years of age.[60] Of note in their study was the finding that mortality was not related to age when based on the ASA classification. This supports the concept

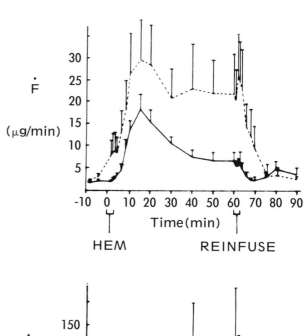
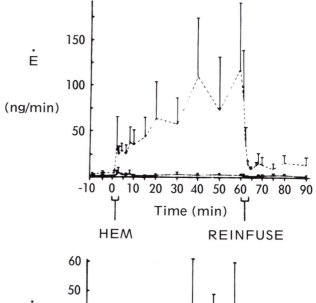
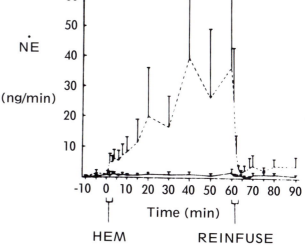

Fig. 4-6. Potentiation of the secretory rates of epinephrine (E), norepinephrine (NE), and cortisol (F) to a 7.5 ml/kg hemorrhage in dogs when a hemorrhage of the same magnitude was performed on the previous day. The pattern of response between E and NE is the same, but that for NE is at a lower absolute rate than that for E. Hemorrhages took place at 0 min; reinfusion occurred at 60 min. ___ = mean response on day 1; ----- = mean response on day 2. (From Lilly MP et al: *Endocrinology* 111:1917, 1982, and 112:681, 1983.)

of physical status rather than age as the more important factor in determining mortality.

Although patients of any age are at a greater risk of morbidity and mortality when they undergo an emergency procedure, elderly patients are particularly at risk, presumably because of their diminished physiologic reserve.[57] In fact, procedures done on an emergency basis in the elderly are associated, on the average, with three to four times the mortality they would have as elective procedures.[47] It is apparent from these data that surgical intervention should be performed on an elective basis in elderly patients whenever possible, rather than waiting for an emergency to force one's hand. The patient can be maximized physiologically before the planned procedure so that the changes of morbidity and mortality are minimized.

THE EFFERENT OUTPUT

For the most part, in response to an injury the secretion of most neuroendocrine effectors is increased (see box below). Simplistically, one may consider all catabolic or counterregulatory hormones (cortisol, catecholamines, glucagon) to increase and anabolic hormones (insulin) to remain unchanged or decrease. Thus, it is no surprise that the neuroendocrine response is associated with net tissue breakdown and energy expenditure.

There are three major branches to the efferent limb of the reflex neuroendocrine response to injury: (1) the autonomic response, (2) the hormonal response, and (3) the local tissue response. The first two arise in two distinct areas of the brain: the autonomic regions of the brainstem and the hypothalamic-pituitary axis. Output from the former changes the activities of the sympathetic and parasympathetic nervous systems, whereas output from both areas changes the rates of hormonal secretion. As such, the endocrine response may be divided into hormones whose secretion is primarily under hypothalamic-pituitary control (cortisol, thyroxine, growth hormone, and vasopressin) and hormones whose secretion is primarily under autonomic control (insulin, glucagon, and catecholamines). The mediators of local tissue response are numerous small peptides (tissue factors, monokines, and autocoids) whose release may be initiated by the local inflammatory response in an injured area or by the injured tissue itself.

The secretion rate and plasma concentration of many of the hormones that increase after injury do so in proportion to the severity of the injury.[20,23,28,40] The actions of cortisol and catecholamines are well-documented in this regard (Figs. 4-7 and 4-8). Despite this well-characterized response, it has not been possible to ascribe all the physiologic responses observed after injury to the actions of individual hormones. Although simple alterations of the endocrine system in healthy people may produce changes in the same direction as those seen after injury, they are not of the same magnitude. Rather, the effects observed after injury appear to depend on the effects of multiple hormones simultaneously. A well-studied example in this regard is the triple hormone infusion of glucagon, cortisol, and catecholamines. In both animals and normal human volunteers, this combination of hormones can produce an increase in metabolic, pulse, and respiratory rates; an increase in glucose production, insulin resistance, negative nitrogen and potassium balance; and sodium and water retention (Fig. 4-9).[14,36,38] However, the triple hormone infusion does not explain the net skeletal muscle proteolysis noted after injury. This, as well as other features of the metabolic response, may rest in the inflammatory-cytokine response to injury.

Inflammatory mediators are usually small molecules released at the site of injury by white cells and platelets. These agents destroy bacteria and other foreign material and frequently act in a nonspecific fashion. Important cytokines derived from monocytes and macrophages include interleukin-1, interleukin-6, interleukin-8, tumor necrosis factor, and interferon.[32] They have broad and overlapping, usually local, metabolic effects. Furthermore, tumor necrosis factor and interleukin-1 reproduce many of the features of sepsis and shock when given intravenously. These effects are augmented by the addition of interferon. Thus, the cytokines appear to act as links between the inflammatory and metabolic responses. Furthermore, they appear to exert an important role in the mediation of pathological conditions that result from injury such as sepsis, shock, and adult respiratory distress syndrome.

METABOLIC RESPONSE

The immediate postsurgical period is characterized by starvation, immobilization, restoration of homeostasis, and repair. The metabolic events consequent to injury are the result of stimuli associated with the injury and starvation and are presumably directed at restoration of homeostasis and at repair. For example, the negative nitrogen balance and weight loss that follow injury appear to be, in large part, the result of the starvation that accompanies the injury.[76] Evidence also suggests that the metabolic response to injury may be altered to some degree by the inflammatory response to the injury. For example, temporal alterations in plasma ketone body and lactate concentrations of wounded animals appear to correlate with the inflamma-

---

Neuroendocrine response		
Increased release		*Decreased release or unchanged*
Epinephrine	Beta-endorphin	Insulin
Norepinephrine	Growth hormone	Estrogen
Dopamine	Prolactin	Testosterone
Glucagon	Somatostatin	Thyroxine
Renin	Eicosanoids	T_3
Angiotensin	Histamine	TSH
Vasopressin	Kinins	FSH
ACTH	Serotonin	LH
Cortisol	Interleukin-1	IGF
Aldosterone	TNF	

tory infiltrate of wounded tissue.[6] A large portion of the increased glucose uptake of wounded tissue is attributable to the inflammatory infiltrate, and tumor necrosis factor appears to be responsible for many of the manifestations of endotoxemia.[82] Thus, an understanding of the metabolic response consequent to starvation and the metabolic alterations produced by the inflammatory infiltrate is central to an understanding of the metabolic response to injury.

Metabolic response consequent to starvation

The average resting, 70-kg man using 1800 kcal/day of energy requires 180 g of glucose—144 g for the metabolism of the nervous tissue and 36 g for other glycolytic tissue (red blood cells, white blood cells, renal medulla) (Fig. 4-10); energy for obligate daily activity; amino acids for protein synthesis; and fatty acids for lipid synthesis.[21] In the absence of oral intake of food, these substrates must be supplied from existing body stores.

Glucose and fuel can be obtained from the 75 g of glycogen stored in the normal fed liver (Table 4-1). However, this is insufficient for either the fuel or glucose requirements of fasting patients. The largest portion of the body's glycogen stores (150 g) is in skeletal muscle. Although this source can be broken down to lactate, it cannot pro-

vide free glucose. Skeletal muscle lacks glucose-6-phosphatase, the enzyme necessary for the release of free glucose from a cell. Thus, the primary stimulus to the metabolic events that occur during fasting and starvation is a reduction in the serum glucose concentration that occurs as the glucose needs of glucose-dependent tissues can no longer be met by the breakdown of glycogen. The reduction in serum glucose, in turn, results in a decrease in the secretion of insulin and an increase in the secretion of glucagon, cortisol, growth hormone, and catecholamines, changes that stimulate an increase in hepatic gluconeogenesis and glycogenolysis. The changes in insulin and glucagon secretion are the primary ones. Indeed, changes in the secretion of catecholamines, growth hormone, and cortisol are not necessary and occur only during severe hypoglycemia.

The production of glucose by glycogenolysis and gluconeogenesis requires the provision of gluconeogenic precursors to the liver. Three primary gluconeogenic precursors are used by the liver and, to a lesser extent, by the kidney for the synthesis of glucose. These are lactate, glycerol, and amino acids such as alanine and glutamine (Table 4-2). There are two main sources for lactate. The first is from the metabolism of glucose by erythrocytes and

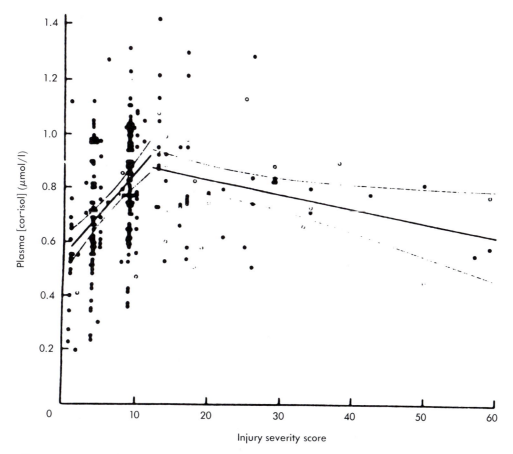

Fig. 4-7. The relationship between plasma cortisol and injury severity score in initial samples from multiply-injured patients studied within 8 hours of injury. The regression lines and their 95% confidence limits between ISS 1 to 12 and ISS 13 to 59 are shown for ethanol negative (●) and ethanol positive (○) patients combined. (From Stoner HB et al: *Clin Sci* 56:563, 1979.)

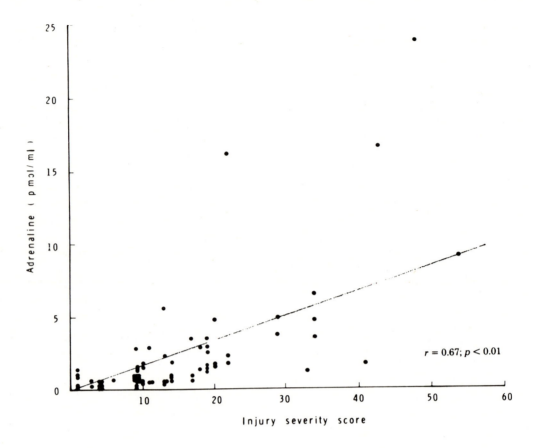

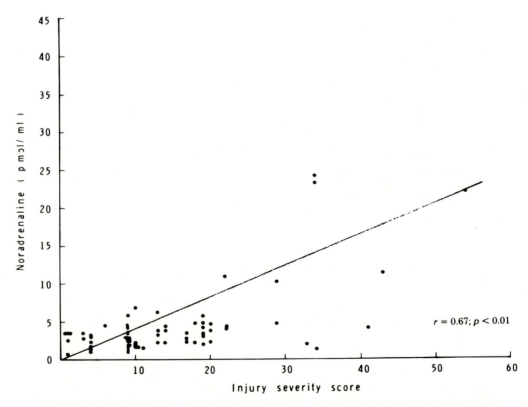

Fig. 4-8. The relationship between plasma concentrations of norepinephrine and of epinephrine with injury severity score in 40 multiply-injured patients. There was a positive correlation between injury severity score, plasma norepinephrine, and plasma epinephrine. (From Frayn KN et al: *Circ Shock* 16:229, 1985.)

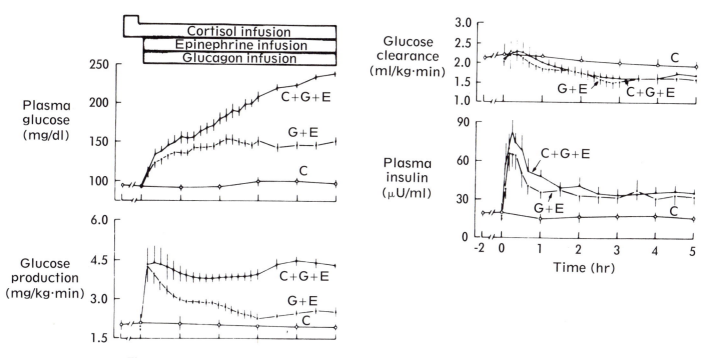

Fig. 4-9. The influence of cortisol *(C)* on the response of plasma glucose and glucose production to glucagon *(G)* or epinephrine *(E)*. Cortisol, which by itself did not alter plasma glucose or glucose production, had the effect of increasing and, more importantly, prolonging the stimulatory effects of glucagon and epinephrine on glucose production. As a result, the effects of the combined hormone infusions on plasma glucose were more than additive. (From Eigler NJ et al: *Clin Invest* 63:114, 1979.)

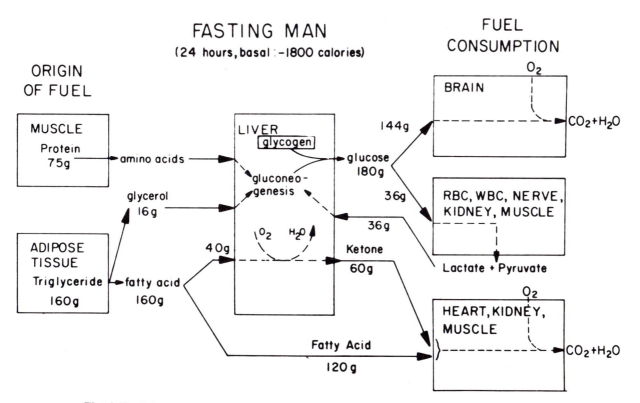

Fig. 4-10. Scheme of fuel utilization in a normal fasted man. The two primary sources are muscle protein and fat. The brain oxidizes glucose completely, the glycolyzers break down glucose by aerobic or anaerobic glycolysis into lactate and pyruvate, which are then remade in the liver in glucose, and the rest of the body burns fatty acids and ketones. (Adapted from Cahill GF: *N Engl J Med* 282:668, 1970.)

Table 4-1. Fuel composition of normal 70-kg man

Fuel	Kilograms	Calories
Tissues		
Fat (adipose triglyceride)	15.0	141,000
Protein (mainly muscle)	6.0	24,000
Glycogen (muscle)	0.150	600
Glycogen (liver)	0.075	300
TOTAL		165,900
Circulating fuels		
Glucose (extracellular fluid)	0.020	80
Free fatty acids (plasma)	0.0003	3
Triglycerides (plasma)	0.003	30
Plasma proteins	0.210	840
TOTAL		953

Table 4-2. Glucose available in early starvation state in a 70-kg man

Origin	Amount of glucose, g/24 hr
New glucose (gluconeogenesis):	
Fat (glycerol)	16
Protein	43
Stored or recycled glucose:	
Glycogen	85
Recycled glucose	36
TOTAL	180

white cells, which do not oxidize the glucose completely to carbon dioxide and water. Instead, they convert glucose to lactate by aerobic glycolysis and release the newly formed lactate into the circulation. This lactate can be reconverted to glucose in the liver and again made available for use by peripheral tissues. This process is known as the Cori cycle (Fig. 4-11). The lactate made available from these sources, however, does not provide any new carbon skeleton for glucose synthesis, because the carbon is derived from preexisting glucose molecules. If glucose demand increases, glucose must be provided from another carbon source. In part, this need may be met by release of lactate from the second major source in the body, skeletal muscle, which cannot release free glucose but can convert glycogen to lactate.

Glycogen stores of skeletal muscle are also limited and not sufficient to maintain glucose homeostasis. As a result, approximately 75 g of protein are degraded daily during fasting and starvation to provide the required gluconeogenic amino acids to the liver (see box on p. 89). This proteolysis results in a rapid increase in the urinary nitrogen excretion from the normal 5 to 7 g/day to approximately 8 to 11 g during the first 2 to 4 days of fasting. Despite the large amount of protein mobilized in starvation from skeletal muscle, the loss of protein from other organs (liver, pancreas, gastrointestinal [GI] tract, and kidneys) is proportionately much greater. In the liver, this protein loss appears to be somewhat selective because the enzymes necessary for gluconeogenesis and lipolysis are spared, whereas those required for the synthesis of urea and serum proteins are not. In the pancreas, exocrine function is lost by a reduction in the production of GI hormones and enzymes; in the GI tract, digestive function is impaired by a reduction in the production of digestive enzymes and in the regeneration of epithelial cells. For these reasons, starved patients often become paradoxically food intolerant as manifested by the development of diarrhea and malabsorption when small amounts of food or enteral feedings are given.

The kidney also assumes an increasing role in gluconeo-

genesis because glutamine and glutamate serve as the primary amino acids for transport of the amino groups to the kidney for ammonia formation and for gluconeogenesis in the kidney. In fact, the kidney may account for up to 45% of glucose production during late starvation.

It is apparent that the rapid proteolysis of body protein cannot proceed at a rate of 75 g/day for very long. First, the total amount of protein in a 70-kg man is approximately 6000 g, and, second, the continued degregation of protein results in continued loss of function, and death will ensue well before all the protein is broken down. Fortunately, proteolysis does slow down by about the fifth day of starvation, eventually reaching a nadir of 20 g of protein per day. This is reflected in a decline in urinary excretion of nitrogen to a minimum of approximately 2 to 4 g of nitrogen per day. This process, in large part, is made possible through ketoadaptation of the brain.[68] Although the brain can metabolize ketone bodies, the limited transport of ketone bodies through the blood-brain barrier under normal conditions limits their utilization. During starvation, transport systems in the blood-brain barrier increase the rate of ketone body transport, and the metabolism of the brain is adapted to use ketone bodies. This results in a significant reduction in the amount of glucose needed by the brain and, therefore, in the amount of protein that must be degraded for gluconeogenesis (Fig. 4-12; Table 4-3).

The synthesis of glucose, like necessary enzymatic and muscular functions such as neural transmission and cardiac contraction, requires energy. These energy requirements in a resting, fasting, 70-kg man can be met by the mobilization of approximately 160 g of triglycerides from adipose tissue in the form of free fatty acids. The release of free fatty acids from adipose tissue and production of ketone bodies by the liver are stimulated by a reduction in the serum insulin concentration and an absolute or relative increase in the concentrations of glucagon and other counterregulatory hormones. The free fatty acids and ketone bodies are used throughout the body by nonglycolytic tissues such as the heart, kidney, muscle, and liver as a source of energy.[22] The main fuel during starvation is fat.

The use of lipids during starvation also provides glucose from the 16 g of glycerol released in the breakdown of 160 g of triglycerides and decreases the amount of glu-

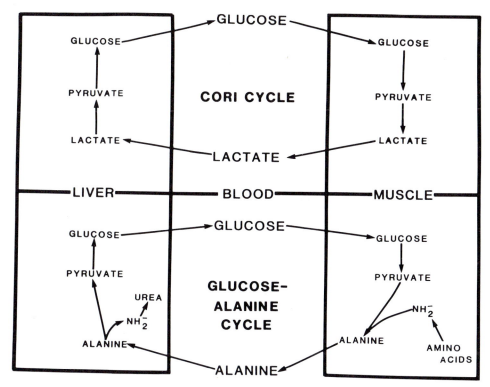

Fig. 4-11. The Cori cycle *(top)* provides for the transfer of energy from the liver to the periphery. Glucose gives up energy to the periphery by anaerobic or aerobic glycolysis to lactate and pyruvate. The latter are remade into glucose in the liver, using energy derived from the metabolism of fatty acids. In the glucose-to-alanine cycle *(bottom)* described by Felig et al, glucose is metabolized to pyruvate in muscle; pyruvate is then converted to alanine, which is transported to the liver where it is remade into glucose.

cose required by skeletal and cardiac muscle by providing fatty acids for fuel (the Randle effect).[77] Similarly, the use of ketone bodies inhibits glucose uptake in most tissues by inhibiting pyruvate dehydrogenase. Thus, the switch to fat as a main fuel source decreases the amount of glucose used and, therefore, the amount of gluconeogenesis and protein degradation required.

Concurrent with these alterations in metabolism, resting energy expenditure is reduced by up to 31%. This is exemplified by the classic studies of total starvation of Benedict,[11] in which energy expenditure decreased from an average of 1650 calories/day in the first week to an average of 1290 calories in the third week. The reduction in resting energy expenditure is multifactorial, deriving from a decrease in lean body cell mass, voluntary work, body temperature, cardiac work, sympathetic nervous system activity, and metabolic activity of muscle. Thus, through reducing resting energy expenditure, using protein for gluconeogenesis, using lipid for energy, and ketoadapting the brain, people are able to survive during prolonged periods of starvation.[62] However, survival during adaptation eventually results in the impairment or loss of important body functions. Ultimately, if starvation persists to a point at which 30% to 40% of the body weight has been lost, death ensues.

METABOLISM IN INJURY

The alterations in substrate metabolism that occur after injury are divided into three phases.[27,63] The first, or ebb, phase occurs during the first several hours after injury. It is characterized by hyperglycemia and by the restoration of circulating volume and tissue perfusion. The second, or flow, phase occurs after tissue perfusion has been restored and may last from days to weeks, depending on the severity of injury, previous health of the injured person, and medical intervention. It is characterized by generalized catabolism, negative nitrogen balance, hyperglycemia, and heat production. The third, or convalescent, phase occurs once volume deficits have been corrected, infection has been controlled, pain has been eliminated, and complete oxygenation has been restored. It is characterized by a

Gluconeogenesis	*Ketogenesis*	*Gluconeogenesis and ketogenesis*
Alanine	Leucine	Isoleucine
Arginine		Lysine
Aspartic acid		Phenylalanine
Aspargine		Tyrosine
Cystine		Tryptophan
Glutamic acid		
Glycine		
Histidine		
Hydroxyproline		
Methionine		
Proline		
Serine		
Threonine		
Valine		

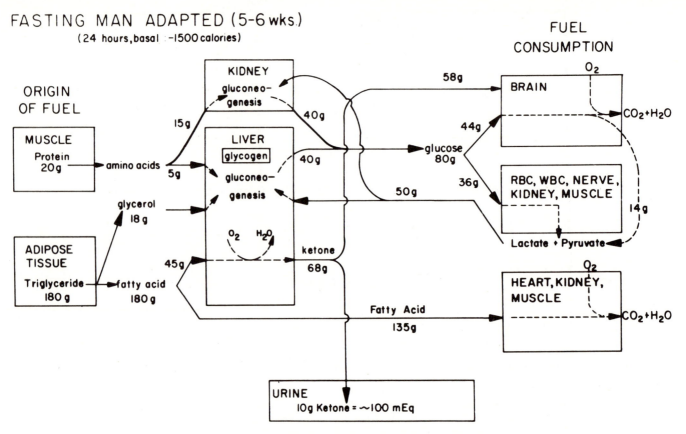

FASTING MAN ADAPTED (5-6 wks.)
(24 hours, basal -1500 calories)

FUEL CONSUMPTION

ORIGIN OF FUEL

Fig. 4-12. Schema of fuel metabolism after 5 to 6 weeks of starvation. Liver glycogen sources are depleted, there is a diminished utilization of muscle protein, the brain is burning ketones, and gluconeogenesis from amino acids is taking place to a large extent in the kidney. (Adapted from Cahill GF: *N Engl J Med* 282:668, 1970.)

Table 4-3. Glucose available in late starvation state in a 70-kg man

Origin	Amount of glucose, g/24 hr
New glucose (gluconeogenesis):	
Fat (glycerol)	18
Protein	12
Stored or recycled glucose:	
Glycogen	0
Recycled glucose	50
TOTAL	80

slow, progressive reaccumulation of protein followed by reaccumulation of body fat. It is considerably longer than the catabolic phase because the rate of protein synthesis cannot exceed 3 to 5 g/day.

Energy metabolism after injury

Energy expenditure. Despite immobilization and starvation, the energy requirements of injured persons are increased. This is reflected in the characteristic loss of body weight and increase in basal metabolic rate seen after surgery. The increase in the energy needed varies directly with the severity of injury.[51] For example, healthy persons undergoing an uncomplicated elective operation demonstrate no greater than a 10% increase in their resting energy expenditure (Fig. 4-13). This increases to 10% to 25% in patients with multiple skeletal injuries and to 20% to 75% in patients with severe infections, such as peritonitis or intraabdominal abscesses. This increase in sepsis is greater than one would predict on the basis of temperature elevation alone, because febrile complications increase the resting energy expenditure by approximately 7% for each degree Fahrenheit of fever. This appears to be related to the inflammatory process because the increase in resting energy expenditure persists for as long as inflammation is present. In this regard, the most severe injury is a thermal burn, in which sustained increases in resting energy expenditure of greater than 100% have been noted.

The relationship between energy expenditure and injury severity is explained, in part, by the increased activity of the sympathetic nervous system and the increased circulating concentrations of catecholamines.[87] However, other factors are important. For example, the increase in resting energy expenditure also depends on the size of the person and, to some extent, on the environmental temperature. The largest increases in energy expenditure are seen in heavily muscled, well-nourished, young men who have large body cell masses; the smallest are seen in elderly, poorly nourished women who have small body cell

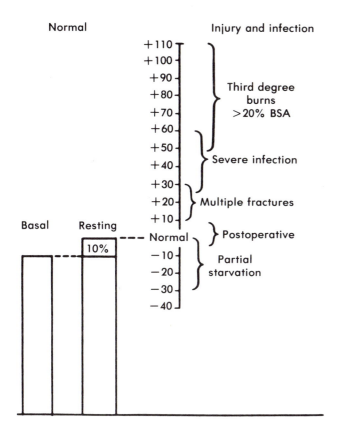

Normal

Injury and infection

Third degree burns >20% BSA

Severe infection

Multiple fractures

Postoperative

Partial starvation

Basal   Resting

10%

Fig. 4-13. Resting energy expenditure of adult patients during injury, stress, and starvation. The highest resting energy expenditures are seen after thermal injuries and severe infections. (From Kinney JM: *The application of indirect calorimetry to clinical studies. In Assessment of energy metabolism in health and disease.* Columbus, OH, 1980, Ross Laboratories, p 42.).

masses.[51] This is a reflection of the linear relationship between body cell mass and resting energy expenditure.

After injury, the available stores of carbohydrate are small, nutritional intake of carbohydrates and proteins is reduced or absent, glucose is required for glucose-dependent tissues, and the degradation of protein for energy results in a loss or reduction of some body functions. As a result, the primary source for energy during injury, as in starvation, becomes fat. This is documented in the low respiratory quotients (0.7 to 0.8) noted after injury and sepsis.[88] These findings argue in favor of the use of intralipids during parenteral nutrition.

Lipid metabolism during injury

Lipolysis. Because the primary source of energy after injury is lipids, it is not surprising that rate of lipolysis is generally increased immediately after injury and during the reparative phase. Immediately after injury, elevated concentrations of the counterregulatory hormones, increased sympathetic nervous system activity, and depressed concentrations of insulin favor lipolysis. Among these agents, the best known stimulus for hormone-sensitive lipase is catecholamines. In fact, the sympathetic nervous system is of paramount importance in the lipolytic response to stress

because adrenergic blockade produces a marked reduction in lipolysis.

Net lipolysis during the ebb phase results in increased glycerol and free fatty acid concentrations in plasma.[3,78] However, if the reduction in effective circulating volume is severe, as in hemorrhagic shock, increased plasma free fatty acid concentrations may not be seen. In part, this may result from intense vasoconstriction occurring in peripheral tissues, which minimizes blood flow to adipose tissue and, therefore, the delivery of neuroendocrine agents. Because the net production of free fatty acids depends on the balance between lipolysis and reesterification of fatty acids, an increase in the reesterification rate may also decrease net free fatty acid release. This occurs in the presence of high concentrations of plasma lactate, such as might occur during shock and sepsis. The mobilization of lipids after injury may also be altered by a decrease in pH, hyperglycemia, and the anesthesia received.[89]

During the flow and reparative phases, net lipolysis persists despite an increase in the concentration of insulin. This is reflected by an increased concentration and clearance of plasma free fatty acids.[66] In the presence of oxygen, the fatty acids released can be oxidized by most tissues in the body, including cardiac and skeletal muscle, to produce energy. Normal or elevated rates of fatty acid oxidation are usually noted during sepsis, endotoxemia, wounding, and thermal injury. However, plasma fatty acid concentrations may not always be elevated if the rate of clearance of fatty acids is equal to or greater than the rate of their appearance.

Ketogenesis. The high concentrations of intracellular fatty acids and the elevated concentration of glucagon during the ebb and flow phases inhibit fatty acid synthesis.[66,81] In hepatocytes, this also stimulates the transport of acetyl CO-A into the mitochondria for oxidation and ketogenesis. The activity of ketogenesis after shock, injury, and sepsis is variable and correlates inversely with the severity of injury. After major injury, severe shock, and sepsis, ketogenesis is low or absent, whereas after minor injury or mild infection, it is increased but to a lesser extent than that seen during nonstressed starvation. Injuries in which ketogenesis is low also appear to be associated with a small or absent increase in plasma free fatty acid concentrations suggesting that the absence of ketogenesis in these situations results from the absence of an increase in the intracellular concentrations of free fatty acids.

Carbohydrate metabolism during injury

Glucose metabolism. Hyperglycemia after hemorrhage was first reported by Claude Bernard in 1877 and has subsequently been confirmed in different species such as the dog, cat, pig, and rat, in humans, and for different injuries such as sepsis, trauma, surgery, and thermal injury.[9,39,56,61] Therefore, in contrast to fasting and starvation, which are characterized by hypoglycemia, injury, sepsis and surgery stress are characterized by hyperglycemia.

Hyperglycemia occurs immediately after injury and frequently persists into the reparative period. The increase in plasma glucose is proportional to the severity of injury as reflected in a positive correlation between injury severity score and glucose concentration in trauma victims (Fig. 4-14). Hyperglycemia provides a ready source of energy to the brain. It also appears possible that, as suggested by Jarhult and by Gann,[44,50,85] a major homeostatic significance of increased plasma glucose concentrations may be the resulting osmotic transfer of fluids from cells to the interstitium that it induces, leading to the restitution of blood volume. Elevated concentrations of glucose are also necessary for adequate delivery of this substrate to wounded tissue.

The alterations in carbohydrate metabolism that occur after injury leading to hyperglycemia include an increase in hepatic glucose production and an impairment in peripheral uptake of glucose. These events result from an increase in the secretion of catecholamines, cortisol, glucagon, growth hormone, vasopressin, angiotensin II, and somatostatin and a reduction in the secretion of insulin. Immediately after injury, the primary source of glucose is hepatic glycogen. However, this is a limited source rapidly depleted within hours. Therefore, glucose production during the flow phase appears to result primarily from hepatic and renal gluconeogenesis.

Differences exist in the mechanism through which these alterations occur. Most studies of glucagon metabolism after nonthermal injury and hypovolemia have noted no increase in the plasma concentration of glucagon immediately after injury. This suggests that an increase in the peripheral concentration of glucagon or in the delivery of glucagon to the liver is not required for the initial hyperglycemia after hemorrhage and injury. This observation is supported by the studies of Lautt, Dwan, and Singh[55] who demonstrated the abolition of the hyperglycemic response to hemorrhage in adrenalectomized and hepatic denervated cats and the restitution of this response when either the adrenals or the liver were left intact. Thus, the immediate hyperglycemia that occurs after injury appears to be related primarily to the actions of catecholamines and cortisol with little contribution from glucagon. However, during the flow phase, glucagon becomes more important and increased concentrations and secretion rates are noted in most studies by 12 to 24 hours after injury.

Insulin resistance. Another important difference in the mechanism of hyperglycemia after injury is related to insulin secretion. Immediately after injury, the plasma insulin concentration is depressed in relation to the degree of hyperglycemia. This results from a reduction in beta islet cell sensitivity to glucose mediated by catecholamines, somatostatin, reduced pancreatic blood flow, and the increased activity of the sympathetic nervous system. An intact adrenal gland is also necessary for this response because the blunting of insulin secretion can be eliminated by adrenalectomy. However, during the flow phase, beta islet cell sensitivity returns to normal, and insulin concentrations rise to more appropriate values despite persistent hyperglycemia.

In part, this is related to the delayed rate of assimilation of a glucose load, glucosuria, and a resistance to exogenously administered insulin noted in both the ebb and flow phases of injury.[3,17] However, this diabetes of injury should not be interpreted as an actual reduction in glucose uptake and utilization, because glucose uptake and utilization by peripheral tissues in both the ebb and the flow phases are consistently greater than under normal circumstances. Instead the resistance to insulin is manifested in a decreased glucose clearance. Therefore, the high plasma glucose concentration appears to overcome the resistance of peripheral tissues to glucose entry, thereby allowing for normal or increased rates of glucose uptake in peripheral tissues.

During the flow phase, gluconeogenesis persists despite near normal concentrations of insulin, another manifestation of the insulin resistance that occurs with injury.[86] Therefore, the hyperglycemia that occurs after injury results from a combination of increased hepatic glucose production and release and from a peripheral resistance to the entrance of glucose. Because production supersedes utilization, hyperglycemia persists. However, if the rate of

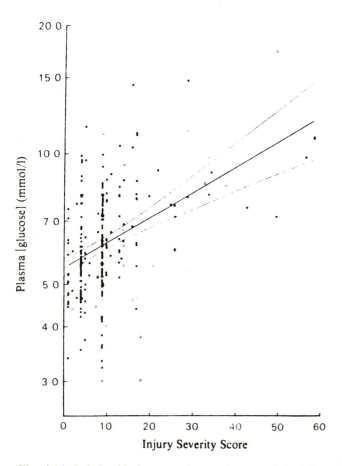

Fig. 4-14. Relationship between plasma glucose and the injury severity score in multiply-injured patients. There was a positive correlation between ISS and plasma glucose both in patients who had ingested ethanol (○) and those that had not (●). (From Stoner HB et al: *Clin Sci* 56:563, 1979.)

gluconeogenesis decreases through a reduction either in gluconeogenic precursors or in gluconeogenic enzymatic function, hepatic glucose production will decrease and hypoglycemia will ensue, a finding in terminal injuries and prolonged sepsis.

Glucose metabolism in wounded tissue. Glucose must be provided not only to red cells, white cells, renal medulla, and neural tissues after injury, but also to wounded tissue. In fact, glucose uptake and lactate production in wounded tissue are increased by up to 100% and are proportional to the circulating concentration of glucose present. Despite the increase in glucose uptake, wounded and burned tissues demonstrate a lack of insulin sensitivity and do not increase their glucose uptake or glycogenesis in response to insulin.[41]

The accelerated glucose uptake in wounded and burned tissue correlates with the degree of inflammatory cellular infiltrate present. Much of the increase above the resting rate of glucose uptake in nonwounded muscle can be explained by glucose uptake in the inflammatory cells. Furthermore, the inflammatory infiltrate may actually mediate an increase in glucose uptake of the wounded noninflammatory tissue itself because the uptake of glucose by nonwounded tissue in the presence of the inflammatory cellular infiltrate is greater than that nonwounded tissue not exposed to the infiltrate.[5]

Lactate metabolism. There is an increase in the plasma concentration of lactate after most injuries that correlates with the severity of injury (Fig. 4-15). The accumulation of lactate after shock accounts in part for the progressive acidosis of shock and derives from anaerobic metabolism in ischemic tissues. Under these circumstances, the likelihood of survival of patients in profound shock can be estimated from the excess levels of lactate present in the blood. For example, Broder and Weil noted an 82% survival in patients in shock with an initial excess lactate concentration of 1 mmol/L, a 60% survival with 2 mmol/L, and a 26% survival when the excess lactate was 2 to 4 mmol/L. A better prognosticator of survival appears to be the serial change in total plasma lactate. In this regard, excess lactate should not be confused with total plasma lactate because the excess lactate is the amount of lactate present in the blood that increases the lactate/pyruvate ratio from normal.

Elevated plasma lactate concentrations may result from local tissue ischemia as mesenteric infarction, from diminished hepatic clearance of lactate as in shock or hepatic dysfunction, and from increased lactate production by inflammatory cells. Thus, the differential diagnosis of any patient with hyperlacticacidemia should include systemic hypoperfusion, regional hypoperfusion, hepatic dysfunction, and severe inflammation.

Protein metabolism during injury

Nitrogen balance. The daily intake of protein for a healthy young adult is usually about 80 to 120 g, or 13 to 20 g of nitrogen. About 2 to 3 g of this nitrogen is ex-

creted per day in the stool, and 13 to 20 g are excreted in the urine. However, after injury, nitrogen excretion in the urine increases greatly and rises to 30 to 50 g of nitrogen per day.[1,26,63] This is nearly all in the form of urea nitrogen and results from net proteolysis because nitrogen intake immediately after injury is minimal or absent. Despite the large amount of protein that is broken down, only 20% is used for calories even with major increases in nitrogen excretion.[34] The remainder is used by the liver and the kidneys to produce glucose and is reflected in the accelerated ureagenesis that is noted after injury.[63]

The increased excretion of urea after injury is also associated with the urinary loss of sulfur, phosphorus, potassium, magnesium, and creatinine.[26] This suggests cellular breakdown and excretion of intracellular components. Isotope dilution studies point to a decrease in cell mass rather than in cell number as the source of the protein breakdown. The nitrogen-sulfur and nitrogen-potassium ratios suggest that this loss occurs mainly from muscle. Analysis

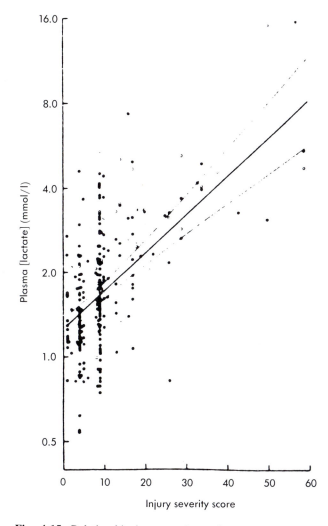

Fig. 4-15. Relationship between plasma lactate and the injury severity score in multiply-injured patients. There was a positive correlation between ISS and plasma lactate both in patients who had ingested ethanol (○) and those that had not (●). (From Stoner HB et al: *Clin Sci* 56:563, 1979.)

of the protein content and the incorporation of radiolabeled amino acids in visceral tissues and skeletal muscle confirm that it is skeletal muscle that is depleted whereas visceral tissues (liver, kidney) are spared, a finding contrary to starvation in which visceral protein are used to a greater extent than muscle.[52]

The net catabolism of protein can result from either increased catabolism, decreased synthesis, or a combination of these factors. Available data on total body protein turnover suggest that after injury net changes in catabolism and synthesis depend on the severity of the injury.[16,80] Elective operations and minor injury appear to result in a decreased rate of synthesis with a normal rate of protein catabolism. Severe trauma, burns, and sepsis appear to be associated with increases in both synthesis and catabolism, but a greater increase in the catabolism occurs, resulting in net catabolism. In this regard, it is important to note that accelerated proteolysis and a high rate of gluconeogenesis persist after major injury and during sepsis. This appears to result from an inhibition of ketoadaptation after major injury and sepsis because, unlike starvation, ketogenesis is not prominent and it does not fuel the brain in significant amounts. As a result, a high requirement for glucose and, therefore, for gluconeogenesis persists. The mechanisms for inhibition of ketoadaptation are not known, but Barocos et al,[8] based on in vitro muscle incubations, have proposed that interleukin-1 may be responsible for the accelerated proteolysis that accompanies fever and sepsis and Clowes et al[25] have presented evidence suggesting the involvement of a circulating peptide (proteolysis-inducing factor [PIF]) containing 33 amino acids in this response that may also represent interleukin-1. More recent data suggest that tumor necrosis factor is also involved in this process and that neither agent by itself is sufficient to explain the accelerated proteolysis observed after injury.

The rise in urinary nitrogen and negative nitrogen balance begins shortly after injury, reaches a peak about the first week, and may continue for 3 to 7 weeks. The degree and duration of negative nitrogen balance are related to the severity of injury. Elective operative procedures have a brief period of minimal negative nitrogen balance, whereas thermal injuries have long periods of major negative nitrogen balance. In addition to injury severity, the degree of negative nitrogen balance and net protein catabolism depends on the age, sex, and physical condition of the patient. Young healthy males lose more protein in response to an injury than do women or the elderly, presumably as a result of the smaller body cell mass present in the latter group. In addition, the urinary excretion of nitrogen is less after a second operation if it closely follows the first, presumably the result of a reduction in available protein stores consequent to the first operation. Finally, negative nitrogen balance can be reduced or virtually eliminated by high caloric nitrogen supplementation as with enteral or parenteral nutrition. Thus, the loss of protein that occurs after injury is not entirely obligatory to the injury, and it is, in large part, a manifestation of acute starvation and the increased need for gluconeogenic precursors during periods of stress.

Amino acid metabolism. The alterations in plasma amino acids in response to injury are not well-defined.[2,7,84] In large part, this may be the result of varying levels of nutrition before the insult, of hypoperfusion, of starvation, and of varying levels of pre-injury physical activity. During the flow phase of injury, alterations in plasma amino acids also appear to be related to the time from injury they are measured. For example, plasma alanine concentrations are increased early in the flow phase but decreased as the flow phase persists. This presumably is the result of lack of alanine availability in peripheral tissues and its continued hepatic uptake for gluconeogenesis.

The type and severity of injury may also have an effect on the alterations seen in amino acid metabolism, although no consensus is established. On the one hand, the direction of changes in the plasma concentrations of specific amino acids are similar in many studies of thermal injury, elective operations, trauma, and sepsis, but the degree of their magnitude is often greater in sepsis. This suggests that changes in amino acid metabolism do not depend on the type or the severity of injury. In contrast, other studies have noted marked differences in plasma and muscle amino acid patterns during sepsis and other injuries that suggest the changes seen are related to the severity of the injury or infection and to the offending microorganism.

Despite these opposing points of view, the intracellular muscle concentrations and the muscle-plasma ratios of glutamine are reduced markedly in most studies of sepsis, wounding, and thermal injury. In general, the release of glutamine is greater than can be predicted from its relative abundance in muscle tissue protein, and evidence for its synthesis in muscle has been presented. However, glutamine release from wounded and nonwounded muscle is not different and, if the release of glutamine is expressed as a ratio to the phenylalanine released, there is a lower release rate in wounded than nonwounded tissue. Because phenylalanine is neither catabolized nor synthesized in muscle, a lower glutamine-phenylalanine ratio suggests that either the synthesis of glutamine in wounded tissue is reduced or that the local catabolism in wounded muscle is increased. In this regard, it is of note that glutamine is a major energy source for lymphocytes and fibroblasts. As a result, the accelerated utilization of glutamine by the cellular infiltrate in wounded or in septic tissue can explain the decreased concentrations noted at the site of injury and in the plasma.

It is also of note that Wilmore, Souba, and others[65,79] have documented the gastrointestinal tract as a major consumer of glutamine after injury. The increased use of glutamine by the gastrointestinal tract not only may contribute to further reductions in plasma glutamine concentrations during injury, it raises important questions as to the function of the gastrointestinal tract during periods when plasma glutamine is low. In this regard, it is noteworthy that Dietch and others[30,31] have implicated translocation of intestinal bacteria after injury as a possible mechanism for postinjury sepsis in general and multiple organ failure in particular. Current speculation ties the translocation of bacteria during these stressful periods to reductions in plasma glutamine; that is, with severe injuries such as thermal injuries or prolonged shock, glutamine delivery to the gut is not adequate or maintained. As a consequence, there is an intestinal energy deficit, which results in loss of intestinal mucosal integrity and, ultimately, in translocation of bacteria into the portal circulation. Fortunately, it appears that this glutamine deficit and the attendant risks of postinjury sepsis can be avoided by providing enteral or parenteral glutamine. This lends further credence to the surgical dogma of using the gut whenever possible.

In conclusion, the stress of surgery results from alterations in homeostasis produced by the injury. The response to these alterations is directed at an integrated attempt to restore cardiovascular stability, preserve oxygen delivery, mobilize energy substrates, mobilize the supply of critical substrates, and minimize pain through the activation of the neuroendocrine, inflammatory, and metabolic systems. These responses are modified by a variety of conditions unique to each patient that are present before the injury, such as the ingestion of ethanol and other recreational drugs, or concurrent medications, the presence of drug withdrawal, or preexisting illness, and the age of the person.

The stress of surgery may also be minimized by careful perioperative management directed at minimizing the surgical stressors incident to the operation. In this regard, effective circulating volume and oxygen delivery to tissues should be maximized before, during, and after surgery. Where indicated because of known concurrent illness, such as cardiac disease, invasive monitoring should be used. Urine output should be maintained in the range of 25 to 50 ml/hr to ensure adequate renal perfusion. Attention should be given to prophylaxis of venous thrombosis and pulmonary embolism, and aggressive pulmonary therapy and ambulation should be instituted immediately to avoid postoperative respiratory complications leading to hypoxia and impaired oxygen delivery. Nutritional support should be instituted as early as possible to ensure provision of critical substrates necessary for wound healing and repair. This should be given through the enteral route whenever possible. Pain should be minimized to avoid emotional stressors and to reduce the activation of the neuroendocrine response. Hypothermia should be avoided not only because of its effects on the neuroendocrine response but also because of its deleterious effects on the coagulation and cardiac systems. Careful attention should be paid to a thorough preoperative history and physical exam to identify risk factors and modifiers that may increase the stress of the surgical procedure. Finally, patients should be monitored closely for the development of postoperative complications, particularly septic ones, which greatly increase the stress of the surgery and its mortality.

REFERENCES

1. Abbott NE, Anderson K: The effect of starvation, infection and injury on the metabolic processes and body composition, *Ann NY Acad Sci* 110:941, 1963.
2. Albina JE et al: Amino acid metabolism following λ-carrageenan injury to rat skeletal muscle, *Am J Physiol* 250:E24, 1986.
3. Allison SP, Hinton P, Chamberlain MJ: Intravenous glucose tolerance, insulin and free fatty acid levels in burn patients, *Lancet* 2:1118, 1968.
4. Amaral JF, Greenburg AG: The surgical treatment of elderly patients, *Problems in General Surgery* 5:296, 1988.
5. Amaral JF et al: Can lactate be used as a fuel by wounded tissue? *Surgery* 100:252, 1986.
6. Amaral JF et al: The temporal characteristics of the metabolic and endocrine response to trauma, *J Trauma* 27:455, 1987.
7. Askanazi I et al: Muscle and plasma amino acids following injury: influence of intercurrent infection, *Ann Surg* 182:78, 1980.
8. Barakos V et al: Stimulation of muscle protein degradation and prostaglandin E2 release by leukocyte pyrogen (interleukin-1), *N Engl J Med* 308:553, 1983.
9. Barton RN: Neuroendocrine mobilization of body fuels after injury, *Br Med Bull* 41:218, 1985.
10. Baylis PH, Zepre RL, Robertson GL: Arginine vasopressin response to insulin-induced hypoglycemia in man, *J Clin Endocrinol Metab* 53:935, 1981.
11. Benedict FG: *A study of prolonged fasting*, pub no. 280, Washington, DC, 1915, Carnegie Institute of Washington.
12. Bereiter DA, Plotsky PM, Gann DS: Tooth pulp stimulation potentiates the ACTH response to hemorrhage in cats, *Endocrinology* 111:1127, 1982.
13. Bereiter DA, Zaid AM, Gann DS: The effect of rate of hemorrhage on sympathoadrenal catecholamine release in the cat, *Am J Physiol* 250:E69, 1985.
14. Bessey PQ et al: Combined hormonal infusion simulates the metabolic response to injury, *Ann Surg* 200:264, 1984.
15. Bie P: Osmoreceptors, vasopressin, and control of renal water excretion, *Physiol Rev* 60:961, 1980.
16. Birkhain RH et al: Effects of major skeletal trauma on whole body protein turnover in man measured by [14C] leucine, *Surgery* 888:294, 1980.
17. Black PR et al: Mechanisms of insulin resistance following injury. *Ann Surg* 196:420, 1982.
18. Bonnet F et al: Suppression of antidiuretic hormone hypersecretion during surgery by extradural anaesthesia, *Br J Anesth* 54:30, 1982.
19. Boyd JB, Bradford B, Walme AL: Operative risk factors of colon resection in the elderly, *Ann Surg* 192:743, 1980.
20. Buckingham J: Hypothalamic-pituitary responses to trauma, *Br Med Bull* 41:203, 1985.
21. Cahill GF: Starvation in man, *N Engl J Med* 235:668, 1970.
22. Cahill GF: Ketosis, *J Parenter Enter Nutr* 5:281, 1981.
23. Charters AC, O'Dell MWD, Thompson JC: Anterior pituitary function during surgical stress and convalescence, *J Clin Endocrinol Metab* 29:63, 1969.
24. Claybaugh JR, Share L: Vasopressin, renin, and cardiovascular responses to continuous slow hemorrhage, *Am J Physiol* 224:519, 1973.
25. Clowes GHA et al: Muscle proteolysis induced by a circulating peptide in patients with sepsis or trauma, *N Engl J Med* 308:545, 1983.
26. Cuthbertson DP: Observations on the disturbances of metabolism by injury to the limbs, *Q J Med* 1:233, 1932.
27. Cuthbertson DP: The metabolic response to injury and its nutritional implications: retrospect and prospect, *J Parenter Enter Nutr* 3:108, 1979.
28. Davies CL et al: The relationship between plasma catecholamines and severity of injury in man, *J Trauma* 24:99, 1984.

29. Del Guercio LRM, Cohn JD: Monitoring operative risk in the elderly, *JAMA* 243:1350, 1980.

30. Dietch EA, Berg R, Specian R: Endotoxin promotes the translocation of bacteria from the gut, *Arch Surg* 122:185, 1987.

31. Dietch EA et al: The gut as a portal of entry for bacteremia: role of protein malnutrition, *Ann Surg* 205:681, 1987.

32. Dinarello CA: Interleukin-1 and the pathogenesis of the acute phase response, *N Engl J Med* 311:1413, 1984.

33. Dripps RD, Lamont A, Eckenhoff JE: The role of anesthesia in surgical mortality, *JAMA* 178:261, 1961.

34. Duke JH et al: Contribution of protein to caloric expenditure following injury, *Surgery* 68:168, 1970.

35. Egdahl RH: Pituitary-adrenal response following trauma to the isolated leg, *Surgery* 46:9, 1959.

36. Eigler N, Sacca L, Sherwin RS: Synergistic interactions of physiologic increments of glucagon, epinephrine and cortisol in the dog, *J Clin Invest* 63:114, 1979.

37. Engeland WC, Byrnes GJ, Gann DS: The pituitary adrenocortical response to hemorrhage depends on the time of day, *Endocrinology* 110:1856, 1982.

38. Felig P et al: Hormonal interactions in the regulation of blood glucose, *Recent Prog Horm Res* 35:501, 1979.

39. Frayn KN: Substrate turnover after injury, *Br Med Bull* 41:232, 1985.

40. Frayn KN et al: The relationship of plasma catecholamines to acute metabolic and hormonal responses to injury in man, *Circ Shock* 16:229, 1985.

41. Gann DS, Amaral JF: *Endocrine and metabolic responses to injury.* In Schwartz SI, Shires GT, Spencer FC, editors: *Principles of surgery,* 1989, McGraw-Hill.

42. Gann DS, Cryer GL, Pirkle JC, Jr: Physiological inhibition and facilitation of adrenocortical response to hemorrhage, *Am J Physiol* 232:R5, 1977.

43. Gann DS et al: Neural control of ACTH release in response to hemorrhage, *Ann NY Acad Sci* 297:477, 1977.

44. Gann DS et al: Role of solute in the early restitution of blood volume after hemorrhage, *Surgery* 94:439, 1983.

45. Goldman L et al: Multifactorial index of cardiac risk in noncardiac surgical procedures, *N Engl J Med* 297:845, 1977.

46. Greenburg AG, Saik RP, Pridham D: Influence of age on mortality of colon surgery, *Am J Surg* 150:65, 1985.

47. Greenburg AG et al: Mortality and gastrointestinal surgery in the aged: elective vs emergency procedures, *Arch Surg* 116:788, 1981.

48. Hume DM, Bell CL, Bartter F: Direct measurement of adrenal secretion during operative trauma and convalescence, *Surgery* 52:174, 1962.

49. Hume DM, Egdahl RH: Effect of hypothermia and of cold exposure on adrenal cortical and medullary secretion, *Ann NY Acad Sci* 80:435, 1959.

50. Jarhult J et al: Osmolar control of plasma volume during hemorrhagic hypotension, *Acta Physiol Scand* 85:142, 1972.

51. Kinney JM: Energy metabolism. In Fischer JE, editor: *Surgical nutrition,* Boston, 1983, Little, Brown.

52. Kinney JM, Elwyn DH: Protein metabolism and injury, *Annu Rev Nutr* 3:433, 1983.

53. Kircheim HR: Systemic arterial baroreceptor reflexes, *Physiol Rev* 56:100, 1976.

54. Lambertson CJ: Neural control of respiration. In Mountcastle VB, editor: *Medical physiology,* St Louis, 1980, Mosby–Year Book.

55. Lautt WN, Dwan PD, Singh RR: Control of the hyperglycemic response to hemorrhage in cats, *Can J Physiol Pharmacol* 60:1630, 1982.

56. Lilly MP, Engeland WC, Gann DS: Adrenomedullary responses to repeated hemorrhage in the anesthetized dog, *Endocrinology* 111:1917, 1982.

57. Lilly MP, Engeland WC, Gann DS: Responses of cortisol secretion to repeated hemorrhage in the anesthetized dog, *Endocrinology* 112:681, 1983.

58. Linn BS, Linn MW, Wallen N: Evaluation of results of surgical procedures in the elderly, *Ann Surg* 195:90, 1982.

59. Long CL et al: Carbohydrate metabolism in men: effect of elective operations and major injury, *J Applied Physiol* 31:110, 1971.

60. Marx GF, Mateo CV, Orkin LR: Computer analysis of postanesthetic deaths, *Anesthesiology* 39:54, 1973.

61. Meguid MM et al: Hormone-substrate interrelationships following trauma, *Arch Surg* 109:776, 1974.

62. Moore FD: Energy and the maintenance of the body cell, *J Parenter Enter Nutr* 4:22, 1980.

63. Moore FD, Brennan MF: *Surgical injury: Body composition, protein metabolism and neuroendocrinology.* In Ballanger WF, Collins JA, Drucker WR, editors: *Manual of surgical nutrition,* Philadelphia, 1975, WB Saunders.

64. Newsholme EA, Start C: *Regulation in metabolism,* New York, 1973, Wiley and Sons.

65. O'Dwyer ST, Smith RJ, Scott T: Glutamine enriched nutrition decreases intestinal injury and increases nitrogen retention, *Br J Surg* 74:1162, 1987.

66. Oppenheim W, Williamson D, Smith R: Early biochemical changes and severity of injury in man, *J Trauma* 20:135, 1980.

67. Overman RR, Wang SG: The contributory role of the afferent nervous factor in experimental shock: sublethal hemorrhage and sciatic nerve stimulation, *Am J Physiol* 148:289, 1947.

68. Owen OE et al: Brain metabolism during fasting, *J Clin Invest* 46:1589, 1967.

69. Owens WD, Felds JA, Spitznagel EL Jr: ASA physical status classifications: a study of consistency ratings, *Anesthesiology* 49:239, 1978.

70. Palmberg S, Hirsjarvi E: Mortality in geriatric surgery: with special reference to the type of surgery, anaesthesia, complicating disease, and prophylaxis of thrombosis, *Gerontology* 25:103, 1979.

71. Raff H, Shinsako J, Dallman MF: Surgery potentiates adrenocortical responses to hypoxia in dogs, *Proc Soc Exp Bio Med* 172:400, 1983.

72. Rankin FW, Johnson CC: Major operations in elderly patients, *Surgery* 5:763, 1939.

73. Redding M, Mueller CB: Effect of ambient temperature upon responses to hypovolemic insult in the unanesthetized unrestrained albino rat, *Surgery* 64:110, 1968.

74. Reiss R, Deutsch AA, Eliashiv A: Decision making process in abdominal surgery in the geriatric patient, *World J Surg* 7:522-526, 1983.

75. Schrier RW, Berl WT, Anderson RJ: Osmotic and non-osmotic control of vasopressin release, *Am J Physiol* 236:F321, 1979.

76. Shearer JD et al: Effect of starvation on the local and metabolic effects of the lambda carrageenan wound, *Am J Surg* 147:456-451, 1984.

77. Siegel JH et al: Physiological and metabolic correlations in human sepsis, *Surgery* 86:163, 1979.

78. Skillman JJ, Hedley-White J, Pallotta JA: Hormonal, fuel and respiratory relationships after acute blood loss in man, *Surg Forum* 21:23, 1970.

79. Souba WW, Wilmore DW: Postoperative alteration of arteriovenous exchange of amino acids across the gastrointestinal tract, *Surgery* 94:342, 1983.

80. Stein TP et al: Changes in protein synthesis after trauma: importance of nutrition, *Am J Physiol* 233:E348, 1976.

81. Stoner HB et al: The relationships between plasma substrates and hormones and the severity of injury in 277 recently injured patients, *Clin Sci* 56:563, 1979.

82. Tracey KJ et al: Cachectin/tumor necrosis factor mediates changes of skeletal muscle plasma membrane potential, *J Exp Med* 164:1368, 1986.

83. US Bureau of the Census, Current population reports, Special studies, ser P-23, no. 59, May 1976, p 9.

84. Vinnars E, Bergstrom J, Furst P: Influence of postoperative state in the intracellular free amino acids in human muscle tissue, *Ann Surg* 182:665, 1975.

85. Ware J et al: Osmolar changes in hemorrhage. The effect of an altered nutritional status, *Acta Chir Scand* 148:8, 1982.

86. Wilmore DW: Hormonal responses and their effect on metabolism, *Surg Clin North Am* 56:999, 1976.

87. Wilmore DW et al: Catecholamines: mediators of the hypermetabolic response to thermal injury, *Am Surg* 180:653, 1974.

88. Wilmore DW et al: Influence of the burn wound on local and systemic responses to injury, *Ann Surg* 186:444, 1977.

89. Wolfe RR, Shaw HF, Durkot MJ: *Energy metabolism in trauma and sepsis: the role of fat.* In *Molecular and cellular aspects of shock and trauma,* New York, 1983, AR Liss Inc.

Part II

PERIOPERATIVE CARE

General Considerations

Chapter 5

ESTABLISHING A DIAGNOSIS
The history, physical examination, and other studies

William J. Dignam

It is clear that surgical procedures will be chosen most appropriately if an accurate diagnosis is made. The most important elements in reaching the correct diagnosis are the history and physical examination. When properly done, these are time-consuming but well worth the effort.

All patients have some apprehension when visiting a physician, particularly for the first time. It is important to remember this and to spend a minute or two putting the patient at ease. Some patients are so apprehensive that they start talking before they are seated, and they should be permitted to do so without interruption. Patients should never be given the impression that they are being rushed.

Certain data are essential because they will direct the physician's thinking about the incidence of certain conditions in certain groups of patients, so these data should be obtained early in the interview. They include age, ancestry, marital status, and occupation. It is also important to inquire about emotional stress at the beginning of the interview. If this inquiry is postponed until later on, the patient may gain the impression that the physician is having difficulty in making a diagnosis and is therefore considering emotional causes for the symptoms as a last resort rather than considering them on an impartial and unprejudiced basis along with all the other causes for symptoms.

CHIEF COMPLAINT

Clearly the chief complaint is a very important feature of the history. It is best if this is expressed spontaneously by the patient and recorded in her own words as a quotation. Some young patients are brought to the physician by parents, but it is still a good idea to have the patient express the problem. At times parents have concerns that are not shared by patients.

PRESENT ILLNESS

Again it is important to have the patient voice her complaints spontaneously in her own words and without interruption. In this manner one gains an impression of the patient's personality and how much she dwells on minor symptoms. Patients who are unable to describe their symptoms in precise terms are less likely to have specific causes for the symptoms.

When the patient has finished describing her problem, it is well to ask if she is worried about the possibility of any specific disease. Some patients are worried about the possibility of cancer or of having acquired a sexually transmitted disease, AIDS in particular. Others are worried that they may have lost their sexual attractiveness or suffered major emotional or mental changes. In general, these patients are primarily seeking reassurance.

Once the patient has completed her presentation it will be necessary to amplify the information by asking her appropriate questions. There is a natural temptation to steer the conversation to a consideration of gynecologic problems, but that temptation must be resisted if the patient's primary concern lies in other areas. It is, of course, important to know about symptoms related to neighboring organs such as the bowel or bladder. Information concerning sexual activity and satisfaction is important, but often this discussion is best deferred until the time when the menstrual history is obtained and the patient can be led more gracefully into a discussion of sexual function. When patients do not answer the questions asked or if they give very vague answers, the physician may question the relative importance of the symptoms and whether these patients simply enjoy talking about themselves. Specific problems are likely to cause specific symptoms.

Gynecologic symptoms

It is not possible in this chapter to adequately discuss the appropriate evaluation of all gynecologic symptoms, but a few comments about some of the more common symptoms are in order.

Abdominal pain. This pain can be acute, recurringly acute, or chronic. Pain that develops abruptly may be due to irritation of the peritoneum by infection, chemical irritation, or stretching. Distension of an intraabdominal structure by blood or gas will also cause the acute onset of pain. Pain for which the patient can state the time of onset in exact terms is likely to be due to a vascular accident such as hemorrhage into a closed space or sudden occlusion of the venous drainage from an organ with resultant engorgement of that organ.

Acute infection produces localized pain that gradually increases over a period of hours and is commonly associated with other manifestations such as fever and leukocytosis. Patients with acute intraabdominal infection prefer not to move, as this increases the pain. They will assume positions that relax the abdominal muscles, generally positions in which the legs are flexed at the hips. If the infection is severe, bowel motility will also be inhibited. Distension and, finally, nausea and vomiting will occur.

Referred pain is an important phenomenon to bear in mind. When pain is referred, it is usually noted in an area that developed from the same embryonic segment or dermatome as the structure in which the pain originates. For example, as the diaphragm migrates during embryonic development it carries the phrenic nerve with it; therefore pain originating in the diaphragm may be appreciated in the tip or superior aspect of the shoulder. Pain originating in the ovaries may be felt in the anterior thigh. Pain originating in the area of the obturator nerve may be noted in the upper inner thigh. When pain originating in a viscus is appreciated both in that location and in a referred location, it seems to spread from the local to the distant site; this is referred to as radiation of the pain.

The relation of the pain to the menstrual cycle is important to ascertain. Pain that occurs 2 weeks before an expected period may be related to ovulation. Pain that occurs when a menstrual period is overdue clearly indicates the possibility of pregnancy complications. Pain associated with menses indicates the possibility of tuboovarian infection, endometriosis, or intraluminal uterine tumors. Cramping suprapubic pain is characteristic of intrauterine problems, including the presence of an intrauterine device, the beginning expulsion of a pregnancy, or the presence of a large endometrial polyp or pedunculated submucous myoma.

It is important to elucidate associated symptoms, such as those involving the bowel or bladder. If present, they indicate the possibility of problems intrinsic to those structures or of gynecologic processes that have involved the adjacent bladder or lower bowel. The presence of fever or symptoms of pregnancy are similarly important.

Chronic pelvic pain is more likely to be due to large pelvic tumors or to pelvic relaxation. Patients with these conditions, particularly those with pelvic relaxation, commonly indicate that they feel better after lying down for a period of time. They therefore have little discomfort in early morning, but as the day progresses they have a steadily increasing sense of pressure in the pelvic area. As genital prolapse progresses, traction on the uterosacral ligaments and on the cardinal ligaments increases throughout the day. Therefore patients may complain of sacral backache in addition to generalized pelvic pressure.

Patients who complain spiritedly about abdominal pain and insist that something be done about it, particularly something surgical, are very difficult to evaluate. For example, some patients hold the strong conviction that hysterectomy will relieve all their symptoms, and clearly this is not always the case. It is important that the physician see these patients on several occasions before making any decisions about treatment in order to accurately evaluate the patient's personality and behavior.

Abnormal bleeding. Abnormal bleeding is another common gynecologic complaint. If the patient describes abnormal bleeding in the chief complaint it is helpful to elicit the entire menstrual history in order to be aware of the background leading up to the abnormal episode. Likely causes for abnormal bleeding are clearly different in patients in different age groups. The age of the patient, therefore, should be kept in mind as the history is elaborated.

Some patients complain of profuse or prolonged menses. It is important to obtain some quantitative impression of the amount of bleeding by having the patient describe the number of pads or tampons that are employed during these episodes. The passage of clots and their approximate size are important because the formation of clots confirms the fact that the bleeding has been so rapid that proteolysis could not take place. Prominent among the causes for profuse menses are submucous myomata, which tend to occur in women over the age of 35.

Perimenstrual spotting is sometimes difficult to interpret. A number of patients develop spotting just before or just after menses with no accompanying abnormality. However, this symptom may be caused by endometriosis.

Posttraumatic bleeding such as that occuring after intercourse or the use of a diaphragm is an important symptom. This indicates the possibility of cervical lesions, including malignancies.

Irregular bleeding is commonly hormonal in origin. This may vary from mild spotting to profuse flooding. The latter is particularly bothersome to patients because it occurs without the warning of premenstrual symptoms and can be a source of great embarrassment. To interpret irregular bleeding it is helpful to know the exact occurrence of the days of bleeding and the amount of bleeding on each day. A menstrual calendar helps to document this information accurately.

Postmenopausal bleeding, particularly in patients who are not having estrogen replacement therapy, is a very important symptom and must always be evaluated by sampling of the endometrium.

Discharge. Vaginal discharge is another common gynecologic symptom. It is important to learn about any relevant antecedent incidents such as casual sexual contacts, antibiotic therapy, use of medicated douches, or recent obstetrical, surgical, or radiation events. The physician should ascertain the amount and color of the discharge and whether it is liquid or contains particulate matter. Whether the discharge is associated with irritation or reddening of the vulva is also important.

Vulvar symptoms. Pressure or protrusion at the vulva is another common gynecologic symptom, particularly in the elderly. For patients with this complaint it is important to know the history of gravidity and parity, particularly difficult deliveries of large babies. Some patients experience relaxation of the pelvic supports without having had pregnancies, but this is uncommon. It is important to know if this symptom is related to standing or activities involving increased intraabdominal pressure. Further, the physician needs to know whether it is necessary to replace the tissues in order to permit voiding or defecation. Any associated urinary incontinence should also be noted.

Incontinence. Urinary incontinence is a very common gynecologic complaint. It is important to know if this is constant or intermittent and whether or not it is related to straining. Any associated urgency is also an important symptom.

Masses. Abdominal tumors are occasionally the presenting complaint in gynecologic patients. Commonly, large abdominal tumors are due to the presence of either uterine myomata or ovarian carcinoma, and, of course, it is extremely important to differentiate between these two entities. Patients who cite the presence of a tumor as a chief complaint are unlikely to have many associated symptoms of great severity, but the possible existence of ovarian carcinoma is so important that they must be thoroughly and promptly investigated.

MENSTRUAL HISTORY

The *menstrual history* should be obtained when the history of the present illness has been completed. Important features include the age of onset of menstruation, the regularity or irregularity of the menstrual cycle, and the length of a typical cycle. A quantitative idea of the amount of bleeding should be obtained and the date of the last menstrual period recorded.

Once the patient has become accustomed to talking about her menstrual history, it is easier to bring up the matter of her sexual activity. The physician should ask about the patient's sexual preference in a straightforward and nonjudgmental way, as patients may not volunteer information about their homosexuality or heterosexuality unless invited to do so. Because of the mounting evidence of

the relationship between sexual activity and tumors of the cervix, it is important to learn the patient's age at first episode of intercourse and the number of sexual partners. The history of sexually transmitted diseases is important in the investigation of abdominal pain and in consideration of possible neoplastic lesions of the cervix. The patient should be asked whether intercourse is satisfactory for her because here again patients may not volunteer complaints of dissatisfaction unless invited to do so. A detailed history of pregnancies is important along with information about contraception and plans for future pregnancies.

FAMILY HISTORY

The *family history* must be recorded for all patients. Commonly patients wish to mention the occurrence of similar complaints among family members, and although this is not always relevant, patients should be permitted to voice their observations and have them recorded. It is difficult to be certain about the familial occurrence of many gynecologic lesions, but certain conditions, such as carcinoma of the ovary, do have an unusual prevalence in certain families. It is clearly important to know about relatives having diabetes, cancer, asthma, hypertension, bleeding abnormalities, tuberculosis, communicable diseases, and AIDS.

PAST HISTORY

In eliciting the *past history*, the physician must be aware that patients may neglect to mention even very important events and should therefore be given sufficient time to reflect on the matter. Elderly patients in particular may require prompting to recall significant events. It will help to refresh their memories if they are asked whether they have ever been a hospital patient and whether they have ever required prolonged care at home for a major illness. It may be helpful to ask if they have any abnormality of the major organs, such as the heart, lungs, blood, liver, kidneys, or nervous system. It is important to obtain specific details about prior care, particularly previous surgical procedures, and pathology reports on any specimens obtained. Copying machines have markedly improved our ability to obtain relevant information and it is important that information be requested from the institutions in which the patient has had medical care.

SYSTEM REVIEW

The *system review* is helpful in eliciting information about related symptoms that the patient has neglected to mention during her description of the present illness. It also serves to remind patients of significant events in their medical history. It is therefore important to ask specific questions about each organ rather than accepting the patient's statement that she has had no problems pertinent to that particular organ. In addition, information should be obtained concerning habits such as smoking and exercise, and a detailed history of any medicines or drugs taken by the patient should be gathered. It is important to know about allergies and changes in weight. Finally, the patient should be asked to describe her emotional makeup. This question commonly triggers comments that are very helpful in understanding the patient's symptoms.

When the history has been completed, an appropriate physical examination should be conducted.

PHYSICAL EXAMINATION

First, a general inspection of the patient is important. Particular attention should be paid to the patient's demeanor and any signs of anxiety or pain. An observation of obesity or evidence of recent weight loss is important. If present, pallor or cyanosis should be noted, as should any difficulty in breathing or discomfort associated with the movements necessary for the physical examination. The vital signs should be recorded. The patient's weight, blood pressure, pulse, and respiratory rate are all important in determining whether she is a suitable operative candidate.

Next, a careful and detailed general physical examination is conducted. Of particular importance are the condition of the skin at the operative site and in the vulvar area and the competence of the connective tissue in general. A detailed examination of the optic fundi produces some evidence about the condition of the vascular system. Since the heart and lungs are critical to the patient's welfare during and after surgery, examination of these organs is also important. When performing the pelvic examination, one must look for evidences of arthritis, which may inhibit placing the patient in the lithotomy position.

Examination of the breasts must be carried out meticulously. Patients depend on their gynecologists for the detection of breast disease. During this examination patients can be instructed in the proper technique for self-examination and can be reminded of the necessity for periodic mammography at appropriate ages.

It is also important, particularly in operative candidates, to note the presence of varices, which may predispose to thrombosis at the time of operative procedures. A careful palpation of the peripheral arterial pulses is also important.

Pelvic examination

The patient must be as relaxed as possible under the circumstances, and therefore gentleness is most important. Patients of all ages can have pelvic examinations. These may be more difficult for children and young women, but with proper attention to gentleness and the avoidance of sudden moves these examinations can be carried out without undue discomfort.

A careful examination of the external genitalia is important, particularly in older patients who may never examine their own genitalia and may not be aware of potential dangers such as pigmented lesions of the vulva. An inspection of the vagina, particularly the degree of estrogen effect in the vaginal epithelium, should be made. The amount of support for the vaginal walls should be recorded, while the patient is relaxed and while straining. The cervix should be carefully inspected. Of particular importance are granulating or ulcerating lesions.

The support for the uterus as evidenced by the descent of the cervix with straining should be recorded. To assess this matter accurately, it is necessary to examine the patient while she is erect.

The position and outline of the uterus should be determined carefully. It is helpful to keep the abdominal hand still while moving the uterus with the vaginal hand. This causes the fundus to move against the abdominal hand and provides good information about its position, size, and outline.

Inexperienced examiners commonly ignore the posterior pelvis, a significant oversight. Conditions such as endometriosis commonly involve the area of the cul-de-sac or posterior portions of the broad ligaments, and evidence must be sought in these areas if the patient's symptoms suggest the presence of endometriosis. This examination can be performed particularly well when approached rectovaginally, which permits an exploration of the cul-de-sac area and posterior surface of the uterus. The pelvic walls should also be palpated carefully to detect the thickening indicative of lymphadenopathy in these areas. In determining tenderness it is important that the examination be carried out gently. Most patients complain of some discomfort if the uterus is manipulated too vigorously. As the uterus is moved with the vaginal hand, particularly during the rectovaginal examination, one is able to determine whether the uterus is separable from other masses in the pelvis. Intrinsic lesions of the rectum such as carcinoma may also be detected during the rectovaginal examination.

Pelvic sonogram

A growing body of opinion holds that pelvic sonography is more accurate than pelvic examination in determining the status of the internal genitalia. With the development of the vaginal transducer for pelvic ultrasound examinations, many gynecologists believe this should be a routine part of a pelvic examination.

This evaluation is of particular importance in determining the size and composition of the ovaries and in measuring the thickness of the endometrium, particularly in postmenopausal women. Even small tumors of the ovary, if they have mixed solid and cystic components, require further evaluation. There is a growing body of evidence that further investigation should be carried out if the endometrium is greater than 5 or 6 mm in thickness.

At the conclusion of the examination it is important to tell the patient that the examination is normal if such is the case. Patients will be relieved to know that no gross abnormality has been detected. On occasion the sole reason for a patient to visit a physician is to hear this statement.

DIAGNOSIS

After completion of the history and physical examination, a specific diagnosis should be recorded. A repetition of the patient's symptoms, such as pelvic pain, is not adequate and indicates that the physician has not considered the diagnosis with sufficient thoroughness. Similarly, general terms such as pelvic inflammatory disease are not adequate. A specific diagnosis such as acute salpingooophoritis or tuboovarian abscess should be recorded, because the treatment for these conditions varies. In stating the diagnosis, it is important for the physician to try to visualize the pathology that is present in order to incorporate these considerations into his or her diagnosis. Thus, if the patient has large endometriomata on the posterior surface of the broad ligaments or abscesses in that same location, large tumors projecting between the leaves of the broad ligaments, or freely movable ovarian cysts in an anterior location, it is important to include this fact in the diagnosis.

DIFFERENTIAL DIAGNOSIS

After recording the diagnosis, some consideration must be given to other possible diagnoses and a brief discussion of these possibilities should be recorded. This keeps the physician from being too narrow in his or her thinking and from jumping too quickly to make an apparently obvious diagnosis. The latter tendency occasionally results in an embarrassing situation.

It is important that all of the patient's medical problems be recorded with the diagnosis. Other significant problems such as hypertension, diabetes, heart disease, pulmonary disease, renal disease, anemia, and significant reactions to anesthetic agents or other drugs should be noted, along with a record of previous surgical complications.

LABORATORY STUDIES

It is difficult to say which laboratory studies should be ordered for all gynecologic patients. Since many patients do not consult any physician other than their gynecologist, it is important to accept some responsibility for preventive health care. Clearly patients depend on their gynecologist for cancer detection. Therefore it seems wise to order complete blood counts and urinalysis for all patients. For patients over the age of 50, a chemistry panel and an assessment of cardiovascular status by means of measuring cholesterol, high- and low-density lipoproteins, and triglycerides are advisable.

To facilitate cancer detection, all patients should have vaginal and cervical smears. A test for blood in the stool should be carried out at the time of each rectal examination. Mammograms should be ordered at appropriate ages, with a screening mammogram for patients between the ages of 35 and 40 and a repeat study every 2 years between the ages of 40 and 50 and annually thereafter. Chest films should be obtained periodically. These tests generally can detect the four most common sites of cancer in women.

PREOPERATIVE PREPARATION
Instructions

If the patient is an appropriate candidate for a surgical procedure, the physician must carefully discuss with her the indications, alternatives, risks, possible complications, and expectations associated with surgery. It is particularly important to discuss the long-term expectations and any foreseeable effects on sexual function. If there is a question of blood transfusion, it is important to discuss the appropriate use of blood products and to introduce the subject of autologous blood transfusion.

Additional laboratory studies

Patients who are to have operative procedures may require additional laboratory studies. The most common of these is a pelvic ultrasound examination.

Pelvic sonogram. Whether or not such a test should be a routine part of the preoperative evaluation of a patient who is to undergo a pelvic laparotomy is still debatable. Sonograms are of value in determining the nature of adnexal masses. If the findings suggest carcinoma of the ovary, a vertical incision is preferable to permit sampling of the peritoneum in several areas in the abdomen and to permit biopsies in the area of the diaphragm.

Other radiologic studies. The use of intravenous pyelograms or barium enemas to help delineate pelvic masses has been recommended by some authorities. Their principal use is in their detecting intrinsic lesions of the urinary or intestinal system. Distortion of the ureters, bladder, or rectosigmoid by pelvic masses is not of great importance unless the process invades those adjacent organs. Appropriate surgical technique and care permit the surgeon to deal effectively with the gynecologic lesion without injury to the adjacent organs.

Many experienced surgeons feel that a bowel preparation is an essential part of the preoperative management of all patients with extensive gynecologic lesions, but in any case it is helpful to know whether or not the process originates in the intestinal system. Therefore, if suspicion of a primary lesion in the rectosigmoid area is high, performance of an endoscopic examination and a barium enema are advisable.

Blood studies. With the current emphasis on cost control, the number of required preoperative blood studies has been reduced. Whereas formerly these studies were required on the day before surgery, it has now been demonstrated that they can be performed as much as 2 weeks before the operation and still be valid.

The American Society of Anesthesiologists has published lists of minimum studies considered essential for uncomplicated patients from their point of view. They are as follows.

Age	Women
Under 40	Hemoglobin or hematocrit
40-59	Hemoglobin or hematocrit
	Electrocardiogram
	Glucose/BUN (or creatinine)
Over 60	Hemoglobin or hematocrit
	Electrocardiogram
	Chest film
	Glucose/BUN (or creatinine)

Clearly the surgeon must think carefully about each patient and order additional studies as indicated. Coagulation studies or tumor markers, for example, may be appropriate in certain patients.

SUMMARY

Generally, no patient should be considered routine, nor should any operative procedure be considered routine. The surgeon must remain alert to all possibilities and variations in the evaluation of patients, their preparation for surgery, and the selection of the appropriate procedure.

Chapter 6

PREOPERATIVE AND POSTOPERATIVE CARE

David H. Nichols

PREOPERATIVE CARE
Philosophic and psychologic considerations

The surgeon should pause periodically for a sober reexamination of his or her surgical policies. When the benefits and risks of current therapy are counterbalanced, the benefits should decisively outweigh the risks. If they do not, then the surgeon's philosophy of practice should be modified to fit the facts. Physicians are constantly weighing the good and bad points of a treatment policy to arrive at the best course of action for the individual patient. We must avoid taking an overzealous approach to surgical treatment without first weighing the risks involved.

Too little attention has been given to the environmental and inner tensions that influence the outcome of a surgical procedure. Pressures created by an unrealistic schedule, by nervous or unhappy associates, and by preoccupations of the surgeon with other problems may result in poor or hasty judgment at the operating table. A serene operating room and competent surgical nurse have much to do with the quality of surgery.

Speed at the operating table too often has been equated with surgical skill. When such speed reflects a masterful organization of surgical techniques, it may be an asset. However, too often such speed reflects the need to meet a later appointment, a desire to impress younger physicians and nurses, or just the inner restlessness of the surgeon. It is believed that uncontrolled speed at the operating table is the foremost cause of surgical complications.

Fatigue of the surgeon and major surgery are a bad combination. If a surgeon has been obliged to go without rest for a long time, it may be wise to defer an operation. If an extensive, radical, or tedious operation is to be performed, it is better to start such a procedure early in the morning when the operating team is physically and mentally alert.

A depressed or anxious or emotionally unstable person breeds disaster in the operating room. Psychologic well-being of the operating room team and good surgery go hand in hand.

Preoperative and postoperative evaluation and care . . . involve liberal use of medical consultants, for it is better to prevent a medical or surgical complication than to manage one.[11]

The gynecologic surgeon should always be mindful of the whole patient, particularly during the preoperative evaluation of her problem. In addition to the inevitable focus on gynecologic conditions, it is essential to investigate the patient's medical history; to consider any current systemic problems, especially any cardiac, blood pressure, or endocrine abnormality; and to determine whether the patient has a history of mental instability or any adverse experience with previous surgery or anesthesia.

Individuals over 65 years of age account for 21% of the total number of inpatient operative procedures and 38.4% of total hospital days. As the population continues to age, these percentages will increase. According to the Bureau of Census, the total number of 25.2 million women in the United States in 1990 who were between the ages of 45 and 65 are expected to increase in number to 41.8 million by 2010. Pulmonary function and renal and hepatic blood flow are reduced in the elderly consequent, in part, to reduced cardiac output. Since hepatic metabolic systems are reduced, drugs dependent on hepatic metabolism will have a longer half-life, leading to a prolonged duration of action. Careful attention to the predictable changes can safely eliminate chronologic age alone as a deterrent to anesthesia and surgery. Very elderly patients (those over 90) having elective surgery tend to fare far better in terms of operative morbidity and mortality than those having emergency operations. Cardiac and respiratory diseases have little impact on short-term morbidity or mortality, but preexistent deficit of the central nervous system is the most powerful predictor of poor outcome and survival, partly because of late referral for surgery and decreased and late diagnostic services and evaluation.[21,22] Emergency surgery with its higher morbidity is thus more frequent among the very elderly.

Medical history and review of laboratory tests

The patient's history and symptoms determine the thoroughness necessary in the preoperative assessment of the genitourinary system. The dictated surgical history of any previous pelvic surgery should be requested and reviewed. If the patient's cervix is still present and she has had a Papanicolaou smear taken and evaluated within the preceding year, the surgeon should obtain the report before surgery. If no smear was done or a report is unavailable, a fresh smear should be obtained and the report reviewed preoperatively. Any recent abnormal uterine bleeding must be assessed. It is also necessary to determine whether there is a family history of gynecologic disorders.

It is essential for the surgeon to consult with the patient's internist or family physician before surgery, particularly if the patient has a history of heart disease, angina, or arrhythmia; has been taking antihypertensive medication; or has a history of rheumatism. A consultation is equally important if the patient is a diabetic, in which case the surgeon needs to know the duration, severity, and current management of the disease. It is often helpful to invite the patient's internist or family physician to participate in the management of the medical aspects of her postoperative care.

The presence of any disease not currently under control warrants reevaluation and reconfirmation of the indications and benefits of recommended surgery, and the patient should be carefully and conscientiously examined for any contraindication to elective surgery. The surgeon should always consider the life expectancy of the patient and the longevity of her ancestors, for to ignore the patient's overall welfare ultimately discredits both the surgeon and the procedure performed.

Preoperative laboratory screening should include a complete blood count, coagulation studies, a blood type and screening determination, and a biochemical profile. If the patient is more than 50 years old or if there is any reason to suspect cardiac abnormality, an electrocardiogram is advisable, not only for the information that it can supply preoperatively but also as a baseline for comparison with any postoperative study that may be required. Any tendency to abnormality in bleeding, any history or suspicion of phlebitis or diabetes, or the probability of an excessive use of alcohol should be investigated. A history or evidence of pulmonary disease, asthma, emphysema, or smoking is also important. The patient should be urged to decrease or stop smoking for a few days or, preferably, weeks before scheduled surgery. A preoperative chest roentgenogram is desirable. If the patient has emphysema or other important respiratory symptoms, spirometric and blood gas studies are also advisable. The surgeon should record the results of all these procedures on the patient's chart and review them before she is taken to the operating room.

The most common electrolyte abnormality is hypokalemia, which is generally secondary to diuretic therapy.

When it was thought that patients in their eighties had a limited life span they were often encouraged not to proceed with elective surgery, but were supported with less than optimal medical care. Today it is fully recognized that a 70- or 75-year-old woman has a life expectancy of at least another 10 to 15 years, and therefore age per se is no reason not to proceed with surgical intervention when indicated in otherwise healthy patients.

Proper preoperative and postoperative remedy of any dietary nutritional deficiencies may help the patient to return to a normal performance level sooner after surgery.

A decline in short-term memory, and hearing, and other senses such as vision make it somewhat more difficult for the patient to clearly understand options as well as preoperative and postoperative instructions. Dementia can be a major risk factor.[8]

It can no longer be assumed that the elderly patient is sexually inactive. For that reason care must be taken in vaginal support and reconstructive operations to not reduce the caliber of the vagina beyond a normal size. Although the vagina of the young estrogen stimulated woman is somewhat elastic, this is less true of those in the postmenopausal age group, and a relatively small amount of postoperative scarring and contraction may produce marked and unexpected dyspareunia in those patients with a smaller vagina.

An interesting report by Narr, Hansen, and Warner[30] of the Department of Anesthesia at the Mayo Clinic concerns preoperative screening laboratory tests in asymptomatic healthy patients who underwent elective surgical procedures at the Mayo Clinic in 1988. Three thousand seven hundred and eighty-two (3,782) patients were studied; routine preoperative screening tests included a complete blood count, creatinine, electrolytes, aspartate aminotransferase, and glucose. Substantially abnormal results were found in 160 of these patients, in 30 of whom the results were predictable on the basis of the history or physical examination. The abnormal test results prompted further assessment in 47 patients. No surgical procedure was delayed, and no association was noted between adverse outcome and any preoperative laboratory abnormality. The anesthesia department at the Mayo Clinic no longer requires preoperative laboratory screening for most patients under 40. Their guidelines for patients of all ages are listed in Table 6-1. For those between the ages of 40 and 59, electrocardiography and the measurement of creatinine and blood glucose are required, and for those over 60 a complete blood count and chest roentenography are required as well. *All* patients have a preoperative review by a staff anesthesiologist of medications, an assessment of allergic and systemic disorders or symptoms, and a physical examination with emphasis on cardiopulmonary status performed 1 to 2 days before the scheduled surgical procedure.

The cost of routine laboratory screening tests is substantial, and false-positive test results and subsequent additional studies may unnecessarily escalate the perioperative costs for healthy patients. Blue Cross and Blue Shield estimate that a total of more than $30 billion dollars was spent in the United States health care system in 1984 to

Table 6-1. Minimal preoperative test requirements at the Mayo Clinic[30]

Age (yr)	Tests required
<40	None
40-59	Electrocardiography, measurement of creatinine and glucose
≥60	Complete blood cell count, electrocardiography, chest roentgenography, measurement of creatinine and glucose

In addition, the following guidelines apply:

A complete blood cell count is indicated in all patients who undergo blood typing and who are screened or cross-matched.

Measurement of potassium is indicated in patients taking diuretics or undergoing bowel preparation.

Chest roentgenography is indicated in patients with a history of cardiac or pulmonary disease or with recent respiratory symptoms.

A history of cigarette smoking in patients older than 40 years of age who are scheduled for an upper abdominal or thoracic surgical procedure is an indication for spirometry (forced vital capacity).

pay for preoperative evaluations.[36] As a consequence of the savings to be realized, the anesthesia department at the Mayo Clinic has determined a considerable cost effectiveness in the reduction of preoperative laboratory work-up of young healthy patients. All of the larger institutions that require each elective surgical patient to have a preoperative review and consultation with a staff anesthesiologist may wish to examine their policies in regard to preoperative laboratory testing to see if significant savings might not be effected by elimination of some routine but apparently superfluous preoperative testing of healthy patients under the age of 40.

Platelet transfusion. When preoperative estimate of blood platelets is less than 50,000 per ml³, platelet transfusion is indicated prior to major surgery. The therapeutic dose of platelets is 1 unit per 10 kg of body weight. Six units are generally adequate to achieve hemostasis in the adult. The use of a standard 170 μm filter is recommended for the administration of platelets. Infections that may be transmitted by platelet transfusion are similar to those associated with the use of other blood products.

Routine IVP. If 650,000 hysterectomies are performed per year, and each patient is given a preoperative intravenous pyelogram for a nominal charge of $100 each, the cost will be $65,000,000. One out of 40,000 will develop a reaction to the intravenous medication, and 16 women per year will die of the reaction. If each patient who had a preoperative pyelogram were to get a postoperative one as well to check on "silent" injury, it would cost the public an additional $65,000,000, or a total of $130,000,000 per year. Routine IVP is not recommended.

Mechanical preparation of the lower bowel. Major pelvic surgery will be facilitated if the large intestine is reasonably empty of its usual content during the operation. Placing the patient on a diet of clear liquids the day before admission to the hospital is worthwhile. The frequency with which patients are admitted the same day as surgery is to be performed requires that the patient take an active role in her preoperative mechanical bowel preparation.

Ingestion of a polyethylene glycol–electrolyte lavage solution (GOLYTELY, NuLYTELY, CoLyte) is most effective for this purpose.[15] The powder is mixed with water and refrigerated the night before it is to be taken. Starting at 8:00 AM the day before surgery, it is consumed as a drink at the rate of 1 L per hour until it is gone. Two tablets of bisacodyl are taken at 6:00 PM the evening before surgery.

For those patients for whom this routine is unacceptable or impossible, an alternative is for the patient to give herself or be given an enema at bedtime the night before surgery and another early on the morning of surgery if time permits. Disposable enema units are effective.

Patient use of medications

The surgeon should review any medications the patient has taken within the preceding year and evaluate their present effect. Some patients may have become so accustomed to taking certain drugs routinely that, unless asked, they may forget to mention them to the surgeon. Therefore, in developing the medical history the physician should ask specifically about the frequent or regular use of aspirin, tranquilizers, antihypertensive agents, antibiotics, birth control pills, and steroids used in the treatment of acne, arthritis, or rheumatism. It is also wise to ask whether the patient remembers any allergy or hypersensitivity to drugs taken previously, sometimes long ago. Both the surgeon and the anesthesiologist should be aware of any allergies, particularly to medications.

If the patient has been taking anticonvulsant drugs and diuretics, any potassium or chloride depletion should be corrected preoperatively. Whenever possible the patient should discontinue all steroids at least a month before surgery to minimize the risk of pulmonary, coronary, or cerebral thrombosis and embolism. Because cortisone and prednisone inhibit the formation of collagen and thus delay wound healing, a patient who is taking one of these drugs should stop taking it 10 days before surgery and should not resume taking it until 4 or 5 days postoperatively. In such patients, the surgeon may be wise to use nonabsorbable suture in buried tissue layers that are subject to tension. If a temporary suspension of the drug is not safe for the patient, massive doses of vitamin A (i.e., 50,000 to 100,000 U daily) may reverse the drug's effects.[23]

Preoperative psychologic preparation

In addition to the usual physiologic and anatomic preparations for surgery, psychologic preparation is necessary. The preoperative period is the poorest of times for a surgeon to appear impatient, hurried, or indifferent. A quiet, personal conversation does much to dispel a patient's fears; no matter how busy, the surgeon must find the time to answer the patient's questions carefully and unhurriedly. In fact, it is always good to encourage the patient to ask questions and to express any fears that she may have, because it is as important for the surgeon to understand the patient's perception of her problem and its treatment as it is for her to understand the surgeon's view of her condition and the surgery that has been recommended.[19] When developed preoperatively, the patient's understanding and confidence increase her anticipation of a successful outcome, help ensure her cooperation, reduce her dismay at postoperative discomforts and the time required for complete recovery, improve the postoperative course, and allow for a more optimistic long-term prognosis. The most desirable one-to-one relationship is that of a considerate surgeon and an informed, confident patient.

Predisposing factors to postoperative psychiatric disturbances that may prolong the period of disability include an absence of demonstrable pelvic disease; a history of previous psychiatric care, especially depression; and marital discord, particularly in a young patient. The surgeon should attempt to recognize and assess such factors and to place them in proper perspective before the surgery, if possible, because doing so preoperatively spares both the patient and her surgeon hours of postoperative apprehension, indecision, and lack of progress. For the patient who needs it, professional psychiatric support is most effective if available well ahead of time so that the psychiatrist, too, can develop a rapport with the patient before the strain of postoperative discomfort complicates any preexisting psychiatric problems.

There are several signs that help the gynecologic surgeon to identify a patient who is likely to have postoperative psychologic difficulties. The surgery addict, often a hysterical neurotic with the scars of many operations, usually reports intense, but ill-defined, pains and often harbors a need to suffer. A surprising indifference should also be a warning, because such an attitude is often a facade that hides an immature refusal to even think about the operation; an infantile type of emotional response to all postoperative discomforts and dysfunctions is likely to follow such a repression of anxiety and denial of the trauma to come. In sharp contrast, the overanxious patient worries about technical details, about the site and size of her incision, about the type of anesthesia, and about the postoperative visiting hours. Such a patient is a good candidate for postoperative unhappiness and perhaps severe emotional instability. Still another problem arises with the would-be seductive patient, whose fantasies in regard to the physician-patient relationship may clearly transcend the usual bounds of professional responsibility.

Some appreciation of the patient's relationships with her family and her husband is usually very important. For example, awareness of a patient's chronically ill child or parent, a husband's current employment crisis, or other pressing problems in the patient's immediate family can enable the surgeon to understand a patient's seemingly unreasonable anxiety. If the patient has a genuine neurosis, the surgeon must honestly question whether the planned operative measures will bring about the desired gynecologic cure. In such tragic situations, a patient only too often blames her marital disharmony on the effects of her surgery. With continued failure to recognize the shortcomings in her relationship with her husband, such a patient may believe that an operative procedure that was indicated and satisfactorily performed has actually made her situation worse.

In considering a particular patient's perception of the likely results of a recommended hysterectomy, the physician must understand the implications of this surgical procedure for the individual patient.[33] For some women, fear of losing their femininity may entirely offset relief at their escape from the concerns surrounding conception. In such instances, the surgeon is well advised to search for and dispel myths and fears that may long have been repressed. The surgeon should reassure the patient that she will remain feminine, giving due consideration to any traditional and deeply ingrained ethnic attitudes she may have about the occurrence of menstruation and the importance of preserving the uterus. The patient should know that being freed from the inconveniences of menometrorrhagia and dysmenorrhea spares many patients predictable disabilities. Finally, the gynecologist should explain clearly to the patient that her freedom from the fear of pregnancy is likely to enhance the quality of her response to her husband.

Patients who seem neurotic preoperatively are certain to be manifestly neurotic postoperatively. An adequate preoperative psychologic evaluation provides an insight into the probabilities of the patient's mental and emotional stability after surgery. This may help to prevent medically unexpected and surgically unwarranted complications, which all too frequently make the surgical experience unpleasant and unsatisfactory for all concerned.

Care in the immediate preoperative period

A final consultation room discussion or hospital visit by the surgeon on the day or evening before a scheduled operation is of inestimable value in providing the patient with an opportunity to raise any last-minute questions and discuss problems that have been troubling her, thus strengthening surgeon-patient rapport. The surgeon who expects to be away or unavailable during a portion of the patient's postoperative stay should explain the absence clearly to the patient in order to dispel any fear she may have of being abandoned during her stay in the unfamiliar hospital room. Such an explanation should include the arrangements that have been made for her care during the absence, clearly indicating who will be responsible for her care, how this individual can be reached, and when the surgeon expects to return to resume personal supervision of her care.

Preparation of the surgeon's hands. Dineen[13] reported equivalent bacterial skin counts after a 5-minute compared with a 10-minute scrub of the surgeon's hands using either povidone-iodine or hexachlorophene solution. Cruse and Foond[12] found no increase in clean wound infections when a 3- to 5-minute hand scrub was used for the first scrub of the day and a 2- to 3-minute scrub before succeeding operations the same day. Shorter scrub periods are as good as longer scrubs in suppressing infection and are cost effective because they reduce operating room time. It goes without saying that the fingernails of the surgical team should be kept short and clean, and all rings, bandages, and adhesive tape removed from the surgeon's fingers. If the surgeon's hands are the site of infection or purulent drainage, the surgeon should refrain from operating until the inflammation has cleared.

Preoperative hair removal. Not only does preoperative shaving of the surgical site offer no advantage to the patient, but the abrasion of the skin that results from shaving may precipitate an increased incidence of wound infection.[1] Patients are no longer shaved routinely, but long hairs may be clipped, if desired, to keep them out of the surgical field. Unshaven patients are much more comfortable during the later recovery phase.

Although preoperative shaving to remove hair at the operative site was once considered essential as a means of reducing operative infection, it is now recognized that this is not the case, particularly if the patient is shaved on the day prior to surgery when bacterial colonization rapidly evolves as a consequence of microscopic abrasion to the skin. If shaving is to be used, it is best employed immediately preoperatively. Depilatories may be used, applied the night before surgery. They are expensive but may be useful in spots inaccessible or not suitable for shaving.

The primary goal of hair removal is to keep hair out of the wound closure. This can be accomplished very effectively by clipping hairs with scissors or the electric clipper immediately before surgery.

A shower or bath the night before surgery removes superficial skin dirt and sweat. Painting the abdominal skin and the vagina with chlorhexidine gluconate (Hibiclens) is effective as a disinfectant, as is polyvinylpyrrolidone-iodine (povidone-iodine, Betadine), applied and preferably allowed to dry and followed immediately by sterile draping of the operative field. Walton and Baker[43] have provided an excellent review of the contemporary literature supporting the above recommendations.

Efforts to prevent embolism and thrombosis. Deep venous thrombosis of the lower extremity is the most frequent vascular complication of pelvic surgery. Consequent lethal pulmonary embolism secondary to deep venous thrombosis occurs in 0.01% to 0.87% of pelvic surgical patients and accounts for about 40% of the postoperative deaths. Prevention of this thrombosis affords the best opportunity for reducing this surgical and postoperative mortality.

The clinical and laboratory effects of low-dose heparin prophylaxis were prospectively studied in a controlled trial of 182 patients undergoing major surgery for gynecologic malignancy.[9] Low-dose heparin was given in 5000-unit subcutaneous doses 2 hours preoperatively and every 12 hours thereafter for 7 days postoperatively. These patients had a significantly increased daily retroperitoneal hemovac drainage. Low-dose heparin was associated with increased

estimated intraoperative blood loss, transfusion requirements, and wound hematomas. All patients had significantly prolonged activated partial thromboplastin time and lower final platelet counts as compared with the control group of patients. There was no significant reduction in thromboembolic complications in the treated group.

Defibrotide (Prociclide, CRINOS) is a natural polydesoxyribonucleotide extracted from animal tissues. It is a compound with antithrombinogenetic activity mediated by an increased liberation of tissue plasminogen activator which does not modify the parameters of blood coagulation. It is given in a dose of 400 mg bid for seven days starting one day before surgery. Because its use is characterized by antithrombotic and profibrinolytic activity but it is free of anticoagulant effects, it can effectively replace the use of calcium heparin in a program of prophylaxis against surgically induced deep venous thrombosis without increasing the risk of excessive intraoperative and postoperative bleeding associated with "low-dose" heparin administration.[2,7,14,41] Defibrotide is not currently available for use in the United States.

On the other hand, Wille-Jorgensen et al[46] studied 245 patients who underwent acute extensive abdominal operations and were studied by ^{125}I-fibrinogen for 7 days. Of 81 patients receiving low-dose heparin, 12 had thromboembolism. Of 79 receiving a combination of low-dose heparin and graded compression stockings, two had thromboembolism, and of 85 receiving a combination of Dextran and graded compression stockings, 13 had this complication. They concluded that the combination of low-dose heparin and graded compression stockings is an effective way to prevent thromboembolism after acute abdominal operations. In an effort, then, to find some common denominator as to the type of patient most likely to benefit from low-dose heparin therapy, it may be that this combination of low-dose heparin and graduated compression stockings should be offered to all patients with a history of previous phlebitis or thrombophlebitis.

Although some surgeons administer subcutaneous minidoses of heparin preoperatively in the hope of reducing the incidence of embolization, its effectiveness seems insufficient to offset the risk of a significant increase in intraoperative and postoperative bleeding.[7]

It is advisable preoperatively, to apply elastic stockings, of graduated compression if available, from the feet to the midthigh, particularly if the patient has appreciable varices or a history of phlebitis or thrombosis. Alternatively, they may be applied after an operation in which the patient has been in the lithotomy or a marked Trendelenburg position, before the legs are lowered and the head is raised. Whether this practice reduces the risk of embolism is debatable, but it does effectively reduce the incidence of thrombosis[39] and the size of the venous bed into which blood will pool as soon as the patient's body is leveled or her feet have been taken down from the stirrups. Under such circumstances the prophylactic use of elastic stockings decreases the degree of postoperative hypotension, which predisposes some patients to cardiac or cerebral thrombosis and may at the very least confuse the recovery room phase of the patient's postoperative course.

Prophylactic administration of antibiotics. Postoperative wound infections affect at least 920,000 of the 23 million patients who undergo surgery each year in the United States.[17] Furthermore, this does not include the postoperative evaluation of the vast number of patients having their surgery in out-patient settings.[44] Among inpatients, wound infections are thought to double the expected postoperative stay with an enormous increase in costs of hospitalization. The vagina is chronically contaminated by multiple bacteria. The bacterial types and numbers in the vaginal canal vary, however, depending on the time of the woman's life, her environment and sexual activity, and, in premenopausal women, even the time of the menstrual cycle.[2] Cleansing the vagina by douching and scrubbing with antibacterial soaps, such as those containing povidone-iodine (Betadine) or chlorhexidine gluconate (Hibiclens), reduces the bacterial quantity significantly, but this procedure in itself does not "sterilize" the vagina.

The risk of postoperative infection seems to be significant when an operative procedure combines surgical manipulation and dissection of the vagina with a large opening of the peritoneal cavity and, at its conclusion, leaves areas of surgically traumatized and devascularized tissue crushed by forceps and tied into pedicles. Burke[6] noted that the presence of an appropriate broad spectrum antibiotic in the tissue being operated on reduces this clinical risk considerably. Like many others,[20,29,34,45] Ledger, Gee, and Lewis[27] found the risk of clinical infection to be especially high in premenopausal patients who undergo vaginal hysterectomy. As a result, they formulated a useful set of guidelines for antibiotic prophylaxis in gynecology, including in these guidelines Burke's recommendation that the "antibiotic must be circulating in the patient's tissue before the operation begins and should be promptly discontinued if there is no specific reason for continuing it after the patient recovers normal physiology." Burke emphasized, however, that preoperative preventive antibiotics will not eliminate all postoperative septic complications. There will be situations in which the level of bacterial resistance, extent of trauma, size of inoculum of bacteria, or combination will be such that antibiotics will be of little use. Antibiotics are but an adjunct to the natural resistance to bacterial invasion. They by no means replace it. Thus although the preventive administration of antibiotics can indeed be useful, there is no substitute for meticulousness and efficiency in technique and hemostasis to minimize tissue trauma.

The use of prophylactic antibiotics has decreased febrile morbidity impressively in patients who have undergone major vaginal surgery and, because it shortens their hospital stays, has been cost-effective. Prophylactic antibiotics are particularly useful when preliminary infiltration of tissue with a vasoconstrictor has augmented local hemosta-

sis. An initial intramuscular injection of an antibiotic 1 hour before the start of surgery "on call to the operating room" seems to provide an effective tissue level when needed; the time period between "on call to the operating room" and the initial incision often varies unpredictably from $\frac{1}{2}$ to 3 hours, however. If it is impossible to anticipate the precise time of surgery, the intravenous administration of an antibiotic appears to provide an effective level of the antibiotic in the tissues within 20 to 30 minutes when it is given in the operating room immediately before the onset of anesthesia. If the operation is to be less than 2 hours in total duration, a single dose of the antibiotic is sufficient. If the operation is likely to be longer than 2 hours, the intravenous dose should be repeated 2 hours after the beginning of the operation.

The first choice of antibiotic is 2 g of a first-generation cephalosporin, such as cefazolin (Ancef or Kefzol), which has a half-life of 80 minutes; if a second dose is given 2 hours after the first, the half-life totals 120 minutes. Although cephalosporins are generally contraindicated for the patient with a history of penicillin allergy, a single preoperative dose may occasionally be warranted if the surgeon feels that the risk-benefit ratio is favorable and if the allergic reaction to penicillin injection was in the nature of a mild skin rash. On the other hand, any previous anaphylactic reaction to penicillin must be thoroughly respected and an alternative such as minocycline, metronidazole,[24] or clindamycin and gentamicin chosen.

A study by Bates et al[3] has concluded that beginning prophylactic antibiotics intraoperatively may be just as effective as starting them preoperatively. Pratt[35] noticed a significant increase in postoperative body temperature morbidity in his vaginal hysterectomy patients between the time he was operating at St. Mary's Hospital (24%), and the Methodist Hospital in Rochester (36%). Upon examination, he determined that St. Mary's Hospital routinely took postoperative temperatures twice a day, but Methodist Hospital took temperatures four times a day, so the same patients receiving the same treatment who had their temperatures taken more frequently demonstrated a morbidity that otherwise would not have been recognized.

There has been a great deal of speculation about why the use of antibiotics, to which anaerobic organisms are not sensitive, reduces postoperative morbidity. Perhaps the antibiotics suppress the aerobic flora, permitting the body to concentrate its defensive energy on the surviving anaerobes, even though the latter are not sensitive to the antibiotic. Another possibility is that an anaerobic infection may require a coincident aerobic colonization. The reverse of this situation, selective suppression of anaerobes, may explain the similar effectiveness of metronidazole (Flagyl) when it is administered preoperatively.[18,24]

POSTOPERATIVE CARE

Postoperative care begins the minute the patient enters the recovery room. The patient's loved ones should be promptly informed of the details of surgery and told when it is likely that they may see the patient, and what to expect. The surgeon should make daily unhurried visits to the patient with assessment of her response to healing and therapy. Recognize and respond to her psychological concerns, and begin the process of discharge planning with notice of the surgeon's availability for advice and detailed notification of changes after discharge from the hospital, such as unexpected bleeding and fever that should be brought to the surgeon's attention. The patient should be told how to find her surgeon after discharge from the hospital. The duration of convalescence should be outlined, with questions solicited and a plan made for postoperative examination. Verbal instructions are so often forgotten that written communications or instructions, even if brief, are desirable.

Each surgeon should develop a plan for long-term follow-up and analysis of each individual and overall series of cases, so that the end results and effectiveness in reaching the surgical goals may be correlated with the techniques performed. The desired benefits of future modifications in care will become obvious and can be implemented, the foundation of the dynamic and evolutionary character of our discipline.

Extended visits with the patient should be discouraged during the first few postoperative days, when the patient needs ample opportunity to rest. Pain relief should be offered as necessary, preferably by means of small doses of medication repeated at frequent intervals to avoid a cumulative effect that can result in systemic or respiratory depression. Because periods of rest should be carefully interspersed with periods of ambulation and physical activity, it is important to avoid oversedation. Regular periods of deliberately deepened breathing should be encouraged as soon as the patient becomes conscious, and frequent repetition of forced inspiration or incentive spirometry has proved effective in reducing postoperative pulmonary problems.

Little seems to be gained by having a patient dangle her legs over the edge of the bed the evening following surgery; in fact, this may even increase venous stasis. The patient should be encouraged to begin flexing her legs, bending her ankles, and gently moving from side to side and changing position in bed soon after awakening from surgery, however, and to continue these movements throughout the entire postoperative period. Beginning the day after surgery, she should be helped to a bedside chair for a few minutes three or four times daily. This may improve the transit time of intestinal gas.[37] Sitting on a rubber doughnut is not recommended, because stretching of unsupported tissues through the hole in the center may strain new sutures. However, a soft pillow is an acceptable substitute. If the patient is willing, warm sitz baths or showers can be started on the second or third postoperative day. When elastic stockings have been applied preoperatively and the patient is resuming physical activity in a satisfactory manner, the stockings can be removed, usually by the third or fourth postoperative day.

The postoperative administration of intravenous fluids should continue until the patient can take and retain sufficient fluids by mouth. It is usually permissible for the patient to take liquids, preferably tea or tap water; by mouth as soon as she has recovered from the anesthesia, but in sips rather than glassfuls. Carbonated beverages, milk products, and fruit juices should be avoided initially to decrease the production of intestinal gas.[34] When repeated frequently, this regimen usually ensures the ingestion of an adequate 2 quarts of liquid per day. The patient may have solid foods as soon as she wants them, but she is unlikely to take more than an occasional nibble until her appetite returns, usually on the second or third postoperative day. There are exceptions, of course. For example, the patient who has had a rectovaginal fistula or an old fourth-degree laceration repaired is best maintained on an initial clear liquid nonresidue diet followed the second week after surgery by a low-residue diet.

If the patient is postmenopausal and sexually active, she can begin oral ingestion of an estrogen as soon as she is taking fluids by mouth. This can be supplemented by nightly and later weekly instillations of an intravaginal estrogen to aid wound epithelialization, help preserve vaginal blood supply and elasticity, and reduce the vaginal atrophy that accompanies postoperative contraction of the vaginal incision. Caution is necessary in the use of estrogen supplementation in these postmenopausal patients, however. The mechanics of intravaginal insertion of the application itself may inhibit the development of postoperative adhesions between the anterior and posterior walls of the vagina.

The surgeon should order appropriate blood studies before discharging a postoperative patient from the hospital. Determination of the patient's hemoglobin level and hematocrit on the third or fourth postoperative day is often adequate if her condition seems satisfactory at that time. A postoperative hemoglobin level of 9 g/ml or greater and a hematocrit of at least 27 in a patient without cardiovascular disease will respond to oral iron therapy, and transfusion is unnecessary.

Postoperative blood transfusion

Of 35 deaths per year nationally from transfusion reaction, one half are the consequence of clerical error (including provider errors, wrong sample being tested, technical errors in the laboratory, and administration of the wrong blood) are therefore presumably preventable. The incidence of transfusion reaction is as follows: one recipient per 100 may develop chills, fever, or urticaria; one in 6000 may develop a hemolytic reaction; and one in 100,000 may develop a fatal hemolytic reaction. In addition, there is the chance for the development of infection as a consequence of transfusion, specifically hepatitis, HIV, cytomegalic virus infection, and Howan T-cell lymphotropic virus infection. It should be remembered that transfusion does tend to suppress temporarily the body's immunologic system, compromising to some small extent the patient's ability to respond to the challenge of postoperative infection and physiologic stress.

Transfusion may disturb a patient's immunosuppressive mechanism and, thus, this potential risk can be avoided if unnecessary transfusion is avoided.

Because transfusion even of the patient's own blood carries a small but definable risk, it should not be employed without significant indication. Single-unit transfusion is but rarely indicated. Nonprogressive iron deficiency anemia can be effectively remedied by iron therapy using the oral route.

Postoperative hemoglobin and hematocrit in the older patient. Many patients over the age of 65 have lost their sense of thirst and consequently are relatively dehydrated most of the time, resulting in some hemoconcentration that may be observed during their preoperative evaluation. At surgery they are hydrated by the anesthesiologist during the course of surgery, and postoperative hemoglobin and hematocrit determinations may reflect this temporary hemodilution by an unusually low reading. By the third or fourth day of an uncomplicated postoperative course, as a consequence of some reinstitution of chronic dehydration due to habitual fluid restriction on the part of the patient, the numerical readings of the hemoglobin and hematocrit will often have risen.

Risk of hepatitis and AIDS associated with postoperative blood transfusion. The Centers for Disease Control estimate that approximately 12,000 people now living in the United States harbor transfusion-acquired infection. It is estimated[32] that there may eventually be as many as 2000 cases of AIDS resulting from transfusions received between 1978 and 1984. There is reason to believe that some people who are infectious do not have a positive test for antibodies to HIV. If the incidence of detected positive donations is 100 per million (1 in 10,000), it is possible that as many as four infected donations will be undetected in each million tested. Thus, the current incidence may be about one in 250,000. Nevertheless, the current risk of acquiring AIDS as a result of transfusion at the present time is extremely low. The incidence of non-A, non-B hepatitis after transfusion is estimated at between 4% and 18%, and appears to be falling.[5]

Homologous transfusion—banked blood. One need not encourage patients to bank 1 pint of their own blood against transfusion during their coming surgery unless a major blood loss (>1000 cc) is anticipated. Like as not a 1-unit (pint) transfusion will not be used and will then not be given back to the patient, and she will have compromised her own iron storage. Also, if she had bled enough to require transfusion, more than 1 unit will be needed, in which case her own unit of blood will not be adequate to meet her needs. It is better for the surgeon to develop a system of precise anatomic dissection and hemostasis for which blood loss does not require transfusion.

During the patient's postoperative course, all the medications she is ingesting should be reviewed frequently to identify any conflicting or unnecessary orders and facilitate their correction in a timely manner. Any preexisting medical conditions under treatment (e.g., hypertension) should be frequently reevaluated, the postoperative routine modified, and appropriate therapy reinstituted as necessary.

The surgeon should see the patient at least once daily during her hospitalization. In addition, a staff physician should visit her daily at a different time of day and more frequently when necessary.

Resumption of bowel function

Bowel movements should be resumed by the third postoperative day. The administration of a gentle laxative with a stool softener, (such as casanthranol and dioctyl sodium sulfosuccinate [Peri-Colace]), beginning when the patient starts to eat solid food is often helpful. If no movement has occurred by the evening of the third postoperative day, 30 ml of milk of magnesia and 4 ml of cascara are given; if this is ineffective, an irritant suppository, such as bisacodyl (Dulcolax), or a saline enema is ordered. If this does not bring about a bowel movement, a gentle rectal examination is necessary to rule out a fecal impaction. Any fecal impaction is gently broken digitally, and an oil retention enema is given, followed by a saline enema.

The withdrawal of nicotine in a postoperative patient who smoked until the day of her surgery may inhibit intestinal peristalsis, so the surgeon should anticipate some problems with hypotonic bowel function in such a patient. Stool softeners and laxatives may be particularly appropriate for patients who have undergone a posterior colporrhaphy or perineorrhaphy.

Under no circumstances should the woman who is recovering from gynecologic surgery be permitted to sit up to strain on a bedpan in an effort to have a bowel movement without an enema. Surgery in the female pelvis is not infrequently followed by thrombosis in the relatively large veins that communicate with the internal iliacs and vena cava. The suddenly increased intraabdominal pressure that occurs when a patient tries to accomplish a bowel movement may lead to thromboembolism in the iliacs and vena cava, with occasionally disastrous results. This risk can be reduced by (1) early ambulation of the patient, (2) prohibition of any major postoperative straining efforts to accomplish a bowel movement, and (3) use of stool softeners and enemas to ensure a postoperative bowel movement without exertion or strain.

Problems with postoperative voiding

The bladder has a triple nerve supply—somatic, sympathetic, and parasympathetic—and the perception of and balance between these sometimes opposing influences vary from patient to patient and from time to time. Even minor physiologic and psychologic events can disturb the harmony of these influences. Therefore difficulty in the resumption of voiding after a major event such as surgery is a rather common problem, although it is not often predictable with any degree of certainty. Such difficulty may occur after any surgical procedure, but it is most likely to occur after procedures involving the abdomen and pelvis (e.g., episiotomy, colporrhaphy, hysterectomy, herniorrhaphy, hemorrhoidectomy, and laparotomy).

Prevention of difficulties in voiding. Facilitating the patient's postoperative resumption of voiding is of primary importance. The circumstances under which the patient is expected to void must be as private and comfortable as possible, and the patient's attendants must be prompt and calm when assisting. Years ago, von Peham and Amreich[42] noted that some patients encounter difficulty when they try to void in the recumbent position. If at all possible, the patient should be permitted to void while sitting in a natural position, using a nearby toilet if feasible, a portable commode if not, or a bedpan if confined to bed. Some postoperative patients can void more comfortably at first from a semistanding position, however, probably because it reduces the likelihood of levator spasm. Others may find manual suprapubic compression over the bladder helpful once voiding has begun, and this technique is more effective when the patient leans somewhat forward during the voiding process.

Overdistention of the bladder (urine volume of over 500 cc) is to be avoided at all costs. Not only is overdistention painful, but it also appears to interfere temporarily with the blood supply of the bladder and thus to reduce local resistance to infection.[26] In addition, overdistention may cause a transient paralysis of the detrusor that can require days to overcome.

The use of synthetic absorbable sutures, such as those made of polyglycolic acid (e.g., Dexon, Vicryl), instead of catgut appears to decrease postoperative intravaginal adhesions, and swelling and edema of the pelvic tissues. This is particularly noteworthy after colporrhaphy that includes any reconstructive plication or support of the vesical neck, where longer lasting monofilament absorbable synthetic sutures of polydiaxanone (PDS) or polygluconate (Maxon) are used. The surgeon should instruct patients who have undergone a suprapubic sling procedure and who have been accustomed to emptying their bladders by tightening the rectus muscles to increase intraabdominal pressure, not to do so in the future, since voluntary rectus muscle contraction may tighten the sling sufficiently to occlude the urethra. When transurethral drainage is necessary, a silicone-coated Foley catheter (which is undoubtedly less irritating to the urethral mucosa than is the uncoated rubber of the standard catheter) reduces mucosal edema and thus decreases the risk of urethral obstruction.

If the patient has an extensive history of bladder decompensation, as may be associated with a long-standing or massive cystocele, some intrinsic detrusor hypotonia can be predicted. Bladder tone can be increased by the judicious administration of bethanechol chloride (Urecholine) initially 10 mg three times daily, and depending on the patient's response, may be increased progressively to 25 mg

four times daily before removal of the catheter and for several days thereafter until the patient can again void comfortably. In obviously anxious patients, preliminary sedation with barbiturates and judicious use of analgesics in doses tailored to the individual patient's needs can be very helpful.

Although stimulation of beta-adrenergic receptors tends to relax the bladder neck and trigone in the presence of low amounts of noradrenaline, stimulation of alpha-adrenergic receptors tends to cause smooth muscle contractions.[38] Because the bladder neck is well supplied with alpha-adrenergic receptors, alpha-adrenergic blocking agents such as phenoxybenzamine hydrochloride (Dibenzyline) or prazosin (Minipres) selectively prevent spasms caused by stimulation of these receptors. The alpha-adrenergic blocking agent phenoxybenzamine hydrochloride (Dibenzyline) in a dose of 10 mg by mouth 4 to 5 hours after surgery and repeated, if necessary, once or twice during the first 24 hours has been effective.[28,31] Any beta-blockers, such as propranolol hydrochloride (Inderal), may not only induce hypertonia by stimulating detrusor tone but also induce some spasm of the bladder neck by selective blocking.

Gentle percussion of the costovertebral angles should be done the evening after surgery and repeated each day for the next several days. Unexpected or pronounced unilateral tenderness should be promptly investigated by infusion intravenous pyelography to exclude ureteral obstruction.

Causes and treatment of inability to void. It is known that a postoperative voiding difficulty can result from several causative factors.[25] There are almost certain to be additional factors that influence the process of voiding but cannot yet be predictably or accurately understood or measured. Not the least of these is the patient's motivation. There are some whose confidence in the function of their own bladders is sufficient to overcome almost any disturbance. For those who are experiencing difficulty, however, the calm, optimistic, and serene understanding of their attendants is of utmost importance during the brief time that for them constitutes a disquieting and disabling crisis.

Anxiety. A powerful cause of inability to void is anxiety on the part of the patient or her attendant staff. Sometimes this is preconditioned by fear, conversation with other patients, hearsay, or observation of other patients. Treatment includes appropriate counseling, gentle calmness, cheerful confidence, and empathy from the attendant staff, as well as appropriate sedation and pain relief. Some authorities recommend the administration of tea to induce some detrusor hyperactivity or beer to provide some general body sedation.

Mechanical interference. Local physical factors, such as the presence of vaginal packing, local edema, rectal fullness, or any obstruction of the urethra or ureters, may interfere with the physiology of voiding in the postoperative patient. Any mechanical factors that interfere with the opening of the internal urethral sphincter during attempts to void may play a role, especially those factors that inhibit the physiologic obliteration of the posterior vesicourethral angle. For example, very few women can void while a tight vaginal packing is in place. Treatment in this circumstance is the removal of any mechanical obstruction of the vagina or urethra; gentle urethral dilation can relieve any urethral stricture that is obstructing normal flow. Overhydration must be avoided when an indwelling catheter is to be removed; it not only exaggerates any difficulties that may be present but also causes rapid and unnecessary overdistention of the bladder.

Reflex interferences. Neurologic reflex interference with the normal physiology of voiding, as often seen after parturition, episiotomy, and hemorrhoidectomy, may be coincident with a levator spasm that causes a reflex spastic contraction in both the internal and external urethral sphincters. Patient nervousness and embarrassment accentuate this problem, of course. Sitz baths, analgesia, and time are of the greatest help, because the bladder and urethral sphincters will once again begin to relax when the painful but temporary levator spasm has finally been overcome. Similarly, pain in the rectus abdominus muscles as a result of a laparotomy incision often reflexly induces levator spasm, interfering with the physiologic descent of the vesical neck during the voiding process. Again, patience, analgesia, and the temporary use of an alpha-adrenergic blocker (e.g., phenoxybenzamine) are often helpful.

As mentioned earlier, overdistention of the bladder can result in a temporary detrusor paralysis and is therefore to be avoided at all costs. It can develop insidiously in the oversedated and overhydrated patient who may fail to perceive or respond to bladder fullness. Once overdistention has become pathologic, the treatment is primarily expectant; bladder tone generally returns several days after continuous decompression by an indwelling catheter. It is essential to prevent additional or future episodes of overdistention, however.

Neurologic abnormality. A primary neurologic defect may lead to chronic bladder hypotonia. Because such a defect may be associated with diabetes, central nervous system lues, or multiple sclerosis, the patient's medical history may suggest the correlation. Neuropathy resulting from a herniated intervertebral disk may be evident; in this instance there is coincident constipation and usually a history of sudden onset. Herniated low disks that involve the cauda equina but are too far caudal to be evident on a myelogram may be present. Skillful neurologic evaluation is required for appropriate diagnosis.

Surgeons often recognize hypotonia preoperatively and may plan to stimulate the detrusor subtly by administering bethanechol (Urecholine) postoperatively. The initial dosage may be as low as 10 mg three times a day, but in order to obtain clinical effectiveness it may be necessary to increase the dosage rapidly to as much as 50 to 75 mg three times daily.

Drug-induced detrusor hypotonia. Coincident and often long-term consumption of common tranquilizing agents may be associated with unexpected and sometimes chronic detrusor hypotonia. Surgeons should suspect this effect among patients who take daily doses of diazepam (Valium), chlordiazepoxide hydrochloride (Librium), thioridazine hydrochloride (Mellaril), chlorpromazine hydrochloride (Thorazine), prochlorperazine maleate (Compazine), and meprobamate (Miltown). In many instances other physicians may have prescribed these drugs, and the patient may have become so accustomed to taking them that she forgets to include her consumption of them in her medical history. Discontinuation of such a drug, when it is a contributing factor to detrusor hypotonia, may result in a rather prompt reappearance of normal bladder tone.

The induction of detrusor hyperactivity by the deliberate creation of a chemical cystitis (e.g., by instilling merbromin [Mercurochrome] or ether in the bladder) is neither popular nor recommended. Not only are the results unpredictable, but the procedure may unexpectedly lead to a long-standing, chemical cystitis, sometimes of massive degree.

Bladder management after removal of the catheter

The administration of antibiotics or antibacterials to "cover" the bacteria often associated with an indwelling bladder catheter need not begin until the day the catheter is removed. A urine culture and sensitivity study should be obtained at this time; if the culture reveals the presence of an infection, the most effective antibiotic should be prescribed until a subsequent culture shows that the infection has been eradicated. Delaying the administration of antibiotics until this time seems to prevent or retard the development of antibiotic resistance in potential infecting organisms, as often occurs when antibacterial coverage is instituted in the immediate postoperative period and continued through the patient's postoperative course. After urinary fistula repair, however, the immediate administration of antibiotics is appropriate in order to decontaminate the urine and mucosal layer of the freshly repaired bladder wound during the early healing phase.

Transurethral catheter. After the removal of a transurethral catheter, a urine culture should be obtained (at bedtime or between 7:00 and 8:00 AM) and an antibacterial, such as 50 mg of nitrofurantoin (Macrodantin) three times daily, 1 g of methenamine three times daily,[40] or trimethoprim sulfa, should be administered. The patient should also take 10 mg of an alpha-adrenergic blocker, such as phenoxybenzamine, by mouth.

The surgeon should instruct the nursing staff to catheterize the patient as necessary if she is unable to void after the indwelling catheter has been removed. (Infinite gentleness is essential in catheterizing these already apprehensive individuals, whose tissues are understandably tender.) An alternative is to catheterize the patient two or three times daily, immediately after she voids but a small amount, until the postvoiding residual volume is no more than 100 ml on two consecutive occasions. The amount that the patient voids is usually of prognostic significance, even when the initial residual volume is undesirably high. It is much more encouraging if a patient is voiding 100 to 200 ml with a residual volume of 200 to 250 ml, for example, than if she is voiding only 10 to 20 ml with the same residual volume. The prognosis for early resumption of adequate voiding is good. In the first situation, the amount voided can be expected to increase as the amount of residual urine decreases. In the second situation, it should be expected that resumption of adequate voiding will require a significantly longer time, often several weeks.

The patient who cannot void in adequate amounts after the catheter has been removed may be taught the technique of self-catheterization with the soft plastic 14 Fr Mentor female catheter (see Chapter 21), or she may be discharged with a Foley catheter in place and clamped, the clamp to be opened and the bladder drained periodically as necessary. The surgeon should explain clearly that the inability to void postoperatively is temporary, that it is by no means rare or unusual, and that it is unlikely to lengthen or change the patient's convalescence in any way. Giving the patient a handout sheet concerning the use of the catheter (see below) is often quite helpful.

USE OF THE TRANSURETHRAL CATHETER

The bladder must be given time to rest so that the swelling and irritation caused by the surgery can subside. The length of time needed for recovery varies from person to person; it may take anywhere from a few days to several weeks. The greater the need for the repair and thus the greater the scope of the repair, the longer the period of recovery of comfortable bladder function.

During this recovery period, a person's kidney system continues to work, of course, and it is necessary to drain the urine from the bladder until functional recovery of the bladder has been completed. This drainage is provided by an indwelling catheter that is inserted through the urethra, the usual canal between the vulva and the bladder, at the time of surgery. This catheter can be clamped to stop the flow of urine until there is a sufficient amount in the bladder to produce a sense of urgency and a desire to void. At that time, the clamp can be removed, the bladder emptied, and the clamp reapplied.

After approximately 2 weeks of bladder rest, the catheter is removed by cutting it across with clean scissors sometime during the midmorning hours. Please call the office that weekday afternoon to tell us how the bladder is functioning. If you are passing adequate amounts of urine and the intervals between voidings are longer than 2 hours, it is likely that comfortable bladder function has returned. There may be a mild sensation of burning or irritation during voiding until the swelling in the urethra from the catheter has subsided, usually within 1 or 2 days. Should urinary burning and frequency increase instead of decrease, be sure to call the office.

Suprapubic catheter. Surgeons may consider using a suprapubic catheter in two particular instances: (1) after repair of a fistula at the vesical neck, as a means of keeping the catheter away from the site of the fistula repair, and (2) after the creation of a neovagina that requires the use of a vaginal obturator postoperatively. Should the surgeon be an advocate of suprapubic catheterization, patients may find a handout concerning the use of the suprapubic catheter informative.

USE OF THE SUPRAPUBIC CATHETER

The physician who wishes to put the recently repaired tissues around the urethra, bladder, and vagina at complete rest while they recover from surgery may place a catheter into the bladder through a tiny incision in the skin of the lower abdomen. This is a temporary way of diverting the urine until the patient's own bladder is able to function again. Furthermore, it saves a patient the nuisance, discomfort, and irritation associated with repeated catheterizations during the healing process.

By the time preliminary healing is under way, usually after the fourth postoperative day, this catheter may be fitted with a screw-type clamp that, when tightened, stops the flow of urine through the catheter and permits the bladder to fill. When the bladder is full and the patient feels a desire to void, she is encouraged to do so; after she has voided or has tried to void through the urethra, the screw clamp is opened and the bladder drained through the suprapubic catheter. This procedure is continued on a regular basis until the patient is able to pass most of the urine naturally through the urethra and less than 2 ounces is drained from the suprapubic catheter after each voiding. Therefore, it is important to keep a running account of the amount of urine voided naturally each time and the amount obtained from the catheter after each voiding.

When the residual volume of urine in the bladder after each voiding has remained less than 2 ounces, the suprapubic catheter clamp should be left firmly applied for a full 1 or 2 days to see whether regular urinary voiding is well established. If so, the catheter is removed by simply cutting across its midpoint. The Foley bulb rapidly decompresses, and the internal portion of the catheter is quietly and easily extracted by gentle traction. The opening left by the catheter usually closes within a day or two, although a small amount of urine often drips from this opening at first so that a small dressing is necessary until the opening has closed.

Discharge from the hospital

The surgeon should discuss the patient's probable date of discharge from the hospital with her a day or two ahead of time so that she and her family can make arrangements and preparations. Taking into account what was learned about the patient's home situation preoperatively, the surgeon should give the patient very specific instructions about what she may and may not do during her convalescence. Written or printed postoperative instructions, as shown in the box on p. 118, can be extremely useful.

The surgeon should also explain the circumstances (e.g., fever, excessive bleeding) in which the patient should call for help postoperatively. Many patients appreciate a summary and an interpretation of the results of laboratory studies performed while they were in the hospital, and every patient should be given specific directions about when to return to the surgeon's office for postoperative examination.

The patient's care after discharge from the hospital may

Instructions on going home

1. Go directly home and rest for the remainder of the day.
2. During the first week at home, rest several times daily. Increase activity gradually. Expect tiredness, and let no day's activities become an endurance contest.
3. Beginning the third week, you may go outdoors, and if you are able, you may drive at the end of the month.
4. Please call the office within the first week to arrange for a postoperative appointment.
5. Do not hesitate to call for further advice if you have any questions.

Activities

Gradually increase activity for the first 2 weeks. Do *not* engage in heavy lifting, scrubbing, douching, or intercourse until you have been checked at the office. A program of perineal resistive exercises (isometric squeezes of the pubococcygeal muscles) is often helpful in restoration of bowel and bladder control. Try to squeeze these muscles 15 times in a row, 3 seconds each squeeze, 6 times a day.

Diet

You may return to your usual diet. For constipation, drink some prune juice or extra water, or take 1 ounce of milk of magnesia, as necessary. Bran with breakfast is often helpful.

Baths

You may shower, take tub baths, and wash your hair at any time.

---

be just as important as her care during hospitalization. Home visits are seldom necessary, however, and assuring the patient before she leaves the hospital that her gynecologist and her surgeon will be available for telephoned questions and consultation while she is convalescing at home reduces the apprehensions that most frequently account for a home visit request. Such assurances maintain the patient's cooperation and confidence until her recovery is complete and her activities are no longer restricted. A routine telephone call at home from the surgeon or the office nurse a few days after discharge is appreciated and invites relevant questions and appropriate discussion of any concerns.

The wise and considerate surgeon does not permit the delicate and at times very personal relationship with the patient to extend inappropriately beyond the time frame of her convalescence. Although a patient's sense of dependence on her surgeon is highly desirable during the perioperative period, the surgeon should consciously discourage the continuation of such a relationship as the patient resumes her private life and personal responsibilities. Ensuring a successful transition and termination requires intelligent and purposeful application of practical psychology and good patient care. The details are likely to be different

for almost every patient. Much of the success of a surgeon's practice is predicated on the development of skills that elevate the surgeon from the role of mere technical craftsman to the intended and more effective role of the physician.

REFERENCES

1. Alexander JW et al: The influence of hair removal methods on wound infections, *Arch Surg* 118:347, 1983.
2. Ballard RM et al: Low doses of subcutaneous heparin in the prevention of deep vein thrombosis after gynecological surgery, *J Obstet Gynaecol Br Commonw* 80:469-472, 1973.
3. Bates T et al: Timing of prophylactic antibiotics in abdominal surgery, *Br J Surg* 76:52-56, 1989.
4. Bonnar J: Venous thromboembolism and gynecologic surgery, *Clin Obstet Gynecol* 28(2):432-446, 1985.
5. Bove, RJ: Transfusion associated hepatitis and AIDS, *N Engl J Med* 317:242-245, 1987.
6. Burke JF: Use of preventive antibiotics in clinical surgery, *Am Surg* 39:6, 1973.
7. Butterman GJ et al: Optimisation of postoperative prophylaxis of thrombosis in gynecology, *Geburtsh Frauen* 38:98, 1978.
8. Capen CV: Gynecologic surgery: pre-operative evaluation, *Clin Obstet Gynecol* 31:673-685, 1988.
9. Clarke-Pearson DL et al: Complications of low-dose heparin prophylaxis in gynecologic oncology surgery, *Obstet Gynecol* 64:689, 1984.
10. Classen DC et al: The timing of prophylactic administration of antibiotics and the risk of surgical-wound infection, *N Engl J Med* 326:281-286, 1992.
11. Copenhaver EH: *Surgery of the vulva and vagina,* Philadelphia, 1981, WB Saunders.
12. Cruse PJE, Foord R: A 5-year prospective study of 23,649 surgical wounds, *Arch Surg* 107:206-210, 1973.
13. Dineen P: An evaluation of the duration of the surgical scrub, *Surg Gynecol Obstet* 129:1181-1184, 1969.
14. Ferrari A, Dindelli M, Sellaroli CM: Personal communication, 1988.
15. Fleites RA et al: The efficacy of polyethylene glycol–electrolyte lavage solution versus traditional mechanical bowel preparation for elective colonic surgery, *Surgery* 98:708-715, 1985.
16. Galask RP, Larsen B, Ohm MJ: Vaginal flora and its role in disease entities, *Clin Obstet Gynecol* 19:61, 1976.
17. Haley RW et al: Identifying patients at high risk of surgical wound infection, *Am J Epidemiol* 121:206-215, 1985.
18. Hamod KA et al: Single-dose and multidose prophylaxis in vaginal hysterectomy, *Am J Obstet Gynecol* 136:976, 1980.
19. Harwood A: The hot-cold theory of disease, *JAMA* 216:1153, 1971.
20. Hemsell DL et al: Cefoxitin for prophylaxis in premenopausal women undergoing vaginal hysterectomy, *Obstet Gynecol* 56:629, 1980.
21. Hosking MP et al: Outcomes of surgery in patients 90 years of age and older, *JAMA* 261:1909-1915, 1989.
22. Hosking MP, Warner MA: Preoperative evaluation and prognosis after surgery in elderly patients, *Geriat Med Today* 9:19-26, 1990.
23. Hunt TK et al: Effect of vitamin A on reversing the inhibitory effect of cortisone on healing of open wounds in animals and man, *Ann Surg* 170:633, 1969.
24. Jackson P, Ridley WJ: Simplified antibiotic prophylaxis for vaginal hysterectomy, *Aust N Z J Obstet Gynaecol* 19:225, 1979.
25. Jeffcoate TNA: *Principles of gynecology,* New York, 1967, Appleton-Century-Crofts.
26. Lapides J: Neurogenic bladder: principles of treatment, *Urol Clin North Am* 1:81, 1974.
27. Ledger WL, Gee C, Lewis WF: Guidelines for antibiotic prophylaxis in gynecology, *Am J Obstet Gynecol* 121:1038, 1975.
28. Leventhal A, Pfau A: Pharmacologic management of postoperative overdistention of the bladder, *Surg Gynecol Obstet* 146:347, 1978.

29. Mickal A, Curole D, Lewis C: Cefoxitin sodium: double-blind vaginal hysterectomy prophylaxis in premenopausal patients, *Obstet Gynecol* 56:222, 1980.

30. Narr BJ, Hansen TR, Warner MA: Pre-operative laboratory screening in healthy Mayo patients: cost effective elimination of tests and unchanged outcomes, *Mayo Clin Proc* 66:155-159, 1991.

31. Nichols DH: Getting the postoperative patient to void, *Contemp Obstet Gynecol* 12:41, 1978.

32. Peterman TA et al: Estimating the risks of transfusion-associated AIDS and HIV infection, *Transfusion* 27:371-374, 1987.

33. Polivy J: Psychological reactions to hysterectomy: a critical review, *Am J Obstet Gynecol* 118:417, 1974.

34. Polk BF et al: Randomised clinical trial of perioperative cefazolin in preventing infection after hysterectomy, *Lancet* 1:437, 1980.

35. Pratt J: Personal communication, 1983.

36. Roizen MF et al: The relative roles of the history and physical examination, and laboratory testing in preoperative evaluation for outpatient surgery: the "Starling" curve of preoperative laboratory testing, *Anesth Clin North Am* 5:15-34, 1987.

37. Sawyers JL: Questions and answers, *JAMA* 253:705, 1985.

38. Stanton SL: *Female urinary incontinence*, London, 1977, Lloyd-Luke (Medical Books).

39. Turner GM, Cole SE, Brooks JH: The efficacy of graduated compression stockings in the prevention of deep vein thrombosis after major gynecological surgery, *Br J Obstet Gynaecol* 91:588, 1984.

40. Tyreman NO et al: Urinary tract infection after vaginal surgery: effect of prophylactic treatment with methenamine hippurate, *Acta Obstet Gynecol Scand* 65:731, 1986.

41. U.S. National Institutes of Health: Consensus conference—prevention of deep thrombosis and pulmonary embolism, *Lancet* 1202-1204, May 1986.

42. von Peham H, Amreich J: *Operative gynecology,* Philadelphia, 1934, JB Lippincott.

43. Walton LA, Baker VV: *Mechanical and chemical preparation of the abdomen and vagina.* In Buchsbaum HJ, Walton LA, editors: *Strategies in gynecologic surgery,* New York, 1986, Springer-Verlag.

44. Wenzel RP: Preoperative antibiotic prophylaxis, *N Engl J Med* 326:337-339, 1992.

45. Whelton A et al: Therapeutic implications of doxycycline and cephalothin concentrations in the female genital tract, *Obstet Gynecol* 55:28, 1980.

46. Wille-Jørgensen P et al: Prophylaxis of deep venous thrombosis after acute abdominal operation. *Surg Gynecol Obstet* 172:44-48, 1991.

Chapter 7

INSTRUMENTS AND SUTURES

David H. Nichols

Although the success of surgery depends more on the surgeon's judgment and technical competence than on the design of the instruments or the quality of the sutures used, the right choices of equipment and materials enable the surgeon to accomplish the best of which he or she is capable with greater ease and efficiency. Furthermore, ensuring that the special instruments or sutures that may be needed are on hand before the start of surgery avoids delays and permits the effective use of each minute of operative time.

OPERATING ROOM AND EQUIPMENT

The operating room should be in a quiet location and should be large enough to provide not only elbow room and moving space for the surgeon and assistants, the anesthesiologist, and the nursing staff but also convenient access to equipment and instrument tables (Fig. 7-1). Appropriate amounts of suture material, any special instruments that might be used, and sterile supplies, including any packing that may be needed, should be immediately at hand. Modern anesthesia equipment that permits continuous monitoring of the patient's pulmonary and cardiac status should also be in the operating room. Continuous suction equipment, including one weighted speculum equipped with a suction tip, is desirable. A separate suction apparatus with a hand-held tube should be available. A trap for each suction device permits a quick and accurate estimate of the amount of blood lost during the surgery.

Lighting

Because most operating room lighting has been designed to illuminate the operative field during procedures such as a laparotomy, it does not always furnish adequate illumination into the horizontal axis of a relatively deep pelvic cavity such as the vagina. Lighting directed over the right-handed surgeon's left shoulder (and vice versa) should provide shadow-free illumination. When the overhead lighting cannot be adapted for vaginal surgery, movable spotlights are necessary; these often have an annoying tendency to move or slide out of focus as a result of the movements of operating room personnel, however. A surgeon may find it advantageous to wear a fiberoptic or tungsten headlight, which will provide a shadowless spot of from 2 to 4 inches of very bright light in the center of the operative field (Fig. 7-2). Because the wearer is in control of the position of the light at all times, it can be quite helpful.

Operating table

For vaginal surgery, the operating table should be equipped with "candy cane" stirrups that can be extended at least a foot so that they can be adjusted to the length of the patient's legs. These should be placed in such a fashion that when the patient's ankles are suspended from the stirrups, acute angulation of the legs does not obstruct venous return. The patient should be so positioned on the operating table that an imaginary line drawn between the two stirrups will intersect each acetabulum, or hip socket. Allen universal supports should be used instead when it is anticipated that the patient will be in the lithotomy position for longer than 2½ hours, to lessen the chance for postoperative femoral neuropathy.

The operating table should also permit rapid adjustment into varying degrees of Trendelenburg and reverse Trendelenburg positions, as needed for individual and emergency circumstances. The table height should be sufficiently adjustable to permit the operator either to stand or to sit down during the operative procedure.

A lithotomy sheet should have ample casings for the feet so that it can be placed in position readily even though the patient's legs are placed somewhat vertically in the extended leg holders or stirrups. Alternatively, the patient and her legs may be draped with sterile sheets.

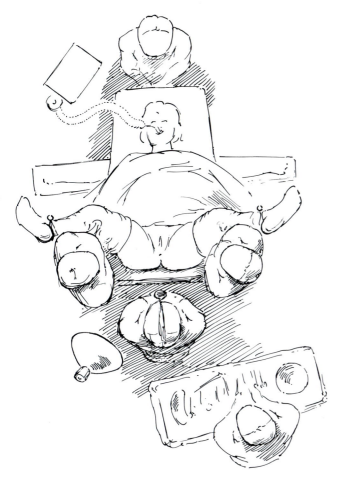

Fig. 7-1. Arrangement of personnel within the operating room when a transvaginal surgical route has been chosen. Surgeon in central position at foot of operating table with second assistant to the right and first assistant to the left. A spotlight over a right-handed surgeon's shoulder illuminates the perineum. Instrument table to the surgeon's back and somewhat to the right. Instrument nurse behind the instrument table, facing surgeon's back and sharing a full view of operative field so as to follow progress of the surgical procedure visually. Positions of spotlight, nurse, and instrument table are reversed if surgeon is left-handed. (From *Instruments and sutures. In Nichols DH, Randall CL: Vaginal surgery,* ed 3, Baltimore, 1989, Williams & Wilkins.)

Thigh-high elastic stockings for the patient are advisable, and they should be in place before administration of the anesthesia. Their usefulness in significantly decreasing the risk of postoperative pulmonary embolism may be debatable, but they certainly provide venous compression and thus reduce the rapid pooling of blood into the large venous beds of the patient's legs that occurs when the legs are taken out of the stirrups and lowered into the horizontal recumbent position at the conclusion of the operative procedure. Lowering the legs without such compression may result in a precipitous and major drop in blood pressure because of what, in effect, is a sudden increase in the size of the venous pool into which a fixed volume of blood is circulating. Intermittent compression boots are useful

when there are extensive varicosities or a history of previous thrombophlebitis or of pulmonary embolus.

Special instruments

Vaginal surgeons usually prefer a few special instruments that are well designed for vaginal procedures. Instruments available for vaginal surgery in standard operating room setups often include

Sharpened curved Mayo scissors
Narrow Deaver retractors
Curved and straight Kocher's forceps
Allis clamps
Rochester or curved Kelly hemostats
Crile hemostats
Lahey thyroid or Gordon uterine vulsella
Double-toothed Jacobs-type tenacula

For vaginal hysterectomy, the setup should include, in addition to the standard instruments, several Heaney-type hysterectomy forceps and a Heaney-type needleholder. Bonney and Russian forceps are desirable. Long straight-bladed retractors are useful, such as the Breisky-Navratil in various sizes.

Although ideal, it is not always possible for the surgeon who is performing a vaginal operation to have two assistants. When the surgeon must work with a single assistant, a large Rigby retractor (Fig. 7-3, *H*) is extremely useful because it frees the assistant's hands for knot cutting, sponging, and holding the movable retractors. A weighted speculum is usually quite helpful when, as often happens, the surgeon must accomplish virtually all the surgical dissection within the vagina. A modification of the standard weighted speculum permits continuous suction (Fig. 7-3, *A*). The suction tubing may be built into the retractor blade, further increasing operative exposure (Fig. 7-4). A wall-mounted trap on the suction apparatus makes it possible to estimate blood loss during surgery at a glance.

The instruments of N. Sproat Heaney were especially designed for use within the vagina. The Heaney needle-holder is particularly valuable, because the considerable range of angles at which the needle can be grasped permits the surgeon to place curved needles and sutures deep within the pelvis at almost any conceivable angle with relative ease (Figs. 7-5, *C* and 7-6). The Heaney hemostats have a "pelvic curve" that ensures proper placement and a secure grip on tissues with minimal risk of slippage. For use in a hysterectomy in which the prolapse may not be severe at the start of the operation, the Heaney-Glenner hysterectomy forceps is valuable (Fig. 7-5, *A*); this instrument has both an upward curve and a lateral curve adapted to the right and left sides of the patient, as stamped on the forceps. The Heaney-Ballantine hysterectomy forceps is also useful (Fig. 7-5, *B*) as are the Masterson and the Maingot forceps. The latter is useful for clamping the mesovarium during oophorectomy because it neither slips nor tears tissue, even when traction is needed.

During the performance of a vaginectomy or a Schauta

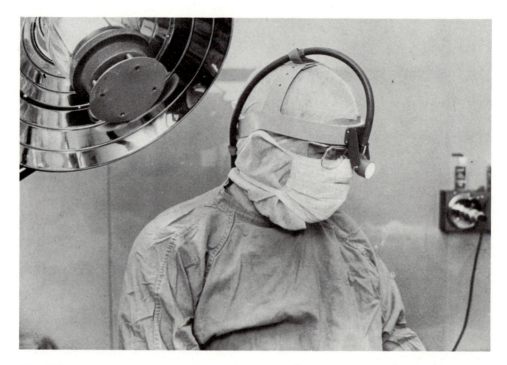

Fig. 7-2. Fiberoptic headlight, which will provide literally shadow-free bright illumination into the depths of a body cavity, even in a horizontal plane. (From *Instruments and sutures*. In Nichols DH, Randall CL: *Vaginal surgery*, ed 3, Baltimore, 1989, Williams & Wilkins.)

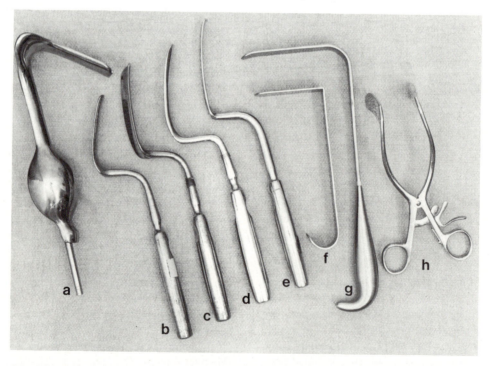

Fig. 7-3. Various retractors. **A,** Remine weighted suction speculum. **B, C, D, E,** Various shapes and sizes of Briesky-Navratil vaginal retractors. **F,** Small Heaney retractor. **G,** Long-handled Heaney retractor. **H,** Large-sized Rigby self-retaining retractor. (From Nichols DH, Randall CL: *Vaginal surgery,* ed 3, Baltimore, 1989, Wiliams & Wilkins.)

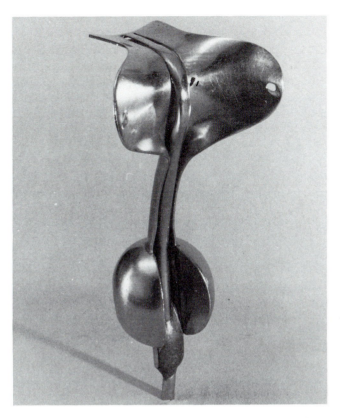

Fig. 7-4. Weighted suction speculum for posterior wall of vagina. Suction tubing has been buried in retractor's posterior blade, improving exposure in the operative field. Available from custom order department, Mr. William Merz, Baxter V. Mueller, Chicago, IL 60648. (From *Instruments and sutures.* In Nichols DH, Randall CL: *Vaginal surgery,* ed 3, Baltimore, 1989, Williams & Wilkins.)

radical vaginal hysterectomy, the long mouse-toothed forceps of Krobach is effective in occluding the vagina temporarily (Fig. 7-5, *D*). Once the operator is familiar with the use of this instrument, one or two of them can be of considerable help during a perineorrhaphy and posterior colporrhaphy.

The Bonney forceps is highly recommended (Fig. 7-7), because it has both a rat tooth for holding the tissues and occlusive serrated edges for grasping a needle that is deeply placed in tissues. The long Singley forceps is particularly useful for handling the peritoneum and intraabdominal organs with minimal trauma (Fig. 7-7). The so-called Russian forceps is an excellent choice for use on the vaginal surface of the bladder during anterior colporrhaphy because it distributes the compression of the tissue within its grasp equally over a wide area (Fig. 7-7).

Most surgeons find it easier to hold a small Heaney retractor (see Fig. 7-3, *F*) than the narrower Deaver retractor. The small Heaney retractor is lightweight, has a short, unobtrusive handle, and can be very helpful during colporrhaphy. The long-handled Heaney retractor can be particularly helpful during vaginal hysterectomy, however, in holding the bladder safely out of harm's way after the anterior vesicouterine peritoneal fold has been identified and opened (Fig. 7-3, *G*).

There are Breisky-Navratil retractors in an almost infinite assortment of sizes (Fig. 7-3, *B, C, D, E*). They are commonly used in vaginal surgery on the European continent but are not as well known in the United States. Having an assortment of these retractors in varying widths and depths immediately available helps to ensure effective retraction in a wide variety of clinical circumstances.

When the handle of a retractor is parallel to the blade, it may be grasped easily and securely, much like a dagger.

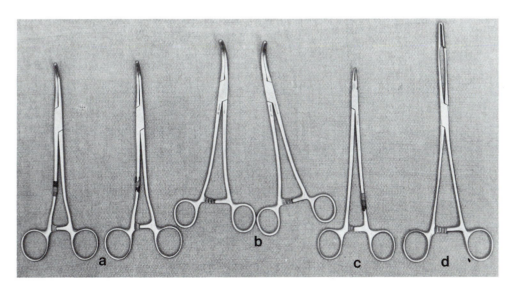

Fig. 7-5. Clamps and needleholders. **A,** Heaney-Ballantine hysterectomy forceps. **B,** Pair of Heaney-Glenner hysterectomy forceps, with right and left curve. **C,** Heaney needleholder. **D,** Krobach mouse-toothed clamp. (From *Instruments and sutures.* In Nichols DH, Randall CL: *Vaginal surgery,* ed 3, Baltimore, 1989, Williams & Wilkins.)

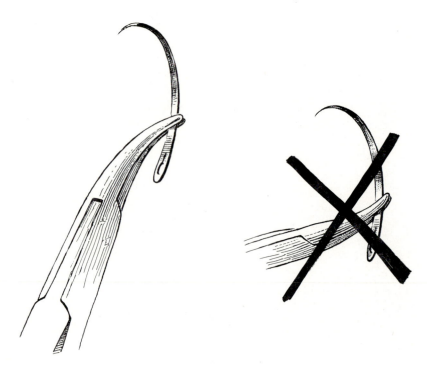

Fig. 7-6. Correct *(left)* and incorrect *(right)* ways to grasp the needle with a Heaney needleholder. (From *Instruments and sutures.* In Nichols DH, Randall CL: *Vaginal surgery,* ed 3, Baltimore, 1989, Williams & Wilkins.)

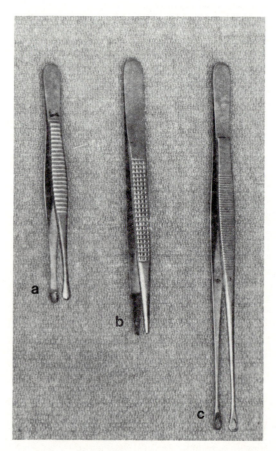

Fig. 7-7. Tissue forceps. **A,** Russian. **B,** Bonney. **C,** Singley. (From *Instruments and sutures.* In Nichols DH, Randall CL: *Vaginal surgery,* ed 3, Baltimore, 1989, Williams & Wilkins.)

Moreover, such a grasp is comfortable, reduces the tendency toward retractor slippage or wandering, and does not obstruct the surgical team's view of the operative field. The use of a flat-bladed retractor, which should be held as shown in Fig. 7-8, may provide even greater exposure into the depths of the wound (Fig. 7-9).

Although the 28-cm Deschamps ligature carrier for the right hand is particularly useful during a right sacrospinous colpopexy procedure, it is also useful during oophorectomy. Its tip curves in a clockwise direction. The tip of a left-handed Deschamps carrier, useful for a left sacrospinous colpopexy curves in a counterclockwise direction. The blunt point tends to push adjacent blood vessels to one side and is less likely to cause lacerations than is a sharp-pointed needle. It is wise to have as an accessory a long hook to grasp the suture after it has penetrated the tissue.

Like the tips of a pair of scissors, the blade of the scalpel should function as if it were an extension of the operator's fingers. A proper position for holding the scalpel to make an incision is noted in Fig. 7-10. For fine dissection, in contrast, the scalpel can be held between the thumb and the first and second fingers, much in the fashion by which a pencil would be held. Delicacy in applying the scalpel blade to the tissue being dissected requires that the cutting surface of the blade be passed over the tissue many times until the precise separation between tissues has been achieved.

Because the average operating room setup is far more likely to have right-handed surgeons and therefore, right-handed scissors than it is to have left-handed surgeons and

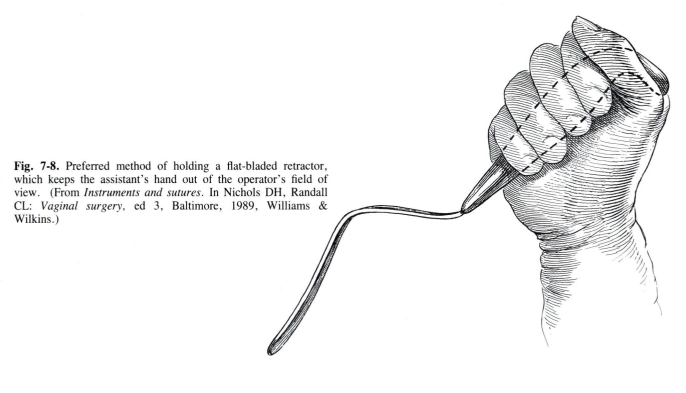

Fig. 7-8. Preferred method of holding a flat-bladed retractor, which keeps the assistant's hand out of the operator's field of view. (From *Instruments and sutures.* In Nichols DH, Randall CL: *Vaginal surgery,* ed 3, Baltimore, 1989, Williams & Wilkins.)

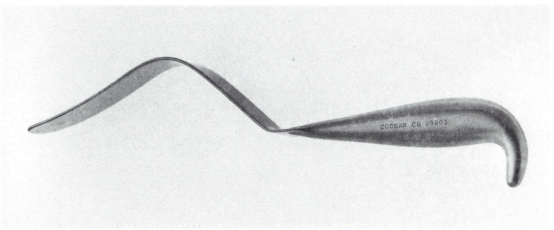

Fig. 7-9. Flat-bladed vaginal retractor CD 1106 or 098034, available in various sizes from custom order department, Codman-Shurtleff, New Bedford, MA 02745, or from Mr. William Merz, Baxter V Mueller, Chicago, IL 60648. (From *Instruments and sutures.* In Nichols DH, Randall CL: *Vaginal surgery,* ed 3, Baltimore, 1989, Williams & Wilkins.)

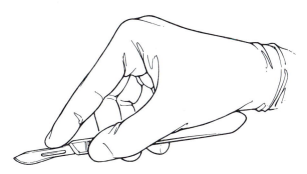

Fig 7-10. A proper position for holding the scalpel to make an incision is identified. The index finger makes pressure against the blade.

scissors, it is more important for the left-handed surgeon to learn to cut with right-handed scissors, which are always available, than for the right-handed surgeon to learn to cut with left-handed scissors, which are rarely available.

SUTURES

Hermann described the basic requirements for sutures to be used in the closing of surgical wounds as follows[1]:

The purpose of a surgical suture is to maintain approximation of tissues until the healing process has progressed to the point where artificial support is no longer necessary for the wound to resist normal stresses. Beyond this point, the sutures serve no useful purpose, and may, in fact, be the source of irritation or serve as a nidus for persistent infection. Thus, the ideal suture should persist and maintain tensile strength until the tissue has healed sufficiently, and then disappear.

Suture materials

Chromic catgut has been the traditional choice for suture material in the past, but the delayed absorption of the new synthetic suture materials (e.g., polyglycolic acid [Dexon] and polyglactin [Vicryl]) makes them clearly superior to similar sizes of chromic catgut. The newer synthetic sutures are strong, which enables the surgeon to use smaller sizes, and they appear to remain stable, even when infection occurs. Braided polyglycolic acid–type sutures retain much of their tensile strength for up to a month postoperatively, and the even newer longer-lasting absorbable sutures (e.g., monofilament polydioxanone [PDS] or polyglyconate [Maxon]) seem to remain strong for up to 3 months. Because these synthetic sutures remain strong in the tissue in which they are placed longer than catgut does, wound healing progresses further before they are absorbed. In addition, there is less tissue reaction to synthetic suture during healing, resulting in a stronger scar. Finally, there is a marked reduction in the formation of postoperative vaginal granulation tissue when synthetic sutures are used.

Polybutester (Novafil) is a unique copolymer monofilament nonabsorbable synthetic suture material that has the unique qualities of high breaking strength, similar to that of similar-sized nylon, combined with stretchability proportional to the force applied, and prompt elastic recovery. It is twice as flexible as nylon or polypropylene of similar size, yet secure knots can be formed with three or four throws. These qualities, particularly that of elastic stretching once it is in place, make it ideal for wound closure, especially when a single buried layer technique is chosen. As postoperative edema and swelling develop in the tissues in which the suture is placed, the suture stretches temporarily up to 10% to 15% of its length, to lessen the chance that it will tear or strangulate the tissues in which it has been placed. As postoperative edema and swelling subside, the suture stretching contracts, taking up any slack that was produced, and holding the tissues in approximation during their long healing phase. This should lessen the chance of postoperative wound dehiscence. Dehiscence unrelated to suture breakage occurs not at the suture site itself, but lateral to the suture line.[5,6]

The knot pull strength of suture material is important (Fig. 7-11) because it takes valuable time to replace sutures that break while being tied. Routine use of the larger,

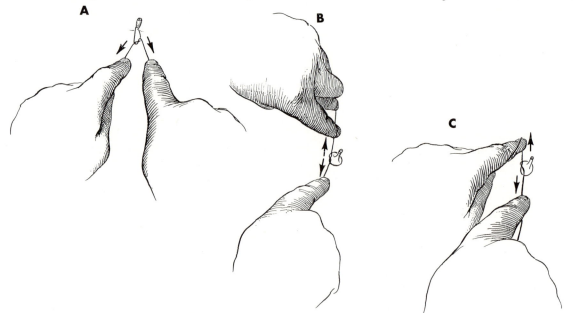

Fig. 7-11. Knot tying. **A,** Traction to both ends of suture toward operator and against point to be ligated is incorrect and dangerous because there is considerable risk of pulling thread and knot off point or vessel being tied. **B,** Instead, traction should be applied to each thread in an equal and opposite direction around the point of ligation. **C,** Deep within a body cavity, tips of index fingers safely provide the fulcrum, lessening the chance of slippage or avulsion. (From *Instruments and sutures.* In Nichols DH, Randall CL: *Vaginal surgery,* ed 3, Baltimore, 1989, Williams & Wilkins.)

stronger sizes of suture material has distinct disadvantages, however. Not only does its greater strength increase the risk of tissue injury—because it permits the knots to be tied too tightly without breaking—but because the larger sizes incite more intensive phagocytic activity, they may not retain their tensile strength any longer than do the smaller sizes. Thus the use of larger sizes of suture may actually result in a weaker scar than that associated with the use of smaller sizes. In most situations, 0 or 2-0 suture is sufficient, although 3-0 or 4-0 suture is occasionally preferable, particularly in fistula repair.

Technique of suturing

There are various methods of suture placement in bringing two edges together. The surgeon may use either a curved needle or a straight needle. The choice depends both on the tension to which the layer is likely to be subjected and on the importance of the layer in providing essential wound support. Some methods clearly take up greater tissue slack than others and thus influence vaginal size when used during colporrhaphy.

When a curved needle has been passed through the patient's tissue, it should be grasped proximal to the point with a tissue forceps or hemostat. If the needle is curved, it should not be pulled straight through, but rather pulled in the direction of the curve of the needle. This avoids bending or breaking the needle and, equally important, avoids inflicting unnecessary damage or tearing of the soft tissue through which the needle has been placed. This pull-through in a curve is accomplished by a twist of the wrist in the direction of the curve, a maneuver similar in concept to that of the follow through of the arm following a golf or tennis swing.

Surgical glove perforation places the surgeon at risk for blood-borne infectious diseases. In one study[8] the overall perforation rate was measured at 13.3%, 62% of which were unrecognized during the surgical procedure. Most perforations occurred in the gloved fingers of the nondominant hand, suggesting perforation due to direct grasping of the needle. More frequent use of tissue forceps to grasp the needle should reduce this incidence. Among 2166 operations in another study[4] there was an incidence of 5.5% inadvertent injuries, of which 95% were a result of needle sticks. Most occurred at the time of wound closing, and 72.3% occurred on the left hand. Visible blood has been reported found on the hands of 38% of gynecologic surgeons wearing single gloves, but on only 2% of double-gloved surgeons.[1] Double gloving does offer significantly increased protection against needle puncture during surgery, and thus offers some measure of protection against exposure to unexpected AIDS or hepatitis infection.

When double gloves are worn it is more comfortable for the surgeon if one of the pairs is a half size larger than that regularly worn. The larger sized glove is donned first, over which the surgeon puts on the glove of the usual size.

A cut-resistant glove liner made of extended-chain polyethylene has been developed to be worn between two layers of sterile latex gloves, and has been recommended for surgeons who are at high risk of injury from cuts and abrasions, though the liner did not provide protection against needle puncture.[2]

The epithelial trauma of through-and-through suture placement, which penetrates the full thickness of the wound, may release collagenase and interfere with healing.[7] Ascorbic acid antagonizes the elaboration of collagenase, so the systemic administration of vitamin C will favor healing and strong wound scarring. The subepithelial placement of sutures probably reduces this trauma, which is one reason that subcuticular closure of the vaginal wall and of the perineal skin is recommended. Another reason is that subcuticular sutures are less likely to be associated with postoperative granulation tissue than are through-and-through sutures. There are two methods of subcuticular suture placement (Fig. 7-12); the method chosen depends on

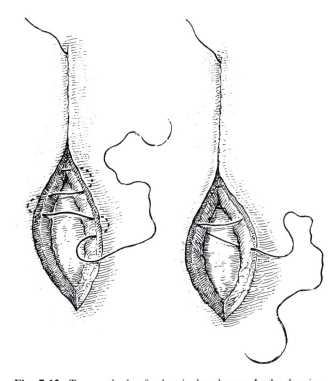

Fig. 7-12. Two methods of subcuticular closure. In the drawing to the right, the full thickness of the subepithelial layer is used by a spiral-type suture placement. This is particularly useful within the walls of the vagina, where maximum strength of this fibromuscular layer will provide essential support to a healing colporrhaphy. In the drawing to the left, a snakelike or zigzag suture placement is used immediately beneath the epithelial layer, which produces a superior cosmetic result. This is useful when subepithelial tissue layer strength is not a specific requirement and is particularly helpful in closing perineal skin or epithelial incisions elsewhere in the body. To avoid overlaps or wrinkling of skin edges, make each point of entry beneath the epithelial layer accurately opposite the point of emergence of the last suture on the opposite side of the incision. (From *Instruments and sutures.* In Nichols DH, Randall CL: *Vaginal surgery,* ed 3, Baltimore, 1989, Williams & Wilkins.)

whether the full thickness of the subepithelial tissue is to be used to provide maximum strength or whether the goal is close approximation of the most superficial layer for the best cosmetic effect.

It is important to pull up the slack in the suture before tying the knot in order to ensure the precise apposition of the tissues. Any failure to approximate the tissues properly creates a suture bridge and greatly weakens the scar (Fig. 7-13). The knots must be tied square, beginning with the first cast, or the suture may fray and break. In tying a square knot, the first cast may loosen, but the second cast

will slide down and remain in place if the operator applies tension on one end of the suture, during knot tying.

In a surgeon's knot, a double turn with the first cast will remain in place; after the second cast the knot will slide down no farther. A third cast for safety is common. Learning to use the newer synthetic sutures may require some knot-tying practice. For example, monofilament sutures need an extra turn to the first cast for knot security, plus three or four additional standard casts.

When closing a hollow viscus such as the bladder or the bowel, the surgeon may place sutures either into the wall

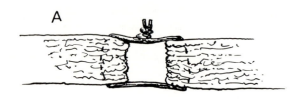

Fig. 7-13. Failure to approximate tissue layers directly during reconstruction gives rise to a suture bridge, often productive of a weak scar, particularly when there is any tension upon layers being approximated **(A). B,** Desirable result of layer approximation, which provides opportunity for strong scar development between edges of closely approximated tissues. (From *Instruments and sutures.* In Nichols DH, Randall CL: *Vaginal surgery,* ed 3, Baltimore, 1989, Williams & Wilkins.)

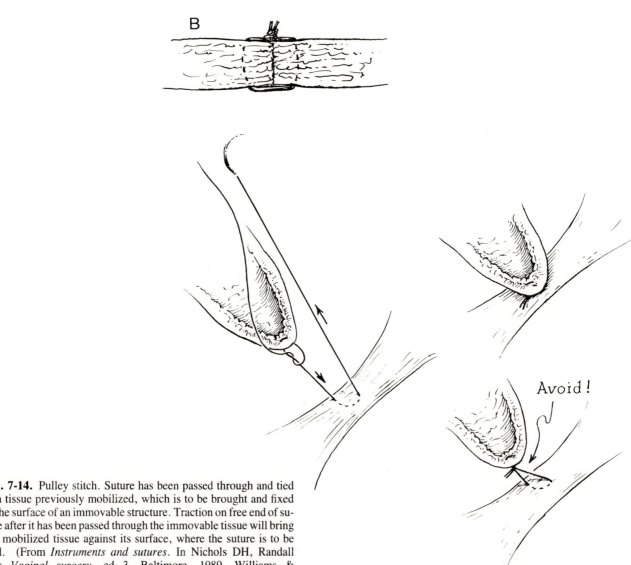

Fig. 7-14. Pulley stitch. Suture has been passed through and tied to a tissue previously mobilized, which is to be brought and fixed to the surface of an immovable structure. Traction on free end of suture after it has been passed through the immovable tissue will bring the mobilized tissue against its surface, where the suture is to be tied. (From *Instruments and sutures.* In Nichols DH, Randall CL: *Vaginal surgery,* ed 3, Baltimore, 1989, Williams & Wilkins.)

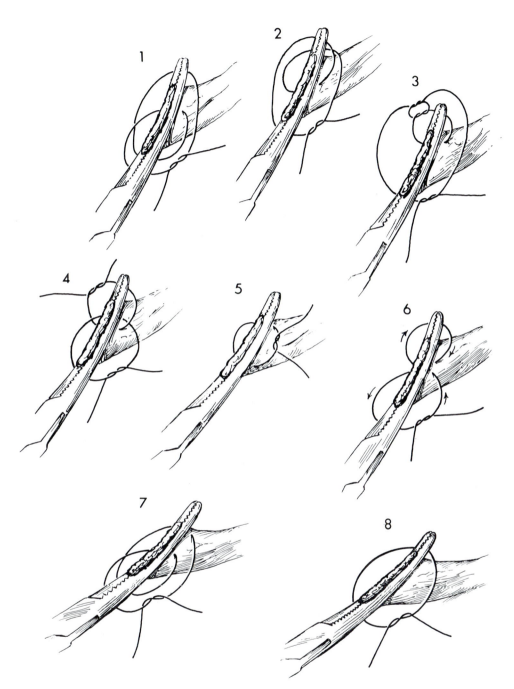

Fig. 7-15. Suture ligation of a pedicle. *1*, There is a single needle penetration of the pedicle, but the base is doubly ligated; *2*, toe is doubly ligated (recommended for the infundibulopelvic ligament, reinforced by a free tie); *3*, after a small loop over toe of hemostat has been tied, a second loop goes around entire pedicle; *4*, interlocking loops provide security but require a double penetration of pedicle by needle; *5*, double penetration leaves a small portion unligated; *6*, provides security but also requires a double penetration; *7*, the Heaney stitch fixes the suture at two points—the Heaney stitch is especially useful for the cardinal or uterosacral ligament and is unlikely to slip, but requires a double penetration of the pedicle; *8*, a single free tie, which is most likely to slip under certain circumstances. (Reproduced with permission of the American College of Surgeons from Nichols DH: A technique for vaginal oophorectomy, *Surg Gynecol Obstet* 147:765, 1978.)

or through the wall and may tie the knots either inside (bladder) or outside (rectum) the lumen. A second intramural layer of suture serves to reduce tension on the first layer. The mucosal layer may be included or excluded. Separate sutures may be used in the mucosa if mucosal hemostasis is required.

A pulley stitch is appropriate when it is necessary to bring one fixed tissue and one movable tissue together within a cavity or confined space (Fig. 7-14). Traction on the free end of the pulley stitch, which must be through the fixed tissue, will bring the movable tissue (through which the suture has been passed and tied) to the fixed tissue. Bringing the tissues into direct contact with one another results in a firm, strong scar.

There are several methods for the suture ligation of a pedicle (Fig. 7-15). Factors such as the contents of the pedicle, the risk of slippage, the tension to which the suture will be subject, and its surgical accessibility determine the appropriate method in a particular instance.

Surgeons improve their technical facility in surgery if they learn to use both hands equally well. An acquired skill that requires frequent practice, this technical ambidexterity is especially helpful in the placement of sutures, the application and removal of hemostatic forceps, and knot tying.

Relationship of sutures to wound healing

Although tissue reaction to a suture material is proportional to the bulk of the suture material in the wound, this reaction does not determine the strength of a surgical wound closure. The strength of a closure is equal to the strength of the scar plus the strength of the suture material. Immediately after closure of the wound and for the next 3 or 4 days, however, the suture material provides all the strength. This strength is approximately 40% of the strength of the tissues before surgery. As healing continues and scar tissue forms, the strength increases. The suture material becomes superfluous when the wound has healed and a strong scar has formed.

A wound that does not become infected is approximately one third healed by the sixth postoperative day, two thirds by the tenth. The remaining one third of healing may require several months. Many factors, including the degree of tension applied to the margins of the wound, the biochemistry and physical condition of the particular patient, and the type of suture material used, may produce variances from these generalizations.[7]

If infection occurs, sutures may be absorbed with unusual speed; in fact, they may be absorbed so quickly that they fail to provide adequate support during the initial, critical healing period. When the suture material is nonabsorbable, infection may lead to postoperative formation of a sinus. The suture behaves as an infected foreign body, and the sinus closes only after the suture is extruded or surgically removed.

REFERENCES

1. Cohn GM, Seifer DB: Blood exposure in single versus double gloving during pelvic surgery. *Am J Obstet Gynecol* 162:715, 1990.
2. Diaz-Buxo JA: Cut resistant glove liner for medical use. *Surg Gynecol Obstet* 172:312, 1991.
3. Hermann JB: Changes in tensile strength and knot security of surgical procedures in vivo. *Arch Surg* 106:707, 1973.
4. Hussain SA, Latif ABA, Choudhary AA: Risks to surgeons: a survey of accidental injuries during operations. *Br J Surg* 75:324, 1988.
5. Rodeheaver GT, Nesbit WS, Edlich RF: Novafil—a dynamic suture for wound closure. *Ann Surg* 204:193, 1986.
6. Rodeheaver GT et al: Unique performance characteristics of Novafil. *Surg Gynecol Obstet* 164:230, 1987.
7. Sanz L, Smith S: *Mechanisms of wound healing, suture material, and wound closure*. In Sanz LE, editor: *Gynecologic surgery*, Oradell, NJ, 1988, Medical Economics Books.
8. Serrano CW, Wright JW, Newton ER: Surgical glove perforation in obstetrics. *Obstet Gynecol* 77:525, 1991.

Chapter 8

INTRAOPERATIVE AND POSTOPERATIVE COMPLICATIONS

David H. Nichols

Efforts to prevent intraoperative and postoperative complications must begin preoperatively. Immediately before the start of a surgical procedure, the surgeon should review the hospital record to refresh his or her memory about significant points in the patient's history, preoperative laboratory findings, and the recommendations of consultants. This review should include the findings of medical students, house officers, fellows, and referring physicians. When specific changes in the usual preoperative preparation of the patient are indicated, the surgeon should confirm that they have been performed.

There are three general categories of complications: intraoperative, early postoperative, and late postoperative complications.

INTRAOPERATIVE COMPLICATIONS

Aside from the problems that may arise in association with the administration of anesthesia, intraoperative complications are related principally to hemorrhage or to accidental injury of adjacent organs or tissues.

Intraoperative hemorrhage

In the evaluation and control of hemorrhage, the operator must first differentiate between venous bleeding, which can usually be controlled by extrinsic pressure, and arterial bleeding, which requires prompt and accurate ligation or electrocoagulation. When ligation at the point of bleeding is not possible, ligation should be performed at a site proximal to the site of bleeding. The operator should inform the anesthesiologist that transfusion may be necessary if blood loss becomes excessive. Because blood loss tends to be directly proportional to the duration of the operative procedure, time-saving surgical efficiency is obviously important.

There are three most probable sites for the development of intraoperative pelvic hemorrhage. The first is from the ovarian pedicle. When an ovarian arterial tie is effective, the vessel bleeds. As a retroperitoneal hematoma forms, the stump of the artery retracts. To secure hemostasis the ovarian artery should be reclamped and tied at a high level within the pelvis, often just below the origin of the renal artery. Another source of intraoperative hemorrhage is from the cut edge of the vaginal vault following hysterectomy. If this occurs following transabdominal hysterectomy, one should study the vaginal cuff by applying upward tension and traction to it. A bleeding vessel can be identified and clamped and tied. Following vaginal hysterectomy, traction to the adnexal pedicle upward and laterally simultaneously with downward traction to the cardinal-uterosacral pedicle of the opposite side in the opposite direction will reveal the bleeding point which can be clamped and tied. If it is not obvious, traction is released and is then applied in an opposite direction to the contralateral pedicles. The third site of bleeding in the pelvis is from a branch of the internal iliac artery. A hematoma forms rapidly, and hemostasis is best achieved by ligation of the internal iliac artery lateral to the hematoma.

The treatment of uncontrolled genital hemorrhage involves tamponade and packing. In rare circumstances, the umbrella pack (Logothetopolous tampon) may be necessary.[6] A gauze veil is filled with packing, and the tails of the veil are lead through the vagina to the vulva. They are inserted through the central opening of a ring pessary and considerable traction applied to the tails sufficient for the body of the "tampon" to compress any bleeding vessels against the pelvic side wall. A clamp across the tails just outside the ring sustains the pressure against the side wall. The ring and clamp used in an umbrella pack are removed in 12 hours. The surface veil may be left in place for several days, although the gradual removal of its interior packing may begin 24 hours after insertion of the pack. Often, the application of traction by means of a twisting motion facilitates the removal of the remaining packing or "veil" after several days.

Accidental injury to adjacent structures

Operative injuries to the bladder will be described and their treatment detailed in Chapter 51.

When the urine is grossly bloody postoperatively and there was no apparent injury of the bladder, the operator should decompress the bladder by catheter drainage. Generally speaking, unless there has been significant damage to the bladder wall, hematuria clears grossly within 48 hours and microscopically within 72 hours. If the urine is not clear after 72 hours, the patient should be examined cystoscopically to investigate the possibility of bladder laceration or trauma, such as unrecognized suture penetration of the bladder wall, and to arrange for surgical removal of the suture, or for it to be cut through the operating cystoscope. Because an empty bladder has a remarkable capacity to heal itself, even after unrepaired cystotomy, continuous catheter drainage usually permits a fresh wound to heal spontaneously when adequate surgical exposure is not feasible. If the traumatized bladder is permitted to distend, however, a pinpoint opening may fail to close or may even enlarge and, when epithelialized, give rise to a fistula.

The operator who suspects that the mucosa or wall of the rectum has been penetrated should immediately insert a finger in the rectum to determine whether such a penetration has indeed occurred. Any demonstrable defect should be repaired. After the repair, 3 days of clear liquid postoperative diet followed by a low-residue diet may be desirable during the first postoperative week, with a rectal tube gently inserted if gas pains or distention develop. The patient should use a stool softener and a gentle laxative for several weeks postoperatively.

In all instances of accidental trauma, the patient should be informed of the unexpected injury and its repair so that she understands the important details of her operation and the need for special postoperative care, perhaps making her convalescence different from others thought by the patient to have had "the same operation."

EARLY POSTOPERATIVE COMPLICATIONS

The operator should perform a gentle bimanual examination at the completion of every vaginal operation, not only to detect swelling or hematoma, but also to determine if the reconstruction has been successful. It is necessary to correct any undesirable ridge in the posterior vaginal wall immediately, even if correcting it requires reopening the posterior vaginal incision. Such a ridge is likely to become more fibrotic and more tender as time goes on, causing discomfort or dyspareunia in the future. Similarly, the operator should approach any undesirable vaginal stricture or stenosis aggressively and immediately. These complications result either from the excision of too much vaginal membrane at the time of surgery or from excessive plication of slack in the subepithelial fibromuscular connective tissues.

Relaxing incisions in the lateral walls of the vagina on one or both sides will correct vaginal stenosis. If simple incisions do not provide adequate relaxation, the vaginal wall may be undermined for a distance of 1 cm along the margins of each incision.. The epithelium need not be closed, but it is advisable to insert a secure intravaginal pack and to leave it in place for 2 days; then, the regular insertion of a vaginal obturator is helpful until healing is satisfactory. If, on the other hand, the relaxation provided by the incisions appears excessive, the defect created in the lateral walls of the vagina may be filled with a full-thickness portion of the patient's own vaginal wall that was excised at the time of colporrhaphy, wrapped in sterile sponges soaked with saline, and retained on the nurse's instrument stand for possible grafting later in the procedure

If the inspection carried out at the conclusion of a vaginal operation reveals that persistent blood loss is excessive, hemostasis is necessary. If venous oozing is significant during the first 24 postoperative hours, the vagina should be packed with gauze. This packing not only acts as a wick in soaking up the blood or serum that would otherwise accumulate, but also gently tamponades the operative site and compresses the connective tissue spaces. Appreciable bleeding through a pack usually indicates unsecured hemostasis of some significance and should be investigated by examination of the patient in the lithotomy position with good lighting and suitable relaxation. When the bleeding point is found, it should be promptly ligated.

The patient who has a vaginal pack in place usually experiences some difficulty in voiding and needs an indwelling Foley catheter. Unless the bladder has undergone some trauma or surgical repair, the catheter should be removed at the same time that the intravaginal packing is removed. The patient may use the bathroom then, but daily palpation of the lower abdomen and careful recording of the patient's voiding pattern should continue during the early postoperative period.

As a last step of a vaginal operation, the operator should perform a gentle rectal examination, before the patient has left the operating table and before she is fully awake, to identify any unsuspected damage that requires repair. It is essential to search carefully for any stitches that may have penetrated the rectal mucosa. Any such penetrating stitch that is found should be exposed with adequate retraction and cut on the luminal side so that the loose ends retract into the wall of the rectum, where they are unlikely to cause any postoperative difficulty.

Finally, the operator should dictate a description of the surgical procedure promptly—before the details that may later assume considerable importance become less clear or are forgotten.

Intestinal paralysis

Significant intestinal paralysis is more common after abdominal surgery than after vaginal surgery. Patients who have undergone a vaginal procedure generally resume a normal fluid intake and a regular diet soon after postoperative nausea subsides. Moving about, both in and out of bed; taking frequent sips of water; and, although the patient is seldom hungry, eating small amounts of solid food from time to time usually initiate peristalsis. If postoperative distention and ileus develop, several additional days are required for a return to normal. If gastric dilation with nausea and vomiting develops, treatment involves nasogastric decompression with an appropriate increase in intravenous fluids. As long as the abdomen is tympanitic, distended, and relatively silent to auscultation, intravenous feedings should continue. Peristalsis eventually returns, coincident with the expulsion of flatus.

Intestinal obstruction

In a peritoneal cavity, local adhesions create a fixed point for torsion and subsequent obstruction of the intestine. Small adhesions may be divided to prevent subsequent small bowel obstruction, but peritoneal adhesions with extensive matting of the small bowel should be left alone if obstruction has not occured, lest injury of the bowel wall occur, with fistula formation.[42]

Generally, a small bowel obstruction results from a pathologic fixation and kinking of a loop of small intestine, sometimes because of a misplaced stitch, but more often because of an attachment of the small intestine to a devitalized tissue surface. Kinking from traction on an unfreed adhesion of bowel to adnexa can also produce an obstruction of the small bowel. Obstruction is more common when intraperitoneal manipulations have been extensive or when the patient has adhesions from previous intraabdominal surgery. Therefore, patients who have undergone surgery in the past should be watched with particular concern during the first postoperative week, even after the resumption of normal peristalsis and bowel function.

At first, postoperative obstruction is usually partial, and the patient may complain only of anorexia and intermittent colicky pain. Tachycardia may occur with only a mild temperature elevation, but peristalsis is usually hyperactive. A radiograph (flat plate) of the abdomen is desirable at this point, and the attending physician should consider intravenous feeding and intestinal decompression. Partial obstruction that is aggravated by postoperative edema responds to conservative management, and bowel function gradually returns to normal; improvement is evident within 2 or 3 days in the majority of cases.

When intestinal obstruction does not improve spontaneously, the condition of the patient soon changes and complete obstruction may supervene. Symptoms include projectile vomiting, more frequent and severe crampy abdominal pain, and waves of audible hyperperistalsis coincident with the height of the crampy pain. The patient appears acutely ill, becomes mildly shocky, and develops severe electrolyte disturbances. Radiographic studies are diagnostic, and laparotomy must be performed for surgical relief as soon as intravenous feeding and gastric decompression have resolved the patient's electrolyte imbalance and dehydration. Clinical deterioration can occur within hours. Thus, a 1- or 2-day delay in the diagnosis and treatment of complete intestinal obstruction may result in the patient's death.

Usually, the site of the obstruction is readily apparent at laparotomy, and the operator can dissect the bowel from the point to which it has become adherent by simple finger separation. The operator should carefully inspect the involved loop of bowel to ensure its viability, however, and should observe the tissue for several minutes to be certain that both color and peristalsis return. If they do not, resection of the loop may be necessary. If the obstruction cannot be found with ease, the operator should perform a running inspection of the intestines, beginning with the distal segment of collapsed bowel.

If excessive balloonlike intestinal dilation is obscuring the operative field, the operator may need to decompress the intestine by means of a large-bore hypodermic needle to which suction tubing has been attached. After decompression, the operator removes the needle and closes the point of penetration with a pursestring suture of fine chromic catgut or polyglycolic suture on an atraumatic or intestinal needle.[14] When, because of the critical nature of the patient's condition, there is no time for adequate exploration and possible resection, an enterostomy proximal to the point of obstruction may be indicated. The surgeon should avoid extensive handling of the multiple loops of distended bowel during this procedure.

Postoperative Oliguria

The usual postoperative urinary output is 1 cc per minute; output less than ½ cc per minute (30 ml per hour) should be investigated and a determination made as to whether the cause of the oliguria is *prerenal* (hypovolemia due secondarily to decreased renal perfusion), *renal* (acute tubular necrosis), or *postrenal* (ureteral obstruction).

In prerenal oliguria, the urine specific gravity is high and the urine sodium is very low. With acute tubular necrosis, the ability to concentrate urine is lost and the specific gravity is 10.10 or lower with a rising urine sodium. The treatment of the former is to add parenteral fluids immediately, and if this is not rapidly successful, a dose of 100 ml of 20% Mannitol. If this is not effective, 40 mg of Furosemide can be given intravenously in an attempt to generate some urinary output. The use of Mannitol may decrease intrarenal vascular spasms and prevent the onset of acute tubular necrosis.

With acute tubular necrosis, one must not flood the patient with parenteral fluids lest one risk acute pulmonary edema. The serum potassium gradually rises with progressive oliguria, and any urinary tract infection should be evaluated with cultures and treated appropriately. If the patient fails to respond indicating renal failure, hemodialysis may be required.[36] Postrenal oliguria is generally caused by ureteral obstruction, which should promptly be diagnosed by an immediate infusion intravenous pyelogram and placement of retrograde ureteral catheters with deligation as necessary,[16] or at the least, a percutaneous nephrostomy.

Older patients tend to lose their sense of thirst with ageing and may thus live in a state of chronic dehydration and hemoconcentration. At the time of surgery this is overcome by hydration during anesthesia, and in the immediate postoperative period this may give rise to a hemodilution reflected as a drop in hemoglobin and hematocrit noted on the first or second postoperative day. After a few days and the resumption of the usual reduced voluntary fluid intake, the hemoconcentration tends to return producing an unexpected rise in the recorded values of hemoglobin and hematocrit of specimens taken beyond the fourth postoperative day.

Postoperative fever

Most often, postoperative fever originates from the problem areas called the "five Ws": wind (pulmonary), water (urinary), wound (abscess), walk (phlebitis), and wonder drugs (drug reactions). As Cruse[9] noted, a major temperature elevation during the first 48 postoperative hours suggests atelectasis, especially if the patient is a heavy smoker. Prompt physiotherapy with an emphasis on incentive spirometry and prolonged inspiration is the backbone of early treatment. Onset of fever during the third postoperative day is usually the result of a urinary infection. Fever beginning between the third and fifth day is likely caused by infection of the wound at the time of surgery. Septic thrombophlebitis may be the explanation for fever arising between the third and seventh postoperative day; pulmonary embolism is a likely possibility for fever that appears between the tenth and fourteenth day.

Fever that persists beyond the first and second postoperative days is likely to be from an infection within the pelvis, often within the site of an unsuspected pelvic hematoma. Prompt, gentle daily palpation of the abdomen for tenderness or masses and gentle bimanual examination of the pelvis are indicated.

Postoperative infection

Antibiotics are not substitutes for sloppy surgical technique. The peritoneal cavity may resist infection, but the subcutaneous fat in the incision is susceptible to infection. The surgeon must protect subcutaneous tissues against contamination.

The occurrence of postoperative infection is directly proportional to the length of the operative procedure; the risk of infection generally increases when the duration of surgery exceeds 2 hours. Careful anatomic dissection (which minimizes trauma), adequate hemostasis, and pro-

vision for drainage (when indicated) can help to minimize the risk of infection. When the surgeon expects to enter the peritoneal cavity during the course of the transvaginal operation or, less commonly, to involve connective tissue spaces (e.g., the pararectal, prevesical, or retrorectal spaces) that, although extraperitoneal, are relatively inaccessible and have no natural path of drainage to the outside, the use of an appropriate broad-spectrum antibiotic, given an hour before surgery and repeated if the operation is longer than 2 hours in duration, is also helpful. Postoperative lavage appears to be of no value even when conducted with antibiotics.

Infection may follow inappropriate timing for the administration of preoperative "prophylactic" antibiotics in which the administration was either too soon or too late, resulting in an inadequate serum and tissue level at the time of surgery.[10,11]

The incidence of posthysterectomy abscess of the vaginal cuff is less if the cuff is left open at the time of hysterectomy.

An elevation in the patient's evening temperature may be the earliest objective evidence that an infection is developing. The attending physician should begin daily percussion of the costovertebral angles the evening of the day of surgery and should promptly investigate any unilateral discrepancy by infusion pyelography. If there are no other findings, unexplained ileus suggests unilateral ureteral ligation, and the physician should order an intravenous pyelogram immediately. Patients with a history of urinary tract infections are at particular risk of developing an infection that involves the urinary system after a surgical procedure.

Premenopausal women have a greater risk of infection after vaginal surgery than do postmenopausal women, probably because of the greater vascularity of the premenopausal woman's tissues and, thus, the greater probability of a hematoma that may become a focus of infection. In addition, premenopausal women are likely to be more active sexually, which increases vaginal bacterial contamination. As a result, the vaginal flora includes more types of organisms that can proliferate under the conditions present after vaginal surgery in the premenopausal woman.

Abscess formation. The physician who suspects that an abscess has formed, which is a common occurrence, can investigate by rectal examination and gentle digital exploration of the vaginal vault. Most abscesses point to and drain into the vault, as evidenced by a sudden seropurulent discharge followed by almost immediate clinical improvement. Gentle digital probing of the suture lines in the vagina over a period of several days facilitates drainage of those that do not drain spontaneously. A culture and sensitivity study of any appreciable exudate is desirable.

Incisional abscesses should be drained as soon as they are fluctuant. The wound will usually cleanse itself within four days of drainage, favoring early closure and a faster convalescence. Once these have been drained, an early closure is recommended without subcutaneous approximation. When a wound has broken down, and after any debridement that was necessary has been accomplished, the surgeon may be waiting for healing by secondary intention. This process of healing can be speeded by daily applications to the open wound of grocery store honey, which is clearly bacteriostatic and will hasten considerably the process of healing.[8,24]

When an abscess cavity involves or is adjacent to the pelvic peritoneum, signs of pelvic peritonitis such as lower abdominal distention, lower abdominal pain, anorexia, and depressed peristalsis may appear. Although an adnexal abscess seldom develops after vaginal surgery, the presence of a unilateral pelvic mass in a patient who has been ovulating regularly suggests this possibility. Relatively late development, sometimes days or weeks after discharge from the hospital, is almost characteristic of this complication. Ledger and associates[20] emphasized that the "diagnostic possibility of an adnexal abscess should be considered in any febrile patient readmitted after a recent pelvic operation." Such adnexal abscesses localize relatively high in the pelvis and may not be palpable; however, they may be identified by ultrasound or compute tomography (CT) scan.[18] Spontaneous drainage through the vaginal vault is unlikely, and transabdominal salpingo-oophorectomy is usually required.

Infection is of particular concern when the patient has a body temperature of 103° F or higher, together with a white blood cell count higher than 15,000 or less than 4000/mm³. Under such circumstances, any purulent exudate should be cultured for both aerobic and anaerobic organisms, and serious consideration should be given to the administration of antibiotics or antibacterials with anaerobic coverage. Usually, anaerobic bacterioid infections are foul-smelling and produce characteristic systemic reactions. Antibiotics that will penetrate an abscess include clindamycin, cefamandole, cefoxitin, and metronidazole.

Septic shock. When a patient goes into a shocklike state postoperatively, even though there is no sign of blood loss, the physician should consider the possibility of septic shock. Peripheral vascular collapse from endotoxins often results in subnormal temperature, hypotension, metabolic acidosis, oliguria, and mental confusion. Transfusion produces no response. Once the intravenous infusion of fluids has overcome the peripheral circulatory collapse—ideally, monitored by central venous pressure or pulmonary wedge pressure measurements—treatment may include the administration of norepinephrine, dopamine, and large doses of an appropriate antibiotic. The physician should search for an abscess cavity. Ultrasound or CT scan studies may be helpful.[18] When found, an abscess should be cultured and excised or drained.

Necrotizing fasciitis. Rare, serious, virulent, and toxic infections, necrotizing fasciitis and synergistic bacterial gangrene can develop subcutaneously at any time.[22,23,30] The overlying skin becomes dark, bullae may be present, and thrombosis of nearby blood vessels may precipitate edema of the skin, rendering it anesthetic. Prompt recognition is essential. The primary treatment is surgical debridement, as extensive as is necessary to excise the bacterial inoculum completely. The infection may cause extensive subcutaneous fascial damage, but may spare the muscle.[4,5,21,37]

Hemorrhage in the early postoperative period

When postoperative bleeding occurs within the first 24 hours postoperatively, there will be signs of internal hemorrhage with dropping of the hematocrit. External bleeding will be obvious, but concealed internal bleeding will generally be from either the ovarian artery or a branch of the internal iliac. The patient should be promptly reoperated upon, and the bleeding vessel found and ligated. Be especially mindful of the position of the ureter, which may not be in its usual position, it should be separately identified to avoid its ligation.

When evidence of postoperative intraperitoneal bleeding is first found after the initial 24 hours from surgery, the patient can generally be treated by careful observation to determine possible progression of the hematoma, and the patient transfused and given antibiotics as necessary. A CT scan is a useful method of measuring the size of the hematoma, and an ultrasound evaluation will identify whether the mass is cystic or not. A persistant cystic mass that is retroperitoneal and has become infected can often be drained percutaneously under realtime ultrasound guidance.

Careful observation of the patient's vital signs during the first 2 postoperative days should reveal any intraperitoneal bleeding. It is important to monitor the patient's hemoglobin and hematocrit. The physician should suspect a coagulation defect if the patient shows unexpected ecchymoses or if a sample of venous blood fails to form a firm clot. The patient whose external blood loss is insignificant, but who seems to be bleeding persistently and is unusually restless should undergo laparotomy. Bleeding points should be identified and ligated, any hematoma should be evacuated, and the source of bleeding should be sought.

If intraabdominal hemorrhage has stabilized at the end of the first postoperative 24 hours and there is no evidence of further bleeding, operative intervention is seldom necessary unless a presumed hematoma becomes infected and requires drainage. Under unusual circumstances, such as the presence of shock due to blood loss or evidence of massive postoperative hemorrhage within the bases of the cardinal ligaments, aggressive surgery may be required. For example, although bilateral ligation of the hypogastric and ovarian arteries is not usually time-consuming, it can arrest an alarming rate of hemorrhage dramatically.[29]

Every gynecologic surgeon should have experience with the technique of transperitoneal bilateral hypogastric artery ligation, particularly when the technique can be readily learned by isolation of the hypogastric arteries on fresh autopsy material. Once the arteries have been found, the relevant surgical anatomy has been identified, the position of the ureter and the hypogastric vein has been clearly distinguished, and these structures have been excluded from the operative field, the surgeon places sutures for ligation around the hypogastric artery and below the origin of the superior gluteal artery. The surgeon then closes the overlying peritoneum with fine absorbable suture, taking care to avoid the nearby ureter.[29] Practice makes it convenient and easy to learn or to teach this procedure so that the operator is ready to use this technique when such a ligation is necessary in an emergency. Should this fail, percutaneous transcatheter embolization performed by a radiologist experienced in this technique may control massive hemorrhage.[15]

Externally evident hemorrhage after vaginal surgery is usually of extraperitoneal origin. When the blood loss approximates that seen with the menstrual period, firm vaginal packing is usually sufficient to achieve control. Surgical intervention may be necessary if such tamponade is inadequate and blood loss continues or accelerates, however. If hemorrhage occurs during the first postoperative day, the rapidity of blood loss is a reliable indication of the size of the vessel involved. Any suspicion that sustained intraperitoneal bleeding comes from an unsecured uterine or ovarian artery mandates a prompt surgical approach. Persistent transvaginal bleeding after a vaginal repair usually arises from a small artery in the edge of a vaginal incision.

When evidence of retroperitoneal bleeding is first noted 10 to 14 days after surgery, the patient generally should be readmitted to the hospital for observation. An examination under anesthesia may be useful. If there is evidence of continued bleeding but time is not of the essence, selective embolization may control the bleeding at its source[34] (see Chapter 14), or laparotomy may be required.

It is often difficult for the surgeon to accept postoperative bleeding to be the result of technical problems, and this may prolong the delay in reoperation for its control. One should set a limit on the number of transfusions for a given period of time while hematologic causes are ruled out. The decision to reoperate is best made during daylight hours.

Blood loss that occurs from the sixth to perhaps the fourteenth postoperative day most commonly results from a local infection that has hastened suture absorption or an abscess under pressure has eroded into an adjacent vascular bed. At this stage, tissues are edematous and friable, and any additional sutures placed will not be secure. Dissection destroys tissue planes and breaks up established barriers of "inflammatory membrane," thereby both disseminating the infection and increasing its clinical virulence. The possibility of undiagnosed diabetes should be investigated, and appropriate measures should be employed if the disease is found. Tight vaginal packing may control such bleeding, even in the presence of infection, and broad-spectrum antibiotics should be administered.

Local application of the microfibrillar collagen, Avitene, may be effective. It exerts its hemostatic effect by attracting functioning blood platelets that adhere to the microfibrils, triggering the formation of thrombi in the adjacent tissue. Because it can cause fibrosis that leads to ureteral obstruction, Avitene should not be used near the ureter. The bladder should be put at rest by the insertion of an indwelling catheter. If vaginal packing is not effective and a coagulopathy has been excluded, the patient should be returned to the operating room.

Hematomas may form intraperitoneally or extraperitoneally. The occasional retroperitoneal hematoma is ominous, however, because it affords an excellent culture medium in proximity to the vaginal or rectal flora and is likely to account for postoperative abscess formation. A palpable hematoma that is increasing significantly in size should probably be evacuated. Again, a coagulopathy must be excluded.

Small hematomas in the vault of the vagina or beneath a reapproximated tissue plane generally liquefy, and, although they may become infected, they usually drain spontaneously through the vaginal suture line. Because these hematomas are common in the vaginal vault, many surgeons leave a small opening in the very center of the vault for drainage after hysterectomy.

Thrombophlebitis

The importance of taking every measure possible to prevent thrombophlebitis cannot be overemphasized. Every patient should be instructed to move her extremities frequently and encouraged to move about in bed freely, starting from the time of recovery from anesthesia. She should sit up in a chair two or three times daily, beginning on the first postoperative day, and she should clearly understand that moving her legs will aid her circulation. Oversedation should be avoided.

The patient should continue to wear the elastic stockings that she wore during the operative procedure and for the initial 3 or 4 postoperative days until she is comfortably ambulatory. On daily rounds, the attending physician should palpate the patient's calves and investigate any complaint of leg pain, particularly if unilateral. Elastic stocking compression of the extremity, elevation, and external heat are appropriate treatment for superficial thrombophlebitis. The administration of phenylbutazone (Butazolidin Alka) three times daily for 7 to 10 days may increase the patient's comfort. Anticoagulation is desirable only when there is evidence of upward expansion of the thrombophlebitis despite the use of these measures.

Obesity or a history of thrombophlebitis predisposes a patient to this potentially dangerous development. A preoperative determination of partial thromboplastin time (PTT) helps considerably to identify any unsuspected bleeding disorders that may result in thrombophlebitis postoperatively. If partial heparinization is desired, 5000 units of heparin are given subcutaneously three times daily, beginning the day before the operation and continuing through the first 4 or 5 postoperative days. Because operative and postoperative bleeding is likely to be increased in these patients, surgical hemostasis must be meticulous. Defibrotide may prove to be a safer antithrombotic than heparin. Although available and used in Europe, it is not available yet in the United States.

Pelvic thrombophlebitis. Thrombophlebitis in the pelvic veins is an uncommon development associated with somewhat ambiguous physical findings. Lower quadrant abdominal pain and tenderness to deep palpation are usually present without any change in hematocrit and without the palpable lower pelvic mass that may be associated with a hematoma. The lack of any apparently related activity in the overlying bowel suggests the extraperitoneal character of the problem. A sense of fullness may be perceived by the fingers of the examiner, but, because there is some muscle guarding, this finding is not specific and certainly not pathognomonic. The most characteristic features of the clinical picture are shaking chills and a high spiking fever. A sustained tachycardia does not change, even with the abrupt fall in temperature. Pelvic thrombophlebitis is somewhat ominous; it is surprisingly resistant to antibiotic therapy, but responds dramatically to anticoagulation with heparin.

It is important to distinguish infected pelvic thrombophlebitis from pelvic cellulitis, because treatment of the two conditions differs in some respects. In pelvic cellulitis, the pelvic floor is noticeably ligneous and diffusely painful. The patient usually has no chills, and her temperature remains elevated. As her temperature gradually subsides, her pulse rate decreases as well. Blood cultures are desirable, but they are not always conclusive; fortunately, however, broad-spectrum antibiotics are indicated in both situations. The role of anticoagulants in pelvic thrombophlebitis is debatable, and many clinicians use anticoagulants only when embolization develops or when the patient's condition fails to respond favorably to intensive antibiotic therapy of several days' duration.

Areas of thrombosis that occur without infection are equally life-threatening and are often totally asymptomatic until uninfected, large, soft thrombi become dislodged and form massive pulmonary emboli. It is well-known, for example, that enormous, bland phlebothrombosis may occur a week or so after pelvic surgery when an in-bed patient is having a bowel movement on a bedpan. For this reason, both early ambulation and frequent administration of stool softeners, laxatives, or enemas are recommended during postoperative convalescence. The indications for vena cava ligation are often debated, but the certainty of the immediate result in blocking the transit of emboli from the distal veins keeps this procedure from being forgotten.

Acute inflammatory thrombophlebitis of the leg. When massive thrombosis occludes practically all the veins of the leg, the entire leg becomes deeply cyanotic and extremely painful. Total heparinization should be accomplished promptly, and thrombectomy should be considered.

Deep vein thrombosis. Total heparinization is the treatment of choice for a deep vein thrombosis of the pelvis or lower extremity. After the intravenous administration of 7500 to 10,000 units of aqueous heparin solution in a loading dose, the patient is infused with a continuous heparin drip that provides 5000 units of heparin every 4 to 6 hours by way of a heparin-well and extends the PTT from two to two and one-half times normal. Not only does a continuous heparin drip have the advantage of making it possible to obtain a PTT at any time, but also it eliminates the worry about peaks and valleys in anticoagulation. Generally, the infusion continues for 6 to 7 days, until oral anticoagulant therapy has been started. Medical consultation and follow-up are needed for 3 to 6 months. If embolism occurs despite heparinization, thrombectomy or vena cava ligation may be necessary.

Atelectasis and pneumonia

The most common postoperative pulmonary complication is atelectasis which occurs between 10% and 20% of patients. Collapse of the alveolar spaces results in hypoxia. The most sensitive test for early detection of microatelectasis is from examination of arterial blood gas, which usually reveals a lowered PO_2 and O_2 saturation with a normal PCO_2.[33]

Because it involves no abdominal incision that can interfere with deep respiration and movement, vaginal surgery is less likely to lead to atelectasis and pneumonia than is pelvic laparotomy. Routine deep inspiration should be encouraged after any type of pelvic surgery, however, beginning the day of operation. Incentive spirometry provides good pulmonary aeration and is preferable to the use of intermittent positive pressure breathing devices, which, unless the patient forcefully inhales, often do not provide adequate aeration and may even increase small airway obstruction. It is important to avoid oversedation, which tends both to depress the respiratory center and to inhibit the sensorium so that the patient's voluntary efforts may noticeably decrease.

Usually occurring early in the postoperative course, atelectasis results from the occlusion of a part of the bronchial tree because of hypoventilation, circulatory stasis, and the accumulation of intrabronchial secretions that are often associated with a preexisting acute or chronic bronchitis. Recent or concurrent upper respiratory infections are distinct contraindications to anesthesia and, thus, to elective surgery, because infection leads to bronchial obstruction which is followed by absorption of trapped gases, with collapse of the distal segment of lung involved. A chest roentgenogram is usually of limited value in making an early diagnosis; the initial symptoms include fever, tachycardia, and a noticeable increase in respiratory rate. Cyanosis and air hunger are less common unless the degree of pulmonary collapse is massive. If unresolved by good pulmonary toilet, atelectasis leads rapidly to bronchial pneumonia and consolidation.

The gradual development of pleural respiratory pain, together with a severe nonproductive cough, suggests pneumonia. There are two principal types: aspiration pneumonia, which develops if the patient inhales foreign matter into her lungs during the phase of immediate recovery from anesthesia; and bacterial pneumonia, which may develop in the later postoperative period if pulmonary ventilation is inadequate or if atelectasis has gone unrecognized and untreated. Treatment for both types of pneumonia must be prompt. For aspiration pneumonia, treatment involves clearing the airway of aspirate, correcting hypoxia, administering steroids (e.g., Solu-Cortef) to diminish pulmonary inflammatory reaction, and administering prophylactic antibiotics. Until the specific pathogen has been identified, bacterial pneumonia is best treated by an aminoglycoside and clindamycin. Inadequate treatment of either type of pneumonia may result in a lung abscess, although it may not be obvious for several weeks. A diagnosis of lung abscess mandates prompt, intensive antibiotic therapy. Failure of resolution requires bronchoscopy and, rarely, lobectomy.

Pulmonary embolism

Efforts to prevent pulmonary embolism begin with the preoperative identification of the patients most likely to develop this complication. The patients at greatest risk are those who have antecedent peripheral venous disease, those who are more than 50 years of age, those who are obese, and those who have cardiac or pulmonary disease. Because a clinically demonstrable pulmonary infarction may be associated with pulmonary embolism, a patient with pneumonia, atelectasis, or pleurisy with or without effusion requires particularly close observation.

Prophylactic heparinization is, of course, contraindicated in patients with a history of stroke, subarachnoid hemorrhage, peptic ulcer, bleeding diathesis, and hypertension. Moreover, it should be used only with great caution in the diabetic patient, because the resultant prolonged elevation of plasma-free fatty acid levels in the diabetic may induce hypercoagulability and cardiac arrhythmia, with increased risk of acute myocardial infarction. Phenobarbital and chloral hydrate have been shown to antagonize anticoagulants and may be contraindicated. Oral contraceptives are strongly suspect of promoting thrombosis and should, therefore, be discontinued a month or two before elective surgery.

Intermittent passive venous compression, as by the Kendall boot, may begin at the time of surgery for the patient at particular risk of pulmonary embolism. It is important to maintain an effective circulating blood volume during surgery to prevent the development of hypotension. Coincidental dehydration leads to hemoconcentration and affects heparin activity. Postoperatively, regular active and passive motion of the lower extremities, and the use of elastic stockings until the patient is ambulatory are of proved prophylactic value. In addition, oversedation should be avoided, and a positive program of voluntary deep breathing exercises should begin on the first postoperative day.

When calf pain and tenderness that are localized to the deep venous system accompany the swelling of an extremity, thrombosis is more likely than when the pain and tenderness are diffuse. If in doubt, the physician should consider x-ray venography, impedance plethysmography, or leg scanning with the use of radioactive iodine-labeled human fibrinogen to confirm suspected thrombosis.[15,25]

The physician who seriously suspects pulmonary embolism, even though it is unconfirmed, may order a single intravenous injection of 10,000 units of aqueous heparin, followed by 5000 units given subcutaneously every 6 hours for 7 to 10 days or until the patient is ambulatory. According to Hirsh,[12] a massive pulmonary embolism that develops after the tenth postoperative day[3] may be an indication for the use of a thrombolytic enzyme such as streptokinase[1] (250,000 IU in a continuous infusion by syringe pump over 30 minutes, followed by 100,000 units per hour for the remainder of the 24-hour period). Because its intense lytic activity may interfere with wound healing and initiate bleeding at the surgical site, streptokinase may be contraindicated during the first 10 postoperative days. Vena cava ligation may be necessary if showers of recurrent or septic emboli occur. Hirsh recommended ambulation 5 or 6 days after the initiation of treatment. When pain-free, the patient may be gradually switched to oral anticoagulants, which should be continued for some weeks. Cardiac arrest or a second major embolism during treatment may be indicators for pulmonary embolectomy.[12]

Early diagnosis and aggressive treatment by adequate anticoagulation have significantly reduced the mortality associated with pulmonary embolism. Fatal pulmonary embolism occurs after major gynecologic surgery approximately once per 1500 major procedures. Prophylactic low-dose anticoagulation, although possibly reducing the risk of fatal pulmonary embolism, increases the otherwise low incidence of significant postoperative bleeding. For this reason alone, anticoagulants are usually employed only if the history or the findings suggest a patient at high risk.

Intraabdominal complications

The patient who has just undergone vaginal surgery is certainly not immune to an attack of appendicitis, cholecystitis, or diverticulitis, and the characteristic symptoms should never be ignored. Indicated surgery should not be delayed.

Evisceration

Dehiscence of the apex of the vagina with extrusion of omentum, intestine, or both generally suggests that the reconstruction of the supports of the vault or the reconstitution of the levator plate at the time of surgery was inadequate, resulting in a faulty vaginal axis. Evisceration occurs only rarely after vaginal hysterectomy and seems independent of whether the vaginal vault is left opened or closed. It may be that a pathologically long (greater than 15 cm) small bowel mesentery permits the intraabdominal contents to exert unusual pressure on the surface of the cul-de-sac in the pelvic floor and vaginal vault. On the other hand, it may be that sudden massive increases in intraabdominal pressure (e.g., violent coughing or postoperative retching) or extreme overexertions (e.g., heavy lifting) in which the entire force of increased intraabdominal pressure is directed to the long axis of the vagina lead to evisceration.

The viability and integrity of the protruding structure determine the appropriate treatment. Protruding loops of intestine should be cleansed, drawn back into the peritoneal cavity by means of laparotomy, and fully inspected. If the tissues have remained viable, the pelvic defect can be repaired—with special care taken to obliterate the cul-de-sac and any enterocele that may be present. Any question about intestinal viability or the condition of the base of the mesentery is an indication for bowel resection, followed immediately by the trimming of any necrotic vaginal tissue and transabdominal closure of the vaginal vault defect. If the vaginal portion of the bowel is perforated or necrotic, the operator may remove that portion by resection per vaginum and then, after redraping, accomplish the transabdominal anastomosis.[17,28]

Forgotten foreign bodies

Seldom are instruments left behind or lost during vaginal surgery. Although an uncommon occurrence, a sponge or pack may occasionally be left in the cul-de-sac or in a tissue plane. A sponge that has been saturated with blood quickly assumes the color of the surrounding tissues and may easily be buried in a line of cleavage or beneath a flap or fold of plicated tissues. Sponges should be counted periodically during the course of a procedure, especially before the peritoneum is closed and again at the conclusion of the operation while the patient is still anesthetized and draped. If a missing sponge is not found in the vagina or in the folds of drapes, a roentgenogram of the pelvis should be obtained while the patient is still on the operating table. (It may be necessary to obtain separate films of the lower and upper abdomen if the patient is obese.) Only sponges with radiopaque marking should be used in surgery, and they can generally be seen on x-ray films. Under no circumstances should a sponge be cut in half during the course of an operative procedure, lest a missing, unmarked half be invisible on a postoperative roentgenogram. Because they are so easily lost, small pushers or swabs in the surgical field are never separated from their holding forceps. Although there are reports of foreign bodies having been found incidentally months or years after they have been left behind, most make themselves known through clinical infection within a few days.

A foreign body forgotten during surgery generally causes a septic fever that is unresponsive to any antibiotic combination. An abscess that points into the vagina may form, and probing of this abscess may bring forth a few threads of the offending foreign body. Signs of local peritonitis indicate that the foreign body is intraperitoneal; if transvaginal removal cannot be accomplished easily, abdominal laparotomy with drainage and culture of the purulent material may be necessary. When there are signs of extraperitoneal infection, such as localized subepithelial fluctuation the surgeon should gently open into the tissue planes near the site of the suspected abscess. In the presence of the local infection, the surgeon should space the sutures of a secondary closure, if any, so that they do not interfere with drainage from the infected area.

A vaginal examination shortly before discharge from the hospital permits the identification of any unsuspected hematoma, the separation of any intravaginal adhesions, and the removal of any overlooked intravaginal sponges or packing. A forgotten intravaginal sponge or packing invariably results in a profuse and offensive vaginal discharge that causes the patient considerable distress. Fortunately, a forgotten sponge or packing in the vagina rarely does any serious damage, and the discharge subsides promptly after removal.

Cerebral changes

It is essential to watch hypertensive patients postoperatively for any signs of cerebral thrombosis, which, if significant, may include paralysis and coincident discrepancy in pupillary size. More often, however, there are minor degrees of cerebral insufficiency that only careful interpretation of the patient's postoperative course can detect. A slight slurring of speech, a fuzziness of thinking, or a minor memory impairment may initially appear to be the effects of postoperative sedation, but those close to the patient are certain to recognize such changes in the later postoperative weeks.

Coronary occlusion

Unexplained postoperative tachycardia, especially when combined with dyspnea and substernal pressure, suggests coronary occlusion, especially in a patient who has a history of angina or findings of arteriosclerosis. Any patient with preoperative clinical or cardiographic evidence of coronary insufficiency should have a postoperative electrocardiogram and serial enzyme determinations, even if she has no additional symptoms.

Unexpected malignancy

The surgeon should carefully review the pathologist's report on the tissues removed in vaginal surgery as soon as the report is available, preferably before the patient's discharge from the hospital. Occasionally, laboratory examination of the surgical specimen reveals an unsuspected or a more advanced than anticipated stage of a recognized malignancy. The patient or a responsible member of her family should be advised promptly of these findings so that appropriate additional therapy can be instituted when indicated and the advisability and nature of recommended follow-up studies can be explained. Consultation with an oncologic team is often desirable at this time.

LATE POSTOPERATIVE COMPLICATIONS

Although genital fistulae may become evident at almost any stage of convalescence, a very small fistula may not be recognizable until weeks or even months after surgery. Iatrogenic urinary stress incontinence may also occur, usually because inadequate attention was paid to the urethral supports or to the preservation of a good posterior urethrovesical angle in the correction of a cystocele. If the patient finds this socially disturbing, additional surgery may be necessary. Eversion of the vaginal vault, postoperative shortening of the vagina, and vaginal stricture are other sequelae that may require surgical correction at a later time.

Whenever a premenopausal woman undergoes a colporrhaphy, the atrophic effects of postoperative estrogen withdrawal some years after a satisfactory repair must be anticipated. During a lifetime of periodic pelvic examinations, atrophy of the vaginal membrane can be detected, reversed, slowed, or prevented by the long-term regular instillation of supplemental estrogen cream once a week, particularly in patients who are sexually active.

Prolapse of the fallopian tube

When the vault of the vagina has been left open or partly open following hysterectomy, there is a watery drainage for the first 2 days postoperatively. Unless there is an unexpected urinary fistula present, the drainage is of other body fluids. It may consist of serum, lymph, pus or a combination of all three. Should it persist beyond 6 weeks, the possibility of prolapse of one end of a fallopian tube should be investigated.[26,35]

A rare complication of vaginal hysterectomy, prolapse of the fallopian tube through the apex of the vagina results in a peritoneal fistula. Such a prolapse is generally a consequence of leaving the vaginal vault open at the conclusion of a hysterectomy and suturing the cut ends of the tube along a cut edge of the vault, or of prolapse of the fimbriated end of the tube through the peritoneal opening unexpectedly and undetected as the peritoneum is being closed. Closing most of the vault in layers is the recommended procedure because it securely buries the transected ends of the tubes beneath the wall of the vagina, well away from all vaginal edges, and prevents the development of a peritoneal fistula. Indications of the uncommon peritoneal fistula include a watery discharge and a friable soft tissue vaginal vault excrescence that bleeds easily and, at first, appears to be granulation tissue, but fails to heal after simple cauterization or attempts to curette the suspected granulations away. If local excision fails and discharge persists, salpingectomy may be necessary for cure; otherwise, the patient is likely to experience intermittent hydrorrhea, and the fistula provides a potential route for ascending infection.

In a useful transvaginal technique of total salpingectomy for a posthysterectomy fallopian tube prolapse, the operator begins by making a horizontal incision through the full thickness of the vagina posterior to the prolapsed tube and the vaginal scar.[17] The operator incises the peritoneal cavity horizontally and carefully inspects the peritoneal side of the prolapsed tube. Mobilizing the tube, the operator makes another horizontal vaginal incision anterior to the prolapsed tube, removes the entire tube and a collar of vagina between the two incisions, and completes the procedure by closing the peritoneum and vagina separately. Alternatively, the salpingectomy may be performed laparoscopically or by laparotomy if there are many adhesions to surrounding tissues.

Colporrhaphy after previous treatment for cervical or vaginal carcinoma

Gynecologic surgeons must be cautious in recommending vaginal repair or reconstruction in patients clinically "cured" of a cervical or vaginal carcinoma by radiation treatment. Cutting through and opening into tissues that contain trapped and inactive nests of clinically "dormant," but histologically recognizable, cancer cells may seem to risk the reactivation of a quiescent malignant neoplasia. Fortunately, this occurrence is rare, and "cancerocidal" radiation usually produces sufficient fibrosis, scarring, and shrinkage of the vagina to have arrested the progress of an earlier degree of genital prolapse.

Neurologic and psychiatric sequelae

Sciatic, peroneal and femoral nerve injury. Sciatic, peroneal, and femoral nerve injury can occur as a complication of vaginal surgery.

Peroneal nerve injury is characterized by postoperative foot drop, difficulty walking, and inability to abduct or evert the foot.[7,13] There may be numbness of the lateral surface of the leg and dorsal surface of the foot.

Patients with sciatic nerve injury demonstrate weakness of the hamstring muscles coincident with difficulty walking. Treatment is by physiotherapy, including massage and galvanic electrical stimulation of the peroneal nerve. The prognosis for recovery is good, but slow, often requiring several weeks or even months.

Prevention of neuropathy is centered on giving much attention to the proper position of the patients legs in the stirrups, requiring flexion of the knees and hips and ensuring minimal external rotation of the latter.

Excessive external rotation of the thigh of the patient with legs in "candy-cane" stirrups for operations longer than 1½ hours invites femoral neuropathy. This is identified postoperatively by the discovery of numbness and paresthesias of the thigh. The knee buckles when the patient stands, and often she cannot walk without assistance.[38]

Treatment of femoral neuropathy is primarily by physiotherapy, including massage, active and passive quadriceps exercises, and the liberal use of a great deal of patience. Femoral neuropathy in the patient having vaginal surgery may be prevented by placement of lateral supports to the thigh of each leg in stirrups, inhibiting excessive abduction and exaggerated external rotation.[31]

Femoral neuropathy also is seen following laparotomy, usually in a thin patient in whom a self-retaining retractor had been used and there had been pressure from the lateral retractor blades upon the femoral nerve or psoas muscles. The type of abdominal incision used seems to have been of no importance.[19]

Prevention of this neuropathy is by most careful placement of the lateral retractor blades, use of the smallest blade that is effective, and placement of a folded laparotomy pad beneath the tip of the blade to cushion the lateral pelvic wall. The prognosis for recovery is good, but over a period of several weeks.

Compartment syndrome. Prolonged gynecologic surgery—usually over 3 hours' duration—upon a patient in the lithotomy position risks compromise of circulation and neurologic function within the legs, if external pressure to a fascial compartment is sustained by the position of the supporting stirrups, elevating the pressure within the compartment sufficient to obstruct arteriolar circulation within the contained muscles. Ischemia promotes edema, which furrther compresses the contained nerves, with resultant compromise of function.[1] Compression syndrome may be suspected following prolonged surgery if the patient complains of cramping in the lower legs, which are found to be firm and tense although pulsations of the pedal arteries are palpable. Accentuation of the pain is elicited upon passive stretching of the muscles within the fascial compartment. These symptoms may progress, often rapidly, to numbness, burning, and difficulty moving the legs. This may be followed by foot drop and decreased sensation over the feet.

Prompt consultation with a vascular or orthopedic surgeon is desirable. Muscle pressure measurements should be obtained without delay,[41] and if elevated and within the first 12 hours postoperatively, surgical fasciotomy should be performed promptly to decompress the compartment inhibiting further damage to its contents. After 12 hours the risk of infection in tissue now partially necrotic or with circulatory compromise is accentuated and may outweigh the benefits of decompression. To aid circulation within the compartment the patient's legs should be positioned at the level of her heart.

Prevention of compartment syndrome in surgical cases of long duration in which stirrups are used requires that both legs and thighs be carefully supported by padded stirrups with special attention to position of the patients feet, avoiding passive dorsiflexion of the ankle. Passive repositioning of the legs is recommended during the surgical procedure.

The prognosis for recovery is good if permanent nerve and muscular damage has not occured, although recovery may take several weeks. Significant neuromuscular damage can be suspected in the patient with compression syndrome who develops foot drop.

Some patients develop a significant degree of depression postoperatively[2]. This is attributed to the consequence of a psychological perception of loss or threatened loss of feminity or sexuality, or in the case following hysterectomy, loss of fertility in addition. Preoperative discussion

and postoperative counseling are valuable. Most psychoses will have been present and demonstrable preoperatively.

Anemia

The patient who has experienced hemorrhage should have daily, more frequent if the values are dropping, postoperative measurements of hemoglobin and hematocrit. For the patient who had no operative hemorrhage and has no visible postoperative bleeding, hemoglobin and hematocrit determinations should be made on the second postoperative day; if these are unexpectedly low in comparison to her preoperative values, readings should be repeated twice daily during the postoperative period until levels have stabilized or begun to improve. Some patients may need oral iron supplementation both during the course of hospitalization and as part of the posthospital postoperative care. Hemoconcentration during the first and second postoperative days may result in normal or elevated hemoglobin and hematocrit values and give a false sense of security; significantly depressed values at this time should arouse immediate suspicion and require further investigation.

Arthritis

Acute postoperative monoarticular arthritis strongly suggests exacerbation of unexpected gout and should respond to appropriate treatment.

REFERENCES

1. Adler LM et al: Bilateral compartment syndrome after a long gynecologic operation in the lithotomy position, *Am J Obstet Gynecol* 162:1271, 1990.
2. Bachman GA: Psychosexual aspects of hysterectomy; *WHI* 1:41, 1990.
3. Bell WR: Thrombolytic agents: a better way to treat pulmonary embolism, *Consultant* 16:39, 1976.
4. Borkowf HI: Bacterial gangrene associated with pelvic surgery, *Clin Obstet Gynecol* 16(2):40, 1973.
5. Borkowf HI, Mattingly RF: *Bacterial gangrenous infection.* In Schaefer G, Graber EA, editors: *Complications in obstetric and gynecologic surgery,* Hagerstown, 1981, Harper & Row, pp 140-156.
6. Burchell C: The umbrella pack to control pelvic hemorrhage, *Conn Med* 32:734, 1968.
7. Burkhart FL, Daly JW: Sciatic and Peroneal Nerve Injury: A Complication of Vaginal Operations. Obstet Gynecol 28:99-102, 1966.
8. Cavanagh D, Beazley J, Ostapowicz F: Radical operation for carcinoma of the vulva: a new approach to wound healing, *J Obstet Gynaecol Brit Commonw* 77:1037, 1970.
9. Cruse PJE: *Complications.* In Beahrs OH, Beart RW, editors: *General surgery.* Media, PA, 1992, Harwal.
10. Geller PL, Jaffe BM: *Reoperation for intra-abdominal infection.* In Tomkins RK, editor: *Reoperative Surgery,* Philadelphia, 1988, JB Lippincott, pp 281-297.
11. Hildebrand JR, Merrill DL, Vernick JJ: Defining appropriate timing of surgical antibiotic prophylaxis, *Infect Surgery* 5:444, 1986.
12. Hirsh J: Venous thromboembolism: Diagnosis, treatment, prevention, *Hosp Pract* 10:53, 1975.
13. Hopper CL: Bilateral femoral neuropathy complicating vaginal hysterectomy. *Obstet Gynecol* 32:543, 1968.
14. Howkins J, Stallworthy J: *Bonney's gynecologic surgery,* Baltimore, 1974, Williams & Wilkins.

15. Jacobson HG, Heitzman ER: Pulmonary thromboembolism—update, *JAMA* 243:2229, 1980.

16. Janisch H, Palmrich AH, Pecherstorfer M: *Selected urologic operations in gynecology,* p. 21, Berlin, 1979, Walter de Gruyter.

17. Kambouris AA, Drukker BH, Barron J: Vaginal evisceration: a case report and brief review of the literature, *Arch Surg* 116:949, 1981.

18. Koehler PR, Moss AA: Diagnosis of intra-abdominal and pelvic abscesses by computerized tomography, *JAMA* 244:49, 1980.

19. Kvist-Poulsen H, Borel J: Iatrogenic femoral neuropathy subsequent to abdominal hysterectomy: incidence and prevention, *Obstet Gynecol* 60:516-520, 1982.

20. Ledger WJ et al: Adnexal abscess as a late complication of pelvic operations, *Surg Gynecol Obstet* 129:963, 1969.

21. Lee RA: *Postoperative necrotizing fasciitis.* In Nichols DH, editor: Clinical problems, injuries and complications of gynecologic surgery, Baltimore, 1988, Williams & Wilkins, pp 1-4.

22. Meleney FL: Bacterial synergism in disease processes with a confirmation of the synergistic bacterial etiology for a certain type of gangrene of the abdominal wall, *Ann Surg* 94:961, 1931.

23. Meleny FL: A differential diagnosis between certain types of infectious gangrene of the skin with particular reference to hemolytic streptococcus gangrene and bacterial synergistic gangrene, *Surg Gynecol Obstet* 56:847, 1933.

24. Morley GW: Carcinoma of the vulva with postoperative inguinal wound breakdown. In Nichols DH, editor: Clinical problems, injuries, and complications of gynecologic surgery, ed 2, Baltimore, 1988, Williams & Wilkins, pp 226-230.

25. Moser KM, Brach BB, Dolan GF: Clinically suspected deep venous thrombosis of the lower extremities, *JAMA* 237:2195, 1977.

26. Muntz HG, Falkenberry S, Fuller AF Jr: Fallopian tube prolapse after hysterectomy, *J Reprod Med* 33:467, 1988.

27. Nichols DH, Randall CL: *Vaginal surgery,* ed 3, Baltimore, 1989, Williams & Wilkins.

28. Powell JL: Vaginal evisceration following vaginal hysterectomy, *Am J Obstet Gynecol* 115:276, 1973.

29. Reich WJ, Nechtow MJ: Ligation of the internal iliac arteries, *J Int Coll Surg* 36:157, 1971.

30. Roberts DB, Hester LL Jr: Progressive synergistic bacterial gangrene arising from abscesses of the vulva and Bartholin's gland duct, *Am J Obstet Gynecol* 114:285, 1972.

31. Roblee MA: Femoral neuropathy from the lithotomy position: Case report and new leg holder for prevention, *Am J Obstet Gynecol* 97:871, 1967.

32. Rosenthal DM, Colapinto R: Angiographic arterial embolization in the management of postoperative vaginal hemorrhage, *Am J Obstet Gynecol* 151:227, 1985.

33. Schleuter DP: *Pulmonary evaluation.* In Rock JA, Thompson JD, editors: *TeLinde's operative gynecology,* ed 7, Philadelphia, 1992, JB Lippincott.

34. Smith DG, Wyatt JR: Embolization of the hypogastric arteries in the control of massive vaginal hemorrhage, *Obstet Gynecol* 49:317, 1977.

35. Sumathy V, Baucom K: Prolapse of the fallopian tube following abdominal hysterectomy, *Int J Gynaecol Obstet* 13:273, 1975.

36. Surwit EA: Postoperative care of the surgical patient. In Garcia C-R, Mikuta JJ, Rosenblum NG, editors: *Current therapy in surgical gynecology,* Philadelphia, 1987, BC Decker, pp 10-13.

37. Stone HH, Martin JD Jr: Synergistic necrotizing cellulitis, *Ann Surg* 175:702, 1972.

38. Tondara AS et al: Femoral neuropathy: a complication of lithotomy position under spinal anaesthesia, *Can Anaesth Soc J* 30:84, 1983.

39. Wetchler SJ, Hurt WG: A technique for surgical correction of fallopian tube prolapse, *Obstet Gynecol* 67:747, 1986.

40. Wheeless CR Jr: *Vaginal evisceration following pelvic surgery:* In Nichols DH: *Clinical problems, injuries and complications of gynecologic surgery,* ed 2, Baltimore, 1988, Williams & Wilkins, pp 121-129.

41. Whitesides TE et al: A simple method for tissue pressure determination, *Arch Surg* 110:1311, 1975.

42. Zollinger RM: *Some principles of reoperative surgery.* In Tompkins RK, editor: *Reoperative surgery,* Philadelphia, 1988, JB Lippincott, pp 1-7.

Chapter 9

LEGAL CONSIDERATIONS FOR THE GYNECOLOGIC SURGEON

Daniel K. Roberts

Many factors have combined to create the malpractice crisis. As it has evolved from the 1970s until now, the crisis has never been one of decreasing medical competency or increasing negligence, but rather involves factors such as changing patient expectations, an increasingly litigious society, a court system that encourages high dollar awards, rising insurance premiums, and the corresponding rise in the practice of "defensive" medicine. The cost of health care, the quality of health care, and the availability of health care are all being adversely affected by the malpractice crisis.

Because lawsuits are so common and because courts of law operate on principles and ethics sometimes at odds with the principles and ethics of medicine, it is important to take note of legal precepts in general as well as specifically in cases of medical malpractice. The underlying principle in law is the adversarial system, in which attorneys are bound to reveal only the evidence that benefits their clients, instead of the whole truth. This system is thought to be the fairest way to ensure that each attorney's client gets the best possible representation.

To prevail in a case, the plaintiff's attorney must provide four pieces of evidence for the court:

1. A standard of care must be established for the particular procedure or practice.
2. A deviation from that standard must be established.
3. An identifiable injury must be proved.
4. The specified deviation or negligence must be proved the cause of the identified injury.

All four conditions must be fulfilled for a verdict of malpractice to be pronounced.

Overall, a chapter on legal considerations is a chapter about patient management. Appropriate interaction with a patient is paramount to minimizing legal repercussions.

Rather than limiting interaction with the patient, it is often prudent to expand communication.

In an effort to partially cover the many areas of physician-patient interaction that might be effectively managed to reduce lawsuits, this chapter is written pragmatically and organized chronologically in the order of a typical patient's course of treatment, starting with the office visit and continuing through preoperative evaluation, surgery, and postoperative care. Case abstracts are used to illustrate points.

OFFICE

Because an office visit usually precedes a surgical operation, a discussion regarding the office environment is imperative to good medicolegal practice. Many elements may seem small at first, but can become very significant. For example, carefully examine the attitude of your personnel. Do they project caring and sensitivity? This is not only important for nurses, but also, in particular, for your receptionist, who is the first person your patients encounter. This sensitivity should carry over into telephone communications. Make sure your patient waiting room is comfortable, and keep the waiting time to a minimum. Your billing and collecting service should be "patient-friendly." In addition, never turn over a patient's account for collection until you have reviewed the chart for potential exposure to malpractice litigation.

In following the previous recommendations, one lays the foundation for a good doctor-patient relationship. Remember that all patients are not good matches for all doctors and vice versa. Dissatisfied patients are often predisposed to file lawsuits. Furthermore, remember that you do not have to accept every patient who comes to your office. If you find yourself incompatible with a patient before surgery, chances are you will also be uncomfortable postoperatively, and if the outcome is disappointing, a lawsuit is in the making. In such a situation, the sooner you dissolve the relationship with the minimum of procedures, the better. However, once you have accepted a patient and wish to dismiss her, you must take special steps to find care for her elsewhere, and you must continue your care until a new physician takes her case or until a reasonable period of time passes. To determine what this time requirement is, it is necessary to check with attorneys in your area. Local legal custom plays a prominent role in many areas of the law, and local legal consultation should always be sought.

INFORMED CONSENT

An important part of the doctor–patient relationship in a surgical practice is informed consent. In establishing both the relationship and informed consent, communication is paramount. To maximize communications, the doctor must assume greater than 50% of the responsibility. Contrary to the past, when doctors told the patient what to do, we now are in true partnership with the patient, collectively determining what is best for her. Adequacy of informed consent depends on various standards.

Different states have different rules to determine whether the information given in a particular case is considered sufficient. Some states use the "professional medical standard," which is based on what a reasonable physician would disclose under the same or similar circumstances.

Other states use the "patient materiality standard," which is based on the informational needs of the patient. There are two subtypes of this standard. The *objective* subtype applies the response of a reasonable person given the same risks of treatment. In the *subjective* subtype, the patient must convince the jury what she would have accepted had she been informed of the treatment risk that came to pass in her case. It is important to find out which standard is applied by the courts in your state.

Ultimately, through personal discussion and patient literature, videotapes, and other teaching devices, the patient should feel comfortable with your impression of her diagnosis; what you plan to do and what the alternatives might be; what risks might reasonably occur including those from anesthesia; the anticipated outcome including sterility or nonsterility; and the anticipated time sequence of the procedure, postoperative hospitalization, and estimated recuperation time.

Because, in spite of best efforts, patients tend to forget, it is important that you document this information. The author believes that a brief handwritten note is an adequate format. This note can be simply stated, "I have explained to the patient my impressions and judgment, the planned procedure, alternatives, and risks to include but not limited to infection, hemorrhage, injury to bowel or genitourinary tract with subsequent fistulas and rarely even death. Timed events discussed. Patient states she accepts and has no further questions."

There have been numerous debates about long forms and obtaining patient signatures. The author believes that the longer the form the more likely a possible risk will be omitted, and that omission might be construed as an admission of surgical error. Also, the longer the form, the more likely the patient will deny either reading or understanding it. Again, local custom plays a part in the interpretation of issues, and adherence to these customs is advised. In some states, informed consent papers have been drawn up by legislatures, and their use is required by law. Their use provides protection from lawsuits in this matter.

Finally, there are very rare occasions when informed consent is not necessary. These exceptions include emergencies, patient waivers, patient incompetence, therapeutic privilege, and risks that are common knowledge. These are beyond the scope of this chapter, and the author leaves them with two comments: (1) confer with your attorney; and (2) determine the validity of these exceptions before, not after, the procedure is performed.

A brief comment is necessary regarding the doctrine of "battery" or unauthorized touching. Whenever a procedure is done without informed consent and does not fall under the exceptions previously listed, a physician is exposed not only to the tort of negligence, but also to the doctrine of battery, which is a criminal act. The author recently reviewed two closed claims in which the patient in the first case was scheduled for a tuboplasty and the patient in the second case for lysis of adhesions. Because of the severity of adhesions, in each case a hysterectomy was performed. Both plaintiffs claimed that they had not given consent for a hysterectomy. In both cases, it was shown that, ultimately, hysterectomy would have been the appropriate therapy, but each plaintiff claimed she was not psychologically ready to lose her uterus. One patient would have waited until the completion of her final semester in college. The other would have waited until a slower time in her business.

Although each doctor claimed the procedure was an emergency because otherwise the patient would have to be exposed to a second anesthesia, the juries disagreed and found for the plaintiffs. Fortunately, these cases were tried under the tort of negligence, a civil offense, rather than prosecuted under battery, a criminal offense. Although attorneys have been known to file charges of battery in informed consent cases, judges seldom consider the doctor's actions to be criminal in nature.

Recently, a new concern accompanies the removal of a uterus. With the wonders of in vitro fertilization and other assisted reproductive technologies, a physician must be sure to justify the removal of any tissue that is not diseased.

MEDICAL RECORDS

Records can be a lifeline or a hangman's noose in a lawsuit. If given due attention, they can be a physician's best witness. On the other hand, poorly kept records can make it nearly impossible to prove that appropriate, timely care was given.

Records have multiple purposes. They are, of course, principally for the physician's own use in consultations or patient referrals. However, in court, they can be used to show what actions were or were not taken in light of the observed conditions, depending on what the record states or omits.

Logically, a record should contain a complete history, results of physical examination, laboratory results, medication prescribed, procedures proposed, informed consent, and other related documentation. It is particularly important to list laboratory data and the clinical response to those data. Known allergies to medications should be in a special identifiable place, preferably in color or otherwise highlighted for easy retrieval and reference. Do not forget to record any telephone conversations you or your personnel have with patients.

The completeness of the record is crucial. Progress notes commensurate with the condition of the patient should be written. They not only document your evaluation and care of the patient, but the fact that you were present. Make sure you mark both the date and the time of the progress note. If you call the floor, make sure the nurse documents the time and nature of your call. Review the nurse's notes daily. If a misleading entry exists, an objective corrective comment in the progress notes should be made.

Timeliness of completion of records and, in particular, operative notes is imperative. Discharge summaries should be completed within a reasonable period of time. Review these or any other documents carefully before signing because you will be held responsible for their contents.

Legibility is a significant problem in medical records. If a physician feels too hurried to write legibly, entries should be dictated and then transcribed into the record. A complete but illegible record is of negative value to the physician.

When making any entries, it is important to state facts rather than conclusions. Objective observations, rather than subjective ones, should be made. Refrain from inappropriate comments regarding colleagues, hospital personnel, or procedures. Do not make statements with an obvious vested interest. Do not mention incident reports.

If a record must be changed, the proper procedure should be observed. First, draw a line through the incorrect information, then make any necessary changes in a separate area, and finally date and initial the changes. Once a record has been requested or a suit filed, *do not* alter the record. Juries frequently interpret changes made after a record is requested as conclusive proof that negligent behavior was covered up.

Also, avoid the use of certain words that suggest inappropriate actions were taken, such as *mistakenly, improperly, negligently, thoughtlessly, inadvertently,* and *unsatisfactorily.* Do not use the absolutes *never* and *always,* because there are exceptions to any medical event.

In the management of records, confidentiality is paramount, and unless the patient has signed a release, no one else should be allowed access. The physician's record is physically owned by the physician, but the information also belongs to the patient. If the patient signs a release, a copy or summaries of the record may be given to another treating physician, an attorney, or other authorized person. In most jurisdictions, the patient has similar access to her records.

The length of time records must be retained varies sufficiently from one locality to the next that consultation with a local attorney is advised. For certain, whenever records are considered out-of-date, they should be shredded, not simply discarded.

PREOPERATIVE EVALUATION

Problems in the arena of failure to diagnose, a delay in diagnosis, or misdiagnosis constitute a high number of lawsuits against physicians. For gynecologists, two such problem diagnoses quickly come to mind: ectopic pregnancy and breast cancer.

The lawsuits in ectopic pregnancy result from cases that involve incidences of both too much aggressiveness and too little. With the advent of the vaginal sonographic probe and the widespread availability of beta human chorionic gonadotropin (HCG) evaluation, we can hope to see a reduction in the numbers of these lawsuits. The index of suspicion should stay high, and the use of these tools and others associated with the operative laparoscope allows a much better approach. If the patient desires to preserve future fertility, proper management of the ectopic pregnancy must include considering techniques such as "milking" a distal ectopic pregnancy, and the use of linear salpingostomy or limited salpingectomy instead of total salpingectomy in more proximal tubal locations.

Breast disease is another major concern, not only diagnostically but also in terms of management. Three symptoms with breast disease are pain, mass, and nipple discharge. When any of these symptoms are present, they must be aggressively investigated.

When the breast is being evaluated, all quadrants and the axillary tail must be systematically examined with the flat of the hand. Methods of breast self-examination should be reinforced, and monthly use should be encouraged. Nipple retraction, unless congenital, must always be investigated.

The major consideration is the presence or absence of a dominant mass. When a patient states she feels a mass, even if you do not find one, proceed as if a mass exists until you conclusively prove otherwise by thorough examination and mammography. A consultative examination is advisable if the patient continues to assert the existence of an undetected mass. Also, become familiar with the various tools available in the diagnosis of breast disease, including mammography, ultrasonography to define cysts, the hooked wire for location, and fine needle aspiration. These tools and the guidelines for their use are described in other chapters and should be followed. In the management of patients with breast disease, all the treatment alternatives must be explained and made available.

In managing biopsy diagnoses, the following facts are significant:

1. The use of the all-inclusive term *fibrocystic disease* should be discouraged.
2. The following diagnoses or biopsies carry no greater risk for cancer than a negative pathology report: adenosis, apocrine metaplasia, cysts, duct ectasia, fibroadenoma, fibrosis, mild hyperplasia, mastitis, and squamous metaplasia.
3. A slightly increased risk (1.5 to 2 times normal risk) occurs in diagnoses of moderate or florid hyperplasia, and papilloma with fibrovascular core.
4. A moderately increased risk (5 times normal risk) occurs with atypical hyperplasia (borderline lesion), ductal and lobular.[1]

PREOPERATIVE PREPARATION

This topic is covered in other chapters, but a few areas of high potential risk are mentioned here. In addition to procedures for specific surgeries such as cancer, make sure that all older patients receive an electrocardiogram (ECG) and chest x-ray evaluation. Evaluate and discuss with them the use of preoperative and postoperative estrogen. Check bleeding time if they have been using low-dose aspirin for arthritis or the popular self-prevention of heart attacks. Check for other bleeding disorders. Similarly, do not overlook the advantages of low-dose heparin where indicated. The appropriate use of prophylactic antibiotics should be followed. If the ureteral anatomy might be distorted, consider an intravenous pyelogram. Last, if the procedure has a chance of entering the bowel, order a bowel prep.

SURGICAL PROBLEMS

Having taken all the appropriate preoperative steps including informed consent, a surgical problem may still occur and may precipitate a lawsuit.

Dr. Charles Ward of Emory University School of Medicine has reviewed 500 closed claims and ranks their order of occurrence as follows:[16]

1. Sterilization
2. Injury to genitourinary tract
3. Other postoperative injuries
4. Ectopic pregnancy
5. Laparoscopy complications
6. Dilation and curettage
7. Nerve injury
8. Appendicitis
9. Rectovaginal fistula
10. Bowel injury

The author's personal experience and research echo Dr. Ward's conclusions. It is beyond the scope of this chapter to discuss all these; however, a few representative examples have been selected and some general, pragmatic guidelines are presented below.

Case Abstract 1. The gynecologist performed an abdominal hysterectomy for leiomyoma and menorrhagia. On or about the fourteenth postoperative day, the patient began to drain urine through her vagina. Immediate referral to a urologist diagnosed a vesicovaginal fistula, which was subsequently successfully repaired. The plaintiff brought suit on the basis of negligent performance and res ipsa loquitur. Expert witnesses testified that this was a known complication of the procedure and could be caused by factors (such as abscess) other than negligent performance of the procedure. The defendant gynecologist maintained that he followed the standard of care in his methodology of performing the hysterectomy. The jury returned a defendant's verdict on the issue of negligence. A higher court also confirmed that the doctrine of res ipsa loquitur did not apply and upheld the verdict.[15]

This precedent-setting case clarified that res ipsa loquitur cannot be claimed if the identified injury is a known complication and might have been caused by something other than negligence. Res ipsa loquitur, meaning "the thing speaks for itself," describes events that are so clearly obvious that a lay person would not require an explanation from medical experts. An example would be operating on the wrong body part or the wrong patient. Leaving instruments or sponges in a patient after an operation also falls in this category. If an adequate count is recorded by hospital personnel, the liability question may be debated. Most consider the liability to rest with the hospital, but in some cases the "captain of the ship" doctrine may be applied and, therefore, the doctor is included in the liability.

The second principle to be learned from this case is that a maloccurrence does not equal negligence. An injury that occurs to the genitourinary tract, in and of itself, is not negligence. If a physician has followed standard procedure, and appropriately recognizes and responds to the injury, it is not malpractice. In this case, the gynecologist followed standard procedure and the jury exonerated him.

Other principles may be extracted from two more cases involving hysterectomies.

Case Abstract 2. After a hysterectomy, the patient developed a limp, allegedly from femoral nerve damage during surgery. The defendant ob/gyn claimed the leg condition resulted from an unforeseeable postoperative complication. A settlement of $160,000 was reached during trial.[7]

Great care must be taken during hysterectomies that nerve injuries do not occur. The lateral blades of self-retaining retractors (or any lateral retractors) must not rest heavily on or below the psoas muscles. This pressure can damage the femoral nerve, causing motor paralysis of the quadriceps muscle, which inhibits knee extension and can result in a limp. The sciatic nerve can be injured by a badly placed injection in the gluteal region. This may result in the motor paralysis of the hamstring muscles, causing only weak flexion of the knee. Often, the common peroneal nerve is also affected in this injury. Furthermore, the common peroneal nerve is exposed as it leaves the popliteal fossa and may be injured in prolonged vaginal procedures with the patient in stirrups. This causes the foot to be plantar-flexed (foot drop) and inverted, an attitude referred to as *equinovarus*. Attention to the placement of the surgical instruments and the patient during surgery will prevent these types of nerve injuries.[12,13]

Case Abstract 3. The patient underwent a hysterectomy after an abnormal Pap smear showed early squamous cell carcinoma. After the operation, the patient had several Pap smears. The patient was then seen by the defendant family practitioner, who she alleged told her no further Pap smears were necessary because of her hysterectomy. Four years later, she was diagnosed with advanced squamous cell carcinoma. The defendant physician responded that the patient clearly knew the value of continued Pap smears and had told him she was regularly seeing a gynecologist. A settlement of $470,000 for the plaintiff was reached.[8]

After hysterectomy, many women question the need for a Pap smear. When the hysterectomy is done for benign disease, most gynecologists follow up with a Pap smear and, if the result is negative, then schedule a Pap smear every 2 to 5 years. However, after removal for precancerous disease or early squamous cell cancer, as was the case here, Pap smears should be done every 3 months for 2 years and, if negative, then every 6 months thereafter. Vaginal carcinoma, although rare, is more common in such patients.

Tubal ligation procedures, like hysterectomies, also rank high on the list of claims frequency. Following are two typical examples.

Case Abstract 4. The defendant gynecologic surgeon performed a tubal ligation with Hulka clips. After the procedure, the patient was informed that she could no longer bear children. However, the patient later became pregnant and delivered a child. A verdict of $64,552.91 was awarded to the patient.[10]

Case Abstract 5. Before undergoing a tubal ligation, the patient asked her gynecologist about the chances of a reversal of the procedure. She was allegedly informed that the chances were 60% to 80%. Several years later, she sought to reverse the procedure and found that the chances were small. Although she signed an informed consent form stating that she understood that the procedure would render her incapable of bearing children, she claimed her consulting gynecologist and the gynecologic surgeon failed to advise her properly of the permanence of the procedure. The jury returned a defense verdict for the physicians.[9]

Numerous issues are raised by these cases. Although informed consent plays a part in all surgical cases, with sterilization procedures it is particularly important. Each patient should be evaluated carefully. Spousal consent should be obtained if the patient is married. Young unmarried women and women who simultaneously ask about the possibility of reversal should clearly be suspect. Remember the adage "never say 'never' or 'always' " because there are exceptions. Patients should be told the possible risk of postoperative conception. The usual figure given is that 5 procedures in 1000 fail, and this failure usually occurs in the first 2½ years.[14] Furthermore, it is necessary to discuss

the medical risks of the procedure, including the possibility of death secondary to anesthesia. Alternative methods of contraception should also be explained.

Occasionally, the uncomfortable situation arises when the successful obstruction of a fallopian tube is uncertain. In such cases, explain the problem to the patient postoperatively, reminding her that this possibility was discussed preoperatively. Advise the patient to continue to use of her contraceptive. In 6 weeks, perform a hysterosalpingography. If the tube is open, offer to redo the surgery in whatever manner is appropriate without an additional fee.

Another claim that arises in sterilization cases is "wrongful birth," in which a child is born after an unsuccessful procedure. Before the late 1960s, there was no such legal cause of action. Subsequently, numerous courts have treated the problem in different ways. Nineteen states either prohibit all wrongful birth actions or are introducing legislation to that effect. Thirty-one states allow wrongful birth actions but limit recovery to cost of prenatal care and delivery. Six states now allow recovery of all costs involved, including the costs of raising the child to maturity. Interestingly enough, the maximum amount of settlement the author has seen in these liberal cases is $150,000.[5]

The second case speaks specifically to miscommunication. It is doubtful a physician knowledgeable in tubal ligations would ever suggest a potential of 60% to 80% reversal. This usually manifests as the patient misremembering information, but may result in fabrication. The latter is likely to result in a defense verdict, especially if records can verify the physician's statements.

Inadequate care sometimes begins with inadequate preoperative procedures. The case that follows was compounded by inadequate intraoperative procedures, postoperative negligence, and a subsequent attempt to cover up the negligence.

Case Abstract 6. A preoperative ultrasound detected an enlarged, cystic ovary in a patient admitted with intense abdominal pain. No preoperative x-rays were obtained. The ovary was removed, but no further exploratory surgery was performed. Copious amounts of serosanguineous fluid were noted both during surgery and postoperatively, but no action was taken. After some time, a treating gynecologist found signs of severe shock and small bowel obstruction, but left the hospital without ordering immediate surgery. The patient died before surgery was initiated. The medical investigator's office was informed that death was from natural causes, and the patient's husband was told that her death was unavoidable. When the records were requested for the trial, they were found to have been "sanitized." Crucial evidence was later revealed by repeated time-line analysis. A settlement of over $1.4 million was reached before trial commenced.[6]

This case is obviously an example of badly mismanaged care. The preoperative work-up is questionable. Exploration of the abdomen seems to have been inadequate. Inattentiveness and nonresponsiveness postoperatively made matters even worse. An attempt at cover-up was evidenced by the statements attributing the death to unavoidable natural causes. This case emphasizes a very serious point about the handling of records. Numerous methods are available to detect "altered" or "sanitized" records, and any tampering with records is usually seen as confirmation of negligent practice. Do *not* alter records after they have been requested.

This is the kind of case people present as an example when they talk about "bad" doctors. Although such cases occur, they are few, and actions such as continuing medical education and peer review keep them rare.

Not all problems occur during surgery. The postoperative period also contributes to claims filed.

Case Abstract 7. After a surgically uneventful hysterectomy, the abdominal incision developed an infection. The physician left an elastic adhesive bandage in place for 6 days without checking the wound, despite patient complaints and indications of infection recorded in the nurses' notes. Follow-up surgeries, debridement of the wound, and a herniorrhaphy were eventually required. The jury returned a verdict against the physician for $250,000.[4]

Obviously, postoperative care includes close monitoring of all parameters, including the site of incision. A wound must be visually inspected and palpated to monitor it, and because a bandage serves little purpose after 24 to 36 hours, it should be removed. Ignoring nurses' notes is a common failing. Nurses' notes need to be scrutinized closely on a daily basis both for information pertinent to treatment and to prevent possible misinterpretations from entering the written record.

The subsequent problems this patient experienced, eventually necessitating a ventral herniorrhaphy, demonstrate the domino effect. Seemingly minor circumstances must be treated before they cause multiple complications.

The final abstracts included here describe cases in which diagnoses have been missed.

Case Abstract 8. Two Pap smears showing carcinoma-in-situ were misread by the pathologist as benign. Despite a suspicious mass that grew rapidly, the gynecologist relied on the false-negative pathology reports and did not perform a biopsy. A settlement of $500,000 was reached before the case came to trial.[11]

In the above case both the pathologist and gynecologist were sued. It is best to remember that a Pap smear on an obvious cancer frequently results in an erroneous reading. In such cases, the biopsy is the best method for definitive answers.

In cases in which malignancy is not obvious, especially if lumps in the breasts are involved, it is important to document that appropriate investigation was either performed or recommended. This prevents a maloccurrence from being mistaken for malpractice.

Case Abstract 9. During a single office visit, the defendant physician palpated a small lump in the patient's breast, but did not believe the lump to be malignant. The patient contended that she was advised no further investigation was necessary. Six months later, breast cancer was detected, requiring a mastectomy and chemotherapy. Although the physician stated that the patient

was advised to seek a mammogram, the records held no indication that this recommendation was made. The case was settled for $350,000.[3]

The following case shows how, under similar medical circumstances as the previous case, well-kept records produced a better legal outcome for the physician.

Case Abstract 10. A painful breast growth was initially diagnosed as fibrous growth disease. Over time, the growth developed, and a biopsy determined its malignancy. The patient contended that she had kept her physician apprised of her worsening condition and had kept her regularly scheduled appointments. The records showed missed appointments, no relevant communication, and that the lump was in a different location from the diagnosed fibrous growth. A defense verdict for the physician was pronounced.[2]

THE RESPONSE TO A SURGICAL COMPLICATION

Whenever a complication is recognized, treat it appropriately and immediately if possible. Immediately inform the patient and her family. Remind the patient that this complication had been discussed with her preoperatively. Visit the patient daily or more frequently if needed. On a successive visit, remind the patient again of your preoperative discussion of this complication. Write progress notes with date and time as indicated. Closely observe the nurse's notes, and stay attuned to what the nurse is observing.

Be quick to call a consultant to help you. However, if you do not choose to follow a consultant's advice, be sure you justify not doing so. If indicated, turn over the majority of care to a specialist or another physician, but do not avoid the patient. The author has seen numerous cases in which the patient equates the absence of her doctor with proof of a guilty conscience over "bad" surgery. It is imperative to *not avoid the patient.*

You must disclose to the patient an unwelcome event or maloccurrence, but do not admit you have made a mistake, and do not mention that you have malpractice insurance. Physicians tend to feel personal guilt if a less-than-perfect result is achieved, even if it is not their actions that caused the problem. Remember that a maloccurrence is not malpractice.

Do not criticize colleagues. If another physician's patient presents with complications, do not make critical remarks such as, "Who did this to you?" or "What a mess this is." Plaintiff patients often say that a comment by another physician caused them to think about a lawsuit.

CONCLUSION

A caring physician communicates well with patients and makes them partners in their care. Good dialogue with your patients concerning informed consent, appropriate responses to surgical complications, good record keeping, and the general practice of good medicine will stand you in good stead as you proceed with your career.

REFERENCES

1. Consensus Meeting: Is "fibrocystic disease" of the breast precancerous? *Arch Pathol Lab Med* 110:171, March 1986.

2. *Medical Malpractice Verdicts, Settlements & Experts,* 4(9):24, September 1988.

3. *Medical Malpractice Verdicts, Settlements & Experts,* 5(2):27, February 1989.

4. *Medical Malpractice Verdicts, Settlements & Experts,* 5(8):28, August 1989.

5. *Medical Malpractice Verdicts, Settlements & Experts,* 5(9):24, September 1989.

6. *Medical Malpractice Verdicts, Settlements & Experts,* 5(11):24, November 1989.

7. *Medical Malpractice Verdicts, Settlements & Experts,* 5(11):27, November 1989.

8. *Medical Malpractice Verdicts, Settlements & Experts,* 6(2):26, February 1990.

9. *Medical Malpractice Verdicts, Settlements & Experts,* 6(3):31, March 1990.

10. *Medical Malpractice Verdicts, Settlements & Experts,* 6(6):33, June 1990.

11. *Medical Malpractice Verdicts, Settlements & Experts,* 6(9):22, September 1990.

12. Ridley JH, editor: *Gynecologic surgery: errors, safeguards, salvage,* ed 2, Baltimore, 1981, Williams & Wilkins, p 42.

13. Snell RS: *Clinical anatomy for medical students,* ed 3, Boston, 1986, Little, Brown, p 680.

14. Soderstrom RM: How to avoid trouble with tubal sterilization. *OBG Management* 2(12):16-22, December 1990.

15. *Tatro v Lueken,* 212 Kan.606 P.2d 529 (1973)

16. Ward CJ: Prepublished data, Department of Obstetrics-Gynecology, Emory University School of Medicine, Decatur, GA, 1991.

Chapter 10

THE ETHICS OF GYNECOLOGIC SURGERY

Thomas E. Elkins
Douglas Brown

The purpose of this chapter is to explore the ethics of gynecologic surgery. Ethics has to do with the determination of what ought to be done, all things considered.[3] This definition distinguishes what is done from what ought to be done and calls for thorough consideration of nonprofessional factors. Ethical discourse concentrates on who decides and by what means decisions are made. Participants attempt to interpret accounts of experiences in the context of societal wisdom about human behavior.

Medical ethics focuses on decision-making situations involving health care. Until the 1960s, the Hippocratic tradition provided the background for ethical reflection about medicine in the United States.[7,37] Patients did not yet have reason to believe that physicians could significantly alter the course of events. Minorities did not yet fully benefit from the democratic promotion of individual rights. Physicians were measured by the standard of compassion and were trusted to "do no harm" when they made paternalistically beneficent decisions "in the patient's best interests."

Technologic and cultural revolutions had combined by the 1960s to radically restructure the discussion of medical ethics. Patient expectations shifted from care to cure and from acquiescence to self-determination. Ethical principles (with autonomy and justice added to nonmaleficence and beneficence) provided the core vocabulary for physicians, philosophers, and theologians.[4] These principles were seen as ends by some (i.e., deontologists) and as means by others (i.e., utilitarians).[16]

Each pillar principle initially enjoyed prima facie standing. Given the affirmation of pluralism and individual rights, however, the principle of patient autonomy rose to trump status in societal, and eventually in medical ethical, discourse.[18,33] Since case-by-case decisions were accordingly thought to originate from within the privacy of individual or familial traditions, attention to values increased.[1,46]

Most recently, perceived deficiencies have been identified amid the strengths of such innovations in medical ethics. Revised affirmations of physician autonomy, accountability, and character relative to the decision-making process have become common.[13,14,41] Also, the range of participants in medical ethical deliberations, frequently organized as ethics committees, has expanded to include lawyers, economists, minority advocates, politicians, and lay persons.

On many issues, the ethical concerns of gynecologic surgery overlap with the ethical concerns of all surgery. The starting point for such general reflections about surgery is the disposition toward the human body. Kass,[28] in "Thinking about the Body," has probed the medical student's initial but fleeting sense of awe[40] when a cadaver is first encountered, noting the difficulty physicians have in recovering and sustaining that sense of awe. Hauerwas[24] has argued that the medical task has fundamentally to do with dispensing "the wisdom of the body," which includes educating patients about decline and death. Beyond most other surgery, gynecologic surgery invades the privacy of a patient's self-image and social relationships, making the gynecologic surgeon's attention to patient dignity particularly important (e.g., clothing that puts the patient at ease, a limit on the number of persons in the hospital or operating room, restrictions on the number of educational pelvic examinations done before beginning the operation).

Among the ethical issues gynecologic surgery shares with surgery in general* are: balancing the patient's autonomy and the attending physician's beneficence; communi-

---

*References 1, 21, 25, 31, 45, 53, 55.

cating preoperative and postoperative information in light of commitment to truth-telling; developing an accessible and available delivery system; and purging the adversarial ethics of litigation from the doctor-patient relationship. Within the discipline of gynecologic surgery, two divisions—oncology[22,63] and infertility*—have specific ethical concerns that are beyond the scope of this chapter. Here we want to comment on three matters: surgical training, informed consent, and future trends.

ETHICAL CONCERNS IN SURGICAL TRAINING[27,38]

Medicine promotes itself as a humanistically motivated profession. Under close scrutiny, does a trainee's experience verify this self-image? Among the multiple motivations and goals, how evident is day-after-day commitment to "the best interests of the patient"?

More often than not in training, the patient is indigent. University-based medical centers in urban areas of the United States have become the primary centers for indigent care. This population has historically borne the burden of providing the clinical experience necessary to the training of surgeons. Health care illustrates that having choices distinguishes the economically privileged from the poor; indigent patients seldom have choices about the location at which medical care is provided or the level of training of those who treat them.

Though subject to many legitimate criticisms, the Hippocratic tradition has called physicians to a sense of obligation toward the community that provides the resources for training. Accordingly, physicians acknowledge by oath their debt to society, ideally leading to a demonstration of covenantal accountability to society.[39] For those still loyal to this component of the Hippocratic tradition, it is distressing to see so many physicians, once trained, contradict the spirit of their oaths by refusing to include indigent patients in their practices. Are they contradicting the spirit of their training experience?

As long as our health care system is two-tiered, indigent patients will receive health care in training environments. Trainees have the necessary energy and liberty for such work. Beyond experience, they need role models and supervision designed to deepen a compassionate regard for such responsibilities. With such encouragement, participation in the care of the indigent would then more likely be trainees' first, rather than only, show of concern in this population's best interests.

After training, the most obvious way for physicians to demonstrate gratitude toward those who contribute so personally to the continuation of the medical profession is to include indigent patients in their practices. However, other ways of expressing a sense of obligation exist. As Folkman[20] explained in a Harvard Medical School class day address:

In the long run, it is better if we come to terms with the uncer-

*References 2, 8, 9, 12, 19, 61.

tainty of medical practice. Once we recognize that all our efforts to relieve suffering might on occasion cause suffering, we are in a position to learn from our mistakes and appreciate the debt we owe our patients for our education. It is a debt which we must repay—it is like tithing. . . . I doubt the debt we accumulate can be repaid our patients . . . by refusing to see medicaid patients when the state can't afford to pay for them temporarily. . . . But we can repay the debt in many ways. We can attend postgraduate courses and seminars, be available to patients at all hours, teach, take recertification examinations; maybe in the future even volunteer for national services; or, most difficult of all, carry out investigation or research.

The need to convey a positive regard for patients manifests itself in many ways in the learning and practice of gynecologic surgery. An analysis of the patient's status in a training context should give special attention to the fact that many gynecologic surgeons-in-training do not have the benefits of a surgical laboratory in which to gain an understanding of pelvic anatomy, particular operative procedures, and even standard surgical equipment. The lack of practice prior to entering the center stage of the operating room contributes to expressed concerns about gynecologic surgical training in the United States. Few surgical specialties expect initiates to perform with graduate-level skill and expertise on their first assignment, when the recipient is a fellow member of the moral community. Some physicians-in-training even expect to participate in operations when they have obviously made no preparation before surgery—no study of the patient's "story," no review of medical texts, and no search for current approaches to the problem creating the need for surgery.

A consistent failure to prepare devalues the patient. For ethical reasons, training programs should ensure the opportunity for laboratory and cadaver experience before actual operating room activities, whenever possible, and should insist upon appropriate preoperative reading at all times.

This emphasis on patient interests in training programs must be clearly and safely balanced with resident interests in surgical experience. Concern for training experience that "maximizes resident benefits" may innocently draw an operative surgeon's attention away from the patient's best interests. To illustrate the tension that can exist, residents in gynecology must now disclose the number of vaginal hysterectomy operations they have performed in their training years, in spite of extended debate about the adequacy of evaluating surgical training by such numbers. With an eye toward private practice, surgical trainees can be impatient to acquire adequate surgical experience in innovative procedures and technologies. Accordingly, operative techniques might be selected in residency training years that reflect the needs of resident trainees rather than the needs of the particular patient undergoing surgery. Complementing attention to the ethical responsibility of providing society with technically dependable surgeons, the training years should also be distinguished by special efforts to develop a respect for patient autonomy and appropriate medically based decision-making guidelines before suggesting invasive surgery to a fellow human being.

Perhaps the recent move to legislate limits to residency working hours can be interpreted in light of the need to balance attention to patient and trainee interests.[49] Should a surgeon who has been up for over 24 hours be expected to operate? Do we want residents to leave their training years with a deeply ingrained habit of disregarding fatigue? We suggest that both patient and physician interests are best served when the option exists to cancel or refer a case (with patient approval) because of impairing fatigue.

Finally, gynecologic surgery training, more than many other types of surgery training, requires special consideration for psychosomatic and psychosexual realities as well as anatomic abnormalities.[44] The classic gynecologic example is the patient with chronic pelvic pain whose pelvic examination by laparoscopy is normal. The simple solution for the surgically oriented gynecologist is to remove everything from the pelvis, hoping that all pain symptomatology will dissolve. In actuality, this approach is seldom effective in pain relief unless coupled with intensive psychotherapy and often sexual therapy.[5,32,58] Scheduling hysterectomy procedures is easy. Taking a history that divulges information about preoperative sexual dysfunction or postoperative fears about marital and family intimacy and individual inadequacy is both difficult and time-consuming.

Whether it be a sterilization procedure, a disfiguring procedure involving vulvar tissue, or a minor operation that could result in major discomfort, concerns for preoperative and postoperative psychosexual function remain the cornerstone of ethical decision-making in gynecologic surgery. Gynecologic surgeons should first and foremost be gynecologists concerned for the "total patient."

ETHICAL CONCERNS ABOUT INFORMED CONSENT[15]

In the contemporary United States, many barriers discourage the accomplishment of truly informed consent before a major operation. First, most patients are being encouraged, if not required, by third-party payers to enter the hospital on the day of surgery. The cost reduction is obvious. However, the time available to develop a trusting physician-patient relationship is severely abbreviated. Same-day admission almost completely eliminates the opportunity for patients to form a preoperative bond with any of the nursing staff and resident house staff before surgery. Such humane considerations are sacrificed in the effort to provide cost-effective medical care.[62]

Second, fear of litigation keeps many gynecologists aloof and as objective as possible while preoperatively discussing surgical options and potential complications with patients. Sensitivity and openness are lost.[47] Any ambiguity about a surgical procedure's outcome may be glossed over for fear that the patient will be suspicious of the surgeon's ability to perform the procedure faultlessly.

Surgical informed consent is at its best a conversation

between two people who share the aim of approximating the best interests of the patient through a surgical procedure. May[34] has effectively explained the many differences between *contractual* informed consent (now so prevalent in the United States) and the more traditional *covenantal* informed consent. The notion of the physician as contractor has some obvious appeals:

First, it breaks with more authoritarian models. It emphasizes informed consent rather than blind trust. Second, a contract provides for the legal enforcement of terms on both parties and thus offers each some protection and recourse under the law to make the other accountable under the contract. Finally, a contract does not rely on the pose of philanthropy or condescend as charity. It presupposes frankly that self-interest primarily governs people. When two parties enter into a contract, they do so because each cuts a deal that serves his or her own advantage.[34]

However, May[34] has also singled out marked problems in this contractual relationship:

First, the notion of contract suppresses the element of gift in human relationships. Second, the contractual approach tends to reduce professional obligation to self-interested minimalism. Do no more for your patients than what the contract calls for: specified services for established fees. Third, professionals in the so-called helping professions serve unpredictable needs. The professional deals with the sickness, ills, crimes, needs, and tragedies of human kind. No contract can exhaustively specify in advance for each patient or client. The professional must be ready to cope with the contingent and the unexpected. Finally, in spirit, contract and covenant differ markedly. Contracts are external; covenants are internal to the parties involved. We sign contracts to discharge them expediently. Covenants cut deeper into personal identity. A contract has a limited duration, but the religious covenant imposes changes on all moments.

Informed consent in a contractual relationship, while underscoring patient autonomy, tends to draw attention away from the physician's role as a responsible moral agent in medical decision-making. Contemporary gynecologic surgeons are confronted with patient demands that stretch the limits of medical reasonableness. Examples include the patient who agrees to surgery at age 49 for a 15-cm adnexal mass "if only the ovary, *and nothing else*, is removed or injured," and the patient who demands the use of laser technology, even if the operation is not one usually benefited by such equipment (e.g., hysterectomy). Adding liposuction, laser adhesiolysis, or scar revision to procedures may unnecessarily increase patient risks and costs as well as physician profits and marketing values. To passively cater to the "consumer" preferences of a highly literate and relatively wealthy patient population is to open the door for abuse. Only a beneficent concern for the patient's best interests and a respect for medically proven indications and approaches will diminish practices that represent self-serving appeals to "autonomy."

Finally, conscientious gynecologic surgeons face issues of honesty and coercion in informed consent. A 1% chance of success in tubal surgery, for example, may be perceived as a 50:50 chance for the one patient, desperate for fertility, undergoing the surgery. Similar outcome ratios frame conversations between surgeons and patients in gynecologic oncology. Reoperations in such settings are especially troublesome. For instance, a patient with chronic pain, recently seen by the author, had a history of 20 laparoscopic procedures in the past 5 years for "minimal endometriosis."

Learning when it is appropriate *not to operate* may now be the test of integrity for gynecologic surgeons.[26,48,56] Only combining concerns for patient autonomy with concerns for beneficence in health care will lead to truly informed consent in gynecologic surgery.

CENTRAL ISSUES OF THE 1990s

Five central issues crystalize the need to focus on the ethics of gynecologic surgery in the 1990s: (1) technological advancements in surgery, (2) the growth of the geriatric population, (3) the increasing number of medically indigent Americans and the associated question of health care financing, (4) the increasing number of developmentally disabled adults, and (5) the acquired immunodeficiency syndrome (AIDS) crisis.

First, laser technology, pelviscopy, urodynamic equipment, and newer colposcopic instrumentation only highlight the expanding technologies available to gynecologic surgeons.[6,30,60] How will surgeons be taught to use this equipment? What research will verify the use of such technologies and who will sponsor it? What financial incentives will encourage surgeons to use such technologies? At what burden of cost and with what proof of benefit will patients be encouraged to seek such technology?

Second, in the 1990s, the largest population group in the United States will be persons over age 65. The women in this age group represent unique ethical issues in gynecologic surgery. Will age alone become a reason to avoid surgery for problems usually surgically managed?[29,50,54] How is informed consent obtained in the face of diminishing mental capacity? As magnified by the Cruzan decision,[23,36] to what degree will living wills, durable power-of-attorney arrangements, and predetermined health care plans control geriatric care? Will repeat operations be discouraged or prohibited? Also, will ethical guidelines be needed to focus attention on the problem of aging surgeons who continue to practice beyond the point when their services are in their patients' best interests?

Third, escalating health care costs have made resource allocation an ethical urgency.[51] Questions of justice demand attention when one person cannot obtain what another person takes for granted in a health care system that prides itself on trying to meet all citizens' needs. Gynecologic surgeons will be pressured more and more frequently to offer not only the most medically effective health care, but also the most cost-effective health care. Will it be deemed unnecessary, or even unreasonable, to order computed tomography (CT) or magnetic resonance imaging (MRI) scans on all patients with an adnexal mass before proceeding to surgery? How much urodynamic evaluation will be required before surgery is performed for stress urinary incontinence, readily discernable in a patient's history? Will obvious leiomyomas require ultrasonographic confirmation before removal?

Fourth, advances in and regionalization of neonatal care in the United States have improved the odds of survival for prematurely born infants. As these infants pass through adolescence into adulthood, the number of patients with developmental disabilities, and especially mental retardation, will increase. Gynecologic surgeons of the 1990s must be familiar with state and federal laws governing sterilization procedures for this patient population. Ethical concerns about ascertaining decision-making capacity, maximizing individual patient well-being, reflecting societal concerns for disabled patients and their families, and offering routine, as well as surgical, care for persons with mental retardation will become more prominent.[17,35]

Fifth, perhaps the overriding source of ethical concern for gynecologic surgeons in the 1990s will stem from the AIDS crisis.[10,42,52,57,59] Will services be denied in any way to persons with AIDS? For gynecologic surgeons, will it become ethically acceptable to treat a patient with a 12-cm tuboovarian abscess for 21 days with intravenous antibiotics when non-HIV-positive patients receive surgical management? Will a hematocrit of 25% or less, now debated, replace 30% as the standard for postoperative blood transfusions? Will invasive procedures become procedures of last resort in an AIDS era?

Questions also remain unresolved about patient and physician testing for high-risk persons in both groups. The relatively high false-positive rate of most routine tests for HIV and the devastating effects of a positive result make most surgical patients and practicing surgeons reluctant to consider mandatory testing for either group. However, 1991 American Medical Association statements concerning testing issues leave little doubt that, as anxiety about the epidemic deepens, some form of mandatory testing awaits both patients and their surgeons.

SUMMARY AND CONCLUSIONS

In this chapter, we have attempted to introduce and organize the discussion of the ethics of gynecologic surgery. Special attention has been given to ethical concerns pertaining to surgical training and to informed consent. A plea has been issued for a vigorous pursuit of biomedical ethics as a component of gynecologic training, research, and practice. Many of the vast number of serious ethical concerns that face gynecologists fall beyond the scope of this chapter. In the final analysis, the ethical practice of gynecologic surgery will serve the patients' best interests "as long as we maintain our integrity."[43]

REFERENCES

1. American College of Obstetricians and Gynecologists: *Patient choice: maternal-fetal conflict.* ACOG policy statement, Washington, DC, 1987, ACOG.
2. Andrews L: Legal and ethical aspects of new reproductive technologies, *Clin Obstet Gynecol* 29:190, March 1986.

3. Association of Professors of Gynecology and Obstetrics Task Force on Medical Ethics: *Exploring issues in obstetrics and gynecologic medical ethics,* Washington, DC, 1990, the Association.

4. Beauchamp T, Childress J: *Principles of biomedical ethics,* ed 3, New York, 1989, Oxford University Press.

5. Bernal E: Hysterectomy and autonomy, *Theor Med* 9:73, Feb 1988.

6. Braine D, Lesser H, editors: *Ethics, technology, and medicine,* Brookfield, Vt, 1988, Gower Publishing Co.

7. Bulger R, editor: *In search of the modern Hippocrates,* Iowa City, 1987, University of Iowa Press.

8. Callahan S: The ethical challenge of the new reproductive technology. In Monagle J, Thomasma D, editors: *Medical ethics: a guide for health professionals,* Rockville, Md, 1988, Aspen Pubs, Inc.

9. Caplan A: The new technologies in reproduction: new ethical problems. In Callahan D, Dunstan G, editors: *Biomedical ethics: an Anglo-American dialogue,* New York, 1988, New York Academy of Sciences.

10. Cooper A: Treating HIV-infected children: the surgeon's role, *Bull Am Coll Surg* 76:13, June 1991.

11. Culver G, Gert B: Basic ethical concepts in neurologic surgery, *Semin Neurol* 4:1, March 1984.

12. US Department of Health and Social Security's Committee of Inquiry into Human Fertilization and Embryology: *A question of life: the Warnock report on human fertilization and embryology,* New York, 1985, Basil Blackwell.

13. Drane J: *Becoming a good doctor: the place of virtue and character in medical ethics,* Kansas City, Mo, 1988, Sheed & Ward.

14. Dunstan G, Shinebourne E, editors: *Doctor's decisions: ethical conflicts in medical practice,* New York, 1989, Oxford University Press.

15. Edwards W, Yahne C: Surgical informed consent: what it is and is not, *Amer J Surg* 154:574 Dec 1987.

16. Elkins T: Introductory course in biomedical ethics in the obstetrics-gynecology residency, *J Med Educ* 63:294, April 1988.

17. Elkins T: Providing gynecologic care for women with mental retardation, *Med Asp Human Sexuality* 56, June 1991.

18. Engelhardt T: *The foundations of bioethics,* New York, 1986, Oxford University Press.

19. *Fertil Steril* 53 (suppl 2):1S, June 1990.

20. Folkman J: Harvard Medical School address, in *The New York Times,* Op-Ed page, June 6, 1975.

21. Gale R et al: Ethical problems in cardiac surgery for lethal, congenital malformation, *J Perinatol* 8:137, Spring 1988.

22. Gallup D, Labudovich M, Zambito P: The gynecologist and the dying cancer patient, *Am J Obstet Gynecol* 144:154, 1982.

23. Harris C, Bostrom B: Is the continued provision of food and fluids in Nancy Cruzan's best interests? *Iss Law Med* 5:415, Spring 1990.

24. Hauerwas S: Authority and the profession of medicine. In Agich G, editor: *Responsibility and health care,* Dordrecht, 1982, D Reidel.

25. Herter F, et al, editors: *Human and ethical issues in the surgical care of patients with life-threatening disease,* Springfield, Ill, 1986, Charles C. Thomas.

26. Jecker N: Knowing when to stop: the limits of medicine, *Hastings Cent Rep* 21:5, May-June 1991.

27. Kane W: Ethics and surgical clerkships, *Bull Am Coll Surg* 69:6, May 1984.

28. Kass L: Thinking about the body, *Hastings Cent Rep* 15:20, Feb 1985.

29. Kilner J: Age criteria in medicine: are medical justifications ethical? *Arch Intern Med* 149:2343, Oct 1989.

30. Kjellstrand C: Giving life, giving death: ethical problems of high-technology medicine, *Acta Med Scand* Suppl 725:1, 1988.

31. Kugel R: Surgery and the rights of children with handicaps, *NY Med Quart* 5:7, 1985.

32. Leppert P: Hysterectomy: a brief look at psychosocial aspects. In Herter F, et al, editors: *Human and ethical issues in the surgical care of patients with life-threatening disease,* Springfield, Ill, 1986, Charles C Thomas.

33. MacIntyre A: *After virtue,* Notre Dame, Ind, 1983, University of Notre Dame Press.

34. May W: *The physician's covenant,*

35. McNeeley G, Elkins T: Gynecologic surgery and surgical morbidity in mentally handicapped women, *Obstet Gynecol* 74:155, Aug 1989.

36. Meisel A: Lessons from Cruzan, *J Clin Ethics* 1:245, Fall 1990.

37. Moffic S, Coverdale J, Bayer T: The Hippocratic oath and clinical ethics, *J Clin Ethics* 1:287, Winter 1990.

38. Nora P: Ethics in house-staff training, *Bull Am Coll Surg* 69:3, May 1984.

39. Oath of Hippocrates. In Hippocrates, Loeb Classical Library, Cambridge, Mass, 1982, Harvard University Press (Translated by W Jones).

40. Otto R: *The idea of the holy,* London, 1926, Oxford University Press.

41. Pellegrino E, Thomasma D: *For the patient's good: the restoration of beneficence in health care,* New York, 1988, Oxford University Press.

42. Peterson L: AIDS and surgical care: a challenge for the 1990s, *Bull Am Coll Surg* 75:20, Nov 1990.

43. Pillsbury H: Challenge for the year 2000: worthy to serve the suffering, *Bull Am Coll Surg* 76:6, March 1991.

44. Press I: The predisposition to file claims: the patient's perspective, *Law, Medicine, and Health Care*:53, April 1984.

45. Pringle K: Ethical implications of fetal surgery. In Brooks B, editor: *Controversies in pediatric surgery,* Austin, 1984, University of Texas Press.

46. Reich W: Caring for life in the first of it: moral paradigms for perinatal and neonatal ethics, *Semin Perinatol* 11:279, July 1987.

47. Sassower R, Grodin M: Scientific uncertainty and medical responsibility, *Theor Med* 8:221, June 1987.

48. Schacht P, Pemberton A: What is unnecessary surgery? who shall decide? issues of consumer sovereignty, conflict, and self regulation, *Soc Sci Med* 20:199, 1985.

49. Schenk W: The tired surgeon, *Ann Surg* 161:627, April 1965.

50. Schofield J: Care of the older person: the ethical challenge to American medicine, *Issues in Law and Medicine* 4:53, Summer 1988.

51. Schwartz W, Aaron H: Rationing hospital care: lessons from Britain, *N Engl J Med* 310:52, 1984.

52. Sheldon M: HIV and the obligation to treat, *Theor Med* 11:201, 1990.

53. Shinebourne E: The ethics of innovative cardiac surgery, *Br Heart J* 52:597, Dec 1984.

54. Siegler M: Should age alone be a criterion in health care? *Hastings Cent Rep* 5:24, 1984.

55. Singer P et al: The ethics of liver transplantation with living donors, *N Engl J Med* 321:620, 1989.

56. Stoll B: Knowing when not to treat, *Baillieres Clin Oncol* 1:443, July 1987.

57. Stotter A: A different slant on surgery and HIV, *Br Med J* 298:536, 1989.

58. Stovall T, Ling F, Crawford D: Hysterectomy for chronic pelvic pain, *Obstet Gynecol* 75:676, 1990.

59. A surgeon won't operate on victims of AIDS, *The New York Times,* p 21A, March 13, 1987.

60. Szawarski Z: Dignity and technology, *J Med Philos* 14:243, June 1989.

61. Walters L: Ethical aspects of the new reproductive technologies. In Jones H, Schrader C, editors: *In vitro fertilization and other assisted reproduction,* New York, 1988, New York Academy of Sciences.

62. Weaver J: A physician's indications for admission the night before surgery, *Gynecol Obstet* 172:227, March 1991.

63. Weiss G, Vanderpool H: Ethics and cancer: an annotated bibliography, Galveston, 1984, University of Texas Medical Branch.

Part III

BASIC TECHNIQUES AND MANAGEMENT OF SURGICAL COMPLICATIONS IN GYNECOLOGIC OPERATIONS

Chapter 11

THE ROLE OF THE SURGICAL ASSISTANT

David H. Nichols

To some, the handling of tools and tissues comes easily—almost without their conscious realization. Others must laboriously learn the many subtle ways that surgeons use their hands to support, expose, remove, manipulate, and repair the tissues of the human body. These movements must be efficient, time-saving, and gentle enough to avoid undue damage to living cells. They require the almost unconscious integration of rather complex movements of both hands.

The hands of the principal surgeon are usually engaged in accomplishing the primary objectives of the operation. The hands of the assistant surgeons must expedite that surgeon's work. This interplay of cooperating hands can produce a flowing and beautiful pattern of teamwork—or, if done badly, it can result in a rough, halting, awkward, and time-consuming exercise. . . .

Good surgical teamwork requires that the assistant be constantly alert. He [she] must anticipate the sequence of surgical steps and try to stay ahead of the surgeon in planning the next phase of the operation. He should take pride in seeing how often he can be in position and ready to facilitate the operation without being given specific instructions. When surgeons work together over a period of time, teamwork becomes much more efficient and few words need be spoken. . . . The key words are to *anticipate and facilitate*. There is no place at the operating table for an assistant who periodically develops the glazed look of someone in a "catatonic trance." An assistant should feel embarrassed if the surgeon frequently needs to take the initiative in many of these support maneuvers. . . .

The assistant would do well to read about the operation the night before if he is unfamiliar with the condition or planned operation. He should always review the regional anatomy before each procedure. The alert and informed assistant will usually be given more operative responsibilities at an early stage of his training than one who is only 'doing his job.'[4]

Working with a good team of surgical assistants can be one of the great joys of a surgeon's life. The smoothness and precision of a surgical operation is directly dependent on the individual attention, resourcefulness, experience, and skill of the surgeon's assistants. Each member of the surgical team must know and understand his or her individual role, as well as that of every other member of the team. Experience and knowledge of the operative principles to be followed ensure that unexpected surgical events are rare; conscientious anticipation makes it possible to predict each operative step with accuracy. Advances in modern surgical technology have made this harmony among the surgical team even more important than it has been in the past. Each step during an operation should be performed correctly the first time if the patient is to obtain maximum benefit.

In the large metropolitan hospitals of Europe, as well as in the small hospitals of the United States, a surgeon may have the privilege of working with the same first assistant or operative team for many years. In the large teaching hospitals of the United States, however, the academic rotation of their training programs makes it necessary for many house officers to seek in succession a maximum exposure to the art and craft of each attending surgeon's operating room activity. This approach to training places a great burden on the senior members of the operating team to ensure not only that the operation is well performed, but also that it has been a learning experience for each member of the team—regardless of their individual levels of experience. "To the mature surgeon, the teaching of the minutiae of surgical technique can become tedious, with the lingering hope that trainees may have a natural sixth sense or an inherent prompt grasp without repeated admonitions."[1] Although it is a serious additional responsibility for the surgeon in the clinical environment, such training leads inevitably to an academic model of surgical perfection that becomes a major part of the heritage of the next generation of surgeons. The consequence of any break, accidental or intentional, in the continuity of this careful system destroys its harmony and compromises the end result.

Most books on surgical technique make operations look easy. Those who are not part of a progressive training program that exposes them to a considerable volume of surgery will not see a surgeon in trouble often enough to know how to avoid problems nor how to resolve the problems that do occur.[3] Experience with many operations makes it possible for surgeons and their assistants to think clearly and to make proper decisions under pressure. Like the surgeon, the surgical assistant must be aware that most serious postoperative complications in otherwise good-risk patients have their genesis in errors of commission or omission during the operative procedure.[5] Both must note countless details, including the patient's general condition and the readiness of suitable equipment. "A good first assistant can make a clumsy surgeon look great, but a poor first assistant can make a competent surgeon look bad."[1]

BEFORE SURGERY

The assistant should know the surgeon's protocol for preoperative and postoperative care and should discuss with the surgeon any possible deviation to be followed in a particular case. If the planned operation is an uncommon one, the surgical assistant should describe to the scrub nurse well ahead of time the goals of the operation and any unusual technical features so that the nurse can locate and prepare rarely used instruments and sutures. "A good scrub nurse must have a flair for organization and be well trained, fast thinking and meticulous."[7] Like every other member of the operative team, the scrub nurse should be calm and not easily "rattled." Furthermore, team members should be well rested, if possible, and in good physical condition.

Before using the brush, all members of the surgical team should wash their hands and forearms with soap and water to remove superficial dirt and grease that would contaminate the brush. Scrubbing should include the forearms, and the fingernails require particular attention. After scrubbing, the team should rinse their hands and forearms thoroughly, holding the hands above the level of the elbow so water does not run from the elbows toward the hands. When the hands are being dried, no part of the towel that has touched the forearm should touch the hand, and there should never be a stroke from the forearm to the hand.

In the operating room before the surgery begins, the assistants and each member of the surgical team should maintain some distance from the others. The nurse should apply the gloves; after the final application, the surgeon may adjust the fingers and wrists. Powder should now be rinsed from the gloves with sterile water.

The assistant should look at the instrument table, observing the instruments on it and the placement of each. In an emergency, an awareness of this layout may be valuable.

DURING SURGERY

The duty of the assistants during surgery is to help the operating surgeon. The first assistant's functions are to anticipate the needs and moves of the surgeon, try to facilitate them, and help to create maximum exposure of the operative site with proper retraction and a clear field of unobstructed vision. The second assistant carries out the wishes of the first assistant and the surgeon, restricting activities to holding instruments or retractors as instructed.

The first assistant has the responsibility of providing hemostasis with the least possible interruption as the operation proceeds. Therefore, the assistant should have suction devices, clamps, scissors, ties, or the electrocautery ready for use. Tamponade of any bleeding surfaces with simple pressure should be an almost reflex motion. Sponging, which should be concentrated at the actual site of cutting, clamping, or sewing, should be by quick blotting rather than by dabbing or wiping. Suction is useful in removing blood or secretions that have accumulated away from the center of the operative site.

In clamping vessels that the surgeon has transected by the incision, the assistant should place hemostatic clamps quickly, but carefully, to include only the vessel and a minimum of its surrounding tissues. As vessels are ligated, the clamps holding them should be opened slowly while the ligature is tightened. Generally, clamped vessels are tied off or coagulated beginning with the last one clamped. When the surgeon ties off a clamped vessel, the assistant holds up the handle of the hemostat so the surgeon can pass the ligature around it, then drops the hand and elevates the tip of the hemostat. As soon as the hemostat has been taken off and the knot has been tied, the assistant cuts the long ends of the ligature.

In general, suture ends are cut ½ to 1 cm from the knot, as the surgeon instructs. Knots are usually square, requiring three throws if a synthetic suture is used or six if a monofilament suture is used. If the ends of a tie or suture are cut too short, the knot may slip; if the ends are left too long, they become the risk of a foreign body. If able to "palm" the suture scissors when the operation is in a phase that requires suture cutting, the assistant can continue to use the hand holding the scissors and save time (Fig. 11-1). It is also helpful if the assistant can clamp, cut, and tie with either hand.

"What might be called timing is learned only by experience. A good assistant will so time his sponging that the operator experiences the minimum of interference."[3] When vessels are cut, the assistant should wait until the surgeon's hand goes back before sponging. The assistant should not grab for bleeders, but should apply pressure with the sponge and apply the hemostat to the bleeding point accurately as the sponge is removed. As far as possible, only the tip of the hemostat should be applied. When the tie keeps slipping from beneath the tip of the hemostat, another hemostat may be applied from the opposite direction just underneath the tip. The suture should be tied

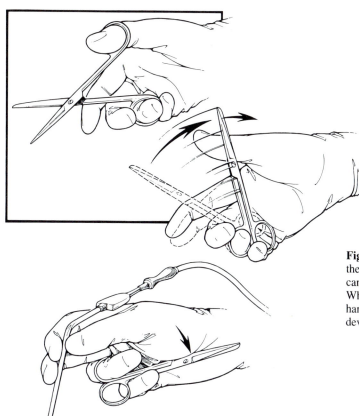

Fig. 11-1. A method of palming the scissors is shown, whereby the scissors, grasped by the fourth finger and thumb as shown, can be quickly flipped back and forth as indicated in the drawing. When these have been palmed, the medial three fingers of the hand are available for other purposes, such as holding a suction device as shown or perhaps in tying knots.

around both, and the second hemostat should be removed first.

It is not necessary for one assistant to do all the clamping, another to do all the tying, and a third to do all the cutting. As a rule, it is easier for the assistant to tie off hemostats on the operator's side, and vice versa. Usually, the one who holds the hemostat can cut sutures much faster and more accurately than can a second assistant who must come into the operative field at arm's length.

The handle of a retractor should generally be low, and the assistant should always know where the tip of the retractor is. Assistants should not move retractors without the surgeon's request or permission, not only because the retractors may then fail to provide sustained exposure of the operative field, but also because they may innocently inflict considerable damage to the structures with which they were in contact.

Instruments should be passed in a firm and decisive manner. The scrub nurse who is watching the operative field will probably know what the surgeon is likely to want next and will be prepared for the surgeon's request. Hand signals are particularly useful both for avoiding unnecessary conversation and for saving time. Some of the widely accepted hand signals in operating rooms are illustrated in Figs. 11-2 through 11-7.

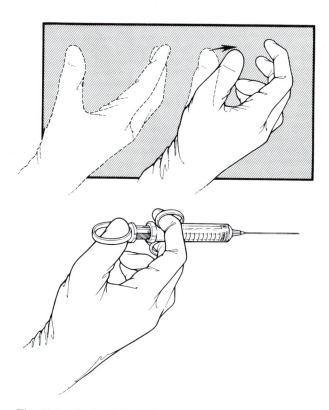

Fig. 11-2. The hand signal for requesting a hand syringe is identified, as if the syringe were already present in the empty hand. The index and middle finger fit the rings of the pressure syringe, and the thumb fits the end of the barrel, and as the thumb moves toward the index finger, the injection of a solution is suggested.

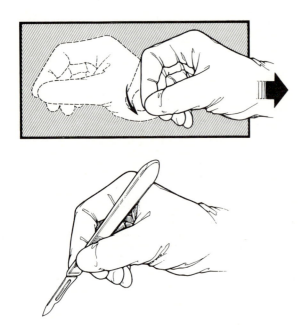

Fig. 11-3. A proper hand signal for requesting a scalpel is shown. The fingers are in the position in which the scalpel would normally be held, and the act of cutting is indicated by bending the wrist and thumb and forefinger as shown.

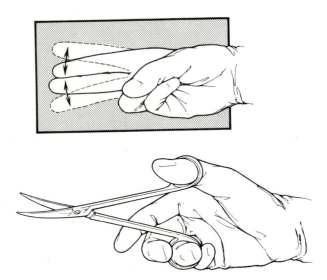

Fig. 11-5. A maneuver for requesting scissors is shown whereby the index and middle finger are spread in a scissorlike fashion, following which the palm is opened to receive the scissors that have been placed within it.

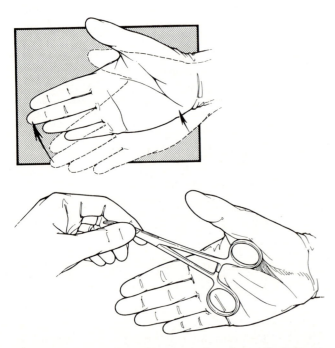

Fig. 11-4. A hand signal for requesting a hemostatic forceps is shown. The operator extends the hand with open palm, moving it up and down as shown, so the forceps can be placed with the rings in the palm of the hand.

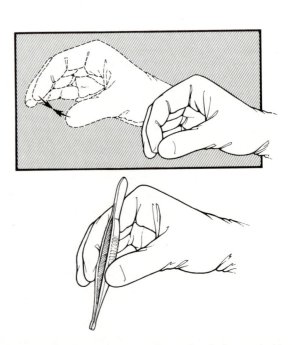

Fig. 11-6. The figure for requesting a thumb forceps is identified. The hand is positioned as if it had a forceps within it and, by bringing the thumb and index finger together, the movement or motion of the forceps is suggested. The hand is then opened to receive the forceps.

As dissection proceeds to the deeper tissues, the assistant can often provide helpful countertraction. It is often necessary to redirect the surgical spotlights at different angles to better illuminate the wound; this can be the responsibility of the assistant. As the operation proceeds, the surgeon may wish to shift or reposition the second assistant's retractors.

Surgical assistants should keep their hands as low as possible and well back from the incision when not in use. Furthermore, an assistant who must reach to the other side of any incision should reach to the side of the operative field rather than across it so as to keep from obstructing the surgeon's view. It is also essential for the assistant to avoid becoming so interested in the operation that he or she bends over and obstructs the surgeon's view of the operative field. The assistant should not take his or her eyes off the wound any more than absolutely necessary, however, especially when holding some piece of tissue or instrument with which the surgeon is working.

Both the surgeon and the assistant learn with experience the importance of gentleness in handling tissues. Roughness may prolong the operation by causing organ damage that requires repair; it may cause an injury that subsequently reveals itself in postoperative complications or sluggish convalescence; it may render anastomoses less than perfect; and it may precipitate immediate or delayed hemorrhage, which is perennially a major cause of avoidable morbidity.

The surgical assistant must be careful not to lean on the patient. Shifting the weight frequently and keeping the lumbar spine as straight as possible prevent the fatigue that leads to carelessness. When tying sutures, the assistant braces the arms, elbows, forearms, and wrists to prevent the hand holding one end of a tie from jerking in the opposite direction should the tie break.

The operative field must be kept orderly and neat; sponges, loose instruments, and cut suture ends should not be left lying about. They should be removed from the field whenever a pause permits.

Noise is distracting to a surgical team in the operating room, and unnecessary noise can be counterproductive. Silence encourages a high level of concentration, and there is less chance of inoculating the surgical wound with the team's respiratory bacteria if they are not talking. Important observations concerning the operative plan or changes should be verbalized, especially when the more experienced surgeon is serving as assistant to the junior, but unimportant observations are best left for another time.

Excellence in the performance of one's duties must receive one's undivided concentration. Usually the best of surgeons were formerly the best of assistants.

While the wound is being closed, the assistant should review with the surgeon the plans for postoperative care and any special routines to be implemented.

In a surgical training program, the surgeon may turn a case over to the assistant, particularly if the assistant has demonstrated interest and ability while assisting the surgeon on similar cases in the past. Expecting the assistant to be aware of the patient's clinical circumstances and the details of the technique to be followed, the surgeon generally plans to become the first assistant in such a delegated case, although he or she must remain acutely observant, highly helpful, and constructively critical. The assistant should never hesitate to ask questions concerning any phase of the operation and the appropriate aftercare.

If problems arise that the assistant doing the surgery feels are beyond his or her ability to handle without compromising patient care, the assistant must instantly convey this concern to the surgeon; if the assistant would like the surgeon to take over the operation or any portion thereof, he or she must not hesitate to say so. Often, the surgeon takes care of the presumably difficult steps and, if still confident of the assistant's ability, permits the latter to resume the surgical operation. When the senior surgeon perceives that a particular maneuver is not going well and asks the assistant who is operating to stop, the assistant must obey instantly—with the hands literally frozen in mid-air, not after the movement or incision in progress has been completed. A scheduled assistant who has been invited to operate on the patient of a private attending surgeon must always remember that such an opportunity is a privilege, not a right.

AFTER SURGERY

Even when surgical assistants are tired from having been up the night before, a shower and a clean uniform do

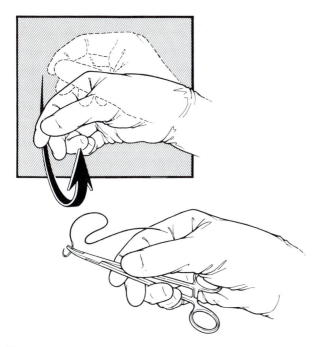

Fig. 11-7. A hand signal for requesting a needle holder and suture is shown. The hand is poised as if it held a ligature carrier, and, with a rotary motion of the wrist in a clockwise direction, the path of the needle is indicated, then the palm is flattened to receive the ligature carrier.

a lot to revive their spirit. Male house officers should be freshly shaven each morning.

On postoperative rounds, the surgical assistant should check for sweating and pallor, which may indicate internal hemorrhage; restlessness and disorientation, which may suggest cyanosis of hypoxia; and an anxious facies, which may reflect serious sepsis.

The patient's costovertebral angles should be gently jabbed, and any pain or asymmetry of discomfort should be noted and brought to the surgeon's attention lest any possible compromise of ureteral patency go undetected.

Auscultation and percussion of the chest help exclude atelectasis. Auscultation of the abdomen, listening for bowel sounds, should be routine, as should palpation of the patient's calves; any departure from normal should be noted and followed. Records of fluid intake, urinary output, and the patient's temperature should be examined.

The patient's questions and complaints should be listened to patiently and attentively, and it should be determined that all of the postoperative orders have been followed, and new ones have been written as healing progresses. Every patient should be seen at least once each day, preferably in the morning, and any difficult questions or clinical departure from normal should be discussed with the senior house officer or the attending surgeon. Patients who are ill or are not doing well should be seen more frequently during the day; when the house officer is going off duty, a report should be given personally to the incoming house officer. A legible note should be written after each visit.

TRAINING

There is a conceptual difference between an assistant who is a fully trained professional associate and an assistant who is participating in an operation as part of a postgraduate training program. Both must have a detailed knowledge of the surgical details of the anticipated procedure and its possible complications. The professional associate, however, is also expected to be familiar by personal experience with the particular operation and to know the operator's preferential or usual approach to this surgical remedy; the individual patient may be preoperatively unknown to this assistant. In contrast, the trainee is expected to have learned the history and clinical findings that have led to surgery, to have grasped the details of the decision-making process for this particular patient, and to understand the specific reasons that this operation was chosen for this patient over alternate procedures. Furthermore, the trainee follows the patient's progress postoperatively.

Surgical internship

"The purpose of a surgical internship is to provide interns with the opportunity to learn firsthand the surgical methods and techniques of dealing with patients employed by the most respected surgeons in the community. The intern should respond promptly to all calls regarding patients within the hospital, no matter how trivial they may seem,

even if he or she is not on duty at the time. The intern should make every effort to understand all the procedures that are employed, taking care to read or inquire about those that are unfamiliar. Tact is as essential as is good judgment. Interns can acquire the latter by continually anticipating all types of situations that may arise.

If possible, an intern who is to assist a surgeon should arrive in the operating room slightly ahead of time to review the patient's chart, introduce one's self to the patient, and supervise the transport of the patient to the operating table, to have the patient prepared and draped for the start of the operation, and to become familiar with the instruments lying on the instrument stand. When the operation begins, the intern should take a place opposite the surgeon. If there is a second intern, he or she should be at the right hand of the first intern; if there is a third intern, he or she takes a position at the surgeon's left hand or between the patient's legs, depending on the patient's position on the operating table.

The attending surgeon's first duty to the intern is to provide systematic instructions. Every patient in the [teaching] hospital should be accessible to the intern. The surgeon should make it a point to show the intern interesting pathologic conditions and to explain fully the reasons for the various therapeutic measures employed. The surgeon should try to have the intern perform all the operations that he or she is capable of handling and should take pains to guide and encourage the intern's first surgical efforts. A surgeon working at high tension may be unjustly impatient with the surgical team, however, and the intern should strive to be patient and self-contained under such circumstances. In no event can the surgeon subordinate the patient's welfare.

Outside the operating room, the surgeon should use questions to stimulate the intern's interests and should encourage the intern to undertake collateral reading, to attend conferences, and to conduct original investigations. The surgeon should strive to set a good example for the intern in an intellectual approach to surgical problems and in a compassionate attitude toward patients. The attending surgeon should endeavor to delegate responsibilities as far as possible and should introduce the intern to patients as a colleague. It is important for the surgeon to take the time to read all the records and orders that the intern has written and criticize them, if necessary. Above all, the surgeon must remember that the intern is human, subject to all the natural human frailties, and, therefore, susceptible to fatigue.

The intern should be loyal to the attending surgeon, even though their opinions about patient care may differ. These differences can be resolved privately—never within earshot of the patient or nurses. In addition, the intern should be loyal to the hospital, particularly in conversation with the patients, and should endeavor to explain satisfactorily circumstances that the patient does not understand.

It is to an intern's benefit to be uniformly courteous and respectful to nurses and to address them by name. Treatment suggestions made by older, experienced nurses may well deserve careful consideration; when certain that the orders given are appropriate, however, the intern should maintain authority and not modify the orders to suit the nurse. An intern should never criticize a nurse within hearing distance of a patient.

The intern should make rounds in the evening and write orders that are consistent with patient comfort and safety and with the intern's understanding of the ideas of the attending surgeon. The intern should anticipate the needs of the patient during the night as far as possible. Inexperienced nurses may call an intern needlessly in the middle of the night, based on what the nurse considers to be a serious responsibility to the patient; interns should answer such calls patiently and courteously—never sarcastically."[2]

Surgical residency

"The surgical resident usually aspires to become an outstanding clinical surgeon. He may begin by acquiring a solid and wide base of knowledge and understanding of basic surgical philosophy and facts. Concurrently, he should develop strong compassion for the sick and a strong surgical conscience. Compassion does not replace the need for an accurate knowledge and application of modern technique, physiology and biochemistry. . . . but in the long run, compassion does much for the total human experience, for the young surgeon's personal growth and for the general stature of the profession. A strong surgical conscience will prevent the resident from embarking unaided upon operations with which he is unprepared to cope. The resident will bear in mind that his senior surgeon is held accountable for all complications or deaths. Often the senior surgeon will silently share the responsibility for a resident's error made entirely without his presence or knowledge. Not only does a staff surgeon have a responsibility to support the resident, but the resident has a responsibility to support his surgical senior. The resident should learn early on to accept responsibility for the patients' welfares and survival. It should be assumed that a junior resident will take longer to perform a given operation than his chief, but when the operation is completed, it must be first-class. If at any point the operation is proceeding unsatisfactorily, the resident with the proper surgical conscience will consult his superior at once, before the clinical situation has been damaged or deteriorated. To do this may require a high order of courage and interpersonal relationships. It definitely requires a combination of objective honesty and genuine humility. Thus, the trainee will strive to achieve nothing less than perfection in each instance, for he will come to realize that in accepting anything less than the perfection possible under the circumstances is to subtract something from another person's life."[5]

The residency program must last several years if it is to provide the extended experience necessary for the development of a degree of surgical maturity. In a year, a bright high school graduate can learn to perform most of the common operations expeditiously in the animal laboratory and to achieve an acceptable mortality in dogs. Such a person knows nothing of diagnosis, operative risks, alternatives, the physiologic management of complications, the exercise of sound surgical judgment, and the management

of worried human beings, however. Senior residents finish their years of formative experience with a lifetime of learning ahead, confident because of their operative experience, but clearly aware of their limitations. These residents have established a firm foundation toward becoming superior clinical surgeons.[5]

BLOOD EXPOSURE IN THE OPERATING ROOM

No member of the surgical team can afford to be indifferent to the possibility of exposure to transmissible infections in the operating room. Of surgeons, 25% have been infected with hepatitis B, and nearly 50% are at risk of infection because they have not received the highly effective hepatitis B vaccine.[8] The uniformly fatal outcome of clinical acquired immunodeficiency syndrome (AIDS) mandates the development of a line of defense against blood exposure that includes strong barriers to contact with patient blood and body fluids, improved operating room techniques, and prompt response to a blood contact or exposure event.

Surgical techniques in which it is necessary to pass the curved surgical needle through tissues require constant vigilance; blind suturing techniques in which the tip of the needle must be palpated for localization should be avoided. The passage of sharp instruments and needle-loaded ligature carriers back and forth between the instrument technician and the surgeon is hazardous. Stapled anastomoses and the use of the cautery instead of the sharp scalpel may be helpful.

A recent study showed that a blood contact event took place in 28% of 684 operations, involving a total of 293 operating room personnel.[9] One third of these blood contact events involved percutaneous injury, mucous membrane contact, or blood contact with nonintact skin! Most incidents were preventable. Precautions should be selected according to procedure variables such as anticipated blood loss and length of operation.

Punctures and tears of surgical gloves are the most common reasons for blood contact in the operating room. Double gloving has been shown to reduce blood contact with the hands.[6,9] Placing a glove that is a half-size larger than needed over the hand with the correct size glove as a second, outer glove seems to optimize dexterity and minimize constriction of the hand. A lightweight apron worn under the gown minimizes the blood contact with the operator's trunk that results from barrier failure associated with major abdominal operations such as cesarean sections. Wearing protective eye shields also reduces blood exposure risks.

When blood contact does occur, the application of isopropyl alcohol or povidone-iodine solution and regloving seem useful, given the virucidal effects of these two solutions.

REFERENCES

1. Cannon B: *Foreword* In Edgerton MT: *The art of surgical technique,* Baltimore, 1988, Williams & Wilkins.

2. Christopher F: *Minor surgery,* ed 5, Philadelphia, 1944, WB Saunders.
3. Dudley DG: The surgical assistant, *Surg Gynecol Obstet* 115:245, 1962.
4. Edgerton MT: *The art of surgical technique,* Baltimore, 1988, Williams & Wilkins.
5. Hardy JD: The superior clinical surgeon, *Surg Gynecol Obstet* 124:1075, 1967.
6. Matta H, Thompson AM, Rainey JB: Does wearing two pairs of gloves protect operating theatre staff from skin contamination? *Br J Med* 297:597, 1988.
7. Novak F: *Surgical gynecologic techniques,* New York, 1978, John Wiley and Sons.
8. Palmer D et al: Hepatitis among hospital employees, *West J Med* 138:519, 1983.
9. Popejoy SL, Fry DE: Blood contact and exposure in the operating room, *Surg Gynecol Obstet* 172:480, 1991.

Chapter 12

INCISIONS

David H. Nichols

Although a wide range of abdominal incisions are available to the gynecologic surgeon, the fundamental guiding precept is that there be adequate exposure of the entire operative field. This must take into account the many likely ramifications of extension of the original planned surgery. For example, surgery performed on a postmenopausal woman to remove a 5-cm adnexal mass, although quickly performed through a cosmetically attractive Pfannenstiel's incision, may reveal that the lesion is malignant, and a thorough exploration of the abdomen is indicated in the course of staging the disease, including the possibility of paraaortic node dissection, further pelvic surgery, and occasionally omentectomy. Similarly, the incision for total abdominal hysterectomy in a patient being treated for adenocarcinoma of the endometrium should permit adequate exposure for pelvic node sampling if the latter is desired consequent to an unexpectedly greater depth of myometrial invasion by the tumor. An incision that is most effective surgically may not be the one that is most attractive cosmetically. If the latter consideration is critical for the patient requiring hysterectomy, perhaps hysterectomy by the vaginal route should be done safely, avoiding an abdominal incision altogether.

Operative exposure for abdominal surgery involving the anterior surface of the sacrum, such as sacral colpopexy or presacral neurectomy, must provide sufficient exposure for surgery to be done safely.

The tiny incisions used with laparoscopy are considered in the appropriate chapters.[39,45]

GENERAL PRINCIPLES

The surgeon should be able to extend the chosen incision if circumstances are found during the course of operation that require a larger operative exposure.

Most pelvic surgery can be performed effectively through a lower midline incision. This can be extended easily if necessary, often alongside the umbilicus, and re-

paired effectively with a minimal risk of postoperative development of evisceration or wound hernia.

The Maylard or transverse incision provides excellent exposure of the pelvis, although it does take a little longer to perform and to repair. The exposure for coincident surgery of the upper abdomen may be compromised (i.e., hepatic or diaphragmatic biopsy, omentectomy, or paraaortic node dissection), so the surgeon should have carefully evaluated the potential for this need preoperatively. The Cherney incision, which avoids transecting the rectus muscles by temporarily detaching them from their insertion on the pubis, provides effective exposure of the pelvis and retropubic areas, but not as broad an exposure as that provided by the Maylard or midline incision. It can be employed to convert a Pfannenstiel's incision into a surgical exposure that is more effective should circumstances require.

Pfannenstiel's incision is the most cosmetically attractive abdominal incision for the patient, but provides access for the least amount of exposure of the pelvis when compared to the midline or Maylard transverse incision. Pfannenstiel's incision is least likely to present a risk of postoperative wound herniation, and is suitable for tubal ligation, hysterectomy for benign disease when the uterus is small, ovarian cystectomy, and certain instances of tubal or adnexal reconstructive surgery.

ANATOMY OF THE ANTERIOR ABDOMINAL WALL

The muscular layers of the anterior abdominal wall must be considered individually because of the differences in the direction in which their fibers run; an incision should traverse each layer separately. The most superficial muscular layer is that of the external oblique (Fig. 12-1). The underlying internal oblique, with fibers almost at right angles to those of the external oblique, is shown in Fig. 12-2; the deepest layer, the transversus abdominus, is

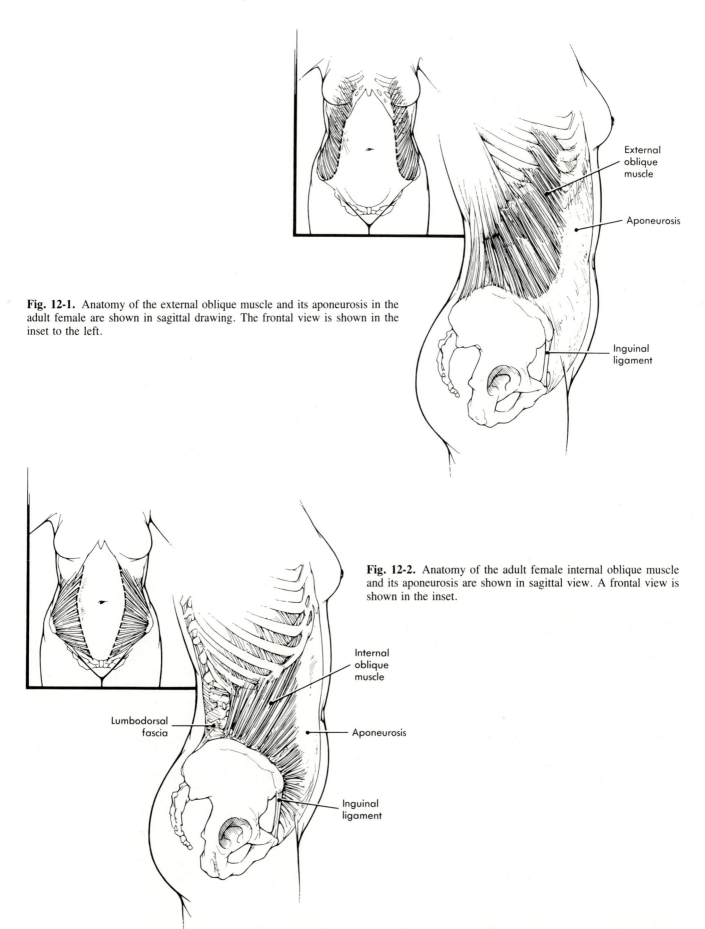

Fig. 12-1. Anatomy of the external oblique muscle and its aponeurosis in the adult female are shown in sagittal drawing. The frontal view is shown in the inset to the left.

Fig. 12-2. Anatomy of the adult female internal oblique muscle and its aponeurosis are shown in sagittal view. A frontal view is shown in the inset.

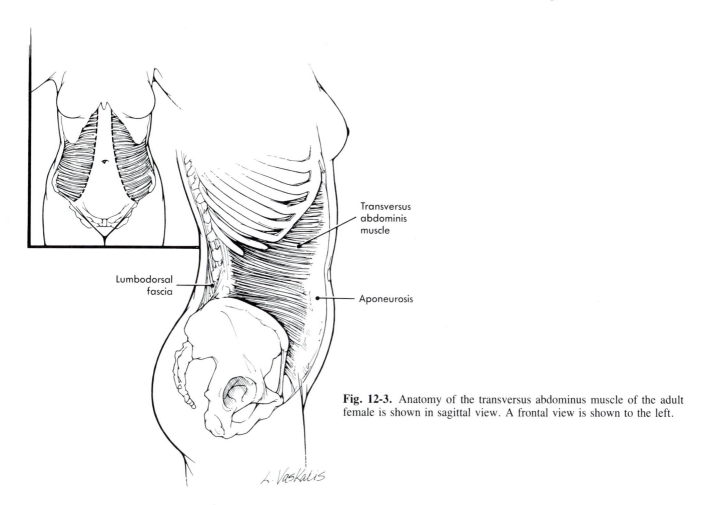

Fig. 12-3. Anatomy of the transversus abdominus muscle of the adult female is shown in sagittal view. A frontal view is shown to the left.

shown in both frontal and side view in Fig. 12-3. Because these muscles function synergistically, a cut-away drawing of their positions relative to one another is shown in Fig. 12-4. The cutaneous nerves arise from the seventh to twelfth thoracic nerves, the anterior cutaneous branch of the iliohypogastric nerve, and the ilioinguinal nerve. These nerves curve forward and downward between the internal oblique and transversalis muscles. The anterior cutaneous branch of the iliohypogastric nerve terminates after piercing the aponeurosis of the external oblique muscle just above the subcutaneous inguinal ring. The ilioinguinal nerve passes through the subcutaneous ring to innervate the skin of the labia majora and medial aspect of the thigh. The anterior branches supply the internal oblique and transverse abdominal muscles as they pass forward between them, and the terminal anterior cutaneous branches supply the rectus muscles, entering from their lateral side.

The superficial and deep nerves of the anterior abdominal wall enter the muscles laterally (Fig. 12-5). If an incision can spare transection of these nerves, muscular function will be preserved, but the surgeon must be careful not to include entrapped nerve tissue in a suture line, which can cause severe postoperative pain. The latter phenomenon is poorly understood because it resembles the response pattern of receptor fiber subjected to chronic stimulation. Sippo and Gomez[43] hypothesize that, unlike other sensory receptors, pain receptors are nonadaptive to continuous or repeated stimulation and can even lower their threshold for excitation when continuously stimulated, as by entrapment in an incisional closure. Until this stimulus is removed by either interruption using local anesthetic infiltration of the site of nerve trauma or, failing this, resection of the nerve, the cascade of transmissions from the receptor continues and the perceived intensity of the pain increases.[17,34,44] The mechanism of this pain relief after local anesthetic injection is not well understood, but it has been hypothesized that the nerve block allows the threshold of stimulation to reset to its original level at a time when ongoing stimulation is subliminal. Although the stimulation is still present, it does not trigger the conduction of a pain impulse.

The arterial blood supply of the anterior abdominal wall to its various layers is shown in Fig. 12-6. Although the superior and inferior epigastric arteries are continuous with one another in 50% of people, there is much individual variation in this relationship, and in many people there is not a common pathway between these vessels. In the presence of obliterative disease of the femoral artery, it is possible for the flow of blood in the inferior epigastric artery to be in the opposite direction and it may supply considerable collateral circulation to the lower extremity. In such patients, it is important to palpate the pulsations of the

Fig. 12-4. A composite of the muscles of the anterior abdominal wall of the adult female is shown. The superficial muscles are to be noted to the left of the drawing. In the illustration to the right of the drawing, the rectus abdominus muscle, external and internal oblique muscles, and lower half of the rectus abdominus have been removed to show the structures underneath. Notice the position of the arcuate line. Above the arcuate line, the posterior leaf of the internal aponeurosis and the aponeurosis of the transversalis unite to form the posterior wall of the rectus sheath. Below the arcuate line, a posterior wall of the rectus sheath is formed only by the muscular plate of the transversalis.

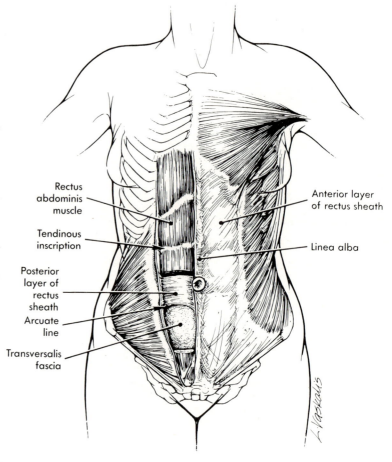

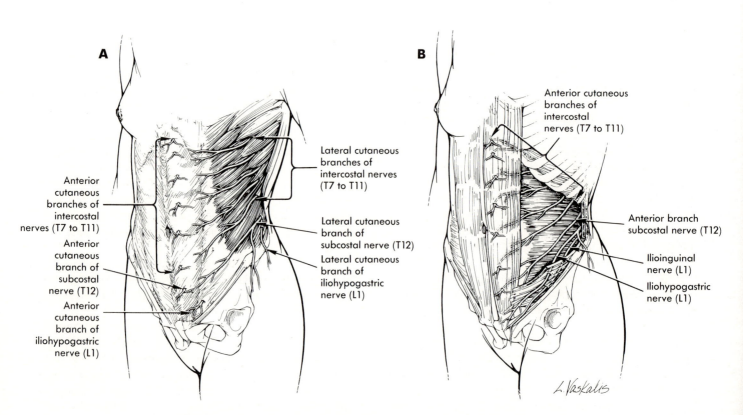

Fig. 12-5. Superficial (**A**) and deep (**B**) nerves of the anterior abdominal wall.

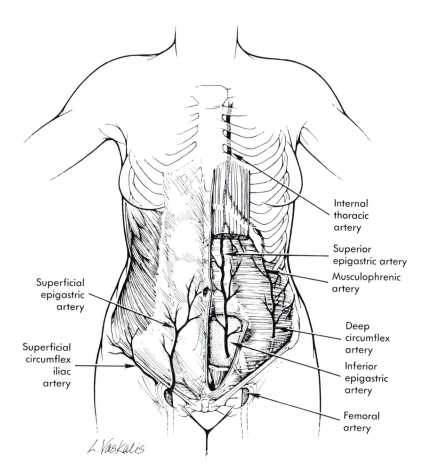

Fig. 12-6. Arterial blood supply of the anterior abdominal wall. The superficial arteries should be noted to the left of the drawing, the deep arteries to the right. Although there is frequently direct continuity between the superior and inferior epigastric artery, it is subject to considerable variation and at times there is no anastomosis between the two.

dorsalis pedis artery after the inferior epigastric artery has been temporarily occluded but before it is transected so there is no risk to the circulation of the lower extremity.

The basic bony landmarks are shown, along with the site for the principal incisions used in transabdominal pelvic surgery: midline, the Mackenrodt-Maylard, and Pfannenstiel's. The muscular components involve the rectus abdominis, the external oblique, the internal oblique, and the transversus abdominus muscles; the fibers of each run in a different direction.[12] Tendinous inscriptions of the muscle can be identified, and the blood supply is from the superior and inferior epigastric artery on each side. These arteries anastomose on each side in 50% of patients. The nerve supply enters the muscles laterally, as shown.

The sites of the usual incisions in the lower anterior abdominal wall are shown in Fig. 12-7, particularly as they relate to the bony landmarks of the pelvis, the pubic symphysis and the anterior superior iliac spine, and to the rectus abdominus muscle and umbilicus.

Cranial to the arcuate line, there is a useful posterior fascia to the rectus sheath, but caudal to the arcuate line, this fascia has disappeared, leaving only a relatively weak transversalis fascia in its place.[50] This is shown in transverse section of the anterior abdominal wall in Fig. 12-8.

Internal access to the organs of the pelvis is affected by the position of the patient on the operating table (Fig. 12-9). Exposure of the pelvis during laparotomy is improved by tilting the head of the operating table downward 30 degrees.[24]

PREPARATION FOR THE OPERATION

In preparing for surgery, the operator scrubs the hands thoroughly with povidone-iodine solution. Because most glove puncture sites are at the fingertip, the surgeon should shorten and clean the fingernails preoperatively. The iodophors and chlorhexidine gluconate solution are stable and without toxicity. Chlorhexidine has shown continued disinfection of hands gloved for 3 hours, whereas 10% povidone-iodine detergent has demonstrated a less persistent effect.[2] Although the Centers for Disease Control recommend a 5-minute scrub from the hands and arms to elbows before each operation, 2 to 5 minutes of scrubbing seems adequate between operations.[28] Lowbury reported a 98% reduction in skin bacterial counts after a 2-minute scrub.[26] After surgery, the hands should be washed to remove blood and other contaminants, with particular attention to the area beneath the fingernails.[28] An alcohol solution (46% to 70% ethyl or isopropyl alcohol) appears to be virucidal.

To lessen trauma to the skin and reduce the incidence of incisional infection, any hair that may interfere with the performance of an incision should be removed either by clipping with scissors or occasionally with an electric trimmer. Leaving the skin of the vulva unshaved does not in-

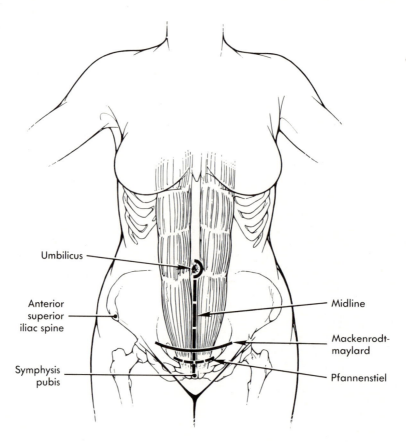

Fig. 12-7. The frequent incisions of the anterior abdominal wall are shown in relation to the anterior superior iliac spines.

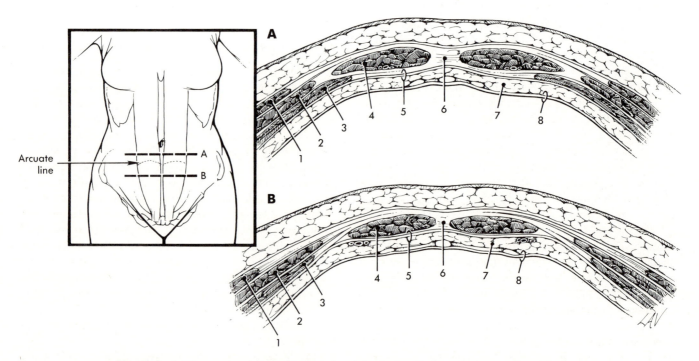

Fig. 12-8. A, Transverse section of the anterior abdominal wall above the arcuate line. The posterior leaf of the aponeurosis of the internal oblique muscle and the aponeurosis of the transversus abdominus muscle unite to form the posterior wall of the rectus sheath. **B,** A transverse section through the anterior abdominal wall below the arcuate line, the posterior wall of the rectus sheath is formed only by the transversalis fascia.

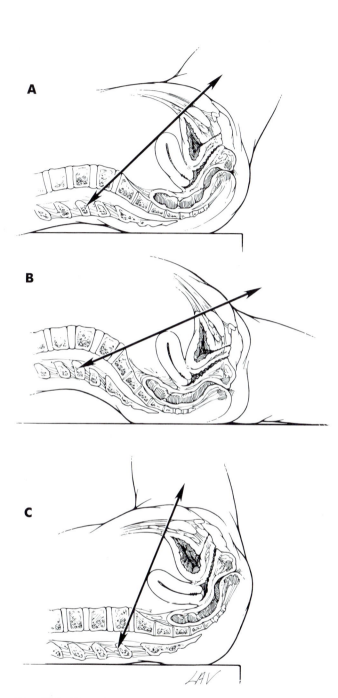

Fig. 12-9. The axis of the pelvic inlet is shown in relation to the various surgical positions. These have a relation to the operative exposure that can be expected during transabdominal surgery according to the position of the patient and her legs on the operating table. When the legs are supported at an angle of 45 degrees in relation to that of the body, as during laparoscopy of combined abdominal-pelvic surgery, the transabdominal exposure of the pelvic organs is as shown in **A.** When the body axis and the legs are both horizontal and parallel to the surface of the operating table, as during laparotomy, the transabdominal view is as shown in **B.** When the legs are in stirrups, as during transvaginal surgery, and the thighs are at about right angles to the horizontal axis of the body and the operating table, the relationship is shown in **C.** Note the differences in arching of the lower back in relation to the three positions.

crease the incidence of wound infection and makes the patient much more comfortable postoperatively. If necessary, the site of the incision may be shaved in the operating room immediately before surgery.

Because iodine is a broad-spectrum antimicrobial, the iodophor complex with the nonsurfactant polyvinyl pyrrolidine (Betadine) is appropriate for use on intact skin; it is not suitable for use in an open wound, however, because it could be absorbed and its high molecular weight would make it difficult for the kidneys to excrete it.[13] After any foreign material has been scrubbed from the incisional site, the skin is painted with povidone-iodine solution and allowed to dry. Traditionally, the vagina is similarly painted with the same antiseptic solution, although Amstey and Jones[1] found no benefits from this procedure beyond those obtained by washing the vagina with saline preoperatively, provided the patient received a prophylactic antibiotic.

CHOICE OF SUTURE FOR CLOSING THE WOUND

Sanz and associates[39] reported that polyglyconate (Maxon) and polyglactin (Vicryl) exhibited consistently better tensile strength than polydioxanone (PDS) and chromic catgut during the late postoperative period, and thought this to be beneficial in situations where wound healing might be delayed, as in corticosteroid therapy, infection, chemotherapy, and in diabetic patients.

Bourne and associates[5] determined that the in-vivo half-life tensile strength of polyglycolic acid (Dexon Plus) and polyglactin 9, 10 (Vicryl) is 2 weeks, whereas those of polyglyconate (Maxon) and polydioxanone (PDS) are 3 and 6 weeks, respectively.

For low-risk patients, continuous fascia closure with a no. 0 polyglactin suture has been reported to be effective. Leaper, Pollack, and Evans[23] showed that 1-cm bites have a suture-holding capacity twice as strong as 0.5-cm bites. When a continuous suture is employed and the bites are 1 cm from the cut edge of the fascia and placed at 1-cm intervals, a suture length four times the length of the incision is recommended.

A study of Smead-Jones closure comparing no. 1 polyglycolic acid suture (Dexon) to continuous muscular fascial closure using no. 1 Prolene demonstrated that the permanent suture group had one third of the frequency of incisional hernias on follow-up as the absorbable suture group. As Morrow points out,[32] vertical subumbilical incisions at risk for dehiscence or delayed healing should be closed with a mass running permanent suture. He identifies those at risk to include women who are elderly, diabetic, malnourished, those who have pulmonary disease, take steroids, have ascites, will receive postoperative radiation or chemotherapy, are very muscular, or have never been pregnant.[25]

Polybutester (Novafil) is a unique copolymer monofilament nonabsorbable synthetic suture material that has the unique qualities of high breaking strength, similar to that of nylon of the same suture size, combined with stretchable elasticity proportional to the force applied, and exhibiting prompt elastic recovery. It is twice as flexible as nylon or polypropylene of similar size, and yet secure knots can be formed with three or four throws. These qualities, particularly that of elastic stretching once it is in place, make it ideal for wound closure, especially when a single buries layer technique is chosen. As postoperative edema and swelling develop in the tissues in which the suture has been placed, the suture stretches temporarily up to 10% or 15% of its length, to lessen the chance that it will tear or strangulate the tissues in which it has been placed. As postoperative edema and swelling subside, the suture contracts to the degree that it had been stretched, taking up any slack that was produced and holding the tissues in approximation during their long healing phase. This should lessen the chance of postoperative wound dehiscence. Dehiscence unrelated to suture breakage occurs not at the suture site, but lateral to the suture line.[37,38]

The use of permanent monofilament absorbable suture is recommended for the closure of most midline incisions. In the very thin patient, however, the suture knots at the ends and midpoint of the fascial closure may remain permanently palpable, to the distress of the patient. In thin patients, therefore, the use of a monofilament delayed absorption suture material such as polydioxanone (PDS) or polyglyconate (Maxon) should be employed. Metz and associates[31] reported that polydioxanone (PDS) retained its integrity in the wound for at least 35 days but found that glycolic acid-trimethylene carbonate (Maxon) became fragile and disintegrated easily 14 days after implantation.

Loosely applied sutures, not intended for hemostasis, promote stronger wound formation because they do not unnecessarily disturb tissue vascularity. The knot, however, should be tied snugly. Although polyglycolic acid sutures are strong and recommended for incisional closure, catgut is most useful for tying smaller bleeders because it is supple and easy to handle.

When using synthetic sutures, the surgeon must be careful not to puncture the outer surface of the suture, as by forceps, needle tips, or ligature carriers, because trauma to the suture may inhibit its strength considerably, or cause it to fracture or break.[29]

Synthetic sutures should be tied with multiple casts, usually a surgeon's knot followed by three square knots.

Subcutaneous sutures are used frequently in a thin abdomen but never in a fat one. A few interrupted stitches placed subcutaneously in the fascia of Camper of a thin woman prevent postoperative scar depression during and after the healing phase.[11]

EXCISION OF OLD SCAR

Careful excision of scars is important in approaching the peritoneal cavity through a previous surgical incision. The excision of unsightly scars with subsequent meticulous closure of the skin by subcutaneous sutures ensures a better cosmetic appearance. Consideration should be given to making the new incision away from the scar of the previous operation when there is reason to suspect the presence of underlying attached intestine. However, reopening a previous incision may be appropriate if it is placed to ensure adequate exposure for the management of the anticipated diagnosis or if it is weakened by a postoperative hernia, which should be repaired.

MIDLINE INCISION

Using a scalpel, the operator incises the skin exactly in the midline from a point just below the umbilicus to a point just caudal to the upper margin of the symphysis pubis (Fig. 12-10, A). If the incision is ended earlier, the lateral retraction of the skin margins pull the lower end of the incision above the pubis, limiting exposure.[12] Making the incision quickly tends to put the smaller arteriolar blood vessels in spasm and, thus, to reduce blood loss during the procedure.

After quickly incising the subcutaneous tissue, the operator identifies the linea alba in the midline between the rectus abdominis muscles (Fig. 12-10, B) and incises it either with scissors or with the needlepoint tip of the electrosurgical scalpel (Fig. 12-10, C). The underlying peritoneum is identified and picked up between two forceps at the cranial end of the incision to avoid any inadvertent penetration of the bladder (Fig. 12-10, D). Usually, the dome of the bladder lies behind the pubis (Fig. 12-10, E), but some intraabdominal pathology (e.g., a retropubic leiomyoma (Figs. 12-10, F and 12-11) or adhesion from previous surgery) occasionally displaces it cranially.

While small Richardson retractors hold the edges of the rectus muscles apart, the operator and the first assistant each insert an index finger into the peritoneal cavity to elevate the peritoneum so that it can be cut between the two fingers (Fig. 12-10, G). The thickness of the layer can be estimated by transillumination against the overhead surgical spotlight, which outlines the upper pole of the bladder beneath the peritoneum. As the incision approaches the bladder, the number of blood vessels transected increases; indicating the proximity of the bladder; great caution is essential to prevent accidental cystotomy.

Peritoneal washings are taken, if desired, and the abdomen is explored. A Bookwalter or Balfour self-retaining retractor is inserted. If the patient is unusually thin, the lateral margins of the retractor blades are padded to protect the underlying femoral nerve and lessen the risk of postoperative femoral neuropathy.

If necessary to provide adequate exposure, the incision may be extended cranially to the left of the umbilicus. Angling the incision in this direction makes it possible to avoid the right-sided ligamentum teres (Fig. 12-10, H). The operator may stitch the peritoneum to the cut edge of the incisional skin, if desired to improve exposure or limit subcutaneous inoculation by bacteria from the pelvis, or may sew wound towels in place to protect the exposed subcutaneous tissue.

At the completion of the procedure, the operator may

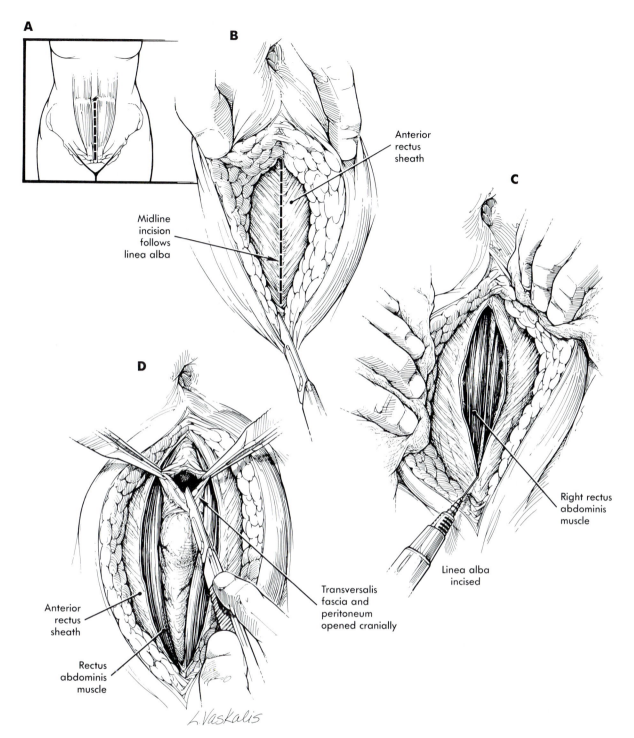

A

B

Anterior
rectus
sheath

Midline
incision
follows
linea alba

C

Right rectus
abdominis
muscle

Linea alba
incised

D

Anterior
rectus
sheath

Rectus
abdominis
muscle

Transversalis
fascia and
peritoneum
opened cranially

L. Vaskalis

Fig. 12-10. The technique of a midline incision in the lower abdomen is shown. **A,** Site of the incision between the umbilicus and pubis. **B,** The midline incision continues through the subcutaneous tissue to expose the linea alba of the anterior rectus sheath. **C,** This sheath is incised, and, **D,** the peritoneum and transversalis fascia are grasped between forceps and opened at the cranial end of the incision. **E,** The usual position of the apex of the bladder within the anterior abdominal wall extends just above the superior margin of the symphysis pubis. **F,** Not infrequently, and particularly when there is a leiomyoma in the anterior portion of the uterus, the apex of the bladder may be displaced cranially. One finger of the operator and one of the operator's assistant are inserted into the peritoneal cavity, and the incision is carried downward toward the pubis. Transillumination of this flap by looking through its peritoneal side discloses the outline of the apex of the bladder, marking the caudal limit of the pubic peritoneal dissection (**G).** When in order to obtain additional exposure it is necessary to extend the midline incision cranially, it should be performed around the left side of the umbilicus to avoid the ligamentum teres. **I,** The transversalis fascia and peritoneum may be closed by a continuous suture at the option of the surgeon, and the rectus aponeurosis may be closed by interrupted or running sutures placed 1 to 1.5 cm apart, and 1 to 1.5 cm away from the fascial margin. Stitches are not usually placed in the subcutaneous tissues, and the skin is closed by clips or a running subcuticular suture.

Continued.

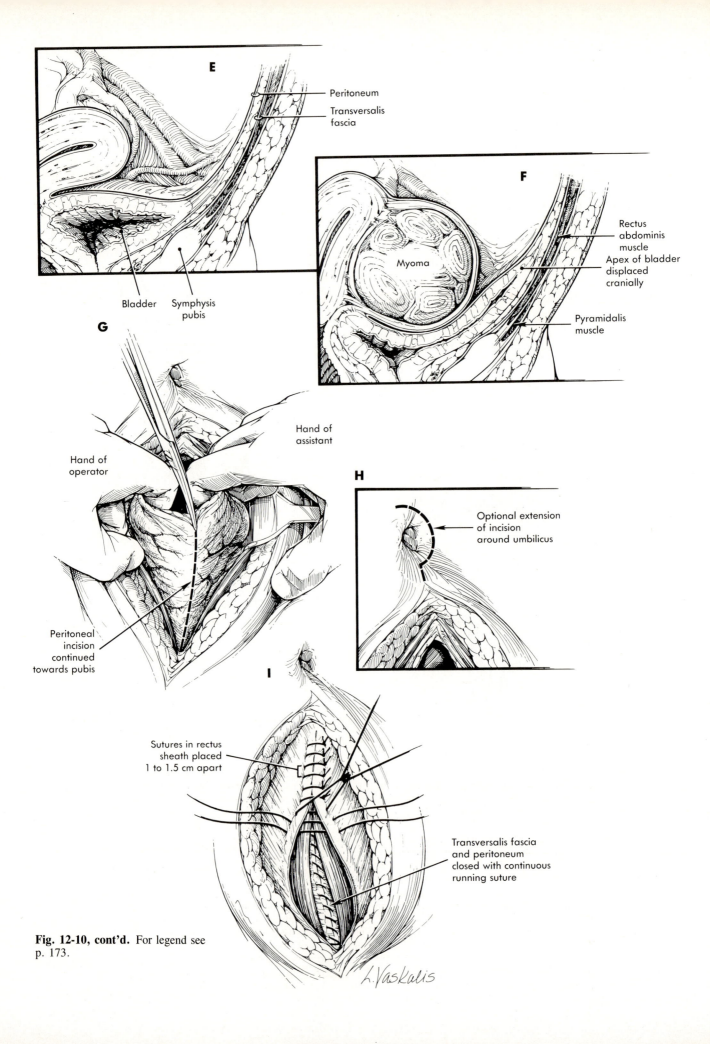

E

Peritoneum

Transversalis fascia

Bladder   Symphysis pubis

F

Myoma

Rectus abdominis muscle

Apex of bladder displaced cranially

Pyramidalis muscle

G

Hand of assistant

Hand of operator

Peritoneal incision continued towards pubis

H

Optional extension of incision around umbilicus

I

Sutures in rectus sheath placed 1 to 1.5 cm apart

Transversalis fascia and peritoneum closed with continuous running suture

Fig. 12-10, cont'd. For legend see p. 173.

L. Vaskalis

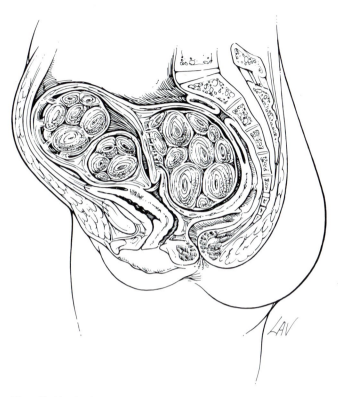

Fig. 12-11. Sagittal section through the pelvis of a patient with multiple myomata is shown. Note the ascent of the bladder fundus onto the anterior abdominal wall where it must be specifically identified by careful dissection when making the incision for abdominal hysterectomy.

close the incision in the older traditional fashion: (1) closing the peritoneum and transversalis fascia with a running absorbable suture; (2) closing the fascia with interrupted synthetic absorbable suture (Fig. 12-10, *I*); and (3) approximating the skin with staples, running or interrupted silk mattress sutures, or a running subcuticular suture. Subcutaneous tissues are not regularly approximated by a separate suture layer because the blood supply of this fatty layer is so poor that suture material may induce necrosis and postoperative subcutaneous infection.

Generally speaking, an old abdominal scar should be excised to provide a fresh area of vital tissue during postoperative wound healing, except possibly when there is reason to suspect that intestine is adherent to the undersurface of an old incision.

It is important to place the stitches in the fascia at least 1 to 1.5 cm lateral to the cut edge of the incision and at least 1 or 1.5 cm distant from one another to reduce the risk of devascularization and necrosis from suture pressure. If the operator decides to use interrupted sutures in the deep musculofascial layer, a Smead-Jones deep-deep-shallow-shallow configuration or a modified deep-shallow-shallow-deep configuration that involves fascia, muscle, and peritoneum may be appropriate (Fig. 12-12).

Alternately, the operator may close the incision by a single buried through-and-through layer of long-lasting monofilament polyglycolic acid-type suture material[14,19] or a synthetic monofilament permanent suture (Fig. 12-13). The one-layer closure of the deeper tissues makes a special effort to close the parietal peritoneum unnecessary, al-

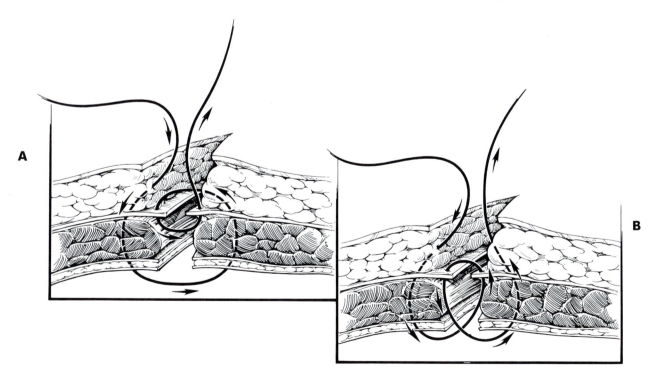

Fig. 12-12. The Smead-Jones single layer closure is illustrated in which the interrupted sutures are placed through the full thickness of the rectus fascia, muscle, and peritoneum in a deep-shallow-shallow configuration as shown in **A.** An alternate deep-shallow-shallow-deep placement is illustrated in **B.**

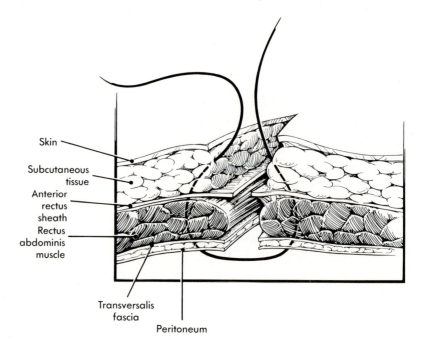

Fig. 12-13. Placement of a through-and-through suture through the rectus fascia, muscle, and transversalis fascia and peritoneum are shown. The sutures are placed 1.5 cm lateral to the fascial incision, and 1.5 cm apart. Inclusion of the peritoneum and transversalis fascia, as shown, is optional. This suture may be of interrupted stitches or over-end-over technique, according to the surgeon's preference.

Skin

Subcutaneous tissue

Anterior rectus sheath

Rectus abdominis muscle

Transversalis fascia

Peritoneum

though some surgeons prefer to close this peritoneum. The synthetic nonabsorbable, but slightly elastic, tissue suture polybutester (Novafil) can be used to great advantage in this one-layer full-thickness closure.[37,38] Its capacity to stretch between 10% and 15% postoperatively accommodates wound swelling and edema, yet its inherent elasticity takes up the slack as the swelling and edema subside. As a result, the tension in the tissues in which the suture has been placed remains more constant, theoretically reducing the risk of devascularization, necrosis, and subsequent incisional hernia. In placing these stitches, the operator may find it useful with better exposure to start suturing at each end of the wound and have the stitches ultimately meet in the middle of the incision.

These sutures, which may include fascia and muscle, are snugly placed but not so tightly as to devascularize the tissues in which they are located.

PARAMEDIAN INCISION

Like the midline incision, the paramedian incision avoids the nerve supply of the rectus muscles that enter from the lateral side. Although the paramedian incision transects more blood vessels, it heals well. Should it someday be necessary to reenter the abdomen of a patient who has had a paramedian incision, the surgeon should not make a midline or contralateral paramedian incision because these incisions may interfere with the blood supply of the tissue being incised and risk wound hernia. The surgeon who reenters a previous paramedian incision will find that the muscle is adherent to its sheath and must be split other than dissected free.

A paramedian incision involves making a vertical incision through the skin and subcutaneous tissue 1 inch lateral to the midline (Fig. 12-14, *A*). The rectus sheath is incised 1 inch lateral to the midline (Fig. 12-14, *B*). The op-

erator reflects the medial flap of the rectus sheath from the muscle and retracts the muscle laterally, separating it from the midline (Fig. 12-14, *C*). Then, the operator incises the transversalis fascia and peritoneum beneath the muscle and 1 inch lateral to the midline (Fig. 12-14, *D*).

The pararectus incision, in which the muscle is retracted medially, is not regularly used because of damage to the nerve supply of the muscle that enters from its lateral border. For the same reason, a transrectus incision is not recommended.

TRANSVERSE INCISIONS

Because they are made in the direction of Langer's lines, transverse incisions produce cosmetically more attractive scars. Wound herniation is rare after transverse incisions, and the incisions seldom cause any permanent damage to the strategic nerve or blood supply of the musculature of the anterior abdominal wall.[7]

Pfannenstiel's incision

The principal disadvantage of Pfannenstiel's incision is that exposure is limited when compared with the midline or Maylard incision and is not useful when upper abdominal exposure may be anticipated. Similarly, because it opens more tissue planes at a larger exposed surface area of subcutaneous tissue, it should not be used in the presence of active infection or abscess formation to prevent increased risk of inoculation of the subcutaneous tissue wound abscess. Because Pfannenstiel's incision takes longer to perform, it is contraindicated when speed is necessary. If after Pfannenstiel's incision has been made and it becomes clear that better operative exposure is required, the incision can be converted to a Cherney incision.

Turner-Warwick[46-49] developed a "supra-pubic-cross" incision that enabled him to repair the great majority of ab-

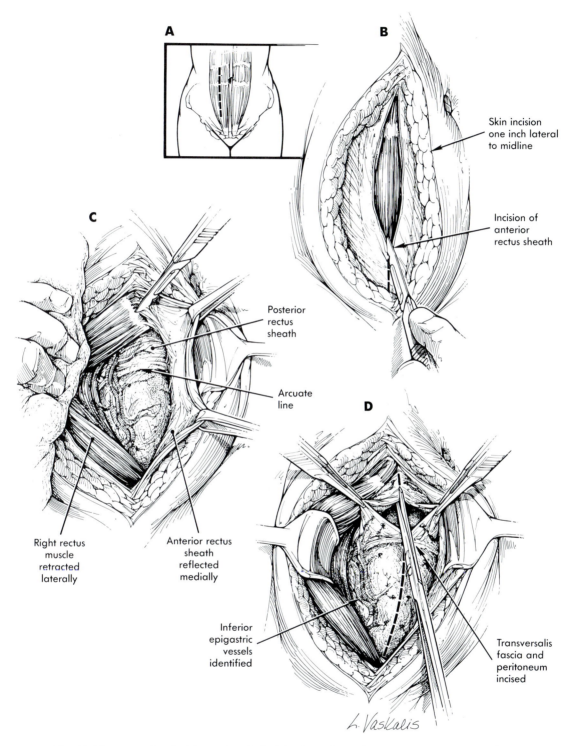

A

B

Skin incision
one inch lateral
to midline

Incision of
anterior
rectus sheath

C

Posterior
rectus
sheath

Arcuate
line

D

Right rectus
muscle
retracted
laterally

Anterior rectus
sheath
reflected
medially

Inferior
epigastric
vessels
identified

Transversalis
fascia and
peritoneum
incised

L. Vaskalis

Fig. 12-14. Paramedian incision. The skin incision is made on either the right or left side of the abdomen along the path of the dashed line as shown in **A,** 1 inch lateral to the midline, as shown. The anterior rectus sheath is incised over the midportion of the underlying rectus muscle **(B),** and retracted laterally while the anterior rectus sheath is reflected immediately **(C).** The posterior rectus sheath, transversalis fascia, and peritoneum are incised in the bed temporarily vacated by the muscle **(D).**

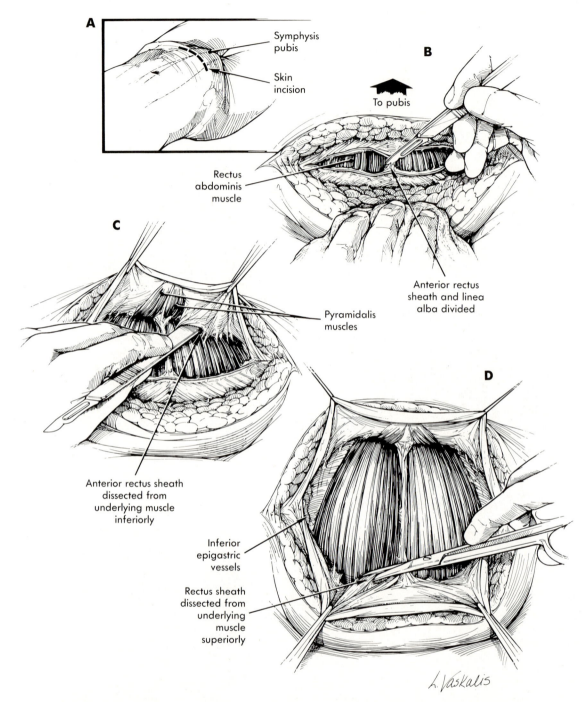

Fig. 12-15. Pfannenstiel's incision. **A,** A transverse eliptical skin incision is made in the suprapubic area. **B,** Subcutaneous tissue is incised exposing the anterior rectus sheath, which is incised exposing the underlying rectus abdominis muscle. The anterior sheath is separated from the muscle by sharp and blunt dissection **(C),** first in the caudal portion of the incision, and then beneath the cranial portion of the anterior rectus sheath **(D).** The peritoneum is identified between the bellies of the rectus muscles, and the transversalis fascia and peritoneum are grasped with forceps and incised in the midline at the cranial margin of the exposure **(E). F,** The operator's fingertips are inserted caudally beneath the peritoneum, and the incision is extended downward between the operator's fingers, with care being taken to recognize and avoid the cranial margin of the apex of the bladder at the inferior pole of the incision. At the completion of surgery, it is optional whether the parietal peritoneum and transversalis fascia are closed. **G,** The rectus muscles are approximated by a series of loosely tied interrupted stitches to relieve any diastasis. **H,** The rectus aponeurosis is closed with a continuous running suture, and the skin incision is closed with staples or a subcuticular suture. *Continued.*

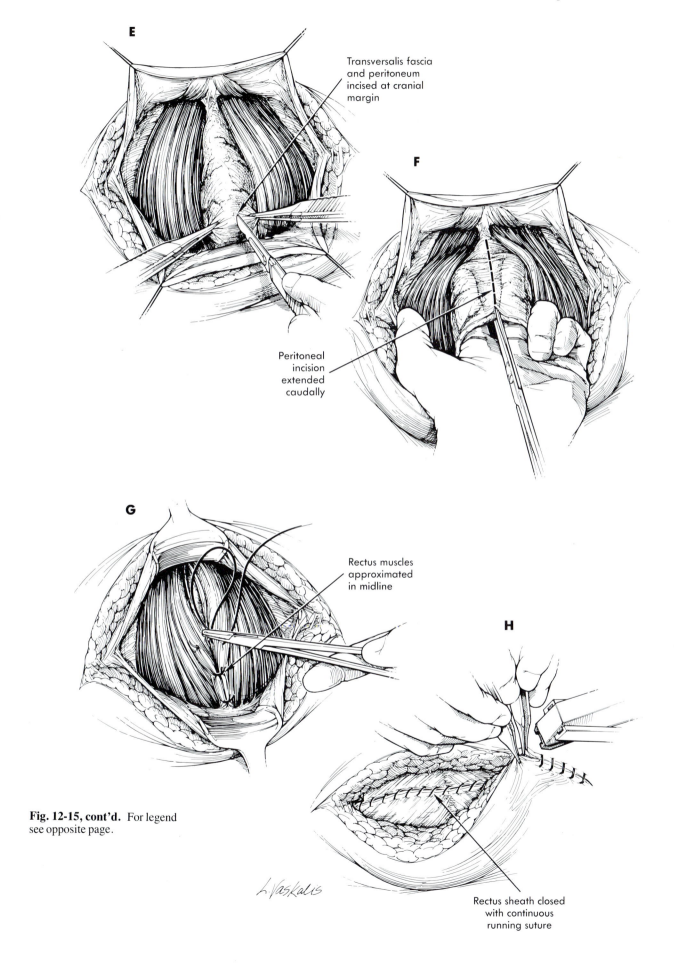

E

Transversalis fascia
and peritoneum
incised at cranial
margin

F

Peritoneal
incision
extended
caudally

G

Rectus muscles
approximated
in midline

H

Fig. 12-15, cont'd. For legend
see opposite page.

L. Vaskalis

Rectus sheath closed
with continuous
running suture

dominal approach fistula repairs to be completed through the original horizontal Pfannenstiel's skin incision. The upper and lower skin flaps were appropriately mobilized to enable a midline abdominal wall incision to be made up to the level of the umbilicus, leaving the original horizontal Pfannenstiel's rectus sheath closure intact.

For the same reason, a transrectus incision is not recommended.

In performing Pfannenstiel's incision,[35] the operator places a transverse incision, convex curve downward, in the skinfold two fingerbreadths above the upper margin of the symphysis pubis and carries it through skin and subcutaneous tissue to the rectus sheath (Fig. 12-15, *A*). Incising the sheath transversely over the belly of each rectus muscle, the operator continues laterally beyond the lateral margins of the rectus muscle and the medial borders of the external and internal oblique muscles. The two incisions in the rectus fascia join in the middle (Fig. 12-15, *B*).

A Kocher clamp is placed on each side, and, with traction applied anteriorly, the rectus aponeurosis is separated from the underlying rectus muscle by sharp and blunt dissection. Usually, the pyramidalis remains firmly attached to the underside of the aponeurosis (Fig. 12-15, *C*). At this point, the operator removes the Kocher clamps from their original placement, applies them to the upper cut edge of fascia, and similarly dissects the fascia from the muscle far enough to permit a midline incision of adequate length through the parietal peritoneum at the cranial end of the exposure (Fig. 12-15, *D*). Picking up the peritoneum between two hemostats, the operator opens it in the midline (Fig. 12-15, *E* and *F*). The incision is extended cranially, between the operator's fingers. Caudal transillumination of the thickness of the peritoneal flap will avoid penetration of the fundus of the attached bladder.

In closing the Pfannenstiel's incision, it appears to make little difference whether the parietal peritoneum is closed or not. The operator may bring the central bellies of the rectus muscles together with a few loosely tied interrupted sutures of polyglycolic acid if there is any diastasis present[36] (Fig. 12-15, *G*) and may close the transverse fascial incision with a 2-0 or 1-0 synthetic absorbable suture (polyglycolic acid-type). Subcutaneous tissues are not approximated, and the skin is closed with either staples, which are left in place for 5 postoperative days, or a subcuticular closure with 4-0 undyed polyglycolic acid-type sutures. The latter is particularly useful if the patient must be discharged before the fifth postoperative day.

For the patient in whom a minimally visible, cosmetically attractive skin incision is essential, the surgeon may elect the "low Pfannenstiel's incision" in which the transverse skin incision is made a fingersbreadth below the pubic hairline, and the abdominal wall and subcutaneous tissue are dissected cranially from the rectus fascia, which can then be opened transversely in classic Pfannenstiel fashion (Fig. 12-16).

The principal disadvantage of Pfannenstiel's incision is that it provides a more limited exposure than does a mid-line or Maylard incision and, therefore, is not useful when upper abdominal exposure may be necessary. In addition, because it opens more tissue planes, exposing a larger surface area of subcutaneous tissue, it should not be used in the presence of active infection or abscess formation; any such infectious condition may inoculate the subcutaneous tissue, inviting wound abscess. Because Pfannenstiel's incision requires more time, it is also contraindicated when speed is necessary.

Küstner's incision[21,22] is not recommended. It differs from Pfannenstiel's incision in that the skin and subcutaneous tissue are dissected from the anterior rectus sheath, which is then opened in the midline. It provides very limited exposure, even less than that provided by Pfannenstiel's incision, but does not reduce the risk of postoperative wound herniation.

Küstner's incision can be considered in a patient who has had a previous Pfannenstiel's incision when, for cosmetic appearance of the skin of the lower abdomen, reoperation requiring greater exposure made possible by a midline incision is required, as suggested by Turner-Warwick.

If, after Pfannenstiel's incision has been made, it becomes clear that better operative exposure is required, the incision can be converted to a Cherney incision.

One should not convert a Pfannenstiel's incision to a Maylard incision because with the Pfannenstiel's the anterior surface of the rectus muscle has been dissected from the undersurface of the rectus fascia and after a secondary Maylard muscle transection the cut ends of the muscle no longer come together with simple reapproximation of the rectus fascial layer. For this reason, converting an inadequately exposing Pfannenstiel's incision to a Cherney incision is a better choice, because with healing after the Cherney it is not essential that the muscle be firmly adherent to the underside of the rectus fascia.[45]

Cherney incision

In 1940, Cherney[8] described a transverse incision in the fold above the pubis. The tendons of the rectus abdominus muscles, provided that they are well developed, are bluntly dissected from the underlying bladder and vesicouterine fold of the peritoneum, and transected near their insertion on the pubic symphysis (Fig. 12-17, *A*). When the tendons have been reflected cranially, the transversalis fascia and peritoneum can be incised transversely beneath them (Fig. 12-17, *B*).

The Cherney incision requires less time to perform than the Maylard and does not require drainage because there is no bleeding from the transected tendon. Poor development of the tendon, however, contraindicates this incision.[6]

At the conclusion of the operation, the surgeon carefully reattaches the transected ends of the tendinous sheath to the undersurface of the rectus sheath and pubic periosteum with interrupted sutures, and closes the transverse incision in the rectus aponeurosis with a running suture similar to that used in a Pfannenstiel's closure (Fig. 12-17, *C*). The Cherney incision supplies better exposure than

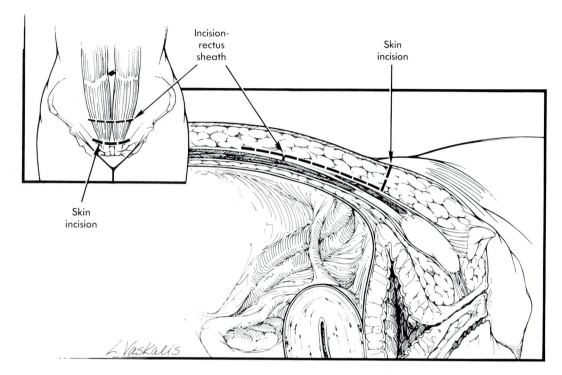

Fig. 12-16. "Low" Pfannenstiel's incision. A transverse skin incision is made a fingerbreadth beneath the upper border of the pubic hairline, and the skin and subcutaneous tissue are dissected from the anterior rectus aponeurosis as shown in the path of the broken line and reflected cranially. A transverse incision in the rectus sheath is made at a more cranial level as shown.

does Pfannenstiel's incision, and it is particularly useful when some of the surgery must be accomplished in the space of Retzius.

V-shaped incision

Turner-Warwick[49] described a V-shaped 4-cm horizontal incision in the rectus sheath 2 cm *below* the upper margin of the pubis (Fig. 12-18, *A* and *B*). The operator angles this V-shaped incision sharply upward so that the edges of the consequent flap remain within the lateral margins of the rectus muscle. The rectus sheath is reflected cranially, and the abdomen is opened in the midline between the rectus muscles (Fig. 12-18, *C*). Because there is no distal rectus sheath margin to retract, the exposure of the retropubic space is unusually good.

For the patient who is concerned with the cosmetic appearance of the scar, the surgeon can make the initial skin incision as if it were to be a low Pfannenstiel's modification. The lateral extension of the rectus sheath incision without transection of the rectus muscle provides additional operative exposure, if necessary.

Mackenrodt-Maylard incision

In 1901, Mackenrodt[27] developed the transverse muscle-cutting abdominal incision that Maylard[30] modified in 1907 by restricting it to the area below the umbilicus. Because the incision is transverse, it does not disturb the innervation of the abdominal musculature. Furthermore, because the tension from the lateral abdominal muscles is

parallel to the line of incision, there is no unusual tension on the suture line. It provides excellent exposure of the pelvis (but not of the upper abdomen).

The incidence of postoperative incisional hernia is increased in the patient with chronic respiratory disease. The transverse Maylard incision, which is similar to the elliptical transverse incision of Bardenheuer,[4] is a better choice for such a patient than is the midline incision because the resultant incisional scar will be stronger.

Beginning approximately 2 inches above the upper border of the symphysis pubis, the operator makes a suprapubic transverse skin incision down to the anterior rectus sheath, incises the sheath transversely over the belly of each rectus muscle, unites the two incisions in the rectus sheath (Fig. 12-19, *A* and *B*), and cuts across the muscle bellies of each rectus abdominis muscle with the electrosurgical scalpel[11] or (Premium poly CS-57) stapler (Fig. 12-19, *C*). Any blood vessels encountered are clamped and tied. As there is no sheath at this level, the operator attaches the transected muscle by interrupted mattress stitches to the rectus sheath at the upper margin of the incision to keep the transected muscle from retracting beneath the incision (Fig. 12-19, *D*). Then, picking up the peritoneum, the operator incises it transversely. If additional exposure is necessary, the operator identifies, clamps, cuts, and ligates the inferior epigastric vessels (Fig. 12-19, *E*).

In closure, because of the raw surfaces offered by the transected bellies of the rectus muscles, the parietal perito-

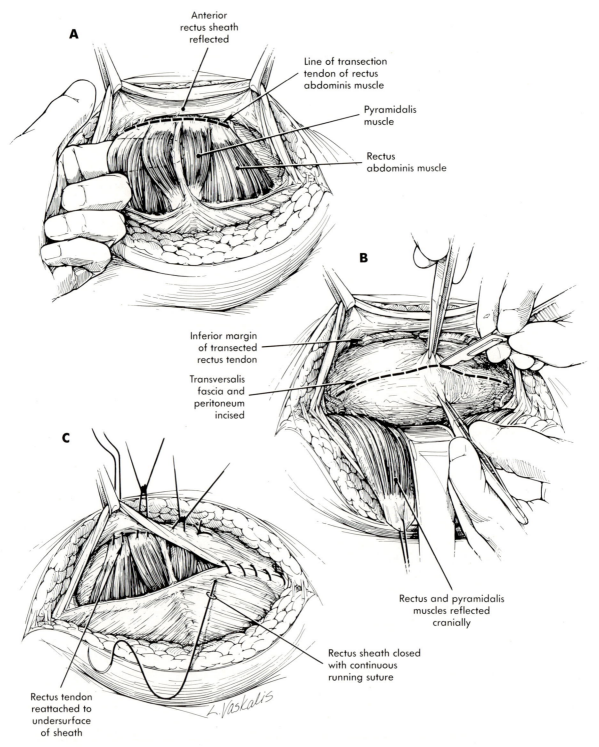

Anterior
rectus sheath
reflected

Line of transection
tendon of rectus
abdominis muscle

Pyramidalis
muscle

Rectus
abdominis muscle

A

B

Inferior margin
of transected
rectus tendon

Transversalis
fascia and
peritoneum
incised

C

Rectus and pyramidalis
muscles reflected
cranially

Rectus sheath closed
with continuous
running suture

Rectus tendon
reattached to
undersurface
of sheath

L. Vaskalis

Fig. 12-17. The Cherney incision. **A,** A transverse elliptical skin incision is made through the skin and subcutaneous tissue. The tendon of the rectus abdominus muscle and pyramidalis is transsected on each side as shown by the broken line. **B,** The muscles are reflected cranially, and the peritoneum and transversalis fascia are picked up between forceps and incised transversely. **C,** At the conclusion of surgery, the tendon of the rectus muscle is attached to the undersurface of the rectus sheath by several interrupted stitches, and the original incision in the rectus aponeurosis is closed with a continuous running suture. The skin incision is closed with staples or a subcuticular closure.

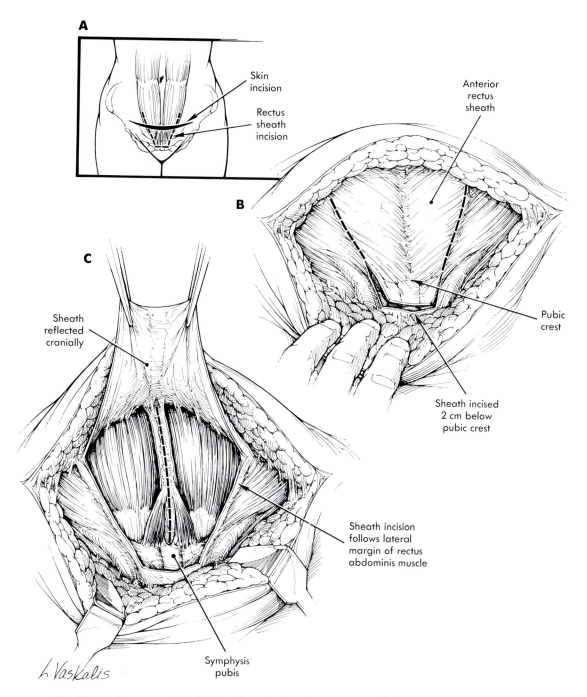

A

Skin
incision

Rectus
sheath
incision

Anterior
rectus
sheath

B

Pubic
crest

Sheath incised
2 cm below
pubic crest

C

Sheath
reflected
cranially

Sheath
incision
follows lateral
margin of rectus
abdominis muscle

Symphysis
pubis

L. Vaskalis

Fig. 12-18. The suprapubic "V" incision. **A,** Excellent exposure of the space of Retzius is provided when a transverse skin incision is made just above the pubic hairline. **B,** The skin and subcutaneous tissues are dissected from the anterior rectus sheath, which is incised 2 cm below the pubic crest and along the path of the broken line. **C,** The rectus sheath is reflected cranially, and the transversalis fascia and peritoneum are incised in the midline as shown by the broken line.

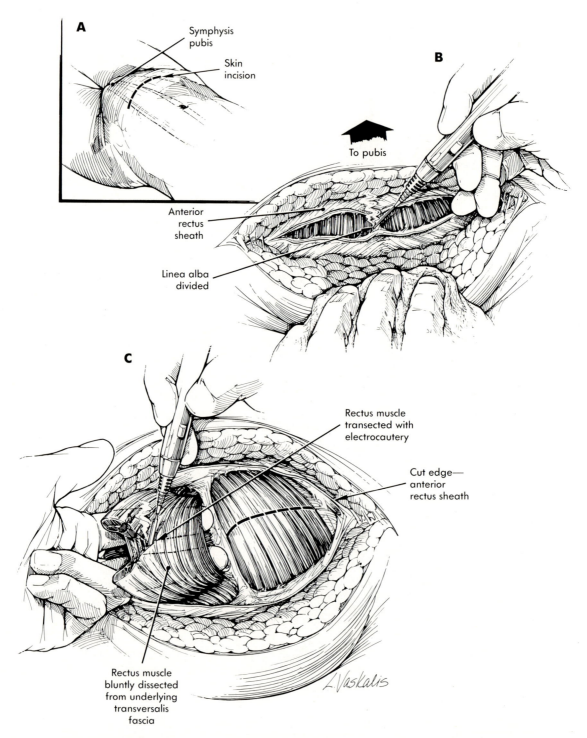

Fig. 12-19. The Maylard incision. **A,** A transverse skin incision is made 5 cm above the superior border of the pubis. **B,** The anterior rectus sheath is incised in the same line, exposing the bellies of the rectus abdominis muscles. The muscle is bluntly dissected from the underlying transversalis fascia and incised transversely on each side, along the path of the broken side, using the electrosurgical scalpel **(C). D,** The transversalis fascia and peritoneum are opened, and the superior cut edge of the rectus abdominus is secured to the anterior sheath with mattress sutures. **E,** The peritoneal incision is extended laterally, and the inferior epigastric vessels must usually be ligated and cut. *Continued.*

neum beneath them should be closed as a separate layer (Fig. 12-19, *F*). The possibility of oozing from the transected rectus muscles under the fascia makes it necessary to place a subfascial 10-mm flat Jackson-Pratt drain (Fig. 12-19, *G*). Making traction the mattress sutures previously placed through the muscle and fascia of the upper wound, the operator places an additional mattress stitch from upper fascia through upper muscle, lower muscle, and lower fascial edge on one side, and the same structures in reverse order on the opposite side. Finally, the operator closes the fascial layers with either interrupted or continuous sutures of 1-0 synthetic material and the skin with either staples or running subcuticular sutures of 3-0 polyglycolic acid-type material (Fig. 12-19, *H*).

If the patient has any obstruction of her common iliac vessels, the direction of blood flow in the inferior epigastric arteries may be cranial instead of caudal. In such a circumstance, ligation of these vessels could interfere with the circulation to the patient's legs.[20] To obviate this misfortune, the operator should make certain to palpate the dorsalis pedis artery and determine the direction of blood flow before clamping and cutting the epigastric vessels.

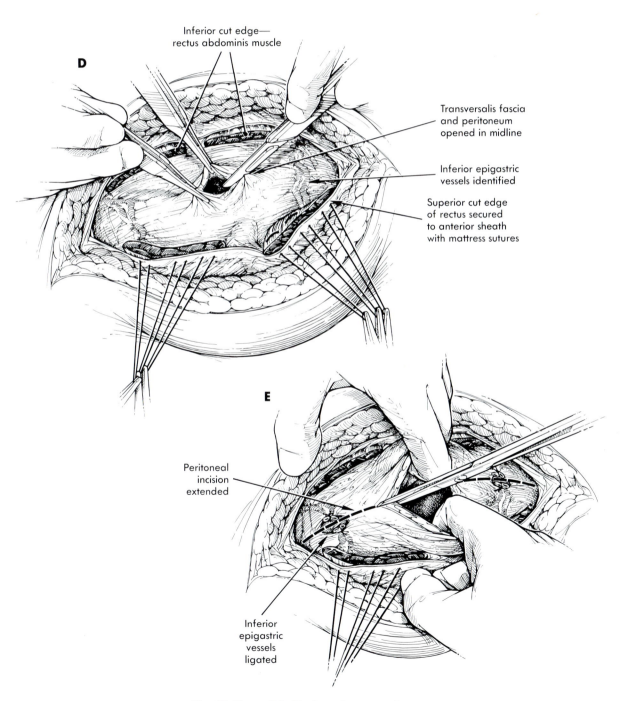

Fig. 12-19, cont'd. For legend see opposite page.
Continued.

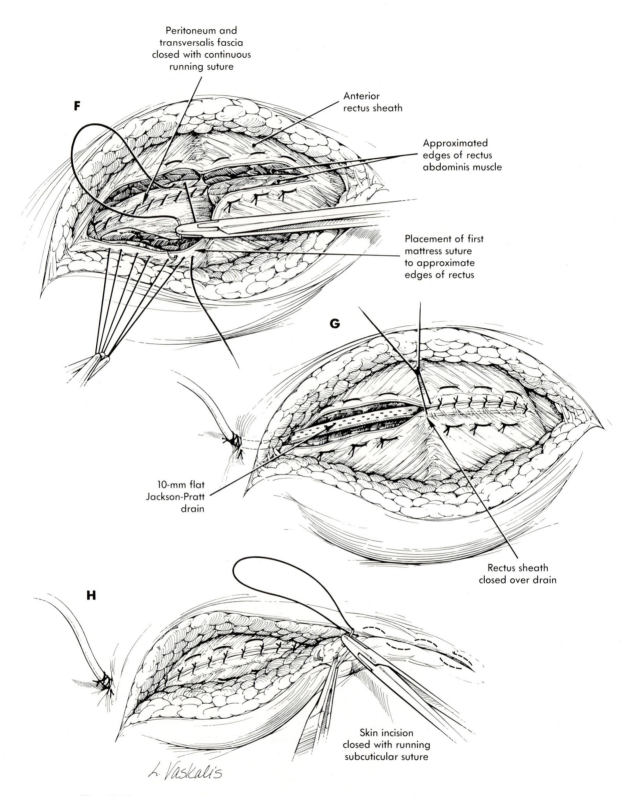

Fig. 12-19, cont'd. F, To close the incision, the peritoneum and transversalis fascia should be approximated with a continuous running suture, and the gap between the edges of fascia and muscle is approximated by a series of mattress stitches placed as shown. **G,** A Jackson-Pratt drain is placed beneath the fascial edges, and the rectus sheath is closed with interrupted sutures. The skin incision is closed with either a running subcuticular suture (**H**) or staples.

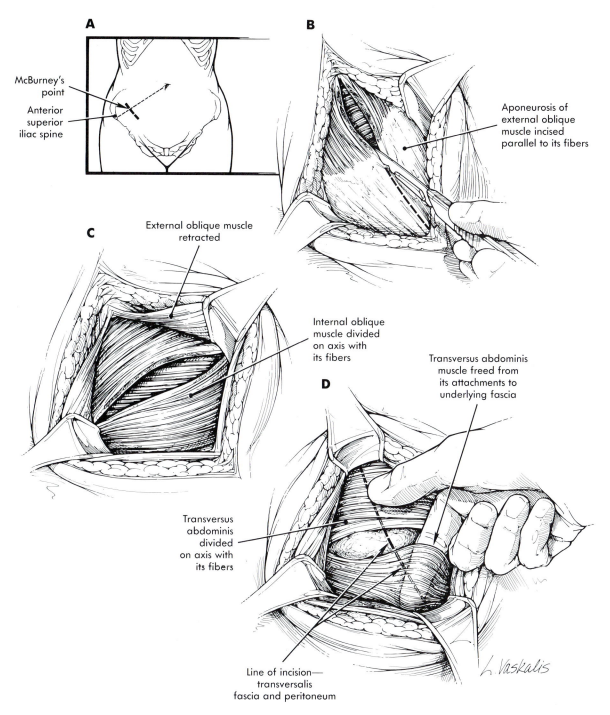

Labels in figure:

A
McBurney's point
Anterior superior iliac spine

B
Aponeurosis of external oblique muscle incised parallel to its fibers

C
External oblique muscle retracted
Internal oblique muscle divided on axis with its fibers

D
Transversus abdominis muscle freed from its attachments to underlying fascia
Transversus abdominis divided on axis with its fibers
Line of incision—transversalis fascia and peritoneum

L. Vaskalis

Fig. 12-20. The Gridiron muscle splitting incision. This is most frequently used for appendectomy or for drainage of the pelvic abscess that is pointed to the inguinal area. McBurney's point for locating the appendix is noted by the dashed line in **A,** which intersects a line between the umbilicus and the anterior superior iliac spine as shown by the dotted line. The skin incision is made along the path of the dashed line. The subcutaneous tissue is incised similarly, and the aponeurosis of the external oblique muscle is incised parallel to its fibers **(B).** The external oblique muscle is retracted, exposing the underlying internal oblique muscle, which is divided on an axis parallel with its fibers **(C).** This, in turn, exposes the underlying transversus abdominis, which is divided on an axis in the direction of its fibers, and the muscle is freed from its attachments to the underlying transversalis fascia and peritoneum as shown in **D.** The muscle is retracted, exposing the underlying peritoneum, which is incised along the site of the heavy broken line as shown **(D).**

Muscle-splitting incisions

The gridiron incision is used primarily for uncomplicated appendectomy, although it may be used to drain a large pelvic or abdominal abscess that does not point into the cul-de-sac or anterior wall of the rectum.[18] The operator first makes an incision over McBurney's point to expose the aponeurosis of the external oblique muscle, incises the muscle parallel to its fibers, and retracts it (Fig. 12-20, *A* and *B*). The fibers of the internal oblique and transversalis muscles run perpendicular to the incision, and the operator divides these muscles along their axis (Fig. 12-20, *C*). This exposes the transversalis fascia and peritoneum, which are incised (Fig. 12-20, *D*). After completing the surgical procedure required, the operator closes the incision in layers.

MANAGEMENT OF THE OBESE PATIENT

Abdominal incisions in the obese patient generally need drainage. As mentioned earlier, a Maylard incision generally requires the placement of a subfascial drain, which prevents the development of a hematoma from the cut edge of the rectus muscle. The obese patient who has had a midline incision needs a subcutaneous, self-contained suction apparatus to inhibit the development of a postoperative seroma to which she is predisposed because of the larger subcutaneous surface area.

Morrow and associates[33] pointed out the dangers of making a transverse incision under the panniculus. They demonstrated that better exposure can be obtained by a midline vertical incision, providing the panniculus is drawn downward below the superior margin of pubis, which can be palpated as the incision is made. This avoids buttonholing the skin beneath the panniculus. Shepherd and associates[40] demonstrated the strength of a continuous one-layer closure for midline incisions using a non-absorbable single-layer technique.

Gallup and associates[15] emphasize the importance of subcutaneous drainage by a closed system for the first 72 hours postoperatively, or until the drainage is less than 50 ml for 24 hours.

Subcutaneous tissue of the markedly obese patient should be drained by a self-contained suction apparatus (Jackson-Pratt, not a Penrose drain), which should be removed in about 72 hours.

In the very obese woman with a large pendulous panniculus, the operator may sometimes make an incision above the umbilicus, away from the panniculus, and use a Bookwalter retractor secured to the operating room table to displace the incision inferiorly and provide adequate exposure[16] (Fig. 12-21). Gallup[14] advocated making a midline incision in these patients, usually extended around the umbilicus rather than passed through it; closing the fascia

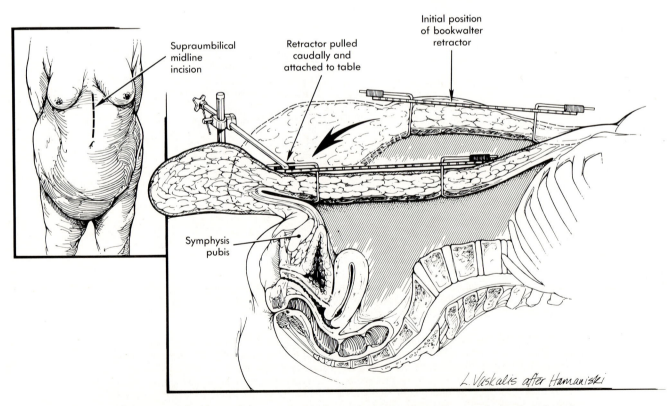

Initial position of bookwalter retractor

Supraumbilical midline incision

Retractor pulled caudally and attached to table

Symphysis pubis

L. Vaskalis after Hamaniski

Fig. 12-21. Transabdominal incision for a morbidly obese patient. The panniculus is reflected downward, and a supraumbilical midline incision is shown along the path of the dashed line. The Bookwalter retractor is inserted into the peritoneal cavity as shown, displacing the panniculus caudally.

with a nonabsorbable monofilament suture; and using a su-
prafascial closed drainage system. The drain should remain in place for 72 hours or until the drainage is less than
50 ml during a 24-hour period. In obese patients, the skin
staples should remain in place for 2 weeks postoperatively.[9]

Although surgeons may be tempted to perform a panniculectomy on the disfigured woman, they seldom do so.
This cosmetic addition to laparotomy not only may involve
considerations of salvage, sacrifice, or physical relocation
of the umbilicus, but also may result in considerable blood
loss and a remarkably longer period of convalescence. In
the multipara, the procedure often coincidentally stretches
and weakens the fascia of the anterior abdominal wall and
causes some significant diastasis of the rectus muscle. Not
uncommonly, there is an associated umbilical hernia. As
alternatives to panniculectomy, rigid dietary discretion or
liposuction can dissipate subcutaneous fat, but they may
only accentuate the faulty appearance that is the consequence of fascial weakness.

Panniculectomy

When the surgeon and patient have decided that a panniculectomy is desirable, the next decision necessary is
whether to use a midline subumbilical skin incision or a
transverse one; the former does not usually require umbilical relocation, but the latter generally does if the umbilicus is to be preserved (Fig. 12-22). Fascial "pants over
vest" layering[36] reinforces the deeper weakness of the anterior abdominal wall (Fig. 12-23). Precise surgical hemostasis is essential, and the residual subcutaneous fat layer
must be dissected free of the underlying fascia and the
wound must be drained through a separate stab wound.

When a great deal of postoperative overdistention is anticipated, or coughing or nausea and vomiting, midline incisions can be supported temporarily by the use of retention stitches. A maximum of strength can be given to the
approximation of the fascial layers by sutures of monofilament nonabsorbable material placed lateral to the incision,
through each side of the fascial incision, and brought back
adjacent to the original incision (Fig. 12-24). Usually three
sets can be placed on each side, and, at the conclusion of
repair of the incision, they are tied against the bolster of a
4 × 4 rolled compress.

COINCIDENT HERNIA

When the abdominal cavity has been opened for surgery
through an incision in the anterior abdominal wall, any
symptomatic hernia of the abdominal wall or pelvis should
be repaired before the abdomen is closed.[3] The repair of
enterocele and prolapse of the vaginal vault are discussed
in Chapters 26 and 27, respectively. The repair of umbilical hernia is discussed in Chapter 13. It is possible to repair inguinal and femoral hernias by the intra-abdominal
route, if surgical exposure can be obtained at the site of
weakness by using an appropriate initial surgical incision.
Techniques for intraabdominal indirect inguinal hernior-

rhaphy and intraabdominal femoral herniorrhaphy are
shown in Fig. 12-25. A direct inguinal hernia can also be
repaired intraabdominally. It represents a congenital defect
or weakness at the medial edge at the line of origin of the
transversalis and internal oblique muscles. The hernia is
reduced and the sac inverted and excised in the same manner as the indirect hernia. The transversalis fascia and the
edges of the transversalis and internal oblique muscles are
sutured to the inguinal ligament or the superior pubic ligament, which is the extension of the inguinal ligament toward the symphysis. An unusually weak or difficult internal hernial orifice may be occluded by the use of a synthetic plastic patch sewn in place beneath the peritoneal incision.

POSTOPERATIVE CARE

In the course of normal healing, the skin incision becomes watertight 48 hours after surgery. It is best kept dry
during that initial period, so bacteria that can cause postoperative infection does not enter the incision. The patient
can obtain the soothing effects of heat through the use of a
heat lamp or a blow-type hair dryer.

Ultrasound examination, if not clinical findings, can
confirm postoperative incisional sepsis. The appropriate
investigation of an abscess cavity includes incision, drainage, and culture of the cavity contents.[18] The incision,
which communicates with the abscess cavity, may be
packed open, and the skin incision can be loosely closed
by a series of interrupted sutures placed approximately 4
inches apart. Between these stitches, some additional sutures can be placed approximately 1 inch apart, but not
tied. The wound will heal more rapidly if the operator
waits until the purulence of the abscess has subsided and a
layer of healthy granulation tissue has covered the base of
the raw wound, usually about 4 days, before tying these
sutures.

The entrapment of the iliohypogastric nerve during the
closure of Pfannenstiel's incision can give rise to a most
disabling postoperative pain that runs from the incisional
site down into the labia or inner aspect of the thigh. Occasionally, a neuroma is palpable, or reexploration of the
wound reveals the nerve trapped within the scar; if so, the
surgeon excises the nerve and ligates the ends.[42] This injury is more likely to occur when the transverse fascial incision extends beyond the lateral edge of the rectus sheath
into the substance of the internal oblique muscle or when
the sutures at the corners of this fascial incision are so
widely placed that they incorporate branches of the nerve
in the closure.

In consideration of nerve entrapment after Pfannenstiel's incision, Sippo[41] has found in his patients that the
right side is most often involved and occasionally more
than one nerve is involved.

When the iliohypogastric nerve is entrapped, pain management may require an ilioinguinal or iliohypogastric
nerve block established by infiltrating the tissue with 10 ml
of a 2:1 mixture of 0.5% bupivacaine (Marcaine) and 1%

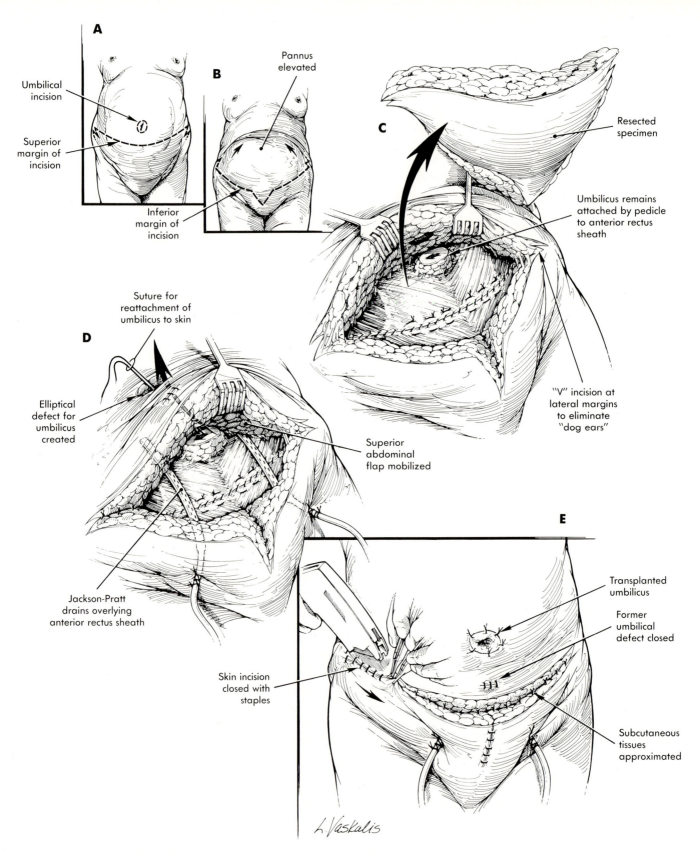

A, Umbilical incision

Superior margin of incision

Inferior margin of incision

B, Pannus elevated

C, Resected specimen

Umbilicus remains attached by pedicle to anterior rectus sheath

"V" incision at lateral margins to eliminate "dog ears"

D, Suture for reattachment of umbilicus to skin

Elliptical defect for umbilicus created

Superior abdominal flap mobilized

Jackson-Pratt drains overlying anterior rectus sheath

Skin incision closed with staples

E, Transplanted umbilicus

Former umbilical defect closed

Subcutaneous tissues approximated

L. Vaskalis

Fig. 12-22. Panniculectomy, using a transverse elliptical incision. **A,** The skin and subcutaneous tissues are incised along the path of the dashed line, and an incision is made around the umbilicus as shown. **B,** The pannus is elevated, and the inferior margin of the incision is made as shown, with a V-shaped extension in the center. **C,** The specimen is removed, and V incisions to eliminate "dog ears" are made at the lateral margins of the incision. **D,** Hemostasis is obtained, an elliptical incision is made for reimplantation of the umbilicus, subcutaneous drains are placed on each side, and closure of the skin incision is begun. **E,** The umbilicus is fixed in its new position by some interrupted sutures, the former umbilical defect is closed, and the skin incision is closed with staples.

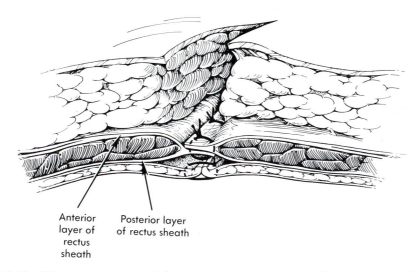

Anterior
layer of
rectus
sheath

Posterior layer
of rectus sheath

Fig. 12-23. When there is a marked diastasis between the rectus muscles, they may be brought closer together and the incision can be made stronger by a "pants-over-vest" closure using interrupted stitches as shown. It is optional whether the peritoneum should be closed.

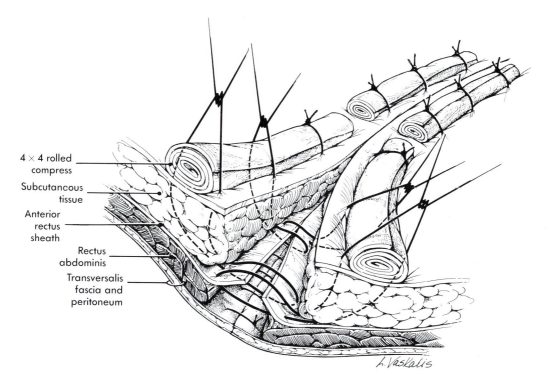

4 × 4 rolled
compress

Subcutaneous
tissue

Anterior
rectus
sheath

Rectus
abdominis

Transversalis
fascia and
peritoneum

Fig. 12-24. Retention sutures. Anticipated excess of postoperative overdistention, coughing, or vomiting may place an extra strain on a midline incision, and retention stitches may give additional support. A maximum of this strength can be given to the approximation of the fascial layers by sutures of monofilament nonabsorbable material placed lateral to the incision, through each side of the fascial incision, and brought back adjacent to the original incision, as shown. Usually, three sets can be placed on each side. After the fascia and skin incisions have been separately repaired, these retention sutures are tied against the bolsters of 4 × 4 rolled compresses as shown.

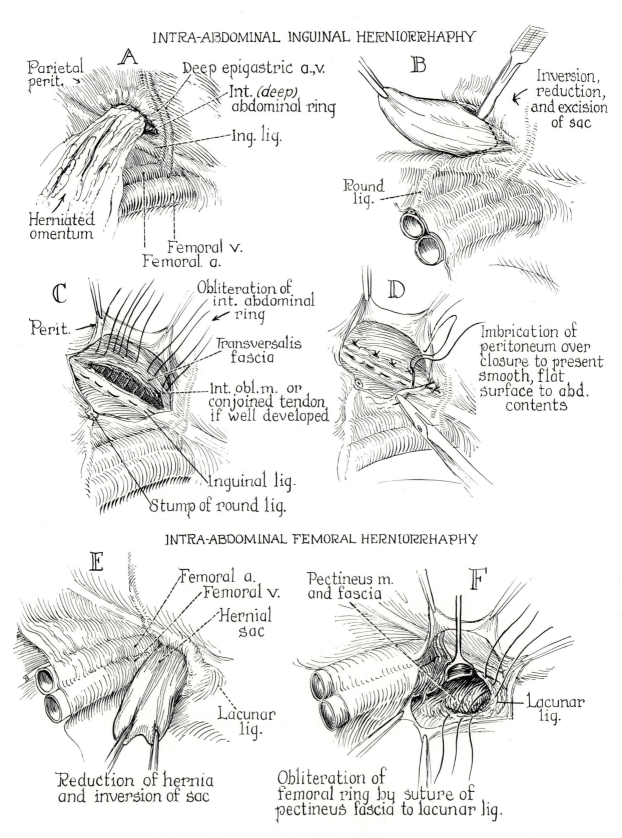

INTRA-ABDOMINAL INGUINAL HERNIORRHAPHY

A
Parietal perit.
Deep epigastric a.,v.
Int. *(deep)* abdominal ring
Ing. lig.
Herniated omentum
Femoral v.
Femoral. a.

B
Inversion, reduction, and excision of sac
Round lig.

C
Perit.
Obliteration of int. abdominal ring
Transversalis fascia
Int. obl.m. or conjoined tendon if well developed
Inguinal lig.
Stump of round lig.

D
Imbrication of peritoneum over closure to present smooth, flat surface to abd. contents

INTRA-ABDOMINAL FEMORAL HERNIORRHAPHY

E
Femoral a.
Femoral v.
Hernial sac
Lacunar lig.
Reduction of hernia and inversion of sac

F
Pectineus m. and fascia
Lacunar lig.
Obliteration of femoral ring by suture of pectineus fascia to lacunar lig.

Fig. 12-25. For legend see opposite page.

Fig. 12-25. The anatomy for intraabdominal inguinal and femoral herniorrhaphy is shown. The anatomy and repair of intraabdominal inguinal herniorrhaphy are shown in **A** through **D. A,** Abdominal view of the inguinal hernia and its contents are noted as a defect in the parietal peritoneum between the inguinal ligament and the deep epigastric artery and vein. The contents are reduced by gentle traction, and the sac is inverted into the abdominal cavity. An incision is made through the peritoneum at the base of the sac in the direction noted by the dashed line. **C,** The round ligament is ligated, permitting the internal ring to be closed completely. The inguinal ligament is sewn to the internal oblique muscle or conjoined tendon and transversalis fascia using permanent suture material or staples. **D,** The peritoneum is closed over the inguinal ligament, if desired. **E** and **F,** The details of intraabdominal femoral herniorrhaphy are shown. Notice that the hernia displaces the femoral artery and vein somewhat laterally. **E,** The hernia is reduced, the sac is inverted into the abdomen, and the sac is excised. **F,** The lacunar ligament is sutured to the pectineus fascia to obliterate the femoral canal. The sutures are started medially and continued toward the femoral vein until the femoral ring is obliterated except for an adequate exit for the femoral vessels and nerve. It may be necessary to remove some of the deep inguinal lymphatics, nodes, and areolar tissue to ensure a secure closure. (From Ball TL: *Gynecologic surgery and urology,* ed 2, St Louis, 1963, Mosby–Year Book, p 575.)

---

lidocaine (Xylocaine) without epinephrine. The operator inserts the tip of a 3-inch 25-gauge spinal needle beneath the external oblique aponeurosis at a point 1 inch medial and 1 inch inferior to the anterior superior iliac spine, advances the needle toward the pubic tubercle, and injects the solution with steady, even pressure. Without removing the needle, the operator redirects it in a fan-shaped fashion to inject the solution in increments, making the last deposition almost perpendicular to the midline. The surgeon may repeat the injection weekly two or three times; if

symptoms recur after a third injection, however, surgical exploration of the wound may be necessary.

If the patient is taking corticosteroids, the daily administration of 50,000 U of vitamin A postoperatively decreases the risk of premature suture absorption. Dermal injury apparently stimulates the elaboration of collagenase, which is hostile to the development of a strong scar. The daily postoperative administration of 500 mg of vitamin C, at least theoretically, may inhibit this collagenase elaboration. Most patients are willing to continue taking vitamin C for 2 or 3 months postoperatively.

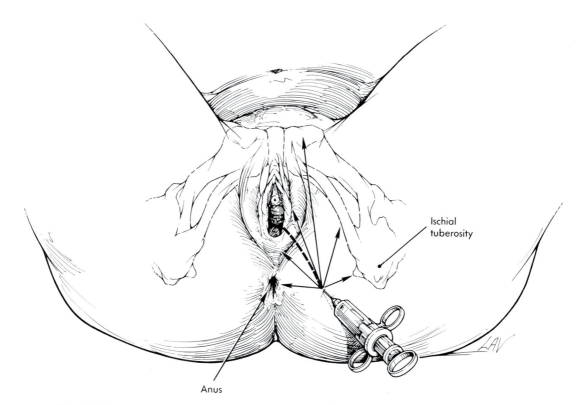

Fig. 12-26. Perineal infiltration by a "liquid tourniquet." From a point midway between the anus and the ischial tuberosity, and using a no. 22 spinal needle, the tissues are thoroughly infiltrated by a solution of dilute epinephrine (1:200,000) along the pathways shown by the arrows. The site of Schuchardt's incision is shown by the path of the heavy broken line.

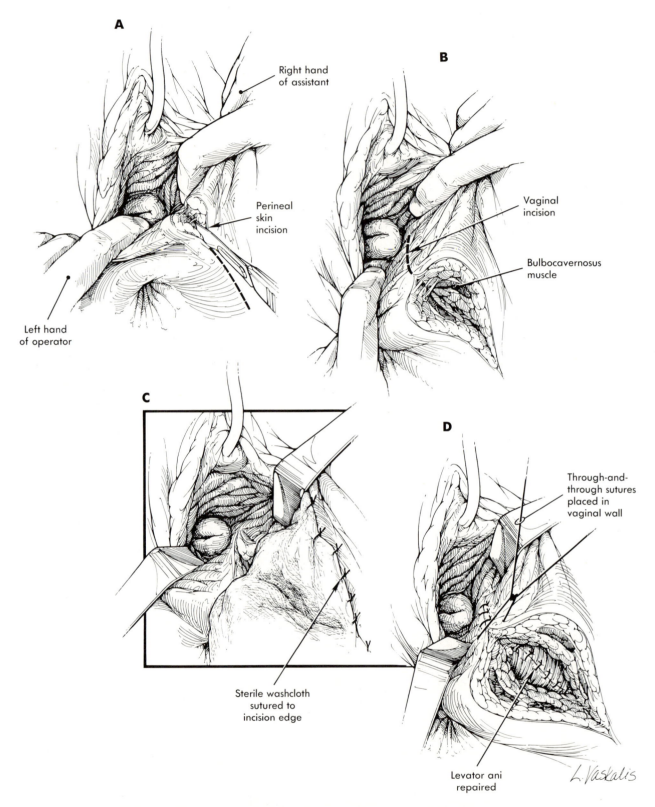

Fig. 12-27. Schuchardt's perineal incision. **A,** With the finger of the operator and the operator's assistant making traction in opposite directions, a skin incision is made along the path of the dashed line, midway between the anus and the ischial tuberosity. **B,** The incision is carried into the vagina. The cut edges of the bulbocavernosus are seen in the depths of the wound. **C,** A sterile washcloth may be sutured to the upper edge of the Schuchardt's incision. The incision is closed by interrupted sutures through the vaginal wall. **D,** The edges of the levator ani are approximated with interrupted sutures, as are those of the bulbocavernosus muscle, and the perineal skin is closed with interrupted sutures.

SCHUCHARDT'S PERINEAL INCISION

A deep incision through the skin of the vulva, vagina, and perineum, Schuchardt's incision markedly increases the surgical access to the vaginal vault when it has been compromised. The tissue in this area is intensely vascular, but a preliminary infiltration of the site by bupivacaine (Marcaine) or lidocaine (Xylocaine), 0.5% in 1:200,000 epinephrine solution, suppresses the blood loss (Fig. 12-26). This "liquid tourniquet" is not a substitute for surgical hemostasis, but a complement to it. Although the transected blood vessels still bleed, they do not bleed as much, and the operator can readily grasp and tie or coagulate them with the electrosurgical unit.

Schuchardt's incision is unilateral. If the patient's left side is to be the site of the incision, the operator should begin at approximately the 4-o'clock position on the hymenal ring. The perineal skin incision is made on a line from the 4-o'clock position on the vulva to a point midway between the anus and the left ischial tuberosity. To increase exposure, the right-handed operator may insert the index finger of the left hand into the wound, establishing traction to the patient's right, while the first assistant may use an index finger to establish countertraction to the patient's left; this maneuver effectively stretches the tissues to be incised (Fig. 12-27, A). The vaginal incision is made similarly in the 4-o'clock position (Fig. 12-27, B). The levator ani often appears in the depths of the wound. The distal portion of the levator may be incised to aid in the exposure of the vaginal vault.

Using a series of temporary interrupted sutures, the operator may sew a sterile washcloth to the upper cut edge of the incision to isolate the raw surfaces of the incision temporarily from the remaining surgery (Fig. 12-27, C). At the conclusion of the intended surgery, the operator cuts the washcloth free and closes the incision with a series of interrupted absorbable through-and-through sutures placed in the full thickness of the vaginal wall (Fig. 12-27, D). The incision in the levator ani may be closed by separate interrupted stitches, or the cut edges of the levator may be included in the stitches placed through the wall of the vagina in its depth. The perineal skin is similarly closed with interrupted absorbable sutures.

REFERENCES

1. Amstey MS, Jones AP: Preparation of the vagina for surgery, *JAMA* 245:839, 1981.
2. Ayliffe GAJ: Surgical scrub and skin disinfection, *Infect Control* 5:23, 1984.
3. Ball TL: *Gynecologic surgery and urology,* ed 2, St Louis, 1963, Mosby–Year Book, p 575.
4. *Bardenheuer's incision.* In Graves WP: Gynecology, ed 4, Philadelphia, 1928, WB Saunders, p 905.
5. Bourne RB et al: In-vivo comparison of four absorbable sutures: Vicryl, Dexon plus, Maxon, and PDS, *Can J Surg* 31:43, 1988.
6. Brand E: Letter to the editor, *Am J Obstet Gynecol* 165:235, 1991.
7. Breen JL: Transverse incisions and the total abdominal hysterectomy, New York, Gynecol Surg Film Festival, Sept 1987.
8. Cherney LS: A modified transverse incision for low abdominal operations, *Surg Gynecol Obstet* 72:92, 1940.
9. Chez RA, Gallup DG: Mass midline closure to avoid wound disruption, *Contemp Ob/Gyn* Oct 1989, p 62.
10. Chez RA, Krebs HB: Steps in performing the Maylard incision, *Contemp Ob/Gyn* Sept 1991, p 39.
11. Chez RA, McDuff HC: The Pfannenstiel incision, *Contemp Ob/Gyn* 7:55, 1976.
12. Christopherson WA: *Surgical incisions and their anatomic basis.* In Buchsbaum HJ, Walton LA, editors: *Strategies in gynecologic surgery,* New York, 1986, Springer-Verlag, p 29.
13. Edgerton MT: Fundamentals of wound management in surgery: technical factors in wound management, South Plainfield, NJ, 1977, Chirurgecom, p 39.
14. Gallup DG, Nolan TE: How to reduce surgery risks, *Contemp Ob/Gyn* 1990, p 172.
15. Gallup DG, Talledo OE, King LA: Primary mass closure of midline incisions with a continuous running monofilament suture in gynecologic patients, *Obstet Gynecol* 73:675, 1989.
16. Greer BE et al: Supraumbilical upper abdominal incision for pelvic surgery in the morbidly obese patient, *Obstet Gynecol* 76:471, 1990.
17. Guyton AC: *Textbook of medical physiology,* Philadelphia, 1976, WB Saunders, p 665.
18. Hajj SN, Mercer LJ, Ismail MA: Surgical approaches to pelvic infections in women, *J Reprod Med* 33:159, 1988.
19. Hoffman MS et al: Mass closure of the abdominal wound with delayed absorbable suture in surgery for gynecologic cancer, *J Reprod Med* 36:356, 1991.
20. Krupski WC et al: The importance of abdominal wall collateral blood vessels, *Arch Surg* 119:854, 1984.
21. Kustner O: Der suprasymphysare kreuzschnitt, eine methode der coeliotomie bei wenig umfanglichen affektioen der weiblichen beckenorgane, *Monatsschr Geburtsh Gynakol* 4:197, 1896.
22. Kustner O: Methodik der gynaekologischen Laparotomie, *Verh Dtsch Ges Gynäkol* (9 Kongr). ix:580, 1901.
23. Leaper DJ, Pollack AV, Evans M: Abdominal wound closure: a trial of nylon, polyglycolic acid and steel sutures, *Br J Surg* 64:603, 1977.
24. Lee RA: *Atlas of gynecologic surgery,* Philadelphia, 1992, WB Saunders.
25. Lewis RT, Wiegand FM: Natural history of vertical abdominal parietal closure: Prolene versus Dexon, *Can J Surg* 32:196, 1989.
26. Lowbury EJL: Skin disinfection, *J Clin Pathol* 14:85, 1961.
27. Mackenrodt A: Die Radikaloperation des Gebärmutterscheidenkrebses mit. Ausräumung des Beckens, *Verh Dtsch Gynokol* ix:139, 1901.
28. Masterson BJ: Skin preparation, *Clin Obstet Gynecol* 31:736, 1988.
29. Masterson BJ: Selection of incisions for gynecologic procedures, *Surg Clin North Am* 71:1041, 1991.
30. Maylard AE: Direction of abdominal incisions, *Br Med J* 2:895, 1907.
31. Metz SA, Chenqini N, Masterson BJ: In-vivo tissue reactivity and degradation of suture materials: a comparison of Maxon and PDS, *J Gynecol Surg* 5:37, 1989.
32. Morrow CP: Discussion of Lewis RT et al: *Yearbook of obstetrics and gynecology, 1991,* St Louis, 1991, Mosby–Year Book, p 240.
33. Morrow CP et al: Pelvic celiotomy in the obese patient, *Am J Obstet Gynecol* 127:335, 1977.
34. Mountcastle VB: *Medical physiology,* ed 13, St Louis, 1974, Mosby–Year Book, p 351.
35. Pfannenstiel J: Ueber die Vortheile des suprasymphysaren Fascienquerschnitts für die gynäkologischen Koliotomien zugleich ein Beitrag zu der Indikationsstellung der Operationswege, *Samml Klin Vortr (Leipzig),* 268:1735, 1900.
36. Ranney B: Diastasis recti and umbilical hernia: causes, recognition, and repair, *So Dakota J Med* 43:5, 1990.
37. Rodeheaver GT, Nesbit WS, Edlich RF: Novafil—a dynamic suture for wound closure, *Ann Surg* 204:193, 1986.
38. Rodeheaver GT et al: Unique performance characteristics of Novafil, *Surg Gynecol Obstet* 164:230, 1987.

39. Sanz LE et al: Comparison of Maxon suture with Vicryl, chromic catgut, and PDS in fascial closure in rats, *Obstet Gynecol* 71:418, 1988.

40. Shepherd JH et al: Abdominal wound closure using a nonabsorbable single-layer closure, *Obstet Gynecol* 61:248, 1983.

41. Sippo WC: Personal communication, March 1990.

42. Sippo WC, Burghardt A, Gomez AC: Nerve entrapment after Pfannenstiel incision, *Am J Obstet Gynecol* 157:420, 1987.

43. Sippo WC, Gomez A: Nerve-entrapment syndromes from lower abdominal surgery, *J Fam Pract* 25:585, 1987.

44. Sola AE: Myofascial trigger point therapy, *Res Staff Physic* Aug 1981, p 38.

45. Thompson JD: *Incisions for gynecologic surgery.* In Thompson JD, Rock JA, editors: *TeLindes Operative Gynecology,* ed 7, Philadelphia, 1992, JB Lippincott, p 261.

46. Turner-Warwick R: *Vesico-vaginal fistula: the resolution of the "frozen pelvis" by caeco-vaginoplasty.* In Robb C, Smith R, editors: *Operative Surgery,* 1986, Butterworth.

47. Turner-Warwick R: *The functional anatomy of the urethra.* In Droller MJ, editor: *The surgical management of urologic disease,* St Louis, 1992, Mosby–Year Book.

48. Turner-Warwick R: *Obstetric and gynaecological injuries of the urinary tract—their prevention and management.* In Bonnar J, editor: *Recent advances in obstetrics and gynaecology,* 18, London, Churchill Livingstone (in press).

49. Turner-Warwick R et al: The 'supra-pubic V' incision, *Br J Urol* 46:39, 1974.

50. von Peham H, Amreich J: *Operative gynecology* (translated by Ferguson LK), Philadelphia, 1934, JB Lippincott, p 131.

Chapter 13

EVISCERATION AND REPAIR OF VENTRAL HERNIAS

George W. Mitchell, Jr.

EVISCERATION

The term *evisceration* implies the extrusion of abdominal contents. In gynecologic practice, this serious accident occurs after abdominal wound disruption or as a result of vaginal operations, trauma, or prolapse. In both instances, immediate surgery is indicated, but even prompt treatment is associated with significant mortality.

Abdominal evisceration

The term *dehiscence* is synonymous with wound separation; the most common form involves only the skin and subcutaneous tissues and is usually caused by infection. When this occurs, the wound is packed open with gauze moistened with sterile saline and is inspected daily. Necrotic tissue is debrided at the time of each inspection, and the wound is repacked by the nursing service three times a day. Available evidence does not indicate that the use of Dakin's solution, hydrogen peroxide, enzymes, povidone-iodine, whirlpool baths, or scrubbing the edges is of any additional value. Cultures often show the presence of multiple organisms and are frequently not helpful, but hyperbaric oxygen treatments may speed the healing process if anaerobic organisms predominate. Granulation tissue forms rapidly, and on about the fourth or fifth day after separation, when the wound has a healthy red color throughout, it should be reclosed with through-and-through interrupted sutures about 1 inch apart, including the skin and subcutaneous tissues as well as a bite in the intact underlying fascia. Reports have shown an 80% success rate for reclosure if the proper initial precautions noted above are taken. In the event of failure, a second attempt may be considered, or the wound may be left to close by second intention, a process involving many weeks or months of continuing home care with nursing supervision.

When wound separation involves the anterior fascia of the abdominal wall, the possibility of the extrusion of abdominal contents must be considered. This is best explored by careful inspection, using a good light, and by gloved finger palpation of the entire length of the incision. If there is no protrusion, the wound may be treated as noted above, but reclosure must include the fascia. Interrupted sutures set far back from the fascial edge and 1 cm apart are placed first, and the skin and subcutaneous tissues are united as noted above.

Dehiscence that results in protrusion of any part of the intestinal tract is called evisceration and constitutes a surgical emergency of the first order. The possible causes of evisceration are listed below.

Factors Predisposing to Wound Disruption
1. *Preoperative*
   Age
   Systemic disease
      Diabetes, cancer pulmonary disease, jaundice, cardiovascular disease, anemia
   Nutrition
      Obesity, hypoproteinemia
   Previous abdominal surgery
   Irradiation of the abdomen
   Drugs
      Chemotherapy, steroids
2. *Operative*
   Imperfect technical closure
   Length of incision
   Length of operation
   Hemostasis
   Necrotic tissue
   Type of closure
   Suture material

3. *Postoperative*
    Wound infection
        Hematomas, seromas
    Distention
        Ileus, ascites
    Exertion
        Coughing, vomiting, hiccups

Although any one or combination of these may play a role, there is some difference of opinion in the literature regarding the relative seriousness of some of the conditions on the list. All agree that age, advanced disease, previous surgery through the same wound, and surgical technique are of the utmost importance, but there is a modern tendency to discount such things as obesity, chemotherapy, and the chronic use of steroids. Bearing in mind all factors that might complicate recovery, including wound disruption, the decision to perform elective surgery must be based on the degree of need relative to those risks. When abdominal surgery is deemed essential, the surgeon is obligated to make and close the incision in a manner calculated to provide maximum wound strength.

The closure of abdominal incisions requires knowledge, care, and skill, and unsupervised neophytes should not be left alone to complete the closure at the end of a major operation. The difference in statistics reflecting the success or failure of different types of closure may be caused in part by the tendency in some institutions to allow residents at a low level to close the incision. Much has been written about the various types of incision, but there is reasonable consensus that vertical (especially midline) and transverse incisions have about the same tensile strength. Rectus splitting incisions incur the risk of devascularization or denervation of the mid-portion of the rectus muscle, and pararectal incisions, where the transversus abdominis muscle joins the fascia of the oblique muscles, are inherently weak. The length of the incision is important; adequate exposure of the abdominal contents is essential, but extended incisions into the upper abdomen increase the likelihood of future dehiscence and evisceration. Difficult cases require prolonged operating time, but routine cases should be accomplished without unnecessary delay, because long operations cause postoperative ileus and distention and increase the infection rate, one of the primary causes of dehiscence.

The method of closure and the suture material to be used vary from one institution to another and among individual surgeons of great experience. These biases are understandable, because the clinical data in the literature are largely uncontrolled and retrospective, and the animal data cannot be extrapolated to humans. It is safe to say that the general trend in recent years has been toward a form of mass closure, using either the interrupted Smead-Jones or modified Smead-Jones technique, or a continuous suture. In the hands of their respective advocates, either of these methods is highly successful in reducing the incidence of postoperative wound disruption. The further addition of

through-and-through interrupted stay sutures in difficult cases, long and vigorously recommended by senior surgeons, has not stood the test of time in providing a better defense against disruption and may increase the likelihood of infection.

The many new types of suture material coming on the market in the last 20 years have offered surgeons a more difficult choice than they faced in the past, when only cotton, silk, catgut, and wire were available. Three of the former favorites are popular enough to remain on the market, but, when applied to wound closure, each has drawbacks that should limit its use. Although flexible and easy to handle, silk is braided and reactive in tissue, with a tendency to give rise to infection and require removal. Wire has good tensile strength initially and is relatively unreactive but tends to undergo work fracture with time, to cut through tissue, and to press upward into dermal nerves producing pain. Catgut is highly reactive, has inconstant initial tensile strength, and gives way between 10 and 20 days when the wound is still in the maturation phase; it should not be used for closure either in obstetrics or gynecology. Many new synthetic sutures have reasonably comparable effectiveness. In making a choice, the following principles are useful:

1. Monofilament sutures are less likely than braided sutures to be associated with infection.
2. Nonabsorbable sutures retain their tensile strength longer than absorbable sutures but not indefinitely.
3. Interrupted sutures may be either absorbable or nonabsorbable.
4. Running sutures for mass closure should be nonabsorbable.
5. Suture size should be zero or above to reduce the likelihood of breakage and cutting through tissue.
6. All sutures should be placed a centimeter or more lateral to the cut edge.
7. The first throw in the knot should be a double pass with four throws above it.

As stated above, the closure is only as competent as the tissues of the patient, and additional protective factors should be kept in mind for each individual. These include the appropriate use of prophylactic antibiotics, especially before operations that are expected to be infected or prolonged; leaving the skin and subcutaneous tissues open when there has been gross contamination; placing suction drains in large dead spaces; inserting nasogastric tubes when ileus is anticipated or distention is encountered; and using abdominal binders to support the wound in obese patients or when mechanical stress is likely.

The incidence of wound disruption through all layers, with exposure or protrusion of the intestine, is between 1% and 3% after all abdominal surgery, but after purely gynecologic surgery the rate is much lower. Mortality was reported to be as high as 50% when this occurs, but recently has dropped below 10% overall, with gynecologic surgery again falling well below this level. The continuing downward trend, both in evisceration and mortality, is most probably due to the increasing use of modern suture material and advances in maintaining the patients' general condition at the best possible level, but the event remains serious and necessitates prompt action.

The classic sign of imminent evisceration, occurring in 85% of cases, is a sudden ooze or gush of serosanguineous fluid, usually from the fourth to the eighth postoperative day. This may be associated with the patient's having the sensation of the wound breaking apart; when this happens, it is often after some undue strain on the abdominal wall. Because it may be a manifestation of a minor dehiscence due to infection or a seroma, the opening should be probed with a sterile gloved finger to determine whether the fascia and peritoneum are intact. The use of clamps, cotton-tipped applicators, or other instruments is more dangerous and not as informative. In the majority of instances when the fascia has actually separated, the wound should be lightly packed with moist sterile gauze and covered with a moist towel, while preparations are made to return the patient to the operating room for secondary closure (Fig. 13-1). When the wound is obviously involved in gross infection and there is no protrusion of the intestine, it may be debrided and packed and the patient may be started on antibiotics in an attempt to delay secondary closure to a more favorable time. If the bowel is visible or palpable at the fascial level or above, however, regardless of infection, further delay in repair is contraindicated. Occasionally, there is doubt about the diagnosis because of the patient's obesity, the poor condition of the tissues, or the presence of an exudative infection. Both computed tomography (CT) scans and ultrasound have been used to make or confirm the diagnosis, but these require moving the patient and running further risk of evisceration. It is safer to assume the worst and proceed accordingly. In the operating room before attempted closure, the bowel is carefully inspected for possible injury or bleeding.

For many years, closure of completely disrupted wounds has been done with through-and-through stay sutures, most often with stainless steel but more recently with nylon, and many surgeons continue to adhere to this technique (Fig. 13-2). Recent literature suggests the use of an interrupted mass closure of the Smead-Jones type, with nonabsorbable suture material (Fig. 13-3). This seems logical, especially in the presence of infection, when one or two sutures may have to be removed subsequently without opening the entire incision. No matter how accurately the sutures are placed and anchored, the closure is only as strong as the surrounding tissues. For this reason, debridement of grossly infected or devitalized subcutaneous tissue, fascia, or muscle must be accomplished before closure is attempted (Fig. 13-4). If debridement leaves a tissue deficiency so that the residual fascia cannot be approximated, some type of prosthesis must be used. The best material is a nonabsorbable synthetic mesh, which can be laid across the defect in direct apposition to the intestine and sutured to the fascia at points at least 2 cm lateral to the fascial edge. Even in infected wounds where the mesh constitutes an additional threat as a foreign body, it must be used in a delaying action in the hope that the patient

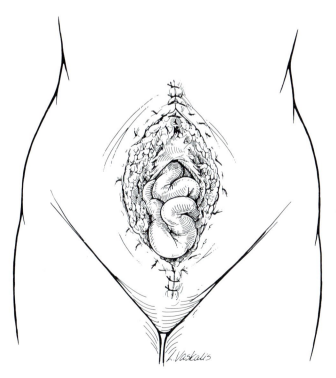

Fig. 13-1. Wound evisceration. The skin, fascia, and peritoneum have separated along almost the entire length of the wound, exposing the underlying small intestine.

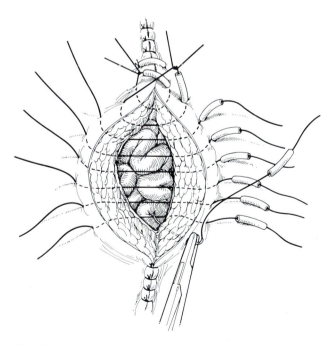

Fig. 13-2. Through-and-through closure of wound evisceration. This traditional method is still in use but has been largely superseded by a Smead-Jones technique.

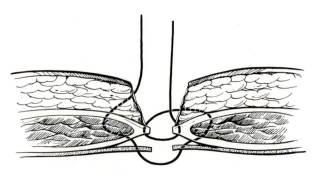

Fig. 13-3. Modified Smead-Jones closure. The modified Smead-Jones far-far-near-near closure includes all layers except the skin. (From Nichols DH: *Reoperative gynecologic surgery,* St Louis, 1991, Mosby–Year Book.)

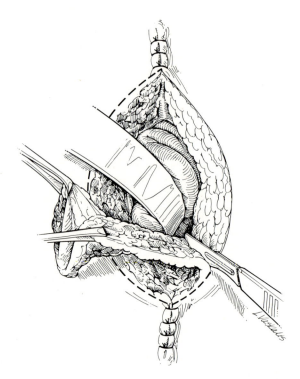

Fig. 13-4. Debridement of wound. Devitalized tissue is resected prior to closure. The bowel is protected and complete hemostasis achieved.

survives the acute emergency and is in better condition for repair on a later day. At the upper level, there is the question of whether the skin should be left open, as would be the case when gross infection is present, or closed without drainage. The decision depends on the estimated degree of contamination. Although there is evidence that metal clips are more desirable than sutures in the skin because they are less likely to be foci of infection, the skin may be the ultimate layer protecting the patient if the fascia separates again, and it is safer to close it with interrupted end-on mattress sutures, set well back from the edge, using the most inert nonabsorbable suture material available.

As previously noted, wounds that are left open should be packed with moist gauze and covered with a loose dressing; the final closure may be delayed for 3 or 4 days. After massive resection of the abdominal wall necessitated by necrotizing fasciitis, split thickness skin and myocutaneous grafts have been used to cover the defect, but this cannot be done until the wound is granulating cleanly.

Even if the bowel is not distended at the time of reclosure of the incision, ileus is likely to supervene, and a prophylactic nasogastric tube is essential. To promote healing, serum proteins must be augmented by hyperalimentation or total parenteral nutrition when the patient is unable to tolerate or absorb an adequate diet. Wound care by the physician, with proper debridement and redressing, should take place at least once daily, and the wound should be inspected and redressed by the nursing service on at least two other occasions during the day. Cultures rarely give the information necessary to determine which antibiotics to select, and a shotgun approach with triple antibiotics should cover most of the commonly responsible organisms.

Evisceration rarely occurs after laparoscopy, but the condition cannot be overlooked if the patient develops a lump at the site of puncture, symptoms and signs of acute entrapment of the bowel, or failure to resume normal bowel function within 48 to 72 hours. When the correct diagnosis is in doubt, CT scans and ultrasonography are helpful. The appropriate treatment is laparotomy, assessment of the condition of the bowel, and firm closure.

This complication is prevented by releasing the gas before withdrawing the laparoscope, visualization as the laparoscope is being withdrawn, and finger palpation of the defect before closing the skin.

Vaginal evisceration

The protrusion of abdominal and pelvic viscera through the vagina has been reported after trauma, surgery, coitus, radiation, the presence of foreign bodies, and the development of enterocele. The involved organs have included the small and large bowel, the omentum, the fallopian tubes, and the ovaries. Approximately 44 cases of bowel evisceration have been reported, and two thirds of these occurred as a result of enterocele or previous surgery for relaxed pelvic floor. The systemic factors contributing to abdominal wound dehiscence are obviously operational in vaginal cases as well. Because 17 of the 44 cases had had vaginal hysterectomies and 3 had had abdominal hysterectomies, it may be assumed that surgical technique was one of the most important etiologic factors leading to the complication. Third-degree unrepaired enteroceles, especially those in postmenopausal women and those with vaginal ulcers, may also rupture as a result of the fragile local tissue, the elongation of the bowel mesentery permitting descent into the sac, and increased intraabdominal pressure.

The patient often experiences lower abdominal pain at the time of the accident and serosanguineous fluid escapes. Prolapse of viscera beyond the introitus is an obvious symptom and may be followed shortly by acute abdominal pain if the blood supply to the prolapsed bowel has been

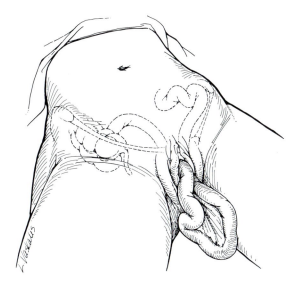

Fig. 13-5. Vaginal evisceration. Rupture of an enterocele in a postmenopausal woman has permitted a loop of ileum with an elongated mesentery to escape through the vagina.

interrupted. The accident often occurs at home, and, when the patient is brought into the emergency room, the likelihood of bacterial contamination is high (Fig. 13-5).

As the patient's general condition is being attended to, she should be prepared for the operating room as rapidly as possible. Although a few surgeons in the past have elected to replace the bowel in the abdominal cavity and close and pack the vagina, some with success, an abdominal approach is definitely indicated in all such cases. The prolapsed intestine is rinsed with sterile saline and gradually replaced into the abdominal cavity by a combination of gentle pressure from below and traction from above. Because of possible injury to the bowel or its blood supply, the small bowel must be run and the omentum and rectosigmoid must be carefully inspected. All visible damage is repaired, and infarcted or severely injured areas are resected. The vaginal defect is closed from above with interrupted sutures, and the posterior cul-de-sac is obliterated either by the Moschowitz or Halban technique. The operation is done under appropriate antibiotic coverage, and soon after surgery the postmenopausal patient is started on estrogen therapy to promote vaginal healing.

Another type of evisceration with prolapse of the intestine through the vagina occurs as a result of surgical injury to the uterus and is not often reported because it most frequently happens during or immediately after abortion, especially in second-trimester pregnancy. The majority of uterine perforations, even those producing large defects, go unrecognized at the time of curettage, but, when suction is used, it is quite possible to trap bowel or omentum in the suction tip and draw it down into the vagina. This same accident may occur during sharp curettage or with grasping instruments, when the operator believes he or she has made contact with the products of conception but in-

stead brings down abdominal viscera (Fig. 13-6). Most diagnostic and therapeutic curettages are done in an outpatient setting poorly equipped to manage complications of this kind, and the patients are almost always transported to an emergency room. The approach to the problem is abdominal, as with other vaginal eviscerations, but the patient may be young, and future fertility may be important. Before being medicated, the patient must be counseled about the possible necessity to perform a hysterectomy, and her wishes with regard to future pregnancy must be kept in mind. The consent form must clearly outline the possibilities and risks inherent in the situation, and the note in the record should be comprehensive. The surgeon responsible for the injury should be notified and urged to visit the patient during convalescence.

At operation, which is always transabdominal, the prolapsed intestine must be carefully replaced in the abdomen by a combination of traction from above and pressure from below. Unless there is obvious gross spillage of fecal material, which must, of course, immediately be controlled, attention is first directed to the uterine laceration, where there is likely to be profuse bleeding and the formation of a hematoma in the broad ligament. After evacuation of the hematoma, bleeding vessels are ligated and the site of perforation is inspected to determine whether the uterus can be salvaged with a reasonable expectation of future successful pregnancies. This is strictly a judgment call, and the outcome depends on the severity of the injury. Because the pregnancy for which the termination was attempted might remain in the fundus, the surgeon must also decide whether to attempt to remove it through the laceration or to monitor from the laparotomy site another effort to perform transcervical curettage. Should the laceration appear incompatible with future successful pregnancy, as would be the case when it extends from the lower uterine segment down the length of the cervix or when there is significant loss of cervical tissue, a hysterectomy is indicated. As noted before, the patient should have been counseled for this possibility. Simple loss of the uterine or ovarian blood supply on one side, however, is not an indication for hysterectomy when the laceration can be repaired with a reasonable expectation of remaining intact in a future third trimester.

When bleeding has been controlled, the entire ileum must be run, and the mesentery, omentum rectosigmoid, and cecum must be carefully inspected. Lacerations are carefully repaired, and extensively damaged areas are resected. The abdominal cavity is liberally irrigated, and the abdomen is closed with the usual care.

VENTRAL HERNIA

The incidence of ventral, or incisional, hernia through abdominal wounds is generally estimated at between 1% and 3%. In gynecologic surgery, in which concomitant trauma and infection are less likely to be present, the incidence is far lower but by no means negligible. Predisposing factors parallel those listed on p. 197 for dehiscence,

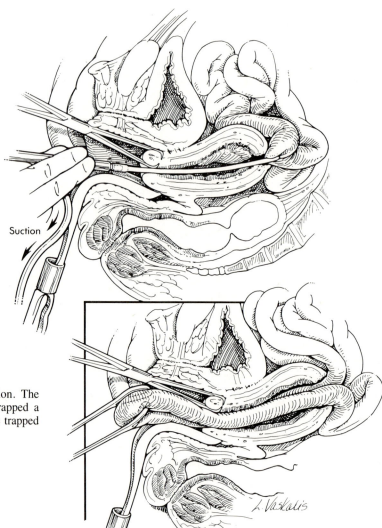

Suction

Fig. 13-6. Uterine perforation during therapeutic abortion. The suction curette has perforated the uterine fundus and trapped a loop of ileum. *Insert,* Placental forceps have grasped the trapped loop, pulling it down through the cervix.

and, of course, previous dehiscence and repair occupy a prominent place in the list.

Diagnosis

The patient's history is the most important single clue to the diagnosis; she complains of lower abdominal pressure and discomfort, particularly after standing for long periods of time or when straining or coughing, and feels relief when lying supine. The symptom often gradually becomes worse, especially when daily activities require considerable exertion, and, depending on the degree of protrusion of the abdominal contents and the thickness of the abdominal wall, she may palpate a definite lump. If there is a palpable lump that recedes when the patient is horizontal, the history alone is pathognomonic of the presence of a hernia. Incisional hernias are seldom the site of acute intestinal incarceration or infarction, but that danger must be kept in mind as an outside possibility.

In the classic case, careful palpation of the abdominal wall reveals a distinct fascial defect, with the edges easily palpable, often in a round or oval configuration. Having

the patient raise her head from the table or increase intraabdominal pressure may or may not reveal the lump of which she originally complained, but, when it is present, the diagnosis is confirmed. In obese patients, grand multiparas, and those with marked diastasis of the rectus muscles, it is often very difficult to determine whether a true hernia is present or whether the fascia is merely thin and attenuated. Additional evidence can sometimes be obtained by the use of ultrasound or CT scan, both of which, in expert hands, can be very helpful. The combination of history, physical examination, and radiologic techniques almost always lead to the correct diagnosis, and positive findings in any two of these should be present before resorting to surgical repair. Even so, mistakes are still possible.

Hernias are often larger than they seem on physical examination because bowel can protrude through a relatively small defect and spread across the abdominal wall beneath the skin and subcutaneous tissues; in some instances, it seems as if most of the gastrointestinal tract is within the hernia sac. It is remarkable that, even under these circumstances, when the hernia has been of long duration, many patients have learned to tolerate the discomfort and manage their affairs reasonably well. Such sufferers tend to be old, obese, or sick and, not infrequently, a combination of all three. Some may have had irradiation to the abdominal wall and numerous previous attempts to repair the defect; when this is the case, the likelihood that future surgery will fail is high. Large hernias require large procedures and prolonged anesthesia time, leading inevitably to an increased risk of postoperative complications. The wise surgeon does not operate on a patient with a chronic hernia when her condition suggests that a poor outcome is likely and when her symptoms can be treated palliatively. Symptomatic relief can often be obtained by the use of abdominal binders and modification of the patient's lifestyle to prevent undue exertion. When the hernia can be reduced, trusses tailored to the patient's anatomic defect can be obtained from medical supply houses.

Preoperative care

Before surgery every effort is made to ensure that the patient is in optimal condition. This means control of diabetes, treatment of local or systemic infections, and normalizing electrolytes, proteins, and hematocrit. It is useless to defer operation until the patient loses weight because this practically never happens. Although insurance companies may dictate otherwise, the patient's best interest is served by admission to the hospital the day before surgery so that her body can be properly cleansed and her bowel can be prepped and decompressed. The appropriate regimen for immediate preoperative care is listed below.

Preoperative Care before Hernia Repair
1. Bathe patient preceding evening
2. Bathe and cleanse abdomen morning of surgery
3. Avoid shaving if possible
4. Nasogastric tube night before
5. Bowel prep
   Cathartic day before
   Enema in AM
   Neomycin, 1 g four times in 24 hr
   Erythromycin, 1 g four times in 24 hr
6. Prophylactic antibiotic <2 hr before surgery

Bowel decompression greatly facilitates the dissection of adherent loops that are almost invariably present in hernias, and reduction of the bacterial content of the bowel to some extent protects the patient from serious sepsis in the event there is bowel perforation. The skin of the abdominal wall should be thoroughly cleansed the night before and the day of surgery but not scrubbed in such a way as to damage the epidermis. Shaving is often unnecessary, but if it is to be done, the best time is immediately before making the incision so bacterial invasion of skin breaks and cuts can be avoided. Prophylactic antibiotics are most effective when given within the 2-hour period before operation and need not be continued beyond 24 hours postoperatively.

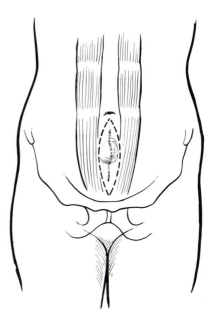

Fig. 13-7. Elliptical incision to excise previous scar and redundant skin over the hernia. (From Nichols DH: *Reoperative gynecologic surgery,* St Louis, 1991, Mosby–Year Book.)

Surgical repair

The basic principles of hernia repair have changed little during the past 100 years. It is essential to dissect free the entire peritoneal sac and excise it. White fascia must be united with white fascia across the defect without the interposition of scar or defective tissue. The edges must meet without tension. Absolute hemostasis must be obtained. After closure of the fascial defect, excess skin and subcutaneous tissue are resected to provide a neat cosmetic closure.

The old skin scar is completely resected, leaving a margin of healthy skin on either side, and a wedge of subcutaneous tissue beneath the scar is removed with it down to the level of the fascia and the hernia sac (Fig. 13-7). The entire hernia sac is freed from its attachments to the subcutaneous tissue above and the fascia below so that it can be visualized in its fullest extent (Fig. 13-8). Before proceeding with further dissection, the sac should be opened with care to avoid injuring adherent bowel. Finger exploration reveals to what extent the opening in the peritoneum can be enlarged (Fig. 13-9), and once it has been opened as far as possible, the peritoneum is retracted upward with multiple clamps to prevent tearing while countertraction on the intestine permits dissection of adherent loops and omentum from the side walls of the sac (Fig. 13-10). This process is continued until the abdominal contents have been completely released and returned to the abdominal cavity. At this point, the omentum and previously incarcerated intestine should be examined thoroughly for bleeding points, nicks, or lacerations, and acute twists or turns in the small intestine should be released. It is tempting to continue to cut away adhesions, wherever they may be, with the object of reconstituting the entire small intestine, but this is

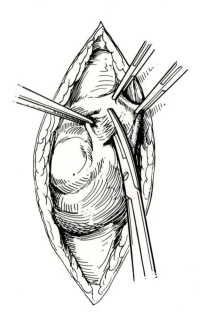

Fig. 13-8. Dissecting hernia sac. While traction is maintained on the fascial edge, the peritoneal covering of the hernia sac is cut away from its undersurface. (From Nichols DH: *Reoperative gynecologic surgery,* St Louis, 1991, Mosby–Year Book.)

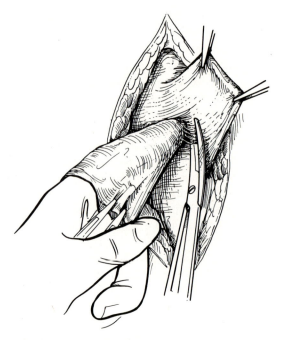

Fig. 13-9. Opening the hernia sac. The hernia sac is opened and kept on traction while a finger inside guides the dissection downward to the origin of the hernia. (From Nichols DH: *Reoperative gynecologic surgery,* St Louis, 1991, Mosby–Year Book.)

an exercise in futility because of the rapid recurrence of such adhesions and the possibility that the new arrangement may be even less favorable. The excess peritoneum constituting the sac is resected down to the level of the surrounding fascia, where, in many instances, it may be fused with the fascial undersurface and the rectus muscle. The fascia is often attenuated and scarred, especially if there has been a previous attempt at repair, and it is absolutely imperative to resect such weakened tissue before attempting repair, regardless of the size of the defect thus created. To do this, the rectus muscle compartment must be opened and the muscle mobilized without disturbing its blood supply from the inferior epigastric artery. To attempt to close the defect with fragmented, thin, or devitalized fascia is to court failure.

When only a well-defined and competent anterior fascia remains, the opposing edges are drawn toward the midline of the incision to see whether they can be joined without tension. If this is possible, the fascia and underlying peritoneum, whether fused or separate, are closed with interrupted, synthetic, monofilament, nonabsorbable sutures placed 1 to 2 cm back from the edge (Fig. 13-11). These may be either straight across, figure-of-eight, or mattress type sutures, and number one caliber is preferable to avoid its pulling through. The overlapping imbricated method that provides a double layer of fascia at the point of closure was popular for many years and is still depicted in textbooks, but it requires redundant fascia, takes more time, leaves more suture material in the wound, and does not improve the results over a simple side-to-side technique.

When the defect is too large to approximate the residual fascial edges, mobilization of the subcutaneous tissues lat-

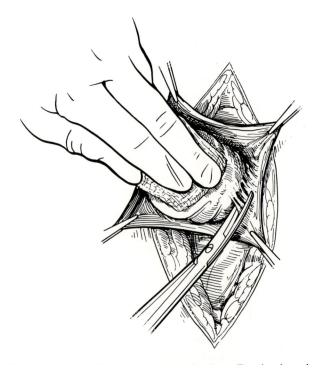

Fig. 13-10. Releasing the intestinal adhesions. Traction is maintained on the peritoneum and counter traction on the contents of the hernia while internal adhesions are lysed to permit return of the intestines and omentum to the general abdominal cavity. (From Nichols DH: *Reoperative gynecologic surgery,* St Louis, 1991, Mosby–Year Book.)

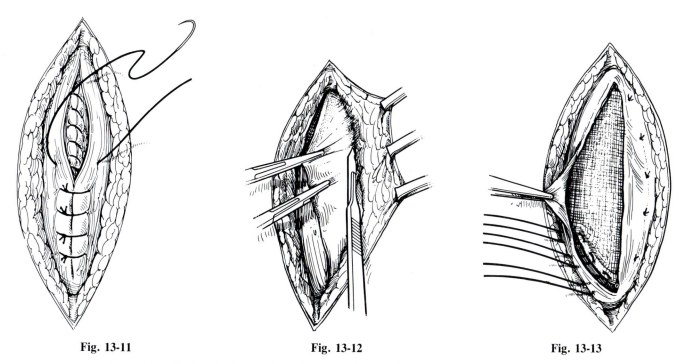

Fig. 13-11.   **Fig. 13-12.**   **Fig. 13-13.**

Fig. 13-11. Closing the fascia. The underlying peritoneum has been closed with a running suture, and the fascia is being closed with straight interrupted sutures. This traditional method is gradually being replaced by a running suture including all layers except the skin. (From Nichols DH: *Reoperative gynecologic surgery,* St Louis, 1991, Mosby–Year Book.)

Fig. 13-12. Undercutting subcutaneous tissue. The subcutaneous tissues are mobilized from the superior surface of the fascia so that it can be resected as necessary and closed without tension. (From Nichols DH: *Reoperative gynecologic surgery,* St Louis, 1991, Mosby–Year Book.)

Fig. 13-13. Suturing the mesh beneath the fascia. The synthetic mesh has been tailored and placed beneath the fascia to support the closure. The folded edge of the mesh is being drawn beneath the fascia with pulley sutures placed well back from the edge. (From Nichols DH: *Reoperative gynecologic surgery,* St Louis, 1991, Mosby–Year Book.)

erally away from the fascial surface on both sides with concomitant mobilization of the rectus muscles beneath may permit union without tension (Fig. 13-12). Vertical relaxing incisions in the fascia lateral to the rectus muscle near the semilunar line where the transversus abdominis muscle joins the oblique muscles leave a weak point in the abdominal wall that may give rise to a future spigelian hernia, and the use of prostheses has largely superseded this technique.

To bridge an absolute tissue deficiency in the abdominal wall, a large variety of different materials have been used for many years; until the modern era, these efforts met with little success. In the 1940s, tantalum mesh was found to be well tolerated, and subsequent sampling of the long-term scar showed that it was eventually replaced by connective tissue. Because of its tendency to undergo work fracture, it could not be placed in direct contact with the intestine, and broken fragments tended to migrate upward into the skin. Coincident with the development of stronger and more durable suture material during the past 25 years, flexible gauze meshes of the same material have been prepared, and these have been found to be inert in wounds, to retain their tensile strength until the wound has matured, and to permit a thick ingrowth of connective tissue. Al-

though absorbable meshes have been tried experimentally, they are inferior to the nonabsorbable type, and polyethylene and polypropylene are the most commonly used.

The mesh is tailored with scissors, usually in an oval configuration, slightly larger than the size of the defect, and sutured beneath the retracted fascial edges, using a pulley stitch inserted from above downward through the fascia approximately 2 cm from its edge, taking a bite in the mesh lying below and coming up again through the fascia to be tied above (Fig. 13-13). When the closure has been completed all around the defect, the mesh lies in direct apposition to the intestine and neatly bridges the gap. Even when the fascial edges can be closed side-to-side without tension, the mesh can be used to strengthen what might be considered a relatively weak closure. It can also be placed and sutured above the fascia, but this is not quite as satisfactory because it leaves more mesh exposed in an area where infection is likely, due to the accumulation of serous fluid in the subcutaneous dead space. In either position, the mesh is eventually infiltrated by a thick layer of connective tissue.

Once the principal layer of the closure has been secured, with or without a prosthesis, attention is directed to the skin and the subcutaneous tissue that has been exten-

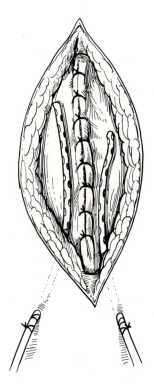

Fig. 13-14. Placement of drains. Suction drains are inserted through separate stab wounds in the dead space left by undercutting the subcutaneous tissues and are sutured at the skin level. (From Nichols DH: *Reoperative gynecologic surgery,* St Louis, 1991, Mosby–Year Book.)

sively undercut and is, therefore, redundant. Meticulous hemostasis is essential, and all bleeding points, however small, should be fulgurated with as little damage to the surrounding area as possible. Excess and necrotic fat is resected, and the skin is trimmed to provide as cosmetic a straight line closure as possible. One or two suction drains are left in the subcutaneous dead space and brought out through lateral stab wounds, where they are carefully secured to the skin so that they cannot be inadvertently pulled out (Fig. 13-14). A dry dressing is applied along with an abdominal binder, which should be tight enough to provide support and assist with hemostasis without unduly compromising diaphragmatic movement.

Postoperative care

Postoperatively, the binder can be removed after 24 hours. The nasogastric tube remains in place until the patient begins to pass gas per rectum. Intravenous feeding is continued for at least 24 hours, and a liquid diet is begun only after there is evidence of returning bowel function. After progression to a regular diet, it is still possible for abdominal distention to occur; if this happens, the nasogastric tube should be immediately replaced. The wound is inspected after 24 hours, and if intact and in good condition, a light dressing is continued from then on, enabling quick daily observation. The drains are removed after approximately 48 hours unless the volume of drainage remains above 100 ml; leaving them in longer invites bacte-

rial contamination of the repair. When the patient is discharged, she is warned that strenuous physical activity is contraindicated for at least 1 month and is told to return without delay if there is swelling in, or discharge from, the wound. Persistent accumulation of fluid in the subcutaneous space is occasionally a long-term complication, especially when a prosthesis has been used; this is treated with periodic aspiration or the introduction of constant drainage. Serious infections rarely occur, but, when they do, they are treated as with any other wound; occasionally, removal of the foreign body prosthesis may become necessary, forcing the surgeon to begin all over again. The prognosis of hernia repair is difficult to ascertain because each one is different and because long-term follow-up is almost impossible. With careful selection of cases and the exercise of skillful surgical technique, a 90% cure rate should be obtained.

BIBLIOGRAPHY

Banerjee SR et al: Abdominal wound evisceration, *Curr Surg* 40:432, 1983.

Boisell P et al: A new technique for closing abdominal incisions in patients with poor wound healing, *Am J Surg* 143:380, 1982.

Brown SE, Allen HH, Robins RN: The use of delayed primary wound closure in preventing wound infections, *Am J Obstet Gynecol* 127:713, 1977.

Bucknall TE, Teare L, Ellis H: The choice of a suture to close abdominal incisions, *Eur Surg Res* 15:59, 1983.

Chan STF, Esufali ST: Extended indications for polypropylene mesh closure of the abdominal wall, *Br J Surg* 73:3, 1986.

Chez RA: Mass midline closure to avoid wound disruption (Clinical dialogue), *Contemp Ob Gyn* 34:62, 1989.

Daly JW: Dehiscence, evisceration, and other complications, *Clin Obstet Gynecol* 31:754, 1988.

Duff JH, Moffat J: Abdominal sepsis managed by leaving abdomen open, *Surgery* 90:774, 1981.

Edlich RF, Rodeheaver GR, Thacker JG: Considerations in the choice of sutures for wound closure of the genitourinary tract, *J Urol* 137:373, 1987.

Farrell SA et al: Massive evisceration: a complication following sacrospinous vaginal vault fixation, *Obstet Gynecol* 73:560, 1991.

Gallup DG, Nolan TE, Smith RP: Primary mass closure of midline incisions with a continuous polyglyconate monofilament absorbable suture, *Obstet Gynecol* 76:872, 1990.

Gilsdorf RB, Shea MM: Repair of massive septic abdominal wall defects with Marlex mesh, *Am J Surg* 130:634, 1975.

Halevy A, Oland Y, Adam YG: Stainless steel wire for closure of abdominal operative wounds, *Am Surg* 44:342, 1978.

Jenkins SD et al: A comparison of prosthetic materials used to repair abdominal wall defects, *Surgery* 94:392, 1983.

Katz S, Izhar M, Mirelman D: Bacterial adherence to surgical sutures: a possible factor in suture induced infection, *Ann Surg* 194:35, 1981.

Kenady DE: Management of abdominal wounds, *Surg Clin North Am* 64:803, 1984.

Kon ND et al: Abdominal wound closure: a comparison of polydioxanone, polypropylene, and Teflon®-coated braided Dacron® sutures, *Am Surg* 50:549, 1984.

Lewis RT: Knitted polypropylele (Marlex) mesh in the repair of incisional hernias, *Can J Surg* 27:155, 1984.

Murray DH, Blaisdell FW: Use of synthetic absorbable sutures for abdominal and chest wound closure, *Arch Surg* 113:477, 1978.

Nehme AE: Repair of large incisional hernias with Marlex mesh, *Int Surg* 67:398, 1982.

Nichols DH: *Reoperative gynecologic surgery,* St Louis, 1991, Mosby–Year Book.

Nichols RL: Postoperative wound infection, *N Engl J Med* 307:1701, 1982.

Orr JW et al: Continuous or interrupted fascial closure: a prospective evaluation of No. 1 Maxon suture in 402 gynecologic procedures, *Am J Obstet* 163:1485, 1990.

Rubin LD, Maplesden DC: Suturing with stainless steel wire, *Vet Med* 72:1431, 1977.

Rubio PA: New technique for repairing large ventral incisional hernias with Marlex mesh, *Surg Gynecol Obstet* 162:275, 1986.

Sabiston D: *Textbook of surgery,* ed 13, Philadelphia, 1986, WB Saunders.

Sanz LE: Wound management—matching materials and methods for best results, *Contemp Ob Gyn* 30:86, 1987.

Schoetz DJ, Coller JA, Veidenheimer: Closure of abdominal wounds with polydioxanone: a prospective study, *Arch Surg* 123:72, 1988.

Schwartz SI, Shires TG, Spencer FC: *Principles of surgery,* ed 5, New York, 1989, McGraw-Hill.

Shapiro M et al: Risk factors for infection at the operative site after abdominal or vaginal hysterectomy, *N Engl J Med* 307:1661, 1982.

Shepherd JH et al: Abdominal wound closure using a nonabsorbable single-layer technique, *Obstet Gynecol* 61:248, 1983.

Shields LE, Diaz K, Mitchell GW: Vaginal evisceration of the small bowel (submitted).

Sloop RD: Running synthetic absorbable suture in abdominal wound closure, *Am J Surg* 141:572, 1981.

Smith SRG, Gilmore OJA: Surgical drainage, *Br J Hosp Med* 33:308, 1985.

Sowa DE et al: Effects of thermal knives on wound healing, *Obstet Gynecol* 66:436, 1985.

Stillman RM, Marino CA, Seligman SJ: Skin staples in potentially contaminated wounds, *Arch Surg* 119:821, 1984.

Stone HH et al: Management of acute full-thickness losses of the abdominal wall, *Ann Surg* 193:612, 1981.

Tyrell J et al: Absorbable versus permanent mesh in abdominal operations, *Surg Gynecol Obstet* 168:227, 1989.

Wallace D et al: Prevention of abdominal wound disruption utilizing the Smead-Jones closure technique, *Obstet Gynecol* 56:226, 1980.

Walters MD et al: Reclosure of disrupted abdominal incisions, *Obstet Gynecol* 76:597, 1990.

Wheeless CR: *Atlas of pelvic surgery,* Philadelphia, 1981, Lea & Febiger.

Chapter 14

HEMORRHAGE AND SHOCK

Beth E. Nelson
Peter E. Schwartz

Massive hemorrhage and its attendant complications occur predominately in the intraoperative or postpartum state in gynecology and obstetrics. Hemorrhage accounts for 13% of maternal deaths in the United States.[25] The best preventive measures are anticipation of situations in which hemorrhage may occur and use of meticulous surgical technique. Careful medical histories to identify patients with coagulopathies, review of prior operative reports to identify difficult sites of dissection, and assessment of prior obstetric complications allow preparation for potential bleeding complications. Immediate action at the initial occurrence of significant bleeding may prevent the escalation of its severity. The steps to be taken in control of hemorrhage depend on the individual situation. This chapter reviews the management of bleeding complications in obstetrics and gynecology and describes techniques employed by the authors in controlling massive hemorrhage in a busy obstetrics and gynecology service.

PREOPERATIVE EVALUATION
Coagulopathies

A history of easy bruising or coagulation difficulties, particularly at a prior operation, or a known coagulopathy in a preoperative surgical patient requires a hematologic evaluation before surgery because simple measures may prevent the complication of significant intraoperative bleeding.[42] Coagulation factor deficiencies or platelet dysfunction may be a contributing factor in the etiology of hemorrhage, and replacement therapy may obviate severe complications. Knowledge of the coagulation system with its intrinsic and extrinsic pathways is important in appropriate preventive therapy.[3,34] The coagulation system is presented in Fig. 14-1. The intrinsic system requires no extravascular component for initiation, whereas the extrinsic pathway is activated by tissue factor (thromboplastin) found only when vascular integrity has been violated. The two pathways have been shown to have multiple sites of interaction.

In patients with platelet abnormalities, a platelet count and bleeding time should be obtained to assess quantitative and qualitative defects. The bleeding time is elevated in thrombocytopenia; after aspirin or nonsteroidal antiinflammatory drug ingestion; after use of some penicillins and cephalosporins; and in cyclooxygenase deficiency, factor V or VIII deficiency, uremia, liver failure, congenital afibrinogenemia, and Bernard-Soulier syndrome.[12,21,37] Patients with these conditions may be asymptomatic until intraoperative or postoperative bleeding occurs.

The prothrombin time (PT) and partial thromboplastin time (PTT) are usually deranged in patients with a coagulation factor deficiency, and specific factor levels may be measured in the work-up of such patients.[41] Factor VIII deficiency is the most common hereditary hemorrhagic disorder.[3] Absence of factor VIII, an x-linked genetic disorder which is therefore rarely seen in women, causes hemophilia A. Deficient von Willebrand's factor, closely related to factor VIII levels, results in decreased factor VIII and platelet dysfunction. Patients with von Willebrand's disease usually experience immediate hemorrhage after injury. In contrast, hemophiliacs have delayed bleeding and develop spontaneous, deep-tissue hemorrhage. In both diseases, the PT is normal and the PTT is increased. Specific factor levels and the clinical picture allow differentiation.[41] Factor IX deficiency, an x-linked trait known as hemophilia B, is less common than hemophilia A.[3] Carriers may exhibit deficiency states. Factor XI deficiency occurs most commonly in patients of Ashkenazi Jewish backgrounds, and levels are further decreased in pregnancy.[40] Inheritance is autosomal recessive, and the bleeding defect is usually mild. The PTT is elevated in patients with deficiency of factors IX and XI, and patients with hemophilia B may have an increased PT as well.[3,41] Factors II (pro-

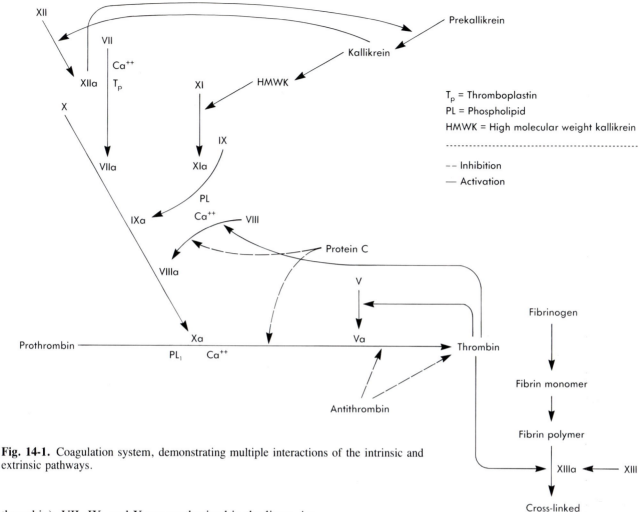

Fig. 14-1. Coagulation system, demonstrating multiple interactions of the intrinsic and extrinsic pathways.

thrombin), VII, IX, and X are synthesized in the liver. An elevated PT occurs in factor VII deficiency, vitamin K deficiency, and mild liver dysfunction. In the setting of severe vitamin K deficiency or liver disease, the PTT may also become abnormal. Inherited deficiencies of factors II, V, and X, while unusual, result in elevated PT and PTT as well.[42] Acquired coagulation factor inhibitors may also contribute to hemorrhage.[35]

Disseminated intravascular coagulation (DIC) may develop as a result of intraoperative or postoperative hemorrhage or as a complication of abruptio placentae. Preeclampsia, sepsis, and amniotic fluid embolism may also precede DIC. DIC is initially characterized by thrombosis in the microvasculature, followed by fibrinolysis and consumptive coagulopathy with resultant bleeding.[5] Oozing may occur at the operative site and from venous or arterial punctures. A laboratory profile typically reveals a falling platelet count and fibrinogen and elevated fibrin split products. Because fibrinogen is elevated in pregnancy, hypofibrinogenemia may not always be evident. Correction of the underlying problem, such as evacuation of retained fetal or placental tissue or treatment of gram-negative sepsis, reverses the process. Replacement of coagulation factors with fresh frozen plasma, repletion of fibrinogen with cryoprecipitate, and platelet transfusions are necessary to

support the patient.[15] Therapy with blood products is often massive but must be tailored to the specific deficit.

SUPPORTIVE CARE OF A HEMORRHAGING PATIENT

The initial evaluation and supportive therapy of any patient experiencing massive hemorrhage must begin by attaining suitable intravenous access with multiple large-bore catheters. Laboratory data including a hemoglobin and hematocrit, platelet count, PT and PTT, fibrinogen, fibrin split products, and serum calcium should be obtained to guide appropriate replacement. Blood bank personnel should be notified of the nature of the situation in order to obtain and cross-match adequate supplies of blood products. Invasive hemodynamic monitoring including Swan-Ganz catheterization should be instituted. A Foley catheter should be placed in the urinary bladder, and urine output should be carefully monitored. Large volumes of crystalloid and blood expanders are often required in addition to packed red blood cells, fresh frozen plasma, and other blood products. Normal saline or lactated Ringer's solution should be infused at a ratio of 3 ml of crystalloid per 1 ml of blood lost.

Gynecologic hemorrhage

Intraoperative hemorrhage. In the author's experience, intraoperative hemorrhage during gynecologic surgery is most frequently encountered in the region of the ureter or infundibulopelvic ligament and the venous plexus along the pelvic sidewall deep to the uterosacral ligaments. Bleeding most often occurs in difficult pelvic surgery for such conditions as extensive endometriosis or broad ligament leiomyomata. However, hemorrhage may occur with routine cases as well. Preventive techniques include use of small tissue pedicles and double ligatures for ovarian and uterine vascular pedicles.

The key to controlling pelvic sidewall hemorrhage intraoperatively often involves exposure of the ureter to avoid ureteric injury. The ureter may be readily exposed as it crosses the common iliac artery and descends into the pelvis by sweeping the medial leaf of the broad ligament with a tonsil suction (Fig. 14-2). The ureter is freed along its course in the broad and cardinal ligaments by applying gentle traction to the areolar tissue surrounding the ureter and dissecting in the ureteric plane with a Mixter clamp. In the patient who is bleeding after complications from a hysterectomy, it may be helpful to redivide the round ligament closer to the pelvic sidewall if the ovary and fallopian tube have been left in place before attempting to expose the ureter. Once the course of the ureter is delineated, it may be retracted to provide improved exposure of the bleeding vessels for ligature placement.

Arterial ligation may be required for control of hemorrhage that occurs during pelvic surgery. Ligation of the anterior division of the hypogastric (internal iliac) artery is a classic surgical technique; uterine or ovarian arterial ligature, however, may be more appropriate at times, particularly in obstetric hemorrhage.[10,11,13] Figure 14-3 demonstrates the site of ligature in each of these instances. The anterior division of the hypogastric artery encompasses the uterine, vaginal, superior vesicle, and middle hemorrhoidal arteries. A position 2.5 to 3 cm distal to the bifurcation of the common iliac artery should be chosen to preserve the posterior division of the hypogastric artery.

The hypogastric artery may be readily exposed by incising the pelvic sidewall peritoneum. This is accomplished by dividing the round ligament (Fig. 14-4) and extending the peritoneal incision cephalad and parallel to the infundibulopelvic ligament (Fig. 14-5). The soft tissue of the pelvic sidewall is swept away with the tonsil sucker exposing the hypogastric artery. A Mixter clamp is gently placed around the hypogastric artery, starting from the lateral side and progressing medially (Fig. 14-6). Lesser angled clamps should not be used because they may perforate the underlying hypogastric vein, resulting in massive bleeding. The artery is then doubly ligated, but not divided. Because of collateral vessels, ligation of the hypogastric artery rarely stops all bleeding.[9] It usually reduces the flow of blood so that identification of the bleeding site is possible. In addition, by reducing pulse pressure, thrombosis occurs more readily. Uterine artery ligation is carried out by taking large "bites" through the uterine wall to encompass the artery at the cervical isthmus just above the

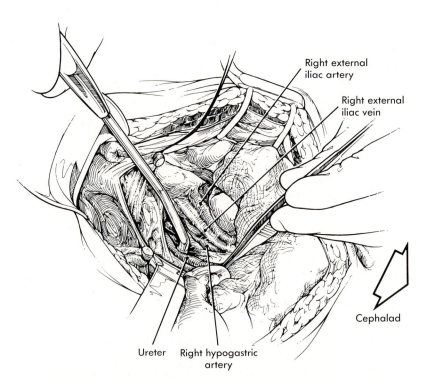

Right external iliac artery

Right external iliac vein

Cephalad

Ureter   Right hypogastric artery

Fig. 14-2. Sweeping the medial leaf of the broad ligament with a tonsil sucker to expose the ureter.

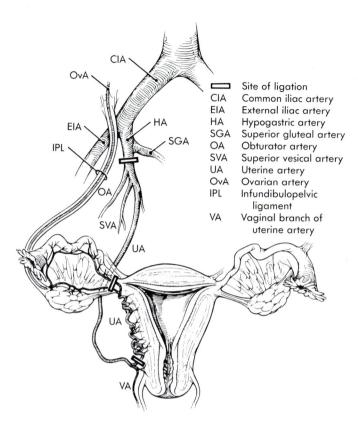

	Site of ligation
CIA	Common iliac artery
EIA	External iliac artery
HA	Hypogastric artery
SGA	Superior gluteal artery
OA	Obturator artery
SVA	Superior vesical artery
UA	Uterine artery
OvA	Ovarian artery
IPL	Infundibulopelvic ligament
VA	Vaginal branch of uterine artery

Fig. 14-3. Site of ligation of the hypogastric, uterine, and ovarian arteries.

bladder flap and near the anastomosis between the uterine and ovarian blood supplies at the ovarian ligament.[14] Selective ligation of the uterine artery at its origin from the hypogastric artery is usually not practical owing to the hypervascularity in this area associated with pregnancy.

Massive gynecologic hemorrhage may also be encountered with arteriovenous malformations, in gestational trophoblastic disease, and in extensive malignancies, particularly when the lateral pelvic wall is invaded.[4,16,39] Occasionally, intraligamentous leiomyomata, ovarian remnants, or endometriomas may extend to the pelvic sidewall and venous injury may occur lateral to the hypogastric artery. In such an event it may be necessary to resect a segment of the anterior division of the artery to expose the bleeding site. If uncontrollable bleeding occurs, particularly with hemorrhage secondary to a malignancy infiltrating the pelvic sidewall, it is possible to pack the sidewall with large operating room sponges to control the bleeding. The tails of the sponges are brought out the abdominal wall through a separate incision. The sponges may be removed when the patient is stable.

A new approach to the management of persistent bleeding in gynecologic patients—fibrin glue—was reported to be successful in two patients with gynecologic malignancies and in a postpartum patient.[27] Fibrin glue is composed of equal parts of cryoprecipitate and bovine thrombin (1000 U/ml) simultaneously sprayed from plastic syringes onto the bleeding site. It is extremely important to have the surgical field as dry as possible. Fibrin glue may be applied in a wet field in conjunction with an absorbable surgical gelatin sponge (Gelfoam) or Avitene. The biochemi-

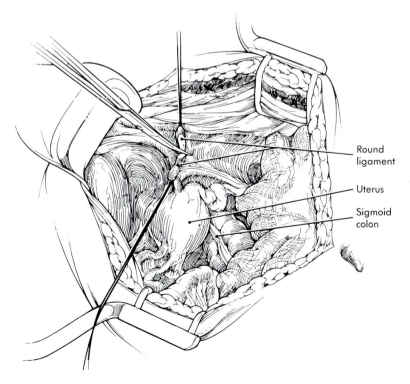

Round ligament

Uterus

Sigmoid colon

Fig. 14-4. In preparation for exposing the pelvic sidewall vascular structures, the round ligament has been doubly suture ligated and then divided.

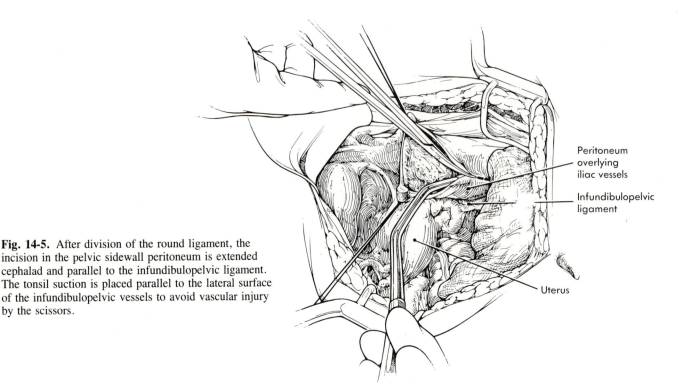

Peritoneum
overlying
iliac vessels

Infundibulopelvic
ligament

Fig. 14-5. After division of the round ligament, the incision in the pelvic sidewall peritoneum is extended cephalad and parallel to the infundibulopelvic ligament. The tonsil suction is placed parallel to the lateral surface of the infundibulopelvic vessels to avoid vascular injury by the scissors.

Uterus

cal principle of the fibrin glue approach is that thrombin converts the fibrinogen in cryoprecipate into fibrin monomer. Factor XIII then converts the fibrin monomer into a fibrin polymer that acts as a hemostatic mesh. The process takes approximately 2 minutes to be completed. Use of cryoparticipate prepared from pooled human blood sources carries with it the risk of infectious complications including hepatitis B and acquired immunodeficiency syndrome (AIDS). Infectious complications may be obviated through the use of autologous blood if one anticipates preoperatively a strong likelihood for hemorrhagic complications. Unfortunately, one cannot routinely anticipate this complication. Fibrin glue is not a substitute for meticulous surgical techniques.

Postoperative hemorrhage. Postoperative patients who have undergone gynecologic surgery develop hemorrhage most commonly from bleeding sites at the vaginal cuff or from retroperitoneal hematomas. The latter may be an occult site of massive blood loss. After hysterectomy, significant bleeding occurs in 0.3% to 2.9% of cases.[19,44] Careful inspection of the vaginal cuff with appropriate suturing under anesthesia often controls bleeding. If bleeding persists, angiographic embolization is often successful and avoids a return to the operating room.[36] Surgical exploration with evacuation and arterial ligation may be required if interventional angiographic techniques are unsuccessful.

Intraoperative obstetric hemorrhage

Intraoperative obstetric hemorrhage is most often related to cervical or vaginal lacerations, abnormal placentation, or uterine atony. Cesarean section performed for placenta previa may precede the development of massive in-

traoperative hemorrhage at the time of placental removal. In the setting of multiple previous cesarean sections, placenta accreta, increta, or percreta, likewise, may lead to hemorrhage. McShane and co-workers reported 147 patients with placenta previa of whom 11 had placenta accreta.[28] Five required hysterectomy for control of hemorrhage. In this study, 27% of women with placenta previa who had previously undergone cesarean section had placenta accreta.

When hemorrhage is anticipated, following placental removal manipulations to correct uterine atony should be immediately instituted. Uterine massage, intravenous infusion of Pitocin, intravenous or intramuscular methylergonovine, and intramuscular or intramyometrial prostaglandin F_2 alpha analogues ($PgF_2\alpha$) may be used. Inspection for lacerations into the uterine vasculature or extension into the lower uterine segment should be performed. When these measures fail, bilateral hypogastric artery ligation should be considered as the next step.

In the author's experience, many obstetricians are uncomfortable performing hypogastric artery ligations at the time of cesarean section to control massive hemorrhage. They often prefer to perform a supracervical or total abdominal hysterectomy to achieve this goal. However, a hysterectomy does not always achieve hemostasis. When the authors have been asked to assist in controlling massive bleeding after the latter surgeries, bilateral hypogastric artery ligations are promptly performed to reduce the amount of blood flow to identify sites of active bleeding, which then may be controlled by mechanical techniques. Normally, clot must first be removed from a blood-filled pelvis using large sponges. After bilateral hypogastric ar-

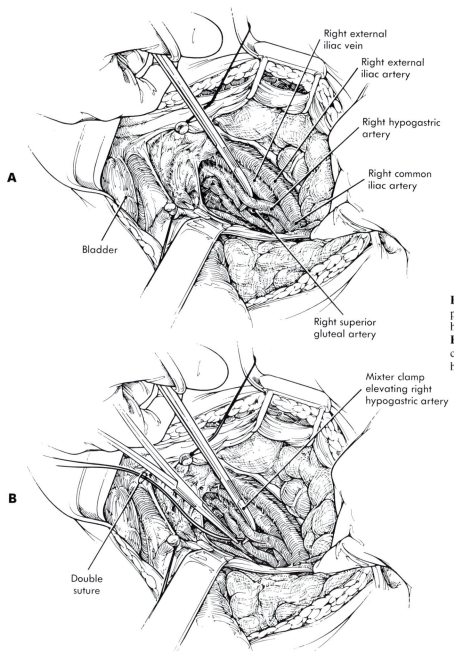

Right external
iliac vein

Right external
iliac artery

Right hypogastric
artery

Right common
iliac artery

A

Bladder

Right superior
gluteal artery

Mixter clamp
elevating right
hypogastric artery

B

Double
suture

Fig. 14-6. A, A Mixter clamp has been gently placed from the superior-lateral surface of the hypogastric artery to the inferior-medial aspect. **B,** A double suture is placed in the jaws of the clamp, and the clamp is withdrawn to ligate the hypogastric artery.

tery ligation, meticulous inspection must be employed to identify bleeding sites that may be controlled with sutures or surgical clips. The technique of ligation is discussed in the preceding section.

An alternative to hypogastric artery ligation for the management of uterine bleeding at the time of cesarean section is to perform a bilateral uterine artery ligation. This is done to save the uterus. If bleeding persists after uterine artery ligation, the ovarian arterial supply may be ligated at the utero-ovarian ligament (Fig. 14-3). By selecting the utero-ovarian ligament rather than the infundibulopelvic ligament, ovarian function is not disturbed. Indeed, a successful pregnancy has been reported in a woman in whom postpartum hemorrhage at the time of a previous cesarean section was controlled by bilateral uterine and ovarian artery ligations.[29]

Diffuse oozing from cut tissue edges is usually due to a coagulopathy accompanying the massive hemorrhage and associated massive transfusions. Because of the massive blood loss commonly incurred at the time of an obstetric hemorrhage, the development of DIC is always a possibility and should be treated immediately. Once mechanically controllable bleeding has been attended to, the abdomen should be closed and the coagulopathy managed with blood replacement products.

Some physicians have advocated uterine packing to control bleeding at the time of cesarean section. However, this is a measure of last resort and has generally been abandoned. Packing may obscure continued hemorrhage and delay definitive therapy. Transcatheter arterial embolization techniques may be required if none of these measures is successful. These techniques are discussed in a later section.

Postpartum hemorrhage

Postpartum hemorrhage is most often related to uterine atony.[1] Conditions that predispose to atony include hydramnios, multiple gestation, macrosomia, high parity, intrauterine infection, precipitous or prolonged labor, use of halogenated anesthetics, preeclampsia, and uterine relaxants such as magnesium sulfate or tocolytics. Hemorrhage immediately after vaginal delivery should prompt an assessment of uterine tone. Bimanual massage of the uterus simultaneously with administration of oxytocics or prostaglandin analogues often control uterine atony and should be promptly initiated. Postpartum hemorrhage was controlled in 22 of 26 patients receiving intramuscular 15-methyl-prostaglandin F_2.[8] Side effects include fever, nausea, vomiting, diarrhea, and hypertension. Prostaglandin E_2 (PgE_2) intravaginal suppositories have also been used in the treatment of postpartum hemorrhage.[23] Continuous intrauterine irrigation with PgE_2 has recently been reported in 22 women, with success in all.[33]

Uterine atony may be a result of retained placental fragments or products of conception. Manual exploration of the uterus should be routinely performed in instances of postpartum hemorrhage. Inspection of the placenta should be done at each delivery to ensure placental fragments or succenturiate lobes are not retained in the uterus. Placental implantation in the noncontractile lower uterine segment may result in hemorrhage nonresponsive to oxytocics. Tamponade of this area using a large Foley catheter balloon has been successful.[7] Even if ultimately unsuccessful, this maneuver may allow preparation of the patient for transarterial catheter embolization or surgery.

Pelvic ultrasound may be useful to evaluate uterine contents and to identify the presence of intraperitoneal free fluid, suggesting uterine rupture.[26] The ultrasound examination may also delineate an intrauterine clot or retained placental fragments. Gentle sharp curettage of the uterus is the next step if placenta remnants are present, taking great care not to perforate the uterine wall.

If atony is not present, a careful inspection of the cervix and vagina to identify mucosal lacerations should be carried out. Rapid delivery, macrosomia, and forceps delivery are factors associated with occurrence of lacerations. Cervical and vaginal lacerations should be repaired with a running absorbable suture. Uterine rupture should be considered, particularly in women who have undergone vaginal delivery after cesarean section or after uterine surgery such as myomectomy. Uterine inversion may also result in postpartum hemorrhage. After abortion, similar etiologies of hemorrhage must be considered including uterine atony, vaginal or cervical lacerations, and uterine perforation. Arterial embolization in the angiography suite may avert sur-

gical exploration. Arterial ligation or hysterectomy may be required if less invasive techniques are unsuccessful. Alternative therapies such as local infusions of vasopressors through fluoroscopically placed arterial catheters have been described.[30,39]

MANAGEMENT OF MASSIVE HEMORRHAGE
Treatment options

Interventional radiology. Interventional radiologic techniques were first used in the management of massive hemorrhage in desperately ill gynecologic cancer patients.[38,39] These patients often were bone marrow–suppressed or had previously been irradiated in the region of the bleeding and were not amenable to immediate operation to control the hemorrhage because of cardiovascular instability. Interventional radiologic techniques were not initially recognized to be of value in benign gynecology or obstetrics because massive hemorrhage was an uncommon complication. However, during the past decade angiographic techniques have been introduced into the successful management of massive postpartum hemorrhage and benign gynecologic processes that have led to such hemorrhage.[17,20,24] The application of these techniques may allow women to avoid hysterectomy and preserve reproductive function.

Selective arteriography. Selective arteriography was initially used to identify bleeding sites so that surgical strategies could be employed to control the hemorrhage. Subsequently, it was recognized that the same arterial catheters placed into the vessels that led to the bleeding site could be used as vehicles for delivery of vasoactive agents to control the bleeding. Vasopressin became the most commonly used vasoactive agent and was infused through selective arterial catheter techniques to control bleeding secondary to esophageal varices, gastric ulcers, and intestinal anastamosis sites.[43] The complications from vasopressin infusion included systemic effects from the pharmacologic agent and ischemic damage to bowel. Thrombosis or infection at the catheter site occurred because these catheters often had to be left in place several days with the infusion running to control the bleeding. The combination of regional intraarterial infusion of a vasoconstrictor (dopamine, norepinephrine) with transcatheter embolization and use of a military anti-shock trousers (MAST) suit has been applied recently with success in control of pelvic hemorrhage.

Catheterization. Balloon catheters were subsequently developed that could be inserted into larger blood vessels under fluoroscopic guidance. Inflation of the balloon obstructed the vessel proximal to the bleeding site and controlled the hemorrhage.[39,45] This technique has had little use in gynecologic oncology. Stainless steel coils (e.g., Gianturco coils) have also been developed and can be placed through selective arterial catheterization techniques into bleeding vessels. The stainless steel coils are most valuable when the vessel is short (e.g., the renal vessels), which would make arterial embolization techniques dangerous to carry out because embolized material might reflux into the aorta leading to distant embolization and ischemic complications. Finally, liquid tissue adhesives have been developed that can be passed through arterial catheters and that congeal on entry into the bloodstream. Liquid tissue adhesives have found limited application in the management of hemorrhage secondary to obstetric and gynecologic processes.

Transcatheter embolization. The most frequently used technique for the management of massive hemorrhage in obstetrics and gynecology has been transcatheter embolization of synthetic material. This technique initially began with embolization of autologous tissue or autologous blood clot for management of massive hemorrhage.[18,39] Because patients with massive hemorrhage frequently have an associated coagulopathy, it was necessary to add pharmacologic agents to make the blood clot rapidly.[6] The development of an absorbable surgical gelatin sponge (Gelfoam) shows that synthetic material may be safely employed in the transcatheter management of massive hemorrhage. At Yale-New Haven Hospital, Gelfoam particles formed by dicing Gelfoam pads into small pieces are routinely used rather than Gelfoam powder because the latter may obstruct the vasa nervorum, causing nerve injury.[20]

SELECTIVE ARTERIOGRAPHY AND EMBOLIZATION TECHNIQUES

For selective arteriography to identify a bleeding site it is necessary that the patient be bleeding at a rate of greater than 0.5 ml/min.[31] If the patient is not actively bleeding at the time of arteriography, the bleeding site will not be recognized. The performance of arteriography is based on the Seldinger technique. A hollow needle with a stent is placed in a major artery. The stent is then removed and a flexible stainless steel guidewire is advanced through the needle into the artery. For obstetric and gynecologic patients, the femoral artery is commonly accessed. The guidewire is advanced into the abdominal aorta under fluoroscopic control. The needle is removed over the guidewire, and a flexible polyethylene catheter is inserted over the guidewire and advanced into the aorta. Usually the tip of the catheter is preformed so that it may be guided into divisions of the abdominal aorta. Once the guidewire is removed, a lower abdominal arteriogram is performed to identify the bleeding sites in the pelvis.

After the aortogram has identified the most likely bleeding sites, the arterial catheter is selectively inserted under fluoroscopy into one of the major arteries supplying the bleeding site. The most common sources for bleeding in the pelvis in the author's experience have been the hypogastric arteries, the fourth lumbar artery, and the median circumflex femoral artery. Less commonly, the bleeding may originate from the ovarian artery or the inferior epigastric artery. It is always necessary to consider dual blood supply to bleeding sites.[9] Certainly, the intact uterus has multiple sources of blood supply including two uterine and ovarian arteries. In dealing with complications in gynecologic cancer management, the dual blood supply of the stomach and the duodenum must also be considered.

Limitations of selective arteriography to determine the arterial source for bleeding include the fact that massive hemorrhage leads to severe volume depletion and resultant arterial spasm, producing a false-negative result on arteriographic examination. It may be necessary to give glucagon intraarterially to dilate the vessels to establish the bleeding source.

Individual physician experience in performing selective arteriography and transcatheter embolization of synthetic material is critical for the technique to be successful. The circumstances of massive hemorrhage require that the most experienced personnel be actively involved in the selective arteriography and embolization techniques. Unilateral embolization of pelvic sidewall vessels including the hypogastric artery is insufficient treatment for the successful control of massive hemorrhage in the pelvis. One must evaluate arteriographically the blood supply to both pelvic sidewalls and routinely embolize both hypogastric arteries when intact to stop the bleeding. The procedure must not be abandoned after a cursory arteriographic examination has been performed. The source of the massive bleeding is frequently small vessels that require selective arteriographic approaches.[32] The fourth lumbar and the medium circumflex arteries and at times accessory obturator vessels arising from the inferior epigastric artery may be injured and may not be associated with obvious bleeding on a screening aortogram.

Patient support during the procedure must be extensive. At Yale-New Haven Hospital, a shock team that includes anesthesiologists, interventional radiologists, and gynecologic oncologists actively participate in the management of massive hemorrhage in the obstetric or gynecologic patient. A team effort is required to successfully take the very sick patient in hemorrhagic shock through interventional radiologic techniques.

Case studies

Some examples in which we have been successful in using this technique in massive bleeding in gynecologic surgical situations include a patient who underwent a cone biopsy for evaluation of a carcinoma in situ of the cervix. She hemorrhaged at the time of the biopsy; the hemorrhage was apparently controlled with suture ligatures, but the patient developed recurrent postoperative bleeding twice during the ensuing month requiring suture ligation in the operating room. A hysterectomy appeared to be the next appropriate step to control the massive bleeding because it was not permanently controllable by suture ligation on the two prior occasions. Figure 14-7, *A* shows a selective hypogastric arteriogram revealing that the source of this patient's bleeding was the left uterine artery. After selective embolization of that vessel (Fig. 14-7, *B*), the bleeding was completely controlled. The patient subsequently had a normal full-term pregnancy.

This technique was also successfully employed for a bi-

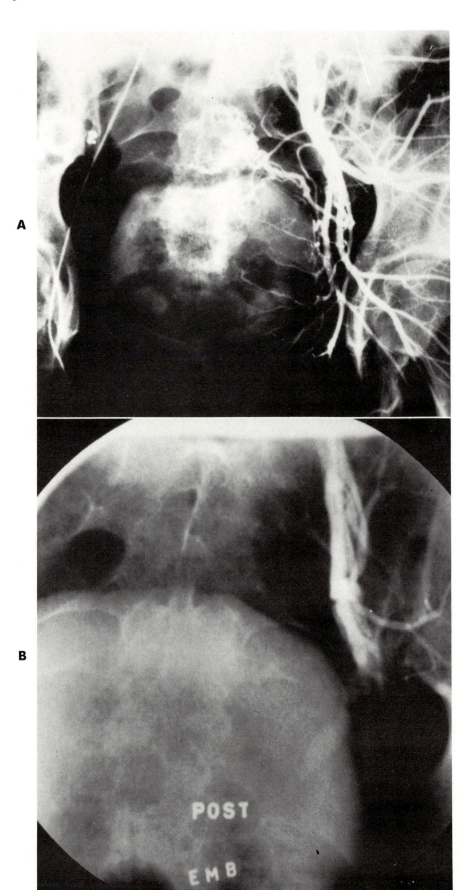

Fig. 14-7. A, Selective left hypogastric arteriogram, demonstrating that the source of uterine bleeding after a cone biopsy is the left uterine artery. **B,** Complete control of bleeding achieved after transcatheter embolization of Gelfoam.

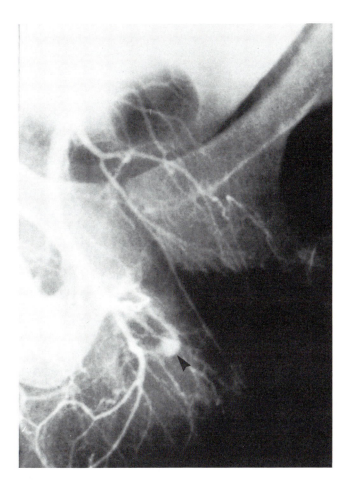

Fig. 14-8. Bleeding into labia from an injured right pudendal artery after a bicycle straddle injury. The arrow indicates the bleeding site.

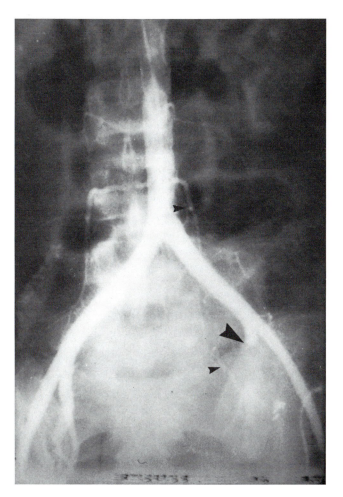

Fig. 14-9. A lower abdominal aortogram revealing the presence of a ligated left hypogastric artery *(large arrow)* in a patient massively bleeding intraabdominally after removal of an intraabdominal pregnancy, the placenta having implanted on the left pelvic sidewall. A unilateral hypogastric artery ligation was performed at the time of surgery to control bleeding. Collateral circulation between the left fourth lumbar artery *(small arrows)* and the left hypogastric vessels *(large arrow)* was controlled by selective arteriography and Gelfoam embolization of the lumbar artery.

cycle straddle injury in a 27-year-old woman. The patient presented with a 15-cm right labial hematoma. Figure 14-8 shows the source of the bleeding, a branch of the right pudendal artery. Rather than performing an evacuation in the operating room and packing this extensive hematoma, the patient underwent a Gelfoam embolization of the right internal pudendal artery with no untoward effects.

A patient with von Willebrand's disease underwent an elective pregnancy termination at 8 weeks gestation.[22] The patient received preoperative and postoperative cryoprecipitate at the time of suction dilation and curettage (D and C). However, massive hemorrhage occurred 16 days later and was unresponsive to cryoprecipitate, D and C, uterine packing, antibiotics, and oxytocin administration. This patient underwent bilateral hypogastric arterial embolization, and the bleeding was completely controlled.

These approaches have been used in the management of massive postpartum hemorrhage. Figure 14-9 shows a lower abdominal aortogram revealing the presence of a ligated left hypogastric artery. The patient had undergone a laparotomy for what proved to be an unsuspected intraabdominal pregnancy. When the pregnancy was recognized

to be intraabdominal, a hysterectomy and removal of the placenta from the left pelvic sidewall were performed. Because of massive hemorrhage, a vascular surgeon was asked to ligate the left hypogastric artery. The ligation initially controlled the bleeding, but the patient subsequently required a total of 33 units of blood to replace intraabdominal blood loss. The patient was taken to the interventional radiography suite rather than the operating room because she was hemodynamically unstable. An aortogram confirmed that the patient was bleeding from the hypogastric artery distal to the ligation site. The patient first underwent an embolization of the right hypogastric artery. Subsequent selective arteriography revealed a communication between the left fourth lumbar artery and the left hypogastric vessels (Fig. 14-9). This vessel was embolized. A subsequent selective arteriogram identified the presence of collateral circulation to the left pelvic sidewall through the left median circumflex femoral artery, which was also embolized, and all bleeding ceased.

Abnormal placentation is the most common reason for massive hemorrhage in obstetric patients. A patient underwent an elective cesarean hysterectomy for delivery of her third child after having two pregnancies complicated by placenta accreta. The patient underwent an uncomplicated

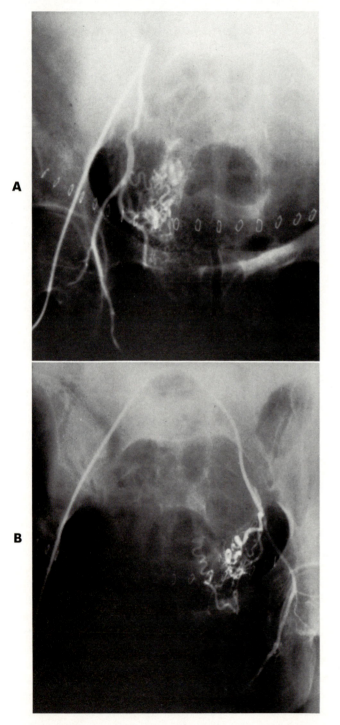

Fig. 14-10. A, Abnormal vascular pattern involving the right pelvic sidewall in a patient hemorrhaging after a cesarean hysterectomy. **B,** Abnormal vascular pattern involving the left pelvic sidewall.

cesarean hysterectomy but was found to be in shock in the recovery room. She remained hemodynamically unstable despite 10 units of blood replacement. The patient was taken to the angiography suite where a hypogastric arteriogram revealed abnormal venous structures involving the right (Fig. 14-10, *A*) and left pelvic sidewalls (Fig. 14-10, *B*). After bilateral hypogastric artery embolization, the patient stopped bleeding and required no further blood replacement. Her postoperative course was uncomplicated.

Hypogastric artery ligation to control bleeding at the time of surgery can be a very effective technique. However, once a hypogastric artery ligation has been performed and bleeding persists, the opportunity to perform selective arteriography and transcatheter embolization rapidly is limited because alternative access through the rich collateral circulation of the postpartum pelvis must be sought. For example, a 24-year-old primigravida underwent a cesarean section for failure to progress.[20] The cesarean section was complicated by a uterine artery laceration at surgery and a subsequent vaginal hemorrhage and fever 6 days postoperatively. The patient was hospitalized and responded to the transfusions of 2 units of blood and 3 days of intravenous antibiotics. She was discharged home where she went into hypovolemic shock on the twelfth postoperative day. The patient returned to the hospital and underwent a prompt exploratory laparotomy, subtotal hysterectomy, and bilateral hypogastric artery ligations because of persistent bleeding. However, she continued to bleed "briskly." She received 10 units of blood and 4 units of fresh frozen plasma, at which point the community hospital's blood bank reported to the surgeon that all blood had been exhausted. The patient was transferred to Yale-New Haven Hospital in a MAST suit. She was stable on admission, and an initial emergency arteriogram revealed no active bleeding. However, 2 hours later, the patient hemorrhaged. The preembolization arteriogram (Fig. 14-11, *A*) shows no obvious site of bleeding. A late-phase arteriogram (Fig. 14-11, *B*) revealed bleeding from the right pelvic sidewall. Selective arteriography confirmed the right median circumflex femoral artery as the source of hemorrhage (Fig. 14-11, *C*). Following embolization of this vessel, all bleeding stopped.

The first disadvantage of selective pelvic arterial embolization is that it may take from 1 to 6 hours to be accomplished successfully. Second, the embolized material might be dislodged, embolize further into other parts of the arterial tree, and cause complications.[20] However, the long length of the hypogastric artery and most of the other vessels involved in routine pelvic hemorrhage are such that the problem of secondary particle embolization is unlikely. Third, necrosis of normal tissue is always a concern.[24] This is more likely to occur as a result of embolizing vessels that supply the intestine. The rich vascular supply of the postpartum pelvis and, indeed, the blood to the pelvis in general are such that necrosis of normal tissue is not a routine complication when bleeding is from pelvic sites.

The advantages of selective pelvic embolization techniques are:

1. The bleeding site is often extremely difficult or impossible to identify at surgery. Huge clots may be present in the pelvis and in the retroperitoneum after massive hemorrhage, making it extraordinarily difficult to identify normal anatomic structures.
2. Injury to the ureters, bladder, or bowel may occur during a surgical attempt to identify the site of bleeding.
3. The rich collateral circulation associated with pregnancy may negate the effects of hypogastric ligation in that circumstance.
4. If one is successful in using selective arterial embolization techniques, a hysterectomy may be avoided and fertility may be preserved.

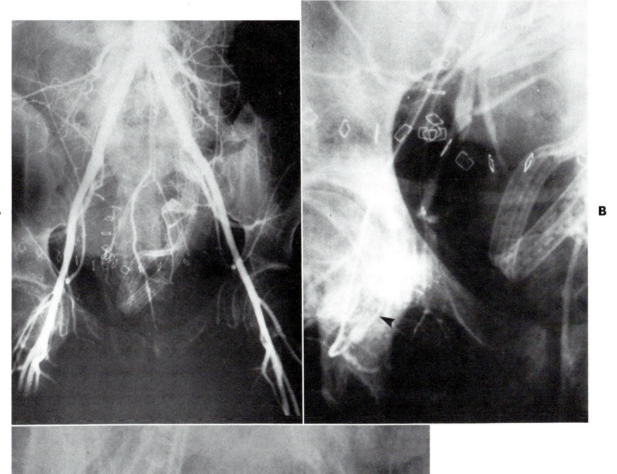

Fig. 14-11. A, Aortogram revealing no evidence of extravasation of contrast in patient who had undergone a subtotal hysterectomy and bilateral hypogastric artery ligations for massive postpartum hemorrhage. No active bleeding was clinically evident at the time of this study. **B,** A late-phase arteriogram revealing bleeding from the right pelvic sidewall *(arrow)* 2 hours after Fig. 14-11, *A,* was taken. The patient was now vigorously bleeding per vagina. **C,** The source of the bleeding *(arrow)* was the right median circumflex femoral artery, which was then embolized to control the bleeding.

5. It is much easier to identify and embolize branches of the hypogastric artery before surgical intervention than after hypogastric artery ligation has failed to control the bleeding. The tiny Gelfoam particles that are embolized through the arterial catheter travel further down the arterial tree than the site where the hypogastric artery is routinely ligated surgically. These particles often go beyond the sites where the collateral circulation enters into the arterial tree. Thus, a transcatheter hypogastric artery Gelfoam particle embolization is far more effective in most circumstances than an exploratory laparotomy and ligation of the hypogastric artery for the control of massive pelvic hemorrhage.[2]

Selective arteriography and embolization techniques can be performed in community hospital diagnostic imaging departments. Most departments have angiographers routinely performing these techniques in the management of trauma patients and evaluation of cardiac and other disorders. Gynecologists and obstetricians should alert the angiographer to be on stand-by when a patient is likely to have massive hemorrhage. Interventional radiologic techniques may avert significant complications associated with surgery in a hemodynamically unstable patient in whom one is trying to control massive hemorrhage.

CONCLUSION

Methods for control of hemorrhage in the obstetric and gynecologic patient have been reviewed. The best of these is prevention. Preparation in anticipation of hemorrhagic complications may minimize the severity of bleeding and allow preservation of reproductive ability in selected patients.

Prompt action to control hemorrhage must be instituted in each instance. The cause of bleeding, whether anatomic or hematologic, must be sought and corrected. Knowledge of the broad armamentarium available to the practitioner and of the facilities and individual consultants in one's own institution is vital when facing a hemorrhagic complication.

REFERENCES

1. American College of Obstetricians and Gynecologists: *Diagnosis and management of post partum hemorrhage,* Technical bulletin no. 143, July 1990.
2. Athanasoulis CA: Therapeutic applications of angiography, *N Engl J Med* 302:1117, 1980.
3. Beck WS, editor: *Hematology,* ed 4, Cambridge, Mass, 1985, MIT Press.
4. Beller U et al: Congential arteriovenous malformation of the female pelvis: a gynecologic perspective, *Am J Obstet Gynecol* 159:1153, 1988.
5. Bick RL: *Disseminated intravascular coagulation and related syndrome,* Boca Raton, Fla, 1983, CRC Press, Inc.
6. Bookstein JJ et al: Transcatheter hemostasis of gastrointestinal bleeding using modified autologous clot, *Radiology* 113:277, 1974.
7. Bowen LW, Beeson JH: Use of a large Foley catheter balloon to control postpartum hemorrhage resulting from a low placental implantation, *J Reprod Med* 30:623, 1985.
8. Buttino L, Garite TJ: The use of 15 methyl F_{2x} prostaglandin (prostin 15m) for the control of post partum hemorrhage, *Am J Perinatol* 3:241, 1986.
9. Chait A, Moltz A, Nelson JH: The collateral arterial circulation in the pelvis: an angiographic study, *Am J Roentgenol* 102:392, 1968.
10. Clark SL et al: Hypogastric artery ligation for obstetric hemorrhage, *Obstet Gynecol* 66:353, 1985.
11. Cruikshank SH, Stoelk EM: Surgical control of pelvic hemorrhage: bilateral hypogastric artery ligation and method of ovarian artery ligation, *South Med J* 78:539, 1985.
12. Day HJ, Rao AK: Evaluation of platelet function, *Semin Hematol* 23:89, 1986.
13. Evans S, McShane P: The efficacy of internal iliac artery ligation in obstetric hemorrhage, *Surg Gynecol Obstet* 160:250, 1985.
14. Fahmy K: Uterine artery ligation to control postpartum hemorrhage, *Int J Gynecol Obstet* 25:363, 1987.
15. Feinstein DI: Diagnosis and management of disseminated intravascular coagulation: the role of heparin therapy, *Blood* 60:284, 1982.
16. Forssman L, Lundberg J, Schersten T: Conservative treatment of uterine arteriovenous fistula, *Acta Obstet Gynecol Scand* 61:85, 1982.
17. Glickman MG: *Pelvic artery embolization.* In Berkowitz RL, editor: *Critical care of the obstetric patient.* New York, 1983, Churchill Livingstone.
18. Goldstein HM et al: Transcatheter arterial embolization in the management of bleeding in the cancer patient, *Radiology* 115:603, 1975.
19. Gray LA: Open cuff method of abdominal hysterectomy, *Obstet Gynecol* 46:42, 1975.
20. Greenwood LH et al: Obstetric and nonmalignant gynecologic bleeding: treatment with angiographic embolization, *Radiology* 164:155, 1987.
21. Harker LA, Slichter SJ: The bleeding time as a screening test for evaluation of platelet function, *N Engl J Med* 287:155, 1972.
22. Haseltine FP et al: Uterine embolization in a patient with postabortal hemorrhage, *Obstet Gynecol* 63(suppl):78S, 1984.
23. Hertz RH, Sokol RJ, Dierker LJ: Treatment of post partum uterine atony with prostaglandin E_2 vaginal suppositories, *Obstet Gynecol* 56:129, 1980.
24. Jander HP, Russinovich NAE: Transcatheter Gelfoam embolization in abdominal, retroperitoneal and pelvic hemorrhage, *Radiology* 136:337, 1980.
25. Kaunitz AM et al: Causes of maternal mortality in the United States, *Obstet Gynecol* 65:605, 1985.
26. Lee CY, Madrazo B, Brukker BH: Ultrasonic evaluation of the post partum uterus in the management of post partum bleeding, *Obstet Gynecol* 58:227, 1981.
27. Malviya VK, Deppe G: Control of intraoperative hemorrhage in gynecology with the use of fibrin glue, *Obstet Gynecol* 73:284, 1989.
28. McShane PM, Heyl PS, Epstein MF: Maternal and perinatal morbidity resulting from placenta previa, *Obstet Gynecol* 65:176, 1985.
29. Mengert WF et al: Pregnancy after bilateral ligation of the internal iliac and ovarian arteries, *Obstet Gynecol* 34:664, 1969.
30. Mud HJ et al: Nonsurgical treatment of pelvic hemorrhage in obstetric and gynecologic patients, *Crit Care Med* 15:534, 1987.
31. Nusbaum M, Baum S: Radiographic demonstration of unknown sites gastrointestinal bleeding, *Surg Forum* 14:374, 1963.
32. O'Hanlan KA et al: Arterial embolization in the management of abdominal and retroperitoneal hemorrhage, *Gynecol Oncol* 34:131, 1989.
33. Peyser MR, Kuptermine MJ: Management of severe postpartum hemorrhage by intrauterine irrigation with prostaglandin E_2, *Am J Obstet Gynecol* 162:694, 1990.
34. Prydz H: *Triggering of the extrinsic blood coagulation system.* In Thornsom JM, editor: *Blood coagulation and haemostasis,* ed 3, New York, 1985, Churchill.
35. Reece EA, Fox HE, Rappaport F: Factor VIII inhibitor: a cause of severe postpartum hemorrhage, *Am J Obstet Gynecol* 144:985, 1982.
36. Rosenthal DM, Colapinto R: Angiographic arterial embolization in

the management of postoperative vaginal hemorrhage, *Am J Obstet Gynecol* 151:227, 1985.

37. Sattler FR, Weitekamp MR, Ballard JO: Potential for bleeding with the new beta-lactam antibiotics, *Ann Intern Med* 105:924, 1986.

38. Schwartz PE: *Arterial hemorrhage in gynecologic malignancies*. In Delgado G, Smith JP, editors: *Management of complications in gynecologic oncology*. New York, 1982, John Wiley.

39. Schwartz PE et al: Control of arterial hemorrhage using percutaneous arterial catheter techniques in patients with gynecologic malignancies, *Gynecol Oncol* 3:276, 1975.

40. Steinberg MH et al: Management of factor XI deficiency in gynecologic and obstetrics patients, *Obstet Gynecol* 68:130, 1986.

41. Suchman AL, Griner PF: Diagnostic uses of the activated partial thromboplatin time and prothrombin time, *Ann Intern Med* 104:810, 1986.

42. Wallerstein RO: Laboratory evaluation of a bleeding patient, *West J Med* 150:51, 1989.

43. Waltman AC et al: Pyhloroduodenal bleeding and intra-arterial vasopressin: clinical results, *Am J Roentgenol* 133:643, 1979.

44. White SC, Wartel LJ, Wade ME: Comparison of abdominal and vaginal hysterectomies: a review of 600 operations, *Obstet Gynecol* 37:530, 1971.

45. Wholey MH, Stockdale R, Hung TK: A percutaneous balloon catheter for the immediate control of hemorrhage, *Radiology* 95:65, 1970.

Chapter 15

POSTOPERATIVE INFECTIONS AND THROMBOPHLEBITIS

Sebastian Faro

POSTOPERATIVE INFECTIONS
Epidemiology

Postoperative infections continue to be an important cause of patient morbidity and mortality and add considerably to overall hospital costs. Infection rates vary among populations, depending on variables such as nutritional status and circumstances surrounding the operative procedure. Overall, the incidence of postpartum endometritis following vaginal delivery ranges from 1% to 3%; the rate following nonelective cesarean section has been reported to range from a low of 5% to a high of 85%.[1,32] The latter occurs among high-risk patients; that is, individuals who received no prenatal care, who have anemia, whose dentition is poor, and whose nutritional status is inadequate, placing them in a state of negative nitrogen balance. Wound infection rates for patients undergoing obstetric or gynecologic operative procedures range from 3% to 9%.[15,31,51,52] Following vaginal or abdominal hysterectomy the most frequent infection is pelvic cellulitis, which occurs in approximately 10% to 30% of patients.[24,48]

An uncommon but not infrequent complication in the surgical patient is deep vein thrombosis, which is of concern because it may lead to septic or aseptic pelvic vein thrombosis and/or pulmonary embolism with or without infarction.[43,53] The occurrence of pelvic vein thrombosis results in a prolonged hospital stay, which increases cost and also increases the potential for further adverse reactions associated with the combined use of antibiotics and anticoagulant therapy. Embolization, particularly in the pulmonary system, is associated not only with significant morbidity but also with mortality. The complication of pelvic vein thrombosis is usually a diagnosis made late in the postoperative course, usually around day 4 to 6, depending on the sequencing of antibiotic use.

Infection in the postoperative patient can be divided into two major categories: (1) that involving the operative site and adjacent tissues and (2) that occurring distant from the operative site. Infections involving the operative site include the abdominal incision, the vaginal incision, and tissues adjacent to the operative site, for example, the parametrium, the pelvic peritoneum, and the upper one third of the vaginal canal and urinary tract. In discussing infection complications associated with pelvic surgery, the urinary tract must also be included, since almost all patients are catheterized via a straight or an indwelling catheter. The bladder is usually manipulated during the operative procedure and is easily traumatized. Since asymptomatic bacteria may be present, especially in geriatric patients, bacteremia may result from manipulation of the bladder.[29,42,60] Bacteriuria may be the leading contributor to the nosocomial infection rate, especially among elderly patients.

Patients undergoing pelvic surgery have an indwelling catheter for approximately 2 to 4 days, and about 10% to 30% of these patients develop bacteriuria.[35] The complications attending nosocomial bacteriuria are acute cystitis, fever, pyelonephritis, bacteremia, and death.[58] Also, individuals whose bladder is traumatized during the operative procedure experience difficulty voiding because of the edema and inflammation that occur, resulting in transient bladder atony. Commonly, the catheter is placed and removed in 24 hours. However, the patient may have difficulty voiding and develop a distended bladder, retaining several hundred milliliters of urine. This results in pain and may cause reflux of the urine, which contains bacteria, leading to the development of pyelonephritis.

Incisional or wound infection occurs in approximately 3% to 9% of patients, with an average rate of about

$5\%.^{15,31,51,52}$ Patients who have an abdominal hysterectomy have two incisions: one in the abdominal wall and the other at the vaginal apex; patients who undergo a vaginal hysterectomy have a single incision. Vaginal incision infections and the accompanying pelvic cellulitis are usually a polymicrobial infection involving aerobic and anaerobic bacteria derived from the lower genital tract. The abdominal incision infection may be due to bacteria from the lower genital tract or from the skin flora or both.

Other infections associated with the operative site are postpartum endomyometritis, pelvic cellulitis, salpingitis, pelvic abscess, and tuboovarian abscess. The incidence of these infections can be approximated by reviewing data from antibiotic prophylaxis studies and examining the failures. In earlier studies, antibiotics were compared to placebos, and infection rates could be estimated. Postpartum endometritis rates in a low-risk population average between 5% and 10%.[11,30] In high-risk settings, rates up to 85% have been reported.[32] The incidence of pelvic cellulitis following hysterectomy ranges up to 30%.[48] However, these rates have been significantly lowered with the use of antibiotic prophylaxis.

Pathophysiology

The underlying mechanism responsible for postoperative soft tissue pelvic and operative site infection is contamination, mainly by bacteria from the lower genital tract. The operative procedures that place the patient at greatest risk for postoperative infection are nonelective and emergency cesarean section and vaginal hysterectomy. Abdominal hysterectomy also places the patient at risk for infection but to a lesser degree than the vaginal hysterectomy. Other surgical procedures associated with a risk for postoperative infection are cervical cerclage at gestation greater than 18 weeks and elective abortion.

The procedures that may be associated with a significant risk of postoperative infection are as follows:

Dilation and curettage of the uterus
Endometrial biopsy
Hysterosalpingography
Chromopertubation at the time of laparoscopy
Hysteroscopy
Fourth-degree extension of an episiotomy
Abdominal cerclage
Tubal reconstructive surgery
Ovarian cystectomy
Forceps delivery

Although there are few data to support antibiotic prophylaxis for these procedures, it is common practice to find patients receiving prophylaxis. However, the indiscriminate use of antibiotics is not without adverse effects in the form of toxic reactions or notable alteration in the host flora.

Cesarean section. The procedure placing the patient at greatest risk for developing postpartum endomyometritis is cesarean section. Although no studies have been published

that explain the pathophysiology leading to the establishment of infection, there has been much speculation. The patient who has an uncomplicated labor and delivers within a reasonable time without the use of instruments (or, if forceps are used, without excessive manual manipulation) usually does not develop endomyometritis. The individual who delivers vaginally is at risk for postpartum endomyometritis if the labor is prolonged, membranes are ruptured for more than 6 hours, intrauterine monitoring is placed, numerous vaginal examinations are carried out, and, finally, if difficult instrumentation is required to effect vaginal delivery. In either case, if the individual is delivered by cesarean section, a postpartum infection is more likely to develop. The uterus of individuals who have had a prolonged labor often exhibits a dysfunctional pattern in which the uterus no longer contracts efficiently because of an unequal distribution of forces, causing the muscle to begin undergoing anaerobic metabolism. During inefficient labor, the presenting part forms a tight seal with the birth canal. When the uterus relaxes, the presenting part is drawn back up into the uterus, creating a suction that draws the vaginal fluid containing bacteria into the uterine cavity, which allows bacterial colonization to take place.

The basic mechanism preceding infection is the same for those who deliver vaginally or by cesarean section. Essentially, it is during the laboring process that bacteria have an opportunity to advance up into the uterine cavity and enter the myometrium. If membranes are ruptured, the bacteria are more likely to ascend between the uterus and amniotic membranes colonizing the decidual layer. Exposure of even a portion of the decidua may allow bacteria to enter the lymphatic and vascular network of the uterus, resulting in dissemination of bacteria, for example, *Streptococcus agalactiae,* throughout the myometrium and the potential for bacteremia. Apparently, one of two factors must be present for infection to occur, based on a comparison of uterine and abdominal wound infection: either a large inoculum must be present (more than 1,000,000 bacteria per mg of tissue) or a foreign body, such as suture. It has been shown that if suture is present in the wound, the requirement for a large inoculum is reduced by 10,000 bacteria per mg of tissue.[14] It can be theorized that during a successful labor, descent of the presenting part is progressive. The presenting part is closely applied to the walls of the birth canal, forming a tight seal and compressing the myometrium, thereby limiting the opportunity for bacteria to ascend into the uterine cavity and colonize the decidual layer. In addition, the uterus tends to be maintained in an aerobic state of metabolism. On the other hand, in the individual who undergoes a cesarean section because of cephalopelvic disproportion, the presenting part may not be tightly oppressed to the walls of the birth canal. This allows the vaginal fluid containing the endogenous microflora to ascend into the uterine cavity. During the delivery, the uterine and the abdominal incisions become traumatized and heavily contaminated as the surgeon's hand reaches down into the vagina to elevate and deliver the fetus. It is during this process that the abdominal incision may become contaminated, as the hand scoops up vaginal fluid and brings it directly into the operative field. The surgeon's hand and delivery of the fetus can easily traumatize the subcutaneous tissue and myometrium, abrading and dislodging microclots from arterioles as well as venules. The final contributing factor is the placement of suture, which frequently is pulled tightly to approximate the opposing cut surfaces of the myometrium. This process strangulates the fragile muscle fibers causing devascularization and necrosis. The presence of necrotic tissue and the seepage of blood and serum in this devascularized tissue contribute to the infectious process. Because bleeding often occurs at this suture line, the inexperienced surgeon may place stitch after stitch at the site of bleeding. A hematoma may then form over the suture line, which in turn is covered by bladder peritoneum, resulting in a retroperitoneal hematoma. This area is very likely to be colonized by bacteria, setting the stage for infection.

The layers of the abdominal wall may also become contaminated by bacteria of the lower female genital tract. Placement of suture in the subcutaneous tissue serves not only as a foreign body but also traumatizes the tissue and disrupts the vascularity. The needle and suture can cause breaks in fragile vessels, allowing blood and serum to leak into the incision.

Vaginal hysterectomy. The vaginal hysterectomy is probably a unique operative procedure from an infectious disease point of view. This operation must be classified as a clean-contaminated procedure. The operation is carried out through the vagina, an area heavily contaminated with a large variety of potentially pathogenic bacteria. Tissue that is bathed in this vaginal discharge is clamped, incised, and sutured continuously throughout the operation. In addition, vaginal fluid and blood are allowed to drain into the pelvic cavity, providing an opportunity for the bacteria to adhere to the pedicles and pelvic peritoneum. The peritoneum is often abraded by sponge sticks, used to provide better exposure. Thus the abraded peritoneum secretes fluid and also serves as an anchoring point for the bacteria, establishing the initial infectious process of bacteria adherence.

As the pelvic peritoneum is closed, the pedicles are brought into this retroperitoneal space. The vaginal cuff may be closed or sutured open, creating retrovaginal and retroperitoneal space, ideal for the growth of bacteria. Serum, lymphatic fluid, and blood collects in the retroperitoneal space and is an ideal incubator, containing the necessary nutrients for bacterial growth (aerobes, facultative and obligate anaerobes).

The incision at the vaginal apex reacts as does any wound, and an infection, namely a cellulitis or abscess, can occur. Here again, both conditions exist for the development of a wound infection; the presence of a large inoculum and the placement of suture, which serves as a foreign body.

A cul-de-sac, tubal, tuboovarian, or interloop abscess can form because the infecting fluid drains into the cul-de-sac. The vaginal fluid containing significant numbers of bacteria can also drain along the colonic gutters, establishing the potential for a localized infection, which may lead to an abscess in the subphrenic, subhepatic, or subsplenic spaces. However, these types of infections are unlikely to occur. If a vaginal cuff cellulitis develops, the infecting organisms can traverse the retrovaginal space, infecting the pedicles and permitting infection to reach the fallopian tubes to cause an abscess. Thus, the anatomic relationships of devitalized tissue to healthy tissue allow for the potential of serious infection.

Abdominal hysterectomy. An abdominal hysterectomy does not expose the patient to the same potential for development of an intrapelvic infection as does the vaginal hysterectomy. The reason for the decreased risk of infection is that the greatest part of the operation is carried out without exposing the individual to microflora of the lower genital tract. However, once the vagina is incised, the patient is at risk for infection. Incision of the vagina for the removal of the cervix allows the bacteria of the vaginal canal access to the pelvic cavity. In addition, the vaginal cuff may be clamped, crushing tissue and causing devascularization. Suture material is placed in the vaginal cuff, again creating all the conditions that favor bacterial growth.

Opening the vaginal cuff also allows bacteria from the lower genital tract to contaminate the abdominal incision. It is not unusual to find bacteria endogenous to the lower genital tract in wound abscesses.[14] This situation is similar to that in patients delivered by cesarean section.

Cervical cerclage. Antibiotic prophylaxis is often administered to patients having a cervical cerclage placed. This procedure is now performed at 10 to 12 weeks gestation, as compared to 14 to 18 weeks. However, there are no data to support the use of antibiotic prophylaxis for these patients. In fact, the more logical approach would be to screen patients for the presence of potential pathogens and treat accordingly. A study by Charles and co-workers[7] found that antibiotic prophylaxis was indicated for patients who had achieved 18 weeks gestation or more at the time a cerclage was placed. The reason for the greater risk of infection at that time is not known.

One could theorize that at the latter gestational ages, the cervix is engorged with blood and lymph. These dilated vessels provide bacteria easier access to tissues and also provide routes for dissemination. The presence of suture in the cervix may also contribute to infection at these later gestational times, but the presence of suture should act as a nidus for infection regardless of gestational age.

Abortion. Elective termination of pregnancy may be associated with an increased risk of postabortal infection, ectopic pregnancy, endometritis, salpingitis, septic shock, and death.[6,13,34,36,37] The organisms of concern are *S. agalactiae, Neisseria gonorrhoeae,* and perhaps *Chlamydia trachomatis.* During the operative procedure, the cervix is dilated, and both the cervix and the uterus are instrumented, resulting in destruction of the decidual layer and exposing the basalis layer of the uterus. This permits bacteria to gain entrance to the deeper myometrium. The mechanical placement of bacteria into the uterine cavity, along with the potential lymphatic and vascular spread of bacteria, enhances the opportunity for infection. The initial infection is an endometritis, but because of the instrumentation and enlarged vascular channels, bacteremia easily occurs. If the initial infection is not recognized, or if perforation of the uterus occurs, septicemia can result, eventually leading to septic shock.

PREVENTION

Postoperative infection can be prevented. Proper evaluation of the patient is critical to determine characteristics that may predispose to infection. In addition, it is important to understand the events that may increase the patient's risk. These two factors are intertwined but will be discussed separately.

Host factors, either exogenous or endogenous, that may contribute to the risk of postoperative infection are as follows:

Exogenous	Endogenous
Antibiotic	Obesity
Infection	Chronic illness
Prehospital stay	Abnormal vaginal flora
Preparation of operative site	History of repeated infection
Handwashing	
Scrub attire	
Surgical technique	

A careful preoperative survey of the patient often reveals the presence of one or more risk factors. Since the great majority of surgery is elective or nonemergent, ample time is usually available to correct some of the potentially adverse conditions.

Thus, the screening process begins with obtaining a thorough patient history. It is important to determine if the patient has had surgery in the past. If so, did any adverse anesthetic reaction or postoperative infection occur, and where was the infection located? Individuals who have had repeated infections are at risk for postoperative infection. This suggests a deficiency in their immunologic makeup. It also indicates that even in the presence of a small inoculum, they may become easily infected.

The use of antibiotics, even a single maintenance dose for suppression, such as for control of bacteriuria or acne, is important since it can alter the flora of the lower genital tract. Selection of resistant bacteria may take place, and if the patient develops a postoperative infection, it may be more difficult to treat.

Since postoperative infection in the obstetric or gynecologic patient has its origin usually in the lower genital microflora, it is important to determine if the vagina is microbiologically healthy. Although it has not been demonstrated that there is a direct causal relationship between such entities as "bacterial vaginosis" and postoperative pelvic infection, it is known, for instance, that if *S. aga-*

lactiae is present, the patient is at greater risk for infection.

Determining if the vaginal microflora are abnormal is not a difficult task, nor is it expensive or time-consuming. In the healthy state, the vaginal discharge is slate-gray to white in color, has a pH of 3.8 to 4.2, has no odor, does not give off an amine odor when mixed with concentrated potassium hydroxide (KOH Whiff test), and is homogeneous in consistency. Microscopic examination reveals the presence of squamous epithelial cells that are not cluttered with adherent bacteria. It is easy to discern the cell membrane and nucleus, bacteria are usually not overabundant, and bacillary forms usually predominate. White blood cells are rarely present.

The bacteriology of the healthy vagina is dominated by *Lactobacillus,* mainly *L. acidophilus.*[2,59] This bacterium is responsible for maintaining the equilibrium of the vaginal environment by keeping the pH between 3.8 and 4.2 and by the production of lactic acid. Lactobacilli also have the capability of producing hydrogen peroxide. These metabolic characteristics are detrimental to the growth of obligate anaerobic bacteria. The constituents that make up the vaginal microflora include gram-positive, gram-negative, aerobic, facultative, and obligate anaerobic bacteria (see box). Many other bacteria not listed in the box can be isolated, but their numbers are extremely small and their significance is not known. In the healthy state, *Lactobacillus* is usually present in a concentration of 10,000 or more bacteria per cubic centimeter of vaginal fluid, whereas the potentially pathogenic bacteria will be present in a concentration of 100 or more bacteria per cubic centimeter. Other commensal bacteria will be present in a concentration of 1000 or more bacteria per cubic centimeter.

The abnormal or unhealthy vaginal state is characterized by a pH of greater than 4.5 and the presence of clue cells and a variety of gram-positive and gram-negative bacteria. Lactobacilli are not dominant, and their concentration tends to fall well below 10,000 bacteria per cubic centimeter of vaginal fluid. The potentially pathogenic bacteria increase their numbers dramatically, some exceeding 100,000 bacteria per cubic centimeter of vaginal fluid. White blood cells may or may not be present. Their presence indicates that an inflammatory condition exists (e.g., vaginitis), whereas their absence implies that an inflamma-

---

Endogenous bacterial flora of the lower genital tract

Commensals	*Potential pathogens*	
Lactobacillus	Staphylococcus	Bacteroides
Corynebacterium	Streptococcus	Fusobacterium
Streptococcus	Enterococcus	Clostridium
Diphtheroids	Escherichia	Peptostreptococcus
	Enterobacter	
	Klebsiella	
	Proteus	

Table 15-1. Treatments for vaginitis

Disease	Antimicrobial	Dosage
C. albicans	Monistat Terazol Femstat Gyne-Lotrimin	Creams or suppositories for 3-7 days
T. vaginalis	Metronidazole	2 g as single dose 250 mg TID × 7 days
Bacterial	Metronidazole Augmentin Ceftin Clindamycin	250-500 mg TID × 7 days 500 mg TID × 7 days 500 mg BID × 7 days 1% cream QD × 7 days

tory state is not present (e.g., bacterial vaginosis).[17,61] However, both these states imply that the flora of the vagina are abnormal. Therefore, the presence of an abnormal vaginal microflora may place the patient who is to have pelvic surgery at risk for a postoperative infection.

These vaginal conditions can easily be detected without high cost. The pH of the vagina can be determined by testing a few drops of vaginal discharge with litmus paper; a result of 4.5 or higher is considered abnormal. A few drops of the discharge should be mixed with concentrated KOH to determine if amines are released, which can be detected by the presence of a fishlike odor (the Whiff test). The discharge should then be examined microscopically by diluting a drop of the discharge with one to two drops of saline to test for the presence of clue cells, numerous bacteria, both bacilli and cocci. White blood cells may or may not be present. These findings definitely indicate that the vaginal flora are abnormal. There is likely to be a preponderance of Enterobacteriaceae and anaerobes. In addition, microscopic examination of the vaginal discharge will, for the most part, identify other abnormal conditions such as *Trichomonas vaginalis,* which is also associated with an abnormal vaginal flora, and *Candida albicans* or other related species.

These conditions should be treated and the patient reexamined before surgery is undertaken. An abnormal bacterial vaginal microflora, be it bacterial vaginitis or vaginosis, can be treated with agents such as those listed in Table 15-1. Treatments for other conditions are also listed. In treating an abnormal bacterial vaginal condition, a gram stain may be helpful. If the gram stain reveals the presence of only gram-negative bacillary forms with a relatively uniform morphologic appearance suggesting mainly the presence of *Enterobacteriaceae,* then an agent such as Ceftin can be used. If the organisms are a mixture of gram-positive and gram-negative bacteria with a uniform morphologic appearance suggesting predominantly aerobes and facultative anaerobes, then an agent such as Augmentin can be used. If the organisms are mixed and the morphologic appearance quite varied, then anaerobes would be suspected, and Augmentin, clindamycin, or metronidazole can be used. No form of antibiotic treatment has proven

completely satisfactory in the treatment of an abnormal vaginal flora. A simple scheme as given above allows for the logical use of antibiotics, without necessarily resulting in the selection of resistant bacteria. Following treatment, the vaginal discharge should be reexamined microscopically. The pH alone is not reliable, since it may be abnormal following treatment while the microscopic characteristics are completely normal. Eliminating the abnormal state of the vagina, if possible, would tend to allow the antibiotic chosen for prophylaxis to be more effective. A reduction in the inoculum load would not overburden a single dose of antibiotic administered for prophylaxis. A single dose of even a parenterally administered antimicrobial is not sufficient to handle the large numbers of bacteria present in patients with bacterial vaginitis. A single dose of an antibiotic administered to an individual with a normal vaginal flora will probably exert a lesser effect for selecting a resistant bacterium. If the agent chosen does not cause a reduction in the numbers of normal flora (e.g., lactobacilli), it may prevent the selection of resistant strains.

The most common approach to the prevention of postoperative infection is the use of antibiotic prophylaxis. This is defined as the administration of an antibiotic for an extremely short period of time to an individual who is not infected but is to experience an operative procedure that is associated with a significant risk of postoperative infection. Antibiotic prophylaxis has become routine in most surgical procedures. The risk factors for postoperative infection are either endogenous or exogenous to the host. In order for antibiotic prophylaxis to be effective, the agent should achieve serum and tissue levels that will provide activity against most of the organisms that are commonly involved in the infection. In microbiological terminology, the potency of an antimicrobial agent is referred to as its minimal inhibitory concentration (MIC). MIC_{90} is the minimal inhibitory concentration that will prevent survival of 90% of the bacteria being tested. Antibiotics used for prophylaxis should be given as a one-time dose, administered shortly before the operative procedure begins or immediately after the umbilical cord is clamped in the case of cesarean section.[3-5,16,38] Additional doses of antibiotic should be given if the operative procedure exceeds 3 hours or if the blood loss is greater than 1500 cc. Obviously, each patient and set of circumstances should be considered individually. If the operative procedure requires more than 3 hours but produces much less than 1500 cc of blood loss, perhaps additional doses of antibiotic can be withheld, especially if the patient has been stable and has experienced no adverse effects intraoperatively (i.e., hypoxia or hypotension).

Until recently, selecting an agent for antibiotic prophylaxis could be accomplished by random choice since all the studies published revealed no differences in the agents tested. Comparative studies between first and second generation cephalosporins and between penicillins and cephalosporins demonstrated that these agents were equal in their ability to reduce the incidence of postoperative infec-

Table 15-2. Antibiotic comparison for prophylaxis in cesarean section

Antibiotic	Dose (g)
Cefazolin	1 x 3
Cefazolin	1
Cefazolin	2
Cefonicid	1
Cefotetan	1
Cefoxitin	1
Cefoxitin	2
Ceftizoxime	1
Ampicillin	2
Piperacillin	4

tion.[3,5,16,38] These data are difficult to understand since the agents' spectra of activity are quite different. Recently, a study was published in which seven antibiotics were compared in a randomized open trial.[26] They were administered for prophylaxis for the prevention of postpartum endometritis in patients having cesarean sections (Table 15-2). Cefotetan and piperacillin were found to be significantly more efficacious in reducing the incidence of postpartum endometritis.

Antibiotics administered for prophylaxis, even when administered in a single dose, have a profound effect on the vaginal microflora. Several investigators have demonstrated that cephalosporin prophylaxis tends to select for resistant bacteria, for example, *Enterococcus faecalis* and *Enterobacter cloacae*.[18,20,26,57] This is manifested in an approximately sixfold increase in the recovery of *E. faecalis* and a twofold increase in the recovery of *E. cloacae* following exposure to cefazolin, cefotetan, and cefoxitin. The penicillins, such as mezlocillin and piperacillin, have a selective effect, although not as dramatic as the cephalosporins, on the *Enterobacteriaceae*. This selection process may be important in the patient who develops postpartum endometritis following exposure to antibiotic prophylaxis, especially if the patient fails to respond to initial therapeutic therapy.

MANAGEMENT

The approach to the patient who develops a postoperative infection can be divided into three basic phases: (1) a review of the chart and history, (2) a physical examination with appropriate methods of obtaining specimens for the culture and identification of microorganisms, and (3) the selection of appropriate therapy. It is important when evaluating the patient that the operative site be examined last, to ensure that the examination is objective.

A review of the patient's chart, including a detailed history, is extremely important. Especially important are past surgical history and incidence of infection. A positive history may alert the physician to an underlying immunological defect that becomes manifest when the individual is stressed. It is important to determine if the patient has

been taking any medications that might have an immunosuppressive effect, such as steroids. The individual may be taking prednisone, which may have been overlooked. Has the patient been on antibiotics within the 2 weeks preceding the surgery? If so, what agent and dosage were used? The purpose of antibiotic therapy preoperatively should also be determined. The surgical procedure should be reviewed in detail. If this information is not readily available, then a discussion should be held with the operating surgeon before the patient is interviewed. Did any adverse effects occur during the operative procedure (e.g., difficult intubation with possible hypoxia, aspiration of stomach contents, significant hypotension, significant blood loss, or an obvious break in sterile technique)? Laboratory values of the patient's hematologic and physiologic status must be reviewed, including iron status, nitrogen balance, blood urea nitrogen and creatinine, liver enzymes, and acid-base balance. These are important since markedly anemic patients may have difficulty with oxygenation of tissues, tachycardia, and orthostatic hypotension. Kidney and liver status are important because many antibiotics are excreted by the kidney and/or liver. Individuals with kidney impairment will require alterations in their dosage of antibiotics. If there is an indication of liver dysfunction, antibiotics that are metabolized via the liver should be avoided.

The physical examination should be preceded by a brief account by the patient of the events preceding the surgical procedure, her understanding of the operation, and the events that took place following surgery. The physician should ask the patient to describe her symptoms and localize any areas of pain. The physical examination should be inclusive, from head to toe. The sites of possible infection (e.g., IV sites, central lines) should be examined closely. The lungs should be carefully auscultated, and even if clear lung fields are heard, a chest x-ray should be obtained including anterior-posterior and lateral views. This is extremely important to rule out the presence of atelectasis, aspiration, pneumonia, or the presence of interstitial or pleural fluid. Again, the chart should be reviewed to determine if the patient had a heart murmur preceding surgery. Auscultation of the heart should be carefully performed. If a murmur is noted that was not present preoperatively, then an echocardiogram should be obtained to rule out acute endocarditis.

The abdominal examination begins with inspecting the contour and skin of the abdomen. Skin changes such as edema, erythema, or induration should be noted. Asymmetry to the abdominal wall should be noted, as this may indicate the presence of a fluid collection (e.g., hematoma, seroma, or abscess). The abdomen should be auscultated, and if it appears distended and no bowel sounds can be heard, the patient most likely has an ileus. If the patient has rebound tenderness and states that it is painful to walk, then peritonitis is likely to be present. A maneuver that sometimes helps is to rock the patient by her hips while she is lying in bed. If pain is elicited, then peritonitis is present. This finding suggests that a pelvic infection is present and has spread to the peritoneal cavity. Gentle palpation of the upper abdomen, well above the umbilicus, will elicit a painful response if the bowel is markedly dilated. This is easily accomplished by gently palpating with one finger and using a quick release. The suspicion of an ileus merits obtaining x-rays (a flat plate of the abdomen and upright views). In addition to determining if air-fluid levels are present, the gas pattern can be detected. Movement of the gas in the bowel can be determined by obtaining serial x-rays. These also allow measurement of the cecum, which should not exceed 10 cm in diameter. If it does, a mechanical obstruction may be present and an exploratory laparotomy should be performed.

If the abdomen is asymmetrical, it is possible that a hematoma, seroma, or purulent collection of fluid is present within the abdominal wall. An ultrasound examination of the abdominal wall can facilitate localization of the fluid collection and permit safe aspiration of the fluid. If a collection of fluid is present, it is usually closely associated with the incision. It is best to cleanse the incision line and adjacent area with either betadine or alcohol before inserting the aspiration needle into this pocket of fluid. Entering through the incision will not cause the patient any pain or require the use of an anesthetizing agent. The fluid should be placed into an anaerobic transport vial and gram stained for the isolation of *Mycoplasma,* aerobic, and anaerobic bacteria. If an attempt at aspiration is made and no fluid is obtained, this may indicate that an organized hematoma is present. If the fluid is dark brown, this suggests a liquefying hematoma; bright red indicates continuing bleeding or a mixture of both. Serous fluid to brownish fluid may indicate a seroma or perhaps a mycoplasma infection. Blackish fluid may indicate a necrotizing infection. The presence of frankly purulent fluid suggests an abscess. The gram stain can be of particular aid in establishing the presence of infection and assist in choosing an appropriate antibiotic.

If the gram stain does not reveal the presence of bacteria or white cells, the possibility of infection decreases, although it is not completely ruled out. The fluid should always be cultured for bacteria since their absence on gram stain indicates that their numbers are below 10,000 per cubic centimeter of fluid and does not necessarily mean that the fluid is sterile. The presence of white blood cells and the absence of bacteria on a gram-stained specimen of a wound aspirate suggests the presence of *Mycoplasma.*[55] This necessitates the use of an antibiotic such as clindamycin or a tetracycline. Since the penicillins, cephalosporins, and metronidazole are not active against *Mycoplasma,* the gram stain can be used to guide the selection of antibiotics if bacteria are present. If only gram-positive cocci are present, then *Staphylococcus aureus* should be suspected and an antibiotic against this organism, for example, naficillin, should be used until an identification and sensitivity are known. Antibiotic changes can be made based on sensitivity determinations. An appropriate choice would be an antibiotic that has good activity, is able to achieve good serum and tissue levels when taken orally, and is inexpensive. If the gram stain reveals only gram-negative rods, then a broad spectrum cephalosporin should be utilized (e.g., cefotetan, ceftizoxime, cefoxitin) or perhaps an oral agent, cephalothin. If the specimen contains a mixture of gram-positive and gram-negative bacteria, then an agent such as ampicillin/sulbactam, piperacillin/tazobactam, or ticarcillin/clavulanic acid can be used. These antibiotics provide excellent activity against gram-positive and gram-negative aerobic and obligate anaerobic bacteria. These agents also provide activity against facultative anaerobic bacteria that is comparable to that of the aminoglycosides.

Ultrasonography can be used to guide the aspirating needle. If no fluid returns upon initial entry, it is best to wait a few seconds because there may be gas present, which will be aspirated first and followed by fluid. The presence of gas indicates a mixed infection involving a variety of bacteria, which may include facultative and obligate anaerobes. If no fluid is present and the patient is developing signs of a wound infection, there is usually an area of erythema and induration. The border of the erythema should be outlined on the abdominal wall with a ballpoint pen. The time of placement of this line should be noted on the chart along with all characteristics of the wound. The patient should be reexamined the same day, within 6 hours, in the same manner as the earlier examination, and this should be repeated daily until her condition returns to normal. If the border of induration or erythema has advanced beyond the line demarcated earlier, then an advancing cellulitis is present and an active infection is ongoing. Since aspiration of the wound is usually of no benefit, antibiotics can be started empirically. If the patient is able to tolerate oral liquids and solids and does not appear to have a systemic infection, an agent such as Augmentin (500 mg every 8 hours) can be given. If the patient cannot tolerate oral nourishment, then ceftizoxime, cefotetan, or cefoxitin should be administered intravenously.

If fluid is aspirated and is serous to brownish in color but does not contain white blood cells or bacteria, all the fluid should be aspirated. A tight pressure dressing may be applied in an attempt to inhibit the recollection of fluid. If the patient's temperature or white blood cell count rises and no other focus of infection can be found, the wound should be reexamined. If fluid has reaccumulated, the wound must be reopened. Also, if blood or purulent material was noted on the initial examination, the wound must be reopened.

Recommendations on opening the wound vary from institution to institution, but a logical approach is first to decide upon the cause of the defect. For example, if it is a hematoma, then perhaps only the area containing the hematoma has not healed and therefore only that portion of the incision requires being opened and cleaned. If purulent material is present, it is best to open the entire wound. Another factor that will impinge on management of the complicated wound is how the incision was closed. At my institution, incisions are usually closed by suturing the peritoneum with a 3-0 absorbable suture. The subcutaneous tissue is not routinely sutured; the skin is approximated and closed with stainless steel staples. Thus, when a wound complication arises that requires opening, the staples are removed. On some occasions the wound will open spontaneously. If not, very gentle traction is applied in an opposing fashion adjacent to the incision line if healing is not progressing normally. Incisions that contain suture in the subcutaneous tissue and/or skin will require their removal. Even in these cases, separation can be noted, as well as the spontaneous release of fluid from the incision.

Where to perform the examination and opening of the wound depends upon the complication suspected. First, attempt to determine the extent of the dehiscence. If there is a strong suspicion that a wound is not healing, probe gently between opposing skin edges with a sterile cotton-tipped applicator, which may slip between the edges of opposing subcutaneous tissue and may reveal a fascial defect. If there is spontaneous drainage of serous fluid, have the patient attempt to sit up, and note if the fluid exits under pressure between the opposing skin edges. If this occurs, a fascial dehiscence should be suspected and the patient should be taken back to the operating room and the wound opened under a general anesthetic. If a fascial dehiscence is not suspected or detected and the patient has a transverse abdominal incision, the patient need not be taken back to the operating room unless there is an extensive collection of pus and the entire subcutaneous area cannot be explored or unless the pus is seen to originate beneath the fascial layer. The patient should be taken back to the operating room if there is any evidence of evisceration, regardless of how small a defect is initially noted. The extent of the evisceration cannot be appreciated by a cursory examination, nor can proper management be carried out.

THE POSTPARTUM PATIENT

The postcesarian section patient should also be taken back to the operating room if there is purulence exiting the incision and a bimanual examination reveals pus exiting the vagina or if a defect can be palpated in the uterine incision line by a digit placed through the cervical canal. This indicates that there is a communication between the uterine and skin incisions. These findings indicate that the uterine lower segment has necrosed along the incision line and formed a communication with the abdominal incision.

In order to determine if the patient has endomyometritis, it is necessary to perform a thorough pelvic examination. There is sometimes a reluctance to do pelvic examinations on patients who have had pelvic surgery, because of tenderness from the surgery. However, a pelvic infection cannot be detected by palpating the abdomen since the pelvic organs usually are positioned deep in the pelvis. The abdominal examination can reveal pertinent information about the wound, the bowel, and the peritoneum. Palpation of the abdomen may elicit pain or tenderness, thus suggesting peritonitis or distended bowel. If the uterus has

subinvoluted, then it may be possible to palpate the fundus abdominally.

A critical observation of the infected wound is whether there is crepitance, blackening of the skin or skin edges, suggesting the presence of a necrotizing infection.[40,56,62] This requires immediate surgical debridement if the patient is to survive. The debridement should be thorough, including all necrotic tissue and a margin of healthy tissue. A satisfactory debridement is accomplished by excising the involved tissue back to an area of normal tissue that is detected by brisk bleeding, encompassing a margin of normal tissue that completely surrounds the infected and involved tissue. In all cases where tissue is removed, specimens containing infected tissue at the margin between the infected and noninfected areas should be sent in separate, well-labelled, anaerobic transport vials. This is important not only for the isolation, identification, and antibiotic sensitivity testing of the infecting organism(s), but for determining the extent of involvement.

The pelvic examination begins with inspection of the vulva. The episiotomy is a wound just like any other surgical wound and should be treated as such. It should be examined for the presence of pus, ecchymosis, blackening of the tissue, crepitance, edema, and bullous edema. A speculum should be inserted into the vagina. If the patient was delivered vaginally or by cesarean section, the uterus should be involuted and the cervix should not be greatly dilated. A ring forceps with a 4-by-4-inch gauze sponge folded to form a sponge stick can be introduced into the uterine cavity. The sponge stick manipulated in a circumferential manner will dislodge the intrauterine contents. The uterus should be emptied of lochia, clots, and any fragments of placental tissue before obtaining a specimen for culture. This may enable the patient to overcome the initial attack by the bacteria and eliminate the infection.

A specimen should be obtained from the inner aspect of the uterus with a Pipelle placed against the inner uterine lining. This instrument is an intrauterine biopsy device that has been shown in comparative studies to be as effective as any other device in retrieving a specimen from the endometrial cavity.[46] The specimen should be transported in an anaerobic vial and processed for the culture of *Mycoplasma, Ureaplasma, Chlamydia,* and aerobic and anaerobic bacteria.

A bimanual examination should be conducted to determine if there is tenderness, induration, and extension into the parametrial areas (e.g., whether the degree of inflammation extends out to the pelvic side walls). If the tissue is markedly indurated, does it have a woody texture, so-called ligneous cellulitis, or phlegmon, or is there a fluctuant mass present suggesting an abscess or hematoma? When performing a bimanual examination, it is best not to palpate the uterus along the incision since this will obviously be tender. The size of the uterus can be ascertained and the consistency (firm, soft, or boggy). A boggy or markedly soft uterus in a febrile patient is consistent with a degree of intrauterine or myometrial infection. Determining the status of the uterus begins by knowing the type of uterine incision. If a transverse lower uterine segment incision was used, the fundus can be palpated and, if pain is present, it should not reflect incisional pain but that associated with infection. If a mass is suspected, then an ultrasonogram or CAT scan should be obtained to delineate the location and determine if percutaneous drainage or aspiration is indicated. If a vertical uterine incision was used, the uterus should be palpated along its lateral borders. If pain is elicited when the uterus is gently moved, it should be considered significant. If the uterus is subinvoluting, boggy, tender, and the cervix remains dilated in a patient who is febrile, then a diagnosis of endomyometritis is likely. If there is tenderness and perhaps induration of the parametrial tissues, then a diagnosis of endomyoparametritis is probable, and the infection should be considered serious. The individual with adynamic ileus, abdominal distention, and rebound tenderness has a serious endomyoparametritis and requires aggressive medical management to prevent suppurative myometritis and complications such as uterine myonecrosis and septic pelvic vein thrombosis.

ANTIBIOTIC CHOICE

If the patient receives an antibiotic for prophylaxis, it is most likely to be an expanded spectrum or beta-lactam cephalosporin (e.g., cefotetan, cefoxitin, or ceftizoxime). These agents will select out for resistant bacteria, such as *Enterococcus faecalis, Enterobacter agglomerans, Enterobacter aerogenes,* or *Enterobacter cloacae.*[18,20,26,57] This is an important consideration since *Enterobacter cloacae* are resistant to most beta-lactam cephalosporins and penicillins. *Enterococcus faecalis* is resistant to cephalosporins, and not all penicillins are equally effective against this bacterium.

Antibiotics for prophylaxis are primarily administered as a single dose, although it is not uncommon to find a variety of dosing schedules used (e.g., 3 doses per day for 2 to 3 days). Antibiotics administered even for a single dose have the effect of altering the vaginal flora, suppressing sensitive bacteria and thereby allowing the resistant strains to dominate. This possible effect should be considered when treating a patient for a postoperative infection who has received antibiotic prophylaxis. Single agent antimicrobial therapy is becoming more acceptable for the treatment of female soft tissue pelvic infections. The beta-lactam agents (i.e., mezlocillin, piperacillin, ticarcillin, ampicillin/sulbactam, ticarcillin/clavulanic acid, cefotetan, cefoxitin, and ceftizoxime) have been found as effective as the combination of clindamycin or metronidazole plus gentamicin for the treatment of postpartum endomyometritis, pelvic cellulitis, and pelvic inflammatory disease.*

When instituting antibiotic therapy, one should not expect to see an immediate response but should allow 48 hours to elapse from administration of the first dose of antibiotic before deciding that the chosen regimen has failed.

It is important to begin from the time the initial dose of antibiotic is actually administered, not from the time the order specifies for administration, since a considerable amount of time may elapse between these two events. For example, the order for antibiotics may specify administration at 6 PM and the agent may not be given until 12 AM. Therefore, it is best to order that the initial dose be given immediately as a loading dose. This will prevent a delay that allows the bacteria to increase in number.

If after 48 hours the patient's condition is not improving, the patient should be reevaluated and new specimens obtained for the isolation of bacteria. The specimens obtained at the initial evaluation should, after 48 hours, reveal the presence of aerobic bacteria. The laboratory can provide important information; for example, if growth is present, a gram stain can be performed to determine if the bacteria are gram-positive or gram-negative. If the patient is receiving a cephalosporin (e.g., cefotetan, ceftizoxime, or cefoxitin) and if the bacteria are gram-positive, the likely organism is *Enterococcus.* Then ampicillin can be added to the present agent. If the organism is gram-negative, then an aminoglycoside can be added. If the patient is receiving a penicillin (e.g., Unasyn, Timentin, piperacillin, or piperacillin/tazobactam), an aminoglycoside should be added. Appropriate dosages for the most frequently used antibiotics are listed in Table 15-3.

The beta-lactam antimicrobial agents are all excreted by the kidney, and therefore it is important that the patient's renal function be assessed before, during, and after administration of these antibiotics. It is not necessary to perform serum peak and trough levels for the beta-lactam agents, but obtaining an initial blood urea nitrogen and creatinine

Table 15-3. Beta-lactam antibiotics suitable for treatment of soft tissue pelvic infections

Antibiotic	Dosage
Single agent therapy	
Mezlocillin	4 g q 6 hr
Piperacillin	4 g q 6 hr
Ticarcillin	4 g q 6 hr
Ampicillin/sulbactam	2/1 g q 6 hr
Ticarcillin/clavulanic	3/1 g q 6 hr
Cefotetan	2 g q 12 hr
Cefoxitin	2 g q 8 hr
Ceftizoxime	2 g q 8 hr
Combination therapy	
Clindamycin or	900 mg q 8 hr
metronidazole	500 mg q 8 hr
with	
Gentamicin*	4-5 mg/kg body wt/day
Tobramycin*	given in 3 divided doses
Amikacin* or	7.5 mg/kg q 12 hr
aztreonam*	1-2 g q 12 hr
	2 g q 6 hr for seriously ill patients
Cefuroxime*	0.5-2 g q 8 hr

*Dosage must be adjusted in patients with renal impairment.

---

*References 19, 21-23, 25, 33, 45, 49.

before starting therapy is prudent. It is not necessary to repeat these tests serially, but a repeat value during or at the termination of therapy would establish that kidney function has not changed because of antibiotic therapy.

Antibiotic combinations are currently used either as empirical therapy or as additions to the agent currently employed. The most popular combination is clindamycin plus gentamicin and the most frequently added antibiotic is an aminoglycoside. The use of an aminoglycoside is logical since these agents continue to provide excellent activity against facultative gram-negative bacteria. Controversy exists over whether it is necessary to obtain serum trough and peak levels of aminoglycosides and vancomycin. Aside from the medicolegal concerns, it is not good practice to administer an antibiotic that is improperly dosed and has the potential for toxicity. It is best to obtain a serum peak level 30 to 60 minutes after a dose has been administered. The trough level should be obtained just before instituting the next dose of aminoglycoside. Thus the serum peak and trough levels should be obtained within an 8-hour period between doses of drug. One should not obtain a trough value, administer antibiotic, then obtain a peak value. This does not reflect the status of kidney function during an antibiotic administration period. The acceptable peak and trough levels for the various aminoglycosides are listed in Table 15-4. If the patient's peak values are too high, then the dosage should be decreased. If the peak values are acceptable but the trough values are high, the time between administration of doses can be increased. If serial trough values indicate the value is rising, even though it is below the toxic range, this may signify that the individual is becoming sensitized to the antibiotic and it may be best to change antibiotics. If the aminoglycoside is needed because of the presence of a suspected gram-negative bacterium, suboptimal dosing will not only be ineffective but may encourage the selection of a resistant strain.

Another important consideration in postoperative infection is the possibility of bacteremia. Approximately 10% to 20% of the infected patients become bacteremic. Two specimens of 10 cc of venous blood should be obtained at least fifteen minutes apart. Each specimen should be divided into two equal portions and used to inoculate an anaerobic and an aerobic blood culture bottle. If the aerobic blood culture bottles are not indicating growth after 48

hours, the bottles should be subcultured on A7 medium for the detection of *Mycoplasma* and *Ureaplasma*.[54,55] If growth is present at the end of 48 hours, the bacteria should be gram stained to determine if they are gram-positive or gram-negative. If gram-positive cocci are present, the most likely choices are *Enterococcus* and *Staphylococcus,* the former being most likely, and therefore ampicillin and gentamicin should be used. If the patient is allergic to penicillin, vancomycin should be used with gentamicin. There is no synergy between a cephalosporin and an aminoglycoside against *Enterococcus,* and therefore a cephalosporin alone or in combination with an aminoglycoside should not be used. Although erythromycin may exhibit activity against *Enterococcus* in vitro, this is not a suitable choice in treating bacteremia due to this particular bacterium. The objectives for treating bacteremia are to eradicate the organisms from the blood stream and to prevent endocarditis and disseminated infection such as brain abscess, kidney abscess, and osteomyelitis. Therefore, bactericidal activity is needed, which is best achieved with the combination of ampicillin or vancomycin plus an aminoglycoside. If gram-negative bacteria are present, then a beta-lactam cephalosporin can be used. However, it is best to initiate therapy with vancomycin plus an aminoglycoside or a penicillinase-resistant penicillin, such as methicillin, initially. Once the organism has been identified and its antibiotic sensitivity pattern is known, a change in antibiotic therapy can be made. It is important that antibiotic therapy be continued until the patient has been truly afebrile for 72 hours. In addition, the pulse rate and white blood cell count should be normal. A negative set of blood cultures should also be obtained. The heart should be auscultated daily, and if a murmur is detected or is more intense than before the onset of the bacteremia, an echocardiogram must be obtained to rule out the presence of vegetations.

THROMBOPHLEBITIS

Thrombosis is the formation of a blood clot in a blood vessel or in the heart that remains at the point of origin. Thrombophlebitis is a condition in which inflammation occurs in the wall of a vein before development of a blood clot. Approximately 20% to 30% of patients undergoing general surgery have deep-vein thrombosis.[39,41,50] Most patients are asymptomatic and do not develop any sequelae, the thrombosis resolving when the patient becomes ambulatory. However, the possibility or suspicion of a deep-vein thrombosis of the lower extremity should not be ignored in either the preoperative or postoperative patient. Although the majority of patients remain asymptomatic, approximately 300,000 cases of pulmonary emboli occur each year in the United States.[44] Pulmonary embolus is responsible for 100,000 deaths and is a contributing factor to an additional 100,000 deaths annually.[28] Autopsy studies have indicated that pulmonary emboli are undiagnosed at death in 40% to 70% of patients who have them.[12,27]

Postpartum pelvic vein thrombosis, sometimes referred

Table 15-4. Normal serum aminoglycoside peak and trough levels

Antibiotic	Collection	Therapeutic range
Gentamicin Tobramycin	30-60 min after infusion	Peak >4 μg <10 μg/ml Trough >0.5 μg <2 μg/ml*
Amikacin	30-60 min after infusion	Peak <30 μg/ml Trough <10 μg/ml*

*Trough levels should be obtained just before administering a therapeutic dose.

to as septic pelvic vein thrombosis, is rare. It is estimated to occur in 1 out of 10,000 deliveries, but the actual incidence is not known since this is a diagnosis that is made by exclusion. Rarely are any definitive tests performed to establish this diagnosis, although a computed tomography (CT) scan can be of assistance in establishing the presence of pelvic vein thrombosis. Although not well understood, the disease was intensely studied at Charity Hospital in New Orleans.[8-10] Thrombophlebitis in the obstetric and gynecologic patient is most likely to occur in the upper extremities, is usually superficial, and is secondary to the use of a intravenous catheter. This is likely to occur when irritant solutions are infused (e.g., magnesium sulfate, doxycycline, erythromycin). Thrombosis or thrombophlebitis of the lower extremity is not commonplace in the obstetric or gynecologic patient, but when it occurs, it has the potential for life-threatening sequelae. It is most likely to occur in the geriatric gynecologic patient or the patient who is bedridden for a prolonged postoperative period. The most likely reason for the decrease in lower extremity thrombosis in the obstetric and gynecologic population is the decrease in ambulation that occurs with periods of prolonged prehospitalization. Today, same-day admissions for surgery and early ambulation postoperatively are major reasons for the decrease in thromboembolic occurrences.

Diagnosis

Thrombophlebitis of the upper extremities, secondary to intravenous infusion, usually involves a superficial vein and rarely has important sequelae. It is first noted by the patient who complains of a painful knot at or adjacent to the intravenous site. If the area contains a palpable knot in the vein, it is likely that the patient has a thrombus. Not uncommonly, these are uncomplicated, the thrombus does not grow, there is no swelling of the extremity, and no evidence of cellulitis. There is no need to conduct vascular flow studies since involvement of the superficial system is not usually responsible for morbidity. If there is an associated erythema with the thrombus, along with pain and fever, the patient probably has thrombophlebitis. It is important to monitor the situation by noting growth of the thrombus, advancing erythema, and increase in size of the extremity. If the patient's extremity is developing any of these signs, it is no longer a superficial thrombosis but serious thrombophlebitis. It is best to obtain consultation from a vascular surgeon if there is any doubt.

The patient most likely to develop pelvic vein thrombosis or thrombophlebitis is the postpartum, as opposed to the postoperative, gynecologic patient. The reason is that the pregnant patient has poor venous return from the lower extremities and the pelvic veins are usually engorged and drain slowly. Pelvic vein engorgement is easily noted at the time of cesarean section as compared to the pelvic vasculature in the gynecologic patient at the time of pelvic surgery. Rarely does one find pelvic vein engorgement or decreased flow in the patient undergoing hysterectomy. However, if either the obstetric or the gynecologic patient has deep vein thrombosis of the lower extremity, she should be considered to be at risk for the development of nonseptic or septic pelvic vein thrombosis. This would be a potential complication if the patient developed a postoperative soft-tissue pelvic infection, which, in turn, may cause peritonitis and/or a paralytic ileus. This usually results in the prolonged administration of intravenous solutions. Because the patient is reluctant to ambulate, there is a decrease in circulation. Often the intravenous site must be changed because of infiltration or time requirements. The intravenous infusion increases the possibility of thrombophlebitis of the upper extremity. The patient's reluctance to ambulate increases the risk for pelvic vein thrombosis or thrombophlebitis.

Thrombosis or thrombophlebitis of the pelvic veins is most likely to occur in the patient who develops a pelvic infection (e.g., postpartum endometritis or perhaps tuboovarian abscesses). The preceding events are usually as follows: The patient develops postpartum endometritis, which may or may not create the impression that the patient may resolve the situation without the aid of antimicrobial agents. Within the next day or so, antibiotic therapy is begun, but the patient does not appear to be responding. The patient is now postpartum day 3 and a single antibiotic is administered (e.g., one of the following: cefoxitin, cefotetan, ceftizoxime, Timentin, or Unasyn). After 48 to 72 hours, there is no response. A second antibiotic may be added or the regimen may be changed completely to clindamycin plus an aminoglycoside or triple agent therapy (e.g., clindamycin, gentamicin, and ampicillin). After an additional 48 hours, there is still no sign of improvement. However, the physical and pelvic examination findings that lead to a diagnosis of endomyometritis are no longer present and the patient has no identifiable focus of infection. Although the pelvic examination is totally benign and unremarkable, the oral body temperature is characterized by a high spiking pattern, usually over 101° F, and a tachycardia is present whose course parallels that of the temperature plot. The white blood cell count is usually elevated and out of proportion to the clinical findings, often greater than 20,000. These findings present a confusing clinical picture since the patient usually feels fine and is asymptomatic except for the elevated temperature, pulse rate, and white blood cell count. The diagnoses to consider at this point are pelvic abscess, septic pelvic vein thrombosis, or drug fever.

Even though the pelvic examination is unremarkable, this does not rule out the presence of a pelvic abscess, which may or may not involve the uterus. In addition, the patient may have an infected hematoma that was not palpable. A pelvic ultrasonogram or CT scan may be extremely helpful. (An ultrasonogram may not be particularly helpful in detecting pelvic vein thrombosis, and therefore a CT scan should be obtained.) The latter will allow detection and localization of a pelvic vein thrombosis and any other mass that may be present. In addition, if a mass is present, it may be aspirated and a catheter placed to facilitate drainage. This permits establishing a diagnosis, determining the microbial pathogens, antibiotic management, and perhaps effective management without the need for exploratory laparotomy.

The unique characteristic of the patient with septic pelvic vein thrombophlebitis is that the thrombi contain bacteria. The bacteria predominantly involved are members of the vaginal microflora that were primarily responsible for initiating the pelvic infection that preceded the development of pelvic vein thrombosis. The most commonly involved bacteria are *Escherichia coli, Bacteroides, Peptostreptococcus,* and perhaps the hemolytic streptococci. The bacteria can cause liquefaction and fragmentation of the thrombus, thus resulting in embolization. This process can produce repeated showers of emboli and lead to dissemination of infection to the lung, kidneys, brain, and elsewhere.

In the past, the diagnosis was established by the institution of heparin in conjunction with antibiotics. Usually heparin would be added to the antimicrobial regimen if antibiotic therapy failed to resolve the patient's fever. Today a more definitive approach can be taken by using computerized tomography. This diagnostic aide can differentiate between the specific veins involved (e.g., the pelvic veins of the pelvic floor versus the ovarian veins). This is important because of the potential for the thrombus involving the inferior vena cava below and at the level above the renal veins. Involvement of the vena cava is even more important because of the increased likelihood of a pulmonary embolus. CT is also an excellent diagnostic aide in determining the presence of other pelvic abnormalities. The scan will delineate the uterus and permit the determination of size, contents, and the presence or absence of gas. It will also facilitate defining associated structures, both normal and abnormal. A thrombosed vessel will appear as a low-density defect that can be followed in sequential images, thus allowing the extent of the thrombus to be traced. The thrombus can be identified as a structure with a central filling defect. A newer imaging technique, magnetic resonance imaging (MRI), has also been used to diagnose this condition, but experience is limited.[47]

The one complication that has significant potential for mortality is pulmonary embolus. The patient's symptoms usually include acute onset of chest pain, tachycardia, and tachypnea and may or may not include elevated body temperature. Patients with recurrent septic emboli have a hectic fever pattern; 35% of the cases have positive blood culture; 46% have an abnormal chest radiograph and a mortality rate of 50%.[54] The most common problem associated with pulmonary embolism is delay in making a diagnosis. The postoperative patient who complains of chest pain should immediately be evaluated for the possibility of pulmonary embolus. Auscultation of the lungs is usually unrewarding but should always be done. If decreased breath sounds are noted, whereas previous examinations did not reveal this finding, then an embolus may have occurred. Similarly, a new murmur should be regarded as highly sig-

nificant. Arterial blood gas should be obtained immediately; a Po_2 less than 80 indicates high likelihood of a pulmonary embolus. An electrocardiogram (ECG) should be obtained to rule out a myocardial infarction. The most common ECG changes are nonspecific t-wave changes and RST-segment abnormalities. A ventilation-perfusion scan with xenon workout should be obtained to determine if any defects are found that would be consistent with a pulmonary embolus. If the test is not definitive, then a pulmonary angiogram should be obtained to establish a definitive diagnosis.[50]

Management

The patient with an uncomplicated thrombus of the upper extremity will respond to discontinuance of the intravenous infusion, removal of the intravenous catheter, and local application of hot compresses. The patient should be advised that a knot is likely to remain and will take several weeks to resolve. In addition to these conservative measures, antibiotic therapy may be necessary, especially if there is an advancing cellulitis, which may indicate the presence of hemolytic streptococci. Heparin therapy is not usually necessary unless the thrombus appears to be increasing in size. If heparin is necessary, a loading dose of 10,000 units is administered intravenously. The patient usually complains of pain, even with the extremity at rest, if followed by a maintenance dose of 1,000 units/hour. A partial thromboplastin time (PTT) should be obtained before instituting therapy to rule out any abnormality in coagulation factors. A PTT should also be obtained after the maintenance dose has been in effect for 2 to 3 hours to ensure that the patient is not hyperanticoagulated.[49] Patients with severe thrombophlebitis of the upper extremities rarely require anticoagulant levels of heparin. If there is an associated cellulitis and fever, then antibiotic therapy is indicated. The organisms usually associated with septic superficial thrombophlebitis are derived from the skin flora, the staphylococci and streptococci. If a methicillin staphylococci has been identified or is suspected, then an agent such as methicillin or dicloxacillin can be used. An alternative is a cephalosporin such as cefazolin. If the patient's vein becomes markedly distended because of the clot and is associated with severe pain, there is a possibility of suppuration. Consultation with a vascular surgeon may be prudent to determine if vein stripping is indicated.

Deep vein thrombosis or thrombophlebitis should, for the present, be managed with the combined use of intravenous antibiotics and heparin. Until the pathophysiology and natural history of this complication of pelvic infection is better understood, it is in the patient's best interest to treat the disease aggressively. One confusing aspect of this disease is that the patient need not be fully anticoagulated to resolve the condition. On the contrary, one standard regimen is as follows: intravenous clindamycin (900 mg every 8 hours), gentamicin dosed independent upon serum peak and trough levels, ampicillin (2 g every 6 hours), and heparin (10,000 units loading dose followed by 1000 units per hour). This regimen is continued until the patient's temperature, pulse rate, and white blood cell count return to normal. Therapy is continued until the patient has remained afebrile for 72 hours.

Individuals who develop pulmonary emboli require doses of heparin that achieve anticoagulent levels, and PTT monitoring. Following the completion of heparin, further anticoagulation is achieved with administration of coumadin for 6 months. The patient's coumadin therapy requires monitoring by the prothrombin time and maintaining the value at 2½ times the normal value. Patients require approximately 6 months of anticoagulant therapy.

REFERENCES

1. Amstey MT, Sheldon GE, Blyth JF: Infectious morbidity after primary cesarean sections in a private institution, *Am J Obstet Gynecol* 136:205, 1980.
2. Barefoot SF, Klaenhammer TR: Detection and activity of lactacin beta, a bacteriocin produced by *Lactobacillus acidophilus, Appl Environ Microbiol* 45:1808, 1983.
3. Benigno BB et al: A double-blind, controlled comparison of piperacillin and cefoxitin in the prevention of postoperative infection in patients undergoing cesarean section, *Surg Gynecol Obstet* 162:1, 1986.
4. Benigno BB et al: A comparison of piperacillin cephalothin and cefoxitin in prevention of postoperative infections in patients undergoing vaginal hysterectomy, *Surg Gynecol Obstet* 163:421, 1986.
5. Carlson C, Duff P: Antibiotic prophylaxis for cesarean delivery: is an extended spectrum agent necessary? *Obstet Gynecol* 76:343, 1990.
6. Castodot RG: Pregnancy termination: techniques, risks, and complications and management, *Fertil Steril* 45:5, 1981.
7. Charles D, Edwards WR: Infectious complications of cervical cerclage, *Am J Obstet Gynecol* 41:1065, 1981.
8. Cohen MP et al: Septic pelvic thrombophlebitis: an update, *Obstet Gynecol* 62:839, 1983.
9. Collins CG: Suppurative pelvic thrombophlebitis: a study of 202 cases in which the disease was treated by ligation of the vena cava and ovarian vein, *Am J Obstet Gynecol* 108:681, 1970.
10. Collins CG et al: Suppurative pelvic thrombophlebitis. I. incidence, pathology, etiology. II. symptomatology and diagnosis. III. surgical technique: a study of 70 patients treated by ligation of the inferior vena cava and ovarian vein, *Surgery* 50:198, 1951.
11. Cox SM, Gilstrap LC: Postpartum endometritis, *Obstet Gynecol Clin North Am* 16:363, 1989.
12. Dalen JE, Alpert JS: Natural history of pulmonary emboli, *Prog Cardiovasc Dis* 17:259, 1975.
13. Darling JR et al: Ectopic pregnancy in relation to previous induced abortion, *JAMA* 253:1005, 1985.
14. Elek SD, Conen PE: The virulence of *Staphylococcus pyogenes* for man: a study of the problems of wound infection, *Br J Exp Pathol* 38:573, 1987.
15. Emmons SL et al: Development of wound infections among women undergoing cesarean section, *Obstet Gynecol* 72:559, 1988.
16. Faro S: Antibiotic prophylaxis, *Obstet Gynecol Clin North Am* 16:27999, 1988.
17. Faro S, Phillips LE: Non-specific vaginitis or vaginitis of undetermined etiology, *Int J Tissue React* 9:173, 1987.
18. Faro S, Phillips LE, Martens MG: Perspectives on the bacteriology of postoperative obstetric-gynecologic infections, *Am J Obstet Gynecol* 158:694, 1988.
19. Faro S et al: Use of single agent antimicrobial therapy in the treatment of polymicrobial female pelvic infection, *Obstet Gynecol* 60:232, 1982.
20. Faro S et al: Influence of antibiotic prophylaxis on vaginal microflora, *J Obstet Gynecol* 6:51, 1986.
21. Faro S et al: Comparative efficacy and safety of mezlocillin, cefoxitin, and clindamycin plus gentamicin in postpartum endometritis, *Obstet Gynecol* 69:760, 1987.
22. Faro S et al: Piperacillin versus clindamycin plus gentamicin in the treatment of postpartum endometritis, *Curr Therap Res* 42:995, 1987.
23. Faro S et al: Ceftizoxime versus cefotaxime in the treatment of hospitalized patients with pelvic inflammatory disease, *Curr Therap Res* 43:349, 1988.
24. Faro S et al: Randomized double-blind comparison of mezlocillin versus cefoxitin prophylaxis for vaginal hysterectomy, *Surg Gynecol Obstet* 166:431, 1988.
25. Faro S et al: Ticarcillin/clavulanic acid versus clindamycin and gentamicin in the treatment of postpartum endometritis following antibiotic prophylaxis, *Obstet Gynecol* 73:808, 1989.
26. Faro S et al: Antibiotic prophylaxis: is there a difference? *Am J Obstet Gynecol* 162:900, 1990.
27. Freiman DG, Suyemoto J, Wessler S: Frequency of pulmonary thromboembolism in man, *N Engl J Med* 272:1278, 1965.
28. Fulkerson WJ et al: Diagnosis of pulmonary embolism, *Arch Intern Med* 146:961, 1986.
29. Garibaldi RA et al: Factors predisposing to bacteriuria during indwelling urethral catheterization, *N Engl J Med* 291:215, 1974.
30. Gibbs RS: Infection after cesarean section, *Clin Obstet Gynecol* 28:697, 1985.
31. Gil-Egea MJ et al: Surgical wound infections: prospective study of 4,468 clean wounds, *Infect Control* 8:277, 1987.
32. Gilstrap LC III and Cunningham FG: The bacterial pathogenesis of infection following cesarean section, *Obstet Gynecol* 53:545, 1979.
33. Gilstrap LC et al: Piperacillin versus clindamycin plus gentamicin for pelvic infection, *Obstet Gynecol* 64:762, 1984.
34. Grimes DA and Schulz KF: Morbidity and mortality from second trimester abortions, *J Reprod Med* 30:505, 1985.
35. Harstein AL et al: Nosocomial urinary tract infections: a prospective evaluation of 108 catheterized patients, *Inf Cont* 2:380, 1981.
36. Heisterberg L, Kringelbach M: Early complications after induced first trimester abortion, *Acta Obstet Gynecol Scand* 66:201, 1988.
37. Heisterberg L et al: Sequelae of induced first trimester abortion: a prospective study assessing the role of postabortal pelvic inflammatory disease and prophylactic antibiotics, *Am J Obstet Gynecol* 155:76, 1986.
38. Hemsell D et al: Preoperative cefoxitin prophylaxis for elective abdominal hysterectomy, *Am J Gynecol* 153:225, 1985.
39. Hull RD et al: Effectiveness of intermittent pneumatic leg compression for preventing deep vein thrombosis after total hip replacement, *JAMA* 263:2313, 1990.
40. Kaiser RE, Cerra FB: Progressive necrotizing surgical infections—a unified approach, *J Trauma* 21:349, 1981.
41. Kakkar VV et al: Natural history of post-operative deep vein thrombosis, *Lancet* 2:230, 1969.
42. Kunin CM, McCormack RC: Prevention of catheter-induced urinary tract infections by sterile closed drainage, *N Engl J Med* 274:1155, 1986.
43. Landefield CS, McGuire E, Cohen AM: Clinical findings associated with acute proximal deep vein thrombosis: a basis for quantifying clinical judgment, *Am J Med* 88:382, 1990.
44. Lensing AWA et al: Diagnosis of deep-vein thrombosis using an objective doppler method, *Ann Intern Med* 113:9, 1990.
45. Martens MG et al: Sulbactam/ampicillin versus metronidazole/gentamicin in the treatment of post-cesarean section endometritis, *Diagn Microbiol Infect Dis* 12:1895, 1989.
46. Martens MG et al: Transcervical uterine cultures with a new endometrial suction curette: a comparison of three sampling methods in postpartum endometritis, *Obstet Gynecol* 74:484, 1989.
47. Martens MG et al: Ampicillin/sulbactam versus clindamycin/gentamicin in the treatment of postpartum endometritis, *Am J Gynecol Health* 4:11, 1990.

48. Mical A, Cureole E, Lewis C: Cefoxitin sodium: double blind vaginal hysterectomy prophylaxis in premenopausal patients, *Obstet Gynecol* 56:222, 1979.

49. Mohr DN et al: Recent advances in the management of venous thromboembolism, *Mayo Clin Proc* 63:281, 1988.

50. Moser KM, LeMoine JR: Is embolic risk conditioned by location of deep venous thrombosis, *Ann Intern Med* 94:439, 1981.

51. Ortona L et al: A study of the incidence of postoperative infections and surgical sepsis in a university hospital, *Infect Control* 8:320, 1987.

52. Pelle H et al: Wound infection rate after cesarean section, *Infect Control* 7:456, 1986.

53. Philbrick JT, Becker DM: Calf deep vein thrombosis: a wolf in sheep's clothing? *Arch Intern Med* 148:2131, 1988.

54. Phillips LE et al: Isolation of *Mycoplasma* species and *Ureaplasma urealyticum* from obstetrical and gynecological patients by using commercially available medium formulations, *J Clin Microbiol* 24:377, 1986.

55. Phillips LE et al: Postcesarean wound infection by *Mycoplasma hominis* in a patient with persistent postpartum fever, *Diagn Microbiol Infect Dis* 7:193, 1987.

56. Rouse TM, Malangoni MA, and Schulte WJ: Necrotizing fasciitis: a preventable disaster, *Surgery* 92:762, 1982.

57. Stiver HG et al: Comparative cervical microflora shifts after cefoxitin or cefazolin prophylaxis against infection following cesarean section, *Am J Obstet Gynecol* 149:718, 1984.

58. Sullivan NM et al: Clinical aspects of bacteremia after manipulation of the genitourinary tract, *J Infect Dis* 127:49, 1973.

59. Tramer J: Inhibitory effect of *Lactobacillus acidophilus, Nature* 211:204, 1966.

60. Warren JW: Catheter-associated urinary tract infections, *Infect Dis Clin North Am* 1:823, 1987.

61. Westrom L et al: *Taxonomy of vaginosis—a definition.* In Mardh PA and Taylor-Robinson D, editors: *Bacterial vaginosis,* Uppsala, 1984, Almquist & Wiksell.

62. Wilson B: Necrotizing fasciitis, *Am J Surg* 18:416, 1975.

Part IV

SURGERY OF THE LOWER GENITAL TRACT

Chapter 16

MINOR AND AMBULATORY SURGERY

David H. Nichols

Surgeons may regularly perform minor gynecologic surgery in an office setting, although they generally perform procedures that require any significant surgical dissection in the operating room of an ambulatory care center or a hospital. Patients may not need anesthesia for the simplest maneuvers, such as endometrial biopsy, but if the discomfort is likely to be severe or more than momentary, they should receive effective anesthesia, often by local infiltration.

BIOPSY OF THE VULVA

Local anesthesia is appropriate for a patient undergoing biopsy of a suspicious lesion of the vulva. The surgeon can obtain a sample of the full thickness of the vulvar skin by using the Keyes skin biopsy drill (Fig. 16-1). Alternatively, a sharp biopsy punch can be used to obtain one or more specimens. Then the base of the donor site should be coagulated to minimize bleeding.

SURGERY OF BARTHOLIN'S GLAND

Although a Bartholin's cyst usually compresses Bartholin's gland around its deep periphery so that the gland may not be visible to the naked eye, the cyst is actually a cyst of the duct rather than of the gland. The surgical excision of such a cyst is often a formidable procedure because the vascularity of the tissues in this area may result in an unexpectedly high blood loss. Unless there is an opening to the external skin, the future secretions of the remaining buried but functional glandular tissue can reaccumulate and create a new and often symptomatic cyst that requires reexcision.

An acute Bartholin's abscess can be treated initially by aspiration through a no. 19 needle and syringe. The aspirate should be sent for bacteriologic identification, culture, and sensitivity testing. Cultures may show pure anaerobic,

aerobic, or mixed bacteria. Bacteriodes of various groups and Peptostreptococci are the most common anerobes, while *Escherichia coli* and *Neisseria gonorrhea* are predominant aerobes.[5] Meanwhile, the patient should begin a regimen of 400 mg of metronidazole 2 times daily and 250 mg of penicillin 4 times daily, both for 7 days. If the infecting organism is found to be *Neisseria gonorrhea*, the patient should be given 1 g of probenecid and 3.5 g of ampicillin. When tissue edema subsides, the patency and function of the duct return to normal in approximately 80% of cases.[8]

Incision and drainage of a Bartholin's abscess can be performed in the vestibular area close to the hymen through an area of fluctuation. The surgeon should make the incision between 1 and 2 cm in length and insert a drain or wick, which should remain in place for 24 hours. Because the skin heals and seals itself rapidly, recurrence is not uncommon, particularly if the infection has damaged the duct.

A simple alternative treatment of a Bartholin's cyst is to create a new duct by inserting a Word catheter through a stab wound into the cyst cavity, inflating the bulb with saline, and allowing it to remain in place for 3 to 4 weeks until the track of the wound has become epithelialized, forming the new duct (Fig. 16-2).[24] The surgeon should always inflate the bulb by using saline rather than air because the latter may permit premature deflation. While the small catheter is in place, the protruding proximal end can be tucked out of the way into the vagina. At the end of the 3- to 4-week period, the bulb on the catheter is deflated and the catheter removed. This procedure is particularly useful in the presence of infection.

A small Foley catheter can also be used to create a new duct. The surgeon inflates the bulb and tightly ligates the entire catheter approximately 3 inches from the site at

239

Fig. 16-1. Biopsy of vulvar skin using a Keyes punch. Site has been infiltrated with local anesthetic, and cutting end of punch is applied to site selected for biopsy. **A,** Pressure is applied lightly and the punch rotated back and forth *(arrows),* drilling a hole through full thickness of skin. **B,** Specimen disk is elevated with fine pointed forceps and cut away from subcutaneous tissue. Wound is cauterized for hemostasis. (With permission from Nichols DH, Evrard JR, editors: *Ambulatory gynecology,* Philadelphia, 1985, Harper & Row.)

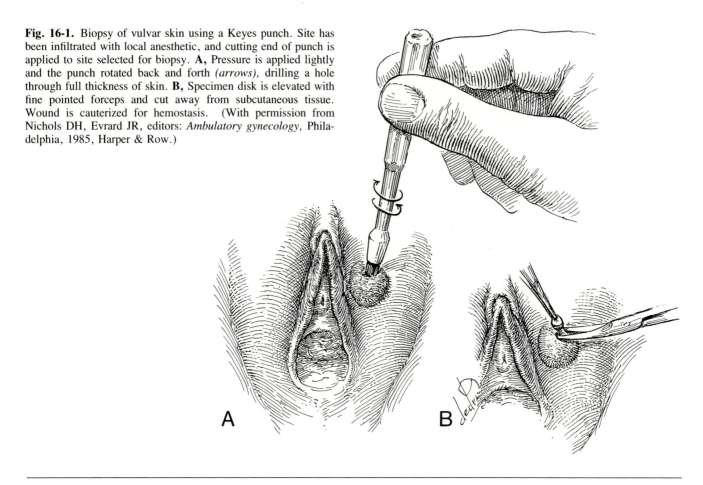

Fig. 16-2. Marsupialization of a Bartholin's cyst using a Word catheter. **A,** A stab wound is made through full thickness of right Bartholin's cyst at site chosen for the new duct. **B,** A Word catheter has been attached to a syringe containing 2 ml of sterile saline, and tip of catheter is quietly introduced into cyst cavity. **C,** Catheter bulb is inflated with saline, syringe removed, and free end of catheter tucked back into the vagina. Catheter should remain in place for several weeks, until the new duct has become epithelialized. Then bulb is deflated and catheter removed. (With permission from Nichols DH, Evrard JR, editors: *Ambulatory gynecology,* Philadelphia, 1985, Harper & Row.)

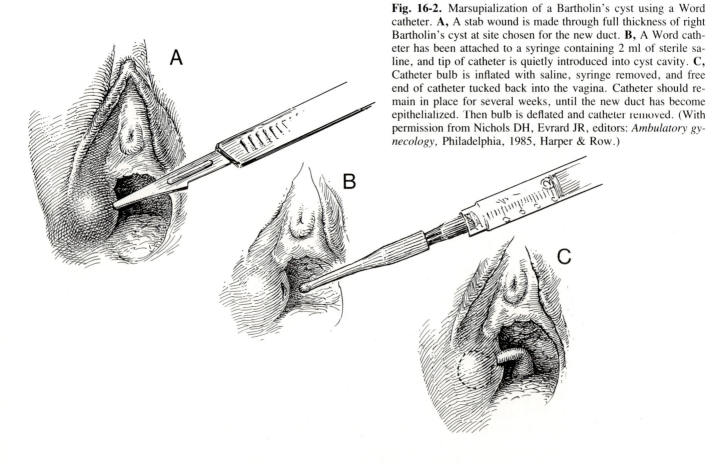

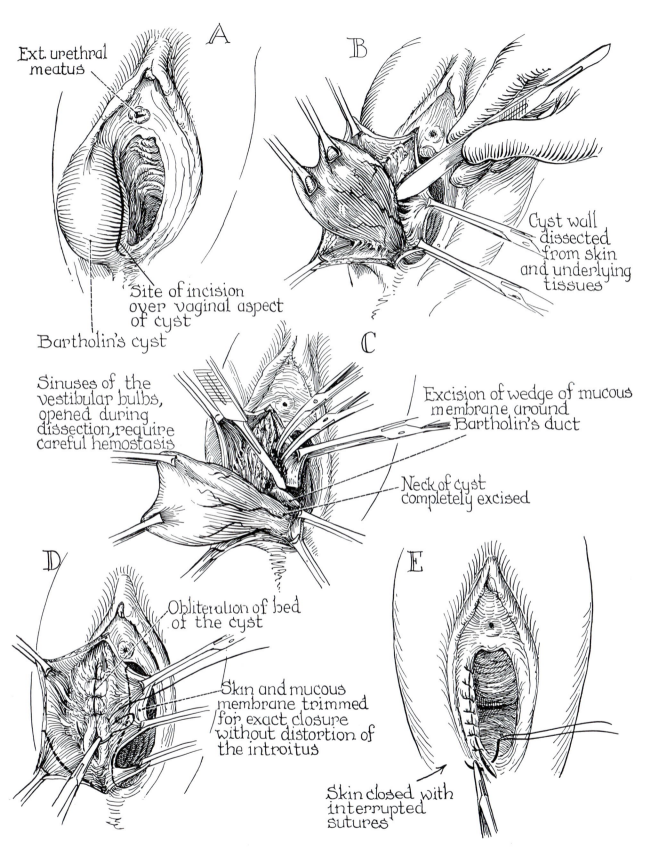

Fig. 16-3. Excision of a recurrent Bartholin's cyst. **A,** An incision is made near the hymenal margin, and **B,** the cyst dissected from the skin and underlying tissues, but **C,** leaving the flattened gland attached to the cyst wall. **D,** Excess skin is trimmed and the deeper tissues approximated with interrupted stitches. **E,** The skin is also closed with interrupted sutures. (From Ball TL: *Gynecologic surgery and urology*, ed 2, St Louis, 1963, Mosby–Year Book.)

which it enters the skin. The catheter may be transected just distal to the point of ligation, which should occlude both the central and side lumina. Again, the free end of the catheter can be tucked into the vagina.

A noninfected Bartholin's cyst that is recurrent following previous marsupialization may be treated by laser or by excision. If the gynecologist is comfortable with the use of the CO_2 laser, it is an effective and quick method of creating a new duct into a Bartholin's cyst.[22] A 1.5-cm oval defect is created by a circular incision with the laser from the vulvar skin into the cyst cavity at the site of the original duct tract. Antibiotics are not necessary, and healing is complete in about a month.[9] Retreatment can be offered if necessary, and the cyst wall vaporized with a defocused laser beam.[19]

Surgical excision of the cyst should be accomplished under general anesthesia, with great care taken to extirpate the Bartholin's gland itself. The gland is usually compressed beneath the wall of the cyst. It is flattened by the adjacent cyst and may be difficult to distinguish from the surrounding tissue, but if any fragment of gland remains behind, it will ultimately begin to secrete mucus, which, lacking a duct to the skin, will accumulate and form another cyst which may have to be retreated. The operation of excision is shown in Figure 16-3.

A large, uninfected Bartholin's cyst may be marsupialized. The surgeon cuts a window from the vestibular skin that includes the cyst wall and then sews the edge of the residual cyst lining to the vestibular skin by a series of interrupted through-and-through stitches. Healing leaves a permanent fistula between the cyst cavity and the skin, which essentially becomes a new duct. The ostium gradually contracts over a period of months so that in time it is scarcely visible, although it continues to be functional (Fig. 16-4).

A solid lesion within Bartholin's gland requires needle biopsy or surgical excision to exclude malignancy.[1] A tumor of the gland may be adenocarcinoma; a tumor of the duct, transitional or squamous cell carcinoma. Bartholin's carcinoma is serious and is generally treated by radical vulvectomy and bilateral groin dissection.

Excision of a benign vulvar fibroma is illustrated in Fig. 16-5.

LESIONS OF THE URETHRA

Prolapse of the urethra is common, particularly in postmenopausal women, although it occasionally occurs in newborns. It rarely causes bleeding, and if asymptomatic it need not be treated. Should it become a source of annoyance to the patient, it may be treated by excising the circular area and sewing the cut edge of wall of the urethra to the cut edge of the circumferential skin of the vulva by a series of interrupted sutures (Fig. 16-6).

When a lesion of the distal urethra causes bleeding, it is essential to differentiate the benign and relatively harmless urethral caruncle from the more ominous invasive carcinoma of the urethra. The carcinoma tends to be somewhat more friable and harder when palpated, but histologic examination of biopsy material is necessary to confirm the diagnosis. The treatment of caruncle is simple excision, but the treatment of carcinoma varies between interstitial radiation and radical surgery, depending on the circumstances of the particular case.

SURGERY OF THE HYMEN

Incision and hymenectomy are curative for an imperforate hymen. (Fig. 16-6). A small but rigid hymen that obstructs the vagina may be treated by hymenotomy at the 4 and 8 o'clock position; digital stretching by the patient maintains the opening during the healing phase. Midline perineotomy, sufficient to admit three fingerbreadths into the vagina, is the treatment of choice for a rigid, inelastic perineum. The edges of the incision should be sewn to the perineal skin transversely, at right angles to the original incision.

A patient who has recurrent postcoital cystitis may have a congenital anomaly of thick lateral bands connecting the urethral meatus to the hymenal margin. Urethrolysis at this site is curative (Fig. 16-7). Perineotomy does not always relieve introital stenosis (Fig. 16-8), which occurs most often in postmenopausal women, but Z-plasty is curative (Fig. 16-9).

VULVAR VESTIBULAR SYNDROME (FOCAL VULVITIS)

The abrupt onset of severe dyspareunia, usually in a young Caucasian patient with no visible outlet obstruction or palpable endopelvic pathology, suggests vulvar vestibular syndrome (focal vulvitis). The patient may have one or more areas of exquisite tenderness in the vestibule, most commonly in the posterior portion between the hymen and the vulvar skin. Gently touching this area with the end of a cotton-tipped applicator produces instant discomfort, and the site can be sharply demarcated. The condition has been identified from time to time for more than 100 years,[31] but it has received increased attention since 1981.[13-15,23,26,37-39]

The gynecologist may suggest alternative or noncoital means of sexual gratification for the couple, but 4% aqueous lidocaine (Xylocaine) saturating a cotton ball applied to the vestibular area some 15 minutes before coitus often provides sufficient temporary anesthesia for sexual relations. For the nonacetowhite lesion not associated with coincident human papillomavirus infection, a course of treatment may be initiated using 15 minute applications of these lidocaine-soaked cotton balls four times daily for a period of 6 months, if relief of symptoms is obtained. Xylocaine ointment may be applied to the area for temporary relief during the day. Because the use of oral contraceptives may exacerbate the condition, for reasons unknown, the patient should stop taking them for at least 6 months. Remission occurs in approximately 50% of cases.

If the syndrome persists after 6 months of observation and treatment, vestibulectomy and perineoplasty provides

Text continued on p. 248.

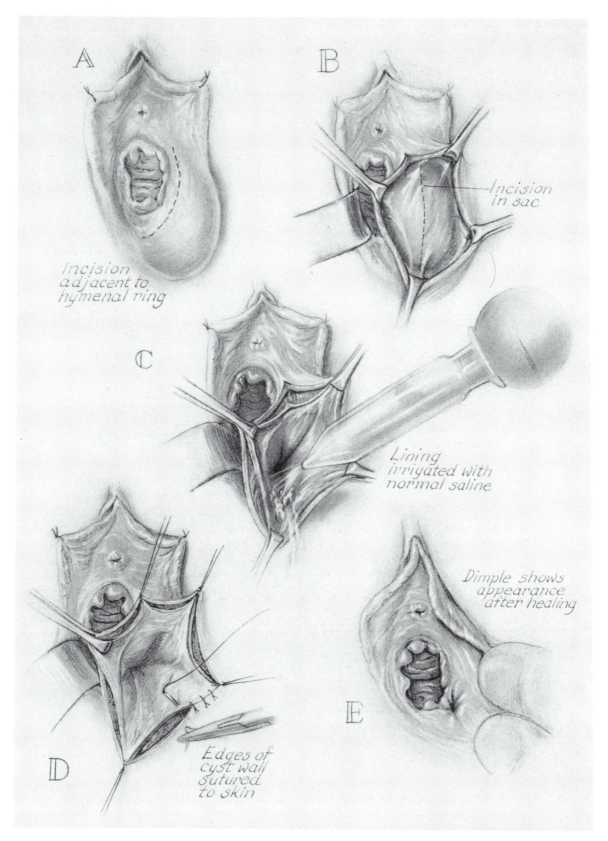

Fig. 16-4. Marsupilization of a Bartholin's cyst. **A,** An incision is made near the site of Bartholin's duct. The wall of the cyst is incised **(B)** and irrigated **(C),** and **D,** the edges of the cyst wall are sutured to the skin. **E,** The new orifice contracts with healing and is represented as a dimple at the site of the original duct. (From Ball TL: *Gynecologic surgery and urology,* ed 2, St. Louis, 1963, Mosby–Year Book.)

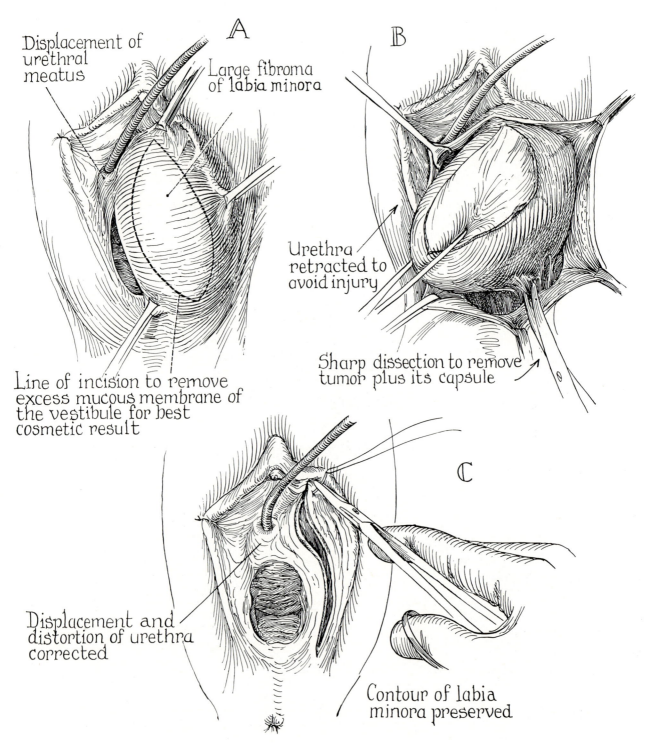

Displacement of urethral meatus

Large fibroma of labia minora

Line of incision to remove excess mucous membrane of the vestibule for best cosmetic result

Urethra retracted to avoid injury

Sharp dissection to remove tumor plus its capsule

Displacement and distortion of urethra corrected

Contour of labia minora preserved

Fig. 16-5. Excision of a labial fibroma. **A,** A large fibroma beneath the left labia is shown. It displaces the urethra to the patient's right. The skin incision to be made is shown by the dashed line. **B,** The tumor is removed using sharp dissection, and **C,** the incision closed using interrupted stitches. (From Ball TL: *Gynecologic surgery and urology*, ed 2, St Louis, 1963, Mosby–Year Book.)

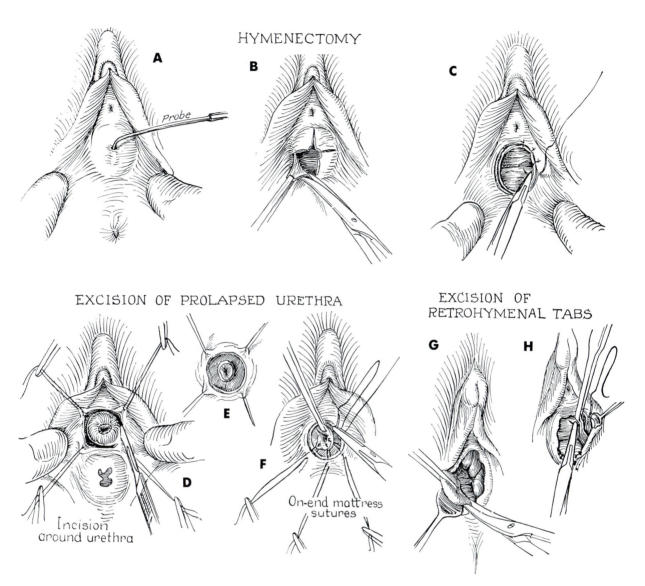

HYMENECTOMY

A

B *Probe*

C

EXCISION OF PROLAPSED URETHRA

EXCISION OF
RETROHYMENAL TABS

D

E

F

G

H

*Incision
around urethra*

*On-end mattress
sutures*

Fig. 16-6. Hymenectomy. **A,** The pinhole-sized hymenal opening is probed to determine the presence of a vaginal canal. A cruciate incision is made, and the hymen excised in quadrants (**B**) and the new edges approximated by interrupted sutures (**C**). Excision of prolapsed urethra. Guide sutures are placed and a circular incision made around the prolapsed urethra as shown (**D**). The prolapsed mucosa is excised (**E**), and interrupted mattress sutures are placed as shown (**F**) sewing the urethral mucosa to the skin of the vestibule. Excision of retrohymenal tabs. Painful retrohymenal tabs are grasped and excised at their base (**G**). Interrupted sutures bring the vaginal wall to the hymenal margin (**H**). Examination assures the surgeon that there is no postoperative introital obstruction. (From Ball TL: *Gynecologic surgery and urology*, ed 2, St Louis, 1963, Mosby–Year Book.)

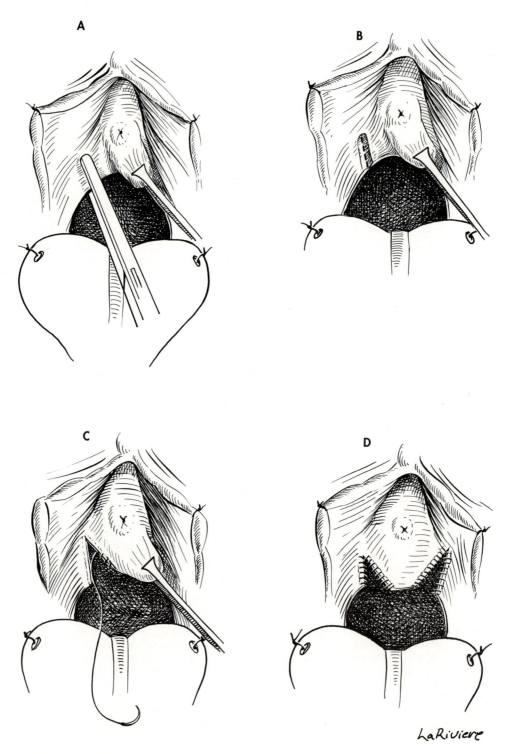

Fig. 16-7. Urethrolysis. **A,** Site of hymenal attachment to urethra is crushed in a forceps, first on one side and then the other. **B,** Incision to be made through crushed tissue is shown by broken line. **C,** Cut edge of incision is overcast by a running locked suture. **D,** End result. (After C Wood, Mason Clinic, Seattle, Wash.)

PLASTIC REPAIR OF CONSTRICTED INTROITUS

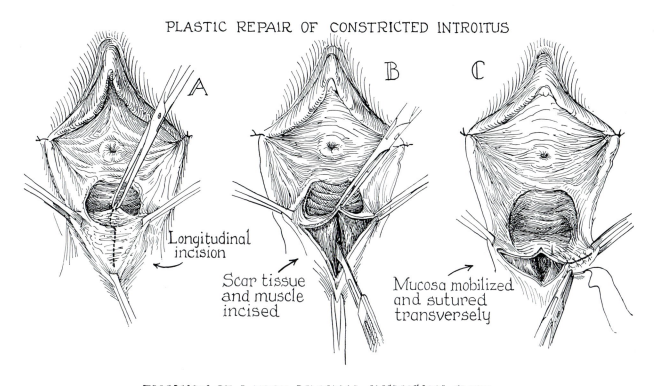

A

Longitudinal incision

B

Scar tissue and muscle incised

C

Mucosa mobilized and sutured transversely

EXCISION OF LARGE VAGINAL INCLUSION CYST

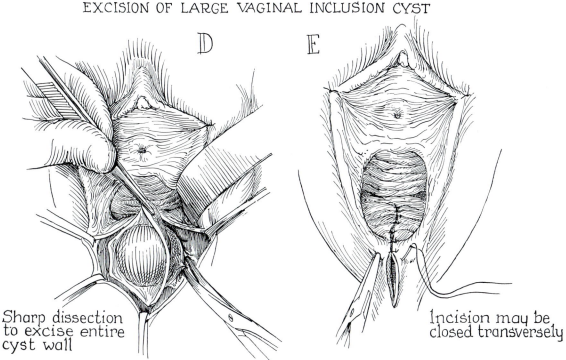

D

Sharp dissection to excise entire cyst wall

E

Incision may be closed transversely

Fig. 16-8. Plastic repair of constricted introitus. **A,** A midline incision is made in the skin of the perineum, and the extent of the subepithelial fibrosis is determined. Obstructive scar tissue, muscle, and fibrosis are incised **(B),** the flaps undermined, and the incision closed transversely using interrupted stitches. Excision of large vaginal inclusion cyst. When an inclusion cyst is the source of obstructive dyspareunia, it should be excised. **D,** A midline longitudinal incision is made and the cyst and its complete squamous epithelial lining are removed by sharp dissection. **E,** The incision is closed, but if the perineum is still obstructive, it may be closed transversely. (From Ball TL: *Gynecologic surgery and urology*, ed 2, St Louis, 1963, Mosby–Year Book.)

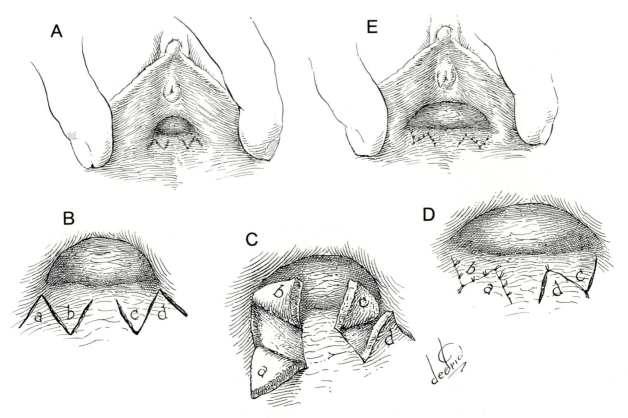

Fig. 16-9. Z-plasty. **A,** Preoperative introital stenosis, showing lines of incision. **B, C, D,** Full-thickness flaps are undermined, rotated, and sewn in place. **E,** Introital enlargement at conclusion of procedure. (With permission from Nichols DH, Randall CL: *Vaginal surgery*, ed 3, Baltimore, 1989, Williams & Wilkins.)

relief in most cases. The gynecologic surgeon should reconfirm the diagnosis preoperatively by examining the vestibule with a magnifying glass or low-power colposcope. There is often a cluster of raised pinkish or yellowish papules in the area of pain, and this specific site of pain may be carefully delineated with a marking pen immediately before the administration of anesthesia to ensure that the affected area is totally excised (Fig. 16-10). The full epithelial thickness, including the adjacent hymen of this sensitive area within the vestibule, should be excised. The full thickness of the posterior vaginal wall should be mobilized for 2 or 3 cm so that at the conclusion of the operation it can be brought down to cover this raw area; it is attached to the skin of the perineum by two layers of interrupted sutures.[37] Because postoperative oozing at this site is common, the patient may be kept in the hospital for a day or two postoperatively.

TREATMENT OF AN OBSTRUCTED VAGINA

A hemivagina associated with a didelphic uterus, or a bicornuate or septate vagina may be totally or partially obstructed. When the obstruction is complete, the patient has dysmenorrhea, and the monthly blood accumulates as a palpable mass in the lateral wall of the vagina.[36] The patient may also have congenital abnormalities of the urinary tract. The gynecologist can confirm the diagnosis by aspiration of old blood from the mass. Treatment is prompt marsupialization to create a large vaginal window that connects the two vaginal cavities.

EXCISION OF THE VAGINAL APEX

A precancerous lesion of the vaginal apex may be treated by full-thickness excisional biopsy (Fig. 16-11). Such a lesion may indicate vaginal intraepithelial neoplasia in a patient who had cervical intraepithelial neoplasia that was treated previously by hysterectomy, but the tissue must be studied in the laboratory to exclude possible unexpected invasion of the subepithelial tissues.

CULDOCENTESIS AND CULPOTOMY

Usually performed at a site in the midline of the upper posterior vaginal wall between the uterosacral ligaments, culdocentesis is useful in identifying the nature and character of any fluid that is distending the cul-de-sac of Douglas (Fig. 16-12). With the unanesthetized patient in the lithotomy position and the cul-de-sac exposed, the needle with syringe attached is against the cul-de-sac, and the patient is asked to cough. At the moment of the cough, the tip of the needle is quickly thrust through the vaginal wall into the cul-de-sac, and a sample of fluid aspirated. If

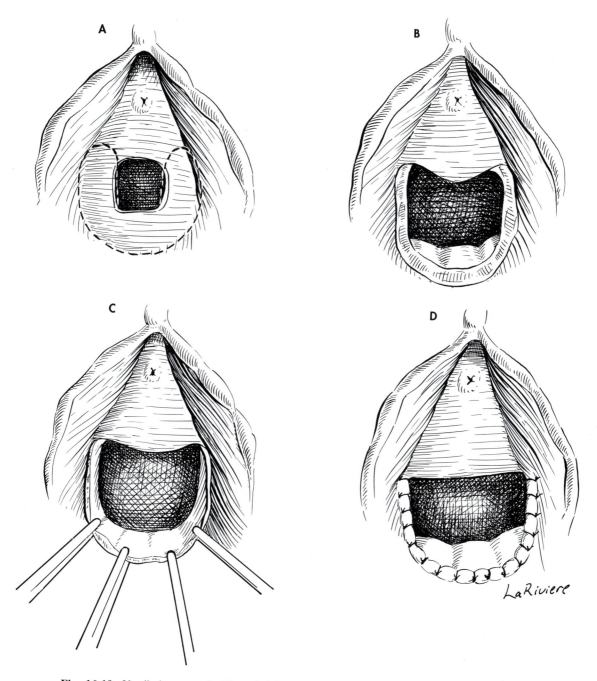

Fig. 16-10. Vestibulectomy. **A,** The painful area of vestibular skin is carefully demarcated preoperatively and an incision made lateral to this line of demarcation as shown by broken line. **B,** Full thickness of skin including adjacent hymen has been removed and any bleeding vessels clamped and ligated or electrocoagulated. **C,** Posterior vaginal wall has been mobilized and pulled down *(arrows)* to cover raw area. **D,** Full thickness of vagina is sewn to skin of vulva by two layers of interrupted synthetic absorbable sutures. Raw areas anterior or lateral to urethra may be left open to granulate in and avoid stricture.

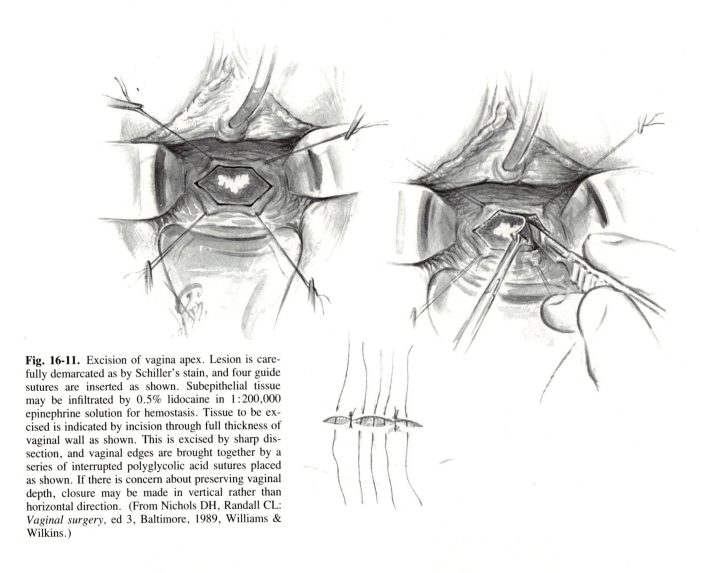

Fig. 16-11. Excision of vagina apex. Lesion is carefully demarcated as by Schiller's stain, and four guide sutures are inserted as shown. Subepithelial tissue may be infiltrated by 0.5% lidocaine in 1:200,000 epinephrine solution for hemostasis. Tissue to be excised is indicated by incision through full thickness of vaginal wall as shown. This is excised by sharp dissection, and vaginal edges are brought together by a series of interrupted polyglycolic acid sutures placed as shown. If there is concern about preserving vaginal depth, closure may be made in vertical rather than horizontal direction. (From Nichols DH, Randall CL: *Vaginal surgery,* ed 3, Baltimore, 1989, Williams & Wilkins.)

Fig. 16-12. Culdocentesis. Cervix has been steadied with a tenaculum, and a sharp pointed no. 18 needle attached to a syringe is inserted directly into the bulging cul-de-sac. The fluid is then aspirated and examined. (With permission from Nichols DH, Evrard JR, editors: *Ambulatory gynecology,* Philadelphia, 1985, Harper & Row.)

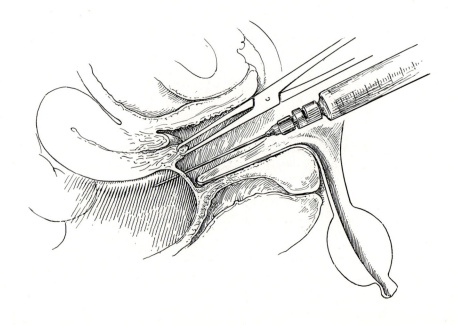

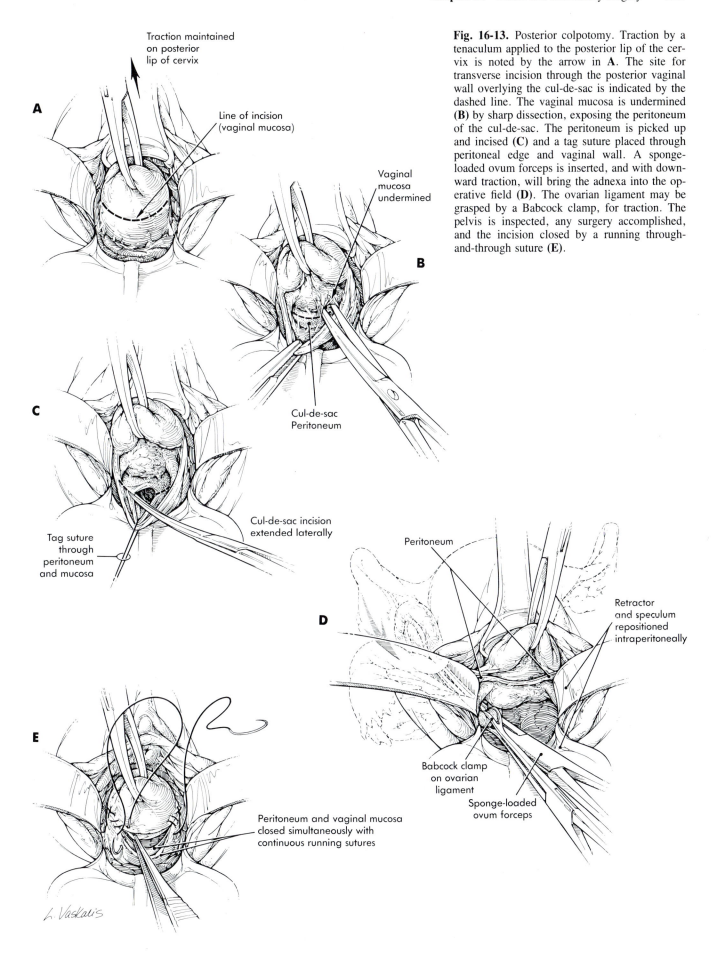

A Traction maintained on posterior lip of cervix

Line of incision (vaginal mucosa)

B Vaginal mucosa undermined

Cul-de-sac Peritoneum

C Tag suture through peritoneum and mucosa

Cul-de-sac incision extended laterally

D Peritoneum

Retractor and speculum repositioned intraperitoneally

Babcock clamp on ovarian ligament

Sponge-loaded ovum forceps

E Peritoneum and vaginal mucosa closed simultaneously with continuous running sutures

L. Vaskalis

Fig. 16-13. Posterior colpotomy. Traction by a tenaculum applied to the posterior lip of the cervix is noted by the arrow in **A**. The site for transverse incision through the posterior vaginal wall overlying the cul-de-sac is indicated by the dashed line. The vaginal mucosa is undermined (**B**) by sharp dissection, exposing the peritoneum of the cul-de-sac. The peritoneum is picked up and incised (**C**) and a tag suture placed through peritoneal edge and vaginal wall. A sponge-loaded ovum forceps is inserted, and with downward traction, will bring the adnexa into the operative field (**D**). The ovarian ligament may be grasped by a Babcock clamp, for traction. The pelvis is inspected, any surgery accomplished, and the incision closed by a running through-and-through suture (**E**).

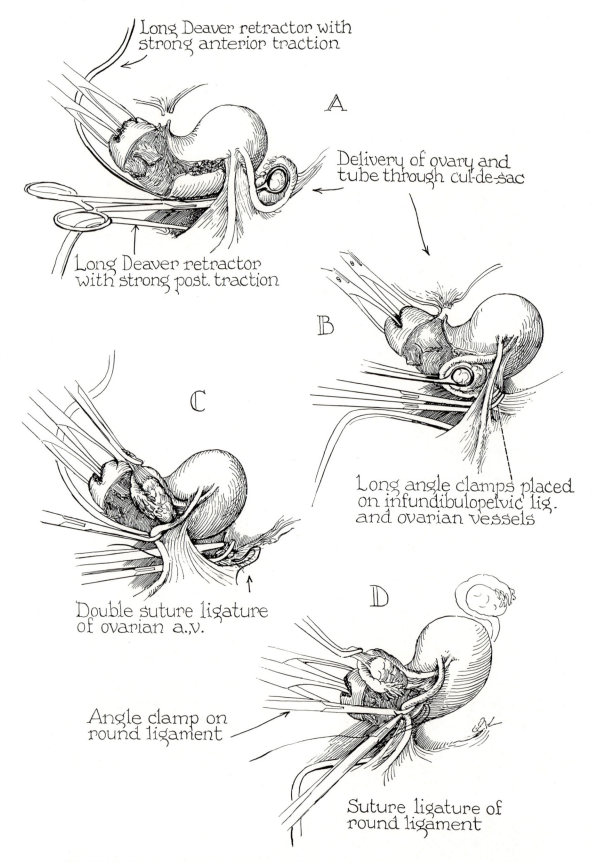

Fig. 16-14. Posterior colpotomy seen in sagittal section. A colpotomy has been made, and the left ovary grasped by a ring forceps (**A**). If ovary and the tube are to be removed, the infundibule pelvic ligament is clamped (**B**) and cut (**C**). Transfixion sutures replace the clamps. The round ligament may be clamped and ligated for additional exposure if necessary (**D**). (From Ball TL: *Gynecologic surgery and urology*, ed 2, St Louis, 1963, Mosby–Year Book.)

blood-tinged serous fluid is obtained, it may represent the presence of a follicle cyst, but if pure unclotted blood is aspirated, an ectopic pregnancy may be assumed.

When an abscess is suspected, the culdocentesis should take place in an operating room, and the needle should be inserted at the site of fluctuation, as determined by bimanual abdominal-rectal-vaginal palpation. If the fluid distending the cul-de-sac of Douglas is purulent, the surgeon should leave the needle in place, enlarge the entry into the cavity by surgical colpotomy, and institute drainage promptly. The abscess contents require prompt bacterial identification, culture, and sensitivity testing. Other aspirates are treated appropriately. Posterior culpotomy may permit direct examination and treatment of the adnexa. The technique is shown in Figure 16-13 and in sagittal section in Figure 16-14. If central dysmenorrhea is a significant complaint, the uterosacral ligaments may be clamped, and a segment resected to interrupt the nerve supply that runs through them to the uterus. A fold of peritoneum should be interposed between the cut ends of each ligament, to prevent nerve regeneration, and the tissues reunited[12] (Fig. 16-15).

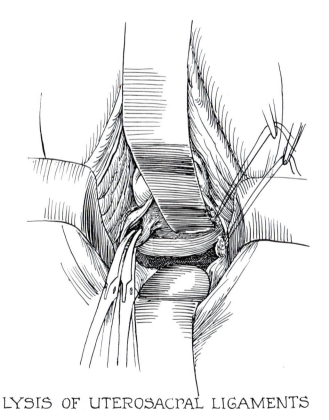

LYSIS OF UTEROSACRAL LIGAMENTS

Fig. 16-15. The Doyle procedure. The posterior cul-de-sac has been opened. The uterosacral ligaments may be clamped, cut, and tied. A fold of peritoneum is placed between the cut ends of each ligament, and they are reattached to the vagina and the incision closed. (From Ball TL: *Gynecologic surgery and urology*, ed 2, St Louis, 1963, Mosby–Year Book.)

EXCISION OF AN ENDOMETRIAL OR ENDOCERVICAL POLYP

The surgeon should excise in its entirety any polyp that protrudes through the external cervix and send it for prompt laboratory study. If the polyp is small, its base can be grasped within the jaws of a small hemostat and the polyp twisted off; it is better to remove a larger polyp by excision of its entire stalk. Because the site of the larger polyp's origin and attachment to the endocervix or endometrium is not usually visible, the polyp can be fed through the loop of a tonsil snare, the loop advanced within the endocervical or endometrial cavity until its progress stops, and the snare then slowly tightened to crush and transect the pedicle of the polyp (Fig. 16-16, *A* through *E*). If the stalk is so firm that it resists cutting by the snare, an electrosurgical cautery can be applied to the snare at the same time as pressure to the snare is made, and the stalk will be transected. A prolapsed submucous myoma or adenomyoma may be similarly excised. The procedure is simple and quick, and as the prolapsed tissue is usually infected, safer than hysterectomy.[4] Rarely, anterior vaginal hysterotomy may be employed (Fig. 16-16, *F* and *G*). A vaginal fibroma may be excised by sharp dissection (Fig. 16-17, *A* through *D*). The patient should be reexamined after a month to determine whether she has other polyps that should also be removed and studied.

TREATMENT OF A WOLFFIAN DUCT CYST

Large Wolffian duct cysts occasionally appear along the side walls or beneath the lateral surface of the vaginal apex. Filled with clear mucus,[28] they are anatomically separate from the urethra and bladder. If they are enlarging or causing dyspareunia, they should be treated, preferably by marsupialization. Excision sometimes leads to unexpectedly profuse bleeding, and there is a risk of ureteral ligation when deep sutures are placed at the base of the cyst cavity to control the bleeding (Fig. 16-17, *E* through *G*).

TREATMENT OF CERVICAL INTRAEPITHELIAL NEOPLASIA

Coincident with careful cytologic interpretation of the screening Papanicolaou smear, colposcopy permits gynecologists to locate the exact site of any epithelial abnormalities of the cervix, vagina, or vulva and to perform a biopsy on these suspicious areas for histologic study. Obviously invasive malignancy should be confirmed by the examination of tissue obtained by punch biopsy.

Cryosurgery and laser therapy

When the surgeon has identified a premalignant condition and can visualize the entire lesion colposcopically, a spectrum of definitive treatment is available to the patient. For example, premalignant lesions can be treated by cryosurgery[25,32,34] or laser vaporization* as alternatives to sur-

*References 2, 3, 6, 7, 21, 27, 30, 33, 34, 40.

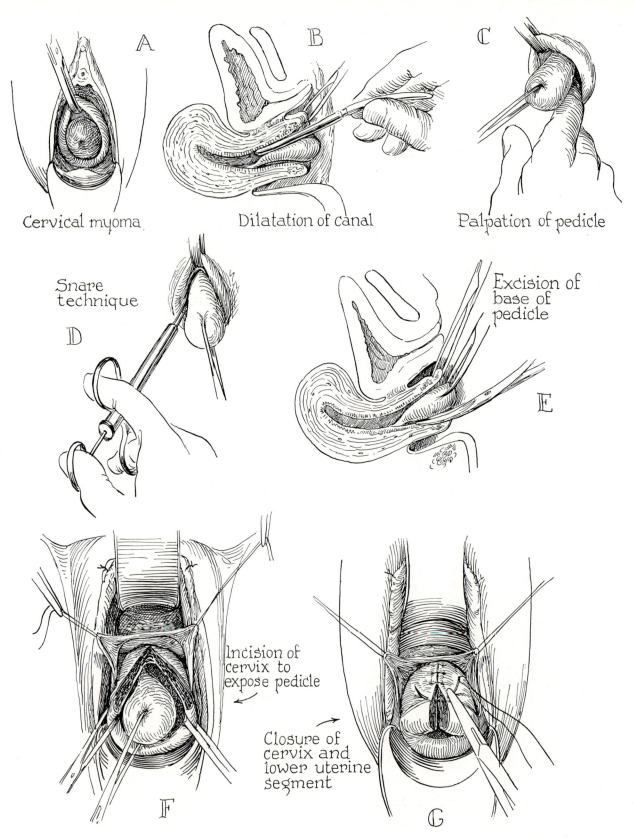

A
Cervical myoma

B
Dilatation of canal

C
Palpation of pedicle

Snare
technique

D

Excision of
base of
pedicle

E

Incision of
cervix to
expose pedicle

F

Closure of
cervix and
lower uterine
segment

G

Fig. 16-16. Pedunculated cervical myoma. **A,** The prolapsed cervical myoma is shown protruding through the external cervical os. **B,** The canal is dilated, and **C,** the pedicle palpated. **D,** The loop of a tonsil snare is passed around the myoma or polyp and advanced as far as it will go; the base is then crushed and transected by tightening the wire snare, and the lesion removed. Alternatively, the pedicle may be transected with scissors (**E**). Anterior vaginal hysterotomy. When the prolapsed polyp or fibroid is too large to be delivered, a transverse incision may be made in the anterior vaginal wall, the bladder dissected from the cervix and retracted out of harm's way, and a longitudinal incision made in the cervix anteriorly (**F**). The myoma is removed, and the incision in the cervix closed by interrupted sutures (**G**), and the transverse vaginal incision closed separately. (From Ball TL: *Gynecologic surgery and urology*, ed 2, St Louis, 1963, Mosby–Year Book.)

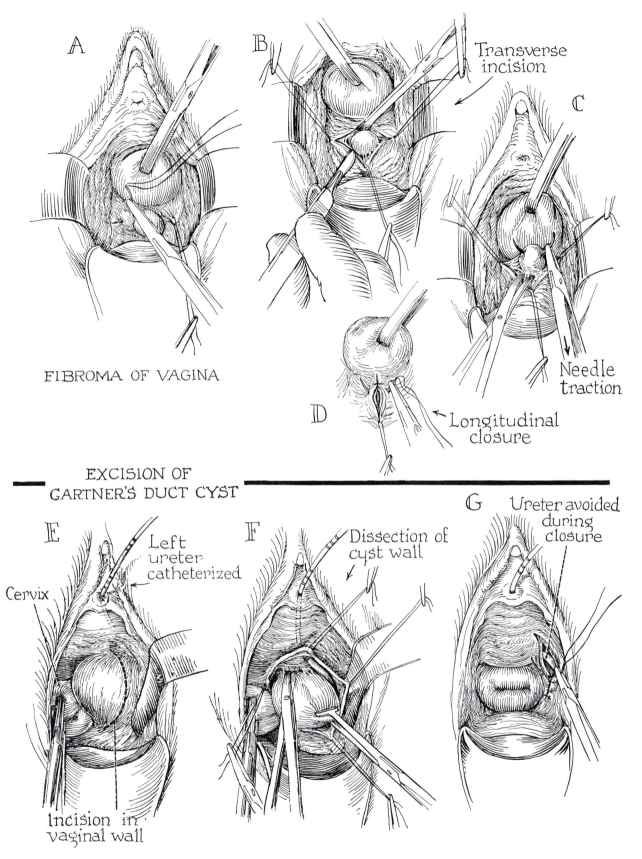

A

B Transverse incision

C

Needle traction

FIBROMA OF VAGINA

D Longitudinal closure

EXCISION OF
GARTNER'S DUCT CYST

G Ureter avoided during closure

E Left ureter catheterized

Cervix

Incision in vaginal wall

F Dissection of cyst wall

Fig. 16-17. Excision of a vaginal fibroma. **A,** Guide sutures are placed lateral to each side of the fibroma, and **B,** a transverse incision through the vagina made between them, exposing the fibroma. It may be fixed with a needle for traction, and removed by sharp dissection (**C**), and the vaginal incision closed longitudinally (**D**). Excision of Gartner's duct cyst. **E,** An incision is made as shown by the dashed line overlying the cyst. A ureteral catheter has been placed in the left ureter to aid in its identification during the operation. **F,** The cyst is removed by sharp dissection, and **G,** the incision closed after hemostasis has been obtained; the ureter is avoided scrupulously. The catheter is then removed. (From Ball TL: *Gynecologic surgery and urology*, ed 2, St Louis, 1963, Mosby–Year Book.)

gical excision. This subject is discussed more fully in Chapter 18.

When a patient with cervical intraepithelial neoplasia wishes to preserve her uterus so that she can become pregnant, among the options for treatment of her condition are (1) cryosurgery, (2) laser surgery, (3) electrodissection (LEEP), and (4) electrocoagulation. A treatment other than hysterectomy is permissible, however, only if the following conditions are met:

1. The surgeon must be able to visualize the abnormal epithelium completely.
2. The result of endocervical curettage must be negative.
3. The findings of cytology must be consistent with the findings of colposcopy.
4. The patient must be willing to participate in long-term follow-up.

Conization of the cervix

When it is not possible to estimate the endocervical extent of a lesion with certainty and the findings of endocervical curettage are inconclusive—or when a colposcopically directed biopsy shows microinvasion, or possible microinvasion, of a malignancy—conization becomes necessary for study of the entire lesion. When this condition is discovered during pregnancy, when the squamocolumnar junction everts, a shallow "coin biopsy"–type conization avoids the potentially dangerous excision of the endocervix.[10] The placement of six purse-string sutures close to the vaginal reflection reduces eversion of the squamocolumnar junction and prevents excessive blood loss.[11]

Although diagnostic conization has been largely replaced by colposcopically directed biopsy, conization continues to be valuable in the investigation required by discovery of a malignant noninvasive lesion or an abnormal result on a Papanicolaou smear when the squamocolumnar junction is so high that it cannot be visualized and a biopsy cannot be performed. The procedure is primarily diagnostic, but it may be therapeutic under certain circumstances, such as when the gynecologist can visualize the entire lesion and can include it within the surgical specimen. Because intraepithelial neoplasia is commonly multicentric, excision of the entire lesion does not preclude future development of other areas of dysplasia or carcinoma in situ, however.

Technique of conization. In recent years, most gynecologists have discontinued the practice of routine preoperative shaving of vulvar and suprapubic hair before a conization, although it is sometimes helpful to clip long hair to keep it out of the way.[35]

A simple technique of conization that provides adequate hemostasis consists of infiltration of the cervical stroma with not more than 50 ml of 0.5% lidocaine (Xylocaine) in 1:200,000 epinephrine solution. This causes a marked spasm of cervical blood vessels that produces a visible blanching of the cervix. With a no. 11 pointed scalpel, a cone of tissue of the proper size is removed, up to but not

including the internal cervical os. (Although some gynecologists prefer laser conization, the so-called cold-knife conization is entirely effective.) It is absolutely essential that the axis of the cone parallel the axis of the vagina and cervix; perforation of the uterus at the apex of the cone can damage the neighboring organs and tissues.

The 12 o'clock position on the surgical specimen may be marked by a suture. Bleeding or oozing points should be coagulated with the electrosurgical unit. As an alternative procedure for preliminary hemostasis, deep hemostatic sutures of absorbable material may be placed in the 3 and 9 o'clock positions. If significant oozing occurs immediately, which happens only rarely, a more hemostatic "hot" electroconization may follow. This procedure is not performed routinely, because if the initial conization does not remove the entire lesion, electroconization leaves no fresh adjacent tissue to study by immediate biopsy. In addition, the tissue destruction causes significant postoperative cervical scarring. Once the cone of cervical tissue has been obtained and the numerous bleeding points coagulated, the cervix is packed for 24 to 48 hours with ¼-inch iodoform gauze. The subject of conization is discussed more fully in Chapter 17.

Complications of conization. Hemorrhage may occur either at the time of conization or within the first postoperative weeks. Visible bleeding points should be electrocoagulated; if there is a general ooze, the area should be suture-ligated. Mild bleeding may be stopped by application of the tip of a silver nitrate stick or a cotton applicator soaked in negatol (Negatan) or Monsel's solution. If this is not successful, packing the affected area with microfibrillar collagen (Avitene) is generally effective. (Avitene attracts functioning blood platelets, which adhere to the microfibrils and thus trigger the formation of thrombi in the adjacent tissue. Although more expensive, it is more effective than either Gel-Foam or Surgicel.) A "pulsating" ooze should be treated by a carefully placed suture. If bleeding recurs, bilateral transvaginal ligation of the uterine artery may be required. Rarely, hysterectomy or internal iliac ligation may be required to control excessive recurrent postoperative bleeding, particularly if the conization has transected a major branch of the uterine artery and the artery has retracted into the substance of the cervix or lower uterine segment.

Cervical stenosis is the principal long-range complication of inadvertent resection or trauma to the internal cervical os. After conization, the cervix heals by scar formation; contraction of the scar tissue may reduce the diameter of the canal and lead to a stenosis or stricture. The gynecologist who performs a conization of the cervix must make certain that the patient's cervical canal does not become stenotic after the operation because stenosis may progress to occlusion and then to amenorrhea, hematometra, and possibly endometriosis. The patient must be advised to return for postoperative examinations at regular intervals for at least 6 months. At each visit, the gynecologist should test the patency of the cervical canal by carefully passing a small dilator or sound through the canal and inner os.

The cervix tending to stenosis cannot always be dilated sufficiently without anesthesia to alter the progressive tightening of scar tissue. In this case, the use of a laminaria tent for 24 hours has been recommended.[17] The operator must not allow the laminaria tent to slip into the uterine cavity, however, for it will swell, making it difficult to remove from the uterus without the insertion of a second laminaria tent to dilate the cervix. If a stenosis does develop, dilating the canal while the patient is under anesthesia and suturing an old-fashioned stem pessary into the canal to be worn for several months (or until it falls out) may be preferable to occasional, usually futile, sounding or dilation in the office or clinic. A stenosis may require long-term treatment by periodic endocervical dilation until the surface of the cervix has been reepithelialized, the scar stabilized, and healing completed.

"Hot" conization has little place in the treatment of chronic cervicitis. The procedure is not cost-effective in such cases. Moreover, it carries additional risks, including the formation of scar tissue and its troublesome sequelae. When endocervicitis causes a chronic leukorrhea that distresses the patient enough to require treatment, strip cauterization or electrocoagulation of the affected area of the cervix may be the procedure of choice. Because infection often involves the depths of the endocervical glands, superficial cauterization of the cervix by local applications of a caustic or silver nitrate is not indicated.

Conization and curettage: preferred sequence. The indications for conization and fractional curettage do not often coexist, but the procedures are not mutually exclusive. If the conization that precedes curettage is carefully done, the results of the fractional curettage can be satisfactory.[20] Identity of the source of the tissue specimens is generally better, however, if the conization takes place after the cervix and uterus have been sounded but before the curette is used in the canal or uterine cavity. An external mucocutaneous junction around the margin of an erosion can, of course, be removed with a large biopsy loop without coagulating the endocervix. Even when the conization involves the excision of 1 or 2 cm of the endocervix, as it usually does, the gynecologist can use the small, sharp curette to determine if there is any friable tissue or a softened area in the lower uterine segment adjacent to the inner os that suggests malignancy. When such curettage of the endocervix does not suggest carcinoma, it will probably be necessary to dilate the inner os in order to admit a larger curette and polyp forceps to the uterine cavity.

When a dilation and curettage (D and C) and conization are to be performed on the same patient at the same time, the D and C is done immediately *after* the conization—never before.

DILATION AND CURETTAGE

A most frequently performed surgical procedure in gynecology is cervical dilation and uterine curettage. Referred to universally as D and C, this operation is often the first surgical procedure to be undertaken by the physician who is preparing to specialize in obstetrics and/or gynecology. The technique of D and C is not difficult to learn; in fact, few surgical procedures are as straightforward or routine.[16]

Conventional D and C of the uterus is performed for the following reasons:

1. To evaluate abnormal uterine bleeding when the cervical os is so tight that an endometrial biopsy cannot be performed
2. To evaluate and diagnose the cause of postmenopausal uterine bleeding when endometrial biopsy has not made the diagnosis clear
3. Immediately preceding hysterectomy in a patient with abnormal uterine bleeding, to uncover positive or suspicious endometrial findings that may influence the operative decision
4. To empty the uterus of its contents when unwanted products of conception remain, as after an incomplete abortion
5. In the patient with intractable menorrhagia and an enlarged uterus, to distinguish between adenomyosis interna and uterine leiomyomata, particularly submucous leiomyomata, and thus to determine the appropriate treatment
6. To complete the work-up of an infertility patient with leiomyomata when a hysterogram has not revealed the location and types of leiomyomata present (e.g., submucous)
7. To evaluate the condition of a patient with an abnormal Papanicolaou smear when there is no gross or colposcopically visible lesion of the cervix
8. To free adhesions and possibly insert an intrauterine device to keep the walls of the uterine cavity apart during the healing process in a patient with known or suspected intrauterine synechiae (Asherman's syndrome)

Although a D and C may be performed with the patient under analgesia only or under local anesthesia (i.e., paracervical block), it is generally performed with the patient under brief general or regional anesthesia so that the gynecologist can carefully examine the internal genitalia without causing the patient any discomfort.

Operating room procedure manuals create both dogma and confusion regarding the degree of surgical preparation that a patient needs for a D and C. Recommendations seem to be based principally on the site at which the procedure will take place. In all instances, cleansing or bacteriostatic douches, pubic shaving, and enemas are not only unnecessary but add to the patient's discomfort.

Setting for D and C

A D and C is ideally suited to an ambulatory setting. For a D and C in this setting, the vagina and cervix are painted with a solution of povidone iodine (Betadine). Instruments are sterile, draping is minimal, and the surgeon, whose hands have been washed but not necessarily scrubbed, wears sterile gloves.

In the hospital operating room, a D and C is generally done under maximum aseptic techniques because the gravid, atrophic, or cancerous uterus is easily perforated and may become infected. After the patient has been prepared with nonabrasive perineal and vaginal wash, the operative area is painted with povidone iodine (Betadine). The patient is fully draped, and instruments are sterile. The surgeon is fully gowned, masked, capped, and gloved.[18]

Technique of D and C

Suction curettage may be used to complete an abortion (see Chapter 62). If suction curettage is not available, conventional curettage may be used to remove retained products of conception (Fig. 16-18). When curettage is to be performed on a recently pregnant uterus, an oxytocic should be administered either intramuscularly or intravenously; such an injection produces a firm contraction of the myometrium, thus increasing its resistance to perforation. Often a *dull* curette will be used in the uterus of pregnancy to avoid the removal of too much endometrium.

Outpatient curettage of the nonpregnant uterus with the Vabra suction apparatus can be preceded by the administration of analgesia or a paracervical block. In the majority of diagnostic cases, uterine curettage should be done fractionally with a sharp curette.

When the patient is under anesthesia, the gynecologist should first perform a careful examination. This always provides vital information, sometimes unexpected, that is useful in diagnosis and future clinical management. It may also provide valuable information about the appropriate route and technical details of a possible future hysterectomy. The size, shape, and mobility of the uterus; the location and size of the cul-de-sac; and the strength and elasticity of the uterosacral ligaments, the cardinal ligaments, and the urogenital diaphragm should all be noted.

After determining the axis and size of the uterus, the operator grasps the anterior cervical lip with a tenaculum for traction and carefully scrapes the endocervical canal with a small, sharp curette (e.g., the Duncan) up to, but not beyond, the internal cervical os. Curettage may begin at the 12-o'clock position and proceed in a careful clockwise or counterclockwise direction around the circumference of the cavity. The curettings are saved on a piece of Telfa or gauze to be examined separately from the curettings obtained later from the endometrial cavity.

A blunt-tipped, malleable Simpson uterine sound should then be bent to accommodate the anteflexion, anteversion, retroflexion, or retroversion of the uterus. It is best to grasp the sound at its round shaft. Holding it firmly by the flat part of the end impedes the tendency of the sound to follow the path of least resistance, the axis of the uterus. The force exerted on both sound and curette during their introduction into the uterine cavity should be mini-

mal, similar to that required to hold a pencil for writing; forceful insertion increases the risk of perforation.

After the sound has been gently inserted into the uterine cavity, the depth of the cavity from the external cervical os to the top of the fundus should be carefully measured. Establishing the size of the endometrial cavity tells the operator the precise depth to which the curette may be passed during the curettage. The cervical canal and internal cervical os are then expanded by the passage of graduated dilators until they are large enough to permit introduction of the largest size curette or polyp forceps that will be used during the procedure. Gradual dilation with the patient under anesthesia markedly reduces the risk of rupture or permanent damage to the musculature of the cervix.

Gently introducing a sharp curette into the endometrial cavity until it reaches the top of the fundus, the operator grasps the handle firmly and, by traction against the resisting uterus, scrapes the endometrial cavity with the curette down to, but not through, the presumed basal layer. In an orderly clockwise or counterclockwise direction, the operator scrapes all segments and quadrants of the endometrium. Scraping is stopped when the passage of the sharp edge of the curette across the surface of the endometrium produces the delicate sensation of a "grating" resistance, characteristic of the basal layer.

After the endometrium has been curetted in this orderly fashion and any submucous irregularities, diverticula, or septa in the uterine cavity have been noted, the separate curettings of the endometrium and the endocervix (which have been saved on a separate piece of Telfa or gauze) are carefully examined and palpated. The experienced clinician often recognizes evidence of the difference between malignancy and endocrine dysfunction by the gross appearance of the endometrial fragments. (No therapy should be initiated, however, before histologic confirmation.) Benign tissue is soft and spongy; when squeezed, it is somewhat elastic and resists shattering. Fragments of normal endometrium, both proliferative and premenstrual, or secretory, can usually be smoothed out on a sponge, where they appear to be fragments of relatively thin or thick membrane. In contrast, malignant tissue tends to be hard and rather fragile; if squeezed gently, it fragments and shatters. When placed on a sponge, these fragments appear to be bits of tissue that have more of a third dimension and are unlikely to smooth out as a membrane would.

The operator should then explore the cavity of the uterus with polyp or kidney stone forceps because the curette may miss an endometrial polyp of almost any size, particularly if the polyp has a narrow base. After the polyp forceps has been introduced, the jaws are opened and then closed in various quadrants of the uterine cavity; after each closing, a tug is made to see if any resistance is encountered. If this procedure locates a narrow-based polyp of a size that permits it to negotiate the dilated cervical canal, it can be removed safely by twisting the forceps.

After the removal of all instruments, the operator should carefully inspect the uterus and cervix. If there is

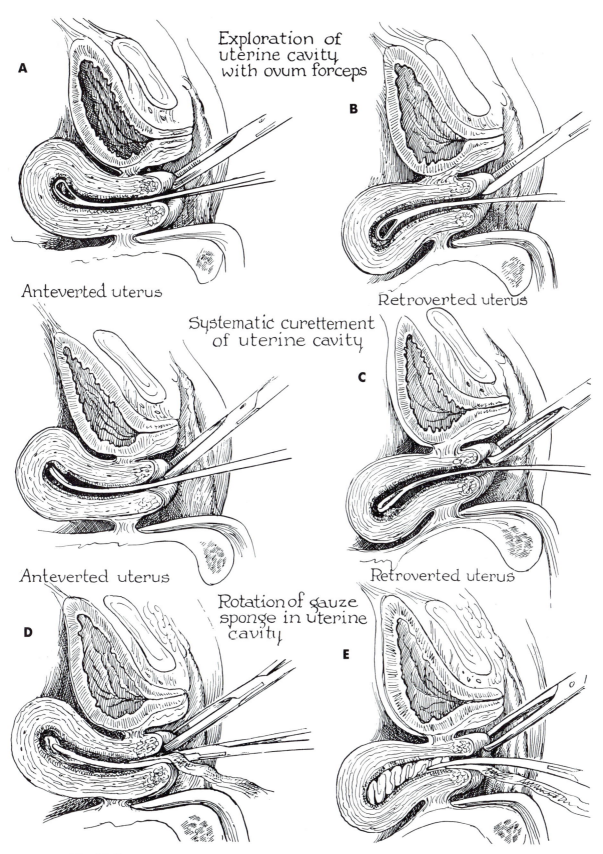

Exploration of uterine cavity with ovum forceps

A Anteverted uterus

B Retroverted uterus

Systematic curettement of uterine cavity

C Retroverted uterus

Anteverted uterus

Rotation of gauze sponge in uterine cavity

D Anteverted uterus

E Retroverted uterus

Fig. 16-18. Dilation and curettage for incomplete abortion. The cervix is grasped with a clamp, and the canal gently and progressively dilated. If the uterus is retroverted, the curve of the dilation is reversed. The uterine cavity may be explored digitally, and the retained products of conception extracted by an ovum forceps (**A**), introduced in reverse direction if the uterus is retroverted (**B**). Other fragments are gently removed. The uterine cavity may be *lightly* curetted by a large dull curette (**C**), and **D**, the cavity packed with a saline soaked sponge, which is rotated and extracted (**E**). (From Ball TL: *Gynecologic surgery and urology*, ed 2, St Louis, 1963, Mosby–Year Book.)

much fresh bleeding from the endometrial cavity, the uterine cavity should be carefully sounded to ensure that the uterus was not perforated nor was the endocervix lacerated. Should either of these events have occurred, appropriate observation and treatment should be instituted. Excessive bleeding from tenaculum marks on the cervix can be cauterized, or a gentle and temporary packing can be placed against the face of the cervix.

The operative report should be dictated immediately, while all the details of each procedure are fresh in the surgeon's mind. A plan should be made for the removal of any packing that was used. The patient or her family should be informed of the operative findings and discharge instructions, and arrangements should be made for postoperative evaluation and follow-up.

Complications of D and C

Although a minor surgical procedure, a D and C must be performed with delicacy and precision if it is to be effective. Done carelessly, forcefully, or thoughtlessly, the procedure can cause serious harm to the patient.

Uterine perforation. If the length of the sound or curette that has passed into the uterine cavity is longer than the measured length of that cavity, the uterine wall has been perforated. When such a perforation has occurred, the instrument may be introduced all the way to its handle without any resistance. Uterine perforation generally results from a failure to identify the axis of the cavity of the uterus, which may often be in anteflexion or retroflexion, and the subsequent use of force in introducing the instrument into the uterine cavity, often on the presumption that it is negotiating a somewhat stenotic internal os. The myometrium that is soft because of pregnancy or invasion by malignant tumor can be perforated quite easily (Fig. 16-19).

When the *sound* has perforated the uterus, the operator should promptly withdraw the instrument. Little of consequence will usually follow. The position of the uterus should be carefully determined by bimanual examination and the sound bent so as to negotiate the uterine cavity safely. If the sound has been reinserted along the axis of the uterine cavity, the insertion will generally stop when the tip of the instrument has reached the fundus of the uterus. The operator can then continue the procedure to completion.

If, following perforation of the uterine wall with the sound, the proper axis of the uterus cannot be determined, it is best to discontinue the procedure and reschedule it for some future date, at which time the myometrium will have had an opportunity to heal. The patient should be told postoperatively of the perforation and should be watched for tachycardia, hypotension, abdominal tenderness, fever, and other signs of intraperitoneal bleeding or of uterine or pelvic infection. Any of these signs will be evident within 24 hours.

If the tip of the sharp curette has perforated the uterus and the surgeon does not realize it, curettage may cause serious damage to the visceral contents of the pelvis. If the curettings contain evidence of perforation (e.g., intestinal epithelium, bowel wall tissue, or bowel contents), immediate laparotomy is essential to repair the damage. If the operator strongly suspects that the intestine has been damaged, but the character of the curettings fails to confirm this suspicion, a preliminary diagnostic laparoscopy may be of value. If it appears that the bowel has not been damaged, the patient may be observed only.

Curettage and Asherman's syndrome. In carefully, thoroughly, and systematically removing the tissue that lines the uterine cavity, the operator must always be mindful of the possibility that an overthorough curettage can remove literally all of the endometrium and thus result in amenorrhea. This most unfortunate result of a curettage, known as Asherman's syndrome, most commonly occurs after a particularly thorough effort to clean out an aborting uterus.

It is not the technique of curetting so much as the status of the myometrium that largely determines the risk of removing too much endometrium. The deeper invaginations of endometrial tissue into the myometrium are not usually removed during even a thorough curettage of the nonpregnant uterus, and these undisturbed portions of endometrium generally proliferate rapidly after a curettage. Because the myometrium of the pregnant or aborting uterus is relatively soft and relaxed, however, the curette tends to spread the myometrial fibers more readily; as a result, curetting removes endometrial tissue at a much greater depth than it would if the myometrial tone was that of a nonpregnant uterus. Therefore, when curettage of an aborting uterus is indicated, an operator should avoid overvigorous curettage to decrease the risk of removing too much endometrium. Intravenous or intramuscular injection of an oxytocic (e.g., Ergotrate, Methergine, Pitocin) 2 or 3 minutes before curettage of the uterine cavity should ensure firm contraction of the myometrium.

Endocervical stenosis. If endocervical stenosis in a patient who is about to undergo a D and C is so severe that it is possible to insert only a small and very narrow sound or probe and not possible to dilate the endocervical canal significantly, the surgeon may insert a small laminaria tent along the path of the sound and reschedule the D and C 24 hours later. At that time the laminaria tent may be removed; the cervix will be sufficiently dilated to permit insertion of a small curette. For the diagnosis of abnormal uterine bleeding, aspiration biopsy is a faster and less costly alternative to D and C.[29]

OFFICE ENDOMETRIAL BIOPSY FOR AMBULATORY PATIENTS

Endometrial biopsy done as an office procedure on a fully ambulatory patient often identifies a malignancy in the endocervix or in the uterine cavity. It is best, however, to depend on the result of biopsy and to plan therapy for endocervical or endometrial malignancy only when the pathology report identifies it. As the first step of therapy, the

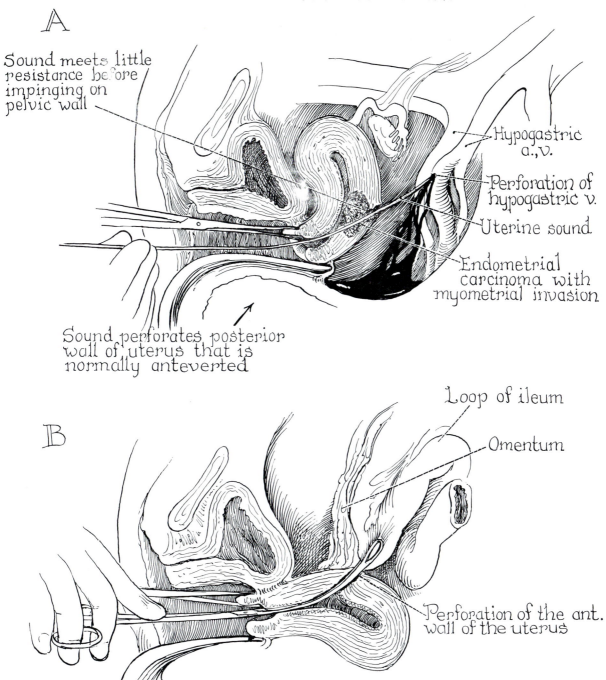

PERFORATION OF THE UTERUS
WITH LACERATION OF A MAJOR VESSEL

A

Sound meets little
resistance before
impinging on
pelvic wall

Hypogastric
a., v.

Perforation of
hypogastric v.

Uterine sound

Endometrial
carcinoma with
myometrial invasion

Sound perforates posterior
wall of uterus that is
normally anteverted

B

Loop of ileum

Omentum

Perforation of the ant.
wall of the uterus

PERFORATION OF A RETROVERTED UTERUS
BY OVUM FORCEPS WITH CRUSHING INJURY
TO BOWEL AND OMENTUM

Fig. 16-19. Perforation of uterus at curettage. **A,** Failure to recognize axis of a markedly anti-flexed uterus may lead the curette to perforate the posterior wall of the uterus. **B,** Similarly, perforation of the anterior wall of the uterus may occur when retroflexion is present. (With permission from Ball TL: *Gynecologic surgery and urology*, ed 2, St Louis, 1963, Mosby–Year Book.)

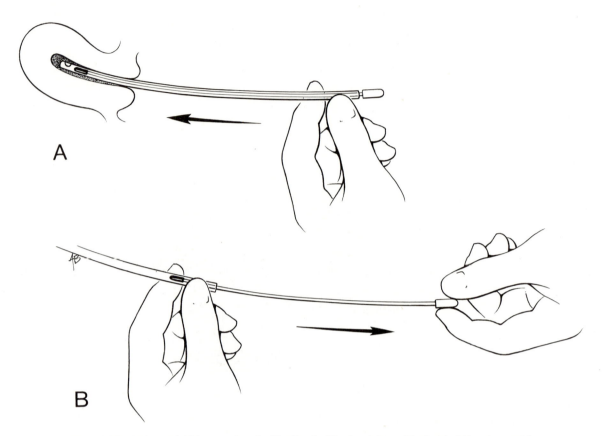

Fig. 16-20. Endometrial biopsy using the Pipelle. **A,** Plastic curette with sheath fully advanced is inserted through cervix into full depth of endometrial cavity. A tenaculum may be used to steady the cervix if necessary. **B,** While holding sheath, piston is quickly and fully withdrawn from it until it is stopped and locked in position. Sheath is rotated as it is moved back and forth several times to sample the endometrium. Then it is withdrawn and the tip cut off and discarded. Contents of the hollow tube are expressed into a specimen jar by pushing plunger to its original position. (With permission from Nichols DH, Randall CL: *Vaginal surgery*, ed 3, Baltimore, 1989, Williams & Wilkins.)

gynecologist should make a careful appraisal of the clinical stage of the malignancy based on findings on examination under anesthesia and during a prehysterectomy fractional curettage of the cervix and uterine cavity.

It is equally important to perform operating room fractional curettage when the results of biopsies taken in the office or clinic are negative and there is a clinical suspicion of malignancy. Preliminary hysteroscopy may help to identify and localize any suspicious areas or sites of the endometrium. First the endocervical canal and then the uterine cavity must be thoroughly explored. In the uterus, the use of both the polyp forceps and a curette, usually larger than that employed in the cervix, ensures detection of a pedunculated polyp or an infiltrating malignancy. When a patient experiences recurrent abnormal or postmenopausal bleeding despite a benign or negative sampling, hysteroscopy may help establish the diagnosis.

Many gynecologists are no longer using rigid, hollow steel curettes of varying sizes for endometrial biopsy; instead they are using a flexible plastic Pipelle-type curette, which is an inexpensive and disposable unit (Fig. 16-20).

Because it is only 3.1 mm in outer diameter, its insertion is virtually painless and can be done without preliminary dilation or anesthesia. After the insertion of its tip into the uterine cavity, suction is applied by traction on a built-in plunger, and the tip is moved back and forth several times within the cavity as the hollow tube is rotated. In this way, the four quadrants of the endometrial cavity are sampled quickly. The curette is removed from the uterus and the tip is cut off. By pushing the plunger to its original position, the contents of the hollow tube are expressed into a specimen jar.

REFERENCES

1. Axe S et al: Adenomas in minor vestibular glands, *Obstet Gynecol* 68:16, 1986.
2. Baggish MS, Dorsey JH: CO$_2$ laser for the treatment of vulvar carcinoma-in-situ, *Obstet Gynecol* 57:371, 1981.
3. Baggish MS: Management of cervical intra-epithelial neoplasia by CO$_2$ laser, *Obstet Gynecol* 60:378, 1982.
4. Ben-Baruch G et al: Immediate and late outcome of vaginal myomectomy for prolapsed pedunculated submucous myoma, *Obstet Gynecol* 72:858, 1988.

5. Brook I: Aerobic and anaerobic microbiology of Bartholin's abscess, *Surg Gynecol and Obstet* 169:32, 1989.

6. Burke L: The use of carbon dioxide laser in the therapy of cervical intra-epithelial neoplasia, *Am J Obstet Gynecol* 144:337, 1982.

7. Capen CV et al: Laser therapy of vaginal intra-epithelial neoplasia, *Am J Obstet Gynecol* 142:973, 1982.

8. Cheetham DR: Bartholin's cyst: marsupialization or aspiration? *Am J Obstet Gynecol* 152:569, 1985.

9. Davis GD: Management of Bartholin duct cysts with the carbon dioxide laser, *Obstet Gynecol* 65:279, 1985.

10. DiSaia PJ: *Microinvasive cancer of the cervix in pregnancy.* In Nichols DH, editor: *Clinical problems, injuries and complications of gynecologic surgery,* ed 2, Baltimore, 1988, Williams & Wilkins.

11. DiSaia PJ, Creasman WT: *Clinical gynecologic oncology,* ed 2, St Louis, 1984, Mosby–Year Book.

12. Doyle JB: Paracervical uterine denervation of the cervical plexus for relief of dysmenorrhea, *Am J Obstet Gynecol* 70:1, 1955.

13. Friedrich EG: The vulvar vestibule, *J Reprod Med* 28:773, 1983.

14. Friedrich EG: Vulvar vestibulitis syndrome, *J Reprod Med* 32:110, 1987.

15. Goetsch MF: Vulvar vestibulitis: prevalence and historic features in a general gynecologic practice population, *Am J Obstet Gynecol* 164:1609, 1991.

16. Grimes DA: Diagnostic dilation and curettage: a reappraisal, *Am J Obstet Gynecol* 142:1, 1982.

17. Hale RW, Pion RJ: Laminaria: an underutilized clinical adjunct, *Clin Obstet Gynecol* 15:829, 1972.

18. Haskins A: Questions and answers, *JAMA* 241:623, 1979.

19. Heah J: Methods of treatment for cysts and abscesses of Bartholin's gland, *Br J Obstet Gynaecol* 195:321, 1988.

20. Helmkamp GF et al: Cervical conization: when is uterine dilatation and curettage also indicated? *Am J Obstet Gynecol* 146:893, 1983.

21. Kaufman RH, Friedrich EG: The carbon dioxide laser in the treatment of vulvar disease, *Clin Obstet Gynecol* 28:220, 1985.

22. Lashgari M, Keene M: Excision of Bartholin duct cysts using the CO_2 laser, *Obstet Gynecol* 67:735, 1986.

23. McKay M et al: Vulvar vestibulitis and vestibular papillomatosis—report of the ISSVD Committee on Vulvodynia, *J Reprod Med* 36:413, 1991.

24. Nichols DH, McGoldrick KL: *Minor and ambulatory surgery.* In Nichols DH, Evrard JR, editors: *Ambulatory gynecology,* Philadelphia, 1985, Harper & Row.

25. Ostergard DR: Cryosurgical treatment of cervical intra-epithelial neoplasia, *Obstet Gynecol* 56:231, 1980.

26. Peckham BM et al: Focal vulvitis: a characteristic syndrome and cause of dyspareunia, *Am J Obstet Gynecol* 154:855, 1986.

27. Raphael SI, Burke L: *Laser and cryosurgery.* In Nichols DH, Evrard JR, editors: *Ambulatory gynecology,* Philadelphia, 1985, Harper & Row.

28. Rock JA, Azziz R: *Wolffian duct cyst at the vaginal vault.* In Nichols DH, editor: *Clinical problems, injuries and complications of gynecologic surgery,* ed 2, Baltimore, 1988, Williams & Wilkins.

29. Smith JJ, Schulman H: Current dilation and curettage practice: a need for revision, *Obstet Gynecol* 65:516, 1985.

30. Stafl A, Wilkinson EJ, Mattingly RF: Laser treatment of cervical and vaginal neoplasia, *Am J Obstet Gynecol* 128:128, 1977.

31. Thomas TG: *Hyperaesthesia of the vulva.* In *The diseases of women,* Philadelphia, 1880, Henry C Lea.

32. Townsend DE: Cryosurgery for CIN, *Obstet Gynecol Surv* 34:828, 1979.

33. Townsend DE, Richart RM: Cryotherapy and the carbon dioxide laser management of cervical intra-epithelial neoplasia: a control comparison, *Obstet Gynecol* 61:75, 1983.

34. Townsend DE et al: Treatment of vaginal carcinoma-in-situ with the CO_2 laser, *Am J Obstet Gynecol* 143:565, 1982.

35. Walton LA, Baker VV: *Mechanical and chemical preparation of the abdomen and vagina.* In Buchsbaum HJ, Walton LA, editors: *Strategies in gynecologic surgery,* New York, 1986, Springer-Verlag.

36. Wiser WL: *Mass in the lateral wall of the vagina.* In Nichols DH, editor: *Clinical problems, injuries and complications of gynecologic surgery,* ed 2, Baltimore, 1988, Williams & Wilkins.

37. Woodruff JD, Friedrich EG: The vestibule, *Clin Obstet Gynecol* 28:134, 1985.

38. Woodruff JD, Genadry R, Poliakoff S: Treatment of dyspareunia and vaginal outlet distortions by perineoplasty, *Obstet Gynecol* 57:750, 1981.

39. Woodruff JD, Parmley THG: Infection of the minor vestibular gland, *Obstet Gynecol* 62:609, 1983.

40. Wright CV, Cavies E, Riopelle MA: Laser surgery for cervical intra-epithelial neoplasia: principles and results, *Am J Obstet Gynecol* 145:181, 1983.

Chapter 17

CONIZATION OF THE UTERINE CERVIX

Erich Burghardt
Frank Girardi

The new ablative techniques were once considered a major advance of modern gynecology. Today, the pendulum is swinging back. It again seems better to remove a premalignant or malignant lesion in such a manner that it can be subjected to histology for an accurate diagnosis rather than to ablate or vaporize it. Whether excision is performed with a diathermy loop, laser, or scalpel is of secondary importance.

The poor reputation of conization stemmed neither from an absent rationale for the procedure nor from inevitable complications or consequences. Wrong indications, poor technique, poor histologic processing of the specimen, and economic pressure brought the technique into disfavor. Many conizations were performed because of abnormal cervical cytology[7,29]; suspect findings at colposcopy[6,16]; or mild and possibly reversible cervical intraepithelial neoplasia (CIN).[45] Too much or too little tissue was removed for the lesion present.[2,46,52] Incorrect technique led to an inordinate number of complications.[29,46,48] Cursory histologic processing meant that incomplete excision of CIN was not recognized[1] and that invasive lesions were missed or their extent was underestimated.[9,47,51] Cold knife conization, which usually requires hospitalization, came under economic pressure because superficial, ablative techniques could be performed on an outpatient basis.[41] These factors led to the opinion that conization was a procedure to be performed only for a few indications, such as lesions extending into the cervical canal.

INDICATIONS

Strictly, there are only two, albeit related, indications for conization.

1. Complete excision of histologically verified epithelial atypia for a definitive diagnosis.
2. An attempt at cure by complete excision of the lesion.

Conization should be performed only when a directed biopsy has revealed CIN III or persisting CIN II, or CIN I.[41] Persistence should have been demonstrated by repeated colposcopically guided biopsies of the lesion, positive cytology, or both at intervals of 6 months to 1 year. Endocervical curettage should be performed in patients with abnormal cytology but a colposcopically normal ectocervix. In patients with abnormal cervical cytology and negative biopsy, cytology should be repeated after 3 to 4 months; biopsy should be repeated if cytology remains abnormal.

The goal of these indications is to avoid unnecessary conizations. In countries with no tradition of colposcopy, the method was advocated with the slogan "colposcopy saves conizations."[16] This slogan betrays that many conizations were performed without a true substrate and without an adequate indication.

A suspicion of microinvasive carcinoma (FIGO stage Ia) is a third, albeit rare, indication for conization. If a directed biopsy has led to the suspicion of invasion, but colposcopy shows no more than the suspicion of microcarcinoma,[11,12] conization is indicated because appropriate histology can evaluate and stage the lesion accurately.

FUNDAMENTAL PATHOLOGY OF THE CERVICAL EPITHELIUM

Physicians performing conizations should have a working knowledge of colposcopy and the pathology of the cervix. Discussions of a possible viral genesis of cervical lesions including carcinoma have again moved into the foreground theories that postulate that cervical cancer originates from a single transformed cell.[5,56] Such concepts are based more on theory than on the natural history of cervical cancer. Step-serial sections of conization specimens permit detailed studies of the pathologic processes of the cervix and their relationship to their surroundings. Such studies have led to the following findings:

1. CIN always develops in sharply demarcated fields.
2. CIN never exceeds the boundaries of the fields in the sense of superficial spread.
3. Numerous fields containing different variations of CIN can occur on the same cervix.
4. Invasion happens after a cell or cell clone within the field of CIN realizes the potential for invasive growth. This is where the unicellular origin of carcinoma begins.
5. Invasion generally occurs only after large areas of the cervix have been occupied by CIN.

A conization specimen can have different angles. Its axis will be longer the more acute the angle. How to shape the cone depends on the extent and location of the lesion to be removed. Lesions occupying a large area on the ectocervix but reaching into the cervical canal (thus obscuring the squamocolumnar junction) can be expected to involve only the lower part of the canal; a flat cone should be obtained in such a case (Fig. 17-1, *A*). A lesion close around the external os may reach far up the canal, in which case a steep cone should be obtained (Fig. 17-1, *B*).

Gland involvement usually occurs only in CIN III and can only occur where CIN III arose in the gland field.[10] This can be within the transformation zone after extensive ectopy or in the cervical canal. In the first case, colposcopy usually shows cuffed gland openings or ovula nabothi within the fields of CIN.[12] Also, a mosaic or punctated area commonly occurs outside of the transformation zone; in this case, gland involvement is not possible. It is

thus contradictory to state that these lesions develop "within an atypical transformation zone."[17] This has been accounted for in the 1990 colposcopy terminology determined by the Nomenclature Committee of the International Federation of Cervical Pathology and Colposcopy.[49]

COLD-KNIFE CONIZATION
Technique

Cold-knife conization is performed with the patient under general anesthesia. The cervix is grasped with two pairs of tenaculum forceps at the 3 o'clock and 9 o'clock positions and pulled outward (Fig. 17-2, *A*). Excision of the cone is made much easier by first infiltrating the cervix with saline to which ornipressin, a synthetic vasopressin, has been added (5 IU per 200 ml saline). Depending on the size of the cervix, 30 to 70 ml of the solution are infiltrated. The cervix swells during infiltration, and the mucosa pales markedly (Fig. 17-2, *B*). Staining the glycogen-containing squamous epithelium dark brown with iodine solution sharply demarcates the suspicious area, which is almost always iodine-negative (Fig. 17-2, *C*). When the cone is excised, the cervical stroma that has been infiltrated with ornipressin is white and rarely bleeds (Fig. 17-2, *D*). Once the cone has been circumcized and only the apex of the cone remains to be divided, the tenaculum forceps are applied to the wound (to avoid disrupting the epithelium) and pulled outward, and the apex is severed. The wound is coagulated with a ball electrode of an electrocoagulation device; special attention is paid to point bleeders (Fig. 17-2, *E*). This contributes to hemostasis and contracts the surface of the wound by vaporizing the ornipressin solution (Fig. 17-2, *F*). The wound is tamponaded with a gauze strip for 24 to 48 hours.

Six weeks after conization, the cervix looks like that of a nullipara. Only bimanual palpation of the uterus reveals some effacement. Colposcopy typically shows circumoral streaks (subepithelial scars) around the external os (Fig. 17-3).

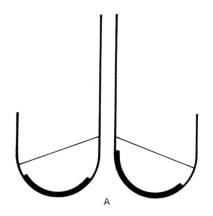 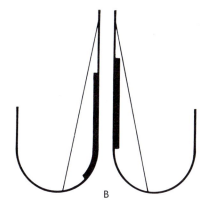

Fig. 17-1. Schematic representation of different types of cones. **A,** A shallow cone suffices for lesions primarily on the ectocervix. **B,** A long, narrow cone is required for lesions in the cervical canal.

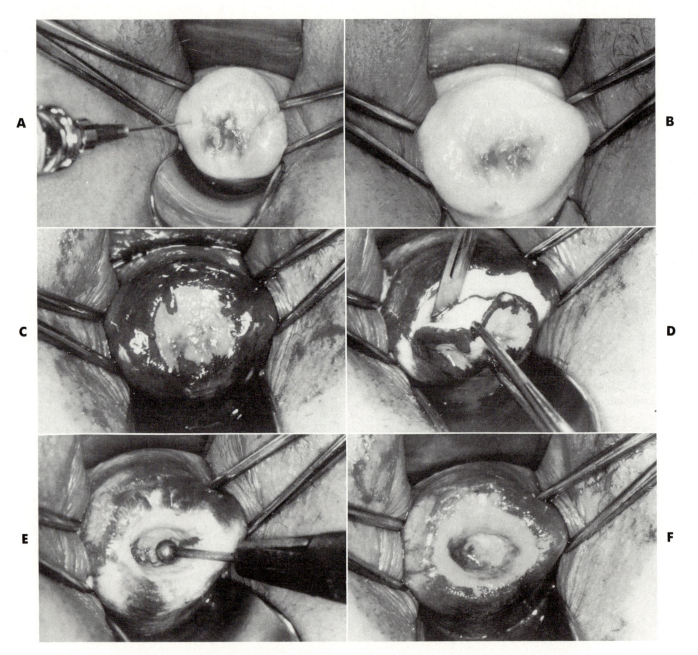

Fig. 17-2. Technique of cold-knife conization. **A,** The cervix is grasped with two pairs of tenaculum forceps at the 3 o'clock and 9 o'clock positions and pulled outward. The needle for infiltration is inserted outside the lesion. **B,** After injection at several points, the cervix is swollen and pale. **C,** After application of iodine (Schiller's test), the suspicious area, which is almost always iodine-negative, is sharply demarcated. **D,** During excision of the cone, the cervical stroma that has been infiltrated with ornipressin is white and rarely bleeds. Once only the apex of the cone remains to be divided, the tenaculum forceps are applied to the wound (to avoid disrupting the epithelium), pulled outward, and the apex is severed. **E,** The wound is coagulated with the ball electrode of an electrocoagulation device. **F,** The cervix after coagulation. See Color Plate 1, facing pp. 274 and 275.

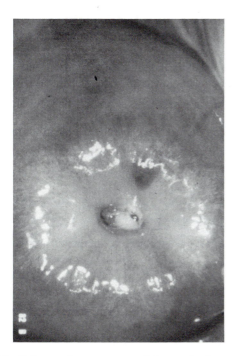

Fig. 17-3. Colposcopic appearance of the cervix 2 months after conization. The external os resembles that of a nullipara. See Color Plate 2, facing p. 275.

Table 17-1. Complications of conization in 5234 patients between 1958 and 1984

Complication	No.	%
Perforation	3	0.05
Hemorrhage	329	6.3
Transfusion	56	1.0
Infection	12	0.2
Stenosis	38	0.7

Table 17-2. Hemorrhage after conization in 1119 patients between 1981 and 1988

	No.	%
Hemorrhage	55	5
Treatment		
Conservative	13	24
Gauze tamponade	25	45
Electrocoagulation	7	13
Suture	10	18

Table 17-3. Outcome after conization during pregnancy in 91 patients

Outcome	No.	%
Term delivery	64	70
Preterm delivery	8	9
First trimester abortion	2	2
Second trimester abortion	7	8
Legal abortion	8	9
Stillborn infant	2	2
TOTAL	91	100

Complications

The complications associated with the technique described above are shown in Table 17-1. Postoperative bleeding is the most common complication, usually occurring between 6 and 8 days after surgery and rarely exceeding the strength of a menstrual period. In the authors' experience, 69% of bleeding complications have been managed conservatively; 31% required electrocoagulation or suture (Table 17-2). One percent of the patients required blood transfusion. Sturmdorf (inverting) sutures should be avoided because of the scarring and stenosis of the cervical canal they cause. With the technique described above, fewer than 1% of the patients developed cervical stenosis, which is easily treated by dilation.

CONIZATION DURING PREGNANCY

For technical reasons, conization should be performed only in early pregnancy.[26,52] During pregnancy, lesions are usually located on the ectocervix and a flat cone is appropriate. Some authors perform conization during pregnancy only rarely and in selected patients[19,24]; others see no danger for the pregnancy.[29,53] Nine (10%) of 91 patients at our institution undergoing conization during pregnancy had a spontaneous abortion between the sixth and twelfth weeks of gestation; eight (9%) were delivered prematurely (Table 17-3). If CIN is discovered in the second trimester or later, we prefer to defer conization until about 6 weeks after delivery.

PREGNANCY AFTER CONIZATION

The evidence to date does not indicate that technically correct conization negatively influences subsequent fertility or pregnancies,[7,25,30] even though a somewhat higher risk of second trimester abortion and premature delivery have been reported.[8,36] Weber and Obel[54] related the rate of abortion after conization to the size of the excised cone but did not consider all factors influencing fertility. Of 376 women under 40 years of age at our institution, 128 (34%) became pregnant after conization. The fertility rate according to age (51% for patients aged 30 years or less and 24% for patients older than 30 years) corresponded to that of normal women.

Forty-four (25%) of 174 intrauterine pregnancies followed at our institution ended as a spontaneous abortion; 20% of these women had had a spontaneous abortion in a previous pregnancy. An increased incidence of abortion was seen only in women who had had three or more children before the conization. Eighteen (14%) of 130 deliveries were premature; 19% of these women had had a premature delivery before the conization. These data suggest that conization does not weaken the cervix and increase the probability of subsequent delivery or premature delivery. Ninety of 101 deliveries at term were spontaneous. Three women were delivered by cesarean section because of failure of a scarred cervix to dilate; the remaining eight patients had indications for forceps or cesarean delivery unrelated to conization.

Some authors have recommended routine prophylactic cerclage according to McDonald for patients undergoing conization during pregnancy or patients who are pregnant after conization.[21,37,52] Other authors consider cerclage indicated only in the presence of manifest cervical insufficiency.[28] Our results suggest a reduced rate of second trimester abortion after McDonald cerclage. However, increased bedrest and reduced physical activity were not included in the analysis because they could not be evaluated in patients without cerclage. All in all, the questionable benefit of cerclage stands opposed to the risks of manipulating a gravid uterus and anesthesia. A pessary may be an alternative to cerclage to prevent premature dilation and effacement of the cervix.[20,23]

CONIZATION VERSUS HYSTERECTOMY

Hysterectomy does not represent a more radical measure than conization to treat CIN or stage Ia1 microinvasive carcinoma of the cervix. The outer layers of the cervix and the body of the uterus have no role in the spread of microinvasive cervical cancer. Thus, primary or secondary hysterectomy does not provide an additional therapeutic benefit.

If primary hysterectomy is performed (e.g., because of findings at directed biopsy or only because of abnormal cytology results) there is a risk of missing major lesions. In an analysis of 1609 patients with carcinoma in situ, Burghardt and Holzer[13] reported two invasive recurrences among 166 patients who underwent primary hysterectomy.

Vaginal hysterectomy is preferable if hysterectomy is performed because the margins of a cone were not free of disease. The vaginal approach permits accurate circumcision of suspicious areas after staining with iodine. Residual disease in the vagina has been found more rarely after vaginal than after abdominal hysterectomy.[13]

REPEATED CONIZATION

If the margins of a cone contain atypical epithelium, this does not necessarily mean that abnormal epithelium has remained in situ. Further management depends on whether the affected margin was at the ectocervix or in the cervical canal and whether the patient wishes to preserve her uterus. In the latter case, management can be expectant. Residual lesions on the ectocervix can easily be seen colposcopically.[12] If the margin containing abnormal epi-

thelium is in the canal, cytology at 3-month intervals and endocervical curettage at 6-month intervals should be performed.

Residual abnormal epithelium, or a suspicion thereof, is not a reason for immediate hysterectomy. The residual cervix is usually large enough that a repeat conization can be performed. The shape and size of the cone depend on the location of the residual lesion. The first author has performed a third conization in one patient. Although hardly any cervix was palpable afterwards, two subsequent pregnancies ended with vaginal deliveries of healthy newborns at term.

HISTOLOGIC PROCESSING OF THE CONE

Histology of the specimen obtained at conization should evaluate the nature of the lesion and whether it has been removed completely. These issues require precise histologic examination. The boundary of the lesion can cross or abut the margins of the cone at short stretches, which may be missed by cursory histology. This may explain so-called recurrences after reportedly complete excision of the lesions.[35]

The accuracy of histologic diagnosis depends on the handling of the specimen, the plane of sectioning, and the number of sections.[10] Optimal fixation of the specimen is important. We divide the fixated specimen in a median sagittal plane and embed the halves separately (Fig. 17-4). Step-serial sections of the entire specimen at intervals of 300-μm intervals produce 60 to 80 sections per cone, each of which offers an excellent survey of the cervical epithelium (Fig. 17-5). The cone can also be sagittally divided into four to five blocks, which are embedded separately (Fig. 17-6). If 3 to 4 sections are made of each block, a loose series of 12 to 20 sections is obtained.[12]

RESULTS OF CONIZATION

Results of treating CIN by conization depend primarily on whether the lesion was removed completely. Conization can be considered therapeutic only if the margins of the cone are free of disease and invasion exceeding FIGO stage Ia2 can be ruled out. However, we have treated 16 patients with tumors between 350 and 500 mm^3 (stage Ib according to the current FIGO classification) with conization or simple hysterectomy only; none of these patients developed recurrent disease.[14] Overall, recurrence develops in only 0.3% to 6.3% of patients, depending on the thoroughness of histology.* Residual disease found a short time after reportedly complete conization results from margins of the specimen being examined at too large intervals. Similarly, numerous sections are required to rule out invasion.[10]

A study of 761 patients at our institution yielded two cases of CIN II in the cervical canal and one case of CIN III 4 to 11 years after conization with margins free of disease. Persistence of the primary lesion can be ruled out by

---

*References 1, 7, 11, 27, 31, 32, 40.

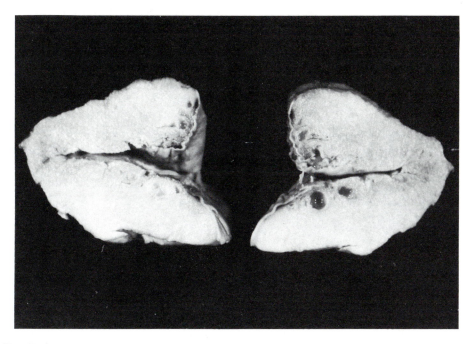

Fig. 17-4. The fixed cone is halved. Each half is embedded in toto for processing as serial sections.

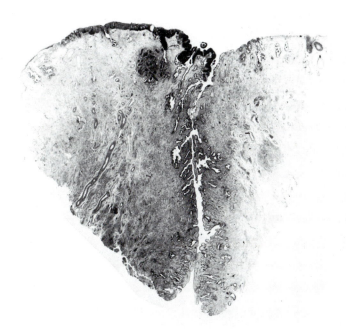

Fig. 17-5. Conization specimen containing a small invasive carcinoma 3 mm in diameter as well as CIN III on the surface and in some ectopic cervical glands. The margins are free of disease.

the long interval, and these lesions most likely represent new disease. Other authors have reported higher rates of recurrences, including invasive carcinoma, after conizations with margins reportedly free of disease.[7,9,32,51] Because most reports did not describe the histologic processing of the cone it cannot be determined whether persisting disease was missed or whether the recurrences represent de novo disease.

If the margins of a cone contain disease, residual atypical epithelium may have been left in situ. Conization should then be considered a diagnostic (as opposed to a primary curative) measure. Further management should be individualized and depends on whether the patient wishes to keep her uterus. The patient may be followed with colposcopy, cytology, and endocervical curettage; she can undergo a second cone biopsy or a hysterectomy. Expec-

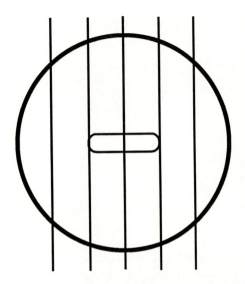

Fig. 17-6. Processing of the conization specimen in serial sagittal sections.

tant management is appropriate especially when only the outer margins of the cone are not free of CIN and residual lesions are thus easily accessible to colposcopy and cytology. If the suspicious margin is in the cervical canal, management should be conservative only if the patient strongly desires to preserve fertility and is reliable. Such patients should undergo follow-up examinations with colposcopy and endocervical cytology and curettage. A decision for conservative management is made easier by the fact that residual disease in hysterectomy specimens after apparently incomplete conization is rarer than expected. At our hospital, 308 patients underwent hysterectomy within 1 year of incomplete conization. Only 30% of the uteri contained residual disease that we could find.[11] In some patients, the resection margin apparently runs very close to the margins of the lesion without disease actually remaining in situ. Small residuals may also be destroyed by electrocoagulation of the wound surface or may deteriorate during necrosis.

At our hospital, 314 patients with margins containing disease were followed conservatively. After 6 or more years of follow-up, only 11% had residual findings; 1.3% had stage Ib carcinoma.[13] Other authors have reported recurrences in 16% to 27% of patients after conservative treatment of patients with incomplete conization.[7,32]

Preinvasive and invasive lesions can occur after incomplete but also after complete conization. This underlines the need for regular follow-up examinations with colposcopy and cytology. Suspicious areas should be biopsied; an endocervical curettage should be performed in patients with a suspicious cytology result but a colposcopically normal cervix. We examine patients at 3-month intervals during the first and second years, at 4-month intervals during the third and fourth years, at 6-month intervals during the fifth year after conization, and yearly thereafter.

ELECTROCONIZATION

Electroconization is performed with an electric knife or a diathermy loop.[39] The procedure can be performed using general or local anesthesia. It is advisable to infiltrate the cervix as described above for cold-knife conization. After staining the cervix with iodine to identify the lesion to be excised, a cone is cut out of the cervix as in cold-knife conization. Heat application to the cervix destroys tissue as well as providing hemostasis of small vessels. Thermal damage affects the cervix as well as the specimen. Histology, particularly evaluation of the margins, is more difficult than after cold-knife conization.[15]

Diathermy loops are used to reduce the thermal damage. Biopsy specimens up to 5 mm in diameter (larger than those obtained by conventional biopsy) can be obtained under colposcopic vision without prior infiltration of the cervix. There is little bleeding or patient discomfort.[3]

Large, high-frequency loops permit excision of the entire lesion with one or two trawls through the cervix.[42,55] The cervix should be infiltrated with dilute ornipressin as described above for cold-knife conization. Local anesthesia can be used. The essential part of the technique is to follow rather than push the loop through the cervix. Dragging the loop produces a shallow cut. If the loop is followed, a deeper cone can be easily removed. Thermal damage is less the shorter the duration of application (i.e., the quicker the procedure is performed). However, speed decreases the hemostatic effect of the procedure, and electrocoagulation may be necessary after the specimen has been excised. Tamponade is usually not necessary. Cones obtained with the diathermy loop should also be processed as giant sections.

LASER CONIZATION

Conization with the carbon dioxide (CO_2) laser became widely used after the reports by Dorsey and Diggs.[18] The procedure requires a CO_2 laser with sufficient power and a colposcope with a focal length of 300 mm and a micromanipulator. A smoke extractor with a inbuilt filter system removes smoke from the surgical field. Standard safety precautions for laser operations are mandatory.[43]

The operation can be performed using local or general anesthesia. The cervix is infiltrated with a dilute ornipressin solution as described above for cold-knife conization. The surgeon should be an experienced colposcopist familiar with cervical pathology and the fundamentals of laser surgery.

After staining the cervix with iodine, a cone appropriate to the lesion is excised with a focused laser beam at a power of 1000 to 2500 W/cm². Excision of the specimen is facilitated by suitable hooks or tenaculum forceps. Hemostasis is obtained with the defocused beam at a power of 650 to 1000 W/cm².

The excision of a cylinder of tissue is recommended in the presence of CIN III in the cervical canal or suspected involvement of endocervical glands. The focused beam is used to cut a 2-cm tall cylinder out of the cervix; the cranial pole of the cylinder is divided with a scalpel. The wound can be coagulated with the laser or with an electrocoagulator.[44]

The advantages of the laser include "no-touch" surgery, microsurgical precision, minimal effects on adjacent tissue, concomitant hemostasis, prompt healing with little wound edema and minimal scarring, and little postoperative pain. However, histology of the specimen, particularly of the margins, is made difficult by thermal artifacts caused by the laser. With optimal surgical technique, this zone of necrosis is no wider than 100 μm.[44] That this is occasionally a problem is indicated by the fact that some authors recommend dividing the apex of the cone with a scalpel.[4] Postoperative bleeding is about as frequent as after cold-knife or diathermy loop conization.[22,34,38,50]

REFERENCES

1. Abdul-Karim FW, Nuñez C: Cervical intraepithelial neoplasia after conization: a study of 522 consecutive cervical cones, *Obstet Gynecol* 65:77, 1985.
2. Ahlgren M et al: Conization as treatment of carcinoma in situ of the uterine cervix, *Obstet Gynecol* 46:135, 1975.
3. Atkinson K: Symposium on cervical neoplasia in diathermy loop excision, *Colp Gynecol Las Surg* 1:285, 1984.
4. Baggish MS, Dorsey JH: Carbon dioxide laser for combination excisional-vaporization conisation, *Am J Obstet Gynecol* 151:23, 1985.
5. Bauer KH: *Die Mutationstheorie der Geschwulstentstehung,* Berlin, 1928, Springer-Verlag.
6. Benedet JF, Anderson GH, Boyes DA: Colposcopic accuracy in the diagnosis of microinvasive and occult invasive carcinoma of the cervix, *Obstet Gynecol* 65:557, 1985.
7. Bjerre B et al: Conization as only treatment of carcinoma in situ of the uterine cervix, *Am J Obstet Gynecol* 125:143, 1976.
8. Breinl H, Piroth H, Schuhmann R: Zur aktuellen Stellung der Konisation im Rahmen von Onkoprävention und Geschwulstdiagnostik an der Cervix uteri, *Geburtshilfe Frauenheilkd* 36:507, 1976.
9. Brown JV, Peters WA, Corwin DJ: Invasive carcinoma after cone biopsy for cervical intraepithelial neoplasia, *Gynecol Oncol* 40:25, 1991.
10. Burghardt E: *Early histological diagnosis of cervical cancer. Textbook and atlas,* Stuttgart, 1973, George Thieme Verlag.
11. Burghardt E: *Behandlung der intraepithelialen Neoplasie des Zervixkarzinoms.* In Burghardt E, editor: *Spezielle Gynäkolgie und Geburtshilfe,* Vienna, 1984, Springer-Verlag.
12. Burghardt E: *Colposcopy and cervical pathology. Textbook and atlas,* ed 2, Stuttgart, 1991, Georg Thieme Verlag.
13. Burghardt E, Holzer E: Treatment of carcinoma in situ: evaluation of 1609 cases, *Obstet Gynecol* 55:539, 1980.
14. Burghardt E et al: Microinvasive carcinoma of the uterine cervix (FIGO stage IA), *Cancer* 67:1037, 1991.
15. Cartier R: *Practical colposcopy,* Paris, 1984, Laboratoire Cartier.
16. Chanen W, Hollyock VE: Colposcopy and the conservative management of cervical dysplasia and carcinoma in situ, *Obstet Gynecol* 43:527, 1974.
17. Coppleson M, Pixley E, Reid B: *Colposcopy,* Springfield, Ill, 1978, Charles C Thomas.
18. Dorsey JH, Diggs ES: Microsurgical conization of the cervix by carbon dioxide laser, *Obstet Gynecol* 54:565, 1979.
19. Ferguson JH, Brown C: Cervical conization during pregnancy, *Surgery* 111:603, 1960.
20. Girardi F et al: *Das Stützpessar—eine Therapiemöglichkeit bei vorzeitiger Eröffnung des Verschlußapparates, Gynäkol Rundsch* 25:236, 1985.
21. Goldberg GL, Altaras MM, Bloch B: Cone cerclage in pregnancy, *Obstet Gynecol* 77:315, 1991.
22. Gunasekera PC, Phipps JH, Lewis BV: Large loop excision of the transformation zone (LLETZ) compared to carbon dioxide laser in the treatment of CIN: a superior mode of treatment, *Br J Obstet Gynaecol* 97:995, 1990.
23. Hamann B, Jorde A, Löffler CH: Erfahrungsbericht über die Anwendung von Stützpessaren als unblutige Cerclageoperation bei Zervixinsuffizienz, *Gynakol Rundsch* 24(suppl 2):124, 1984.
24. Hannigan EV et al: Cone biopsy during pregnancy, *Obstet Gynecol* 60:450, 1982.
25. Holzer E: Fertilität, Schwangerschaft und Geburtsverlauf nach Konisation der Portio vaginalis uteri, *Geburtshilfe Frauenheilkd* 32:950, 1972.
26. Holzer E: Die diagnostische Konisation der Portio vaginalis uteri während der Schwangerschaft, *Geburtshilfe Frauenheilkd* 33:361, 1973.
27. Holzer E: Ergebnisse der konservativen Behandlung des Carcinoma in situ durch Konisation, *Geburtshilfe Frauenheilkd* 36:630, 1976.
28. Holzer E, Kömetter R, Hofmann H: Die Wertigkeit der Cerclage in der Prophylaxe der Frühgeburtlichkeit, *Geburtshilfe Frauenheilkd* 41:615, 1981.
29. Jones HW III, Buller RE: The treatment of cervical intraepithelial neoplasia by cone biopsy, *Am J Obstet Gynecol* 137:882, 1980.
30. Kofler E, Philipp K: Schwangerschaft nach Konisation wegen atypischer Epithelprozesse der Cervix uteri, *Geburtshilfe Frauenheilkd* 37:942, 1977.
31. Kolstad P: Follow-up study of 232 patients with stage Ia1 and 411 patients with stage Ia2 squamous cell carcinoma of the cervix (microinvasive carcinoma), *Gynecol Oncol* 33:265, 1989.
32. Kolstad P, Klem V: Long term follow-up of 1121 cases of carcinoma in situ, *Obstet Gynecol* 48:125, 1976.
33. Krebs HP: Outpatient cervical conization, *Obstet Gynecol* 63:430, 1984.
34. Kristensen GB, Jensen LK, Holund B: A randomized trial comparing two methods of cold knife conization with laser conization, *Obstet Gynecol* 76:1009, 1990.
35. Larsson G: Conization for cervical dysplasia and carcinoma in situ: long term follow-up of 1013 women, *Ann Chir Gynaecol* 70:79, 1981.
36. Leiman G, Harrison NA, Rubin A: Pregnancy following conization of the cervix: complications related to cone size. *Am J Obstet Gynecol* 136:14, 1980.
37. McDonald IA: Suture of the cervix for inevitable miscarriage, *J Obstet Gynaecol Br Emp* 64:346, 1957.
38. Meandzija MP, Locher G, Jackson JD: CO_2 laser conization versus conventional conization, *Lasers Surg Med* 4:139, 1984.
39. Monaghan JMM, Burghardt E: *Cervical intraepithelial neoplasia (preinvasive cancer).* In Burghardt E et al, editors: *Surgical gynecologic oncology,* Stuttgart, Georg Thieme Verlag (in press).
40. Ostergard DR: Cryosurgical treatment of cervical intraepithelial neoplasia, *Obstet Gynecol* 56:231, 1980.
41. Peckham BM, Sonek MG, Carr WF: Outpatient therapy: success and failure with dysplasia and carcinoma in situ, *Am J Obstet Gynecol* 142:323, 1982.
42. Prendiville W, Cullimore J, Norman S: Large loop excision of the transformation zone (LLETZ). A new method of management for women with cervical intraepithelial neoplasia, *Br J Obstet Gynaecol* 96:1054, 1989.
43. Reid R: Laser safety I. Avoidance of surgical misadventure with the CO_2 laser, *Colp Gynecol Las Surg* 1:117, 1984.
44. Reid R: Symposium on cervical neoplasia. V. Carbon dioxide laser ablation, *Colp Gynecol Las Surg* 1:291, 1984.
45. Richart RM: Natural history of cervical intraepithelial neoplasia, *Clin Obstet Gynecol* 10:748, 1967.
46. Rubio CA, Thomassen P, Kock Y: Influence of the size of cone specimens on postoperative hemorrhage, *Am J Obstet Gynecol* 122:939, 1975.
47. Sevin BU et al: Invasive cancer of the cervix after cryosurgery, *Obstet Gynecol* 53:465, 1979.

48. Sprang ML, Isaacs JH, Boraca CT: Management of carcinoma in situ of the cervix, *Am J Obstet Gynecol* 129:47, 1977.

49. Stafl A, Wilbanks GD: An international terminology of colposcopy: report of the Nomenclature Committee of the International Federation of Cervical Pathology and Colposcopy, *Obstet Gynecol* 77:313, 1991.

50. Tabor A, Berget A: Cold-knife and laser conization for cervical intraepithelial neoplasia, *Obstet Gynecol* 76:633, 1990.

51. Townsend DE et al: Invasive cancer following outpatient evaluation and therapy for cervical disease, *Obstet Gynecol* 57:145, 1981.

52. van Nagell JR et al: Diagnostic and therapeutic efficacy of cervical conization, *Am J Obstet Gynecol* 124:134, 1976.

53. Wanless JF: Carcinoma of the cervix in pregnancy, *Am J Obstet Gynecol* 110:173, 1971.

54. Weber T, Obel E: Pregnancy complications following conization of the uterine cervix, *Acta Obstet Gynecol Scand* 58:259, 1979.

55. Whiteley PF, Olah KS: Treatment of cervical intraepithelial neoplasia: experience with the low-voltage diathermy loop, *Am J Obstet Gynecol* 162:1272, 1990.

56. zur Hausen H: Human genital cancer: synergism between two virus infections or synergism between a virus infection and initiating events? *Lancet* 1370, 1982.

Chapter 18

EXTRAPERITONEAL LASER SURGERY

Michael S. Baggish

CERVIX

Cervical intraepithelial neoplasia

The carbon dioxide (CO_2) laser, the dominant method for treating cervical intraepithelial neoplasia (CIN) during the 1980s, has now been displaced by large loop electrical excision.[20,42,44]

Compared to other ablative techniques, the laser had advantages of producing conelike defects precisely and rapidly. The therapeutic results for laser vaporization performed during the decade from 1982 to 1992 revealed a high degree of efficacy with cure rates for high-grade lesions ranging from 90% to 96%, preservation of the anatomical integrity of the cervix, and a visible squamocolumnar junction postoperatively.[1,6,19,28] The series of Baggish, Dorsey, and Adelson reported 10-year results in more than 3000 women with elimination of CIN in all grade categories with a single laser treatment in 94% of cases. Nevertheless, the major overriding disadvantage dogging all ablation techniques is the absence of a histologic specimen for the pathologist to view.[15]

Clearly, it is always better to obtain a suitable specimen to determine the adequacy of resection margins and whether invasive disease is present.

Laser vaporization is an easily learned operation performed through the colposcope. The laser micromanipulator is coupled to the objective of the colposcope rendering both lenses identically focused.

Vaporization is performed based on the following facts:

1. Endocervical glands (clefts) may plunge into the underlying stroma to a depth of up to 6 to 7 mm, but involvement of the cleft with extension of CIN rarely exceeds a depth of 3 mm.[2]

2. Advanced grades of CIN tend to spread out not only onto the portio but upwards into the canal. CIN rarely extends beyond 1 cm (measured from the squamocolumnar junction).[33,45]

Using these data, vaporization is performed by marking out a 3-mm peripheral margin beyond the atypical transformation zone and vaporizing down to a *maximal* depth of 1 cm (Fig. 18-1). The deepest part of the vaporization zone is in juxtaposition to the endocervical canal. The defect is gently graded to produce a funnel-shaped crater (Fig. 18-2). The finished product is identical to a small cone. This operation, performed at 30 to 40 W of power with a 2-mm spot (beam diameter), should be completed in 5 minutes with or without local anesthesia. Ten percent (10%) or fewer patients experience some bleeding postoperatively, usually occurring 4 to 7 days.[4] The bleeding is self-limited and usually stops spontaneously. Only a small minority of patients require treatment, typically an application of Monsel's paste. If arteriolar bleeding occurs, the bleeding vessel should be sutured.

Vaginal discharge ceases within a week or two, and healing is complete within 4 weeks with a visible squamocolumnar junction located at the anatomical external as (Figs. 18-3 and 18-4).

Compared to the laser vaporization, the laser excisional cone requires excellent hand-eye coordination and skill. The laser cone employs a manipulating hook to place traction on the tissue as it is cut to obtain sharp margins and to limit thermal artifact. The specifications for laser cone include a beam diameter smaller than 0.5 mm, a power density of at least 16,000 W/cm^2, and special handling of the endocervical margin (superpulse resection or sharp sec-

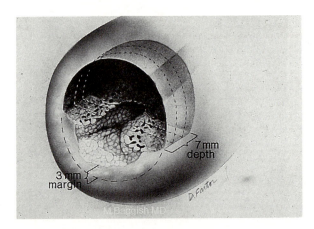

Fig. 18-1. Vaporization is carried out plane after plane to a maximum central depth of 10 mm. The margin around the ATZ is 3 mm.

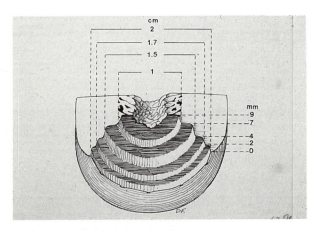

Fig. 18-2. The defect created is a gently sloping funnel shape.

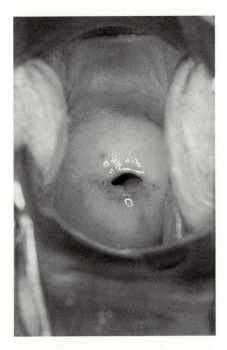

Fig. 18-3. Postoperative multiparous cervix.

tion). Properly trained personnel should complete the cone within 10 to 12 minutes with a mean blood loss of less than 10 ml.[10] When the procedure is skillfully performed, tissue margins show thermal injury of less than 160 μm. Excessive thermal injury to the specimen can only be attributed to faulty technique.[34] The loop electrical excision cone (LEEC) requires less technical skill and cuts through tissue by identical methodology (i.e., vaporization). Because the 0.2-mm wire electrode may range from 5 mm to 2.0 cm in diameter, this vaporization is very rapid compared to the 0.3- to 0.5-mm spot obtained by the laser, which, in turn, must be connected by sweeping across the tissue field to produce an incision (Figs. 18-5 and 18-6). Baggish et al[18] compared thermal injury zones between electrical loop and superpulsed laser. Accurate measurement showed that thermal artifact was not significantly different between the two techniques. The tissue margins were acceptable from the standpoint of pathologic interpretation. Baggish, Dorsey, and Adelson reported a series of 954 laser excisional cones with 97% showing no evidence of persistent or recurrent disease. Four cases of invasive carcinoma were picked up, which might have otherwise been missed (if an ablative procedure had been done). Seventy-three women had disease extending to the margin; of these, 44 had no further treatment and remained free of disease. Twenty-five women with persisting atypia under-

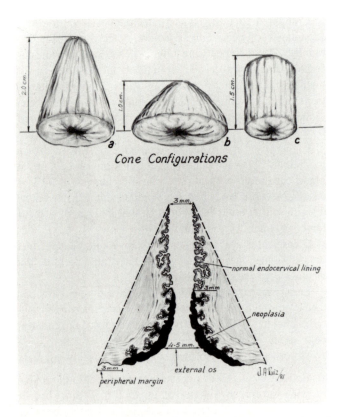

Fig. 18-4. Cone configurations based on laser geography of ATZ.

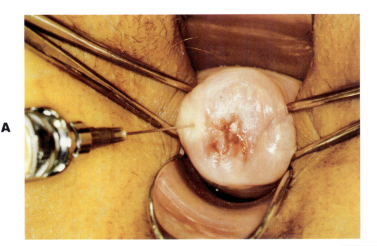

A

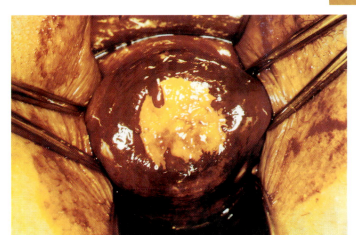

C

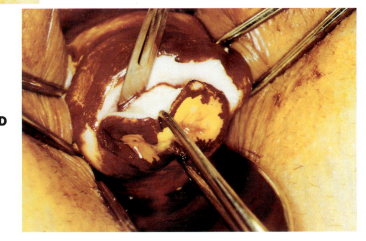

B

D

Color Plate 1. Technique of cold-knife conization. **A,** The cervix is grasped with two pairs of tenaculum forceps at the 3 o'clock and 9 o'clock positions and pulled outward. The needle for infiltration is inserted outside the lesion. **B,** After injection at several points, the cervix is swollen and pale. **C,** After application of iodine (Schiller's test), the suspicious area, which is almost always iodine-negative, is sharply demarcated. **D,** During excision of the cone, the cervical stroma that has been infiltrated with ornipressin is white and rarely bleeds. Once only the apex of the cone remains to be divided, the tenaculum forceps are applied to the wound (to avoid disrupting the epithelium), pulled outward, and the apex is severed.   *Continued.*

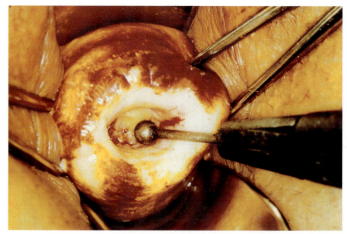

E

Color Plate 1, cont'd. E, The wound is coagulated with the ball electrode of an electrocoagulation device. **F,** The cervix after coagulation.

F

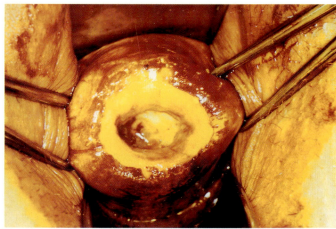

Color Plate 2. Colposcopic appearance of the cervix 2 months after conization. The external os resembles that of a nullipara.

went repeat cone or hysterectomy.[15] Comparing morbidity, time to complete the operation, and healing results, there is no rational reason *not* to perform an excisional operation.[16]

The lessons learned with laser excisional cone may be directly applied to LEEC. The operations are performed

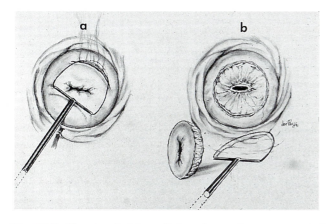

Fig. 18-5. The electrical loop (0.2 mm) vaporizes across at 1.5 to 2.0 cm front; therefore, it cuts more rapidly than a laser.

under local anesthesia. Hemostasis is acquired by combining a vasoconstrictor with the local anesthesia. Mixing 0.5 ml of vasopressin with 50 ml of 1% xylocaine produces 1/100 diluted solution. Ten to 12 ml of this solution injected with a 25 to 27-gauge needle directly into the cervix produces excellent anesthesia and vasospasm. The objective is to place the needle just beneath the mucosa, inject under pressure, and blanch the cervix white.[16] When the needle is removed, no bleeding is seen. Injecting circumferentially with a 2- to 3-mm margin outside the abnormal transformation zone produces a visible landmark demarcating the peripheral extent of the cone (Fig. 18-7).

Complications after laser operations to the cervix have been acceptably low compared to other techniques.[36,39] Cervical stenosis has been reported in 1.3% of cases. Cervical incompetence is a rarity as is pelvic inflammatory disease (0.05%).[15] Excessively large excisional cones effectively remove a substantial volume of cervical stroma as well as endocervical mucosa and result in cervical stenosis and infertility. Cervical substance can also be removed by degree by performing multiple cervical operative procedures over a period of time. The additive result is a shrunken, stenotic, functionless remnant flush with the vaginal vault. Table 18-1 lists the specifications for exci-

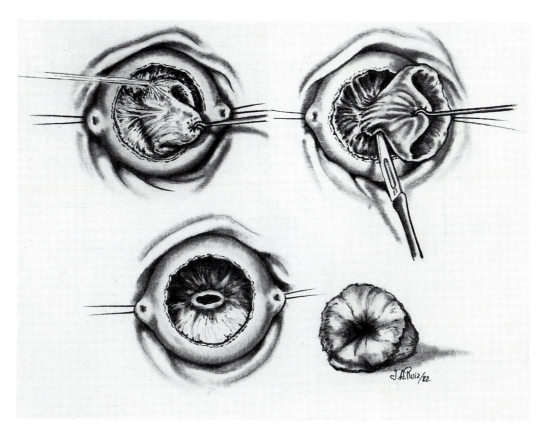

Fig. 18-6. The laser creates a 0.3 to 0.5-mm spot, which cuts as it is swept across the tissue plane. A hook provides traction as the laser cuts and permits shaping of the cone.

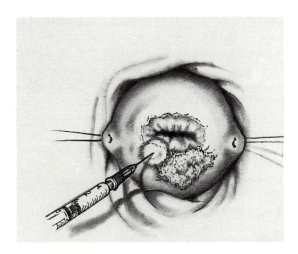

Fig. 18-7. A dilute vasopressin solution (mixed with 1% lidocaine) is injected just beneath the mucosa. The injection sites are placed peripheral to the ATZ.

Table 18-1. Specifications for excisional cone

Peripheral margin*	3.0 mm
Height (ATZ at level external os)	1.5 cm
Height (ATZ on portio)	1.0 cm
Height (ATZ in canal)	2.0 cm

*Around atypical transformation zone (ATZ)

sional conization performed either by laser or loop electrical excision (LEEC).

Perhaps the single operation for which the CO_2 laser maintains an advantage compared to the electrical loop is the combination cone. The technique for the laser combination cone has been amply described in the literature.[14,26,59] This technique is ideally suited for geographically extensive CIN (i.e., involving three or four quadrants and extending into the vaginal fornices. Briefly, the ectocervical portion of the lesion is vaporized to sculpled depths (e.g., <1 mm in the vagina, 1 to 2 mm on the ectocervix, 3 to 4 mm in proximity to the canal). A narrow (1 cm or less) cylindrical excisional cone removes the portion of the lesion extending into the endocervical canal (Fig. 18-8). The advantages of the combination cone versus a conventional excisional cone are apparent by measuring volume of tissue removed with each procedure. The combination cone conserves at least twice as much cervical stroma compared to a large excisional cone.

Cervical stenosis

Cervical stenosis regardless of its etiology is best treated by means of the CO_2 laser. *Only* lasers equipped with superpulse are acceptable instruments for this operation. Superpulsing delivers laser energy to tissue in intermittent bursts with very high peak powers (Fig. 18-9). The peak powers exceed the highest continuous power output of the laser by a factor of five to ten times. The duty cycles of such lasers are very low (i.e., 10%, which trans-

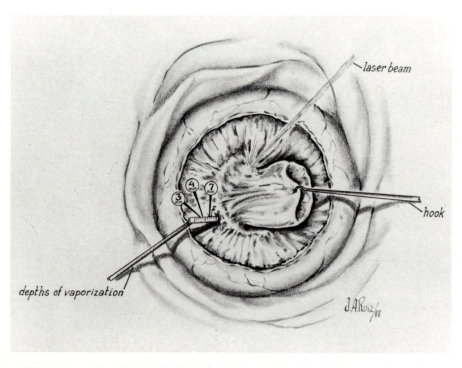

Fig. 18-8. The combination cone consists of selective vaporization of the ectocervix and a narrow cylindrical cone to remove the endocervical extension.

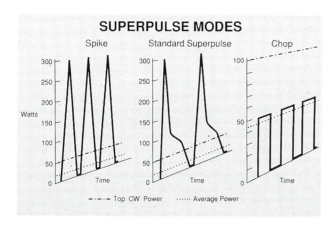

Fig. 18-9. Superpulsing produces very high peaks of power for an instantaneous part of a second followed by a refractory interval. During the latter, tissue cools and diminishes thermal injury.

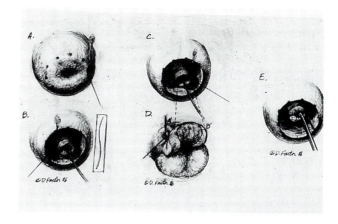

Fig. 18-10. Scar tissue is vaporized away; then the endocervical canal is split by a superpulsed beam. The remaining endocervical canal is everted.

lates into laser time off tissue 0.9 second and on tissue 0.1 second). During the pulse interval, the tissue cools down sufficiently to reduce thermal damage significantly. The principle for alleviation of cervical stenosis relies on carefully vaporizing away the fibrotic tissue constricting the cervical canal layer by layer until visible (reddish) endocervical tissue is identified. A baby Hegar sound is then placed into the canal. The beam diameter is narrowed from 1.5 mm to less than 0.5 mm. This is accomplished by the variable focusing mechanism located on the laser micromanipulator. The remnant on the endocervical canal is cut along a single axis. After this maneuver, an immediate relief of stenosis allows progressively larger dilators to be placed through the canal. The procedure is finished by everting the endocervical mucosa by enlarging the beam to 1 mm and gently placing it just peripheral to the mucosal margin (buttoning; Fig. 18-10). This operation is the only reliable method for relieving cervical stenosis. If any endocervical mucosa is present, the degree of success for this operation is 80%.[12,41] Postoperatively, conjugated estrogen is administered in doses of 5 mg daily. The patient is seen weekly to keep the canal dilated. This combination should be continued for 6 to 8 weeks postoperatively; invariably some rescarring occurs.

Cervical myoma

Cervical myomas of any size may be excised by the CO_2 laser using a superpulsed beam. The aim of this operation is to preserve the structural integrity of the cervix and to spare more or less completely normal cervical tissue. The greatest risk of this operation is cervical incompetence. The latter results from inexact excision. The margin of the myoma is identified, and a 1:100 vasopressin solution is injected into the periphery of the myoma. The myoma is cut along the line where it joins normal cervix either on the anterior or posterior cervical lip. A laser hook device is placed into the myoma, placing the tissue on tension. The

laser sharply excises the myoma free. This is repeated at all attached margins. For large myomas, the cervix may be split along its anterior or posterior axis to gain exposure. After the myoma has been removed, the cervical wound is sewn with 3-0 polyglycolic acid-type (Dexon or Vicryl) suture. Rosenzweig et al[50] reported eight excisions of moderate and large cervical tumors with restoration of normal anatomy in every case. No immediate or delayed bleeding was observed.

VULVA
Vulvar intraepithelial neoplasia

In recent years, vulvar intraepithelial neoplasia (VIN) has occurred with increasing frequency in a younger population.[52] The peak age of this disorder is now 35 to 54 years.[53] Vulvar intraepithelial neoplasia may be classified together with cervical intraepithelial neoplasia and vaginal intraepithelial neoplasia to comprise a triad of disorders known as intraepithelial neoplasia of the lower genital tract. Several articles have recorded a coexistence of VIN and human papilloma virus infections, particularly human papilloma virus types 16 and 18.[21,56] Several series of cases treated by CO_2 laser have been reported in the literature during the past 10 years.[13,29,40,54,57] Although the natural history of this disorder, particularly its relationship to invasive squamous cell carcinoma, is by no means clear, recent data suggest that VIN may be two distinct diseases, that occurring in the population below the age of 40 and a more aggressive entity occurring after the age of 50.[9] In the latter group, there does seem to be a more linear relationship between intraepithelial disease and subsequent invasive cancer. In the below-40 group, spontaneous remissions have been reported and progression from the intraepithelial stage to invasive disease is uncommon. Therapy for VIN emphasizes conservative versus radical treatment. Although in the past simple vulvectomy and skinning vulvectomy have been standards of therapy, these have largely been replaced by local excision and ablative procedures. The difficulty encountered with ablative procedures in the treatment of this disorder relate, again, to the lack of a tissue specimen for the pathologist and the determination of whether invasive disease is present or whether margins of excision are involved with intraepithelial neoplasia. Regardless of the therapeutic regimen, conservative or radical, a substantial number of cases persist or recur.

The CO_2 laser has proved to be as efficacious as more radical procedures for the treatment of VIN. Newer therapeutic techniques employing this device and obtaining a tissue specimen for the pathologist effectively blunt the objections to laser vaporization, particularly relating to missing invasive cancer.

Any treatment regimen must emphasize the principal that VIN is part of a regional disease rather than a focal disorder. Careful evaluation of both the vagina and the cervix is imperative to the therapeutic regimen. Additionally, with any conservative therapy, follow-up is extremely important. This must include colposcopic examination of the vulva after the application of 4% acetic acid and the acquisition of directed biopsies when suspicious skin changes are seen.

Baggish et al have quantified the depth of involvement of epidermis as well as skin appendages associated with VIN.[17] Any therapeutic program that does not take into consideration the contiguous spread of neoplasia to skin appendages will fail to remove the disease completely. In an evaluation of over 1000 sections, 38% of patients with vulvar carcinoma in situ were found to have skin appendage involvement. The appendages most frequently involved were the pilosebaceous apparatus, hair follicles, and sebaceous glands (Fig. 18-11). Clearly, a differential depth of treatment must be considered in any schema that seeks to preserve normal anatomy while eliminating VIN. Treatment in hair-bearing areas of the labia majora, the perineum, and perianal areas requires vaporization to a depth of 2.5 mm. Treatment of the labia minora requires treatment to a depth not exceeding 1 mm. Treatment of periclitoral skin should be tailored individually and based on biopsy measurement of the depth of the neoplasia. Equally important to depth of treatment are the peripheral margins. A minimum circumferential boundary of 3 mm beyond from any single or contiguous lesion is required. Wide peripheral margins and adequate depth are the key elements to eliminating disease with a single treatment. Multiple staged treatment schedules may be required for geographically extensive disorders. Diagnosis must be made with the aid of magnification in a fashion analogous

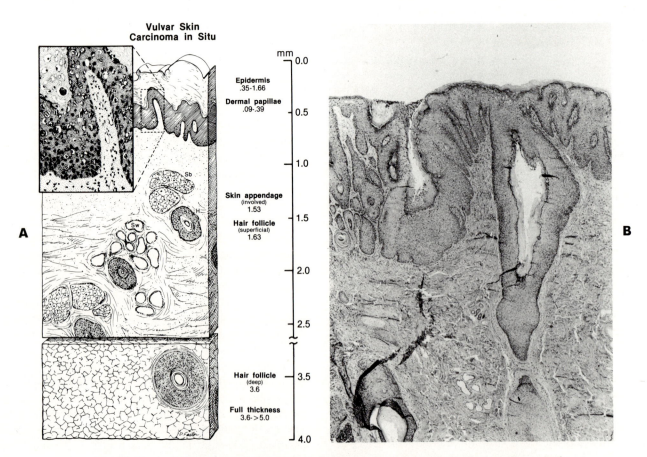

Fig. 18-11. **A,** Schema for epithelial thickening with vulvar carcinoma in situ and involvement of skin appendages (mean depth 1.53 mm). **B,** Carcinoma in situ extending down hair shaft.

to CIN. Colposcopic examination and organized mapping of all lesions followed by multiple biopsies must precede any treatment program. Depending on the extent of disease, therapy may be performed under local or general anesthesia.

The CO_2 laser is the most appropriate device to use for vulvar intraepithelial disease. The reasons for this relate to the fact that the CO_2 laser is heavily absorbed by water, is primarily a vaporizing laser, and creates mainly surface injury rather than deep coagulative injury. All vulvar laser treatments should be performed with a superpulsed beam. Superpulsing minimizes thermal injury. Baggish et al[17] and Reid et al[25,46,47] have identified the various anatomical layers of vulvar skin based on gross, colposcopic evaluation. Thermal artifact always occurs with laser vaporization because of its heating action. This creates an identifiable yellowish hue to the dermis. The normal appearance of vulvar dermis is rosy pink. With superpulse beams, this pink appearance is frequently seen because thermal artifact is diminished. Thermal artifact injury in skin may penetrate to a depth of approximately 500 μm. This zone of thermal injury, which will subsequently slough, should be included in any specification for treatment.

All laser treatment to the vulva requires some form of anesthesia. For extensive disease, which will be either ablated or excised in a single sitting, general anesthesia is indicated. When local anesthesia is used, treatment may be staged depending on the extent of the disease. The main disadvantage to local anesthesia is pain at the anesthetic injection site. The volume of local anesthesia injected must be carefully limited to avoid toxicity.

Once the appropriate anesthetic has been administered, the laser beam should be adjusted to deliver a spot of approximately 0.5 mm. Trace spots outline the extent of vaporization or excision to be done. This is most conveniently carried out by setting the timing interval at approximately 0.2 seconds and setting the power meter to approximately 10 W. If a superpulsed beam is to be used, the most convenient setting is 300 pulses per second at a 0.3-ms pulse width. Tracing may be carried out either with the free hand piece using magnifying loops or directing the laser by a micromanipulator attached to a colposcope. The optical loops should deliver a magnification of approximately 2.5 to 3 times.

The preferred method for treating VIN is by laser thin section (Fig. 18-12). Laser thin section permits intradermal removal of strips of vulvar skin such that the tissue may be analyzed by the pathologist for both the presence of invasive disease and adequacy of surgical margins.[17] Thin section is carried out in the following manner: using a 27-gauge needle, an intradermal injection of either saline or local anesthesia plus 1:100 diluted vasopressin is placed within the area to be treated. Several injections may be required. The purpose of the injection is to create a heat sink within the dermis to absorb heat and minimize thermal damage. The laser beam diameter is set at 0.5 mm or less. An average superpulse power of approximately 22 W

is obtained. The previously marked trace spots are connected by means of a slow sweeping movement of the laser beam. A laser hook is placed at a margin of the incision, and a tissue plane is developed in the superficial reticular dermis. With constant traction being placed upward, the thin section is completed by removing strips of epithelium to depths ranging between 1 and 2 mm (Fig. 18-13). No sutures or grafting is required. The laser-treated area will heal in a manner analogous to a laser vaporization. After excision but still using the superpulse setting previously noted, the laser beam's diameter is increased to 1 to 1.5 mm. Superficial vaporization is carried out to a 3-mm peripheral margin. The char material is swabbed away with 4% acetic acid.

Although there are disadvantages to vaporization compared to thin section, occasionally this may be indicated, especially in strategic locations such as the clitoris and labia minora, which have been previously adequately biopsied. Vaporization should be carried out to the appropriate skin level depending on the location of the lesion. Vaporization is best done with a superpulsed beam and a beam diameter of approximately 1.5 mm to 2 mm. In all cases in which perianal skin involvement occurs, a laser speculum should be placed into the anus and the rectal mucosa should be swabbed with 4% acetic acid. A moist 4 × 4 sponge should be placed in the anus above the intraepithelial lesion to prevent methane gas explosion during laser treatment. Vaporization in the anus should be carried to a depth not exceeding 0.5 mm.

All skin wounds created by the laser vaporization or excision will be painful. Frequently, this pain occurs on a delayed basis with the maximal discomfort coming 3 to 4 days after laser treatment. Covering the wounds ameliorates the severity of the pain. Bio-occlusive dressings should be applied immediately after surgery if possible. When these wounds are covered, they are virtually painless. Covered wounds also heal more rapidly than undressed wounds because they retain moisture. Dressings

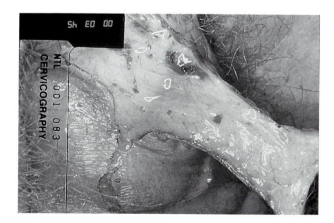

Fig. 18-12. CO_2 laser thin section peals away neoplastic epithelium. The 1- to 2-mm-deep sample provides the pathologist with a sample of tissue and at the same time removes the diseased epithelium and dermis.

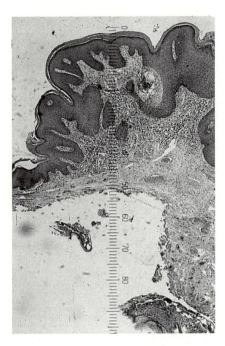

Fig. 18-13. Section of vulvar skin removed by thin section.

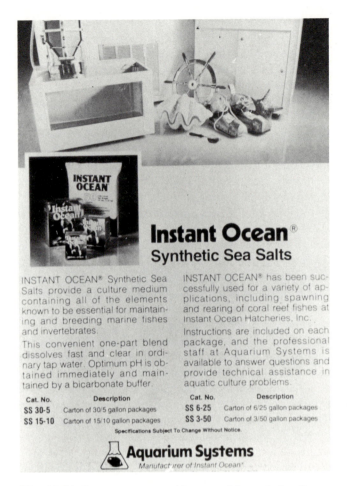

Fig. 18-14. Instant ocean provides a soothing solution for patients to diminish their discomfort after vulvar laser surgery. It additionally debrides the wounds.

are allowed to fall off, which they usually do several days after treatment. For extensive laser wounds, patients are asked to take sitz baths using Instant Ocean (Fig. 18-14). Ocean water can be reconstituted by dissolving Instant Ocean (sea salts) in tap water. The Ocean water is more comfortable for the patients than are saline sitz baths and tend to debride the wounds, thereby enhancing healing.[43] Patients should take seawater sitz baths approximately four to six times per day. A 1:4 diluted solution of Betadine provided in a plastic bottle is squirted on the perineum after urination or defecation. After bathing or irrigation, the areas are dried using an electric hair dryer on the air cycle.

Alternatively, the skin may be thoroughly covered with Silvadene cream. This should be reapplied several times per day. All patients are instructed to wear oversized cotton pants to provide adequate circulation of air to the vulva and also to provide a barrier for the Silvadene cream. Healing is usually complete in approximately 6 weeks. The patient should be seen at approximately 2-week intervals until healing is complete and thereafter every 6 months.

Most patients experience little immediate pain. The explanation for this relative anesthesia relates to the nerve-sealing action of the laser resulting in a clublike nerve ending compared to the shaving brush pattern seen after a knife cut. Delayed bleeding is rare after laser vaporization or thin section. When full-thickness excision occurs, scarring invariably results. Great care must be taken during any excision or vaporization treatment to avoid extending beyond the reticular dermis. Deeper vaporization can be identified by the visualization of fine white subvulvar fat. In our series of 51 cases, no infections have occurred. An-

other concern is coaptation of the labia. This may be avoided by having patients manually separate their labia during sitz baths.

Several series in the literature report cure rates of approximately 80%.[13,54,58] With thin section, these cure rates may exceed 90%. Careful long-term follow-up is imperative.

Because vulvar carcinoma in situ is a disease predominantly of younger women, conservative methods of treatment that preserve functional anatomy should be offered to every patient. Even with extensive lesions, laser therapy compares favorably to other methods of treatment. Paget's disease may be the exception; recurrent disease is quite common after laser therapy.

Condylomata acuminata

The single most frequent indication for CO_2 laser surgery in the lower genital tract during the past decade was condylomata acuminata.[3,5] Unfortunately, the greatest abuse of the laser as a therapeutic tool was the elimination of condylomata acuminata. The recent history of this disorder has been hallmarked by overdiagnosis, overtreatment, and overreaction by the gynecologic community. The acme of this frenzy to treat the human papilloma virus (HPV) was reached when a group of unfortunate women were submitted to more or less total ablation of the vulva, vagina, and cervix.[49] The results of this type of unsubstantiated therapeutic adventurism are predictable: the subclinical HPV infection was not eliminated, the number of complications were excessive, the postoperative pain inflicted on the patient was unnecessary.

Genital warts are ugly and may cause some discomfort for the patient. They spread principally by autoinoculation and may undergo spontaneous regression. HPV is an opportunistic invader that preys on an immunocompromised host. Several factors provide ample opportunity for accelerated growth of genital warts and include: immunosuppressive drugs, corticosteroids, oral contraceptives, pregnancy, diabetes mellitus, cigarette smoking, and human immunodeficiency virus infections. The only potentially significant danger associated with warts occurs in children and young adults who are afflicted with laryngeal papillomas. Genital warts by themselves are associated with no significant risk for the patient with the possible exception of misdiagnosis.[11] For the latter reason, a representative biopsy or even multiple biopsies should be performed before the performance of any laser operation.

The indication for CO_2 laser ablation of genital warts is the presence of gross disease. Subclinical HPV infections, koilocytosis, and papillosis are not indications for treatment. Other than for research purposes, HPV typing is not advantageous and adds unnecessary expense to the workup of these patients. It is prudent to reserve laser vaporization for severe disease and attempt to eliminate mild infections with less draconian measures.

The goal of laser vaporization is to eliminate all visible condylomata. The colposcope should be employed in all cases to pick up small warts not visible to the naked eye and to provide the best means to examine the anal canal, vestibule, urethra, vagina, and cervix properly. Every patient should have extragenital sites examined for the presence of warts. Although the role of the male in the transmission of this disease to his female partner is not clear, nevertheless, he should be examined and treated if warts are present on his genitalia.[31]

Although local anesthesia may be used, most patients require general or regional anesthesia to permit laser vaporization. Skill and precision result in the removal of warts while preserving normal surrounding tissues. In this circumstance, depth of vaporization does not improve results. In fact, no wart should be vaporized deeper than the level of the surrounding skin surface (Fig. 18-15). Power levels should be set at 40 to 60 W, and beam diameter should be set at 3 mm. Experienced surgeons may use even higher powers to shorten the laser exposure. When vaporization has been completed, the laser beam should be defocused and the power should be dropped to less than 10 W. The defocused beam is carried across the surrounding skin, blanching it white but producing no vaporization or

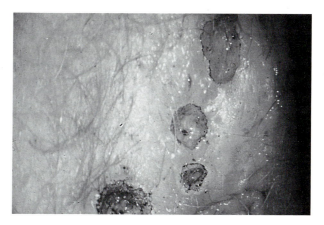

Fig. 18-15. Genital warts are vaporized no deeper than to a level of the surrounding normal skin.

charring. This technique raises surface skin temperatures to approximately 50° C and results in sloughing of the epidermis while preserving undisturbed the underlying papillary dermis. This peripheral blanching or brushing should take in skin to a radius of 1 to 2 cm around to the vaporized warts.[8,32] Anal warts are vaporized by inserting a laser speculum into the anus in a manner analogous to the technique described for VIN except vaporization is more superficial (i.e., to the level of the surrounding anal mucosa). A nasal speculum is inserted into the urethra, and the laser beam is directed to vaporize urethral warts superficially at a power setting of 10 to 15 W, beam diameter 1.5 mm. Finally, a speculum is placed into the vagina, a laser hook is used to provide exposure, and all visible warts are eliminated; similarly, the cervix is inspected and treated as necessary. All treated areas are thoroughly swabbed with 4% acetic acid to clean off all carbon. A pudendal nerve block is done to eliminate immediate postoperative pain. Silvadene cream is liberally applied to the treated area. Oral contraceptives should be discontinued. Patients should be advised to use condoms for a minimum of 6 months after surgery. The postoperative treatment regimen is identical to that described for VIN. It is preferable to see these patients within 1 week after surgery. The labia should be separated to prevent coaptation. The operative site should be irrigated with saline, and Silvadene cream should be reapplied. Several studies following the above routine have reported elimination of warts after one or two laser treatments in over 90% of patients. For those patients who are immunologically compromised, supplemental and chronic applications of 5-fluorouracil cream have been recommended.[38] Long-term data about this routine are lacking, and possible mutagenic effects of these applications on surrounding tissues are unknown. Recently, Reid et al have diminished recurrent warts after laser debulking by administering recombinant interferon.[48]

Laser vaporization of warts during pregnancy has produced varying results.[7,30] High numbers of failures are uniformly observed in early pregnancy. Treatment during

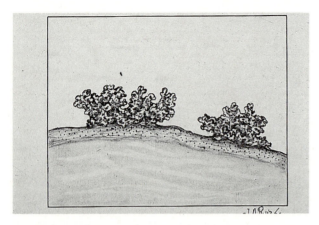

Fig. 18-16. Human papillomavirus is present in both the gross wart and the normal-appearing surrounding skin.

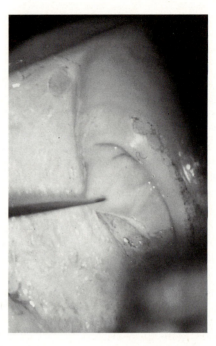

Fig. 18-17. A titanium laser hook exposes a vaginal vault tunnel in a woman who has previously undergone hysterectomy.

the third trimester produces better results, but the elimination of warts may also relate to the subsequent termination of the pregnancy state. I prefer not to treat beyond 34 gestational weeks because of the increased risk of bleeding and also to allow sufficient time for healing of the operative site before delivery.

The laser does not remove all viable HPV from the lower genital tract. It is likely that large volumes of replicating virus are destroyed as the warts are vaporized, however it is most probable the patient's own immune system plays an important role in the final outcome (Fig. 18-16).

VAGINA
Vaginal intraepithelial neoplasia

The vagina is more difficult to treat than either the vulva or cervix because of its very large surface area, its numerous folds and fornices, its limited maneuvering space, and its laborious exposure. Most women find stretching of the vagina extremely uncomfortable and reflexly resist this by contracting their levator ani muscles, which, in turn, increases the pain. Because of the above-cited factors, conventional surgery is difficult to perform and good assistance is problematical to render. The operating microscope with multiple magnification options and consistently bright light is the most useful tool for facilitating vaginal surgery. An 11-inch-long titanium laser hook permits examination of vaginal folds and the posthysterectomy vaginal tunnels located at the vaginal vault (Fig. 18-17). Control of bleeding in the vagina is crucial because, as stated above, the view of the operative site particularly in the upper and middle thirds of the vagina is tenuous under the best circumstances. As with other locations in the lower genital tract, the CO_2 laser is best suited for surgery in the vagina. The ability to operate without directly touching the tissue and at the same time to obtain thermally based hemostasis are real advantages in this location. Electrosurgical cutting and cryosurgical instruments are ill-suited and even hazardous to use in the vagina.[24]

The vaginal mucosa in a menstruating women is less than 500 μm in thickness. A postmenopausal women's epithelium is 100 to 200 μm deep, and the entire wall may be only 2 to 3 mm thick. With the exception of girls and women with adenosis, the vagina does not contain glands or crypts, therefore intraepithelial neoplasia is limited to the vaginal mucous membrane; the neoplastic process does not project into the underlying stroma unless invasion is present.

Vaginal intraepithelial neoplasia (VAIN) is the least common of the group of lower genital tract premalignancies (i.e., an annual incidence of 0.2 per 100,000 women).[23] It is more common in women who have had CIN and/or VIN. The disorder most often is located in the upper third of the vagina and is multifocal. The lesions are best identified by colposcopic examination after generous swabbing of the vagina with 4% acetic acid. The VAIN appears as white, flat or raised foci usually devoid of abnormal vessels (Fig. 18-18). Occasionally, a pigskinlike punctuation is visualized, but mosaic patterns are a rarity. Confluent papillomatous growths may also be seen particularly in the anterior and posterior fornices. These wartlike lesions are difficult to grade on the basis of colposcopic appearance alone and should be plentifully biopsied before undertaking laser treatment. Typically, these lesions are initially picked up as a result of routine cytology. Patients who have undergone hysterectomy should continue to undergo annual cytologic sampling of the vagina for this reason.

Adequate examination and mapping of the vagina is not an easy task and will not be completed in 5 or 10 minutes. I find it consumes the better part of 30 minutes to do this

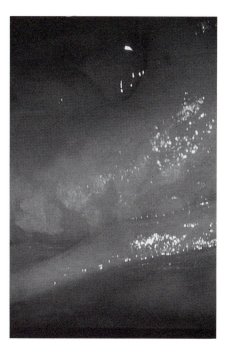

Fig. 18-18. Plaques of white vaginal intraepithelial neoplasia located in the upper, posterior third of the vagina.

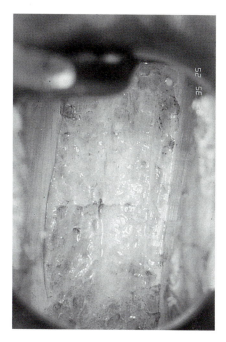

Fig. 18-19. Superpulse vaporization of upper vagina. Note the clean appearance of the superficial ablation of the vagina (less than 1 mm depth).

examination adequately. Most failures of therapy are related to inadequate preoperative evaluation. Invasive cancer after treatment for intraepithelial neoplasia invariably was present at the time of the initial treatment.[57] Women who develop VAIN after hysterectomy demand scrupulous attention to diagnosis and sampling before embanking on laser treatment. Elderly women who show cytologic atypia and who have confirmation of VAIN on directed biopsy should be given a 30-day course of estrogen cream into the vagina and then be reevaluated by cytology and colposcopy. It is not uncommon for such women to revert to normal findings after the intense local steroid therapy. Additionally, if no reversion to normal is observed, the vagina is in much better condition to undergo the laser surgery and heals infinitely better than an unprepared atrophic vagina. We have witnessed this fact time and again and now routinely prepare all postmenopausal women with topical estrogen.

The key to laser vaporization of the vagina is to use power densities of approximately 500 W/cm^2 and a beam diameter of 2 mm. All laser treatments *must* be performed with the aid of a laser hook, otherwise significant areas of the vagina will be missed and disease will persist. Vaporization should be carried to a depth of 1 mm or less. Deeper vaporization adds nothing to cure rates, but will surely increase complications. Very wide peripheral margins are required to eliminate this multifocal disease. Disease in the upper third of the vagina should be treated by vaporizing the entire upper third of the vagina. If the disease spreads into the middle third, then, the entire upper two thirds are vaporized. When VAIN is found to involve

upper, middle, and lower thirds of the vagina, the entire vagina should be vaporized in two planned, staged sessions. It is preferred to carry out the operation using a superpulsed laser at settings varying from 100 to 300 pulses per second with pulse interval at 0.1 to 0.3 ms (Fig. 18-19). This preserves underlying stromal tissue and shortens healing time. Properly performed laser vaporization results in no scar formation, rapid healing, and no reduction in vaginal capacity. As stated above, all surgery should be done with the CO_2 laser coupled to the operating microscope (colposcope) under general or regional anesthesia. Attempting this surgery under local block is the shortest route to therapeutic failure. After the vaporization, the treated area is thoroughly swabbed with 4% acetic acid and the vagina is flushed two times with sterile chilled water. This water irrigation is accomplished by means of an asepto syringe. Finally, using a vaginal applicator, the vagina is filled with triple sulfa cream. The vaginal cream is employed mainly as a vehicle to prevent the opposing vaginal walls from coapting during the healing phase.

Postoperative bleeding is not a problem after vaginal laser vaporization, and it makes no sense to apply routinely caustic solutions such as ferric subsulfate (Monsel's solution).

Results with laser treatment of VAIN have varied from 65% elimination of disease up to 90%.[22,55] More than one treatment may be required. Jobson and Homesly treated the entire vagina at a single setting and achieved cures above 90%.[37] The group in Birmingham, England, reported high failure rates and a number of invasive carcinomas after laser vaporization in women who had previous hysterectomies.[57] A report from the United States advocates excision of the vaginal vault in such cases.[35] The question again arises as to the accuracy of preoperative diagnosis and whether similar advocated techniques were used, accessory hooks, and extensiveness of peripheral vaporization. Sharp and Sanders reported a technique in the vagina analogous to the laser thin section used in the vulva.[51] These same authors reported 24 cases of VAIN, 16 of whom were treated by CO_2 laser ablation. Four have required other therapy to deal with recurrent VAIN.

Dorsey and Baggish reported 111 cases of VAIN of whom 83 were treated by laser only; 6 by laser plus excision; 5 by laser plus 5-fluorouracil cream. The remaining 17 cases were treated by total vaginectomy or partial vaginectomy.[27] The cure rates using laser in this large series was 80%, however, 40% of the cases required more than one laser exposure.[27]

The CO_2 laser remains an exceedingly precise and useful instrument for the treatment of lower genital tract disease. In this period of rising medical costs, instruments with such diversified uses, particularly by more than one surgical specialty, are cost effective and worthy of maximal usage.

REFERENCES

1. Anderson MC: Treatment of cervical intraepithelial neoplasia with the carbon dioxide laser: Report of 543 patients, *Obstet Gynecol* 59:720, 1982.
2. Anderson MC, Hartley RB: Cervical crypt involvement by intraepithelial neoplasia, *Obstet Gynecol* 55:546, 1980.
3. Baggish MS: Carbon dioxide laser treatment for condylomata acuminata venereal infections, *Obstet Gynecol* 55:711, 1980.
4. Baggish MS: Complications associated with carbon dioxide laser surgery in gynecology, *Am J Obstet Gynecol* 139:568, 1981.
5. Baggish MS: Treating viral venereal infections with the CO_2 laser, *J Reprod Med* 27:737, 1982.
6. Baggish MS: Laser management of cervical intraepithelial neoplasia, *Clin Obstet Gynecol* 26:980, 1983.
7. Baggish MS: *Condylomata acuminata genital infections treated by the CO_2 laser*. In Baggish MS, editor: *Basic and advanced laser surgery in gynecology*, Norwalk, 1985, Appleton-Crofts-Century.
8. Baggish MS: Improved laser techniques for the elimination of genital and extragenital warts, *Am J Obstet Gynecol* 153:545, 1985.
9. Baggish MS: *Laser for the treatment of vulvar intraepithelial neoplasia*. In Baggish MS, editor: *Basic and advanced laser surgery in gynecology*, Norwalk, 1985, Appleton-Century-Crofts.
10. Baggish MS: A comparsion between laser excisional conization and laser vaporization for the treatment of cervical intraepithelial neoplasia, *Am J Obstet Gynecol* 155:39, 1986.
11. Baggish MS: *Laser therapy for genital warts*. In Winkler B, Richart RM, editors: *Clinical practice of gynecology: Human papillomavirus infections*, 1:187, 1989.
12. Baggish MS, Baltoyannis P: Carbon dioxide laser treatment of cervical stenosis, *Fertil Steril* 48:24, 1987.
13. Baggish MS, Dorsey JH: CO_2 laser for the treatment of vulvar carcinoma in situ, *Obstet Gynecol* 57:371, 1981.
14. Baggish MS, Dorsey JH: Carbon dioxide laser for combination excisional vaporization conization, *Am J Obstet Gynecol* 151:23, 1985.
15. Baggish MS, Dorsey JH, Adelson M: A ten-year experience treating intraepithelial neoplasia with the CO_2 laser, *Am J Obstet Gynecol* 161:60, 1989.
16. Baggish MS, Noel Y, Brooks M: Electrosurgical thin loop conization by selective double excision, *J Gynecol Surg* 7:83, 1991.
17. Baggish MS et al: Quantitative evaluation of the skin and accessory appendages in vulvar carcinoma-in-situ, *Obstet Gynecol* 74:169, 1989.
18. Baggish MS et al: Comparison of thermal injury zones in loop electrical and laser cervical excisional conization, *Am J Obstet Gynecol* 166:545, 1992.
19. Benedet JL, Miller DM, Nickerson KG: Results of conservative management of cervical intraepithelial neoplasia, *Obstet Gynecol* 79:105, 1992.
20. Bigrigg MA et al: Colposcopic diagnosis and treatment of cervical dysplasia at a single clinic visit, *Lancet* 336:229, 1990.
21. Buscema J et al: Carcinoma in situ of the vulva, *Obstet Gynecol* 55:695, 1980.
22. Capen CV et al: Laser therapy of vaginal intraepithelial neoplasia, *Am J Obstet Gynecol* 62:90, 1982.
23. Cramer DN, Cutler SJ: Incidence and histo-pathology of malignancies of the female genital organs in the US, *Am J Obstet Gynecol* 118:443, 1976.
24. Dini MM, Jajag K: Lliovaginal fistula following cryosurgery for vaginal dysplasia, *Am J Obstet Gynecol* 136:692, 1980.
25. Dorsey JH: Understanding CO_2 laser surgery of the vulva, *Colpo Gynecol Laser Surg* 1:205, 1984.
26. Dorsey JH: *Excisional conization of the cervix by CO_2 laser*. In Baggish MS, editor: *Basic and advanced laser surgery in gynecology*, Norwalk, 1985, Appleton-Century-Crofts.
27. Dorsey JH, Baggish MS: *Multifocal vaginal intraepithelial neoplasia with uterus in situ*. In Sharp F, Jordan J, editors: *Gynecological laser surgery. Proceedings of the Fifteenth Study Group of the Royal College of Obstetricians and Gynecologists*, Ithaca, NY, 1986, Perinatology Press.
28. Evans AS, Monaghan JM: Treatment of cervical intraepithelial neoplasia using the carbon dioxide laser, *Br J Obstet Gynecol* 90:553, 1983.
29. Ferenczy A: Using the laser to treat vulvar condylomata acuminata and intraepithelial neoplasia, *Can Med Assoc J* 128:135, 1983.
30. Ferenczy A: Treating genital condyloma during pregnancy with the carbon dioxide laser, *Am J Obstet Gynecol* 148:9, 1984.
31. Ferenczy A: Evaluation and management of male partners of condyloma patients, *Colpo Gynecol Laser Surg* 2:15, 1986.
32. Ferenczy A, Mitao M, Silverstein SP: Latent papillomavirus and its relationship to recurrence of genital warts following laser surgery, *N Engl J Med* 313:784, 1985.
33. Fluhmann FC: *Ther cervix uteri its disease*, Philadephia 1961, WB Saunders.
34. Fowler JM et al: Effect of CO_2 laser conization of the uterine cervix on pathological interpretation of cervical intraepithelial neoplasia, *Obstet Gynecol* 79:693, 1992.
35. Hoffman MS et al: Laser vaporization of grade 3 vaginal intraepithelia neoplasia, *Am J Obstet Gynecol* 165:1342, 1991.
36. Indman PD, Arndt BC: Laser treatment of cervical intraepithelial neoplasia in an office setting, *Am J Obstet Gynecol* 152:674, 1985.
37. Johson VW, Homesley HD: Treatment of vaginal intraepithelial neoplasia with the carbon dioxide laser, *Obstet Gynecol* 62:90, 1983.
38. Krebs HB: Prophylactic topical 5-fluorouracil for the treatment of human papillomavirus associated lesions of the vulva and vagina, *Obstet Gynecol* 68:837, 1989.
39. Larsson G, Gullberg B, Grundsell H: A comparison of complication of laser and cold knife conization, *Obstet Gynecol* 62:213, 1983.
40. Leuchter RS et al: Treatment of vulvar carcinoma in situ with the CO_2 laser, *Gynecol Oncol* 19:314, 1984.
41. Luesley DM et al: Management of postconization cervical stenosis by laser vaporization, *Obstet Gynecol* 67:126, 1986.
42. Luesley DM et al: Loop diathermy excision of the cervical transformation zone in patients with abnormal cervical smears, *Br Med J* 300:1690, 1990.
43. McCullough AM, MacLean AB: Healing of the vulvar epithelium after laser treatment, *J Gynecol Surg* 6:33, 1990.
44. Prendiville W, Cullimore J, Normans: Large loop excision of the transformation zone (LLETZ). A new method of management for

women with cervical intraepithelial neoplasia, *Br J Obstet Gynecol* 96:1054, 1989.

45. Przybora LA, Plutowa A: Histological topography of carcinoma in situ of the cervix uteri, *Cancer* 12:263, 1959.

46. Reid R: Superficial laser vulvectomy III, *Am J Obstet Gynecol* 152:504, 1985.

47. Reid R et al: Superficial laser vulvectomy II, *Am J Obstet Gynecol* 152:261, 1985.

48. Reid R et al: Superficial laser vulvectomy V, *Am J Obstet Gynecol* 166:815, 1992.

49. Riva JM et al: Extended carbon dioxide laser vaporization in the treatment of subclinical papillomavirus infection of the lower genital tract, *Obstet Gynecol* 73:25, 1989.

50. Rosenzweig BA, Baggish, MS, Sze EHM: Carbon dioxide laser therapy for benign cervical tumors, *J Gynecol Surg* 6:97, 1990.

51. Sharp F, Saunders N: The treatment of vaginal premalignancy, *Clinical Practice of Gynecology* 2:211, 1990.

52. Singer A: The treatment of vulvar premalignancy, *Clinical Practice of* Gynecology, 2:231, 1990.

53. Sturgeon SR et al: In situ and invasive vulvar cancer incidence trends (1973-1987), *Am J Obstet Gynecol* 166:1482, 1992.

54. Townsend DE et al: Management of vulvar intraepithelia neoplasia by carbon dioxide laser, *Obstet Gynecol* 60:49, 1982.

55. Townsend DE et al: Treatment of vaginal carcinoma in situ of the vagina, *Am J Obstet Gynecol* 43:565, 1982.

56. Wolcott HD, Gallup DG: Wide local excision in the treatment of vulvar carcinoma in situ: A reappraisal, *Am J Obstet Gynecol* 150:695, 1984.

57. Woodman CBJ, Jordan JA, Wade-Evan T: The management of VAIN after hysterectomy, *Br J Obstet Gynecol* 91:707, 1984.

58. Wright VC, Davies E: Laser surgery for vulvar intraepithelial neoplasia: Principles and results, *Am J Obstet Gynecol* 156:374, 1987.

59. Wright VC, Davies E, Riopelle MA: Laser cylindrical excision to replace conization, *Am J Obstet Gynecol* 150:704, 1984.

Chapter 19

SURGERY FOR VULVAR CANCER

George W. Morley

Cancer of the vulva is one of the less frequently encountered malignancies of the female genital tract with a reported incidence of 4% among all gynecologic tumors. Vulvar malignancy usually affects women of advanced years; more than two thirds of the cases occur in women between 60 and 80 years of age. Invasive carcinoma of the vulva is seen in about 2 per 100,000 women per year.

While the exact causes remain unknown, this lesion is frequently associated with some type of chronic vulvar dystrophy, which is present in approximately 40% to 50% of the cases. These patients are almost always Caucasian. Diabetes mellitus and/or hypertension is seen in over 25% of patients with cancer of the vulva, but a cause-effect relationship has not yet been established and the incidence may merely be related to the patient's ages.

There have been many advances in the treatment of carcinoma of the vulva over the past 25 years. Previously, basically three forms of therapy were used in the treatment of this malignant lesion: a total vulvectomy was considered the treatment of choice for preinvasive disease; radical vulvectomy and regional lymphadenectomy were the treatment for invasive disease; and palliative vulvectomy was reserved for treatment of the unresectable or incurable condition. In a comparative study reported from the University of Michigan Medical Center covering a 40-year period from 1935 to 1975, there was a 20% incidence of lesions too extensive to be treated therapeutically as a curative procedure.[16] In a more recent series reported from the University of Michigan, the incidence of palliative vulvectomy had decreased to approximately 5%.[11]

During the past few decades, patients have sought medical attention much earlier than previously after once noting some physical abnormality. This is because the lesion has ceased to be thought a symptom of a sexually transmitted disease or to reflect a lack of cleanliness or laxity in personal hygiene.

CLASSIFICATION OF VULVAR CANCER

Following is the 1989 revision of the International Federation of Gynecology and Obstetrics (FIGO) definitions of the surgical staging of carcinoma of the vulva.[6]

Stage 0

T_{is} — Carcinoma in situ, intraepithelial carcinoma

Stage I

$T_1 N_0 M_0$ — Tumor confined to the vulva and/or perineum—2 cm or less in greatest dimension, nodes not palpable

Stage II

$T_2 N_0 M_0$ — Tumor confined to the vulva and/or perineum—more than 2 cm in greatest dimension, nodes not palpable

Stage III

$T_3 N_0 M_0$
$T_3 N_1 M_0$ — Tumor of any size with:
(1) adjacent spread to the lower urethra and/or the vagina, or the anus, and/or
(2) unilateral regional (groin) lymph node metastasis

$T_1 N_1 M_0$
$T_2 N_1 M_0$

Stage IVa

$T_1 N_2 M_0$
$T_2 N_2 M_0$ — Tumor invades any of the following: upper urethra, bladder mucosa, rectal mucosa, pelvic bone and/or bilateral regional (groin) lymph node metastasis

$T_3 N_2 M_0$
T_4 Any N M_0

Stage IVb

Any T, Any N, M1 — Any distant metastasis including pelvic lymph nodes

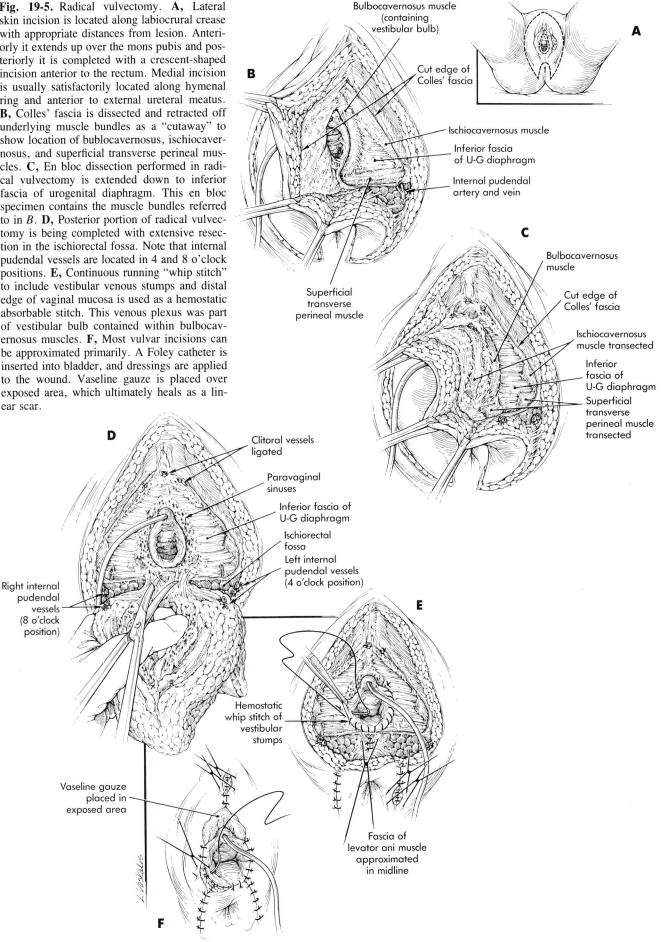

Fig. 19-5. Radical vulvectomy. **A,** Lateral skin incision is located along labiocrural crease with appropriate distances from lesion. Anteriorly it extends up over the mons pubis and posteriorly it is completed with a crescent-shaped incision anterior to the rectum. Medial incision is usually satisfactorily located along hymenal ring and anterior to external ureteral meatus. **B,** Colles' fascia is dissected and retracted off underlying muscle bundles as a "cutaway" to show location of bublocavernosus, ischiocavernosus, and superficial transverse perineal muscles. **C,** En bloc dissection performed in radical vulvectomy is extended down to inferior fascia of urogenital diaphragm. This en bloc specimen contains the muscle bundles referred to in *B*. **D,** Posterior portion of radical vulvectomy is being completed with extensive resection in the ischiorectal fossa. Note that internal pudendal vessels are located in 4 and 8 o'clock positions. **E,** Continuous running "whip stitch" to include vestibular venous stumps and distal edge of vaginal mucosa is used as a hemostatic absorbable stitch. This venous plexus was part of vestibular bulb contained within bulbocavernosus muscles. **F,** Most vulvar incisions can be approximated primarily. A Foley catheter is inserted into bladder, and dressings are applied to the wound. Vaseline gauze is placed over exposed area, which ultimately heals as a linear scar.

Bulbocavernosus muscle (containing vestibular bulb)

Cut edge of Colles' fascia

Ischiocavernosus muscle

Inferior fascia of U-G diaphragm

Internal pudendal artery and vein

Superficial transverse perineal muscle

Bulbocavernosus muscle

Cut edge of Colles' fascia

Ischiocavernosus muscle transected

Inferior fascia of U-G diaphragm

Superficial transverse perineal muscle transected

Clitoral vessels ligated

Paravaginal sinuses

Inferior fascia of U-G diaphragm

Ischiorectal fossa

Left internal pudendal vessels (4 o'clock position)

Right internal pudendal vessels (8 o'clock position)

Hemostatic whip stitch of vestibular stumps

Vaseline gauze placed in exposed area

Fascia of levator ani muscle approximated in midline

member, mapping and identification of margins is required before sending the specimen to the pathologist.

POSTOPERATIVE CARE AND COMPLICATIONS

Once the immediate postoperative and postanesthetic periods have passed, patients undergoing this type of surgery usually have a progressively satisfactory course. Most of these patients are continued on prophylactic anticoagulant and antibiotic therapy for a reasonable period of time, and they remain strictly confined to bed for approximately 48 hours assuming a modified semi-Fowler's position to avoid tension on the wound edges. Conservative measures such as "log rolling" and intermittent movement of the lower extremities are permissible during this period as a method of improving their circulation. Sequential compression devices applied to the lower extremities may be used in place of anticoagulation therapy. Subsequently patients are allowed progressive ambulation, and the indwelling catheter is removed on the fourth or fifth postoperative day.

The most common postoperative complication seen in these patients is some degree of wound cellulitis and wound disruption, which occurs to some degree in approximately 30% to 40% of the patients. Usually these separations are not great and are treated conservatively with debridement and open packing. An attempt to reapproximate the wound edges at a later date is considered unwise since these wounds heal secondarily with a normal-appearing linear scar as their end point.

One must be aware that hemorrhage as a complication, although occurring infrequently, can be the result of anticoagulants prescribed prophylactically or of frequent, long-term self-administration of salicylates and similar drugs, as used by many elderly people. Pulmonary embolization itself is rarely reported as a complication of this procedure.

Not infrequently a lymphocyst will appear in the groin region. This complication occurs in less than 10% of the cases, and its incidence can be further reduced by careful attention to ligation of the lymphatic vessels in both the superficial and deep groin compartments. The presence of a lymphocyst requires frequent aspiration followed by local compression to the area. Only on rare occasions does one have to surgically isolate and ligate the causative lymphatic vessel. The usual postoperative complications, which are unrelated to the procedure itself, must also be kept in mind by the attending surgical team throughout the remainder of the hospitalization.

Late complications are of a more permanent nature and have primarily to do with alterations of the vaginal introitus, the urinary tract system, and the lower extremities. Introital stenosis of the vagina may give rise to dyspareunia; however, this can easily be corrected using relaxing incisions at the introitus or by performing a reversed perineorrhaphy. Fissuring or "cracking" of the perineum is not un-

common, and a vitamin A and D ointment or other non-medicated skin softener applied 1 to 2 times daily to this area will often soften up this inelastic tissue.

Now that less advanced malignant lesions of the vulva are being seen, postsurgical disfigurement is less frequently encountered, even though there is obvious alteration of the local anatomy and appearance of the operative site. Infrequently, one may see a far advanced lesion requiring extensive therapeutic surgical intervention, which may necessitate reconstructive vulvoplasty. A number of techniques have been described, which include the classic Z-plasty approach, the myocutaneous gracilis flap technique, and the rhomboid skin flap mobilization.[2,13,18,22] Again, these procedures are seldom indicated. Finally, if sexual function is satisfactory following primary healing and only local appearance is of concern, patients should probably receive sexual counseling rather than undergo surgical correction of these changes.

A number of patients complain of misdirection of the urinary stream during micturition. Embarrassment can be avoided by the patient repositioning herself on the toilet seat or through the use of a plastic deflector attached to the commode. This annoyance can be prevented at the time of surgery by repositioning the external urethral meatus in a more proximal position on the anterior vaginal wall 1 to 2 cm in from the introitus. If an external urethral stenosis is encountered as a late complication, an external urethral meatotomy may be the only corrective step required.

Not uncommonly, pelvic relaxation with the appearance of a cystocele and/or rectocele or symptoms of stress urinary incontinence are reported during a follow-up examination. These changes may or may not be related to the radical surgery itself but are easily corrected through well-known nonsurgical or surgical approaches.

Probably the most annoying late complication to the patient and the most frustrating complication to the physician is swelling of the lower extremities. Much of this can be avoided if the patient is instructed to use elastic stockings prophylactically for the first 6 months following surgery. In spite of this preventive measure, a number of patients will develop leg edema, which must then be treated therapeutically with compression stockings worn almost continuously when ambulatory. To date, surgical intervention has not been successful. Preservation of the saphenous vein at the time of groin lymph node dissection may help in reducing this complication, without any compromise of survival. The overall mortality reported of 1% to 2% following radical pelvic surgery for carcinoma of the vulva seems reasonable when one realizes that this is a disease of the elderly.

RESULTS

The results of collective experience over a 50-year period (1935 to 1988) at the University of Michigan Medical Center are similar to those reported in the literature.[11,14] During this time, almost 500 patients with invasive carcinoma of the vulva were treated with some type of radical vulvar surgery in this institution.

From a review of a collected series over a 20-year literature search,[1,7,14,21] there is a 35% incidence of groin lymph node involvement when all stages of the disease are analyzed; the nodes being involved in 12% to 15% of the cases with stage I disease and in 90% with stage IV disease. The overall 5-year survival rate for all stages approximates 60%, with almost 85% survival in patients with stage I disease. Only a 12% to 15% survival is to be expected in stage IV disease. Given that the regional lymph nodes are negative for metastases, an overall 5-year survival rate of 85% for all stages can be anticipated. The absolute 5-year survival rate for patients with stage I disease and negative lymph nodes approximates 95%. If the regional lymph nodes are positive for metastatic disease, the overall 5-year survival rate drops to around 40%. Again, the lymph node status significantly influences survival; however, it has been shown that the survival rates for patients having only one groin node involvement is essentially equal to the survival of patients with no regional lymph node involvement.

Patients with advanced vulvar cancer are still seen in our clinics, and they present a unique and difficult problem. A surgical approach to advanced vulvar cancer usually involves some type of pelvic exenteration, especially when the primary lesion is geographically located in close proximity to the bladder anteriorly or to the bowel posteriorly. Often these patients respond quite satisfactorily to this radical pelvic surgery, and although the series at Michigan[17] is small, the overall survival approximates 60%. Recently, Boronow and others[3,19] have reported on preoperative irradiation for patients with an advanced lesion. They found that lesser surgery could be anticipated following preoperative irradiation, thus satisfying the goal of preservation of the visceral organs. Boronow reported a 72% 5-year survival rate using this type of combination therapy in patients with stage III and IV carcinoma of the vulva.[4] Radiation therapy alone and postoperative pelvic irradiation are other options still being considered.[9,12]

Approximately 10% of patients will experience a recurrence of the vulvar malignancy at the primary site.[8,10] The mainstay of therapy for this recurrent disease is wide local excision with or without radiation therapy depending on the surgical margins and the presence or absence of metastatic disease to the regional lymph nodes. Again, the status of the lymph nodes is a significant prognostic factor. When the recurrences remain localized to the vulva, surgical resection of the involved area with wide and deep margins can provide an excellent survival rate for these patients.

CONCLUSION

Medicine has always been in transition, and it will continue to be so. Results of the treatment of invasive carcinoma of the vulva in the next several years should reflect the current knowledge gleaned from a variety of facts, which include: (1) a 25% to 35% inaccurate clinical assessment of groin lymph nodes; (2) a threefold increase in groin lymph node involvement in clitoral/perineal lesions; (3) an essentially equal 5-year survival rate for patients with negative groin lymph nodes versus patients with one positive groin lymph node; (4) a 5-year survival rate for all patients in all stages dropping approximately 50% when groin lymph nodes are positive; (5) an ipsilateral groin lymph node dissection only in a unilateral lesion if the lymph nodes are negative; (6) a preservation of body image and sexual response through conservation of normal tissue through a partial or hemiradical vulvectomy when feasible; and (7) a frequently satisfactory survival rate when recurrences are usually treated with radical local excision and supplemental regional lymph node dissection when required.

In closing, it was Mr. Stanley Way of Newcastle-on-Tyne, England, a noted gynecologic oncologist, who once said, "Surgery will one day become obsolete in the treatment of cancer of the vulva." It is hoped that through a better understanding of the biology of the disease and through continued advances in radiation therapy, chemotherapy, and immunotherapy or their combinations, we may be able to provide a new and better direction in the treatment of invasive carcinoma of the vulva in the future.

REFERENCES

1. Annual Report: International Federation of Gynecology and Obstetrics. vol 18, 1988.
2. Barnhill DR, Hoskins WJ, Metz P: Use of the rhomboid flap after partial vulvectomy, *Obstet Gynecol* 62:444, 1983.
3. Boronow RC: Therapeutic alternative to primary exenteration for advanced vulvovaginal cancer, *Cancer* 1:233, 1973.
4. Boronow RC et al: Combined therapy as an alternative to exenteration for locally advanced vulvovaginal cancer. II. Results, complications, and dosimetric and surgical considerations, *Am J Clin Oncol* 10:171, 1987.
5. Burrell MO et al: The modified radical vulvectomy with groin dissection: an eight-year experience, *Am J Obstet Gynecol* 159:715, 1988.
6. FIGO staging for carcinoma of the vulva: annual report on the results of treatment in gynecologic cancer, *Int J Gynaecol Obstet* 28:189, 1989.
7. Hacker NF et al: Individualization of treatment for Stage I squamous cell vulvar carcinoma, *Obstet Gynecol* 63:155, 1984.
8. Heaps JM et al: Surgical-pathologic variables predictive of local recurrence in squamous cell carcinoma of the vulva, *Gynecol Oncol* 38:309, 1990.
9. Homesley HD et al: Radiation therapy versus pelvic node resection for carcinoma of the vulva with positive groin nodes, *Obstet Gynecol* 68:733, 1986.
10. Hopkins MP, Reid GC, Morley GW: The surgical management of recurrent squamous cell carcinoma of the vulva, *Obstet Gynecol* 75:1001, 1990.
11. Hopkins MP et al: Squamous cell carcinoma of the vulva: prognostic factors influencing survival, *Gynecol Oncol* 43:113, 1991.
12. Jafari K, Magdotti M: Radiation therapy in carcinoma of the vulva, *Cancer* 47:686, 1981.
13. Julian CG, Callison J, Woodruff JD: Plastic management of extensive vulvar defects, *Obstet Gynecol* 38:193, 1971.

14. Malfetano J, Piver MS, Tsukada Y: Stage III and IV squamous cell carcinoma of the vulva, *Gynecol Oncol* 23:192, 1986.

15. Microinvasive cancer of the vulva. Report of the ISSVD Task Force. *J Reprod Med* 29:454, 1984.

16. Morley GW: Infiltrative carcinoma of the vulva: results of surgical management. *Am J Obstet Gynecol* 124:874, 1976.

17. Morley GW et al: Pelvic exenteration, University of Michigan: 100 patients at five years, *Obstet Gynecol* 74:934, 1989.

18. Rankin R, Pinkney Jr: The use of Z-plasty in gynecologic operations, *Am J Obstet Gynecol* 117:231, 1973.

19. Rotmensch J et al: Preoperative radiotherapy followed by radical vulvectomy with inguinal lymphadenectomy for advanced vulvar carcinomas, *Gynecol Oncol* 36:181, 1990.

20. Rutledge F, Sinclair M: Treatment of intraepithelial carcinoma of the vulva by skin excision and graft, *Am J Obstet Gynecol* 102:806, 1968.

21. Trelford JD et al: Ten-year prospective study in a management change of vulvar carcinoma, *Am J Obstet Gynecol* 150:288, 1984.

22. Wheeless CR Jr et al: Gracilis myocutaneous flap in reconstruction of the vulva and female perineum, *Obstet Gynecol* 54:97, 1979.

Chapter 20

VAGINAL HYSTERECTOMY

David H. Nichols

About 650,000 hysterectomies are performed annually in the United States, a number somewhat fewer than in previous years;[39] about 70% will be done transabdominally and 30% transvaginally. At present less than one third of hysterectomies are performed by the vaginal route. Welch and Randall[49] reported in 1958 that 50% of the hysterectomies at the Mayo Clinic were done vaginally. A similar figure was obtained at the Lahey Clinic[5,6] and 60.9% of 9967 hysterectomies were performed by the vaginal route at the University of Vienna.[11]

The complications of 1851 abdominal and vaginal hysterectomies performed between September 1978 and August 1981 were studied in detail at nine institutions by the Collaborative Review of Sterilization, an observational study coordinated by the Centers for Disease Control. This review concluded that "women who underwent vaginal hysterectomy experienced significantly fewer complications than women who had undergone abdominal hysterectomy" and went on to recommend that "vaginal hysterectomy with prophylactic antibiotics should be 'strongly considered' for those women of reproductive age for whom either surgical approach is clinically appropriate."[7]

In the selection of an operative procedure for hysterectomy, there is no place for surgical histrionics or dogmatic pronouncements. The gynecologic surgeon should try to gain by personal experience equal confidence in the transabdominal and transvaginal procedures for hysterectomy. With this confidence, the surgeon can choose the approach that seems to be in the best interests of each patient.

The performance of hysterectomy requires of the surgeons:
1. Proper and effective training and experience.
2. Awareness of possible complications, including intraoperative ones, and their treatment.
3. Three-dimensional thinking[21] and the necessary psychomotor skills.

Following the initial careful preoperative pelvic examination, first with the patient standing, then supine, and a decision that hysterectomy is in the patient's best interests, that conclusion as well as the alternatives to hysterectomy should be given to the patient thoughtfully and with abundant opportunity for the patient to discuss any questions or details. She should be made aware of the possible complications of surgery and the details of the usual convalescence, and she should be given the opportunity to formulate and express her own views as to what has been proposed. It is valuable for the surgeon to know how the patient perceives her problem and its proposed remedy and the effect it is likely to have upon her future life and relationships.

Ultimately the indications for abdominal hysterectomy may evolve as the contraindications for vaginal hysterectomy, for instance, presence of a suspicious adnexal mass, uterine immobility, invasive cancer, very large uterine leiomyomata, or lack of operator experience, enthusiasm, and confidence. Indications relating to the choice of operative route are listed in Table 20-1.

The goals of reconstructive surgery, whether performed transvaginally or transabdominally, are as follows:

1. Relief of symptoms
2. Restoration of normal anatomic relationships
3. Restoration of function

The operation chosen for a particular patient should make it possible for all of these goals to be achieved.

It is with the second of these goals that the professional may encounter conflict and controversy. Standard anatomic texts describe in detail the anatomic and organ relationships of the cadaver, but these observations may be in sharp contrast to those of the living, in whom voluntary muscle tone permits the vagina to lie upon a normally empty rectum, which in turn lies upon an intact levator

Table 20-1. Vaginal versus abdominal approach to possible hysterectomy

Indication	Approach		
	Vaginal	Laparoscopically assisted vaginal hysterectomy	Abdominal
Myomata uteri	Occasionally	Occasionally	Usually
Pelvic inflammatory disease	Rarely	Occasionally	Always, except for posterior colpotomy
Recurrent dysfunctional uterine bleeding	Usually		Occasionally
Endometriosis	Rarely	Occasionally	Usually
Adenomyosis	Usually	Occasionally	Occasionally
Symptomatic pelvic relaxation	Usually	Occasionally	Occasionally
Adnexal mass	Rarely	Occasionally	Always
Pelvic pain	Rarely	Occasionally	Usually
Cancer of cervix			
Stage 0 and Ia	Usually	Rarely	Occasionally
Stage IA, IB, IIA	Occasionally	Rarely	Usually
Cancer corpus	Occasionally	Occasionally	Usually

Modified from Thompson JD: *Clin Obstet Gynecol* 24:1255, 1981.

plate[32,41] (see Chapter 3). The normal upper vaginal axis of the standing woman is thus horizontal and not vertical as it is shown in textbook descriptions of cadaver anatomy. Restoration, support, and suspension of the vaginal vault into the hollow of the sacrum and over an intact levator plate is a major goal of reconstruction if the vault is to remain postoperatively where it is intended to be. This is most easily accomplished by the transvaginal approach to the patient's surgery, as a New Orleans or McCall-type cul-de-plasty can be added easily. A deep cul-de-sac should be sought, and if found excised or obliterated. If the anatomic support of the vault is found wanting, it should be provided by coincident colpopexy, either transvaginal or transabdominal. The surgeon should be familiar and experienced with the techniques of each (see Chapter 27). Reduction in operative time and surgical blood loss is directly dependent on precision in the knowledge of each patient's connective tissue septae, planes, and potential spaces. The blood vessels run within the septae, which should be clamped and cut before blood is lost. In general the patient's convalescence is more comfortable after a vaginal than after an abdominal hysterectomy. Moreover, the surgeon can correct any problems of pelvic relaxation, which are often present in a patient whose condition requires a hysterectomy, during a vaginal operative procedure.

The gynecoid pelvis provides the most room for successful transvaginal hysterectomy, while the android type may compromise exposure. The slant that the vulva makes with the body axis frequently suggests the type of pelvis. The operator can determine whether the width of the vaginal outlet is adequate for transvaginal hysterectomy by inserting a closed fist between the ischial tuberosities during the pelvic examination; if the fist fits comfortably, the width of the bony pelvis is adequate.

The most important single observation in evaluating the feasibility of vaginal rather than abdominal hysterectomy may well be the demonstrable mobility of the uterus. Generally, a movable uterus can readily be removed in a vaginal procedure. Conversely, a uterus that is not movable should rarely be approached transvaginally, even when the vaginal operation seems otherwise indicated, as when the patient is extremely obese or when a vaginal or perineal repair is necessary. The phenomenon of pseudoprolapse can demonstrate the degree of uterine mobility; with the pelvic musculature effectively relaxed under anesthesia, if moderate traction brings an ordinarily well-supported cervix nearly to the introitus, the uterus is sufficiently mobile to permit a vaginal hysterectomy.

VAGINAL HYSTERECTOMY FOR THE PATIENT WITHOUT PROLAPSE

The vagina is often the appropriate route for hysterectomy when the uterus is movable, whether it is prolapsed or not. This is the easiest of vaginal hysterectomies to perform because the anatomy of the uterine supports is constant and unaltered by disease. Hospitalization can be shortened, and the patient is often home by the second or third postoperative day. Vaginal hysterectomy can be performed easily on the nulligravida patient.

Provided that the uterus is movable, the less the prolapse, the easier the hysterectomy; the greater the prolapse, the more difficult the hysterectomy. Anatomic differences are fewer in patients without prolapse, greater and less predictable in patients with some degree of prolapse. In fact massive vaginal eversion with procidentia can be among the most challenging of all gynecologic surgical cases because each progressive step requires precise surgical judgment and the resolution of the problems that arise requires creative resourcefulness. In a hundred such operations in which there is a significant degree of prolapse, the anatomic challenges, findings, and solutions will be identical in no two procedures.

In some cases the anus seems to be the most dependent portion of the perineum, and the patient literally sits on her anus. This uncommon finding usually indicates a major defect in the integrity of the levator ani. Such a defect may be associated with postmenopausal estrogen deficiency and loss of tissue tone, but it is more likely to result from major trauma to the levator ani and pelvic diaphragm, an acquired or congenital deficiency of innervation, or a degenerative neurologic disease. This syndrome is discussed further in Chapter 30.

CONSERVATION VERSUS PROPHYLACTIC REMOVAL OF THE OVARIES

From a theoretical standpoint, the criteria that determine the desirability of removing the ovaries at the time of vaginal hysterectomy are the same as those that apply during an abdominal operation.[4,44] Because the ovaries are not technically as readily accessible during a vaginal hysterectomy as during an abdominal laparotomy, however, prophylactic ovarian removal is less common when hysterectomy is accomplished by the vaginal approach. They may be removed, however, by coincident operative laparoscopy.

Indications for oophorectomy

When evaluating the indications for oophorectomy, the surgeon should balance the effects of removing the ovaries against the relatively low risk (in most cases) that the patient may in the future develop an ovarian neoplasm if the ovaries are preserved.[37,38] For example, the patient who has a family history of ovarian cancer may be considered a candidate for prophylactic oophorectomy at the time of vaginal hysterectomy. She should be told that oophorectomy would reduce her risk of developing carcinoma of the ovary but that it would not eliminate the risk, because the disease seems to have certain potential general coelomic manifestations. Elective oophorectomy in the premenopausal patient is a preoperative decision in which the patient should be a participant.

In their studies of steroidogenesis in the postmenopausal ovary, Mattingly and Huang[28] demonstrated that stromal steroid production persists for a long time after the menopause, even though estrogen production falls precipitously when menstruation ceases; therefore the postmenopausal ovary continues to have an important metabolic function. The authors noted that in reported studies of 7,765 patients whose ovaries had been conserved at the time of hysterectomy (and presumably inspected and found to be grossly normal) and who had been followed for varying intervals after surgery, only 12 women were known to have developed cancer in the preserved ovaries, an incidence of only 0.15%. The overall general incidence of ovarian malignancy suggests that the eventual frequency of ovarian cancer is likely to approximate 1 per 100 patients; however, this estimate includes the whole population, most of whose ovaries had never been previously inspected.

Although castration should not be routine at any arbitrarily designated age, it appears that so-called prophylactic oophorectomy should be considered after the age of true ovarian senescence, whether that be demonstrable at 40 or 70 years of age, because the tendency of the ovaries to neoplasia does not disappear when steroidogenesis ceases. As a general rule, transvaginal removal of the grossly normal ovary may be encouraged in the patient who is older than 55 and discouraged in the patient who is younger than 40; the operator's advice to those patients in between may be somewhat flexible, depending more on the present degree of ovarian activity than on the chronologic age of the patient. The surgeon must take into account the fact that oophorectomy in the younger patient will accelerate the onset of osteoporosis and other degenerative changes. Because there seems to be no arbitrary age at which all ovaries must be removed, the view of the surgeon who elects not to perform routine oophorectomy is defensible.

Estrogen replacement therapy

Although estrogen can be readily replaced after oophorectomy, many authorities argue that the usual replacement therapy only relieves the subjective vasomotor symptoms of the menopause and, unless long continued, does not prevent the degenerative changes that may follow castration. Furthermore, Randall[32,38] noted that patients for whom estrogen supplementation or replacement had been prescribed after a surgical menopause tended to discontinue the medication after 1 or 2 years. He suggested that because the more significant of the degenerative effects that may follow estrogen withdrawal may not appear for years, patients do not immediately associate cause and effect.

To be effective, estrogen replacement therapy must be given prophylactically. The particularly undesirable bony changes are preventable, but once developed they are apparently not reversible. Moreover, as Robinson, Cohen, and Higano[42] pointed out, the standard postmenopausal daily dose of 1.25 mg of conjugated estrogen is only partially successful in altering postmenopausal blood serum lipid levels. A dose of 2.5 mg per day is somewhat more effective. The optimal effect may require 5 mg per day or more, however, and this dosage is likely to produce such distressing secondary effects as breast tenderness, fluid retention, and weight gain.

PROCEDURE FOR VAGINAL HYSTERECTOMY

As surgeons develop their own techniques through personal experience and comparisons with the procedures described by other operators, they usually identify and embrace a large group of fundamental principles. They do not merely memorize a sequence of operative steps. Step four need not follow step three; it may follow step six or seven or even be skipped altogether depending on the characteristics of a particular patient's tissues and the operator's development of tissue relationships. The "whys" of doing something are every bit as important as the "whats." Illustrations enhanced by sagittal drawings can help surgeons visualize important operative details by adding a third dimensional or spatial geometric concept to their surgical thinking; for example, they can show that only in cases of advanced prolapse does the surgery start in tissues that actually protrude from the pelvis.

Obstetrician-gynecologists who prefer to stand while they do episiotomy repairs are likely to prefer to stand during vaginal hysterectomy and repair as well. This position seems to give the operator desirable mobility with minimal muscle tension. If the operator chooses to stand, it will be necessary to elevate the operating table almost to its maximum height. Regardless of operative technique, some operators prefer to be seated.

Horizontal light sources are always desirable for surgical procedures within the pelvis. Because operating room spotlights tend to wander during the course of a procedure, some operators use a fiberoptic forehead lamp (see Fig. 7-2), which provides a readily directed, shadowless illumination into the very depths of the wound and into the hollow of the sacrum. The operator and all assistants must keep their visual attention on the operative field; no one but the anesthesiologist needs to watch the patient, and no one at all needs to watch the nurse, clock, technician, or one another. A retractor can cause an injury if held by an uninterested assistant who allows it to wander, or it may obscure the telltale spurt of a small unsecured artery. When tension upon a pedicle or adjacent structure is relaxed, bleeding from a momentarily exposed vessel may remain undetected if the operator and the assistants have not been closely watching the operative field.

Initial procedures

Approximately 8 hours before surgery (or the night before)—not just shortly before surgery—the rectum should be carefully cleansed by either enema or an oral electrolyte bowel preparation (Go-Lytely, Nu-Lytely, CoLyte). The patient should be instructed to void just before coming to the operating room. A single dose of a "prophylactic" antibiotic, usually a cephalosporin, is given either intramuscularly or intravenously when the patient is ready for transit to the operating room.[13,46] Only if the bladder is palpably distended must it be catheterized at the beginning of surgery because a bladder that contains a little urine is easier to identify during surgery than one that is empty. If desired, 60 ml of dilute indigo carmine, methylene blue solution, or sterile evaporated milk can be instilled into the bladder preoperatively to facilitate recognition of any unanticipated bladder opening, which occasionally occurs during the course of a gynecologic operative procedure. This should be done routinely for every patient who has undergone a cesarean section in the past.

As soon as the patient is under anesthesia, the surgeon should perform a careful preoperative bimanual pelvic reexamination to decide whether to proceed with the hysterectomy vaginally or to perform the hysterectomy abdominally. The size, position, shape, and especially the mobility of the uterus should be carefully assessed. The freedom

and position of the cul-de-sac should be noted and the thickness and length of the uterosacral ligaments evaluated. Elongation of the cervix should be noted because any cervical elongation affects the point at which the incision through the vagina should begin. The direction and depth of the vaginal axis at rest should also be noted.

A preliminary dilation and curettage (D and C) should be performed if the patient has any history of abnormal bleeding. This procedure usually suggests the cause of the bleeding. Furthermore, it provides additional information about the size, mobility, consistency, position, and internal architecture of the uterus. The position of the uterus is particularly important. A prolapsed uterus is rarely in anteversion unless a suspension or fixation procedure was performed earlier. A retroverted uterus is usually accompanied by pathologic elongation of the infundibulopelvic ligaments; in this case, the ovaries are generally in the cul-de-sac, which makes them much more accessible if they are to be removed through the vaginal incision during the course of the operation.

Following examination under anesthesia and preliminary curettage of the uterus, traction is established by applying a double-toothed tenaculum to the anterior lip of the cervix, and the integrity of the urogenital diaphragm and the anterior vaginal wall is assessed. This evaluation indicates whether suspension or support of the urethra and lower vagina should accompany the repair and whether the planned reconstruction is likely to restore the normal vaginal axis and depth. Another tenaculum is applied to the posterior lip of the cervix and used to evaluate the location and size of the cul-de-sac of Douglas, as well as the strength and size of the uterosacral ligaments that become more readily demonstrable as they are stretched by traction. (Fig. 20-1). The attachment of the cul-de-sac to the cervix then usually becomes more obvious, which helps the operator determine the appropriate site for the initial incision to circumscribe the cervix. Having been grasped anteriorly and posteriorly with two double-toothed tenacula, the cervix is drawn downward so that both the cervix and the upper vagina can be adequately exposed with the use of vaginal retractors. (If the labia minora are large enough to obstruct exposure of the vagina, they should be temporarily fixed to the skin lateral to the labia majora by one or two sutures on each side.)

The selective paracervical infiltration of not more than 50 ml of 0.5% lidocaine (Xylocaine) or bupivacaine (Marcaine) in 1:200,000 epinephrine (Adrenaline) solution,[12,32] the so-called liquid tourniquet, considerably decreases blood loss during surgery, particularly in premenopausal, nonhypertensive women. In addition, the use of this agent seems to lessen the amount of additional anesthesia that is necessary and the need for postoperative analgesia, and it facilitates the identification of cleavage planes as they are developed and separated. Because it produces a temporary ischemia, the infiltration of lidocaine may reduce the immediate resistance to infection[8], but if prophylactic antibiotics have been started preoperatively, a

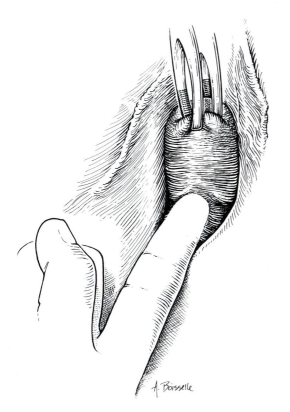

Fig. 20-1. Traction is made to a tenaculum applied to posterior lip of cervix and site of cul-de-sac of Douglas, palpated as shown. Length and strength of uterosacral ligaments are noted. (From Nichols DH, Randall CL: *Vaginal surgery,* ed 3, Baltimore, 1989, Williams & Wilkins.)

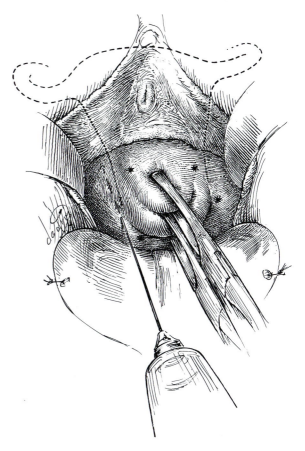

Fig. 20-2. Cervix is grasped with two double-toothed tenacula, one anterior and one posterior to the external os, and downward traction is applied. Vaginal retractors of adequate length and proper design then provide satisfactory exposure of cervix and upper vagina. In a premenopausal patient who has received preventive antibiotics, the circumference of the cervix, along a line where a circumcisionlike incision is about to be made, may be first carefully infiltrated with a mixture of 1:200,000 epinephrine (Adrenaline) and 0.5% lidocaine (Xylocaine) or bupivacaine (Marcaine). This is readily accomplished using a pressure syringe and a long 22-gauge spinal needle. Before injecting solution at each puncture site, traction is applied to plunger of syringe to make certain no blood is obtained and thus prevent intravenous or intraarterial injection of the solution. If a bloody aspirate is obtained, needle is repositioned. The cervical insertions of the uterosacral ligaments, or paracervical portions of the cardinal ligaments, and the bladder pillars (as noted by asterisks) should be the objectives of this infiltration. About 50 ml of this solution, half into either side and 8 ml at each injection site, usually provides adequate infiltration. (From Nichols DH, Randall CL: *Vaginal surgery,* ed 3, Baltimore, 1989, Williams & Wilkins.)

therapeutic concentration should already have been disseminated within the pelvic tissues, and there should be no increase in morbidity. When a patient is receiving halothane or cyclopropane anesthesia, has been taking a beta-blocker (e.g., propranolol), or has unstable or severe hypertension or coronary heart disease, normal saline solutions may be substituted for the epinephrine solution. However, a much larger volume of fluid is needed, which may tend to distort the anatomy a bit.

The anesthetist should be informed before the injection is given. The actual infiltration is most easily accomplished with the use of a pressure syringe and a 22-gauge spinal needle (Fig. 20-2). Before injecting the solution, the operator should pull and release the plunger of the syringe to make certain that no blood is obtained; if there is blood in the aspirate, the operator must reposition the needle to avoid intravenous or intraarterial injection of the solution. The solution is not injected into the cervical tissue itself but into the tissues to which the cervix is attached and the tissues around the cervix, such as the bladder pillars, the lower cardinal ligaments, and the insertions of the uterosacral ligaments. A wait of 15 minutes from the time of completion of the injection until the start of surgery permits wider dissemination of the fluid into the intercellular connective tissue,[33] but this time is a luxury that not all

operating room schedules permit. Although the use of the "liquid tourniquet" may reduce blood loss significantly, it is a complement and not a substitute for careful dissection and meticulous surgical hemostasis.

Operative technique

Making the initial incision. The correct spot for circumcision of the vagina before hysterectomy is often at some distance from the external cervical os.[10] As Bandler[2] pointed out, the closer the initial incision to the external cervical os, the greater the bleeding and the more dissection of the cervical branches of the uterine blood vessels is required to reach the cul-de-sac. Conversely, there is less bleeding when the incision is made farther above the external cervical os, but the risk of inadvertently opening the bladder or rectum is greater. Most surgeons compromise, based in large part on their estimate of the length of the cervix and the palpable level of the peritoneum of the posterior cul-de-sac. The initial incision should be at the level of the base of the cul-de-sac of Douglas.

Using either curved Mayo scissors or a scalpel, the operator opens the vagina by making a circumcisionlike incision around the cervix along the grooved depression noticeable in the transverse rugae through the full thickness of the vaginal membrane. At the upper limits of the vagina, there are fewer rugae as the vagina blends with the epithelial layer of the cervix, which has no rugae. Posteriorly the incision exposes the uterosacral ligaments and peritoneum of the cul-de-sac, but the initial incision should not cut the ligaments or actually open the peritoneum into the cul-de-sac.

Dissecting the vagina. After making the initial incision around the cervix, the operator may remove the double-toothed tenacula and reapply them so as to pull the cut edge of the vagina over the lower cervix and external os. It

is critical for the operator to continue the dissection in the correct cleavage plane because dissection in the wrong plane greatly increases blood loss and, even more important, jeopardizes the blood supply of the tissue flaps on which the success of the repair depends. The full thickness of the vaginal membrane should be peeled back from all underlying connective tissue but only for a short distance unless the uterosacral ligaments are markedly elongated. In this case, the tips of only partially opened scissors may be used in a "cut and push" maneuver to "skin" the vagina over a considerable distance from the external surfaces of the connective tissue plane that covers these ligaments.

If unexpected infection is discovered in the cervix, the operator may free the cervix from the surrounding tissues to the level of the internal os and then amputate it from the fundus before opening the peritoneum either anteriorly or posteriorly, thereby reducing the risk of contamination and postoperative peritonitis. Shortening the cervix in this manner occasionally makes it easier for the operator to hook a finger around the fundus of the uterus to facilitate opening the anterior peritoneum.

Opening the posterior peritoneum. The operator can usually identify the cul-de-sac of Douglas readily after pulling the subvaginal tissue layer taut with forceps (Fig. 20-3). If the peritoneum is not evident, the full thickness

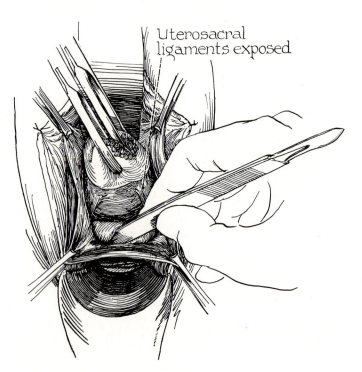

Fig. 20-3. The incision is now carried completely around the cervix, and the posterior vaginal wall is grasped with Allis clamps. The uterosacral ligaments are identified, and the dissection is continued until the peritoneum of the cul-de-sac is evident. The degree of herniation of the cul-de-sac will vary but must inevitably exist coincident with prolapse. The larger the herniation, the more extensive the dissection and exposure at this time. (From Ball TL: *Gynecologic surgery and urology*, ed 2, St. Louis, 1963, Mosby–Year Book.)

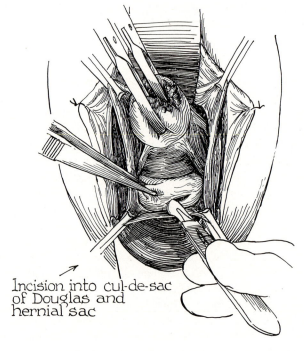

Fig. 20-4. The cul-de-sac peritoneum is now picked up with a thumb forceps and the peritoneal cavity entered. An exploration of the pelvis is carried out with one finger while strong traction is made on the uterus in an anterior direction. The status of the ovaries and tubes, as well as the presence of any bowel or omentum adhesions to the uterus, is determined. (From Ball TL: *Gynecologic surgery and urology*, ed 2, St. Louis, 1963, Mosby–Year Book.)

of the posterior vaginal membrane is undermined for several centimeters, then incised vertically, exposing the peritoneum of the cul-de-sac of Douglas, which can then be entered under direct vision (Fig. 20-4).

If the dissection has been in the wrong plane or if adhesions have obliterated the cul-de-sac of Douglas, the operator may be unable to identify the posterior peritoneal fold, which lines the cul-de-sac, after circumcising the cervix and stripping back the wall of the vagina. In this event, it is often best to begin the hysterectomy extraperitoneally by clamping and ligating the uterosacral and caudal portions of the cardinal ligaments close to the cervix (Fig. 20-5). Unless abnormally restrained (e.g., by adhesions), the uterus will be brought closer to the operator and will bring with it both its posterior and anterior peritoneal attachments. Later in the procedure, the peritoneum can be identified and opened under direct vision.[3,13,22,32] This procedure, the same as the "climb-up" maneuver recommended by Krige,[24] is infinitely preferable to stabbing blindly in the hope of opening into the peritoneum, which involves considerable risk of inadvertent penetration of any adherent bowel or the rectum.

The operator can easily open the peritoneum but should open it no more than is necessary to admit an examining finger or two. Keeping the opening as small as possible not only reduces unnecessary bleeding but also prevents an incision that could detach an unsecured uterosacral liga-

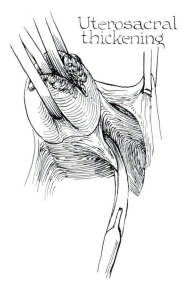

Fig. 20-5. The uterosacral thickenings are cut. This connective tissue is useful in reestablishing the vaginal obturator, obliterating the cul-de-sac, and suspending the vaginal vault. As with any hernia, tissue useful in the herniorrhaphy should not be sacrificed. A curved Heaney or Kocher clamp is used to grasp the tissue. The uterosacral ligaments are ligated and the ends of the ligatures left long and tagged. Resection of the uterosacral thickenings permits further descensus of the uterus. Palpation of the cul-de-sac can be carried higher in the pelvis and the size of the fundus more accurately determined. The operator may start planning for the correction of the cul-de-sac hernia and resection of excess peritoneum that will be part of the posterior repair. (From Ball TL: *Gynecologic surgery and urology,* ed 2, St. Louis, 1963, Mosby–Year Book.)

ment from the uterus. The operator then explores the interior intraabdominal surface of the cul-de-sac with one or two fingers to identify any enterocele or potential enterocele for later excision. Any pathologic adhesions, any cul-de-sac irregularity, and the nature of any intraperitoneal fluid should be noted. The operator should also sweep the posterior surface of the uterus with an index finger superiorly to ensure that the uterus is free, confirm the size of the uterus, and determine the position of any fibroids or other pathology. Although the uterosacral ligaments should not be included in this preliminary incision into the cul-de-sac of Douglas, their thickness and possible elongation should be noted at this time.

If possible, it is preferable to avoid joining the peritoneum to the vaginal cuff at this stage by placing interrupted sutures for hemostasis, even when oozing persists. Such sutures increase the risk of future enterocele if later in the operation the operator fails to resect any excess of peritoneum in the cul-de-sac before placing the purse-string closure of peritoneum cranial to these sutures.

Cutting the uterosacral ligaments. The uterosacral ligaments are clamped and, if elongated and strong, shortened, after which they are cut from the uterus. (Double clamping "for safety" is elective, according to the surgeon's preference.) The tip of the clamp should include the uterosacral and the lower portion of the cardinal ligaments. In placing a suture around this pedicle, the flexibility of the operator's wrist is important because it permits the operator to push and pull the needle through the tissues along the course of the needle's curved direction and thus to avoid the laceration of tissue more likely to occur when the needle is pushed through in a straight line. Just as the follow-through of a golfer's swing affects the accuracy of the ball's flight, the flexibility of the surgeon's wrist minimizes the size of the opening and the trauma to tissues that can result from each placement of a hemostatic suture around each pedicle.

The uterosacral ligaments are secured by transfixion ligature to the posterolateral surface of the vagina at approximately the 4 and 8 o'clock positions. These sutures should include the full thickness of the vaginal wall so that the ligaments will be firmly and permanently reattached to the vagina at this point (Fig. 20-6). These uterosacral sutures should not yet be cut so they can be used for later identification of the ligaments which possibly will be included in the repair.

Entering the vesicovaginal space. Anteriorly the full thickness of the cut edge of the vagina may be identified between forceps at either side of the 12 o'clock position. Using Mayo scissors—with the points directed away from the bladder—the operator makes an inverted V-shaped incision in the anterior vaginal wall, having entered the vesicovaginal space (Fig. 20-7). The opening may be enlarged by spreading the tips of the Mayo scissors, which are then withdrawn without being closed

The full thickness of the vaginal wall is now separated from the bladder (Fig. 20-8). If the position of the cervix

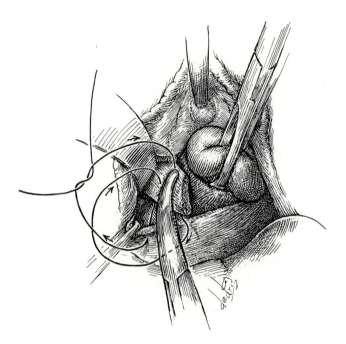

Fig. 20-6. Cut ends of uterosacral ligaments are secured to posterolateral surface of vagina by transfixion ligature at about the 4 and 8 o'clock positions. These sutures include full thickness of vaginal wall, and by this means the ligaments should be firmly and permanently reattached to the vagina at this point. Ends of these uterosacral sutures are left long to facilitate later identification and probable involvement of the ligaments in closure of the repair. (From Nichols DH, Randall CL: *Vaginal surgery*, ed 3, Baltimore, 1989, Williams & Wilkins.)

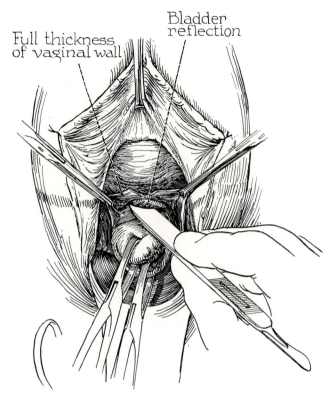

Fig. 20-7. An inverted V incision is made anteriorly through the full thickness of the vaginal wall and extended laterally around the cervix for a short distance. The bladder is pushed off the cervix by the knife handle entering the fragile areolar tissue between these organs. The vesicouterine reflection of the peritoneum appears between the bladder and upper part of the cervix. Any active bleeding is controlled by ties. The remainder of the anterior vaginal wall will be opened retrograde after the hysterectomy. This sequence in the steps of the operation avoids unnecessary bleeding from the incised anterior vaginal wall during the hysterectomy. The extent of this first incision is shown in this figure. (From Ball TL: *Gynecologic surgery and urology*, ed 2, St. Louis, 1963, Mosby–Year Book.)

at this point suggests that the prolapse is not as great as the operator had suspected, the inverted T incision becomes especially advantageous in exposing the undersurface of the bladder. On the other hand, if the prolapse appears to be greater than the operator had expected (increased somewhat because the hold of the uterosacral ligaments on the uterus has been released), a horizontal vaginal incision alone may be sufficient to permit dissection of bladder from cervix because the vesicouterine peritoneal fold becomes closer to the surgeon's hand and vision.

The bladder, readily identified by its looseness, may be picked up in the midline with forceps and some gentle tension placed on it. The supravaginal septum is incised and entered in the midline with the points of the curved Mayo scissors pointing downward or posteriorly. The plane of separation follows the line of fusion between the posterior layer of the connective tissue of the anterior vaginal wall and the encapsulation of the cervix. The operator should elevate the handles of the Mayo scissors during this maneuver to ensure that the tips of the scissors are pointed away from the undersurface of the bladder. The operator separates the bladder from the cervix by meticulously snipping the fine fibers that bind the connective tissue capsule of the bladder to that of the cervix. This sharp dissection is much safer than bluntly stripping the bladder away from the cervix, either with the finger or with a sponge, because

blunt stripping may lacerate the lowest section of the bladder fundus.[19]

Dissecting along the proper cleavage plane. As the scissors approach the vesicouterine peritoneal fold, the tissues usually become readily distinguishable. The operator can generally ensure a bloodless and safe entry into the proper cleavage plane by pressing firmly against the cervix with the closed curved tips of the Mayo scissors pointing toward the cervix and, while elevating the handles of the scissors above the horizontal, spreading apart the tips of the scissors and withdrawing them while maintaining pressure of the scissor tips against the cervix. After this maneuver, the opening may be readily enlarged. This dissection is carried upward until the anterior vesicouterine peritoneal fold is free. The fold is recognized by its almost frictionless smoothness to palpation or visualized as the white line of a double fold of peritoneum. Once the desired opening has been established along the proper cleavage plane, a retractor is placed beneath the bladder to hold it away from the cervix (Fig. 20-9). The anterior vesico-

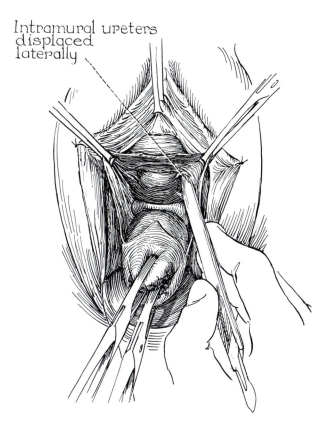

Intramural ureters displaced laterally

Fig. 20-8. Shows the dissection carried farther and the landmarks of importance. The bladder base, vesicouterine peritoneal fold, and cervix should be clearly evident if the correct tissue plane was entered. Previous surgery or scarring may make this diffucult at times. A sound placed in the bladder can help differentiate the tissue of the bladder base from the cervix when they are unusually adherent. (From Ball TL: *Gynecologic surgery and urology,* ed 2, St. Louis, 1963, Mosby – Year Book.)

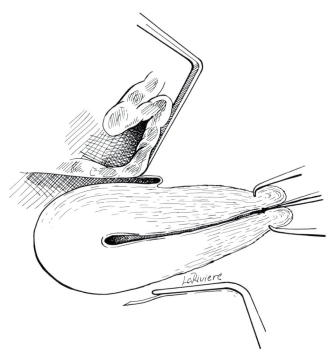

Fig. 20-9. Exposure of anterior peritoneum is now facilitated by displacing bladder anteriorly and holding it out of harm's way with a retractor. Anterior vesicouterine peritoneal fold is now much easier to observe, and it may be brought closer to the operator after detachment of the cardinal ligaments. Usually it can be identified by a somewhat frictionless sensation imparted to the ·operator's examining finger, or it may appear as a whitish fold of tissue because of the doubled thickness of peritoneum where it folds back upon itself to extend over the bladder. (Modified from Nichols DH, Randall CL: *Vaginal surgery,* ed 3, Baltimore, 1989, Williams & Wilkins.)

uterine peritoneal fold may be opened at this time (Figs. 20-10 and 20-11) and a long-handled retractor inserted.

Either immediately before or after retraction of the bladder superiorly, the so-called bladder pillars may be clamped, cut, and ligated near their attachments to the cervix. These pillars are never as strong as they may appear, and they usually contain portions of the cervical capsule. This surgical maneuver provides considerable protection to the ureters by ensuring that the subsequent dissection will be closer to the cervix and relatively distant from the ureteral knees.

Although a gauze-covered thumb may strip the bladder capsule from that of the cervix along a cleavage plane up to the anterior peritoneal fold, this procedure risks tearing the bladder if the operator has not entered the correct plane. Adhesions and fibrosis following previous low cervical cesarean section may have obscured the proper plane, and careful sharp dissection reduces the risk of bladder penetration. Occasionally the operator's readiness to dissect and desire to avoid penetrating the bladder cause him or her to incise within the connective tissue capsule of the cervix, particularly if the initial incision around the cervix was too close to the external cervical os. Because

the operator did not enter the anatomic plane between the bladder and the cervix, continuing sharp dissection may lead beneath the peritoneum that covers the anterior uterine segment. The smooth undersurface of the peritoneum may be recognized by palpation, but if it is not readily and actually visualized, it should not be opened; it is difficult to determine the actual site of the peritoneal reflection from the superior surface of the bladder unless the area is under direct vision. Failure to proceed with caution at this stage is one of the most common reasons for unintentional bladder penetration. Fortunately, any bladder injury that occurs at this point will be well above the bladder trigone and relatively easy to repair after the uterus has been removed.

Opening the anterior peritoneal fold. The proper time to open the peritoneum during the course of mobilization and identification of the bladder is soon after the smooth, thin layer of peritoneum has been visualized, usually as a fold or double reflection that appears after the cardinal and uterosacral ligaments and the bladder pillars have all been separated from the uterus. Because all pedicles have been cut close to the cervix, the uterus has further descended, bringing the peritoneum down with it. After the anterior peritoneal fold has been recognized by palpation and visualized but not yet

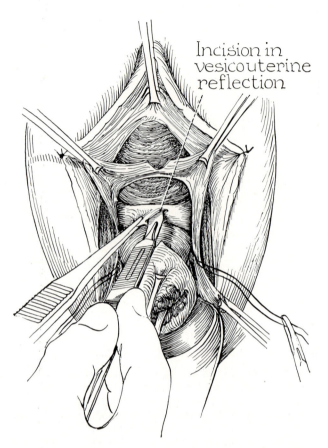

Incision in vesicouterine reflection

Fig. 20-10. Attention is directed toward opening into the peritoneal cavity anteriorly. To this end the uterus is now drawn strongly downward. Assistants who can anticipate and sense the steps of this operation make matters easy by drawing the uterus in just the right direction. A retractor may be used to retract the bladder if it seems to facilitate the exposure of the peritoneum. The bulge of the vesicouterine fold of peritoneum is picked up with thumb forceps and sharply incised. Frequently this is not as simple as illustrated, and the surgeon finds himself too close to the cervix and lower uterine segment of the uterus, with the cleavage plane entering the superficial layers of fibromuscular tissue. An excessive amount of bleeding indicates that the wrong cleavage plane has been entered and the surgeon should try dissecting closer to the bladder. In elderly patients the bladder wall is thin and in a procidentia the musculature is further attenuated. In such patients the bladder may be inadvertently entered. This is not a serious complication. If it does happen, the bladder should be closed in two layers with interrupted 0000 or 000 polyglycolic acid-type sutures and the operation continued. (From Ball TL: *Gynecologic surgery and urology*, ed 2, St. Louis, 1963, Mosby–Year Book.)

opened, the portion of the bladder pillars closest to the cervix may be included in the clamp across the adjacent portion of the cardinal ligament. A small, rather superficial artery in the bladder pillar often bleeds as the vaginal membrane is reflected from the midline over the cervix, however. When such bleeding occurs, it is advisable to clamp and ligate or coagulate the vessel and adjacent bladder pillar separately on each side close to the cervix. Similarly, the surgeon should identify the cardinal ligament tissue to each side of the cervix and make an effort to clamp, cut, and ligate

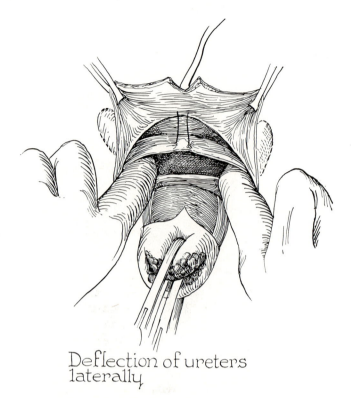

Deflection of ureters laterally

Fig. 20-11. The vesicouterine reflection of the peritoneum may now be tagged by a suture passing through the anterior vaginal wall. Both index fingers are passed within the peritoneal cavity, and, with a lateral rolling motion, the opening is enlarged, while at the same time the ureters, together with their surrounding areolar tissue, are displaced laterally. This maneuver aids in keeping the ureters out of the field of operation and simulates the same method used to displace the ureters during an abdominal hysterectomy. (From Ball TL: *Gynecologic surgery and urology*, ed 2, St. Louis, 1963, Mosby–Year Book.)

that structure without picking up the uterine vessels separately.

Clamping and ligating the uterine vessels. In a vaginal hysterectomy, one non-slipping clamp at a time may be used on each cardinal ligament. With the vaginal approach, traction applied to the cervix brings the uterine artery down, which pulls the ureter down. The use of a second clamp decreases the distance of safety between the clamp and the ureter, thus putting the ureter at some degree of risk. With a total abdominal hysterectomy, however, two clamps may be used simultaneously on each portion of the cardinal ligament detached from the uterus, because upward traction on the uterus pulls the uterine artery *away* from the ureter.

An intermediate or advanced degree of uterine prolapse may occasionally allow the surgeon to use a clampless technique, in which uterine pedicles are ligated by primary passage of the needle without preliminary clamping. The operator who uses this technique must be careful *not* to cut the pedicle until after the first cast of the stitch has been placed and tightened. Then the pedicle of the ligated tissue should be cut, the first cast of the knot tightened *again*, and the second cast placed and tightened.

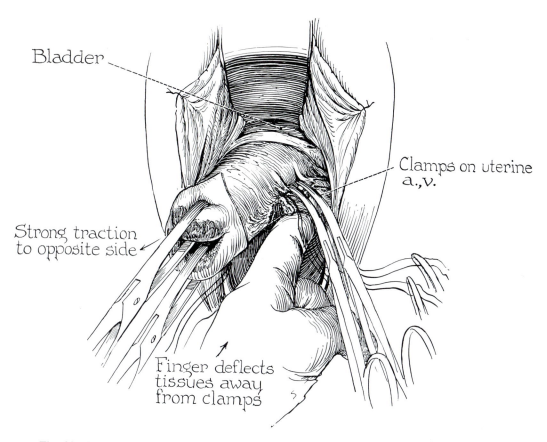

Bladder

Clamps on uterine a.,v.

Strong traction to opposite side

Finger deflects tissues away from clamps

Fig. 20-12. The uterine arteries are now doubly clamped as shown. The index finger in the peritoneal cavity pushes laterally as the clamps are applied. Double suture ligatures are placed around the vessels, and the distal ligature is left long and tagged. This procedure is repeated for the right uterine artery and veins. (From Ball TL: *Gynecologic surgery and urology,* ed 2, St. Louis, 1963, Mosby–Year Book.)

If separately identified, the uterine vessels should be safely clamped and ligated with a tie that is cut short so that it will not be used for subsequent traction (Fig. 20-12). When the uterus is large or when an irregular or intraligamentous fibroid has distorted the usual anatomic relationships, however, it may be more difficult to locate the uterine artery and adjacent veins in the cardinal ligament tissue caught in the initial clamp. At this point, a cautious, deliberate push or pull on the clamped tissues along the axis of the ascending branch of the uterine artery invariably separates the anterior and posterior layers of ligament attached to the lower uterine segment sufficiently to disclose an underlying segment of the uterine vessels; usually these vessels promptly and literally bulge into the operator's view. (This maneuver may tear a small vein, but the vein can easily be clamped along with the uterine artery.) The uterine vessels can then be clamped (extraperitoneally, without including the peritoneum either anteriorly or posteriorly), cut, and ligated with a minimal amount of ligamentous tissue. After the uterine vessels have been ligated, the remaining superior portions of the broad ligament, including the adjacent peritoneum both anteriorly and posteriorly, may be clamped and caught in a transfixing ligature without risk of disturbing or jeopardizing the ligation of the uterine vessels.

Delayed entry into the peritoneal cavity. A variety of techniques permit safe entry into the peritoneal cavity through the anterior vesicouterine peritoneal fold. In selecting the appropriate technique, the operator must consider the specific degree and type of prolapse involved, the presence of a coexistent cystocele that the operator intends to repair, the size of that cystocele, the extent of cervical descent, the degree of cervical mobility (i.e., whether the cervix can be brought closer to the operator by traction on the tenaculum), and the length of the cervix. Often the site of the anterior vesicouterine peritoneal reflection is at the same level as the site of the posterior peritoneal reflection (within the cul-de-sac of Douglas) to the uterus.

The anterior peritoneal fold should be opened only under direct vision—never blindly—because a blind entry could easily damage the bladder. If the operator was earlier unable to identify the anterior peritoneal plication with certainty and postponed further attempts at an anterior opening into the peritoneal cavity, a point of safe opening can now be positively identified either by longitudinal section of the cervix or by inserting the operator's first and second left fingertips through the posterior peritoneal opening over the fundus of the uterus[6,22,32] and spreading them beneath the vesicouterine peritoneal fold, making it both palpable and visible. If identification of the peritoneum is still uncertain, a Sims uterine sound may be bent

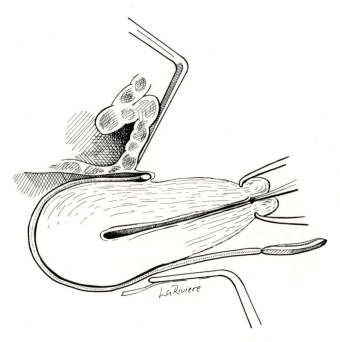

Fig. 20-13. When the anterior cul-de-sac is difficult to identify particularly in the patient with previous cesarean section, a Sims uterine sound bent in the shape of a U may be inserted through the posterior peritoneal opening and over the uterine fundus, as shown. The tip can be palpated, and dissection *beneath* the tip will expose the peritoneum of the anterior cul-de-sac, which can be safely opened.

in the shape of a U and inserted through the posterior peritoneal opening over the top of the fundus, and the tip made to distend the anterior cul-de-sac, which may be dissected beneath the tip and opened under direct vision[15](Fig. 20-13). Grasped with forceps and tented as a vertical fold, the peritoneum may be opened readily with the scissors. To facilitate later identification of the edges of the peritoneum, some surgeons tag the midline of both the anterior and the posterior edges with a suture left long so as to be easily retrievable when it is time to close the peritoneum (Fig. 20-14).

The operator explores the anterior cul-de-sac with an index finger, noting any pathology or adhesions and making certain that the incision has properly entered the peritoneal cavity anteriorly. The operator may then insert both index fingers into this anterior peritoneal opening, enlarging it by spreading the fingers laterally. A long-handled Heaney or Deaver retractor may be inserted to keep the bladder up and out of the operative field. The relationship of the ureter to the uterine artery during hysterectomy is shown in Figure 20-15.

Ligating the cardinal-uterosacral ligament complex. With the peritoneum opened both posterior and anterior to the uterine fundus, the operator clamps, cuts, and ligates the upper cardinal and lower broad ligaments. Clamps should be applied from the cornual angles downward, and the tips of the hemostats should be placed so that each is within the peritoneal cavity, both anteriorly and posteriorly. This placement seals off the broad ligament by com-

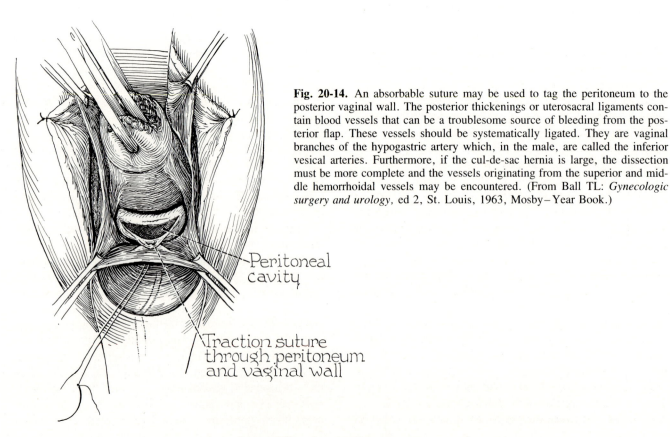

Fig. 20-14. An absorbable suture may be used to tag the peritoneum to the posterior vaginal wall. The posterior thickenings or uterosacral ligaments contain blood vessels that can be a troublesome source of bleeding from the posterior flap. These vessels should be systematically ligated. They are vaginal branches of the hypogastric artery which, in the male, are called the inferior vesical arteries. Furthermore, if the cul-de-sac hernia is large, the dissection must be more complete and the vessels originating from the superior and middle hemorrhoidal vessels may be encountered. (From Ball TL: *Gynecologic surgery and urology,* ed 2, St. Louis, 1963, Mosby–Year Book.)

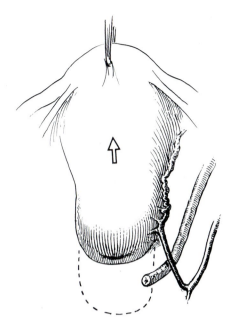
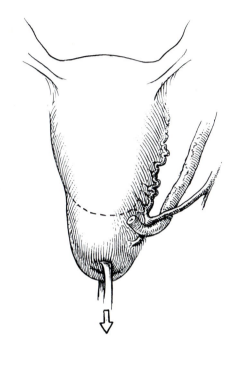

Fig. 20-15. Relationship of ureter to uterine artery during hysterectomy. Dashed line represents a usual position of the uterus. *Left,* relationship between uterine artery and ureter when upward traction is applied to uterine fundus as in abdominal hysterectomy; *right,* change in this relationship when downward traction is applied as during vaginal hysterectomy. (From Nichols DH, Randall CL: *Vaginal Surgery,* ed 3, Baltimore, 1989, Williams & Wilkins.)

pressing both its anterior and its posterior peritoneal leaves between the jaws of the hemostat. This step effectively prevents the extension of any laceration into the very vascular venous plexus located within layers of the broad ligaments. The hemostats should be immediately replaced by transfixing ligatures.

Removing the uterus

Failure of the uterus to descend. After the cardinal-uterosacral ligament complex has been ligated and the cul-de-sac opened both anteriorly and posteriorly, the operator may find that traction applied to the cervix fails to move the uterus any further down. This event requires investigation, for the broad ligament and its contents, including both round and ovarian ligaments, offer little resistance to downward traction under normal circumstances. The operator should suspect and must determine with certainty whether the patient has in the past undergone a ventral fixation or Gilliam-type uterine suspension or whether adhesions are binding the uterus to other intraabdominal organs. Any one or more of the following conditions could also be interfering with the descent of the uterus: (1) parametrial and broad ligament fibrosis from previous or chronic infection, (2) pelvic endometriosis, (3) undiagnosed pelvic carcinoma, extending either from the uterus or from an extrauterine site.

Another possibility is a mechanical obstruction to the further descent of the uterus. For example, the patient may have a large fibroid uterus with leiomyomata situated so as to interfere with the delivery of the uterus. The operator is then faced with a choice among several alternate procedures. The first is to abandon the vaginal approach to hysterectomy at this point and finish the operation through a transabdominal incision. As Allen[1] cautioned,

I do not believe that large tumors should be attacked through the vagina. How large a tumor one should attack depends on one's experience and skill, but also on the location of the tumor in the uterus. Relatively small tumors immediately beneath the bladder or extending out into the broad ligament, where the uterine blood supply is reached with difficulty, are much more important as contraindications than large tumors if they are in the fundus. Once the lower blood supply is secured, these upper tumors can be reached and morcellated with, shall I say, impunity.

A possible alternative is amputation of the cervix and morcellation of any fibroid tumors of the uterus (Fig. 20-16), provided that they can be grasped safely through the vagina.[9] Werner and Sederl,[50] as well as other authorities, have recommended bisection of the noncancerous uterus and removal of first one side and then the other. The operator should choose the option that is consistent with the patient's best interests and the operator's confidence, experience, and technical ability.

Delivery of the uterus. If there is no interference with the descent of the uterus, the operator continues to apply traction on the cervix, drawing it further down. It may be necessary in avoiding hematoma to clamp, cut, and ligate the middle portion of the broad ligament separately, again

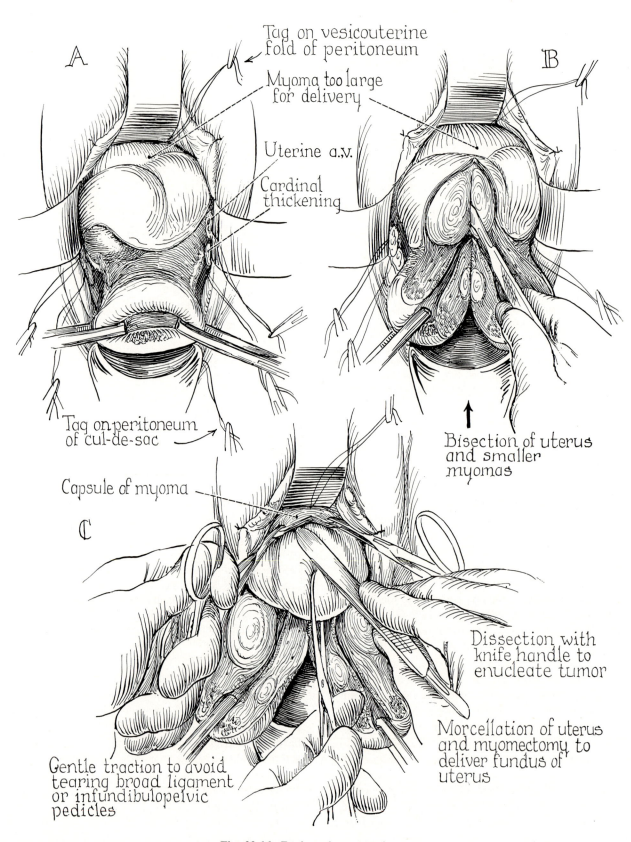

A

Tag on vesicouterine
fold of peritoneum

Myoma too large
for delivery

Uterine a.v.

Cardinal
thickening

B

Tag on peritoneum
of cul-de-sac

Bisection of uterus
and smaller
myomas

Capsule of myoma

C

Dissection with
knife handle to
enucleate tumor

Morcellation of uterus
and myomectomy to
deliver fundus of
uterus

Gentle traction to avoid
tearing broad ligament
or infundibulopelvic
pedicles

Fig. 20-16. For legend see opposite page.

with care to ensure that both the anterior and posterior leaves of the broad ligament peritoneum are included within the grasp of the hemostat on either side. Transfixion ligatures on the uterine blood vessels, including both the ascending and descending branches of the uterine artery, should by now have secured the blood supply to the uterus.

When the fundus of the uterus is low in the pelvis, the operator may deliver it through either the anterior or the posterior peritoneal opening (Fig. 20-17). If the fundus is freely movable and readily visualized, however, it need not be "flipped" either anteriorly or posteriorly for delivery. Hemostats are applied to the cornual angle of the uterus on either side, and the uterus is removed. The cavity is opened immediately and the endometrium and endocervical canal carefully inspected to determine if there is any grossly visible but unsuspected pathology present that might alter the surgical plan. Frozen section is requested if there is doubt as to the possibility of malignancy.

Removing the uterus without flipping it decreases the risk of contaminating the peritoneal surfaces through contact with a bacteriologically dirty cervix. Because retroperitoneal infection in the cellular tissues is responsible for posthysterectomy morbidity much more frequently than is peritonitis, prophylactic amputation of the external cervix may be indicated whenever the size or relative immobility of the uterus seems likely to necessitate more than the usual manipulation of the uterus as the fundus is being freed and removed.

If the body of the uterus is movable but too large to permit comfortable delivery through either the anterior or posterior peritoneal opening and morcellation is not desired, the operator may incise the myometrium. Such an incision should be carried symmetrically around the full circumference of the uterus, through the myometrium, parallel to the axis of the uterine cavity and just beneath the serosa.[23,32] The uterus is freed by this procedure much as a banana is peeled by turning the skin inside out. The procedure brings the cervix closer to the operator but does not violate the integrity of the endometrial cavity (Fig. 20-18). Incision of the lateral portions of myometrium medial to the remaining attachment of the broad ligament results in considerable additional descent and mobility of the as yet unremoved fundus (Fig. 20-19).

At this point the operator replaces the cornual angle hemostats with transfixion ligatures. After these are tied, an additional bite is taken through the round ligament on each side, and the suture is tied again. Any traction on the adnexal pedicles will then be borne principally by the round ligament, which has been ligated higher than the infundibulopelvic ligament by virtue of the extra bite.

Performing an oophorectomy. The adnexa should be carefully inspected on each side. If they are to be removed, particular care must be taken to ensure ligation of the ovarian vessels (Figs. 20-20 and 20-21).[4,32,33,35,44] When performing a vaginal oophorectomy of an obviously benign ovarian tumor, the operator should first doubly clamp the mesovarium, cut between the clamps and then remove the ovary, using the clamp on the mesovarium as a handle so that the ovarian tumor does not fill the vagina and obstruct the operator's vision of its pedicle.

Alternatively, if the ovaries appear to be reasonably accessible but removal by clamp technique is not feasible, oophorectomy using the endoloop technique may be employed after the hysterectomy described by Heffman.[15] The ovary is grasped with a long Babcock clamp and pulled into the vagina. The endoloop suture is brought around the clamp and ovary and tightened at the mesovarium, and a second loop fixed close to the first. The ovary is then excised under direct vision and the process repeated on the opposite side.

The operator may decide to spare the tube and mesosalpinx, which may aid appreciably in subsequent peritonealization of the intraperitoneal mesovarium stump. In this case, the operator must be careful to preserve the tubal blood supply when ligating the ovarian pedicle. When the tube and ovary are to be removed, the round ligament is clamped, cut and ligated.[44] The slanted Deschamps liga-

Text continued on p. 316.

Fig. 20-16. The operation proceeds as in any vaginal hysterectomy until the uterine artery and veins have been identified, doubly clamped, cut, and ligated. At this time the vesicouterine fold of peritoneum, as well as the peritoneum of the cul-de-sac, will have been entered. Both of the peritoneal reflections have been tagged with a suture ligature. The cardinal thickenings and the uterosacral thickenings will have been cut, clamped, and ligated and appropriately identified for closure of the vaginal vault at the conclusion of the operation. Two Jacobs tenaculi are placed on the cervix at the lateral angles in preparation for dissecting the uterus (**A**).

Strong traction is made downward and outward, and a knife is used to bisect the cervix in the mid-sagittal plane. Small fibroids that are encountered may be bisected together with the uterus itself (**B**) rather than a myomectomy performed.

As shown in **C,** a large myoma that could not be delivered under the symphysis is grasped with a tenaculum. A vaginal myomectomy is performed by grasping the capsule of the myoma with Allis clamps. The operator cautions his assistants to exert only gentle traction from now on, since with the delivery of the uterus, considerable strain is placed on the infundibulopelvic pedicles. They may be torn and the ovarian vessels ruptured. The myoma is enucleated either by the knife handle technique (**C**) or by the use of scissors, leaving the capsule intact. After removal of the large myoma the remainder of the uterus is delivered to the outside and the bisection continued.

Continued.

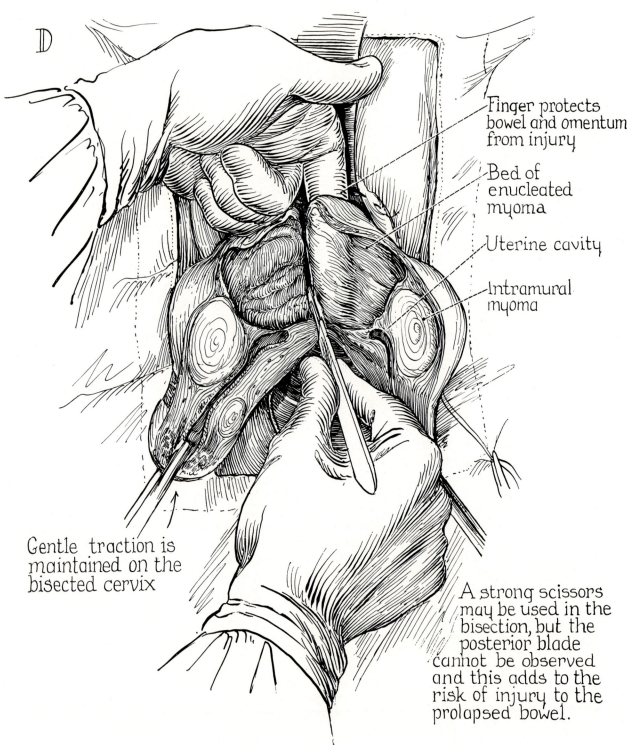

D

Finger protects
bowel and omentum
from injury

Bed of
enucleated
myoma

Uterine cavity

Intramural
myoma

Gentle traction is
maintained on the
bisected cervix

A strong scissors
may be used in the
bisection, but the
posterior blade
cannot be observed
and this adds to the
risk of injury to the
prolapsed bowel.

The myomectomized uterus can now be delivered
and the bisection completed

Fig. 20-16, cont'd. For legend see opposite page.

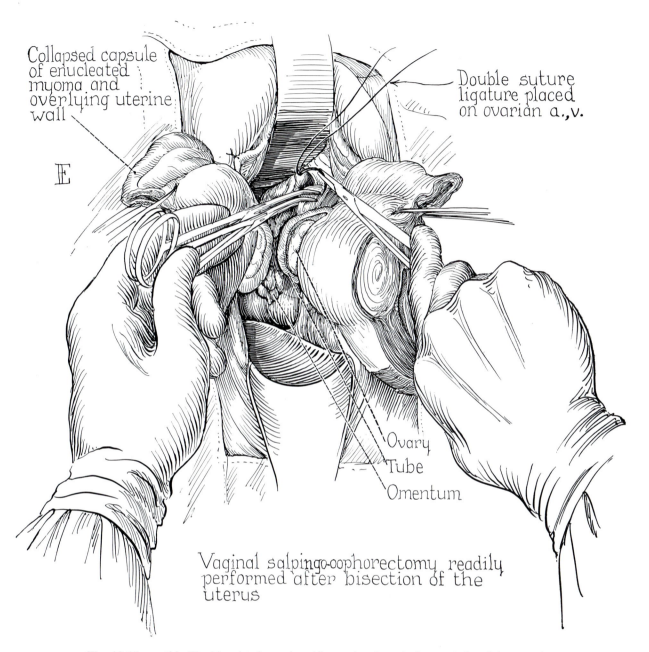

Collapsed capsule
of enucleated
myoma and
overlying uterine
wall

E

Double suture
ligature placed
on ovarian a.,v.

Ovary
Tube
Omentum

Vaginal salpingo-oophorectomy readily
performed after bisection of the
uterus

Fig. 20-16, cont'd. The bisection is continued by cutting through the remainder of the posterior portion of the capsule of the myoma that was removed. As shown in **D,** a finger should be placed behind the uterus to protect bowel or omentum from injury. Small laparotomy pads are used to pack off the bowel and omentum. In performing the bisection a strong scissors may be used; a crushing instrument, particularly when the posterior blade cannot be observed, adds to the risk of injury to prolapsed bowel or omentum.

The two halves of the bisected uterus, together with tubes and ovaries, are delivered out of the pelvis. Traction is made on the capsule of the enucleated myoma and, together with gentle traction on the cervix, the infundibulopelvic pedicles are visualized. Angle clamps are used to clamp the infundibulopelvic pedicle, and this is double ligated with 0 PGA suture **(E).** The round ligament is double clamped, cut, and ligated and the left half of the uterus is removed together with the tube and ovary on that side attached to the specimen. An identical procedure is carried out on the right side, completing the removal of the uterus, tubes, and ovaries. The surgeon further explores the pelvis for other pelvic pathology. The closure of the vaginal vault and the anterior and posterior colporrhaphies are completed in the same manner as a routine vaginal hysterectomy. (From Ball TL: *Gynecologic surgery and urology,* ed 3, St Louis, 1963, Mosby–Year Book, pp 137-140.)

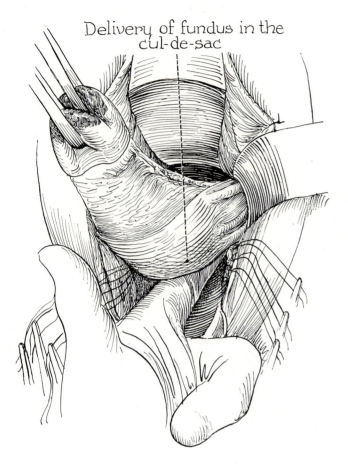

Delivery of fundus in the cul-de-sac

Fig. 20-17. The vesicouterine reflection of the peritoneum is smaller in all dimensions than the rectovaginal reflection or pouch of Douglas. The fundus of the uterus is thus more easily delivered posteriorly than by forcibly extracting it through a hiatus artificially created between the vagina and bladder. Some local pathology may cause a variation in this rule. In this type of surgery one does not create bigger openings when such can be avoided. The basic objectives (namely, to decrease the size of the genital hiatus and to strengthen the obturators filling this outlet) make logical the delivery of the uterus posteriorly.

The uterus is now mobile except for the resistance offered by the round ligaments, tubes, and infundibulopelvic vessels and their connective tissue thickenings. The fundus is now delivered through the posterior route by applying bullet tenaculi alternately along the posterior aspect of the uterus. This sometimes is accomplished by a finger alone. If it does not come out without difficulty, make traction on the fundus and push the cervix back up under the symphysis; this has the effect of rotating the organ about its last remaining attachments. This maneuver is usually successful unless abnormal attachments exist. In this event the anterior Deaver retractor is manipulated to see the reason for resistance and any structures adherent to the uterus or adnexa. Failure to deliver the uterus by this technique is rare.

Following this dissection the bladder neck is plicated prophylactically and the vaginal wall appropriately resected to correct any cystocele. The incision is carried toward the vault to meet the upper incision that was previously tagged. Any posterior colporrhaphy is completed and a high perineorraphy is done to complete the reconstruction of the pelvic floor as necessary. (From Ball TL: *Gynecologic surgery and urology,* ed 2, St Louis, 1963, Mosby–Year Book, pp 127-136.)

Fig. 20-18. Lash incision into the myometrium. Operator has already secured by transfixion ligature inferior and major blood supply of uterus (ascending and descending branches of uterine artery) and has determined that uterus is not being deviated or fixed by any previously unsuspected adhesions. If it is now determined that body of uterus is too big to permit delivery, outer superficial myometrium can be incised circumferentially. If circumferential incision has been properly placed, the bulk of the uterus can be enucleated without transgressing the endocervical or endometrial cavity. The large bulky uterus is thereby increased in length and decreased in width, which in essence "makes the cork smaller than the neck of the bottle." (From Nichols DH, Randall CL: *Vaginal surgery,* ed 3, Baltimore, 1989, Williams & Wilkins.)

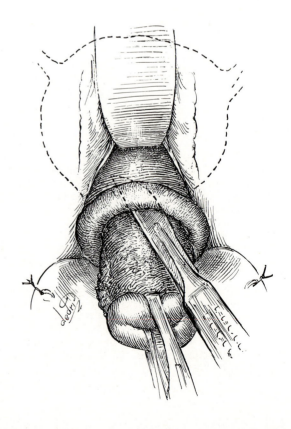

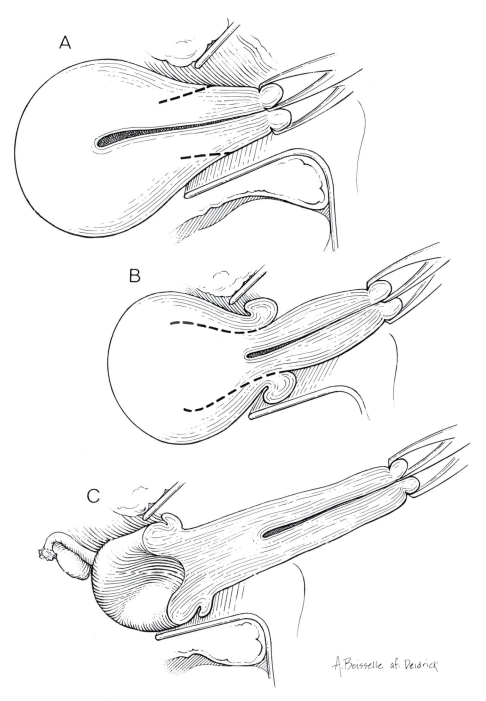

Fig. 20-19. A, Sagittal drawing of a large bulky uterus. Cardinal and uterosacral ligaments have been separated from sides of uterus, but delivery of the body is difficult because of its size. Pathway for incision into myometrium parallel to axis of uterus is identified by broken line. **B,** Incision has been deepened, as traction further exteriorizes the cervix. Myometrial incision will be extended further as indicated by broken line. **C,** Uterus can now be delivered outside the pelvis. Its length has increased as its diameter has decreased, as shown. Cornual angle can now be clamped under direct visualization and the uterus cut free. (Modified from Nichols DH, Randall CL: *Vaginal surgery,* ed 3, Baltimore, 1989, Williams & Wilkins.)

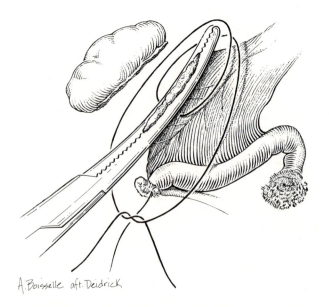

A. Boisselle aft. Deidrick

Fig. 20-20. When infundibulopelvic ligament is short, transvaginal oophorectomy may be accomplished as shown. Mesovarium has been clamped and ovary removed. There is a single penetration of the mesovarium at its midpoint, and each end of the suture is passed around distal tip of hemostat and tied beneath heel of clamp. (From Nichols DH, Randall CL: *Vaginal surgery,* ed 3, Baltimore, 1989, Williams & Wilkins.)

ture carrier with its blunt point is good for ligation of the infundibulopelvic ligament. After the cornual angle stitches have been tied, the uncut ends of the sutures can be secured in a clamp and kept long for use later in the procedure. If there are a great many adhesions, the leaves of the broad ligament may be spread by funneling with the scissor tips for mobilization of the components that have been ligated separately.[4]

Recognizing and preventing an enterocele. The operator may identify an enterocele, enterocele sac, or potential enterocele at this time by exploring the cul-de-sac with a finger (Fig. 20-22). At times, packing the interior of the sac with a moistened gauze sponge facilitates identification and aids dissection. Because the patient should already be in a 5- or 10-degree Trendelenburg position, the contents of the abdomen can usually be readily packed away from the operative field with a little gauze packing. An enterocele sac can be easily separated from the surrounding connective tissue by alternating sharp and blunt dissection as far down as the anterior surface of the rectum, which is identified by the small condensations of fat adherent to the peritoneum and by the noticeably longitudinal muscle layer of the outer rectal wall.

Inspecting the anterior or vesicouterine peritoneum, the operator should excise any excess or redundant peritoneum

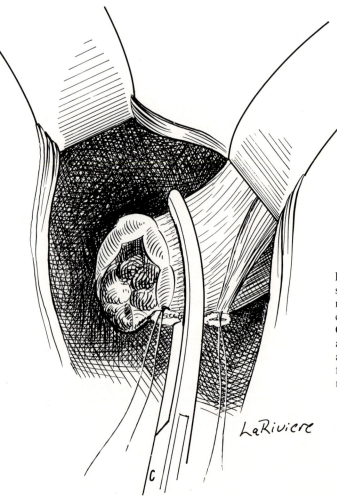

LaRiviere

Fig. 20-21. If adnexal removal or resection is desirable, it should be performed at this time. Vaginal salpingooophorectomy may be accomplished as follows: The ligament is clamped and cut. Downward traction is applied to round ligament suture. Ovary may be grasped in a spongeholder and a forceps applied across infundibulopelvic ligament. Ovary and tube are excised, and a transfixion suture of medium thickness is placed. (Modified from Nichols DH, Randall CL: *Vaginal surgery,* ed 3, Baltimore, 1989, Williams & Wilkins.)

left after the opening and dissection of the anterior peritoneal cul-de-sac to decrease the possibility of an anterior postoperative enterocele. The bladder, if at all distended, should now be emptied of urine by catheter because this seems to facilitate reperitonealization by making the anterior cut edge of the peritoneum more readily visible and accessible. Should it be difficult to locate the anterior peritoneum, the operator may grasp the tissues inferior to the anterior peritoneum lightly with successive gentle bites of an unlocked hemostat so as to "walk" or roll these tissues toward the operator until the anterior peritoneal edge can be identified. When unmistakably visible, the peritoneal

edge is grasped by a hemostat, and sutures are placed to close the peritoneal opening.

Closing the peritoneum. The primary purpose of peritoneal closure following vaginal hysterectomy is to incorporate the strength of the subperitoneal connective tissue retinaculum into a firm scar at the bottom of the pelvis that will resist increases in intraabdominal pressure. The mesothelial lining of the peritoneal cavity per se has little supportive value.

The operator begins peritoneal closure with a full length of suture: polydiaxonone absorbable 0 suture. Traction on the previously clamped and held transfixion ligature

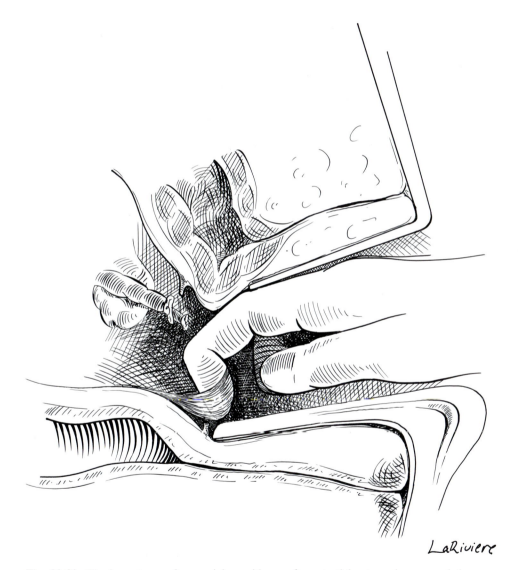

Fig. 20-22. The importance of recognizing evidence of a potential enterocele or an existing enterocele sac always warrants careful exploration of cul-de-sac by operator's fingers, as shown in this sagittal section. For demonstration or identification purposes, a suspected sac can be packed with a gauze sponge to facilitate demonstration of excess peritoneal connective tissue by both sharp and blunt dissection down to a point where excision of excess peritoneum will extend across anterior surface of rectum. Any fat that is present belongs on rectal side of dissection. Rectum should be recognized promptly during this dissection either by characteristic condensations of fat or by longitudinal muscle fibers of outer layer of rectal wall. In the same manner, anterior peritoneum should be inspected. If there is excessive redundant peritoneum anteriorly, it should be excised at this time, lessening the postoperative possibility of an anterior enterocele. (Modified from Nichols DH, Randall CL: *Vaginal surgery*, ed 3, Baltimore, 1989, Williams & Wilkins.)

readily identifies the uterosacral ligament. After placing a stitch through the peritoneal surface and into the peritoneal side of the left uterosacral ligament, the operator reefs the posterior peritoneum in a linear fashion by a series of bites until the same level on the opposite uterosacral ligament location is reached. This posterior peritoneal reefing should be along the level of the reflection of the peritoneum from the anterior wall of the rectum. Reefing sutures placed any higher than this level would displace an excessive amount of rectum into the vaginal space.

The purse-string sutures[6,24,32] placed to close the peritoneum and any suture placed to bring the uterosacral or infundibulopelvic and round ligaments together should be above or proximal to the ligature on the pedicles. The purpose of the suture that brings the ligamentous structures together is twofold: (1) to promote a firm tissue union and (2) to ensure that all ligated pedicles will be extraperitonealized. The ligatures on the uterine vessels are not caught up on an approximating suture. Although the vessels will retract into the parametria, their ligated pedicles remain extraperitonealized.

After passing the peritoneal closure stitch through the uterosacral ligament and adjacent peritoneum (Fig. 20-23), first on one side and then on the other, the operator relaxes traction on the previously held uterosacral transfixing ligatures. Grasping the homolateral adnexal pedicle suture on the patient's right side, the operator again applies gentle traction to bring the round ligament into view. The operator then passes the peritoneal closure stitch through the round ligament proximal and medial to the previously placed pedicle ligation. The round ligaments do not support the vagina; they are incorporated in the purse-string stitch only to enhance peritonealization of the pelvis. The anterior peritoneum is then identified, and any excess is excised and the remainder reefed by a series of bites that continue to and through the opposite round ligament. At this point the operator has continued the stitch entirely around the peritoneal opening, through the round and uterosacral ligaments on each side (Fig. 20-24).

After carefully removing all intraabdominal, intraperitoneal packing, the operator takes up all slack in the purse-string peritoneal suture[6,24,32] by reefing the tissues fairly

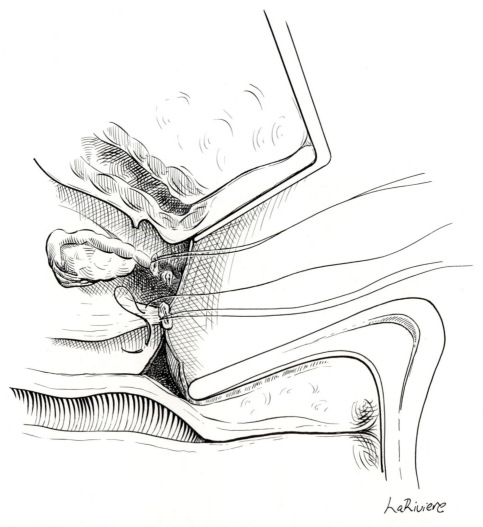

Fig. 20-23. Beginning of high peritoneal closure stitch through peritoneal surface of uterosacral ligament, and posterior peritoneum just above its cut edge. (Modified from Nichols DH, Randall CL: *Vaginal surgery,* ed 3, Baltimore, 1989, Williams & Wilkins.)

snugly along the suture, both anteriorly and posteriorly. Only after such reefing should the operator tie the purse-string suture, closing the peritoneum; to be effective, all reefing should be accomplished before—not as—this stitch is tied. This plication of tissues at the bases of the uterosacral ligaments actually draws the pubococcygei and their fasciae together,[26,27] narrowing the genital hiatus. After the purse-string peritoneal closure stitch has been tied, both ends of the stitch should be left long and held for later use.

Because the uterosacral ligaments are relatively fixed in position, this suturing technique brings the movable round ligaments that are also included in the purse-string suture to the semifixed uterosacral ligaments. This technique tends to reestablish the horizontal axis of the upper vagina and appreciably decreases the likelihood of a postoperative enterocele.

Closing the vaginal wall. The round ligament pedicle stitches may be tied together beneath the base of the blad-

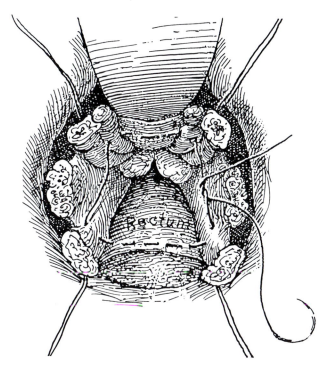

Fig. 20-24. If a marking suture has not been placed and difficulty is experienced in locating anterior peritoneum, tissue caudal to anterior peritoneum is lightly grasped with successive gentle bites of an unlocked hemostat in such fashion as to "walk up" this area until anterior peritoneum is recognized and grasped in forceps. Peritonealization is accomplished using a full length of absorbable 0 or 2/0 suture held in a light hemostat for identification later. I prefer to begin this stitch on peritoneal side of left uterosacral ligament. Traction is made on previously clamped and held transfixion ligature of uterosacral ligament, but putting the ligament on tension, it is readily identified. Posterior peritoneum is reefed by a series of bites until opposite uterosacral ligament location is reached. Suture passes through right round ligament, anterior peritoneum, and left round ligament and is ready to be tied. (From Nichols DH, Randall CL: *Vaginal surgery,* ed 3, Baltimore, 1989, Williams & Wilkins.)

der to provide auxiliary support to the intraabdominal contents should the peritoneal sutures be broken or come untied. The retracting sutures in the labia minora may now be cut and the vagina prepared for closure. If no colporrhaphy is to be done and maximal vaginal depth is to be preserved, the vagina is closed in a sagittal direction.[6,32]

After completion of any anterior colporrhaphy, the operator begins closing the anterior vaginal wall by passing the needle on one end of the preserved peritoneal closure stitch through each side of the uppermost portion of the anterior vaginal wall, from the inside out on one side and the outside in on the other, at precisely the level of the vault that corresponds to the previous sutures in the uterosacral ligaments, which were held for tying later. The operator then ties the end of the previously tied peritoneal closure stitch (sewn beneath the anterior vaginal wall at its apex, as noted earlier) to its other held end, taking care (as when preparing to tie the peritoneal purse-string suture) to reef the tissues to be tied rather snugly together before seating and tying the knot. This suture fixes the anterior vault to the edge and level of the peritoneal purse-string suture, effectively lengthening the anterior vaginal wall and aiding in the support of the vaginal vault.

Tying the held end of the peritoneal closure stitch to an uppermost stitch in the anterior vaginal wall with a bite or two to either side of the midline effectively unites the anterior connective tissue capsule of the vagina to the area in which the peritoneal stitch brought the uterosacral ligaments together. Because each uterosacral ligament has in effect been joined to the posterolateral surface of the vaginal wall, this unites the tissue capsule of the anterior vaginal wall to that of the posterior vaginal wall.[10]

The anterior vaginal wall is closed by either running or interrupted subcuticular sutures placed from side to side. A subcuticular closure provides a more exact, smoother approximation of the epithelial layers. This alignment not only reduces postoperative development of foci of granulation tissue in the suture line and thus the likelihood of future development of an enterocele but also appreciably strengthens the vault.[3,35] Closing the vagina from side to side in a longitudinal direction rather than from front to back provides an additional 2 or 3 cm of vaginal length, which at times may mean the difference between a depth that contains the sexual partner and a depth that does not.

Performing a cul-de-plasty. When the cardinal-uterosacral ligaments are elongated but strong, as they usually are with uterovaginal prolapse, and the vagina is obviously shortened or telescoped, the operator can increase the vaginal depth by fixing the vagina posterior to this ligament complex. One method of doing this is to use the McCall[29,32,36] cul-de-plasty or a modification of it. In one modification the operator excises most of the peritoneum of any coexistent enterocele before placing the polyglycolic acid–type cul-de-plasty stitches, thus repairing the enterocele while reducing the size of the subsequent cul-de-sac (Figs. 20-25 through 20-27). If the vault is unusually wide, an appropriate wedge should be removed and

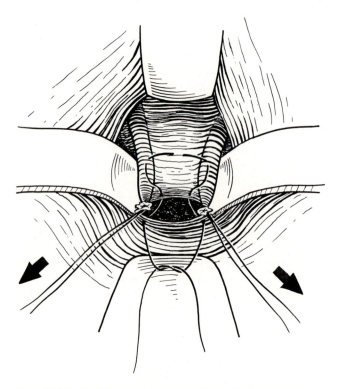

Fig. 20-25. Modified cul-de-plasty stitch. Enterocele sac has been resected, and a bite of absorbable long-lasting polyglycolic acid type suture has been placed through full thickness of posterior vaginal wall at a spot selected to become highest point of reconstructed vaginal vault. Traction is made on uterosacral ligament pedicles, and suture picks up cut edge of peritoneum and peritoneal site of each uterosacral ligament at the level to which vaginal vault will be fixed. Suture is returned through the peritoneum between the uterosacral ligaments, then the uterosacral ligament, peritoneum, and vaginal vault of the opposite side. (Modified from Nichols DH, Randall CL: *Vaginal surgery,* ed 3, Baltimore, 1989, Williams & Wilkins.)

the edges approximated (Figs. 20-28 and 20-29). The cul-de-plasty stitch should be tied under direct vision to eliminate the chance that the now buried proximal end of a fallopian tube will prolapse postoperatively into the line of the vaginal incision.

If the posterior vault is wide, as it may be after an enterocele repair, the operator may dissect a V-shaped wedge of excess vaginal membrane free and remove it and sew the cut edges of the V together from side to side (Fig. 20-30). This maneuver brings the vaginal attachments of the uterosacral ligaments still closer together toward the midline. It is entirely consistent with the purse-string peritonealization and surgical narrowing or V-shaped wedging of a voluminous vaginal vault, as described. The operator should tie the purse-string peritonealization stitch under direct visualization to avoid the possibility of trapping any intraabdominal structure, such as an ovary, a knuckle of tube, or bowel, in the stitch.

Rarely, usually in a patient with procidentia, the uterosacral ligament may have no palpable, usable strength. In this circumstance, the operator must find an alternate method of fixing and stabilizing the vaginal vault; otherwise the unfixed vault may later telescope and evert. In such a patient the operator may sew the vault to the fascia of the pelvic diaphragm[18] or to the sacrospinous[32] or sacrotuberous ligament after the peritoneal cavity has been closed (see Chapter 27).

The Manchester operation

When the patient with symptomatic prolapse desires surgical treatment that will preserve her uterus or her fertility and has the combination of cervical elongation coincident with strong though elongated cardinal-uterosacral ligaments, cystocele, and rectocele, the Manchester[43] (or

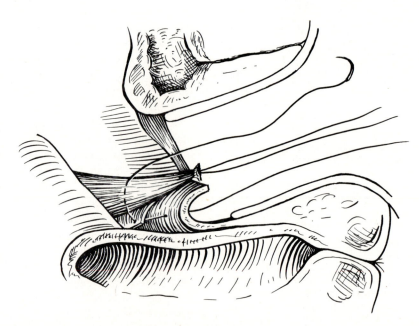

Fig. 20-26. First half of this stitch is seen in sagittal section before tying. (Modified from Nichols DH, Randall CL: *Vaginal surgery,* ed 3, Baltimore, 1989, Williams & Wilkins.)

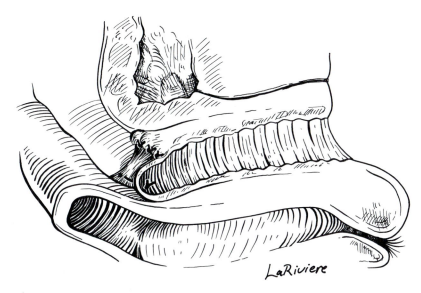

Fig. 20-27. First half of this stitch is seen in sagittal section after tying and subsequent closure of peritoneal cavity and vaginal vault, demonstrating that apex of vagina is now cranial and posterior to new peritoneal cul-de-sac. (Modified from Nichols DH, Randall CL: *Vaginal surgery,* ed 3, Baltimore, 1989, Williams & Wilkins.)

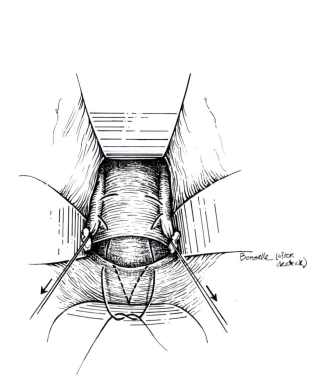

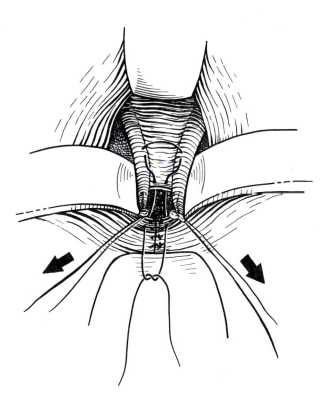

Fig. 20-28. Even with cul-de-plasty, a pathologically wide vaginal vault can be narrowed by excision of an appropriate V-shaped wedge posteriorly and this defect closed from side to side by interrupted sutures. (From Nichols DH, Randall CL: *Vaginal surgery,* ed 3, Baltimore 1989, Williams & Wilkins.)

Fig. 20-29. The posterior vault has been narrowed by excision of the V-shaped wedge and the defect closed with interrupted stitches. (Modified from Nichols DH, Randall CL: *Vaginal surgery,* ed 3, Baltimore, 1989, Williams & Wilkins.)

Donald-Fothergill) operation can be considered. In the previous generation it was the the surgical treatment of choice for most patients with symptomatic uterine prolapse, but with the more widespread use of postmenopausal estrogen replacement therapy, and its tendency to prolong the years of uterine bleeding, the operation has lost much of its favor and has largely been replaced by vaginal hysterectomy with colporrhaphy. The latter operation, of course, by its very nature removes the uterus as a source for future bleeding.

There are some additional potential difficulties concerning the Manchester operation with which the surgeon must be prepared to contend. If the cardinal-uterosacral ligament complex is of unusually poor quality, it may be inadequate to support the vaginal vault postoperatively. If there is no significant elongation of the cervix, amputation of a normal-sized cervix as a means of mobilizing the cardinal-uterosacral ligaments may disturb the integrity of the internal cervical os, causing the risk of postoperative cervical incompetence. The diminished size or caliber of the vagina following colporrhaphy will interfere with vaginal dilation during subsequent labor and delivery damaging the vaginal repair which by virtue of the scarring already present from the colporrhaphy will make future re-repair more difficult. Post-Manchester cervical stenosis may lead to mechanical dysmenorrhea and to secondary infertility.

All things considered, the Manchester operation is a worthy one and the surgeon who chooses to perform it should be equally adept at vaginal hysterectomy, should the operative change be found necessary during the course of the procedure. The technique is well illustrated in Figure 20-31. Coincident enterocele is often present and should be sought and if found, corrected to avoid future progression or recurrence of the prolapse.

The technique is illustrated and described in Fig. 20-31.

Trachelectomy. The cervix remaining after a subtotal or supracervical hysterectomy will occasionally require surgical removal, or trachelectomy. Most frequently this will be required as part of the reparative surgery to relieve a symptomatic prolapse,and because cystocele and recto-

Text continued on p. 328.

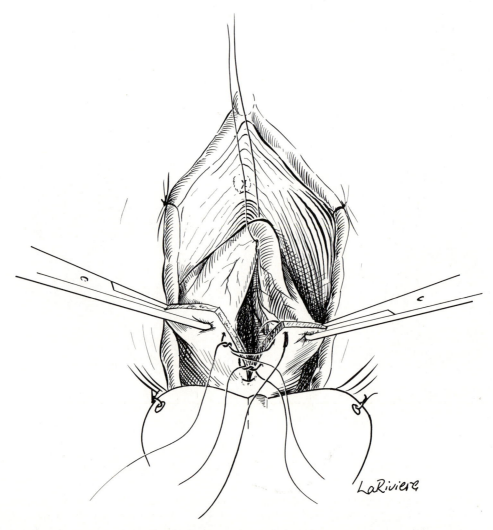

Fig. 20-30. Whenever the vaginal vault is excessively wide, it can be easily narrowed by excision of a V-shaped wedge and the defect closed by interrupted through-and-through sutures, as shown.

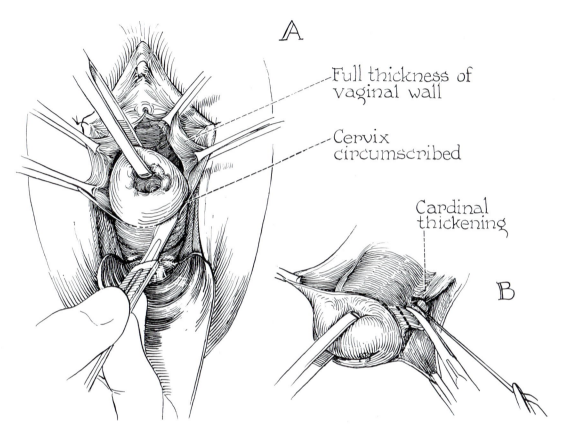

Fig. 20-31. A dilatation and curettage are done. the cervix should be dilated to a no. 10 Hegar dilator and the length of the cervial canal measured.

The full thickness of the vaginal wall is opened from the bladder reflection with an inverted V incision, and then the incision is continued to the urethral meatus in the same manner as illustrated for a simple anterior repair. The bladder is pushed off the cervix at its natural line of cleavage and the urethra mobilized for future plication. Bleeding points are ligated, and then attention is directed to the cervical amputation. The inverted V incision at the bladder reflection is now extended around the cervix **(A).** The degree of hypertrophy of the cervix, the extent of the prolapse, and the elongation of the visceral connective tissue determine the site of amputation of the cervix. The internal os is the guiding landmark in describing descensus. In general, a distance of 3 cm from the internal os to the point of amputation will allow for shortening of the ligaments and correction of the cystocele and rectocele, both of which strengthen the vagina as an obturator and contribute to correction of the prolapse.

The flaps are now developed laterally and posteriorly to demonstrate the cardinal and uterosacral ligaments. The extent of this dissection is governed by the amount of cervix to be amputated. The ligaments should be cut, clamped, and tied close to the cervix in order to permit suture in the midline **(B).** By suture of these thickenings, anterior to the amputated cervix for the cardinal structures and posterior for the uterosacral thickenings, the vagina is restored as a competent obturator.

Continued.

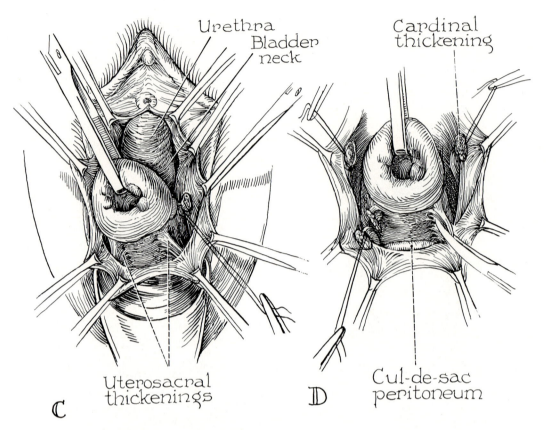

Urethra
Bladder neck
Cardinal thickening

Uterosacral thickenings

C

Cul-de-sac peritoneum

D

Fig. 20-31, cont'd. The cardinal ligaments, which at this level contain the descending branch of the uterine artery, are secured with two suture ligatures of 0 PGA **(B).** They are mobilized to a sufficient length to be brought together in the midline after the cervical amputation **(C).**

The posterior thickenings, the uterosacral ligaments, are cut, clamped, and tied **(D).** In these thickenings are vaginal branches of the inferior vesical arteries, and failure to respect this fact can give rise to postoperative bleeding and a hematoma of the rectovaginal septum.

The cervix is amputated and coned **(E).** Active bleeding points are secured and ligated. A bullet tenaculum is attached to the anterior lip of the cervix, which is drawn anteriorly **(F).**

Following the principle of correcting the pelvic floor as a whole, attention is now directed to obliteration of the cul-de-sac since some degree of herniation inevitably exists because of the nature of uterine prolapse **(E and F).** This is done by dissecting the full thickness of the vaginal wall from the cul-de-sac peritoneum and subsequently from the rectum in retrograde fashion. It is continued until the posterior thickenings (uterosacral ligaments) fan out and lose their identify as their vessels approach their origins from the hypogastric artery. Hemostasis is important as the ligaments are approximated. Realize the proximity of the ureters so that they are not ligated nor distorted.

The uterosacral ligaments are now united in the midline **(F).** If a definitive hernial sac is evident, the peritoneum is opened prior to this and the neck of the sac transfixed and amputated. Retrograde dissection is continued, stopping periodically to unite the uterosacral thickenings and control bleeding.

Depending on the size of the cul-de-sac herniation, the rectovaginal septum is soon reached. The dissection goes remarkably well if it is in the right plane. Simultaneous correction of the upper portion of the rectocele is started. No part of the composite picture of the pathologic anatomy of prolapse is thus neglected **(F and G).**

G shows this retrograde method of dissection. Consecutive wedge-shaped sections of the posterior vaginal wall are removed, the uterosacral thickenings are approximated, and the field is kept free of active bleeding. The connective tissue fanning out toward the sacrum gradually thins out and its identity is lost in the perirectal connective tissue.

H shows the appearance of this dissection and line of trimming if folded back and seen from the vaginal aspect. This line of incision will be met from below upward when the perineorrhaphy is done and the lower part of the rectocele is corrected.

Continued.

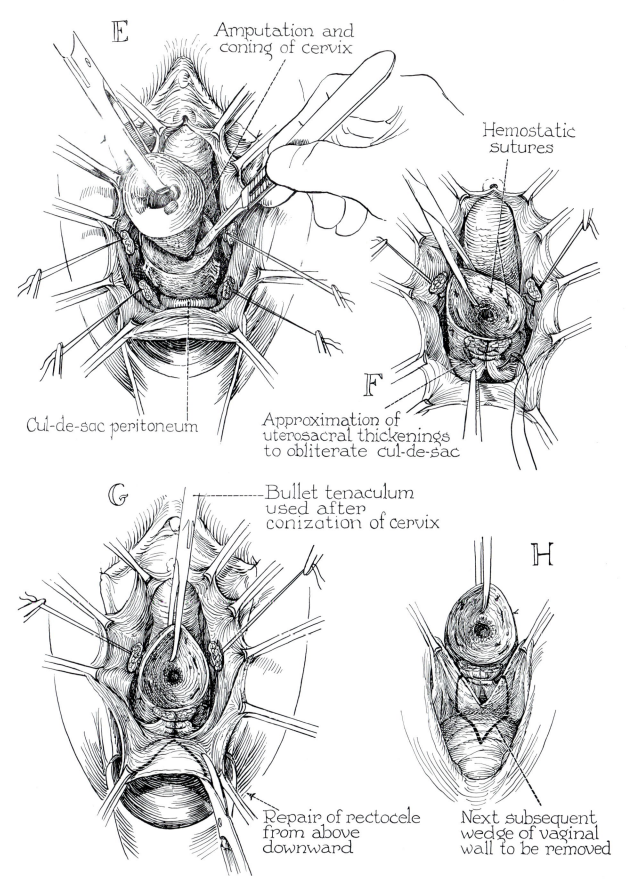

E

Amputation and
coning of cervix

Hemostatic
sutures

F

Cul-de-sac peritoneum

Approximation of
uterosacral thickenings
to obliterate cul-de-sac

G

Bullet tenaculum
used after
conization of cervix

H

Repair of rectocele
from above
downward

Next subsequent
wedge of vaginal
wall to be removed

Fig. 20-31, cont'd. For legend see opposite page.

Fig. 20-31, cont'd. An inverting suture, commonly known as a Sturmdorf, is used to slide the flaps of the vagina over the raw fibromuscular tissue of the cervix **(I)**. As illustrated, this has the effect of drawing the edges into the new external os and recreating the posterior fornix.

Interrupted sutures of 00 PGA are now inserted to approximate the posterior wall. The last suture is left long and is tagged as a landmark to be used later when the reconstruction of the perineal body and completion of the rectocele repair are done from below upward **(J)**.

A full-length plication of the urethra, bladder neck, and bladder base is done in the same manner as illustrated for a simple anterior repair **(E to L)**. This plication is done regardless of the pre-existence of stress incontinence. The anatomic arrangement that results in incontinence can easily be fabricated in repair of the anterior wall by the surgeon intent upon curing the protuberances of a cystocele and rectocele but neglecting a prophylactic plication of the bladder neck. Once again, the importance of attacking the herniation as a whole is apparent **(J)**.

The cardinal thickenings are then sutured in the midline by several interrupted sutures **(K)**. This feature of the operation has the effect of shortening these extensions of the parietal connective tissue and enhancing their contribution to the support of the pelvic floor.

An anterior Sturmdorf-type suture is placed and left untied pending a study of the flaps of the anterior wall **(L)**. The original inverted V incision will have reconstructed a few centimeters of the anterior vaginal wall comprising the anterior fornix. The remainder of the walls are developed by the following method: Push the cervix toward the sacrum with the tenaculum and observe the flaps of the anterior vaginal wall. Cross the Allis clamps so that one flap overlaps the other. Observe the amount of vaginal wall to be resected on each side and then do the resection with the Metzenbaum scissors as it is done in a simple anterior repair.

The anterior vaginal wall is now closed with interrupted sutures of 00 PGA suture, beginning at the anterior fornix. As the walls are approximated, more vaginal wall can be resected if this seems indicated. The anterior Sturmdorf suture, when tied, will complete the reconstruction of the anterior vaginal wall **(M)**.

The lateral or crown sutures which bring together the vaginal wall in the lateral fornices are placed as shown in **M**. These sutures should include some of the superficial layers of the fibromuscular structure of the cervix since their purpose is to epithelize all raw areas.

As in the posterior repair previously illustrated for a simple vaginal plastic operation, a butterfly section of skin and mucous membrane is outlined on the perineum **(M)**. The landmarks are the skin just anterior to the anus, the mucocutaneous junction laterally, and above this the hymenal ring or its remnants **(M)**. The genital hiatus must now be closed at one of its crucial areas. Its anteroposterior length must be decreased and the width of its transverse slit narrowed. This cannot be done by a routine method of placing sutures in the hiatus. Descriptions of the placing of "levator sutures" are as unrealistic as the frequent illustrations of this anatomic forgery. The levator muscles (specifically, the puborectali) are centimeters away from the perineum. One should not place heavy sutures and forcibly draw the insertions of a group of paired, laterally placed muscles to an abnormal position in the midline. The plastic reconstruction of the genital aperture requires more selective surgery if a functional vagina is desired.

From the hymenal ring the butterfly pattern is advanced by incisions up to the traction suture left from the retrograde dissection and repair of the rectocele **(M)**. This proceeds without the usual difficulty in locating the proper line of cleavage between vagina and rectum since this has already been identified from above.

The last phase of this operation, the formation of a strong obturator and a narrow hiatus, is now begun. By using interrupted sutures of 0 PGA-type suture the musculature of the perineum is built up. Multiple sutures are placed without strangulation to build up the perineum so that the approximation of the bulbocavernosi and remnants of the transverse perineal muscles decreases the genital aperture and adds to the support of the pelvic viscera. The anterior edges of the puborectalis may be drawn to the midline to decrease the pelvic aperture, but this must be done with caution or a stricture will result despite the fact that adequate vaginal wall remains. Repeated palpation of the lower third of the vagina is necessary during the reconstruction of the perineum. Individualize with each operation, for the depth of the pelvic floor varies and the extent of the musculature support remaining varies in each patient. The vaginal wall is closed with interrupted sutures of 00 PGA suture. (From Ball TL: *Gynecologic surgery and urology,* ed 2, St Louis, 1963, Mosby–Year Book.)

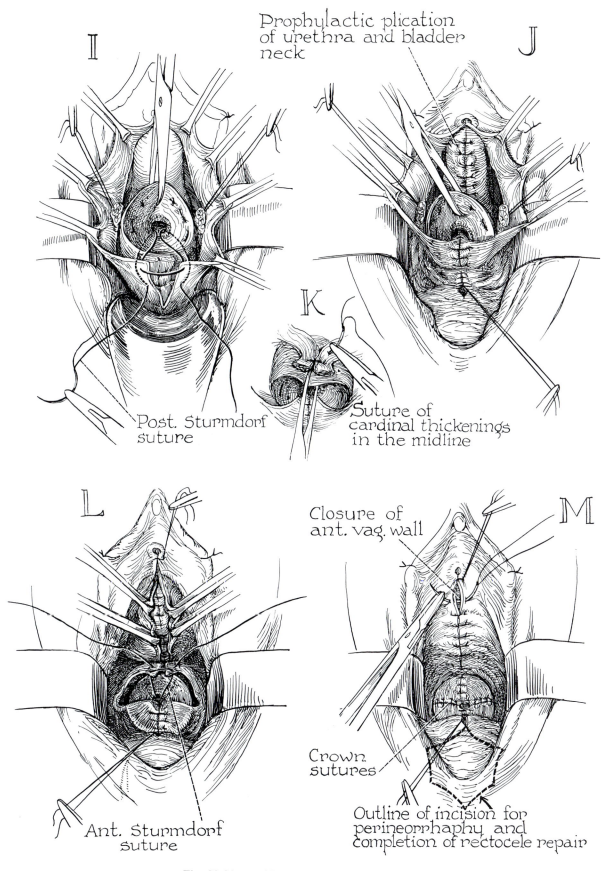

I

Prophylactic plication of urethra and bladder neck

J

K

Post. Sturmdorf suture

Suture of cardinal thickenings in the midline

L

Ant. Sturmdorf suture

Closure of ant. vag. wall

M

Crown sutures

Outline of incision for perineorrhaphy and completion of rectocele repair

Fig. 20-31, cont'd. For legend see opposite page.

cele usually coexist, a coincident anterior and posterior colporrhaphy are performed.

Occasionally, the remaining cervix will be the site of severe dysplasia or intraepithelial neoplasia, for which trachelectomy would be an appropriate remedy—with or without coincident colporrhaphy, depending on the presence of cystocele and rectocele. Trachelectomy is most easily accomplished by the transvaginal approach, but there is little indication for "prophylactic" removal of the retained cervix,[34] but in any patient with a retained cervix it is most important that it be evaluated regularly, with cytologic study and colposcopy as necessary, as any cervix may harbor future neoplasia.

Ikedife[17] reported a high incidence of primary infertility in women with a long (4 to 6.5 cm) cervix in the absence of uterine or vault prolapse with no other explanation for their lack of fertility.

Laparoscopy and hysterectomy

For the hysterectomy candidate in whom there is uncertainty about the condition of the adnexa, and adnexal or pelvic adhesions that might compromise the ability to safely perform vaginal hysterectomy, a preliminary diagnostic laparoscopy should clarify whether or not it is safe to perform vaginal hysterectomy. This is the diagnostic contribution of laparoscopy to the planned surgery.

When troublesome adhesions have been identified before hysterectomy, they can be severed during preliminary laparoscopy, and the adnexa freed or removed thus making vaginal hysterectomy safely possible in this particular patient and permitting surgical attention to support of the vault postoperatively as well as coincident repair of any other features of pelvic relaxation through the same transvaginal operative exposure. This, then, is laparoscopic-assisted vaginal hysterectomy. Portions of the hysterectomy may be added to that which is done laparoscopically (e.g., transection of the round ligaments, broad ligaments, preparation of the bladder flap).[31] On occasion it has been shown that the entire hysterectomy can be done through the laparoscope[40]—the so-called "laparoscopic hysterectomy," though even then the specimen is usually removed by way of the vagina rather than by morcellation through the laparoscope.

A difficulty with a totally laparoscopic hysterectomy concept is that little or no provision is made for effectively reattaching the transected ligamentous supports of the uterus to the vagina to aid in vaginal support after hysterectomy. Now that it has been shown that total laparoscopic hysterectomy is possible in the hands of a very experienced laparoscopist, it must be proven that the method is as safe or safer than the traditional approach and is cost-effective.

Laparoscopically *assisted* vaginal hysterectomy, on the other hand, may increase the numbers of patients who can safely enjoy the reduced pain and shorter hospitalization afforded by vaginal hysterectomy.

Final procedures

After surgery the vaginal cavity may be lightly packed for 24 hours with 2-inch plain or iodoform gauze, and a silicone-coated transurethral Foley catheter may be inserted. Packing not only provides hemostatic pressure and obliterates potential spaces but also bolsters the new sutures in the vaginal vault and soaks up secretions, removing blood and serum and preventing pooling.[24] Unless there is considerable oozing, it is usually unnecessary to pack the vagina, however, and the presence of vaginal packing makes it difficult for some patients to initiate voiding. Similarly, routine insertion of an indwelling transurethral catheter is not recommended, particularly if no colporrhaphy has been done and no packing used, because the risk of subsequent cystitis appears to be much less if the patient is able to void by herself.

Before the operation is complete, the surgeon should perform a rectal examination to check for anal stricture and to confirm rectal integrity. If a stitch passes through the rectal mucosa, it should be visualized on the rectal side and cut, and the ends permitted to retract into the perirectal tissues.

VAGINAL HYSTERECTOMY AND PARTIAL VAGINECTOMY

In the hands of a surgeon experienced in the procedures, vaginal hysterectomy with partial vaginectomy seems to have several advantages for the definitive treatment of in situ carcinoma of the uterine cervix when the disease has extended to or involves the vagina, as determined by preoperative colposcopically directed biopsy.[47] For example, this approach permits specific preoperative and intraoperative delineation of the lesion to be removed, which is not possible with other techniques. The operation itself consists of vaginal hysterectomy and removal of a predetermined amount of vaginal cuff. Simon et al[45] have suggested that vaginal hysterectomy can be performed for the cervix cancer patient with microinvasion (i.e., less than 3 mm).

As part of the preparation for surgery, the vagina is lightly painted with tincture of iodine or freshly prepared Schiller's solution. The nonglycogen-containing areas of the cervix and vagina, which should be removed because of their pathologic and precancerous nature, are then clearly established, because they do not take up the iodine stain. Furthermore, the multicentric origin of the disease can be appreciated. With this type of visualization, the operator can readily determine the level at which the cuff, along with a comfortable margin of uninvolved tissue, should be amputated—a determination that can only be estimated or surmised during an abdominal hysterectomy.

Because a vaginal hysterectomy is essentially an extrafascial procedure, it permits additional mobilization of the parametrium and the removal of more tissue with the operative specimen than does the standard intrafascial total abdominal hysterectomy. This may be a particular advantage if the pathology report discloses superficial unsuspected microinvasion of the carcinoma to a less than 3-mm depth (which by probability has not yet progressed to the point of lymphatic extension).

It is easier to measure the amount of vagina being removed during a vaginal hysterectomy than during an abdominal hysterectomy. In the vaginal operation, the operator cuts the cardinal ligament support system from the uterus after the vagina has been "measured and cut," and the vagina is much less stretched. In an abdominal hysterectomy, however, the stretch of the vagina is greater because the cardinal ligaments are cut before the vagina is measured and cut, and traction on the uterus during its removal stretches the vagina. An apparent 1-inch cuff of (stretched) vagina with a uterus removed abdominally may, as the previously stretched tissue contracts, prove to be only ⅓ or ½ inch of vagina.

Finally, as mentioned earlier, the patient who has undergone vaginal surgery generally has a distinctly less complicated, more comfortable postoperative course and a shorter recovery period than does the patient who has undergone abdominal surgery.

Schuchardt perineal incision

When transvaginal exposure is awkward and accessibility seems limited, the operator may use the Schuchardt perineal incision for hysterectomy or fistula repair. It is usually desirable for the right-handed operator to make the incision on the patient's left side and vice versa. When the case is difficult or the operator not yet experienced in this procedure, instillation of 60 ml of sterile evaporated milk or a solution of methylene blue into the bladder before the procedure permits prompt recognition of any inadvertent bladder penetration.

The tissues to be incised may be infiltrated thoroughly with a solution of 0.5% lidocaine (Xylocaine) or bupivacaine (Marcaine) in 1:200,000 epinephrine (Adrenaline) in a fanlike fashion by inserting a 22-gauge spinal needle through the skin of the perineum midway between the anus and the left ischial tuberosity.[24] To reduce blood loss fur-

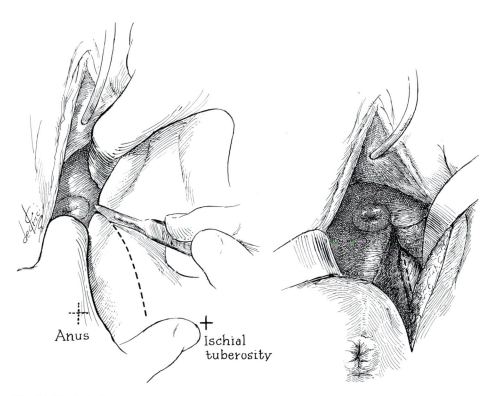

Fig. 20-32. *Left,* Schuchardt incision is started immediately behind site of hymenal margin and continued posterolaterally in a gentle curve around anus to end at a point midway between anus and left ischial tuberosity. Surgeon and assistant introduce their index fingers deeper into the vagina, maintaining tension, and vaginal portion of incision is continued in a posterolateral direction as high as is necessary to provide desired exposure of vaginal vault. *Right,* Lowermost fat tissue of ischiorectal fossa has been divided, and in depths of the wound the medial portion of pubococcygeus muscle is visible. A portion of this may be divided if necessary *(dashed line).* Bleeding points are clamped as they are encountered and coagulated with electrosurgical unit, care being taken not to coagulate surface of rectum should it be visible within the wound. At conclusion of operation, Schuchardt incision is closed in layers. (From Nichols DH, Randall CL: *Vaginal surgery,* ed 3, Baltimore, 1989, Williams & Wilkins.)

ther, the operator should use the electrosurgical scalpel to make the incision. The skin incision follows a curved line from the 4 o'clock position at the hymenal margin to a point halfway between the anus and the ischial tuberosity (Fig. 20-32).

To protect the nearby rectum from damage during this incision, the right-handed operator inserts the index finger of the left hand into the vagina, depressing the perineum and rectum, while the assistant on the right simultaneously inserts an index finger into the vagina to provide pressure in an anterolateral direction and keep the tissues taut. The operator begins the incision immediately behind the site of the hymenal margin and continues it posterolaterally in a gentle curve around the anus, ending it at a point midway between the anus and the left ischial tuberosity. To maintain tension, the surgeon and the assistant insert their index fingers more deeply into the vagina, and the surgeon continues the vaginal portion of the incision in a posterolateral direction as high as is necessary to provide the desired exposure of the vaginal vault. This incision divides the lowermost fatty tissue of the ischiorectal fossa.

In the depths of the wound, the medial portion of the pubococcygeus muscle is visible, and a portion of it may be divided if necessary. Bleeding points are clamped as they are encountered and are coagulated with the electrosurgical unit; care must be taken not to coagulate the surface of the rectum, however, as it tends to remain prominently in the wound. At the conclusion of the operation, the Schuchardt incision is closed in layers. The vaginal stitches may include and unite the severed portions of the pubococcygeus muscle, bringing them together beneath the edges of the vaginal incision.

If an incision of this depth is not necessary, the operator may make a classic mediolateral episiotomy incision on one or both sides, which should be carefully closed by reapproximation of all incised tissue layers.

Procedure for partial vaginectomy with hysterectomy

The first step in performing a partial vaginectomy with hysterectomy is to apply iodine to the cervix and upper half of the vagina and to note any areas that do not take the stain. The operator then applies a rim of colpohemostats to a fold of the vagina at least 1.5 inches away from the lateral margin of the cervix and lateral to any nonstained tissue within the vagina (Fig. 20-33), tucks the cervix into this fold, and makes an incision through the full thickness of the vagina with Mayo scissors or an electrosurgical scalpel (Fig. 20-34). The counterpressure from

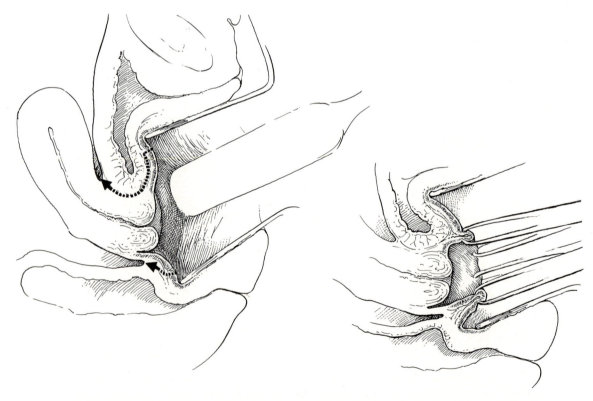

Fig. 20-33. Partial vaginectomy with hysterectomy. Vagina and cervix are carefully exposed and thoroughly examined, and amount of vagina to be removed with specimen is determined with precision. *Left,* Lines of proposed dissection are shown in sagittal drawing. Infiltration here by 1:200,000 epinephrine (Adrenaline) in 0.5% lidocaine (Xylocaine) solution aids hemostasis and later identification of connective tissue planes and spaces. *Right,* Distal to this point, vagina is grasped circumferentially by a series of single-toothed tenacula. (From Nichols DH, Randall CL: *Vaginal surgery,* ed 3, Baltimore, 1989, Williams & Wilkins.)

anterior, posterior, and lateral retractors permits the bladder and its fascia to recede promptly from the point at which the vagina was held by the colpohemostats. After establishing the vaginal flap circumferentially and carefully noting the position of the ureters, the operator clamps, cuts, and ligates the lateral fascial bundles on either side. The operator then separates the rectum from the tissues to be removed by gentle dissection; identifies the posterior cul-de-sac; makes an opening into it; and clamps, cuts, and ligates the posterior and lateral portions of the uterosacral ligaments.

The fundus of the uterus can be brought through either the anterior or the posterior colpotomy. The adnexa are then inspected and, if necessary, removed. Hemostats are applied over the cornual angles of the uterus, and the uterus, cervix, and parametrial tissues are removed en masse, after which the hemostats are replaced by transfixion ligatures. There may be areas of venous oozing around the base of the bladder, but there should be no active

bleeding. The vaginal vault can then be closed with an absorbable suture on each side that goes through the anterior vault, round ligament, and anterior peritoneum on each side. A second set of sutures is placed through the posterolateral vault, uterosacral ligament pedicle, posterior peritoneum, and the same structures on the opposite side, as suggested by Durfee (Fig. 20-35).

If, after hysterectomy, the vagina seems too short for marital comfort, the operator may perform an anterior or posterior colporrhaphy before closing the Schuchardt incision. A sheath of mobilized peritoneum can be sewn to the distal cut edge of the vagina and the peritoneal cavity closed cranially. The patient should wear an obturator postoperatively during the period of vaginal reepithelialization. Distal length can be added by using the Williams vulvovaginoplasty or a perineorrhaphy if the perineum is inadequate.

The technique of the Schauta-Amreich operation, the radical vaginal hysterectomy, is the subject of Chapter 23.

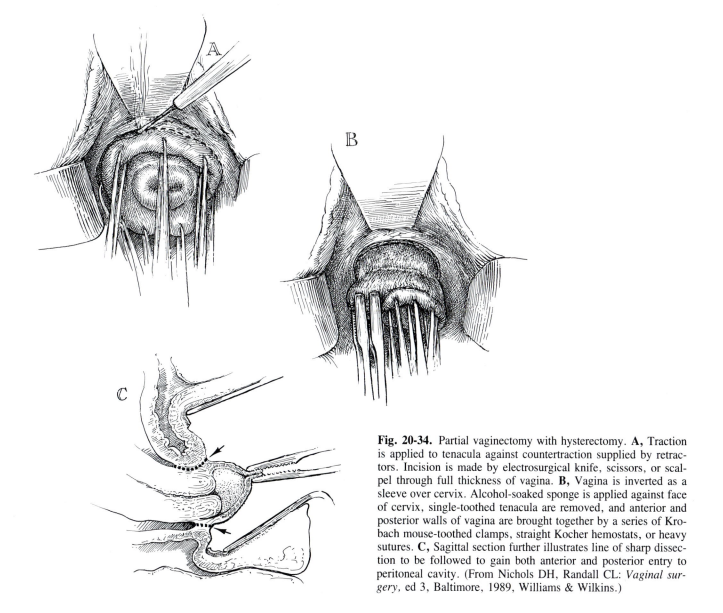

Fig. 20-34. Partial vaginectomy with hysterectomy. **A,** Traction is applied to tenacula against countertraction supplied by retractors. Incision is made by electrosurgical knife, scissors, or scalpel through full thickness of vagina. **B,** Vagina is inverted as a sleeve over cervix. Alcohol-soaked sponge is applied against face of cervix, single-toothed tenacula are removed, and anterior and posterior walls of vagina are brought together by a series of Krobach mouse-toothed clamps, straight Kocher hemostats, or heavy sutures. **C,** Sagittal section further illustrates line of sharp dissection to be followed to gain both anterior and posterior entry to peritoneal cavity. (From Nichols DH, Randall CL: *Vaginal surgery,* ed 3, Baltimore, 1989, Williams & Wilkins.)

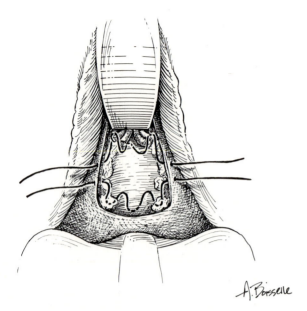

A.Borselle

Fig. 20-35. When there has been no coincident prolapse of vaginal vault, depth may be preserved by closure from side to side. A stitch of polyglycolic acid–type suture is passed through full thickness of lateral vaginal wall and peritoneum, round ligament portion of adnexal pedicle, a reefing of anterior peritoneum, and the same structures in reverse order on the opposite side. A second stitch is placed through full thickness of posterolateral vaginal wall, uterosacral ligament stump, a reefing of posterior peritoneum, and the same structures in reverse order on the opposite side. Any remaining gaps in vaginal wall may be closed by interrupted sutures. (From Nichols DH, Randall CL: *Vaginal surgery,* ed 3, Baltimore, 1989, Williams & Wilkins.)

POSTHYSTERECTOMY FALLOPIAN TUBE PROLAPSE

Posthysterectomy prolapse of the fallopian tube is sporadically encountered. At first it is mistaken for some granulation tissue at the vaginal vault, but its true nature becomes evident when it fails to heal after curettement and office cauterization. Because it is a source of chronic vaginal discharge, often blood tinged, it requires surgical treatment by salpingectomy, preferably total, so as to reduce long-term postoperative pain.

Although salpingectomy can be treated by laparotomy, a less formidable approach can be either by operative laparoscopy[25] or by transvaginal excision. An excellent technique has been described by Wetchler and Hurt.[51] Allis clamps are placed just below the lateral angle of the cuff and a transverse incision is made in the vault just posterior to the prolapsed tube and vaginal scar. By sharp and blunt dissection the vaginal wall is freed from the underlying peritoneum, which is opened, and the cul-de-sac is explored. Adhesions are freed and a separate horizontal incision is made in the vagina *anterior* to the prolapsed tube and vaginal cuff to remove a portion of the vagina wall around the prolapsed tube. The mesosalpinx is clamped and cut, the specimen removed, pedicles are ligated, and the peritoneum and vaginal cuff closed separately.

Combined abdominovaginal procedures

For those women in whom vascular or lymphatic penetration has been established preoperatively by biopsy study or lymphography, a combined vaginal-abdominal hysterocolpectomy, including lymphadenectomy, can have certain advantages. The surgeon can plan an operative procedure for these patients that combines the best features of both the vaginal and the abdominal operations into a single or composite operative procedure. In order to shorten operating time, minimize the risks to the patient as much as possible, and promote surgical efficiency, such a composite procedure may best be performed with the simultaneous use of two operating teams.

The vaginal portion of the operation permits the widest possible excision of parametrium, rectal pillars, and uterosacral ligaments, as well as the removal of a predetermined amount of vagina or vaginal cuff at the time of the initial operative procedure, under the direct vision and control of the operator. The vaginal approach ensures vastly improved dissection of the paracolpium, the inferior portion of the horizontal connective tissue ground bundle, the inferior portion of the rectal pillars, and the vesicouterine ligaments. Ureteral exposure and dissection can best be accomplished during the vaginal portion of the operation. Meanwhile, through an appropriate incision, the abdominal team will have begun the bilateral extraperitoneal or intraperitoneal lymphadenectomy, which may be completed while the vaginal team is closing the Schuchardt incision. Combined synchronous operation has been reported by Mitra,[30] Howkins,[16] and Vidakovic,[48] among others, in various sequential modifications. The combined operation should be of particular value for those in whom vascular or lymphatic penetration has been established preoperatively by biopsy study or lymphography. However, it remains to be seen whether such a combined operation will provide an improved prognosis.

REFERENCES

1. Allen E: Discussion, *Am J Obstet Gynecol* 61A (suppl):219, 1951.
2. Bandler SW: *Vaginal celiotomy,* Philadelphia, 1911, WB Saunders.
3. Candiani GB, Ferrari AG: *Isterectomia vaginale,* Milano, 1986, Masson.
4. Capen CV et al: Vaginal removal of the ovaries in association with vaginal hysterectomy, *J Reprod Med* 28:589, 1983.
5. Copenhaver EH: Vaginal hysterectomy. An analysis of indications and complications among 1,000 operations, *Am J Obstet Gynecol* 84:123-128, 1962.
6. Copenhaver EH: Hysterectomy: vaginal versus adbominal; *Surg Clin North Am* 45:751-763, 1965.
7. Dicker RC et al: Complications of abdominal and vaginal hysterectomy among women of reproductive age in the United States, *Am J Obstet Gynecol* 144:841-848, 1982.
8. England GT, Randall HW, Graves WL: Impairment of tissue defenses by vasocontrictors in vaginal hysterectomies, *Obstet Gynecol* 61:271, 1983.
9. Gigliotti B: Isterectomia vaginale per morecellement. Considerazion di tecnica chirurgica e casistics personale, *Riv di Ostetrics e Ginecologia* II 1:18-21, 1989.
10. Gitsch E, Palmrich AH: *Gynecological operative anatomy,* Berlin, 1977, Walter de Gruyter.

11. Gitsch G, Berger E, Tatra G: Trends in thirty years of vaginal hysterectomy, *Surg Gynecol Obstet* 172:207-210, 1991.

12. Gray LA: *Vaginal hysterectomy,* ed 3, Springfield, Ill, 1983, Charles C Thomas.

13. Hemsell DL et al: Single-dose cephalosporin for prevention of major pelvic infection after vaginal hysterectomy: cephazolin versus cefoxitan versus cefotaxime, *Am J Obstet Gynecol* 156:1201-1205, 1987.

14. Hemsell DL et al: Cephazolin for hysterectomy prophylaxis, *Obstet Gynecol* 76:603-606, 1990.

15. Hoffman MS: Transvaginal removal of ovaries with endoloop sutures at the time of vaginal hysterectomy, *Am J Obstet Gynecol* 165:407-408, 1991.

16. Howkins J: Synchronous combined abdomino-vaginal hysterocolpectomy for cancer of the cervix: a report of fifty patients, *J Obstet Gynaecol Br Emp* 66:212, 1959.

17. Ikedife D: Long vaginal cervix: a clinical entity, *J Obstet Gynaecol* 10:333-334, 1990.

18. Inmon WB: Pelvic relaxation and repair including prolapse of vagina following hysterectomy, *South Med J* 56:577, 1963.

19. Janisch H, Palmrich AH, Pecherstorfer M: *Selected urologic operations in gynecology,* Berlin, 1979, Walter de Gruyter.

20. Jaszczak SE, Evans TN: Vaginal morphology following hysterectomy, *Int J Gynaecol Obstet* 19:41, 1981.

21. Kamina P: From anatomy to the technique of vaginal hysterectomy, *Rev Fr Gynecol Obstet* 85:434-444, 1990.

22. Käser O, Iklé FA, Hirsch HH: *Atlas of gynecologic surgery,* ed 2, New York, 1985, Thieme-Stratton.

23. Kovac SR: Intramyometrial coring as an adjunct to vaginal hysterectomy, *Obstet Gynecol* 67:131-136, 1986.

24. Krige CF: *Vaginal hysterectomy and genital prolapse repair,* Johannesburg, 1965, Witwatersrand University Press.

25. Letteria GS et al: Laparoscopic management of fallopian tube prolapse, *Obstet Gynecol* 72:508-510, 1988.

26. Malpas P: *The choice of operation for genital prolapse. In Meigs JV, Sturgis SH, editors: Progress in gynecology,* vol 3, New York, 1957, Grune & Stratton.

27. Malpas P: *Genital prolapse. In Claye A, Bourne A, editors: British obstetric and gynaecological practice,* ed 3, London, 1963, William Heinemann.

28. Mattingly RF, Huang WY: Steroidogenesis of the menopausal and postmenopausal ovary, *Am J Obstet Gynecol* 103:679, 1969.

29. McCall ML: Posterior culdeplasty: surgical correction of enterocele during vaginal hysterectomy: a preliminary report, *Obstet Gynecol* 10:595, 1957.

30. Mitra S: *Mitra operation for cancer of the cervix,* Springfield, Ill, 1960, Charles C Thomas.

31. Nezhat C, Nezhat F, Silfen S: Laparoscopic hysterectomy and bilateral salpingocophorectomy using multifire GIA surgical stapler, *J Gynecol Surg* 6:285, 1990.

32. Nichols DH, Randall CL: *Vaginal hysterectomy,* ed 3, Baltimore, 1989, Williams & Wilkins, pp 182-238.

33. Novak F: *Surgical gynecologic techniques,* New York, 1978, John Wiley & Sons.

34. Pasley WW, Leigh RW: Trachelectomy: a review of fifty-five cases, *Am J Obstet Gynecol* 159:728-732, 1988.

35. Philipp K: Ergebnisse der routinemaBigen entfernung der Ovarien und/oder Tuben im Rahmen der vaginalen Hysterektomie, *Geburtshilfe Frauenheilkd* 40:159, 1980.

36. Piura B: *Am J Obstet Gynecol* 155:685, 1986 (letter to the editor).

37. Pratt JH: Technique of vaginal hysterectomy, *Clin Obstet Gynecol* 2:1125, 1959.

38. Randall CL: The risks of gynecologic malignancies in older women, *Clin Obstet Gynecol* 7:545, 1964.

39. Ranney B: Decreasing numbers for vaginal hysterectomy and plasty, *South Dakota J Med* 43:7-12, 1990.

40. Reich H, DeCaprio J, McGlynn F: Laparoscopic hysterectomy, *J Gynecol Surg* 5:213-216, 1989.

41. Reiffenstuhl G, Platzer W: *Atlas of vaginal surgery,* Philadelphia, 1975, WB Saunders.

42. Robinson RW, Cohen WD, Higano N: Estrogen replacement therapy in women with coronary atherosclerosis, *Ann Intern Med* 48:95, 1958.

43. Shaw WF: *Plastic vaginal surgery.* In Kerr JMM, Johnstone RW, Phillips MH, editors: *Historical review of British obstetrics and gynaecology,* Edinburgh, 1954, Livingstone, pp 372-376.

44. Sheth SS: The place of oophorectomy at vaginal hysterectomy, *Br Obstet Gynaecol* 98:662-666, 1991.

45. Simon NL et al: Study of superficially invasive carcinoma of the cervix, *Obstet Gynecol* 68:19-24, 198.

46. Soper DE, Yarwood RL: Single-dose antibiotic prophylaxis in women undergoing vaginal hysterectomy, *Obstet Gynecol* 69:879-882, 1987.

47. Thompson JD, Lyon JB: Vaginal hysterectomy, *Clin Obstet Gynecol* 9:1033, 1964.

48. Vidakovic S: The vagino-abdominal approach to the extended operation, *Arch Gynakol* 186:420, 1955.

49. Welch JS, Randall LM: Vaginal hysterectomy at the Mayo Clinic, *Obstet Gynecol* 4:199-209, 1961.

50. Werner P, Sederl J: *Abdominal operations by the vaginal route,* Philadelphia, 1958, JB Lippincott.

51. Wetchler SJ, Hurt WG: A technique for surgical correction of fallopian tube prolapse, *Obstet Gynecol* 67:747-749, 1986.

Chapter 21

CYSTOCELE

David H. Nichols

When considering the indications for surgical repair of damage to the anterior vaginal wall, the gynecologist must first correlate the damage with the patient's symptoms. Thus it is necessary both to investigate the patient's history and to check carefully for evidence of coexistent prolapse of the uterus, vaginal vault, or rectum, and for signs of enterocele.

Any history of urinary stress incontinence, which may have been relieved as the prolapse progressed, is important.[39] The supports of the urethra, even though attenuated, may have more strength than do those of the bladder because of their continuity with the urogenital diaphragm. Predictably, therefore, the degree of bladder descent when the prolapse is advanced usually exceeds the degree of accompanying urethral descent, resulting in an angulation or kinking of the urethra at its junction with the bladder.

Contraindications to transvaginal surgery for urinary stress incontinence include:

1. Chronic respiratory disease.
2. Socially disabling recurrent urinary stress incontinence.
3. Lifestyle embracing the necessity for performing regular heavy lifting, i.e. nurses in nursing homes.

Although the bladder itself is not suspended, it receives support from the vagina and its attachments (Fig. 21-1). Thus damage to the vaginal wall itself, the connective tissue to which the vagina is attached, or both may affect the bladder supports and lead to cystocele. When a cystocele is large, increases in intraabdominal and intravesical pressure are greater in the dependent portion of the cystocele than in the attenuated urethrovesical junction. Hodgkinson[21] observed that the hydrostatic pressure within the bladder is always greater at the bottom of this column of fluid than midway up or at the top. The presence of a coexistent defect in the posterior vaginal wall, of course, aggravates this tendency toward bladder distension. Because of the absence of adequate posterior vaginal or perineal support, the elasticity of the sagging bladder when filling is relatively unrestrained.

Preoperative evaluation of the presence or absence of urinary stress incontinence generally indicates whether the anterior genital segment has been damaged. Since there are various types of incontinence and they often occur simultaneously in a single patient, it is essential to determine the precise nature of the problem in a particular patient—whether the problem is primarily one of stress, overflow, urgency incontinence, or a combination of these. A proper diagnosis is required for the identification and selection of an appropriate surgical remedy.

The gynecologist who is selecting an operation for the repair of the anterior vaginal wall must consider the future functions and strains to which that wall may be subjected—not only coitus but also future pregnancy and parturition and not infrequently heavy physical work. All these factors must be correlated with current findings, which may partially be the result of earlier attempts at surgical repair. Furthermore, allowances must be made for any atrophic changes that have occurred or are expected to occur after the patient's menopause.

ASYMPTOMATIC CYSTOCELE

Repair of an asymptomatic cystocele is seldom indicated unless it is coincident with pelvic repair performed for other reasons or unless the gynecologist has observed unmistakable evidence of the cystocele's progressive protrusion into the vagina over a period of time. Within limitations, the larger the cystocele and the more advanced its progression, the more complicated its repair and the less certain the restoration of normal bladder function because there may be some permanent impairment to a properly balanced nerve supply. The primary advantage of reexamination by the same gynecologist over a period of years is that of following evidence of progression to a degree that

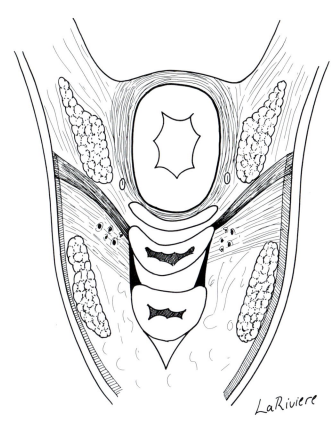

Fig. 21-1. The female pelvis is shown in coronal section. Notice the tissue condensations. They extend from each anterior vaginal fornix to the pelvic side wall. These, plus the vaginal wall between them, form a hammock for the bladder, which is separated from the vagina by the vesicovaginal space. The paravesical and pararectal "spaces" are filled with loose areolar tissue, however.

requires operative repair and being able to make that recommendation before increased medical risks associated with the patient's advancing age preclude elective surgery. At each examination the gynecologist should record his or her impression of the size of the lesion in a manner that permits reliable comparison with findings on subsequent reexaminations.

The degree of vaginal cornification demonstrable on cytologic examination often indicates the extent of postmenopausal atrophy. This index should correlate at least roughly with the persistence of lateral wall rugal folds. If there is little cornification, an estrogen deficiency should be suspected. The gynecologist should estimate the relevance of this deficiency to the development of the cystocele and should consider the advisability of estrogen replacement.

Should the gynecologist and the patient decide that surgery is indicated for an asymptomatic cystocele, a primary objective is the restoration of normal anatomic relationships, with attention to contributing causative factors, all in a conscious effort to reduce the risks of recurrence in later years.

Low urethral compliance is one of the causes of postop-

erative urinary incontinence.[7] It may be present but unidentified, particularly in the postmenopausal patient, and especially the one with massive eversion of the vagina. A simple method of detecting this potential is that of inserting a pediatric-sized Foley catheter (no. 8 or 10 with a 3-cc bulb) and only partly inflating the bulb with but 0.5 cc of saline followed by gentle traction to the catheter to see whether or not it can be drawn easily through the urethra. If the catheter is drawn readily through, the urethra should be tightened by appropriate plication to the extent that the partly inflated bulb can no longer be drawn through the urethra. Marking the catheter at 1-cm intervals from the bulb will provide a "ruler" to measure urethral length as well as the point of low urethral pressure.[5]

SYMPTOMS OF CYSTOCELE

Cystocele is often asymptomatic, and coincident urinary stress incontinence is infrequent. The patient may describe feelings of pelvic pressure and "falling out," sensations often related to a coexistent uterine or vault prolapse. Descent of the uterus seems to annoy the patient in a degree proportional to the time it takes the condition to develop. Patients appear to notice a rapidly developing prolapse fairly quickly and to make an early request for reconstruction and relief, but they may accept a slowly progressive descensus without comment or complaint. A patient with a large cystocele may or may not be aware of a mass protruding from the vagina associated with a bearing-down sensation, but she generally notices a sense of pelvic heaviness after she has been standing for a time.

Some patients have learned to elevate a large cystocele manually to facilitate voiding. Surprisingly, only the larger cystoceles are associated with any significant amount of residual urine. The large dumbbell-shaped bladder that is often evident with complete procidentia, for example, frequently leads to a degree of persistent urinary stasis that contributes both to infection and to stone formation. Presumptive chronic cystitis is not the inevitable result of supposedly "stagnant urine," however. Often women with residual urine complain that when they stand after apparently emptying their bladders, they immediately feel a desire to void again, but they find that they can void very little additional urine when they sit down the second time. The reason for these sensations is that the hydrodynamics associated with the standing position differ from those of the sitting position. When the bladder contains a great volume of residual urine, some overflow incontinence may occur.

Urinary stress incontinence is not a characteristic or even frequent experience of a majority of the women with cystocele—unless there has been a rotational descent of the bladder neck. Urinary stress incontinence usually requires coincident and specific repair of coexistent damage to the supports of the bladder neck and urethra.

Some patients with cystocele may have coincident urinary dysfunction that can be assessed urodynamically but is clinically masked by the vesicourethral kinking coincident with cystocele. This dysfunction sometimes includes the potential for urinary stress incontinence,[18] and if anterior colporrhaphy fails to include specific surgical steps to provide adequate support or elevation of the vesicourethral junction, postoperative urinary stress incontinence may become evident,[39] to the distress of both patient and surgeon. Prevention of this unwelcome development requires full-vaginal-length anterior colporrhaphy that includes special attention to restoring the supports of the vesical neck. With full-length anterior colporrhaphy, whether the patient has had preoperative urodynamic studies or not, the incidence of postoperative urinary stress incontinence will be reduced.[6]

TYPES AND CAUSES OF CYSTOCELE

Two anatomic systems maintain the vesicourethral junction and urethra in position. The pubourethral "ligament" portion of the urogenital diaphragm suspends it, and the vaginal wall and its attachments support it. Damage to either or both systems may alter the pelvic location of the urethra and affect its function.

Cystocele has been described according to its position anterior to the interureteric ridge or posterior to it.[4] These conditions may coexist, and both must be recognized and corrected if surgery is to be effective.

Anterior cystocele (pseudocystocele)

In patients who have only an anterior cystocele (pseudocystocele or pseudourethrocele), a straining effort causes the downward bulging or rotational descent of the urethra. This descent is permitted by the separation of the urethra from the urogenital diaphragm and the pubourethral ligament portion of the urogenital diaphragm that binds it to the pubis,[28] or separation of the vagina from its intermediate connective tissue attachment to the arcus tendineus.[36,47] The rotational descent of the urethrovesical junction may be of varying degrees, and the bladder may

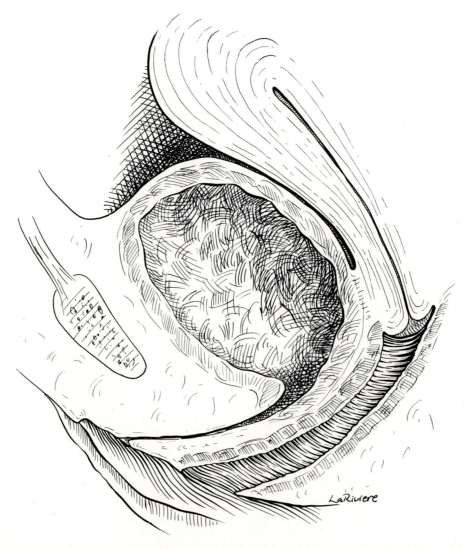

Fig. 21-2. The partly filled bladder is shown in the center of this sagittal drawing of the pelvis. There is both rotational descent of the vesicourethral junction as well as funneling of the urethra. This is an "anterior" cystocele, as it is located anterior to the interureteric ridge (Mercier's Bar).

or may not herniate behind the urethrovesical junction. The condition is often associated with urinary stress incontinence. This type of damage is usually postobstetric and is often associated with a wide subpubic arch.

With anterior cystocele, the diameter of the urethra is unchanged except at its proximal end, where the diameter may be increased if funneling or vesicalization of the urethra has occurred (Fig. 21-2). Pathologic dilation of the midportion or distal urethra (true urethrocele) is quite uncommon, but it can result from pathologic stretching from within the urethra, occasionally digital or manipulative, or, rarely, from necrosis of the internal wall of a preexisting infected urethral diverticulum. However, a *routine* full-length plication of a normal, *undilated* urethral wall may itself be followed by later stricture and "postmenopausal stenosis," creating an iatrogenic obstructive uropathy that sometimes requires a lifetime of troublesome periodic urethral dilation.

True or posterior cystocele (distention cystocele)

Almost without exception, a true cystocele results either from a stretching of the anterior vaginal wall during parturition beyond its ability to involute postpartum, possible even during "normal" vaginal delivery or from the atrophic changes of aging on the intrinsic structural components of the vaginal wall, even if they have not been damaged earlier (Fig. 21-3). The most common type of cystocele is merely the late result of an overstretching and subsequent eversion of the wall of the vagina. Rugal folds of the anterior vaginal epithelium decrease and may disappear as the weakness within the vaginal wall allows the bladder to bulge into the vagina. The lateral attachments of the vagina and bladder may be relatively undamaged if they are merely compressed against the side wall of the pelvis during labor.

Usually, the cystocele does not become clinically evident until after the menopause. With the postmenopausal

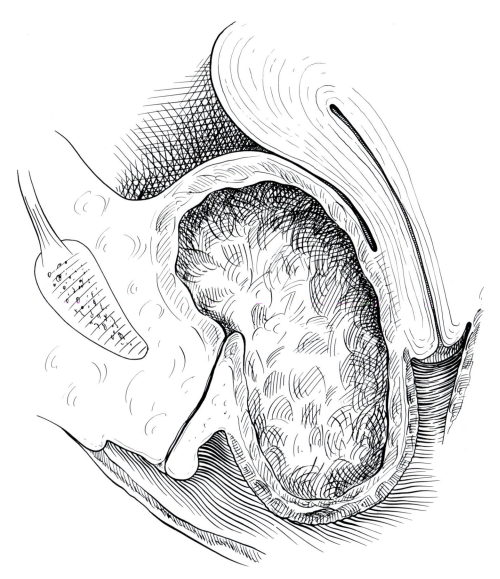

Fig. 21-3. Posterior cystocele. A large cystocele is seen *posterior* to Mercier's Bar.

loss of estrogen-related elastic tissue and smooth muscle tone, the relaxation and redundancy associated with weakened connective tissue support increase, and symptoms develop. In such instances, the vaginal walls, especially the anterior and posterior walls, may remain pathologically thinned. Later, as a result of circulatory stasis and chronic hyperemia, the vagina may become hypertrophic in appearance. Some women appear to have a basic congenital defect in the elastic tissue and smooth muscle components of the vagina that contributes to the condition.

Displacement cystocele

Because it results from a primary and pathologic elongation of the lateral or "ligamentous" attachment and support of the vagina, a displacement cystocele is quite different from that produced by simple overstretching of the connective tissues within a previously normal vaginal wall. Damage to the lateral vaginal supporting tissues may be the result of either of two mechanisms: (1) damage to attached tissues, such as the supports of the cervix and (2) damage to the vaginal wall itself that results from the forces of labor.

The cervix is attached to the upper anterior vaginal wall, and the tissues that support both the vagina and the cervix are component parts of the cardinal ligaments. Because these tissues tend to function as an anatomic unit, the displacement of one component often leads to similar displacement of the other. Like eversion or prolapse of the upper vagina, a displacement cystocele may develop rapidly when it is the result of obstetric injury to the cardinal-uterosacral ligament complex, or it may occur more insidiously in older women as a result of long-standing increased intraabdominal pressure.

When, because of inadequate dilation during parturition, a segment of the vaginal wall becomes a soft tissue obstruction to the passage of a rapidly descending presenting part, slowing the descent until the segment gives way, the supporting tissues attached to the rolled-up, telescoping segment of the vagina become overstretched and avulsed as the presenting part descends. This mechanism may not have damaged the integrity of the vaginal wall itself, however, so eventual repair should shorten the lateral attachments of the vagina and cervix with reestablishment of the vaginal length. In its pure form, this type of cystocele is an eversion of the vagina with relatively well-preserved rugal folds, although the sulci disappear to some extent.

Rugae of comparable size on both the anterior and lateral vaginal walls suggest displacement cystocele, while diminished rugae on the anterior wall in the presence of more clearly defined rugae on the lateral walls suggest distention cystocele. The surgeon must identify the cause of the recurrent cystocele as displacement, overdistention, or a combination of the two—with demonstrable defects in the midline supporting structures, the lateral supporting structures, or both—and must note the relationship of the cystocele to the urethrovesical junction or urogenital diaphragm.

If one has determined that a cystocele should be repaired, it is essential, in order to achieve the best optimal result, to decide whether or not the vaginal vault is partially prolapsed so that this element too can be surgically corrected as part of the same operative procedure. Examination of the patient when she is standing, and reexamination under anesthesia when the pelvis muscles are relaxed and pain is not present is important. Especially think of the displacement type of cystocele when considering a repair of a recurrent cystocele, or one that is seen in a nullipara.

Postmenopausal bladder urgency may be associated with an atrophic "urethritis and trigonitis." The atrophic changes that occur after the menopause result in a significant thinning of the epithelial and subepithelial layers of the urethra and the bladder trigone, making them oversusceptible to stimulation and irritation. When this can be demonstrated or is even suspected, estrogen replacement therapy is likely to reduce the patient's symptoms promptly. If the therapy is effective, surgical repair should be deferred for a month or two until the beneficial results and symptomatology have stabilized and can be reevaluated.

Cystocele that results from a combination of factors

Sometimes a cystocele results from a combination of the factors that have been discussed. The importance of each component may be noticeable at different levels within the vagina. The gynecologist who is contemplating a repair must take into consideration the mechanism—or combination of mechanisms—that accounts for the pathology demonstrable in the individual patient.

In at least one fourth of the instances of symptomatic genital prolapse, both the upper and the lower vagina are everted. Because the relative significance of these factors differs from patient to patient, the technique selected for repair must be based on an appraisal of the relative importance of the etiologic factors in each patient.

Paravaginal defect

When there are no anterior sulci, the gynecologist should examine the patient for lateral detachment of the urethral paravaginal tissues. According to Baden and Walker,[2] such a detachment should be suspected when the anterior vaginal wall is relaxed. If there is no elevation of the anterior vaginal wall when the patient squeezes her pelvic muscles tightly (i.e., in a "holding" position), the connective tissue and vascular supports of the anterior vaginal wall may have been detached from the arcus tendineus.

The vagina itself is not attached directly to the arcus tendineus,[9,11,34,43] but the anterior vaginal fornix is attached to the arcus tendineus by a meshwork of intervening connective tissue that may be subject to various strains and stretching or even partial avulsion. Because this type of strain is usually a consequence of trauma during labor and delivery, detachment of these tissues is more common in parous patients. It may also be related to life-style, however, and may occasionally follow the pull of massive vaginal eversion, even in the nullipara. Therefore direct surgical attachment of the vaginal fornix to the arcus tendineus may to some extent correct the widening of the anterior vaginal wall that occurs with certain types of cystocele.[11,36,47,48] Bilateral attachment is generally necessary when stretching or avulsion of the lateral supports has resulted in a cystocele.[47] Large midline defects of the vaginal wall are much more common and are remedied by the standard midline plications and colporrhaphy. The existence or coexistence of the less common lateral defects should be determined preoperatively for appropriate planning of surgical technique.

RECURRENT CYSTOCELE

When a cystocele has recurred after an initial repair, the gynecologist who is contemplating reoperation must first try to determine the reason(s) that the result of the earlier surgery was unsatisfactory. The gynecologist should review the hospital surgical record of the previous operation, relate the earlier procedure to the current findings, and then take these considerations into account in choosing the technique and sutures for a reoperation for this particular patient.

During the physical examination of a patient with recurrent cystocele, the gynecologist should check the position of the vaginal vault when the patient is standing and bearing down, as by a Valsalva's maneuver. This procedure discloses any coincident partial eversion of the vaginal vault that brings the bladder with it. It is essential to determine and surgically remedy any coincident prolapse of the vaginal vault.

Voluntary isometric pubococcygeal perineal resistance exercises (15 three second squeezes 6 times a day) may be recommended preoperatively if the patient has coincident urinary stress incontinence or has weak voluntary contractions of her pubococcygei. The program may be resumed with benefit starting the day after surgery and continued for six months postoperatively to aid in reestablishment of continence. A program of voluntary pubococcygeal resistance exercises will be of great help to the patient.[10,25]

TECHNIQUES OF COLPORRHAPHY

If the gynecologist has determined that a cystocele repair is necessary, it is essential to determine whether the vaginal vault is partially prolapsed so that this condition can be surgically corrected during the same operative procedure. Examination of the patient while she is *standing,* and preoperative reexamination while she is in the lithotomy position (after the administration of anesthesia, when the pelvic muscles are relaxed and the patient has no pain) are confirmatory, and appropriate surgical steps can then be planned to restore vaginal length (i.e., sacrospinous

colpopexy). It is especially important to consider vaginal vault descent when planning the repair of a recurrent cystocele or of a cystocele in a nullipara.

In a postmenopausal patient with greater than usual atrophic changes, surgery may be preceded and followed by estrogen replacement therapy to restore the vascularity, elasticity, thickness, and cellular integrity of the vaginal wall.

Because cystocele results primarily from damage to the vagina—either to its supports or to the vaginal wall itself—the primary site for reconstructive surgery for cystocele must be the vagina. Many operations designed to restore a defective posterior urethrovesical angle also elevate the proximal urethra to a position that once again permits a normal response to changes in intraabdominal pressure. Only when these surgical changes affect the proximal urethra, as well as the bladder, is this important aid to continence restored.[22]

The technique appropriate for dissection and repair of the anterior vaginal wall in an individual patient depends on many factors, including the presence of vaginal telescoping or coexistent vault eversion. A short vagina due to telescoping may be surgically lengthened by a coincident procedure, such as a vaginal hysterectomy or a Manchester operation (see Chapter 20), by shortening of the cardinal or uterosacral supports, by a transvaginal sacrospinous colpopexy, or by transabdominal sacrocolpopexy (see Chapter 27). Restoration of vaginal depth by returning the vagina, with the bladder, to the pelvis is the essence of surgical treatment for the displacement cystocele.

In procidentia, as defined by Ricci and Thom,[35] the entire uterus protrudes from the pelvis. As a rule, the eversion of the vagina is complete and an enterocele is present, and there may be only a minimal or secondary rectocele. The supporting vaginal and uterine portions of the cardinal ligaments are markedly elongated and often attenuated. Therefore the displacement is greatest and most apparent in relation to the anterior vaginal wall and the cervix, which function as an anatomic unit because they are attached by continuity to each other and to the pelvic side walls. With massive prolapse, both suffer severe circulatory changes, resulting not only from stasis due to their compression against the sides of the genital hiatus, but also from congestion aggravated by gravity. The degree of chronic congestion apparently stimulates corresponding lymphangiectasia, which in turn stimulates considerable fibroblastic proliferation within the anterior vaginal wall. Chronic edema leads to hypertrophy and fibrosis, which thicken the anterior vaginal wall. These tissues elongate with advancing age and sag noticeably because they are deficient and defective in other components, especially elastic tissue.

After mobilizing the full thickness of the anterior vaginal wall, including the epithelium and the underlying fibromuscular connective tissue layer, the gynecologic surgeon can enter the desired plane most readily by opening directly into the vesicovaginal space.[38] Sharp dissection should be used to enter the proper pelvic spaces, although the spaces may be developed safely by blunt dissection after they have been entered. It takes longer to locate the correct plane after an initial dissection in the wrong plane than to locate it correctly the first time. This initial direct approach to the vesicovaginal space is equally useful for anterior colporrhaphy when a cystocele is to be repaired without coincident hysterectomy or cervical amputation and when there has been previous hysterectomy or cervical amputation. Ricci and Thom[35] described a useful technique:

The anterior vaginal wall is placed on moderate tension by grasping each lip of the cervix with short tenacula and pulling the prolapsed vagina completely outward and downward. That part of the anterior vaginal wall above the point of fusion above the cervix is rolled or massaged between the index finger and thumb several times to accentuate planes of separation between bladder and cervix and vaginal wall. At the point where the fusion between the vaginal wall and the cervix ends and the avascular space begins, smooth and lacking in rugae, and usually about ¾ inch above the orifice of the cervix, the reduplicated layers of the entire thickness of the vaginal wall are grasped between two Allis clamps. The full thickness of the vaginal wall is cut between these two instruments with a curved scissors, the tip of the scissors pointing perpendicular to the axis of the cervix, exposing an

avascular space and bringing the bladder musculature into view [Fig. 21-4]. The cut surfaces of the vaginal wall are grasped with Allis clamps, and with a straight scissors the vaginal wall is cut upward exactly in midline (Fig. 21-5). This incision is continued to the urethrovaginal junction where the cleavage plane ends. The bladder wall is displaced from both lateral flaps of the incised vaginal wall and cut from the cervix, exposing the vesicouterine peritoneal fold, which may be incised, the index finger introduced, and the pelvis explored.

Reconstruction of the anterior vaginal wall

Cystocele is commonly associated with a degree of uterine prolapse less than procidentia. A transurethral Foley catheter is inserted, and the bladder is emptied. Any resistance to the passage of the catheter suggests that there is a urethral stricture. Under this circumstance, the surgeon must be careful to avoid urethral plication at this point, which would only make the stricture worse. In fact it may be wise to dilate the urethra while the patient is still asleep in the operating room.

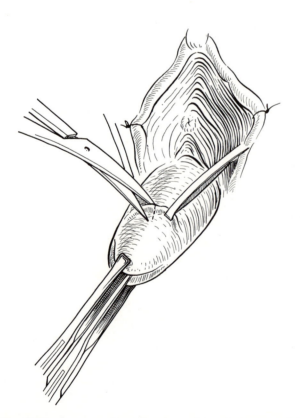

Fig. 21-4. A means of entering the vesicovaginal space of the patient not receiving coincident hysterectomy is shown. The anterior vaginal wall is grasped between two Allis clamps overlying the vesicovaginal space as shown, and an incision made between them directly into the vesicovaginal space.

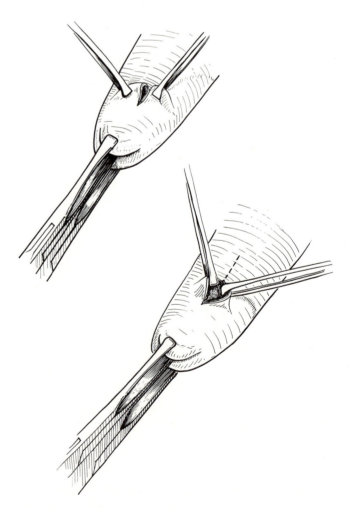

Fig. 21-5. The incision directly into the vesicovaginal space is shown in the drawing on the left. The full thickness of the vaginal wall is grasped by repositioning the Allis clamps as shown in the drawing to the right, and the incision continued both cranially and caudally.

Alternatively, the avascular space may be entered through the full thickness of the anterior vaginal wall by means of an inverted T-shaped incision at the point where the vagina meets the cervix. The midpoint of the anterior vaginal cuff incision is grasped between two forceps and incised exactly in the midline and directly into the avascular vesicovaginal space (Figs. 21-6 to 21-8). The incision is then carried superiorly to the point of fusion of urethra with vagina. (Fig. 21-9)

The remainder of the suburethral anterior vaginal wall is incised in the midline to within 1 or 1.5 cm of the external urethral meatus. The extent of the earlier damage to the supports of the urethrovesical junction, the degree of attenuation, and the integrity of the tissue available for plication determine the amount of bolstering necessary for the urethrovesical junction.

In performing an anterior colporrhaphy, the surgeon should reconstruct the full length of the anterior vaginal wall, including the urethrovesical junction and the supports of the urethra. Such a reconstruction involves separating the urogenital diaphragm from the vagina, plicating it, and reattaching it to the vagina. This procedure is sometimes associated with temporary postoperative diffi-

culty in voiding, but it is far preferable to straightening the neck of the bladder and obliterating the urethrovesical angle, which may lead to iatrogenic urinary stress incontinence (Fig. 21-10).

Because the patient being operated on is in the lithotomy position and under anesthesia, the tissue relationships that prevail differ from those that prevail when she is conscious and standing. Vulnerability to urinary continence is greatest when the fully conscious patient is in the standing position. Surgical repair of a large hypotonic "decompensated" cystocele probably restores some intravesical pressure, reducing the incontinence. Surgical support of the urethrovesical junction should strengthen the anatomic and physiologic factors that contribute to postoperative continence.

By sharp dissection with either scissors or scalpel (see Fig. 21-11) the operator separates the full thickness of the anterior vaginal wall from the bladder laterally and anteriorly as far as the lateral limits of the vesicovaginal space, sometimes almost to the pubic rami, in a line of cleavage that preserves the attachment between the subepithelial fibromuscular connective tissue layer and the vaginal epithelium. As the dissection proceeds laterally, a possibly in-

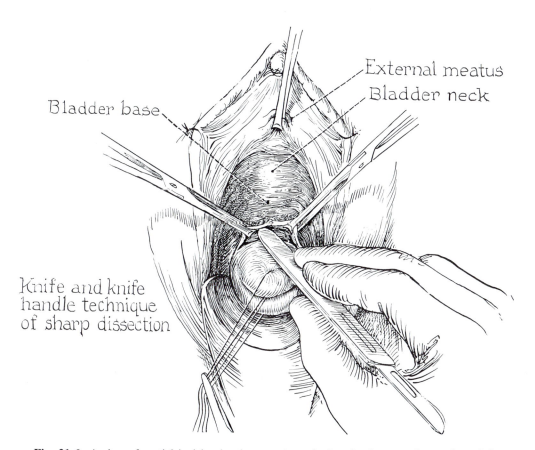

Fig. 21-6. A circumferential incision has been made at the junction between the cervix and the anterior vaginal wall, two Allis clamps 1 cm apart are placed as shown, and a short midline incision is made through the full thickness of the anterior vaginal wall, creating an inverted T incision. By blunt dissection the tissues are separated from the underside of the vagina. (From Ball TL: *Gynecologic surgery and urology*, ed 2, St. Louis, 1963, Mosby–Year Book.)

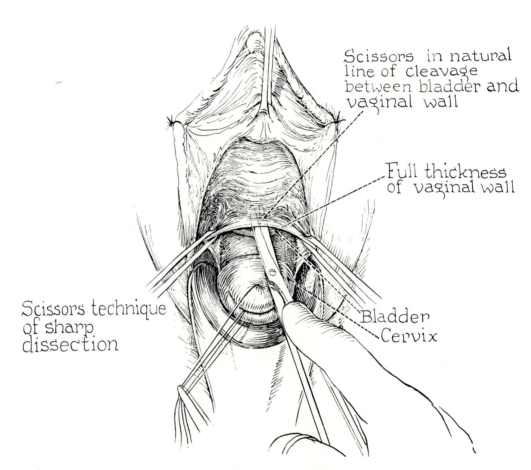

Scissors in natural line of cleavage between bladder and vaginal wall

Full thickness of vaginal wall

Scissors technique of sharp dissection

Bladder
Cervix

Fig. 21-7. Using curved Mayo scissors with the curve directed anteriorly, the scissors are inserted into the vesicovaginal space beneath the anterior vaginal wall, spread and withdrawn enlarging the width of this dissection.

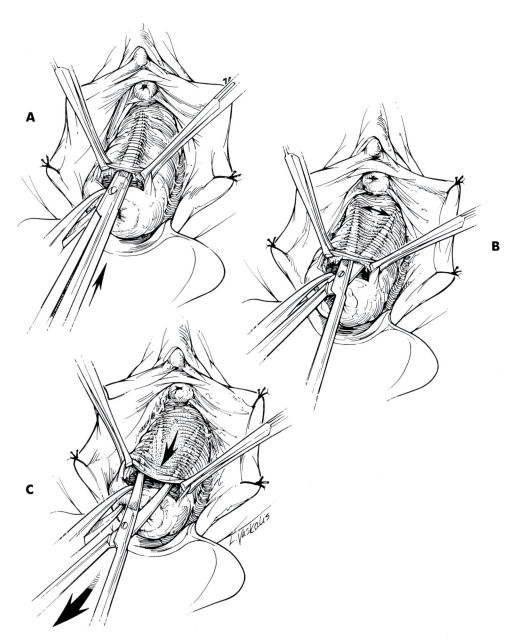

Fig. 21-8. Hilton's maneuver in the use of scissors. To avoid cutting a viscus or unidentified blood vessel, the closed tip of the dissecting scissors may be used to establish a plane as in **A.** Once the scissors have been inserted, the tips may be spread as in **B,** and the opened scissors withdrawn as shown by the arrow in **C.** Thus, the connective tissue plane is successfully widened without risk to the underlying viscus.

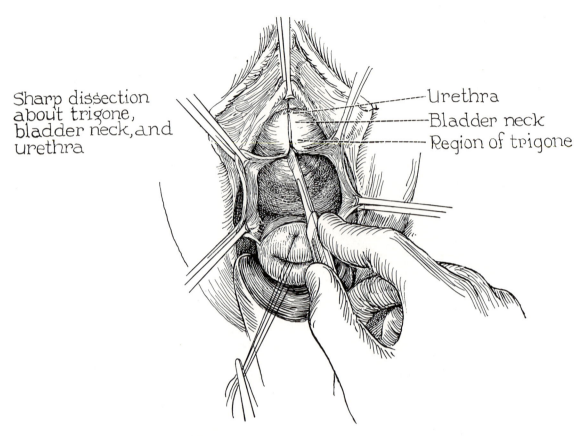

Sharp dissection about trigone, bladder neck, and urethra

Urethra
Bladder neck
Region of trigone

Fig. 21-9. The incision is continued in the anterior vaginal wall to the external urethral meatus. (From Ball TL: *Gynecologic surgery and urology*, ed 2, St. Louis, 1963, Mosby–Year Book.)

complete but identifiable musculoconnective tissue may be freed between the connective tissue left attached to the vaginal epithelium and the predominantly muscular bladder wall. Ideally it is possible to establish such lines of cleavage without compromising the blood supply of these supporting tissues; great care must be taken to open along tissue planes because simply slicing tissue into arbitrary layers is likely to damage the tissue planes that usually harbor blood supply.

A simpler technique that does not require dissection and therefore does not disturb the vaginal blood supply leaves the entire thickness of the vaginal wall intact and retains the attachment of all musculoconnective tissue to the vaginal epithelium. In this technique the surgeon excises a carefully measured ovoid or wedge of the redundant full thickness of thinned vaginal wall.[38] Unless the entire full thickness of the anterior vaginal wall has been correctly mobilized, however, only the superficial epithelial layer may be excised, and such an operative procedure would be as inadequate in the treatment of cystocele as the simple excision of an ellipse of overlying skin would be in the treatment of an inguinal hernia.

As a first step in correcting cystocele, the operator may plicate the entire length of the bladder's fibromuscular connective tissue capsule longitudinally by placing a series of running or interrupted 2-0 or 3-0 long lasting but ab-

sorbable sutures from the connective tissue capsule at the vault of the vagina all the way to the urogenital diaphragm (Figs. 21-12 and 21-13). It is essential to avoid overcorrecting the cystocele because overcorrection may obliterate the posterior urethrovesical angle and, by making the urethra the most dependent portion of the bladder, result in postoperative stress incontinence.[39] A pathologically dilated urethra may be plicated (Fig. 21-14) with special attention to lateral plication of the urethrovesical angle (Figs. 21-15 to 21-17).

Long-term results will be improved by using longlasting synthetic absorbable suture, such as polydiaxone (PDS) or polyglyconate (Maxon), of small diameter in subepithelial layers.

A common error in the performance of anterior colporrhaphy is to separate the vaginal epithelium from the fibromuscular layer of the vagina, plicate the fibromuscular tissue in the midline, trim the vaginal epithelium, and close without ever entering the vesicovaginal space. This repair is ineffective and can be associated with a high incidence of recurrent cystocele or persistent stress incontinence.

The Gersuny "tobacco pouch" purse-string suture may be used in reducing or inverting the bladder wall size of a very large cystocele, but this stitch provides little intrinsic strength. It must always be reinforced by a layer of side-to-side plication stitches. Reconstruction of any defect in

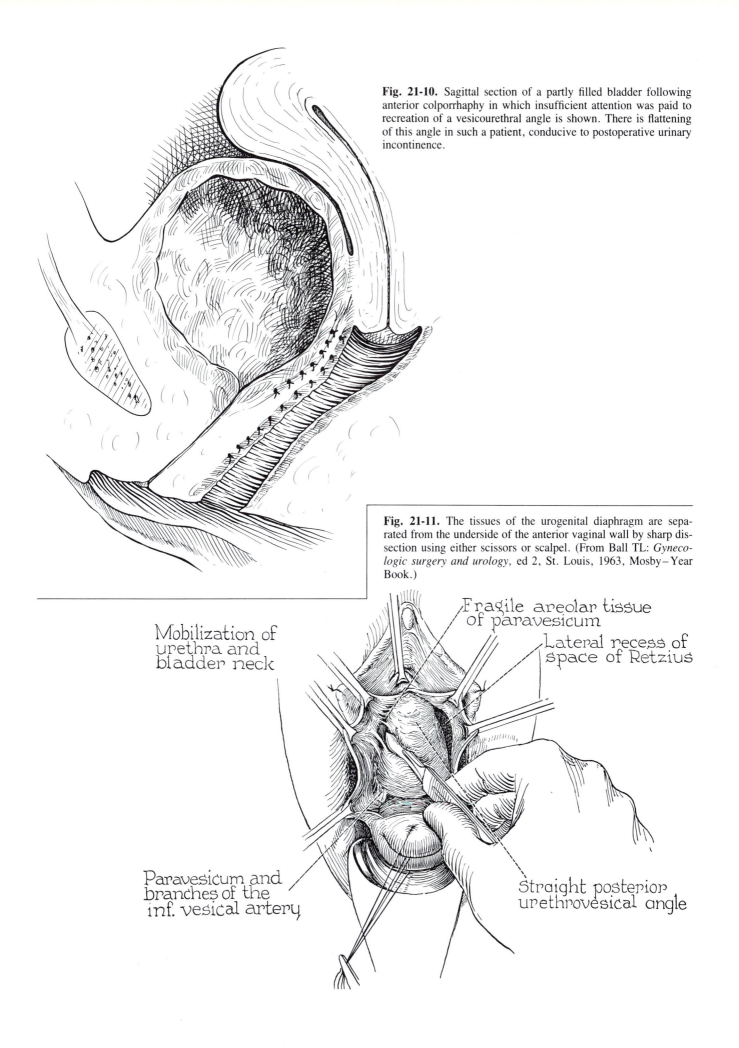

Fig. 21-10. Sagittal section of a partly filled bladder following anterior colporrhaphy in which insufficient attention was paid to recreation of a vesicourethral angle is shown. There is flattening of this angle in such a patient, conducive to postoperative urinary incontinence.

Fig. 21-11. The tissues of the urogenital diaphragm are separated from the underside of the anterior vaginal wall by sharp dissection using either scissors or scalpel. (From Ball TL: *Gynecologic surgery and urology,* ed 2, St. Louis, 1963, Mosby–Year Book.)

Mobilization of urethra and bladder neck

Fragile areolar tissue of paravesicum

Lateral recess of space of Retzius

Paravesicum and branches of the inf. vesical artery

Straight posterior urethrovesical angle

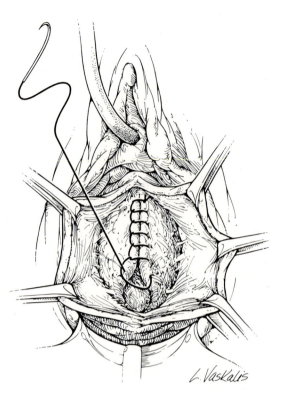

Fig. 21-12. The fibromuscular capsule of the bladder of a patient with cystocele is reduced in width by a suture of running locked long-lasting thread placed as shown. Tension on the suture is such that the tissues are approximated but not strangulated.

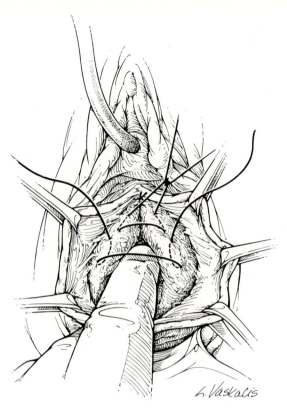

Fig. 21-13. For the patient with larger cystocele the operator's index finger depresses the bladder in the midline and the fibromuscular capsule of the bladder is reduced by one or more layers of interrupted mattress sutures placed in a rhomboid configuration. A very large cystocele may receive preliminary reduction by a purse string suture, the neck of which must be carefully supported by additional side-to-side stitches of absorbable suture material placed in the fibromuscular capsule of the bladder.

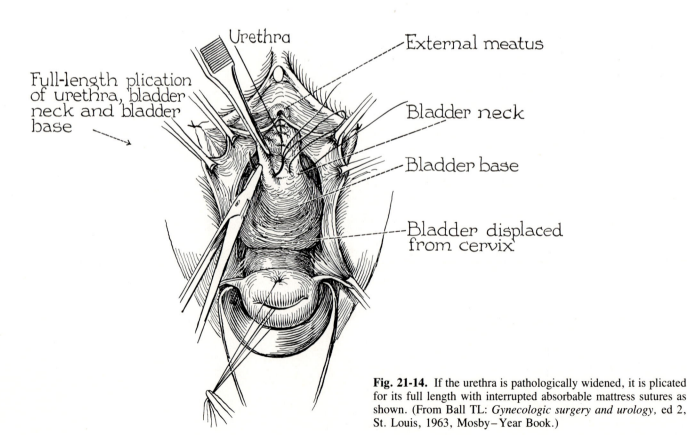

Urethra

External meatus

Full-length plication of urethra, bladder neck and bladder base

Bladder neck

Bladder base

Bladder displaced from cervix

Fig. 21-14. If the urethra is pathologically widened, it is plicated for its full length with interrupted absorbable mattress sutures as shown. (From Ball TL: *Gynecologic surgery and urology*, ed 2, St. Louis, 1963, Mosby–Year Book.)

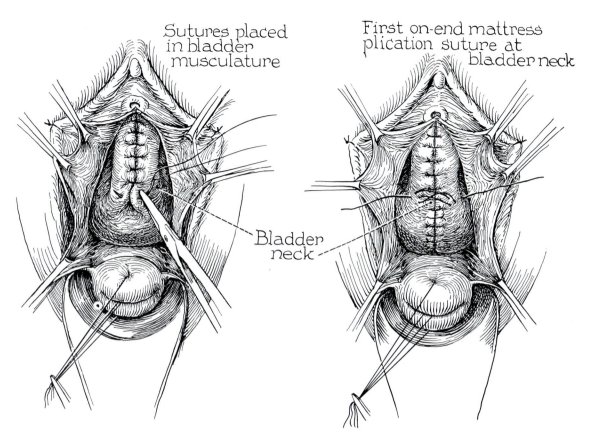

Sutures placed in bladder musculature

First on-end mattress plication suture at bladder neck

Bladder neck

Fig. 21-15. This plication extends beyond the vesicourethral junction onto the muscularis of the bladder, if the trigone is widened, as is seen with a large cystocele. (From Ball TL: *Gynecologic surgery and urology,* ed 2, St. Louis, 1963, Mosby–Year Book.)

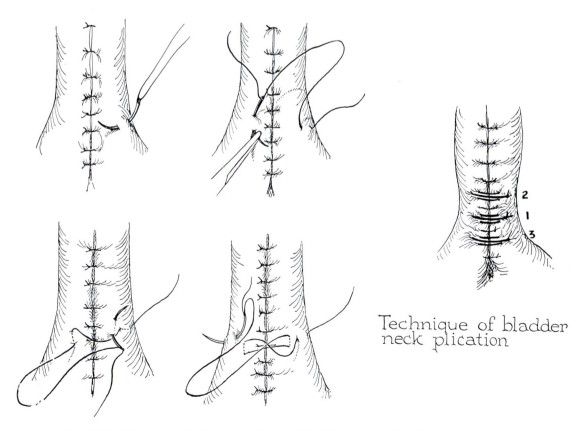

Technique of bladder neck plication

Fig. 21-16. The urogenital diaphragm is plicated at the vesicourethral junction using a far-near-near-far suture. This may be applied to correction of any funneling of the bladder neck, as shown.

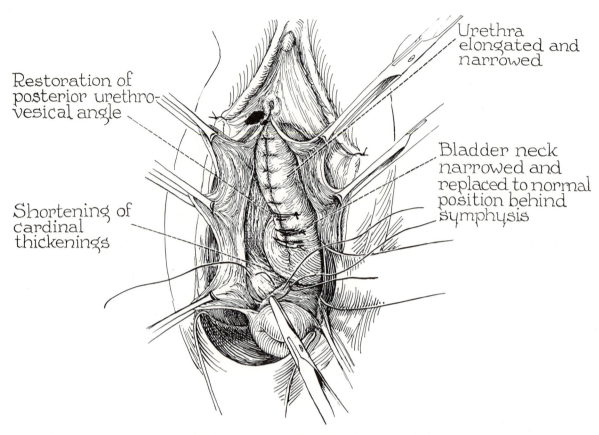

Restoration of
posterior urethro-
vesical angle

Shortening of
cardinal
thickenings

Urethra
elongated and
narrowed

Bladder neck
narrowed and
replaced to normal
position behind
symphysis

Fig. 21-17. The urethrovesical angle has been restored as shown, the bladder neck and any funneling have been corrected, and the vesicourethral junction is now near its regular position at the junction of the upper two thirds of the lower third of the back of the pubis. (From Ball TL: *Gynecologic surgery and urology,* ed 2, St. Louis, 1963, Mosby–Year Book.)

the posterior vaginal wall and its supporting tissues is desirable.

Urethrovesical junction. Funneling of the vesical neck physiologically shortens the urethra to a degree equal to the lengthening of the physiologic bladder neck. As a result the effective urethrovesical junction is often displaced to a more distal segment of the urethra, where it is further removed from and less responsive to changes in intraabdominal pressure. When the location of the junction is below the inferior margin of the pubis, there is a disturbing tendency toward urinary stress incontinence. Such a development is not surprising, however, because funneling of the vesical neck usually reflects damage to the supports of both bladder and urethra and contributes markedly toward a functional break in the "bladder base plate" of Uhlenhuth[40] and Hutch.[19]

Although Green[22] noted the importance of both the posterior urethrovesical angle and the urethral inclination, others have emphasized vesicourethral funneling as an anatomic defect that by physiologically "shortening" the effective urethral length favors the direct hydrostatic transmission of bladder pressure to the urine inside the funnel (Figs. 21-18). Such funneling should be corrected by the placement of a number of vertical mattress Kelly-type su-

tures in a way that plicates the funnel and restores the normal tone, configuration, and caliber of the urethral segment (Fig. 21-19). Kelly[26] stitches are subvesical urethral plication stitches that correct funneling and its associated stress incontinence, even though they were originally developed to strengthen a presumed internal urethral sphincter.

Some elongation of the bladder trigone and some lateral displacement of the ureterovesical orifices are likely to occur with massive cystocele.[41,42] This condition disturbs the physiology of continence and may be remedied by the insertion of a U-shaped suture, which is intended not only to shorten the trigone but also to narrow it.[37]

Urethral supports. Studies[28,49,50] have shown that the urethra is normally suspended from or supported by the pubic bone by means of bilaterally symmetrical, anterior, posterior, and intermediate pubourethral "ligaments." Because these bands of muscle and connective tissues pass from the pubic bone to the urethra—not to the bladder—they are comparable to the puboprostatic ligaments in the male. It has been established[28] that these ligamentous supports are continuous with the urogenital diaphragm. Although the posterior "ligament" elongates physiologically during the normal voiding process (Fig. 21-20), any defect

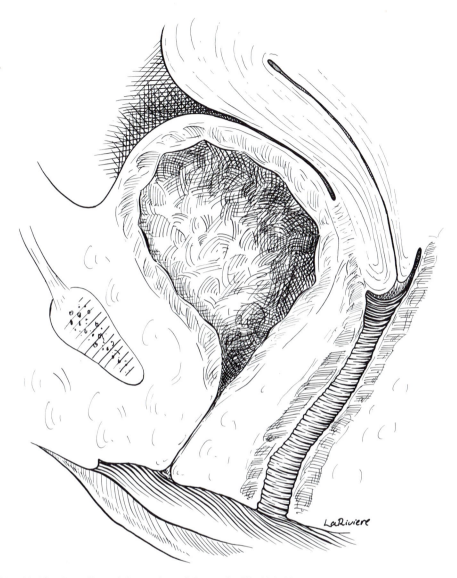

Fig. 21-18. Funneling of the urethra of the partly filled bladder is shown. Although this is normal during the voiding process, it is pathological at all other times, and effectively shortens the functional urethra as well as displacing the vesicourethral junction.

or injury that lengthens or loosens the pubourethral ligaments contributes strongly to the occurrence and persistence of urinary stress incontinence.

With marked degrees of prolapse and with procidentia, the pubourethral ligaments may be very much elongated, and they may sometimes be found quite far laterally. It is essential to elevate and support the urethrovesical junction to the most cranial position possible behind the pubis in order to restore normal relationships and ensure that sudden increases in intraabdominal pressure will register in the proximal urethra, as well as in the bladder. It is particularly important to shorten the pubourethral ligaments in the patient with massive prolapse lest the patient suffer a postoperative iatrogenic urinary stress incontinence that is more distressing and disabling than the prolapse for which she originally sought relief.[39]

The vaginal ends of the pubourethral ligament portion of the urogenital diaphragm can be identified transvaginally and plicated beneath the urethrovesical junction (Fig. 21-21).[33] The operator incises the vagina in the midline and then dissects laterally to the pubic rami, clearly exposing the tissues of the urethrovesical junction. Although these ligaments are not discrete anatomic structures, they can be recognized as paired tissue condensations or thickenings in the sheetlike tissue of the urogenital diaphragm.

Palpation of the inflated bulb of the transurethral Foley catheter demonstrates the urethrovesical junction, but as Gardiner[17] noted, excessive traction on the catheter may draw the bulb of the Foley catheter into a pathologically widened and funneled urethra. To avoid forceful traction on the catheter, small straight Kocher hemostatic forceps can be applied to the periurethral tissue 1.5 to 2 cm on ei-

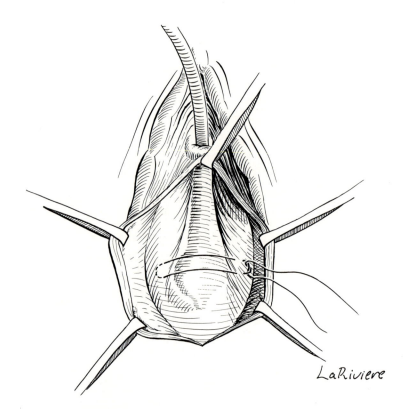

LaRiviere

Fig. 21-19. A traditional Kelly stitch for reducing the size of a urethral funnel is shown. It is essentially a three-point mattress stitch placed as indicated. If one stitch is insufficient to relieve urethral funneling, additional stitches may be placed both lateral to the original stitch and cranial and caudal as well. This repair is generally done while an adult-sized Foley catheter is in the bladder, so as to lessen the possibility of creating a urethral stricture. (Modified from Nichols DH, Randall CL: *Vaginal surgery,* ed 3, Baltimore, 1989, Williams & Wilkins.)

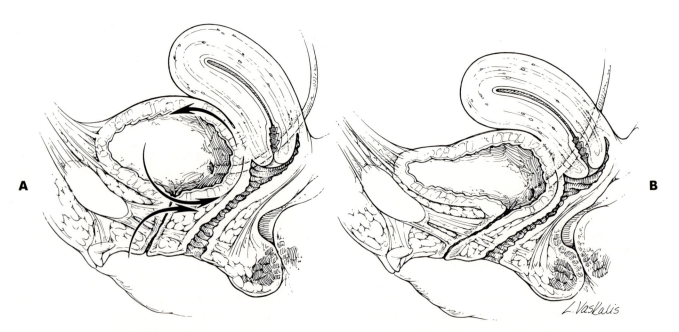

L. Vaskalis

Fig. 21-20. "Wheeling" of the vesicourethral junction is identified in drawing **A.** This occurs physiologically during the voiding process, to permit temporary flattening of the urethrovesical angle, but when it is present, in the patient who is not voiding (as shown in drawing **B**), the anatomic relationship is pathologic, and is conducive to the development of urinary stress incontinence.

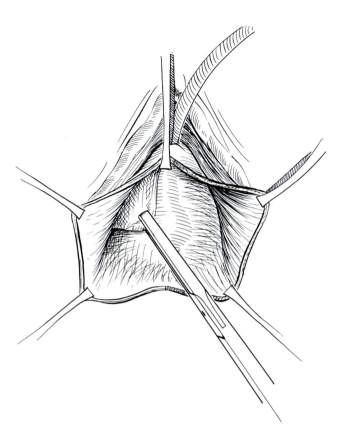

Fig. 21-21. The tissues lateral to the urethra and just anterior to the inflated bulb of a Foley catheter are grasped with the tip of a Kocher hemostat, first on one side and then on the other.

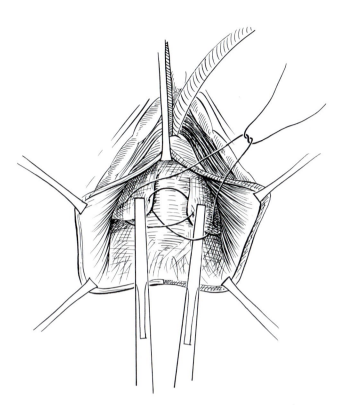

Fig. 21-22. These are plicated with a far-near-near-far suture of polyglycolic acid as shown.

ther side of its fusion to the urethra, as recommended by Gainey[15] and Frank.[12]

After the ligamentous condensations have been identified, the ligaments are further shortened by means of a more lateral bite into an often thicker portion. If the retropubic attachments of these ligaments are intact and the Kocher forceps have been properly placed, downward ventral traction toward the coccyx *in the direction in which the fibers of the ligament run to the pubis* actually moves the patient slightly on the operating table. The degree of resistance to this pull indicates whether the strength and length of the ligament are sufficient to permit a suburethral plication that elevates the urethrovesical junction. The same procedure of verification and evaluation should be repeated on the opposite side, after which the tips of the forceps may be brought together in the midline to ensure that the plication will indeed elevate the urethra. Mattress-type sutures of a size 2-0 long-lasting synthetic absorbable material, such as polydiaxonone (PDS), are then placed lateral and medial to the hemostats (Figs. 21-22).

It is usually possible to achieve the desired retropubic elevation of the urethrovesical junction by means of the essential sutures described. Should these sutures fail to raise the urethrovesical junction cranial to the inferior border of the pubis, the operator should place second pubourethral ligament stitches lateral to the first until a proper degree of

elevation has been obtained. Such pubourethral sutures should always be placed lateral to the urethra, not in the urethral wall. Because they are placed more laterally than are urethral plication stitches, paraurethral stitches can be inserted directly into the urethral attachment of the pubourethral ligament portion of the urogenital diaphragm, which makes them even more effective in elevating the urethrovesical junction. (Any second stitches also bury and reduce the tension of the initial sutures.) The ends of such buried stitches are sewn to the underside of the trimmed anterior vaginal wall to reestablish a normal site of fusion of the vagina to the urogenital diaphragm (Fig. 21-23). After they have been tied, they should neither reduce the urethral diameter nor produce subsequent stricture, which would certainly be accentuated after the menopause.

When stress incontinence is the patient's sole problem, a buried, nonabsorbable suture may be used in the plication of pubourethral ligaments (Fig. 21-24). The surgeon must ensure that the suture does not penetrate the lumen of either urethra or bladder lest it form a nidus for future infection or stone formation. When the urethrovesical junction has been elevated to a spot cranial to the inferior margin of the pubis, any appreciable funneling of the bladder neck or urethra should be corrected by plication with interrupted sutures of 2-0 absorbable sutures placed directly in the wall of the urethral funnel itself. These can be placed

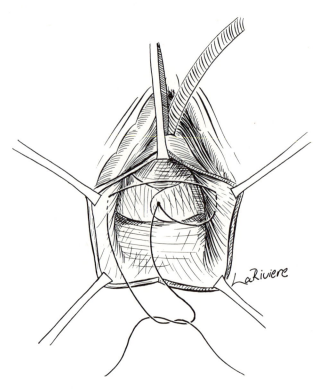

Fig. 21-23. When this suture has been tied, effectively elevating the vesicourethral junction but without compromising the lumen of the urethra, the stitch is passed through the underside of the anterior vaginal wall as shown. When this stitch has been tied, fusion of the anterior vaginal wall and urogenital diaphragm has been restored.

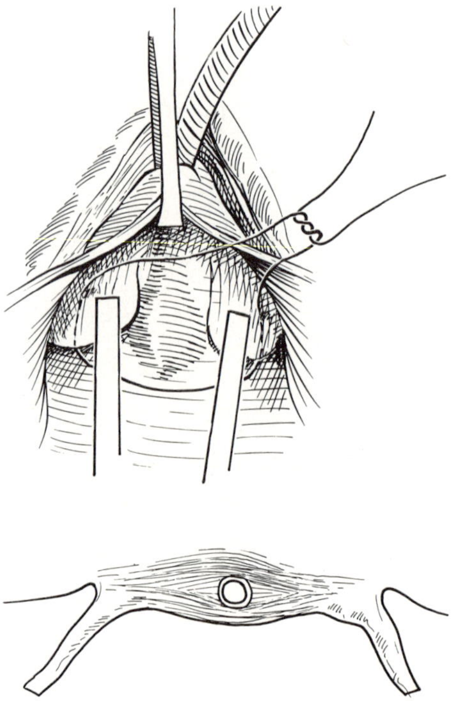

Fig. 21-24. When the tissues of the pubourethral portion of the urogenital diaphragm are markedly scarred, a single mattress stitch may be placed in the tissues lateral to the tips of the Kocher hemostat as shown, generally using a monofilament delayed absorption synthetic suture.

from side to side by the mattress-type suture of Kelly.[26] The stitches of Royston and Rose[37] may be used to shorten a pathologically elongated trigone.

In the presence of a pathologically dilated or funneled urethra, Kelly-type stitches used for urethral plication may be deliberately placed in the wall to reduce its lumen. When Kelly-type plication stitches are placed in the periurethral supporting tissues, they may not only correct funneling but also unintentionally approximate the paraurethral portions of the posterior pubourethral ligaments. The more laterally placed pubourethral ligament sutures, on the other hand, are inserted directly into the urethral attachment of the posterior pubourethral ligament portion of the urogenital diaphragm.[20,27] This placement seems to explain the greater success of this procedure.

Because Kelly plication stitches are particularly useful in the presence of funneling or vesicalization of the urethra and bladder neck, the surgeon may sometimes choose to use both pubourethral plication stitches *and* Kelly plication stitches in a particular clinical situation (e.g., rotational descent of the urethrovesical junction with simultaneous urethral funneling). The merits of these techniques for each case must be decided individually.

Alternate transvaginal methods of support. Obviously several important factors may contribute to urinary stress incontinence. For example, the pubococcygeus muscle

may be attached to the lateral paraurethral and paravaginal connective tissues, as has been pointed out by Muellner.[31] Sometimes these factors require the surgeon to use different procedures for anterior colporrhaphy.

When traction on the Kocher hemostatic forceps applied to the paraurethral tissue shows no evidence of pubic fixation of the tissue to which the hemostat has been applied (i.e., failure of traction to move the patient a small bit), the paraurethral or paravaginal tissues have been either avulsed or detached on one or both sides of the pelvis, and the pubourethral ligament support is insufficient for reconstruction. In this instance it is necessary to consider alternative methods of support, such as a transplant of the pubococcygeus muscle,[8,13,23] lateral (or paravaginal fixation) sutures, or the use of buried plastic synthetic mesh.

Pubococcygeus muscle transplant of Ingelman-Sundberg. The operator isolates the finger-thick medial pedicle of the pubococcygeus on each side by dissection and transects it in the midportion of the vagina at the level of the urethrovesical junction. Sewing the two pedicles together by transfixion suture provides useful support after the repair of a cystocele, as after the repair of a urethrovaginal fistula. In fact failure to provide such support after the repair of a fistula at the urethrovesical junction is likely to result in postoperative urinary stress incontinence.

The first step in performing a pubococcygeus muscle

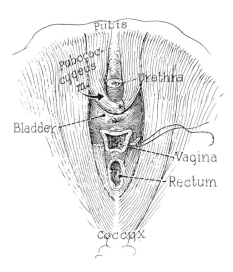

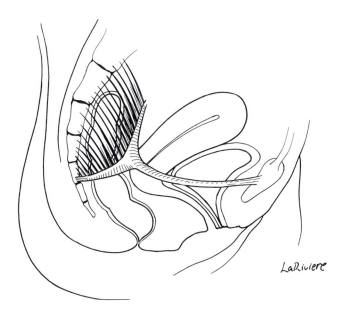

Fig. 21-25. When the tissues of the urogenital diaphragm are pathologically weak at the vesicourethral junction, an alternate method of support of this tissue is that of the pubococcygeus muscle transplant. The dissection in the vesicovaginal space is carried laterally until the pubococcygei are identified. Each pubococcygeus is transected as shown by the dashed line, and approximated in an overlapping fashion beneath the vesicourethral junction. The posterior cut end of each pubococcygeus is fixed to the adjacent ileococcygeus muscles to inhibit subsequent development of rectocele. (From Nichols DH, Randall CL: *Vaginal surgery,* ed 3, Baltimore, 1989, Williams & Wilkins.)

Fig. 21-26. Sagittal drawing showing the pelvic sidewall. The arcus tendineus of the levator ani is noted as it passes from the ischial spine to the back of the pubis. Notice that although this orientation is almost horizontal, it is oriented in the same direction as the axis of the vagina, as shown, although it is not parallel.

transplant is to open the vagina in the midline into the vesicovaginal space. The operator then mobilizes the full thickness of the walls laterally almost to the pubic rami, through the lateral limits of the vesicovaginal space, if necessary. Palpation of the upper two thirds of the lateral vaginal wall permits identification of the medial borders of the pubococcygei, which can be visualized with a little dissection. Alternately, some operators prefer to make an inverted U-shaped incision through the full thickness of the anterior vaginal wall to expose the full length of the urethra, most of the bladder, and laterally the pubococcygei at the point where they cross the urethra and the vagina.

The operator mobilizes a finger-sized pedicle of the pubococcygeus muscle on each side and separates it laterally from the remainder of the muscle (Figs. 21-25). When transected posteriorly, this muscle graft is suspended because of its continuity with the superior extremity of the rest of the muscle. The portion mobilized should be long enough to permit it to be joined to the pedicle from the other side snugly, but without tension, by means of a series of transfixion sutures placed in a side-to-side fashion beneath the urethrovesical junction.

In order to prevent its retraction and loss of support, the free segment of the posterior pubococcygeus from which the upper muscle was cut is now sewn by a mattress suture to the main body of the levator ani on its respective side. If there is a prominent rectocele, however, these fibers may be mobilized and fixed beneath the posterior vaginal wall during the subsequent posterior repair.

Lateral or paravaginal fixation. When midline plication is not an effective treatment of rotational descent of the urethrovesical junction, lateral or paravaginal fixation on one or both sides may be necessary. If a patient has both a lateral defect and a midline lesion that should have been diagnosed preoperatively, a midline incision in the anterior vaginal wall provides operative exposure for the repair of each of these elements (i.e., pubourethral ligament plication and paravaginal fixation). An interesting approach is to attach the paraurethral connective tissue to the arcus tendineus on the undersurface of the pubis[2,11,36,47,48] (Fig. 21-26).

The Baden vaginal analyzer is shown in Fig. 21-27. On the tips of a sponge forceps, it is inserted into the vagina of the cystocele patient who is in the lithotomy position. The handles are spread and the blades made to occupy the position of the arcus tendineus on each side of the pelvis. The gynecologist observes the presence or absence of residual cystocele. Considerable remaining cystocele indicates the presence of a defect in the central or midline supporting tissues of the bladder and anterior vaginal wall, whereas virtual disappearance of the cystocele indicates a defect in the paravaginal supporting tissues. The instrument is removed, and the surgeon notes what happens to the anterior vaginal wall. Some patients have defects in both the midline and paravaginal supporting tissues, both of which should be repaired. (The examiner must separately support the vaginal vault, as with a sponge forceps, during these maneuvers lest an unsuspected and undiag-

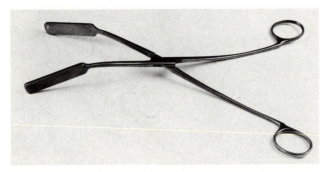

Fig. 21-27. Baden vaginal analysing forceps. When they are inserted into the vagina and opened, they press each anterior vaginal fornix against the arcus tendineus. The observer should note what happens to the cystocele in this circumstance. If it disappears, there is probably a defect in the paravaginal supporting tissue. If it does not, there is a midline defect. Occasionally both are present. The instrument is available from the Special Order Department, Codman-Shurtleff Inc., New Bedford, MA 02745. (From Nichols DH: *Reoperative gynecologic surgery,* St Louis, 1990, Mosby–Year–Book.)

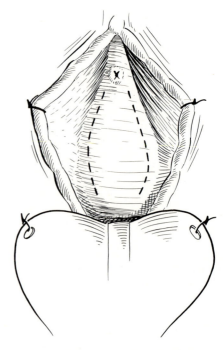

Fig. 21-28. When only paravaginal reattachment is to be made, symmetrical incisions are made along the site of the anterior fornix as shown by the dashed line. (Modified from Nichols DH, Randall CL: *Vaginal surgery,* ed 3, Baltimore, 1989, Williams & Wilkins.)

nosed partial eversion of the vaginal vault masquerade as a cystocele.)

A bent uterine sound may be inserted as a probe into the bladder to identify its lateral margins by palpation of the tip of the probe, first on one side and then on the other. A guide stitch may be placed in the vaginal wall at each site where the lateral margin has been determined.

TECHNIQUE OF TRANSVAGINAL PARAVAGINAL REATTACHMENT

1. A sponge forceps or vaginal analyzer is inserted and spread to confirm paravaginal defect.
2. With indelible marking pencil draw violet line on each side along the upper margin of the tips of the analyzer (Fig. 21-28)
3. Insert guide sutures on each side along the violet line
   a. in front of the ischial spine
   b. halfway to the urethrovesical junction
   c. one at the urethrovesical junction
4. Instill 60 cc of indigo-carmine in saline through a transurethral catheter and clamp the catheter.
5. Inject 50 cc of sterile saline solution lateral to the violet colored line on each side of the patient's pelvis.
6. Pick up the anterior vaginal wall between Allis clamps placed at the vesicourethral junction.
7. Open the anterior vaginal wall between Allis clamps placed to either side of the violet line, and insert an index finger to separate the tissues from the pelvic side wall (Fig. 21-29).
8. Extend the incision the full length of the violet line.
9. Peel, push, and dissect the bladder from the underside of the medial flap for a distance of about 1.5 cm from the cut edge of the vagina.
10. Peel and dissect the undersurface of the lateral flap of vagina from the obturator fascia for a distance of about 1 cm.

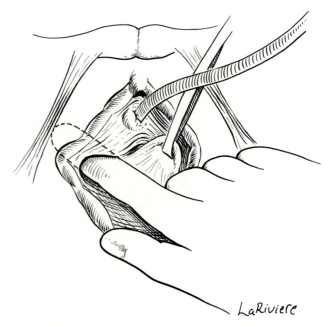

Fig. 21-29. Access to the obturator fascia and arcus tendineus is made by an incision lateral to the urethra with dissection directly into the paravaginal space palpating the obturator fascia, as shown, and the arcus tendineus of the pelvic diaphragm. This incision is then carried upwards in the vagina to the site near the ischial spine. (Modified from Nichols DH, Randall CL: *Vaginal surgery,* ed 3, Baltimore, 1989, Williams & Wilkins.)

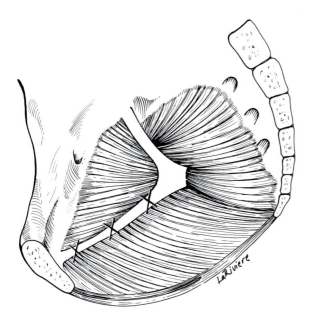

Fig. 21-30. The points along the arcus tendineus or the underlying obturator fascia to which the anterior vaginal fornix may be attached on each side of the pelvis during a bilateral paravaginal repair are indicated by the **X**s. The most posterior is near the ischial spine, the most anterior is at the back of the pubis, and the point in between approximates the vesicourethral junction.

11. Further develop the space of Retzius and more fully dissect and expose the obturator fascia, the arcus tendineus, and the levator fascia.

12. Penetrate the obturator fascia at the site of the arcus tendineus with a Deschamp's ligature carrier holding 00 synthetic monofilament suture in three places (Figs. 21-30 and 21-31):
    a. anterior to the ischial spine
    b. midway to the urethrovesical junction
    c. at the urethrovesical junction
    d. an extra suture may be placed along the way if the vagina is long.

13. Starting with the deepest suture (i.e., at the ischial spine) sew one end of the monofilament suture to the underside of the medial flap of the vaginal wall 1 cm from the cut edge tie as a pulley stitch.

14. Then, place the middle suture similarly adjacent to the middle guide suture, and then the urethrovesical junction suture (Fig. 21-32)—one free end tied to the underside of the flap adjacent to the guide suture, to be tied later as a pulley stitch (See Chapter 27). Meanwhile hold all sutures.

15. Do the same thing on the other side of the pelvis.

16. Close each vaginal wall fornix incision with a running horizontal mattress stitch of 00 Dexon or Vicryl allowing the held sutures to penetrate the incision line at each end and in the middle at the site of the respective guide sutures.

17. Do the same thing on the other side.

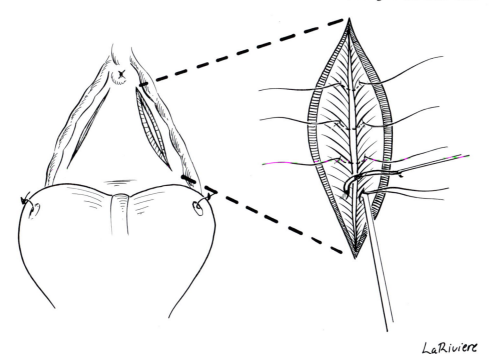

Fig. 21-31. Bilateral incisions for paravaginal colpopexy are shown in the drawing to the left. In the drawing to the right, the obturator fascia, and arcus tendineus if available, are grasped with interrupted sutures of long-acting absorbable material placed as shown. A tug on each suture after it has been placed, if accompanied by effective resistance of the tissues is identified. One may use the Deschamps ligature carrier as shown, or a swedged-on needle. (Modified from Nichols DH, Randall CL: *Vaginal surgery,* ed 3, Baltimore, 1989, Williams & Wilkins.)

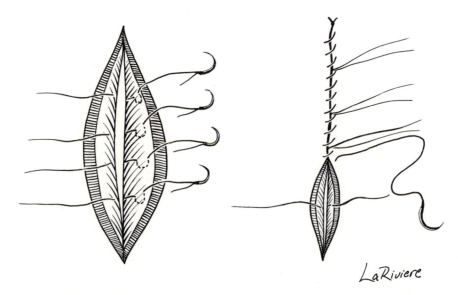

Fig. 21-32. Each of the interrupted stitches are attached to the undersurface of the medial flap of the vaginal incision as shown in the drawing to the left, but are not yet tied. The vaginal incision is closed by a running suture of polyglycolic acid suture, and the incisional line is penetrated by the ends of the untied paravaginal fixation stitches as in the drawing to the right. When the vaginal incisions have been reapproximated, the colpopexy stitches are tied drawing the anterior fornix to the site of the obturator fascia and/or arcus tendineus.

18. Remove the guide sutures.
19. Tie the pulley stitches, first one side then the other, and cut them short to allow the suture ends to retract beneath the cut edges of the vaginal wall.
20. Complete any other necessary colporrhaphy including anterior midline, or posterior as needed.
21. Excise any enterocele and perform a sacrospinous colpopexy as needed—finish the posterior colporrhaphy and perineorrhaphy.
22. Check the rectal examination for integrity.
23. Pack the vagina overnight with iodoform gauze.
24. At bedtime the next day, start nightly installations of estrogen vaginal cream.
25. Remove Foley on the third postoperative day after giving the patient a single dose of 10 mg of Phenoxybenzamine, catheterize only if necessary, and stimulate bowel movement as necessary.

ALTERNATE METHOD OF TRANSVAGINAL PARAVAGINAL REATTACHMENT IN THE PATIENT WITH AN OBVIOUS COEXISTENT DEFECT IN THE MIDLINE SUPPORTING TISSUES

1. Insert a transurethral Foley catheter into the bladder.
2. Open between two Allis clamps directly into the vesicovaginal space. An inverted V- or U-shaped incision may be used if desired (Fig. 21-33). Excess anterior vaginal wall may be excised (Fig. 21-34).
3. Open the full-length of the anterior vaginal wall including an exposure of the bladder base and tissue under the urethra.

4. Dissect the full lateral limits of the vesicovaginal space.
5. Plicate the pubourethral ligament portion of the urogenital diaphragm, and if there is any funneling

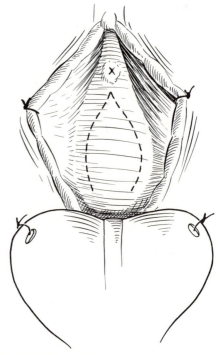

Fig. 21-33. For the patient with both paravaginal and midline defects in support, an incision may be made along the dashed line as shown. In essence this may represent an inverted V or U configuration. (Modified from Nichols DH, Randall CL: *Vaginal surgery,* ed 3, Baltimore, 1989, Williams & Wilkins.)

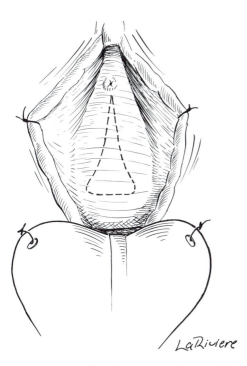

Fig. 21-34. When a portion of excess anterior vaginal wall is to be excised, coincident with anterior colporrhaphy and paravaginal fixation, an appropriate incision is made as shown by the dashed line, and the tissue removed. (Modified from Nichols DH, Randall CL: *Vaginal surgery,* ed 3, Baltimore, 1989, Williams & Wilkins.)

present, insert Kelly stitches using Maxon or PDS suture.

6. Plicate the underside of the bladder using one or more layers of 00 polyglycolic acid mattress stitches.

7. Instill 60 cc of indigo-carmine colored saline into the bladder and clamp.

8. Inject 50 cc of sterile saline between the lateral limits of the vesicovaginal space in the pelvic sidewall.

9. Go through the latter limits of the vesicovaginal space to the space of Retzius and the pelvic sidewall, exposing the obturator fascia, arcus tendoneus, and fascia of the pelvic diaphragm.

10. With a Deschamp's ligature carrier, place three or more sutures of synthetic monofilament material through the obturator fascia at the site of arcus tendineus, start the first such stitch just in front of the ischial spine, the second and third half way to the urethrovesical junction, and the last at the urethrovesical junction.

11. Hold the vaginal vault in a proper desired postoperative position. Insert the vaginal elevating forceps into the vagina and note where the fold of the dissected anterior vaginal wall crosses the blade of this elevator. Using a free end of the suture in the obturator fascia, insert it subcutaneously through the full thickness of the underside of the fibromuscular layer of the anterior vaginal wall flaps (Fig. 21-35).

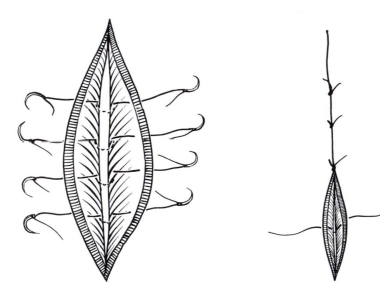

Fig. 21-35. When long-acting absorbable sutures are used, such as polydiaxanone (PDS), the stitches are placed through each edge of each incision in the anterior vaginal wall, first on one side and then on the other, as shown. When all have been placed, they are tied, as shown in the drawing on the right, bringing the anterior fornix to the desired position on the pelvic sidewall. (Modified from Nichols DH, Randall CL: *Vaginal surgery,* ed 3, Baltimore, 1989, Williams & Wilkins.)

12. Perform the same procedures in the opposite side of the pelvis.
13. Tie the lateral colpopexy stitches, first on one side then the other.
14. Bring the cut edges of the vagina together to effect a tension free closure.
15. Complete any posterior colporrhaphy that may be necessary.
16. Lightly pack the vagina overnight.

Plastic mesh support. When a large cystocele is associated with an abnormal thinning of the vaginal wall, a single-layered, porous plastic mesh insert may be used to encourage the formation of an adequately strong, satisfactorily functional vaginal wall.[29,32] The operator sews a layer of Mersilene mesh gauze into the vesicovaginal space, covering the entire surface of the exposed bladder surface that had previously been in contact with the anterior vagina. Fibroelastic connective tissue infiltrates and fixes the anterior vaginal wall after implantation. This type of foreign material is best used on postmenopausal or previously sterilized patients because the stretching and dilation of labor in a fertile patient would probably disrupt the attachments and result in avulsion of the mesh.

Mersilene mesh appears to be particularly effective when used to support the anterior vaginal wall because it is flexible, permanent, porous, and only a single layer in thickness. Perhaps most important, connective tissue readily infiltrates it, forming a permanently thickened, pli-

able tissue layer between the mesh and the undersurface of the vagina. The procedure used to place a Mersilene mesh insert is similar to that used to place a Tantalum patch, introduced for the same purpose by Moore, Armstrong, and Will.[30] Moore has abandoned the use of tantalum, however, because it may fragment in an area where it is subject to repeated bending. (Friedman and Meltzer[14] used a somewhat similar but absorbable collagen mesh prothesis successfully.) Supplemental reinforcement and insulation of this Mersilene mesh patch may be provided by the vaginal lapping operation or by a wide bulbocavernosus fat pad transplant.[27]

After opening the vesicovaginal space and reflecting the full thickness of the anterior vaginal wall from the midline laterally for the full extent of the vesicovaginal space, the operator cuts a pattern of sterile cardboard to fit the estimated size of the defect. From this pattern, a rhomboid-shaped piece of Mersilene gauze is fashioned. The operator then tacks the mesh to the capsular connective tissue underlying the bladder by placing three or four sutures on either side along the lateral margins of the vesicovaginal space, from as high in the vaginal vault as can be reached to the area beneath the urethrovesical junction. In unusual cases the operator may extend the mesh patch anteriorly to reinforce the urethra as well. Sutures should also be placed anteriorly into each pubourethral ligament. Laterally the mesh can be attached to the firm tissues of the lateral wall of the perivesical spaces, to the obturator fascia, and to the pelvic diaphragm. The prosthesis should be insulated by

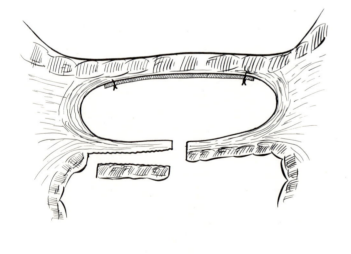
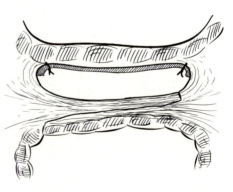

LaRiviere

Fig. 21-36. When there is a very large cystocele, and a very thin vagina with which to support its repair, a piece of Mersilene mesh cut to size, may be fixed into position to the bladder capsule, but this should be buried beneath the vagina by a vaginal lapping operation. One flap of vagina is split, separating the epithelium from the underlying fibromuscular layer, and the excess epithelium is excised as shown in the drawing on the left. The tip of this fibromuscular layer is then sewn to the underside of the unsplit flap of the opposite side, as shown in the drawing to the right, and the unsplit cut edge of the opposite side sewn to the point from which the epithelium was excised as noted in the drawing to the right, effectively doubling the thickness of the fibromuscular wall of the vagina at this point. (Modified from Nichols DH, Randall CL: *Vaginal surgery,* ed 3, Baltimore, 1989, Williams & Wilkins.)

the vaginal lapping procedure (Fig. 21-36) or a bulbocavernosus fat pad transplant.

This type of mesh should be used only as a subepithelial prosthesis. Inmon[24] has successfully buttressed the urethrovesical junction when supporting tissues are defective by imbedding a short hammock of Mersilene mesh transvaginally, sewing it to the urethrovesical supporting tissues of first one side and then the other. The material must always be carefully buried beneath a two-layered closure, however, and must not be allowed to come into contact with an epithelial surface.

Necrosis of the covering vaginal flap could result from ischemia; for this reason the cut edges of the vagina must be united without tension. Zacharin[51] has reported success using a free full thickness patch of excised vaginal skin buried beneath the vaginal flaps, tacked in place and in place of the synthetic plastic mesh.

Closure of vaginal wall. When vaginal hysterectomy has immediately preceded anterior colporrhaphy, the residual inverted T-shaped flaps of the upper vagina should be carefully trimmed to an inverted V (Figs. 21-37 and 21-38). If a functional vagina is not an objective of surgery, attenuated vaginal walls can effectively support a cystocele repair; the operator can deliberately excise wide flaps of vaginal wall, thereby narrowing the vagina to a finger-breadth caliber. This does not appreciably improve incontinence, however; it simply narrows the vagina.

For those patients who wish to preserve a functional vagina, it is essential to avoid the overenthusiastic or careless excision of too much of the anterior vaginal wall. Furthermore, in trimming the vaginal flaps to provide a desirable contour for the vault of the vagina, the operator must remember that the greater the amount of anterior wall flap that is removed, the less the amount of posterior wall flap that can be removed. The operator's failure to make this type of adjustment in procedure may also narrow the vagina, and dyspareunia may follow.

When closed under too much tension, the vaginal membrane may later separate or slough, thereby inviting recurrence. If there is evidence of flap tension, the operator should make simple longitudinal "relaxing incisions" that undermine 1 cm of the full thickness of the lateral vaginal walls at the 3 and 9 o'clock positions to release the tension and increase the caliber of a narrowed vagina. Such lateral relaxing incisions may be left open and the "raw" bases allowed to granulate in, and they are usually reepithelialized within 2 to 3 weeks. In colporrhaphy, the reapproximation of the subepithelial fibromuscular tissues produces the desired repair—not the reapproximation of the superficial vaginal skin.

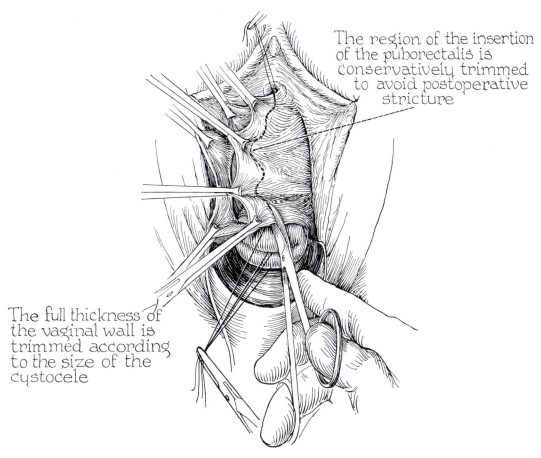

Fig. 21-37. Excess but unsplit vaginal wall is trimmed appropriately. (From Ball TL: *Gynecologic surgery and urology*, ed 2, St. Louis, 1963, Mosby–Year Book.)

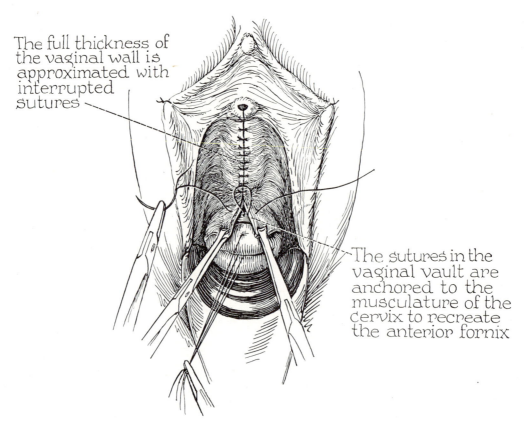

The full thickness of the vaginal wall is approximated with interrupted sutures

The sutures in the vaginal vault are anchored to the musculature of the cervix to recreate the anterior fornix

Fig. 21-38. The full thickness of the anterior vaginal wall is approximated from side to side, using a running subcuticular suture if the vaginal wall is thick, through-and-through interrupted sutures if it is not. (From Ball TL: *Gynecologic surgery and urology,* ed 2, St. Louis, 1963, Mosby–Year Book.)

In some patients, the separation of a thin layer of connective tissue from the vaginal membrane, mobilization, and plication, often by means of multiple, somewhat incomplete rows of fine synthetic absorbable or nonabsorbable sutures, may produce a satisfactory long-term result. The redundant sling of the fibromuscular tissues is shortened and strengthened by the duplication because the supporting layer of vaginal membrane fits the newly formed plane of the anterior vaginal wall with much less excision of vaginal membrane than may have been expected.

Aldridge[1] suggested that after the removal of a properly sized, somewhat V-shaped wedge from the vaginal flap beneath the urethra, full-thickness vaginal wall approximation is more important in supporting the urethra than is plication of the urethral wall itself. The operator should close the suburethral vaginal wall with running or interrupted 2-0 absorbable stitches, often placed subcuticularly, through the full thickness of the underlying fibromuscular layer. The first stitch should be near the urethral meatus. If hysterectomy has immediately preceded the repair, the operator should sew the ends of the tied peritoneal closure stitch to the undersurface of the now trimmed upper vault margins of the anterior vaginal wall near the attachment of the bladder pillars to ensure maximal elongation of the wall when these stitches have been tied. It is best to slide the index finger down the suture strand of the peritoneal closure stitch to a point below the knot while bringing the vaginal wall to the point of peritoneal closure. Because the peritoneal closure stitch includes the uterosacral ligaments, this procedure effectively though indirectly attaches the anterior vaginal wall to the uterosacral ligaments, helps to lengthen the anterior vaginal wall, and directs the vaginal axis posteriorly.

As the reconstruction of the anterior vaginal wall continues, the operator places subcuticular stitches approximately 1 cm apart. If not previously accomplished, the ends of the pubourethral ligament suture may be sewn and tied to the undersurface of the vaginal wall at the site of the previous attachment of the vagina to the urogenital diaphragm (Fig. 21-16), which reestablishes the fusion normally found in this area between the vaginal wall and the urethra. Finally, the operator closes the remainder of the full thickness of the vaginal wall beneath the urethra with subcuticularly placed 2-0 absorbable sutures.

A program of voluntary perineal resistive exercises will enhance the continence mechanism[10,25] both preoperatively and for some months postoperatively.

Simultaneous perineorrhaphy

Because the lower anterior wall rests on the perineal body for the length of the urethra, perineal support should also be provided whenever urethral support has been the major objective of vaginal reconstruction. Coincident perineorrhaphy not only reinforces the external genital sphincter system but also improves the long-term results of repair for the cure of urinary stress incontinence (see Chapter 22).

The Watkins-Wertheim[44,45,46] interposition type of operation in which the uterine fundus is interposed between the bladder and the anterior vaginal wall is not recommended for the treatment of cystocele because there is a risk of future bleeding from the retained uterus. In addition, should pathology that requires hysterectomy subsequently develop, the extensive adhesions to the uterine fundus and the proximity of the lower ureters and the bladder trigone to the adherent fundus that result from such an operation make hysterectomy appreciably more difficult. Rarely, if the vaginal wall is very thin and the uterine cervix is well supported, transposition using the Ocejo modification in which the uterus is opened and the entire endometrium excised may be used.[16]

INABILITY TO VOID POSTOPERATIVELY

Relaxation of the muscular component of the pubourethral ligaments and the urethral attachment to the levator ani (muscular, fascial, or both) is an integral part of the physiologic voiding process, and significant surgical plication of these ligaments beneath the urethrovesical junction may inhibit the normal voiding process until healing is well under way and spasms have ceased. A temporary suprapubic cystostomy may be helpful if the surgeon suspects that the patient (e.g., a patient with unusual anxiety or with a very large hypotonic bladder) will be unable to void after anterior colporrhaphy. Suprapubic cystostomy should be used routinely after repair of a fistula at the vesical neck (see Chapter 51).

At the time the silicone-coated no. 16 transurethral Foley catheter is removed, the patient may be given a single dose of an alpha-adrenergic blocker such as phenoxybenzamine [Dibenzyline] (10 mg) to relax urethral spasm. An order is left for the patient to be catheterized only if unable to void. If after a day of unsuccessful trying the patient is still unable to void, she may be taught the technique of self-catheterization, to be used as necessary even after discharge from the hospital. Use of the plastic flexible "Mentor" 14 Fr female catheter facilitates this procedure considerably. Its use can be discontinued as soon as the patient is able to void adequate amounts spontaneously and there is but little (less than 60 cc) residual urine obtained. The patient may be given a printed hand-out of the technique which is as follows:

Instructions to patient for intermittent self-catheterization*

Self-catheterization can be accomplished several times a day, as frequently as someone normally voids. It is impor-

tant to be sure that the bladder never holds more than 500 cc (1 pint) of urine at one time. If the bladder is allowed to hold more than 500 cc for any length of time the urine can stretch the bladder muscle to the point where it won't work as well as it should, and if the bladder becomes too stretched, it cannot receive a proper blood supply, which can precipitate a bladder infection. To avoid these problems make sure that the bladder is emptied every few hours during the day. Some people do the procedure while standing, some sitting on the toilet, and some lying down. Which ever is the easiest for you is the method you should use.

Procedure

1. Wash hands and then wash the perineal area. Spread the labia with one hand, and with the other hand wash the opening from where the urine comes, and the surrounding area, from front to back, using a povidone iodine (Betadine) packet, or a wash-and-wipe disposable towelette. Use one wipe to wash down the left side of the non–hair bearing inner vaginal lips, then wipe down the inner surface of the right side, and another one to wash down the urethral meatus (the opening from which the urine comes).

2. Hold the labia open with one hand, and grasp the Mentor plastic disposable catheter 2 to 3 inches from the tip, inserting it slowly into the meatus (urethral opening) until the urine begins to drain. Leave it in place until the urine stops coming, and slowly pull the catheter out. If urine begins to drain again, stop and wait until the flow stops before removing the tube. The catheter can be allowed to drain directly into the toilet or container. When the flow of urine is finished, remove the catheter.

3. The catheter should be washed well with soap and water after each use, and then rinsed with clear water.

4. Each day boil the catheters for 3 to 5 minutes, empty the water, and let them dry. They may be stored in a clean towel, an aluminum foil packet, a "Baggie" ziplock, or a sterilized jar. You should carry a catheter with you wherever you go. Clearly, the catheters can be reused for an almost indefinite period of time if the above procedure is followed. Should you need a new supply, do not hesitate to request this of your physician, who can prescribe a new supply from a surgical supply house.

REFERENCES

1. Aldridge AH: Personal communication, 1965.
2. Baden WF, Walker TA: Evaluation of the stress incontinent patient. In Cantor EB, editor: *Female urinary stress incontinence* Springfield, Ill, 1979, Charles C Thomas.
3. Ball TL: *Gynecologic surgery and urology,* St. Louis, 1963, Mosby–Year Book.
4. Ball TL: Anterior and posterior cystocele, *Clin Obstet Gynec* 9:1062, 1966.
5. Beck RP: Personal communication.
6. Beck RP, McCormick S: Treatment of urinary stress incontinence with anterior colporrhaphy, *Obstet Gynecol* 59:269, 1982.

*Adapted from Ebrady SM, Yale-New Haven Hospital, New Haven, Conn.

7. Borstad E, Rud T: The risk of developing urinary stress incontinence after vaginal repair in continent women: a clinical and urodynamic follow-up study, *Acta Obstet Gynecol Scan* 68: 545, 1989.

8. Copenhaver EH: *Surgery of the vulva and vagina: a practical guide,* Philadelphia, 1981, WB Saunders.

8. DeLancy JOL: Corrective study of paraurethral anatomy, *Obstet Gynecol* 68:91, 1986.

9. DeLancy JOL: Anatomic aspects of vaginal eversion after hysterectomy, *Am J Obstet Gynecol* 166:1717, 1992.

10. Ferguson KL et al: Stress urinary incontinence: effect of pelvic muscle exercise, *Obstet Gynecol* 75:671, 1990.

11. Figurnov KM: Surgical treatment of urinary incontinence in women, *Akush Ginekol* 6:7, 1949.

12. Frank RT: Operation for cure of incontinence of urine in the female, *Am J Obstet Gynecol* 55:618, 1947.

13. Franz R: Levator plastik bei relativen Harn inkontinenz, *Gynakologe* 137:393, 1954.

14. Friedman EA, Meltzer RN: Collagen mesh prosthesis for repair of endopelvic fascial defect, *Am J Obstet Gynecol* 106:430, 1970.

15. Gainey HL: Motion picture and personal communication.

16. Gallo D: *Ocejo modification of interposition operation. In Urologica ginecologica,* Guadalajara, 1969, Gallo.

17. Gardiner SH: Vaginal surgery for stress incontinence, *Clin Obstet Gynecol* 6:178, 1963.

18. Gardy M et al: Stress incontinence and cystoceles; *J Urol* 145:1211, 1991.

19. Green TH: Development of a plan for the diagnosis and treatment of urinary stress incontinence, *Am J Obstet Gynecol* 83:632, 1962.

20. Halban J: *Gynakologische operationslehre,* Berlin-Vienna, 1932, Urban & Schwarzenberg.

21. Hodgkinson CP: Stress urinary incontinence, *Am J Obstet Gynecol* 108:1141, 1970.

22. Hutch, JA: A new theory of the anatomy of the internal urinary sphincter and the physiology of micturition, *Obstet Gynecol* 30:309, 1967.

23. Ingelman-Sundberg A: Stress incontinence of urine, *J Obstet Gynaecol Br Emp* 59:699, 1952.

24. Inmon WB: Personal communication, 1976.

25. Kegel A: Progressive resistance exercise in the functional restoration of the perineal muscles, *Am J Obstet Gynecol* 56:238, 1948.

26. Kelly HA: Incontinence of urine in women, *Urol Cutan Rev* 1:291, 1913.

27. Martius H: *Martius' gynecological operations,* Boston, 1956, Little, Brown (Translated by McCall M, Bolten K).

28. Milley PS, Nichols DH: The relationships between the pubourethral ligaments and urogenital diaphragm in the human female, *Anat Rec* 163:433, 1969.

29. Moir JC: The gauze-hammock operation, *J Obstet Gynaecol Br Commonw* 75:1, 1968.

30. Moore J, Armstrong JT, Wills SH: The use of tantalum mesh in cystocele with critical report of ten cases, *Am J Obstet Gynecol* 69:1127, 1955.

31. Muellner SR: The anatomies of the female urethra, *Obstet Gynecol* 14:429, 1959.

32. Nichols DH: The Mersilene mesh gauze-hammock in repair of severe recurrent urinary stress incontinence. In Taymor ML, Green TH, editors: *Progress in gynecology,* vol 6, New York, 1975, Grune & Stratton.

33. Nichols DH, Milley PS: Identification of pubourethral ligaments and their role in transvaginal surgical correction of stress incontinence, *Am J Obstet Gynecol* 115:123, 1973.

34. Reiffenstuhl G: The clinical significance of the connective tissue planes and spaces, *Clin Obstet Gynecol* 25:811, 1982.

35. Ricci JV, Thom CH: Uterovaginal extirpation for procidentia, *Am J Surg* 83:192, 1952.

36. Richardson AC, Lyons JB, Williams NL: A new look at pelvic relaxation, *Am J Obstet Gynecol* 126:568, 1976.

37. Royston GD, Rose DK: A new operation for cystocele, *Am J Obstet Gynecol* 33:421, 1937.

38. Sims JM: *Clinical notes on uterine surgery,* London, 1866, Robert Hardwicke.

39. Symmonds RE, Jordan LT: Iatrogenic stress incontinence of urine, *Am J Obstet Gynecol* 82:1231, 1961.

40. Uhlenhuth E, Hunter DT: *Problems in the anatomy of the pelvis,* Philadelphia, 1953, JB Lippincott.

41. Van Duzen RE: The cystoscopic appearance of various types of cystoceles, *South Med J* 23:580, 1930.

42. Van Rooyen AJL, Liebenberg HC: Clinical approach to urinary incontinence in females, *Obstet Gynecol* 53:1, 1979.

43. Von Peham H, Amreich J: *Operative gynecology,* Philadelphia, 1934, JB Lippincott, (Translated by Ferguson LK).

44. Watkins TJ: The treatment of cystocele and uterine prolapse after the menopause. *Am Gyn Obstet J,* 15:420-23, 1899.

45. Watkins TJ: Treatment of cases of extensive cystocele and uterine prolapse. *Surg Gyn Obstet* 2:659-67, 1906.

46. Wertheim E: Zur plastischen Verwendung des Uterus bei Prolapsen. *Centralbl f Gynäk,* 23:369-72, 1899.

47. White GR: Cystocele—a radical cure by suturing lateral sulci of vagina to the white line of pelvic fascia, *JAMA* 53:1707, 1909.

48. Word BH Jr, Montgomery HA: *Paravaginal fascial repair,* Motion picture and personal communications, 1989.

49. Zacharin RF: The suspensory mechanism of the female urethra, *J Anat* 97:423, 1963.

50. Zacharin RF: A Chinese anatomy—the pelvic supporting tissues of the chinese and Occidental female compared and contrasted, *Aust NZ Obstet Gynecol* 17:11, 1977.

51. Zacharin RF: Free full thickness vaginal epithelium graft in correction of recurrent genital prolapse. Presented at 42nd Annual Meeting of the Society of Pelvic Surgeons, Munich, Germany, Sept, 1992.

Chapter 22

RECTOCELE AND PERINEAL DEFECT

David H. Nichols

Damage to the structures of the posterior vaginal wall or their supporting attachments may result from one or more types of injury. A carefully taken history and a thorough physical examination in the office should clarify the type of injury, the site, and the degree of damage to all demonstrable components of the posterior vaginal wall. The examination should include an evaluation of vaginal caliber, tone, and support with the patient not only prone and relaxed on the examining table, but also erect, both with and without voluntary bearing-down efforts. The strength of voluntary contraction of the pubococcygei and external anal sphincter muscles should be noted. Only by considering the findings under all conditions is it possible for a surgeon to select the operative procedure most likely to restore normal relationships and functions.

Posterior colporrhaphy and perineorrhaphy are separate and distinct surgical operations.[23,26] Some patients require one of the operations, some the other, and many both (Fig. 22-1). Satisfactory correction of only one defect when more than one is present may compound the patient's symptoms and functional problems. Each defect should be recognized and surgically corrected by an appropriate combination of operative procedures in order to achieve an optimal postoperative result.

The goal of treatment of rectocele is to reduce to normal the size of an overly large and usually asymmetrical rectal reservoir, not to eliminate the reservoir altogether. In most instances of rectocele, transvaginal plication of the rectovaginal septum, the muscularis of the anterior rectal wall and an appropriate perineal reconstruction will correct the problem.

An unexpectedly shortened and persistently uncomfortable vagina after posterior colporrhaphy can result in dyspareunia. To minimize this complication, a full-length posterior vaginal wall reconstruction may be used in selected cases. Furthermore, if a patient has developed a weakness and thinning throughout the posterior wall of the vagina and the surgeon elects to repair only the lower part of that weakness by standard perineorrhaphy without colporrhaphy, the persistence of disturbed function or an early recurrence, probably with a troublesome exacerbation of symptoms, is predictable; full-length posterior colporrhaphy is necessary in this instance. The normal support that the voluntary pelvic muscles give to the pelvic organs is effectively paralyzed by anesthia, and pelvic examination under anesthesia may lead to an erroneous diagnosis of rectocele and perineal defect. As Jeffcoate[14] and Porges[24] noted, the need for and the extent of a posterior vaginal wall repair can best be determined preoperatively by examining the *unanesthetized* patient.

POSTERIOR VAGINAL WALL WEAKNESS

For the most part, weakness of the posterior vaginal wall is a late effect of the trauma of labor and delivery. Marks[20] described rectocele in terms of postobstetric dehiscence of the rectovaginal septal tissues permitting overdistension and thinning of the adjacent anterior rectal wall. As the perineal body and lower rectovaginal fascial supports weaken, the apex of the defect moves inferiorly and anteriorly relative to the sphincter and abdominal straining during defecation compounds the problem by pushing the bolus of stool farther from the anal opening.[6] This funnel-like distortion of the lower rectum is thus concentrated on the anterior rectal wall.

Rectocele and its associated symptoms of incomplete bowel movements, often requiring manual expression to achieve evacuation, usually becomes worse with the relaxation of pelvic supportive tissues coincident with aging. Aging and loss of hormone support reduce vaginal elasticity, which may lead to damage from overdistension of the

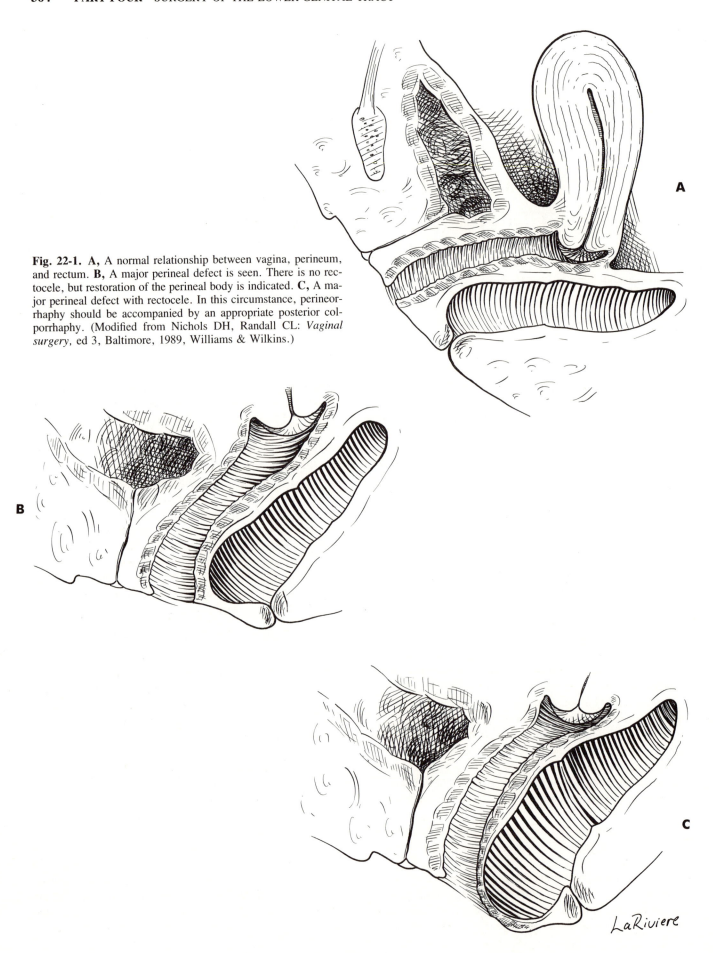

Fig. 22-1. A, A normal relationship between vagina, perineum, and rectum. **B,** A major perineal defect is seen. There is no rectocele, but restoration of the perineal body is indicated. **C,** A major perineal defect with rectocele. In this circumstance, perineorrhaphy should be accompanied by an appropriate posterior colporrhaphy. (Modified from Nichols DH, Randall CL: *Vaginal surgery*, ed 3, Baltimore, 1989, Williams & Wilkins.)

vagina. There may be a congenital underdevelopment of the perineal musculature and elastic tissues, often because of associated abnormal innervation (as may be suspected with a coexistent spina bifida occulta). The attachments of the perineal body to the rectovaginal septum may have been avulsed by trauma, or the perineal body, vagina, and rectum may have been separated from the fibrous attachments of the levator ani-pelvic diaphragm complex. Laceration of the rectovaginal septum and Denonvilliers' fascia may obliterate the rectovaginal space, resulting in fusion of the anterior capsule of the rectum to the capsule of the posterior wall of the vagina. In addition, a rectocele (i.e., a herniation or ballooning of the rectum and posterior vaginal wall into the lumen of the vagina) may result from the traction associated with progressive procidentia of a general prolapse.

Sullivan and associates[31] and Capps[6] have also noted that plication of the anal sphincter without correction of coincident and asymptomatic rectocele will increase anal outlet resistance and may convert an asymptomatic rectocele to a symptomatic one requiring future secondary repair. Thus, if an anal sphincter plication is to be done, even an asymptomatic rectocele should be repaired simultaneously.

Proper repair providing freedom from unexpected rectal outlet obstruction will decrease the venous stasis in the terminal hemorrhoidal vessels (coincident to straining at stool), reducing the reformation, progression, and severity of coincident hemorrhoidal disease.

The straining efforts associated with chronic constipation can aggravate minor degrees of damage to the rectal wall and its connective tissue supports. Repeated interference with the progress of the fecal stream may prevent the normal completion of defecation, resulting in physiologic or functional obstruction as the redundant sacculation of the rectum becomes larger and the residual stool stimulates more ineffectual straining. A rectocele may be caused by pulsion or by repeatedly increased intraabdominal pressure, a factor more often evident during a patient's postmenopausal years when atrophic changes decrease the elasticity of the vaginal wall and the integrity of the supporting tissues.

Anatomic types of rectocele

Many women who have a rectocele are not constipated, and many women who do not have a rectocele are constipated. The primary symptoms of rectocele, however, are aching after a bowel movement and such difficulty in evacuating the bowel completely that manual expression may be necessary. Effective posterior colporrhaphy should relieve these symptoms but is likely to relieve constipation only if the constipation results from the presence of a pocket of the rectal wall that repeatedly traps stool, precluding complete emptying of the bowel.

The gynecologist who is planning the repair of a rectocele must first determine which type of rectocele is present.[22] The posterior vaginal wall may exhibit three basic types of damage:

1. The full thickness of the vaginal wall may be stretched and attenuated, usually as a result of overdistention during childbirth, and some of the intrinsic elasticity of the fibromuscular vaginal tube may be permanently lost. The damage is greatest where the vaginal wall is furthest removed from its anchoring attachments; damage to the anterior and posterior walls is greater than is damage to the lateral vaginal walls, because the vagina is fixed or attached to the lateral walls. Like cystoceles, a rectocele is associated with the flattening of the rugal folds over its site and is likely to be progressive in its development.

2. The lateral attachments of the vagina to the pelvic side wall, particularly the vaginal portion of the cardinal ligament, may be stretched as a result of increased intraabdominal pressure or as a result of the vagina's slowness to dilate adequately during labor so that a roll of undilating vaginal wall was pushed along during the descent of the presenting part, much as a coat sleeve is turned inside out. Vaginal rugae are generally preserved in the redundant vaginal wall involved in such a rectocele.

3. The lateral attachments of the vagina may have been not only stretched, but also torn from the lateral vaginal walls, only to reunite by scarring and fibrosis at a lower level in the pelvis. Because the refusion is often quite dense and fibrous, this is probably the origin of the nonprogressive, postobstetric prolapse described by Malpas.[19]

All types of damage may coexist in the same patient, producing a combination defect. In addition, each is frequently associated with a defective perineum.

Sites of damage

Damage may occur to the lower, middle, or upper portions of the posterior vaginal wall in any combination. Damage to the midvagina, which has been referred to as the rectal portion of the posterior vaginal wall, is perhaps the most common. This may be the only lesion that requires repair. Damage in the upper vagina may be noted either as a high rectocele, an enterocele, a potential enterocele, or a widened posterior fornix that may subsequently be narrowed by surgery.

True low rectocele. A rather major and inadequately repaired obstetric laceration of the perineum that disrupts the attachments of the levator ani (fascia of the pubococcygeal portion) or the bulbospongiosus muscles to the perineal body and lower vagina may result in a true low rectocele. Either injury may occur without producing a midvaginal or high rectocele. When there are additional etiologic factors, such as a defective or absent Denonvilliers' fascia, as may occur if enterocele has divided its layers, a coexistent middle or high vaginal rectocele may develop.

Most frequently, the injury that produces a low rectocele is a shearing of the lower attachments of the rectovaginal septum and Denonvilliers' fascia from their attachment to the superior portion of the perineal body. A marked gaping or eversion of the introitus is usually evident. Although this causes some loss of support to the sides of the urethra, bladder function is only slightly disturbed unless the urogenital diaphragm has also been torn or the pelvis denervated.[28,29,32] A low rectocele aggravates any tendency to constipation because of the decreased effectiveness and correspondingly increased bearing-down effort during defecation.

Midvaginal rectocele. Although a midvaginal rectocele is also a late result of obstetric injury, the damage does not usually involve the levator ani; the vaginal attachment and effective support of the pelvic diaphragm are below this area of involvement. The pathologic stretching and laceration of the connective tissues between the vagina and the rectum not only leave these tissues pathologically thin, but also lead to adhesions that fuse the rectal and vaginal capsules to the rectovaginal septum. Such a fusion tends to eliminate the ability of the rectum and the vagina to function independently; the vaginal wall must not only follow the contour of the rectal wall but must, to some extent, participate in rectal function as well. This is likely to result in persistent difficulties with constipation and defecation. A bearing-down sensation, discomfort after a bowel movement, and inability to empty the bowel completely are the usual symptoms.

A midvaginal rectocele often coexists with a high rectocele, and, if planning to repair one, the surgeon should repair both. As emphasized by Bullard and by Goff,[10] surgery in the midvaginal area should be designed to preserve or restore independent movement of the posterior vaginal and the anterior rectal walls; only at the level of the perineal body should the vaginal and rectal walls be fused in the reconstruction of the posterior vaginal wall. To accomplish this goal, the surgeon must carefully identify and preserve the relatively avascular tissue relationships in the rectovaginal space.

High rectocele. Like the midvaginal rectocele, a high rectocele is usually the result of a pathologic overstretching of the posterior vaginal wall. In this instance, however, the anterolateral attachments of the cardinal ligaments (hypogastric sheath) bind the vagina and cervix together to such an extent that the cervix functions almost as a part or extension of the anterior vaginal wall.[9,22]

The length of the anterior vaginal wall plus the diameter of the cervix normally equals the length of the posterior vaginal wall. The cranial envelope of the rectovaginal space terminates at the most caudal portion of the pouch of Douglas. This ensures flexibility and mobility but also, with the rectovaginal space, forms a more or less frictionless inclined plane down which the structures anterior to the rectovaginal space can slide without disturbing those

primarily rectal structures posterior to the rectovaginal space. Thus, although classic procidentia begins as an eversion of the upper vagina, it usually permits the entire uterus and much of the bladder to extend outside the bony pelvis. An enterocele develops, and the cervix, uterus, and bladder may drop as though in a sliding hernia. (All this often occurs without an accompanying rectocele.)

Such a descensus, noticeably involving the bladder, has been considered evidence of primarily anterior segment damage and is usually the result of chronically increased intraperitoneal pressure. It could result from damage sustained during the first stage of labor, however, if there have been bearing-down efforts or attempts to accomplish delivery before the cervix is fully dilated. Therefore, anterior segment damage per se may not be mechanistically related to damage to the levator ani or its sheath.

In discussing enteroceles, Malpas[19] described prolapse of the vaginal vault with an obvious peritoneal sac, the bulge usually containing omentum or a loop of intestine. The upper rectum forms the posterior wall of the sac, and a high rectocele may coexist with such a prolapse. Because the peritoneal fusion of Denonvilliers' fascia is missing from the posterior vaginal wall that covers an enterocele, there is a loss of support to both the anterior rectal wall and the posterior vaginal wall in this area, and a high rectocele may develop. Similarly, a high rectocele may be associated with a congenital deepening of the pouch of Douglas, because there is no Denonvilliers' fascia to support the anterior rectal wall in this situation either.

On the other hand, a uterovaginal or sliding prolapse does not involve the high rectum, so the peritoneal descent affects only the anterior wall of the pouch of Douglas, usually without dilation of the peritoneal sac. A high posterior colporrhaphy with careful excision of all of the peritoneal pouch is an essential part of the repair of a total vault prolapse, but, because a uterovaginal prolapse may not compromise the integrity of the rectum itself, the major objective of repair is to shorten the cardinal-uterosacral ligament complex and reattach it to the vault of the vagina. When the strength of the cardinal-uterosacral ligament complex is inadequate, sacrospinous colpopexy may be used to support the vaginal vault (see Chapter 27).

POSTERIOR COLPORRHAPHY AND THE RECTOVAGINAL SEPTUM

When a full-length posterior vaginal reconstruction is performed immediately after vaginal hysterectomy, the progress of blunt finger dissection of the "avascular rectovaginal space" is consistently obstructed at the vaginal apex near the cut edge of the vaginal vault by a thin, but firm, membrane. This membrane usually requires a distinct incision for penetration.

Existence of the rectovaginal septum

Tobin and Benjamin[33] concluded that the tissue described by Denonvilliers in the male included two layers: (1) the ventral peritoneal fusion layer and (2) a dorsal or posterior layer composed of rectal fascia. After studying the gynecologic relevance of this information, Ricci and Thom,[25] and Uhlenhuth and Nolley[34] reached almost diametrically opposed conclusions; however, their differences in methodology may explain their differences of opinion. The evidence that led Ricci and Thom to deny the existence of "fascial tissue" in the integrity of the vaginal walls was based entirely on the study of hematoxylin–eosin-stained histologic preparations and involved no correlation with gross anatomic dissections. Uhlenhuth and Nolley, on the other hand, based their conclusion solely on gross dissection and made no attempt at histologic correlation or confirmation.

To reconcile these controversial reports, Milley and Nichols conducted simultaneous studies of both the gross anatomy and related histologic specimens.[21] These studies demonstrated a rectovaginal septum that can be identified as a distinct and relatively strong connective tissue layer between the vagina and the rectal walls (Fig. 22-2). Extending in a curved coronal plane, somewhat in conformity with the curvature of the bony pelvis, this septal structure is attached cranially to the caudal peritoneum and the rectouterine pouch of Douglas and extends inferiorly to its caudal fusion with the perineal body. The tissues of this septum are always adherent to the posterior aspect of the vaginal connective tissue, but may easily be separated from it by blunt dissection. The demonstrable adherence of the septum to the "vaginal wall" explains, at least partially, why its existence has, at times, been denied.

In transverse and coronal dissections, this septum was found to curve posterolaterally, paralleling the course of the paracolpium and blending laterally with the parietal layer of the pelvic fascia. It varies in character from a thin, readily perforated, translucent membrane to a tougher layer of almost leathery consistency. A septum can be identified during dissection, but only when a definite effort to do so is made.

Histologic studies showed that this septum consists of a fibromuscular elastic tissue, including dense collagen, abundant smooth muscle, and coarse elastic fibers that are all readily separable from the fibromuscular elastic tissue of the posterior vaginal wall. In sections stained by orcein, the elastic fibers in the area of the rectovaginal septum appeared larger and coarser than those in the connective tissue within the vaginal wall proper. It is possible that such differences in elastic tissue fibers give the septum its demonstrable integrity during dissection. Appropriate tissue stains are necessary to demonstrate the presence of a septum. The difficulty of demonstrating a rectovaginal septum histologically with standard hematoxylin-eosin staining may be another reason that the existence of this important structure has often been denied.

These observations are of more than academic interest, because the strength and integrity of this membrane are clinically significant and surgically useful. The rectovaginal septum normally facilitates the independent mobility of the rectal and vaginal walls and, as a result, ensures their functional independence. It also acts as a protective barrier

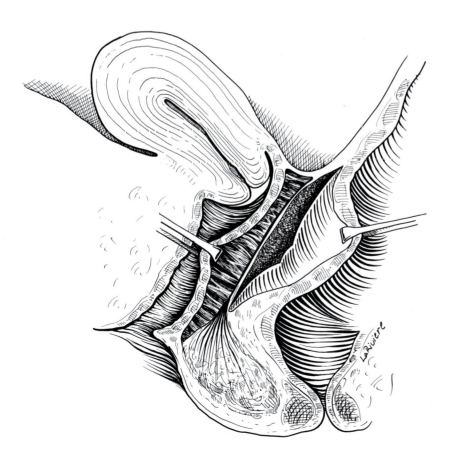

Fig. 22-2. The rectovaginal septum is shown. It forms the anterior border of the rectovaginal space and has been partly dissected from the underside of the posterior vaginal wall to which it is normally adherent. Note that it is fused to the cranial margin of the perineal body from which it may be torn during labor and delivery.

to the spread of neoplasia or infection between the rectum and the vagina, as Uhlenhuth and Nolley suggested.[34]

Surgical significance of the rectovaginal septum

Although not emphasized as an identifiable or significant structural entity, the rectovaginal septum appears to have been recognized and carefully restored in the New York Woman's Hospital type of posterior colporrhaphy described by Goff[10] and later in Bullard's modification of Goff's technique.[22] Uhlenhuth and Nolley suggest an explanation for this lack of emphasis or recognition.[34]

It has been mentioned that the rectovaginal septum adheres closely to the vagina; it is, therefore, probable that the surgeon, in performing a posterior colporrhaphy, does not get into the space between the vaginal fascia and rectovaginal septum, but into the space between the rectovaginal septum and rectal fascia.

Generally, the surgeon can easily break down a pathologic thickening of the rectovaginal septum during the preliminary dissection. This thickening is caused by scarring within the posterior avascular rectovaginal space and usually is demonstrable during a preoperative rectovaginal examination to determine whether the posterior vaginal wall can be moved independently of the anterior rectal wall. Rupture of the septum, even in the presence of an apparently intact vagina, may result in adhesions that fix the vaginal wall to the underlying rectal wall. This injury can, in turn, lead to uninhibited distention of the rectum, distention of the posterior vaginal wall, formation of a high or midvaginal rectocele, and symptomatic interference with function.

Because the rectovaginal septum normally curves posterolaterally as it becomes attached to the fascia overlying the levator ani, decreasing the vaginal width by approximating the cut edges after the excision of a midportion of the septum increases the pull on the lateral attachments of the septum that tend to direct the vagina posteriorly toward the sacrum. This tension is likely to restore the original and proper upper horizontal vaginal axis. The excision of an upper vaginal wedge of tissue may also be helpful (Fig. 22-3).

In the repair of an obstetric or surgical episiotomy, restoration of the rectovaginal septum as a distinct layer at the apex of the wound not only provides better support, but also ensures better function and increased comfort. This restoration can be readily accomplished by substituting running subcuticular stitches for the usual through-and-through epithelial stitches. In addition to decreasing the patient's postoperative and postpartum discomfort, this procedure effectively prevents epithelial inclusion cysts.

The tissues normally supporting the upper third of the vagina are different from those supporting the middle and lower thirds. Harrison and McDonagh wrote that "by far the most commonly neglected step in vaginal plastic procedures is reconstruction of the upper posterior vagina."[12] A low colporrhaphy sund perineorrhaphy cannot be expected to provide an anatomically adequate repair of a

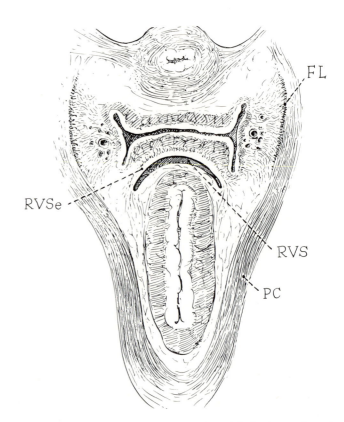

Fig. 22-3. Cross-section of the female pelvis is shown through the lower midportion of the vagina. Note the convex configuration of the pubococcygeus *(PC)*. The rectovaginal space *(RVS)* is indicated between the rectum and vagina, as well as the position of the rectovaginal septum *(RVSe)*. The blood vessels in the connective tissue lateral to the vagina are shown. The fibers of Luschka *(FL)* are shown as they attach the paravaginal connective tissue to the sheaths of the pubococcygei. These connections tend to give the vagina an H-shaped configuration. (From Nichols DH, Milley PS: *Clinical anatomy of the vulva, vagina, lower pelvis, and perineum.* In Sciarra J, editor: *Gynecology and obstetrics,* New York, 1993, Harper & Row. Reproduced with permission of Harper & Row.)

weakness in the upper third of the vagina. When high rectocele and enterocele coexist, as they frequently do, each must be recognized and repaired separately.

POSTERIOR COLPORRHAPHY WITHOUT PERINEORRHAPHY

When the defect to be repaired involves only the perineal body, reflection and mobilization of the perineal skin and the vaginal membrane should stop at the cranial margin of the perineal body on its vaginal face. When there is a coexistent rectocele of the middle or upper vagina, however, the surgeon should extend the reflection of the vaginal membrane by dissection into the rectovaginal space to a point above the bulge of the rectocele. Any adhesions that bind the anterior wall of the rectum to the full-thickness flap of the posterior vaginal wall should be divided by blunt and, when necessary, sharp dissection.

A patient who has previously undergone an otherwise

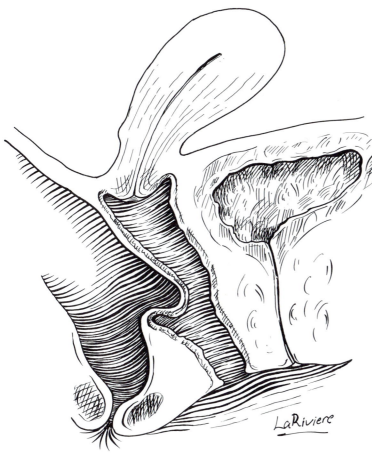

Fig. 22-4. A perineorrhaphy may hide an unrepaired midvaginal rectocele. Effective repair must always begin proximal to the point of weakness. (Modified from Nichols DH, Randall CL: *Vaginal surgery,* ed 3, Baltimore, 1989, Williams & Wilkins.)

adequate perineorrhaphy may develop a symptomatic rectocele that may not have been evident at the time of the initial surgery (Fig. 22-4). This herniation may appear to be an enterocele. When the perineal body does not require repair, the surgeon may simply open the posterior vaginal wall directly into the rectovaginal space through either a transverse (Fig. 22-5) or longitudinal incision into the vagina. This procedure can be performed without denuding or opening the perineum.

With lateral traction on sutures or clamps at the hymenal margin, the surgeon may open the rectovaginal space and establish a line of cleavage between the anterior rectal wall and the connective tissues of the rectovaginal septum, taking care not to open the often attenuated or thinned rectal wall. When episiotomy repairs have resulted in excessive scar tissue, the preliminary insertion of the surgeon's double-gloved finger into the rectum may be advisable for identification and guidance. The surgeon should carry the dissection to free the rectum from the posterior vaginal wall and its adherent septal tissues to a level somewhat superior or cranial to any demonstrable rectocele (Fig. 22-6).

The estimated amount of excess vaginal wall determines the amount of vaginal membrane that should be removed; the excision should involve just enough to permit a normal three-fingerbreadth vaginal introitus and vaginal caliber without demonstrable tightness and stenosis. In deciding the amount of vagina to be removed, the surgeon

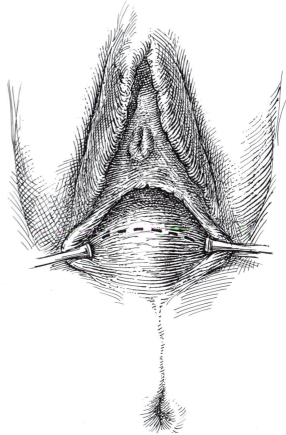

Fig. 22-5. When posterior colporrhaphy without perineorrhaphy is desired, the rectovaginal space may be entered through a transverse incision through the posterior vaginal wall proximal to the perineal body. (Modified from Nichols DH, Randall CL: *Vaginal surgery,* ed 3, Baltimore, 1989, Williams & Wilkins.)

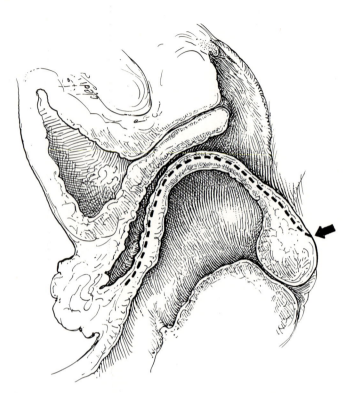

Fig. 22-6. Sagittal section demonstrating the initial line of dissection exposing the full perineum and rectocele. Above the perineum, the dissection enters the rectovaginal space and continues proximal to the highest point of the rectocele. (Modified from Nichols DH, Randall CL: *Vaginal surgery*, ed 3, Baltimore, 1989, Williams & Wilkins.)

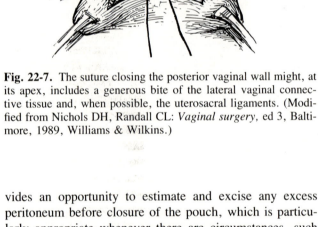

Fig. 22-7. The suture closing the posterior vaginal wall might, at its apex, includes a generous bite of the lateral vaginal connective tissue and, when possible, the uterosacral ligaments. (Modified from Nichols DH, Randall CL: *Vaginal surgery*, ed 3, Baltimore, 1989, Williams & Wilkins.)

should take the patient's endocrine age (e.g., future postmenopausal shrinkage and loss of elasticity) into account. DeCosta recommended that the introitus of an older woman be left a little "loose," anticipating that the rigidity of her husband's erection may not be as firm as that in his younger years.[8] In general, it is better to leave too much vaginal skin than too little in a multilayered repair; therefore, it is important not to excise any suspected excess vaginal membrane until the repair is essentially complete, at which time the supposed excess of vaginal epithelium often fits surprisingly well over the restored rectovaginal septum.

With a high rectocele, the vaginal incision, as well as the identification and mobilization of the connective tissue that is to become the rectovaginal septum, should be carried to the very apex of the vagina. It may be necessary to cut through the edge of the vaginal cuff to the attachment of the upper portion of the rectovaginal septum to the cul-de-sac. If the upper margin of the portion of the vaginal wall to be removed proves to be higher than the attachment of the rectovaginal septum to the bottom of the pouch of Douglas, the latter is likely to be entered. An open pouch is actually an advantage because it permits the surgeon to identify, shorten, and suture the uterosacral ligaments together under direct vision, incorporating the ligaments in the top of the posterior colporrhaphy. It also pro-

vides an opportunity to estimate and excise any excess peritoneum before closure of the pouch, which is particularly appropriate whenever there are circumstances, such as an excessively wide vault, that may predispose the patient to the development of an enterocele.

In the presence of an enterocele, when the posterior vaginal wall has less support from Denonvilliers' fascia, the surgeon can often develop support for the rectovaginal septum by bringing the so-called rectal pillars together in the midline anterior to the rectum. If the uterus has not been removed, the uppermost of the approximating sutures may incorporate the uterosacral ligaments and the posterior aspect of the uterine cervix for additional strength and stability (Fig. 22-7).

Although ballooning of the anterior rectal wall appears to be the result of a rectocele rather than the cause, the surgeon may reduce ballooning by placing one or more layers of running locked 00 or 000 absorbable suture, through the rectal muscularis and the strong submucosal layer[10,17] but *not* including the mucosa, sometimes continuing this downward posterior to the level at which the perineal body is to be reconstructed (Fig. 22-8). Then the surgeon closes the full thickness of the posterior vaginal wall from side to side, reconstructs the perineal body, and closes the perineal skin. Even during the performance of a sacrospinous colpopexy, obvious ballooning of the anterior

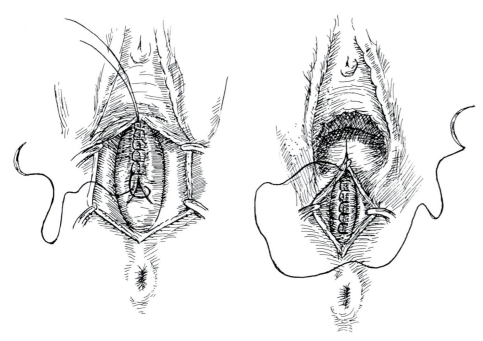

Fig. 22-8. Any ballooning of the anterior rectal wall may be corrected by one or more layers of running, locked, fine absorbable suture commencing proximal to the defect and continuing distally for its full length. Reconstitution may be carried posterior to the site of the new perineal body, yet to be restored. Side-to-side closure of the full thickness of the posterior vaginal wall is accomplished to the proximal margin of the perineal body and fixed at its cranial margin by suture to the tissue of the rectovaginal septum. In addition, reconstruction of the perineal body may be indicated. (Modified from Nichols DH, Randall CL: *Vaginal surgery,* ed 3, Baltimore, 1989, Williams & Wilkins.)

wall of the rectum should be corrected by a running locked stitch of polyglycolic acid suture material.

CLASSIC POSTERIOR COLPORRHAPHY

In performing the classic posterior colporrhaphy described by Goff,[10] the surgeon begins by picking up a bite of the hymen and its subcutaneous tissue at approximately the 3 o'clock and 9 o'clock positions with a clamp or a suture and anchoring these tissues to the perineal skin lateral to the labia majora to provide lateral traction. (Used only for retraction, these lateral sutures or clamps are removed during the final steps in the reconstruction.) The operator then normally makes a narrow V-shaped or wider U-shaped incision through the perineal skin, depending on the size of any perineal defect to be repaired. If an older patient with atrophy and narrowing of the tissues and skin of the perineum wishes to preserve her coital ability, it may be desirable to make only an initial midline skin incision that exposes the subcutaneous tissue of the perineum (Fig. 22-9). Occasionally, an inverted T-shaped incision may be made in the posterior vaginal wall to facilitate access to the rectovaginal space.

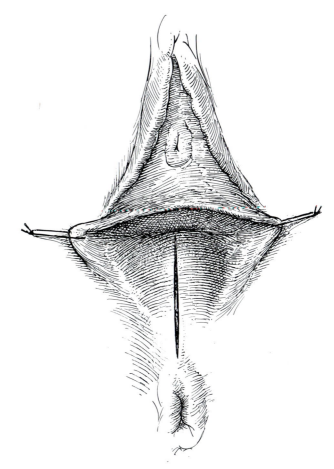

Fig. 22-9. When there is atrophy and narrowing of perineal skin, an initial midline perineal incision may be desirable to expose the base or inferior surface of the perineal body. (Modified from Nichols DH, Randall CL: *Vaginal surgery,* ed 3, Baltimore, 1989, Williams & Wilkins.)

After making the initial opening through the perineal skin, the surgeon dissects a segment of skin from the exposed structures of the perineum and perineal body, then continues upward by undermining beneath the full thickness of the posterior wall. Adhesions that thicken the normal attachments of the vaginal membrane may be the result of earlier obstetric damage, and all such attachments should be freed. In addition, in all repairs of a rectocele, it is essential that the vaginal membrane be freed of all appreciable fixation by scar tissue and be separated from all pathologic adhesions to the perineal body and the rectal wall, to a point well above any demonstrable rectocele. The surgeon undermines and frees the perineal skin flaps, exposing the surfaces of what is usually a distorted or irregularly deficient perineum and displaying the defective segments that are to be reconstructed into a more normal perineal body.

After entering the rectovaginal space, the surgeon corrects any anterior ballooning of the rectum as previously described, using one or more layers of running, locked, fine absorbable interrupted sutures placed in the muscularis and connective tissue of the anterior rectal wall, from points both above and below the area of the demonstrable rectocele.

The rectum may be displaced posteriorly by a retractor; after excision of the estimated excess of vaginal membrane, the cut edges of the full thickness of the posterior vaginal wall, including the still adherent fibers of the rectovaginal septum, are brought together by a running subcuticular suture of 0 or 00 absorbable suture (Fig. 22-10). At the apex, the suture may include a generous bite of the lateral vaginal connective tissue of the paracolpium and, possibly, of the most inferior portion of the uterosacral ligaments (Fig. 22-6), if the incision and dissection were carried into this area. Carefully and purposefully avoiding attachment to the fascia over the levator ani, the surgeon should continue the running subcuticular suture or sutures to the cranial border of the perineal body.

When the use of subcuticular suturing is undesirable because the vaginal wall seems unusually thin, a running locked suture through the full thickness of the posterior vaginal wall, if placed to avoid invagination of the cut edges, may be appropriate to reunite the vaginal membrane in the midline. Although the administration of estrogen for several weeks preoperatively may increase blood loss during the operation, it thickens a vaginal membrane that is noticeably thin (as often occurs after menopause) and facilitates closure and healing. Particularly in the closure of the vaginal membrane, it is important, first, that the sutures bring the tissues together without tension and, second, that the knots be tied loosely enough to avoid blanching the tissues. The risk of tissue strangulation is especially great when interrupted mattress-type sutures are being tied.

In a modification of the frequently used Goff technique, the surgeon may excise a wedge or segment of what is estimated to be the proper size and shape from the whole

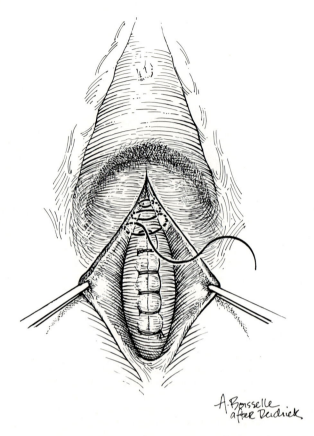

Fig. 22-10. The perirectal fascia has been plicated by a running locked suture, and the excess vaginal wall has been trimmed. The fibromuscular layer of the vaginal wall with the attached fascia of Denonvilliers is being united by a running subcuticular suture.

length and full thickness of the posterior vaginal wall, while leaving the septal layer attached.[22] It is important to estimate carefully the amount to be excised, however, if the vaginal circumference is to be sufficient for satisfactory sexual function. The amount of vaginal wall to be retained and, therefore, the size of the vagina after colporrhaphy vary according to the age of the patient, her parity, and the presence or amount of estrogenic hormones.

The surgeon approximates the lateral cut edges of the vagina, to which the rectovaginal septum has remained fused, by intravaginal subcuticular or interrupted sutures (Fig. 22-11); so they remain capable of natural independent movement, the rectum and its fascial investments should be uninvolved in this suturing. After this phase of posterior repair, the surgeon should be able to insert a finger between the anterior rectal wall and the reconstituted rectovaginal septum throughout the full length of the repair, demonstrating that the functional independence of the rectal and vaginal walls has been restored and that there is no iatrogenic fixation of the rectal wall (Fig. 22-12). The attenuated levator fascia may have been united only in the lower half or third of the vagina, which permits a more normal horizontal tilt to the upper vagina. The surgeon finally restores the subvaginal portion of the perineal body

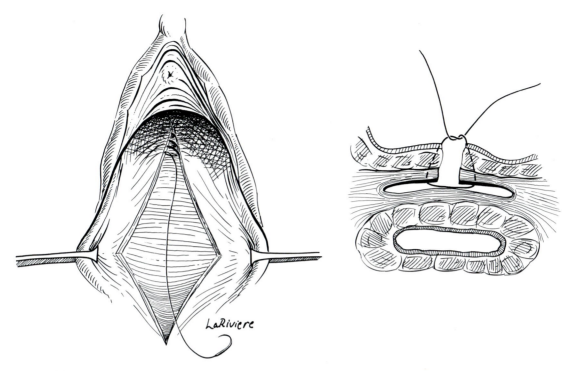

Fig. 22-11. In the Goff method of posterior colporrhaphy, an appropriate full-thickness wedge of posterior vaginal wall is excised and the tissues, including the fused rectovaginal septum, are closed from side-to-side (see upper portion of the illustrations). A subcuticular suture is preferred. (Modified from Nichols DH, Randall CL: *Vaginal surgery,* ed 3, Baltimore, 1989, Williams & Wilkins.)

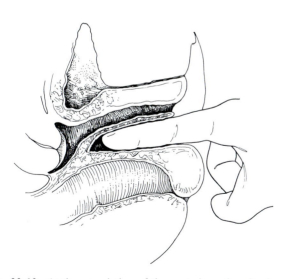

Fig. 22-12. At the completion of the posterior colporrhaphy and before starting the perineorrhaphy, the surgeon should be able to insert an index finger freely between the posterior vaginal wall to which the rectovaginal septum is attached and the anterior surface of the rectum, demonstrating the desired freedom of the plane. (Modified from Nichols DH, Randall CL: *Vaginal surgery,* ed 3, Baltimore, 1989, Williams & Wilkins.)

by interrupted sutures, continuing the suture line down the vaginal wall, over the perineal body, and back to the hymenal margin.

POSTERIOR COLPORRHAPHY BY LAYERS

The Goff technique of posterior colporrhaphy usually ensures an anatomically acceptable result, but it may not restore the integrity and function of a rectovaginal septum as reliably as the layering technique of Bullard does. Essentially, the layering technique consists of (1) separation of the septal tissues, first from the anterior rectal wall and second from the overlying vaginal membrane, and (2) thickening of the resulting layer of loosely arranged musculoconnective tissue and restoration of an appreciable layer of septum by several plicating stitches of fine suture material.

The dissection involves the following steps:

1. The surgeon incises the posterior vaginal wall in the midline to a point well above the rectocele, as far as the apex of the vagina when a high rectocele or enterocele is present.
2. The surgeon identifies the rectovaginal space and separates the rectal wall by blunt dissection from the overlying connective tissue of the rectovaginal septum, which can usually be done without difficulty.
3. By spreading the points of curved Mayo scissors in demonstrable planes of cleavage, more than by cut-

ting into or through tissue layers, the surgeon reflects the vaginal membrane anteriorly and away from the connective tissue.

These procedures result in (1) a thinned and bulging anterior rectal wall that is readily identifiable; (2) a loose and somewhat thinned posterior vaginal wall that appears excessive for the caliber of the vagina that is to be restored; and (3) a loosely incomplete, somewhat fragmented, and partially detached layer, often only sections of intervening connective tissues, all of which should be carefully preserved and incorporated by plication with fine suture material into the restoration of a demonstrably stronger rectovaginal septum.

It should be axiomatic that, as a surgeon should not capriciously discard viable tissue that can be incorporated in the repair of a herniating viscus, the gynecologist should not excise tissue that can be used in restoring a rectovaginal septum simply because it is adherent to an assumed excess of posterior vaginal wall that will probably be excised. Rather, the gynecologist should carefully identify a line of cleavage that separates connective tissue from the redundant posterior vaginal membrane and, after thickening by fine plicating sutures, attempt to use this tissue to restore the integrity of a significant rectovaginal septum between the anterior rectal wall and the posterior vaginal membrane. The objective of restoring a recognizable septal layer is the distinctive characteristic of Bullard's modification of Goff's technique of posterior colporrhaphy.

The tissues of the carefully identified rectovaginal septal layer, throughout a width of approximately 3 cm and a length of 5 to 6 cm, are united in the midline. Although thickened by a few plicating sutures, this septum is not attached by suture to either the underlying rectal wall or to the overlying posterior vaginal membrane (Fig. 22-13). It is possible to demonstrate the integrity of this thickened rectovaginal septum and its nonattachment to either the rectal or vaginal walls after the edges of the vagina have been trimmed and reunited in the midline, but before the perineal body has been sutured, by inserting two fingers simultaneously into the space available on either side of the septum, one finger between septum and vaginal wall, the other between septum and rectal wall. Reduced adhesion between the layers of repair favors independent mobility of the vagina and the rectum, an important objective of a posterior vaginal repair.

At the completion of a vaginal repair, an objective evaluation of the result is critical. If the vaginal depth and axis are not satisfactory, it is certainly preferable to make any necessary correction or modification at the time of the initial operation, provided that the patient's condition permits prolongation of the surgery. A vaginal caliber that is tight at the end of surgery will not enlarge after healing is complete. As a matter of fact, if any change occurs, particularly as the patient grows older, a tight vagina tends to become even smaller.

If the repair is satisfactory, the surgeon may minimize oozing and collection within the spaces between layers by

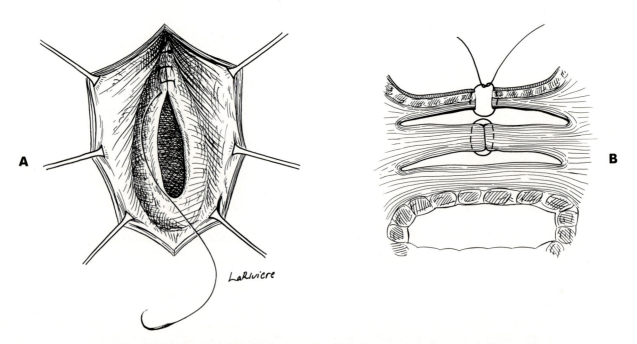

Fig. 22-13. The Bullard modification is shown in which the rectovaginal septum is dissected from the posterior vaginal wall and closed as a separate layer between rectum and vaginal membrane (**A**). When this has been accomplished, excess vaginal membrane is trimmed, and the sides are brought together by interrupted suture (**B**). A running subcuticular suture may be used. (Modified from Nichols DH, Randall CL: *Vaginal surgery,* ed 3, Baltimore, 1989, Williams & Wilkins.)

packing the vagina lightly with 2-inch plain or iodoform gauze, which can be removed the morning of the day after surgery. If the repair has resulted in a vaginal caliber obviously or even suspiciously tight, however, the surgeon may make appropriate relaxing incisions through the thickness of the lateral vaginal walls. When this has been done, the surgeon should pack the vagina rather tightly for a period longer than 24 hours. When necessary, full-thickness grafts obtained from the vaginal membrane previously resected from either the anterior or the posterior vaginal wall may be sewn into incisions parallel to the axis of the vagina made at the point or points of constriction. Portions of the vaginal membrane that have been excised should be kept wrapped in saline-soaked sponges on the nurse's instrument stand until the conclusion of the operation.

Sutures that are palpated or visualized within the lumen of the rectum should be cut immediately to lessen postoperative pain and the risk of rectovaginal or rectoperineal fistula. The cut ends will promptly retract up and out of the rectal lumen; the loss of that single suture should not jeopardize the effectiveness of the repair.

PERINEORRHAPHY

Historically, one objective of perineorrhaphy was to improve the patient's ability to retain a pessary that could be inserted into the vagina much as a cork is inserted into the neck of an inverted bottle. Under this unfortunate, and incorrect but popular, concept, a good perineal repair should prevent not only the progression of an upper vaginal prolapse, but also the development of genital prolapse in general. The fact that genital prolapse is uncommon among women with unrepaired third- and fourth-degree obstetric lacerations who had long suffered a complete loss of any support that the perineal body would have provided to the uterus, cervix, and upper vagina demonstrates the inadequacy of this concept, however.

The basic objective of perineorrhaphy is to realign the muscles and connective tissues of the perineal body to a degree that ensures normal relationships and encourages normal, comfortable function. When a patient's perineum is defective or absent, perineorrhaphy increases the vaginal depth (i.e., the length of the posterior vaginal wall; Fig. 22-14).

Defects in the perineum

A relaxed perineum, which may or may not coexist with a demonstrable rectocele, is rarely due to inadequate innervation of the muscles that contribute to the support of the components of the perineal body[28,29,32]. More commonly, it is the result of overdistention during parturition or, occasionally, the result of a poorly repaired or unrepaired obstetric laceration of the perineum. When the perineum is the sole or major site of damage, the virtual absence of the perineal body exposes an otherwise normal posterior vaginal wall to a pathologic degree, accounting for the condition known as pseudorectocele (see Fig. 22-14). In this case, the insertion of the examining finger into the rectum reveals no abnormality in rectal caliber, angulation, and tone, and no irregular distensibility of the anterior rectal wall; in addition, the posterior vaginal and anterior rectal walls are independently mobile. Symptoms are usually minimal, and the patient is often considered a can-

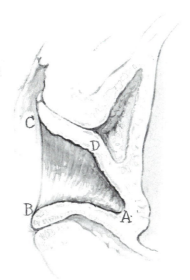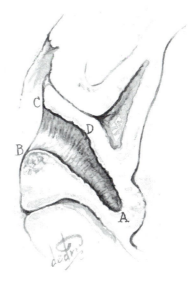

Fig. 22-14. The effect of perineorrhaphy after lengthening the posterior vaginal wall is demonstrated. Sagittal drawing of the pelvis of a patient with a defective perineum is shown on the left. The anterior vaginal wall, ADC, is longer than the posterior wall, AB. The lengthening of the posterior vagina, AB, after perineorrhaphy is shown in the drawing to the right. The length of the anterior vaginal wall, ADC, is unchanged. (Modified from Nichols DH, Randall CL: *Vaginal surgery,* ed 3, Baltimore, 1989, Williams & Wilkins.)

didate for perineal reconstruction or perineorrhaphy only when other surgery, such as vaginal hysterectomy or anterior colporrhaphy, is indicated.

The congenital absence of the perineum leaves the posterior vaginal wall exposed and simulates the appearance of rectocele, which may not be present. This condition, too, may be termed a pseudorectocele. Proper treatment requires surgical reconstruction of the defective perineum with the use of whatever tissues are available. When an acquired defect is repaired, the tissues to be reapproximated were previously in apposition, and innervation can be expected to be normal; when a congenital defect is repaired, however, connective tissues and muscle must be appropriated from the nearest fibromuscular layers.

An incomplete perineal repair leads to lateral retraction of the muscles that are normally attached to the perineal body. Detachment or interruption of the transverse perineum and the bulbospongiosus muscle must be recognized and corrected. Not only does the repair of such a detachment aid in the support of the anterior wall of the rectum, but also it adds considerable support to the anterior wall of the lower vagina and urethra. In this connection, it should be remembered that the length of the perineal body effectively approximates the length of the female urethra, in part because the medial portion of the pubococcygeal muscle, as it passes along the sides of the vagina, urethra, and rectum, sends slips of connective tissue to fuse with the capsule tissue that invests each of these hollow organs. When indicated, perineorrhaphy effectively complements the support of the anterior vaginal wall and the urethra.

In examining the patient before perineorrhaphy, it is important to recognize that, as Davies emphasized,[7]

any perineal laceration which permits the labia minora to retract laterally and expose a gaping vagina harbors the divided and retracted origin of the bulbocavernosus muscle. Such a lesion lowers the efficiency of the voluntary urethral sphincter and should be considered as an etiologic basis for stress incontinence in the female.

The examiner should also carefully note the position of the patient's anus in relation to the most dependent portion of the buttocks, the tip of the coccyx, and the ischial tuberosities. Posterior displacement of the anus strongly suggests that the anal sphincter has been detached from the perineum. This may also occur when there is a defect of the levator ani, either because of an intrinsic fault of the muscle or as a result of defective innervation of this voluntary muscle. In either instance, straining during defecation may, in effect, produce elongation and funneling of the levator ani, with the anus descending to an even more dependent position. The harder the patient strains, the more narrow the stool must become, and the more difficult defecation becomes. Obstipation is often the result. Barrett proposed that this condition be corrected by making an incision *posterior* to the rectum and attaching the separated levators to each other and to the rectal wall.[2]

Perineal body

In a woman, the perineal body is a structure of considerable anatomic and physiologic importance. It may be visualized as roughly pyramidal, and a repair must restore the body in all three dimensions. The base of the pyramid is situated beneath and parallels the perineal skin. The anterior, posterior, and two lateral surfaces converge superiorly to the most inferior limit of the rectovaginal space, fusing with the lowermost margin of the rectovaginal septum (Fig. 22-15).

The principal portion of the levator ani concerned with support of the lower vagina and birth canal attaches to the sides of the vaginal connective tissue through Luschka's fibers rather than to the muscular tissues of the posterior vaginal wall. Although perineal laceration or other obstetric trauma may lengthen, displace laterally, and sometimes detach the levator ani, such damage to the levator ani may produce only a midvaginal rectocele cranial to the perineal body. When examining such a patient, the gynecologist should note whether there is evidence of external hemorrhoids, because weakness of the perineum and anal sphincter may contribute to their development. When the upper vagina and cervix have prolapsed, however, the distention of the genital hiatus caused by the protrusion may have reduced the tone of the introitus musculature by the same mechanism as the dilating wedge of an enterocele in this area may widen the pelvic outlet. An effective repair restores much of the tone of the lateral vaginal walls, largely as a result of the removal of a major causative factor (i.e., the prolapsing cervix, uterus, or enterocele).

Most so-called levator stitches only increase the approximation of thinned or separated layers of the perineal body

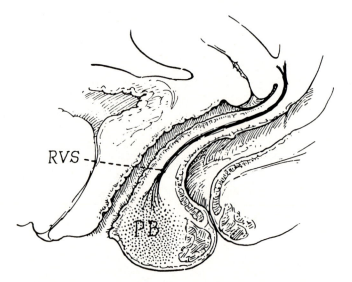

Fig. 22-15. Sagittal section shows the relationship between the rectovaginal septum *(RVS)* and the superior portion of the perineal body *(PB)* with which it blends. (From Nichols DH, Randall CL: *Vaginal surgery,* ed 3, Baltimore, 1989, Williams & Wilkins.)

and do not usually build up the levator itself. If placed far enough laterally to include the fascia of the pelvic diaphragm, they may reinforce a defective pelvic diaphragm; but, if placed directly into the belly of the levator muscle, these sutures may actually destroy portions of the muscle, eventually resulting in a shelflike ridge of nonelastic fibrous tissue within the introitus and immediately beneath the posterior vaginal wall. Superficial, side-to-side stitches are preferable because they usually reconstitute the perineal body and draw the fascia of the pubococcygeal muscles closer to the upper lateral sides of the perineal body. This effectively narrows the widened genital hiatus.

The extent to which reconstruction of a very loose vaginal outlet contributes to coital satisfaction has undoubtedly been overemphasized. Because a noticeable looseness of the vagina is not a common cause of marital incompatibility, prophylactic "tightening up" of the introitus does not necessarily improve marital relations, which are more often frayed by nonanatomic factors. Indicated correction, but not overcorrection, of a damaged or relaxed perineal body can improve coital satisfaction within an otherwise compatible domestic relationship, however.

The elasticity of the premenopausal or estrogen-maintained vagina normally permits it to grasp or contain an erect penis much as an expansible rubber glove grasps a finger. The normal-sized vagina can adapt comfortably and adequately to a large male organ, as well as to a small one. Because the elasticity of the vagina is important in preserving coital harmony, surgeons should avoid unnecessary procedures that tend to result in fibrosis and rigidity in this area.

The argument as to which muscle bundles penetrate the perineal body is, in large part, more academic than practical. The gynecologic surgeon should not regularly attempt to incorporate in the perineal body repair muscle bundles that were not there originally, because such displaced bundles are likely to be replaced by fibrosis, resulting in a loss of elasticity and persistent tenderness. The objective of repair should be based on a fairly definite concept of normal fibromuscular attachments and relationships of the perineal body. A successful restoration of the more essential relationships requires a recognition of the function of each component and attachment, and allowance for individual variation.

Operative procedure

Reconstruction begins with uncovering the perineal body along its base beneath the perineal skin and on the vaginal (anterosuperior) side. The usual transverse incision along the posterior hymenal margin is not recommended for perineorrhaphy unless the surgeon is not planning a significant perineal body reconstruction, but rather intends to direct all efforts to the repair of a rectocele well above the perineal body. Not only may a transverse incision facilitate the development of the ridgelike "dashboard"

perineum that is often associated with dyspareunia, but also it may not provide sufficient exposure of the inferior surface of the base of the perineal body for a complete perineorrhaphy. Without adequate exposure, the surgeon can reconstruct only the anterior and upper portion of the perineal body—the only exposed or denuded area—and cannot involve the equally important middle and posteroinferior portions of the perineal body in the repair. The Krobach clamp, shown in Fig. 22-16, is heavy but relatively atraumatic, providing a good grasp without tearing the tissue to which it is applied. Two of these clamps are useful during perineorrhaphy and posterior colporrhaphy; one is applied to the base of perineal skin that will remain, for which it aids exposure as it will retract by hanging down by itself. The other may be used to grasp in the midline the full thickness of the posterior vaginal wall portion that will be excised.

A V-shaped incision in the perineal skin ensures better access to more of the tissues of the perineal body than is possible with the "standard" transverse incision. Therefore, after applying clamps or traction sutures to the hymenal margin on either side, the surgeon should make a V-shaped incision (Fig. 22-17) in the perineal skin layer (U-shaped for especially large perineal defects). It is important to place the lateral traction sutures or clamps on the hymenal ring rather than on the labia minora (Fig. 22-18); if the placement of the retracting forceps or sutures is too lateral, a superficial transverse ridge or "dashboard" perineum may develop and subsequently obstruct the vagina.

Scar tissue is carefully freed by sharp dissection to mobilize the tissue from which the perineal body will be reconstructed (Fig. 22-19). The desired size of the vaginal introitus determines the appropriate width for the base of this triangle in relation to the hymenal margin. The greater the amount of epithelium removed, the smaller the caliber of the resulting vaginal orifice.

After the mobilization and removal of the excess vaginal wall and skin, the reconstruction is often accomplished

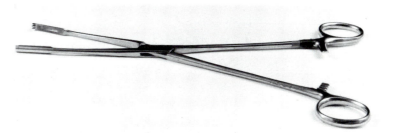

Fig. 22-16. The Krobach (or Chrobach) mouse-toothed clamp is shown. It can be obtained in the United States by special order from the custom order department of Codman-Shurtleff, New Bedford, MA, 02745, or from Mr. William Merz of Baxter–V Mueller, Chicago IL, 60648.

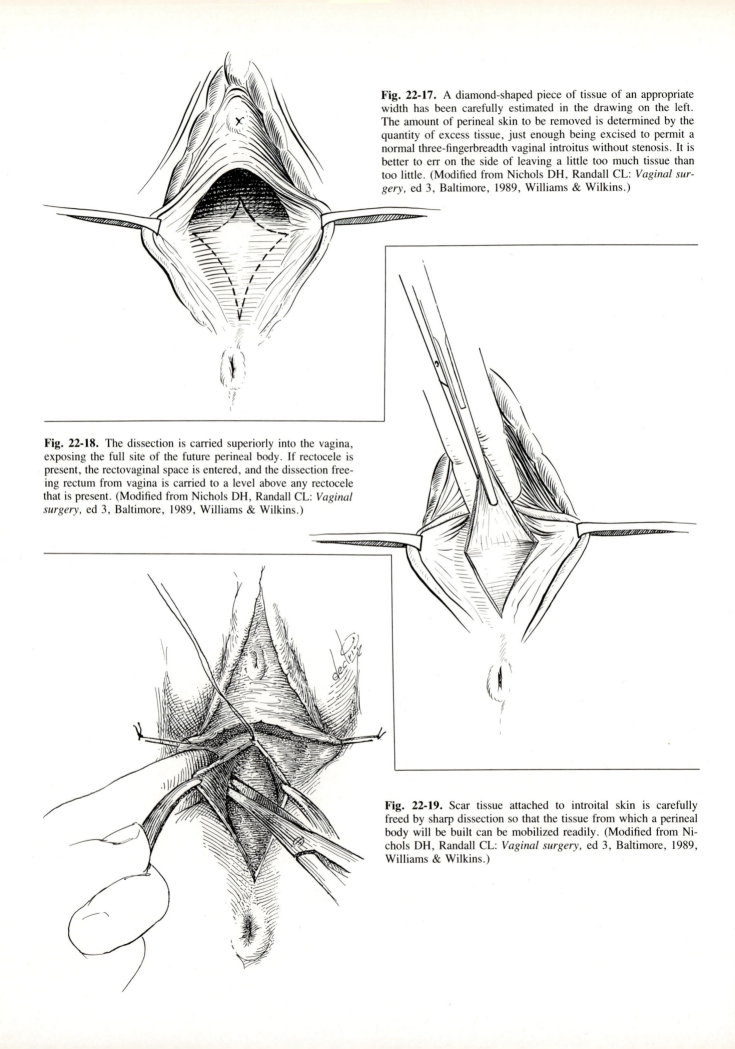

Fig. 22-17. A diamond-shaped piece of tissue of an appropriate width has been carefully estimated in the drawing on the left. The amount of perineal skin to be removed is determined by the quantity of excess tissue, just enough being excised to permit a normal three-fingerbreadth vaginal introitus without stenosis. It is better to err on the side of leaving a little too much tissue than too little. (Modified from Nichols DH, Randall CL: *Vaginal surgery,* ed 3, Baltimore, 1989, Williams & Wilkins.)

Fig. 22-18. The dissection is carried superiorly into the vagina, exposing the full site of the future perineal body. If rectocele is present, the rectovaginal space is entered, and the dissection freeing rectum from vagina is carried to a level above any rectocele that is present. (Modified from Nichols DH, Randall CL: *Vaginal surgery,* ed 3, Baltimore, 1989, Williams & Wilkins.)

Fig. 22-19. Scar tissue attached to introital skin is carefully freed by sharp dissection so that the tissue from which a perineal body will be built can be mobilized readily. (Modified from Nichols DH, Randall CL: *Vaginal surgery,* ed 3, Baltimore, 1989, Williams & Wilkins.)

by side-to-side reapproximation of denuded tissues, both deep and superficial. The upper portion of this side-to-side reapproximation of the perineal body should pull the pubococcygeal muscles closer, although the sutures should not actually include them. This procedure narrows the genital hiatus. Lower placed stitches bring the transverse perinei together, helping to reconstruct the lower portion of the urogenital diaphragm. Similar sutures reattach the bulbospongiosus muscles to the perineal body.

Any detachment of the connective tissue of the rectovaginal septum from the cranial or uppermost portion of the perineal body must be remedied by surgical reattachment to ensure the restoration of normal function, particularly in regard to the role of the perineum and its continuity with the rectovaginal septum during the act of defecation. Because there may be considerable scarring from previous trauma in this vulnerable area, dissection through indistinct cleavage planes should proceed with caution to avoid penetration of the rectum. Reattachment and restoration relieve the problem of incomplete bowel movements, and it is unlikely to recur. To reattach or reinforce the attachment of the fascia of Denonvilliers to the perineal body, the surgeon should carry the dissection for perineorrhaphy higher than the defect to be repaired, always opening into the rectovaginal space and then attaching the underside of the posterior vaginal wall in the rectovaginal space to the most cranial buried stitch of the perineorrhaphy.

During reconstruction of the lower third of the vagina when the perineal defect is extreme and there is little tissue available for the reconstruction, it may be necessary to provide better support to the rectal ampulla; in this instance, the operator may bring the medial margins of the puborectal or pubococcygeal muscles together by a small series of superficially placed and loosely tied interrupted sutures, which, in turn, may at their insertion be attached to a sagging ampulla (Fig. 22-20). Lee[17] describes his satisfaction with the posterior repair that interposes stitches uniting the pubococcygei between the rectum and vagina. In providing such support, it is important to avoid the production of troublesome and inevitably tender ridges beneath the posterior vaginal wall. After placing each stitch and before tying it, the surgeon should cross the ends of the suture and apply traction. If there is a palpable ridge, the operator should promptly remove and replace the stitch, usually closer to the rectum. When perineal surgery is performed under local anesthesia, the voluntary muscle bundles may be more readily identified.

The retracted ends of often long-separated bulbospongiosus muscles should be identified and reattached to the perineal body. Separated segments of the transverse perinei should also be reunited if the medial edge of the levator ani and the puborectal muscle can be identified. In the correction of a low rectocele, the adjacent fascia of the pelvic diaphragm is attached to the posterolateral surface of the vagina, duplicating the original attachment of Luschka's fibers, fixing and holding the vagina in place. The

placement of a few interrupted horizontally placed, loosely tied perineal sutures brings together the smooth muscle of the perineal body (Fig. 22-21), helping to reestablish its integrity.

Although not a common result of perineal injury during childbirth, posterior displacement of the anus must be repaired. It is necessary to reattach the capsule of the external sphincter ani to the perineal body, for example, by using a figure-eight suture (Fig. 22-22) as described by Kennedy and Campbell.[15] This step, which stabilizes the perineum, is similar to reattaching spokes to the hub of a wheel (perineal body).

Operative compression of the veins that communicate with hemorrhoids often temporarily aggravates existing hemorrhoids. As postoperative edema subsides, however, a new tissue equilibrium usually develops. The hemorrhoids may undergo involution and improvement, especially if any sphincter weakness has been corrected. For this reason, hemorrhoidectomy should not be done at the same time as a posterior colporrhaphy. The need for hemorrhoidectomy can be evaluated better several months postoperatively.

The superficial perineal fascia may be brought together, and the perineal skin may be closed with running or interrupted sutures. Subcuticular sutures should be used in the closure of both the vaginal epithelium and the perineal skin, with care to avoid irregularities in the approximation of the edges being united or in invaginations of epithelial edges. Irregular bulging or invaginations in the suture line are likely to cause granulations and irregularities in healing that may account for persistent tenderness in the scar.

In [Figure 22-20, *F*] is shown an instrument under study to be used in an attempt to take some of the guesswork out of the repair of the pelvic floor when a functional vagina is desirable. Some of our predecessors sensed the need for such a device if only to impress upon operators the importance of preoperative study in this surgery. Its inclusion in a text of this type is justified when one realizes that in describing a vaginal plastic operation writers find themselves without some standard object that could be used to tell the reader how big to make the vagina. One wonders how long it may take for the vagina to come into its rightful place among the organs upon which plastic surgery is performed. While moulages are made of future noses, while artists draw ears to guide plastic surgeons, and even simple grafts are planned and plotted days in advance, vaginal plastic surgery is undertaken with a shameful lack of study. Habitually the operators' fingers are unceremoniously poked into the field of operation to determine the ultimate dimensions of the organ. Fat fingers, thin fingers, big fingers, or small fingers—this technique has yet to be replaced by something more esthetic and reliable. While constrictions and dyspareunia, recurrent relaxations and gaping, and scarring and abnormal fixation have been all too frequent results in vaginal surgery, the same postoperative appearance would scarcely be tolerated elsewhere. Should not the guesswork be taken out of this surgery?

While the vaginal surgeon may passionately desire faithfully to restore the virginal dimensions, axis, contour, and markings of his subject, this is not possible. In place of this the objective is resolutely to reconstruct a functional, pain-free, pliable, distensi-

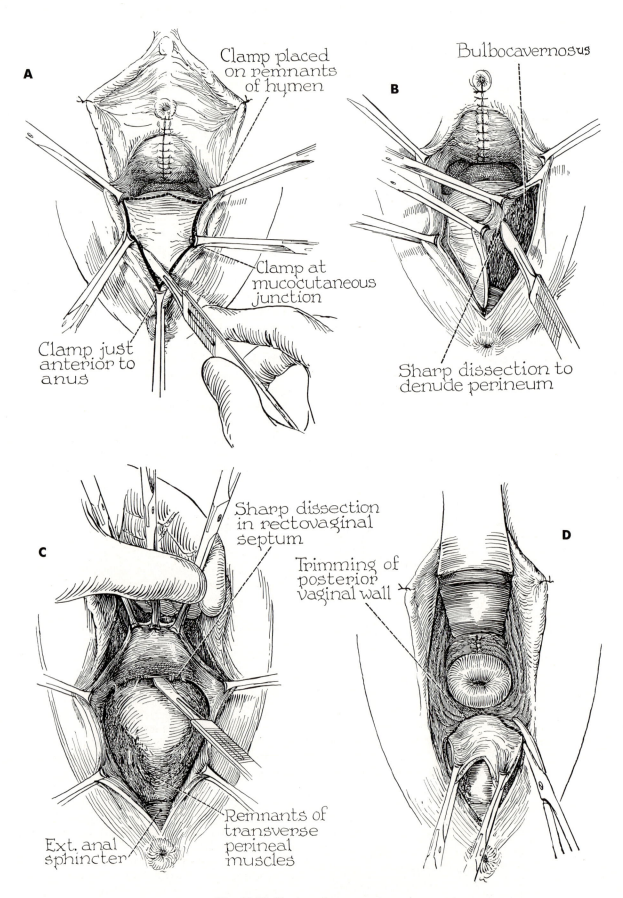

A Clamp placed on remnants of hymen

Clamp at mucocutaneous junction

Clamp just anterior to anus

B Bulbocavernosus

Sharp dissection to denude perineum

C Sharp dissection in rectovaginal septum

Ext. anal sphincter

Remnants of transverse perineal muscles

D Trimming of posterior vaginal wall

Fig. 22-20. For legend see opposite page.

ble, and well-supported structure. The dimensions of the instrument under study are based on the studies of Dickinson, who has made some of the most memorable contributions to the human sex anatomy. He insisted on distinguishing the anatomy of the "quick from the dead," a philosophy vaginal surgeons should devoutly embrace.[1]

ENDORECTAL REPAIR OF RECTOCELE

Block[4] points out that the traditional transvaginal approach to rectocele repair is indispensable when associated with conditions such as cystocele, enterocele, and uterine or vaginal vault prolapse. Sehapayak[27] has emphasized that simultaneous transvaginal posterior repair coincident with endorectal repair of rectocele is contraindicated, since interruption of the natural barriers or mucosal lining on both sides of the rectovaginal septum at the same time may invite infection, abscess formation, and subsequent rectovaginal fistula.

If the size of the rectal reservoir is too large following transvaginal posterior colporrhaphy, and the bowel movements are still incomplete and may still require manual expression, a surgeon finding conditions and scarring unsuitable for reoperation by the vaginal route lest the vagina be made too small for coital comfort may wish to consider endorectal repair.[3-6,16,27,31]

This is a relatively simple operation to correct low or midvaginal rectocele designed to reduce the size of the luminal rectal reservoir.

Sullivan[31] first described the endorectal repair of rectocele permitting, after mucosal incision and dissection of

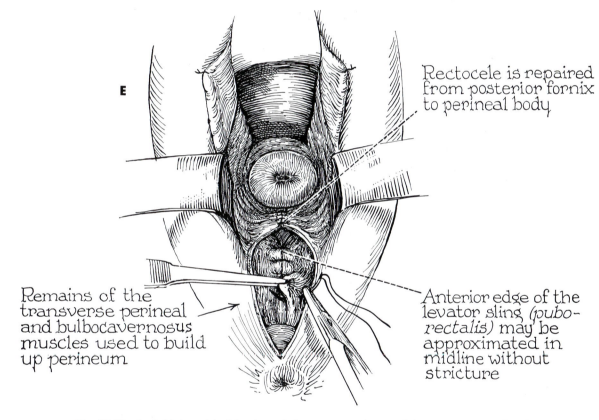

Fig. 22-20. **A,** A V-shaped incision is made between two clamps of the mucocutaneous junction on the posterior vaginal wall as shown, the widths of the V being determined by the extent to which the vagina will be narrowed. This flap is dissected from the underlying perineal body and adjacent scar tissue, and the incision carried in the vagina as indicated by the dashed line of an amount appropriate to the degree by which the vagina will be narrowed postoperatively. **B,** This flap is separated by sharp dissection, using either curved Mayo scissors or a scalpel, from the underlying muscle, scar tissue and connective tissue as shown. **C,** This is carried the full depth of the rectocele, until a point cranial to the rectocele has been reached. If an enterocele is encountered, it is opened and the sac resected and the neck closed. **D,** The excess posterior vaginal wall is trimmed as shown by the dashed line, and reapproximated using a running subcuticular suture that incorporates the full thickness of the posterior vaginal wall. Any ballooning of the anterior rectal wall is corrected by plication, and the pararectal fascia may be reapproximated by running or interrupted subcuticular sutures. Just before the skin of the perineum is closed, it should be possible for the operator to insert a finger between the undersurface of the posterior vaginal wall and the anterior surface of the rectum, indicating the preservation of the rectovaginal space. **E,** If there is little tissue of substance to be used to support this area, the anterior medial edge of the fascia of the puborectalis may be brought together with interrupted stitches, presuming that they are placed close enough to the rectum that no subvaginal ridges are palpable.

Continued.

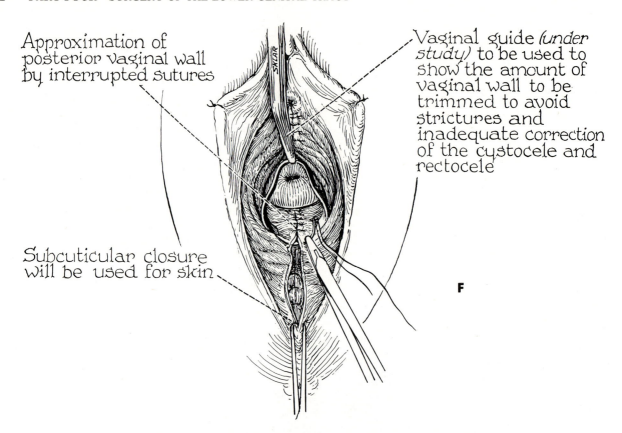

Approximation of
posterior vaginal wall
by interrupted sutures

Vaginal guide *(under study)* to be used to show the amount of vaginal wall to be trimmed to avoid strictures and inadequate correction of the cystocele and rectocele

Subcuticular closure
will be used for skin

F

Fig. 22-20, cont'd. F, The remainder of the posterior vaginal wall is closed, the perineum reconstructed with some interrupted stitches, and the skin closed by a subcuticular suture as shown. (From Ball TL: *Gynecologic surgery and urology,* ed 2, St. Louis, 1963, Mosby Year Book.)

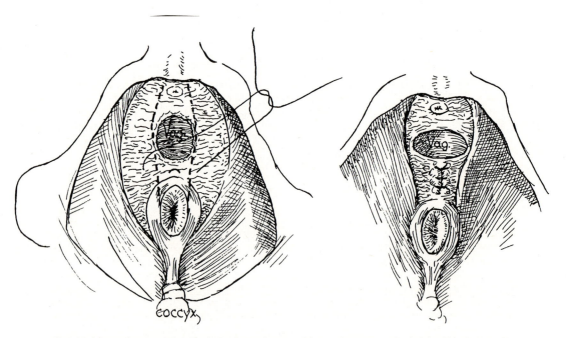

Fig. 22-21. Perineorrhaphy may be accomplished without placement of stitches directly into the bellies of the pubococcygeal muscles, as shown with the wide genital hiatus to the left of the drawing. When the interrupted stitches in the perineal body have been tied, the lateral attachments of this tissue to the fascia of the pubococcygeal muscles bring the latter closer together, narrowing the genital hiatus, to a new position as noted by the dashed line. The end result is illustrated at the right. The genital hiatus has been effectively narrowed. No stitches have been placed directly into the pubococcygi. (Modified from Nichols DH, Randall CL: *Vaginal surgery,* ed 3, Baltimore, 1989, Williams & Wilkins.)

flaps, a transanal exposure and plication of the underside of the rectovaginal septum, excision of redundant or prolapsed rectal mucosa, and correction of any coincident anorectal pathology.

Jansen et al[13] noted the importance of the submucosal layers in intestinal healing first described by Halsted[11] as the strongest part of the intestinal wall. Lord et al[18] demonstrated by scanning electron microscopy that it is a honeycomb of collagen fibers forming a strong skeleton-like cylinder through the entire length of the intestine. It contains a plexus of arterial vascularization.[30] They determined that surgical anastomosis with inversion of the intestinal layers with good submucosal approximation resulted in primary intestinal healing and rapid restoration of villous epithelium, but with bad approximation resulted in secondary healing with a predictably weaker scar.

As emphasized by Capps[6] and by Khubchandani[16] and associates, the endorectal repair can be done under local infiltration anesthesia during a short hospitalization. This approach also permits transrectal reattachment of the puborectalis to the perineal body. They report a high rate of success and low incidence of complications.

Preoperative rectal mechanical cleansing such as by electrolyte solution (Nu-Lytely) given the evening before surgery, or enemas until clear, add but a few minutes to the total preparatory time. The operation is performed as follows:

A Fansler rectal retractor is inserted into the rectum, the obturator removed, and each quadrant of the rectal mucosa carefully examined. The anterior rectal wall at the site of the rectocele and defect in the submucosa is identified and the full thickness of the anterior rectal wall grasped by a suture of absorbable material—either polyglycolic acid or chromic catgut, size 00 (Fig. 22-23). This excess anterior rectal wall is incorporated in a tightly drawn running locked stitch, which closes the weakness in the anterior wall of the rectum in a longitudinal direction cephalad to the initial stitch. As traction is exerted on each stitch as it is placed, the submucosa is tented toward the surgeon, facilitating placement of the succeeding suture. Although the full thickness of the rectal wall is included in this obliterative suture, digital examination of the vagina during the

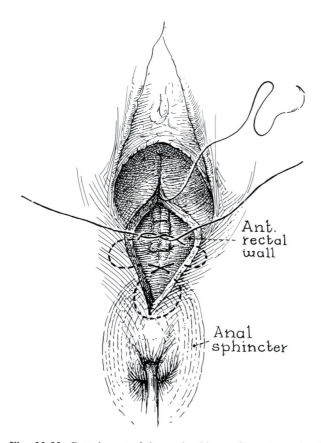

Fig. 22-22. Detachment of the anal sphincter from the perineal body may be restored by a buried figure-eight suture placed as shown. This will stabilize both the anus and the perineal body. (Modified from Nichols DH, Randall CL: *Vaginal surgery,* ed 3, Baltimore, 1989, Williams & Wilkins.)

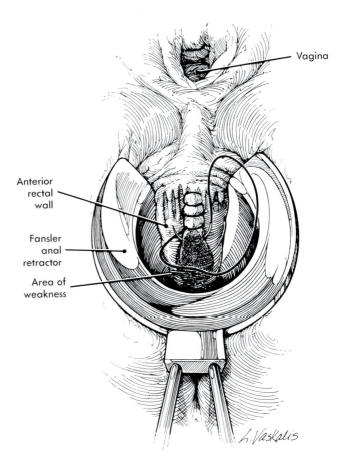

Fig 22-23. Endorectal repair of rectocele. A Fansler rectal retractor has been inserted into the rectum, and the redundant mucosa and submucosa of the weakened anterior rectal wall have been identified. Starting just proximal to the mucocutaneous junction a running locked obliterative suture has been started. The suture is placed through both mucosal and submucosal layers and may include the rectal muscularis. With each stitch the suture is tightly drawn. No portion of the intact vaginal wall is included in the suture. When the rectal tissue of the rectocele has been obliterated to a point cranial to the low or midvaginal rectocele, the direction of the suture is reversed and a second obliterative layer is placed reinforcing the initial layer.

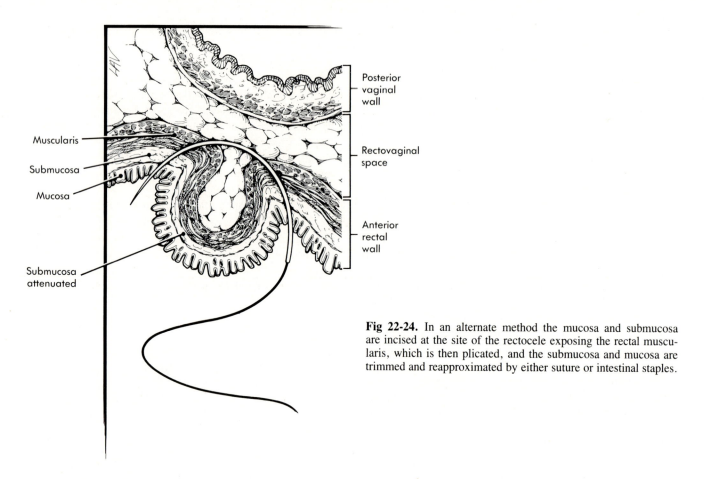

Muscularis

Submucosa

Mucosa

Submucosa
attenuated

Posterior
vaginal
wall

Rectovaginal
space

Anterior
rectal
wall

Fig 22-24. In an alternate method the mucosa and submucosa are incised at the site of the rectocele exposing the rectal muscularis, which is then plicated, and the submucosa and mucosa are trimmed and reapproximated by either suture or intestinal staples.

suturing makes certain that attachment to or penetration of the vagina has not occurred. The suture is carried to a point about 1 cm past the upper edge of the rectocele, then returned as a reinforcing lock-stitch to the beginning of the suture line and tied there. Each stitch must be pulled tightly to exert a strangulating effect on the tissue contained within the suture.

Block[5] describes the obliterative suture as "essentially a tightly drawn running lock-stitch which strangulates and causes to slough the tissues in the grip of each stitch, yet preserves the viability and approximates the tissues at the base of the suture. This surgical maneuver is peculiarly adapted to rectal surgery, since it cannot be used anywhere else in the body, but in the rectum it is an amazingly versatile tool for the surgeon."

Alternatively, in the techniques of Sullivan[31], Capps[6], and Sehapayak[27] the mucosal and submucosal layers are dissected off the underlying rectal muscularis, which is then plicated and the mucosa closed by a separate layer.

At about the 12 o'clock position, the rectal mucosa may be grasped and incised longitudinally from within the rectum, undermined and reflected laterally. The rectal side of the rectal muscularis is plicated,[6,16,,27,31] excess mucosa is trimmed, and the edges sewn or stapled without tension (Fig. 22-24). If desired, a predetermined full thickness of the rectal wall including the muscularis may be excised in its longitudinal axis following endorectal clamping and su-

turing or stapling (GIA endo 30 or 60) with excision of this predetermined full-thickness portion of the rectal wall in its longitudinal axis. Coincident endorectal pathology, such as excision of symptomatic hemorrhoids or mucosal prolapse or removal of any rectal polyps can be undertaken simultaneously if within the operator's area of expertise.

Endorectal repair of rectocele avoids the possibility of vaginal stricture, dyspareunia, or rectovaginal fistula.

REFERENCES
1. Ball TL: *Gynecologic surgery and urology,* ed 2, St Louis, 1963, Mosby–Year Book.
2. Barrett CW: Hernias through the pelvic floor, *Am J Obstet Dis Wom* 59:553, 1909.
3. Bethoux JP: *Traitement chirurgical des rectoceles, Ann Gastroenterol Hepatol* 23:217-220, 1987.
4. Block IR: Transrectal repair of rectocele using obliterative suture, *Dis Colon Rectum* 29:707-711, 1986.
5. Block IR: *Dis Colon Rectum* 30:314, 1987 (letter to the editor).
6. Capps WF: Rectoplasty and perineoplasty for the symptomatic rectocele, *Dis Colon Rectum* 18:237-244, 1975.
7. Davies JW: In Ullery JC, editor: *Stress incontinence in the female,* p 33, New York, 1953, Grune & Stratton.
8. DeCosta EJ: After office hours—"dance me loose," *Obstet Gynecol* 6:120, 1955.
9. Delancey JOL: Anatomic aspects of vaginal eversion after hysterectomy, *Am J Obstet Gynecol* 166:1717-1728, 1992.
10. Goff BH: A practical consideration of the damaged pelvic floor with a technique for its secondary reconstruction, *Surg Gynecol Obstet* 46:866, 1968.

11. Halsted WS: Circular suture of the intestine; an experimental study, *Am J Med Sci* 94:436-461, 1887.
12. Harrison JE, McDonagh JE: Hernia of Douglas' pouch and high rectocele, *Am J Obstet Gynecol* 60:83, 1950.
13. Jansen A et al: The importance of the apposition of the submucosal intestinal layers for primary wound healing of intestinal anastomosis, *Surg Gynecol Obstet* 152:51-58, 1981.
14. Jeffcoate TNA: Posterior colporrhaphy, *Am J Obstet Gynecol* 77:490, 1959.
15. Kennedy JW, Campbell AD: *Vaginal hysterectomy,* Philadelphia, 1942, FA Davis.
16. Khubchandani IT et al: Endorectal repair of rectocele, *Dis Colon Rectum* 26:792-796, 1983.
17. Lee RA: *Atlas of gynecologic surgery,* Philadelphia, 1992, WB Saunders.
18. Lord MG, Valies P, Broughton AC: A morphologic study of of submucosa of the large intestine, *Surg Gynecol Obstet* 145:155-160, 1977.
19. Malpas P: *The choice of operation for genital prolapse.* In Meigs JV, Sturgis SH: *Progress in gynecology, vol 111,* New York, 1957, Grune & Stratton.
20. Marks MM: The rectal side of rectocele, *Dis Colon Rectum* 10:387-388, 1967.
21. Milley PS, Nichols DH: A corrective investigation of the human rectovaginal septum, *Anat Rec* 163:433, 1968.
22. Nichols DH, Randall CL: *Vaginal surgery,* ed 3, Baltimore, 1989, Williams and Wilkins.
23. Nichols DH: Posterior colporrhaphy and perineorrhaphy: separate and distinct operations, *Am J Obstet Gynecol* 164:714-721, 1991.
24. Porges RF: A practical system of diagnosis and classification of pelvic relaxations, *Surg Gynecol Obstet* 117:769, 1963.
25. Ricci JV, Thom CH: The myth of a surgically useful fascia in vaginal plastic reconstructions, *Obstet Gynecol* 7:253, 1954.
26. Richter K: Erkrankungen der Vagina. In Schwalm H, Doderlein G, Wulf KH, editors: *Klinik der Frauenheikunde und Geburtshille,* vol 8, Munich, 1971, Urban & Schwarzenberg.
27. Sehapayak S: Transrectal repair of rectocele: an extended armamentarium of colorectal surgeons, *Dis Colon Rectum* 28:422-433, 1985.
28. Snooks SJ, Burnes PRH, Swash M: Abnormalities of the innervation of the voluntary anal and urethral sphincters in incontinence: an electrophysiological study *J Neurol Neurosurg Pyschiatry* 47:1269-1273, 1984.
29. Snooks SJ et al: Risk factors in childbirth causing damage to the pelvic floor innervation, *Int J Colorectal Dis* 1:20-24, 1986.
30. Spjut HJ: Microangiographic study of gastrointestinal lesions, *Am J Roentgenol* 91:1187, 1974.
31. Sullivan ES, Leaverton GH, Hardwick CE: Transrectal perineal repair: an adjunct to improved function after anorectal surgery, *Dis Colon Rectum* 11:106-114, 1968.
32. Swash M: *Electromyography in pelvic floor disorders.* In Henry MM, Swash M: *Colpoproctology and the Pelvic Floor,* ed 2, Oxford, 1992, Butterworth-Heinemann.
33. Tobin CE, Benjamin JA: Anatomical and surgical restudy of Denonvilliers' fascia, *Surg Gynecol Obstet* 80:373, 1945.
34. Uhlenhuth E, Nolley GW: Vaginal fascia, a myth? *Obstet Gynecol* 10:349, 1957.

Chapter 23

THE SCHAUTA-AMREICH RADICAL VAGINAL HYSTERECTOMY

Luigi Carenza
Flavia Nobili
Ankica Lukic

The operating technique through the vaginal route is a prerogative of gynecologic surgery and is an essential prerequisite in the cultural and surgical training of every qualified gynecologist.

HISTORY

Gynecologic surgery witnessed a revolution in the middle of the last century when surgeons came to realize the huge possibilities open to them following the discovery of anesthesia and antisepsis.

According to research sources, the treatment of cervical cancer by a vaginal technique was introduced in 1829 by J.P. Warren,[63] a surgeon at Harvard University. The first radical vaginal hysterectomy was performed in 1887 by K. Pawlik[40] and later (in 1893) by K. Schuchardt,[49] whose incision technique rendered radical surgery easier to perform. F. Schauta[48] performed his first radical vaginal operation on June 1, 1901, having somewhat altered the existing technique.

At first the technique met with little approval, unlike the radical abdominal hysterectomy introduced in 1898 by E. Wertheim,[66] a pupil of Friedrich Schauta at the University Gynecologic Clinic in Prague, whose technique gained widespread support. However, the initial results achieved with the Wertheim technique revealed an operative mortality rate eight times higher than Schauta's (18.6% versus 2.3%). Schauta highlighted the advantages of the vaginal technique: less stress from surgery, reduced blood loss, and, in particular, a marked drop in septic complications, much feared at that time on account of the high mortality and morbidity associated with them.[48,67] Schauta therefore deserves credit for having developed a systematic radical

procedure in 1901, which was handed down to fellow gynecologists.

In the late 1920s, despite improved methods of anesthesia, the introduction of blood transfusion, and control of the electrolytic balance, the advantages of the vaginal route were evident,[23,41,65] in terms of both primary mortality and 5-year survival rate, probably in part because of the more radical surgery performed at that time to remove the parametria via the vaginal route.

The Schauta surgical technique was subsequently altered by gynecologists like J. Halban,[25] W. Stockel,[55] and, in particular, I. Amreich,[1] whose efforts resulted in an improvement of the technique that made it possible to thoroughly remove pelvic connective tissue, an accomplishment unmatched by previous vaginal procedures. This period, which was marked by important new developments in radical gynecologic surgery, gave way to a less eventful period, which also coincided with the advent of radiotherapy.

In the 1940s, the surgical treatment of cervical carcinoma began to make further progress, while certain forms of this pathology proved to be resistant to radiotherapy. Further progress in medical science greatly reduced the number of patients classified as at high risk for surgery via the abdominal route, thus bridging the gap between the operability rates of both procedures.

ADVANTAGES

For many years, radical vaginal surgery was a selective surgical treatment for early-stage cervical cancer, providing a number of advantages that should not be underestimated today. These advantages include:

Table 23-4. Frequency of lymph node metastasis on the basis of invasion depth

Authors	Years	Depth of invasion ≤ 3.0 mm		Depth of invasion 3.1-5.0 mm	
		No. of patients	No. of patients with positive nodes	No. of patients	No. of patients with positive nodes
Foushee, Greiss, and Lock[19]	1969	16	0	13	1
Roche and Norris[44]	1975	9	0	21	0
Leman et al[32]	1976	32	0	3	0
Seski, Abell, and Morley[50]	1977	37	0	0	0
Taki et al[58]	1979	55	0	0	0
Yajima and Noda[69]	1979	90	0	0	0
Hasumi, Sakamoto, and Sugano[26]	1980	106	1	29	4
Van Nagell et al[61]	1983	52	0	32	3
Creasman et al[13]	1985	24	0	8	0
Simon et al[52]	1986	43	0	26	1
Maiman et al[33]	1988	65	1	30	4
TOTAL		529	2 (0.38%)	162	13 (8.02%)

vasion, and histologic grade—which, especially when correlated to the conditions of the lymph nodes, have highlighted subgroups at risk within FIGO stages. Likewise in the case of microcarcinoma, the depth of the stromal invasion made it possible to distinguish stage Ia1 from stage Ia2.

The almost total absence of lymph node metastases with an invasion depth of 3 mm or less (according to data in the literature) and the extremely low rate of recurrence after surgery have led to a standardization of treatment by simple conization or simple hysterectomy with follow-up in stage Ia1 cases.[20,30] On the other hand, the frequency of lymph node metastases reported in Ia2 cases (Table 23-4) seems to be an indication for pelvic lymphadenectomy in combination with more or less radical hysterectomy.[2,20,30]

In stage Ib, the tumor size (less than, equal to, or greater than 3 cm), which is closely correlated to the condition of the lymph nodes and hence to survival, has determined different forms of therapy.[8,12] Consequently, today radical vaginal hysterectomy is justified only in patients who are at high risk for the abdominal procedure and when the preoperative lymph node trial is negative (e.g., CT, lymphography) in stages Ia2 and small Ib tumors (less than or equal to 3 cm), in the absence of additional adverse prognostic factors. Ovarian conservation and function are thus permitted in premenopausal patients not receiving pelvic radiation.

A thorough preoperative histologic and biologic investigation (on biopsy or cone) might prove, through a multivariant analysis of various prognostic factors, even those studied more recently (e.g., nuclear grading, ploidy, proliferative activity, oncogene and growth factor expression), to be useful for a preoperative identification of less aggressive clinical forms (with a lower incidence of lymph node metastases) that could be treated by radical vaginal surgery.

Surgical treatment of carcinoma of the cervical stump is no longer exclusively confined to the vaginal route but, in our opinion, depends on the clinical stage of the neoplasia and the patient's performance status. We believe that endocervical adenocarcinoma is a contraindication for this surgical procedure because of the evidently greater biologic invasiveness and the greater likelihood of lymph node involvement.

PREOPERATIVE EVALUATION AND PREPARATION OF PATIENT

Once the neoplastic lesion has been ascertained, the patient is carefully examined to evaluate her condition and to effect a correct staging of the disease. Routine diagnostic tests are performed, including complete blood count with platelets, urinalysis, SMA-12, electrocardiogram, chest x-ray, intravenous pyelogram, lymphangiography, cystoscopy, proctoscopy, and pelvic examination under anesthesia. Since 1982, we have also included a preoperative abdominopelvic CT and, more recently, pelvic MRI for certain selected cases.

The patient is put on a low-residue diet 3 to 4 days before surgery and a fully liquid diet 1 day before surgery. Mineral oil is administered 2 days preoperatively, followed by an enema the morning and evening preceding the operation.

The patient is administered antibiotics 24 hours before surgery to reduce the bacterial population in the bowel and is scrubbed with an antibacterial cleanser and two vaginal douches.

INSTRUMENTS

To perform the Schauta-Amreich vaginal operation correctly, specific surgical instruments have to be used in addition to standard operating room instruments. These include a complete set of Schauta retractors (Fig. 23-1), Chrobak (or Krobach) clamps, d'Allaines clamps, Collin clamps, Heaney clamps, Overholt clamps, and Mixter clamps (Fig. 23-2).

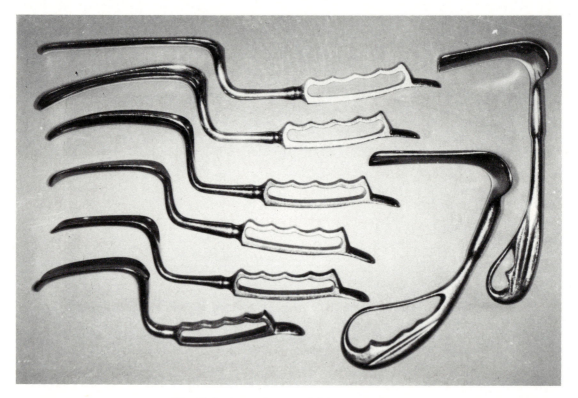

Fig. 23-1. A complete set of Schauta retractors.

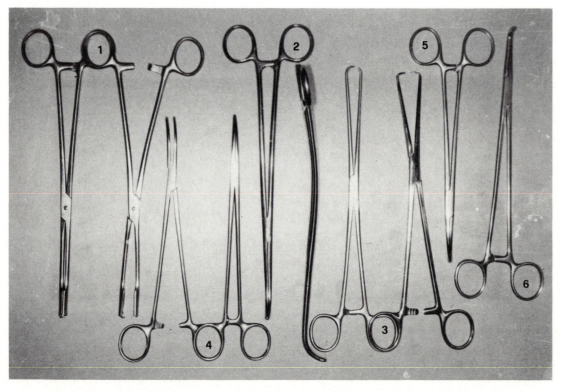

Fig. 23-2. *1*, Chrobak clamps; *2*, d'Allaines clamps; *3*, Collin clamps; *4*, Heaney clamps; *5*, Overholt clamp; and *6*, Mixter clamp.

OPERATIVE TECHNIQUE
Preparatory phase

The patient is placed on the operating table in a lithotomy position to allow easier access to pelvic organs through the vaginal route. The operative field (external genitalia, vagina, vulva, upper thirds of the thighs, and pubic area) is disinfected with Betadine (Purdue Frederick Co, Norwalk, Conn) and enclosed with sterile drapes. A Foley bladder catheter is inserted, and a thorough rectovaginal examination is performed while the patient is under anesthesia. The cervix and upper and middle thirds of the vagina are swabbed with a Schiller iodine solution to determine the extent of the neoplastic lesion.

Schuchardt incision and preparation of left pararectal space

To facilitate dissection and to augment local hemostasis, an ischemizing infiltration of up to 120 ml of 1% carbocaine and adrenalin 1:200,000 diluted in 3:1 normal saline solution is administered. Eighty ml of this solution are injected along the expected course of the incision, and the remaining 40 ml are injected circularly in the paracervical regions (Fig. 23-3). After a 10 to 15 minute interval the surgeon performs the Schuchardt incision. The incision is made at the junction between the posterior wall and the left lateral wall of the vagina, kept under tension respectively by the left index finger of the operator and the right index finger of the second assistant. The apex of the incision will depend on the amount of vaginal cuff to be removed: the base will extend to the borderline of the vulva and to the perineal skin for 3 to 5 cm. The incision is made with a scalpel through the full thickness of the vagina and through subcutaneous tissue as far as the levator ani (Figs. 23-4 and 23-5). The operator then introduces the right index finger at the apex of the incision in the left pararectal space (ischiorectal fossa) above the levator muscle and displaces the rectum medially, pushing the finger repeatedly in a lateromedial direction. The rectum is thus freed from its attachments to the levator. Identification of the ischial spine is a useful anatomic reference to confirm correct performance of this maneuver. Only slight bleeding will occur if the infiltration has been performed and if planes have been identified anatomically.

At this point the levator ani, kept under tension by the operator's left index finger, is dissected sharply as far as its proximal part, which is not severed to facilitate subsequent reconstruction of the muscle (Fig. 23-6). The left pararectal space is now completely exposed.

The Schuchardt incision offers two advantages: it extends the field of operation and affords complete preparation of the left pararectal space.

This phase may be complicated by some troublesome bleeding that can usually be controlled by ligation of the most visible blood vessels. When bleeding is mild and diffuse, it is sufficient to apply a warm gauze packing to the incision.

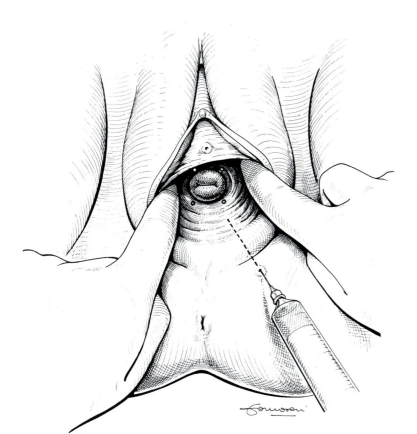

Fig. 23-3. Ischemizing infiltration along the expected course of the Schuchardt incision and in the paracervical regions.

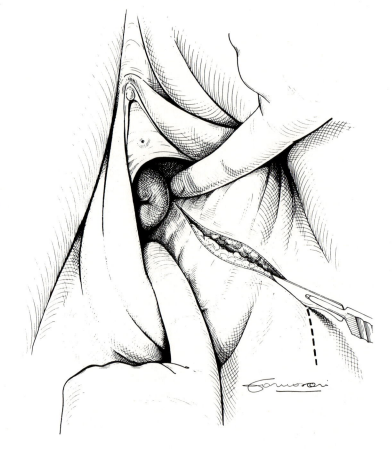

Fig. 23-4. The Schuchardt incision (dissection of vaginal wall and perineal plane).

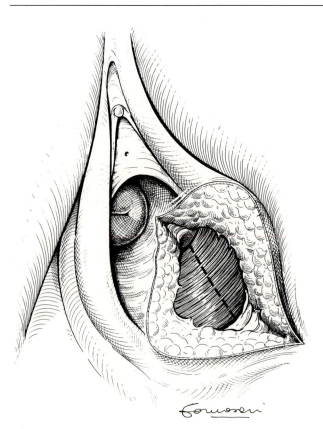

Fig. 23-5. Exposure of levator ani and its line incision.

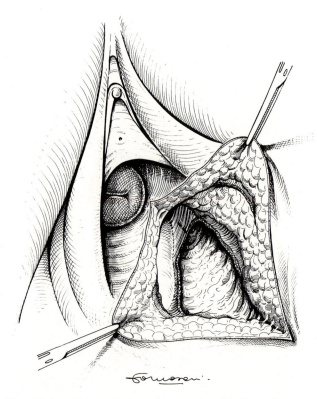

Fig. 23-6. Incision of levator ani with exclusion of extreme proximal part.

Preparation of vaginal cuff and dissection of rectum and bladder

Preparation of the vaginal cuff begins by placing several Collin clamps or single-toothed tenacula around the vaginal fold. The first clamp is applied at a point corresponding to the apex of the Schuchardt incision (Figs. 23-7 and 23-8). Once the part of vagina to be excised is grasped, an upward concave incision is made on the anterior vaginal wall, making sure the tissues to be dissected are kept under tension by exerting a downward pressure upon the Collin clamps and a simultaneous counterpressure upon the retractors. The vaginal dissection is completed with a posterior upward concave incision ending laterally with the anterior incision (Figs. 23-9 and 23-10). Correct pressure facilitates dissection and allows for assessment of the exact depth of the anterior and posterior incisions, which should penetrate all three layers of the vagina: mucosa, muscular layer, and connective tissue.

At this point the rectum is separated from the vagina by pushing the posterior retractor downward and pulling the vaginal stump upward. The peritoneal serosa is thus exposed but not incised.

The operator will then proceed to anteriorly separate the bladder from the uterine cervix. By exerting a moderate downward pressure on the Collin clamps, the gap of the incision is further enlarged and the bladder wall is exposed anteriorly. The anterior retractor is positioned so as to lift up the bladder, thus bringing the vesicocervical fascia into view. The fascia is incised in the midline as far as bladder pillars, which must not be severed (Fig. 23-11). The operator uses the right index finger to separate the bladder completely by blunt dissection. The anterior retractor, when correctly held in place by the second assistant, should suffice to free the bladder.

The Collin clamps are now replaced by Chrobak clamps, which afford a stronger grasp of the vagina. The

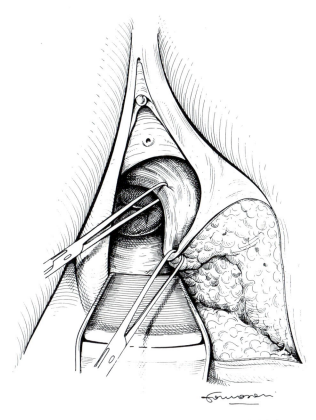

Fig. 23-7. Formation of vaginal cuff by clamps, initiating at a point corresponding to apex of Schuchardt incision.

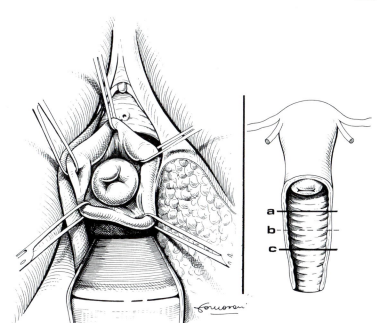

Fig. 23-8. Definition of vaginal cuff whose extent, proportionate to extent of neoplasia, may be fixed at point a, b, or c.

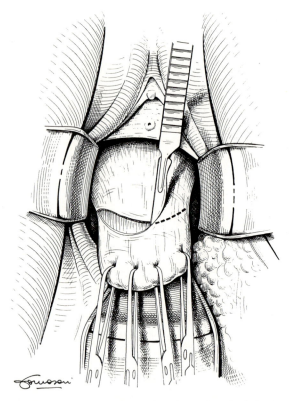

Fig. 23-9. Anterior incision of vagina and vaginal fascia.

anterior and posterior margins of the vaginal cuff are clasped together to enclose the uterine cervix completely within the vaginal tissue and to prevent neoplastic cell diffusion during the subsequent stages of the operation.

On rare occasions, the bladder cleavage plane may not be properly identified and a sudden opening of the bladder may occur. To avoid such complications, it is advisable to instill indigo carmine or sterile milk into the bladder before surgery to permit immediate identification and repair of any such injury as soon as the bladder has been mobilized and isolated.

The following three steps are performed first on the left and then on the right side. Remember that the pararectal space will have to be opened on the right side before proceeding.

Preparation of left paravesical space

The paravesical space is opened by pulling the vaginal cuff clasped by Chrobak clamps to the patient's right and downward; the left lateral retractor exposes the site to be prepared. Using curved scissors with closed tips pointed upward and outward, the operator enters the paravesical space medially to the unsevered portion of the levator and laterally to the left bladder pillar at a point corresponding to the apex of the Schuchardt incision (Fig. 23-12). The scissors are then opened and withdrawn, creating a sufficient gap for the operator's right index finger. It should not meet with resistance but should readily penetrate the loose connective tissue between the bladder and the lateral wall of the paravesical space. A second finger and then the en-

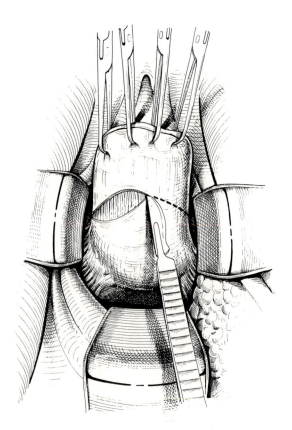

Fig. 23-10. Posterior incision of vagina and vaginal fascia.

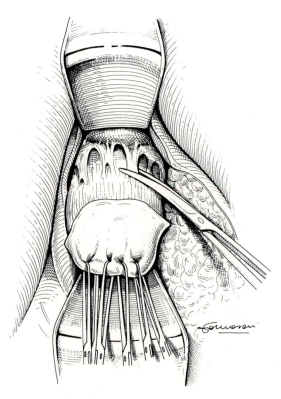

Fig. 23-11. Dissection of vesicocervical fascia.

tire hand are inserted into the space and displace the bladder medially, separating it from its residual attachments to the pelvic wall (Fig. 23-13). The left paravesical space is then opened, and communication is established with the corresponding pararectal space.

If the point of entry into the paravesical space has been properly identified, this step can be performed easily and without significant blood loss. Bleeding may occur if the side of the space has been penetrated by the operator too far laterally (thus interrupting vessels affluent to the hypogastric artery) and too far medially (injuring the uterine vessels), or if penetration is too low (lacerating the cardinal ligament). The hemorrhage may be controlled promptly by exerting pressure with a gauze; then the operator may proceed to the subsequent step.

Isolation of the left ureter

The operator's right hand is withdrawn from the left paravesical space and a large lateral retractor is introduced, while upward and lateral pressure is exerted to fully expose the lateral wall of the bladder pillar. A second retractor placed in the vesicocervical space exerts traction upward and to the right and thus elevates the bladder. The pillar tightened by traction of the two retractors will facilitate access to the ureter.

The operator may locate the ureter by palpation with the thumb and index finger or with both index fingers. As the operator's examining fingers slide along the pillar, he or she will distinctly feel a characteristic "taut cord" being released once located (Fig. 23-14).

An incision of the fibrous layer of the pillar is then made with a scalpel to expose the ureter. The incision courses from back to front, crossing the bend of the ureter 2 to 3 cm from the base of the pillar. Once the ureter has been identified, the tips of the closed scissors are introduced posterolaterally between the ureter and the surrounding tissue. If the ureteral canal has been properly identified, the scissors can enter readily and must penetrate for 3 to 4 cm before being withdrawn with the tips spread apart to widen the canal (Fig. 23-15). The lateral wall of the canal is then cut, and the ureter is pushed upward by a stick sponge to the point where it adheres to the peritoneum (Fig. 23-16).

Certain difficulties may arise in the performance of this step, the most frequent being the presence of residual levator fibers adhering to the pillar or an incomplete mobilization of the bladder. In cases where it is difficult to identify the ureter manually, it may be useful to incise the pillar

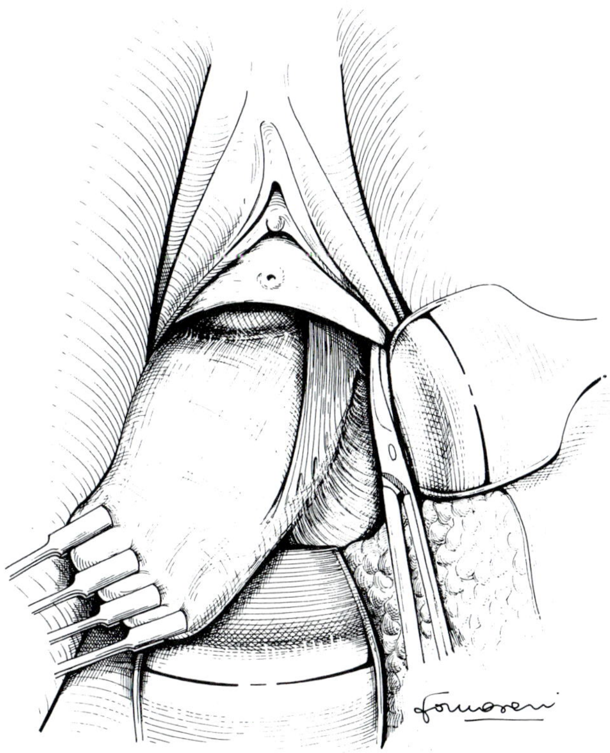

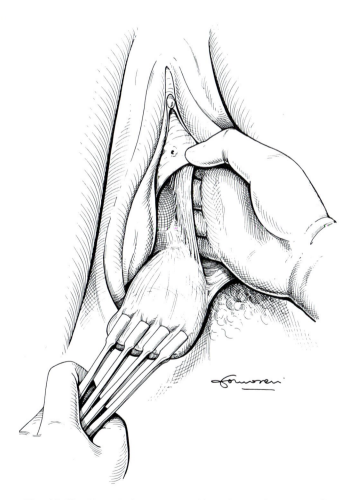

Fig. 23-12. Enclosure of uterine cervix in vaginal cuff clasped by Chrobak clamps under traction; introduction of scissors in upper paravesical space medially to levator ani and laterally to left bladder pillar.

Fig. 23-13. Through the gap created by scissors, the operator introduces one finger, then a second, and finally the entire right hand in the left paravesical space and mobilizes the bladder by a front-to-back maneuver.

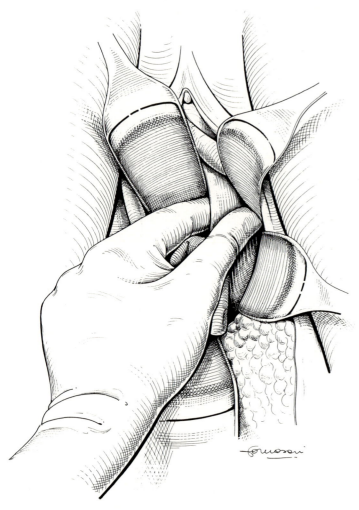

Fig. 23-14. Palpation of left ureter in bladder pillar with left thumb and index finger.

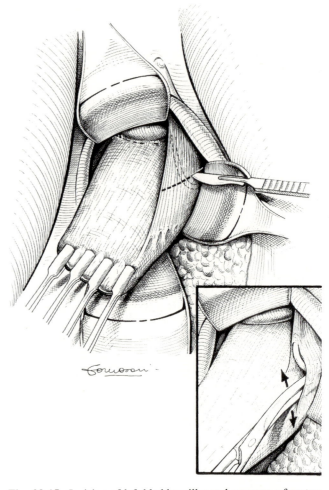

Fig. 23-15. Incision of left bladder pillar and exposure of ureter; identification of ureteral canal widened by scissors and then dissected sharply.

halfway between its starting point in the cardinal ligament and its point of attachment to the bladder. Exposure of the lower vesical vessels extending over the ureter from above is a useful anatomic reference.

Injury to the ureter, although uncommon, must be repaired immediately.

Dissection of left anterior parametrium (pillar) and ligation of left uterine vessels

The ureter and the bladder are displaced upward and further isolated by traction of two retractors in anterior and lateral position, thus exposing the uterine vessels running at the base of the bladder pillar adjacent to the uterus.

Dissection of the anterior pillar generally presents no problems. The entire length of the pillar (tightened by retractors), is cut close to the bladder (Fig. 23-16).

The uterine vessels are fully isolated by means of a Mixter clamp and are doubly ligated and cut. Ligation of the distal pedicle is effected as high as possible, almost where it branches out of the hypogastric artery (Fig. 23-17).

As already mentioned, the same steps are performed on the right side, after preparation of the right pararectal space. At this point the bladder is totally mobilized and is elevated by an anterior retractor. The anterior peritoneum is fully exposed, while the ureters have been pushed away from the operative field and are situated deep in the paravesical spaces.

Opening of posterior peritoneum and dissection of uterosacral ligaments (rectal pillars)

Attention is now turned to the posterior peritoneum. The peritoneal fold is opened extensively (Fig. 23-18), and a catgut stitch is placed on the lower peritoneal edge to facilitate later identification.

Next, the bowel must be pushed away from the operative field. For this purpose it is advisable to place the patient in a moderate Trendelenburg position and to introduce a broad and lengthy gauze tape into the peritoneal cavity to maintain the bowel above the sacrum. The uterus is elevated by a long angular retractor and by upward traction applied to the Chrobak clamps, while the rectum is forcibly lowered by a posterior retractor placed in the pelvic cavity (Fig. 23-19).

The rectal pillars are now clearly in view and are separated from the peritoneum by the surgeon. Proceeding first on the left and then on the right, he or she makes an incision into the peritoneum at the junction between the rectum and rectal pillars. The incision extends upward to the point where the ureter adheres to the peritoneum. The rectum is completely separated from the rectal pillars, which are subsequently resected close to the rectal wall (Figs. 23-20 and 23-21).

Dissection of cardinal ligament (Mackenrodt)

Complete exposure of the cardinal ligament is achieved by the use of retractors on the part of assistants. An anterior retractor protects the bladder upwardly while a lateral retractor brings into view the point of attachment of the cardinal ligament to the pelvic wall. The isolated ligament is grasped by two large Ingiulla or Heaney clamps, the distal clamp being placed as close to the pelvic wall as possible. The ligament is then cut, and its distal pedicle is ligated with no. 2 catgut suture (Fig. 23-22).

The procedure is performed first on the left and then on the right side.

If the pedicle of the severed cardinal ligament escapes ligation, the ensuing bleeding may be controlled by packing. Once the uterus has been removed, the pedicle may be ligated again.

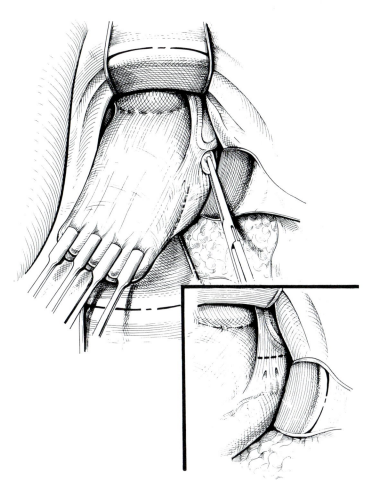

Fig. 23-16. Separation of left ureter by stick sponge; line of incision of left anterior pillar close to the bladder wall.

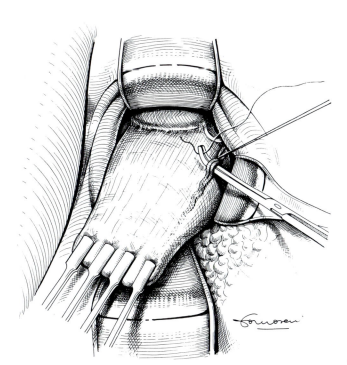

Fig. 23-17. Isolation and ligation of left uterine vessels.

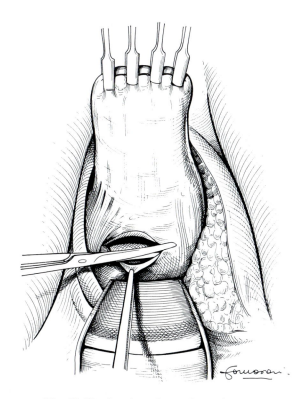

Fig. 23-18. Opening of posterior peritoneum.

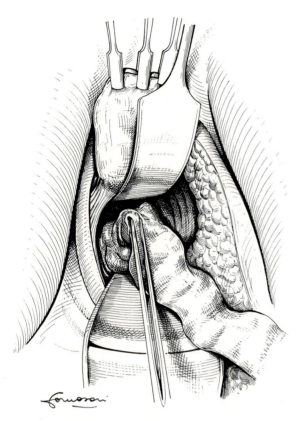

Fig. 23-19. Introduction of lengthy gauze into peritoneal cavity to push bowel away.

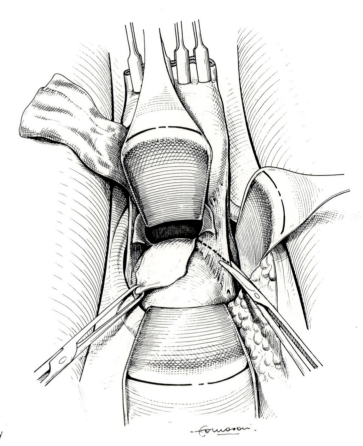

Fig. 23-21. Dissection of left rectal pillar close to rectal wall.

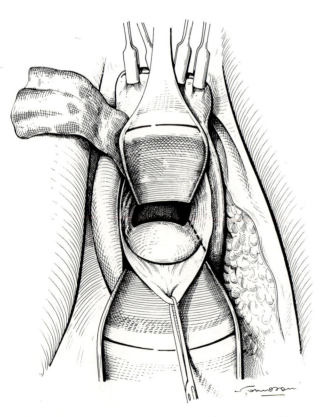

Fig. 23-20. Line of incision of visceral peritoneum while rectal pillars are under tension.

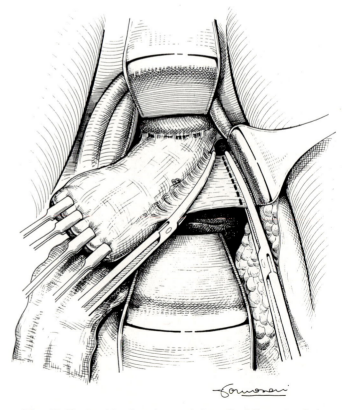

Fig. 23-22. Double clamping on left cardinal ligament close to pelvic wall.

Opening of anterior peritoneum, dissection of round and infundibulopelvic ligaments, and removal of uterus and adnexa

The anterior peritoneum is now opened and an anterior retractor is placed in the peritoneal cavity to push the bladder upward while the uterus is pulled downward (Fig. 23-23). If the adnexa are to be removed, the ovaries are grasped with ovarian clamps and the tubes with straight Klemmer clamps. In this way, the round and infundibulopelvic ligaments are exposed and then secured together by d'Allaines curved clamps and dissected to leave a long pedicle ligated with two loose no. 1 catgut sutures (Fig. 23-24).

The same procedure is carried out on both sides. The uterus, adnexa, and parametria are then removed.

Closure of the peritoneum

By exerting adequate pressure on the anterior and posterior retractors and, if necessary, placing a third retractor laterally, the margins of the peritoneal opening become more accessible. The cut edges of the peritoneum are then closed by a semicircular pursestring suture, which follows a posteroanterior direction on the right side and a reverse direction on the left. Stitches are placed so that the pedicles of the infundibulopelvic and round ligaments and uterine vessels are lying extraperitoneally (Fig. 23-25). The

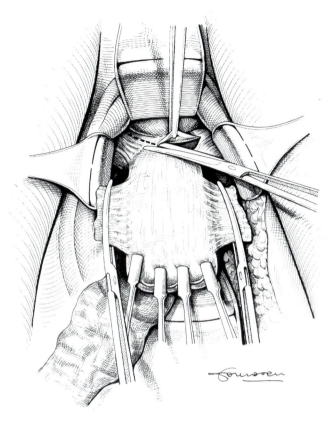

Fig. 23-23. Opening of anterior peritoneum.

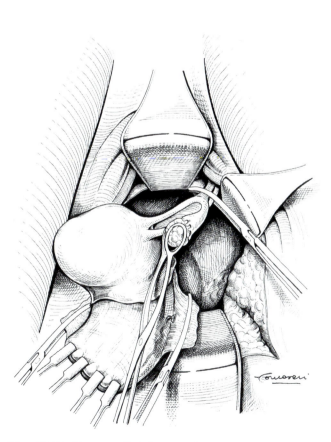

Fig. 23-24. Uterus pulled forward; left round and infundibulopelvic ligaments clamped and then dissected.

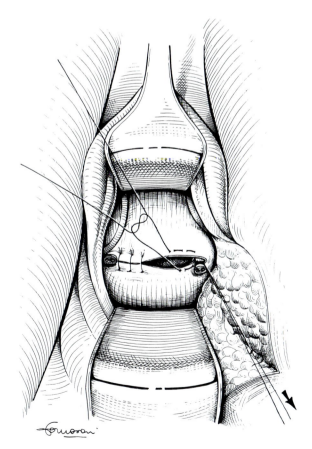

Fig. 23-25. Closure of peritoneum with pedicles of uterine vessels lying extraperitoneally.

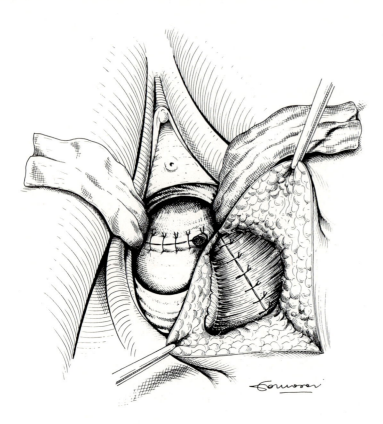

Fig. 23-26. Reconstruction of levator ani by interrupted suture after packing of subperitoneal lateral spaces.

gauze intraabdominal packing must be removed before closing the peritoneum completely with interrupted or continuous sutures. The cut edges of the vagina are not sutured but gauze is introduced as tamponade. In case of prolapse, it is advisable to suture the peritoneum with interrupted stitches, which will be anchored to the edge of the vaginal wall.

Suture of the Schuchardt incision

Before the Schuchardt incision is closed, the subperitoneal lateral spaces are packed to ensure hemostasis at this site. The incision is closed with a first stitch that joins the superior lateral edge of the vagina to the inferior medial edge. The levator plate is then sutured at the proximal and distal parts, with the most proximal part that was not dissected acting as a reference point (Fig. 23-26). Suture of the vaginal part of the Schuchardt incision is completed with interrupted stitches (Fig. 23-27).

POSTOPERATIVE CARE

Postoperative care after Schauta-Amreich surgery does not differ from that after other radical procedures. Antibiotics are administered for 4 to 6 days, fluids for 5 days, and normal intestinal function is restored 4 days after surgery. The packing is completely removed 24 hours after surgery. In cases of mild bleeding, a new packing may be inserted for an additional 24 hours. The indwelling catheter is removed on the seventh to tenth day, and the patient is then catheterized at intervals to determine postvoiding residual volume until complete voiding is recovered. Dis-

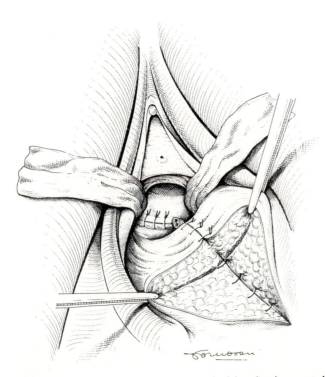

Fig. 23-27. Suture of the Schuchardt incision by interrupted stitches.

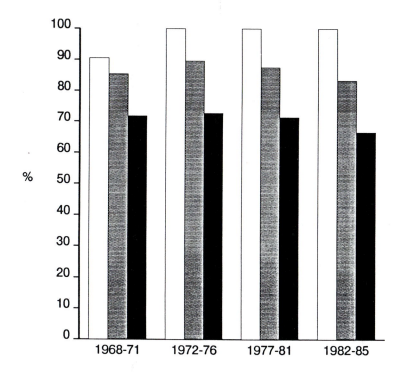

Fig. 23-28. Schauta-Amreich operative 5-year survival rate.

Table 23-5. Schauta-Amreich operation: 5-year survival rate

Years	Stage Ia			Stage Ib			Stage IIa		
	No. operated	No. dead	5-year survival (%)	No. operated	No. dead	5-year survival (%)	No. operated	No. dead	5-year survival (%)
1968-71	21	2	90.5	41	6	85.4	39	11	71.8
						87.1			72.0
1972-76	14	0	100	29	3	89.6	11	3	72.7
1977-81	13	0	100	25*	3	87.5	8*	2	71.4
						86.7			70.2
1982-85	4	0	100	6	1	83.3	3	2	66.6
1986-90	1	—	—	2	—	—	0	—	—

*1 patient lost at follow-up.

infection of the vagina is maintained by douching during the postoperative period. An intravenous pyelogram is generally performed before the patient is discharged. The patient is usually ready to leave the hospital 12 to 14 days after surgery.

PERSONAL EXPERIENCE

From 1968 to 1990, 217 Schauta radical vaginal hysterectomies were performed in patients with stages Ia, Ib and IIa cervical carcinoma. From 1968 to 1971, the Schauta procedure was also performed mistakenly in some patients at stage IIb, but we have not included them in our evaluation.

Since 1972 patients have been selected for the Schauta technique on the basis of lymphographic findings. Therefore, data for the period from 1972 to 1981 only concern patients with negative lymphographies.

The number of patients operated on through the vaginal route has declined substantially since the 1980s (Table 23-

5). This is primarily because of a more careful selection of patients based on the integration of several diagnostic techniques and the biologic characterization of the neoplastic lesion.

The 5-year survival rate of the 217 patients who underwent radical vaginal surgery is shown in Fig. 23-28. There is a good survival rate for patients operated on with the Schauta procedure from 1977 to 1985. This rate is similar to that obtained from 1968 to 1976.[11] The limited number of patients treated since 1982 (Table 23-5) did not permit the use of a statistical method to ascertain whether the variation in the survival rate was correlated to treatment; we expect a better survival rate with the more recent careful selection of patients.

CONCLUSIONS

An excellent "anatomic" operation such as the Schauta-Amreich procedure may be useful in selected cases of cervical carcinoma, as shown by these data.

As greater insight was gained into the mechanisms responsible for neoplastic growth, the use of this surgical procedure became less frequent, since it became more necessary to take account of the lymph node problem.

What about the future? New research of a biologic nature will undoubtedly influence future treatment of cancer. New insights into prognostic factors, their application in the clinical field, and the use of new adjuvant therapeutic methods or multimodal programs based on a combination of surgery, radiotherapy, chemotherapy, and biologic response modifiers may give a new impetus to the use of this operating technique in the future.

Unfortunately, in the meantime the number of surgeons capable of performing this operation properly is declining as a result of the smaller number of patients requiring this form of surgery.

REFERENCES

1. Amreich I: Zur Anatomie und Technik der erweiterten vaginalen Carcinomoperation, *Archiv f. Gynäkologie* 122:497, 1924.
2. Averette HE: Cervical cancer: reflections of the professor, *Gynecol Oncol* 36:157, 1990.
3. Balzer J et al: Die operative Behandling des Zervixkarzinomas, *Geburtshilfe Frauenheilkd* 44:179, 1984.
4. Bandy LC et al: Computed tomography in evaluation of extrapelvic lymphadenopathy in carcinoma of the cervix, *Obstet Gynecol* 65:73, 1985.
5. Berman ML et al: Survival and patterns of recurrence in cervical cancer metastatic to periaortic lymph nodes, *Gynecol Oncol* 19:8, 1984.
6. Boie H et al: Diagnostic value of lymphography in cervical cancer stage I_B, *Eur J Gynaecol Oncol* 10:6, 1989.
7. Brenner DE et al: An evaluation of the computed tomographic scanner for the staging of carcinoma of the cervix, *Cancer* 50:2323, 1982.
8. Burghardt E et al: Prognostic factors and operative treatment of stages I_B to II_B cervical cancer, *Am J Obstet Gynecol* 156:988, 1987.
9. Camilien L et al: Predictive value of computerized tomography in presurgical evaluation of primary carcinoma of the cervix, *Gynecol Oncol* 30:209, 1988.
10. Carenza L, Nobili F: L'apparato urinario dopo chirurgia pelvica radicale per neoplasia della cervice. Atti del convegno: le lesioni iatrogene in ostetricia e ginecologia, Roma, 6-9 giugno 1985.
11. Carenza L, Villani C: Schauta radical vaginal hysterectomy, *Clin Obstet Gynecol* 25:913, 1982.
12. Carenza L, Villani C: Parametria and therapy in stage I_B cervical cancer, *Baillieres Clin Obstet Gynaecol* 2(4), 1988.
13. Creasman WT et al: Management of stage I_A carcinoma of the cervix, *Am J Obstet Gynecol* 153:164, 1985.
14. Dargent D: A new future for Schauta's operation through pre-surgical retroperitoneal pelviscopy? *Eur J Gynaecol Oncol* 8:45, 1987.
15. Dargent D: Personal communication, Nov 1990.
16. De Graaff J: The Mitra Schauta operation in combination with preoperative irradiation as treatment for carcinoma of the cervix, *Gynecol Oncol* 10:267, 1980.
17. Falk V et al: Primary surgical treatment of carcinoma stage I of the uterine cervix, *Acta Obstet Gynecol Scand* 61:481, 1982.
18. Feigen M et al: The value of lymphoscintigraphy, lymphography and computer tomography scanning in the preoperative assessment of the lymph nodes involvement by pelvic malignant conditions, *Surg Gynecol Obstet* 165: Aug 1987.
19. Foushee JHS, Greiss FC, Lock FR: Stage I_A squamous cell carcinoma of the uterine cervix, *Am J Obstet Gynecol* 105:46, 1969.
20. Fu YS, Berek JS: Minimal cervical cancer: definition and histology, Recent Results Cancer Res 106: 1988.
21. Gasparri F et al: Lesioni chirurgiche dell'apparato intestinale nella chirurgia allargata per via vaginale. Atti del convegno: Le lesioni iatrogene in ostetricia e ginecologia, Roma 6, giugno 1985.
22. Gastaldi A: Danni indotti dal trattamento chirurgico addominale in oncologia ginecologica. In *Compicanze dei trattamenti in oncologia ginecologica*. S. Margherita Ligure, 8-10 novembre 1984.
23. Gitsch E: Die I. Universitats-Frauenklinik von Friedrich Schauta bis heute. Wiener klinische Wochenschrift, Jg. 102, Heft 12, 8 juni 1990.
24. Grumbine FC et al: Abdominopelvic computed tomography in the preoperative evaluation of early cervical carcinoma, *Gynecol Oncol* 12:286, 1981.
25. Halban J: *Gynakol Operationslehre*, Berlin, 1932, Urban u. Schwartzenberg.
26. Hasumi K, Sakamoto A, Sugano H: Microinvasive carcinoma of the uterine cervix, *Cancer* 45:928, 1980.
27. Ingiulla W: Five-year results of 327 Schauta-Amreich operations for cervical carcinoma, *Am J Obstet Gynecol* 96:188, 1966.
28. Kindermann G, Gerteis W, Weishaar J: Was leistet die Lymphographie in der Erkennung von Metastasen beim Zervixkarzinom, *Geburtshilfe Fraunheilkd* 30:444, 1970.
29. Kolbenstvedt A: Lymphography in the diagnosis of metastases from carcinoma of the uterine cervix Stage I and II, *Acta Radiol Diagn* 16:81, 1975.
30. Kolstad P: Follow-up study of 232 patients with stage I_{A1} and 411 patients with stage I_{A2} squamous cell carcinoma of the cervix (microinvasive carcinoma), *Gynecol Oncol* 33:265, 1989.
31. Kovacic J et al: The treatment of invasive carcinoma of the cervix at the department of gynecology and obstetrics in Ljubljana, *Eur J Gynaecol Oncol* 1: 1980.
32. Leman MH et al: Microinvasive carcinoma of the cervix, *Obstet Gynecol* 48:571, 1976.
33. Maiman MA et al: Superficially invasive squamous cell carcinoma of the cervix, *Obstet Gynecol* 72(3):399, 1988.
34. McCall ML: A modern evaluation of the radical vaginal operation for carcinoma of the cervix, *Am J Obstet Gynecol* 85:295, 1963.
35. Mitra S: Extraperitoneal lymphadenectomy and radical vaginal hysterectomy for cancer of the cervix (Mitra technique), *Am J Obstet Gynecol* 58:191, 1959.
36. Morgan S, Nelson JH: Surgical treatment of early cervical cancer, *Semin Oncol* 9:312, 1982.
37. Morrow CP: Panel report: is pelvic radiation beneficial in the postoperative management of stage I_B squamous cell carcinoma of the cervix with pelvic node metastasis treated by radical hysterectomy and pelvic lymphadenectomy? *Gynecol Oncol* 10:105, 1980.
38. Muylder De X et al: Value of lymphography in stage I_B cancer of the uterine cervix, *Am J Obstet Gynecol* 148:610, 1984.
39. Navratil E: Indications and results of the Schauta-Amreich operation with and without postoperative roentgen treatment in the epidermoid carcinoma of the cervix of the uterus, *Am J Obstet Gynecol* 86:141, 1963.
40. Novak F: *Gynakologische Operationstechnik*, New York, 1978, Springer-Verlag.
41. Peham HV: Diskussion zu Herrn Stockel, *Zentralbl Gynakol* 51:1992, 1927.
42. Petri E: Urologische Komplikationen, *Gynakologe* 22:39, 1989.
43. Ralph G et al: Funktionelle Storungendes unteren Harntraktes nach der abdominalen und vaginalen Radikaloperation des Zervixkrebses, *Geburtshilfe Frauenheilkd* 47:551, 1987.
44. Roche WD, Norris HJ: Microinvasive carcinoma of the cervix: the significance of lymphatic invasion and confluent patterns of stromal growth, *Cancer* 36:180, 1975.
45. Sall S et al: Surgical treatment of stage I_B invasive carcinoma of the cervix by radical abdominal hysterectomy, *Am J Obstet Gynecol* 135:442, 1979.
46. Salvat J, Vincent-Genod A: Lymphadenectomie pelvienne par retroperitoneoscopie "operatoire" en gynecologie, *Presse Med* 16(20): 1006, 1987.

47. Sarrazin R, Bolla M, Dyon JF: Le retroperitoneoscopie iliaque en cancerologie gynecologique, *Presse Med* 16(42):2130, 1987.

48. Schauta F: Die enveiterte vaginale Totalextirpation der Uterus beim Collumcarzinom, Wien Seipzig, J. Safar, 1908.

49. Schuchardt K: Eine neue Methode der Gebarmutter-extirpation, *Zentralbl Chir* 20:1121, 1893.

50. Seski JC, Abell MR, Morley GW: Microinvasive squamous carcinoma of the cervix—definition, hystologic analysis, late results of treatment, *Obstet Gynecol* 50:410, 1977.

51. Shingleton HM et al: Tumor recurrence and survival in stage I_B cancer of the cervix, *Am J Clin Oncol* 6(3):263, 1983.

52. Simon NL et al: Study of superficial invasive carcinoma of the cervix, Obstet Gynecol 68:19, 1986.

53. Sinistrero G et al: Computed tomography in uterine cervix cancer: staging and management, *Cervix* 8:51, 1990.

54. Stallworthy J: Radical surgery following radiation treatment for cervical cancer, *Ann R Coll Surg Engl* 34:161, 1964.

55. Stockel W: Die vaginale Radikaloperation des Kollumcarzinom, *Zentralbl Gynakol* 39: 1928.

56. Swart E, Bouma J, Schuur K: The clinical value of lymphography in cervical cancer, FIGO stage I_B-II_A, *Eur J Gynaecol Oncol* 10:2, 1989.

57. Szabo BG: *Disseminatie onderzoek bij carcinoma colli uteri*, doctoral dissertation, Groningen, 1980, van Denderen BV.

58. Taki I et al: Treatment of microinvasive carcinoma, *Obstet Gynecol Surv* 34:839, 1979.

59. Van Bouwdijk Bastiaanse MA: Treatment of cancer of the cervix uteri, *Am J Obstet Gynecol* 72:100, 1956.

60. Van Engelshoven JMA et al: Computed tomography in staging untreated patients with cervical cancer, *Gynecol Obstet Invest* 18:289, 1984.

61. Van Nagell JR et al: Microinvasive carcinoma of the cervix, *Am J Obstet Gynecol* 145:981, 1983.

62. Villasanta V et al: Computed tomography in invasive carcinoma of the cervix—an appraisal, *Obstet Gynecol* 62(2):218, 1983.

63. Warren JP: Extirpation of cancer of the uterus, *Am J Med Sci* 4:536, 1829.

64. Webb M, Symmonds R: Wertheim hysterectomy: a reappraisal, *Obstet Gynecol* 54:140, 1979.

65. Weibel W: 25 Jahre "Wertheimscher" Carcinomoperation, *Arch Gynacol* 135:1, 1929.

66. Wertheim E: A discussion on the diagnosis and treatment of cancer of the uterus, *Br Med J* 2:689, 1905.

67. Wertheim E: The extended abdominal operation for carcinoma uteri (based on 500 operative cases), *Am J Obstet Gynecol* 66:169, 1912.

68. Winter R, Petru E, Haas J: Pelvic and para-aortic lymphadenectomy in cervical cancer, *Baillieres Clin Obstet Gynaecol* 2: Dec 1988.

69. Yajima A and Noda K: The results of treatment of microinvasive carcinoma (stage I_A) of the uterine cervix by means of simple and extended hysterectomy, *Am J Obstet Gynecol* 135:685, 1979.

Chapter 24

THE SMALL AND PAINFUL VAGINA

David H. Nichols

Disproportion between the size of a woman's vagina and her partner's penis is a common cause of dyspareunia. Congenital deformities, such as absence of the vagina and uterus, absence of the lower half of the vagina, and obstructive transverse septa at any level, including an imperforate hymen, may result in a vagina that cannot admit or contain the penis comfortably. Some women have a longitudinal vaginal septum that creates a second birth canal that may be coincident with a rudimentary uterine horn, leading to dysmenorrhea as well as dyspareunia. Thick lateral bands connecting the external urethral meatus to the hymenal margin may be a source of dyspareunia. Also, because they drag on the meatus during coitus, they may invite recurrent postcoital cystitis.[3]

Menopausal change may be a factor, especially when the woman has undergone pelvic irradiation or when an unusual degree of progressive atrophy and shrinkage has accompanied the aging process. Some relative flaccidity of the penis of the menopausal woman's partner may compound the coital problem, making vaginal penetration difficult.

There are significant iatrogenic causes of a too small vagina. For example, postepisiotomy scarring may decrease the size of the vagina, or hysterectomy, especially radical surgery with partial vaginectomy, may leave the vagina too short. The vaginal diameter may be left too narrow as a consequence of excessive subepithelial plication or the excision of a more than necessary amount of vaginal membrane with colporrhaphy. Subepithelial ridges that form postoperatively may become more tender as the fibrosis of scarring progresses.

Psychosomatic factors may also contribute to dyspareunia associated with a small vagina by inhibiting relaxation of paravaginal muscles. Some women fear being hurt or becoming pregnant, must overcome the psychologic scar-

ring that follows rape, or lack accurate knowledge concerning sexual practices. Some have an unconscious or conscious desire to inflict punishment on themselves or their marital partners.

These factors may be etiologically grouped in any combination. Successful treatment requires identification and proper attention to each contributing factor.

PREVENTION OF A SMALL VAGINA

The best treatment of a small vagina is prevention. If the patient is postmenopausal, particularly if there are signs of mucosal or vulvar atrophy, more or less permanent estrogen replacement therapy will strengthen, restore, and preserve vaginal elasticity in estrogen-sensitive pelvic tissues.

Proper techniques of either vaginal or abdominal hysterectomy, particularly in patients who had some degree of genital prolapse, require that elongated cardinal and uterosacral ligaments be shortened and firmly attached to the vault of the vagina. When these ligaments are hypertrophic, cul-de-plasty is often helpful in preserving or restoring vaginal length. In principle, cul-de-plasty involves fixing the vaginal vault to the undersurface of strong uterosacral ligaments after bringing them together in front of the vagina, thus reducing any tendency toward enterocele formation (Fig. 24-1). In fact, the surgeon should attempt to identify any actual or potential enterocele and should excise any excess peritoneum before high peritonealization. The excision of any excess width strengthens the vaginal vault. This technique can be successful in conjunction with either vaginal or abdominal hysterectomy, but, with the latter, the surgeon must be especially careful not to allow a ureteral obstruction.

As Amreich has pointed out,[2] a short vagina that ends anterior to the levator plate tends to become even shorter

404

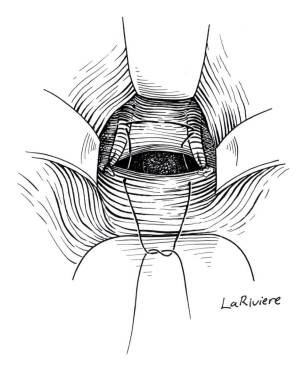

Fig. 24-1. Modified New Orleans cul-de-plasty. The enterocele sac has been mobilized, excised, and a synthetic absorbable suture placed as shown.

with time, as intraabdominal pressure may be transmitted in the axis of the vagina. Fixing the vault above the levator plate preserves vaginal depth and lessens any tendency for telescoping, as increases in intraabdominal pressure compress the vagina against the levator plate. If the cardinal-uterosacral ligaments are not strong and surgically useful, the surgeon must use alternative methods of colpopexy to support the vault (see Chapter 27).

When performing colporrhaphy, the surgeon must carefully calculate the amount of the vagina to be excised to ensure an acceptable postoperative vaginal width. There should be suitable allowance for any shrinkage that is likely to occur with aging and hormone withdrawal; all other things being equal, the surgeon should excise less of the vaginal membrane from a premenopausal patient in whom postmenopausal vaginal shrinkage has yet to occur. In addition, there should be some consideration of the age and genital size of the patient's partner. In the temporary absence of sexual activity, the periodic insertion of a vaginal obturator is helpful if there is any tendency toward stricture or stenosis.

TREATMENT OF A SMALL VAGINA

With lower vaginal agenesis, the surgeon dissects a tunnel through the vestibular area toward the upper vagina. (If a functional uterus accompanies this condition, a rectal examination reveals a hematocolpos.) The surgeon mobilizes the upper vaginal canal, opens it, and stretches it, and sews the upper vaginal skin edge to the skin of the vesti-

bule to cover the raw lower area. It should not be necessary to perform a graft.

A patient with a transverse vaginal septum at any level may have a uterus, which is usually functional. There is no associated urinary tract anomaly, (a significant difference from the Rokitansky-Küster-Hauser syndrome). Appropriate excision is the treatment of choice for a vaginal septum or imperforate hymen.

Correction of a stricture or stenosis

When the vagina is narrow or constricted at a specific point, the appropriate surgical procedure to provide additional width depends on the site of the constriction. The most common site is the perineum, where constriction often follows overenthusiastic perineorrhaphy or hurried, inadequate reapproximation of an episiotomy, particularly when the pubococcygeal muscles have been approximated anterior to the rectum. A midline perineotomy with a suture of the wound placed at a right angle to the incision may be all that is necessary, although this procedure shortens the vagina slightly (Fig. 24-2). If atrophy is present, a bilateral episiotomy with sliding of the skin margins widens the introitus[11] (Fig. 24-3 and 24-4).

Lateral relaxing incisions through the full thickness of the vagina may relieve a stricture of the midportion of the vagina[10] (Figs. 24-5 and 24-6). The margins of the incision are undercut, and the vaginal caliber is maintained by a suitable obturator during epithelialization and healing. If the vaginal wall has been freshly excised, a patch may be cut of a size sufficient to fill the defect in the lateral vaginal wall and sewn in place as a full-thickness graft. These relaxing incisions can be made in a constricted vagina at any time, even years later, although a brief rehospitalization and anesthetic are necessary. The technique and aftercare are precisely the same as they are in the fresh surgical patient, however.

With moderate constriction of the lower vagina, as seen, for example, in the patient with congenital adrenal hyperplasia, the surgeon may develop a fasciocutaneous flap from the labia and swing it into place to bridge the defect created by a fresh episiotomy[9] (Figs. 24-7 to 24-9).

The use of full-thickness skin flaps[7] from the inner thigh, a modification of the Graves operation[5] for construction of a neovagina, may be necessary in patients with extensive constriction of the lower half of the vagina because of either congenital underdevelopment or postoperative stricture. Convalescence requires several weeks of relative rest and several months' use of a vaginal obturator.

Modified Graves procedure. In the Graves procedure,[5] a method of treating the congenital absence of the vagina, the surgeon creates a tunnel between the bladder and rectum and lines it with four full-thickness flaps of skin. Two of these flaps are raised from the medial surface of the thighs; two are raised from the full thickness of the skin medial to the labia majora, including the labia minora, which are spatulated. These are all sewn together,

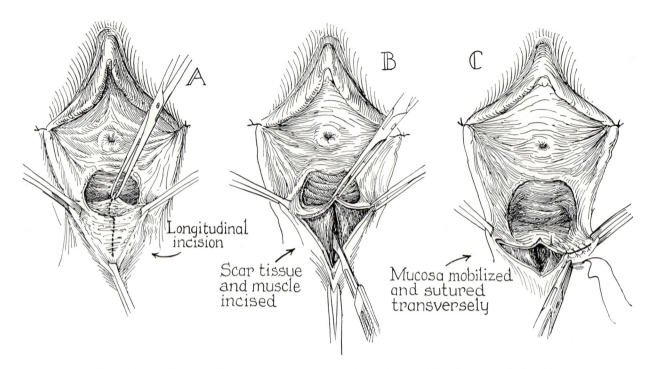

Fig. 24-2. A, The area of contraction and scar tissue is outlined by Allis clamps, and a longitudinal incision made to determine the depth of the scar. **B,** The tissue around the area of contracture is excised. If this extends into the musculature of the perineum or, in the vent of a higher stricture, into the musculature of the vaginal wall, the muscle and scar tissue are incised to release the constriction. **C,** The mucosa and skin of the perineum, if the constriciton is at the introitus, are then mobilized to permit a transverse closure without tension. The vaginal circumference in this operation is reconstructed larger than normal to allow for some postoperative contracture. The incision is closed with interrupted absorbable sutures, and the sutures are tied to approximate the edges without strangulation of the tissues. (From Ball TL: *Gynecologic surgery and urology,* St Louis, 1963, Mosby–Year Book, pp 309-310).

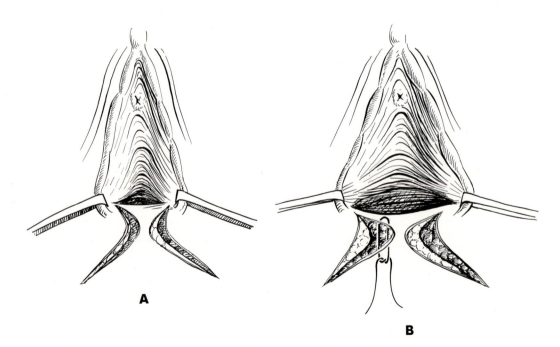

Fig. 24-3. A, Bilateral episiotomy is performed. Repair is begun at the medial edge **(B)** in such a fashion that the original apex is, in fact, moved laterally on each side a distance sufficient to enlarge the introitus as much as is necessary. (From Nichols DH, Randall CL: *Vaginal surgery,* ed 3, Baltimore, 1989, Williams & Wilkins.)

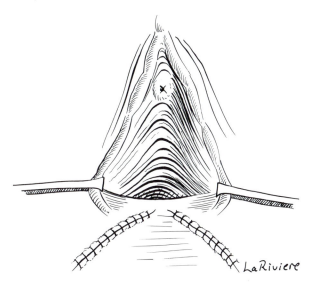

Fig. 24-4. The end result shows the now widened introitus. (From Nichols DH, Randall CL: *Vaginal surgery,* ed 3, Baltimore, 1989, Williams & Wilkins.)

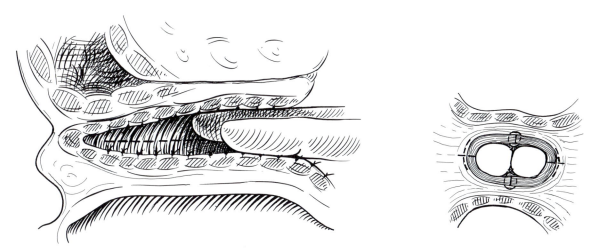

Fig. 24-5. Digital examination of the vagina immediately after colporrhaphy discloses an unexpected stenosis in the upper half that admits only two fingerbreadths. The sites of the lateral relaxing incisions are indicated by the dotted lines. (From Nichols DH, Randall CL: *Vaginal surgery,* ed 3, Baltimore, 1989, Williams & Wilkins.)

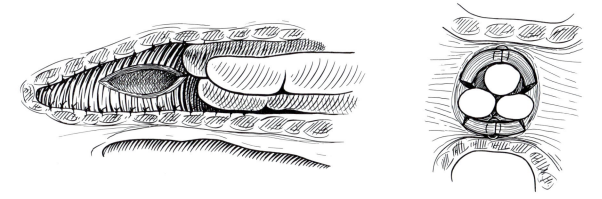

Fig. 24-6. These incisions are made through the lateral wall of the vagina to a depth sufficient for the vagina to admit comfortably three fingerbreadths. The vaginal wall is undercut for a centimeter in each direction. Any obvious bleeding vessels are clamped and tied, and a firm vaginal packing is inserted. This may be replaced within a day or so by a large vaginal obturator or mold to keep the cut edges of the relaxing incisions apart until healing and epithelialization are well underway, usually by the fifth postoperative day, after which the obturator or dilator may be worn only at night for an additional 2 or 3 weeks. Thus, the integrity of the colporrhaphy incisions in the anterior and posterior vaginal walls is not compromised. (From Nichols DH, Randall CL: *Vaginal surgery,* ed 3, Baltimore, 1989, Williams & Wilkins.)

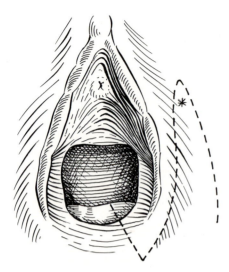

Fig. 24-7. Labial cutaneous flap. At the site of a perineotomy, an incision through the full thickness of the labia skin and subcutaneous fat is made, as shown by the broken line. (From Nichols DH, Randall CL: *Vaginal surgery,* ed 3, Baltimore, 1989, Williams & Wilkins.)

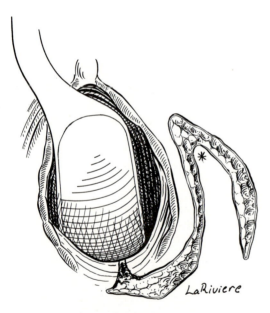

Fig. 24-8. The base of the flap is wider than the apex. (From Nichols DH, Randall CL: *Vaginal surgery,* ed 3, Baltimore, 1989, Williams & Wilkins.)

Fig. 24-9. The flap has been freed from the underlying fascia, swung into the defect created by the perineotomy, and fixed in place by a few interrupted stitches as shown. The labial defect is closed. Note the change in location of the tissue marked with the asterisk. (From Nichols DH, Randall CL: *Vaginal surgery,* ed 3, Baltimore, 1989, Williams & Wilkins.)

inverted into the tunnel of the neovagina, and held there by a glass obturator until fixed to the walls of the cavity.

When a stricture or atresia of the lower half of the vagina is so extensive that a simple midline perineotomy with a transverse closure cannot relieve it, a modification of the Graves procedure is useful. After mobilizing two full-thickness flaps from the medial surface of each thigh, the surgeon swings them into the vagina to cover the site of a fresh midline episiotomy. In performing this procedure, the surgeon

1. Infiltrates the perineum and the medial skin of each thigh subcuticularly with approximately 100 ml of 0.5% lidocaine in 1:200,000 epinephrine solution.
2. Makes a deep midline episiotomy, separating the skin edges enough to establish the desired vaginal diameter.
3. Marks off with indelible stain skin flaps large enough for each to fill half of the space created by the unrepaired episiotomy.
4. Cuts full-thickness flaps all the way to the underlying fascia, leaving the subcutaneous fat attached to the undersurface of each flap.
5. Undermines the residual skin of the thigh to prepare for its approximation.
6. Swings the flaps medially so that they meet in the midline and approximates their medial edges with interrupted sutures of polyglycolic acid-type material.
7. Closes the thigh incisions from side to side and sews the apex of the now united flaps to the apex of the episiotomy with polyglycolic-type suture, trimming any excess adipose tissue from the underside of the flaps.

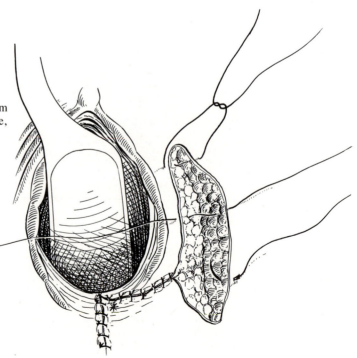

8. Fixes the lateral margins of the flap to the edges of the episiotomy with a few interrupted sutures, again of polyglycolic acid-type material.

9. Inserts a Penrose drain beneath the skin of each thigh, a Foley catheter in the bladder, and a splinting obturator in the vagina.

On the fourth postoperative day, the obturator and the Foley catheter are removed, the flaps and vagina are inspected thoroughly to determine healing, and the obturator is replaced. The patient wears the obturator constantly for 2 or 3 weeks, removing it only when she voids. After this period, she wears the obturator at night for several months until healing has been completed. Long-term postoperative

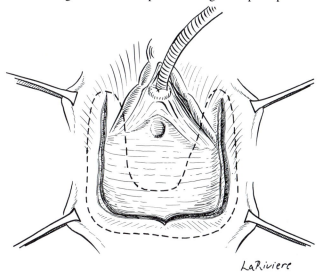

Fig. 24-10. Vulvovaginoplasty. The dimpled area of softening beneath the urethra identifies the site of the missing vagina. Following through infiltration with 0.5% lidocaine in 1:200,000 epinephrine solution, a U-shaped incision is made along the inner surface of the labia majora about 4 cm lateral to the urethra and undermined as indicated by the broken line. (From Nichols DH, Randall CL: *Vaginal surgery,* ed 3, Baltimore, 1989, Williams & Wilkins.)

estrogen replacement therapy may be indicated, and frequent wearing of a suitable obturator is often desirable to maintain both vaginal depth and width.

Williams vulvovaginoplasty. When the vagina is short, for example because of earlier radical pelvic surgery that included partial vaginectomy, the distal vulvovaginoplasty of Williams[12] may add as much as 1 to 3 inches to the length of the vagina. In patients who need more depth, the surgeon may use a partial McIndoe procedure to construct a new upper vagina. The use of appropriate vaginal obturators may create and maintain additional depth.[4,6]

When the vagina is too short, too narrow, and generally inelastic because of fibrosis and scarring from previous surgery, the vulvovaginoplasty of Williams[12] may be useful if the labia are thick and well-developed (Figs. 24-10 to 24-15). If the labia are atrophic and thin, however, vaginectomy followed at the same operation by construction of an Abbe-McIndoe type neovagina is often helpful.

As in the Graves procedure, long-term postoperative estrogen replacement therapy and frequent wearing of a suitable obturator are often indicated after a Williams vulvovaginoplasty.

Everted shortened vagina

In an occasional patient who has undergone multiple surgical procedures, a shortened vagina—sometimes so short, in fact, that it does not reach the sacrospinous ligament—becomes totally everted. The surgeon has several treatment alternatives from which to choose in this case.

1. The use of Ingram-Frank dilators lubricated with estrogen cream may lengthen the vagina until it reaches the sacrospinous ligament so that the surgeon can perform sacrospinous colpopexy.[6]

2. Transabdominal sacrocolpopexy permits the place-

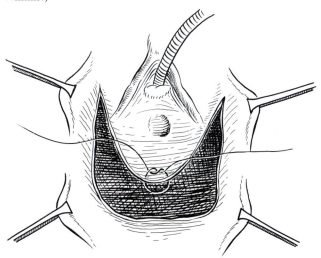

Fig. 24-11. The medial margins of the incision are united by interrupted absorbable suture. (From Nichols DH, Randall CL: *Vaginal surgery,* ed 3, Baltimore, 1989, Williams & Wilkins.)

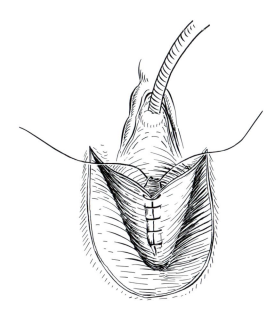

Fig 24-12. Notice that the knots are tied on the *inside of* the new vaginal pouch. (From Nichols DH, Randall CL: *Vaginal surgery,* ed 3, Baltimore, 1989, Williams & Wilkins.)

ment of an intermediate bridge of fascia lata or of a synthetic plastic material.

3. Sacrospinous colpopexy (see Chapter 27) allows the surgeon to use deliberate suture bridges of nonabsorbable synthetic monofilament material, such as Prolene or Surgilene. If the labia are large enough, the surgeon may also perform a Williams vulvovaginoplasty to increase the depth of the vagina by an additional 1.5 or 2 inches.

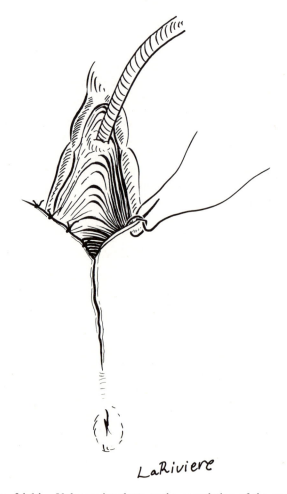

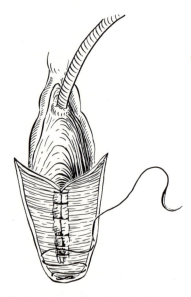

Fig. 24-13. The lateral margins of the incision are approximated separately. (From Nichols DH, Randall CL: *Vaginal surgery,* ed 3, Baltimore, 1989, Williams & Wilkins.)

Fig. 24-14. Vulvovaginoplasty at the completion of the operation is shown in frontal view.

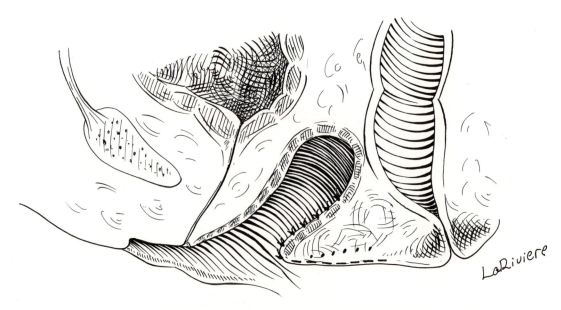

Fig. 24-15. The neovaginal poach is shown in sagittal section. (After Capraro VJ, Capraro EJ: *Obstet Gynecol* 39:544, 1972.)

REFERENCES

1. Abbe R: New method of creating a vagina in a case of congenital absence, *Med Rec* 54:836-838, 1898.
2. Amreich J: Aetiologie und Operation des Scheidenstumpf Prolases, *Wein Klin Wochenschr* 63:74-77 1951.
3. Cummings KG et al: Scientific Exhibit, American College of Obstetricians and Gynecologists, 1976.
4. Frank RT: The formation of an artificial vagina without operation, *Am J Obstet Gynecol* 35:1053, 1938.
5. Graves WP: Operative treatment of atresia of the vagina, *Boston Med Surg J* 163:753, 1910.
6. Ingram JM: The bicycle seat stool in the treatment of vaginal agenesis and stenosis, *Am J Obstet Gynecol* 140:807, 1981.
7. Martin LW, Sutorius DS: An improved method for vaginoplasty, *Arch Surg* 98:716, 1969.
8. McIndoe AH, Banister JB: An operation for the cure of congenital absence of the vagina, *J Obstet Gynaecol Br Commonw* 45:490, 1938.
9. Morton KE, Davies D, Dewhurst J: The use of the fasciocutaneous flap in vaginal reconstruction, *Br J Obstet Gynecol* 93:970, 1986.
10. Nichols DH, Randall CL: *Vaginal surgery, 3rd ed,* Baltimore, 1989, Williams & Wilkins, pp 404-407.
11. West JT, Ketcham AS, Smith RR: Vaginal reconstruction following pelvic exenteration for cancer or postirradiation necrosis, *Surg Gynecol Obstet* 118:788, 1965.
12. Williams EA: Congenital absence of the vagina: a simple operation for its relief, *J Obstet Gynaecol Br Commonw* 71:511, 1964.

Chapter 25

VAGINECTOMY

David H. Nichols

INDICATIONS FOR VAGINECTOMY

Surgical removal of the vagina may be accomplished for many vastly different reasons. When a neovagina has been created, and for one reason or another the patient has failed to keep the vaginal canal open, shrinkage of the neovagina occurs rather rapidly, with contraction of the scar tissue surrounding the vagina at times producing a rather dense fibrosis. That which seemed to be a vagina of normal depth and caliber at the end of neovaginal construction, in the absence of adequate postoperative dilation, may contract both in width and in depth, often to a diameter of less than one fingerwidth, rendering coitus impossible.

Vaginal intraepithelial neoplasia (VAIN) may be suspected from the report of a posthysterectomy Papanicolaou (Pap) smear. This is not only often multifocal, but may occur in the vault of the vagina at a spot where the surface is poorly visualized, making colposcopy and colposcopically directed biopsy difficult and inconclusive.

Removal of the upper portion of the vagina may be coincident with radical hysterectomy and upper vaginectomy for uterine cancer. Removal of the lower portion of the vagina may take place with coincident radical vulvectomy for vulvar cancer that involves the vaginal introitus.

One occasionally sees a patient with total posthysterectomy vaginal eversion whose tissues cannot retain a pessary and who suffers a major disability. When such a patient is also a poor medical and surgical risk, a surgical procedure that will solve her prolapse problem swiftly and safely must be performed. LeFort partial colpocleisis has been recommended in the past but recurrence of the prolapse is sometimes observed along the lateral canals of vaginal epithelium remaining after the procedure. For many, total transvaginal colpectomy is an acceptable procedure and is followed by extensive scarring and total obliteration of the space formerly occupied by the vagina. Coitus, of course, is impossible. These procedures are discussed at some length in Chapter 27.

TYPES OF VAGINECTOMY AND GOALS

Three types of vaginectomy must be considered by the gynecologist: total vaginectomy, partial vaginectomy, and superficial vaginectomy.

Total vaginectomy

Total vaginectomy is generally of two types. The first consists of colpectomy without replacement of the vagina, as mentioned above, and is usually a feature of the treatment of massive genital prolapse in the patient medically and surgically at high risk.

Vaginectomy with creation of replacement neovagina. The second type is vaginectomy followed by replacement with a neovagina of sufficient caliber to permit coitus. For this purpose, there are a wide variety of procedures from which the surgeon may choose.

Abbe-McIndoe vagina. One involves construction of a replacement vagina by the Abbe-McIndoe procedure with a split-thickness skin graft.[2]

Successful vaginal reconstruction can be achieved even years after initial therapy in patients who develop an obliterated vagina from previous radiation or surgery. Stenosis may also be seen after radical hysterectomy and vaginectomy with creation of a neovagina as treatment in patients with cancer of the vagina, or after neovagina formation in patients undergoing pelvic exenteration. The procedure is as follows (Figs. 25-1 and 25-2):

The scarred vagina is excised by scissor dissection beginning lateral and peripheral to the scar, which provides the least chance for inadvertent damage to bowel or bladder.[7,21] When this has proceeded close to the vaginal vault, one of the surgeon's fingers is inserted into the rectum to facilitate posterior dissection, which ultimately is made to communicate with the lateral spaces. A Foley catheter is instilled into the bladder, and 100 cc of saline heavily colored with indigo carmine or methylene blue are instilled into the bladder through the Foley catheter and the dissection is carried anteriorly. Hemostasis is achieved,

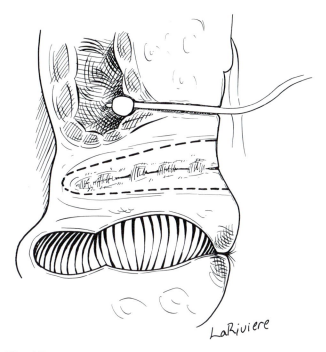

Fig. 25-1. A massively scarred vagina is shown in sagittal section. A Foley catheter is shown within the bladder, which has been partly distended by saline containing a concentrated indigo carmine solution. The entire vagina is excised by sharp dissection, first on each side, and then posteriorly and finally anteriorly beneath the urethra and bladder. Dissection from the rectum may be guided by temporarily placing one of the operator's fingers in the rectum during the dissection.

and an obturator covered by harvested split-thickness skin is inserted.

The donor site may be covered by xeroform or Op-site. The patient is kept at bedrest and given a low-residue diet with prophylactic medication to curb intestinal activity. For further details of the surgical technique, see Chapter 48.

Williams' vulvovaginoplasty. If there are fleshy labia majora present, the patient may be a candidate for the Williams' vulvovaginoplasty[29] as described in Chapter 24. This, however, requires infinite patience on the part of both the patient and her sexual companion and a long process of developing postoperative vaginal width and increased depth both by wearing an obturator as necessary and the employment of frequent coitus.

Davydov peritoneal transplantation. The Davydov procedure[6] is a transplantation of widely mobilized parietal peritoneum to line the cavity of the neovagina (Fig. 25-3). It permits rapid growth of squamous epithelium underneath the transplanted peritoneum. This may be accomplished with particular ease when the patient has just received a radical hysterectomy and vaginectomy as treatment for invasive cervical cancer. The technique of laparoscopically assisted Davydov peritoneal transplantation is considered in some detail in Chapter 73.

Follow-up procedures. Fresh amnion may be used to cover the neovagina,[10,25] permitting rapid ingrowth of squamous epithelium from the cut edges of the remaining vagina and vulva.

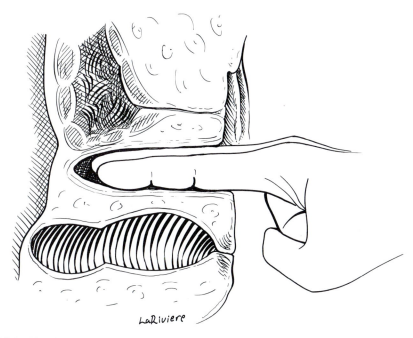

Fig. 25-2. The size and depth of the canal remaining after vaginectomy are carefully estimated by insertion of the operator's fingers. The cavity should accommodate at least three and possibly four fingerwidths and demonstrate an adequate vaginal depth. If the width is inadequate, relaxing incisions can be made in the paravaginal scar tissue at the 3 and 9 o'clock position in the circumference of the vagina.

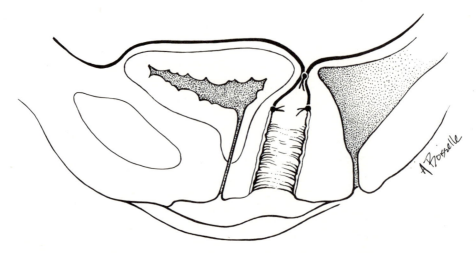

Fig. 25-3. The Davydov operation. Proximal length can be added to a shortened vagina by attaching the margins of the previously dissected parietal peritoneum to the cut edges of the remaining vagina. The peritoneal cavity is securely closed by a separately placed cranial pursestring suture as shown. (From Nichols DH, Randall CL: Vaginal surgery, ed 3, p 229, Baltimore, 1989, Williams & Wilkins.)

Fresh human amnion is a good biologic dressing, if available. It does not convert to epithelium but most effectively resists infection and permits epithelium to grow upward from established epithelial edges. The popularity of this method may be uncertain because of the prevalence of AIDS, because one would not wish to transmit the disease in this fashion.

Because of their length, myocutaneous flaps can be transplanted after vaginectomy because of cancer, if the surgeon has scrupulously determined that all active invasive malignant disease has been extirpated. The gracilis myocutaneous flap is good.[23]

It is possible to use a tissue expander buried beneath the labia minora, which, after some weeks of progressive distention, will provide a surface area sufficient to line the neovaginal canal.[17] Under general anesthesia, tissue expanders are inserted along a bluntly dissected tract to the internal aspect of the labia minora made from an incision over each groin. These buried expanders are connected by flexible plastic tubing to a valve and reservoir in each groin and the skin is closed. Each expander is initially inflated with 40 ml of sterile saline. Expansion is increased by an increment of 10 to 15 cc each day for the next 2 or 3 weeks to an approximate inflation of 120 ml on each side. At the time of construction of a neovagina, each dilator is inflated to 200 ml for 3 minutes at a time, and this is repeated three times. The large folds of essentially hairless labial skin are identified, the labia minora are incised, and large full-thickness flaps are raised by incision along the inner aspect of each enlarged labia minora, and turned into the vagina to line the new cavity. The neovagina is packed for 4 days. The patient is started on the use of a vaginal obturator postoperatively to prevent contraction of the neovagina.

There is a place for the transplantation of a loop of sigmoid colon with which to line the neovagina, particularly in the patient who is neither psychologically nor socially able or willing to use dilators of the neovagina regularly in the postoperative period and who is not sexually active at the time of surgery.[4,12] This may also be useful in the patient who has experienced an exenterative procedure. Because this involves intestinal resection and anastamosis, the patient must be prepared for the possibility of anastamotic leaking and peritonitis and all of its consequences, although the incidence of this complication is low. Sigmoid resection of properly prepared bowel may be performed using the biofragmentable anastamosis ring (BAR)[3,5,9,13,14] (resembling Murphy's[20] steel button; Figs. 25-4 and 25-5). The device fragments after polymer hydrolosis, and it is passed from the body about 18 days after surgery when mechanical support is no longer needed.* The use of the device is easily learned, the technique is accomplished swiftly, and it is cost-effective.

The serosal surface of the bowel should be cleaned for a distance of 1 cm from the point of division. An end-to-end anastomosis (EEA) sizer is inserted into the lumina of the intestinal segments, and the largest sizer the segments accept is selected. Pursestring sutures are placed in the segments, manually or with a pursestring instrument, using a monofilament absorbable suture. The BAR with inserter is advanced into one lumen of the intestinal segment, and a pursestring suture is tightened around the central portion of the BAR. It is tied snugly with a surgeon's knot onto the BAR, but not tightly. The inserter is disengaged from the BAR by bending it back and forth, the opposite end of the BAR is positioned into the other intestinal lumen, and the remaining pursestring is tied down. The BAR is snapped

*Valtrac-Davis & Geck Medical Device Division, American Cyanamid Company, Wayne, NJ.

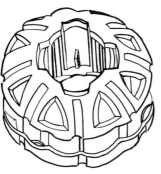

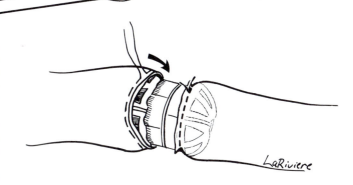

Fig. 25-4. Use of the biofragmentable anastamosis ring (BAR). The ring, composed of polyglycolic acid, is shown in its open position in the drawing at the left. A loop of intestine with an intact blood supply has been resected, and the anastamosis has begun by placement of a hand-sewn pursestring suture around the circumference of the serosal surface of the intestine, the muscularis, and submucosa as shown. At least four passes of the needle for each half of the intestinal circumference are placed, as shown in the central drawing. The pursestring suture is tied snugly but not tightly onto the BAR as shown. The applicator handle is detached from the opposite extremity of the BAR, the proximal BAR is inserted into the distal lumen, and a previously placed pursestring is tied down, as shown in the drawing at the bottom.

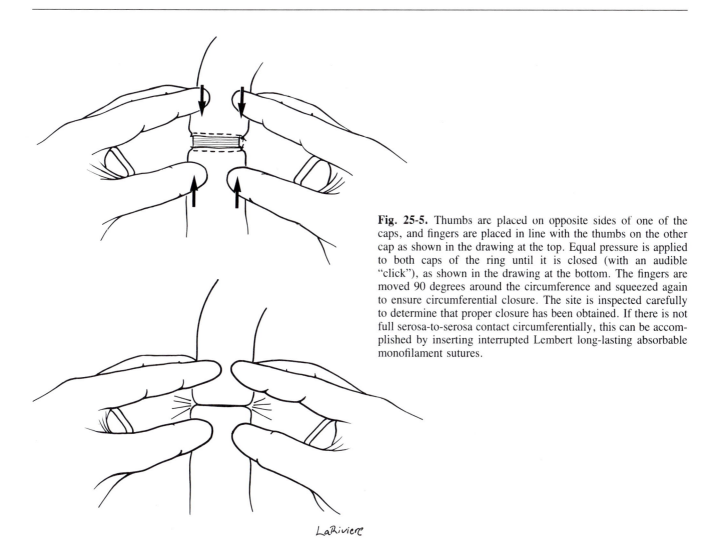

Fig. 25-5. Thumbs are placed on opposite sides of one of the caps, and fingers are placed in line with the thumbs on the other cap as shown in the drawing at the top. Equal pressure is applied to both caps of the ring until it is closed (with an audible "click"), as shown in the drawing at the bottom. The fingers are moved 90 degrees around the circumference and squeezed again to ensure circumferential closure. The site is inspected carefully to determine that proper closure has been obtained. If there is not full serosa-to-serosa contact circumferentially, this can be accomplished by inserting interrupted Lembert long-lasting absorbable monofilament sutures.

shut by even pressure on both sides of the anastamosis forming a serosa-to-serosa inverted sutureless anastamosis.[9] Postoperatively, fluid intake is withheld until bowel sounds are heard, and, once gas has been passed, the diet is advanced as tolerated.

Radical vaginectomy. Radical vaginectomy may be performed as part of the treatment of invasive cancer involving the vagina.

Technique.[19,22] An indwelling Foley catheter is inserted in the bladder, and the vagina is tightly packed. After the abdomen is opened, a traction suture is placed between the residual upper uterosacral ligaments, and the peritoneum is undermined and incised. The bladder is separated from the anterior vagina with gentle sharp dissection, and the posterior dissection divides the peritoneum overlying the psoas muscles to expose the retroperitoneal space and permit identification of the ureter and development of the pararectal and paravesical spaces. The uterine artery is divided at its origin from the internal iliac. The ureter is dissected from the medial leaf of the peritoneum as far as the ureteral tunnel in the anterior parametrium, after which the peritoneum of the cul-de-sac can be safely divided. The rectovaginal space is developed, and the uterosacral ligaments are divided to the level of the pelvic diaphragm. The vagina is dissected from the anterior vaginal wall as far as possible, and, by placing slight tension on the ureter, the tissue covering the most distal ureter is identified and transected. The vagina is removed, which may be made easier if a circumferential incision is made around the introitus at the level of planned amputation. A neovagina can be created by lining the cavity with tissue of various sites as described above.

The vagina may be removed as part of an exenteration (see Chapter 42).

Partial vaginectomy

Partial vaginectomy may occur with radical hysterectomy, either abdominal or vaginal, but, if the cut edge of the peritoneum is sewn to the vaginal cuff, there may be adequate residual depth to permit coitus. If this is not true, parietal peritoneum may be mobilized and sewn to the cut edge as a Davydov operation, as described earlier, and the peritoneum is separately closed by a pursestring suture within the abdominal cavity as shown.

The technique for partial vaginectomy with vaginal hysterectomy is described in Chapter 20.

Partial vaginectomy with hysterectomy, generally done transvaginally, although possible transabdominally, is used when a severe dysplasia of the upper vagina coexists with carcinoma-in-situ of the uterine cervix.

Fresh amnion can be used to coat the raw area of an upper neovaginal dissection.[10,25] A full-thickness skin graft can be used, which may be obtained from the abdomen or from the skin removed between elliptical skin incisions made over the iliac crest.[19]

When a partial vaginectomy has occurred previously

and it is desirable to restore vaginal depth, the following technique is applicable:

Extraperitoneal construction of a neovagina

Full or partial Abbe-McIndoe operation.[1,18,26] When the vagina is too short for coital comfort and the labia majora are not suitably fleshy for a Williams-type vulvovaginoplasty,[29] depth can be added to the proximal vagina by daily applications of obturators of increasing length (the Frank-Ingram[11,15] procedure), which will require an investment of at least 2 hours per day on the part of the patient and supplying forceful pressure to these vaginal obturators, whose length will gradually be increased until the desired vaginal depth has been achieved. When the amount of discomfort that must be borne is unacceptable to the patient during this procedure, or when there is so much scar tissue in the vaginal vault that it cannot be effectively stretched, an alternate procedure is that of surgically creating a cavity at the vault of the vagina, which can be lined with a split-thickness skin graft. The patient must be a given a full description of the procedure and aftercare. The importance of her role in the success of this operation should be discussed. She will be required to wear a vaginal obturator for some months after the operation to make certain that unwanted postoperative shrinkage does not occur.

The procedure is as follows: A wide strip of split-thickness skin is obtained (Braun electric dermatone set at 0.00018 inch). The author's preference is to use the skin of the suprapubic area of the anterior abdominal wall.[8,24] The surface of the skin is shaved, and multiple subcutaneous injections of sterile saline, totaling 200 to 300 cc, are made to flatten the skin surface allowing for a graft of uniform surface dimension and thickness. The skin of the donor site is painted with sterile mineral oil, the graft is removed and wrapped in saline-soaked dressings, and a xeroform dressing is applied to the donor site. Use of this area of donor skin has several advantages:

1. By its anterior location, the patient is not required to endure the pain and discomfort of sitting or resting on the donor site during the long healing phase.
2. Because the graft is cut superficial to the hair follicles, there is prompt regrowth of hair of the escutcheon covering much of the donor site, thus making the donor site more cosmetically acceptable to the patient (there is no hair growth within the graft because the hair follicles are not contained in the split-thickness graft).
3. Pigmentation of the donor site is minimal, and any that is present is mostly covered by pubic hair regrowth.
4. A thicker split-thickness graft is less likely to shrink postoperatively than a thinner graft.

Then 100 cc of sterile milk or infant formula or of sterile saline deeply colored with indigo carmine are instilled into the bladder through an indwelling Foley catheter, which is then clamped. The bladder will be palpable during subsequent dissection of the neovagina. The bulb of the Foley catheter can be palpated, and any unwanted penetration of the bladder is recognized by prompt appearance of dye or milk in the operative field.

In addition, 100 cc of sterile saline is injected beneath the wall of the vaginal vault and upper vagina to compress sites of venous bleeding, and make the dissection of the vagina from the surrounding tissues and scar safer, proceeding in a somewhat conical direction to the peritoneum of the cul-de-sac of Douglas, which may be exposed for no more than 1 to 1.5 cm (lessening the chance for future enterocele development as would be risked if the peritoneal exposure were made greater). Such lateral relaxing incisions in the vestibule or medial border of the pubococcygei are made to permit the patient to contain the obturator postoperatively. Bleeding points are clamped and coagulated or tied. Venous oozing may be controlled with a tight vaginal gauze packing placed for a few minutes.

A precut polyethelene foam cylinder, 5 by 15 cm and rounded or tapered at the proximal end, is prepared.[27]

The edges of the split-thickness graft (raw side out) are draped over the polyethelene foam obturator (no covering condom is needed).

Alternatively, the appropriate sized Heyer-Schulte "inflatable" obturator can be used.

The edges of the graft are approximated with fine absorbable sutures.

The graft-covered obturator* is inserted into the neovagina, and the vaginal orifice is closed temporarily by two or three heavy silk sutures, loosely tied, to hold the mold in place for the next 7 to 8 days. The Foley catheter is connected to a drainage system, and the patient is placed on a low-residue diet and bedrest. Between the seventh and tenth postoperative day, the vestibular stitches are cut and removed, the mold is gently removed, under anesthesia if necessary, and the neovagina is inspected.

A transverse incision is made in the full width of the vaginal vault.

A new obturator made of firm plastic or balsa wood covered by rubber measuring 15 cm in length and 12 cm in circumference is inserted. Alternatively, the Heyer-Schulte mold may be reused. The patient is promptly ambulated and instructed in removal and replacement of the obturator, which may be generously lubricated with estrogen cream. The patient is discharged. The mold should be removed only when the patient goes to the toilet, then promptly replaced. Any help needed holding the obturator in place may be given by the support of a sanitary napkin worn beneath the patient's underpants. After a postoperative month, the vagina is reinspected in the surgeon's office, any granulation tissue is coagulated with silver nitrate, and permission is given to the patient for coital activity, if appropriate. New instructions may be given to the patient to wear the obturator every night during the hours

of sleep and for a total of 2 hours during the day. After 6 postoperative months, if there is no evidence of vaginal stricture, the patient may be asked to wear the obturator nightly three times per week, more frequenty if any obstruction to its insertion is observed.

The transvaginal translaparoscopic modification of the Davydov operation using pelvic peritoneum to cover the raw surfaces of the neovagina is described in Chapter 73.

Alternatively, cecal or ileocecal segments may be transplanted, although this requires an obligatory bowel resection with its small risk of increased morbidity.[4,12]

Length may be added at the distal portion of the vagina by a Williams[29] vulvovaginoplasty as described previously.

Frank-Ingram vaginal dilators. For the patient willing to participate actively in the production of additional vaginal length, several months of daily use of lucite vaginal obturators of progressively increasing depth are useful according to the descriptions of Frank[11] and Ingram.[15] The patient must be willing to devote at least 2 hours per day to this endeavor, survive its discomfort, and pursue this program under her gynecologist's guidance for between 2 and 6 months. The gynecologist may change the obturator at succeeding visits for a progressively larger size. Regular and frequent coitus will aid in the development of increased vaginal depth and ultimate redirection of the vaginal axis toward the hollow of the sacrum.

When the lower half of the vagina needs replacing, full-thickness skin flap transposition as described in Chapter 24 may be employed.

Vecchietti operation. The Vecchietti operation[28] rapidly develops vaginal depth because round-the-clock traction is applied transabdominally to an olive that has been placed within the vaginal vault and threaded to a suture passed from the anterior abdominal wall and attached to a spring supported within a frame, which rests upon the lower abdomen. Additional vaginal length will be evident within 1 to 2 weeks.

Superficial vaginectomy using the CO_2 laser[16]

In the posthysterectomy patient with an abnormal Pap smear, but also in the patient treated by radiation therapy for invasive cervical cancer, an apparent discrepancy may arise between an abnormal cytology report and the difficulties with effective and decisive vaginal colposcopy. Postmenopausal vaginal atrophy and the vaginal deformities after hysterectomy or radiation therapy, for example, account for some of the disparity. Negative reports obtained on specimens received after random vaginal biopsy are not helpful in the face of persistently positive cytology studies. Traditional cervical vaginectomy is often difficult in such cases and requires grafting and a long period of obturator use to permit preservation or restoration of a coitally useful vagina. Superficial partial vaginectomy using the CO_2 laser in the hands of a surgeon experienced in laser surgery and colposcopy has been reported by Julian,

---

*The lucite obturators are available from Faulkner Plastics Incorporated, 4504 East Hillsborough Ave., Tampa, FL 33610.

O'Connell, and Gosewehr[16] as a most useful procedure.

The vagina of the younger patient with a clearly defined small lesion can be studied by direct or colposcopically directed biopsy.

Skillfully performed partial superficial vaginectomy provides a surgical specimen for histologic study, helping to discriminate between vaginal intraepithelial neoplasia (VAIN) and cervical intraepithelial neoplasia (CIN) as well as invasive squamous cancer, in contrast to the use of laser vaporization of the area in question, which does not provide a surgical specimen for diagnosis.

Vaginal epithelial regeneration with minimal scarring has been reported after superficial laser excision, and postoperative healing might be hastened in the postmenopausal patient with the use of vaginal obturators and generous frequent application of intravaginal estrogen cream.

Procedure.[16] After preliminary colposcopy with determination of the amount of vagina to be removed for study, and under general or regional anesthesia, the area is thoroughly infiltrated with a "liquid tourniquet," such as 1:200,000 epinephrine or pitressin solution.

Using the CO_2 laser mounted on a colposcope, and employing a sharply focused beam with power density of 750 to 1200 W/cm^2, the surgeon makes an incision just beneath the 3-mm thickness of vaginal epithelium raising first the posterior flap, then an anterior one, and by traction to an applied Allis clamp, the entire specimen is removed for study. The patient is hospitalized overnight for observation, then discharged with plans for frequent follow-up. Reepithelialization is prompt, but any granulation tissue may be effectively coagulated with silver nitrate. Obturators, dilators, and vaginal estrogen cream are prescribed as necessary.

PREOPERATIVE AND POSTOPERATIVE CARE

It is important that the patient clearly understand the objectives of treatment. A careful and honest prediction concerning the duration of treatment, the duration of disability, and the degree to which the patient must participate in her care is essential to the success of any of these techniques. With the exception of the nonsurgical Frank-Ingram pressure technique, all of the above methods require hospitalization. Most require the wearing of a vaginal obturator postoperatively for varying lengths of time during the day, at night, and for varying weeks or months after surgery, with periodic assessment of residual vaginal size during the interim. Any tendency toward shrinkage or fibrosis of the neovagina must be combated vigorously with reinstitution of dilation and increased number of intervals of wearing the obturator.

For the postmenopausal patient, estrogen replacement therapy in an adequate dose is important in maintaining an adequate vaginal blood supply and vaginal elasticity. The increased thickness it induces in the wall of the vagina will be a barrier against infection and erosion and will improve the patient's coital comfort. The obturators can be generously lubricated with estrogen cream during their use, and,

in the interim, 1 g of estrogen cream instilled at bedtime once or twice a week in the neovagina helps to enhance the healing process and maintain good vaginal health postoperatively. This may be used in addition to oral estrogen administration that may be given in adequate dose to retard the development of osteoporosis and provide protection of the patient's cardiovascular system.

REFERENCES

1. Abbe R: New method of creating a vagina in a case of congenital absence, *Med Rec* 54:836, 1898.
2. Berek JS et al: Delayed vaginal reconstruction in the fibrotic pelvis following radiation or previous reconstruction, *Obstet Gynecol* 61:743, 1983.
3. Bubrick MP et al: Prospective, randomized trial of the biofragmentable anastomosis ring, *Am J Surg* 161:136, 1991.
4. Burger RA et al: Ileocecal vaginal construction, *Am J Obstet Gynecol* 161:162, 1989.
5. Corman ML et al: Comparison of the Valtrac biofragmentable anastomosis ring with conventional suture and stapled anastomosis in colon surgery, *Dis Colon Rectum* 32:183, 1989.
6. Davydov SN: Modifizierte kolpopoese aus peritoneum der excavatio rectouterina, *Obstet Gynecol* (Moscow) 12:55, 1969. Quoted in Käser O, Iklé FA, Hirsch HA: *Atlas der gynäkologischen operationen*, 4 Auflage, Stuttgart, 1983, Georg Thieme Verlag, p. 14.21, 14.22.
7. DiSaia PJ, Rettenmaier MA: *Vaginectomy*. In Sanz LE, editor: *Gynecologic surgery*, Oradell, NJ, 1988, Med Economics.
8. Dudzinski MR, Rader JS: The mons pubis: an excellent graft donor site in gynecologic surgery, *Am J Obstet Gynecol* 162:722, 1990.
9. Dyess DL, Curreri PW, Ferrara JJ: A new technique for sutureless intestinal anastomosis, *Am Surg* 56:71, 1990
10. Feroze RM, Dewhurst CJ, Welply G: Vaginoplasty at the Chelsea Hospital for Women: A comparison of two techniques, *Br J Obstet Gynaecol* 82:536, 1975.
11. Frank RT: The formation of an artifical vagina without operation, *Am J Obstet Gynecol* 35:1053, 1938.
12. Goligher JC: The use of pedicled transplants of sigmoid or other parts of the intestinal tract for vaginal construction, *Ann R Coll Surg Engl* 65:353, 1983.
13. Hardy TG et al: A biofragmentable ring for sutureless bowel anastomosis, *Dis Colon Rectum* 28:484, 1985.
14. Hardy TG, Jr. et al: Initial clinical experience with a biofragmentable ring for sutureless bowel anastomosis, *Dis Colon Rectum* 30:55, 1987.
15. Ingram JM: The bicycle seat in the treatment of vaginal agenesis and stenosis: a preliminary report, *Am J Obstet Gynecol* 1:867, 1981.
16. Julian TM, O'Connell BJ, Gosewehr JA: Indications, techniques and advantages of partial laser vaginectomy, *Obstet Gynecol* 80:140, 1992.
17. Lilford RJ, Sharpe DT, Thomas DFM: Use of tissue expansion techniques to create skin flaps for vaginoplasty, *Br J Obstet Gynaecol* 95:402, 1988.
18. McIndoe AH, Banister JB: An operation for the cure of congenital absence of the vagina, *J Obstet Gynaecol Br Commonw* 45:490, 1938.
19. Morley GW, DeLancey JOL: Full-thickness skin graft vaginoplasty for treatment of the stenotic or foreshortened vagina, *Obstet Gynecol* 77:485, 1991.
20. Murphy JB: Cholecysto-intestinal, gastro-intestinal, entero-intestinal anastomosis, and approximation without sutures, *Med Rec* 42:665, 1892.
21. Nichols DH, Randall CL: *Vaginal surgery,* ed 3, pp. 422, 423, Baltimore, 1989, Williams & Wilkins.
22. Rettenmaier MA, DiSaia PD: Understanding current vaginectomy techniques, *Contemp Obstet Gynecol* 30:109, 1987.
23. Soper JT et al: Short gracilis myocutaneous flaps for vulvovaginal re-

construction after radical pelvic surgery, *Obstet Gynecol* 74:823, 1989.

24. Stal S, Spira M: Mons pubis as a donor site for split-thickness skin grafts, *Plast Reconstr Surg* 75:906, 1985.

25. Tancer ML, Katz M, Veridiano NP: Vaginal epithelialization with human amnion, *Obstet Gynecol* 54:345, 1979.

26. Thompson JD, Wharton LR, TeLinde RW: Congenital absence of the vagina, *Am J Obstet Gynecol* 74:397, 1957.

27. Tolhurst DE, van der Helm TWJS: The treatment of vaginal atresia, *Surg Gynecol Obstet* 172:407, 1991.

28. Vecchietti G: Le neo-vagin dams le syndrome de Rokitansky-Kuster-Hauser. *Rev Med Suisse Romande* 99:593, 1979.

29. Williams EA: Congenital absence of the vagina: a simple operation for its relief, *J Obstet Gynaecol Br Commonw* 71:511, 1964.

Chapter 26

ENTEROCELE

David H. Nichols

The posterior peritoneal cul-de-sac occasionally extends caudally between the rectum and the vagina to varying depths, even as far as the perineal body.[14,21] A deep cul-de-sac becomes an enterocele (a peritoneum-lined sac between the vagina and the rectum) when small bowel mesentery and omentum have lengthened sufficiently to permit them to enter and distend this deep cul-de-sac. Therefore, such a cul-de-sac should be obliterated coincidently whenever it is found at surgery. The question may be asked, however, does a long small bowel mesentery precede an enterocele sac, or does it follow an enterocele sac?

Because not all deep cul-de-sacs have abdominal content, it is necessary to distinguish between those with bowel content and those without. The former are symptomatic, causing backache and a dragging sensation that is accentuated in the erect position and relieved by lying down; the discomfort is probably the result of omental and mesenteric traction. The latter type, without bowel content, is generally asymptomatic. It is not known whether the two are etiologically different and whether the long intestinal mesentery is the cause or the result of the deep cul-de-sac when the two coexist, although the weight of the bowel with a long mesentery may increase the risk of a recurrence of enterocele after treatment.

Despite the frequency with which the vaginal vault is left open at the time of abdominal hysterectomy, postoperative vaginal evisceration is rare. (Is this because the small bowel mesentery is usually too short to permit routine pressure of the small bowel's weight against the vault of the vagina?) Massive eversion of the vagina may occur with or without enterocele (although the former condition is more common), and enterocele may occur with or without massive eversion. Enterocele and massive eversion often coexist, but they are *separate* anatomic and clinical entities, each requiring separate, specific surgical treatment. The gynecologist must make these distinctions, because the treatments are quite different.

A vagina with previously normal depth may become unexpectedly short and poorly supported after the repair of a challenging enterocele, even though the repair was competently performed. The reason for an unacceptable shortening of the vagina is not always immediately apparent. It should be possible to recognize the possibility of such a problem in advance, however, by considering the enterocele's location and etiology, which seem to be directly correlated. Taking these factors into account in the selection of the operative procedure not only reduces the likelihood of a recurrence, but also prevents an undesirable degree of vaginal shortening.

TYPES OF ENTEROCELE

Essentially, an enterocele is a herniation of the lining of the peritoneal cavity, with portions of the abdominal viscera within the herniating sac, that extends into areas of the pelvis where the peritoneum is not usually found. Strictly speaking, the term *enterocele* is a misnomer because a hernia is normally named not according to its contents, but according to its location. A better gynecologic term may be hernia of the cul-de-sac, but the present usage of the term *enterocele* has been accepted for so long that it would be difficult to displace. At any rate, an enterocele that is unrecognized and unrepaired tends to progress and causes increasing discomfort and, eventually, increasing disability.

An enterocele may be either anterior, posterior, or lateral to the vagina,[20] with or without secondary eversion of the vaginal vault. The surgeon should always distinguish an enterocele with an accompanying vault eversion from one without such a complicating factor[19] because the causes, as well as the objectives and techniques of surgical reconstruction, vary for each type of enterocele and are quite different when vaginal eversion is also present.

There are four basic types of enterocele: congenital, pulsion, traction, or iatrogenic. They may occur either singly or in combination. The progression of each of these types of true prolapse may result in massive eversion of the vagina. Not only are these the most frequently encountered enteroceles, but also each represents one of the basic etiologic factors. The significant relationships in the anatomy of the enteroceles suggest the important differences in etiology.

Congenital enterocele

An enterocele posterior to the vault of the vagina is often associated with a congenitally deep pouch of Douglas, but not generally with eversion of the vaginal vault (Fig. 26-1, *A*). An unusually deep peritoneal pouch generally results from failure of normal fusion of the anterior with the posterior peritoneum of the cul-de-sac during late fetal development. If the soft tissue supports of the pelvis are oth-

erwise intact, this type of posterior enterocele may exist quite independently of other lesions.

With the congenital type of enterocele related to a pathologically deep pouch of Douglas, the anterior wall of the sac is attached to the undersurface of the posterior vaginal wall. This attachment is certainly not present when the descent of the vaginal vault occurs coincidently with general postmenopausal prolapse.

Pulsion versus traction enterocele

An enterocele associated with procidentia results from massive anterior segment damage as a result of both pulsion from above and traction from below.[15,21] As the cervix descends, it takes with it the anterior margin of the cul-de-sac, although the posterior peritoneal wall remains in situ and attached to the anterior wall of the rectum. An enterocele that coexists with eversion of the vaginal vault may be the result of *pulsion* from pathologically increased intraabdominal pressure (Fig. 26-1, *B*); such an enterocele is usually associated with the uterovaginal or sliding type of genital prolapse. This is a most massive form of damage, and the descent of the entire upper vaginal suspensory apparatus is a secondary effect. Reconstruction of this type of enterocele involves not only excision of the enterocele sac, but also, more importantly, fixation or suspension of the vaginal vault to some structure capable of supporting it to avoid permanent pathologic shortening of the vagina. Another type of enterocele develops as a result of *traction* on a poorly supported vaginal vault by the other pelvic structures that are already prolapsed (Fig. 26-1, *C*). Although a traction enterocele is preceded by a cystocele and a rectocele, a pulsion enterocele may be followed by them.

Although pudendal[2] or lateral enteroceles are most uncommon (Figs. 26-2 to 26-4), they may develop in sites of

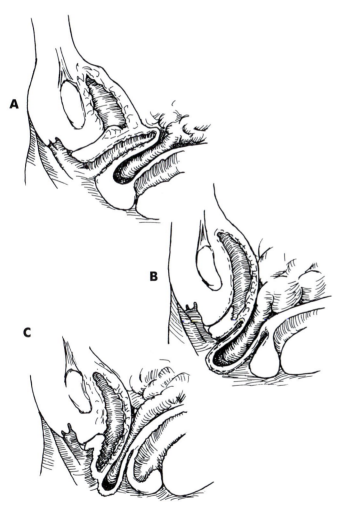

Fig. 26-1. A, Posterior enterocele without eversion of the vagina. **B,** With pulsion enterocele, the upper vagina is everted and the enterocele sac follows the everted vault. Cystocele and rectocele are minimal. **C,** With traction enterocele, there is eversion of the vagina with enterocele, cystocele, and rectocele. (Redrawn and reproduced with permission of American College of Obstetrics and Gynecology from Nichols DH: Types of enterocele and principles underlying the choice of operation for repair, *Obstet Gynecol* 40:257, 1972.)

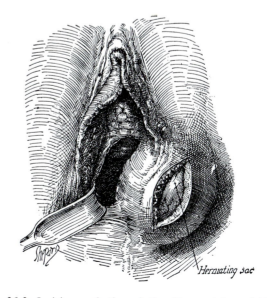

Fig. 26-2. Incision made through the skin overlying a labial or pudendal enterocele, showing the sac of the hernia. (From Watson LF: *Hernia,* St Louis, 1948, Mosby–Year Book.)

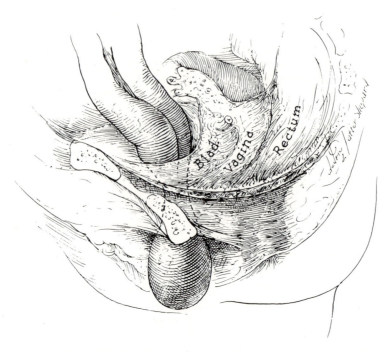

Fig. 26-3. Pudendal or lateral enterocele is shown in sagittal view. (Reproduced with permission of American College of Obstetrics and Gynecology from Nichols DH: Types of enterocele and principles underlying the choice of operation for repair, *Obstet Gynecol* 40:257, 1972.)

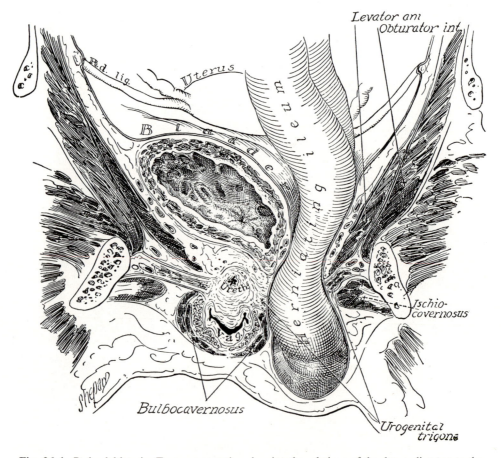

Fig. 26-4. Pudendal hernia. Transverse section showing the relations of the descending sac to the labium majora. (From Watson LF: *Hernia,* St Louis, 1948, Mosby–Year Book.)

unusual weakness within or alongside the pelvic diaphragm or through the pelvic foramina. There may be a history of sudden traumatic increase in intraabdominal pressure, either from the strain of exceedingly heavy lifting or from sudden massive abdominal compression, as from an explosion or blast. This traumatic increase has been noted in a patient whose abdomen had been run over by the wheel of a car and in a patient on whose abdomen a horse had fallen. The patient with a pudendal or lateral enterocele may notice a mass alongside the vagina, especially when standing. Enteroceles of this type that do not appear externally are likely to be diagnosed at the time of laparotomy for intestinal obstruction, as the neck of the pudendal enterocele is found to be the site of the mechanical obstruction.

PUDENDAL HYDROCELE

When a canal persists alongside the round ligament, in a labium majora, and the internal or proximal end of the canal is closed, fluid may collect within the sac producing a pudendal or labial hydrocele. It differs from labial enterocele in that the neck of the hydrocele sac is closed and the fluid content is not reducible, nor is a cough impulse transmitted. Hydrocele is distinguished from a Bartholin's cyst by its location in the anterocranial portion of the labium majora. Occasionally hydrocele is bilateral.

Pudendal hydrocele is harmless, but when painful is treated surgically by opening and extirpation of the sac and suture obliteration of the wound. Simple aspiration of the fluid or balloon marsupialization of the sac usually is followed by prompt recurrence. The treatment of pudendal enterocele requires excision of the sac and careful closure of its neck. If the edges of the neck of the sac are crisp and well-defined it may be closed from below, but if the edges are rounded or ill-defined, transabdominal closure may be more secure and preferable.

Because both pulsion and traction enteroceles are invariably progressive, they tend ultimately to pull with them the organs attached to the sides of the herniating peritoneal sac. As a result, there may be complete eversion of the vaginal vault, usually combined with a degree of lower vaginal eversion. This type of enterocele requires repair.

Iatrogenic enterocele

Iatrogenic alterations in pelvic anatomy may play a role in the development of an enterocele. For example, an anterior enterocele may develop if an unresected excess of anterior peritoneum was not removed at the time of hysterectomy (Fig. 26-5), or a posterior enterocele may develop if a surgical procedure changed the normally horizontal vaginal axis to a vertical inclination (Fig. 26-6). The failure to recognize and correct an unusually deep cul-de-sac at the time of hysterectomy may also lead to the development of a posterior enterocele.

Burch has suggested that enterocele may follow the urethrovesical "pin-up" operation in from 11% to 15% of instances, probably because the operation changes the vaginal axis in a way that may leave the cul-de-sac unprotected and, therefore, subject to unusual stress from changes in intraabdominal pressure.[3] For this reason, the gynecologic surgeon should take specific intraperitoneal operative steps to obliterate the cul-de-sac at the time of a pin-up operation, thus sparing the patient the risk of the secondary difficulty of subsequent enterocele. Such steps may include the use of Moschcowitz[12] or Halban[4] sutures, or even peritonealization after coincident hysterectomy.

The incidence of enterocele subsequent to vaginal hysterectomy can be determined only by long-term follow-up. A postoperative examination at 6 weeks gives no indication of this problem, because it is usually more than 6

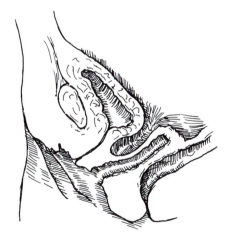

Fig. 26-5. A posthysterectomy anterior enterocele is illustrated. It lies between the bladder and the vagina. (Redrawn and reproduced with permission of American College of Obstetrics and Gynecology from Nichols DH: Types of enterocele and principles underlying the choice of operation for repair, *Obstet Gynecol* 40:257, 1972.)

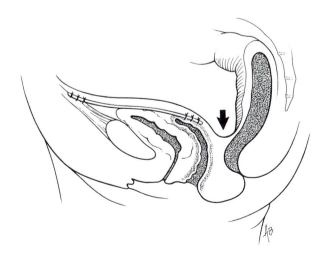

Fig. 26-6. The unprotected cul-de-sac left after ventral fixation of the vagina is noted by the arrow. (Redrawn and reproduced from Nichols DH: *Repair of enterocele and prolapse of the vaginal vault.* In Barber H, editor: *Goldsmith's practice of surgery,* Woodbury, Conn, 1981, Cine-Med, with permission.)

months after surgery before an enterocele occurs; often, it is not until after 1 or more years. At 6-week follow-up examinations of 944 patients after vaginal reconstruction, Hawksworth and Roux noted that only three had symptoms of enteroceles that required subsequent operation.[5] More than 1 year after surgery, however, 26 of 416 such patients had developed enteroceles that required repair.

Anterior and posterior colporrhaphy should follow vaginal hysterectomy whenever there is a significant degree of genital prolapse, as determined by an examination of the unanesthetized patient both while she is supine and while she is standing. Many surgeons elect the vaginal route when hysterectomy is indicated, for example, when there is dysfunctional uterine bleeding, with or without small fibroids. Surgery by this route can often proceed quickly and with a minimum of postoperative discomfort and morbidity. An accompanying vaginal prolapse that is demonstrable, however, is likely to progress in the postoperative years to a point that requires secondary operative reconstruction. A so-called pseudoprolapse (demonstrated *only* when traction is applied to the cervix by a tenaculum) may warrant no other attention than recognition at the time of vaginal hysterectomy.

SYMPTOMS OF ENTEROCELE

Patients with an enterocele and vault prolapse often describe a feeling of pelvic heaviness and a bearing-down sensation, especially when standing; these symptoms occur because the pull of gravity stretches the mesentery of the contents of the sac. If the cardinal and uterosacral ligaments are involved in the prolapse, downward traction on the uterosacral ligaments often causes a backache that may worsen as the day goes on and is quickly relieved by lying down.

The presence of a protruding vulvar mass may cause vaginal discomfort, and coincident dyspareunia, which is accentuated by the dryness of the exteriorized vagina, is common. If the vaginal skin is ulcerated, there may be troublesome discharge and bleeding. When rectocele coexists, the patient may experience difficulty in emptying the bowel, incomplete movements, and postevacuation discomfort. Urinary complaints are uncommon unless displacement cystocele coexists when there is inability to empty the bladder, resulting in stagnation of urine with overflow incontinence. Thoughtful and appropriate reconstructive genital surgery should relieve the discomfort and distress of all these symptoms.

DIAGNOSIS

The descent of the cul-de-sac without an accompanying enterocele is related primarily to a major defect in the pelvic diaphragm. It is usually, although not always, seen in a postmenopausal woman in whom the pelvic diaphragm sags, the levator plate tips, and the horizontal axis of the upper vagina is lost. This condition differs from an enterocele, which is an actual herniation between the rectum and the vagina, and it is important to distinguish between the two conditions before surgery, as the treatment of each is different (see Chapter 30).

An enterocele can coexist with other manifestations of genital prolapse, but it is likely to be unrecognized when the patient is examined only when relieved and in the lithotomy position. The proper time to identify an enterocele is before surgery, because damage that is obvious when the patient is awake and straining is less evident when she is anesthetized and in the recumbent position. Preoperative rectovaginal examination of the unanesthetized patient is, therefore, indicated with the patient both at rest and while straining, in both the lithotomy and standing positions. Contrast radiography occasionally proves helpful.[6,7]

An effective way of distinguishing between enterocele, prolapse of the vaginal vault, rectocele, a defective perineum, and combinations of these weaknesses is by the preoperative examination of the standing, unanesthetized patient. With an index finger in the patient's rectum, the gynecologist inserts the thumb into her vagina. The presence of vault prolapse can be established by replacing the vault of the vagina to its highest level within the pelvis and noting what happens when the patient bears down, as by Valsalva's maneuver. If a peritoneal sac that contains omentum or a palpable loop of bowel comes down between the thumb and the index finger, the woman unquestionably has an enterocele (Fig. 26-7). Because an enterocele splits Denonvilliers' fascia, it weakens the upper posterior vaginal wall. A high rectocele is so often associated with an enterocele that the presence of one should always give rise to a suspicion of the presence of the other; the treatment of both should be coincident and often requires a transvaginal, rather than a transabdominal, surgical procedure for optimal success.

Such a preoperative evaluation is important because many enteroceles thought to have developed after vaginal surgery are actually aggravations of an unrecognized and, therefore, untreated condition that existed at the time of an original pelvic operation.

MANAGEMENT OF ENTEROCELE

The indicated management of enterocele may be prophylactic, nonsurgical, and surgical.

Prophylaxis

Intraabdominal pressure may be decreased and, thus, the development or progression of an enterocele may be prevented by reducing weight, avoiding tight girdles and corsets, and refraining from cigarettes to decrease smoker's cough.

At the time of a vaginal hysterectomy and repair, the surgeon can do a great deal to prevent postoperative enterocele,[8] even though an existing or potential enterocele may not be obvious in a patient who is anesthetized and in Trendelenburg's position, for example, in which the pull of gravity is toward the head of the table. After removing the uterus and before closing the peritoneum, the surgeon

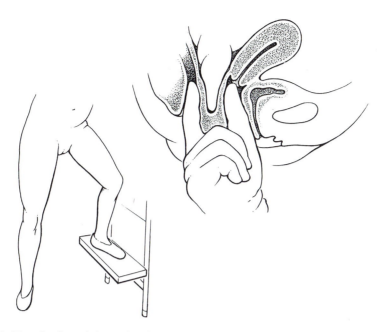

Fig. 26-7. Examination of the patient in a standing position permits the thumb in the vagina to note and replace any descent of the vaginal vault, while the index finger introduced into the rectum permits evaluation of any possible rectocele. When the patient strains, any enterocele present is evidenced by palpation of a bowel-filled sac prolapse dissecting the rectovaginal septum. (Redrawn and reproduced with permission of Cine-Med, Woodburn CT, from Nichols DH: Repair of enterocele and prolapse of the vaginal vault. In Barber H, editor: *Goldsmith's practice of surgery*, Woodbury, Conn, 1981, Cine-Med, with permission.)

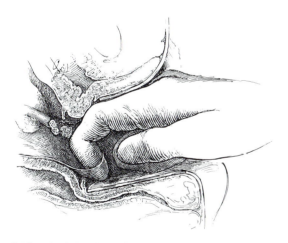

Fig. 26-8. The index finger is hooked into the peritoneum of the cul-de-sac following hysterectomy to identify any enterocele sac that may be present so that it may be excised at this point. (From Nichols DH, Randall CL: *Vaginal surgery*, ed 3, Baltimore, 1989, Williams & Wilkins, p 217.)

should hook a finger in the cul-de-sac to see if it contains any extra peritoneum that should be excised (Fig. 26-8). If the uterosacral ligaments are strong, they should be shortened and used appropriately to help support the vaginal vault. This procedure may involve a cul-de-plasty in which stitches are placed into these shortened uterosacral ligaments to draw the vault of the vagina back into the hollow of the sacrum, cranial and posterior to the point at which the peritoneum has been closed (Fig. 26-9).[11] The same

type of stitches may be placed immediately after abdominal hysterectomy. Coincident excision and side-to-side approximation of an appropriate wedge from the posterior vaginal vault may be performed either transvaginally or transabdominally if it is excessively wide (Figs. 26-10 and 26-11).

After vaginal hysterectomy, a high pursestring closure of the peritoneal cavity is often helpful. Taking good bites of both the uterosacral and the round ligaments, but with care to avoid the ureter, the surgeon approximates the connective tissues to which the peritoneum is attached. If a large enterocele has been resected, the surgeon may place two pursestring sutures, one caudal to the other.

Nonsurgical treatment

Pessaries are occasionally of temporary help in patients with coincident genital prolapse who are not candidates for surgery or whose personal schedule does not permit surgery (e.g., those with small children at home or with an aging relative who requires constant care). Patients are most likely to be able to retain a pessary of the ring type, a rubber doughnut, or sometimes a Gellhorn (see Chapter 27). Isometric pubococcygeal contraction exercises are helpful in restoring muscle tone, but they are not curative.

Surgical treatment

The goals of the surgical repair of an enterocele are (1) to recognize the entity and its probable cause; (2) to expose, dissect, mobilize, and then excise or obliterate the

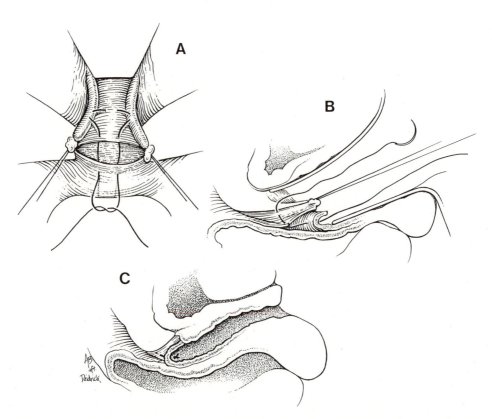

Fig. 26-9. A, Modified cul-de-plasty stitch. The enterocele sac has been resected, and a bite of absorbable polyglycolic-type acid suture has been placed through the full thickness of the posterior vaginal wall at a spot selected to become the highest point of the reconstructed vaginal vault. Traction is made on the uterosacral ligament pedicles and the suture picks up the cut edge of the peritoneum and the peritoneal side of each uterosacral ligament at the level to which the vaginal vault will be fixed. The suture is returned through the peritoneum and vaginal vault of the opposite side. **B,** The first half of this stitch is seen in sagittal section before typing, **C.** After tying and subsequent closure of the peritoneal cavity and vaginal vault, the apex of the vagina is now cranial- and posterior to the new peritoneal cul-de-sac. (Redrawn from Nichols DH, Randall CL: *Vaginal surgery,* ed 3, Baltimore, 1989, Williams & Wilkins, p 223.)

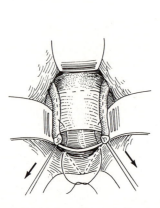

Fig. 26-10. A pathologically wide vaginal vault should be narrowed by excision of a V-shaped wedge (*dashed line*). (Redrawn from Nichols DH, Randall CL: *Vaginal surgery,* ed 3, Baltimore, 1989, Williams & Wilkins, p 223.)

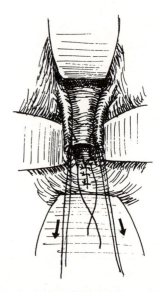

Fig. 26-11. The edges of the V are sewn together, thus narrowing a pathologically wide vaginal vault. (From Nichols DH: *Reoperative gynecology.* St Louis, 1991, Mosby–Year Book, p 118.)

entire sac; (3) to occlude the orifice of the sac by ligation as high as possible; and (4) to perform all indicated repair to provide adequate support from below for the occluded orifice of the sac and to reestablish a normal upper vaginal axis, if the axis is defective, so that the area of previous herniation will be held in place over a horizontal levator plate. The specific objectives of surgical treatment are

1. Restoration of normal anatomy and function
2. Prevention of recurrence as a result of the recognition and consideration of etiologic factors
3. Appropriate surgical treatment of coexistent pelvic disease, when indicated
4. Recognition and treatment of any contributing medical disease

The choice of a surgical procedure for the repair of an enterocele is based on several considerations. There is no one standard corrective operation. The etiology, symptoms, and principles of surgical treatment are considerably different for each of the various sites.

Transvaginal procedures involve recognition and excision of the sac, followed by high ligation of the peritoneum. The transvaginal double pursestring closure of the neck of the sac of an enterocele is essentially a transvaginal Moschcowitz closure. Each of the two pursestring sutures takes some of the strain off the other. In addition, bringing together two areas of peritoneum lining the neck of the sac instead of one produces a stronger scar (Fig. 26-

12). This technique is useful if there is a coincident vault prolapse that is to be treated separately.

The problem with the transabdominal Moschcowitz procedure for enterocele is that the operation was originally developed to repair a prolapsed or sliding rectum by attaching it to a fairly strong vagina and cervix. Gynecologists appropriated the operation and reversed the principle by attaching a sliding vagina to the anterior wall of the rectum. The latter has rather poor structural support, however (Figs. 26-13 and 26-14).

The Halban or Moschcowitz obliteration of the cul-de-sac helps prevent an enterocele, but it is not an effective procedure for the treatment of a vault prolapse. Neither the Halban nor the Moschcowitz procedure per se provides adequate support for the vaginal vault. Both obliterate the cul-de-sac, and neither requires skinning out removal of excess peritoneum (Fig. 26-15). There are several problems with this approach. Tying the top stitch at the pelvic brim is difficult, and any central opening that remains can provide access to a loop of small bowel and may cause intestinal obstruction. Furthermore, because it is placed near the ureter, the top stitch may be close enough to pull or displace the tissue to which the ureter is attached, causing a kink in the ureter on either side and leading to urinary obstruction.

Sagittally placed Halban-type stitches are, literally, vertical Moschcowitz-type of stitches, but they do not disturb the course of the ureter. They are especially useful when

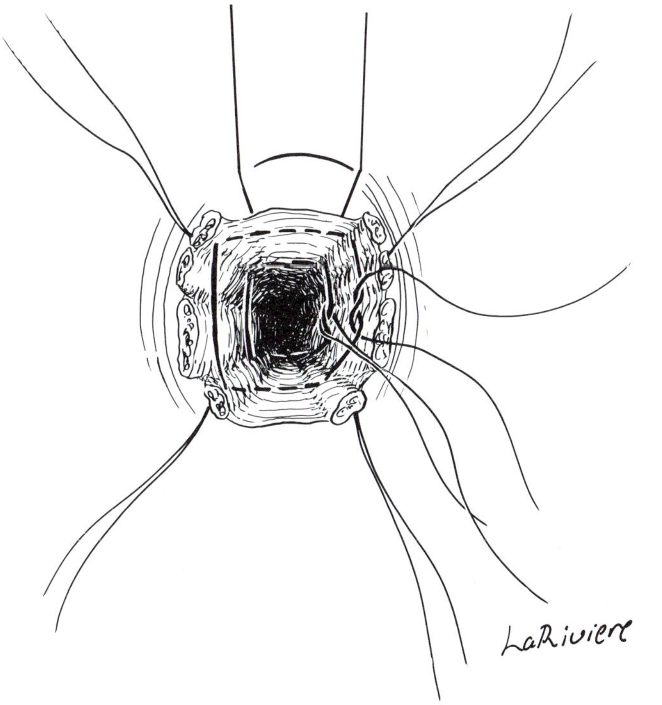

Fig. 26-12. The enterocele sac has been resected, and the peritoneal cavity will be closed by a pursestring suture that incorporates the uterosacral and the round ligaments as shown. After this has been tied, a second pursestring stitch placed 1 cm distal to the first reinforces the closure. (Redrawn from Nichols DH, Randall CL: *Vaginal surgery*, ed 3, Baltimore, 1989, Williams & Wilkins.)

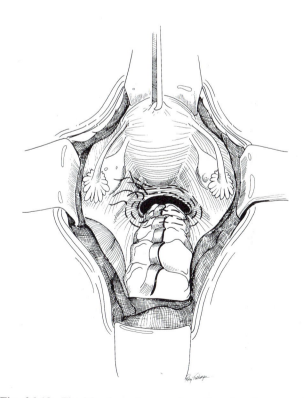

Fig. 26-13. The Moschcowitz procedure. A series of concentric sutures are placed as shown to obliterate the cul-de-sac. (From Corson SL, Sedlacek TV, Hoffman JJ: *Greenhill's surgical gynecology*, ed 5, St Louis, 1986, Mosby–Year Book, p 151.)

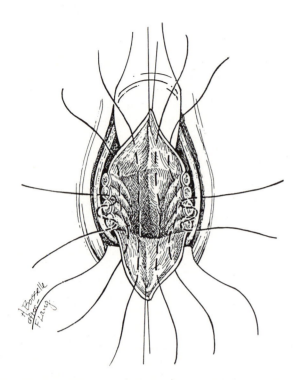

Fig. 26-14. Sagittal obliteration of the cul-de-sac may be performed after vaginal hysterectomy as shown. (From Nichols DH, Randall CL: *Vaginal surgery*, ed 3, Baltimore, 1989, Williams & Wilkins.)

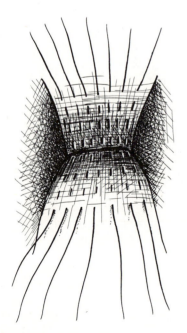

Fig. 26-15. The cul-de-sac is being obliterated by a series of interrupted stitches placed from front to back. (Redrawn from Nichols DH, Randall CL: *Vaginal surgery*, ed 3, Baltimore, 1989, Williams & Wilkins.)

the vault has not prolapsed. They can be placed after either transabdominal or transvaginal operations (Figs. 26-16 and 26-17) but neither type of stitch effectively anchors a poorly supported or unsupported vaginal vault, the latter requiring separate colpopexy. The patient who has a very wide and deep pouch of Douglas and risks chronically increased intraabdominal pressure secondary to obesity or respiratory obstruction from chronic pulmonary disease or vigorous life style, may carry increased risk for reopening of a surgically obliterated or fused cul-de-sac. There are two additional surgical methods of obliterating the pouch of Douglas over a wider area. One is to dissect and resect the entire peritoneal lining of the pouch, and after controlling the many areas of oozing and bleeding by ligature or cautery, sew the raw surfaces together by many interrupted sutures. This method is time consuming, usually bloody, and may expose to possible trauma the surfaces of the larger blood vessels and ureters. Another effective, faster, and safer method that does not involve peritoneal resection is to obliterate such a wide pouch of Douglas by sewing from front to back a transversely placed continuous suture that begins at the very bottom of the cavity. By alternate bites 1 cm apart between the anterior and the posterior cul-de-sac surfaces the suture is continued back and forth from one side of the pelvis to the other using a running locked stitch. The stitch is continued by additional rows a centimeter or so cranial to its predecessor until the brim of the pelvis is reached when the suture is tied. A final row of interrupted sutures 1 cm apart is placed at the pelvic brim. During the course of the procedure the site of the vital structures is kept under observation, and trauma to them is avoided.

An enterocele accompanied by a prolapse of the vault posterior to the cervix in a patient whose uterus has been fixed by a Gilliam suspension or ventral fixation is treated transvaginally by high ligation of the neck of the sac. This includes a deep bite or two into the lower posterior part of the cervix or lower uterine segment, then excision of the sac. If the uterosacral ligaments are strong, they are approximated at the midline and shortened. Any coexistent cystocele or rectocele is repaired, with the rectocele repair including the high, full-length posterior colporrhaphy. If eversion of the upper vagina coexists and the strength of the cardinal and uterosacral ligaments is insufficient to support the vaginal vault securely, the upper vaginal vault may be sewn to the right sacrospinous ligament (see Chapter 27).

Transabdominal procedures that may be used for the repair of an enterocele include excision of redundant cul-de-sac peritoneum with approximation of uterosacral ligaments, transverse obliterative sutures of the Halban type,[4] or circumferential obliterative sutures of the Marion-Moschcowitz type.[9,12] A wide, voluminous posterior vagina should be narrowed by wedging, as suggested by both Waters[18] and Torpin.[17] This procedure, which can be done either transabdominally or transvaginally, tends to approximate the uterosacral ligament attachments closer to the

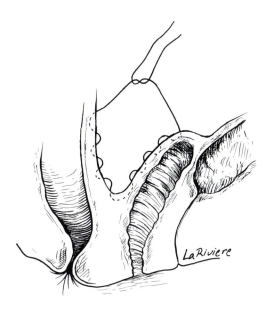

Fig. 26-16. The placement of the stitches is shown in sagittal section. (Redrawn from Nichols DH, Randall CL: *Vaginal surgery*, ed 3, Baltimore, 1989, Williams & Wilkins.)

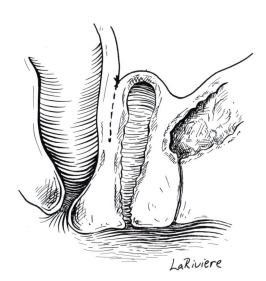

Fig. 26-17. The stitches have been tied, obliterating the cul-de-sac from front to back. (Redrawn from Nichols DH, Randall CL: *Vaginal surgery*, ed 3, Baltimore, 1989, Williams & Wilkins.)

Table 26-1. Correlation between etiology, location, and treatment of enterocele

Cause	Location	Treatment
Congenital	Sac between posterior vaginal wall and anterior rectal wall	Excision of the sac with high ligation of its neck; approximation of uterosacral ligaments
Pulsion (pushed)	With eversion of vaginal vault	Restore vault depth by shortening cardinal-uterosacral ligaments or cul-de-plasty if ligaments are strong: If ligaments are of poor quality, do sacrospinous fixation or sacrocolpopexy: coincident hysterectomy if desirable
Traction (pulled)	Same as congenital, with lower eversion (cystocele and rectocele) pulling vault into eversion	Use same procedure as above plus anterior and posterior colporrhaphy
Iatrogenic	Anterior to vagina, or posterior from change in vaginal axis	Excise or obliterate sac and restore normal vaginal axis if it is defective

From Walters EG: Vaginal prolapse, *Gynecology* 8:432, 1956.

midline. The McCall transvaginal cul-de-plasty may be useful if there are palpably strong uterosacral ligaments, as with the uterovaginal or "sliding" type of prolapse,[11] and can even be employed transabdominally when surgery is by laparotomy.

If eversion of the vagina coexists with enterocele and the abdomen is open, the surgeon may consider transabdominal colposacropexy to preserve vaginal length; however, any coincident cystocele and rectocele must be repaired by a separate procedure at a later date. Any transabdominal procedure that changes the vaginal axis to a more vertical direction (e.g., the Marshall-Marchetti-Krantz procedure[10] or the Burch procedure,[3] ventral suspension, or fixation) necessitates surgical obliteration of the peritoneum-lined cul-de-sac anterior to the rectum to provide adequate protection for the pouch of Douglas. The increased exposure, vulnerability, and risk of enterocele that result from a failure to obliterate a deep anterior or posterior cul-

de-sac should be more widely recognized. An anterior enterocele that develops after hysterectomy is probably best treated by transvaginal resection of the sac and redundant peritoneum, with restoration of the normal upper vaginal axis and correction of any defect in the levator plate.

Anterior enterocele (i.e., anterior to the vagina) rarely can develop following sacrospinous colpopexy if there has been a previous permanent change in the axis of the anterior vaginal wall, as for example from a vaginal "pin-up" procedure such as the Marshall-Marchetti or Burch operation. In this event, the therapeutic approach should be that of obliteration of the peritoneal sac, usually transabdominally and possibly incorporating sagittally placed sutures of the Halban type. These sutures recreate the peritoneal fusion of the fascia of Denonvilliers. They should be placed about 1 cm apart.

A pudendal or lateral enterocele may be approached transvaginally if the margins of the neck of the sac can be readily identified. If these margins are ill-defined, the surgeon should consider either a combined vaginal-abdominal or an abdominal approach.

The simplest treatment of true rectal prolapse with or without coexistent genital prolapse is the insertion of Thiersch wires to reinforce the anal sphincter. More radical procedures for recurrence are the transperineal resection developed by Altemeier, Hoxworth, and Giuseffi[1] or, better yet, the transabdominal operation developed by Ripstein and Lanter,[16] in which a slinglike pararectal replacement of synthetic plastic material is used to replace or supplement attenuated rectal supports. Coincident genital prolapse should be treated by appropriate surgical reconstruction. Anal prolapse may be treated by retrorectal levatorplasty.

It is essential that the gynecologist recognize an enterocele and any condition likely to result in an enterocele and correlate such a condition with its cause, symptoms, progression, and other coexistent pelvic damage. The possible operative procedures should be chosen on the basis of the correlation between etiology, location, and treatment of various types of enterocele (Table 26-1).[13]

REFERENCES

1. Altemeier WA, Hoxworth PI, Giuseffi J: Further experiences with the treatment of prolapse of the rectum, *Surg Clin North Am* 35:1437, 1955.
2. Anderson WR: Pudendal hernia, *Obstet Gynecol* 32:802, 1968.
3. Burch JC: Urethrovaginal fixation to Cooper's ligament for correction of stress incontinence, cystocele, and prolapse, *Am J Obstet Gynecol* 81:281, 1961.
4. Halban J: *Gynakologische Operationslehre,* Berlin, 1932, Urban and Schwarzenberg.
5. Hawksworth W, Roux JP: Vaginal hysterectomy, *J Obstet Gynecol Br Commonw* 63:214, 1958.
6. Lash AF, Levin B: Roentgenographic diagnosis of vaginal vault hernia, *Obstet Gynecol* 20:427, 1962.
7. Lenzi E: *L'Ernia Vaginale del Douglas O Elitrocele,* p 65, Pisa, 1959, Edizioni Omnia Medica.
8. Litschgi M, Käser O: The problem of enterocele, *Geburtshilfe Frauenheilkd* 38:915, 1978.
9. Marion J: Quoted by Read CD: Enterocele, *Am J Obstet Gynecol* 62:743, 1951.
10. Marshall VF, Marchetti AA, Krantz KE: The correction of stress incontinence by simple vesicourethral suspension, *Surg Gynecol Obstet* 88:509, 1949.
11. McCall ML: Posterior culdeplasty: surgical correction of enterocele during vaginal hysterectomy, a preliminary report, *Obstet Gynecol* 10:595, 1957.
12. Moschcowitz AV: The pathogenesis anatomy and cure of prolapse of the rectum, *Surg Gynecol Obstet* 15:7, 1912.
13. Nichols DH: Types of enterocele and principles underlying the choice of operation for repair, *Obstet Gynecol* 40:257, 1972.
14. Pirogoff (Fig. 4, Plate XXI) in Hart DB: *Atlas of female pelvic anatomy,* Edinburgh, 1884, W & AK Johnston.
15. Read CD: Enterocele, *Am J Obstet Gynecol* 62:743, 1951.
16. Ripstein CC, Lanter B: Etiology and surgical therapy of massive prolapse of the rectum, *Ann Surg* 157:259, 1963.
17. Torpin R: Excision of the cul-de-sac of Douglas for the surgical cure of hernias through the female caudal wall: including prolapse of the uterus, *J Med Assoc Ga* 36:396, 1947.
18. Walters EG: Vaginal prolapse, *Gynecology* 8:432, 1956.
19. Weed JC, Tyrone C: Enterocele, *Am J Obstet Gynecol* 60:324, 1950.
20. Wilensky AV, Kaufman PA: Vaginal hernia, *Am J Surg* 49:31, 1940.
21. Zacharin RF: *Pelvic floor anatomy and the surgery of pulsion enterocele,* New York, 1985, Springer-Verlag.

Chapter 27

MASSIVE EVERSION
OF THE VAGINA

David H. Nichols

More women are living longer, and they are interested in maintaining a self-image of femininity and the capacity for sexual activity beyond the menopause. Few maladies are more disruptive to these goals than is massive eversion of the vagina. It is specific, dramatic, obvious, frustrating, embarrassing, and progressive. It may occur with or without prolapse of the uterus, because uterine prolapse is the result, not the cause, of the eversion. Cystocele, rectocele, or enterocele may coexist, and the distinction is surgically important because each, when present, should be repaired (Fig. 27-1). Clearly, massive eversion of the vagina is a complex disorder, but surgery is curative, relieving symptoms and restoring normal anatomic relationships.

Although massive eversion of the vagina is more common in the postmenopausal patient, it can sometimes also occur in the young. It is more common in the white patient than in the black patient for reasons not totally understood. Some cases of massive eversion of the vaginal vault occur in the nullipara—probably related to congenital pelvic tissue weakness, defective innervation, or unusual trauma— but most are seen in parous women. Obstetrically skillful management of labor and delivery reduces the risk of eversion. In some childbirth settings, however, persons other than skilled obstetricians deliver babies, and timely, anatomically repaired episiotomy takes place less frequently in these settings. With resurgence of interest in home delivery, an increase in the incidence of genital prolapse, as well as of the other gynecologic consequences of unattended childbirth, can be expected.

That a "dropped uterus" is the result—not the cause—of genital prolapse has not always been appreciated. Surgeons have performed "routine" abdominal hysterectomy for uterine prolapse in the mistaken belief that the removal of a prolapsed uterus will prevent further genital prolapse (i.e., "no uterus, no dropping"). The vaginal

vault prolapse, which *caused* the uterine prolapse, persists whether or not the uterus has been removed, however. Therefore, these patients may often be seen in consultation some time after their primary surgery, frequently because their initial surgeon referred them.

PREOPERATIVE HISTORY AND EXAMINATION

In taking the patient's history, the gynecologist should ask whether urinary stress incontinence was a problem when the patient was younger and, if so, which symptoms were relieved as the vaginal vault descended. The relief of symptoms under these circumstances suggests a kinking of the urethra coincident with the prolapse. Such a patient is likely to develop a recurrent urinary stress incontinence after the vagina has been repositioned within the pelvis unless special steps are taken during the anterior colporrhaphy to decrease the likelihood of this possibility.

If the patient with massive eversion of the vagina has a history of previous urinary stress incontinence that is no longer present, presumably due to kinking of the urethra coincident with the progression of the prolapse, she should have a urodynamic evaluation, which includes measurement of her urethral pressure profile. If a low compliant or low-pressure urethra (less than 20 cm H_2O) is found, the surgeon can plan how the low-pressure urethra should be treated as part of the original primary procedure. A coincident vesicourethral sling procedure is one choice to lessen the chance of postoperative urinary incontinence.

The chronically increased intraabdominal pressure that is so often the cause of massive eversion of the vagina may also lead to the development of a coincident hiatal hernia. Such a patient often gives a history of heartburn when lying down.

The patient should be examined when she is fully awake and standing. The gynecologist should replace the

431

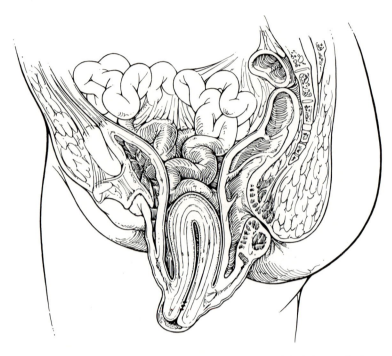

Fig. 27-1. Massive eversion of the vagina and the organs to which it is attached are shown in sagittal section.

vault and note any possible cystocele, rectocele, or enterocele (Fig. 27-2). Generally, if there are any weaknesses in these areas, even of a minor degree, they should be repaired simultaneous with the primary procedure. This improves the overall surgical success of a reconstructive procedure and decreases the likelihood that a separate secondary operation will be necessary in the future.

It is sometimes possible to predict with reasonable accuracy the patient with uterine procidentia who will require coincident sacrospinous colpopexy. This can be achieved by identifying the primary site of weakness in the upper or the lower vaginal supports, with the patient in the lithotomy position on the examining table. The gynecologist should replace the prolapse within the pelvis and have the patient bear down and observe to see which organs appear first. If the cervix and uterus appear first followed by the rest of the vagina and some cystocele and rectocele, the patient has massive damage to the upper supports of the vagina, particularly the cardinal and uterosacral ligaments, and will probably require hysterectomy and colpopexy as part of the primary procedure.

If, on the other hand, the cystocele and rectocele appear first followed by the cervix, the primary damage in all likelihood is concentrated on the supports of the lower pelvis, particularly the pelvic and urogenital diaphragms, and the patient will probably be best treated by a skillful vaginal hysterectomy with colporrhaphy and will not require planning for a probable coincident sacrospinous colpopexy.

The gynecologist should beware of the unsuspected anatomic weaknesses of the patient who has been operated on several times previously without lasting success. Often

there will be an underlying systemic or generalized connective tissue weakness that has been undiagnosed and unappreciated.[17,32]

PREVENTION OF RECURRENT PROLAPSE

When a surgical repair of a genital prolapse is indicated, the skilled surgeon has several techniques from which to choose. There are various etiologic factors, and different surgical procedures are required for correction. As a surgical maxim, the surgeon "should make the operation fit the patient, not make the patient fit the operation." A surgeon tends to use most frequently the operations that he or she performs best, but every surgeon must thoroughly learn the various techniques available to ensure that he or she can perform the procedure that best fits the particular combination of damage in any individual patient. Significant steps can be taken in the operating room to prevent recurrent prolapse.

Posthysterectomy vaginal vault eversion occurs when the support of the vaginal vault is inadequate. After total hysterectomy, the uterosacral-cardiac ligament complex is detached from the uterus and, if not reattached to the vaginal vault, undergoes atrophy. After a few months or years, it may no longer be sufficiently strong to be of much use in surgical reconstruction of any future vault eversion. Furthermore, there are partial degrees of eversion that, if ignored at hysterectomy or otherwise left unattended, generally will progress (Fig. 27-3).

To prevent eversion, the surgeon must determine the strength and length of the patient's uterosacral-cardinal ligaments at the time of hysterectomy (Fig. 27-4). If they are strong and long, they should be shortened before they are

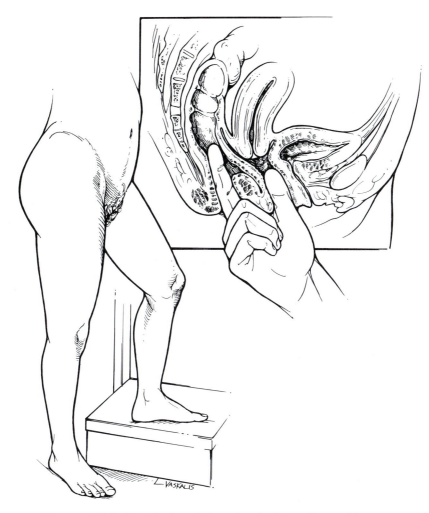

Fig. 27-2. Examination of the patient in the standing position.

attached to the vaginal vault (Fig. 27-5). A wide vaginal vault should be surgically narrowed (Fig. 27-6), the cul-de-sac should be obliterated, and any enterocele should be excised. Sewing the uterosacral ligaments together at the time of posthysterectomy reperitonealization is useful, and the New Orleans or McCall cul-de-plasty can be used (see Chapter 20). When the strength of the uterosacral-cardinal ligaments is insufficient for this technique, as it may be in the patient with total genital procidentia, the surgeon must use an alternate method of colpopexy.

The surgeon should attempt to restore the normal depth and axis of the vagina, particularly after any urethrovesical pin-up operation, such as the Marshall-Marchetti-Krantz[18] or the Burch modification[6] that pulls the vagina anteriorly. Many times, this can be achieved by a perineorrhaphy and posterior colporrhaphy. If the uterosacral-cardinal ligaments are not strong enough to be surgically usable, colpopexy to a nongynecologic structure (e.g., the sacrospinous ligament) may be required to restore vaginal depth.

Amreich[2] noted the importance of preserving vaginal depth after hysterectomy. If, after removal of the uterus, the vagina is otherwise well supported and sits on an intact levator plate, pressure from the pelvic diaphragm will

counter the intra-abdominal pressure applied to the vagina. Compressed between these two pressures, the vagina remains in place. If the vagina is short after hysterectomy, however, it may telescope upon itself, becoming even shorter as intraabdominal pressure is directed along the axis of a vagina that ends anterior to the levator plate (Fig. 27-7). (This is less likely to occur in the patient who has had a Wertheim or Schauta radical hysterectomy, because the scarring in this area after either of these procedures is so great that very little will disturb it.) Although most cases of massive eversion of the vagina are seen in women who have experienced previous hysterectomy, there are some women with procidentia and complete eversion of the vagina who have never experienced previous pelvic surgery. Because in this circumstance the uterus serves as a passenger with the prolapse and not the cause, its influence is therefore more or less passive. The primary defect has to do with the integrity of the connective tissue supports of the vaginal vault and vagina, which, in the presence of massive vault eversion, have been seriously compromised. When the uterus is present in a patient with massive eversion of the vagina, the uterosacral-cardinal ligament complex is always extensively elongated. If these

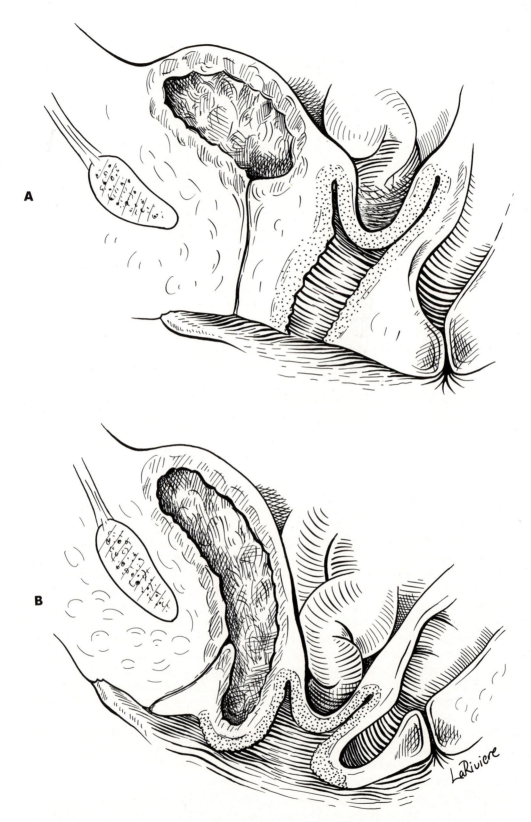

Fig. 27-3. A, Partial eversion of the vagina without cystocele and rectocele is noted after hysterectomy. In **B,** Partial eversion of the vaginal vault after hysterectomy coexists with obvious cystocele and rectocele. (From Nichols DH, Randall CL: *Vaginal surgery,* ed 3, Baltimore, 1989, Williams & Wilkins.)

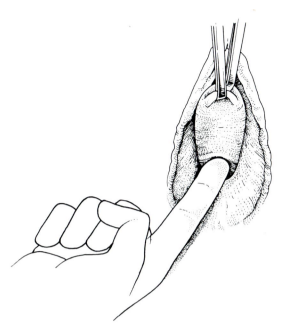

Fig. 27-4. When traction is made to a tenaculum applied to the posterior lip of the cervix, one can palpate both the length and strength of the uterosacral ligaments, as well as the base of the cul-de-sac of Douglas. (Redrawn from Nichols DH, Randall CL: *Vaginal surgery,* ed 3, Baltimore, 1989, Williams & Wilkins, p 188.)

supports are strong, they may be used, after sufficient shortening, to support the vault and hold it in place back within the pelvis where it belongs. The New Orleans or McCall type cul-de-plasty is often helpful as a means of attaching the vault to the mid or upper portion of these strong ligaments as a part of the reconstruction.[24]

With complete procidentia, even in the presence of an enterocele, the uterosacral ligament complex is usually ineffective for postoperative vaginal support, therefore, colpopexy can be planned as part of the primary surgical operation.[21,24] However, when this ligamentous support is inadequate, as is almost invariably the case in the patient who has had previous hysterectomy, an alternate method of support must be found. This should include a colpopexy, either transvaginal as by a sacrospinous fixation, or transabdominal as by sacral colpopexy.

Because a "dropped" uterus is the result and not the cause of genital prolapse, eversion of the vaginal vault can be distinctly independent of the presence or absence of the uterus.

Eversion or protrusion of parts or all of the vagina beyond the hymenal ring may be seen involving various levels of the vagina either singly or in any combination, de-

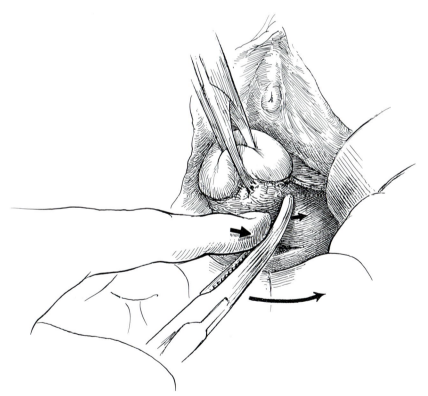

Fig. 27-5. The uterosacral ligaments are identified and clamped, and, if these appear elongated and seem strong, the clamps may be placed to ensure some shortening of the ligaments as they are cut from the uterus. The tip of this clamp usually includes the lower portion of the cardinal ligament. Necessary shortening is accomplished by placement of the *unlocked* clamp across the uncut uterosacral ligament. The operator's finger presses the clamp as shown; the heel is moved a further distance than the tip. A lateral retractor, shown, displaces the vaginal wall, previously stripped from the surface of the ligament. (From Nichols DH, Randall CL: *Vaginal hysterectomy,* ed 3, Baltimore, 1989, Williams & Wilkins.)

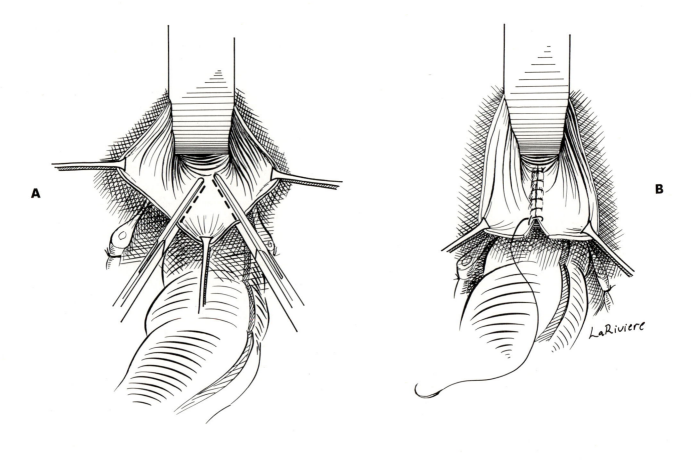

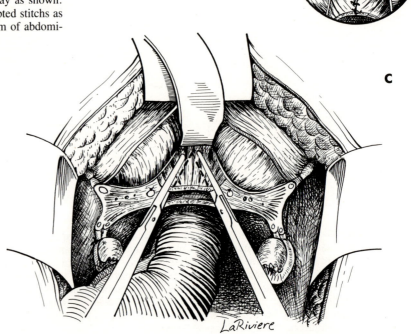

Fig. 27-6. After hysterectomy, a wide vaginal vault can be narrowed by excision of a wedge from the center of the posterior wall as indicated by the broken lines in **A,** and the cut edges united by a running locked stitch shown in **B. C,** If it is too wide, the anterior vaginal wall can be narrowed by excision of a wedge as indicated by the broken line, after the bladder has been dissected down and held out of the way as shown. The cut edges are united by interrupted stitchs as shown in the inset. This is one form of abdominal cystocele repair.

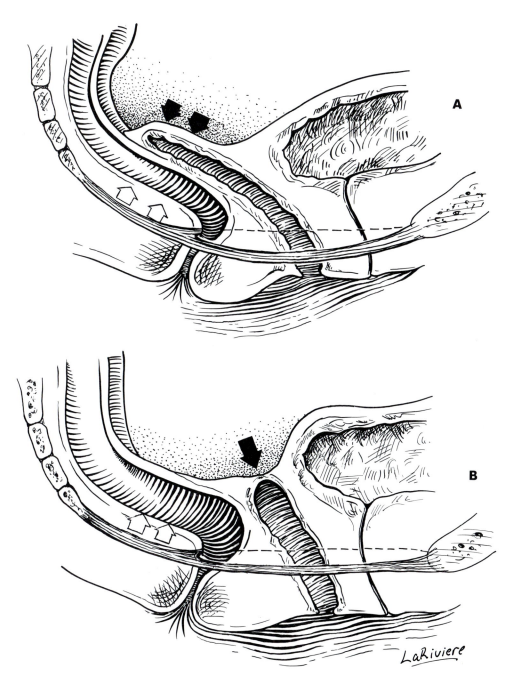

Fig. 27-7. A, The long posthysterectomy vagina in which the vaginal vault is supported above the intact levator plate *(white arrow)* and posterior to its anterior margin. Increases in intraabdominal pressure *(black arrow)* tend to squeeze the vagina against the intact levator plate. In **B,** however, the vault of a shorter posthysterectomy vagina ends anterior to the intact levator plate *(white arrow),* and increases in intraabdominal pressure *(black arrow)* are exerted in the axis of the vagina, tending to cause it to telescope and to become even shorter. (Redrawn from Amreich J: *Wien Klin Wochenschr* 63:74, 1951.)

pending on which of the various supporting structures have been damaged by one means or another. Damage to the vaginal supports at the level of the urogenital diaphragm or below may be associated with perineal defect and urethral hypermobility. Damage to the middle group of supports including the rectovaginal septum, fibromuscular vaginal wall and its lateral attachments to the pelvic side wall, the

levator ani and arcus tendineus in particular, may permit the development of cystocele and rectocele, discussed in their separate chapters, and damage by stretching or avulsion of the uterosacral-cardinal ligament complex may permit eversion of the vaginal vault independent of any coincident enterocele.

The multiplicity of possible anatomic supportive defects

that give rise to the combinations of clinically significant damage that may be encountered in examination of the patient with posthysterectomy vaginal eversion were studied and evaluated in 94 cadavers of various ages.[9] The conclusions were that the upper third of the vagina is supported by vertical fibers of the paracolpium (i.e., cardinal ligament continuations that arise from a broad area on the pelvic side walls). Support of the paracolpium in midvagina arises from attachment to the arcus tendineus, and in the lower vagina by fusion to the perineal body and its muscular and fibrous attachments. This study provides further support of the concept that damage to these support levels may occur singly or in any combination, and the gynecologic surgeon should identify each site of damage preoperatively and incorporate suitable remedial steps in the surgery of reconstruction. Symptomatic patients who are unidentified and untreated may require future reoperation with its attendant risks, suffering, and expense.

The symptoms of vaginal vault eversion include backache, a feeling of vaginal fullness, and presence of a protruding vaginal mass when the patient is standing, because the pull of gravity aggravates the descent of the parts.

Vaginal vault eversion can occur as a consequence of an isolated deficiency in genital support, the vault coming down according to the attenuation of the vaginal portion of the uterosacral-cardinal ligament complex. Vaginal vault eversion is seen far more frequently as the consequence, usually progressive, of damage to the several levels of genital support.[1,4,9,24]

There are three goals of reconstructive surgery:

1. Relieve the symptoms
2. Restore the anatomic relationships between the pelvic organs
3. Restore function of each component organ system

To achieve a perfect surgical reconstruction, the surgeon must determine preoperatively the specific sites of damage,[4,9,24] and, in the operating room, must reaffirm the presence and extent of the damage by a careful examination under anesthesia immediately preceding the operation. Consideration of these observations determines the extent and details of the reconstruction.

There are essential differences between partial eversion of the vaginal vault (often diagnosed by examination of the patient while she is standing and bearing down or straining), subtotal eversion (protrusion of the vagina and organs to which it is attached above or cranial to the urogenital diaphragm), and total eversion of the vagina, which includes the above plus eversion of the vaginal tissues below or caudal to the urogenital diaphragm.

Urinary incontinence coexists more commonly in the postmenopausal patient with total eversion of the vagina. Although it is not frequent, it may be of several types and can be best demonstrated by examination of the awake patient with a partly filled bladder and with the vaginal vault digitally replaced and held in an intrapelvic position. The types of incontinence may include urinary stress incontinence, overflow incontinence from a bladder never completely empty, incontinence from significant detrusor or urethral instability, or incontinence resulting from low urethral pressure (a urethral closing pressure less than 20 cm H_2O). The causes of the latter, related to decreased urethral tone, are hard to pinpoint but may include contributions from decreased estrogen, decreased elasticity of the urethral wall, decreased vascularity, decreased muscle contractility, and a decrease in the effective support of the paraurethral tissues. The consequences, however, are usually obvious (i.e., troublesome postoperative urinary incontinence in spite of coincident anterior colporrhaphy resulting from unrecognized preoperative urethral kinking).

Because effective repair of the coincident low-pressure urethra (vesicourethral sling, periurethral injections, bulbocavernosus fat pad transplant, urethral plication) greatly improves patient satisfaction with surgery, it is vital that its presence should be determined ahead of time. Low urethral pressure or compliance should be suspected in every instance of total vaginal eversion seen in a postmenopausal patient, especially among women who have not been participating in estrogen replacement therapy (ERT). In the author's experience, a low compliant urethra will be found in 5% to 10% of such patients. Its prevalence in postmenopausal patients is a reason for prescribing biweekly vaginal instillations of 1 to 2 g of estrogen cream for a month or two preoperatively and weekly installations during at least the first year postoperatively.

If sophisticated urodynamic laboratory testing is not available to a patient, there is a simple method of demonstrating low urethral compliance. Preoperatively, in the examining room and with the patient's bladder partly full, the vaginal vault is manually replaced, and the patient, previously incontinent or not, is asked to cough and strain, and one observes whether urine is involuntarily lost. This examination is performed with the patient first in the lithotomy position and then standing.

If incontinence is demonstrated while straining, a condition of low compliant urethra is strongly suspected. An inexpensive preliminary test is passing a no. 8 or 10 pediatric Foley catheter into the bladder, partially inflating the Foley bulb with 1 ml of saline, and gently making traction on the catheter to draw the bulb easily through the urethra. If this can be done, the diagnosis of low compliant urethra is likely, and an appropriate surgical remedy should be incorporated in the primary reconstructive repair. If the bulb cannot be pulled through with gentle traction, 0.5 ml of saline is removed from the bulb and again traction is made to the catheter whose bulb is partially inflated with the residual 0.5 ml of saline. If it can be drawn through the urethra with minimal resistance, the diagnosis of low compliant urethra can be seriously entertained. This suspicion can, of course, be more fully "proven" by more sophisticated laboratory assessment if such a facility is available and is affordable.

In the operating room, near the end of the "corrective" surgery, the catheter pull-through "test" using the pediatric

Foley catheter with the partly inflated bulb can be performed. The results can be expected to conform with the patient's future clinical behavior (i.e., correction of pathologically low compliance of the urethra and the prevention or correction of the often-associated urinary incontinence).

Perineal hernia and vaginal prolapse as complications of pelvic exenteration may be treated by transvaginal sacrospinous colpopexy, but coincident perineal hernia anterior to the colpopexy has been effectively remedied by transvaginal placement of a crescent-shaped piece of plastic mesh sutured between the pubic rami and covered by the anterior vaginal wall.[5]

Simultaneous prolapse of the rectum and of the vagina is occasionally encountered (Fig. 27-8).[36] Surgical treatment of one element will not provide benefit to the other. It is possible to treat both simultaneously. One method is transvaginal-transperineal, with colpopexy and repair and resection of the prolapsed rectum, but, if there is need for transabdominal exploration, surgical treatment of both prolapses can be offered by laparotomy. In this instance, the rectal prolapse should be treated first, often by rectopexy with or without intestinal resection according to the amount of redundant bowel present. Sacrocolpopexy will be anterior to the rectal suspension and should be per-

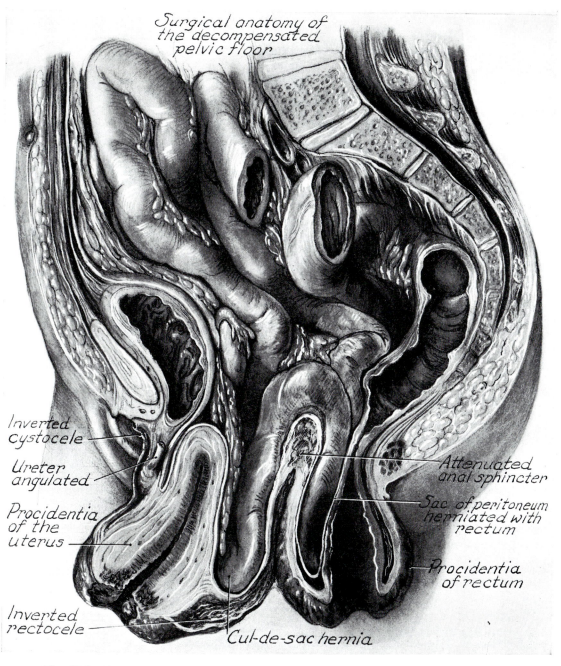

Surgical anatomy of the decompensated pelvic floor

Inverted cystocele

Ureter angulated

Procidentia of the uterus

Inverted rectocele

Cul-de-sac hernia

Attenuated anal sphincter

Sac of peritoneum herniated with rectum

Procidentia of rectum

Fig. 27-8. Simultaneous genital prolapse and rectal prolapse are shown in sagittal section. Because they are each of entirely different cause, each must be repaired separately. (From Ball TL: *Gynecologic surgery and urology,* ed 2, St Louis, 1963, Mosby–Year Book.)

formed as the second procedure. The cul-de-sac should be obliterated before the abdomen is closed. Any necessary transvaginal repair of cystocele or rectocele should be accomplished separately.

When it is necessary to postpone surgery for a symptomatic prolapse, temporary relief of symptoms may be provided by use of an intravaginal pessary such as the Gelhorn (Fig. 27-9) or an inflatable pessary.

There are significant degrees of vaginal vault eversion with which the surgeon should be familiar so that he or she can recognize each example at the initial examination, and again at the beginning of a surgical procedure, and to confirm the end result and absence at the conclusion of surgery and at the follow-up examinations for at least 2 years.

In *partial eversion*, the upper supports are weakened (vaginal portion of the cardinal ligament and the uterosac-

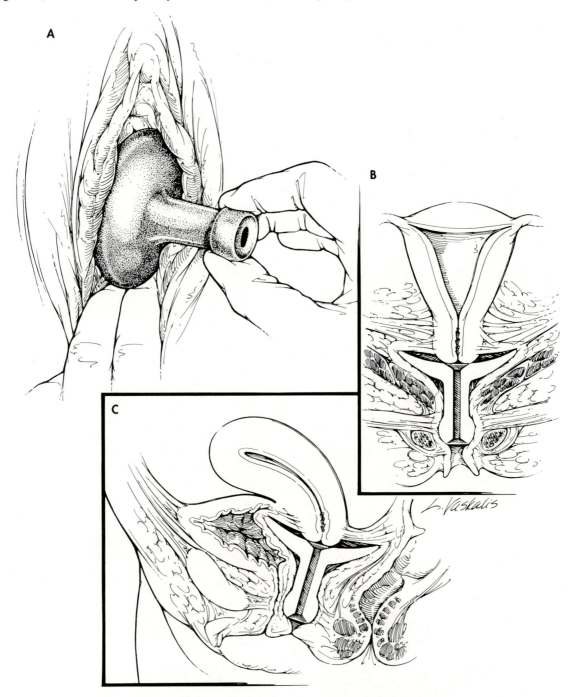

Fig. 27-9. Insertion of a Gellhorn pessary. **A,** The perineum is depressed, and the disc portion of the pessary is inserted. **B,** It should rest comfortably and be retained above the pelvic diaphragm. **C,** Notice in sagittal section that the properly fit pessary elevated the vaginal vault and uterus to a position once again within the pelvis and, at the same time, relieved some of the distention of the cystocele and rectocele.

ral-cardinal ligament complex). This is often but not exclusively associated with a poor or vertically oriented vaginal axis. Enterocele is usually present, but cystocele and rectocele do not always coexist.

In *total eversion,* the entire vagina is inside out, including massive attenuation, stretching or avulsion of the attachments of the vagina to the urogenital diaphragm and the levator ani, and very often a considerable amount of paravaginal detachment. The latter can be identified by examining the patient in the lithotomy position and replacing the vault to its usual position in the hollow of the sacrum and examining the anterior vaginal wall with the patient at rest and again while straining. A sponge forceps or parallel tongue blades of two tongue depressors, or a vaginal elevating forceps can be opened and spread.[4] When these bring the anterior vaginal sulcus into contact with the site of the arcus tendineus on the obturator fascia, the gynecologist should carefully evaluate the presence or absence of residual midline cystocele, because the latter, if present, would indicate a significant and, therefore, surgically repairable defect in the midline supports of the anterior vaginal wall, which should be repaired as well.

The patient with total prolapse of the vagina including tissues of the urogenital diaphragm must be considered to have a clinically significant paravaginal defect until proven otherwise, and the surgeon should be prepared to repair it appropriately at the time of the original operation.[4,24] For those patients with a genital prolapse that occurs cranial to the vesicourethral junction, and in whom the lower part of the vagina does not descend appreciably with the vault or with traction to the vault, a paravaginal defect requiring repair is less common, but it should be measured at the time of surgery by replacement of the vault to a position adjacent to the ischial spine, and by careful examination of the anterior vaginal wall first unsupported, and again when supported by the vaginal elevator or a sponge forceps.

An element of lateral anterior forniceal stretching (or even less commonly detachment) often exists with cystocele. When the "lateral" cystocele is sufficiently symptomatic or progressive as to require surgical correction, the operator may elect the transvaginal White paravaginal reattachment operation.[39] In the presence of coexistent vaginal vault eversion, however, the primary surgical goal should be reconstitution of effective support of the vaginal vault by either transvaginal (sacrospinous colpopexy) or a transabdominal (sacrocolpopexy) surgical route. Reconstitution of vaginal vault support will often "straighten out the sagging clothes line" of anterior vaginal fornix support avoiding the need for direct paravaginal reattachment.

TRANSVAGINAL SURGICAL TREATMENT

The vaginal approach is particularly useful if the patient's general picture includes significantly increased medical risks.

There are several methods of transvaginal surgical treatment:

1. Vaginal hysterectomy and repair
2. Partial (LeFort) colpocleisis or colpectomy
3. Other transvaginal reconstructive procedures, such as sacrospinous colpopexy with treatment of cystocele and rectocele through the same operative exposure

Because no single operation can correct all the pathology that may be present in various types of prolapse, it is often necessary to combine surgical procedures.

Vaginal hysterectomy and repair

Because the pathologic descent of the uterus is the result of genital prolapse, hysterectomy is not as important as the repair, nor should it be the prime objective of surgery for genital prolapse. Hysterectomy may be useful as the means of mobilizing parametrial tissues for use in reconstructive surgery, but it should be an adjunct to repair. For the patient who wishes to retain her uterus, the surgeon may elect to perform colpopexy without hysterectomy.

Vaginal hysterectomy and repair constitute the procedure most often selected for genital prolapse. If the uterosacral-cardinal ligaments are strong, they can be shortened and attached to the vault of the vagina, providing a satisfactory result. When there is a coexisting enterocele, the New Orleans or McCall cul-de-plasty is helpful. If the patient wishes to retain the uterine fundus, a Manchester-Fothergill operation may be considered; however, the possibility of subsequent pregnancy or abnormal uterine bleeding must be understood. For the same reasons, the Watkins-Wertheim transposition operation is not recommended.

Partial colpocleisis or colpectomy

Although partial colpocleisis or colpectomy has, at times, been popular for the aged patient, four problems are specific to this type of operation: (1) it limits or destroys vaginal coital function; (2) because the operation is extraperitoneal, it does not permit the repair of an enterocele; (3) postoperative urinary stress incontinence may result from fusion of the anterior rectal wall to the base of the bladder, flattening the posterior urethrovesical angle; (4) if the uterus is retained, the patient can bleed in the future from a number of causes, including carcinoma. In addition, because the uterus and cervix are hidden behind the new vaginal septum, investigation is difficult. Therefore, colpocleisis is seldom recommended.

Colporrhaphy is preferred to reduce the risk of postoperative urinary stress incontinence, but partial colpocleisis (Fig. 27-10) or total colpectomy can be effective and satisfactory in certain older patients for whom surgery entails greater risks than for most patients and for whom preservation of coital potential may be neither essential nor desirable. This is especially true when the tissues are not strong enough to be used in reconstruction.[7,27,37] Colpectomy

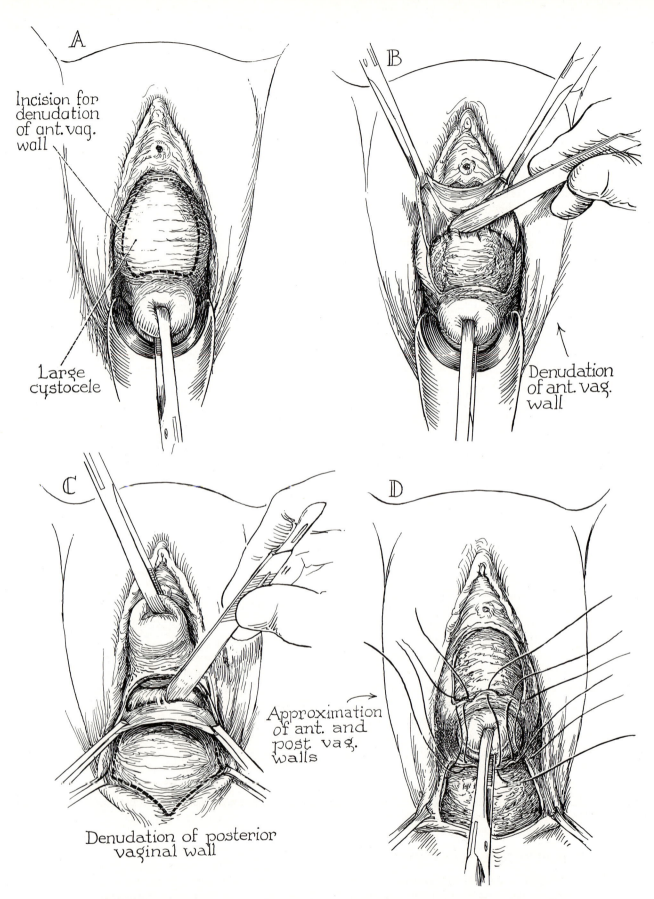

Fig. 27-10. A, An area to be denuded is outlined from the external urinary meatus to the bladder reflection on the cervix. Along the outline, an incision is made that extends through the mucosa and superficial musculature of the vaginal wall. **B,** The area is now denuded of mucosa, leaving as much of the muscular wall as is possible while dissecting in this unnatural line of cleavage. Considerable general oozing may be encountered despite the fact that patients subjected to this procedure are postmenopausal. *Continued.*

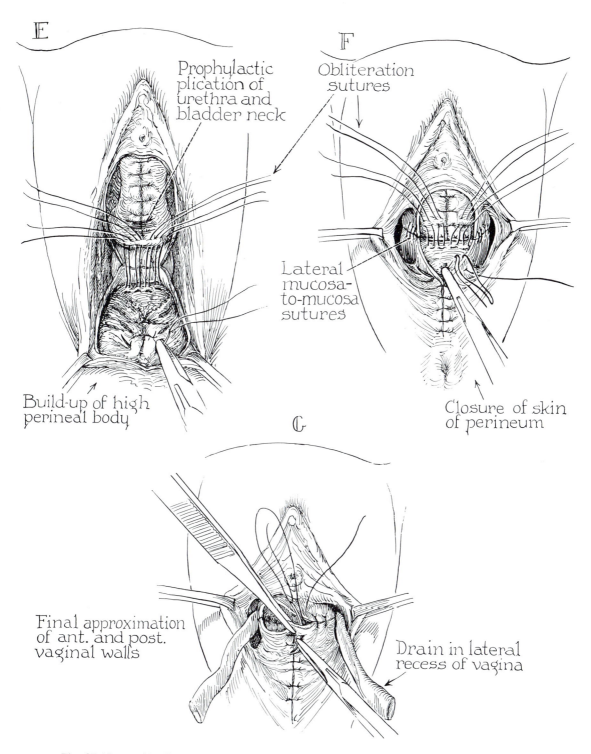

E
Prophylactic plication of urethra and bladder neck

Build-up of high perineal body

F
Obliteration sutures

Lateral mucosa-to-mucosa sutures

Closure of skin of perineum

G
Final approximation of ant. and post. vaginal walls

Drain in lateral recess of vagina

Fig. 27-10, cont'd. C, A similar area is denuded posteriorly but also including a triangular area of the skin of the perineum. Bilateral strips of mucosa are left. **D,** Using interrupted sutures of 00 chromic catgut, the mucosa of the vault is approximated over the cervix. After the anterior wall has been united to the posterior wall, the lateral edges on each side are approximated. **E,** The denuded vaginal wall is approximated anteroposteriorly by a series of mattress sutures in conjunction with the mucosal closure. When the area of the bladder neck is reached, this is plicated not only in the event of stress incontinence, but also for prophylactic purposes. **F,** The musculature of the perineal body is built up with interrupted sutures to aid in the obliteration of the genital aperture. Successive rows of mattress sutures continue the obliteration of the vaginal canal. The skin of the perineum is approximated in the midline by interrupted sutures. **G,** The remainder of the anteroposterior approximation is done, and drains are placed in both of the lateral tunnels of the vagina that result. (From Ball TL: *Gynecologic surgery and urology,* St Louis, 1963, Mosby–Year Book.)

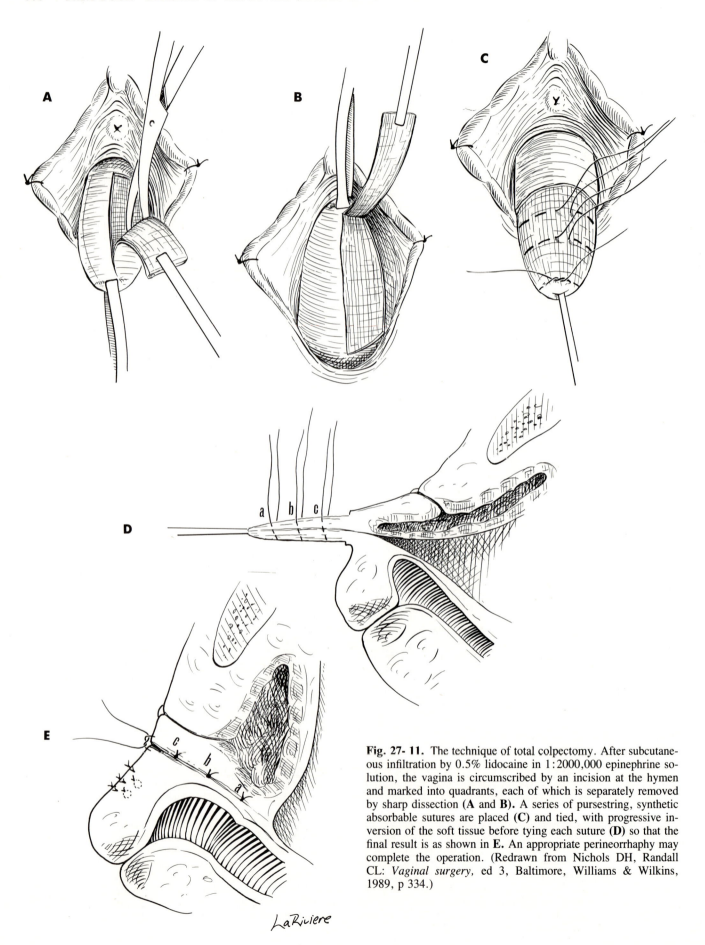

Fig. 27-11. The technique of total colpectomy. After subcutaneous infiltration by 0.5% lidocaine in 1:2000,000 epinephrine solution, the vagina is circumscribed by an incision at the hymen and marked into quadrants, each of which is separately removed by sharp dissection (**A** and **B**). A series of pursestring, synthetic absorbable sutures are placed (**C**) and tied, with progressive inversion of the soft tissue before tying each suture (**D**) so that the final result is as shown in **E**. An appropriate perineorrhaphy may complete the operation. (Redrawn from Nichols DH, Randall CL: *Vaginal surgery,* ed 3, Baltimore, Williams & Wilkins, 1989, p 334.)

LaRiviere

should be considered a destructive rather than a reconstructive operative approach (Fig. 27-11). Because there is no route for subsequent uterine drainage, colpectomy is not appropriate when the uterus has been retained. Furthermore, coexistent enterocele must be recognized and excised. Symptomatic and troublesome vulvar hernias may occur in patients who have undergone total colpectomy as a treatment for prolapse of the vaginal vault, generally as a result of enteroceles that have recurred or were unrecognized and untreated at the time of the original surgery.

Other transvaginal reconstructive procedures

Although obstetric trauma is the most significant and frequent factor in initiating vaginal eversion, the endocrine and nutritional changes during and after the menopause seem to accelerate the progression of vaginal eversion by causing atrophic weakening of muscular and connective tissues. Thus, it is not uncommon to encounter an aging, but sexually active, patient who has vaginal eversion, cystocele, and rectocele, but who cannot retain a vaginal pessary. Genital prolapse may have progressed in association with postmenopausal atrophic changes. The prolapsed uterus can be removed without difficulty; if the cardinal and uterosacral ligaments are strong, they should be shortened and used to support the vaginal vault.[24,35] Sometimes, however, there is nothing of strength to use for support of the everted vagina. This condition usually indicates a major problem with the integrity of all endopelvic soft tissues, particularly of the pelvic diaphragm.

The vault descends without a true enterocele in approximately 20% of patients.[21] Although enterocele and massive eversion of the vagina often coexist, they are *separate* anatomic and clinical entities, each requiring definitive, specific surgical treatment. When eversion of the vagina follows a previous hysterectomy, enterocele coexists two thirds of the time. This disabling and uncomfortable outcome suggests that insufficient attention had been paid during surgery to the reinforcement and correction of weakened genital supports. If strong uterosacral-cardinal ligaments can be found at the sides of the everted vaginal vault, they can be shortened and the vagina can be attached to them for support,[24,35] followed by excision of any enterocele and by high ligation of the peritoneum. As mentioned earlier, however, the remaining uterosacral ligament complex usually undergoes atrophy after total hysterectomy and, after a few months or years, is no longer sufficiently strong to have much usefulness for surgical reconstruction. With minimal or negligible uterosacral strength, alternate methods of restoring vaginal depth and axis must be employed.

A number of alternate techniques have been described. As early as 1892, Zweifel[40] wrote that he had attached a weakened vagina to the sacrotuberous ligament. White[39] described transvaginal suture of the vagina to the arcus tendineus in 1909. Inmon[14] and later Symmonds and associates[35] reported stitching the vagina to the fascia of the pelvic diaphragm. In 1951, Amreich[2] reported his experience using both a transgluteal (Amreich I) and transvaginal (Amreich II) approach to attach an inverted vagina to the sacrotuberous ligament. Sederl[31] sewed the vagina to the sacrospinous ligament (Fig. 27-12). More recently, Richter[29,30] enthusiastically described his success with the use of the sacrospinous ligament, stimulating interest in this operation.

There are certain specific advantages to a transvaginal sacrospinous colpopexy. First, it permits restoration of a functional vagina with a normal, horizontally inclined upper vaginal axis atop the levator plate,[23] thereby decreasing the risk that vault eversion will recur. Second, unlike abdominal sacrocolpopexy, it offers a convenient opportunity to correct cystocele, rectocele, or enterocele simultaneously. Third, it is a shorter procedure than the abdominal operation and, therefore, requires less duration and depth of anesthesia. Finally, because it is principally extraperitoneal, there is a reduced risk of postoperative ileus, intestinal obstruction, incisional pain, and other hazards of transabdominal surgery. For the patient with uterine procidentia and demonstrably weak uterosacral-cardinal ligaments, transvaginal sacrospinous colpopexy can be planned with vaginal hysterectomy and colporrhaphy as part of the primary operative procedure.[8,20,23]

Although the procedure is not commonly done, it is surprisingly easy to perform primary sacrospinous colpopexy immediately after vaginal hysterectomy in a patient with extensive prolapse without a strong, surgically useful uterosacral-cardinal ligament complex. The fact that the patient has undergone no previous surgery to alter tissue planes and spaces facilitates the procedure. The addition of sacrospinous colpopexy to vaginal hysterectomy with anterior and posterior colporrhaphy, between the steps of peritoneal closure and the posterior repair, extends the operating time of the experienced vaginal surgeon only by approximately 15 minutes. This is the time required for penetration of the rectal pillar and identification and placement of the vagina to one sacrospinous ligament. By using this procedure, the surgeon can provide adequate support for the vagina, lengthen the well-supported vagina, restore bladder and rectal function, and preserve normal coital ability.

Technique of transvaginal sacrospinous fixation

For transvaginal sacrospinous colpopexy, the operator should have fingers of at least average length to be able to reach the hollow of the sacrum. An operator with short fingers has a distinct handicap.

With the patient in the dorsal lithotomy position, after the completion of any necessary hysterectomy, the operator makes a V-shaped incision in the perineum and reflects the skin and the posterior vaginal wall from the perineal body until the avascular rectovaginal space has been entered. Development of this space is continued to the vaginal apex. The posterior vaginal wall is incised longitudinally as necessary, or, if the vagina is to be narrowed by planned colporrhaphy, the excess vaginal wall is excised.

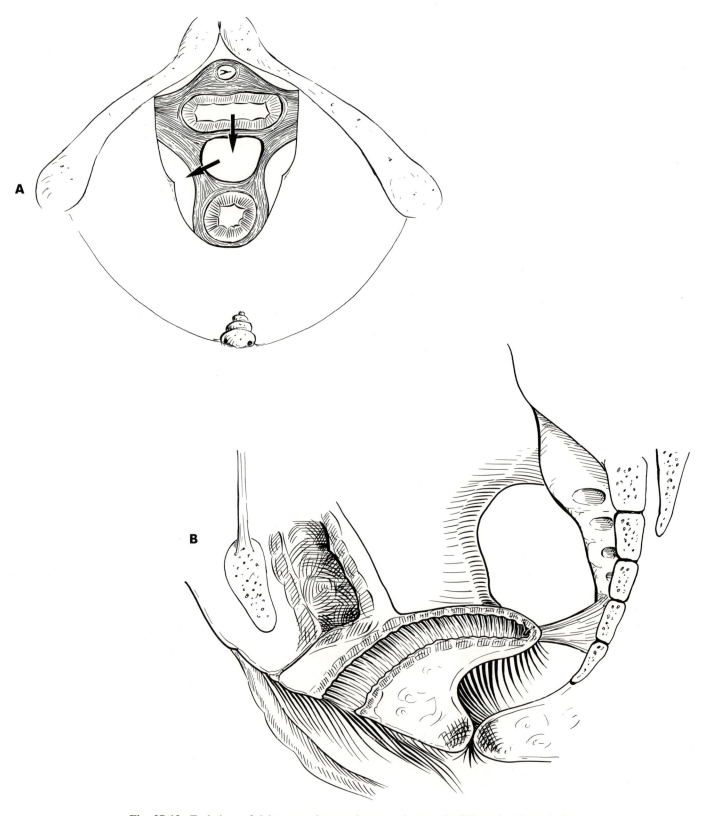

Fig. 27-12. Technique of right sacrospinous colpopexy. **A,** A path of dissection through the posterior vaginal wall into the rectovaginal space and then through a window in the descending rectal septum into the right pararectal space. The dissection always proceeds toward the ischial spine in the lateral wall of the pararectal space. The vagina is sewn to the right sacrospinous ligament-coccygeal muscle complex at a point one and one half fingerbreadths medial to the right ischial spine as shown in **B.** After the fixation stitches have been tied, the attachment of the vagina to the right sacrospinous ligament is shown in **C,** indicating after appropriate colporrhaphy, a fairly normal vaginal depth and axis.

Continued.

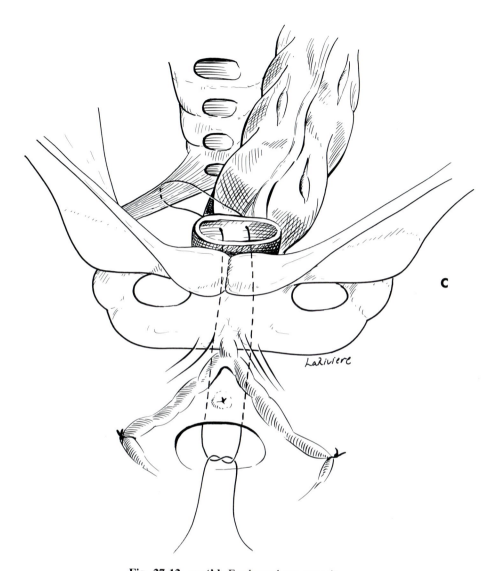

Lariviere

Fig. 27-12, cont'd. For legend see opposite page.

Any enterocele sac is identified and opened.

When the surgeon opens an enterocele coincident with massive eversion of the vagina after previous total abdominal hysterectomy, there is a slightly greater danger of unplanned cystotomy than when the opening and dissection of the enterocele follows total vaginal hysterectomy. The location of the vesical peritoneum after abdominal hysterectomy may be different from its location after vaginal hysterectomy. After total abdominal hysterectomy, the surgeon often brings the bladder peritoneum across the vault of the vagina, whether it is left open or closed, for attachment to the peritoneum of the anterior surface of the rectum. After vaginal hysterectomy, however, the surgeon commonly performs peritonealization by placing one or more pursestring sutures, and the center of the pursestring generally overlies the cut edge of the vaginal vault. Identification of the site at which an enterocele sac meets the bladder may be difficult in a patient with previous hysterectomy. Insertion of a bent blunt uterine sound through the

urethra into the bladder can facilitate identification by palpation of the tip of the bent sound (Fig. 27-13).

Once opened, the sac is mobilized and resected. After determining by palpation that there is no surgically useful uterosacral-cardinal ligament support, the surgeon closes the sac by high, pursestring reperitonealization.

Locating the sacrospinous ligament. It is easier for a right-handed operator to use the patient's right sacrospinous ligament, although the left can be used if desired. (There appears to be no advantage to using both ligaments because this tends to fan out the upper portion of the vagina unnecessarily.) The sacrospinous ligament is an aponeurosis located within the substance of each coccygeal muscle, which extends from each ischial spine to the lower portion of the sacrum (Fig. 27-14). Therefore, with the right index finger introduced into the rectovaginal space, the operator seeks first the ischial spine on either side and traces the fingerlike thickening of the ligament that runs posteriorly from this point to the hollow of the sacrum.

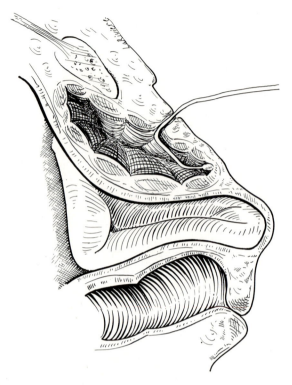

Fig. 27-13. If the limits of a partly filled bladder cannot be determined precisely, palpating the tip of a bent uterine sound can identify at surgery the site where the bladder and the wall of an enterocele sac come together.

The operator then palpates the right ischial spine, usually at the 9-o'clock or 3-o'clock position, and notes the position and size of the right sacrospinous ligament. To find it safely, the operator must understand the nature and boundaries of the connective tissue spaces.

The right rectal pillar separates the rectovaginal space from the right pararectal space. The ease of exposure of the coccygeus muscle-sacrospinous ligament complex depends on how thick the rectal pillar is and whether it exists as one fused or two separate and distinct layers. It is necessary to penetrate *both* layers in proceeding from the rectovaginal space to the pararectal space. Along this path, the surgeon should penetrate the descending rectal septum, which separates the rectovaginal space from the pararectal space, by either sharp or blunt dissection *closer to the undersurface of the vagina* than to the rectum; in doing so, the operator should aim directly at the site at which the ischial spine has been palpated. The length and strength of the descending rectal septum seem to vary inversely with the diameter of the rectum, making the septum easier to penetrate in the patient with a large rectocele.

Proceeding from the rectovaginal space into the right pararectal space, the operator perforates the right rectal pillar at a spot overlying the ischial spine. If the pillar is thin or weak, the operator can penetrate it by blunt dissection with the fingertip; if not, the operator can use the tips of Mayo scissors or a long hemostatic forceps, such as a tonsil forceps (Fig. 27-15). After being inserted through

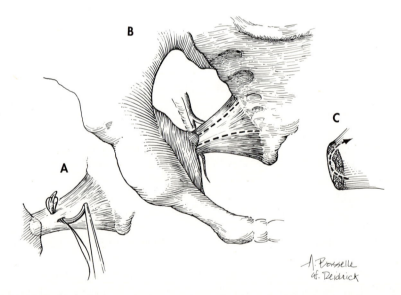

Fig. 27-14. Technique of transvaginal sacrospinous fixation. **A,** After the posterior vaginal wall has been incised and the rectovaginal space has been opened, the operator has perforated the right rectal pillar, proceeding from the rectovaginal space into the pararectal space. A Deschamps ligature carrier has perforated the right sacrospinous ligament, two fingerbreadths medial to the ischial spine. This suture, when passed through the vaginal wall and tied, fixes the vagina to the right sacrospinous ligament. **B,** Sagittal postoperative section showing the attachment of the vagina to the right sacrospinous ligament. **C,** The *dashed line* and *arrow* trace the path of incision from the vagina into the rectovaginal space, and from the rectovaginal space through the right pillar to the right pararectal space, and then to the ischial spine and the sacrospinous ligament. (Reproduced with permission of Harper & Row from Randall CL, Nichols DH: Surgical treatment of vaginal inversion, *Obstet Gynecol* 38:327, 1971.)

the window into the right pillar, the tips of the scissors or the forceps may be opened and spread to enlarge the window and expose the superior surface of the pelvic diaphragm. A long, preferably straight retractor (Fig. 27-16) is inserted into the wound, displacing the rectum to the patient's left; another displaces the cardinal ligament and ureter anteriorly. Similar exposure can be obtained with the use of three narrow Deaver retractors, but they are not as easily applied. The curve of the Deaver retractors offers no advantage, and there is a risk that the tip of a retractor will be pushed across the anterior surface of the sacrum and damage the sacral veins.

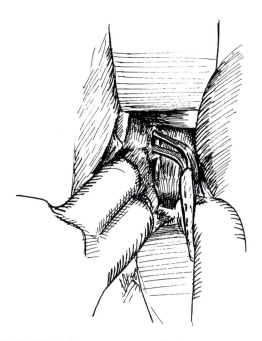

Fig. 27-15. While the upper retractor displaces the cardinal ligament and ureter and the lower retractor holds the rectum to the patient's left, the right rectal pillar has been penetrated by the tips of a long pointed forcep, providing entry to the right pararectal space at a point overlying the right ischial spine. (From Nichols DH: *Reoperative gynecologic surgery,* St Louis, 1991, Mosby–Year Book.)

Direct illumination of this deep area is essential. A spotlight just over the operator's shoulder or a suitable bright fiberoptic forehead lamp can provide the necessary illumination. Loose areolar tissue is pushed to one side, exposing the superior surface of the pelvic diaphragm, and the blunt dissection easily proceeds to the ischial spine. The superior surface of the coccygeal muscle is readily identified, running posterolaterally from the ischial spine. Areolar tissue may be pushed from the surface of the right coccygeal muscle containing the sacrospinous ligament, if desired, using a "rosebud" or wisp sponge. Bleeding within the pararectal space is uncommon; when it does occur, it is usually of anomalous venous origin and is easily controlled by medium-sized vascular clips.

Placing the sutures. If using the right sacrospinous ligament, the operator places the middle finger of the left hand on the medial surface of the ischial spine and, under direct vision, inserts the tip of the long-handled Deschamps ligature carrier (Fig. 27-17) into the coccygeal muscle-sacrospinous ligament at a point one and one half to two fingerbreadths medial to the ischial spine. The carrier tip must go through (not around or under) the ligament. Obvious resistance should be encountered as the tip of the ligature carrier passes through the ligamentous tissue, and the operator must overcome this resistance by persistent forcefulness in the process of rotating the handle of the ligature carrier. Gentle traction on the handle should actually move the patient on the table, confirming proper placement. If there is no resistance, the ligature carrier may be in front of the ligament; or, it may be around the ligament, exposing the structures behind the ligament to potential injury. In either case, the operator should remove the ligature carrier and reinsert it through the substance of the ligament. (Rarely, the nearby sacrotuberous ligament will be found to be stronger and more convenient than the sacrospinous, in which case suture to the sacrotuberous ligament may be substituted.[2,40]

Simultaneous use of nonabsorbable and absorbable suture for colpopexy is generally of value. The use of an absorbable suture permits penetration of a thin vaginal wall with knots tied deliberately on the vaginal side of the incision, from which the knots will ultimately fall as the su-

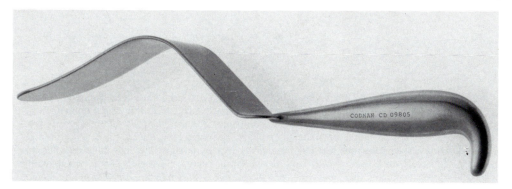

Fig. 27-16. Flat blade retractor CD 09805 available in various sizes from special order department Codman & Shurtleff, New Bedford, MA 02745, or from Mr. William Merz, Baxter V. Mueller, Chicago, IL 60648.

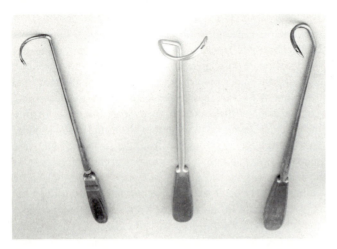

Fig. 27-17. Long Deschamps ligature carriers are shown. An angled Deschamps ligature carrier (modeled after one modified by Rosenshein) noted at the right is useful when the sacrospinous ligament is unusually deep. The handle must be swung through a wide arc. These instruments are available on special order from Codman & Shurtleff, Custom Device Dept., New Bedford, MA 02745, or Mr. William Merz, Baxter V. Mueller, Chicago, IL 60648.

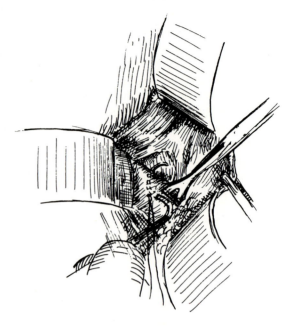

Fig. 27-18. The opening through the right rectal pillar has been enlarged and the sacrospinous ligament-coccygeal muscle complex has been grasped with a long Babcock clamp. At a point about one and one half fingerbreadths medial to the right ischial spine, the sacrospinous ligament and coccygeal muscle have been penetrated by the suture-bearing tip of a long Deschamps ligature carrier. (From Nichols DH: *Reoperative gynecologic surgery,* St Louis, 1991, Mosby–Year Book.)

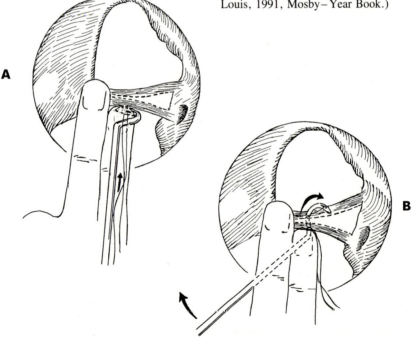

Fig. 27-19. The middle and index fingers of the operator's left hand have been inserted through a "window" in the rectal pillar into the right pararectal space. The lateral side of the tip of the middle finger touches the medial surface of the ischial spine. The Deschamps ligature carrier is positioned as shown and advanced down the index finger, as shown in **A,** until its tip touches the right coccygeal muscle-sacrospinous ligament complex at a point one and one half fingerbreadths medial to the ischial spine, safely away from the pudendal nerves and vessels. As it penetrates the muscle-ligament complex (the ligament within the muscle is shown by the *broken line*) by rotation of the handle, the latter is simultaneously swung to the operator's left *beneath* his or her palm so that the tip of the ligature carrier penetrates the ligament from below upward at right angles to the axis of the ligament, as shown in **B.** (From Nichols DH, Randall CL: *Vaginal surgery,* ed 3, Baltimore, 1989, Williams & Wilkins.)

ture beneath them is absorbed. The buried nonabsorbable suture, on the other hand, permits a long-lasting support of the subepithelial tissues once the preliminary scar formation from the absorbable suture has developed.

The less experienced surgeon should expose the area of fixation for suture placement to direct vision, which requires appropriate anatomic dissection. Suture loop or needle retrieval must always be under direct visualization, however. Grasping the coccygeal muscle and the ligament within it in the tip of a long Babcock clamp often helps to isolate the tissue to be sutured from any underlying vessels or nerves. The sutures in the Deschamps ligature carrier or needle should be inserted directly *through* the substance of the ligament one and one half to two fingerbreadths *medial* to the ischial spine (Fig. 27-18). With increased experience, the operator can place these sutures by touch through a smaller incision into the septum without compromising the accuracy of the suture placement.

If the window made through the descending rectal septum is smaller than 3 cm in diameter, if the operator is certain that the rectum has been displaced medially, and if it is difficult to expose the surface of the muscle, there is a possible alternative approach to the ligament. The operator inserts the tip of the left middle finger through the window and along the inner surface of the pelvic diaphragm until the tip of the ischial spine and the sacrospinous ligament are identified. Keeping the lateral surface of the tip of the middle finger adjacent to the tip of the spine, the operator directs the tip of the long-handled Deschamps or the modified Deschamps ligature carrier along the undersurface of the left index finger until it reaches the coccygeal muscle-sacrospinous ligament complex (Fig. 27-19). At a point clearly one and one half to two fingerbreadths medial to the spine and well away from the underlying pudendal nerve and vessels to avoid trauma to these structures, the operator rotates the tip of the ligature carrier and penetrates the sacrospinous ligament. The fingers of the left hand are then withdrawn, the retractors are suitably repositioned, the tip of the ligature carrier is visualized at this point, the suture is grasped with a hook (Fig. 27-20), and the carrier is removed; then the operation proceeds in the usual fashion.

The tip of the Deschamps ligature carrier is passed through the coccygeal muscle-sacrospinous ligament complex in an almost vertical direction, by swinging the handle of the ligature carrier through a wide arc, once vertical penetration of the ligament has been achieved by distinct pressure from the tip of the ligature carrier, which has been *pushed* beneath the inferior margin of the "ligament" one and one half to two fingerbreadths beneath the ischial spine as shown in Figure 27-19.

The operator grasps the suture material at the tip of the ligature carrier, holds it with the hook, pulls the loop through 2 or 3 inches, and then removes the Deschamps carrier slowly and carefully in a counterclockwise rotation. The blunt point of the Deschamps ligature carrier is less apt to lacerate nearby blood vessels than is the sharp point of the conventional needle. The latter, being brittle because it is made of extruded wire, may break, and the broken tip is hard to find and may be lost. A second suture is similarly placed 1 cm medial to the first and held. Alternatively, after pulling the first suture through, the operator may retain both free ends, cut the loop in its center, pair each end of the cut loop with its respective free suture end, and, thus, obtain two sutures through the ligament with only one penetration by the Deschamps carrier.

Once the operator is comfortable with surgery in the pararectal space and is able to find the coccygeal muscle-sacrospinous ligament easily, it is not necessary to use the special ligature carriers that have been described, and in their place the operator can use a conventional half-curved strong Mayo needle with a tapered point, through which the suture to be used has been threaded. When the needle in the grasp of a conventional needle holder has been passed through the muscle-ligament complex at the desired spot, the now exposed tip is grasped by a Heaney-type needle holder, the original needle holder is removed, and the needle is comfortably extracted following its inherent rotary curve. It is better *not* to use swedged-on needles, because the latter generally are made of extruded wire and are brittle by comparison and subject to fracture and loss!

The free end of the sutures through the ligament are sewn to the underside of the vagina, but not yet tied. Ideally, the operator sews the vagina to the muscle-ligament as a firm tissue-to-tissue approximation. One method of bringing the soft movable vagina to the surface of the coc-

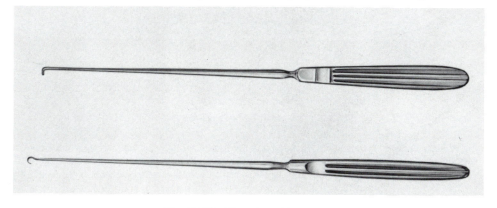

Fig. 27-20. Thread-catching hooks.

cygeal muscle and ligament is by creating a "pulley" stitch (Fig. 27-21) to be used later to pull the vagina directly onto the muscle and ligament. After placing the stitch in the ligament, the operator rethreads one end of the suture on a free needle and ties it by a single half-hitch to the full thickness of the fibromuscular layer of the undersurface of the vaginal apex, keeping the free end of the suture long (Fig. 27-22). This pulley need be created with only one of the suture pairs. The second or "safety" stitch can be inserted through the muscular wall of the vagina, but not tied until later.

Performing the colporrhaphy. If an anterior colporrhaphy has not yet been performed, a full-length repair of the anterior vaginal wall is usually done at this point. The surgeon should replace the prolapsed vaginal vault to its normal position within the pelvis and carefully examine the anterior vaginal wall to determine the size and extent of a cystocele. Allis clamps can be applied to the vaginal wall at the central portion of the cystocele, and approximated in the midline to indicate the extent of vaginal wall that should be resected during the anterior colporrhaphy. These Allis clamps can be replaced with marking sutures to indicate the lateral margins of the planned excision.[19] The operator may also begin the upper part of the posterior colporrhaphy.

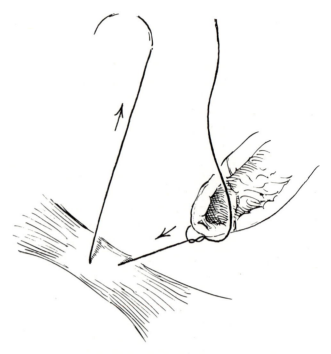

Fig. 27-21. The "pulley stitch." The suture is passed through the fixed structure, and one free end in sewn to the wall of the movable tissue and a single knot fixes it to the latter. When traction is made to the other suture end, as shown by the direction of the arrow, the movable structure is brought to the fixed one, and the suture ends are tied and cut.

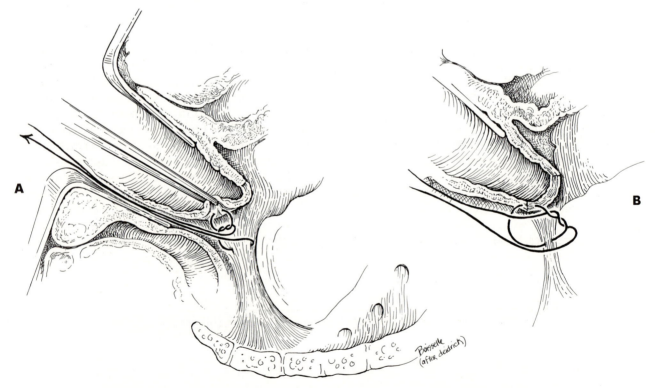

Fig. 27-22. A, The "pulley stitch." One end of the suture through the sacrospinous ligament has been sewn to the undersurface of the cut edge of the vaginal vault. Traction to the other end of the suture draws the vagina up and laterally to the surface of the ligament, and the ends are tied together, fixing the vagina to the ligament at this point. **B,** A second "safety" stitch similarly placed through the ligament is sewn to the subepithelial tissues of the vaginal wall and tied. (From Nichols DH, Randal CL: *Vaginal surgery,* ed 3, Baltimore, 1989, Williams & Wilkins.)

The vagina normally is much wider at the vault. This is particularly evident when the vagina has turned inside-out, as from massive posthysterectomy prolapse. A wide vaginal vault should be deliberately narrowed by the excision of excess vagina (Fig. 27-23). The width and length of the vagina determine the width of posterior vaginal wall to be removed. The vaginal length may be modestly shortened after the excisions of previous operations. Excision of a narrower strip may permit an elastic vagina to be stretched to the region of the ischial spine.

When the vagina is thin or greater vaginal length is desired, each end of the colpopexy stitch may be inserted *through* the vagina (Fig. 27-24). This should be done after an appropriate segment of posterior vaginal wall has been excised as part of the posterior colporrhaphy and after side-to-side approximation with a running subcuticular stitch of polyglycolic acid suture has united the sides of the upper half of the vagina. Tying the fixation stitches before this latter step reduces the visibility of the vaginal vault, making suture of the colporrhaphy more difficult.

Whether a colpopexy should be unilateral or bilateral depends on the width of the vaginal vault. If it is wide and the operator intends to keep it that way, the colpopexy should be bilateral; a unilateral colpopexy allows the unattached side of a wide vault to descend gradually. If the vault is narrow or if the operator has narrowed it, the colpopexy should be unilateral. If a narrow vault is attached bilaterally, the undersurface of the vagina cannot reach the surface of the coccygeal muscle-sacrospinous ligament complex without suture bridges. If the suture material used in these bridges is absorbable, the scar will be weak, and the prolapse is likely to recur; if the material is nonabsorbable polypropylene (Prolene or Surgilene), however, the vault will stay in place. Usually, the results of a unilateral colpopexy are good if a wide vault is resected to convert the shape of the vagina from one resembling a light bulb to that of a cylinder of uniform diameter—because the vagina is now an instrument of coitus, not parturition.

Tying the sacrospinous fixation stitches. When the upper 2 inches of posterior vaginal wall have been approximated, traction on the free end of the pulley stitch (opposite to that which had been fixed to the undersurface of the vagina) takes up all slack and pulls the vagina directly onto the surface of the coccygeal muscle-sacrospinous ligament complex. The pulley stitch and the second or safety stitch are tied with a simple square knot. It is essential to tie the pulley stitch snugly so that there is no void or suture of absorbable suture between the vagina and the ligament (Fig. 27-25). Absorbable suture bridges hinder the formation of strong scar tissue; thus, once the suture is absorbed, the scar tissue may not be able to hold the vagina to the ligament, and the prolapse may recur. Each of the other colpopexy stitches are then tied, fixing the vaginal vault in the hollow of the sacrum. Figure 27-26 shows the effect on the urethrovesical junction of bringing an everted vault of the vagina back into the hollow of the sacrum.

It is best to use no. 2 size polyglycolic acid-type suture

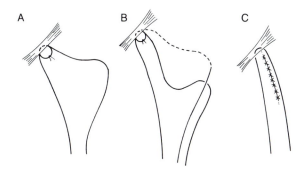

Fig. 27-23. A, A wide vaginal vault after sacrospinous colpopexy. The result of failure to narrow this wide vault is shown in **B** in which there may be prolapse of the left side. **C,** The result of narrowing this wide vault by excision of a proper width tissue from the anterior and posterior vaginal wall, which has converted the shape of the vagina to that of a cylinder of more or less uniform diameter. It is now an instrument of coitus and not parturition. (Redrawn from Nichols DH, Randall CL: *Vaginal surgery,* ed 3, Baltimore, 1989, Williams & Wilkins, p 338.)

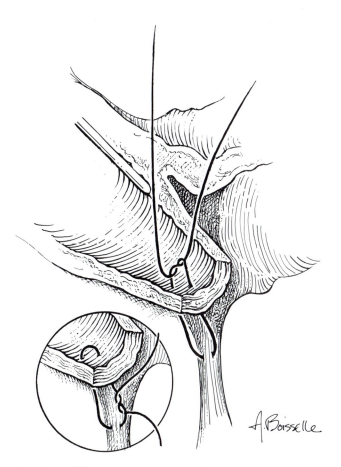

Fig. 27-24. When the vaginal wall is thin, its full thickness may be sewn to the surface of the coccygeal muscle-sacrospinous ligament complex as shown, leaving the knot of an absorbable suture within the lumen of the vagina. If a monofilament nonabsorbable suture has been used, the knot is buried beneath the vagina, as shown in the inset. (From Nichols DH, Randall CL: *Vaginal surgery,* ed 3, Baltimore, 1989, Williams & Wilkins.)

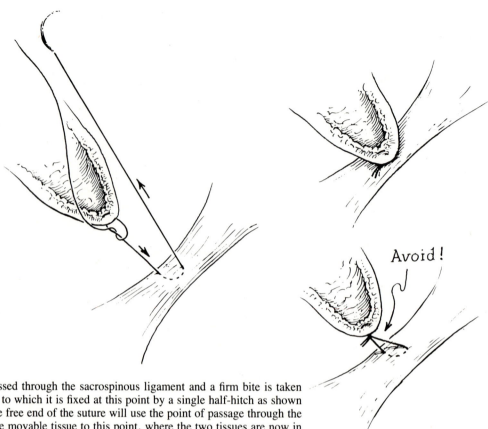

Fig. 27-25. A suture has been passed through the sacrospinous ligament and a firm bite is taken into the tissues of the vaginal wall to which it is fixed at this point by a single half-hitch as shown on the *left*. Traction to the opposite free end of the suture will use the point of passage through the firm tissue as a pulley, bringing the movable tissue to this point, where the two tissues are now in direct contact with one another and a conventional knot is tied, fixing the new relationship, seen in the *upper right*. A suture-bridge, as shown on the *lower right,* should be avoided. (From Nichols DH, Randall CL: *Vaginal surgery,* Baltimore, 1989, Williams & Wilkins.)

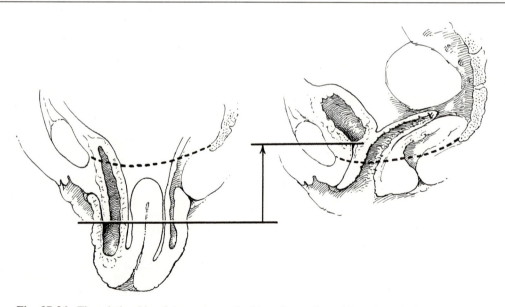

Fig. 27-26. The relationship of the vesicourethral junction to the pubis and pelvis is illustrated in sagittal section. The usual location of the pelvic diaphragm is indicated by the *dotted line.* The vesicourethral junction is indicated by the *solid line.* On the *left,* advanced genital prolapse is depicted showing that eversion of the vagina may pull on tissues supporting the vesicourethral junction, exteriorizing the latter. The effects of restoration of vaginal depth and axis are shown on the *right.* Repositioning of the vagina has provided upward traction to tissues of the vesicourethral junction, helping to restore them to a position within the pelvis. (Reproduced with permission of Harper & Row from Nichols DH: Effects of pelvic relaxation on gynecologic urologic problems, *Clin Obstet Gynecol* 21:759, 1978.)

material (Dexon or Vicryl) in this procedure, because too fine a suture in the sacrospinous ligament may act somewhat like a saw and actually cut through the ligament with tying. The no. 2 size thickness has good knot-tying strength and, because it is of controlled, slow absorbency, will last for several weeks. In contrast, catgut retains its maximal strength and continuity for only 7 to 10 days.

Although the operator must ensure that the knot of any nonabsorbable suture is buried beneath the vagina, permanent sutures such as monofilament synthetic nonabsorbable suture (e.g., size 0 polypropylene [Prolene or Surgilene]) can be recommended as the colpopexy stitches for patients with

1. Recurrent vaginal vault eversion
2. Chronic respiratory disease, which will increase intraabdominal pressure
3. A vagina that is too short to reach the ischial spine. (In this circumstance, the operator may create a deliberate nonabsorbable suture bridge between the top of the vault of the short vagina and the surface of the coccygeal muscle-sacrospinous ligament.)
4. A need to perform heavy lifting after convalescence

The remainder of the posterior colporrhaphy and perineorrhaphy are then completed.

Completing the procedure. The depth of the vagina after sacrospinous colpopexy depends on the distance from the vulva to the point at which the vagina is fixed to the sacrospinous ligament. In most instances, the distance from the vulva to the ligament and, hence, the length of the restored vagina is greater than 4 inches; rarely, the distance may be only 3 or 3-½ inches. When this distance is short, the fixation stitches should be placed closer to the sacrum and a greater effort should be made to build up the thickness and depth of the perineal body at reconstruction; at times, a Williams vaginoplasty is a useful supplement.

The vagina can be packed lightly with iodoform gauze for 24 hours. Postoperatively, the vault of the vagina lies in its normal horizontal axis, although it deviates to the side of the patient to which the attachment was made. Similarly, because the rectal pillar is compressed between the vagina and the sacrospinous ligament to which the vagina was attached, immediate postoperative examination shows the rectum to be pulled to the side of the attachment. Within a few weeks, the pillar must elongate, because by then the rectum is again in the midline.

Postoperatively, many patients notice a transient mild discomfort or pulling sensation deep in the buttock on the side of the attachment, without transmission of discomfort to the thigh. This discomfort regresses within a few days or weeks as the edema subsides.

Postoperative examination usually shows excellent vaginal depth and axis, and increased intraabdominal pressure presses the vagina against the levator plate and accentuates the restored horizontal axis of the vagina. To date, no patient of the author has complained of dyspareunia after this type of vaginal fixation.

Managing operative complications. If a needle tip penetrates the lumen of any adjacent viscus (most likely the rectum), the needle should be withdrawn. Any laceration should be repaired by a standard two-layered closure. If at any time during the procedure a rectal examination indicates that a suture has transgressed the wall of the rectum, the operator should promptly remove the suture and replace it in a proper position outside the rectal lumen.

Immediate, severe postoperative gluteal pain running down the posterior surface of the affected leg indicates pudendal trauma, a rare complication of sacrospinous colpopexy. Sutures placed in error adjacent to the ischial spine risk trauma to the pudendal nerve as it bends around the ischial spine; or the posterior cutaneous nerve of the thigh, which is deep to the spine; or even the sciatic nerve, which is lateral to the spine. Such a complication would be manifest by immediate postoperative pain running down the posterior surface of the thigh, often accompanied by perineal paresthesia or anesthesia. A treatment of choice is immediate reoperation with removal of the offending suture and repositioning of new colpopexy sutures to the sacrospinous ligament either significantly more medial to the spine, or to a medial position in the ligament of the opposite side. Hematoma, although rare, may occur, usually within the pararectal space, and its presence is suggested by a falling hematocrit. The findings of pelvic and rectal examination may not be confirmative as a result of local postoperative discomfort, but a significant collection of extraperitoneal blood will be seen in a pelvic computed tomography (CT) scan. Its progress toward liquifaction or absorption can be followed by subsequent CT scans. Once stabilized, and after any necessary transfusion, most are surprisingly asymptomatic and will absorb over a period of several weeks. Infection within such a hematoma makes itself known by pain and persistent fever, and drainage of the cystic cavity should be considered. Often, this can be accomplished by percutaneous placement of a drain under real-time ultrasound guidance, using local anesthesia.

Postoperative evisceration has been reported in a patient who was straining at stool 3 months after sacrospinous colpopexy and repair.[11] The authors speculated that it may have occurred at the site of a recurrent enterocele to which insufficient attention had been given previously.

Late complications. In spite of the full-length anterior colporrhaphy usually done, an occasional patient develops a mild, usually transient urinary stress incontinence, probably the result of a temporary straightening of the posterior urethrovesical angle. It tends to disappear after several months as a new posterior urethrovesical angle becomes established. Kegel isometric perineal resistive exercises (see Chapter 21) are helpful. Rarely, suprapubic urethrovesical suspension may be recommended.

Recurrent, but asymptomatic, cystocele without stress incontinence is the most frequent complication of colpopexy. Cystocele generally becomes evident within the first 3 months after surgery, but only rarely does it require treatment. In some cases, cystocele probably results from progression after under-repair at the time of surgery; in other cases, from natural progression of disease; in still other cases, from unrecognized and unrepaired lateral (paravaginal) attenuation or avulsion. The presence and degree of the latter, when recognized preoperatively or intraoperatively, can be repaired as part of the reconstructive surgery.

TRANSABDOMINAL SURGICAL TREATMENT

Some abdominal approaches have been used in the treatment of massive eversion of the vagina, but the success of these procedures is variable. A transabdominal approach should be considered if massive vaginal eversion is secondary to a previous ventral fixation of the vagina or uterus or after a vesicourethral pin-up operation such as the Marshall-Marchetti-Kranz or Burch,[4] because it is difficult to return this type of vaginal axis to normal by a transvaginal operation without freeing the vagina or uterus from its attachment to the anterior abdominal wall.

An abdominal route should be considered if there is a history of extensive previous pelvic surgery, pelvic kidney, or a need to investigate an adnexal tumor.

Ventral fixation

Although ventral fixation of the uterine fundus to the anterior abdominal wall was once popular, it does not relieve the cause of the prolapse. The patient may be reasonably comfortable for a while, but, given enough time, continued progression of the prolapse becomes evident. The uterine fundus may remain fixed to the abdominal wall, but the uterus and cervix often elongate until, ultimately, the vagina and those organs to which it is attached again descend. The patient, meanwhile, has often forgotten the nature of her original surgery, which may have taken place many years before; her operative records may have been lost; and the surgeon may no longer be in practice. An operator may begin what is expected to be a routine vaginal hysterectomy and repair only to find on opening the peritoneal cavity that the uterine fundus extends all the way to the anterior abdominal wall (Fig. 27-27). A confirmatory tug on the cervix at that point produces visible dimpling in the anterior abdominal wall.

A drawback of ventral fixation of either the uterine fundus or the vaginal vault (i.e., after hysterectomy or after a vesicourethral pin-up operation) is that it leaves the cul-de-sac exposed. Because the procedure alters the axis of the vagina, the cul-de-sac becomes more directly vulnerable to increases in intraabdominal pressure (Fig. 27-28). This vulnerability of the cul-de-sac may explain the 11% to 15% incidence of enterocele that has been noted after fixation of the vagina to Cooper's ligament in the treatment of stress incontinence, as described by Burch.[6] The cul-de-sac should be clearly obliterated as a separate step with any abdominal surgery that changes the normal horizontal axis of the vagina.

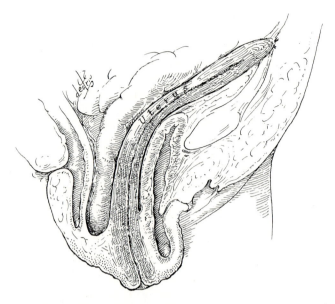

Fig. 27-27. The failure of ventral fixation of the uterus to retard progression of genital prolapse is illustrated. An enterocele has developed. (From Nichols DH, Randall CL: *Vaginal surgery,* Baltimore, 1989, Williams & Wilkins.)

Sacropexy

The transabdominal method of retroperitoneal sacropexy is a satisfactory, but complex, procedure. It is particularly attractive when it is necessary to open the abdomen for an unrelated reason, such as the removal of an ovarian tumor, or when the vagina is too short to be brought to the ischial spine. A transabdominal sacropexy corrects eversion of the vaginal vault, but it does not correct eversion of the lower vagina.

Arthur and Savage[3] and Falk[10] attached the fundus of the uterus to the periosteum of the sacrum. It is even more effective to remove the uterus and attach the vagina to the sacrum by a retroperitoneal bridge of polyester (Mersilene) mesh or fascia lata,[24,35] because this reestablishes a somewhat horizontal vaginal axis. Coexistent intestinal diverticulosis is a relative contraindication to the use of synthetic mesh, however, because there is a risk of future perforation of a diverticulum at the site of the mesh. If the mesh bridge becomes infected, it must be removed. The presence of cystocele or rectocele is also associated with a risk. To attempt a vaginal repair of cystocele or rectocele simultaneously with transabdominal sacral fixation of the vagina appreciably increases the risk of infection at the site of the nonabsorbable sutures and polyester (Mersilene) mesh, and it is not recommended. Any cystocele or rectocele should be repaired at another time.

Massive eversion of the vagina is by no means uncommon after even a single pregnancy in a patient with a history of exstrophy of the bladder, even if the patient's delivery had been by cesarean section. The obvious anatomic weakness of the anterior vaginal wall prevents its use as a

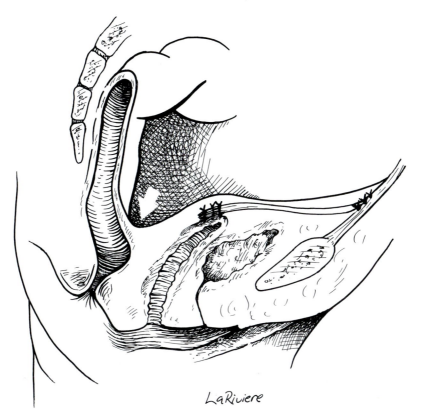

LaRiviere

Fig. 27-28. The unprotected cul-de-sac left after ventral fixation of the vagina is noted by the arrow in the drawing. (Redrawn from Nichols DH: Repair of enterocele and prolapse of the vaginal vault. In Barber H, ed: *Goldsmith's practice of surgery,* Philadelphia, 1981, JB Lippincott.)

basis for surgical support, because so many of these patients have previously undergone a cystectomy. One possibility, should an enormous "cystocele" (i.e., a massive relaxation of the anterior wall of the vagina with bulging accompanied by a subjective feeling of falling out and fullness) appear without uterine descent, is a modification of the Watkins-Wertheim transposition in which the operator sews the fundus of the uterus to the periosteum of the pubic rami. To this may be added the Ocejo modification described by Gallo,[13] in which the operator amputates the cervix and opens the uterus. The entire endometrial cavity is excised before the transposition. The extent of the endometrial cavity may be defined by the intrauterine installation of an ampule of indigo-carmine, which stains all the tissue a deep violet color. The uterine wall is then reunited, and the transposition is finished.

When a procidentia accompanies a prolapse in a patient with a history of bladder exstrophy, the cardinal or uterosacral ligament is often not strong enough to support the vaginal vault. In this case, some surgeons have successfully used an operation developed by Howard Jones.[16] The operator obliterates the cul-de-sac of Douglas by a transabdominal approach and attaches the vagina by an intermediate polyester (Mersilene) strip to the periosteum of the pu-

bis. Alternatively, Jones has performed ventral fixation using the cervical stump remaining after subtotal hysterectomy in such a patient. Because there is no bladder, there is minimal displacement of the ureteral sigmoidostomy that may have been accomplished at the time of the preceding cystectomy, often in the patient's youth.

Technique of transabdominal sacropexy. Because of the possibility of contamination of the operative field by microorganisms from the vagina, a patient who is to undergo transabdominal sacropexy may be given a single dose of an appropriate prophylactic antibiotic preoperatively. A Foley catheter has been inserted into the bladder. The operator opens the lower abdomen through a midline lower incision and explores the abdomen.[10,24,25] Fingers elevating the vagina make it easy to identify the vaginal vault (Fig. 27-29, *A* through *C*). The operator makes a transverse incision in the peritoneum over the uppermost portion of the vagina, reflecting the peritoneum both anteriorly and posteriorly for a distance of 2 to 3 cm. This line of cleavage denudes the musculoconnective tissue wall of the vagina. After identifying the bladder, with its attachment to the anterior peritoneal reflection, the operator identifies any enterocele sac. A longitudinal incision is made through the peritoneum over the sacral promontory, and the incision is extended caudally for 5 to 6 cm below and posterior to the promontory (Fig. 27-29 *D* through *F*). The peritoneal flaps on either side may be caught in retraction sutures left long enough to permit an adequate exposure of the bifurcation of the aorta and the common iliac veins. The midsacral artery and vein generally require ligation or cautery to permit access to a 6- to 8-cm area of clean periosteum over the promontory of the sacrum be-

tween the common iliac veins. The exposed area of periosteum must be freed of all connective tissue, and hemostasis must ensure a dry field where a segment of fascia lata or plastic gauze is to be sutured to the periosteum. Small blood vessels may be electrocoagulated to ensure a dry operative field.

A 00 guide suture is placed on each side of the vaginal apex. Three pairs of 00 coated *nonabsorbable* braided syn-

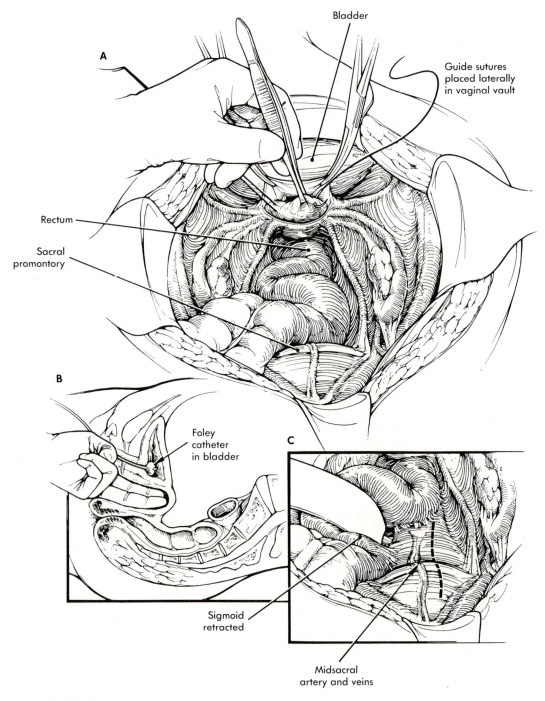

Fig. 27-29. Transabdominal sacrocolpopexy. The abdomen has been opened by a midline incision. The vaginal vault is manually elevated, as shown, and the peritoneum covering it is incised transversely **(A).** Bowel is packed out of the way, and the promontory of the sacrum is exposed. The peritoneum overlying the promontory is incised as shown by the *broken line* **(C).**

Continued.

thetic sutures are placed tranversely 1 cm apart in the central portion of the vaginal vault—through the full subepithelial fibromuscular thickness of the vaginal wall, but not into the vaginal lumen. The midpoint of a 2- to 8-inch piece of polyester (Mersilene) mesh folded longitudinally (alternatively, a large strip of fascia) is brought to the vaginal apex; the braided plastic sutures are threaded through it and tied securely.

Using a long, curved intestinal clamp or kidney stone forceps for dissection, the operator establishes a subperitoneal tunnel that extends from the inferior edge of the incision over the sacral promontory, beneath the peritoneum across the posterolateral aspect of the right side of the cul-de-sac, to the cut edge of the peritoneum overlying the vaginal apex (Fig. 27-29, *G* through *I*). Alternatively, the operator may incise the peritoneum of the cul-de-sac longitudinally and reflect it. With the curved intestinal clamp running through the subperitoneal tunnel, the operator grasps the free end of the mesh (or fascia) now attached to the apex of the vagina and draws it to the promontory of the sacrum by withdrawing the clamp.

Using a strong, but small, half-circle needle with a trochar point, the operator places three pairs of 2-0 braided nonabsorbable sutures in the sacral periosteum and fixes them to the bridge. A little slack is left in the strip; it is not pulled so tightly as to elevate the cul-de-sac of the perito-

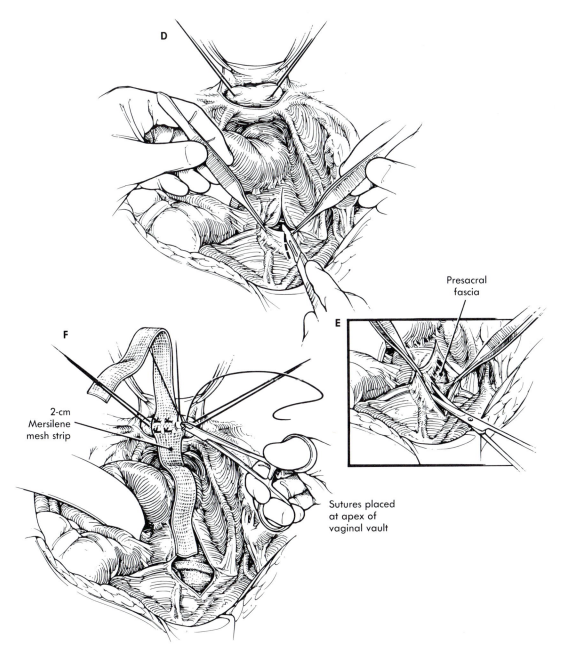

Presacral fascia

2-cm Mersilene mesh strip

Sutures placed at apex of vaginal vault

Fig. 27-29, cont'd. The tissues are carefully separated **(D)**, exposing the presacral fascia **(E).** The central belly of a precut band of polyester (Mersilene) or fascia lata is sewn to the vaginal vault **(F).**   *Continued.*

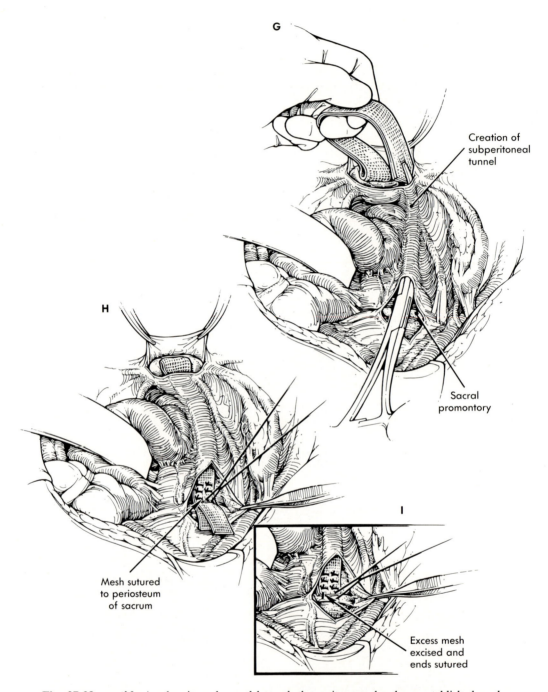

Fig. 27-29, cont'd. A subperitoneal tunnel beneath the peritoneum has been established, and a long Kelly forceps is introduced to grasp the free ends of the polyester or fascia (**G**), which is drawn through the tunnel and sewn to the presacral fascia and periosteum (**H**). The excess mesh is excised (**I**).   *Continued.*

neum appreciably. Excess ends of the bridge are excised, the peritoneum is closed with fine absorbable suture, and the cul-de-sac is obliterated (Fig. 27-29, *J* through *M*). Unless an anterior colporrhaphy has been planned, a suprapubic pin-up of the urethrovesical junction is appropriate to reduce the risk of postoperative urinary stress incontinence. The vagina is distended for 1 or 2 days with a splinting iodoform or gauze pack. The patient is permitted

out of bed on the first postoperative day, and the urinary catheter is removed at the same time as the vaginal packing.

Complications of sacral-colpopexy. Addison and associates[1] have observed an occasional patient with recurrent vaginal vault eversion after abdominal sacral colpopexy and believe that the complication can be avoided by the use of permanent material attached to a

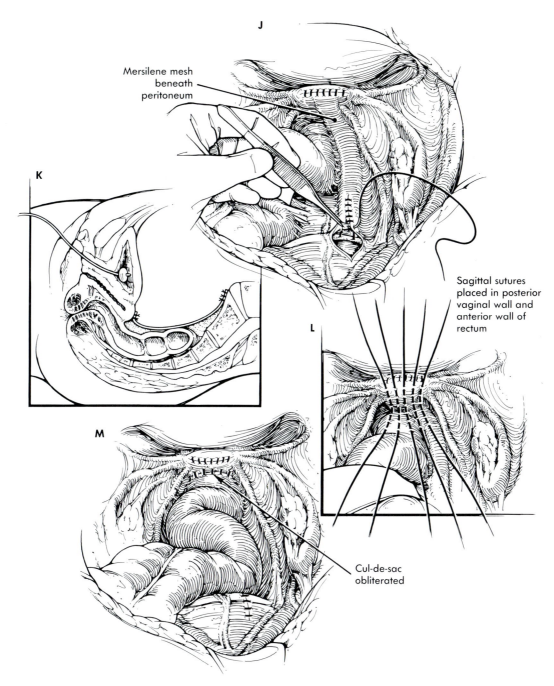

Fig. 27-29, cont'd. The peritoneum is closed **(J).** Sagittal view **(K)** shows the end result of the sacral colpopexy. The surfaces of the cul-de-sac of Douglas are approximated by sagitally placed sutures **(L)** and has thus been obliterated **(M),** and the abdomen is closed.

wide area of the vagina by multiple sutures and a meticulous culdoplasty using permanent sutures brought through the suspensory mesh.

After coincident total abdominal hysterectomy and vault closure, tack the plastic mesh to the posterior vaginal vault with three pairs of polyglycolic acid sutures, tied after all have been placed. This will fix the mesh *posterior* to the cut edge of the vagina, lessening the chance of postoperative erosion of mesh into the vagina.

Hemorrhage from laceration of a vessel entering one of the sacral foramina can be brisk and massive. Suture or coagulation of the torn vessel is rarely successful in controlling the bleeding, nor is the local application of packing or hemostatic agents, because the edge of the injured vein will have retracted into the ostium. Success in controlling such hemorrhage quickly has been reported from placement of a sterile stainless steel thumbtack into the sacrum.[15,26,28,32,34,38,] Pressure with the tip of a long

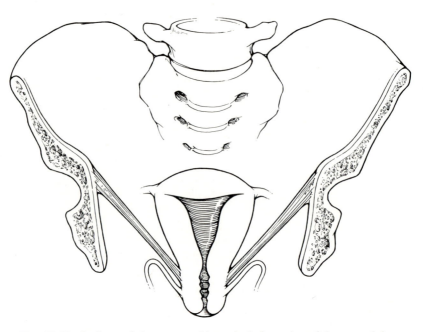

Fig. 27-30. Prolapse of the uterus, with marked elongation of the paracolpium.

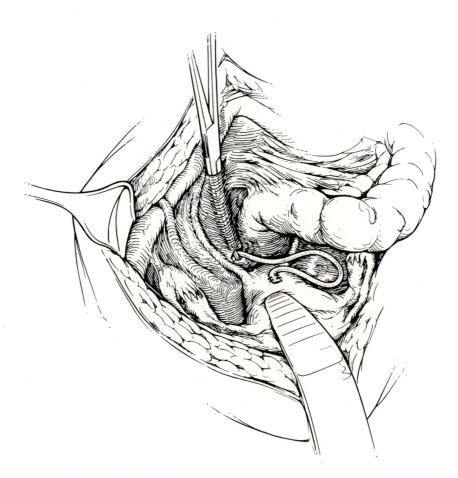

Fig. 27-31. Construction of a sacro-cervical ligament. A strip of fascia lata has been sewn to the posterior cervix and lower uterine segment, and a tunnel has been established beneath the presacral peritoneum.

Kelly hemostat is applied to the center of the head of the tack. A lag screw can be used similarly if a larger opening is encountered. It must, of course, be screwed into place. For a consultant in pelvic surgery or one who performs a good number of transabdominal sacral colpopexy operations or in a clinic where a number of these operations are performed, it may be prudent to have on hand a small supply of such sterile tacks or screws. The occasion to use them will be infrequent, but lifesaving.

Construction of a sacro-cervical ligament. The patient with symptomatic genital prolapse who wishes to retain her fertility (Fig. 27-30) has several options from which to choose. A ring pessary combined with a program of vigorous perineal resistive exercises may be used to support the internal genitalia until childbearing is completed, after which the patient may elect a permanent reconstruction such as vaginal hysterectomy with repair. If there is cervical elongation, and preservation of the uterine corpus is desired, a Manchester-type procedure may be performed, but with the knowledge that menses will continue as usual. Subsequent pregnancy may be complicated by cervical stenosis, however, and should there be cervical incompetence, a risk of premature labor and delivery must be considered. Suspension of the prolapsed uterus by

transvaginal sacrospinous colpopexy can be performed, but coincident colporrhaphy is not recommended at the same time lest a soft tissue obstruction be created that may impede future vaginal delivery. The author is unaware of any reports describing the consequences of pregnancy, labor, and delivery in such a patient. An option that will correct the uterine prolapse while conserving the uterus for reproduction is transabdominal construction of a sacrocervical ligament.[22] This relieves the symptoms of uterine prolapse and permits subsequent labor and vaginal delivery. This operation relieves the symptoms of uterine prolapse while making pregnancy, labor and delivery possible, but does not preclude eventual progression of the other manifestations of prolapse, which might require future reoperation. The operation is shown in Figs. 27-31 through 27-33.

Strips of fascia lata may be used as suture, particularly when fixing fascia lata to the posterior cervix.[12] The Gallie large-eyed needle is useful, and the fixation of the fascia-suture is ensured by the use of a slip-knot arrangement in which the easily frayed ends of the suture are tied with long-lasting ligatures (Fig. 27-33). The suture, having been passed through the point of anchorage, is now passed through its own body, as shown, and the slack is taken up.

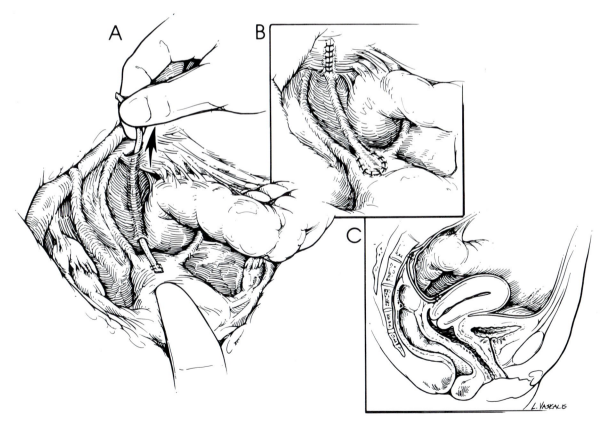

Fig. 27-32. A long forceps is introduced through this tunnel to grasp the free end of the strip. This is drawn through the tunnel **(A)** and sewn to the presacral fascia and periosteum **(B). C,** The final result is shown. The uterus is once again within the pelvis, and there is a horizontal axis to the vagina.

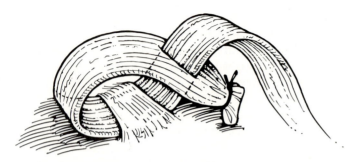

Fig. 27-33. When these strips of fascia lata are to be fixed to another surface, a slip-knot type of arrangement is useful. This can be placed as shown, often using a Gallie needle, which has a very wide eye through which the strip of fascia can be threaded.

CONCLUSION

Vaginal hysterectomy and repair, although usually successful, cannot serve all patients with massive eversion of the vagina equally well. The various causes, tissue strengths, and damages must be identified and correlated with a choice of different surgical procedures. For those patients with vaginal vault prolapse, but without surgically useful uterosacral-cardinal ligament support, the surgeon must add supplemental techniques for support of the vault. The ultimate goals are to relieve symptoms, restore the natural depth and position of the vagina, and effectively treat any coexistent pelvic disease, including cystocele, enterocele, and rectocele. This can be accomplished by using techniques that restore or preserve coital function.

It is usually unnecessary and often a distinct disservice to an active patient with prolapse to leave her with a short vagina or to perform a partial or total colpectomy. When colpectomy is performed, however, the results are better if any coexistent enterocele has been identified and the sac has been excised. Accurate perception and an adequate procedure cannot help but improve the long-term result of the surgery employed.

REFERENCES

1. Addison WA et al: Failed abdominal sacral colpopexy: observations and recommendations, *Obstet Gynecol* 74:480, 1989.
2. Amreich J: Aetiologie und Operation des Scheidenstumpf prolapses, *Wien Klin Wochenschr* 63:74, 1951.
3. Arthur HGE, Savage D: Uterine prolapse and prolapse of the vaginal vault treated by sacral hysteropexy, *J Obstet Gynecol Br Emp* 64:355, 1957.
4. Baden WF, Walker T: *Surgical repair of vaginal defects,* Philadelphia, 1992, JB Lippincott.
5. Barnhill D et al: Repair of vaginal prolapse and perineal hernia after pelvic exenteration, *Obstet Gynecol* 65:764, 1985.
6. Burch JC: Urethrovaginal fixation to Cooper's ligament for stress incontinence, *Am J Obstet Gynecol* 81:2, 1961.
7. Cox OC: Hystero-colpectomy, *Sibley Mem Hosp Alumni Assoc Bull* 1:9, 1958.
8. Cruikshank SH: Sacrospinous fixation—should this be performed at the time of vaginal hysterectomy? *Am J Obstet Gynecol* 164:1072, 1991.
9. DeLancey JOL: Anatomic aspects of vaginal eversion after hysterectomy, *Am J Obstet Gynecol* 166:1717, 1992.
10. Falk HC: Uterine prolapse and prolapse of the vaginal vault treated by sacropexy, *Obstet Gynecol* 18:113, 1961.
11. Farrell SA et al: Massive evisceration: a complication following sacrospinous vaginal vault fixation, *Obstet Gynecol* 78:560, 1991.
12. Gallie WE, LeMesurier AB: A clinical and experimental study of the free transplantation of fascia and tendon, *J Bone Joint Surg* 4:600, 1922.
13. Gallo D: *Ocejo modification of interposition operation.* In *Urologica Ginecologica,* Guadalajare, 1969, Gallo.
14. Inmon WB: Pelvic relaxation and repair including prolapse of vagina following hysterectomy, *South Med J* 56:577, 1963.
15. Khan FA, Fang OT, Nivatvongs S: Management of presacral bleeding during rectal resection, *Surg Gynecol Obstet* 165:272, 1987.
16. Jones HW Jr: Personal communication, 1990.
17. Magdi I: Obstetric injuries to the perineum, *J Obstet Gynaec Br Commonw* 49:687, 1942.
18. Marshall VF, Marchetti AA, Krantz KE: The correction of stress incontinence by simple vesicourethral suspension, *Surg Gynecol Obstet* 88:509, 1949.
19. Miyazaki FS: Miya hook ligature carrier for sacrospinous ligament fixation, *Obstet Gynecol* 70:286, 1987.
20. Morley GW, DeLancey JOL: Sacrospinous ligament fixation for eversion of the vagina, *Am J Obstet Gynecol* 158:872, 1988.
21. Nichols DH: Sacrospinous fixation for massive eversion of the vagina, *Am J Obstet Gynecol* 142:901, 1982.
22. Nichols DH: Fertility retention in the patient with genital prolapse, *Am J Obstet Gynecol* 164:1155, 1991.
23. Nichols DH, Milley PS, Randall CL: Significance of restoration of normal vaginal depth and axis, *Obstet Gynecol* 36:241, 1970.
24. Nichols DH, Randall CL: *Vaginal surgery,* ed 2, Baltimore, 1989, Williams & Wilkins.
25. Parsons L, Ulfelder H: *An atlas of pelvic operations,* ed 2, Philadelphia, 1968, WB Saunders.
26. Patsner B, Orr JW Jr: Intractable venous sacral hemorrhage: use of stainless steel thumbtacks to obtain hemostasis, *Am J Obstet Gynecol* 162:452, 1990.
27. Percy NM, Perl JI: Total colpectomy, *Surg Gynecol Obstet* 113:174, 1961.
28. Qinyao W et al: New concepts in severe presacral hemorrhage during proctectomy, *Arch Surg* 120:1013, 1985.
29. Richter K: Die operative Behandlung des prolabierten Scheidengrundes nach Uterusextirpation Beitrag zur Vaginaefixatio Sacrotuberalis nach Amreich, *Geburtshilfe Frauenheilkd* 27:941, 1967.
30. Richter K, Albrich W: Long term results following fixation of the vagina on the sacrospinal ligament by the vaginal route (vaginaefixatio sacrospinalis vaginalis), *Am J Obstet Gynecol* 141:811, 1981.
31. Sederl J: Zur Operation des Prolapses der blind endigenden Scheide, *Geburtshilfe Frauenheilkd* 18:824, 1958.
32. Stoddard FJ, Myers RE: Connective tissue disorders in obstetrics and gynecology, *Am J Obstet Gynecol* 102:136, 1968.
33. Sutton GP: Thumbtacks (letter to the editors), *Am J Obstet Gynecol* 164:931, 1991.
34. Sutton GP et al: Life-threatening hemorrhage complicating sacral colpopexy, *Am J Obstet Gynecol* 140:836, 1981.
35. Symmonds RE et al: Posthysterectomy enterocele and vaginal vault prolapse, *Am J Obstet Gynecol* 140:852, 1981.
36. Tancer ML, Fleischer M, Berkowitz BJ: Simultaneous colpo-recto-sacropexy, *Obstet Gynecol* 70:951, 1987.
37. Thompson HG, Murphy CJ, Picot H: Hystero-colpectomy for treatment of uterine procidentia, *Am J Obstet Gynecol* 82:743, 1961.
38. Timmons MC, Kohler MF, Addison WA: Thumbtack use for control of presacral bleeding, with description of an instrument for thumbtack application, *Obstet Gynecol* 78:313, 1991.
39. White GR: An anatomical operation for the cure of cystocele, *JAMA* 53:1707, 1909.
40. Zweifel P: *Vorlesungen über klinische gynäkologie,* Berlin, 1892, Hirschwald.

Chapter 28

TRANSABDOMINAL PARAVAGINAL REPAIR

A. Cullen Richardson

All patients who present with the physical finding of a urethrocele or cystocele have some defect in the supporting anatomy that has allowed the bladder or urethra to sag. All cystourethroceles, with or without stress urinary incontinence (SUI), are *not* the result of the same defect in the anatomic supports. There are several places at which the support of the bladder or urethra can break. The most common place for this support to give way is at the pelvic sidewall.

The paravaginal repair is an operative procedure that evolved in the treatment of one specific anatomic defect: a separation of the pubocervical fascia from its attachment to the lateral pelvic sidewall. When this defect is present, the paravaginal repair yields excellent anatomic and functional results. When this defect is accompanied by genuine SUI, the carefully done paravaginal repair will correct the SUI almost uniformly. The procedure is appropriate only in the treatment of this specific anatomic problem.

A knowledge of the anatomy, particularly of those structures around the vesical neck, is essential to understanding the procedure. The mechanism of pelvic support is always from inside out—structures never fall out, they are always pushed out by intraabdominal pressure. Because the mechanism is always from inside out, for any structure to be pushed out, there must be some break in the continuity of support within the innermost layer: the endopelvic fascia.

The bladder rests on and is attached to the pubocervical portion of the endopelvic fascia (Figs. 28-1 and 28-2). This layer of fibromuscular tissue extends from the cardinal ligaments and pericervical tissue in the mid pelvis ventrally to pass under the symphysis and merge with the urogenital diaphragm. Laterally on each side, it fuses into the fascial covering of the muscles of the pelvic sidewall (obturator internus and pubococcygeus) at the arcus tendineus fasciae pelvis (white line or fascial arcus). The urethra traverses this layer tangentially—beginning above it at the vesical neck and terminating below it at the external meatus.

All operations for cystocele have attacked the pubocervical fascia. It has been either plicated from below (as in the classic anterior vaginal repair and Kelly urethroplasty) or pulled upward and reattached to some structure from above (as in the Marshall-Marchetti-Kranz [MMK] pin-up procedure and its many modifications).

RATIONALE FOR PARAVAGINAL REPAIR

What happens to this layer of support under the bladder that allows the bladder to sag as in a cystocele? Traditionally, it had been taught that cystoceles resulted from a generalized stretching or attenuation of the pubocervical fascia and that this attenuated or stretched fascia was to be found beneath the vaginal covering of the bulging mass of the cystocele.

A chance observation over 22 years ago in a single patient caused me to doubt this traditional view. When she strained and pushed out a cystourethrocele, this action also everted the right superior sulcus of her vagina. When this area alone was supported, the bladder and urethra no longer descended. It was clear that the supporting tissue had broken away from its attachment to the lateral pelvic wall.

This observation was incompatible with the two concepts that had always been taught. First, this was clearly an isolated break in the supports, and, second, it was at the pelvic sidewall—not involving the bulging mass that was coming through her vaginal opening.

At the time, I considered this an aberration and just an

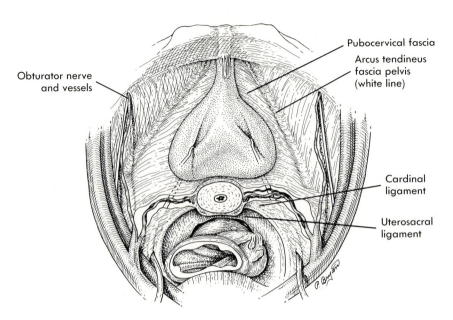

Fig. 28-1. Schematic drawing of the relationship of bladder to pubocervical fascia. (From *Contemp OB/GYN* 35:110, 1990.)

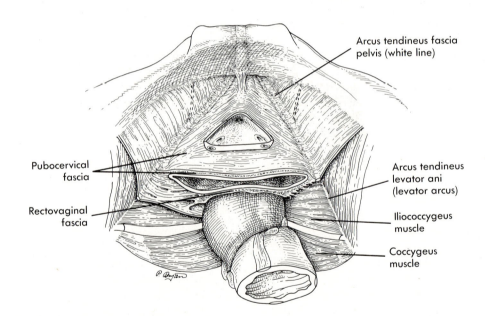

Fig. 28-2. Schematic representation of the various fascial structures to the lateral pelvic wall. (From *Contemp OB/GYN* 35:110, 1990.)

unusual exception; however, it forced me to realize that I had no good mental picture of just where this tissue attached laterally. We began to study this by pelvic dissections at autopsy.

Simultaneously, we began to look more closely at all patients with cystourethrocele. It became clear that the findings in the original patient were not an exception. We found most patients with cystourethrocele to have isolated defects, most often at the pelvic sidewall. Unknown to us, others had made similar observations that led them to operative remedy.

After this first year of autopsy dissections, we operated

on this first patient by reattaching the fascia to the pelvic sidewall on the right side only. This procedure cured her cystourethrocele, and she was relieved of her symptom of SUI.

MECHANICS

Anatomically, clearly this layer of fibromuscular tissue that we call pubocervical fascia is the principal supporting structure of the bladder, vesical neck, and urethra. As noted earlier, it constitutes a hammocklike diaphragm into which the trigone and vesical neck are embedded, and on which the base of the bladder is resting. The urethra

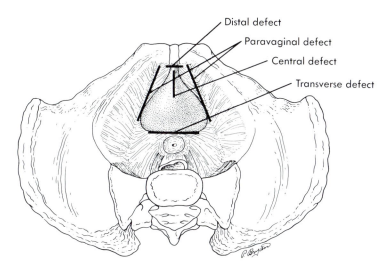

Distal defect
Paravaginal defect
Central defect
Transverse defect

Fig. 28-3. Four areas in which pubocervical fascia can break or separate—the four defects (From *Contemp OB/GYN* 35:110, 1990.)

traverses this layer and is supported by it throughout its entire length. As the urethra passes under the symphysis, it, with the adjacent pubocervical fascia, attaches to the urogenital diaphragm.

Mechanically, when a structure is subjected to stress, areas of stress concentration develop within the stressed structure. There tends to be a concentration of the stress anywhere the lines of force change direction. Structures break or fail where the stress is concentrated. If one looks at the pubocervical fascia, which is attached only peripherally, one can speculate as to where it might break if placed under stress.

In the case of a diaphragmlike configuration, the lines of force would change direction along the lines of this peripheral attachment. When such a structure is subjected to a force equally distributed over its surface, it would generally always break along this line of peripheral attachment. Only with inherent weakness in isolated spots would it break otherwise.

Clinically, our observations of the breaks that do occur follow this pattern. We have been able to distinguish four areas in which this continuity can be interrupted (Fig. 28-3), yielding some loss of support to the bladder. We refer to these as the four "defects" seen with cystocele or urethrocele. Three of the four of these are in the area of the peripheral attachment and only one is away from the periphery.

DIAGNOSIS

The distinction of the various defects is of paramount importance because each anatomic defect requires a different operative procedure for its correction. They can be distinguished only by careful physical examination done with a knowledge of the normal anatomy. The abnormality is detected by careful observation. The findings of each are as follows:

1. Paravaginal defect (Figs. 28-4 and 28-5):

   The lateral attachment of the pubocervical fascia separates from its attachment to the fascial covering of the obturator internus and levator muscles. This separation may be unilateral or bilateral. It usually yields a combined cystocele and urethrocele. Because the vagina is attached to the pubocervical fascia, when the break is in this area, the lateral superior vaginal sulcus descends, the bladder neck becomes hypermobile, and often there is SUI.

   When the superior sulcus is supported on each side, the cystourethrocele disappears. If the defect is unilateral (more often on the right), support of the sulcus on that side alone corrects the cystourethrocele. Paravaginal repair is appropriate for the correction of this defect (and this defect only).

2. Transverse defect:

   There is a transverse separation of the pubocervical fascia from its attachment to the pericervical ring of fibromuscular tissue into which not only the pubocervical fascia but also the cardinal and uterosacral ligaments merge. When it occurs alone, this defect yields a large cystocele, but the vesical neck remains well supported. The bladder dissects downward, obliterating the anterior vaginal fornix. Supporting the lateral sulci of the vagina has little effect on the cystocele.

   This separation of the fascia away from the cervix does not cause SUI. Patients with this anatomic defect usually experience excessive residual urine. This defect is often seen in the patient with total prolapse.

   We prefer the vaginal surgical approach to this problem. It should be emphasized, however, that it is important to close this break in the fascia anteroposteriorly—not with a side-to-side plication.

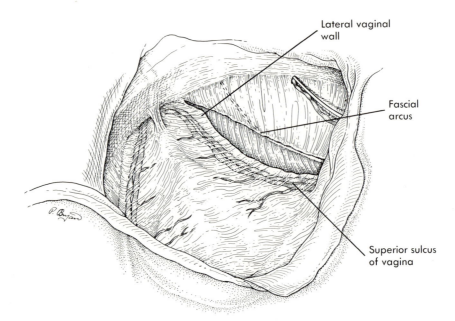

Fig. 28-4. Paravaginal defect. (From *Contemp OB/GYN* 35:110, 1990.)

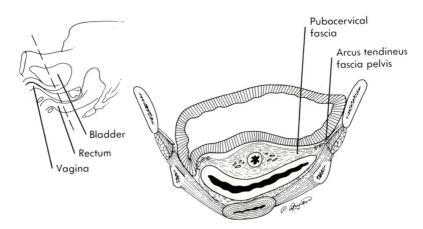

Fig. 28-5. Paravaginal defect in diagrammatic cross-section. (From *Contemp OB/GYN* 35:110, 1990.)

3. Distal defect:

The distal urethra is avulsed or separated from its attachment by way of the urogenital diaphragm (urogenital membrane or compressor urethra portion of the deep transversus perinei muscle) to the overlying symphysis. This would include patients who have had an amputation of the distal urethra as part of a radical vulvectomy. The physical findings are unusual. The vesical neck does not descend, and there is no downward rotation of the urethra with the Q-tip test. Rather, there is direct outward projection of the urethral meatus and the entire urethra. Usually there is a visible tiny bulge in the mucosa above the urethral meatus with Valsalva's maneuver.

These patients have distressing urinary incontinence that is difficult to repair. Fortunately, patients with this defect are rare. Our experience with this defect is too limited to draw any general conclusions, but we have employed one of the sling procedures with moderately good success.

4. Central defect:

This is any break in the central portion of the hammock between its lateral, dorsal, or ventral attachments. For many years, it was assumed that most cystoceles were the result of problems in this area of the support—hence, the popularity of the traditional anterior repair. As we have become aware of the other defects, we have found the central defect to be surprisingly uncommon. On casual inspection, these patients' cystourethroceles look very similar to those accompanying the paravaginal defect. However, with support of the lateral superior sulci of the vagina, the cystocele will persist. On occasion, we have seen scarring of the overlying vaginal mucosa, indicating a direct obstetric tear.

A central separation can develop secondarily after high suspension of the lateral portion of the fascia from above, as in the Burch modification of the MMK. It has been observed on one occasion after paravaginal repair. The defects in these patients are located immediately beneath the vesical neck. When a sound is placed in the urethra, palpation at the vesical neck reveals essentially only vaginal mucosa and urethral mucosa between the examining finger and the sound. There is striking palpable thinning of the tissue beneath the vesical neck.

In the surgical treatment of this defect, a traditional anterior vaginal repair and Kelly-type urethroplasty are necessary. After careful reflection of the vaginal mucosa from the underlying fascia, one can distinguish the edges of the fascial defect and approximate the broken edges.

As mentioned above, combinations of two or more defects do occur. Many patients with complete prolapse have both a transverse defect in front of the cervix and a paravaginal one laterally. When this is found, the patient requires both a repair of the transverse defect and paravaginal repair.

In our patient population, about 80% to 85% of patients with cystoceles have paravaginal defects. About 15% have transverse defects (some in combination with paravaginal ones). Only 1% to 2% have central or distal defects. Of the patients with cystourethrocele accompanied by stress urinary incontinence, over 95% have paravaginal defects. Thus, the paravaginal repair is our operation of choice in about 95% of our patients with SUI.

Because this chapter is focused on the paravaginal repair, we briefly describe the procedure.

TECHNIQUE OF PARAVAGINAL REPAIR

A Pfannenstiel incision is made through skin, subcutaneous tissue, and fascia. The peritoneum is freed from the undersurface of the rectus muscles, and the recti are retracted. (Better exposure can be obtained by detachment of the rectus muscles from the superior pubic ramus as in the Cherney incision, but once experience is gained, the Pfannenstiel is sufficient.) The retropubic space is entered by incising the transversalis fascia at its attachment to the superior pubic ramus. The transversalis fascia is "wiped off" of the superior pubic ramus laterally until the obturator notch can be palpated or seen. The bladder is drawn medially away from the sidewall of the pelvis. The left hand of the operator is inserted into the vagina. While the bladder is held with a sponge stick (Fig. 28-6), the lateral superior sulcus of the vagina is elevated and the prominent veins coursing down the lateral sulcus of the vagina are exposed. The separation of the lateral sulcus (as indicated by the veins in the sulcus) from the pelvic sidewall can be appreciated.

The objective of the procedure is to reattach the lateral sulcus of the vagina with its overlying pubocervical fascia to the pelvic sidewall at the level to which it was originally attached. This is at the level of the arcus tendineus fasciae pelvis (white line), which runs from the back of the lower edge of the symphysis to the ischial spine. At this point, it is well to palpate these two landmarks because that is the level to which the fascia is to be reattached.

Permanent suture should be used. We have principally used silicon-coated Dacron swedged onto a medium gastrointestinal needle (Davis and Geck, 3-0 Tycron, on the T-5 needle). Because this is a coated and very slick suture, at least six throws must be placed for knot security.

The first stitch placed on each side is the "key suture." The placement of this stitch determines where along the pelvic sidewall the vagina is reattached. The vesical neck can be palpated with the vaginal hand. The lateral extent of an imaginary arc (convex toward the symphysis) at the level of the vesical neck is the location of the vaginal bite of this first stitch.

While the lateral superior sulcus is elevated, a stitch is placed for the full thickness of the fibromuscular layer of the vagina through the lateral sulcus *beneath* the prominent veins. (Palpation with the vaginal finger should allow this medial bite to go down to but not through the vaginal mucosa; Fig. 28-7.) Before the needle is released, traction is placed on the needle holder moving its tip toward the ischial spine. While palpating with the vaginal hand, this traction is carried toward the ischial spine until the external meatus of the urethra can be felt to be drawn immediately beneath the middle of the lower edge of the symphysis (Fig. 28-8). The lateral (pelvic wall) bite is taken. This suture is held and not tied.

After placement of this first stitch, additional sutures are placed between the vaginal sulcus with its overlying fascia and the pelvic sidewall. These are placed at about 1-cm intervals—both dorsally (toward the ischial spine) and ventrally (toward the pubic ramus). Dorsally, the last stitch should be about 1 cm in front of the ischial spine. Ventrally, the last stitch should be as close as possible to the pubic ramus. Once all sutures are placed, they are tied (Fig. 28-9).

The procedure is repeated on the opposite side. Generally we do the right side first because most patients have a defect only on the right (the reason for this is unknown). Even if there is no defect on one side, the junction between the vagina and the pelvic sidewall should be reinforced by placing sutures around the junction of the pubocervical fascia to the fascia over the obturator internus as described above.

Many times there is some bleeding around the needle puncture sites as the sutures are placed. This usually ceases as the sutures are tied. The retropubic space is irrigated with warm lactated Ringer's solution, and hemostasis is rechecked. We have rarely (less than 1%) felt it necessary to drain the retropubic space.

Figure 28-3 shows a defect that has occurred by a separation immediately medial to the arcus. This is sometimes

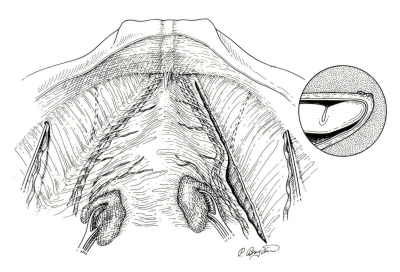

Fig. 28-6. Elevation of lateral superior sulcus of vagina with vaginal hand. (From *Contemp OB/GYN* 35:110, 1990.)

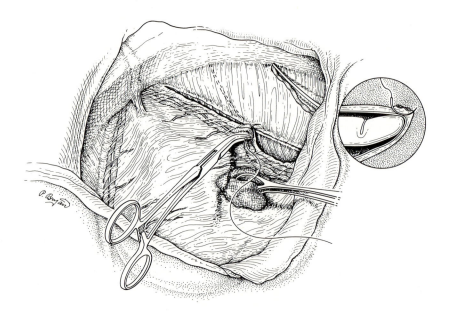

Fig. 28-7. First medial bite of paravaginal repair. (From *Contemp OB/GYN* 35:110, 1990.)

seen, but, more commonly, the entire arcus is separated from the lateral pelvic wall. Rarely, the separation seems to be down the middle of the arcus, and remnants of the arcus can be identified on both the pelvic sidewall and the superior sulcus of the vagina.

When the entire arcus is pulled away, it is necessary to locate the level at which it originally attached, as described above. The arcus extends from a point 1 cm up and 1 cm lateral to the midline of the lower edge of the symphysis back to the ischial spine. For the dorsal two thirds of the way, the fascial arcus (white line) overlies the levator arcus (arcus tendineus levator ani), which is the semitendinous origin of the iliococcygeus muscle from the surface of the obturator internus muscle. Usually when the

fascial arcus has been torn away, careful palpation locates the levator arcus. The vagina is to be reattached along a line between the two points referenced above. This line lies at a 40-degree angle from the lower edge of the superior pubic ramus.

When the fascial arcus is torn away, the levator arcus should be incorporated in the lateral bite of the stitches in the upper two thirds of the repair. The levator arcus is a structure with some strength and ability to hold a suture.

An indwelling urethral catheter is not used during or after the procedure. However, until one gains sufficient experience in the procedure, the indwelling Foley catheter helps as a landmark in locating the urethra and bladder neck.

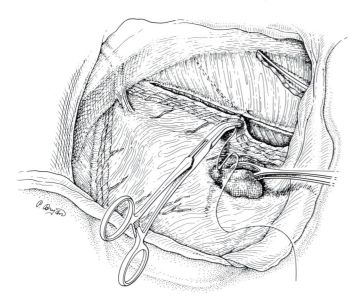

Fig. 28-8. Completed first bite of paravaginal repair. (From *Contemp OB/GYN* 35:110, 1990.)

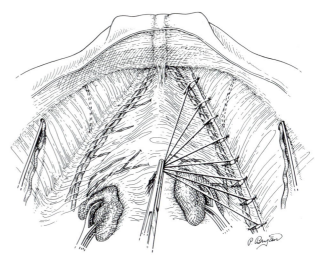

Fig. 28-9. Completed procedure. (From *Contemp OB/GYN* 35:110, 1990.)

Results. We have done this procedure over 800 times, either as a primary operation for cystourethrocele with SUI or as a secondary procedure in those patients who have had failed prior surgery for SUI or cystourethrocele. We continue to see better than 95% satisfactory results. By satisfactory results, we mean:

1. Correction of the cystourethrocele
2. Satisfactory relief of the abnormal urine loss (SUI)
3. Preservation of normal voiding function
4. No persistent postoperative bladder dysfunction.

Similar results have been reported by others who are employing this approach.

Over 80% of patients void immediately after surgery. We use straight catheterization two or three times if necessary; if the patient is still unable to void, an indwelling Foley catheter is left in place for 24 hours. Less than 5% of our patients have required the Foley catheter. Similarly, we have had no patient return postoperatively with an unstable bladder who had no evidence of detrusor instability preoperatively. If one is familiar with the anatomy and dissects gently, there will be few problems with the procedure.

It should be emphasized that this operation is only for patients whose cystourethrocele (with or without SUI) is the result of a paravaginal defect as described above.

Discussion. If defects in pelvic support occur as isolated breaks, it should be possible to approach the defect directly, repair it, and restore the normal anatomy. The paravaginal repair is just that—an attempt to restore normal anatomy.

The paravaginal repair is not an operation for SUI. It is a procedure designed to correct a cystourethrocele result-

ing from a paravaginal defect, which may or may not be accompanied by the symptom of SUI. SUI is not a single disease entity, but is a symptom of an underlying anatomic or functional problem.

By paravaginal repair, the delicate interplay between the passive connective tissue and the striated muscle is restored.

The primary surgical approach to all patients with support defects should be first to assess where the breaks have occurred. It must be determined if they can be approached directly. If so, the operative procedure should be designed to correct each identified defect in an attempt to restore normal anatomy. If this is not possible (and only when it is determined that it is not possible), the surgeon should consider a procedure that creates a compensatory abnormality.

BIBLIOGRAPHY

Durfee RB: Anterior vaginal suspension operation for stress incontinence, *Am J Obstet Gynecol* 92:615, 1965.

Figurnov KM: Surgical treatment of urinary incontinence in women, *Akusherstvo I Ginekologiia* 6, 1948.

Goff BR: The surgical anatomy of cystocele and urethrocele with special reference to the pubocervical fascia, *Surg Gynecol Obstet* 87:725, 1948.

Inman WB: Suspension of the vaginal cuff and posterior repair following vaginal hysterectomy, *Am J Obstet Gynecol* 120:977, 1974.

Richardson AC, Edmonds PB, Williams NL: Treatment of stress urinary incontinence due to paravaginal fascial defect, *Obstet Gynecol* 57:357, 1981.

Richardson AC, Lyon JB, Williams NL: A new look at pelvic relaxation, *Am J Obstet Gynecol* 126:568, 1976.

Shull BL, Baden WF: A six-year experience with paravaginal defect repair for stress urinary incontinence, *Am J Obstet Gynecol* 160:1432, 1989.

White GR: Cystocele, a radical cure by suturing lateral sulci of vagina to white line of pelvic fascia, *JAMA* 53:1707, 1909.

White GR: An anatomic operation for the cure of cystocele, *Am J Obstet Dis Women Child* 65:286, 1912.

Youngblood JP: Paravaginal repair, *Contemp OB/GYN* 35:28, 1990.

Chapter 29

REPAIR OF RECTAL FISTULA AND OF OLD COMPLETE PERINEAL LACERATION

David H. Nichols

RECTAL FISTULA

Although occasionally congenital in origin,[32] the rectovaginal fistula seen in the developed countries of the world is usually the aftermath of trauma—either unrecognized or unrepaired, or inadequately and unsuccessfully repaired. Suture penetration of the rectal mucosa during episiotomy repair or perineorrhaphy; Crohn's disease; infection and necrosis of a vaginal hematoma from hysterectomy, perineorrhaphy, or posterior colporrhaphy; pelvic irradiation, particularly after trauma to the vagina in the presence of endarteritis obliterans; and the growth of residual or recurrent cancer may also cause a rectovaginal fistula.

A rectovaginal fistula may occur at any level within the vagina, but it occurs most commonly in the lower third, generally at the apex of an improperly healed repair of a fourth-degree perineal laceration caused by obstetric trauma. Difficulty expelling the fecal bolus with the first bowel movement after the repair may have caused the patient to strain excessively, thus compromising the repair. Even though the surgeon may have approximated the tissue properly, such strain may result in a breakdown of the initial repair cranial to the perineum, often between the fifth and tenth day after surgery. The liberal use of stool softeners and a low-residue diet for a few weeks postoperatively may prevent this complication.[13] Hauth and associates[13] have recommended early re-repair of rectal mucosal and anal sphincter dehiscence after an unsuccessful repair, but their patients all required a minimum of 10 days hospitalization postoperatively, during which they were maintained on an initial diet of nothing by mouth followed by a no-residue diet for an additional week.

Fistulas may be single or multiple. Moreover, a single fistula may have several connecting tracts that communicate with one another within the subepithelial tissues, occasionally originating from several openings into the rectal lumen. Less commonly, a single opening in the rectal mucosa may communicate with several fistulous openings in the vagina and perineal skin. The relationship of a fistulous tract or tracts to the external anal sphincter is of paramount importance in planning surgical repair.

Observing the following principles in the management of rectovaginal fistula increases the probability of successful surgical treatment:

1. At the time of fistula repair, granulation tissue, infection, and edema should be minimal.
2. The repair must interrupt the continuity of the fistula.
3. The repair need not involve levator plication, with its associated risk of dyspareunia, but the operator should interpose a layer of fresh tissue with an independent blood supply between the layers of repair, if possible, particularly with postirradiation fistulas.
4. The epithelialized fistulous tract should be excised, and the edges should be inverted into the lumen when possible.
5. Closure of the tissues of each organ using two suture layers, usually in a transverse axis, is advisable, because a second layer removes much of the tension from the suture line of the first layer.
6. The vaginal side of the fistula may be left open for drainage. When a rubber drain is used, it should be left in place for 2 to 7 days. The appropriate time for removal depends on how large the fistula was, how

much drainage there is likely to be, and whether an abscess was encountered during the procedure.

Before repair, a relative degree of constipation provides reasonable fecal continence, but the patient is not usually able to control flatus. It is, in fact, the inability to prevent the involuntary loss of flatus that may first make the patient aware of the fistula and often accounts for her decision to seek surgical repair. While awaiting surgery, the patient can use several simple techniques to reduce the quantity of flatus, much of which is related to unabsorbed nitrogen ingested with swallowed air. For example, not talking while there is food in her mouth, chewing her food well, eating slowly without gulping, and finishing and swallowing one mouthful before taking another often reduce considerably the amount of air swallowed and, thus, the amount of gas that is likely to be expelled.

Diagnosis of rectovaginal fistula

Although some rectovaginal fistulas are asymptomatic, most are not. Incontinence of rectal gas or of liquid or solid stool when the perineum is intact and the external anal sphincter is functional suggests the presence of a fistula. When contaminants pass through the vagina, the bacterial concentration may precipitate a chronic, recurrent vaginitis. The patient may experience dyspareunia when infection and fibrosis are present.

If the patient passes liquid stool through the fistula while passing solid stool through the rectum, a gastrointestinal-vaginal fistula in the upper vagina may have arisen from small bowel. The surgeon should also consider such a possibility if the vagina and vulva are excoriated, as may result from contact of the skin with digestive enzymes of the small intestine.

Finding a pin hole-sized fistula. When it is difficult to demonstrate a suspected pinhole-sized rectovaginal fistula, its specific site may be determined by filling the vagina of the recumbent patient with warm water or soapy water sufficient to cover the expected site of the fistula, placing a Foley catheter with a 10-ml bulb into the rectum, and instilling air through the catheter. A stream of air bubbles coming through the vaginal water pool indicates the site of the fistula through which a blunt probe can be placed.

If the vagina will not contain the soapy water, the site of the fistula can be determined by instilling milk or a concentrated solution containing methylene blue or indigo-carmine into the rectal Foley catheter and watching where it appears on the posterior vaginal wall.

In seeking radiographic demonstration of the tract of a small rectovaginal fistula, one can inject a mixture of barium, mashed potato mix, and water into the rectum using a caulking gun. A lateral radiograph is taken while the patient bears down.

Surgical repair should be considered when a fistula has caused troublesome symptoms and when local edema and inflammation have subsided (usually coincident with relief of pain).

Preparation for surgery

Because the standard antibiotic erythromycin-neomycin bowel preparation (1 g of each by mouth at 1:00, 2:00, and 11:00 PM the day before the operation) is associated with a high incidence of troublesome gastrointestinal side effects, it is preferable to administer cefoxitin sodium (Mefoxin). An initial 2-g dose of cefoxitin should be given intravenously when the patient is on call to the operating room; another 2-g dose should be given 2 hours later, during surgery or in the recovery room if surgery is completed in less than 2 hours from the initial dose; and a third 2-g dose may be given 6 to 8 hours later. As Menaker[23] has stated, however, "systemic antibiotics administered preoperatively and for a short perioperative interval . . . have little effect on intestinal colonization . . . antibiotics are not indicated merely to cover breaks in the operative technique." But Hibbard[14] has reported increased surgical success when antibiotic coverage is provided.

The patient should take only clear liquids by mouth for 2 days before admission to the hospital.

As part of the bowel preparation for surgery, drinking 3 or 4 L of chilled polyethylene glycol (PEG) 3350 electrolyte solution (Nulytely, GoLYTELY, Colyte)[3] the afternoon before surgery, followed by two bisacodyl (Dulcolax) tablets to eliminate retained excess water in the bowel, is usually more effective than giving the patient preoperative enemas, because the incontinent patient usually cannot retain the latter. As an alternate, a half bottle of citrate of magnesia or two bisacodyl (Dulcolax) tablets are given the afternoon before admission. Two packaged (Fleet) enemas should be administered an hour apart the day before surgery; on the morning of surgery, plain water or saline enemas should be administered until the return is clear.

Surgical procedure

The gynecologic surgeon must consider several factors in choosing the most appropriate surgical procedure for a patient with a rectovaginal fistula. Foremost among these is the location of the fistula (lower, middle, or upper third of the vagina). Second is the etiology of the fistula (trauma, postirradiation, postsurgery, postepisiotomy, Crohn's disease, active malignant disease). Additional considerations are the age of the patient, the need for preserving or restoring coital function of the vagina, the presence or absence of a perineal body, and the integrity of the exterior anal sphincter.[33] The goals of surgery are, as for all reconstructive surgery, to relieve the symptoms and to restore the anatomy and function to normal.

There are eight basic operative procedures with which the surgeon who is to repair of rectovaginal fistula should be familiar:

1. Closure in layers without disrupting the perineum
2. Closure in layers after episioproctotomy
3. Transperineal mucosal flap transplant dorsal to an intact external sphincter

4. Transperineal mucosal layers and closure ventral to an intact external sphincter
5. Transrectal anterior rectal mucosal flap transplant
6. Noble-Mengert-Fish[24,28] anterior rectal flap operation
7. Transabdominal procedures for a fistula in the vault of an immobile vagina, which, when following radiation, may include temporary transverse colostomy
8. Colpocleisis or colpectomy

The gynecologic surgeon should be capable of performing all these procedures so that a technique or combination of techniques for the surgical treatment of a rectovaginal fistula can be chosen on the basis of what the patient needs. An effective combination must be thoughtfully planned and carefully executed for each patient.

The gynecologic surgeon should perform a fistula repair only when there is no abscess, because the presence of an infection will seriously impede the quality of wound healing. When, at surgery, an abscess is unexpectedly encountered in the tissues between the rectum and the vagina, the operator must modify the intended procedure and perform a simple unroofing operation in which the full thickness of the vaginal wall overlying the abscess is widely excised. This permits immediate and adequate drainage. Such a wound granulates in from the bottom up; in some instances, the granulation of the base of the wound closes the communication with the rectum, and no further surgery is necessary.

When it is necessary to repair coexistent rectovaginal and vesicovaginal fistulas, the vesicovaginal fistula should be repaired first, or postoperative scarring from the rectovaginal fistula repair may compromise the operative exposure. If the vesicorectovaginal fistula followed pelvic irradiation, the surgeon should usually perform a preliminary diverting transverse colostomy, followed in 2 or 3 months by repair of the vesicovaginal fistula in the usual manner, then repair of the rectovaginal fistula 2 months later, which may at times involve a colpocleisis; followed after 2 or 3 additional months by closure of the colostomy.

Rectovaginal fistulas resulting from an earlier obstetric trauma may be closed at the time of a subsequent delivery by episioproctorrhaphy. The excellent blood supply and laxity of the perineal muscles during pregnancy encourage healing. The operator makes a fresh incision to perform an episioproctotomy, "re-creating" a fourth-degree laceration; excises the fistulous tract and scar tissue; and repairs the wound as if it were a new injury. In the nonpregnant patient, however, episioproctorrhaphy in the treatment of rectovaginal fistula may lead to a postoperative infection with abscess formation that can destroy the integrity of the perineal body and external anal sphincter. Even without tissue destruction in abscess formation, infection in this area may initiate chronic painful inflammation, edema, and spasm of the pubococcygeal portion of the levator ani muscle, giving rise to the "levator syndrome" of levator spasm pain and tenderness that is so resistant to effective treatment.

In most cases, proctoscopy should precede rectovaginal or rectoperineal fistula repair. It is occasionally difficult to demonstrate the rectal opening of the fistula, except by gentle probing while the patient is under anesthesia. When the fistula is not demonstrable with certainty, traction applied with an Allis clamp on the external secondary opening, as described by Bacon and Ross,[2] usually produces dimpling at the primary opening, which is often in an anal crypt. If visualization is still unclear, the surgeon may inject the fistulous tract with methylene blue, using a no. 18, 19, or 20 needle that has been cut off approximately 1 cm from its hub. Through an anoscope, the surgeon then looks for the blue dye as it comes through the rectum, as well as for branches of the fistula.[39]

As Corman[8] noted, genital fistulas have a high-pressure side and a low-pressure side. In the presence of a symptomatic fistula, the flow of material from a hollow viscus is always from the high-pressure side to the low-pressure side. With a rectovaginal fistula, the rectum is the high-pressure side and the vagina is the low-pressure side. Material flows from the rectum into the vagina, not from the vagina into the rectum. Primary attention must be given to secure and effective closure of the high-pressure side. Even if unattended, the low-pressure side (the vagina) generally closes spontaneously once the continuity of the fistula has been interrupted and the high-pressure side has been closed. Excising the epithelium that lines the vaginal opening and loosely approximating the sides of the vaginal defect (with the stitches far enough apart to permit postoperative drainage, if there is any) strengthens and hastens the vaginal continuity over the rectum, however.

Because of the high vascularity of the pelvis, meticulous hemostasis in the area of fistula repair is essential to improve wound healing and reduce the chances of hematoma and abscess formation. Infiltration by up to 50 ml of a "liquid tourniquet" (e.g., 0.5% lidocaine in 1:200,000 epinephrine solution) is helpful, although the surgeon may substitute phenylephrine hydrochloride (Neo-Synephrine), vasopressin (Pitressin) or saline solution in patients who have severe hypertension or coronary heart disease.

Effect of location

Lower third of the vagina. Stern and associates[36] have demonstrated that rectovaginal fistulas low in the vagina can be repaired using either a transvaginal or transanal approach. An endorectal approach permits simultaneous correction of coincident anorectal pathology, and, by leaving the vaginal defect open for drainage, postoperative infection is minimized as is painful subvaginal scarring.

For the patient with an intact perineum, an intact external anal sphincter, and a fistula in the lower third of the vagina, the transperineal sliding rectal flap operation is appropriate. It does not disturb the perineal body, but does permit plication of an intact, although lax, external anal sphincter, if desired.

Episioproctotomy. Episioproctotomy permits excision of the entire fistulous tract followed by repair similar to that of a fresh fourth-degree perineal laceration (Fig. 29-1). The technique is generally simple to perform, but because it requires transsection and reunification of the external anal sphincter and the lower part of the internal sphinc-ter, there is a risk of recurrence as well as anal inconti-nence should healing be imperfect, compounding the original problem and requiring more sophisticated future reoperation.

Transperineal rectal flap sliding technique. A sliding rectal flap procedure such as that described with the

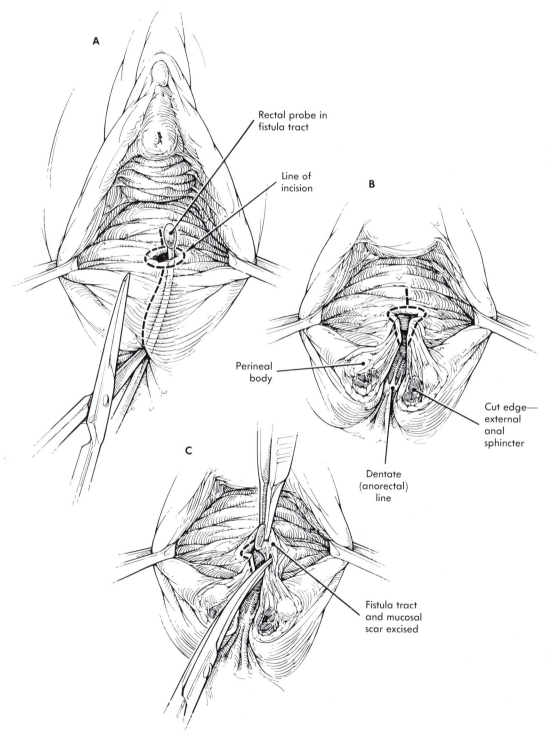

Fig. 29-1. Repair of a fourth-degree perineal laceration with coexistent low rectovaginal fistula. A mallable probe is inserted through the fistula tract as shown in **A,** and an incision along this probe exposes the tissue as shown in **B.** The fistula tract is excised along the site of the dashed line as shown in **B** and **C.**

Continued.

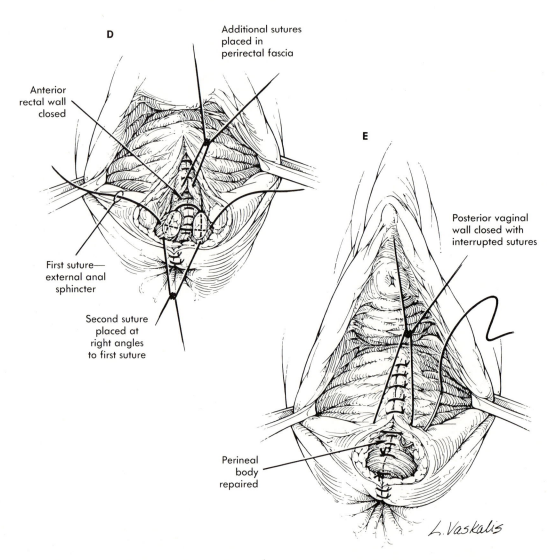

Fig. 29-1, cont'd. The submucosa and muscularis of the anterior rectal wall are closed with interrupted sutures as shown in **D,** and this is inverted by an additional layer of sutures placed in the perirectal fascia. The edges of the external anal sphincter are dissected out and the scar tissue around their severed ends is reapproximated with two interrupted sutures placed at right angles to one another, as shown. As shown in **E,** the full thickness of the posterior vaginal wall is closed with interrupted sutures and the perineal body restored by a few interrupted stitches.

Noble-Mengert-Fish operation[24,28] permits the mobilization and the excision of the portion of the anterior rectal wall that includes the fistula. If the external anal sphincter has been lacerated, its severed ends can be reunified and a perineal body can be constructed (Fig. 29-2).

Middle third of the vagina

Layered closure. When the fistula is in the midvagina and the external anal sphincter and perineal body are intact, a layered closure is useful. The operator incises the full thickness of the vaginal wall (Fig. 29-3, *A*) entering the rectovaginal space, and carefully separates the rectum from the vagina. Transecting the fistulous tract (Fig. 29-3, *B*), the operator excises the rectal tract in its entirety (Fig. 29-3, *C*). Two layers of submucosal interrupted size 3-0 polyglycolic acid-type mattress sutures, placed 2 or 3 mm apart in the rectal wall, are used to close the rectal wall

(Fig. 29-3, *D*). These may be placed transversely or, if there is no risk of compromising the rectal lumen (Fig. 29-3, *E*), longitudinally in the muscular wall of the rectum,[20] depending on available exposure. A second layer not only reinforces the first, but also takes some of the tension from the first layer of closure.

The operator excises the epithelialized tract through the wall of the vagina and loosely approximates the opening in a longitudinal direction by interrupted sutures of polyglycolic acid (Fig. 29-3, *F*) placed at least 1 cm apart to allow for adequate postoperative drainage.

Alternately, after irrigating the wound, the operator may split the posterior vaginal vault (Fig. 29-4) and interpose a layer of rectovaginal septum from side to side; the edges of the vaginal incision are freshened and made symmetrical, and the vagina is closed with interrupted sutures.

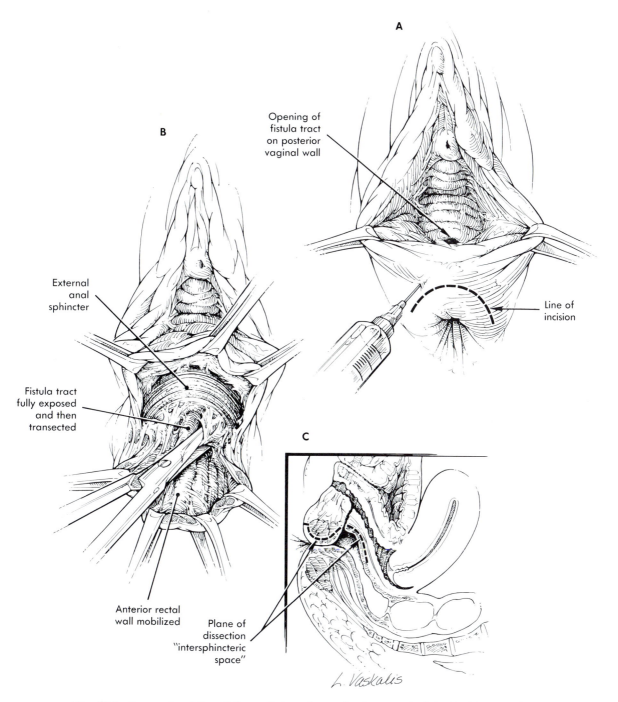

Fig. 29-2. Transperineal flap sliding technique for repair of rectovaginal fistula. The site of the fistula is noted in **A,** and the perineum and perineal body thoroughly infiltrated by 1:200,000 epinephrine in 0.5% lidocaine. A semilunar incision is made around the anus, posterior to the external anal sphincter along the course of the dashed line. Allis clamps grasp the edges of the incision, and by gentle traction to those placed on the anterior portion of anus, the dissection proceeds beneath the capsule of the external anal sphincter into the intersphincteric space as shown in **B.** The fistula tract is fully exposed as the anterior rectal wall is mobilized, and the tract is then transected. The path of dissection beneath the external anal sphincter and into the intersphincteric space is noted in **C.**

Continued.

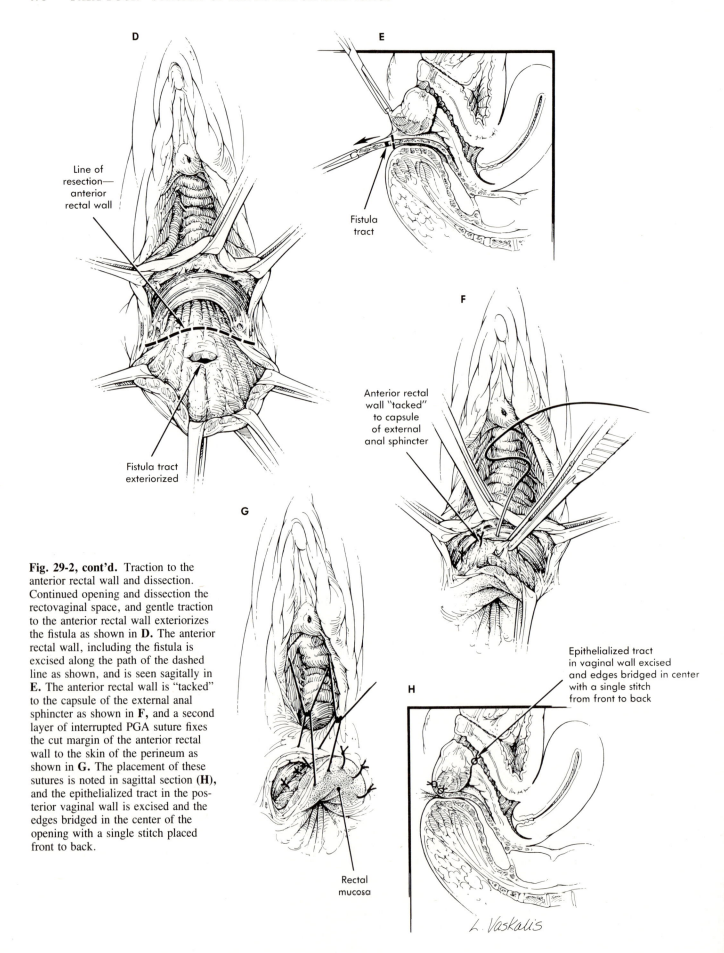

D

Line of resection— anterior rectal wall

Fistula tract exteriorized

E

Fistula tract

F

Anterior rectal wall "tacked" to capsule of external anal sphincter

G

Rectal mucosa

H

Epithelialized tract in vaginal wall excised and edges bridged in center with a single stitch from front to back

Fig. 29-2, cont'd. Traction to the anterior rectal wall and dissection. Continued opening and dissection the rectovaginal space, and gentle traction to the anterior rectal wall exteriorizes the fistula as shown in **D**. The anterior rectal wall, including the fistula is excised along the path of the dashed line as shown, and is seen sagitally in **E**. The anterior rectal wall is "tacked" to the capsule of the external anal sphincter as shown in **F**, and a second layer of interrupted PGA suture fixes the cut margin of the anterior rectal wall to the skin of the perineum as shown in **G**. The placement of these sutures is noted in sagittal section (**H**), and the epithelialized tract in the posterior vaginal wall is excised and the edges bridged in the center of the opening with a single stitch placed front to back.

L. Vaskalis

When the operator has decided to use a layered closure after the excision of the epithelialized fistulous tract has created a fresh third-degree laceration and little other tissue is available for this use, the interposition of some "levator" stitches between the rectum and vagina, placed without palpable ridges, increases the thickness of the perineum and insulates the site of the fistula repair on the rectal side from that on the vaginal side.

Transverse transperineal repair. When the fistula is in the midvagina and the perineal body and external anal sphincter are intact, the transverse transperineal repair, which involves a transverse perineal incision, is also use-

Text continued on p. 484.

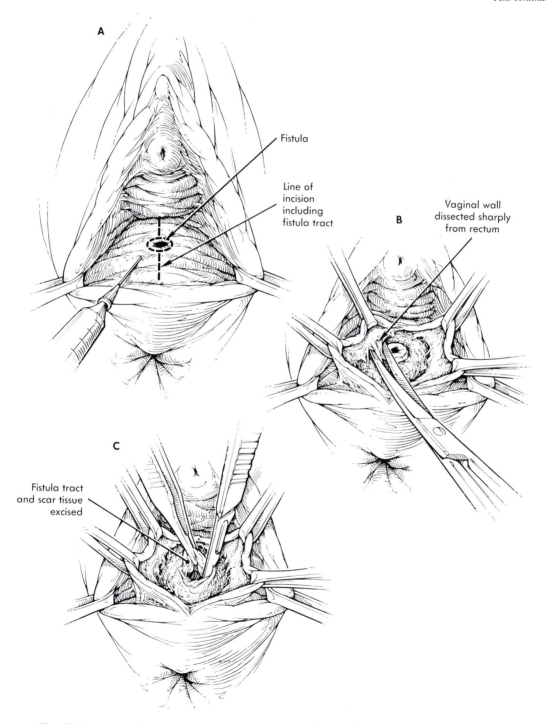

Fig. 29-3. Layered closure of a midvaginal rectovaginal fistula. The tissues around the site of the fistula are thoroughly infiltrated by 1:200,000 epinephrine in 0.5% lidocaine, as shown in **A,** and an incision made along the path indicated by the dashed line. This incision circumscribes the tract of the fistula as shown in **A.** The cut edges of the vagina are grasped by Allis clamps and sharply dissected from the anterior rectal wall, as shown in **B.** The fistula tract in its entirety is excised along with its surrounding scar tissue as shown in **C.**   *Continued.*

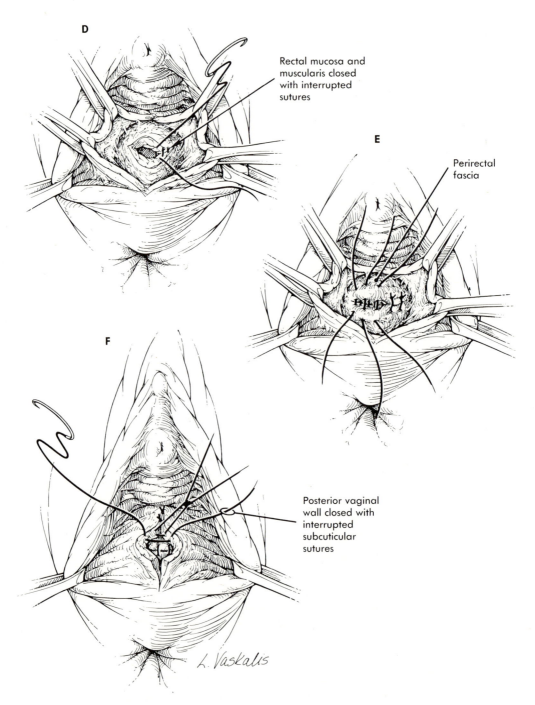

D

Rectal mucosa and muscularis closed with interrupted sutures

E

Perirectal fascia

F

Posterior vaginal wall closed with interrupted subcuticular sutures

L. Vaskalis

Fig. 29-3, cont'd. D-F. The rectal submucosa and muscularis are closed with interrupted sutures as shown in **D**, and this suture line is buried by a second layer of interrupted sutures in the muscularis and perirectal fascia, as shown in **E.** The wound may be thoroughly irrigated with sterile saline solution, and the posterior vaginal wall closed longitudinally and at right angles to the repair in the rectal wall using interrupted subcuticular sutures in the fibromuscular wall of the vagina as shown in **F.**

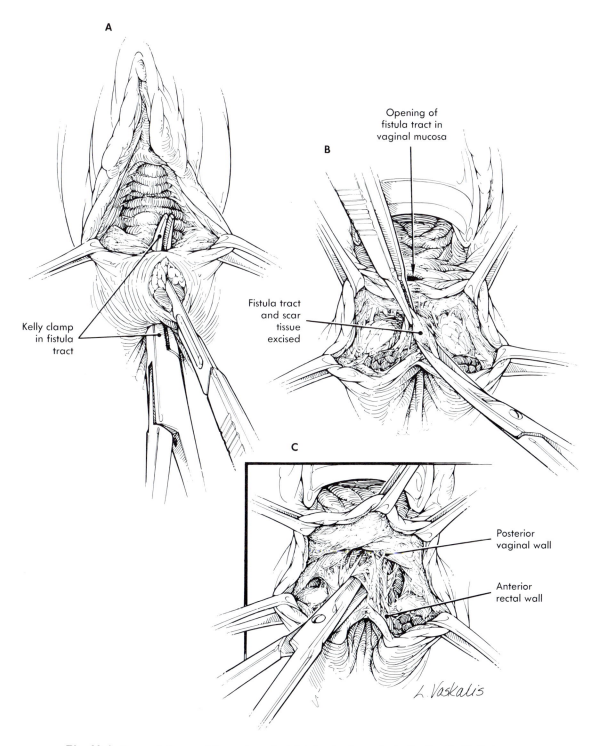

Fig. 29-4. Layered closure of the rectovaginal fistula. As shown in **A,** the tip of a Kelly hemostat is inserted through the fistula tract and an incision made through the perineal body and internal sphincter. The entire fistula tract and scar tissue are excised as shown in **B,** and the anterior rectal wall separated from the under surface of the posterior vaginal wall by sharp dissection as shown in **C.**   *Continued.*

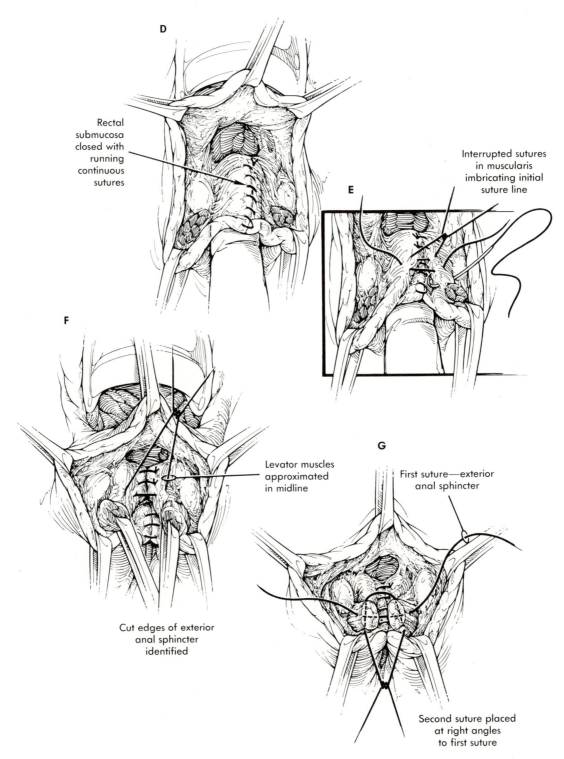

Fig. 29-4, cont'd. The freshened edges of the rectal submucosa are brought together with running continuous sutures placed in the submusoca as shown in **D.** This is covered by a second layer of interrupted sutures in the muscularis of the rectum as shown in **E,** imbricating the initial suture line. As shown in **F,** the medial surfaces of the levator ani are approximated with interrupted sutures and the cut edges of the external anal sphincter are identified and grasped with Allis clamps. The external anal sphincter muscle is reapproximated with two interrupted sutures placed at right angles to each other, as shown in G. *Continued.*

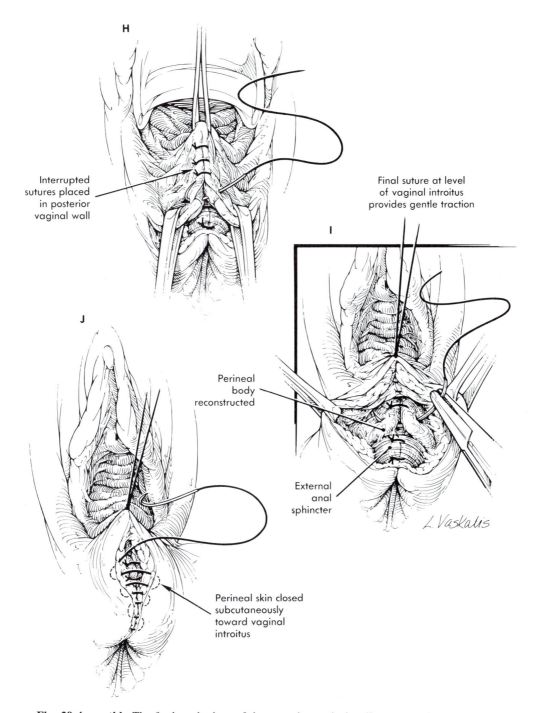

H

Interrupted
sutures placed
in posterior
vaginal wall

Final suture at level
of vaginal introitus
provides gentle traction

I

J

Perineal
body
reconstructed

External
anal
sphincter

L. Vaskalis

Perineal skin closed
subcutaneously
toward vaginal
introitus

Fig. 29-4, cont'd. The freshened edges of the posterior vaginal wall are approximated by interrupted sutures as shown in **H**. Upward traction to the lowermost of these sutures in the vaginal wall exposes the tissues from which the perineal body will be constructed; these are approximated with interrupted sutures as shown in **I**. This takes much of the tension from the stitches placed within the external anal sphincter. The wound may be throughly irrigated with saline solution, and the perineal skin closed subcutaneously as shown in **J**.

ful.[12,39] In this procedure (Fig. 29-5), the operator injects the perineum and, makes a transverse perineal incision, then dissects beneath the posterior vaginal wall ventral or anterior to the external anal sphincter and enters the rectovaginal space. The passage of a malleable probe facilitates the indentification of the fistula during dissection of the vaginal wall. After separating the rectum from the vagina, first laterally, then cranially to the fistula, the operator transects the fistula at its central portion. The transected fistula and the epithelialized tract are excised from both the rectal and vaginal walls.

The operator closes the rectal defect transversely with two layers, one of interrupted submucosal and the other of intramural sutures, and then closes the vaginal wall longitudinally. A single layer of interrupted sutures may be placed in the vagina, rather widely apart to permit possible postoperative drainage. The perineal skin may be closed transversely, but the skin and subcutaneous tissue may be approximated in the midline if the perineal body needs to be lengthened (Fig. 29-5, *K*).

Transrectal mucosal flap transplant technique. When there is considerable fibrosis of the perineum and transvaginal repair would so reduce the caliber of the vagina and the size of the perineum that dyspareunia would be certain to follow surgery, an alternate surgical technique is necessary to preserve the vaginal diameter and the integrity of the external anal sphincter. One such operation is the transrectal sliding mucosal flap operation.[11,17,19,27]

In this procedure, the patient is face down in a jackknife position with small sandbags elevating the hips. The fistula may be evident, and the operator may explore it from the rectal side (Fig. 29-6), using a small malleable blunt probe until the probe is palpable within the vagina. With the use of a Smith self-retaining retractor and a Sims retractor to provide exposure in the vagina, the rectal circumference of the fistula may be infiltrated with dilute vasopressin (Pitressin) 0.5 ml (10 pressor units) in 30 ml normal saline or 0.5% lidocaine (Xylocaine) in 1:200,000 epinephrine (Adrenalin) solution. The rectal ostium is circumscribed by an incision placed 0.5 to 1 cm from the margins of the tract (Fig. 29-6). The operator extends this incision distally onto the perineum and removes an inverted V-shaped wedge of skin and subcutaneous tissue to expose the anal sphincter. Deepening the incision to permit the identification of both the internal and external anal sphincters, the operator may partially divide them to remove any tendency toward a ridge or shelflike effect. The operator identifies the rectovaginal septum close to the posterior wall of the vagina, develops the rectovaginal space, and mobilizes the anterior rectal wall for approximately 3 cm above the site of the fistula.

At this point in the procedure, the operator places a figure-of-eight suture through the rectal opening of the fistula and ties it to the needle eye of the blunt probe. Traction on the probe from the vaginal side inverts the fistulous tract into the vagina, where the operator cuts it off flush with the vaginal skin. A series of interrupted 2-0 absorbable polyglycolic sutures is used to fix the rectal muscularis to the cranial edge of the external anal sphincter, and another layer of sutures is used to fix the mucosal edge of the anterior rectal wall to the posterior surface of the external anal sphincter. A small Malecot or Penrose drain may be placed through the vaginal opening at the site of the previous fistulous tract, sewn in place with a single absorbable suture, and the anal canal is lightly packed with a plug of petroleum jelly gauze. An in-dwelling Foley catheter is inserted into the bladder.

For primary repair of rectovaginal fistulas, Hibbard[14] has recommended proctotomy. But for secondary repair of a layered closure, and for the fistula high in the vagina or for the larger fistula, Hibbard[14] has recommended bringing in a separate and fresh blood supply to this area by performance of a bulbocavernosus fat pad transplant (Martius graft).[15,34]

Upper third of the vagina. Many fresh and unepithelialized fistulas in the upper third of the vagina, which are usually the result of postoperative pelvic abscess after hysterectomy, close spontaneously if the patient is placed on a no-residue, elemental diet with clear liquids for several weeks to inactivate the lower bowel. Several weeks of local estrogen therapy are beneficial to wound healing, even preoperatively, if the patient is postmenopausal. Of the vault fistulas that do not close spontaneously, the small ones may be closed transvaginally by a Latzko partial colpocleisis. Laparotomy may be necessary to close large fistulas, however.

After bowel preparation, the operator separates the rectum and the upper vagina by sharp dissection. After excision of the epithelialized margins, the rectal opening is closed transversely in two layers; the vaginal opening is closed longitudinally in one layer. The operator covers the site of each closure with a layer of mobilized peritoneum. Temporary colostomy is not usually necessary unless the patient has previously undergone therapeutic pelvic irradiation.

Effect of etiology. When fistulas appear after therapeutic pelvic irradiation, usually years later as a result of the reduced blood flow associated with endarteritis obliterans, the gynecologist should first perform a biopsy of viable tissue from the fistula margin to rule out active malignant disease. If there is no evidence of malignancy, the gynecologist prescribes the nightly application of intravaginal estrogen cream to improve the local blood supply and thicken the genital epithelium. Repair should be delayed for approximately 1 year after the fistula is first noticed to permit adequate stabilization of the blood supply and further confirmation that there is no malignancy in the area. If repaired prematurely (before restabilization or arrest of the vascular obliteration), this type of fistula is likely to recur; furthermore, the recurrent fistula may be larger and more difficult to repair than the original.

Boronow's operation of partial colpocleisis of the upper vagina is frequently effective in the repair of a radiation-induced rectovaginal fistula.[7] The operator exposes the

Text continued on p. 489.

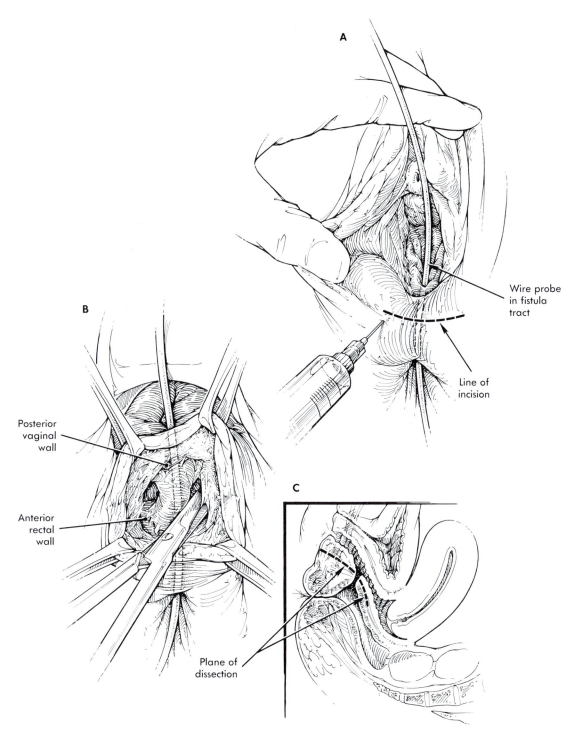

A

Wire probe
in fistula
tract

Line of
incision

B

Posterior
vaginal
wall

Anterior
rectal
wall

C

Plane of
dissection

Fig. 29-5. Transperineal sphincter-sparing repair of rectovaginal fistula. A mallable probe has been inserted through the tract of the fistula as shown in **A,** and the area to be dissected is thoroughly infiltrated by a solution of 1:200,000 epinephrine in 0.5% lidocaine. The perineum is incised transversely as shown. The dissection separates the vagina from the perineal body and by sharp dissection, starting laterally, the entire tract of the fistula is exposed as in **B.** The path of dissection is noted in **C.**   *Continued.*

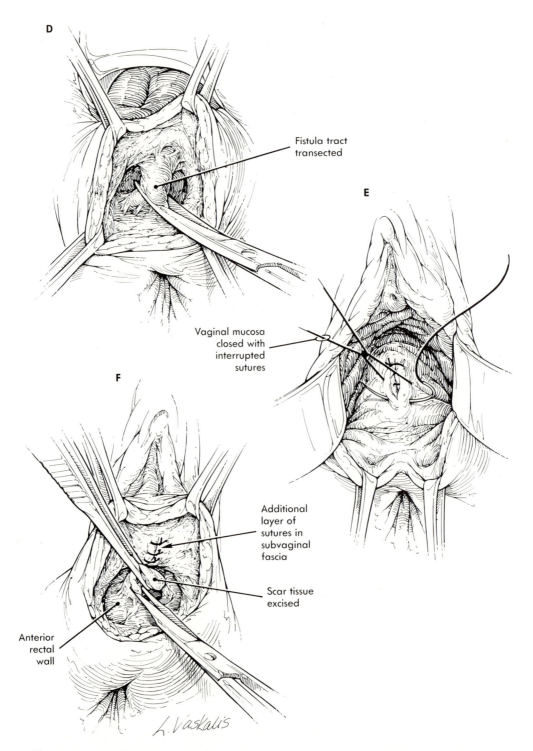

D

Fistula tract
transected

E

Vaginal mucosa
closed with
interrupted
sutures

F

Additional
layer of
sutures in
subvaginal
fascia

Scar tissue
excised

Anterior
rectal
wall

L. Vaskalis

Fig. 29-5, cont'd. After the tract has been isolated from the surrounding tissue, it is transected, as shown in **D.** The Allis clamps attached to the vagina are brought posteriorly, exposing the vaginal surface of the posterior vaginal wall. After the epitheliazed tract of the vaginal side of the fistula has been excised, the defect is closed with a few interrupted stitches of polyglycolic acid suture, as shown in **E.** As shown in **F,** the vaginal wall is again retracted anteriorly and an additional layer of suture is placed in the fibromuscular layer of the vagina on the underside of the posterior vaginal wall. The fistulous tract in the rectum and its surrounding scar tissue are excised.

Continued.

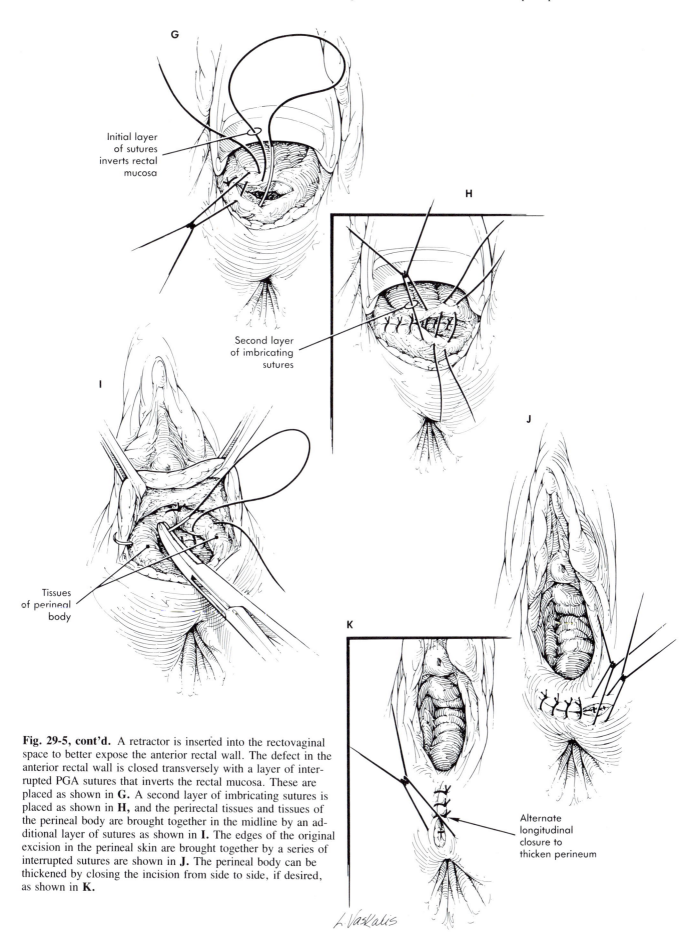

G

Initial layer
of sutures
inverts rectal
mucosa

H

Second layer
of imbricating
sutures

I

Tissues
of perineal
body

J

K

Alternate
longitudinal
closure to
thicken perineum

Fig. 29-5, cont'd. A retractor is inserted into the rectovaginal space to better expose the anterior rectal wall. The defect in the anterior rectal wall is closed transversely with a layer of interrupted PGA sutures that inverts the rectal mucosa. These are placed as shown in **G.** A second layer of imbricating sutures is placed as shown in **H,** and the perirectal tissues and tissues of the perineal body are brought together in the midline by an additional layer of sutures as shown in **I.** The edges of the original excision in the perineal skin are brought together by a series of interrupted sutures are shown in **J.** The perineal body can be thickened by closing the incision from side to side, if desired, as shown in **K.**

L. Vaskalis

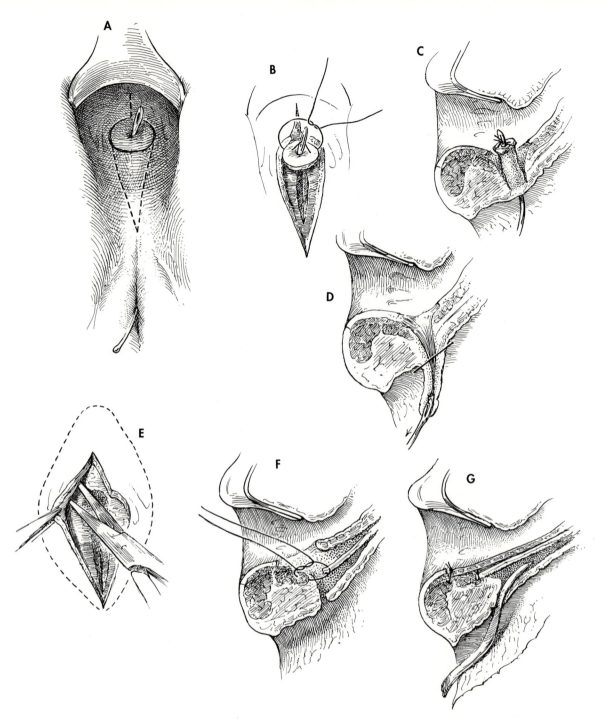

Fig. 29-6. The transrectal mucosal flap transplant is depicted. With the patient face down and in a jackknife position, the posterior rectal wall is displaced by a retractor, and the fistula is explored from the rectal side by a small malleable probe **(A).** The rectal circumference of the fistula is infiltrated by 0.5% lidocaine in 1:200,000 epinephrine solution and the opening circumscribed by an incision placed 1 cm from the margin. This incision is extended distally onto the perineum, and a V-shaped wedge of epithelium is excised as indicated by the dotted line. Sufficient superficial fibers of the rectal side of the anal sphincter are incised as to remove this as an obstruction postoperatively to the passage of stool and gas **(B),** and the mobilized rectal opening of the fistula is sewn to the eye of the malleable probe **(B).** This is shown in sagittal section in **C.** Traction on the vaginal end of the probe is made as shown in **D,** inverting the fistulous tract into the vagina where it is excised as indicated by the dotted line. The anterior rectal wall is separated from the vagina for about 2 cm **(E).** A series of interrupted sutures fixes the rectal wall to the internal anal sphincter **(F),** and another layer of sutures sews the mucosal edge of the anterior rectal wall to the posterior surface of the external sphincter **(G).** A small drain may be placed through the vaginal opening at the site of the previous fistula and fixed in place with a single absorbable stitch. (Modified from Nichols DH, Randall CL: *Vaginal surgery,* ed 3, Baltimore, 1989, Williams & Wilkins.)

somewhat fibrotic vaginal vault fistula by means of Schuchardt's incision (see Chapter 20) and carefully dissects the vagina from the anterior rectal wall for 1 to 2 cm in all directions at the site of the fistula. Hemostasis must be meticulous to prevent postoperative hematoma formation. The defect in the anterior rectal wall, the high-pressure side of the fistula, is closed transversely without tension by a two-layered interrupted fine polyglycolic acid suture technique. A bulbocavernosus fat pad on one or both sides is mobilized, swung beneath the anterior vaginal wall, and sewn in place to cover the site of the fistula repair, and the vagina is closed.

In general, the gynecologic surgeon performs colpocleisis only for the large fistula that is sometimes seen after irradiation, when the viability of the adjacent tissue is so poor that good wound healing is unlikely. It, of course, destroys the function of most or all of the vagina, and the patient must understand and accept this before the surgery takes place.

Sigmoid-vaginal fistula usually results from perforation of a sigmoid diverticulum coincident with abscess formation from diverticulitis. It generally occurs in an older patient with diverticulosis. A transabdominal operation, often combined with partial colectomy, is the proper approach for surgery for this type of fistula.

Transabdominal closure is generally reserved for those rectovaginal fistulas in sites that are relatively inaccessible from below and that are awkward to visualize, making repair of the bowel more difficult once the two organs have been separated. This situation is usually associated with a longstanding epithelialized fistula that developed after hysterectomy and pelvic abscess that may have limited vaginal mobility. When it follows pelvic irradiation, successful closure may require the operator to perform a temporary transverse colostomy and bring into the repair an interposing layer of fresh tissue with an independent blood supply (e.g., the omentum or the bulbocavernosus fat pad) because postirradiation fibrosis has obliterated local blood vessels and has led to endarteritis obliterans, which effectively reduces the blood supply to the irradiated tissues.

Other types of rectal fistula

The appropriate treatment for anoperineal fistula that does not communicate with the anal sphincter is simple excision of a wide area of surrounding skin, at least 1 cm lateral to each side of the fistula (Fig. 29-7). The operator places a probe into the fistulous tract, incises through the full thickness of the overlying skin and subcutaneous tissue, and widely excises the surrounding skin margin, removing the fistulous tract. Any bleeding vessels are tied, and the wound is packed open to granulate in from the bottom. The skin margins should be the last portion of the wound to close. Although healing requires a 4- to 6-week period, the patient remains surprisingly comfortable, and there is little disability.

Because standard surgical techniques do not generally resolve fistulas resulting from Crohn's disease, it is essential to recognize this disorder before recommending surgical repair of a fistula. The gynecologist should suspect Crohn's disease when there has been no mechanical trauma that would explain the origin of the fistula and the patient reports weight loss and frequent loose bowel movements, often accompanied by intestinal cramping. The fistula is invariably quite painful to touch (especially during the active phases of the disease), even when it has been present for a considerable length of time. Its edge has the roughened red appearance of granulation tissue. Biopsy, endoscopy, and study of the films of both upper and lower gastrointestinal radiography confirm the presence of Crohn's disease. The surgeon may consider repairing a Crohn's disease-induced rectovaginal fistula in the lower vagina during a temporary remission of the disease; the use of a sliding rectal flap operation permits the excision of the bowel wall that contains the fistula. The patient must be informed of the high risk of surgical failure or of exacerbation of the disease, however. Preoperative preparation may include the administration of metronidazole (Flagyl), 1000 mg daily along with 20 mg of prednisone daily, for 1 month.[5]

When rectovaginal or anovaginal fistulas are the result of Crohn's disease, success may be achieved with surgical closure providing that the timing is such that the disease is clearly in an inactive phase.[26] A rectal flap sliding technique is the preference of the author, providing that the fistula is low within the vagina and otherwise uncomplicated by stenosis or other fistula.

Although Beecham[4] recommended coincident colostomy, we have not found this to be necessary in most instances.

Unless associated with an invasive neoplasm, rectouterine fistulas are almost invariably the result of coexistent diverticulosis, in which diverticula became adherent to the posterior wall of the uterus and an abscess formed, ultimately eroding into the uterine cavity. The condition produces a profuse, cloudy, watery discharge from the cervix in an amount that is usually sufficient to require the patient to wear sanitary protection. Early in its course, the discharge may be intermittent, coinciding with flare-ups of activity within the abscess cavity, and the patient may be relatively comfortable between spells fo watery leukorrhea. A barium enema and sigmoidoscopy readily confirm the diagnosis. Treatment is surgical, sometimes requiring a preliminary colostomy, a bowel resection and hysterectomy 2 or 3 months later, and closure of the colostomy as a tertiary procedure 2 or 3 months after the hysterectomy.

Vesicorectal fistula is a rare late complication of hysterectomy. Because of its location high within the vault of the vagina, successful repair usually requires a transabdominal approach with dissection followed by separate repair of each organ system. Depending on the size of the fistula and any previous irradiation, a preliminary diverting colostomy may be desirable.

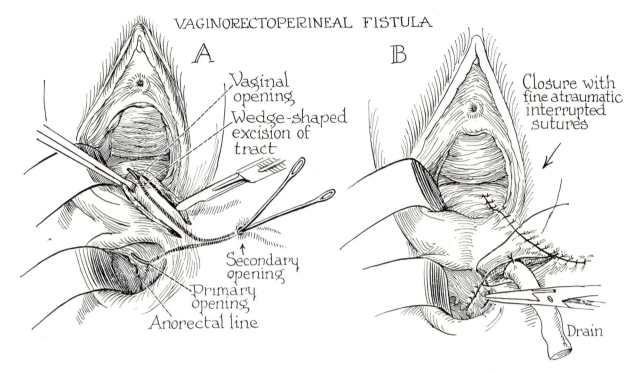

Fig. 29-7. Probes are used to follow the tract and, if possible are passed through its entire length **(A).** The injection of dye in the tract is seldom of any help and obscures the field of operation. If probes can be inserted, a wedge-shaped excision of the tract is carried out. All of the infected tissue between the primary and secondary openings is removed. The excision of the tract going from the vagina to the perineum is shown. Subsequently the entire tract from the primary opening near the anorectal line to the skin of the perineum is excised.

The anterior tract, after thorough and adequate excision from the vagina to the perineum, is closed with attraumatic interrupted sutures **(B).** After excision of the fistula-in-ano, several sutures are used to close the skin of the anoderm and invert it into the anal canal. Remnants of the rectal sphincter that can be approximated without tension are brought together with 00 PGA suture on atraumatic needles. A drain was inserted in the most dependent portion of the skin just lateral to the rectal sphincter. (From Ball TL: *Gynecologic surgery and urology,* ed 2, St Louis, 1963, Mosby–Year Book.)

POSTOPERATIVE CARE AFTER FISTULA REPAIR

Postoperatively, the antibiotic that was administered preoperatively can be continued for a short time unless a significant diarrhea develops, in which case the antibiotic should be promptly discontinued and the diarrhea should be brought under control. The patient should have a clear liquid diet for 3 days; when she is passing gas, she is gradually changed to a low-roughage or bland diet for 3 weeks. Stool softeners should be given, and, if there has been no bowel movement by the seventh day, a gentle laxative should be added. Small doses of GoLYTELY are preferable to an enema at this time.

The vaginal drain should be removed between the fifth and seventh postoperative days, depending on the amount of drainage and the stability of the patient's temperature. Sitz baths given twice daily after the drain has been removed may make the patient more comfortable. Coitus is not permitted until the end of the third postoperative month.

Stool softeners such as docusate sodium (Colace)

should be given for 5 weeks. Tincture of opium, 10 drops in water three times a day for the first 5 days, is often helpful if cramps are troublesome. When a partial colpocleisis has been performed, intravaginal estrogen cream should be instilled nightly for many weeks until healing, followed by long-term weekly use.

Late recurrence of rectovaginal fistula, even 10 or 15 years after the time of an original repair, occasionally occurs. For this reason, it is desirable for the operator to examine the patient periodically for some time.

REPAIR OF OLD COMPLETE PERINEAL LACERATION

Kelly once noted that genital prolapse was only rarely observed in patients with a complete and unrepaired perineal laceration.[18] Because the principal effectiveness of the pubococcygei and levator ani in supporting the birth canal is exerted posterior to the rectum where their fusion forms the levator plate, a laceration through the anterior rectum, perineal body, and posterior vagina is not likely to be the result of forces simultaneously exerted in a way that overstretches the major sources of the uterine support. Although such a laceration disrupts the anal sphincter, many of these patients, by vigorously exercising the pubococcygeus over a long period of time, develop a hypertrophy in this muscle that permits a side-to-side sphincterlike action that helps hold the sides of the fistula in opposition and accomplishes a semblance of anal continence. This mechanism does not restore control of flatus, but it may result in continence of the stool, particularly if the patient is careful to maintain a helpful degree of constipation. To test for fecal incontinence, have a packaged enema given to the patient in the office and see if she can retain it voluntarily.

According to Miller and Brown[25], there are three essential requirements for the successful repair of an old laceration of the perineum: (1) evidence of a good blood supply, (2) absence of infection in the tissues involved, and (3) closure of the repair with no tension on the sutures that reapproximate the tissues. It is equally important to excise all scar tissue to ensure that the tissues being reapproximated are similar to those of a fresh fourth-degree laceration. Layer-by-layer reconstruction of the rectal wall perirectal connective tissue, anal sphincter, and rectovaginal septum before closure of the overlying vaginal floor should be accomplished by means of terraced rows of fine absorbable suture, although such a repair occasionally breaks down, leaving a rectovaginal fistula. This discouraging result is particularly likely in the postmenopausal patient with atrophic tissues and a reduced blood supply.

Particularly in the postmenopausal years, age reduces intestinal peristalsis. Nicotine withdrawal indirectly reduces it in someone who has just stopped smoking, prior to hospitalization, tending to invite postoperative constipation.

The results are best when an obstetric laceration is properly repaired immediately after delivery, when the vascularity of the perineum and perivaginal tissues favors rapid healing. Patients may seek a repair of a complete perineal laceration at any time, however, even years after the original injury. In these patients, scar tissue is appreciable, wound healing is poorer, and the fistula is more likely to recur. Therefore, when the laceration to be repaired is an old one, it is important for the surgeon to choose an operation that provides the optimal chance of success with but one repair procedure.

Partial or total denervation of the external anal sphincter and of the levator ani can result from a combination of many factors.[35,37,38] Occult damage can be measured even after uncomplicated vaginal delivery, although it generally heals rapidly. Straining at stool may contribute to further damage, as may damage to the motor nerve roots of S3 and S4 from coincidental disc disease or spinal canal stenosis from osteoarthritis. Manning and Pratt[22] described their surgical results as best following the first repair; they noted difficulty in finding the frayed ends of the external anal sphincter when they were buried in scar tissue. They thought that the symptomatic improvement following surgery to restore anal incontinence was less when the patient has been clinically diagnosed as having an irritable bowel syndrome. Pezim and associates[31] from the same institution concluded from examination of their own data that because 48% of their incontinent patients had been labelled as having irritable bowel prior to presentation, a much higher percentage than one would find among the normal population, in most cases the diagnosis was unwarranted. Their postsurgical results were equally satisfactory in this group, and they concluded that surgical repair should be offered to such patients with assurance of equal success. Although Fang et al[10] following on the work of Blaisdell[6] report better results with overlapping sphincterplasty, acceptance of this conclusion is by no means universal. Not only may it be surgically difficult to dissect the external anal sphincter from surrounding scar tissue, but excessive dissection may compromise both the blood and the nerve supplies of the sphincter. Classic descriptions of the transected external anal sphincter characterize it as a narrow bundle to be sought just beneath the perianal skin and distinctly caudal to the internal sphincter.[15,30] More recent studies using magnetic resonance imaging (MRI) come to quite a different conclusion. Aronson and colleagues[1] have observed from their MRI studies that the external sphincter normally is a strong ellipsoidal cylinder complex that surrounds the distal portion of the internal anal sphincter in the adult for a distance of 3 to 4 cm and is thicker anteriorly and posteriorly than laterally. They submit that surgical reapproximation of this entire muscular cylinder should be followed by a more effective restoration of sphincter function than that following reapproximation of just the superficial subcutaneous portion of the external anal sphincter. This author believes this is to be true and no longer makes a decisive effort to dissect the external anal sphincter away from its surrounding tissues, nor to separate it from the internal anal sphincter at this level. The free but scarred ends of the lacerated external sphincter should be sought and grasped so that they may be sewn together as a part of the perineal reconstruction, but combining this with full perineal reconstruction will produce the best anatomic and functional result. Fecal continence is the result of effective interaction and support between not only the external and internal anal sphincters, but with the whole of the pelvic diaphragm including its puborectalis portion.[21]

Layered closure

Rectum and vagina are separated by dissection through the dense scar tissue between them. The separation is carried into the rectovaginal space (Fig. 29-8). The scarred ends of the external anal sphincter are identified and grasped in Kocher or Allis clamps or by a towel clip, and held for later reapproximation. The submucosal rectal wall and anoderm are closed (Fig. 29-8, D). A second layer approximates the perirectal fascia and muscularis, and the ends of the external anal sphincter are brought together. The perineal body should be restored by a few buried in-

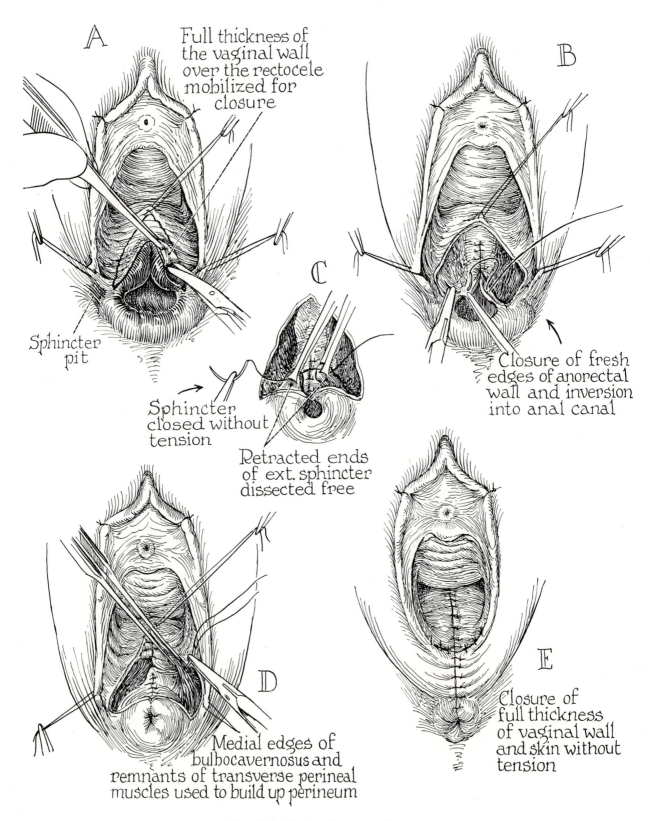

A

Full thickness of
the vaginal wall
over the rectocele
mobilized for
closure

Sphincter
pit

B

Closure of fresh
edges of anorectal
wall and inversion
into anal canal

C

Sphincter
closed without
tension

Retracted ends
of ext. sphincter
dissected free

D

Medial edges of
bulbocavernosus and
remnants of transverse perineal
muscles used to build up perineum

E

Closure of
full thickness
of vaginal wall
and skin without
tension

Fig. 29-8. For legend see opposite page.

terrupted stitches, and the skin of the posterior vaginal wall and perineum closed with interrupted sutures.

The Noble-Mengert-Fish anterior rectal flap operation has often been recommended for the repair of an old perineal laceration[24,28]; primary healing with restoration of function usually follows the Warren-Miller-Brown vaginal flap operation as well.[9,25,40] The surgeon often chooses between the two operations on the basis of the size of the vagina. The rectal flap operation does not remove vaginal membrane and can be used in a patient with a smaller vagina, whereas the vaginal flap operation makes the vagina measurably smaller and, therefore, is appropriate when this is a desired goal.

Rectal flap operation

In principle and usefulness, the rectal flap operation (Noble-Mengert-Fish procedure[24,28]) is not unlike the mucosal flap operations for rectovaginal fistula, but the rectal flap operation is a procedure of choice when the integrity of the external anal sphincter has been disturbed. The rectal flap operation is particularly useful if an old fourth-degree laceration extends no more than 3 or 4 cm into the anal canal. By freeing up and pulling down the anterior rectal wall and suturing the edge of the mobilized segment of anterior rectal mucosa to the anal sphincter and perineal skin outside of the former anal canal, the surgeon can cover the area where the sutures not protected by such a flap are often disrupted postoperatively.

Brief electrical stimulation with an electrosurgical needle electrode not only aids hemostasis, but can also help identify striated muscle. An occasional stitch should include a superficial bite of the anal sphincter. The lower edge of the remaining flap of the anterior rectal wall is fixed to the skin of the perineum by several interrupted 2-0 absorbable polyglycolic acid-type sutures placed not more than 1 to 2 cm apart.

Vaginal flap operation

The bowel is cleansed by an electrolyte purgative[3] such as Nu-Lytely or Co-Lite or by enemas until the return is clear, in preparation for the vaginal flap operation. To begin the procedure, the surgeon makes an inverted V-shaped incision in the posterior vaginal wall. The incision should be of a width that will leave the introitus with the desired caliber when the sides of the vagina are subsequently united[25,40] (Fig. 29-9, A through C). The base of this vaginal flap is continuous with the margin of the anterior rectal wall.

By sharp dissection through any scar tissue, the surgeon develops the avascular space between the rectum and vagina for several inches, mobilizing the anterior rectal wall. Stretching the rectal wall by traction to the free end of the vaginal flap will bring it and the V-shaped vaginal flap to beneath the site of the external anal sphincter. Then, grasping the buried ends of the sphincter, the surgeon places appropriate mattress sutures of 2-0 long-lasting, but absorbable synthetic suture but without tying them just yet.

The perineal body is reconstituted by several side-to-side sutures that are tied. After this, the anal sphincter stitches can be tied, and the perineal skin can be closed from side to side. The undersurface of the vaginal flap is sewn to the external anal sphincter and perineal skin, and the excess tissue in the flap is trimmed and removed.

The anal sphincter fibers will retract and shorten. Therefore, the reconstructed anal canal should admit one fingerbreadth comfortably at the time of the surgery; if not, the operator should make a paradoxical sphincter incision as described by Miller and Brown.[9,25] Such an inci-

---

Fig. 29-8. Traction sutures are placed outlining a triangular area to be denuded. The apex of this triangle is above any scar tissue in the vagina, while the angles of the base are over the sphincter pits (**A**). The incision is carried high enough so the full thickness of the vaginal wall over a rectocele or lateral vaginal wall relaxation can be mobilized to aid in the closure.

The dissection is continued until the full thickness of the vagina is mobilized and separated from the rectal wall and mucosa. The scar tissue in the vaginal and rectal walls is excised so that fresh edges are approximated, and the rectal and anorectal walls are inverted into the canal by interrupted sutures of 00 PGA on atraumatic needles (**B**). These sutures extend just to the submucosa and precisely approximate the tissues.

The retracted ends of the external sphincter are located and mobilized sufficiently for approximation in the midline without tension (**C**). They are sutured together with interrupted sutures of 00 PGA on atraumatic needles.

The medial edges of the bulbocavernosi and remnants of the transverse perineal muscles are used to build up the perineal body over and above the reunited external sphincter (**D**). The anterior edges of the levators are approximated in the midline to give additional support.

The full thickness of the vaginal wall and the skin of the perineum are closed by interrupted sutures (**E**). They are approximated without tension and inspected again so that scar tissue is not incorporated into the wound. (From Ball TL, *Gynecologic surgery and urology,* ed 2, St Louis, 1963, Mosby–Year Book.)

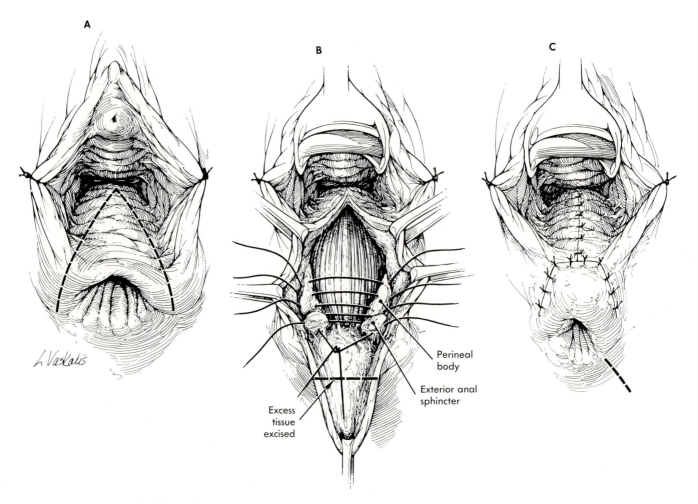

Fig. 29-9. The Warren-Miller-Brown vaginal flap operation. **A,** An inverted V-shaped incision is made through the full thickness of the vagina and skin of the perineum, opening into the rectovaginal space. Traction is applied to the vaginal skin overlying the rectum at the site noted by the asterisk. This is freed laterally from the surrounding scar tissue, exposing the site of the perineal body and the ends of the anal sphincter. **B,** These are united from side to side with a series of interrupted stitches of absorbable polyglycolic acid-type sutures. When the perineal body has been restored and the sphincter ends approximated, the flap is trimmed as shown and turned up to cover the sphincter repair. The posterior vaginal wall and skin of the perineum are closed by a series of interrupted stitches. If the reconstructed anal canal does not admit one fingerbreadth generously, the paradoxical sphincter incision of Miller and Brown can be performed. (See text.) The site is shown by the dotted line at the bottom right of **C.** (Modified from Nichols DH, Randall CL: *Vaginal surgery,* Baltimore, 1989, Williams & Wilkins.)

sion should be made between the 4 o'clock and 5 o'clock positions, cleanly through the perineal skin and anal sphincter and perpendicular to the muscle fibers of the sphincter. The sphincter remains relaxed, and the patient may not be completely continent until the formation of scar tissue reunites the sphincter ends and restores a degree of functional competence. This healing requires between 8 and 12 weeks, and the patient should be so informed.

Restoration of continence by repair of a lacerated anal sphincter

Incompetence of the anal sphincter is almost invariably the result of an obstetric laceration that interrupted the in-

tegrity of the sphincter, generally in the midline near the 12 o'clock position. The anterior wall of the rectum may or may not have been torn as well. If the repair of the fresh injury does not heal properly, various situations may develop. For example, the rectal tear may have healed, but not the sphincter or perineal body; when this occurs, sphincter incontinence results. The perineal body and skin may have healed, but not the rectal laceration. The sphincter repair or some part thereof may or may not have healed. A rectovaginal fistula may form, sometimes, but not always, leading to sphincter incontinence. When the healing process has stabilized after the injury or previous repair and any raw areas have become epithelialized, the defective area should be reconstructed, provided, of course, that the patient is symptomatic and desires a restoration.

Symptoms and etiology. Symptoms of anal sphincter insufficiency are those of rectal incontinence (i.e., inability to control rectal gas or feces, especially when liquid). At times, soiling may precipitate a troublesome vaginitis.

Damage to the nerves, often involving the pudendal nerve, that essentially denervates the pelvic diaphragm and the external anal sphincter may produce the anorectal incontinence.[37] This can be suspected during the preoperative pelvic examination if the patient cannot voluntarily contract her pubococcygeal muscles and her external anal sphincter. The diagnosis can be confirmed by electromyography. Acquired nerve damage usually results from straining at stool or from a difficult or prolonged labor. Myoplasty can tighten a loose external sphincter system, but, if the muscles have been denervated, the prognosis for functional improvement is guarded. The prognosis for postsurgical function is better in the patient with unilateral or partial residual innervation. A good internal (involuntary) sphincter system aids rectal continence.

Other less common causes of anal sphincter incompetence include peripheral neuropathy (e.g., caused by diabetes); diseases of the central nervous system, spinal cord, or cauda equina; and postsurgical trauma (e.g., after laminectomy). The condition may be associated with the perineal descent syndrome or with rectal prolapse. Some patients who complain of chronic diarrhea may really harbor an undiagnosed sphincter incompetence secondary not only to sphincter laceration, but also to sphincter denervation. A sphincter plication is usually ineffective in a patient whose rectal sphincter weakness is not the result of a previous sphincter laceration. Medical treatment, including the administration of loperamide hydrochloride (Imodium), may be helpful.

Operation for restoration of anal sphincter competence. Novak suggested an operation to restore sphincter integrity and anal continence to a patient in whom this has been lost by laceration.[29] Often, the operation is necessary because of the postoperative breakdown of an earlier repair of a fourth-degree obstetric laceration and, occasionally, of the perineum. The operation provides good exposure to the critical areas, particularly the ends of the lacerated anal sphincter and the tissue from which the perineum will be reconstructed. An essential step is the placement of the stitches so that they reinforce or restore the integrity of the perineal body and take much of the tension from the ends of the recently approximated external anal sphincter, splinting or bracing this repair and aiding in the integrity of its healing. If this tissue has been adequately identified and mobilized, it is not necessary to bring the medial borders of the pubococcygeal muscles together in front of the rectum, thus reducing the risk that painful ridges will form in the newly approximated tissue and cause subsequent dyspareunia. Polyglycolic acid-type 1-0 or 2-0 suture is used. When the perineum has "disappeared," it must be

mobilized and reconstructed as an integral part of the repair, which effectively decreases the strain on the sphincter repair during its healing phase.

As in the rectal flap and vaginal flap operations, the bowel should be cleansed by enemas until clear before surgery to restore anal sphincter competence. Traction stitches are placed. The damaged tissues must be mobilized carefully, and scar tissue must be freed by sharp dissection. None of the tissue needs to be discarded. The torn ends of the sphincter will be buried in scar tissue, but they can be identified by the subcutaneous dimples. An incision resembling the letter W is made with the knife through the skin margin between the vagina and rectum and extended upward *lateral* to the cut ends of the sphincter. After the rectovaginal space has been entered, the vagina is carefully separated from the anterior wall of the rectum up to the site of the previously placed traction suture.

When the cut edge of the vagina has been grasped with Allis forceps, the surgeon frees the scar tissue by both sharp and blunt dissection with wide mobilization of the vagina from the rectum. This procedure clearly exposes the caudal portion of the rectovaginal space and the site of the perineum. A traction stitch is placed in the muscularis of the anterior rectal wall. The application of upward tension to this latter suture makes the dimpling that identifies the scar of the torn edges of the external anal sphincter more noticeable, and the edges may be grasped with Allis clamps or Kocher forceps. The scarred ends of the sphincter may be excised from the surrounding scar tissue by sharp dissection, and a polydiaxonone or polyglycolic acid-type suture is placed in the retracted scarred ends of the sphincter. If the freed sphincter is long enough, the ends can be overlapped. For recurrent cases, a suture of a permanent monofilament, Prolene, Novafil, or Surgilene, can be used, provided that it can be effectively buried.

If there is a V-shaped defect in the anterior anal wall, it is approximated by interrupted submucosal polyglycolic acid-type sutures, and a second reinforcing layer is placed to reduce the tension on the first layer.

The perineal body is reinforced or reconstructed by a series of horizontally placed interrupted sutures, the stitch in the anal sphincter is tied, a second and perhaps third reinforcing mattress suture is placed in the muscle itself and tied, and the perineal skin is closed vertically.

Postoperative care

Postoperative care after all these procedures is similar. A clear liquid and nonresidue diet should be employed for 5 days, and constipation should be encouraged during this period. A rectal tube may be used for short intervals, however, to overcome any difficulty in expelling flatus. Stool softeners are administered and a gentle laxative is given on the fourth day, at which time a gradual return to the house diet should begin. An initial bowel movement is usually desirable by the seventh postoperative day. Stool softeners are given for a month postoperatively.

REFERENCES

1. Aronson MP, Lee RA, Berquist TH: Anatomy of anal sphincters and related structures, i, Continent women—studies with magnetic resonance imaging, *Obstet Gynecol* 76:846, 1990.

2. Bacon HE, Ross ST: *Atlas of operative technique: anus, rectum, and colon,* St, Louis, 1954, Mosby–Year Book, p 110.

3. Beck DE, Harford FJ, DiPalma JA: Comparison of cleansing methods in preparation for colonic surgery, *Dis Colon Rectum* 28:491, 1985.

4. Beecham CT: Recurring rectovaginal fistulas, *Obstet Gynecol* 40:323, 1972.

5. Bernstein LH et al.: Healing of perineal Crohn's disease with metronidazole, *Gastroenterology* 79:357, 1980.

6. Blaisdell PC. Repair of the incontinent sphincter ani, *Surg Gynecol Obstet* 70:692, 1940.

7. Boronow RC: Management of radiation-induced vaginal fistulas, *Am J Obstet Gynecol* 1:1, 1971.

8. Corman ML: *Colon and rectal surgery,* Philadelphia, pp 108-110. 1984, JB Lippincott.

9. Crossen HS, Crossen RJ: *Operative gynecology,* ed 6, St Louis, 1948, Mosby–Year Book, pp 455-460.

10. Fang DT et al: Overlapping sphincteroplasty for acquired anal incontinence, *Dis Colon Rectum* 27:720, 1984.

11. Gallagher DM, Scarborough RA: Repair of low rectovaginal fistula, *Dis Colon Rectum* 5:193, 1962.

12. Goligher JC. *Surgery of the anus recrum and colon,* ed 3, London, 1975, Bailliere Tindall, p 246.

13. Hauth JC et al: Early Repair of an external sphincter ani muscle and rectal mucosal dehiscence, *Obstet Gynecol* 67:806, 1986.

14. Hibbard LT: Surgical management of rectovaginal fistulas and complete perineal tears, *J Obstet Gynecol* 130:139, 1977.

15. Hirschman LJ: *Synopsis of Ano-rectal Diseases,* ed 2, St Louis, 1942, Mosby–Year Book, pp 18-19.

16. Hodgkinson CP: Correcting failed rectovaginal fistula repair. In Sanz LE, editor: Gynecologic surgery, Oradell, NJ, Medical Economics Books, 1988, pp 133-139.

17. Jackman RJ: Rectovaginal and anovaginal fistulas: a surgical procedure for treatment of certain types, *J Iowa State Med Soc* 42:435-440, 1952.

18. Kelly HA: *Operative gynecology,* vol I, p 211, New York, 1898, D Appleton.

19. Laird DR: Procedures used in the treatment of complicated fistulas, *Am J Surg* 76:701, 1948.

20. Leacher TC, Pratt JH: Vaginal repair of the simple rectovaginal fistula, *Surg Gynecol Obstet* 124:1317-1321, 1967.

21. Madoff RD, Williams JG, Caushaj PF: Fecal incontinence, *N Engl J Med* 326:1102-1107, 1992.

22. Manning PC, Pratt JH: Fecal incontinence caused by lacerations of the perineum, *Arch Surg* 88:569-576, 1964.

23. Menaker GH: The use of antibiotics in surgical treatment of the colon, *Surg Gynecol Obstet* 164:581-586, 1987.

24. Mengert WF, Fish SA: Anterior rectal wall advancement, *Obstet Gynecol* 5:262, 1955.

25. Miller NF, Brown W: The surgical treatment of complete perineal tears in the female, *Am J Obstet Gynecol* 34:196, 1937.

26. Morrison JG et al: Results of operation for rectovaginal fistula in Crohn's disease, *Dis Colon Rectum* 32:497-499, 1989.

27. Nichols DH, Randall CL: *Vaginal surgery,* ed 3, Baltimore, 1989, Williams & Wilkins, pp 394-398.

28. Noble GH: A new operation for complete laceration of the perineum designed for the purpose of eliminating danger of infection from the rectum, *Trans Am Gynecol Soc* 27:357, 1902.

29. Novak F: *Surgical gynecologic techniques,* p 164, New York, 1978, John Wiley & Sons.

30. Oh C, Kark AE: Anatomy of the external anal sphincter, *Br J Surg* 59:717-723, 1972.

31. Pezim ME et al: Sphincter repair for fecal incontinence after obstetrical or iatrogenic injury, *Dis Colon Rectum* 30:521-525, 1987.

32. Rock JA, Woodruff JD: Surgical correction of a rectovaginal fistula, *Int J Gynaecol Obstet* 20:413-416, 1982.

33. Rosenshein NB, Genadry RR, Woodruff JD: An anatomic classification of rectovaginal septal defects, *Am J Obstet Gynecol* 137:439-442, 1980.

34. Sanz LE, Blank K: The Martius graft technique for rectovaginal fistulas. In Sanz LE, editor: *Gynecologic Surgery,* Oradell, NJ, Medical Economics Books, 1988, pp 125-150.

35. Snooks SJ, Henry MM: Fecal incontinence due to external anal sphincter division in childbirth is associated with damage to the innervation of the pelvic floor musculature: a double pathology, *Br J Obstet Gynaecol* 92:824-828, 1985.

36. Stern H et al: Rectovaginal fistula: initial experience, *Can J Surg* 31:359-362, 1988.

37. Swash M: New concepts in incontinence, *Br Med J* 290:4, 1985.

38. Swash M, Henry MM: Unifying concept of pelvic floor disorders and incontinence, *J Roy Soc Med* 78:906-911, 1985.

39. Thompson JD, Rock JA: TeLinde's operative gynecology, ed 7, Philadelphia, 1992, JB Lippincott, pp 972-977.

40. Warren JC: A new method of operation for the relief of rupture of the perineum through the sphincter and rectum, *Trans Am Gynecol Soc* 7:322, 1882.

Chapter 30

PERINEAL DESCENT, RETRORECTAL LEVATORPLASTY, AND RECTAL PROLAPSE

David H. Nichols

THE PERINEAL DESCENT SYNDROME

The levator plate, formed by the fusion of the bellies of the pubococcygeal muscles, for the most part posterior to the rectum, extends to the insertion of these muscles upon the coccyx and lower portion of the sacrum.[5,28] When the plate is intact, it is more or less horizontal in position; when markedly attenuated, however, it becomes a loose hammock. As the plate sags, it tips (Fig. 30-1) and, with any increases in intraabdominal pressure, may permit those structures that lie on it to slide downward (Fig. 30-2). These structures, principally the vagina and the rectum, not only may descend, but also may occasionally telescope when increases in intraabdominal pressure occur along their axes.

In a rare patient, the pelvic diaphragm and the levator plate may sag to such a degree that the patient actually sits on her anus (Fig. 30-3). The patient may describe an unusual bearing-down sensation and difficulty with evacuation. The harder she strains in attempting evacuation, however, the greater the levator funneling, the smaller the subsequent diameters of the anus and the stool, and, thus, the more difficult evacuation becomes. As a result, the condition may be associated with chronic constipation, obstipation so severe that digital manipulation is necessary for evacuation, or the deliberate abuse of laxatives to achieve an almost chronic state of diarrhea. Some patients may evacuate by sitting on a board with a 3-inch hole, the edges of which exert counterpressure around the sides of the anus.[11]

A pelvic examination with the patient in the lithotomy position reveals a pathologic and almost vertical vaginal and rectal axis, and a short, tipped levator plate posterior to the rectum, but it is easiest to demonstrate this condition while the patient is sitting on the examination table. After

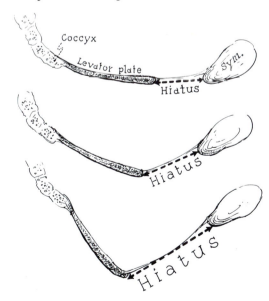

Fig. 30-1. As the levator plate sags, the genital hiatus becomes larger. In addition, the pull of gravity and the forces of intraabdominal pressure accentuate the strain on the pelvic suspensory system. Sym., symphysis pubis. (Modified form Berglas B, Rubin IC: Study of the supportive structures of the uterus by levator myography, *Surg Gynecol Obstet* 97:672, 1953.)

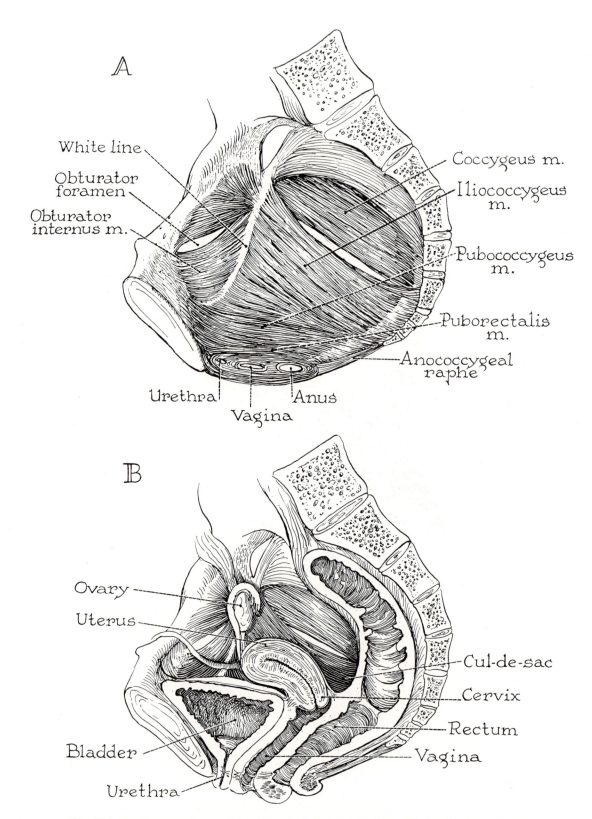

A

White line

Obturator foramen

Obturator internus m.

Coccygeus m.

Iliococcygeus m.

Pubococcygeus m.

Puborectalis m.

Anococcygeal raphe

Urethra

Vagina

Anus

B

Ovary

Uterus

Bladder

Urethra

Cul-de-sac

Cervix

Rectum

Vagina

Fig. 30-2. A, The musculature of the side wall of the pelvis is shown. Notice the almost horizontal inclination of the anococcygeal raphe and the dependent portion of the pubococcygeal muscle just above it, which is called the levator plate. **B,** A side view of the pelvic organs in their normal position is shown. Notice that the vagina rests on the rectum, which, in turn, lies on the almost horizontal levator plate.

Continued.

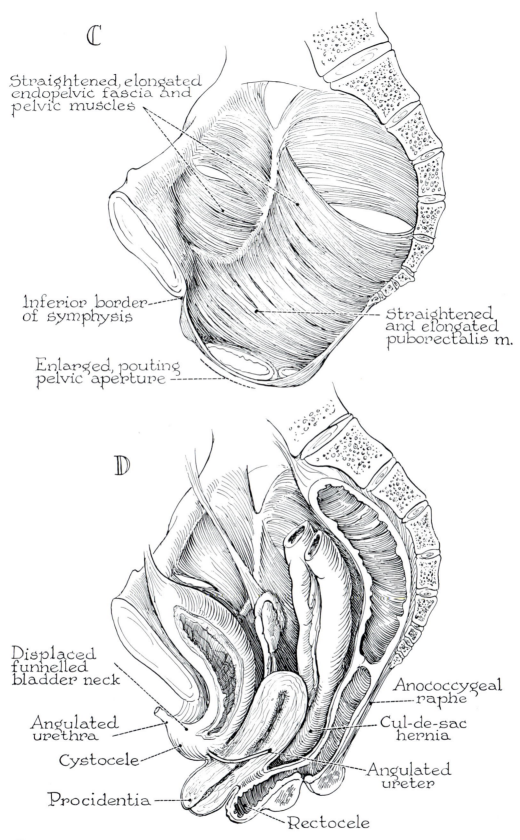

C

Straightened, elongated endopelvic fascia and pelvic muscles

Inferior border of symphysis

Enlarged, pouting pelvic aperture

Straightened and elongated puborectalis m.

D

Displaced funnelled bladder neck

Angulated urethra

Cystocele

Procidentia

Anococcygeal raphe

Cul-de-sac hernia

Angulated ureter

Rectocele

Fig. 30-2, cont'd. C, Side view of the pelvis in which the muscles and their fasciae have become attenuated and are sagging. The pelvic basin is now funnelled, and the levator plate is tipped. **D,** As a consequence of the soft tissue attentuation, a genital prolapse has developed. Notice the protruding bladder, uterus, and vagina, and there is a rectocele and an enterocele. The levator plate is tipped, and the organs above it are literally sliding down hill in their descent. (From Ball TL: *Gynecologic surgery and urology,* ed 2, St. Louis, 1963, Mosby.)

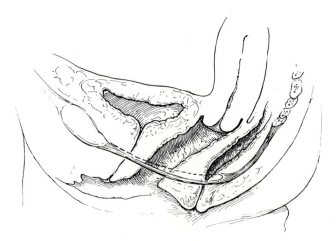

Fig. 30-3. Sagittal section of the pelvis shows elongation and sagging of the levator plate. The usual angle between the anal canal and the rectum has been lost, as well as the horizontal axis of the rectum and the upper vagina. (From Nichols DH, Randall CL: *Vaginal surgery,* 3rd ed., Baltimore, 1989, Williams & Wilkins.)

placing a hand beneath the anus, the examiner can feel the anus descend still further as the patient strains. This descent or prolapse of both anus and perineum must be clearly differentiated from rectal prolapse, which is an actual intussusception of the bowel through the anal sphincter and anus.

At times, the condition produces not only its characteristic symptom complex, but also a feeling of pelvic and rectal pressure or falling out when standing. The patient may occasionally find it very difficult to sit comfortably.

Prolapse of the anus and perineum may result from a variety of causes, including trauma, obstetric damage, defective innervation,[15,17,30,31] aging, and chronically increased intra-abdominal pressure. There appear to be two kinds of perineal prolapse. One is the result of traumatic stretching of the pelvic diaphragm in multiple pregnancies and is associated with constipation or obstipation. The other is neuropathically induced, probably by stretching of the pudendal nerve during labor or consequent to longstanding constipation and straining at stool.[17,31] More common in the parous than in the nonparous patient, this neuropathy may lead to a degeneration of the muscular cells of the levator ani that is histologically demonstrable and more or less irreversible. Urinary stress incontinence may accompany this neuropathic condition.[17] Although neuromuscular activity can be measured electromyographically,* it can be estimated to some degree by the patient's ability or inability to contract her pubococcygei and external anal sphincter voluntarily.

Constipation may be an early symptom of perineal descent. The loss of the integrity of an intact pelvic diaphragm may make voluntary bearing-down efforts more necessary, more regular, and more intense. These efforts may stretch the pudendal nerve,[15,17,30,31] damaging the in-

*References 14, 15, 17, 31, 37, 40.

nervation of both the pelvic diaphragm and the external anal sphincter and, in turn, leading to partial paralysis and atrophy of these muscles. Sometimes, if the protective internal sphincter mechanism becomes overburdened, the result is perineal prolapse with first obstipation and later rectal incontinence. When perineal prolapse correlates with a decreased perception of rectal fullness, some of the neuromuscular receptors within the levator ani may degenerate. In this event, anatomic surgical reconstruction is less likely to be successful.

Provided that the conduct of any labor has been proper, it is possible to prevent perineal prolapse through good bowel habits, even including the use of a mild laxative or suppository, if necessary, and increased bulk in the diet. A greater intake of water (because some degree of systemic dehydration may accompany the diminution of thirst that takes place with aging) and regular pubococcygeal isometric resistive exercises are also helpful.

RETRORECTAL LEVATORPLASTY (SURGICAL REPAIR)

Reconstruction of a damaged levator muscle may produce a functionally more favorable result when the nerve supply is intact than when the nerve supply is significantly defective, whatever the cause. When descent of the anus and rectum and sagging of the normally horizontal levator plate is associated with longstanding severe constipation and marked decrease in the diameter of the stool while straining, retrorectal levatorplasty with colporrhaphy may be curative. The coexistence of rectal incontinence and perineal prolapse suggests severe neuropathology, and the postsurgical prognosis is less favorable. Retrorectal levatorplasty with colporrhaphy or the less extensive Parks postanal repair[30] may recreate a useful anal valve that will help these patients, however.

The Parks postanal repair[30] is a technique designed to restore a defective anorectal angle in patients with fecal incontinence secondary to denervation of the pelvic musculature. Parks attributed its success in such cases primarily to recreation of an effective anorectal flap-valve mechanism, and secondarily to mechanical improvement of puborectalis muscle fiber function resulting from their plication. In this operation, an incision is made between the anus and coccyx, and carried into the intersphincteric "space" between the external and internal anal sphincters. The puborectalis portions of the levatores ani are sewn together *behind* the rectum recreating an anorectal angle.

Uniting the medial portions of the pubococcygei between the vagina and rectum and anterior to the latter thickens the tissues of the perineum by interposing a muscular layer not initially well developed in this area, but it does not shorten the muscles, restore the defective axis of the plate, or correct the pathologic descent of the anus and rectum. The literature on techniques that have been used to achieve these goals is sparse, although there have been reports of lengthening the levator plate by the transperineal approach of Lange[21] and by the transabdominal approach used in various modifications of the operation of Graham.[10,12,13] Barrett[4] suggested a transperineal approach by incision and dissection between the anus and vagina, "posteriorly to the rectum in properly selected cases and the separated levator reunited with attachment of the rectal wall to this muscle," but apparently did not document any effort to pursue his idea. It is possible to plicate the pubococcygeal muscles posterior to the rectum by means of a transabdominal approach; however, it is difficult to obtain adequate exposure deep within the pelvis by means of this technique, and the operator cannot satisfactorily approach pathologic vaginal displacements with associated cystocele and rectocele through the same operative exposure.

Clinical experience with the Kraske or sacral transperineal approach to some surgical lesions of the rectum has reaffirmed the safety of this route,* and this approach has been used to correct levator deficiencies.[25,26] This transperineal retrorectal approach allows the operator to shorten the pubococcygei and puborectalis as necessary, as well as to unite the medial bellies of these muscles in the midline posterior to the rectum, thus lengthening the levator plate and advancing the genital hiatus anteriorly. By attaching the posterior rectal wall to the internal periosteum of the lower sacrum with a series of interrupted sutures, then sewing together the bellies of the pubococcygei together *behind* the rectum, and shortening them as necessary, the operator can also establish a relatively horizontal axis to the rectum and to the vagina overlying it. This procedure makes it possible to suspend the elongated rectum[8,19,35] and, by performing appropriate supplemental anterior and posterior colporrhaphy,[33,38] to correct any coexistent cystocele and rectocele. Any enterocele should be excised.[43]

A preventive antibiotic, usually one dose of a cephalosporin, is given 1 hour preoperatively. A mechanical bowel prep is given the night before.

For the procedure, the patient is usually placed in the Kraske jackknife position (Fig. 30-4), although the standard lithotomy position may be used in those patients with plenty of room in the pelvis and for whom colporrhaphy is also planned. The operator makes a midline incision from the sacrum to the site of the external anal sphincter. After identifying the anococcygeal raphe (which varies significantly in strength and length among individuals), the operator separates it from the coccyx. The latter is grasped in a towel clip but is not removed. Fat is displaced, and the undersurfaces of the pubococcygei and the levator plate are identified. The operator incises the levator plate, usually in the midline, separating the right muscle belly from the left. The rectum is identified and separated from the levator muscles and plate. The rectococcygeal muscle or ligament is identified and, if present, transected. (Like the anococcygeal raphe, this structure also varies in length and strength.) The retrorectal (or presacral) space is thoroughly explored. Then, the undersurface of the sacrum is cleansed

*References 6, 7, 13, 18-20, 22, 23, 27, 41.

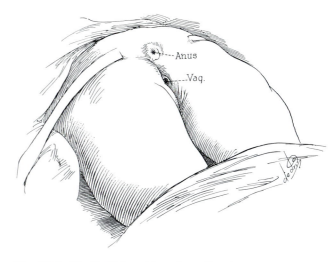

Fig. 30-4. "Jackknife" position. A sandbag has been placed beneath the hips, and the gluteal muscles are pulled apart by wide strips of adhesive tape fastened to the edges of the operating table. (From Nichols DH, Randall CL: *Vaginal surgery,* Baltimore, 1989, Williams & Wilkins.)

of fat and loose connective tissue, exposing the periosteum.

The operator places three plication stitches in the posterior rectal wall 1 cm apart and ties, but does not cut them (Fig. 30-5, *A).* Using an overglove, the operator performs a rectal examination to determine whether any sutures have penetrated the rectal mucosa; if so, they must be replaced lest there be risk of abscess or fistula. These sutures are sewn to the presacral fascia (Fig. 30-5, *B).* Polyglycolic acid-type sutures (Dexon or Vicryl) or longer lasting polyglactin-type (PDS or Maxon) are used throughout the procedure. For patients with chronic respiratory disease and, therefore, likely to have chronically increased intraabdominal pressure, a synthetic nonabsorbable suture such as O Surgilon or a TT22 needle may be used to provide firmer future resistance to recurrent herniation. A large dental mirror and a fiberoptic headlight help the operator visualize the placement of these stitches. After placing all stitches, the operator ties them, beginning with the most cranial suture. The coccyx is not generally removed, and the middle sacral artery is ligated only if required to improve the exposure.

At this point, the operator uses a series of interrupted sutures (Fig. 30-5, *C)* to sew the medial borders of the levators (pubococcygei and puborectalis) together in the midline posterior to the rectum; this procedure restores the integrity and length of the levator plate and displaces the rectum forward. The operator then shortens the undersurface of both right and left limbs of each pubococcygeal muscle (part of the anterior portion of the pelvic diaphragm) with Z-type sutures (Fig. 30-5, *C)* and reattaches the lower rectum to the medial surfaces of the pubococcygei, suspending the rectum higher within the pelvis than it had been suspended preoperatively. The anococcygeal raphe is shortened by resection of the now excess length as

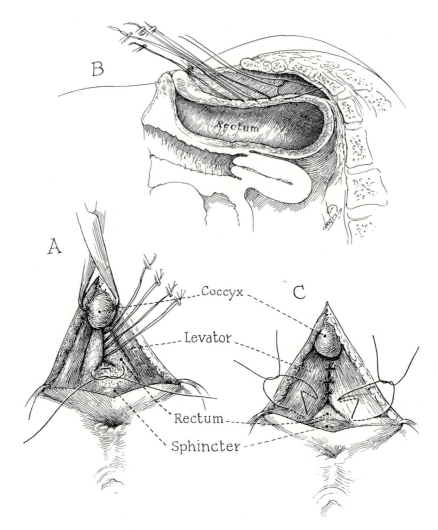

Fig. 30-5. The essential steps of the operation are: **A,** A series of plication stitches have been placed 1 cm apart in the posterior wall of the rectum, tied, and left long. **B,** These are anchored individually to the anterior periosteum of the sacrum. **C,** The levator plate is restored and lengthened by bringing the pubococcygei of each side together in the midline between the coccyx and rectum. The bellies of the pubococcygei may be shortened by a Z stitch placed as shown in **C.** (From Nichols DH: Retrorectal levatorplasty for anal and perineal prolapse, *Surg Gynecol Obstet* 154:251, 1982.)

necessary and reattached to either the coccygeal periosteum or to the gluteal fascia. The subcutaneous tissue and the skin are closed with interrupted sutures.

If coincident anterior and posterior colporrhaphy, vaginal hysterectomy, or excision of any enterocele is to be performed, the patient is repositioned to the conventional lithotomy position. If the perineal body has been separated from the connective tissue of the external anal sphincter, it may be reattached by a figure-8 stitch, which further stabilizes both the perineum and the anus.

A sagittal section of the preoperative findings is shown in the drawing at the left in Fig. 30-6; the postoperative result is shown in the drawing at the right.

RECTAL PROLAPSE

When the patient complains of "hemorrhoids," although none is found at the time of examination, gynecologists must consider a previously undiagnosed intermittent (present only with straining) prolapse of the rectum or a mucosal prolapse. The patient, after the bowel has been given a preliminary mechanical prep, should be asked to squat and to bear down heavily, as by a Valsalva maneuver. The surgeon carefully inspects the anus and confirms either hemorrhoids, mucosal prolapse, or rectal prolapse.

Examination of hemorrhoids show them to be lobular, with a visible sulcus between the masses of tissue. Prolapsing mucous membrane, being a single layer, is thinner to palpation than is the thickness of a true rectal prolapse with its multiple layers. The mucosal folds of a mucosal prolapse are found to be radial in their direction in contrast to those of rectal prolapse, which are arranged concentrically.[36]

To the patient so afflicted, prolapse of the rectum is of overwhelming clinical importance. Fortunately, genital

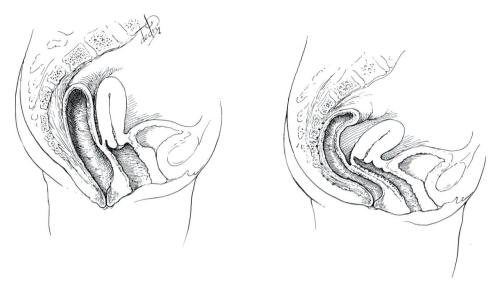

Fig. 30-6. Preoperative prolapse of the anus and perineum with tipping of the levator plate and elongation of the attachment of the rectum to the anterior surface of the sacrum are shown in the drawing to the left. The result of surgery is seen in the drawing to the right. The rectum has been approximated to the anterior periosteum of the sacrum, and the levator plate has been lengthened posterior to the rectum and the pubococcygei shortened as necessary. The axis of the lower rectum and upper vagina are more or less horizontal. An anorectal angulation is present, and the anus is no longer the most dependent portion of the perineum. (From Nichols DH: Retrorectal levatorplasty for anal and perineal prolapse, *Surg Gynecol Obstet* 154:251, 1982.)

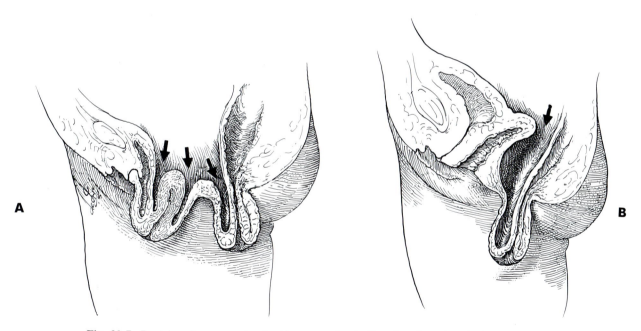

Fig. 30-7. Rectal prolapse associated with enterocele. **A,** Rectal prolapse is coincident with genital procidentia. **B,** The rectal prolapse is posterior to the vagina, which is not involved. (Reproduced with permission of Harper & Row from Nichols DH: Types of enterocele and principles underlying the choice of operation for repair, *Obstet Gynecol* 40:257, 1972.)

prolapse is not often coincident with rectal prolapse, because it has a different etiology (Fig. 30-7). Rectal prolapse is probably the result of a rectorectal intussusception, rather than a sliding hernia.[36] A distended, freely mobile segment of rectal wall may virtually intussuscept into the previously normal caliber of the anal canal. Forcing defecation may be a contributing factor. The anatomic abnormalities noted in conjunction with rectal prolapse are probably the result, not the cause, of the prolapse.

Rectal prolapse occurs predominantly in women who

are thin and elderly; aging may have diminished the tone of the pelvic muscles in these patients. Women with rectal prolapse are more likely to be nulliparous than multiparous, may suffer from chronic constipation, with chronic straining at stool, and may have abused laxatives. There is sometimes a coincident uterine prolapse.[21] Because the pelvic diaphragm and levator plate are tipped, the pelvic basin acts as a funnel, and as it becomes longer, the outlet opening becomes smaller, resulting in almost ribbonlike stools that become increasingly narrowed as the patient strains harder.

The symptoms of rectal prolapse are primarily rectal protrusion with straining or lifting, incomplete bowel movements, and rectal incontinence. As the condition progresses and the prolapsed rectum remains outside a greater portion of the time, bleeding develops. The physical findings are often clear enough to indicate the diagnosis, but the protrusion of the bowel when the patient strains (for example, in a Valsalva maneuver) provides confirmation. The walls of the protruded rectum are thick, especially anteriorly, and there may be an enterocele sac that contains small bowel. The anus is usually patulous up to three or four fingerbreadths in diameter, and the condition is surprisingly painless.[22]

Most successful treatments for rectal prolapse in the otherwise healthy patient have been transabdominal,[25] although some surgeons have used the transperineal approach and combinations of the transabdominal and transperineal approaches. Simple obliteration of the cul-de-sac on the rationale that the rectal prolapse is a sliding hernia has not been consistently effective; the recurrence rate has been about 63%.[32] Intraabdominal and transperineal plication of the levator muscles has been employed, but lasting success has been obtained by transabdominal rectal and sigmoid suspension operations with or without the use of foreign materials.[34,39]

Retrorectal levatorplasty may be used for the early stages of rectal prolapse. Perineal anal encirclement (for example, by the Thiersch technique) has been recommended with hesitation for the elderly or poor-risk patient, although this technique requires the insertion of a foreign body around the anus, which decreases the anal diameter and risks ulceration of the epithelium, requiring removal of the implant.[42] Unless the surgeon has special training and experience in rectal surgery, he or she should enlist the cooperation of an appropriate surgical consultant when planning and performing the necessary reconstruction.

Because prolapse of the rectum is often associated with rectal incontinence, successful treatment of rectal prolapse requires some appreciation of the normal mechanisms of lower bowel function and a knowledge of the possible causes of any pathologic alterations.

Normal lower bowel function

To a large extent, bowel function is the product of habit. The contents of the sigmoid colon are evacuated by first voluntarily relaxing the pelvic diaphragm, unlocking the colic valve, and relaxing the external anal sphincter. When the rectum is full, the internal sphincter opens. Modest increases in intraabdominal pressure obtained, for example, by bearing down force the stool content downward. The gastrocolic reflex pattern regularly assists in this process by promoting intestinal peristalsis. A disorder that affects any of these steps predisposes a person to or causes constipation.

The levator ani and the external anal sphincter differ from the other striated muscles of the body in that they maintain a constant state of tone that is inversely proportional to the quantity of the rectal content. Neuromuscular pressure receptors within the levator ani are responsible for mediating its tone and apparently communicate with the central nervous system by way of the pudendal nerve on each side of the body, which generally arises from S3 and S4. Because intestinal peristalsis continues around the clock, although at apparently various degrees of intensity, this tone is responsible for rectal continence.

The contraction of the levator ani and puborectalis muscles pulls the genital hiatus toward the pubis, placing the rectum at an angle that allows it to function effectively as a valve, according to the observations of Parks.[28,29] There is a reflex reciprocity with the tone of the external anal sphincter. These muscles are innervated by the pudendal nerve and its accessory branches, and they function in synergism. The innervation of the puborectalis is less certain, although it may come from a sacral plexus component.

Pathologic dysfunction of the lower bowel

Constipation may appear as an early symptom of perineal descent. A rectocele does *not* commonly cause constipation, however, although both may occur simultaneously. The primary symptoms of a rectocele are aching after a bowel movement and an inability to empty the bowel completely so that manual expression is often necessary for full evacuation. Posterior colporrhaphy should relieve these primary symptoms, but it will not necessarily relieve constipation other than that produced when stool is caught in a pocket of the rectal wall, precluding complete emptying of the bowel. Many women with a rectocele are not constipated, and many more women without a rectocele are constipated.

Either congenital or acquired pathology of the pudendal nerve can alter its efficiency and, thus, affect the ability of the neuromuscular receptors within the levator ani to influence pressure and maintain the responsive muscular tone of the levator ani. Acquired damage may result from the trauma of the stretching of the pelvic floor during childbirth and quite possibly from chronic excessive straining at stool. Regular and excessive bearing down during defecation may stretch the pudendal nerve, destroying its anatomic integrity, consequently weakening the muscles that it innervates, and occasionally resulting in a permanent loss of muscle tone in the denervated pelvic diaphragm and external anal sphincter. The neuropathic loss of the tone of the anal sphincter permits it to relax at inopportune times, resulting in rectal incontinence that may be most difficult to treat surgically. The Parks group has suggested that this loss of voluntary muscle tone within the pelvic diaphragm may be coincident with urinary stress incontinence.[17]

Henry[16] described the relationship between rectal prolapse and rectal incontinence as follows:

I think the primary pathology is one of neuropathy affecting the pelvic floor—in many patients a consequence of damage to the pudendal nerve, damage inflicted by traumatic childbirth. Incontinence may not develop initially if the internal anal sphincter is functioning normally. Pelvic floor denervation initiates rectal prolapse because of disruption of the anorectal flap valve. The prolapse starts with descent of the anterior rectal wall and at a later stage a circumferential complete prolapse intussuscepts through the anus. The dilatation of the internal anal sphincter caused by the prolapsing rectum then destroys the only mechanism protecting anorectal continence and a major functional problem results. Because the internal sphincter recovers, many patients recover a reasonable degree of control after successful repair of the prolapse. If continence is not recovered within six months, we will offer the patient a transperineal post-anal repair (of the puborectalis and the pelvic diaphragm).

Types and combinations of anorectal prolapse

When a rectal prolapse and massive genital prolapse coexist (Fig. 30-7, *A*), they should be treated simultaneously if possible. The etiology and treatment of each are entirely different from one another.

Often the rectal prolapse involves a pathologically long sigmoid colon and coincident enterocele. After appropriate diagnostic workup, including sigmoidoscopy, barium enema, and other studies on the presence of coexistent rectal incontinence, this can be treated surgically by large bowel resection with low anastamosis, and rectopexy attaching the rectal "stalk" to the periosteum of the sacrum. This is followed by appropriate treatment of the genital prolapse. If the latter is associated with poor cardinal-uterosacral ligament strength and colpopexy to a nongynecologic strong structure is planned, a transvaginal sacrospinous colpopexy with colporrpaphy may be done. If the surgeon and patient prefer a transabdominal route for treatment, an abdominal colposacropexy with Halban-type stitches sagittally obliterating the cul-de-sac should be done at the same operation and, if possible, immediately after the treatment of the bowel prolapse. Because the vagina is anterior to the rectum, the sacrocolpopexy must be performed anterior to the rectopexy. This surgical program is not to be taken lightly, however, use of the circular stapler improves the ease and speed of large intestinal low anastamosis. Overall, there appears to be a small (1%) but significant risk of anastamotic leakage with subsequent peritonitis and all of its problems.[42] Such colporrhaphy as might be necessary should be accomplished by a separate transvaginal route.

For the older patient with massive eversion of the vagina including large cystocele and rectocele and a simultaneous but shorter (less than 5 cm) prolapse of the rectum, the surgeon may elect a transperineal approach to each.

Transvaginal excision of any enterocele, sacrospinous colpopexy, and colphorrhaphy are followed by resection of the prolapsed rectal mucosa, and longitudinal accordian pleating of the muscularis followed by reunification of the mucosa and replacement of the resultant "doughnut" back within the anal canal, essentially the Delorme operation.[24,39]

For the younger patient, transperineal, full-thickness resection of the type recommended by Altemeier[1,2] of the rectal prolapse, may be chosen in anticipation of the patient's longer life span and postoperative perception of discomfort.

Some surgical treatments for rectal prolapse

The Delorme-type mucosal stripping operation.[3,9,24] The combined prolapse is noted in Fig. 30-8, *A.*[3] It is replaced within the pelvis, and the colpopexy and colporrhaphy are accomplished. The rectal procidentia is gently pulled back into the operative field, and an incision is made just distal to the pectinate line down to the superficial layers of the muscularis (Fig. 30-8, *B*). This is the first of two techniques of reducing the rectal procidentia. First is the accordion type of plication. Because the peritoneal sac from the cul-de-sac has already been reduced and retracted upward during the reduction of the hernia vaginally, it is not necessary to locate and deal with the hernial sac as it would be were this an isolated operation for rectal procidentia alone.

The surgeon encounters a general ooze of blood from the operative area during this dissection. Distinct bleeding points are clamped and ligated. Final hemostasis is obtained when the longitudinal plication sutures are tied.

Figure 30-8, *C,* shows a method of denuding the mucosa and underlying muscularis mucosa from the rectal procidentia. Four or five longitudinal segments are selected, and, as the mucosa is separated by sharp dissection, it is rolled on a Halstead clamp. Specific arterial bleeding points are ligated during this denudation. As the denudation is continued distally, the terminal end of the intussusception is reached. This dissection is continued until a small edge of mucosa at the distal end of the prolapse is left for anastomosis (Fig. 30-8, *D*). Figure 30-8, *E,* shows the denudation of the mucosa from the posterior aspect. The blood loss during this dissection is carefully estimated, and one or more units may be needed for replacement.

Accordion pleating sutures are placed longitudinally about 2 cm apart. These should penetrate the muscular coats of the rectal wall but preferably avoid going deep enough to pass through the full thickness of the rectum (Fig. 30-8, *F*). The preferred material is 0 polyglycolic acid-type suture on a fine Ferguson needle. After all the pleating sutures have been placed, they are tied by the operator while the assistants gradually draw up on the untied sutures and reduce the prolapse (Fig. 30-8, *G*).

The mucosal edges should approximate each other without tension. A few additional sutures in the muscularis

Text continued on p. 510.

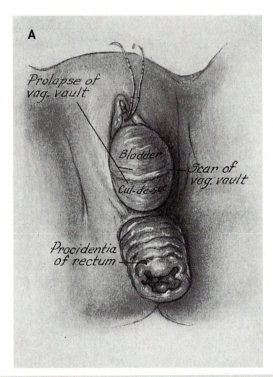

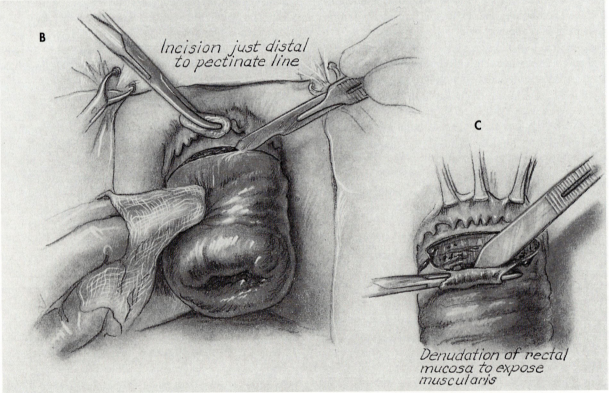

Fig. 30-8. Delorme-type mucosal stripping operation. **A,** A combined genital posthysterectomy prolapse and rectal prolapse. **B,** A circumferential incision is made to remove the protruding rectal mucosa. **C,** The prolapsed rectal mucosa is dissected from the underlying muscularis.

Continued.

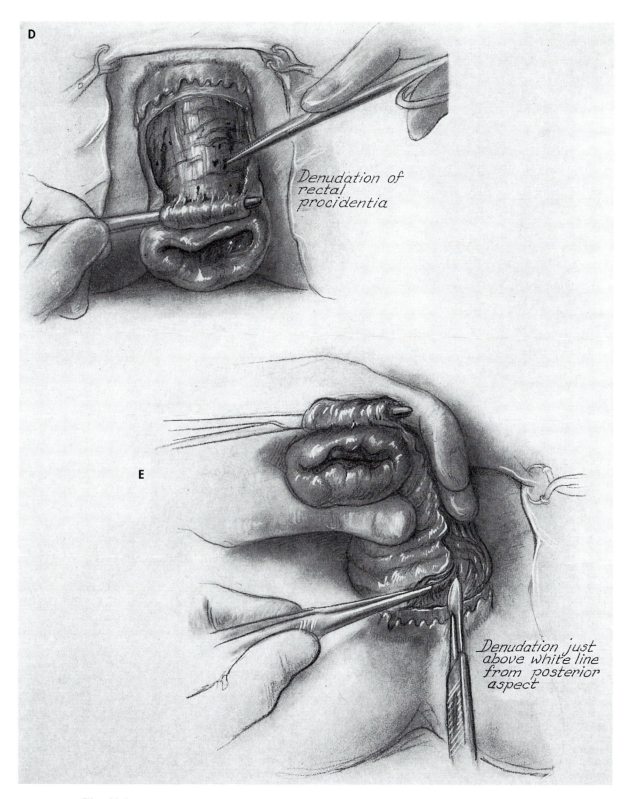

Fig. 30-8, cont'd. D, Mucosa denudation continues. **E,** Denudation progresses posteriorly to a limit just above the white or dentate line.

Continued.

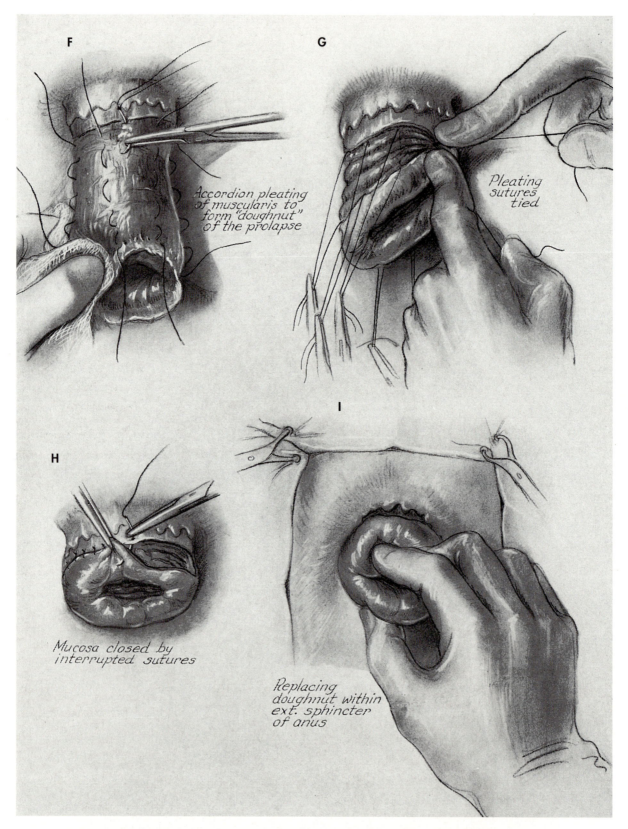

Fig. 30-8, cont'd. F, A series of longitudinally placed pleating stitches is placed in the muscularis. **G,** When all pleating sutures have been placed, they are tied in sequence. **H,** The mucosal edges are closed by interrupted sutures. **I,** The "doughnut" is gently replaced within the anal canal. (From Ball TL: *Gynecologic surgery and urology,* ed 2, St. Louis, 1963, CV Mosby.)

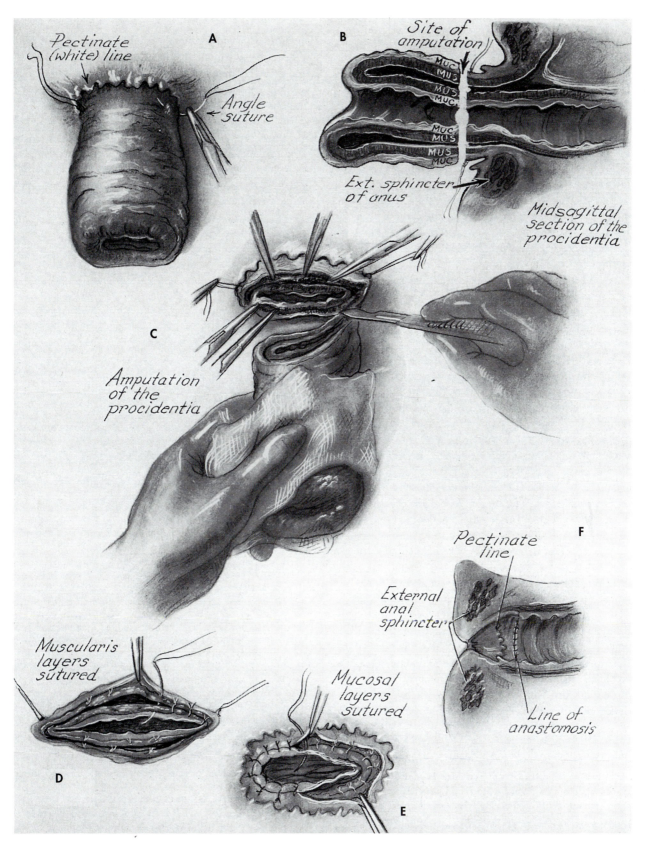

Fig. 30-9. Altemeier-type full-thickness resection. **A,** Angle stitches are placed to each side of the prolapsed rectum. **B,** Sagittal section through the prolapse shows the site of amputation. **C,** Procidentia is amputated. **D,** Muscularis layers are sewn together by interrupted sutures. **E,** Mucosal layers are sutured with interrupted sutures. **F,** Sagittal drawing shows the site of the bowel reanastomosis at the completion of the operation. A petroleum jelly gauze plug is placed in the rectum, and the vagina is packed with gauze. (From Ball TL: *Gynecologic surgery and urology,* ed 2, St. Louis, 1963, CV Mosby.)

may be needed at some points to permit approximation. Sutures of 00 polyglycolic acid on chromic catgut are used to close the mucosa (Fig. 30-8, *H*).

The doughnut formed by the accordion method of pleating is replaced in the pelvis through the dilated rectal sphincter (Fig. 30-8, *I*). Attention is directed to further support of the rectum by the transvaginal approach.

The Altemeier-type full thickness resection. [1-3] The rectal prolapse may be amputated as an alternate method. This is preferred in younger patients for whom the doughnut resulting from the plication technique may impinge on the posterior vaginal wall and cause a constriction. This is unimportant when the vagina need not be a functional organ. Figure 30-9, *A*, shows angle sutures placed just above the white line (distal to the white line as seen with the rectum inverted). These should be placed through all layers to prevent retraction when the procidentia is amputated.

Figure 30-9, *B*, shows the layers in midsagittal section. The layers to be approximated are shown because the intussuscipiens (outer layers) and intussusceptum (inner layers) are best delineated in midsagittal section. The hernial sac of peritoneum that would prolapse between the two anterior layers is missing because it was dissected out and reduced during the mobilization of the cul-de-sac hernia transvaginally.

The prolapsed rectum is then amputated (Fig. 30-9, *C*). The bleeding points are clamped and tied. If the mucosa of the bowel tends to retract, it can be grasped with Allis clamps. The muscularis of the rectum is anastomosed with interrupted sutures of 00 polyglycolic-acid type suture (Fig. 30-9, *D*). A clamp technique, continuous sutures, or the use of other suture materials may be elected according to the preference of the surgeon. The angle sutures are removed if they distort the approximation of either the mucosal or muscular layers during the anastomosis.

Figure 30-9, *E*, shows the approximation of the muscularis of the bowel. This is done with 00 polyglycolic acid-type suture. The line of anastomosis is inverted behind the external sphincter of the anus. Its position, in midsagittal section, is shown in Fig. 30-9, *F*. The "doughnut" is replaced inside the anal canal, and the vagina is packed with plain or iodoform gauze. A Foley catheter is placed into the bladder.

Postoperative care

The vaginal pack and petroleum jelly gauze plug in the rectum are removed in 24 hours. The patient's diet is modified, depending on whether the rectal procidentia was accordion-pleated or resected. With a bowel resection, even though it is retroperitoneal, the patient is maintained on intravenous fluids for the first 2 days. Vitamins and milliequivalents of potassium as indicated are added to the infusions. Blood chemistry studies to include serum potassium and chlorides are made for the first few days. The diet is progressed to clear liquids, then a soft diet as tolerated, and finally to a regular diet by the eighth day or

sooner. This is modified, depending on the postoperative course of the patient. If the rectal procidentia is accordion-pleated, the patient can proceed to a regular diet much sooner. Intubation is seldom necessary, but the usual indications may necessitate this on some occasions.

With a thorough bowel preparation before surgery and the preceding dietary routine, a warm mineral oil enema of 240 ml can be administered about the sixth postoperative day. If the patient is not uncomfortable, a tap water enema can be deferred until the eighth or ninth day. All this must be adapted to the individual patient and situation.

The patient is progressively ambulated, beginning by being out of bed the day after the operation. Urinary antiseptics are administered. Because of the extent of the operation, some surgeons prefer to give combined therapy consisting of one sulfonamide preparation and one wide-spectrum antibiotic. The selection of drugs may be guided by the cultures and sensitivity tests if a bacteriuria was found. The catheter is removed on the fifth postoperative day, and residuals are measured. An average hospital stay would be 14 days.

REFERENCES

1. Altemeier WA, Culbertson WR: Technique for perineal repair of rectal prolapse, *Surgery* 58:758, 1965.
2. Altemier WA et al: Nineteen years' experience with the onestage perineal repair of rectal prolapse, *Ann Surg* 173:993, 1971.
3. Ball TL: *Gynecologic surgery and urology*, ed 2, St. Louis, 1963, CV Mosby.
4. Barrett CW: Hernias through the pelvic floor, *Am J Obstet Dis Women* 59:553, 1909.
5. Berglas B, Rubin IC: Study of the supportive structures of the uterus by levator myography, *Surg Gynecol Obstet* 97:672, 1953.
6. Bevan AD: Carcinoma of rectum—treatment by local excision, *Surg Clin* 1:1233, 1917.
7. Crowley RT, Davis DA: A procedure for total biopsy of doubtful polypoid growths of the lowest bowel segment, *Surg Gynecol Obstet* 93:23, 1951.
8. Davidian UA, Thomas CG: Transsacral repair of rectal prolapse, *Am J Surg* 123:231, 1972.
9. Delorme R: Sur le traitement des prolapsus du rectum totaux part l'excision de la muquese rectale au rectal-colique, *Bull Soc Chir Paris* 26:498, 1900.
10. Efron G: A simple method of posterior rectopexy for rectal procidentia, *Surg Gynecol Obstet* 145:75, 1977.
11. Gallagher DM: Personal communication.
12. Goligher JC: The treatment of complete prolapse of the rectum by the Roscoe Graham operation, *Br J Surg* 46:323, 1958.
13. Graham R: Operative repair of massive rectal prolapse, *Ann Surg* 115:1007, 1942.
14. Haskell B, Rovner H: Electromyography in the management of the incompetent anal sphincter. Proceedings of American Proctologic Society, Cleveland, OH, June 1966.
15. Henry MM: Personal communication, September 2, 1987.
16. Henry MM, Swash M: Assessment of pelvic floor disorders and incontinence by electrophysiological recording of the anal reflex, *Lancet* 17:1290, 1978.
17. Henry MM, Swash M, editor: *Colpoproctology and the pelvic floor*, 2nd ed., London, 1992, Butterworths.
18. Jenkins SG, Thomas CG: An operation for the repair of rectal prolapse, *Surg Gynecol Obstet* 114:381, 1962.
19. Klingensmith W, Dickinson WE, Hays RS: Posterior resection of selected rectal tumors, *Arch Surg* 110:647, 1975.

20. Kraske P: Zur Extirpation Hochsitzender Mastdarmkrebse, *Vehr Dtsch Ges Chir* 14:464, 1885.
21. Lange F: *Intestinal and anal surgery.* Quoted in Hadra BE, editor: *Lesions of the vagina and pelvic floor,* Philadelphia, 1888, McMullin.
22. Lockhart-Mummery JP: Rectal prolapse, *Br Med J* 1:345, 1939.
23. Mason AY: Trans-sphincteric surgery of the rectum, *Prog Surg* 13:66, 1974.
24. McCaffrey JF: Delorme repair for prolapse of the rectum following "failed" Ripstein operation, *Am J Proctol Gastroenterol Colon Rectal Surg* 34:5, 1983.
25. Nichols DH: Retrorectal levatorplasty for anal and perineal prolapse, *Surg Gynecol Obstet* 154:251, 1982.
26. Nichols DH: Retrorectal levatorplasty with colporrhaphy, *Clin Obstet Gynecol* 25:939, 1982.
27. O'Brien PH: Kraske's posterior approach to the rectum, *Surg Gynecol Obstet* 142:412, 1976.
28. Parks AG: Modern concepts of the anatomy of the anorectal region, *Postgrad Med J* 34:360, 1958.
29. Parks AG: Anorectal incontinence, *Proc R Soc Med* 68:681, 1975.
30. Parks AG, Porter NH, Hardcastle J: The syndrome of the descending perineum, *Proc R Soc Med* 59:477, 1966.
31. Parks AG, Swash M, Urich H: Sphincter denervation in anorectal incontinence and rectal prolapse, *J Br Soc Gastroenterol* 18:656, 1977.
32. Pemberton J de J, Stalker LK: Surgical treatment of complete rectal prolapse, *Ann Surg* 109:799, 1939.
33. Redding MD: The relaxed perineum and anorectal disease, *Dis Colon Rectum* 8:279, 1965.
34. Ripstein CB, Lanter B: Etiology and surgical therapy of massive prolapse of the rectum, *Ann Surg* 157:259, 1963.
35. Romer-Torres R: Sacrofixation with Marlex mesh in massive prolapse of the rectum, *Surg Gynecol Obstet* 149:709, 1979.
36. Schoetz DJ Jr, Veidenheimer MC: *Rectal prolapse—pathogenesis and clinical features.* In Henry MM, Swash M, editors: *Culpoproctology and the pelvic floor,* 2nd ed., London, 1992, Butterworths.
37. Sharf B et al: Electromyogram of pelvic floor muscles in genital prolapse, *Int J Gynaecol Obstet* 14:2, 1976.
38. Sullivan ES et al: Transrectal perineal repair; an adjunct to improved function after anorectal surgery. Proceedings of American Proctologic Society, New Orleans, LA, April 1967.
39. Tancer ML, Fleischer M, Berkowitz BJ: Simultaneous colpo-recto-sacropexy, *Obstet Gynecol* 70:951, 1987.
40. Taverner D, Smiddy FG: An electromyographic study of the normal function of the external anal sphincter and pelvic diaphragm, *Dis Colon Rectum* 2:153, 1959.
41. Turner GG: Ideals and the art of surgery, *Surg Gynecol Obstet* 52:273, 1931.
42. Watts JD, Rothenberger DA, Goldberg SM: *Rectal prolapse—treatment.* In Henry MM, Swash M, editors: *Colpoproctology and the pelvic floor,* 2nd ed., London, 1992, Butterworths.
43. Wiersema JS: Treatment of complete prolapse of the rectum by the vaginal approach, *Arch Chir Neerl* 28:25, 1976.

Part V

SURGERY OF THE UPPER GENITAL TRACT

Chapter 31

ABDOMINAL HYSTERECTOMY

Colonel Kunio Miyazawa

TECHNICAL CONSIDERATIONS

The first most refined total abdominal hysterectomy was introduced by Wilhelm Alexander Freund of Breslau, Germany (now Wroclaw, Poland), on January 30, 1878.[17] Since then, many hysterectomy techniques have been introduced with various improvements in mind. Hysterectomy is now considered the most common major surgical procedure next to cesarean section in the United States.[28] Whether we like it or not, the success of a medical practice depends heavily on cost-effective management systems. A quality assurance program is an ongoing process for the hospital and its physicians. Hysterectomy based on a good quality assurance program and cost-effective management is accepted not only by physicians but also patients.[30] Hysterectomy technique has received peer review and various cost-effectiveness considerations for the past 110 years. While various technical methods have been handed down from pelvic surgeon to pelvic surgeon, basic principles and practice relative to pelvic surgery should be emphasized constantly. This is an essential part of the curriculum for medical student teaching and resident education.[12,32] The example of an American hysterectomy technique and a Japanese one will be presented. The latter is not familiar to many English-speaking physicians.

Example of the American technique

After a long clinical practice experience in New York and Los Angeles areas, Thomas L. Ball presented 29 surgical principles and refinements in performing total abdominal hysterectomy in his book, *Gynecologic Surgery, and Urology.*[3] Preoperatively, the following principles are applicable:

- High Trendelenburg's position

- Large, uncomplicated fibroid seldom complicates hysterectomy
- Pfannenstiel's incision adequate for simple surgery
- Incision should be adequate
- Vaginal repair to be performed before abdominal hysterectomy if needed
- Insert ureteral catheter for anticipated difficult hysterectomy due to endometriosis and pelvic inflammation
- Consider the uterine position as possible site of existing adhesion

The following points are applicable during the operative period:

- Watch for the ureter in the presence of old pelvic inflammation, start with uterine artery and base of the broad ligament
- Uterine traction as well as rotation is crucial for exposure
- Be flexible to modify the technique according to any special situation of the case involved
- Do not clutter the field with multiple clamps
- Identify the thin areolar layer of the vesicovaginal septum
- Expect there to be large veins in the broad ligament in the presence of intraligamental fibroid or cysts
- Catheterize the ureter directly at the pelvic brim when ligation, kinking, or perforation of the pelvic ureter is suspected
- Ligate the uterine artery at its origin when multiple bleeding points are encountered
- Palpate the portio vaginalis of the cervix before entering the vagina
- Provide anterior plication and a suprapubic urethral suspension for coexisting mild urinary stress incontinence

The actual operative procedure starts with emptying the bladder by catheter and after preliminary dilatation and

The opinions and assertions herein are those of the author and are not to be construed as official or as representing the views of the Department of the Army or the Department of Defense.

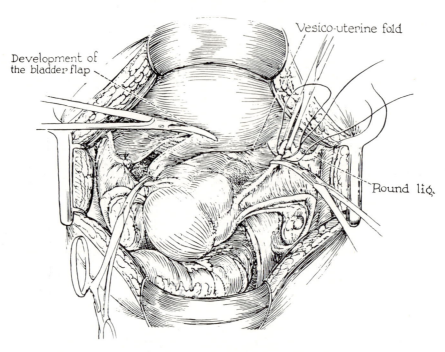

Fig. 31-1. Technique of severing the round ligament and creating a bladder flap. (From Ball TL: *Gynecologic surgery and urology,* ed 2, St Louis, Mosby–Year Book, 1963.)

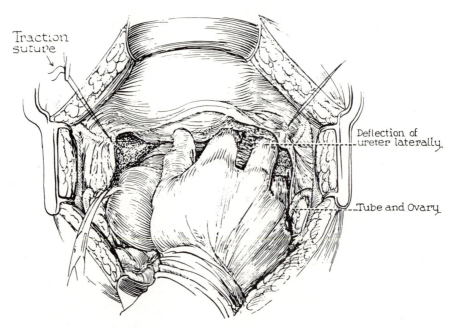

Fig. 31-2. The ureter is displaced laterally by a scissorlike motion of the index and middle fingers. (From Ball TL: *Gynecologic surgery and urology,* ed 2, St Louis, Mosby–Year Book, 1963.)

curettage (D and C). If there are no suspicious findings, the abdomen is opened with the operating pelvic surgeon standing on the patient's left side. The head of the operating table is lowered about 10 degrees at a time, gradually reaching about a 45-degree Trendelenburg's position. The entire abdomen is explored carefully and systematically.

To prevent formation of a large denuded area, only the operative field immediately in advance of the various operative steps is mobilized. The round ligament is grasped with an Allis clamp at a point midway between the uterus and the internal inguinal ring, and a Kelly hemostat is placed about 2 cm from the uterus. A suture with medium silk is

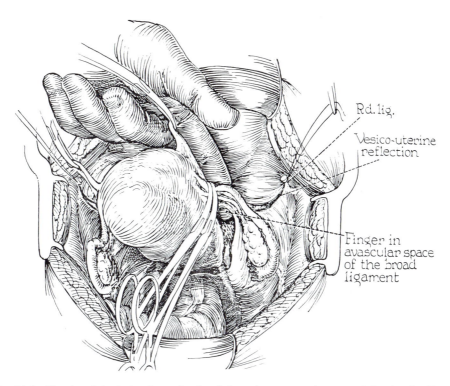

Fig. 31-3. The tip of the index finger is placed through an avascular area of the sheath. (From Ball TL: *Gynecologic surgery and urology,* ed 2, St Louis, Mosby–Year Book, 1963.)

placed between the hemostat and Allis clamp. The round ligament is cut, and the anterior sheath of the broad ligament is incised by the use of Metzenbaum scissors to create a bladder flap (Fig. 31-1). With gentle traction by an assistant on the tagged suture of the round ligament and traction of the uterus to the opposite side by the surgeon, the operator's index and middle fingers are inserted anteriorly under the sheath of the broad ligament to open the sheath by a scissorlike motion. The uterine vessel is seen, and the ureter is displaced laterally (Fig. 31-2). The same procedure is applied to the opposite side. The index finger is inserted through the avascular area of the sheath. While stretched over the operator's index finger, the posterior sheath is cut through (Fig. 31-3). Kelly clamps are placed on the tube and the uteroovarian ligament, which are cut (Fig. 31-4) and a suture ligature is placed as seen in Fig. 31-5. While forward traction to the uterus is maintained, the posterior sheath of the broad ligament is incised at the level of the internal os to skeletonize the uterine vessels and to expose the uterosacral ligaments. These are clamped, cut, and ligated. The posterior vaginal fornix is readily palpable behind the cul-de-sac peritoneum. It is important to place any needle points directed medially because the ureters lie just lateral to the uterosacral thickenings as shown in Fig. 31-6. The uterine vessels are triply clamped with curved Kocher clamps. The vessels are divided, leaving two clamps on the proximal pedicle, which are doubly ligated as demonstrated in Fig. 31-7. The suture should be placed in the grooves created by the clamps (Fig. 31-8). The same procedure is applied to the opposite

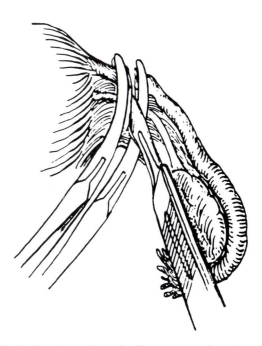

Fig. 31-4. The tube and ovarian ligament are clamped and cut. (From Ball TL: *Gynecologic surgery and urology,* ed 2, St Louis, Mosby–Year Book, 1963.)

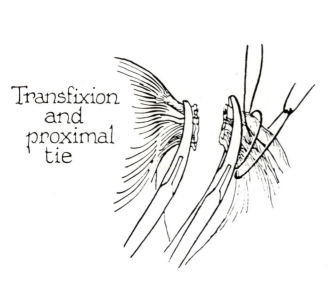

Fig. 31-5. The tube and ovarian ligament are sutured. (From Ball TL: *Gynecologic surgery and urology,* ed 2, St Louis, Mosby–Year Book, 1963.)

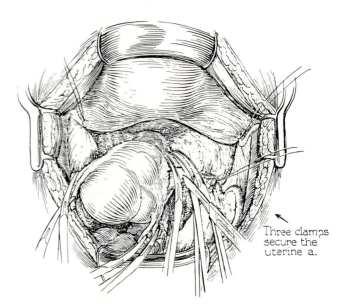

Fig. 31-7. Triple clamps secure the uterine vessels. (From Ball TL: *Gynecologic surgery and urology,* ed 2, St Louis, Mosby–Year Book, 1963.)

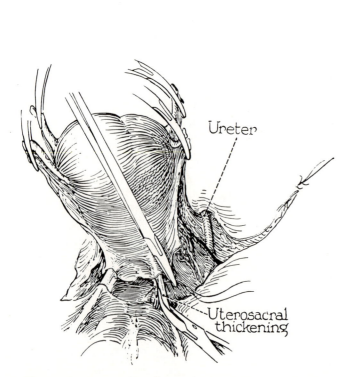

Fig. 31-6. Ureteral injury is avoided by placing a needle medially. (From Ball TL: *Gynecologic surgery and urology,* ed 2, St Louis, Mosby–Year Book, 1963.)

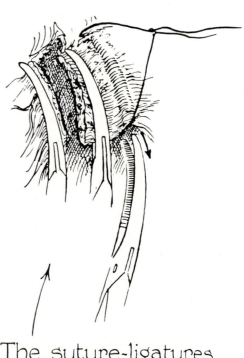

Fig. 31-8. Uterine ligatures are placed in the grooves made by clamps. (From Ball TL: *Gynecologic surgery and urology,* ed 2, St Louis, Mosby–Year Book, 1963.)

side. The bladder is dissected from the cervix and the upper vagina by stroking gently the thin areolar layer and pushing the bladder down and laterally with the knife handle (Fig. 31-9). For excision of the parametrium and paracolpium, with uterine traction toward the opposite side from the operating site, an Ochsner clamp is placed to clamp the cardinal ligament and a portion of paracolpium. The cardinal ligament is cut close to the cervix and the paracolpium close to the lateral vaginal fornix, and the pedicle is ligated (Fig. 31-10). The same is applied to the

opposite side. With a Deaver retractor placed anteriorly for bladder retraction, the upper vagina and cervix are palpated. An Allis clamp is placed on the vagina just below the cervix, and the vagina is incised just above the clamp (Fig. 31-11). The full thickness of the vaginal wall is grasped with Allis clamps, and the cervix is amputated with Metzenbaum scissors (Fig. 31-12). The uterus is opened in the operating room to see if there are any unexpected findings. Clamps are placed at both angles, and an angle suture anchors the cardinal ligament, uterine vessels,

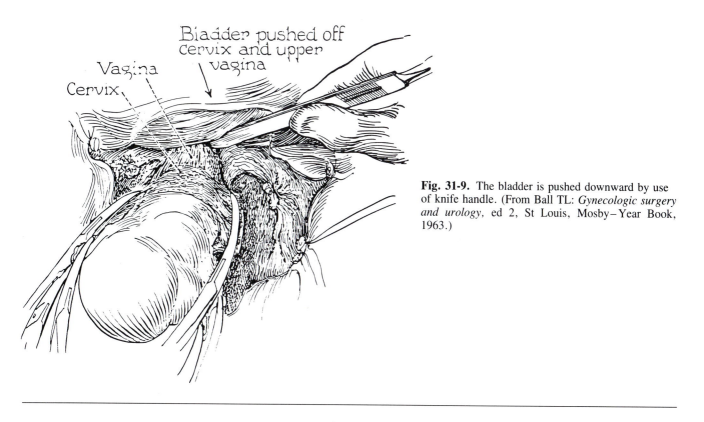

Fig. 31-9. The bladder is pushed downward by use of knife handle. (From Ball TL: *Gynecologic surgery and urology,* ed 2, St Louis, Mosby–Year Book, 1963.)

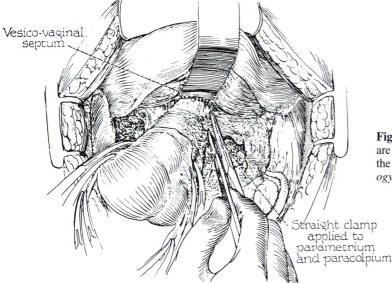

Fig. 31-10. The cardinal ligament and paravaginal tissue are excised by placing an Ochsner clamp and cutting with the knife. (From Ball TL: *Gynecologic surgery and urology,* ed 2, St Louis, Mosby–Year Book, 1963.)

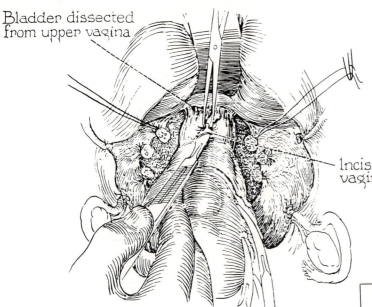

Bladder dissected from upper vagina

Incision into vaginal vault

Fig. 31-11. Technique of entry into the vagina. (From Ball TL: *Gynecologic surgery and urology,* ed 2, St Louis, Mosby–Year Book, 1963.)

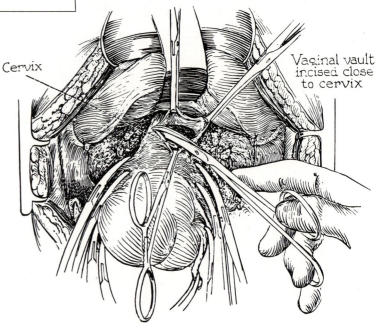

Cervix

Vaginal vault incised close to cervix

Fig. 31-12. Technique of amputating the cervix from the vagina. (From Ball TL: *Gynecologic surgery and urology,* ed 2, St Louis, Mosby–Year Book, 1963.)

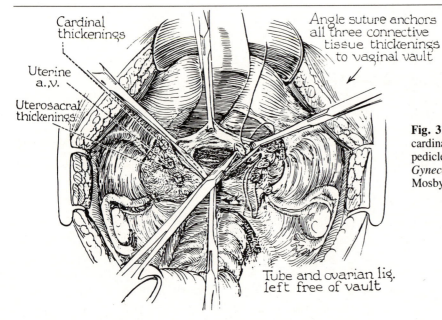

Cardinal thickenings

Uterine a.,v.

Uterosacral thickenings

Angle suture anchors all three connective tissue thickenings to vaginal vault

Tube and ovarian lig. left free of vault

Fig. 31-13. The vagina is supported by anchoring cardinal ligament, uterine vessels, and uterosacral pedicle to the vaginal lateral angle. (From Ball TL: *Gynecologic surgery and urology,* ed 2, St Louis, Mosby–Year Book, 1963.)

and uterosacral pedicle (Fig. 31-13). The same is applied to the opposite angle. Approximating the vaginal wall is accomplished by placing a running suture submucosally to approximate the vaginal mucosa (Figs. 31-14 and 31-15). No drainage is placed. The adnexal pedicle is not anchored to the vaginal angle. The muscular layer of the vagina is closed by figure-of-eight sutures (Fig. 31-16). Tube and ovarian ligament pedicle are inverted behind the peritoneum (Fig. 31-17). The peritoneum is closed by a running suture after the field of operation is free from bleeding (Fig. 31-18). The sigmoid is placed in the pelvis, and the omentum is drawn down over the bowel after the laparotomy pad is removed. Throughout the procedure, medium silk or cotton is used for pedicle ligation except in the presence of pelvic infection and for vaginal cuff closure when chromic catgut suture is used.

Example of the Japanese technique

The Japanese technique of radical hysterectomy and pelvic lymphadenectomy was first published by Okabayashi[26] of Japan in 1921, which was later modified by Yagi[37] in 1950. In 1982, Uchida[35] of Kanazawa, Japan, presented a film in English, entitled "Uchida's Abdominal Simple Hysterectomy," which was based on his own experience of more than 22,000 cases. He emphasized that his technique can accomplish simple hysterectomy in less than 20 minutes with minimal bleeding. His hysterectomy technique is generally unfamiliar to obstetric and gynecologic physicians in the Western world. The author believes it is a very efficient technique that should be shared with the reader who is not familiar with it.

The operating tray should contain minimal essential tools. As seen in Fig. 31-19, Uchida's tray is simple with only essential instruments. He believes pelvic surgeons should use only those instruments with which they are familiar. Usually, the instrument tray in the operating rooms of U.S. hospitals has many items that are rarely used. The abdominal wall is opened first by a transverse skin incision

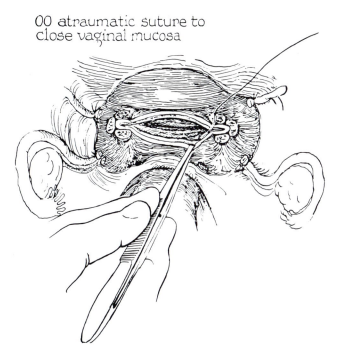

OO atraumatic suture to close vaginal mucosa

Fig. 31-14. Closure of vaginal mucosal edge defect by 00 atraumatic chromic suture. (From Ball TL: *Gynecologic surgery and urology,* ed 2, St Louis, Mosby–Year Book, 1963.)

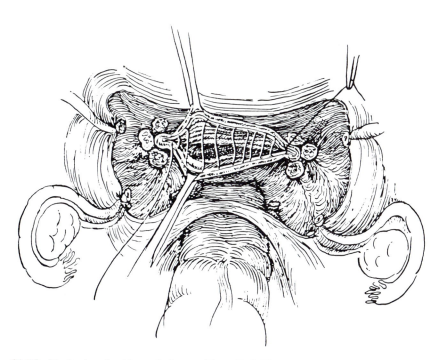

Fig. 31-15. Vault closed without drainage. (From Ball TL: *Gynecologic surgery and oncology,* ed 2, St Louis, Mosby–Year Book, 1963.)

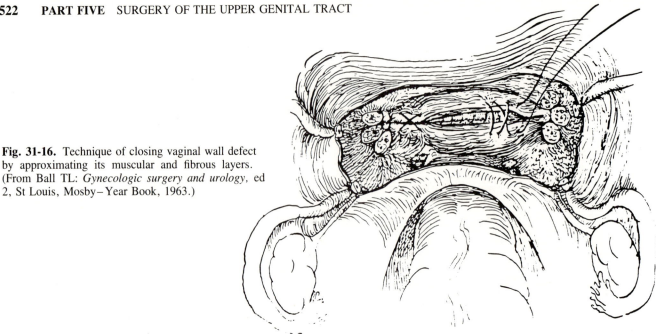

Fig. 31-16. Technique of closing vaginal wall defect by approximating its muscular and fibrous layers. (From Ball TL: *Gynecologic surgery and urology,* ed 2, St Louis, Mosby–Year Book, 1963.)

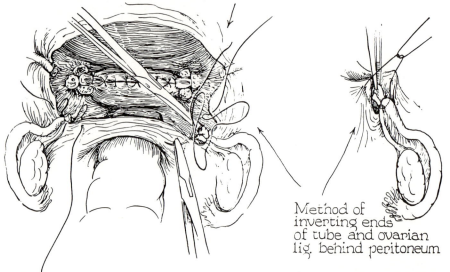

Peritoneum closed with running sutures of plain catgut

Method of inverting ends of tube and ovarian lig. behind peritoneum

Fig. 31-17. Method of inverting the tubal and ovarian ligament pedicles in the retroperitoneal space. (From Ball TL: *Gynecologic surgery and urology,* ed 2, St Louis, Mosby–Year Book, 1963.)

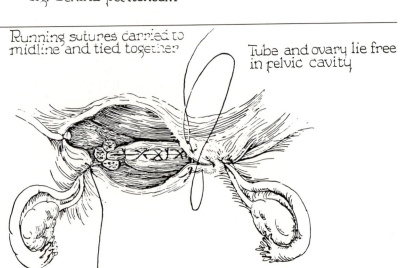

Running sutures carried to midline and tied together

Tube and ovary lie free in pelvic cavity

Fig. 31-18. Closure of the retroperitoneal space. (From Ball TL: *Gynecologic surgery and urology,* ed 2, St Louis, Mosby–Year Book, 1963.)

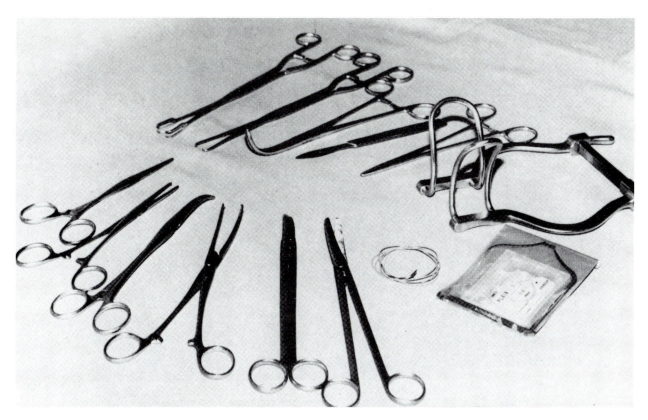

Fig. 31-19. Example of Uchida's simple instrument set in the operating tray. (By courtesy of Dr. Hajime Uchida and permission of Igakutosho Publishing Co. From Uchida H: *Abdominal simple hysterectomy,* Tokyo, 1985, Igakutosho.)

in the lower midabdomen, and, with the fingers, the subcutaneous tissue is separated in the midline from the fascia. A longitudinal incision is made in the fascia, and the peritoneal cavity is entered by a sharp longitudinal incision. There is no hemostatic effort made unless a pumping arterial vessel is present. After careful intraabdominal exploration, a self-retaining retractor is applied and the uterus is brought up by hand into the operating field. The uteroovarian ligament and fallopian tube are doubly ligated with 0 chromic catgut and cut widely after sliding forceps are applied to the uterine side (Figs. 31-20 and 31-21). After the round ligament is doubly ligated with 0 chromic catgut and cut (Fig. 31-22), the broad ligament is widely separated further into two sheets (Fig. 31-23). The lateral side of the uterus is pressed downward with gauze and the index finger through a widely separated leaf of the broad ligament (Fig. 31-24). The same procedure is applied to the opposite side. A curved scissor is pushed through between vesicouterine peritoneum and the uterine cervix and anterior vaginal wall to create an ample avascular space (Fig. 31-25), similar to a pitched tent, by separating the scissor blades to free the bladder (Fig. 31-26), and the vesicouterine peritoneum is incised transversely. The median portion of the uterine cervix is pressed downward with gauze and the index finger (Fig. 31-27). Caution is taken not to involve either side of the bladder pillar to

avoid unnecessary and severe bleeding. Usually there is no bleeding in the center portion of the cervix or anterior vaginal wall (Fig. 31-28). The cardinal ligament, uterine vessels, uterosacral ligament, and vesicouterine ligament are clamped in one entire block, placing the tip of the forceps in the upper fornix of the vagina (Fig. 31-29), and cut by pressing the backside of the scissors along the cervix (Fig. 31-30). Usually, a tympanic sound is audible when the scissors reach the tip of the forceps at the level of the vaginal fornix. The same procedure is applied to the opposite side. The vaginal wall is entered with scissors through the midanterior fornix (Fig. 31-31). A popping sound indicates that the incision has entered the vagina. The vaginal wall is opened by scissors, and the uterus is removed. The vaginal cuff is clamped at the midportion anteriorly and posteriorly. The vaginal cuff is sutured continuously with one long, plain catgut suture. The clamp holding the cardinal ligaments, uterine vessels, uterosacral ligament, and the vesicouterine ligament is stretched medially while the round ligament is stretched laterally and distally and the adnexal stump is stretched laterally and proximally, thus creating a triangular retroperitoneal space (Fig. 31-32), and making it possible to visualize the uterine artery and the ureter (Fig. 31-33). The uterine artery is ligated just outside the ureter (Fig. 31-34). The cardinal ligament, uterine vessels, uterosacral ligaments, and the vesicouter-

Text continued on p. 531.

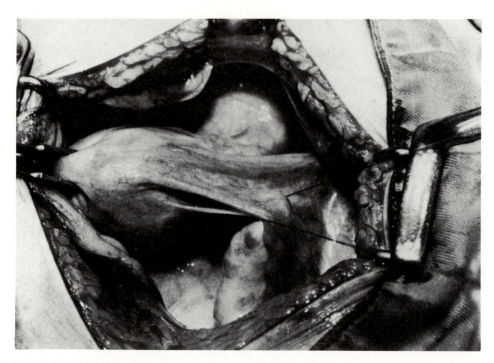

Fig. 31-20. Ligation of the uteroovarian ligament and fallopian tube. (By courtesy of Dr. Hajime Uchida and permission of Igakutosho Publishing Co. From Uchida H: *Abdominal simple hysterectomy*, Tokyo, 1985, Igakutosho.)

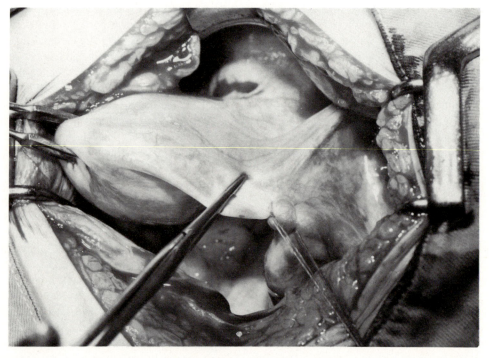

Fig. 31-21. Double ligations of the uteroovarian ligament and fallopian tube. A clamp is placed to the uterine side to create a whitish avascular space. (By courtesy of Dr. Hajime Uchida and permission of Igakutosho Publishing Co. From Uchida H: *Abdominal simple hysterectomy*, Tokyo, 1985, Igakutosho.)

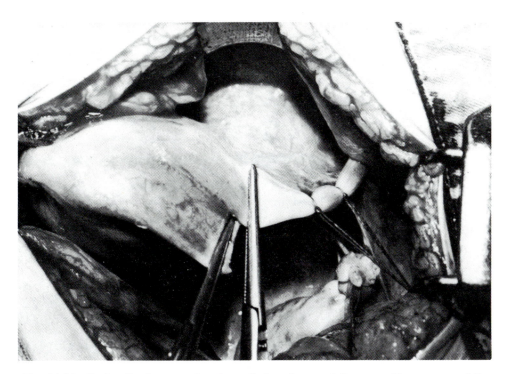

Fig. 31-22. Similar ligation procedure is applied to the round ligament. (By courtesy of Dr. Hajime Uchida and permission of Igakutosho Publishing Co. From Uchida H: *Abdominal simple hysterectomy,* Tokyo, 1985, Igakutosho.)

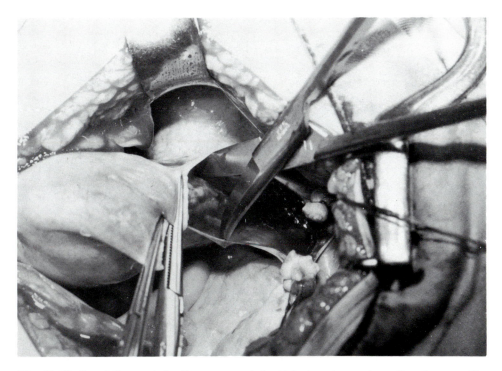

Fig. 31-23. Broad ligament sheaths are separated widely to enter a retroperitoneal space. (By courtesy of Dr. Hajime Uchida and permission of Igakutosho Publishing Co. From Uchida H: *Abdominal simple hysterectomy,* Tokyo, 1985, Igakutosho.)

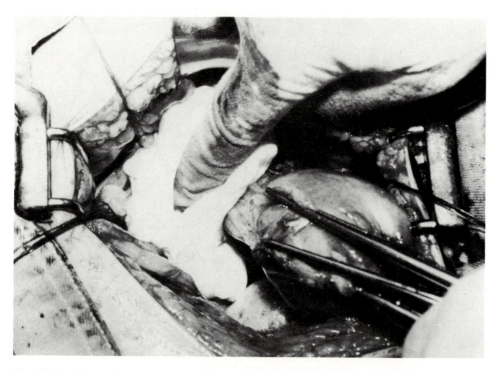

Fig. 31-24. The uterine side is pressed downward with gauze and the index finger through the retroperitoneal space just created. (By courtesy of Dr. Hajime Uchida and permission of Igakutosho Publishing Co. From Uchida H: *Abdominal simple hysterectomy,* Tokyo, 1985, Igakutosho.)

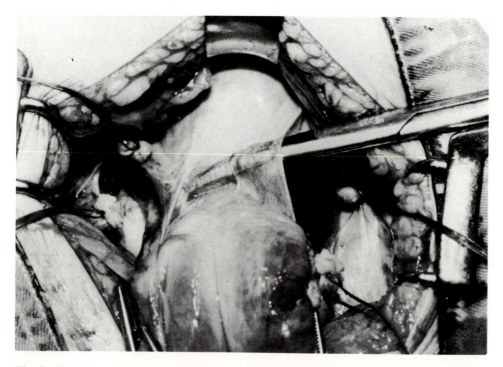

Fig. 31-25. A curved scissors is placed between vesicouterine peritoneum and the cervix and the anterior vaginal wall to create avascular space. (By courtesy of Dr. Hajime Uchida and permission of Igakutosho Publishing Co. From Uchida H: *Abdominal simple hysterectomy,* Tokyo, 1985, Igakutosho.)

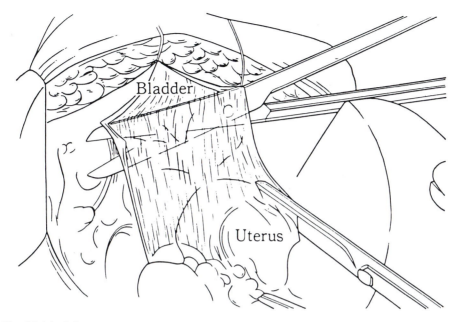

Fig. 31-26. Scissors are separated to create an avascular space like a pitched tent. (By courtesy of Dr. Hajime Uchida and permission of Igakutosho Publishing Co. From Uchida H: *Abdominal simple hysterectomy,* Tokyo, 1985, Igakutosho.)

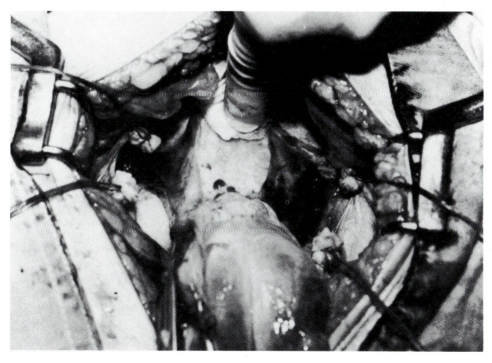

Fig. 31-27. The median portion of the cervix is pushed downward with gauze and the index finger. (By courtesy of Dr. Hajime Uchida and permission of Igakutosho Publishing Co. From Uchida H: *Abdominal simple hysterectomy,* Tokyo, 1985, Igakutosho.)

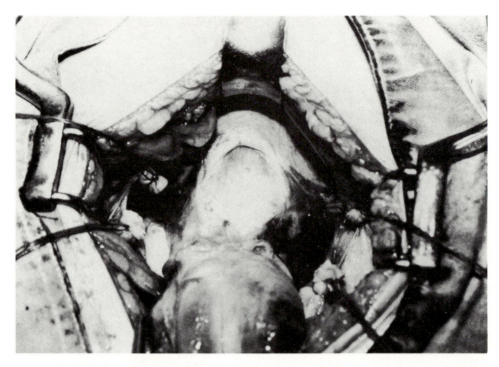

Fig. 31-28. Note avascular anterior portion of the cervix. (By courtesy of Dr. Hajime Uchida and permission of Igakutosho Publishing Co. From Uchida H: *Abdominal simple hysterectomy,* Tokyo, 1985, Igakutosho.)

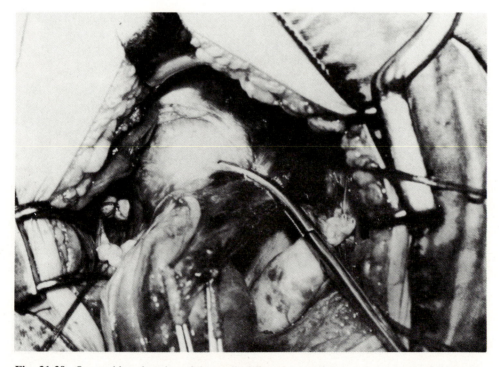

Fig. 31-29. One en-bloc clamping of the cardinal ligament, uterine vessels, uterosacral ligament, and vesicouterine ligament. The tip of the forceps is in the upper fornix of the vagina. (By courtesy of Dr. Hajime Uchida and permission of Igakutosho Publishing Co. From Uchida H: *Abdominal simple hysterectomy,* Tokyo, 1985, Igakutosho.)

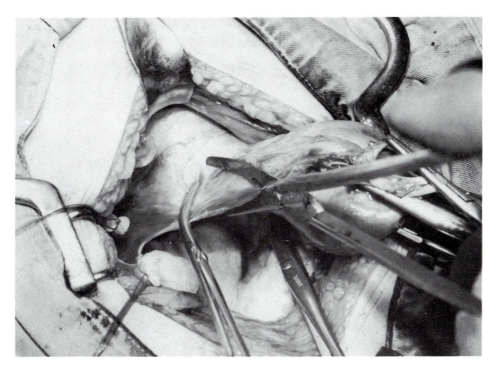

Fig. 31-30. One en-bloc dissection of the cardinal ligament, uterine vessels, uterosacral ligament, and vesicouterine ligament. Note the back side of the scissors along the cervix. (By courtesy of Dr. Hajime Uchida and permission of Igakutosho Publishing Co. From Uchida H: *Abdominal simple hysterectomy,* Tokyo, 1985, Igakutosho.)

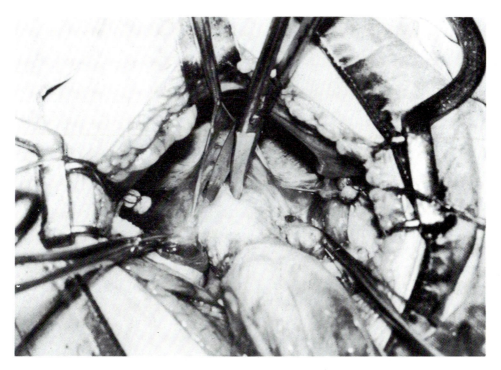

Fig. 31-31. Entry into the midanterior vaginal fornix with the scissors. (By courtesy of Dr. Hajime Uchida and permission of Igakutosho Publishing Co. From Uchida H: *Abdominal simple hysterectomy,* Tokyo, 1985, Igakutosho.)

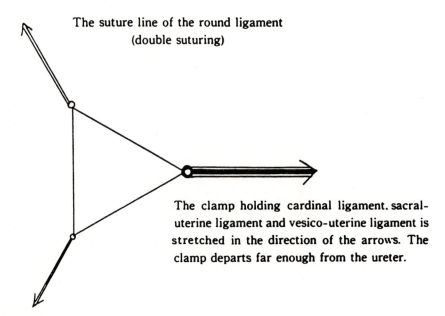

The suture line of the round ligament
(double suturing)

The clamp holding cardinal ligament. sacral-
uterine ligament and vesico-uterine ligament is
stretched in the direction of the arrows. The
clamp departs far enough from the ureter.

The suture line of adnexae.
(double suturing)

Fig. 31-32. Creation of a left-sided triangular retroperitoneal space. (By courtesy of Dr. Hajime Uchida and permission of Igakutosho Publishing Co. From Uchida H: *Abdominal simple hysterectomy,* Tokyo, 1985, Igakutosho.)

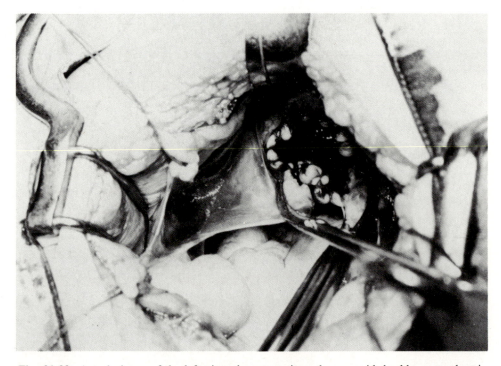

Fig. 31-33. Actual picture of the left triangular retroperitoneal space with healthy ureteral peristalsis and uterine artery in view. (By courtesy of Dr. Hajime Uchida and permission of Igakutosho Publishing Co. From Uchida H: *Abdominal simple hysterectomy,* Tokyo, 1985, Igakutosho.)

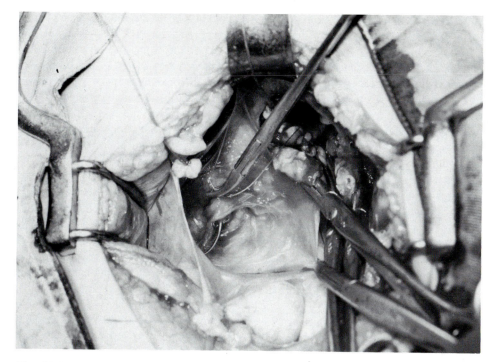

Fig. 31-34. Ligation of the left uterine artery just outside of the ureter after confirming ureteral peristalsis. (By courtesy of Dr. Hajime Uchida and permission of Igakutosho Publishing Co. From Uchida H: *Abdominal simple hysterectomy,* Tokyo, 1985, Igakutosho.)

ine ligament are sutured with interrupted 0 chromic catgut suture to the lateral vaginal wall angle three times to prevent future vaginal prolapse. The ureter is visualized away from the lateral vaginal cuff margin and having good peristalsis. Exactly the same procedure is applied to the opposite side. The pelvic peritoneum is closed with continuous plain catgut suture bringing all stumps into the retroperitoneal space. The abdominal retroperitoneum is closed continuously with plain catgut. The fascia is reapproximated with interrupted stitches of 0 chromic suture. The skin incision is reapproximated with metal clips. The entire procedure takes 10 to 20 minutes, depending on the individual case.

Discussion

Hysterectomy was rarely used for the management of gynecologic diseases 100 years ago, but it has now become the most common major surgical procedure next to cesarean section. It is estimated that the average length of hospital stay for women undergoing hysterectomy has been dropping from 12.2 days in 1965 to 5.7 days in 1987.[29] This change is obviously due to various factors including improved surgical techniques, early ambulation, and use of prophylactic antibiotics. It is crucial that we seek the best techniques for abdominal hysterectomy to provide a challenging method for younger physicians who are learning its technique based on the correct surgical anatomy of the living and knowledge of a respectable scientific technique. Correct pelvic surgical technique remains one of the major objectives in designing obstetric

and gynecologic resident training programs.[16] This surgical and technical importance must be emphasized to maintain basic pelvic surgical skills for future obstetricians and gynecologists who are learning the use of pelvic endoscopy to remove the uterus.[24] To support available techniques for abdominal hysterectomy, several points must be discussed.

First, a patient should be well prepared, not only physically but psychologically. Not only should there exist an adequate indication for hysterectomy based on symptomatology and clinical findings, but women should be given all other necessary options for conservative management. A patient may be cured physically of an enlarging uterine leiomyoma with menometrorrhagia after hysterectomy, but postoperatively she complains of loss of her sexual desire and inability to reach sexual orgasm. This could be easily prevented by careful preoperative counseling, which should include discussion of treatment alternates such as myomectomy. It is not unusual to observe sexual dysfunction such as decrease or loss of sexual desire after major illness or surgery, particularly when body image is affected after such a procedure as mastectomy or hysterectomy.[19] The period after a gynecologic procedure such as hysterectomy is a challenging transition time for a woman.[15] The good outcome of the successful hysterectomy technique depends on a well-prepared patient.

Second, as the older population has been increasing recently with a prolonged life expectancy and enhanced geriatric physical activity, every effort should be made to prevent a future pelvic relaxation and vaginal prolapse at the time of abdominal hysterectomy. Vaginal support becomes a key point for hysterectomy. Ball[3] suggested removing a wedge of peritoneum in the cul-de-sac and uniting the uterosacral ligaments in the midline to avoid subsequent surgery for pelvic repair. Sufficient sutures placed in the muscular layer of the vagina form a firm and muscular vault in appreciation of its function as a supporting structure in the mechanics of the pelvis as a whole. He believes attachment of the round ligaments to the vaginal vault does not contribute to the support but causes a persistent urinary tenesmus in some patients. Uchida believes the attachment of the cardinal ligament, uterine vessels, uterosacral ligament, and vesicouterine ligament to the lateral vaginal wall angle three times will prevent future vaginal prolapse.[22] Further, it is crucial for a pelvic surgeon to obtain a good, deep bite in the vaginal cuff repair because the muscular and fibrous layers tend to retract at the time of amputation of the cervix causing poor vaginal support in the future as mentioned by Jaszczak et al.[18]

Third, although most hysterectomies can be performed intrafascially for benign disease of the uterus, extrafascial technique should be mastered so this can be used for uterine neoplasia such as endometrial carcinoma or uterine sarcoma. Although there are many variations in either technique, Thompson[34] defines it as intrafascial hysterectomy when the clamps are placed on the cardinal ligament beneath the so-called pubovesicocervical fascia, part of endopelvic fascia. Lahey[20] of Boston introduced this technique in 1923 by applying double hooks to the front and back of the thin shell of cervical tissue that was left behind while the uterus was pulled upward and the hooks were pressed downward, by which danger to the ureters was reduced and vaginal support was obtained. Aldridge[1] dissected within the paracervical fascia and transfixed transverse cervical ligaments to the vaginal cuff for better support with a good result. Contrary to intrafascial technique, the extrafascial hysterectomy excises the paracervical fascial tissue without separating the pubovesicocervical fascia from the uterus by placing a clamp not so close to the cervix. An example of the extrafascial approach is the Mayo Clinic (Masson-Counseller) technique,[33] which emphasizes a generous abdominal incision for visualization of the pelvic organs with adequate space to identify the ureters, clear exposure of the base of the bladder and rectum, and meticulous closure of the vaginal cuff. With strong traction on the uterus, Ochsner forceps are placed well down both sides of the cervix at a 45-degree angle, clamping both uterine vessels and the superior portion of the cardinal ligament; the tip of the forceps engages the endopelvic fascia. In the presence of endometrial cancer, clamps can be placed more laterally and the cervical fascia is dissected more laterally.

Fourth, the age at which we should remove normal appearing ovaries at the time of hysterectomy has been a controversial subject. Although most physicians agree with their removal when a woman is in the postmenopausal age, difficulty arises with this decision in a premenopausal woman who is undergoing hysterectomy.[34] When a decision is made to leave the ovaries for her female function, it is important to preserve ovarian blood supply as much as possible. Every effort should be provided not to twist the infundibulopelvic ligament so as to maintain blood supply to the ovaries and not to transfix them to the pelvic side wall for support. The normal fallopian tube should not be removed to avoid compromising the blood supply to ovarian tissue. Burford and Diddle,[7] and Whitelaw[36] demonstrated continued ovarian activity after hysterectomy. Chambers et al[9] have shown the incidence of symptomatic ovarian cysts requiring operative management is greater in radical hysterectomy patients with lateral ovarian transfixation than in those without.

Fifth, when a disease process is so severe that total abdominal hysterectomy cannot be carried out with safety in a case such as severe endometriosis or extensive pelvic inflammatory disease, option should be given to performance of subtotal hysterectomy. Although subtotal hysterectomy is no longer performed frequently, this is an efficient technique to remove the body of the uterus. This technique also may be applied to advanced ovarian carcinoma with diffuse intraabdominal metastasis when the complete removal of the uterus together with adnexal masses is not safe because of tumor involvement in the paracervical, lower broad ligament, and prevesical regions. Maximal tumor debulking can be established swiftly and safely by performing subtotal hysterectomy, especially when the removal of the cervix does not reduce residual tumor volume.

Conclusions

A tremendous change has been made in the technique of abdominal hysterectomy over the past 110 years. History shows that it will continue to change. It is the opinion of the author that the superb and excellent techniques ought be taught and shared together with appreciation for principles such as the details of anatomy of the living, developing avascular spaces, application of proper traction and countertraction, prevention of future vaginal relaxation and prolapse, shorter operating time, fewer complications, and shorter hospital stay.

HYSTERECTOMY FOR ENDOMETRIAL CANCER

Although the older population has been increasing recently, the estimated number of cases of cancer of the endometrium has been gradually declining; in the United States the estimated number of new cases was 1992 of 32,000 compared to 39,000 in 1984.[5,31] However, endometrial carcinoma still remains the most common malignancy of the female genital tract. Its major treatment modality is total abdominal hysterectomy and bilateral salpingo-oophorectomy. Nearly 75% of endometrial cancer is in the stage I category according to the old FIGO (International Federation of Gynecology and Obstetrics) clinical staging system (see the left box).[13] The other box shows the new FIGO surgical staging classification. This new

---

FIGO old clinical staging—carcinoma of the corpus uteri

Stage 1   Carcinoma confined to the corpus
Stage 1A   Uterine cavity 8 cm or less
Stage 1B   Uterine cavity more than 8 cm
  G1   Highly differentiated adenomatous carcinoma
  G2   Moderately differentiated adenomatous carcinoma with partly solid area
  G3   Predominantly solid or entirely undifferentiated carcinoma
Stage 2   Carcinoma involved the corpus and the cervix but not extended outside the uterus
Stage 3   Carcinoma extended outside the uterus, but not outside the true pelvis
Stage 4   Carcinoma extended outside the true pelvis or involved with bladder or rectal mucosa. Bullous edema not counted
Stage 4a   Spread to the adjacent organs
Stage 4b   Spread to distant organs

From Morrow CP, Townsend DE: *Synopsis of gynecologic oncology*, ed 3, New York, 1987, John Wiley & Sons, p 173.

FIGO new surgical staging—carcinoma of the corpus uteri

Stage 1A G123   Tumor confined to endometrium
Stage 1B G123   Invasion <one half myometrium
Stage 1C G123   Invasion > one half myometrium
Stage 2A G123   Endocervical glandular involvement
Stage 2B G123   Cervical stromal invasion
Stage 3A G123   Tumor invades serosa and/or adnexa and/or positive peritoneal cytology
Stage 3B G123   Metastasis to pelvic and/or paraaortic lymph nodes
Stage 4A G123   Tumor invasion of bladder and/or bowel mucosa
Stage 4B   Distant metastasis includes intraabdominal and/or inguinal lymph nodes

Histopathology—degree of differentiation

G1 = 5% or less of a nonsquamous or nonmorular solid growth pattern
G2 = 6% to 50% of a nonsquamous or nonmorular solid growth pattern
G3 = more than 50% of a nonsquamous or nonmorular solid growth pattern

---

From FIGO annual report on the results of treatment in gynecologic cancer, *Int J Gynecol Obstet* 28:189, 1989.

---

surgical pathologic staging system is believed to promise better evaluation of endometrial carcinoma and establish the true extent of the disease. This new system should be understood by all primary care providers and used by general obstetricians and gynecologists to provide the best quality of patient care, especially in areas where a gynecologic oncologist is not readily available. Three questions will be considered on this subject: (1) What kind of hysterectomy? (2) What else should be performed in addition to hysterectomy? (3) Who should be operating?

Kind of hysterectomy

The standard surgical approach for early endometrial adenocarcinoma is total abdominal extrafascial hysterectomy and bilateral salpingo-oophorectomy, and selected cases of stage 2 endometrial carcinoma can be managed by radical abdominal hysterectomy and bilateral salpingo-oophorectomy. In addition to total abdominal hysterectomy and bilateral salpingo-oophorectomy for advanced disease, it is necessary to debulk existing tumor as much as possible to decrease the tumor burden before chemotherapy or radiation therapy. When the primary surgery is performed for such a reason as prolapse of the uterus, unsuspected endometrial adenocarcinoma is sometimes observed after vaginal hysterectomy. Fortunately, most of these lesions are very early cases of well-differentiated adenocarcinoma without myometrial invasion and no additional therapy seems needed. Although all diagnosed endometrial adenocarcinomas should be treated by the abdominal route, some advocate vaginal hysterectomy with possible removal of both adnexal structures to provide less operating time and quick postoperative recovery, particularly for those patients with coincident medical prob-

lems.[4,8] Total abdominal hysterectomy should be done through an extrafascial approach rather than intrafascial approach as stated previously. Undoubtedly, there are many variations of extrafascial hysterectomy technique, but the following technique has been used and is recommended by the author.

The abdominal cavity is entered either through low-mid longitudinal incision or Maylard/Cherney transverse incision. A peritoneal cytology sample is obtained using 100 ml of saline or physiologic solution with heparin. Meticulous abdominal exploration follows. Abnormally palpable pelvic and paraaortic lymph nodes should be sought. The uterus should be palpated gently to locate any abnormal nodularity or irregularity, especially in the lower uterine segment or cornual areas. Both ends of the fallopian tube should be tied or clamped to prevent spillage of the cancer cells from the uterine cavity into the pelvic space (although previous study indicates *any* manipulation or D and C disseminates malignant cells into systemic venous circulation[21]). Use of a single-tooth tenaculum in the uterine fundus for uterine traction should be avoided. Rather, straight clamps are placed along each side of the uterus for traction and manipulation. The round ligament is ligated as distally as possible and cut. The retroperitoneal cavity is entered through an incision in the avascular area of the broad ligament. The sheaths are separated with the index and middle fingers gently through the avascular area. The infundibulopelvic ligament is clamped and severed as proximally as possible, and doubly tied. Gentle separation of the areolar tissue avoids unnecessary bleeding in the retroperitoneal space. Retroperitoneal structures should be identified including the ureters and abnormally palpable lymph nodes. A central peritoneal reflection in the vesicouterine space is sharply incised with scissors, and the bladder is moved away from the cervix and anterior vaginal fornix. It is important to identify the avascular plane between the bladder and the cervix. The lateral paracervical area should not be dissected, because it is very vascular. The peritoneum overlying both uterosacral ligaments in the posterior uterus is incised transversely to enter the avascular space. This space can be enlarged by a curved dorsal movement of the fingers, which allows the uterus, cervix, and posterior vaginal fornix to be separated from the anterior rectal wall. The tip of the cervix can be palpated with the thumb and index finger to confirm that the bladder and the rectum are freed adequately from the uterus. The uterine vessels, uterosacral ligaments, and cardinal ligaments are respectively clamped, severed, and doubly ligated. The tissue is clamped not too close to the uterus and cervix to obtain adequate tissue margins. To remove adequate amounts of paracervical and paravaginal tissue, these are clamped, severed, and ligated as laterally as possible. The use of uterine elevation and palpation of the ureter by thumb and index finger advocated by Burch will prevent ureteral damage.[6] The same procedure is applied to the opposite side, and the uterus is removed with more than 1 cm of vaginal cuff attached. The specimen should be opened in the operating room to search for any gross abnormality. Myometrial invasion of endometrial carcinoma should be assessed grossly, which appears to be reliable according to the data reported.[14] However, in practice, this is not always easy and clearcut. Frozen section should be performed for microscopic evaluation.[25] The vaginal wall is closed with interrupted sutures. The vaginal angle is anchored to the cardinal and uterosacral ligaments for vaginal and pelvic support. An adequate amount of vaginal wall tissue should be reapproximated to include the retracted vaginal muscular and fibrous tissues to avoid future development of anatomic support defects and pelvic relaxation. Good repair of vaginal support defects at the time of hysterectomy should prevent future pelvic relaxation among the elderly population at large.

Additional procedures

The concept of surgical staging began in early 1977, and a significant contribution was made by the Gynecologic Oncology Group.[11] Beyond the standard procedure of extrafascial hysterectomy, bilateral salpingo-oophorectomy, careful abdominal exploration, and peritoneal cytology, bilateral selective pelvic and paraaortic lymphadenectomy has become a cornerstone to accurately assess the extent of the disease process by which the best treatment plan is established to obtain the best survival rate and to prevent any recurrence. If the grade of the tumor is well differentiated and stage 1 disease in old FIGO staging system without any myometrial invasion, no additional procedure is necessary beyond hysterectomy.[2] When the lesion

is grade 1, pelvic and paraaortic node metastasis of endometrial adenocarcinoma with no myometrial invasion is 0%, and, when the inner third is involved, it is 3% and 1%, respectively.[10] There is disagreement on lymph node sampling for all patients with stage 1 endometrial carcinoma, but, if there is any myometrial invasion of more than the inner one third, an additional procedure is required to obtain more information. In all other grades and stages of endometrial carcinoma, pelvic and paraaortic nodes should be sampled accordingly. For the pelvic node sampling procedure, the paravesical and pararectal spaces are identified and opened and the external iliac nodes are removed above the level of the deep circumflex iliac vein. Obturator nodes are removed above the level of the obturator nerve. Hypogastric and common iliac nodes are sampled also. At least 10 lymph nodes are necessary to provide quality staging assessment. Detailed lymph node dissection as seen in treatment of early cervical invasive cancer is not necessary. Paraaortic nodes can be sampled after exposing the area with an appropriate retractor and packing in the upper abdomen. A small incision is made in the peritoneum along the right common iliac artery and lower portion of the aorta. Nodes are obtained from the right side of the periaortic and precaval area toward renal and ovarian vessels. Chain dissection of the left side is difficult because of limited exposure. Meticulous hemostasis is necessary. The peritoneal defect is closed with interrupted stitches of absorbable suture. This surgical procedure adds some additional operating time, but, if done correctly, provides useful information for the best planned treatment without increasing perioperative morbidity.[27] The new FIGO staging system (see box p. 533, right column) should be applied to any case of endometrial carcinoma.

Operating personnel

Extended surgical staging and hysterectomy require that we not only prepare our patients preoperatively but also enforce the teamwork concept. Although this surgical staging procedure promises to produce an accurate knowledge of the extent of the disease and, thus, we can apply the best treatment program, its extended surgical procedure is not within reach of the usual Board-certified general gynecologist. The length of surgical training in many American obstetric-gynecologic residency programs will not produce a pelvic surgeon who is able to independently handle any complication associated with this technique. In some communities, there is an inadequate supply of gynecologic oncologists. Thus, it seems feasible to refer patients with a diagnosis of endometrial cancer to a fully trained gynecologic oncologist. The following guidelines are presented as a feasible policy for any given medical community:
1. Histopathologic diagnosis of endometrial adenocarcinoma should be made based on adequate preoperative sampling from the endometrium and endocervix. The grade of the tumor is based on the classification in the grade concept in the box on p. 533, at right. If there is any question, a full fractional D and C should be per-

formed. When any doubt exists, a consultation with the gynecologic pathologist should be sought.

2. The patient scheduled for surgery should be prepared for a possible extensive staging procedure beyond hysterectomy. The general gynecologist can proceed with the surgical procedure for stage 1 and grade 1 cancer according to the old FIGO staging system, but a pathologist and a gynecologic oncologist should be available in the event of myometrial invasion or any other unexpected findings. Additional staging procedures can be performed by the gynecologic oncologist or surgeon who is familiar with pelvic and paraaortic lymphadenectomy and is able to handle any unexpected complication such as a lacerated inferior vena cava.

3. The pathologist should be thoroughly familiar with the new staging system, especially in the grade of histopathologic criteria, to provide a uniform diagnosis to the pelvic surgeon. Invasion of the myometrium by the endometrial cancer should be accurate not only grossly but also microscopically by frozen section performed at the time of hysterectomy. Accurate gross and microscopic information is provided immediately to the team of surgeons in the operating room setting.

4. Ideally, all gynecologic cancer cases should be handled by a gynecologic oncologist with referring general gynecologist in the team care program so that each patient receives individual attention as well as continuity in care.

Conclusions

The new staging system is time honored and promising, but it seems that some patients will undergo unnecessary extended surgical procedure. This becomes significant because the cancer is more prevalent among the elderly who may have various medical problems that increase surgical risk. Some of these medically complicated patients who have an early stage and well-differentiated lesion can be managed without extensive surgical staging, with less operating time, and a shorter hospital stay. The discipline of surgical oncology has maintained radical excision of the malignant process without any residual disease. We might look carefully and critically at a simpler, less extensive, and more cost-effective procedure including laparoscopy-assisted hysterectomy and lymph node sampling to provide our patients with more comfort, without sacrificing their cure and survival rate.[23,24] The medical technology in the field of pelvic surgery and gynecologic oncology has been drastically changing over the past 30 years. It is our hope that we maintain excellent pelvic surgical practice and training discipline, but we should be open-minded to accommodate the new exciting techniques for a better quality assurance program and superior overall benefit for our patients.

REFERENCES

1. Aldridge AH, Meredith RS: Complete abdominal hysterectomy, a simplified technique and end results in 500 cases, *Am J Obstet Gynecol* 59:748, 1950.

2. Averette HE et al: Surgical staging: the new FIGO definitions, *Contemp Obstet Gynecol* Nov, p 112, 1991.

3. Ball TL: *Gynecologic surgery and urology,* ed 2, St Louis, 1963, Mosby–Year Book p 325.

4. Berek JS, Hacker NF: *Practical gynecologic oncology,* Baltimore, 1989, Williams & Wilkins, p 299.

5. Boring CC, Squires TS, Tong T: Cancer statistics 1992, *CA-Cancer J Clin* 42:19, 1992.

6. Burch JC, Lavely HT: Hysterectomy, *Ann Surg* 136:720, 1952.

7. Burford TH, Diddle AW: Effect of total hysterectomy upon the ovary of the Marcus rhesus, *Surg Gynecol Obstet* 62:701, 1936.

8. Carenza L et al: Does today's vaginal surgery still have a specific role in the treatment of endometrial cancer? *Ann NY Acad Sci* 622:477, 1991.

9. Chambers SK et al: Sequelae of lateral ovarian transposition in unirradiated cervical cancer patients, *Gynecol Oncol* 39:155, 1990.

10. Creasman WT et al: Surgical pathologic spread patterns of endometrial cancer: a Gynecologic Oncology Group study, *Cancer* 60(8 suppl):2035, 1987.

11. Currie JL: *Malignant tumors of the uterine corpus.* In Thompson JD, Rock JA, editors: *Te Linde's operative gynecology,* ed 7, Philadelphia, 1992, JB Lippincott, p 1267.

12. Dilts PV: Pleas on specialty training, *Council news bulletin, Spring 1985, Council on Resident Education in Obstetrics and Gynecology.*

13. DiSaia PJ, Creasman WT: *Clinical gynecologic oncology,* ed 3, St Louis, 1989, Mosby–Year Book, p 161.

14. Doering DL et al: Intraoperative evaluation of the depth of myometrial invasion in stage 1 endometrial adenocarcinoma, *Obstet Gynecol* 37:47, 1990.

15. Droegemuller W: *Postoperative complications.* In Droegemuller W, Herbst AL, Mishell DR, editors: *Comprehensive gynecology,* St Louis, 1987, Mosby–Year Book p 700.

16. *Educational objectives for residents in obstetrics and gynecology,* ed 3, Washington, DC, 1984, Council of Resident Education in Obstetrics and Gynecology.

17. Freund WA: Extirpation of the entire uterus by a new method, *Am J Obstet NY* 12:200, 1879.

18. Jaszczak SE, Evans TN: Intrafascial abdominal and vaginal hysterectomy: a reappraisal, *Obstet Gynecol* 59:435, 1982.

19. Kaplan HI, Sadock BJ: *Synopsis of psychiatry,* ed 6, Baltimore, 1991, Williams & Wilkins, p 448.

20. Lahey FH: A simple method of removing the cervix with the uterus in hysterectomy, *Surg Gynecol Obstet* 46:257, 1928.

21. Merrill JA: Dissemination of cancer cells during surgical curettage, *Am Surg* 29:206, 1963.

22. Miyazawa K: Technique for total abdominal hysterectomy: historical and clinical perspective, *Obstet Gynecol Surv* 47:433, 1992.

23. Nezhat C et al: Laparoscopic radical hysterectomy with periaortic and pelvic node dissection, *Am J Obstet Gynecol* 166:864, 1992.

24. Nezhat F et al: Laparoscopic versus abdominal hysterectomy, *J Reprod Med* 37:247, 1992.

25. Noumoff JS et al: The ability to evaluate prognostic variables on frozen section in hysterectomies performed for endometrial carcinoma, *Gynecol Oncol* 42:202, 1991.

26. Okabayashi H: Radical abdominal hysterectomy for cancer of the cervix uteri, *Surg Gynecol Obstet* 33:335, 1921.

27. Orr JW et al: Surgical staging of uterine cancer: an analysis of perioperative morbidity, *Gynecol Oncol* 42:209, 1991.

28. Pokras R: Hysterectomy: past, present and future, *Stat Bull Metrop Insur Co,* 70:12, 1989.

29. Pokas R, Hufnagal VG: *Hysterectomies in the United States, 1965-84,* Vital and Health Statistics Series 13 No 92 DHHS Pub No. (PHS) 88-1753, National Center for Health Statistics, Washington, DC, 1987, US Government Printing Office.

30. *Quality assurance program in obstetrics and gynecology,* Washington, DC, 1989, American College of Obstetricians and Gynecologists.

31. Silverberg E: Cancer statistics 1984, *CA-Cancer J Clin* 34:7, 1984.

32. *Standards for obstetric-gynecologic services,* ed 6, Washington, DC, 1985, American College of Obstetricians and Gynecologists.
33. Symmonds RE, Pratt JH, Welch JS: Total abdominal hysterectomy by the Mayo Clinic (Masson-Counseller) technique, *Surg Gynecol Obstet* 113:379, 1961.
34. Thompson JD: *Hysterectomy.* In Thompson JD, Rock JA, editors: *Te Linde's operative gynecology,* ed 7, Philadelphia, 1992, JB Lippincott, p 687.
35. Uchida H, Uchida M: Uchida's abdominal simple hysterectomy, film presentation. Tenth World Congress of Gynecology and Obstetrics, Oct 1982, San Francisco, CA
36. Whitelaw RG: Ovarian activity following hysterectomy, *J Obstet Gynecol Br Emp* 65:917, 1958.
37. Yagi H: Treatment of carcinoma of the cervix uteri, *Surg Gynecol Obstet* 95:552, 1950.

Some technical points and indications for hysterectomy

David H. Nichols

Hysterectomy is second only to cesarean section as the most frequently performed major operation in the United States.[4] Data from the National Hospital Discharge Survey indicate that approximately 590,000 hysterectomies are performed annually,[4] and that over one third of women in the United States have undergone hysterectomy by the age of 60.[9]

A composite of the route for hysterectomy related to the indications for the operation is given in Table 31-1. Often more than one indication may be found in the preoperative evaluation of the patient.[10]

INDICATIONS FOR HYSTERECTOMY

The most common indication for a total abdominal hysterectomy is myoma (fibroid) of the uterus.[1,2,7] Of the vast majority of women who have fibroids, only a small fraction ever require a hysterectomy. This percentage depends on the conservative attitude of the surgeon, the position and symptoms caused by the fibroids, and the alternate choice of myomectomy being considered. The more common indications for removal of fibroids are as follows: (1) the presence of bleeding that cannot be controlled by medical or expectant treatment—this constitutes the bulk of the indications for surgery; (2) much less frequently, the presence of pain or urinary and rectal symptoms; (3) an intraligamentary tumor that compresses the ureter on one side or the other and requires removal before a hydronephrosis develops. The postmenopausal uterus may have to be removed if rapid growth of the fibroids suggests that they are undergoing degeneration or hemorrhage if painful, or development of a leiomyosarcoma if not painful. A pedunculated myoma may twist on its pedicle, and some have become parasitic and adherent to bowel or omentum. In some instances, the size and number of the fibroids obscure the pelvic examination, even if done under anesthesia, so that a solid ovarian tumor sometimes cannot be excluded without a laparotomy. The use of radium and x-ray in the management of fibroid tumors has been discarded.

A hysterectomy may be indicated because of endometriosis or adenomyosis that is far advanced in its destructive course. The young patients on whom conservative surgery cannot be done for endometriosis are rare indeed. However, in the older age group or in those patients in whom involvement of the bowel and bladder is seriously impairing the vital functions of the urinary and gastrointestinal tracts, a hysterectomy and bilateral salpingo-oophorectomy may have to be done, despite the desire of the surgeon to preserve the childbearing and menstrual functions.

Chronic pelvic inflammatory disease formerly was a common indication for hysterectomy. The advent of antimicrobial therapy and effective surgical drainage on laparoscopic aspiration have reduced the number of patients requiring this operation for pelvic infection. When recurrent pelvic inflammatory disease has compromised the health of a patient and has involved other vital structures in the pelvis, a total hysterectomy is indicated unless the patient wishes to be a candidate for future in vitro fertilization, in which case salpingectomy alone should be considered, with conservation of ovarian tissue if possible, and if she is premenopausal.

There are a group of indications on the basis of chronic uterine bleeding in which the surgeon is unable to demonstrate the presence of submucous myomas, polyps, hyperplasia, or other organic disease and coagulopathies have been excluded. It is the second most frequent indication for hysterectomy.[7] After failure to control the bleeding by hormonal methods and two or more curettages, a hysterectomy is the last resort for dysfunctional uterine bleeding. In the surgery of malignant ovarian tumors, the uterus and cervix are removed at operation. Some of the less common indications for hysterectomy are as follows: Cesarean hysterectomy is indicated if the uterus fails to contract and the patient continues to bleed. A fibroid uterus in an older multigravida may be removed at the time of section. The cesarean section should be indicated for appropriate obstetric reasons. A hysterectomy may have to be done in the treatment of a septic abortion, for a chronic pyometra, or for chronic inversion of the uterus. The type of operation recommended for fundal malignancy, is described elsewhere.

Intrafascial and extrafascial hysterectomy

Although the terms intrafascial and extrafascial are popular when describing the techniques of hysterectomy, they are basically misnomers—there being no fascia, per se—although the uterus and each organ adjacent to it are surrounded by a connective tissue capsule. (For this reason, a more appropriate choice of description might be intracapsular or extracapsular hysterectomy.)

Table 31-1. Route for hysterectomy

Indication	Vaginal	Abdominal	Combined	Observation laparoscopy plus vaginal hysterectomy	Laser assisted	Laser
Myomata uterus	Occasionally	Usually	Rarely	Occasionally	Occasionally	Occasionally
Pelvic inflammatory disease	Rarely	Usually	Rarely	Occasionally	Occasionally	Rarely
Recurrent-dysfunctional uterine bleeding	Usually	Occasionally	Rarely	Rarely	Rarely	Occasionally
Endometriosis	Rarely	Usually, except for involvement of cervix, vagina, or vulva	Occasionally	Frequently	Frequently	Rarely
Leiomyoma:						
Longer than 12 weeks gestational size	Rarely	Usually	Occasionally	Rarely	Occasionally	Rarely
Less than 12 weeks gestational size	Frequently	Occasionally	Rarely	Occasionally	Occasionally	Occasionally
Adenomyosis	Usually	Occasionally	Rarely	Rarely	Rarely	Rarely
Symptomatic pelvic relaxation	Usually	Occasionally	Occasionally	Rarely	Rarely	Never
Adnexal mass	Never	Usually	Occasionally	Frequently	Occasionally	Rarely
Pelvic pain	Rarely	Occasionally	Rarely	Occasionally	Rarely	Rarely
Cancer of cervix:						
Stage 0 and A	Usually	Occasionally	Rarely	Rarely	Rarely	Never
Stage Ia, Ib, IIa	Occasionally radical vaginal hysterectomy	Usually	Occasionally	Rarely	Rarely	Never
Corpus cancer	Occasionally	Usually	Rarely	Rarely	Rarely	Never
History of previous pelvic surgery	Frequently	Frequently	Occasionally	Occasionally	Occasionally	Rarely
Nulliparity	Frequently	Frequently	Rarely	Rarely	Rarely	Occasionally
Morbid obesity	Usually	Occasionally	Occasionally	Occasionally	Rarely	Rarely

Modified from Thompson JD: *Clin Obstet Gynecol* 24:1255, 1981.

Most hysterectomies, and virtually all vaginal hysterectomies, should be extrafascial, with precise and careful sharp dissection employed to separate the bladder from the lower uterine segment and cervix. This technique is readily learned and, with regular practice, becomes comfortable for the surgeon and safe for the patient.

For the patient requiring an abdominal hysterectomy who has a poorly supported vault, it is particularly important to preserve the identity and integrity of the cardinal-uterosacral ligament complex requiring that these structures, now shortened with hysterectomy, be incorporated in the support of the vaginal vault postoperatively. This may be easier to accomplish by using an "endofascial" hysterectomy than an "extrafascial" hysterectomy.

The extrafascial hysterectomy, however, is probably safer than its endofascial counterpart and is associated with less blood loss and weakness. The cardinal-uterosacral ligament complex is harder to define and mobilize with transabdominal hysterectomy than with with vaginal hysterectomy.[3]

Total vaginal hysterectomy for the patient without prolapse is more likely to be of the extrafascial type, although, for the patient with prolapse, an endofascial dissection might make it possible to more effectively mobilize the cardinal-uterosacral ligament complex for incorporation in the support of the vault after hysterectomy.[3]

Support of the vaginal vault at the time of total abdominal hysterectomy

A deep cul-de-sac may represent an enterocele or potential enterocele and, when seen at the time of laparotomy, should be obliterated. The usual choice of procedure in the past had been a Moschcowitz or Halban procedure (see Chapter 26), but the former risks ureteral kinking and the latter may, when the stitches are tied, shorten the former cul-de-sac although it does not risk disturbance in the pathway of the ureter. Because the goal of obliteration of the cul-de-sac is to oppose the anterior to the posterior surface of the cul-de-sac of Douglas, these faces may be obliterated by a running back-and-forth suture from one side to the other, starting at the bottom of the cul-de-sac. This is continued in ascending levels back and forth, gradually obliterating the cul-de-sac until the pelvic brim is reached. It is not necessary to excise the peritoneum of the cul-de-sac. Either permanent suture or long-lasting absorbable suture may be used.

The surgeon should have determined preoperatively by examination of the pelvis and supporting tissues of the cervix (when traction has been applied to it), in particular whether the cardinal-uterosacral ligament complex has sufficient strength to be used to support the vault of the vagina after hysterectomy. This may be accomplished by shortening and then attaching the cardinal-uterosacral ligament complex to the vaginal vault, or if strong but quite elongated, an abdominal New Orleans or McCall-type cul-de-plasty may be employed.[13] If strong tissues for this purpose are lacking, the surgeon should plan to add colpopexy as an additional step of the primary operative procedure. The need for this should be established first by the preoperative examination (and confirmed later by the examination under anesthesia immediately preceding hysterectomy) so a suitable informed consent form can be given to the patient concerning the possibility of coincident colpopexy, the operating room can be properly notified to prepare for this possible procedure, and the surgeon can refresh his or her knowledge of this technique and, if this is lacking, the surgeon can seek ahead of time to obtain the best surgical assistance available, preferably someone experienced with the techniques of colpopexy.

Prophylactic oophorectomy at time of hysterectomy

Enthusiasm for elective oophorectomy at the time of hysterectomy to reduce the risk of future ovarian cancer in the woman between 35 and 45 years of age must be tempered by the negative effects of lack of compliance in taking estrogen therapy postoperatively.[11] Unless the patient takes the recommended estrogen replacement, the adverse effects on the bones and cardiovascular system outweigh the benefit of preventing ovarian cancer, although the high-risk patient (family history, never pregnant, never took oral contraceptives) may constitute an exception.[8]

If the surgeon has decided to leave the peritoneum open after hysterectomy, the retained ovary may become retroperitoneal or adherent to the vaginal cuff and the subject for future painful symptoms and oophorectomy. Therefore, the surgeon should either suspend the ovary or close the pelvic peritoneum to prevent a residual ovary syndrome.

To suspend a prolapsed ovary transabdominally, it may be sewn to the round ligament, or better a retroperitoneal tunnel can be made through the pelvic sidewall. The peritoneum is opened again, and the ovary is led through this tunnel, and brought back into the body cavity at the site of the second peritoneal perforation.[12]

Laparoscopic hysterectomy

Laparoscopic-assisted vaginal hysterectomy is not a substitute for vaginal hysterectomy but may be a substitute for a total abdominal hysterectomy when the condition and removability of the adnexa are uncertain. The infundibulopelvic ligament (or ovarian ligament if ovarian conservation is elected) may be translaparoscopically transected and secured, as well as the round ligament and upper broad ligament. Peritoneal flaps may be established. If there is no significant attenuation of the paracervical support, other steps of the hysterectomy may be developed, particularly transsection of the paracervical areas and uterosacral ligaments, depending on the skills and experience of the laparoscopist. The uterus is usually removed transvaginally.

If the cardinal-uterosacral ligament support is compromised by stretched or attenuated cardinal and uterosacral ligaments, their detachment from the cervix might be best addressed by using a primary transvaginal approach, which permits a safe New Orleans or McCall-type cul-de-plasty (see Chapter 20), to ensure support of the vaginal vault postoperatively.

Subtotal hysterectomy

Although invasive squamous cell carcinoma of the cervical stump accounted for 5% of the new cervix cancer patients seen at the Roswell Park Memorial Institute in Buffalo, NY, 30 years ago, these occurred, for the most part, among women who had not been receiving regular pelvic examinations, cytology smears, or colposcopy. That observation, similar to those made elsewhere, was a major reason for advocating total hysterectomy whenever removal of the uterus was indicated, and this view went so far as to find subtotal hysterectomy forbidden on certain gynecologic teaching services, influencing the habits and practices of a whole generation of pelvic surgeons.

Prevalent conditions have changed to a degree since the early 1980s. Dogmatic pronouncements have been ameliorated, and the patients' perceptions and views that have challenged this dictum are being discussed and brought into the doctor-patient relationship. The ultimate surgical decision more likely is to be made as much by the patient as by the surgeon, although invariably with the surgeon's advice concerning specific treatment options.

When hysterectomy is required, the surgeon may wish to consider several indications for the subtotal procedure.

For the patient with severe endometriosis, and intractable menometrorrhagia and pain who may require hysterectomy, it is sometimes found at surgery that not only has the cul-de-sac of Douglas been totally obliterated by endometriosis, but that the latter disease has infiltrated the anterior muscular wall of the rectum, uniting it to the uterosacral ligaments, the posterior wall of the bladder and the cervix, without a plane of cleavage. If the cervix is otherwise more physiologically "normal," and the cytology is negative, surgical discretion may suggest that it be left behind at hysterectomy.[1] Although it may be technically feasible to remove the cervix in this instance, the risk:benefit ratio may favor a conservative approach of leaving the otherwise normal cervix in situ, although much of the endocervical canal may be excised with the hysterectomy

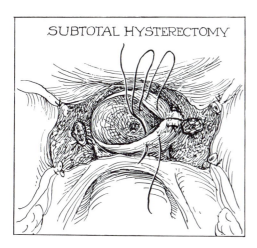

Fig. 31-35. Subtotal abdominal hysterectomy. The infundibulopelvic and round ligaments have been clamped, cut, and ligated, as well as the ascending branches of the uterine artery. The uterine fundus has been amputated from the cervix at the internal os. A reverse "conization" may be performed, if desired, excising the endocervical canal. The edges of the cervical stump are brought together by a series of interrupted sutures. (From Ball TL: *Gynecologic surgery and urology,* ed 2, St Louis, 1963, Mosby–Year Book.)

specimen by dissection using a reverse conization (Fig. 31-35). In this circumstance, the more radical procedure may be to excise the cervix, risking operative injury to the bladder, ureter, or rectum.[1]

The next indication for subtotal hysterectomy concerns meeting, if possible, the medico-social expectations of certain ethnic groups that require the woman to give evidence of monthly menstruation during her reproductive years to demonstrate her femininity to her husband and family. This requirement can be fulfilled by tailoring the patient's hysterectomy to that of a subtotal operation, in which a small bit of normally functioning endometrium is conserved within the retained stump. This social more is seen commonly among women of African descent. If the patient introduces the subject in preoperative conversation, the concept should be thoroughly discussed with the surgeon, and the decision should be understood by both parties.

An uncommon but useful indication for subtotal hysterectomy exists in the parous patient born with bladder exstrophy who has developed a genital prolapse, especially one that involves a large segment of the poorly supported anterior vaginal wall. Jones has remedied this by performing a ventral suspension of the cervical stump after subtotal hysterectomy and attaching the stump with nonabsorbable sutures to the retroperitoneal area of the anterior abdominal wall beneath the lower pole of a rather high midline abdominal incision.[5]

There are times when the uterus must be removed coincident with cesarean section—usually to arrest an immediate postpartum hemorrhage that cannot be otherwise controlled. If the cesarean incision in the uterus had been

made transversely and there is no coincident cervical or vaginal laceration, the obstetrician can easily clamp and cut the broad, round, and ovarian ligaments, and continue the uterine incision transversely and posteriorly to effect a subtotal hysterectomy. When the patient has been in labor before cesarean section, and the cervix is completely effaced and fully dilated, it may be difficult for the obstetrician to determine with precision the exact margin of the cervix, making the otherwise obvious landmarks of the cervix difficult to find, because the lower margins of the cervix blend smoothly into the walls of the vagina.

A vocal minority of women believe that the female sexual response to coitus is related directly to the presence of the cervix and its nerve supply, although there is no objective proof of this observation, and a prevailing concentration of opinion seems overwhelmingly to the contrary.[6]

Prerequisites for subtotal hysterectomy include a negative cytology, absence of a genital prolapse, and preoperative patient consent if the procedure is to be elective.

With total hysterectomy, the ligamentous attachments to the uterus and cervix should be deliberately attached to the vaginal vault providing for its future support. With total hysterectomy, the effective reattachment of the uterine ligaments to the vagina may be overlooked.[3] Although subtotal or total hysterectomy can be done by the laparoscopic approach, the ability to effectively reattach the uterine ligaments to the vagina may be lost.

It was widely believed that the cervix was a principal source of vaginal moisture and lubrication, and without it the vaginal wall would become so dry that comfortable coitus would be impossible. We now know that the vaginal fluid is a direct transudate from the vagina vault, which is reabsorbed distally, creating a circulation of vaginal fluid.

The technique of subtotal hysterectomy is a modification of that for total hysterectomy. The round, broad, and ovarian or infondibulopelvic ligaments are clamped, cut, and ligated, and the peritoneum covering the bladder is incised transversely, permitting the bladder to be dissected from the lower uterine segment. This dissection is carried down to the level of the internal cervical os, and, when the ascending cervical branch of the uterine artery has been secured on each side of the pelvis, the cervix is cut across and the uterus is amputated. If removal of a portion of the endocervical canal is desired, it may be accomplished by a reverse "conization." The anterior and posterior edges of the site of amputation are brought together by a series of interrupted sutures, if desired, and the anterior peritoneum and bladder flap may be brought over the top of the cervical stump and fixed to its posterior peritoneal surface. The strength and length of the uterosacral ligaments and depth of the cul-de-sac are examined, and their strength and surgical usefulness are reaffirmed. The uterosacral ligaments may be sewn to one another at the site of their insertion into the posterior cervix, and any deep cul-de-sac or enterocele that has been identified should be obliterated.

Werner and Sederl[14] have described a technique for vaginal subtotal hysterectomy for consideration if the patient is obese, an abdominal incision is contraindicated, there is good cardinal-uterosacral ligament support, a "normal" cervix is present that is cytologically unremarkable, and the patient wants the cervix preserved, believing that it enhances her sexual fulfillment. Transvaginal subtotal hysterectomy may be performed, the technique for which is as follows: If the patient wishes, the corpus can be amputated about one fingerwidth cranial to the internal cervical os, which preserves sufficient endometrium for a small amount of monthly menstruation. Occasionally, it will be found in a patient for whom transvaginal myomectomy was planned that there is insufficient myometrium left for effective reconstruction, and, if fertility is not an issue, fundectomy or subtotal hysterectomy may be accomplished, provided that the uterine fundus is freely movable and there is no inflammation present. A midline incision is made in the anterior vaginal wall, and the bladder is separated from the lower uterine surface up to the anterior vesicouterine peritoneal fold, which is opened. The surgeon, proceeding bite by bite with a pair of tenacula, proceeds to the fundus of the uterus and, through the opening in the peritoneum anterior to the uterus, draws the corpus down into the vagina. The adnexa are detached, and with the surgeon holding the corpus between the thumb and palmar surfaces of the fingers of one hand, the posterior wall of the uterus is incised horizontally one fingerwidth above the internal cervical os. The incision must go through the entire thickness of the endometrium. The branches of the uterine artery are clamped, cut, and ligated separately. The upper margin of the remaining cervix is grasped by a tenaculum, and the anterior wall of the uterus is cut from the cervix, completing the excision of the fundus.

The cut cranial edges of the remaining cervix are brought together by a series of interrupted stitches. Any enterocele may be excised or obliterated, and the uterosacral ligaments may be brought to one another by transperitoneal plication. The bladder peritoneum is tacked to the posterior wall of the cervical stump, and the cut edge of the vagina is fixed to the anterior remaining cervical stump by a few interrupted sutures. Any necessary colporrhaphy can now be performed.

SUMMARY

Many patients requiring hysterectomy have more than one indication for their surgery, and the decision for hysterectomy is based on a number of circumstances, with care and recommendations individualized for each patient. Length of hospital stay is influenced by its affordability, both by the patient and by the health care delivery system, and, thus, as the daily cost of hospitalization continues to rise, cost effectiveness will become more significant and directly correlated with frequency of performance.

Significant regional variations in the rate and numbers of hysterectomy in the United States have not been thoroughly explained.[2]

REFERENCES

1. Ball TL: *Gynecologic surgery and urology,* ed 2, St Louis, 1963, Mosby–Yearbook, p 325.
2. Carlson KJ, Nichols DH, Schiff I: Indications for hysterectomy, *N Engl J Med* (in press).
3. DeLancey JOL: Anatomic aspects of vaginal eversion after hysterectomy, *Am J Obstet Gynecol* 166:1717, 1992.
4. Graves EJ: National hospital discharge survey: annual summary, 1990, National Center for Health Statistics, *Vital Health Stat* Series 13, No. 112, 1992.
5. Jones HW Jr: Personal communication, July 1990.
6. Kilkku PP: *Total versus subtotal abdominal hysterectomy.* In Garcia C-R, Mikuta JJ, Rosenblum NG, editors: *Current therapy in surgical gynecology,* Philadelphia, 1987, BC Decker, p 58.
7. Lee NC et al: Confirmation of the preoperative diagnoses for hysterectomy, *Am J Obstet Gynecol* 150:283, 1984.
8. Morrow CP, discussing Speroff T, Dawson NV, Speroff L, Haber RJ. A Risk-benefit analysis of elective bilateral oophorectomy: effect of changes in compliance with estrogen therapy on outcome. *Am J Obstet Gynecol* 164:165-174, 1991. In Mishell DR, Kirshbaum TH, Morrow CP (eds), *Yearbook of obstetrics and gynecology,* 1992, p 209.
9. Pokras R, Hufnagel VG: Hysterectomies in the United States, 1965-84, National Center for Health Statistics, *Vital Health Stat* Series 13, No. 92, 1987, DHHS Pub. No. (PHS)87-1753.
10. Ranney B: Multiple diagnoses and procedures during hysterectomy, *Int J Gynecol Obstet* 33:325, 1990.
11. Speroff T et al: A risk-benefit analysis of elective bilateral oophorectomy: effect of changes in compliance with estrogen therapy on outcome, *Am J Obstet Gynecol* 164:165, 1991.
12. Thompson JD: Personal communication, 1990.
13. Thompson JD: *Hysterectomy.* In Thompson JD, Rock JA, editors: *TeLinde's operative gynecology,* ed 7, Philadelphia, 1992, JB Lippincott, p 702.
14. Werner P, Sederl J: *Abdominal operations by the vaginal route* (translated by LM Szamek), Philadelphia, 1958, JB Lippincott, p 79.

Chapter 32

EXTENSIVE PELVIC DISEASE AND THE DIFFICULT HYSTERECTOMY

John J. Mikuta

The term "difficult" hysterectomy may be applied for a variety of reasons. For instance, if a patient is morbidly obese or has significant medical disease such as hypertension, cardiovascular disease, or diabetes, these will add to the complexity and risk of the operation. Likewise, the inability to administer ideal anesthesia to the patient may create problems for the surgeon in achieving adequate exposure, visibility, and working conditions to ensure that the operation goes smoothly. Finally, there are difficulties and anatomical distortions created by diseases of the pelvic reproductive organs and surrounding organs. This chapter identifies various approaches from anatomical and surgical standpoints that may make a difficult hysterectomy feasible and perhaps even easy.

One of the critical issues with respect to the difficult hysterectomy is that the gynecologist identifies the fact that the operation will be a difficult one. Once this is done, the next issue is one of adequate concentration and thought on difficulties that may be encountered so that all potential hazards and the complications that might ensue will be properly considered in advance. A thorough knowledge of pelvic anatomy is essential, more specifically a thorough acquaintance with the retroperitoneal area, where those structures are located that provide the uterine blood and lymphatic supply, the uterine supports and the proximate structures such as the ureters, bladder and rectum, which must be identified. By and large, an atlas of surgical procedures, while in its own way a valuable tool, does not always provide the surgeon with the necessary information to deal with the unexpected vagaries that may be encountered in real life. A thorough knowledge of the anatomy relating to the pelvic organs plus excellent surgical technique provide much better surgical results than a step-by-step rote knowledge of a given operation. Nothing is more greatly appreciated by the surgeon than having had ample experience in dealing with a multitude of problems and in knowing the sight, touch, and feel of various disease processes and how to deal with them. Flexibility, variability, and ability to change one's course at will, and as indicated, are the hallmarks of a confident, experienced, and capable surgeon.

CAUSES OF EXTENSIVE PELVIC DISEASE

The major causes of extensive pelvic disease contributing to the difficult hysterectomy can be generally considered in five categories: prior infections, prior surgery, benign growths, malignant growths, and prior radiation therapy. It is important in the evaluation of the patient to determine which of these possibilities exists. For instance, the type of prior surgery (e.g., cesarean section, tubal reconstruction, and so forth) may be of significance in defining what potential problems may be encountered, whereas infections such as gonoccocal salpingitis, tuboovarian abscess, or ruptured appendix have their own specific impact on the surgical difficulty.

The most common benign growths encountered are uterine myomata, endometriosis, and adenomyosis. Malignant growths of the adnexa, such as ovarian carcinoma, may contribute to the difficulty of a hysterectomy depending on the extent of the disease or size of tumor, but carcinoma of the endometrium and cervix, although usually requiring more extensive or radical surgery, generally do not complicate the operation. One word should be mentioned concerning prior radiation therapy. The procedure may be complicated, first, by the fact that the surrounding structures may be more adherent and, second, the intestinal tract must be treated with great respect because even a minor degree of intraoperative trauma to the radiated intestine may create a tendency for postoperative intestinal wall breakdown resulting in fistula formation or peritonitis.

DIAGNOSTIC EVALUATION

The diagnostic evaluation should always include a thorough history and physical examination. The conditions mentioned above can usually be readily identified. Special attention to the physical examination of the pelvis by the gynecologist should allow the identification of areas that may be a source of trouble in the course of the hysterectomy. The first of these would be the anatomical changes the surgeon will have to face. The pelvic examination should help define the size of the lesion, whether it is fixed or mobile; whether the cul-de-sac is free, obliterated, or "frozen"; whether the uterus can be lifted out of the pelvis; and whether the disease is predominantly uterine, adnexal, or possibly of another nature. Pelvic ultrasound (US), computed tomography (CT) scan, and magnetic resonance imaging (MRI) cannot substitute for this examination.

The assessment of the patient with the history and findings of the potentially difficult hysterectomy should include a pelvic US, and evaluation of the urinary tract as indicated, by intravenous pyelogram, retrograde pyelogram, and cystoscopy. The lower intestinal tract should be evaluated by barium enema and sigmoidoscopy, and, in situations where it is warranted, the use of CT and MRI is of help. The use of preoperative diagnostic laparoscopy may or may not be helpful, depending on the physical findings, the history, and the evaluation just noted.

PREOPERATIVE PREPARATION

As with any operation, the patient should be given as much information as possible with respect to potential problems with the surrounding structures such as ureters, bowel, and bladder. Some procedures such as cystoscopy and sigmoidoscopy may be put off until the time of operation. In anticipation of any possible intestinal complications, a bowel preparation is indicated as a part of the preoperative preparation. There may be a need for ureteral catheterization before the operation. This should be discussed with a urologist or gynecologic oncologist, particularly if there is significant ureteral deviation, constriction, or dilatation.

Another issue deals with the necessity for blood replacement. Today, whenever anticipated blood loss may be significant, it is advisable to suggest to the patient that she set aside one or two units of her own blood for transfusion during or after the procedure. Because many of these procedures are not of an emergency nature, it is possible to have this carried out without any detriment and probably with great benefit to the patient. Designated donors such as family members or friends are also of great help when time is of importance or the patient's condition does not allow her to donate her own blood.

OPERATIVE PLAN
Incision

The type of incision the surgeon selects may be important in the avoidance of injury upon abdominal entry. For instance, if the patient has had a prior paramedian or midline incision, it is conceivable that underlying this area there will be the potential for significant intestinal adhesions that may create problems upon entry into the peritoneal cavity. This could lead to either intestinal injury or loss of valuable time in achieving a clear way into the abdomen. An incision in a different site and direction (e.g., transverse) may be a wise choice. When a vertical incision has been used in the past, a transverse incision may allow the surgeon to find an area laterally where the peritoneum and intestinal tract are not adherent so that under direct visualization the incision can be extended and any adherent bowel close to the midline incision may be more safely dissected (Fig. 32-1). In general, after incising the fascia, I have found it helpful to pick up the fascia with a stout clamp such as a Kocher and then, after entering the peritoneal cavity, to take the peritoneum also into the Kocher to provide ample traction. This allows a delineation of the areas that are adherent to the parietal peritoneal surface and outlines the adherent tissues to be sharply dissected. Ideally, separation of the intestine from the parietal peritoneum or from itself is best done by the use of gentle traction and sharp dissection with fine scissors.

ABDOMINAL EXPLORATION

After achieving abdominal entry, attention is paid to identifying structures and assessing the location of various organs in relation to each other. In patients who had prior surgery or inflammatory disease, the omentum may be found attached loosely or densely to the pelvic structures. If the omental adhesions are filmy and easily resectable, these can be freed without removing any of this structure. If, however, the omentum is found to be densely adherent to the parietal peritoneum or to other areas of the pelvic organs or the bowel, it may be helpful to cut across the omentum leaving a portion attached to the structures that are going to be removed.

IDENTIFICATION OF PELVIC LANDMARKS

After omental or intestinal adhesions have been separated and the small and large intestines have been brought up as much as possible out of the pelvis and packed away, the various pelvic structures are identified. It is usually easy to find the uterine fundus, the round ligaments, the infundibulopelvic ligaments, posterior cul-de-sac, anterior cul-de-sac, the peritoneum over the bladder, and the pelvic brim. However, pathologic distortion of these areas may make the procedure difficult. At this point, it is helpful to assess the intraperitoneal structures in relationship to each

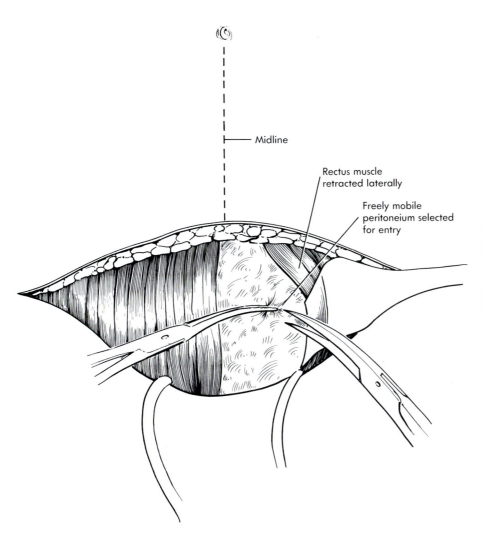

Fig. 32-1. A transverse incision has been made through the skin and rectus fascia and the rectus muscles separated in the midline. The rectus muscle has been displaced laterally, as shown, and the freely mobile peritoneum grasped by the tip of a Kocher hemostat prior to entry.

other and to the disease process. Although the peritoneum is known to be a single-cell, layered structure, when it is distended, stretched, and folded on itself as it might be with uterine fibroids, ovarian masses, retroperitoneal masses and the like, a tensile strength may be present that may impede the mobility of the pelvic structures. At this point, it is wise for the surgeon to select an area for entry into the retroperitoneum because in this area the blood supply to the tubes, ovaries, uterus, bladder, and vagina can be identified and the blood supply is secured here before removal of these structures. In addition, one can identify the ureter as it comes into the pelvis so that it can be kept under direct vision during ligation of the infundibulopelvic ligament and during the dissection of the peritoneum around the uterus.

ENTRY INTO THE RETROPERITONEUM

The retroperitoneum may be entered through several different locations. In ordinary circumstances when the uterus is going to be removed, with or without removal of the adnexa, and when the disease process is limited, several points may be considered for entry. My preference has always been to enter retroperitoneally just below the level

of the pelvic brim if the tube and ovary are to be removed. The infundibulopelvic ligament is elevated with a Babcock clamp about 2 to 3 cm below the pelvic brim and, staying as close as possible to the tube and ovary with the help of forceps and scissors, a small opening is made into the peritoneum on the medial side of the infundibulopelvic ligament (Fig. 32-2). This entrance is enlarged carefully cephalad and caudad, after which the index fingers of each hand may be placed into the retroperitoneal space. The opening is further enlarged, bringing the ureter into view on the medial retroperitoneal surface. If the infundibulopelvic ligament is not going to be ligated, the entry may be more readily accomplished by elevating the infundibulopelvic ligament as just described, bringing it medially, and making an incision into the peritoneum lateral to it from the round ligament in a cephalad direction along the infundibulopelvic ligament. This allows one to separate the peritoneum along with the ureter and the infundibulopelvic ligament from the side of the pelvis, allowing entry into the retroperitoneal area (Fig. 32-3). It is then simple to ligate the round ligament.

A third method of retroperitoneal entry is by clamping, dividing, and ligating the round ligament, which allows

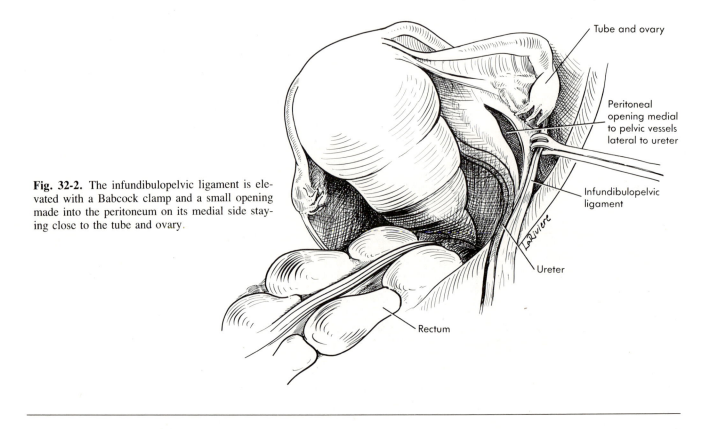

Fig. 32-2. The infundibulopelvic ligament is elevated with a Babcock clamp and a small opening made into the peritoneum on its medial side staying close to the tube and ovary.

Tube and ovary

Peritoneal opening medial to pelvic vessels lateral to ureter

Infundibulopelvic ligament

Ureter

Rectum

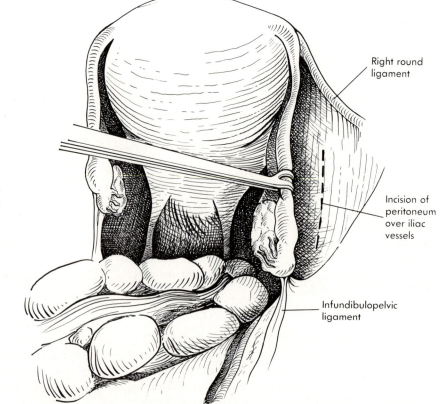

Fig. 32-3. If the ovary is to be preserved, the elevated infunibulopelvic ligament is brought medially and an incision is made into the peritoneum from the round ligament cephalad along the infundibulo ligament, as shown. The round ligament is then easily ligated.

Right round ligament

Incision of peritoneum over iliac vessels

Infundibulopelvic ligament

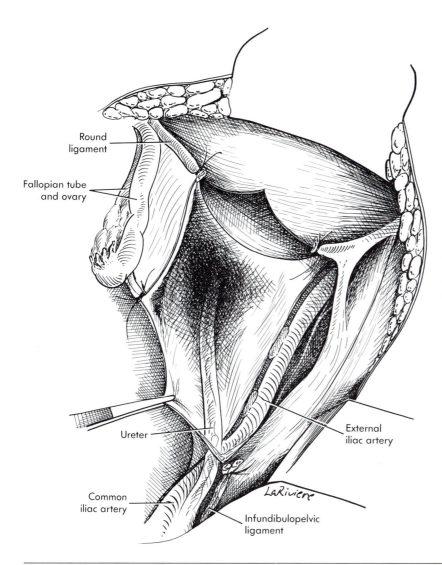

Fig. 32-4. An alternate method of retroperitoneal entry is by dividing the round ligament permitting direct entry into the retrovesical space and broad ligament adjacent to the uterus, as shown. This permits direct separation of the loose areolar tissue around the bladder.

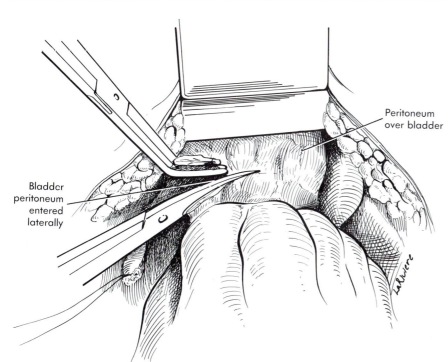

Fig. 32-5. The peritoneal bladder flap is dissected from the cervix by transverse incision, as shown.

Fig. 32-6. Yet another method of entry into the retroperitoneum is by elevating the peritoneum and entering the space beneath it laterally, following which the peritoneum is incised from one side to the other and separated from its remaining attachments to the cervix, as shown.

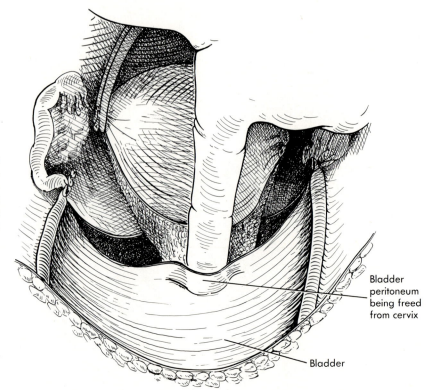

Bladder peritoneum being freed from cervix

Bladder

entry into the retrovesical space and into the area of the broad ligament adjacent to the uterus (Fig. 32-4). This also provides the ability to produce traction on the peritoneum and allows the separation of the areolar tissue around the bladder where it is not densely adherent. Continuation of dissection of the bladder flap from the cervix by going across from one side of the pelvis to the other is then accomplished (Fig. 32-5).

A fourth method of entry into the retroperitoneum is by going directly to the bladder flap and making an entry lateral to the midline with the peritoneum elevated. As the retroperitoneum is entered, the incision in the peritoneum is carried across from one side to the other (Fig. 32-6).

It should be emphasized that retroperitoneal entry is basically the key to the performance of a safe, difficult hysterectomy and, for that matter, any hysterectomy. At times, it is possible to carry out a hysterectomy while seeing very little of the retroperitoneal structures. The use of the retroperitoneal approach, however, provides the surgeon with the ability to reach around structures that are fixed in the pelvis by the peritoneum, to elevate those structures out of the pelvis, to identify the blood supply, and to remove safely and carefully just about any type of pelvic pathology.

THE URETER

The gynecologist's dilemma still tends to be the ureter. When the retroperitoneal area has been entered at any point near the infundibulopelvic ligament from the pelvic brim to the round ligament, the ureter must be identified before anything else is done. Although at times the ureter

may be seen through the thin peritoneum as it comes over the common iliac artery down into the pelvis, it is generally not clearly visible and may be seen only after the peritoneum has been opened. The ureter should be identified in three ways: (1) Direct visualization (the ureter is usually white, nonpulsatile, with fine blood vessels coursing in a longitudinal fashion in the adventitia), (2) peristalsis, and (3) palpation. The ureter should be felt between the thumb and forefinger, and, as the surgeon rolls over this structure on the peritoneal surface, a definite "snap" will be felt (Fig. 32-7). It should also be noted that the left ureter near the level of the pelvic brim will be more ventral (i.e., closer) to the ovarian vessels than it is on the right side. This is due to the location of the sigmoid and its mesentery on the left side, which elevates the ureter in the ventral direction. Once the ureter has been identified, it should be left attached to the peritoneum as much as possible. Where the pathology to be removed is densely adherent to the peritoneum, the ureter may be separated from the retroperitoneal surface as far down into the pelvis as is necessary to allow the removal of the peritoneum along with the pathology, allowing the ureter to be kept safely away from the dissection and under direct vision at all times. The extent of this dissection will vary with the pathology, but occasionally may have to be carried down to the level of the broad ligament and at times even further (Fig. 32-8). The position of the ureter should never be assumed or taken for granted.

The ureter should never be handled excessively, and, when it has been freed, it is best to let it lie free rather than retracting it with either umbilical tapes or Penrose

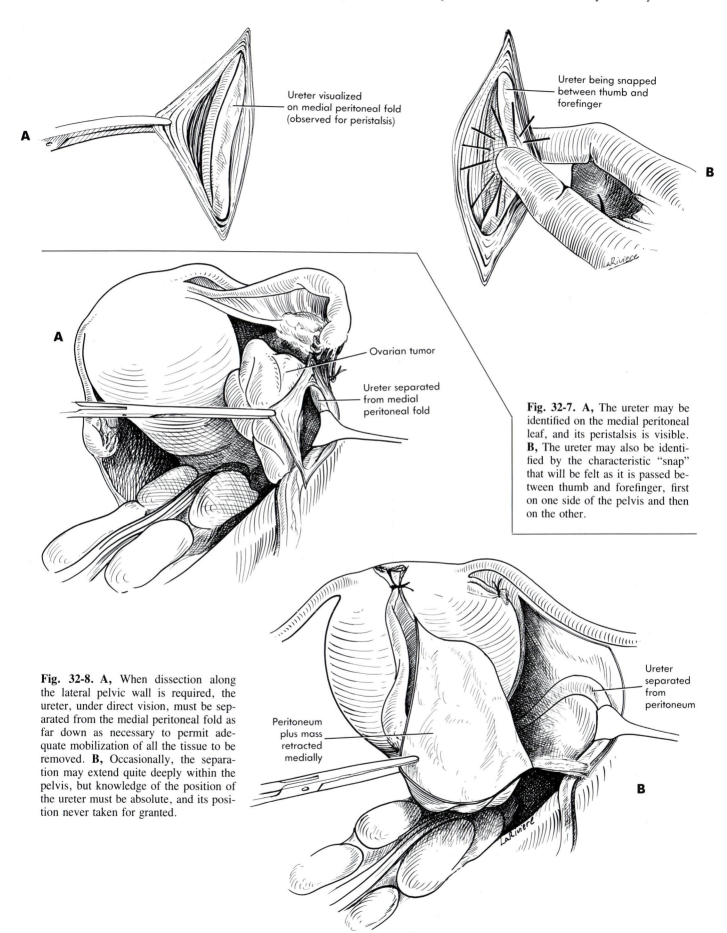

Ureter visualized on medial peritoneal fold (observed for peristalsis)

A

Ureter being snapped between thumb and forefinger

B

A

Ovarian tumor

Ureter separated from medial peritoneal fold

Fig. 32-7. A, The ureter may be identified on the medial peritoneal leaf, and its peristalsis is visible. **B,** The ureter may also be identified by the characteristic "snap" that will be felt as it is passed between thumb and forefinger, first on one side of the pelvis and then on the other.

Fig. 32-8. A, When dissection along the lateral pelvic wall is required, the ureter, under direct vision, must be separated from the medial peritoneal fold as far down as necessary to permit adequate mobilization of all the tissue to be removed. **B,** Occasionally, the separation may extend quite deeply within the pelvis, but knowledge of the position of the ureter must be absolute, and its position never taken for granted.

Peritoneum plus mass retracted medially

Ureter separated from peritoneum

B

drains. These may slide up and down the ureter, causing damage to the vasculature that lies in the adventitia of the ureter. The ureter may be gently held aside by hand or by a small retractor such as a vein retractor or a protected Deaver retractor.

DISSECTION OF THE BLADDER

Prior surgery in the bladder area, such as cesarean section, bladder advancement with uterine suspension, or reperitonealization with the bladder after myomectomy, may make the bladder adherent and hard to separate. Normally, the bladder peritoneum should be flexible, mobile, and easy to free from the cervix and vagina. Disease processes such as endometriosis, prior infection, or tumors of the ovaries or uterus may create difficulty in dissecting the bladder from the underlying uterus and cervix. There are several approaches that help make dissection of the bladder from the cervix and vagina more feasible. The first of these is to enter the retroperitoneal area laterally near the round ligaments because in this location the bladder may not have been involved in the prior dissection and the tissue may be more areolar and less dense than it is in the midline. Once this is accomplished, the bladder may be elevated by coming directly across the pelvis anterior to the cervix and uterus. By rolling one's finger or an instrument cephalad in the anterior leaf of the broad ligament, it can

be sharply separated from the cervix. In instances where the bladder is very densely adherent, the surgeon may be wise to make an incision into the dome of the bladder well away from the cervix so that the interior of the bladder can be visualized (deliberate cystotomy). The index finger is placed into the bladder so that one can identify the bladder reflection and cut through the dense adhesions between it and the cervix and vagina much more safely than doing it blindly.

THE "FROZEN" CUL-DE-SAC OF DOUGLAS

The usual definition of the posterior cul-de-sac bounded laterally by the uterosacral ligaments, posteriorly by the rectum and sacrum, and by vagina caudally may, at times, be totally lost depending on the type of pelvic pathology present. Extensive inflammatory disease, tumors of the tubes and ovaries, extensive pelvic endometriosis, prior infections of the pelvis with diverticular abscess or ruptured appendix all may create a situation in which the cul-de-sac is indefinable. In addition, it may be obliterated by the presence of large uterine myomas, which may fill the pelvic cavity and extend up beyond the sacral promontory into the abdominal cavity, thereby displacing the intestines and creating potential deviation and compression of the ureters (Fig. 32-9).

At times, this appearance may be more apparent than

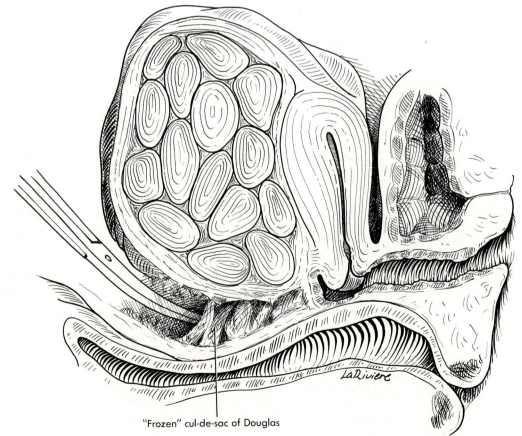

Fig. 32-9. The "frozen" cul-de-sac. The dissection of the cul-de-dac should be as close to the posterior surface of the uterus and cervix as possible, using both sharp and blunt dissection in the midline, until the uterosacral ligaments can be identified, clamped, and divided. Occasionally it is safer to first enter the vagina anteriorially to allow better definition of the relationship between the posterior uterus and cervix and adjacent bowel.

"Frozen" cul-de-sac of Douglas

real. As mentioned earlier, freeing up the peritoneal attachments both anteriorly and posteriorly as well as on the sides of the pelvis may release the pelvic contents to allow the elevation of the uterus into the abdominal cavity from whence the surgeon may proceed with identification of the ureter, the uterine vasculature, and the supporting ligaments. From that point, continuation of the dissection becomes relatively easy. However, when the rectum and uterus are densely adherent in the "frozen" cul-de-sac complex, the dissection becomes a very testy exercise. A basic principle of any approach to removing the uterus is to "hug" the uterus as much as possible, staying close to the posterior surface of the uterus and cervix using both sharp and blunt dissection. This allows one to find eventually a reasonable plane to enter the superior portion of the cul-de-sac between the uterosacral ligaments and at the point where they attach to the uterus. Most of the time, the tissue below this level gives way readily once the uterosacral ligaments have been clamped, divided, and ligated. It is unnecessary to go below this level to any great extent because the cervix has already been passed. Under certain conditions, entry into the vagina anteriorly may allow better definition of the relationship between the posterior uterus and cervix to the adherent bowel.

Although entry into the space between the bowel and vagina is generally safe and feasible, efforts to identify the endopelvic fascia on the posterior surface of the cervix may be attempted. It is my experience that the endopelvic fascia in this location does not have the same quality or integrity as that of the endopelvic fascia lying over the cer-

vix. Therefore, I think the approach described above is probably the safest.

It should be noted, as mentioned earlier, that, if the bowel is prepared, one should not fear a rectal enterotomy during this dissection. If it occurs, closure and drainage are all that is necessary, and a temporary colostomy can be avoided. In some circumstances, it may be necessary, if damage to the bowel is extensive, to carry out a bowel resection, but I have found this to be necessary rarely, and, if the anatomy is identified adequately beforehand, such a problem should not occur.

CONCLUSION

This chapter describes various approaches in the management of the so-called extensive pelvic disease difficult hysterectomy. Success in this kind of surgery depends on a thorough knowledge of the pelvic anatomy and the pathology of the disease processes that create anatomical distortions that the surgeon must surmount. The greatest ally a gynecologic or pelvic surgeon has is the ability to identify and use the retroperitoneal approaches and to understand the location and extent of the anatomy under consideration. Care must be taken to avoid injury to the urinary tract, the ureter and the bladder, to identify the vascular connections and blood supply to the uterus, and to separate the surrounding structures from the peritoneum of the pelvis, from the cervix, and from the rectum. A successful pelvic operation with the problems presented here should cause the patient minimal morbidity and minimal hospital stay if the basic principles described above are followed.

Chapter 33

SURGICAL STAGING OF CERVICAL CANCER

James H. Nelson, Jr.

It is important and fitting to include a chapter on surgical staging of cervical cancer in this compendium of obstetric and gynecologic surgery. It is also important in this discussion to make clear distinctions between clinical and surgical staging of cervical cancer. Clinical staging does not permit any examination or procedure except chest x-ray, which cannot provide absolute evidence of malignancy by histologic evaluation. In addition, it does not permit any examination or procedure that cannot be carried out by "the physicians and surgeons" in any hospital that is able to carry out a chest x-ray, cystoscopy, or proctosigmoidoscopy. The thrust for surgical staging came about as a natural evolution when new information began to emerge about the natural history of not only cervical carcinoma but endometrial carcinoma and ovarian carcinoma as well. An attempt is made here to contrast clinical and surgical staging as well as the values and weaknesses of each.

FIGO CLINICAL STAGING

Table 33-1 gives the FIGO classification of the clinical stages in carcinoma of the cervix.[1] The rules for clinical staging[1] are also reprinted here because herein lies the importance of FIGO classifications both in principle and in reality.

RULES FOR CLINICAL STAGING

The staging should be based on careful clinical examination and should be performed before any definitive therapy. The examination should be performed by an experienced examiner and with the patient under anesthesia.

The clinical stage must under no circumstances be changed on the basis of subsequent findings.

When it is doubtful to which stage a particular case should be allotted, the case must be referred to the earlier stage.

For staging purposes, the following examination methods are permitted: palpation, inspection, colposcopy, endocervical curettage, hysteroscopy, cystoscopy, proctoscopy, intravenous urography, and x-ray examination of the lungs and skeleton. Suspected bladder or rectal involvement should be confirmed by biopsy and histologic evidence.

Findings by examinations such as lymphangiography, arteriography, venography, and laparoscopy, are of value for the planning of therapy, but because these are not yet generally available and also because the interpretation of results is variable, the findings of such studies should not be the basis for changing the clinical staging.

Infrequently, hysterectomy is carried out in the presence of unsuspected extensive invasive cervical carcinoma. Such cases cannot be clinically staged or included in therapeutic statistics, but they should be reported separately.

Only if the rules for clinical staging are strictly observed is it possible to compare results among clinics and by differing modes of therapy.

Discussion of rules

All of the examination methods permitted, except x-ray examination of the lungs and skeleton, permit direct biopsy of tissue and, therefore, histologic proof of malignant tissue present either in the uterus, bladder, or rectum. Today, computed tomography (CT) scanning and magnetic resonance imaging (MRI) are used far more often than lymphangiography, arteriography, venography, or laparoscopy and are very valuable in the planning of therapy, but are not permitted to alter the clinical stage to which a patient's disease is assigned. The clinical stage must not be changed on the basis of subsequent findings. Surgical staging results cannot be allowed to influence the clinical stag-

Table 33-1. Definitions of the clinical stages in carcinoma of the cervix uteri (correlation between the FIGO, UICC, and AJCC nomenclatures)

Stage 0	Carcinoma in situ, intraepithelial carcinoma
	Cases of stage 0 should not be included in any therapeutic statistics for invasive carcinoma.
Stage I	The carcinoma is strictly confined to the cervix (extension of the corpus should be disregarded).
Stage Ia	Preclinical carcinomas of the cervix (i.e., those diagnosed only by microscopy).
Stage Ia1	Minimal microscopically evident stromal invasion.
Stage Ia2	Lesions detected microscopically that can be measured. The upper limit of the measurement should not show a depth of invasion of more than 5 mm taken from the base of the epithelium, either surface or glandular, from which it originates. A second dimension, the horizontal spread, must not exceed 7 mm. Larger lesions should be staged as Ib.
Stage Ib	Lesions of greater dimensions than stage Ia2 whether seen clinically or not. Performed space involvement should not alter the staging but should be specifically recorded so as to determine whether it should affect future treatment decisions.
Stage II	The carcinoma extends beyond the cervix but has not extended onto the pelvic wall. The carcinoma involves the vagina, but not as far as the lower third.
Stage IIa	No obvious parametrial involvement.
Stage IIb	Obvious parametrial involvement.
Stage III	The carcinoma has extended onto the pelvic wall. On rectal examination, there is no cancer-free space between the tumor and the pelvic wall. The tumor involves the lower third of the vagina. All cases with a hydronephrosis or nonfunctioning kidney should be included, unless they are known to be due to other cause.
Stage IIIa	No extension onto the pelvic wall, but involvement of the lower third of the vagina.
Stage IIIb	Extension onto the pelvic wall or hydronephrosis or nonfunctioning kidney.
Stage IV	The carcinoma has extended beyond the true pelvis or has clinically involved the mucosa of the bladder or rectum.
Stage IVa	Spread of the growth to adjacent organs.
Stage IVb	Spread to distant organs.

ing of a patient's disease. Once a stage has been entered in the patient's official medical record and treatment has been instituted, the patient's records concerning what stage her original lesion was should not be altered. If the patient develops recurrent disease, secondary staging is not carried out at that time. Instead, her disease is listed as recurrent disease. It is important to define the extent of recurrent disease for possible treatment, but it is classified as "recurrent disease with metastases" to sites proven. Any subsequent admissions for active disease should also come under the classification of recurrent disease. It is vitally important that these rules be accepted and practiced if gynecologic oncologists around the world are to continue to converse in a common language. This simple principle was the entire thrust of the initiators of the League of Nations Classification in 1928.[8] For the first time, physicians were able to communicate on the same clinical basis to compare methods of treatment. They were talking about patients with the same extent of disease so, when new methods did appear, the results could be compared to previous methods with reasonable speed. The diagnostic studies permitted were very wisely restricted to those procedures that could be done in any hospital. Equally important, however, and not immediately as apparent, was the fact that all of the studies permitted, except the chest and bone x-rays, were ones that permitted direct examination of anatomic areas and permitted biopsies of those areas if suspicious lesions were found. The only place that clinical impressions were permitted was in the bimanual and rectovaginal pelvic examinations done under anesthesia to determine whether nodular induration was present in the car-

dinal ligaments or uterosacral ligaments. Direct extension to the bladder, rectum, or upper vagina could be biopsied directly using the cystoscope, proctoscope, or vaginal speculum and the presence of disease could be proven beyond question.

SURGICAL STAGING

Surgical staging in gynecology originated as a formalized approach when Nelson first reported on staging laparotomy for 13 patients with stages IIb and III carcinoma of the cervix in January 1970, at the first Annual Clinical Meeting of the Society of Gynecologic Oncology.[11] Nelson followed with an overall plan for surgical staging in endometrial, ovarian, and cervical cancer at the National Conference on Gynecologic Cancer sponsored by the American Cancer Society in 1976.[9] The stimulus for this work was a 26-year-old woman with stage IIa carcinoma of the cervix who underwent laparotomy with the intention of carrying out a radical hysterectomy and pelvic node dissection and was found to have a large single paraaortic node replaced by metastatic epidermoid carcinoma. This raised the question: How often do we treat such patients with pelvic irradiation when disease has already extended beyond the pelvis? Of the 13 patients reported in January 1970, 7 had metastatic disease proven histologically in the paraaortic nodes well above the bifurcation of the aorta. In two of the seven patients, the metastases were microscopic foci. Eventually, the experience of Nelson's group at Downstate Medical Center was reported[10] and was confirmed by other investigators who carried out independent studies after hearing the presentation in January 1970[3,5,7]

Table 33-2. Surgical staging—cervical carcinoma stages IIB and III

	Stage IIb		Stage III	
Author	Cases	Positive nodes	Cases	Positive nodes
Nelson	31	5 (16.6%)	28	13 (46.4%)
Buchsbaum	11	1 (9.09%)	20	7 (35%)
Averette	9	2 (22.2%)	10	2 (20%)
LaGasse	52	19 (32.8%)	61	19 (31.1%)

(Table 33-2). Averette extended the idea from advanced stage patients to all patients with invasive cervical cancer.[3] The importance of this new information in the natural history of cervical carcinoma resides partly in the fact that it explained why institutions treating cervical cancer had not been able to improve their results in the preceding three decades. The ultimate importance of the new information was that it ignited a great curiosity in all of the cancer sites in gynecology resulting in a flood of new information about the natural history of ovarian and endometrial cancer.

What is the purpose of surgical staging? First and foremost, surgical staging is the best method available to accurately define the extent of disease before making a decision on treatment. Surgical staging should be aided as much as possible by all of the new technology such as CT scans or MRI. When abnormalities are found, if needle biopsies can be carried out without laparotomy to confirm metastases, so much the better. Surgical staging has made it quite clear that to treat patients without a complete evaluation looking for distant metastases is unacceptable. Is such an extensive evaluation necessary in patients with microinvasive disease or in patients with clear-cut stage IB disease? The answer should be based on the histologic findings in that particular cancer. Most poor prognostic factors can be detected before treatment planning. Boyce and co-workers[4] looked at prognostic factors in stage I carcinoma of the cervix and found the poor prognostic factors to be considered in therapeutic planning are (1) a depth of invasion greater than 10 mm; (2) invasion to more than half the thickness of the cervix; and (3) invasion of lymph-vascular spaces in the cervix. These authors also found spread to the pelvic nodes, the parametria, or the corpus uteri to be poor prognostic factors. The latter two are not as obvious, but the former three factors can be determined by cone biopsy in most situations or by the naked eye if looking for spread to more than half the cervix. In such cases, treatment planners must look for distant spread in the paraaortic nodes as well as the mediastinal nodes and the supraclavicular nodes. It is possible to carry out needle biopsies of many of the paraaortic lymph nodes and mediastinal lymph nodes without mediastinoscopy, and a scalene node biopsy can be carried out for patients in whom the likelihood seems reasonable, namely those in stages III or IV,

or in patients in whom paraaortic nodes have been found positive.

PRACTICAL CONSIDERATIONS IN STAGING

Many tests can be carried out diagnostically but they do not provide absolute evidence of metatastic disease (see list below).

Lymphangiography
Angiography
CT scans
Magnetic resonance imaging
Ultrasound
Bone scans

All of these tests have the same problems. They have a high rate of error, both false-positive and false-negative, and, therefore, require follow-up biopsies for histologic proof of spread of disease. Lymphadenography, for example, has become unavailable in many institutions because of its lack of specificity, but also because it is not being propagated from one generation of radiologists to the next. At best, it always required a radiologist or surgeon or both who were particularly interested in the technique so that they worked very hard at achieving the best possible results. It is simply not valuable and reliable enough to be of great use in staging of cervical cancer. Somewhat the same criticism applies to most of the other examinations listed. CT and MRI examinations have come to the forefront in pretreatment evaluations. These two examinations, while expensive, are more comprehensive and do roughly the same thing that the several individual tests listed above can do, namely, point to areas of possible metastatic disease, which then must be proven. It cannot be emphasized enough that both CT and MRI examinations have limitations on accuracy and sensitivity. It is well known that lymph nodes can be replaced by tumor but, if they are 1 cm in greatest dimension, they will be missed most of the time by both of these diagnostic tests.

The ultimate question becomes, what is the place for surgical staging in cervical cancer? It is important to state emphatically from the outset that, at this point, surgical staging has no place in the FIGO clinical staging system for cervical cancer. On the other hand, it does have an important place in determining patient care. It is an important method in selected cases when planning and carrying out treatment. Perhaps its place can best be reviewed by a stage-by-stage approach.

The notes to the staging of cervical carcinoma developed by FIGO are printed below.[1]

NOTES TO THE STAGING

Stage 0 comprises those cases with full thickness involvement of the epithelium with atypical cells, but with no signs of invasion into the stroma.

Over the last several decades there has been continued confusion about the stages of preclinical invasive carcinoma of the cervix. Several classification systems have been developed which have not been generally satisfactory. The addition of colposcopy in many countries has caused further confusion as to what is a clinical lesion for obvious reasons. There has also been an increased pressure to put measurements into the definition. As a result of the above a new definition is proposed which is as follows:

Stage Ia Carcinoma should include minimal microscopically evident stromal invasion as well as small cancerous tumours of measurable size. Stage Ia should be divided into those lesions with minute foci of invasion visible only microscopically as Stage Ia1, and the macroscopically measurable micro-carcinomas as Stage Ia2 in order to gain further knowledge of the clinical behavior of these lesions. The term Ib Occult should be omitted.

The diagnosis of both Stage Ia1 and Ia2 should be based on microscopic examination of removed tissue, preferably a cone, which must include the entire lesion. As noted above, the lower limit of Stage Ia2 should be that it can be measured macroscopically (even if dots need to be placed on the slide prior to measurement) and the upper limit of Ia2 is given by measurement of the two largest dimensions in any given section. The depth of invasion should not be more than 5 mm taken from the base of the epithelium, either surface or glandular, from which it originates. The second dimension, the horizontal spread, must not exceed 7 mm. Vascular space involvement, either venous or lymphatic, should not alter the staging, but should be specifically recorded as it may affect treatment decisions in the future.

The remaining Stage I cases should be allotted to Stage Ib. As a rule, these cases can be diagnosed by routine clinical examination.

As a rule, it is impossible to estimate clinically whether a cancer of the cervix has extended to the corpus or not. Extension to the corpus should therefore be disregarded.

A patient with a growth fixed to the pelvic wall by a short and indurated but not nodular parametrium should be allotted to Stage IIb. It is impossible, at clinical examination, to decide whether a smooth and indurated parametrium is truly cancerous or only inflammatory. Therefore the case should be placed in Stage III only if the parametrium is nodular out on the pelvic wall or if the growth itself extends out on the pelvic wall.

The presence of hydronephrosis or non-functioning kidney due to stenosis of the ureter by cancer permits a case to be allotted to Stage III even if, according to the other findings, the case should be allotted to Stage I or Stage II.

The presence of bullous oedema, as such, should not permit a case to be allotted to Stage IV. Ridges and furrows into the bladder wall should be interpreted as signs of submucous involvement of the bladder if they remain fixed to the growth at palposcopy (i.e., examination from the vagina or the rectum during cystoscopy). A finding of malignant cells in cytologic washings from the urinary bladder requires further examination and biopsy from the wall of the bladder.

In the notes to staging above, stage Ia is divided into Ia1 and Ia2 depending on whether the lesion is microscopic or macroscopic, respectively. (Stage Ia2 is viewed almost unanimously by U.S. gynecologic oncologists as an error, which ultimately must be corrected.) A stage Ia2 lesion with horizontal spread of 7 mm and a depth of invasion of not more than 5 mm from the basement membrane is a macroscopic lesion and carries with it a significant mortality unless treated aggressively. Add to that vascular

space involvement and the patient is in serious jeopardy unless the treating physician is very aggressive. Finally, many hospitals and pathology laboratories do not have pathologists interested in gynecology or do not have the time and money to carry out the examination required. Therefore, in this country for the most part, although many institutions are following the FIGO classification in an effort to be cooperative and accumulate data, the fact of the matter is that they are using the definition of 3 mm depth of stromal invasion and no lymph vascular space involvement for the criteria to carry out conservative treatment. Any lesions with a depth of stromal involvement greater than 3 mm or with tumor emboli in lymph vascular spaces regardless of the depth of invasion are treated as a stage Ib carcinoma of the cervix. These facts are mentioned because data derived from U.S. institutions have borne out the wisdom of that definition. It also provides an easily determined division where conservative or aggressive therapy can be determined with the simplest of means, namely, a cone biopsy of the cervix. It also provides a sensible division between where radical surgical staging should begin, namely, with lesions of greater than 3 mm depth of stromal invasion, or tumor emboli in lymph vascular spaces. The exception to this would be in the case where the patient's medical condition prohibits major surgery. Certainly, stage Ia2 as defined by FIGO calls for surgical staging. It should be pointed out that before surgical staging laparotomy all of the diagnostic tests available should be carried out, including either a CT or an MRI scan of the pelvis, abdomen, and chest. It has been the author's experience that mediastinal lymph node involvement is significantly more frequent than we are aware. The importance of lymph vascular space involvement cannot be too strongly emphasized. Averette's report[2] demonstrating a lesion in the cervix measuring 0.1 mm depth of stromal invasion with a common iliac lymph node completely replaced by tumor and fixed to the sacrum is an excellent illustration of this fact. The same remarks apply to patients with stage Ib carcinoma of the cervix. Stage Ib lesions are obvious on routine clinical examination and further evaluation should include sigmoidoscopy, cystoscopy, and examination under anesthesia plus CT or MRI examinations of the pelvis, abdomen, and chest. The best approach seems to be MRI of the abdomen and pelvis plus CT scan of the chest. If these examinations are negative for evidence of tumor, a laparotomy should be carried out with the intent of doing a radical hysterectomy and pelvic node dissection along with a thorough staging laparotomy as part of the operative procedure. Biopsies should be done liberally above the pelvic brim to include especially paraaortic lymph nodes. In all of these cases, peritoneal washings should be taken immediately after opening the abdominal cavity; these should be fixed and sent off immediately so that a fresh specimen arrives in the cytology laboratory for evaluation. It is not suggested that any rapid tests should be done on this cytology specimen, but the information can be used postoperatively when all of the information is available concerning the full picture of the extent of the primary cervical carcinoma and the status of the pelvic lymph nodes as well as the status of any other specimens taken during surgery.

Stage IIa carcinoma of the cervix should be evaluated and managed in the same way as stage Ib unless the lesion is a very bulky one, in which case other approaches may be elected. Alternatives could be chemotherapy associated with radiotherapy or radiotherapy followed by exploratory laparotomy. It is important to understand that bulky stage Ib or stage IIa carcinoma of the cervix carries with it an increased probability of metatastic disease in the pelvic and paraaortic lymph nodes. Therefore, a staging laparotomy should be considered at some point in treatment as part of the approach to this patient's disease. The complete surgery illustrated in Fig. 33-1 is an example of radical surgery to include paraaortic and pelvic nodes.

Stage IIb carcinoma of the cervix is treated in the United States by radiation therapy. The author's findings and those of others shown in Table 33-2 have indicated that approximately 12% to 15% of such patients have positive paraaortic lymph nodes. Certainly, the diagnostic evaluation of patients with this stage of disease should have precisely the same work-up as mentioned above, namely, cystoscopy, sigmoidoscopy, and examination under anesthesia, plus CT or MRI examinations of the pelvis, abdomen, and chest. It is the author's experience that with this set of diagnostic studies before treatment a surprisingly large number of patients with stage IIb disease are found to have disease beyond the pelvis. It is difficult, however, to recommend staging laparotomy in patients when the yield is apt to be 12% to 15%. On the other hand, it is equally difficult to recommend paraaortic irradiation with no knowledge except that found on CT or MRI. This is the dilemma clinicians are faced with today. Perhaps the only information one can get to help make a rational decision is the appearance of the primary tumor and the microscopic picture on biopsy. If tumor emboli were frequent findings on biopsy, it would be hard to ignore a

staging laparotomy unless one were to consider the use of an extended field to include the lumbar paraaortic lymph nodes. An obvious shortcoming in this plan is the lack of knowledge concerning the paraaortic lymph nodes in terms of the bearing it has on the true picture in the mediastinal lymph nodes histologically. In such cases, a rather simple aid may be to carry out a scalene node biopsy.

Stage IIIb carcinoma of the cervix is somewhat different in that the reports shown in Table 33-2 have indicated that stage III carcinoma of the cervix will have paraaortic lymph node involvement 35% to 45% of the time. The same pretreatment studies should be carried out as mentioned above for stage IIb. If the patient has abnormal findings on the MRI in the paraaortic area, fine needle biopsy can very often be carried out. If positive, this obviates the need for staging laparotomy. If positive, it compounds somewhat the treatment plan because it strongly suggests that the disease is systemic and mandates consideration of systemic therapy in addition to radiation therapy. If the MRI study of the abdomen is negative, the clinician may feel compelled to carry out a staging laparotomy in an effort to be certain. The staging laparotomy also permits the evaluation of visceral metastases, which Buchsbaum found in a significant number of stage III patients.[6] These questions are not so important with stage IV disease because in stage IVb it is already a systemic disease. Stage IVa presents extremely difficult decisions, but when a patient presents with stage IVa disease and no other evidence of disease on the basic diagnostic evaluation one is probably dealing with a rapidly progressive lesion and, in the few cases providing the dilemma, the patient may not be in condition to tolerate a laparotomy.

REFERENCES

1. Annual report on the results of treatment in gynecological cancer, Vol 20, Ed. Folke Pettersson, Stockholm, 1988, pp 29-31.
2. Averette HE: Microinvasive carcinoma of the cervix: formal discussion, *Am J Obstet Gynecol* 145:989, 1983.
3. Averette HE, Dudan RC, Ford JH: Exploratory celiotomy for surgical staging in cervical carcinoma, *Am J Obstet Gynecol* 113:1090, 1972.
4. Boyce J et al: Prognostic factors in stage I carcinoma of the cervix, *Gynecol Oncol* 12:154, 1981.
5. Buchsbaum H: Para aortic node involvement in cervical carcinoma, *Am J Obstet Gynecol* 113:942, 1972.
6. Buchsbaum HJ: Extrapelvic lymph node metastases in cervical carcinoma, *Am J Obstet Gynecol* 133:814, 1979.
7. LaGasse LD, Ford JH, Blessing JA: Results and complications of operative staging in cervical cancer, *Gynecol Oncol* 9:90, 1980.
8. League of Nations Classification of carcinoma of the cervix. Cancer Commission of the Health Organization of the League of Nations. Heyman J, editor. Stockholm, 1929.
9. Nelson JH Jr, Urcuyo R: Pretreatment staging. Presented at the American Cancer Society's National Conference on Gynecologic Cancer. *Cancer* 38:458, 1976.
10. Nelson JH Jr et al: The incidence, significance and follow-up of para aortic lymph node metastases in late invasive carcinoma of the cervix, *Am J Obstet Gynecol* 128:336, 1977.
11. Pretreatment laparotomy in stages IIB and III carcinoma of the cervix. Presented at 1st Annual Meeting Society of Gynecologic Oncologists, January 1970.

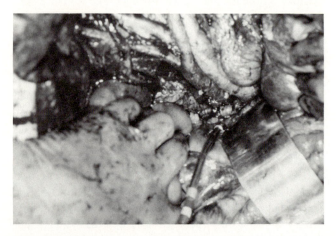

Fig. 33-1. Sample of radical surgery to include paraaortic and pelvic nodes.

Chapter 34

RADICAL HYSTERECTOMY AND PELVIC LYMPHADENECTOMY

Colonel Kunio Miyazawa

The surgical treatment of cervical cancer has a long history. In the early nineteenth century, an attempt was made to treat cervical cancer by simple amputation without success. The use of simple hysterectomy was not successful either. John Clark at Johns Hopkins Hospital undertook a radical abdominal operation for the treatment of invasive cervical cancer in 1895.[19,20] In 1907, Wertheim of Vienna first described 500 patients with cervical cancer treated by radical surgical procedure, which was popularized mainly in Europe.[48] In 1921, Okabayashi introduced his technique of removing the widest parametrium and the cancer-infiltrated area according to Takayama who developed and described his method at the Japanese Gynecological Association Meeting 10 years previously.[31] In May 1934, Bonney of London presented his operative technique of Wertheim's operation at the annual meeting of the American Gynecological Society.[5] Taussig of St. Louis, Missouri, in 1934 published his iliac lymphadenectomy technique for irradiated patients.[39-41] In 1944, Meigs of Boston published an account of his radical surgical procedure,[21] which he called the Wertheim-Clark plus Taussig operation. He proved that the procedure could be carried out by a specially trained gynecologist and yielded a mortality of 1%.[19,21-24] In 1952, Yagi reported his 333 patients treated by Okabayashi's radical hysterectomy and pelvic lymphadenectomy.[50] Since then, various modifications have been introduced by pelvic surgeons to reduce operative morbidity and mortality as well as to bring about a better quality of life.

During the past three to four decades, several advancements and improvements have been made in anesthesia, intensive care, antibiotics, and blood component therapy, as well as surgical techniques, resulting in better operability and improved complication and survival rates. At the same time, the incidence of invasive cervical carcinoma has declined from the most common invasive cancer 30 years ago to the third most common of the female genital tract cancers. Surgical approach to the early invasive cervical carcinoma has been changing gradually from a radical approach to conservative procedures, resulting in decreased mortality and morbidity as well as better functional quality of lifestyle.[2]

PREOPERATIVE CONSIDERATIONS
Indications

The following summarizes the indications for surgical management of early invasive cervical carcinoma:

1. A young patient who needs preservation of ovarian function
2. Any patient who desires preservation of sexual vaginal function
3. Any patient for whom radiation treatment is contraindicated (e.g., because of a history of severe pelvic inflammatory disease or bowel inflammatory disease)
4. Any patient who desires a short treatment time

Contraindications

The following summarizes the contraindications for surgical management of early invasive cervical carcinoma[9]:

1. Significant medical illness
2. Positive paraaortic nodes

The author gives his thanks to Dr. Hajime Uchida for providing the pictures relating to his radical hysterectomy technique.

3. Carcinoma extending to the parametrial region or vesicouterine space
4. Grossly involved multiple pelvic nodes
5. Severe obesity
6. Old age. (However, in a recent report Lawton and co-workers suggest that chronologic age is a poor determinant of surgical risk and elderly patients can go through radical surgery almost as well as younger women.[13])
7. Barrel-shaped cervix (should be treated by radiotherapy and extrafascial hysterectomy, especially when the lesion is larger than 5 cm)

It is extremely important that the pelvic surgeon individualize the approach to the patient and determine whether to use radiation therapy or radical hysterectomy as appropriate given the existing disease and its extent.[9] The patient should be fully aware of the benefits and risks of either treatment in dealing with short- or long-term effects.

Preparation

History and physical examination. A careful history is a sine qua non for preoperative evaluation. Particular attention should be paid to the patient's current general physical status and any history of unusual disorders, such as early bruises and bleeding. Recent ingestion of aspirin-containing drugs should be ruled out. Each organ system should be carefully reviewed. Existing iron deficiency anemia should be corrected in advance with oral iron and multivitamins. Smoking should be stopped to prevent postoperative atelectasis. Determining the degree of cardiovascular tolerance to exercise provides a good indication of the patient's physical stress reserve.

Laboratory studies. In addition to the routine preoperative evaluation of blood count, platelet and differential count, and urinalysis, a renal and hepatic profile, chest x-ray, and electrocardiogram should be ordered. A patient who smokes, is obese, and has an existing lung disorder should undergo an arterial blood gas analysis to be applied postoperatively. An intravenous pyelogram is routinely obtained for staging purposes. Use of computed tomography (CT) scans to detect nodal metastasis is limited in early lesions.[11]

Preoperative orders. Adequate blood should be available. A review of one series indicates a mean blood loss from radical hysterectomy is reported to be 1400 ml.[34] The patient should have a thorough bowel prep using both the mechanical and the antibiotics methods. I use Golytely one day before surgery. Pulmonary toilet should begin with the inspirometer. The patient should ambulate as much as possible on the ward and should be advised to resume this as soon as possible after surgery.

OPERATIVE CONSIDERATIONS
Radical hysterectomy and pelvic lymphadenectomy

Review of Meig's operative technique. Wertheim's paper, "The Extended Abdominal Operation for Carcinoma Uteri," was translated into English and appeared in August 1912.[48] Since this original work, many modifications have appeared. The procedure that became popular in the United States is that of Meigs, first published in 1944.[21] Various modifications have followed. (For details of modifications on this procedure, the reader can refer to various textbooks on pelvic surgery.*) Only the major points are described here for the purpose of review.[25,32]

After a Foley drainage system is placed into the patient's bladder, careful pelvic and rectal examinations are performed to determine the extent of the tumor and its mobility. The vagina and cervix are painted with Schiller's solution, and the unstained area is identified. After the extent of the tumor is determined, the abdominal portion of the surgery begins. The operating surgeon usually stands on the left side of the patient while the patient is kept in Trendelenburg's position. A midline incision is made from the mons pubis to the umbilicus. If this is inadequate, the incision can be extended to the right side of the umbilicus. The pyramidalis muscle at the lower end is preserved. To provide an extra space for pelvic dissection, the fascial incision extends to the symphysis. Exploration of the abdominal cavity and contents is carried out, with special attention given to the paraaortic area. If an enlarged node above the bifurcation is detected, it must be dissected for frozen section evaluation. The abdomen is packed systematically, a self-retaining retractor is placed, and the uterus is grasped with a double hook or tenaculum. With adequate upward tension on the uterus, the pelvic cavity and organs are inspected and palpated for any sign of tumor extension.

The peritoneal reflection on the lower uterine region is entered by a small superficial incision and extended in the peritoneum with the aid of the index finger and scissors. The peritoneal edge is pulled to reflect the median raphe. Fine fibers between the bladder and vagina are incised. The round ligament and infundibulopelvic ligament are ligated and dissected if ovarian preservation is not applicable. Then the same procedure is carried out on the opposite side. Next, the paravesical space and pararectal space are explored bilaterally. Care should be exercised so as not to injure the vein in exploration of the pararectal space because this causes tremendous unnecessary bleeding between the ureter and hypogastric vessels. The cardinal ligament (web) is palpated for any evidence of tumor invasion. It is usually soft bilaterally when free from tumor. Bilateral pelvic lymph nodes are palpated in the entire chain; if any enlarged node is present, it should be removed for frozen section diagnosis. With the uterus pulled to the opposite side, the ureter is identified on the medial flap of the peritoneum and the uterine vessels are noted arising from the hypogastric vessels. The uterine artery is ligated and dissected at the origin bilaterally. It is important to spare the superficial vesical artery at this point. The ureter is separated from the underlying medial leaf of the

*References 17, 20, 28, 32, 33, 42, 49.

peritoneum gently without damaging the ureteral sheath, in which there is a longitudinal arterial blood supply to the ureter. Further dissection is made, separating the bladder from the lower end of the cervix and the anterior vaginal wall. The posterior peritoneum in the rectovaginal space is widely incised transversely, and the rectovaginal space is entered, creating a large retrovaginal space while ensuring that the rectum is away from the cervix and vagina. With the bladder well advanced and the rectum separated, the ureter is dissected away from the tissues that lie above and beneath it. With the ureter under light traction, it is untunneled and the tissue overlying the ureter is divided without any trauma to the ureter. The ureter is freed from all attachments. The most lateral aspect of the bladder is dissected free from the underlying tissue. The same procedure is applied to the opposite side. The deep uterosacral ligament is severed closer to the rectum, and the cardinal ligament is excised as laterally as possible. The same is applied to paracervical and paravaginal tissue. The vagina is removed, including the upper 3- to 4-cm portion, depending on the tumor extension and Schiller's staining. The cuff is closed by interlocking suture.

With the uterus removed and pelvic dissection completed, dissection of the regional lymph nodes follows. It begins lateral to the external iliac vessels along the psoas muscle. With retraction of the external iliac vessels, the obturator space becomes accessible. The genitofemoral nerve is preserved. All tissue is removed from the pelvic wall down to the obturator nerve. Dissection moves upward to the common iliac vessels, and the distal and proximal ends are ligated to prevent lymphocyst formation. All lymphatic and surrounding fat is removed to the lower limit of the level at which the deep circumflex iliac vein crosses the major vessels. For the obturator space nodes, the external iliac artery and vein are retracted and the block of tissue is removed. The lateral tissue along the external iliac vessels is removed. Extreme care should be taken to remove the tissue from the hypogastric vessels and presacral area without injury to the vein.

Complete hemostasis is obtained from the operating site. Ureters and bladder are inspected. Rectal injuries are ruled out. The peritoneum is closed, placing the ureters in the retroperitoneal space, and a hemovac is placed in both retroperitoneal cavities. The abdomen is closed in three layers.

Okabayashi summarizes his technique in the following order[31]:

- Abdominal incision
- Exposure of the pelvic cavity
- Examination to determine operability
- Division of the broad ligaments
- Ligation of the uterine artery
- Freeing the ureter from the posterior layer of the broad ligament
- Separation of the rectum
- Removal of the infiltrated and the loose cellular pelvic tissues

- Separation of the bladder
- Isolation of the ureter
- Completion of the separation of the bladder
- Division of the anterior lateral paravaginal and parametrial tissue
- Division of the lateral paravaginal tissue
- Division of the vagina
- Application of the ligatures
- Removal of the pelvic glands and lymphatic tracts
- Suturing the pelvic floor
- Closure of the abdominal wall

Nakano illustrated a modified Okabayashi's technique in 1981 as follows[27]:

- Abdominal incision
- Examination to determine operability
- Opening the broad ligament
- Exposure of the ureter
- Separation of the bladder from the cervix
- Lymph node dissection
- Exposure of the paravesical space
- Exposure of the pararectal space
- Ligation of the uterine artery
- Mobilization of the ureter
- Separation of the rectum from the cervix
- Cutting the uterosacral ligament
- Cutting the uterovaginal ligament
- Clamping and cutting the cardinal ligament
- Mobilization of the ureter and cutting the superficial layer of the vesicouterine ligament
- Cutting the deep layer of the vesicouterine ligament
- Clamping and cutting the lateral paravaginal tissue
- Transecting the vagina
- Closure of the vagina and pelvic peritoneum
- Closure of the abdominal wall

Uchida's technique of radical hysterectomy and pelvic lymphadenectomy.[43,44] Uchida's technique was born as a result of over 4500 radical hysterectomies he performed over the past 45 years. His technique has been mastered by many Asian gynecologic oncologists, because it originated with Okabayashi's technique, which was later modified by Yagi. The most impressive point of his technique is an average operating time of 75 minutes with minimal blood loss and an excellent 5-year survival rate. There are a few differences between his technique and a standard radical hysterectomy.

After the patient is properly prepped and draped, a low abdominal longitudinal incision is made. After the abdomen is explored, a self-retaining retractor is placed to expose the pelvis widely. Two pairs of Uchida's uterine clamps are applied to the side of the uterus, including the round and infundibulopelvic ligaments to hold the uterus up. Because of the catches on the clamp it is easy to manipulate the uterus during the operative procedure (Fig. 34-1).

The round and infundibulopelvic ligaments are ligated and severed. The broad ligament is widely separated between two sheets (Fig. 34-2). The uterine artery is isolated,

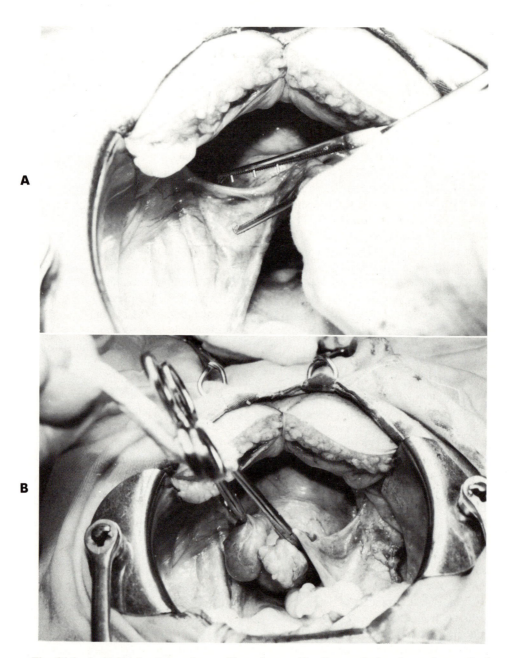

Fig. 34-1. A, Uchida's uterine clamp with catches avoids slippage during the uterine manipulation. **B,** Uchida's uterine clamp is applied to side of uterus including round ligament and adnexa to maintain a proper uterine traction.

ligated, and severed at its origin (Fig. 34-3). The ureter is separated in one stroke by scissors from the posterior leaf of the broad ligament (Fig. 34-4). The same procedure is applied to the opposite side of the pelvis.

Lymphadenectomy starts with the paraaortic region. Along the common iliac and external iliac vessels, lymph nodes and fatty tissue are removed by the "peeling off" technique. The very fine space between the blood vessel and the lymphatic system is detected by peeling off the lymphatic tissue (Fig. 34-5). Lymph tissue should be removed from the external iliac vessels in one block, including the hypogastric chain. It should be noted that the

clamp is used to peel off the lymphatic tissue (Fig. 34-6).

The obturator space is explored next, and the obturator nerve and vessels are identified. The same technique is used to clear the lymphatic system in this area. The obturator nerve is easily visible, appearing denuded and white (Fig. 34-7). The obturator node is removed as an entire block. The same procedure is applied to the opposite side of the lymphatic chain.

Next, the rectovaginal space is opened widely, creating a large rectovaginal sac (Fig. 34-8). The pararectal and paravesical spaces are opened bilaterally. The cardinal ligament is completely isolated now. The lymphatic system

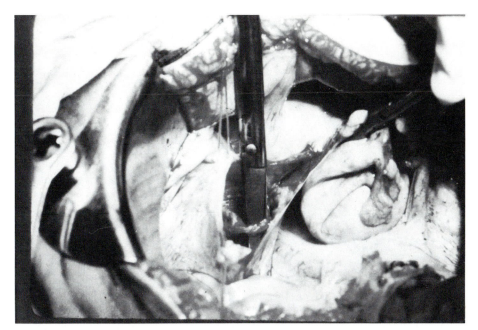

Fig. 34-2. Round and infundibulopelvic ligaments are ligated and severed. Retroperitoneal space is entered by separating between two sheets of broad ligaments.

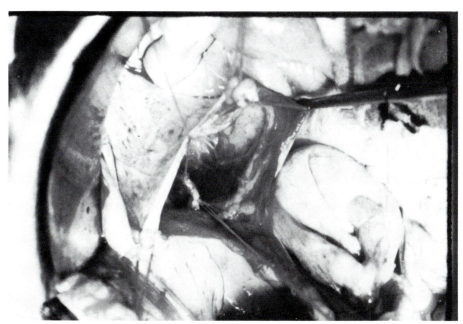

Fig. 34-3. Uterine artery is isolated, ligated, and cut.

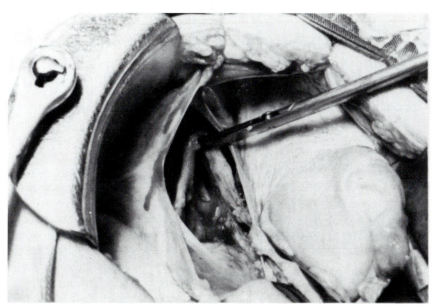

Fig. 34-4. Ureter is separated in one stroke from posterior leaf of broad ligament.

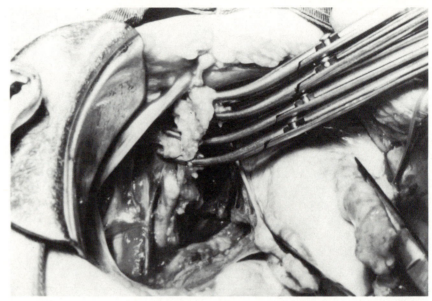

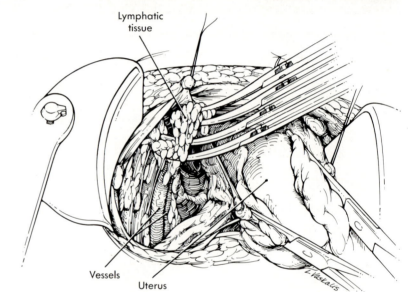

Lymphatic
tissue

Vessels

Uterus

L. Vaskalis

Fig. 34-5. **A,** Lymph nodes and fatty tissue are removed by peeling off lymphatic tissue. **B,** Schematic drawing of **A.**

and blood vessels around the root of the ligament are squeezed and pushed upward to the uterine side. The cardinal ligament is narrow and thin, with remaining denuded thick vessels (Fig. 34-9). This is clamped near the sidewall, cut, and ligated. The deep uterosacral ligament is clamped near the rectum, cut, and sutured.

Next, vesicovaginal exposure starts by placing and pushing a scissors between the vesicouterine peritoneum and the cervix. Use of the scissors is important to create a tentlike space (Fig. 34-10). The peritoneum is cut transversely (Fig. 34-11). It is crucial to note that there is no bleeding when the medial portion of the bladder is separated from the vagina. The lateral margin of the vesicouterine ligament should not be touched because it bleeds excessively. For separating the ureter from this area, a special instrument, Uchida's ureter scoop, is used. It has grooves on both edges. By suspending the portion where the ureter goes into the bladder pillar with two pairs of forceps, a triangular space is produced (Fig. 34-12). The ure-

ter scoop is pushed through the fine space between the anterior portion of the vesicouterine ligament and the ureter, and two pairs of long, thin forceps are inserted just above the ureter (Fig. 34-13). The anterior portion of the vesicouterine ligament is excised along the two long, thin forceps on the uterine side as shown in Fig. 34-14. When the two pairs of forceps are turned over, the ureter appears under the scoop. The forceps are placed away from the bladder (Fig. 34-15). When the two pairs of forceps are further turned aside, departing further from the ureter, a space can be noticed beside the ureter and between the cervix and the bladder. Uchida found that there is no bleeding even if the tissue adjacent to the uterus is not clamped. To separate the ureter from the uterus, this space is pushed through and opened (Fig. 34-16). Figure 34-17 shows how the bladder pillar and the ureter can be manipulated. Two pairs of slim forceps are inserted through this space, and an incision is made between the forceps to separate the ureter from the cervix (Fig. 34-18). The posterior layer is

Text continued on p. 571.

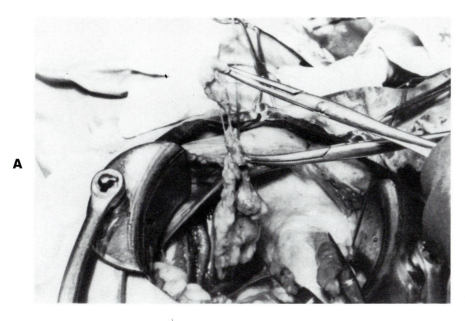

A

Fig. 34-6. A, Clamp is used to peel off lymphatic tissue. **B,** Schematic drawing of **A.**

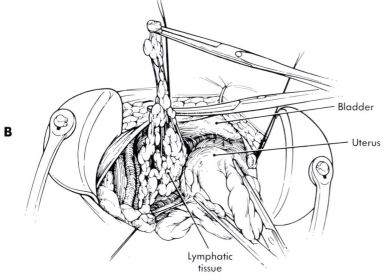

B

Bladder

Uterus

Lymphatic tissue

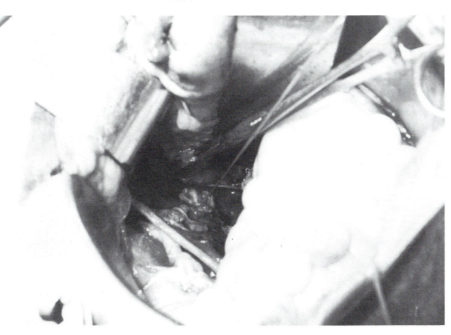

Fig. 34-7. Obturator nerve.

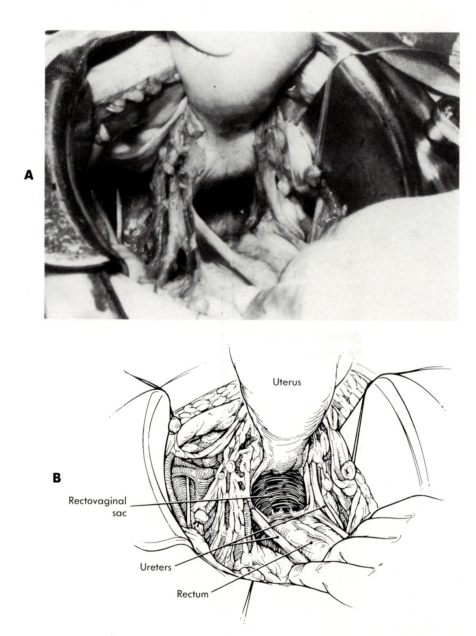

Fig. 34-8. A, Rectovaginal space is opened, creating rectovaginal sac. **B,** Schematic drawing of **A.**

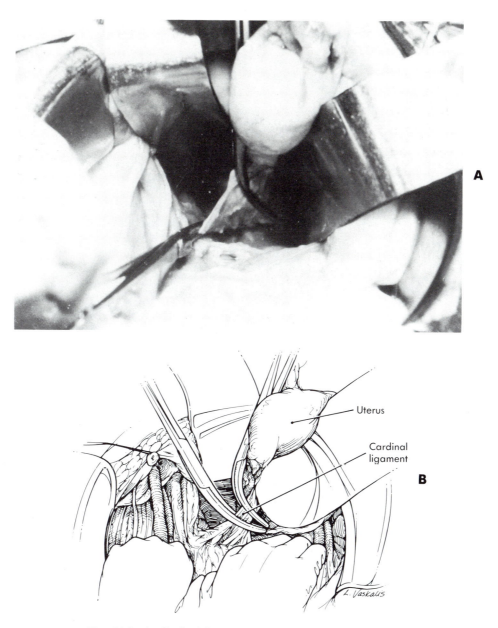

Fig. 34-9. A, Cardinal ligament. **B,** Schematic drawing of **A.**

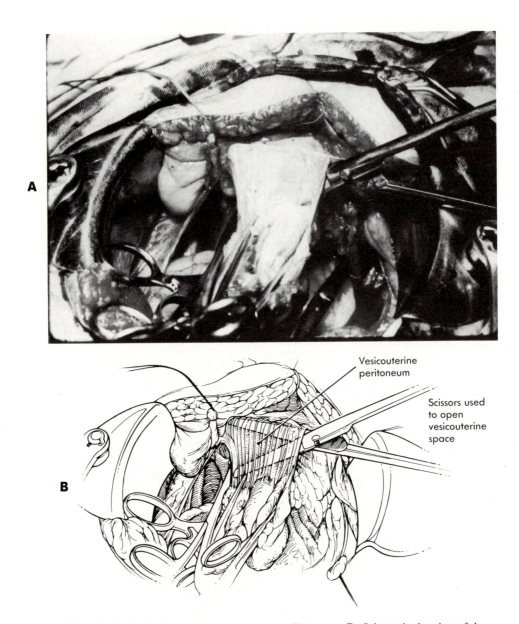

Fig. 34-10. A, Scissors are used to create tentlike space. **B,** Schematic drawing of **A.**

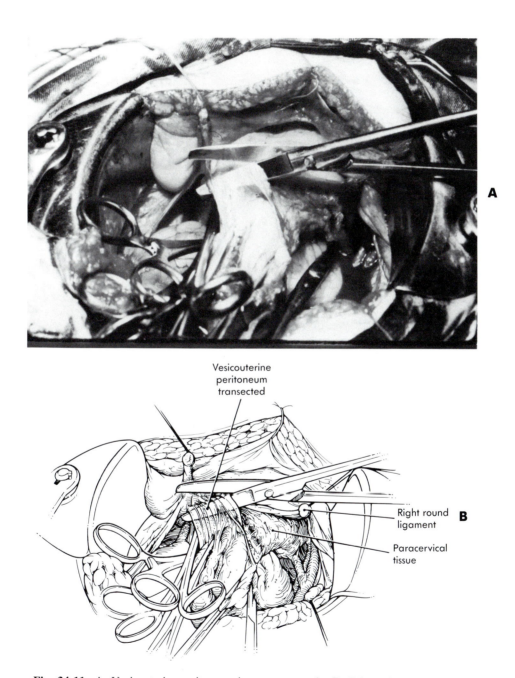

Vesicouterine
peritoneum
transected

Right round
ligament

Paracervical
tissue

A

B

Fig. 34-11. A, Vesicouterine peritoneum is cut transversely. **B,** Schematic drawing of **A.**

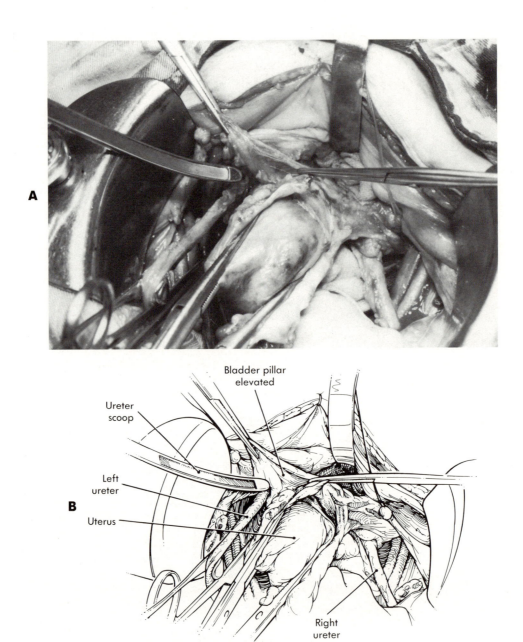

Fig. 34-12. A, Using Uchida's ureter scoop and two pairs of forceps, the bladder pillar is elevated and a triangular space is produced. **B,** Schematic view of **A.**

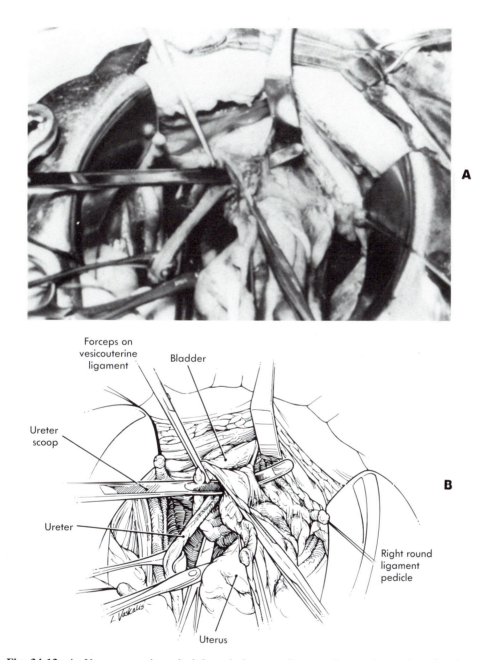

Fig. 34-13. A, Ureter scoop is pushed through the space between the anterior portion of vesico-uterine ligament and ureter, and forceps are inserted above the ureter. **B,** Schematic drawing of **A.**

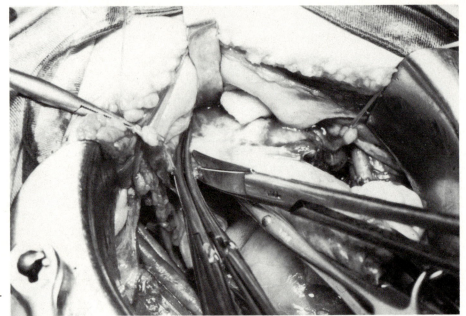

Fig. 34-14. A, Anterior portion of vesi-couterine ligament is excised. **B,** Schematic drawing of **A.**

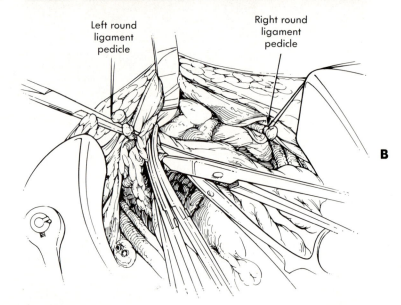

Left round ligament pedicle

Right round ligament pedicle

Fig. 34-15. When two pairs of forceps are turned over, away from bladder, the ureter appears under the scoop.

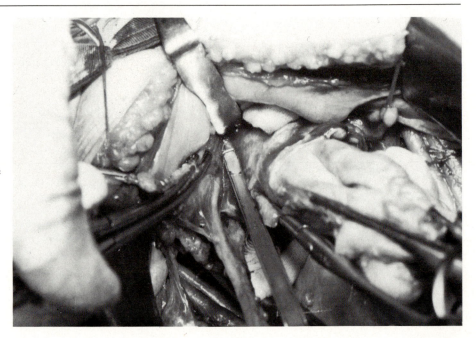

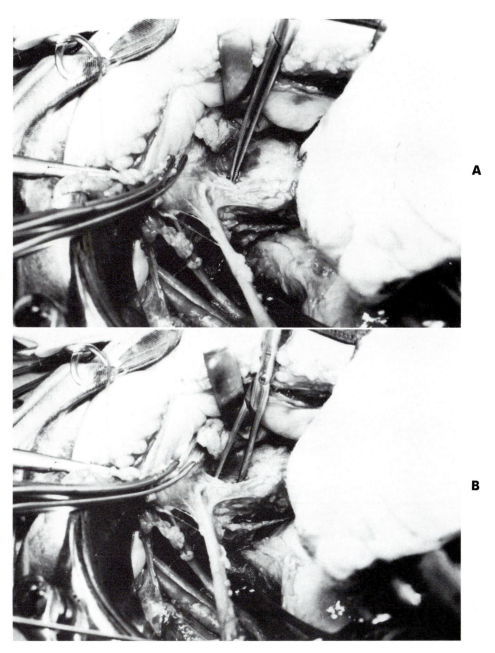

Fig. 34-16. To separate ureter from uterine side, forceps are used to push through **A** and open **B**.

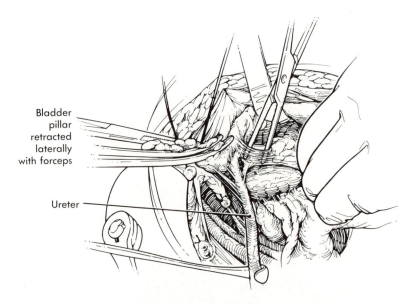

Bladder
pillar
retracted
laterally
with forceps

Ureter

Fig. 34-17. Manipulation of bladder pillar and ureter.

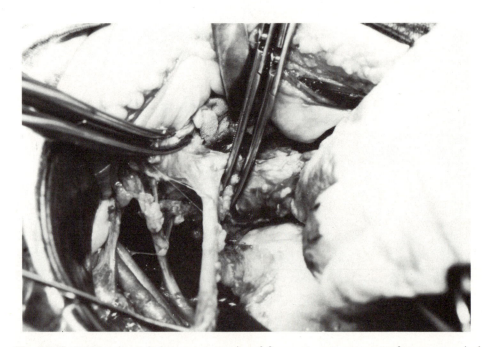

Fig. 34-18. Incision is made between two pairs of forceps to separate ureter from paracervical tissue.

separated and excised. Both layers are ligated with fine suture. The ureter can be noted (Fig. 34-19).

Uchida's paracolpium clamps are used to separate the connecting tissue around the vagina. This clamp has catches on the tip (Fig. 34-20). Two pairs of clamps are placed in the paravaginal tissue (Fig. 34-21). Paravaginal tissue is cut between the two clamps. The catches are very effective for grasping the soft paracolpium tightly without any slippage (Fig. 34-22). The paravaginal tissue is excised between the clamps and ligated. The vagina is clamped bilaterally and amputated, and the uterine specimen is removed (Fig. 34-23). The vaginal cuff is kept open by running a continuous suture to provide and retain enough length of vagina; this also facilitates good postop-

erative drainage. The entire vagina should be inspected before closure of the cuff (Fig. 34-24). Two drains are inserted into the pelvic cavity through the vagina and fixed to the vaginal wall with very fine catgut (Fig. 34-25). The edge of the bladder flap is sutured to the vaginal cuff and rectal peritoneal edge to the cuff with one catgut suture. The ureters are placed in the abdominal cavity by closing the retroperitoneum. This replacement of the ureters in the abdominal cavity can maintain ureters straight to the bladder through the abdominal peritoneal cavity. Uchida believes that such placement of the ureters prevents formation of a ureteral fistula and pyelitis (Fig. 34-26). A complete picture of the removed specimen is seen in Fig. 34-27. The abdominal cavity receives 100 ml of antibiotic

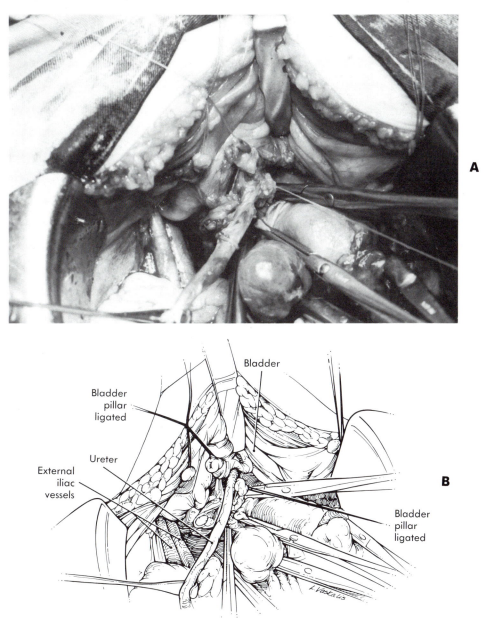

Fig. 34-19. A, Posterior layer is separated and excised, and the bladder pillar is ligated. **B,** Schematic drawing of **A.**

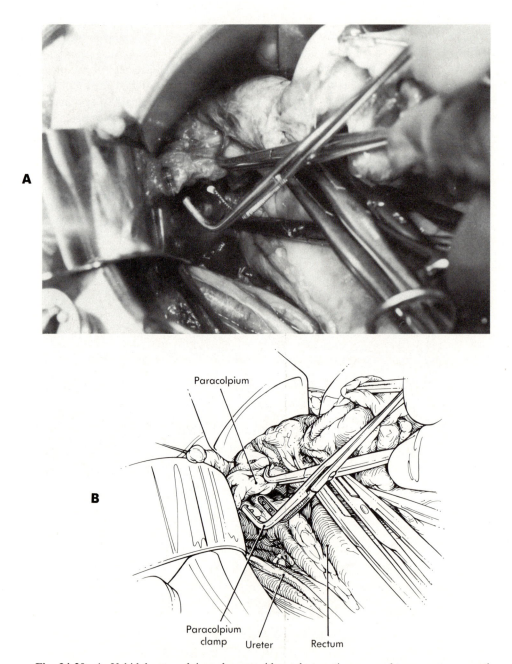

Fig. 34-20. A, Uchida's paracolpium clamps, with catches on tip, are used to separate connecting tissue around vagina. **B,** Schematic drawing of **A.**

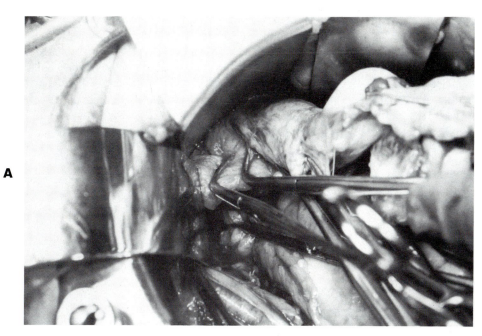

A

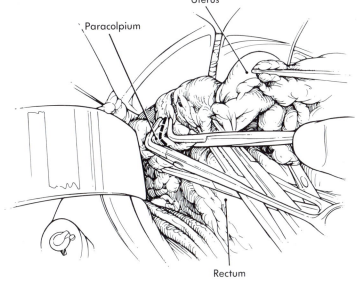

B

Paracolpium

Uterus

Rectum

Fig. 34-21. A, Two pairs of clamps are placed in paravaginal tissue. **B,** Schematic drawing of **A.**

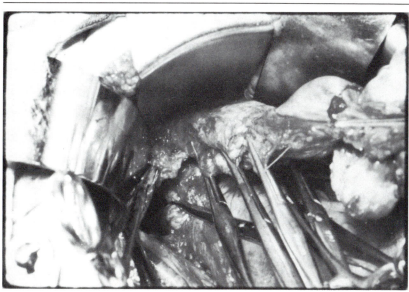

Fig. 34-22. Catches on clamps are effective for grasping paracolpium tightly. Paravaginal tissue is cut between clamps.

solution of Terramycin, and the peritoneum and fascia are closed with catgut continuously. The skin incision is reapproximated with clips.

Before Uchida reached this successful operation he had to overcome innumerable difficulties in conducting this radical procedure. Characteristics of his surgical technique are summarized now. No suction apparatus is used during the procedure, because there is very little bleeding. Only gauze is used for applying pressure to bleeding tissue. During dissection, anatomic avascular fine spaces between tissues or organs are used for the procedure. Uchida emphasizes detecting anatomic fine avascular spaces between tissues or organs and expanding these spaces rather than

making frequent incisions and amputations. This technique reduces blood loss greatly. Successful surgery depends on special instruments, in particular, a uterine clamp with catches at the tip, which can hold up the uterus during the procedure; a paracolpium clamp with catches at the tip, which can grasp the paravaginal tissue firmly, preventing slipping; and a ureteral scoop, used for separating the ureter from the vesicouterine ligaments. Other unique techniques include separating the ureter from the posterior leaf of the broad ligament in one stroke, peeling off lymph nodes and tissue from the arteries and veins in one entire block for lymphadenectomy as if a snake's skin were shed, squeezing the cardinal ligament toward the uterus to make

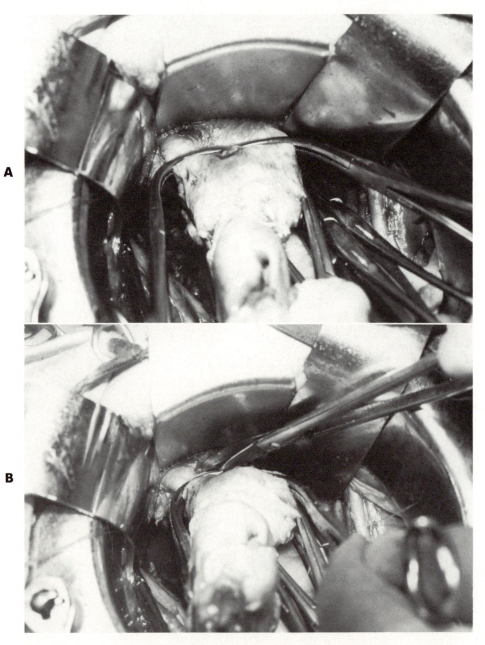

Fig. 34-23. A, Vagina is clamped bilaterally to include adequate vaginal cuff below cervix. **B,** Vagina is amputated, and uterine specimen is removed.

it narrow and thin and incising as close as possible to the pelvic side wall, and separating the ureter by Uchida's ureteral scoop through the small space between the anterior portion of the vesico-uterine ligament and the ureter.

As a result of practicing these principles of radical hysterectomy and lymphadenectomy, no blood transfusion is necessary in most cases. A complete resection of the lesion always brings a favorable cure and plays a principal role, even if the treatment is supplemented by chemotherapy, radiation treatment, and immune therapy. Understanding of living anatomy of the pelvis is absolutely essential.

Miyazawa's modification. Abdominal entry can be accomplished very efficiently by making a sharp, one-stroke, low midline incision down to the fascia level. Hemostasis is obtained by electrocauterization only for arterial bleeding from subcutaneous tissue. An approximately 5-cm sharp fascial incision is made in mid abdomen. Both fascial edges are grasped by straight Kocher clamps, and the abdominal wall is lifted. Both index fingers are used to enter the peritoneal cavity by "digging in" while an assistant keeps lifting the abdominal wall (Fig. 34-28). When the cavity is entered, the left index and middle fingers are placed longitudinally along the middle incision line, and the incision is extended by a sharp knife caudally and distally (Fig. 34-29). Attention is given in the lower end of the incision so as not to injure the bladder. It is a very fast entry without significant blood loss.

After abdominal and pelvic exploration, the peritoneum over the aortic bifurcation is opened longitudinally for ex-

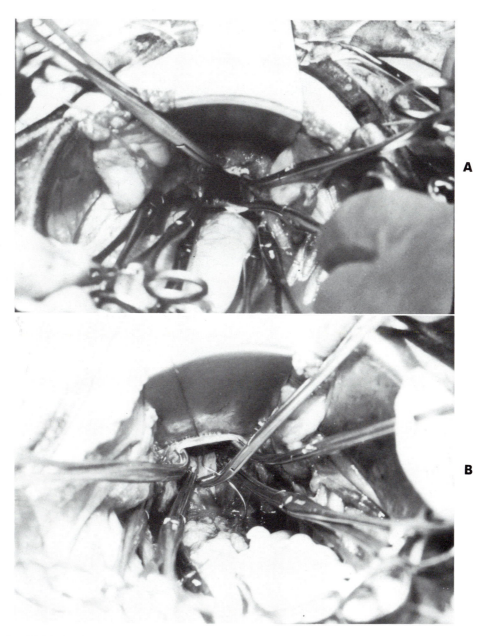

A

B

Fig. 34-24. Vaginal cuff is inspected (**A**) before suturing with one continuous running stitch (**B**).

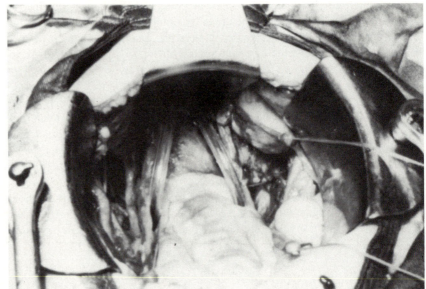

Fig. 34-25. Two drains are inserted into pelvic cavity through vagina.

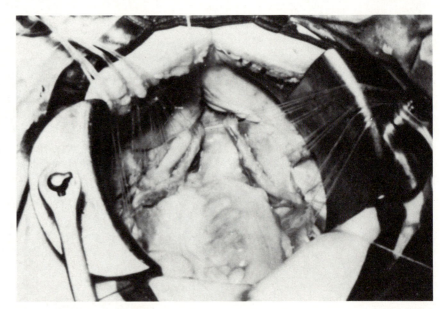

Fig. 34-26. Pelvic peritoneum is closed interruptedly, placing ureters in abdominal cavity.

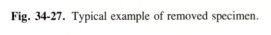
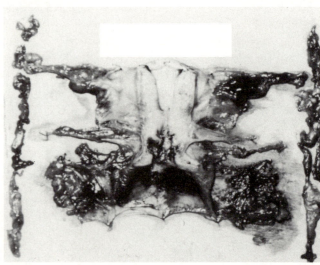

Fig. 34-27. Typical example of removed specimen.

ploration of paraaortic and presacral nodes. Avascular space is extended to search for abnormally enlarged nodes to rule out cervical cancer involvement. Suspicious nodes are removed and sent for frozen section. The peritoneal defect is closed interruptedly with chromic 3-0 sutures. The Brunschwig self-retaining retractor is readjusted if necessary after proper replacement of the abdominal contents. Both sides of the uterus are grasped with Uchida's uterine clamps, and careful palpation of the pelvic structure and lymph nodes follows. The right round ligament is ligated near the pelvic side wall and cut. The peritoneal incision is extended anteromedially to expose the vesicouterine fold, and the posterior leaf incision is extended proximally to enter the retroperitoneal cavity. Pelvic nodes are carefully palpated. The paravesical and pararectal spaces are entered, and the web is palpated to rule out any gross invasion of the cervical tumor. The peritoneal fold of the bladder flap is lifted, and the paravaginal layer is identified to separate the bladder from the cervix and upper anterior vaginal wall. No attempt is made to extend laterally.

The ureter on the medial leaf of the broad ligament is identified. The edge of the medial leaf of the peritoneum is grasped with two right-angle clamps for traction, the ureter is picked up with the thumb and index finger at the midportion, and the avascular space is identified between the

ureteral sheath and peritoneum, which should be cleared with long Metzenbaum scissors. While a gentle lifting tension is applied to the ureter and counter traction is maintained to the posterior leaf of the broad ligament, the avascular area is further cleared from the peritoneum, and the uterine vessels are identified and dissected at their origin. With moderate caudal tension applied to the ureter, the roof of ureter is untunneled step by step distally. The uterovesical ligament is identified, and Uchida's ureteral scoop is placed just above the ureter. The tissue on the groove is clamped on both sides with a fine clamp. After the tissue between is excised, the lateral tissue is tied with a fine catgut. The medial side is usually clamped with a metallic clip. The ureter is now relatively free from the surrounding tissue, and the posterior attachment can be easily freed by separating the avascular space with Metzenbaum scissors while a ureter is kept slightly elevated with tension. The cardinal ligament is palpable at the pelvic side wall, which is squeezed gently with fingers toward the uterine specimen. Essentially the same procedure is performed on the opposite side.

Attention is now directed toward the posterior cul-de-sac. The peritoneal defect is enlarged by identifying a large space between the rectum and vagina. Three fingers (index, middle, and fourth fingers) are placed and by dor-

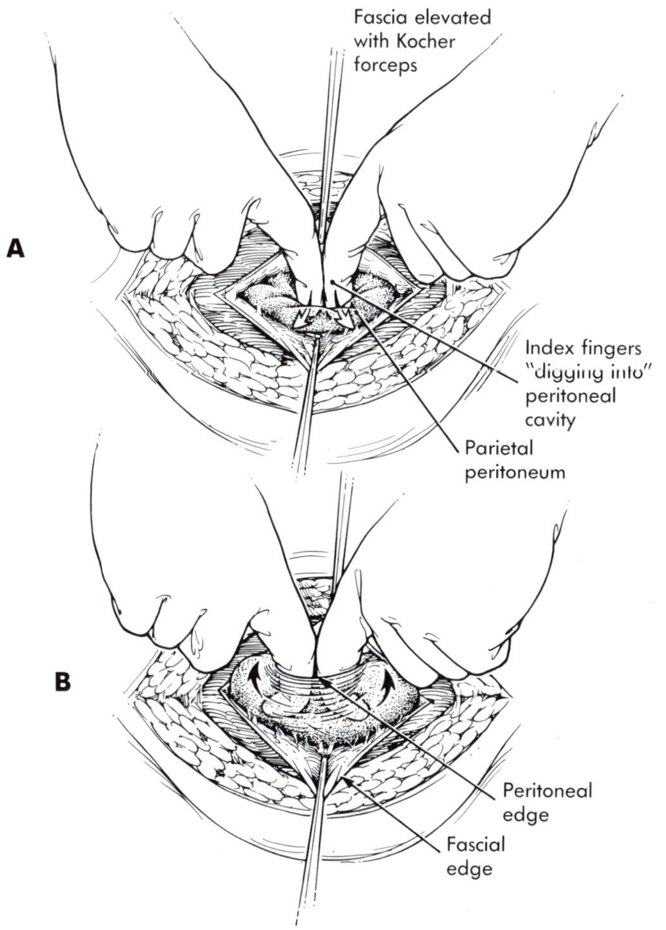

Fascia elevated with Kocher forceps

A

Index fingers "digging into" peritoneal cavity

Parietal peritoneum

B

Peritoneal edge

Fascial edge

Fig. 34-28. **A,** Both index fingers are used for "digging in" method. **B,** Digging into peritoneal cavity.

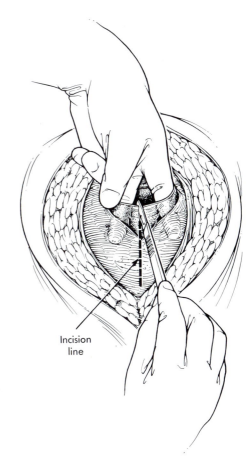

Incision line

Fig. 34-29. Left index and middle fingers are placed longitudinally along middle incision line, and incision is extended caudally and distally.

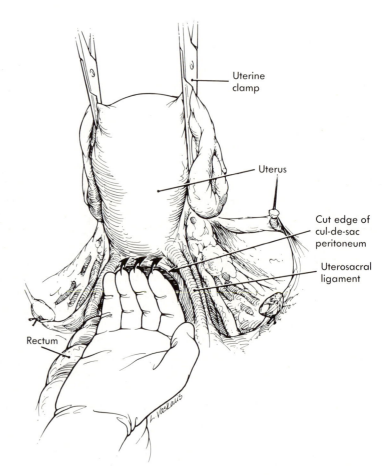

Fig. 34-30. Three fingers (index, middle, fourth) are placed, and by dorsal sweep the space between rectum and vagina will be expanded.

sal sweep, this space is expanded (Fig. 34-30). The uterovesical space is pushed further down anteriorly along the perivaginal avascular space. The cervix and upper vagina are palpated gently by thumb, index, and middle fingers. The deep uterosacral ligament is clamped with Uchida's paracolpium clamp near the rectal side (but not too close), dissected, and sutured. The cardinal ligament is clamped close to the pelvic side wall, dissected, and sutured. The paravaginal tissue and vagina are clamped with Uchida's paracolpium clamp placed horizontally and cut on both sides. With large Mayo scissors, the vagina is dissected anteriorly, and the vaginal cuff is grasped with a straight Kocher forceps while the resected portion of the vaginal cuff is inspected for adequacy of the resection. The same is applied posteriorly. The vaginal angle and remainder of the vaginal cuff are closed interruptedly. At the midpoint of the vaginal cuff, the anterior and posterior peritoneum are sutured together with the vaginal cuff. Before closure, the specimen is inspected and, if necessary, additional vaginal cuff is removed and sent for frozen study.

Pelvic lymphadenectomy begins with the common iliac proximally and moves toward the distal end of the external iliac vessels, including the hypogastric and obturator regions. The proximal and distal ends are held with large metallic clips. Avascular space is identified around and between vessels. Every attempt is made to obtain one block specimen, and it is sent as "pelvic nodes." Care is taken to

avoid genitofemoral and obturator nerve injury during dissection. Also, the superior vesical vessel and hypogastric vein are clearly identified to avoid unnecessary damage. A finger sweep with the thumb and index finger is used to obtain lymphatic tissue from the pelvic side wall in the obturator space. Uchida's peeling off technique is used whenever avascular space is easily obtained, but forcing this technique should be avoided when avascular fine space is not readily available.

The retroperitoneal cavity is irrigated with 1000 ml of normal saline with 2 g of Cefadyl (cephapirin sodium) or Mandol (cefamandole nafate),[26] and two hemovac drains are placed in the retroperitoneal cavity along the dissection site to be brought to both sides of the lower abdomen. The bladder is distended with methylene blue and sterile water for any undetected bladder rent through the bladder drainage system placed before surgery. The ureter is inspected carefully for any change of color or any abnormal peristalsis. Ureters are placed in the retroperitoneal cavity, and the cavity is closed with interrupted 3-0 chromic catgut sutures. The self-retaining retractor and packing are removed. The paraaortic region is inspected, and the abdomen is closed.

The fascial layer is closed with 0-PDS (polydioxanone) continuously starting from the top of the incision downward and from the bottom upward, and sutures are separately tied at the mid-portion of the incision. The wound is irrigated with the same solution used for retroperitoneal ir-

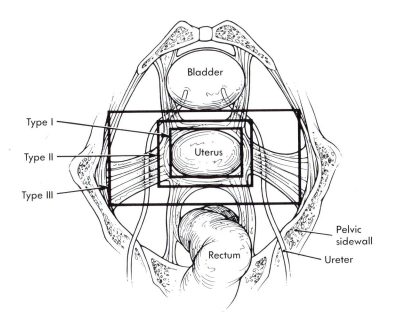

Fig. 34-31. Different types of hysterectomy: type I simple hysterectomy, type II modified radical hysterectomy, type III radical hysterectomy.

rigation; hemostasis is obtained with electrocautery if needed. The skin edge is reapproximated with metallic clips, and the drain site and wound are dressed.

Modified radical hysterectomy

Because carcinoma of the cervix is being diagnosed early, the less than radical procedure is being used more often.[2] Whereas radical hysterectomy and pelvic lymphadenectomy remove the entire cardinal ligament and all lymph nodes in the pelvis (type III hysterectomy), the modified hysterectomy removes only the medial portion of the cardinal ligament with or without lymph nodes, as shown in Fig. 34-31 (type II hysterectomy).[33] The major difference is that the ureter has not been freed from its posterior attachment, as in the radical procedure.[28,33] The ureters are moved laterally, but the blood supply to the ureters is conserved because the uterine vessels are ligated medial to the ureters. The procedure is most commonly used for surgical treatment of microinvasive carcinoma of the cervix. The technique of modified radical hysterectomy is described briefly as an adaptation of Uchida's method.[45]

Uchida's subradical hysterectomy with regressive ureteral separation. After the abdomen is opened through a low mid-subumbilical incision, careful abdominal and pelvic exploration is performed. The uterus is grasped with Uchida's uterine clamps and lifted. The right round ligament is ligated and cut, and the incision is extended to open the broad ligament widely. The uterine vessels are identified, ligated medial to the ureter, and cut. If ovarian preservation is not required, the right infundibulopelvic ligament is clamped, cut, and ligated. The ureter is mobilized laterally in one stroke by using the back portion of the Metzenbaum scissors. The same procedure is applied to the opposite side. The peritoneum of the posterior cul-de-sac is opened transversely, and the rectovaginal space is deeply opened. The uterosacral ligament is clamped, cut, and ligated deeply on the both sides. The

uterovesical peritoneum is excised transversely, and the vesicouterine space is pushed distally to expose paravaginal tissue anteriorly. The vesicouterine ligament of the lateral attachment is identified. A thin clamp is inserted medially along the ureter toward the pelvis from the bladder side against the flow of urine, and it is widely opened. Two fine clamps are placed, and the tissue is cut in the middle and ligated. The ureter is replaced laterally, and parametrial, paracervical, and paravaginal tissue is clamped, cut, and ligated. The vaginal angle is clamped, and the vagina is amputated. The vaginal angle is ligated, and the vaginal cuff is closed by a running interlocking suture. The retroperitoneum is closed by continuous suture. The specimen usually includes 2 to 3 cm of vaginal cuff with partial parametrium, paracervical, and paravaginal tissue attached. The abdomen is closed in three layers.

Extraperitoneal lymphadenectomy

The staging classification for carcinoma of the cervix is based on that of the International Federation of Gynecology and Obstetrics (FIGO), which includes clinical and some radiographic evaluation for assessment of the tumor's extension. It includes cystoscopy, sigmoidoscopy, chest x-ray, intravenous pyelography, and barium enema when indicated. However, this staging system is not quite adequate to reflect the true status of patient's pelvic and paraaortic lymph nodes.[1] Lymphangiography and CT scanning for evaluating the pelvic and paraaortic nodes are not always accurate.[11,46] Because lymph node metastasis of the cervical cancer affects survival of the patient adversely, its accurate evaluation is essential to developing a treatment plan. Transperitoneal pelvic and paraaortic node dissection has been associated with increased intestinal complications when followed by conventional or extended field radiation therapy.[3,47] Berman and co-workers reported a very low morbidity associated with pelvic and paraaortic lymphadenectomy performed extraperitoneally through a lateral J-shaped vertical incision in the left abdominal wall.[4] Lagasse and co-workers reported that their technique confirmed an adequate resection in each level of the periaortic, common iliac, and pelvic node areas reflected by pretreatment lymphangiogram.[12] Downey and associates reported a similar approach through a low midline subumbilical incision.[10] The abdominal entry is made through a lateral J-shaped vertical incision, a low mid-subumbilical incision, or a paramedian incision. This could be adjusted according to the site and extent of the tumor involvement. The fascia is cut in the same line as the skin incision. The peritoneum is rolled medially until the psoas muscle is visible. The round ligament and inferior epigastric vessels can be ligated and cut for a better exposure to the opposite side pelvis. With the help of wide large retractors the left ureter is identified on the peritoneum, and this is pushed medially to expose the vessels. Left paraaortic node dissection begins from the region of the second lumbar spine down to the bifurcation of the aorta. This is followed by dissection of the common iliac, external iliac, hypogastric, and obturator lymph node chains of the left side. For right sided dissection, care should be taken to remove the peritoneum very gently from the underlying great vessels, especially the inferior vena cava. It is also important to identify the right ureter when exposing the right side vessels. The same lymphadenectomy is carried out. The specimen from each chain is sent separately. The currently available protocols suggest making a small peritoneal opening, obtaining a peritoneal washing, and gently exploring to determine a gross tumor extension. Any gross lesion found should be biopsied. A drain is placed in the retroperitoneal cavity, and the wound is closed. For paraaortic node sampling, such structures as the bifurcation of the aorta, inferior vena cava, ovarian vessels, inferior mesenteric artery, and ureters, as well as a portion of the duodenum must be identified. Any enlarged or suspicious nodes are excised, or biopsied if not resectable.

This technique is being used to evaluate lymph node status and tumor extent of the invasive cervical carcinoma before radiation therapy at various medical centers under such collaborative study projects as the Gynecologic Oncology Group (GOG). It is also useful for evaluating and staging other gynecologic cancer on an individual basis, for example, invasive carcinoma of the vulva. It is important that the pelvic surgeon performing this procedure has proper training and experience to handle any associated vascular, intestinal, and genitourinary complications that might occur during the procedure. The position of the patient on the operating table assists an operating team by the ability to tilt her to either side of the table to obtain better exposure of the deeper vessels and nodes. Further details of the technique can be found in the literature.[16,19,27,32]

POSTOPERATIVE CONSIDERATIONS
Prevention and management of complications

Vascular and pulmonary complications. Although it is rare, massive pulmonary embolism remains the most common cause of death postoperatively.[36] The incidence of pulmonary embolism is reported to vary from 0.3% to 3.0%. Because a massive pulmonary embolism is usually fatal, it is crucial to prevent this thromboembolic episode during postoperative care. Venous thrombosis is asymptomatic in 50% of cases. Malignancy is known to be associated with the hypercoagulative vascular system. Postoperative immobility and multiple traumas to the pelvic vessels create a favorable source for development of silent thrombosis and subsequent sudden thromboembolic phenomena. Classical use of miniheparin introduced by Kakkar in 1975 has been challenged by the use of intermittent pneumatic cuff compression and prolonged preoperative use of miniheparin.[6] Clarke-Pearson and associates reported that 5000 units given subcutaneously preoperatively every 8 hours for two to nine doses and continuously postoperatively for 7 days effectively prevented thrombosis without a bleeding problem.[7] It is important to monitor activated thromboplastin times and platelet counts preoperatively and postoperatively.

Pulmonary complications are considered to be the most common cause of morbidity and mortality in a major surgical patient. The most common pulmonary complication, atelectasis, results in hypoxia owing to partial or complete collapse of the alveolar spaces. Prevention should start before surgery by instructing patients on the use of inspirometer, deep breathing, and early ambulation. The most sensitive test for early detection of microatelectasis is arterial blood gas, which usually reveals lowered P_{O_2} and O_2 saturation with normal P_{CO_2}.[20] Chest physiotherapy should be provided early for the patient. She should receive adequate pain medication frequently and stay in a sitting position, often with frequent deep inspiration to avoid other serious pulmonary complications such as pneumonia, hypoventilation, acute ventilatory failure, and adult respiratory distress syndrome.

Urinary complications. Temporary paralysis of the bladder is the most common complication of radical hysterectomy. Interruption of parasympathetic and sympathetic nerve fibers contained in the pelvic nerve plexus produces both temporary and prolonged bladder dysfunction. The degree of bladder dysfunction appears to be directly related to dissection of the inferolateral aspect of the cardinal ligament as well as the deep uterosacral ligament. Sasaki et al reported a surgical technique to preserve the posterior portion of the cardinal ligament that has a beneficial effect on bladder function.[35] Prolonged bladder drainage by a Foley catheter or a suprapubic catheter assists in preventing overdistention of the bladder. Shingleton et al reported an advantage of suprapubic drainage over the transurethral catheters and very few long-term bladder complications without intermittent self-catheterization.[38]

Vesicovaginal fistula is rare even if there is an extensive dissection of the bladder from the anterior cervix and vagina. To detect bladder injury, a bladder irrigation set should be installed before the procedure and the bladder should be distended with sterile water and methylene blue dye before reperitonealization. Immediate repair of the rent on the operating table is the best management of this complication. If found a few days postoperatively, ureteral damage also should be ruled out by injecting 5 ml of 0.8% indigocarmine into a vein. A tampon placed into the vagina should demonstrate the presence of ureteral vaginal fistula. Intravenous pyelography assists in localizing the ureteral fistula.

Ureterovaginal fistula is now found in less than 1% of radical hysterectomies, whereas this complication was a very common problem in the past.[9,13,15,19,38] Suction drainage has made a significant contribution in reducing this complication.[29,38] It is manifested about 1 or 2 weeks postoperatively with a watery vaginal discharge. The history reveals the presence of vague elevated temperature or pelvic discomfort during the postoperative period. A retrograde cystoscopic procedure can identify a fistula, and an attempt should be made to insert a catheter to the involved renal pelvis through a damaged ureter to bring a communication, which could be established in 2 to 3 weeks. A retrograde catheterization can be attempted again later if reduction of tissue edema is expected. Surgical repair is best performed with ureteroneocystostomy if the fistula is in the lower pelvis. End-to-end ureteral anastomosis is indicated for the fistula located 5 cm or more above the ureterovesical junction.[30]

Infectious complications. It is estimated that about 30% of patients will develop febrile morbidity after radical hysterectomy.[38] Significant causes include urinary tract infection, pelvic cellulitis and abscess, wound infection, and pulmonary atelectasis. Prophylactic antibiotics, suction drainage, perioperative care, and surgical technique have resulted in a remarkably low incidence of serious infectious complications.[9] Because of prolonged catheterization, urinary tract infection can be seen after radical hysterectomy in up to 10% of patients despite the use of prophylactic antibiotics. For the high-risk patient, it is advisable to use urinary antiseptics as long as she has a urinary catheter.

Sevin and co-workers advised closure of the vaginal cuff to reduce pelvic infection by avoiding an ascending infection through the vagina; however, others report a few infectious problems with the open vaginal cuff technique.[37] Prophylactic broad-spectrum antibiotics reduce the incidence of pelvic cellulitis to less than 5% of all radical hysterectomies, according to Mattingly.[20] The use of antibiotic irrigation at the time of the procedure seems associated with a significantly lower incidence of pelvic and wound infection.[26] Pelvic infection, if it occurs, should be treated aggressively with antibiotics and drainage.

Care must be taken to prevent a serious wound problem such as dehiscence and evisceration. Skin stands as the first line of defense. Painting the surgical area for 120 seconds with an agent such as aqueous solution of povidone-iodine and air drying is the most effective way to prepare a patient for surgery.[18] Fascial closure with an absorbable monofilament synthetic suture such as polydioxanone (PDS) and polyglyconate (Maxon) results in about 50% strength in 4 weeks.[34] Their tensile strength is greater than that of Dexon and Vicryl. Fascial suture should be placed loosely for single layer closure with at least 1 cm from the edge and 1 cm between bites. Any surgical patient with fever should receive immediate attention to the wound, especially early postoperatively. Early wound infection usually caused by group A beta-hemolytic *Streptococcus* or *Clostridium perfringens* requires immediate antibiotic therapy and excision of necrotic tissue.

Lymphatic complications. Lymphocyst formation has become a very infrequent complication of radical hysterectomy. Most series reveal their incidence to be up to 3%.[29] This is mainly due to the effective function of suction drainage of the pelvis. Shingleton et al report that this complication is very rare even without ligating lymphatics routinely.[38] Although most lymphocysts are not symptomatic, if a symptomatic lymphocyst is found, it can be aspirated usually by a needle, and if required, obliteration of the cavity is obtained by instilling tetracycline through a catheter under ultrasound guidance.[16] Serial ultrasound study may detect a silent progressive lymphocele; this can be corrected by percutaneus catheter drainage on an outpatient basis.[8] Lymphedema of the lower extremities is sometimes seen after radical hysterectomy, especially in patients who received radiation treatment subsequent to the procedure.

Follow-up

Because most recurrences are observed in the first 24 months after the procedure, the patient should be seen every 3 months during this period. If there is no recurrence, then she is seen every 6 months for an additional 3 years. At each visit, a thorough history regarding her general health should be taken. Physical examination includes weighing the patient and carefully examining her for supraclavicular and groin nodes, abdominal mass, and hepatomegaly. The vaginal cuff should be inspected as well as the lower vagina and suburethral region; a Pap smear is also taken. Rectovaginal examination is performed to evaluate any sign of recurrence. Chest x-ray is taken every year, and computed tomography scan may be ordered for any questionable case of recurrence.

CONCLUSION

The key to successful pelvic surgery is to find the avascular space and dissect it swiftly. Because this is not usually found in detail in textbooks, it must be learned through experience. Living anatomy of the pelvic structure is available to any pelvic surgeon through various pelvic surgeries, especially in procedures such as radical hysterectomy and pelvic lymphadenectomy. We must appreciate the three-dimensional pelvic structure each time we operate.

Time efficiency is essential for a prolonged pelvic surgical procedure. Each minute the patient spends on the operating table should be used efficiently. When we encounter difficulties, we can seek an easier area to work first to increase safety for our patients. As long as our goal is clear and focused, we should be able to find a plane to dissect. Although in some cases it seems almost impossible to continue a planned procedure because of various adhesions or dense fibrosis, it should be remembered that by recalling the anatomy of the living and seeking a hidden avascular plane we generally find an easier path to dissect.

REFERENCES

1. Averett HE et al: Exploratory celiotomy for surgical staging of cervical cancer, *Am J Obstet Gynecol* 113:1090, 1972.
2. Averett HE et al: How radical should surgery be for cervical Ca? *Contemp Obstet Gynecol* 91, July 1990.
3. Ballon SC et al: Survival after extraperitoneal pelvic and paraaortic lymphadenectomy and radiation therapy in cervical carcinoma, *Obstet Gynecol* 57:90, 1981.
4. Berman ML et al: The operative evaluation of patients with cervical carcinoma by an extraperitoneal approach, *Obstet Gynecol* 50:658, 1977.
5. Bonney MS: The treatment of carcinoma of the cervix by Wertheim's operation, *Am J Obstet Gynecol* 30:815, 1935.
6. Clarke-Pearson DL et al: Prevention of postoperative venous thromboembolism by external pneumatic calf compression in patients with gynecologic malignancy, *Obstet Gynecol* 63:92, 1984.
7. Clarke-Pearson DL et al: A controlled trial of two low dose heparin regimen for the prevention of postoperative deep vein thrombosis, *Obstet Gynecol* 75:684, 1990.
8. Conte M et al: Pelvic lymphocele following radical paraaortic and pelvic lymphadenectomy for cervical carcinoma: incidence rate and percutaneous management, *Obstet Gynecol* 76:268, 1990.
9. Curry SL: *Surgical treatment of cervical cancer: radical hysterectomy*. In Sciarra JJ, Buchsbaum HJ: *Gynecology and obstetrics*, ed 2, vol 4, Philadelphia, 1986, Harper & Row.
10. Downey GO et al: Pretreatment surgical staging in cervical carcinoma: therapeutic efficacy of pelvic lymph node resection, *Am J Obstet Gynecol* 160:1055, 1989.
11. Hann LE, Crivello MS: Imaging techniques in the staging of gynecologic malignancy, *Clin Obstet Gynecol* 29:715, 1986.
12. Lagasse LD et al: Pretreatment lymphangiography and operative evaluation in carcinoma of the cervix, *Am J Obstet Gynecol* 134:219, 1979.
13. Langley II et al: Radical hysterectomy and pelvic lymph node dissection, *Gynecol Oncol* 9:37, 1980.
14. Lawton FG, Hacker NF: Surgery for invasive gynecologic cancer in the elderly female population, *Obstet Gynecol* 76:287, 1990.
15. Lee YN et al: Radical hysterectomy with pelvic node dissection for treatment of cervical cancer: a clinical review of 954 cases, *Gynecol Oncol* 32:135, 1989.
16. Mann WJ et al: Management of lymphocysts after radical gynecologic surgery, *Gynecol Oncol* 33:248, 1989.
17. Masterson BJ: *Manual of gynecologic surgery*, ed 1, New York, 1979, Springer-Verlag.
18. Masterson BJ: Skin preparation, *Clin Obstet Gynecol* 31:736, 1988.
19. Masterson JG: Radical surgery in early carcinoma of the cervix, *Am J Obstet Gynecol* 87:601, 1963.
20. Mattingly RF, Thompson JD: *Telinde's operative gynecology*, ed 6, Philadelphia, 1985, JB Lippincott.
21. Meigs JV: Carcinoma of the cervix—The Wertheim operation, *Surg Gynecol Obstet* 78:195, 1944.
22. Meigs JV: Gynecology: carcinoma of the cervix, *N Engl J Med* 230:577, 607, 1944.
23. Meigs JV: The Wertheim operation for carcinoma of the cervix, *Am J Obstet Gynecol* 49:542, 1945.
24. Meigs JV: Radical hysterectomy with bilateral pelvic lymph node dissections. A report of 100 patients operated on five or more years ago, *Am J Obstet Gynecol* 62:854, 1951.
25. Meigs JV: *Surgical treatment of cancer of the cervix*, ed 1, New York, 1954, Grune & Stratton.
26. Miyazawa K et al: Prophylactic topical Cefamandole in radical hysterectomy, *Int J Gynecol Obstet* 25:133, 1987.
27. Nakano R: Abdominal radical hysterectomy and bilateral pelvic lymph node dissections for cancer of the cervix, *Gynecol Obstet Invest* 12:281, 1981.
28. Nelson JH: *Atlas of radical pelvic surgery*, ed 2, New York, 1977, Appleton-Century-Crofts.
29. Newton M, Newton ER: Complications of gynecologic and obstetric management, ed 1, Philadelphia, 1988, WB Saunders.
30. Nichols DH: *Clinical problems, injuries and complications of gynecologic surgery*, ed 2, Baltimore, 1988, Williams & Wilkins.
31. Okabayashi H: Radical abdominal hysterectomy for cancer of the cervix uteri, *Surg Gynecol Obstet* 33:335, 1921.
32. Parson L, Ulfelder H: *An atlas of pelvic surgery*, ed 2, Philadelphia, 1968, WB Saunders.
33. Ridley JH: *Gynecologic surgery, error, safeguard, salvage*, ed 2, Baltimore, 1981, Williams & Wilkins.
34. Sanz LE: Wound management—Matching materials and methods for best results, *Contemp Obstet Gynecol* 86, Nov 1987.
35. Sasaki H et al: Urethral pressure profiles following radical hysterectomy, *Obstet Gynecol* 59:101, 1982.
36. Scaffer G, Graber EA: In *Radical hysterectomy. Complications in obstetrics and gynecologic surgery*, ed 1, Hagerstown, MD, 1981, Harper & Row.
37. Sevin BU et al: Antibiotic prevention of infections complicating radical abdominal hysterectomy, *Obstet Gynecol* 64:539, 1984.
38. Shingleton HM, Orr JW: *Cancer of the cervix, diagnosis and treatment*, ed 1, New York, 1987, Churchill Livingstone.
39. Taussig FJ: Iliac lymphadenectomy with irradiation in the treatment of cancer of the cervix, *Am J Obstet Gynecol*, 28:650, 1934.
40. Taussig FJ: The removal of lymph nodes in cancer of the cervix, *Am J Roentgenol Radium Therapy* 34:354, 1935.
41. Taussig FJ: Iliac lymphadenectomy for group II cancer of the cervix, *Am J Obstet Gynecol* 45:733, 1943.
42. Tovell HMM, Dank LD: *Gynecologic operation*, ed 1, Hagerstown, MD, 1978, Harper & Row.
43. Uchida H: Radical operation for cancer of the cervix, presented by film, Nov 1977, Seventh Asian Congress of Obstetrics & Gynecology, Bangkok, Thailand.
44. Uchida H: Radical operation for cancer of the cervix, presented by film, Oct 1982, Tenth World Congress of Gynecology and Obstetrics, San Francisco, CA.
45. Uchida H: Sub-radical hysterectomy with regressive ureter separation, *Obstet Gynecol Therapy*, 59(suppl):44, 1989.
46. Villasanta U et al: Computed tomography in invasive carcinoma of the cervix: an appraisal, *Obstet Gynecol* 62:218, 1983
47. Weiser EB et al: Extraperitoneal versus transperitoneal selective paraaotic lymphadenectomy in the pretreatment surgical staging of advanced cervical carcinoma (a Gynecologic Oncology Group study), *Gynecol Oncol* 33:283, 1989.
48. Wertheim E: The extended abdominal operation for carcinoma uteri (based on 500 operative cases) Grad H (trans), *Am J Obstet* 66:169, 1912.
49. Wheeless CR: *Atlas of pelvic surgery*, ed 1, Philadelphia, 1981, Lee and Febiger.
50. Yagi H: Treatment of carcinoma of the cervix uteri, *Surg Gynecol Obstet* 95:552, 1952.

Chapter 35

PERCUTANEOUS PELVIC LYMPHADENECTOMY UNDER LAPAROSCOPIC GUIDANCE

Daniel Dargent
Pierre Arnould

For decades, the development of cancer therapy has been directed toward a single goal: to improve the power of different weapons and to use them in the most powerful combinations. This direction did not give the expected results in the field of solid tumors. The overall survival rate did not improve, but the rate of different iatrogenic complications increased. A new tendency is to identify high-risk patients, so we can focus the power of the most aggressive therapies on them while sparing the low-risk patients the drawbacks of those therapies.

As the concept of more conservative management was accepted and has even matured, enthusiasm for laparoscopic surgery has grown, starting from simple procedures (treatment of ectopic pregnancy) to more sophisticated ones (treatment of tuboperitoneal infertility, endometriosis, and so forth). The convergence of the two movements led to the design of the endoscopic assessment of regional lymph nodes—the percutaneous pelvic lymphadenectomy (PPL).

The status of the regional lymph nodes is the most significant parameter in the prognosis of solid epithelial tumors. If we know this parameter at the same time as the data concerning the tumor (both qualitative and quantitative), we can classify each case as high-risk or low-risk with great accuracy and make the right decision for its management.

Until recently, staging lymphadenectomy performed for pelvic cancer patients by a laparotomy was the only way to assess the nodes. But such a surgical procedure has many drawbacks. With the endoscopic assessment, a new era begins.

HISTORICAL DEVELOPMENT

Assessing the pelvic nodes without performing a laparotomy was first formally described by Hald and Rasmunssen[6] in 1980. The method, designated "extraperitoneal pelvioscopy," was set up to help the staging of tumors of the lower urinary tract. It was not really a new technique but a transposition of methods designed 10 years before to assess the lumbar retroperitoneal area and named "retroperitoneoskopie" by Bartel[1] or "lomboskopie" by Sommerkamp.[9] Assessment of the lumboaortic nodes, lumbar sympathectomy, renal biopsy, and other procedures could be performed through this approach.

Bartel's retroperitoneoscopy was copied from the mediastinoscopy proposed at the end of the 1950s by Carlens and which is still used in the assessment of the mediastinal space. The instrumentation used is almost the same: a tube, 17 to 27.5 cm in length and 10 to 30 mm in diameter, through which the surgeon can obtain a direct look at the targeted anatomic area, illuminated through a little lateral light. A dissection and biopsies can be performed, using tools introduced directly through the endoscope. The surgical procedure is also the same: minilaparotomy (minicervicotomy for the "mediastinoscopy"), digital preparation of the virtual space until contact with the targeted area is obtained, introduction of the endoscope, and working on the anatomic structures.

The advantages of the mediastinoscopy-derived techniques in assessment of the pelvic nodes are obvious. The technique is simple and the surgical traumatism is low, leaving only two little scars at the site of the inguinal incisions. The accuracy of the evaluation is good as demonstrated by the publications of Hald and Rasmunssen[6] or Wurtz.[10] But the procedure is only a node sampling and a rather blind one. It is not an actual surgical lymphadenectomy. On the contrary, the coelioscopic techniques enable us to perform a true surgical lymphadenectomy while retaining all the advantages of an endoscopic procedure.

LATER DEVELOPMENT

We performed our first retroperitoneal pelviscopy on December 15, 1986. The patient, 6 years after a subtotal hysterectomy, was a 46-year-old woman with a stage Ib adenocarcinoma of the cervical stump. The anatomic characteristics of the tumor made the vaginal approach to treatment preferable. The general conditions (obesity, antecedent thrombophlebitis, and a Wolf-Parkinson-White syndrome) made it mandatory. Having neither a mediastinoscope nor a lumboscope, we performed a bilateral inguinal extraperitoneal pelviscopy using the coelioscope as is done according to the open laparoscopy protocol: minilaparotomy, digital exploration of the space to be assessed, introduction of the coelioscope, insufflation of CO_2 through the sheath of the coelioscope after a suture had been placed around the sheath to avoid leaking of the gas.

The lymph nodes of the first patient were perfectly located during the preliminary palpation, and the consecutive endoscopic assessment identified them clearly together with the vascular and nervous structures of the pelvic wall. A fine-needle aspiration was performed under endoscopic guidance. The collected material, unfortunately, did not contain significant cells. Nevertheless, taking argument from the negativity of the palpatory and endoscopic assessment, we performed a radical trachelectomy through the vaginal route 10 days later. The patient is alive and well 6 years after the operation.

Our first experience was half a failure because the microsopic confirmation of the lymph node status was not obtained. But it was also a success because it was demonstrated that the pelvic wall could be palpated and then inspected as if a laparotomy had been done, but without the drawbacks of the latter. After this first experience, our concern was to modify the technique, to be able to introduce forceps, scissors, and other instruments in the targeted area to perform a surgical preparation and an actual lymphadenectomy. A protocol called "interiliac percutaneous lymphadenectomy under guidance of retroperitoneal pelviscopy" was devised in collaboration with Salvat.[3] The reliability of the procedure was first tested immediately before radical abdominal hysterectomies. Then the procedure was integrated into the therapeutic management as explained later.

Soon after our first publication,[2] other groups working in laparoscopic surgery, Querleu's in Roubaix[8] and Dauplat's[4] in Clermont Ferrand, advocated the classical transperitoneal coelioscopy for the assessment of retroperitoneal lymph nodes. Their way is perfectly acceptable. The coelioscopic procedure is surely easier to perform, and the lymph nodal assessment can be extended to areas other than the pelvis, which is an advantage. But there are drawbacks both in the conceptual and in the technical sense. The transperitoneal coelioscopic approach is, for us, no more than a way to succeed if the retroperitoneal approach fails. In that sense, the transperitoneal coelioscopy will be described here as a useful, complementary second choice.

RATIONALE FOR ENDOSCOPIC INTERILIAC LYMPHADENECTOMY

As was said earlier, the status of the nodes is the main prognostic factor in an epithelial malignant tumor together with certain pathologic characteristics. Figure 35-1 illustrates this assertion on the basis of data obtained by assessment of radical surgery specimens. However, the problem is "how to assess the lymph nodes before scheduling the treatment?"

For patients affected by lymph nodal involvement, the radiotherapy, if given after radical hysterectomy, is given under unfavorable conditions due to the various anatomic and physiologic changes linked with the operation. That is the reason why the majority of the contemporary gynecologic oncologists prefer to first do a staging laparotomy and to perform the radical hysterectomy only for patients not affected by lymph nodal involvement. But the complete lymphadenectomy has no benefit at all for the pN-patients.

The ideal approach would be to use imaging procedures for assessing the lymph nodes before scheduling the treatment. However, the procedures that we have at our disposal (lymphography computed tomography [CT] scan, magnetic resonance imaging [MRI]) are inappropriate for micrometastasis and cannot be used if we intend to select the very low-risk patients. Identification of macrometastasis, on the contrary, is easy, and therefore selection of high-risk patients is possible. But when the patient cannot be identified as high risk, it does not necessarily follow that she is a low-risk patient.

Because surgical assessment is too heavy and imaging assessment is too inaccurate, laparoscopic assessment appears to be a good compromise. If we use a laparoscopic assessment as a mimicry of the surgical one, we will probably avoid postoperative peritoneal adhesions, which are one of the drawbacks of the latter, but the endoscopic operation will be as heavy, dangerous, and, for the pN-patients, useless as a surgical one. The best way to use the laparoscopic assessment is to restrict it to the assessment of the "sentinel lymph nodes."

For carcinoma affecting the pelvic organs (except for the gastrointestinal tract), the lymph nodes to be assessed are well known. They are those located along the pelvic wall between the external iliac vein and the obturator nerve and situated on the medial side of the iliac vein between the two branches of the common iliac artery. These lymph nodes, referred to as "obturator" and "hypogastric" nodes, can also be designated, as proposed by Reiffenstuhl, as the "interiliac lymph nodes." Figure 35-2 illus-

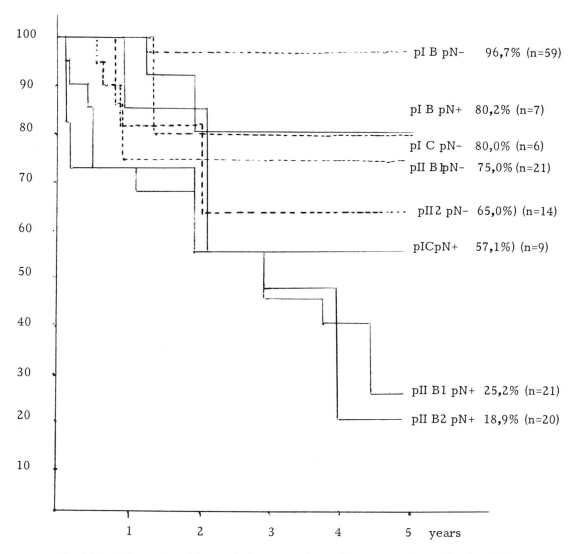

Fig. 35-1. Patients affected by cervical cancer and treated by surgery. Personal series 1979 to 1981. Calculation after Kaplan and Meyer. Chances of survival according to the pathologic status of the lymph nodes (pN) and to the pathologic stages.
Stages pI B = not bulky I B
Stages pI C = massive involvement of the cervix (bulky pI B)
Stages pII B 1 = infiltration of one of the parametrium
Stages pII B 2 = infiltration of both parametrium.

trates the main anatomic presentation of those lymph nodes. A ratio usually exists between the volume of the obturator and hypogastric groups: the obturator is larger two times out of three. The reliability of the assessment of the interiliac lymph nodes to select low-risk patients has been demonstrated in many surgicopathologic surveys. After reviewing the charts of 1000 patients submitted to pelvic and subaortic lymphadenectomy for cancer of the cervix, the first survey was published in 1973 by Pilleron, Durand, and Hamelin.[7] They established that the subaortic nodes were involved in only 5 of 873 observations in which the interiliac lymph nodes are uninvolved. The five cases were stage IIb. Other studies, afterwards, confirmed their findings. As demonstrated in Table 35-1, the rate of involvement of subaortic and aortic nodes is less than 2%

if the interiliac nodes are not involved in patients with cancer of the uterine cervix. It may be lower if we consider only the stages Ib and early IIb. Then the direct involvement of subaortic or aortic lymph nodes seems to be observed mainly in more advanced cancers, which are often the faster growing types. The same phenomenon can be observed with some nuances in patients with cancer of the endometrium, the vagina, the prostate, and the bladder.

Direct involvement of the lymph nodes situated down the interiliac in the usual pattern of extension is not the only problem. We also have to consider the nodes situated upstream (i.e., the microlymph nodes disseminated in the pelvic cellular tissue between the organs and the pelvic wall). Girardi,[5] studying this problem on Burghardt's very large specimens of radical hysterectomy, has demonstrated

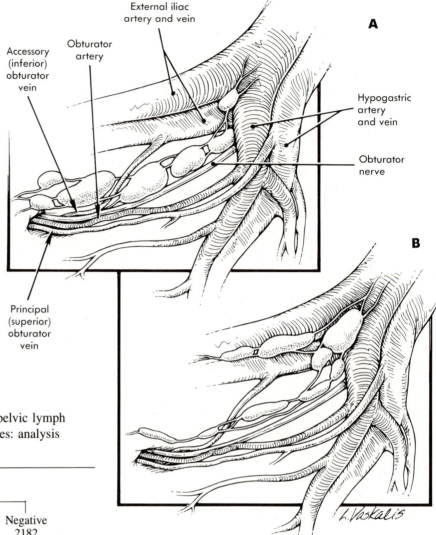

Fig. 35-2. Anatomy of the interiliac obturator, **A,** and hypogastric, **B,** lymph nodes: the first type of pattern (large obturator lymph nodes, small hypogastric lymph nodes) is seen two times out of three.

Table 35-1. Cancer of the cervix uteri pelvic lymph nodes and sub Ao and/or Ao lymph nodes: analysis of the literature—Arnould 1991*

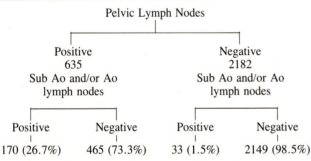

	Pelvic Lymph Nodes		
Positive 635		Negative 2182	
Sub Ao and/or Ao lymph nodes		Sub Ao and/or Ao lymph nodes	
Positive	Negative	Positive	Negative
170 (26.7%)	465 (73.3%)	33 (1.5%)	2149 (98.5%)

*After Pilleron, Wharton, Lagasse, Chung, Dargent, Martimbeau, Inoue, Michel, and Burghardt.

Table 35-2. Frequency of parametrial micrometastasis depending on the status of interiliac lymph nodes (after Girardi[5])

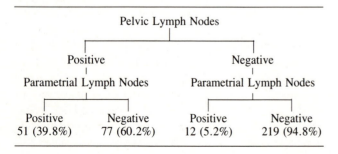

	Pelvic Lymph Nodes		
Positive		Negative	
Parametrial Lymph Nodes		Parametrial Lymph Nodes	
Positive	Negative	Positive	Negative
51 (39.8%)	77 (60.2%)	12 (5.2%)	219 (94.8%)

that those microlymph nodes were numerous and infiltrated in more than 10% of cases of stage Ib cervical cancers. However, there is a correlation between the involvement of those nodes and the status of pelvic wall nodes. Table 35-2 demonstrates that in 95% of cases in which the pelvic wall nodes are uninvolved, the parametrial nodes are also uninvolved. Moreover, the metastasis seen in the parametrial microlymph nodes, in cases of uninvolved pelvic wall nodes, are located as shown in Fig. 35-3 near the uterus in three out of four cases.

If we summarize these data, we observe that the interiliac lymph nodes are really the "sentinel lymph nodes" in the assessment of regional spread of cancers of internal female genital organs (as well as cancer of the prostate and the bladder). The assessment of those nodes can be performed through a "pelvic staging laparotomy" as it is done by the majority of urologists for prostate and bladder cancers. It can also be performed through a mediastinoscopic inguinal approach or a transperitoneal coelioscopic approach. We believe that the best way to do it is by per-

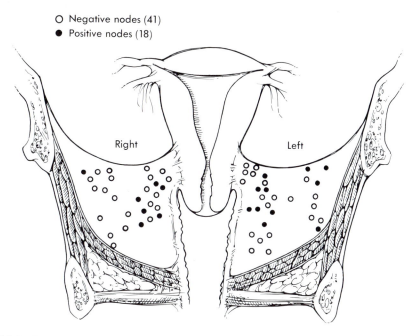

Fig. 35-3. Topography of the parametrial micrometastasis in patients with no pelvic lymph nodal metastasis. (Modified from Girardi F et al: The importance of parametrial lymph nodes in the treatment of cervical cancer, *Gynecol Oncol* 34:206, 1989.)

forming a suprapubic median retroperitoneal pelviscopy (RPP). It is the clearest, the most direct, and the least dangerous approach.

THE INSTRUMENTATION

The instruments we need to perform a transcutaneous lymphadenectomy are the same as for a classical minilaparotomy and coelioscopic surgery. We will not describe them except for the forceps (Figs. 35-4 and 35-5), which include the following:

- H. Mahnes "cobra forceps" (Microfrance Fab: Fig. 35-4, *A*)
- H. Mahnes atraumatic hemostatic forceps with 20-mm jaws (Microfrance Fab: Fig. 35-4, *B*)
- H. Mahnes bipolar coagulation forceps (Microfrance Fab: Fig. 35-4, *C*)
- Lyonese coelioextractor (Lepine Fab: Fig. 35-5).

The first three instruments are introduced through 4-mm tubes. The fourth is introduced through a classic 10-mm coelioscopic tube. It works as a "sugar forceps" operated through to an unpalmable handle. Coelioscopic clips and scissors can be useful. A system allowing washing with cold saline and aspirating at the same time (e.g., aquapurator) is also, in certain circumstances, useful.

Although the endoscopic surgery can be performed under direct optic guidance, it is much more comfortable working under video surveillance. This imposes a certain training on the surgeon but is physicaly better and makes the work of both assistant and nurse much easier and more efficient. Many video transmission systems are available

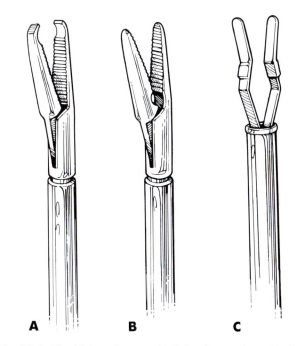

Fig. 35-4. The Mahnes forceps. **A,** Cobra forceps (grasping forceps); **B,** atraumatic hemostatic forceps (dissecting forceps); **C,** bipolar coagulation forceps.

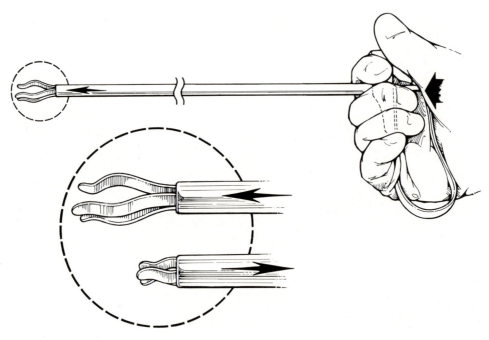

Fig. 35-5. Lyonese "coelioextractor."

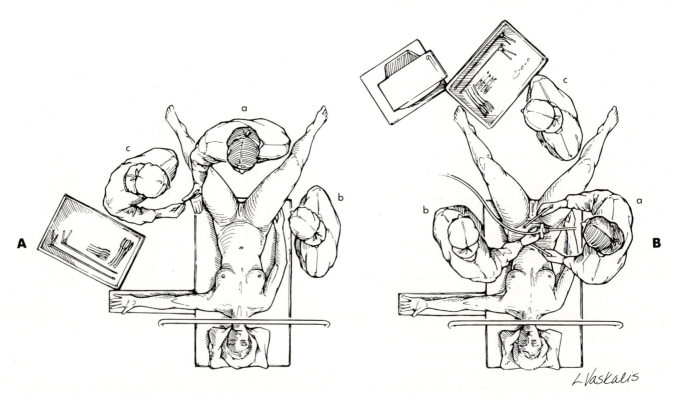

Fig. 35-6. Posture of patient and operative team during the two steps of the surgery. **A,** Suprapubic minilaparotomy; **B,** working endoscopically on the pelvic wall. *a,* Surgeon; *b,* assistant; and *c,* nurse.

on the market. They are compact, sturdy, strong, and inexpensive.

The position of the patient on the operating table is shown in Fig. 35-6. For the retroperitoneal approach, the surgeon has to stay between the legs to do the suprapubic incision (Fig. 35-6, *A*). Then the surgeon moves laterally, standing on the side opposite the pelvic wall to be assessed. The assistant stays between the legs of the patient during this stage of the surgery (Fig. 35-6, *B*).

SUPRAPUBIC MEDIAN RETROPERITONEAL APPROACH TO THE INTERILIAC LYMPH NODES

The suprapubic median retroperitoneal approach to the interiliac lymph nodes is described while answering three questions: (1) which route to choose, (2) how to do it, and (3) what to do in case of failure. The answers are based on our personal experience of 200 operations performed between December 15, 1986 and February 28, 1991:

- Operations done on documentary basis just before a planned laparotomy
- Operations done as "help in decision making" or "staging" operations.

Through which route can it be done?

The interiliac lymph nodes adhere to the blood vessels along which they are located. The peritoneum covers them. If we separate the peritoneum from the pelvic wall, the nodes remain in contact with the blood vessels while the ureter goes aside, keeping its relations with the peritoneum as does the fat pad interposed between the pelvic side wall and the peritoneum. This anatomic detail makes the retroperitoneal approach logical and relatively easy to perform. If we are working on direct contact with the pelvic side wall, all the dangerous or uninteresting structures go away and only the lymph nodes remain in place.

The secret of a correct approach to the lymph nodes is to be in full contact with the side wall of the pelvis. If we use the suprapubic route, it is easy to find this contact if we remember that the adipocellular interface between the peritoneal fascia and the parietal fascia in the suprapubic area is specially broad (space of Retzius). The parietal fascia, on the other hand, is a short distance from the abdominal wall because it is inserted on the dorsal surface of the pubis, whereas the recti abdominal muscles are inserted on the ventral surface. On the median sagittal section a triangular space can be seen that is called the "cavum suprapubicum" (Fig. 35-7). There is no other place where the space between the abdominal fascia and the abdominal wall can be found so easily. The steps to follow are: opening the "cavum suprapubicum," getting in touch with the posterior surface of the abdominal wall, and then laterally following the cranial surface of the pubic bone until contact with the iliac vessels is made.

How to do it

The suprapubic incision is performed in the midline. For cosmetic as well as for mechanical reasons, the skin is

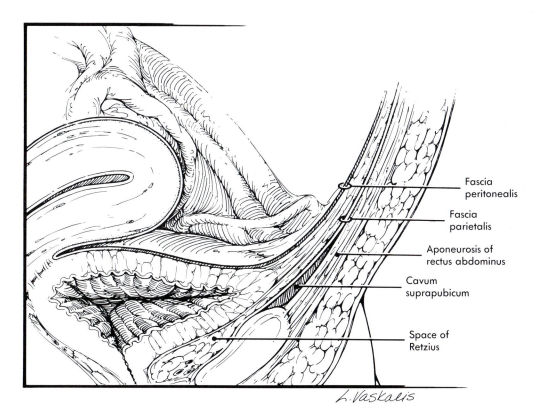

Fascia
peritonealis

Fascia
parietalis

Aponeurosis of
rectus abdominus

Cavum
suprapubicum

Space of
Retzius

L. Vaskalis

Fig. 35-7. Anatomy of the "cavum suprapubicum," the space located between the dorsal surface of the rectus abdominis muscles and the parietal fascia.

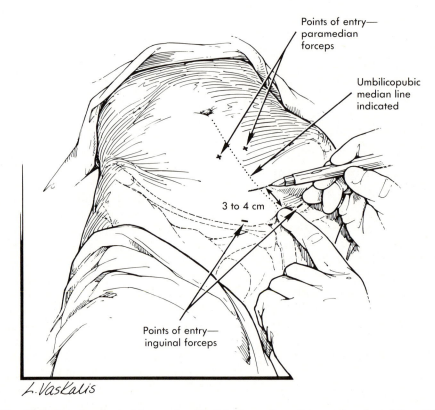

Points of entry—
paramedian
forceps

Umbilicopubic
median line
indicated

3 to 4 cm

Points of entry—
inguinal forceps

L. Vaskalis

Fig. 35-8. Drawing the incision on the skin 3 to 4 cm above the superior edge of the pubis.

cut transversely and the aponeurosis is cut longitudinally on the median line (linea alba abdominalis). The cutaneous scar is located in the pubic hair-bearing area, and we can avoid suturing the aponeurosis because we have two incisions, each done in an opposite direction.

To not lose the midline, we recommend that before cutting the surgeon uses a skin-marking pen to draw the umbilicopubic median line and the area of the suprapubic transverse incision, 3 to 4 cm above the cranial ridge of the pubic bone, 3 to 4 cm in length (Fig. 35-8). After incising the skin, the subcutaneous fat is cut and dissected until contact with the aponeurosis is obtained (Fig. 35-9, *A*). With two retractors in place, the aponeurosis is opened in the midline with a scalpel (Fig. 35-9, *B*). Then the two edges are held with forceps, and, without fear, the retroparietal space is opened with scissors. The cellular tissue is abundant, and the bladder is far (except in the patient who has had a previous operation).

After that space is opened, we must make contact with the posterior surface of the abdominal wall and then the superior surface of the pubic bone. This is done with curved scissors after introducing the second finger of the left hand into the space and working along the curve of the palmar face of the finger (Fig. 35-10). Once contact with the superior face of the pubic bone is reached, it is easy to follow the pectineal crest with the finger and to reach the iliac vessels whose axis has been identified by feeling the pulsations of the iliac artery with the other hand (Fig. 35-11).

Once in contact with the iliac vessels, we know that we are in the right direction. We can progress with the finger along the vascular axis, which is almost vertical because of the position of the patient. This movement is easy to do in most cases. But when patients have antecedent pelvic surgery, one must be careful to stop as soon as resistance is felt. The freeing of the retroperitoneal space will have to be performed later using the forceps under video guidance, as described below.

The first step of the procedure, the "blind" one, enables us to prepare the second, the "open eyed one." It enables us also to obtain immediately a diagnosis if the lymph nodes are enlarged, indurated, and fixed to the pelvic wall. That is one of the great advantages of the suprapubic route. However, before starting with the endoscopic part of the procedure, one has to perform a last preparation: freeing the preperitoneal space of the anterior wall in the paramedian area for an equal distance between the pubis and the umbilicus. This preparation is performed with the finger, as shown in Fig. 35-12. A 4-mm cutaneous incision is done on top of the prepared area. The aim is to prepare for the introduction of one of the dissection forceps.

What can we do if the route is not practical?

The retroperitoneal suprapubic approach to the interiliac lymph nodes is not easy or possible in every case because various difficulties can be encountered. In some cases, the retroparietal space appears completely obliterated. In other cases, the digital dissection is hard, and bleeding suddenly

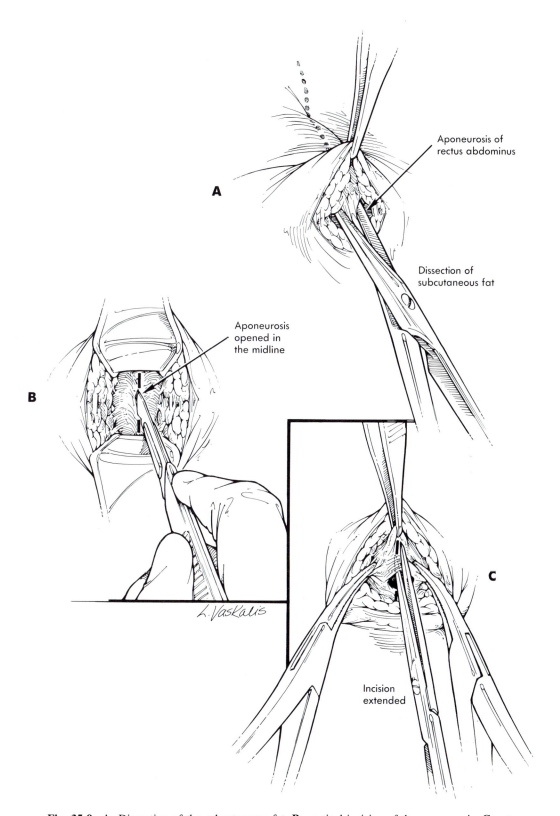

Aponeurosis of
rectus abdominus

Dissection of
subcutaneous fat

Aponeurosis
opened in
the midline

L. Vaskalis

Incision
extended

Fig. 35-9. A, Dissection of the subcutaneous fat; **B,** vertical incision of the aponeurosis; **C,** retroparietal space opened with scissors.

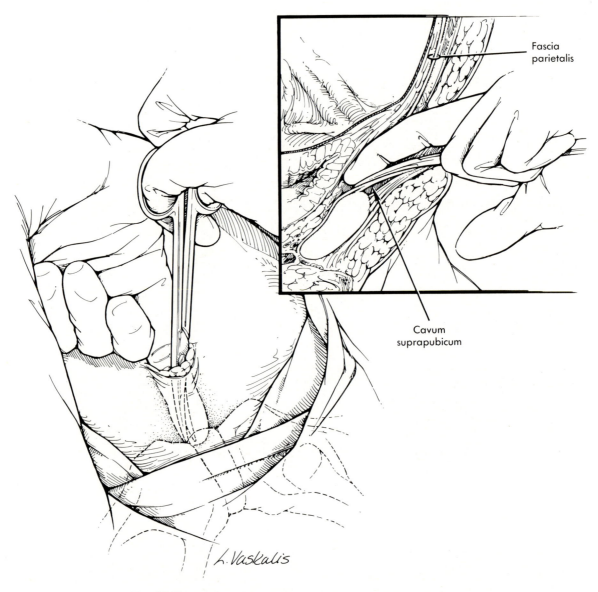

Fig. 35-10. Opening of the retroparietal space (cavum suprapubicum).

occurs, which indicates the tearing of some branch of an artery or vein. Going further, a laceration of the peritoneum can occur, which leads to the fact that the insufflation does not set apart the peritoneal pouch, and the abdomen becomes distended. Less commonly, a laceration of the bladder can occur, which is shown at first by the inflation of the bag collecting the urine. All these incidents or accidents have been observed in our experience. The frequency of the difficulties leading to renounce the suprapubic median retroperitoneal approach was 29% in patients previously operated on ($n = 58$) and 5% for the other subpopulation ($n = 142$).

A first answer to the question "what can we do" is to avoid the median suprapubic approach in patients previously operated on. But in three out of four cases, the suprapubic approach is possible in those patients. Therefore, an attempt by the primary route can be recommended with

the possibility of relying on back-up techniques if necessary. Three back-up procedures are specific for mixed indications and can eventually be used one after the other.

The inguinal alternative is mentioned first because it was the original one we used as an elective procedure. The operation is quite simple: an oblique inguinal incision (3 to 4 cm in length) is made starting from the spine of the pubic bone, opening the aponeurosis of the latissimus abdominalis muscle and penetration of the retroparietal space through the inguinal orifice inside the cross of the epigastric vessels. Access to the targeted area is direct.

However, the drawbacks are obvious. We work so close to the vessels that we lack the distance necessary to operate as well as in coelioscopic surgery (the procedure is more a "mediastinoscopy" improved method than a true coelioscopic method). The failures in previously operated patients, despite the fact that we operate at a certain dis-

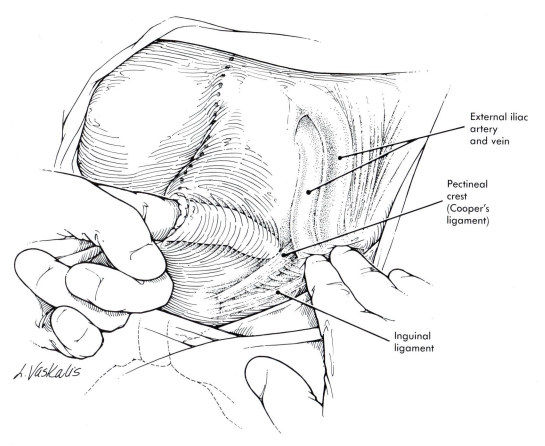

External iliac
artery
and vein

Pectineal
crest
(Cooper's
ligament)

Inguinal
ligament

L. Vaskalis

Fig. 35-11. Digital preparation of the pectineal crest until the contact with the iliac vessels is reached.

tance from the scar, are possible as well as inducing a vascular accident. Of 16 operations in our practice (15 elective operations and 1 alternative operation), we have met with 3 failures in the 8 patients previously operated on.

The laparotomy alternative is a resort that is always available. It is the solution of choice if bleeding occurs during the first step of the suprapubic median procedure. It is also a good alternative in case of failure of the inguinal approach, particularly if bleeding is the cause of the failure. The incision performed is a medium-size curved suprapubic and iliac incision leading to the pelvic inlet without opening the peritoneum. The postoperative course after this extraperitoneal limited laparotomy is generally simple except for retroperitoneal or intraparietal seromas, hematomas, and abscess, which are relatively common. We have had to proceed to laparotomy four times in patients operated on for staging (excluding patients operated on just before a scheduled laparotomy). The postoperative course was simple, and the average postoperative stay was 8 days.

The transperitoneal coelioscopic alternative is surely the best when the retroperitoneal approach appears impracticable (suprapubic retroperitoneal space obliterated in the median area or in the inguinal area) or when the CO_2 distends directly the peritoneal cavity (peritoneal laceration). In the

second event, the abdominal distention enables us to trocard immediately the abdominal wall in the umbilical area. In the first one, the previous insufflation is done as usual (the left subcostal approach is the best for the scarred abdomen). After the pelvic cavity has been freed from the intestinal loops (enterolysis may be necessary), the pelvic peritoneum is opened along the pelvic inlet between the round ligament and the infundibulopelvic ligament. Afterwards, it is easy to enter "the paravesical space" and to treat the lymph nodes in the same manner as in the retroperitoneal procedure. We have used the transumbilical coelioscopic procedure in only one instance, but with success.

The transumbilical coelioscopic procedure is obviously simpler than the retroperitoneal suprapubic pelviscopy (except in cases of peritoneal adhesions, but, in those cases, the retroperitoneal access is also difficult and coelioscopic adhesiolysis, even if time consuming, is always possible). But the coelioscopic approach has important drawbacks either from the anesthetic or from the surgical point of view: hemodynamic hazards due to the compression of the inferior vena cava are possible (compression which does not exist in the retroperitoneal approach), and access to the interiliac lymph nodes following this route may be difficult. Therefore, for us, the transumbilical coelioscopic approach remains only an alternative approach, but it is a better "al-

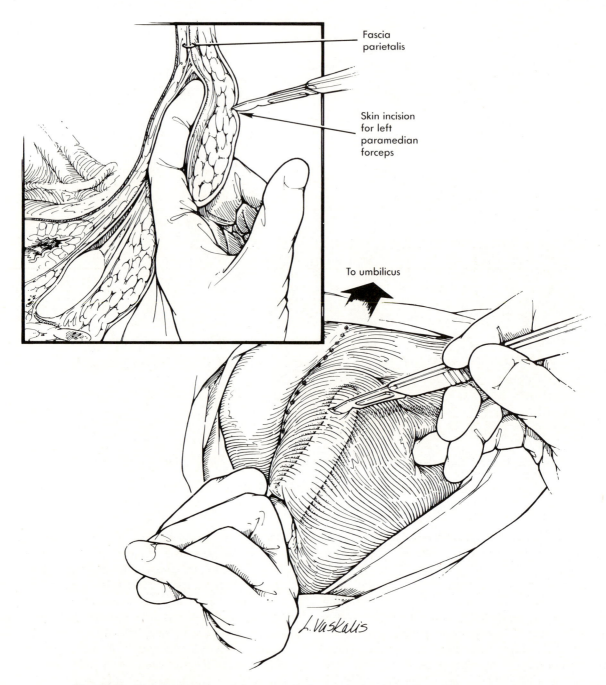

Fascia
parietalis

Skin incision
for left
paramedian
forceps

To umbilicus

L. Vaskalis

Fig. 35-12. Digital preparation of the retroparietal space in the upper paramedian area (to prepare the latter for the introduction of one of the two dissection forceps).

ternative approach" than the suprapubic inguinal retroperitoneal and the laparotomic ones enumerated before.

EXTIRPATION OF THE INTERILIAC LYMPH NODES

Whatever the route of access, the management of the interiliac lymph nodes in the panoramic endoscopic procedure (retroperitoneal pelviscopy or transperitoneal pelviscopy) is done the same way, which is very different from the "mediastinoscopy" technique. A true lymphadenectomy can be performed rather than a simple "picking up."

The technique of endoscopic lymphadenectomy is described while answering three questions: (1) how to prepare the nodes, (2) how to extirpate them, and (3) what to do in case extirpation is not suitable.

How to prepare the interiliac lymph nodes

Preparation of the interiliac nodes is usually easy. It is done by blunt dissection using forceps only. There is no need for hemostasis or lymphostasis. Bleeding and lymph extrusion leading to secondary cyst formation are uncommon when compared with classic surgery due to the baro-

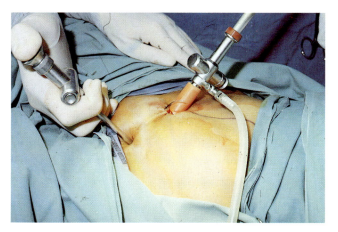

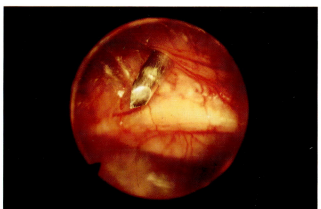

Color Plate 3. Suprapubic trocarization flush to the superior edge of the iliac bone just inside of the epigastric vessels.

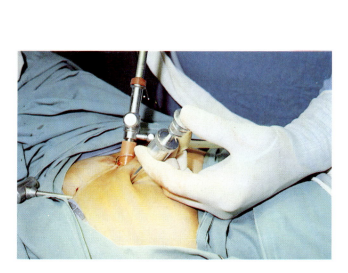

Color Plate 4. Upper paramedian trocarization at the top of the area prepared before.

A

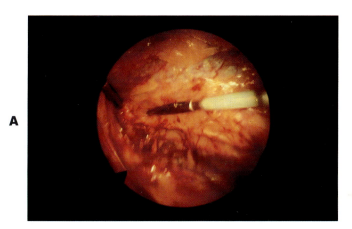

B

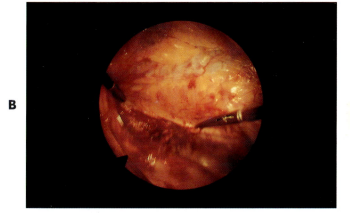

C

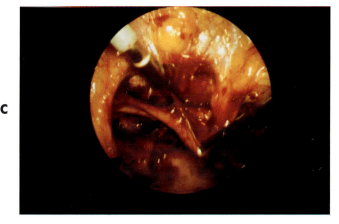

Color Plate 5. Dissection of the interiliac lymph nodes. **A,** Pushing away the round ligament. **B,** Evidencing the obturator nerve. **C,** Detaching the obturator lymph nodes from the iliac vein.

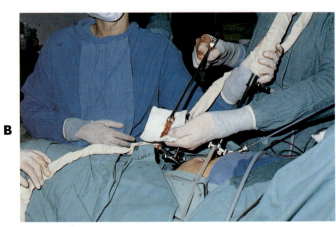

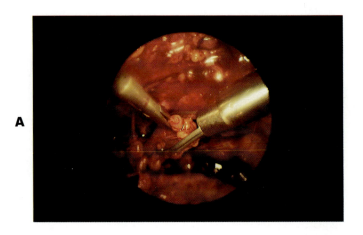

A

B

Color Plate 6. Extraction of the obturator lymph nodes. **A,** Grasping the inferior pole of the lymph nodal group. **B,** Extracting the lymph nodal group.

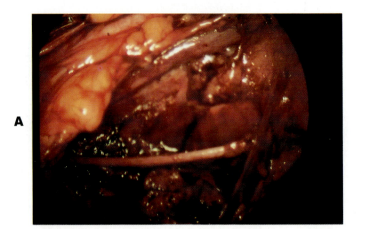

A

Color Plate 7. The pelvic wall after the laparoscopic lymphadenectomy. **A,** Subvenous area. **B,** Hypogastric area.

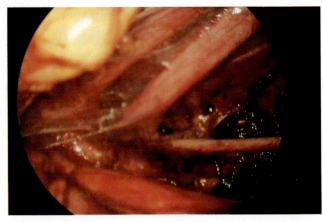

B

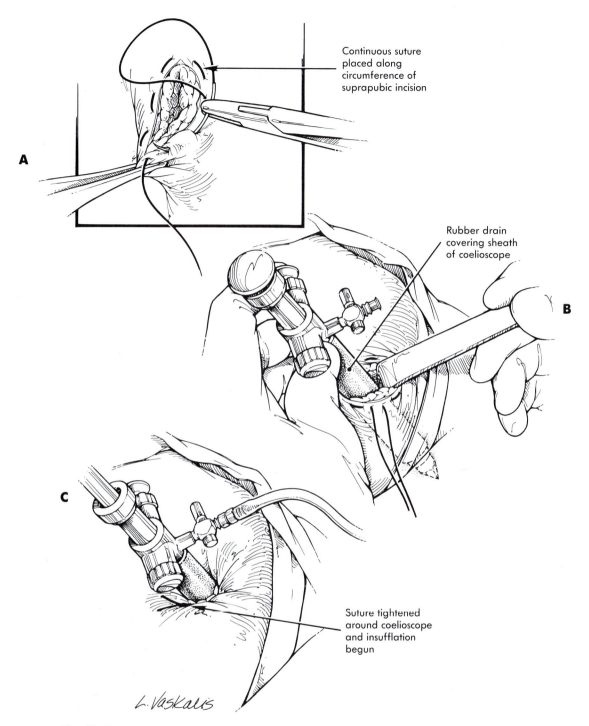

Fig. 35-13. Introduction of the laparoscopic trocar into the prepared space. **A,** A continuous suture has been performed on the margin of the cutaneous incision. **B,** The sheath of the coelioscope has been covered with a rubber drain. **C,** Suture is tightened around coelioscope, and insufflation is begun.

Continuous suture placed along circumference of suprapubic incision

Rubber drain covering sheath of coelioscope

Suture tightened around coelioscope and insufflation begun

L. Vaskalis

hemostatic effect of CO_2 insufflation or to the absence of a real opening of the abdominal wall.

The two forceps are introduced after completion of the insufflation. In retroperitoneal pelviscopy, the insufflation is done directly through the sheath of the coelioscope introduced obliquely in the area prepared before with the finger (Fig. 35-13). To avoid losing gas, two important

"tricks" have to be mentioned: to cover the sheath of the trocar with a rubber drain and to perform continuous suture on the margin of the cutaneous incision once the trocar is introduced to the right depth (not too deep, to keep a good panoramic view of the lateral pelvic wall) (Fig. 35-13, *A* and *B*). Once in place, the sharp axis of the trocar is removed and the CO_2 insufflation is started at a flow rate

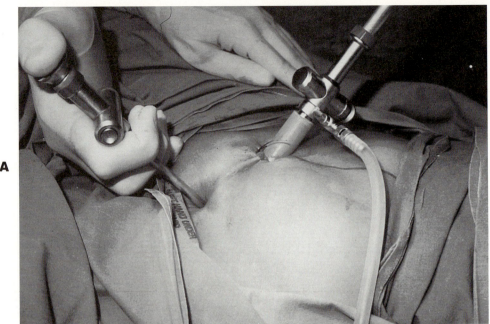

A

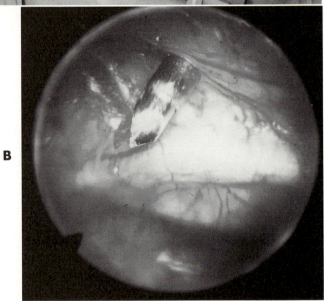

B

Fig. 35-14. Suprapubic trocarization flush to the superior edge of the iliac bone just inside of the epigastric vessels. See Color Plate 3, facing p. 594.

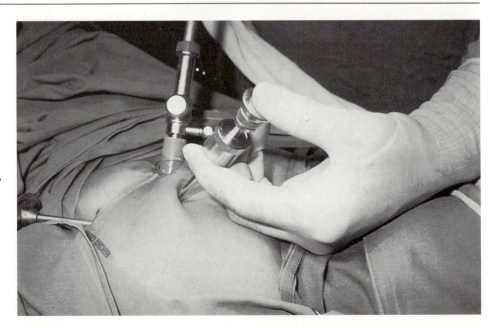

Fig. 35-15. Upper paramedian trocarization at the top of the area prepared before. See Color Plate 4, facing p. 594.

of 3 L/min (Fig. 35-13, *C*). The endoscopic exploration is then started.

The first step of the exploration is identifying the insertion of the abdominal wall on the iliopubic bone in the inguinal area. (In difficult cases, it is helpful to press the abdomen in the targeted area.) Once the pectineal crest is evidenced, the epigastric vessels are identified by means of transillumination (Fig. 35-14). A microincision (4 mm) is performed inside of them, just at the level of the superior edge of the bone, and the trocar is pushed directly from front to back under endoscopic surveillance.

The introduction of the second small trocar is performed in the paramedian area using the microincision done at the end of the last stage of the preliminary digital preparation. The trocar is pushed obliquely in the direction of an ideal point situated at the center of the pelvic cavity. Visual observation is not necessary (Fig. 35-15). The forceps are introduced, and the anatomic preparation can be started (Fig. 35-16).

The first thing to do is to identify the external iliac vein. This is not difficult if we follow, from inside to outside, the pectineal crest identified at the beginning of the procedure. This is achieved by first palpating the pectineal crest with the extremity of the paramedian forceps, then slipping along this structure and at the same time detaching the structures adherent to it. After each progress in the dis-

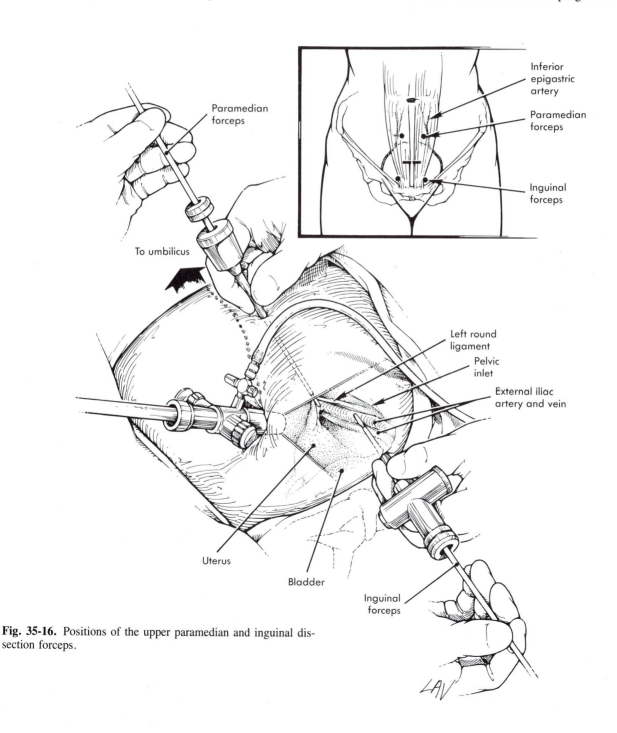

Fig. 35-16. Positions of the upper paramedian and inguinal dissection forceps.

section, the structures set apart are taken in charge by the inguinal forceps, and the paramedian forceps can work one more time until it comes to the end of its run. Then the inguinal forceps takes charge of the structures set apart and so forth. The iliac vein is soon identified at the point where it crosses the pectineal crest.

After the iliac vein has been identified, the moves along the vein are the same we have performed along the pectineal crest. The round ligament is pushed away at the same time as the umbilical artery (Fig. 35-17, *A* and *B*). The procedure becomes progressively less easy, due to the resistance of the round ligament, but one generally arrives

quickly at the level of the bifurcation of the common iliac artery.

The lymph nodes situated inside the bifurcation of the common iliac artery (hypogastric nodes) are the first to prepare. This is achieved by grasping the inferior pole of the nodes or group of nodes with the inguinal forceps and then pulling and pushing it alternately to break the weak connections attaching them laterally. The connections attaching them dorsally (the lymph collectors connecting it to the lymph nodes situated downstream), on the contrary, are respected. Then we progress to the space situated caudally to the iliac vein. The movements in this area are eas-

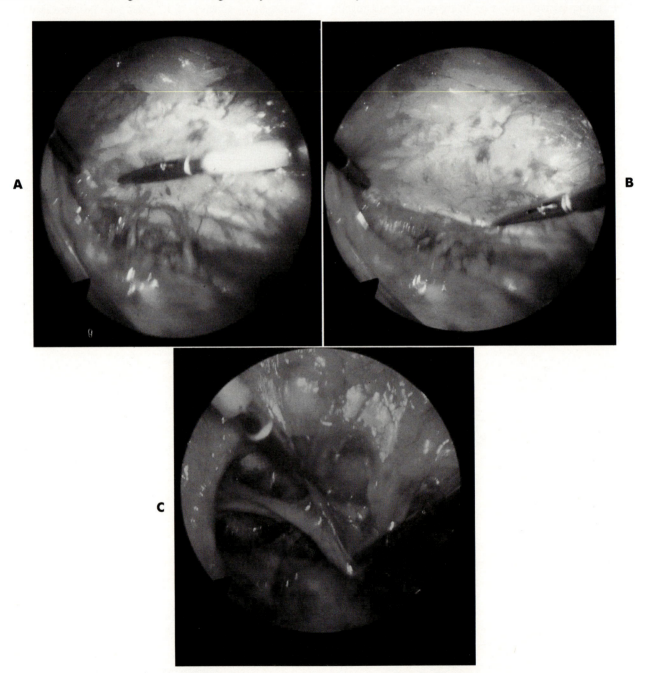

Fig. 35-17. Dissection of the interiliac lymph nodes. **A,** Pushing away the round ligament.
B, Evidencing the obturator nerve. **C,** Detaching the obturator lymph nodes from the iliac vein.
See color Plate 5, facing p. 594.

ier to perform. The two forceps are used alternatively as prehensive and dissecting forceps, and the connections attaching the obturator nodes to the vein are broken from back to front (Fig. 35-17, *C*). The last task is freeing the inferior pole of the internal retrocrural node. Then the preparation ends with the freeing of the caudal side of the obturator group.

The dangers in these sequences of anatomic preparation are theoretically numerous but practically nonexistent. We have never observed a direct injury to the iliac vein even during the sequence when we operate in direct contact with its medial surface (preparation of the hypogastric nodes), nevermore a direct trauma to the iliac artery. The only real danger is tearing the obturator vessels and, more specifically, the veins—the superior one, which follows the obturator nerve caudally and flows into the internal iliac vein, and the inferior one, which flows into the external iliac vein after crossing the obturator nodes. These veins are located in a manner and in a place that cannot be anticipated. Tearing of these vessels is equivalent to a lateral wound to the main vein, and the resultant bleeding can be quite heavy. We have to be careful in the dissection, which can almost always be carried out without cutting the vessels. If we have to cut, we should use biactive bipolar electrocauterization or clips. The lymphatic channels, which are often well identified thanks to endoscopic

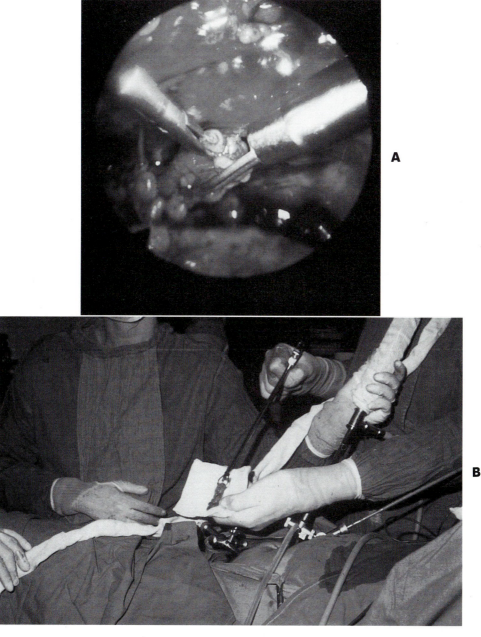

Fig. 35-18. Extraction of the obturator lymph nodes. **A,** Grasping the inferior pole of the lymph nodal group. **B,** Extracting the lymph nodal group. See Color Plate 6, facing p. 595.

magnification, do not have to be coagulated before dissection.

How to extirpate the lymph nodes

The extirpation of the nodes is done just before their complete freedom has been achieved. The remaining connections of the prepared structures keep them in place, so we avoid a time-consuming "fishing out," which has to be done if the nodes fall into the depth of the paravesical space.

The extraction is performed with the device we have named "coelioextractor." To introduce it in the operative field, we widen the inguinal microincision and trocard the abdominal wall with a coelioscopy trocar, which allows the introduction of the device. The obturator nodes are the first to be extracted (Fig. 35-18, *A*). They are grasped by the superior pole and directed into the sheath and removed (Fig. 35-18, *B*). The dorsal connections are usually weak enough, and the whole lymph nodal group comes out. The same procedure is repeated for the hypogastric nodes.

After extirpation of the two main groups of nodes, the neurovascular anatomy of the targeted area appears more clearly, and one can start going after the isolated lymph nodes left in place. These nodes are usually located in the dorsal part of the obturator area and the ventral part of the iliac arteriovenous space.

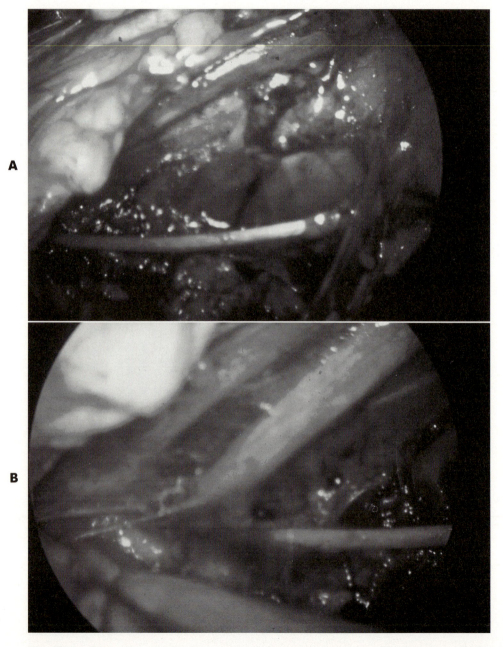

Fig. 35-19. The pelvic wall after the laparoscopic lymphadenectomy. **A,** Subvenous area. **B,** Hypogastric area. See Color Plate 7, facing p. 595.

Search for the posterior obturator nodes must be made along the obturator nerve in the interstice between the internal iliac vein and the pelvic wall. Operating through the suprapubic route, we are in just the right axis to perform this pursuit: that is one of the advantages of this approach when compared to the transumbilical one and even with a classic surgical one (Fig. 35-19). The nodes we are looking for are grasped with the coelioextractor, which works with its three teeth as the three first fingers of the hand, extracting the membranes remaining in the vagina at the last moment of a delivery.

The vascular environment of the posterior obturator nodes is quite dangerous: that is the region where the obturator vein flows into the internal iliac vein along with other parietal and visceral veins. In case of significant bleeding, washing with hot water generally leads quickly to a perfect cleaning and hemostasis of the operative field, thanks to the fact that the vessels are usually torn at a distance from the branch and then retract themselves. This retraction provides the hemostasis. We had to perform a laparotomy in only one case to ensure hemostasis. The only serious difficulties we had during the extraction of the nodes occurred during the period in which we did not use the coelioextractor. The nodes were extracted by fragmentation, and this fragmentation was often long and hard to perform. The extirpation through the abdominal wall twice produced a carcinomatous contamination. In the first case, the contamination was discovered during a laparotomy performed 3 months after PPL. The obturator lymph nodes were involved as demonstrated by partial endoscopic node extraction on the right side. A neoadjuvant chemotherapy was given, which did not hinder the development of a 3-cm^3 tumor within the abdominal wall. The second case of carcinomatous contamination was a little different. The nodes extracted by fragmentation through the inguinal microincision were uninvolved. A Schauta operation was performed. However, 8 months later, a lateral pelvic recurrence was discovered with an intraparietal and subcutaneous invasion in the left inguinal area. That is one of the reasons why we designed the extraction device.

What to do if the lymph nodes cannot be extirpated

In cases in which the lymph nodes are obviously hypertrophic, indurated, and fixed, the extraction and even the attempt of extraction are contraindicated. The lymphadenectomy is a staging procedure more than a therapeutical one. That is the case for all types of lymphadenectomy. The advantage of debulking the lymphodal metastatic masses is always questionable. That is even more the situation with endoscopic lymphadenectomy during which the debulking is impossible and not useful. We only have to see whether the lymph nodes are infiltrated or not. If they are, it is not useful to proceed further.

Evidence for the tumor metastasis to the nodes can be obtained in the first step of the procedure by palpating the pelvic wall with the finger. It can also be shown during the attempt at dissection. In this situation, the dissection has to

be stopped. But we have the duty, using all means at our disposal, to obtain specimens for a microscopic assessment. The false-positive rate of the clinical evaluation is low. We have encountered this fact in one of our observations, which paradoxically is at the same time the only false-negative observation in our practice. All the lymph nodes were hypertrophic and indurated, but they were able to be extirpated. We removed them, except for the hypogastric one on the right side. The proofs of the involvement of the nodes were numerous enough! We were surprised to learn that the extirpated nodes were not carcinomatous, but, 3 months later (the patient treated at first with neoadjuvant chemotherapy), we learned that the only lymph node left in place and whose aspect was not different from the others was, in fact, metastatic.

There are three methods to perform the biopsy: (1) fine-needle aspiration, (2) trucut needle, and (3) biopsy forceps. Although these techniques are easy to perform transcutaneously under endoscopic guidance, the reliability of the gathering is hazardous. We learned from our experience that it is best to perform the three methods successively, because frequently only one of the three types of sampling is significant. It is not exceptional that no one of the three is positive in case of actual metastasis (a very interesting lesson about the reliability of the sampling performed transcutaneously under imaging guidance: how can it work if we know that the sampling performed in the center of a visually assessed lymph node does not work in all cases?).

INTEGRATION OF TRANSCUTANEOUS ENDOSCOPIC INTERILIAC LYMPHADENECTOMY IN THE THERAPEUTIC SCHEDULES

Although the endoscopic assessment of the interiliac lymph nodes obviously has numerous and highly interesting applications in the management of pelvic cancer patients, we have, first of all, to demonstrate that it is both without danger and can be accurate.

RELIABILITY OF THE ENDOSCOPIC ASSESSMENT

The endoscopic procedure, as every invasive medical procedure, cannot be perfectly innocuous, but the risks are low. The accuracy of endoscopic assessment is at a level as high as surgical assessment (i.e., very near perfection). There are obviously no false positives. False negatives, on the contrary, can be seen (i.e., involved lymph nodes kept in place while the extracted lymph nodes are all uninvolved). This phenomenon can be evidenced in two ways: (1) discovering an involved node during a laparotomy performed after negative endoscopy or (2) discovering a lateropelvic recurrence in the follow-up of a patient treated without surgical lymphadenectomy (nor radiotherapy) after a negative endoscopy. The discovery of involved lymph nodes during a laparotomy performed after a negative endoscopic assessment is uncommon. We have encountered this only once for the 91 patients operated on in these conditions. The case was special: there was a fast growing stage IIb epidermoid carcinoma of the cervix, 8 cm in diameter, observed in a 23-year-old patient with a negative endoscopic initial lymphadenectomy (only inflammatory changes in the extirpated nodes), chemotherapy (three courses of BEMP), discovery during the laparotomy performed 12 weeks after the laparoscopy of a single but massive metastasis in an hypogastric lymph node on the right side, which was the only lymph node left behind. One can ask if the "missed" lymph nodal metastasis did not develop during the chemotherapy and in spite of it considering that the response at the level of the cervical cancer was nil.

The discovery of a lateropelvic recurrence during the follow-up of a patient treated without surgical lymphadenectomy (or radiotherapy) after negative endoscopic assessment is, unfortunately, more frequent than the phenomenon mentioned above, but its significance has to be discussed. Lateral pelvic recurrences can also occur in the N-patients treated in the classic manner (i.e., after a protocol including surgical lymphadenectomy or radiotherapy).

These recurrences are roughly equally frequent, at least in the common form of the disease. This assertion is confirmed by Fig. 35-20 where we have juxtaposed the curves of disease-free survival for two groups of patients, 47 patients we have operated on after a Schauta radical vaginal hysterectomy (the negativity of the lymph nodes being demonstrated by a laparoscopic interiliac lymphadenectomy) and a control group of 94 patients operated on after a radical abdominal hysterectomy and selected randomly in our books, the common feature being that the lymph nodes were negative and the tumoral major diameter was precisely assessed. For tumors less than 4 cm in diameter, the chances of disease-free survival are the same. But, for the tumors 4 cm or more in diameter, the chances of disease-free survival are less for the patient operated on after a Schauta procedure. One possible explanation is that tumors of this sort are mostly fast-growing tumors whose lymphatic spread can cross over the sentinel lymph nodes and directly colonize the lymph nodes situated downstream.

Postoperative problems are uncommon: there is no ileus at all and the patient can be discharged after 48 to 72 hours (3 to 5 days in our practice, but in Europe, we are more cautious and more spendthrift than in the United States; the hospital stay can probably be shortened without any danger).

The postoperative complications are limited to the possible consequences of a persisting lymphohematocele in the operative field and its bacterial contamination. These complications are rare. Bleeding and lymph escape end generally just after the deinsufflation when the peritoneal pouch comes back into contact with the pelvic wall. If a draining system has been put in place, the output ends usually in the first hour after the procedure, and it is unusual to have to maintain it more than 24 hours. Therefore, we have few postoperative lymphohematoceles; we have had six cases for retroperitoneal pelviscopy performed as isolated procedures in our practice (one of them observed for the only patient submitted to a prophylactic heparin therapy). The postoperative retroperitoneal suppuration is even more unusual, three cases in our practice.

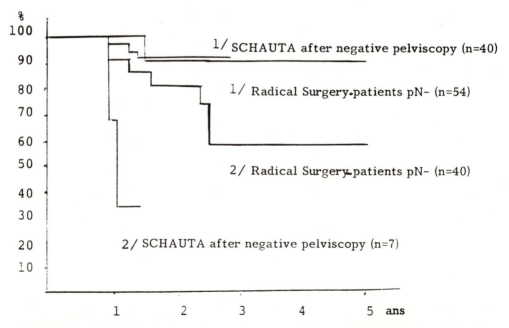

Fig. 35-20. Chances of disease-free survival for patients affected by cervical cancer and treated by Schauta radical vaginal hysterectomy operation after negative pelviscopy or by radical abdominal surgery (Wertheim) including classic lymphadenectomy (pN− patients only). Personal series 1986 to 1991. *1/* = tumoral diameter less than 4 cm; *2/* = tumoral diameter equal or greater than 4 cm.

In summary, it can be assumed that the endoscopic assessment of the interiliac lymph nodes has a level of innocuity and reliability high enough to consider them as a cardinal element in the management of pelvic cancer. The best application in the field of gynecologic cancer concerns cervical cancer stage Ib and early stage II. However, interest in the method is also high in other situations. It is our opinion that RPP is indicated in almost all cases of pelvic cancer as part of the initial staging procedure.

CARCINOMA OF THE CERVIX STAGE Ib AND EARLY STAGE II

Early carcinoma of the cervix may be treated either by surgery, radiotherapy, or a radiosurgical combination. There are a lot of discussions about the point. There are also a lot of discussions about the definition of "early cancer." For some specialists, stage Ib cancer with a diameter of more than 2 cm is not an early cancer; for others, all cancers belonging to stage Ib, IIa, and early IIb (infiltration limited to the medial part of the parametrium) are early cancers. They can be designated as stage Ib and IIp (II proximal) and treated either by surgery or radiotherapy or a combination of both. If we look at the problem from an acute oncologic view, these discussions are untimely and futile because there are, even in the smallest tumors, some high-risk factors, and some very large tumors are low risk. Because tumor volume and local extension are not the only nor the main factors of prognosis, management cannot be based on those two items alone.

All multifactorial studies have demonstrated that the status of the regional nodes is the most important factor in the prognosis of cervical cancer. There is obviously a correlation between this factor and the two others (volume and local extension of the tumor). The three factors act jointly in determining the fate of the patients. From a practical point of view, if we know the tumor volume, its extension (clinical examination and imaging are quite accurate), and the status of the interiliac lymph nodes, we are able to differentiate the low-risk forms of stage Ib and IIp cancers with great accuracy.

Endoscopic assessment of interiliac lymph nodes can be used to separate high-risk and low-risk patients to concentrate the efforts of the integrated therapies on the high-risk patients and to avoid for the low-risk patients (the vast majority) the risks of the most radical therapies. Starting from this basic concept, all sorts of decisions can be made. For us, considering the results presented in Fig. 35-20, we have decided to treat with integrated therapies (chemoradiotherapy with or without surgery) pN+ patients and to do surgery in pN− patients using the vaginal route if the tumor diameter is smaller than 4 cm and the histologic type is epidermoid. The abdominal approach is reserved for the other cases.

The reasons for our preference for Schauta's operation for the low-risk patients are developed in Chapter 23. The surgical risk is at least three times lower than using the abdominal approach. Other therapeutic decisions can be made depending on the general status of the patients or the choice of the physician: brachytherapy alone for high-surgical risk patients having a low-risk cancer, for example, and combined radiotherapy with or without surgery for the others. Whatever the therapeutic choice, we think that endoscopic assessment of the interiliac lymph nodes has to be integrated in the initial staging procedure in stage Ib and IIp cervical cancers.

CARCINOMA OF THE CERVIX LATE STAGE II, AND STAGES III AND IV

A consensus does exist on treatment of late cervical carcinoma that is to be managed by radiotherapy. A consensus also exists on the poor results of the treatment. A great many trials are going on concerning the integration of chemotherapy in the therapeutic schedule. One has also to evaluate the place of surgery.

The results of the first randomized trials about chemoradiotherapy are disappointing. The chances of survival are not improved except when we separate the good from the poor responders. Regarding the place of surgery, the common opinion is still that it is highly dangerous and has to be reserved for some selected patients. Endoscopic assessment of the regional lymph nodes, in this context, can play an important role. In late stages, the N factor is more significant than in early stages. In very large or broadly extended tumors, the negativity of regional lymph nodes, more than in small tumors, indicates a special pattern of growth (local) and can, by hypothesis, be used as an indicator for selecting the therapeutic directions.

It is too soon to assume that late stages with negative regional nodes are not good indications for chemoradiotherapy. It is also too soon to assume that good indications for chemotherapy are those cases with positive regional nodes (all the fast-growing tumors and especially the early stages with positive lymph nodes). But the item of "regional lymph nodes" is certainly to be taken into account in the evaluation of the therapeutic results. The endoscopic evaluation of interiliac lymph nodes must be included in the initial staging of late cervical carcinoma in the context of the therapeutic trials, which must be multiplied if we are to move to a better management of this peculiar situation.

CARCINOMA OF THE ENDOMETRIUM

Most agree that surgery is the treatment for endometrial carcinoma with or without adjuvant therapy (radiotherapy, hormonotherapy, chemotherapy). The initial surgery has to be performed through the abdominal route and has to include at the same time an evaluation of the whole peritoneal cavity, lymphadenectomy with various protocols ranging from sampling of the obturator nodes to a complete pelvic and lumboaortic lymphadenectomy. There is, in this context, no place for endoscopic evaluation of interiliac lymph nodes.

The problem is that the patients affected by endometrial adenocarcinoma are often in bad or very poor medical condition (obesity, hypertension, diabetes) and, therefore, unable to tolerate the risk of a laparotomy. Vaginal hysterectomy, for these patients, can be an alternative to radiotherapy, which is usually indicated for inoperable patients but is not as efficient as surgery. But operating through the vaginal route impedes the lymph nodal assessment, which, in endometrial carcinoma, appears as important as in cervical carcinoma.

The endoscopic evaluation of the interiliac lymph nodes finally has a place in the study of endometrial adenocarcinoma. However, the conditions that can indicate a laparotomy make a laparoscopy difficult and dangerous unless we use the retroperitoneal suprapubic instead of the transperitoneal transumbilical route. This exploration has, in our opinion, to be performed in every case of "inoperable" adenocarcinoma of the endometrium.

CARCINOMA OF THE VULVA

Vulvar carcinoma is a highly lymphotropic cancer, and the status of regional nodes is of great significance in assessing the prognosis and setting up the therapeutic management. Because the regional nodes are mainly inguinal, and the pelvic nodes are rarely and lately involved, there is no place in these conditions for the endoscopic assessment of the interiliac lymph nodes. As a matter of fact, the usual pattern of lymphatic spread in vulvar cancer (starting by the ipsilateral inguinal, then the contralateral inguinal nodes, and, finally, the ipsi or bilateral pelvic nodes) is observed only (and with some exception) in the lateral forms of the disease and exclusively for stages I and II. In central forms and in lateral forms of stages III and IV (which are mostly fast-growing cancers, rather than neglected cancers), one can observe direct involvement of the pelvic lymph nodes, which is of great prognostic significance.

Therefore, one can assume that, in central forms of vulvar carcinoma as in lateral forms of late stages, the endoscopic assessment of pelvic nodes is highly interesting. The retroperitoneal suprapubic approach is, in this context, especially precious when the patients are generally old or very old and the nodes we have to assess preferentially are retrocrural and easier to join through the suprapubic route.

CONCLUSION

Every gynecologist should remember the classic debate between Schauta and Wertheim about the surgical treatment of carcinoma of the cervix: Schauta did not perform a lymphadenectomy and Wertheim did. It was at the beginning of the century (on the 14th and 21st of October 1904 exactly) at the meeting of the Gynecological Society of Vienna. The debate still remains open today because there is no consensus on the actual place of lymphadenectomy.

As a matter of fact, the discussion between Schauta and Wertheim concerned a special kind of lymphadenectomy, which could be named "selective lymphadenectomy." Wertheim extirpated only the enlarged nodes. And this "debulking lymphadenectomy" is certainly of low interest, especially if done in the absence of adjuvant therapy. The number of patients salvaged by the extirpation of lymph node macrometastasis does not significantly exceed the number of patients endangered by the surgery.

The aim of lymphadenectomy developed in the second era of the history of surgical treatment of carcinoma of the cervix (the era of Meigs and followers) is different because it is a "staging lymphadenectomy" more than a therapeutic one. Even if the extirpation of metastatic lymph nodes has, perhaps, a certain value (especially in cases of micrometastasis), the goal is essentially to select the patients for adjuvant therapy. In this perspective, one has to perform a "systematic lymphadenectomy" as completely as possible.

The contemporary "staging lymphadenectomy" is an operation beginning at the level of the left renal vein and going downstream to the femoral rings. Not a single node can escape. In this manner, the efficacy is certainly improved but more hazardous also, both during and after surgery and during and after adjuvant therapy. Although the use of the extraperitoneal route lowers those hazards, they remain high. For cervical cancer, some surgeons advocate the concept of "targeted lymphadenectomy" whose adequacy is already accepted for vulvar cancer.

The "interiliac lymphadenectomy" is the form of targeted lymphadenectomy that suits cervical cancer. The nodes extirpated (i.e., obturator and hypogastric) are the "sentinel lymph nodes." (It is important to underline that the targeted lymphadenectomy is not a "random lymphadenectomy.") We have few extirpated nodes, 10% of the potentially concerned ones, but they are the sentinel nodes (i.e., the lymph nodes whose uninvolvement enables us to say with 99% accuracy that the others are also uninvolved).

The "transcutaneous interilac lymphadenectomy performed under endoscopic guidance" is the best way to perform the staging lymphadenectomy in cervical cancer (but also in endometrial and vaginal ones). The procedure is both accurate and has a low surgical risk, especially if we can use (in 9 out of 10 cases) the retroperitoneal suprapubic route, dissection performed in the right space and along the right axis avoiding the hazards of the pneumoperitoneum. With the procedure, we avoid all the risks of surgical lymphadenectomy while keeping its first interest —selecting the patients who have a good prognosis that we treat with the least traumatic method (i.e., radical surgery, performed through the vaginal route).

Considering that cervical cancers today are mostly diagnosed in stages I and early II and that cases with no lymph node metastasis are the most common (70% to 85%), one can say that the operation of Schauta at the end of the century starts with a new future—an unexpected revolving of history that has to be credited to pelviscopy.

Acknowledgment. We are grateful to Professor Michel Roy for reviewing the manuscript from both oncologic and editorial points of view.

REFERENCES

1. Bartel M: Die retroperitoneoskopie. Eine endoskopische Methode zur Ispektion un bioptischen Untersuchung des retroperitonealen Raumes, *Zentralbl Chir* 94:377, 1969.
2. Dargent D: A new future for Schauta's operation through pre-surgical retroperitoneal pelviscopy, *Eur J Gynecol Oncol* 8:292, 1987.
3. Dargent D, Salvat J: *Envahissement ganglionnaire pelvien. Place de la pelviscopie retroperitoneale,* Medsi, 1989, McGraw-Hill.
4. Dauplat J et al: La lymphadenectomie endoscopique. Indications dans le cancer du col de l'uterus (in press).
5. Giradi F, Lichtenegger W, Tamussino K: The importance of parametrial lymph nodes in the treatment of cervical cancer, *Gynecol Oncol* 34:206, 1989.
6. Hald T, Rasmussen F: Extraperitoneal pelviscopy: a new aid in staging of lower urinary tract tumors. A preliminary report, *J Urol* 124:245, 1980.
7. Pilleron JP, Durand JC, Hamelin JP: Location of lymph node invasion in cancer of the uterine cervix: study of 140 cases treated at the Curie Foundation, *Am J Obstet Gynecol* 119:453, 1974.
8. Querleu D, Leblanc E, Castelain B: Lymphadenectomie pelvienne sous controle coelioscopique, *J Gynecol Obstet Biol Reprod* 19:576, 1990.
9. Sommerkamp H: Lomboskopie: ein neues diagnostisch-therapeutisches Prinzip der Urologie (Vorlaufige Mitteilung), *Aktuel Urol* 5:183, 1974.
10. Wurtz A, Luck H: Reflexions a propos de la retroperitoneoscopie "operatoire" en chiurgie pelvienne, *Presse Med* 16:1865, 1987.

MYOMECTOMY

Celso-Ramón García
Samantha M. Pfeifer

Uterine myomas are among the most common tumors encountered in women. These tumors vary in appearance and specific distortions. Although derived from a single myometrial cell, their histologic composition can be quite varied, depending on how they have been influenced in their progressive development. These tumors may contain primarily smooth muscle but may have varying densities of fibrous elements derived from the interstitial tissues. In addition, there may be varying degrees of degeneration, hemorrhage, and even calcification. The simple tumor is preferentially referred to as a myoma but is often called fibroid, fibromyoma, leiomyoma, leiofibroma, fibroleiomyoma, and so forth, synonymously. Multiple myomas are particularly confusing because they can produce a variety of symptoms depending on the number, the size and location, as well as any associated pathologic condition that may accompany their presence. In light of the clinical variation in symptoms, each woman so afflicted will have different needs, the most important of which is the need to have her symptoms corrected without the loss of reproductive function.

The recent technological advances applied to diagnose and manage this variable tumor entity have been hailed as useful, but, at the same time, their application has clouded the issues. Never have we had the ability to assess the pelvic structures as well as we have at present. At the same time, never have we had so varied an approach to address the management of the problem from both a medical and surgical viewpoint. This pleuralism exists despite the fact that myomectomy, basically, is a simple procedure. However, it does require a dedication to meticulous pursuit of excellence requiring a matured experience in adaptability for dealing with the anatomic variations of the myomas. In addition, it also requires the ability to address the needs of the specific woman. For this reason, it is well to review the various factors that should be considered when deciding what to do and how to counsel each woman in light of her specific situation and considerations.

ANATOMIC CONSIDERATIONS

It is estimated that some 20% to 25% of women of reproductive age have myomas.[8,9] They are seen more commonly during or after the third decade, and are rare before the age of 20. A threefold higher incidence in black compared to white women has been reported.[8,9,12] Myomas are found in various locations within and around the uterus. The subserous and intramural uterine locations are most common (Fig. 36-1). Pedunculated myomas can be seen arising from below the serosal surface but also from the submucosal myometrium. The submucosal myomas have an incidence of 5% to 10%.[5] They may be broad based or may arise on a narrow pedicle as a submucous pedunculated myoma. The latter can be extruded through the endocervix and can be associated with varying degrees of uterine inversion (Fig. 36-2).[31,53] Cervical and intraligamentous myomas (para-uterine) are less common, with an incidence of 5% and 2.4%, respectively.[34] Parametrial and perisalpingeal locations are less frequent.[44] A parasitic myoma can arise from a pedunculated subserosal myoma that undergoes torsion subsequently deriving its blood supply from another source with which it has interacted. Accordingly, they most commonly are found in the omentum.

Myomas can vary considerably in size from small seedlings (millimeters) to enormous tumors, which have been reported reaching more than 100 lb.[37,59] Rates of myoma growth are unpredictably variable, and the explanation for this variability is equally vexing. Myomas are typically benign uterine tumors, occurring as multiple tumors, although, less frequently they may be solitary. It is of interest that rapidly enlarging solitary tumors are more likely malignant than the multiple cohorts. Each myoma tends to be a discrete, elliptically spheroid pseudoencapsulated

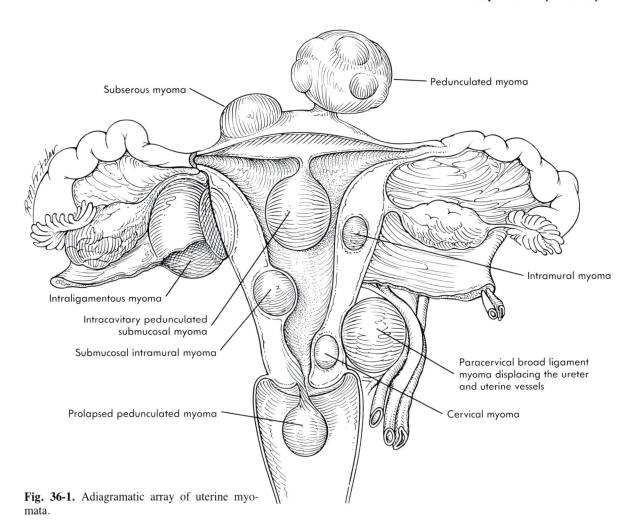

Fig. 36-1. Adiagramatic array of uterine myomata.

Labels on figure:
Subserous myoma
Pedunculated myoma
Intramural myoma
Intraligamentous myoma
Intracavitary pedunculated submucosal myoma
Submucosal intramural myoma
Paracervical broad ligament myoma displacing the ureter and uterine vessels
Prolapsed pedunculated myoma
Cervical myoma

mass, often interlacing with another myoma in the myometrium, producing a lobulated shape of the uterine body. Cut sections disclose a whorl-like pattern of smooth muscle and fibrous connective tissue. The fibrous connective tissue forms a pseudocapsule around the myoma. Hemorrhage and degeneration usually in the central aspect of the tumor are seen when the myoma outgrows its blood supply. Necrosis of myomas can subsequently occur. Hyalinization, fibrosis, and calcification are late sequelae. Infection of a necrotizing myoma (pyomyoma) can also occur, usually after pregnancy, instrumentation of the myomatous uterus, in association with an ascending infection, or by hematogenous spread.[28,66]

SYMPTOMATOLOGY

Symptomatic myomas have been reported in approximately 20% to 50% of cases. The severity of these parallels the degrees of pathology, which are more notable during the latter years of reproductive potential.[8,9] The wide array of symptoms includes abnormal uterine bleeding, which occurs in approximately 30% of patients, seen more often with submucous myomas. Abdominal and pelvic pain, abdominal enlargement, and gastrointestinal pressure symptoms (backache, constipation) are related to the impingement of the tumor on the adjacent organs. These dis-

tortions of the anatomy can also elicit dysfunctions of the urinary bladder (urinary frequency, urinary retention) or, on rare occasion, even obstruction of the ureters. Pedunculated or enlarging myomas arising from the serosal surface can be attached by a thick stalk. On occasion, they may be mistaken for an adnexal mass. Those with a thinner stalk may undergo torsion, giving rise to acute or recurrent abdominal pain. Pedunculated submucous myomas are frequently associated with heavy bleeding and have led to uterine inversion and sepsis when prolapsed through the cervix. Pain due to necrosis of a myoma can be seen in rapidly growing myomas, as well as during pregnancy.

Myomas may cause infertility through mechanisms such as compression of oviducts and distortion of the endometrial cavity, or perhaps as an IUD-like effect seen especially with pedunculated submucous myomas.[12] Pregnancy loss has been attributed to myoma constraint on uterine cavity expansion. Pregnancy loss rates as high as 75% to 80% have been reported; the rate in women without myomas is 30%.[9]

ETIOLOGIC CONSIDERATIONS

Although the etiology of myomas is unknown, several factors have been implicated. Evidence appears to support the fact that myomas, like many other benign tumors, are

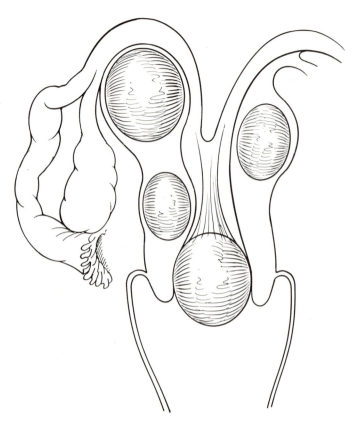

Fig. 36-2. Myomatous uterus with a prolapsing myoma creating a uterine inversion.

monoclonal.[51,63] Cytogenetic studies have found clonal chromosome arrangements in 50% to 60% of myomas studied. The most common abnormalities reported involve a translocation involving chromosomes 12 and 14, specifically, t[12;14].[q14-15,q23-24].[18,43,51,63] The many different cytogenetic abnormalities described support the hypothesis that different genetic loci may be responsible for the development of myomas, and these differences may explain the heterogeneity seen in the clinical presentation. Familial uterine myomas[38] have been reported, however, the actual incidence is unknown.

For years, estrogen has been causatively implicated in the pathophysiology of myomas. This theory is supported by the observation that myomas grow principally during the years of active ovarian function. Myomas are not seen before puberty; after the menopause, they not only do not grow, but are believed to regress in size.

Nelson was the first to demonstrate the association between estrogen and myomas by stimulating myomas to grow in guinea pigs after the administration of large doses of estrogens, which he thought to be a dose-related effect.[47] Estrogen and progesterone receptors have been demonstrated in myoma tissue.[50,60,62,65] It is also of interest that the concentration of estrogen receptors is found to be greater in myoma tissue than in the myometrium.[12]

Epidermal growth factor has been demonstrated in myoma tissue as well as in the myometrium.[31,53] Its receptor is present in low concentrations, and no difference has been demonstrated among endometrium, myometrium, and myomas. However, the role of the epidermal growth factor in myomas is unknown.

MANAGEMENT CONSIDERATIONS

Because the etiology of myomas is not understood, preventing their occurrence is not feasible. Also, it should be recognized that there are no long-term medical therapies available for the treatment of myomata with proven safety. Thus the treatment of myomas is usually surgical and should address the specific symptoms and needs of the woman. As such, conservational versus extirpative treatment must be individualized according to the woman's age, medical status, size, and involvement of the myomatous uterus. This should address the importance of the uterus to the specific woman, including the desire for future reproduction. Selection of appropriate management for each woman is highly subjective and requires careful discussion and counseling on all the issues. Moreover, the surgeon's empathy, experience, and ability play a fundamental role. Careful consideration must ensure the appropriate individualized treatment.

When the myomas are asymptomatic, and particularly if they are 3 months in size or less, most concur that nothing need be done.[8] These patients should be followed by periodic evaluation including pelvic examination and ultrasound evaluation every 6 to 12 months to assess the possible changes in the rate of growth. Rapid growth rate may be suggestive of malignancy and requires more frequent evaluation with possible intervention. Women exhibiting only minimal changes in uterine mass and who remain asymptomatic should be counseled of the need for careful, expectant follow-up, although medical or surgical intervention is not warranted.

The increased effort and experience required to perform myomectomy with limited risks leads many to conclude that there must be a justification for the need to preserve uterine function. Hysterectomy often is looked on as the definitive approach with which many surgeons feel most comfortable. Multiple myomectomy is most compelling when the aim is to improve fertility or to relieve a symptomatic myomatous distortion in the woman desirous of preserving her reproductive function. In general, the risks associated with myomectomy are prolonged operative time, blood loss, and intestinal obstruction secondary to adhesions of bowel to the uterine operative sites as well as the probability of myoma recurrence. These two latter complications of myomectomy, cited for their future potential need for pelvic surgery, are often viewed as outweighing the potential benefit to be gained by myomectomy. Of course, hysterectomy is not without risks and the importance of the uterus to the specific woman must not be underestimated. Sincere, careful counseling of the woman is key, and her desires must be weighed carefully. The woman should be counseled to seek another opinion when a consensus is not reached.

Infertile women with symptomatic myomas deserve every effort needed to preserve their uterine function. Successful pregnancies in women who have undergone myomectomy for intramural, subserosal, and submucosal myomas are reported in the range of 48% to 62%.[8,23,54] Pregnancy rates of 53% have been reported when submucosal myomas exceeding 5 cm in diameter were removed.[2,23,54] The fact that most of the pregnancies occur within the first year (75% to 80%) after myomectomy despite years of prior infertility supports the concept that myomectomy restores fertility. Nonetheless, there is no evidence to support the theory that the excision of small solitary myomas (<5 cm) significantly improves fertility.[7]

The feminist community argues for preservation of the reproductive organs and for myomectomy rather than hysterectomy at any age. This large group believes that not only is hysterectomy a reproductive loss, but that it seriously contributes adversely to their sexual feelings through dyspareunia and of the loss of deep orgasm. Moreover, they also point out that hysterectomy with and without oophorectomy is also associated with myocardial infarction related to estrogen deficiency secondary to premature ovarian failure. Several epidemiologic studies support this contention.[4,11,57] Significant disagreement still exists regarding the advisability of performing a myomectomy, especially in a woman over the age of 40, in whom the reproductive needs may be unrealistic and the distortion extensive. Although it may severely affect some women who perceive it as a loss of their femininity, it is important that the woman be counseled about the recurrence of myomas. There are those who raise concern regarding the appropriateness of myomectomy under these circumstances because subsequent myoma growth may lead to the need for reoperation. Myomas do recur in at least 15% to 20% of women who have undergone myomectomy.

The difficulties associated with making the diagnosis of a leiomyosarcoma, although very rare in occurrence, is another contributing factor of concern. The clinical presentation is not reliable, and the diagnosis may not be made at the time of dilation and curettage (D and C). Radiographic studies, including magnetic resonance imaging (MRI), are not reliable in diagnosing early nonmetastatic uterine sarcomas. The malignant transformation of myomas is viewed with less concern because they are exceedingly rare, occurring in less than 0.1% of women with myomas.[8]

Increased size of myomas, for some, may be associated with a greater risk in performing a myomectomy. Indeed, this need not be. Attention to meticulous hemostasis, careful appropriate dissection, repair with speed of surgery, and so forth facilitate safe restorative surgery. The presence of coexisting pathology, however, can make the surgery prolonged and tedious. In the more severe circumstances with myriads of myomas and for extensive adnexal disease, the "simpler" extirpative approach through hysterectomy might be preferable. For most whose situation may not be as severe, the goal probably should be the removal of all myomas with preservation of reproductive function. Proximity of the myomas to the oviducts and endometrial cavity does not endorse leaving the myomas. Microsurgical dissection techniques may be needed to resect such myomas as well as the repair of the defects. Removal of all myomas to ensure the lowest risk of recurrence should be the aim.

Preoperative evaluation and patient preparation

Before myomectomy, patients should have a complete history and physical examination and all existing medical problems should be addressed. Preoperative screening should include endometrial biopsy or uterine curettage to diagnose a possible chronic endometritis and/or malignancy. Hysterosalpingography is indicated to evaluate the possible uterine cavity distortion as well as tubal distortion or compression by the myomas. Hysteroscopy can also evaluate the uterine cavity but not the oviducts. An abdominal ultrasound or an excretory urogram is helpful in identifying ureteral dilatation, although it may not be routinely requested. Ultrasound and MRI have become useful adjuncts to define the location and size of the myomas and perhaps differentiate between an ovarian mass and a pedunculated myoma.[17,29] Laparoscopy is especially helpful in evaluating the size, location, and number of myomas as well as the presence of additional pelvic pathology that may weigh on the decision to proceed with the myomectomy (e.g., severe endometriosis and chronic pelvic adnexal inflammatory disease). Through such preoperative evaluation review, including the extent of the myomas and the relation to the total clinical features, the physician can more accurately counsel the patient who will feel better informed regarding her surgical options.

Anemia must be corrected before surgery. This can best be accomplished by a high-iron diet and with iron supplementation (e.g., ferrous sulfate, 325 mg, four times daily, after meals). In some cases, when menstrual blood loss has been severe, combinations of estrogen and progestagen or a gonadotropin-releasing hormone (Gn-RH) agonist have been used to stop vaginal bleeding to facilitate the correction of anemia *in conjunction with iron therapy*. Gn-RH agonists have had a recent popularity and can be administered by daily subcutaneous injection (Lupron, 0.5 to 1.0 mg/day), depot IM form (Lupron, 3.75 mg or 7.5 mg IM q month), or by nasal spray (nafarelin or Synarel), one to two puffs per nostril bid. The Gn-RH approaches have not had FDA approval for the management of myomata. Bleeding can be stopped acutely with these regimens. Combinations of estrogens and progestogens such as were used with the high-dose oral contraceptive have long been shown to be effective in the control of uterine bleeding. This was the initial approved indication for Enovid by the U.S. Food and Drug Administration (FDA). Three tablets of Estinyl, (ethinyl estradiol) 0.05 mg (total of 0.15 mg) and Norlutin (norethindrone), 10 mg, is a dosage level of the estrogen-progestagen combination that halts dysfunctional uterine bleeding associated with submucous myomas. It can be used for 6 to 8 weeks together with hematinic therapy to correct the anemia and allow the surgery to be scheduled. It should not be used other than as a short-term approach to stop the bleeding and reverse the anemia before surgery. Prolonged use results in subsequent uterine bleeding requiring increases in dosage of this estrogen-progestogen combination, and also effects increases in uterine and myoma size. However, it does not contribute to an estrogen-deficient menopausal state as with the releasing hormone analogues with their skeletal and other implications.

In all patients planning to have a multiple myomectomy, autologous and directed donor blood donation should be discussed with the patient early on, before scheduling surgery. Presurgical autologous blood donation has been suggested as well as use of a directed donor. Some recommend two units of the autologous blood available for surgery. However, it is not totally convincing that this approach is truly physiologically sound for anemic women. Preoperative donation of blood cannot but detract from the hemic buildup of an iron therapy if the bloods were not donated. Moreover, two units of blood might be inadequate were there significant bleeding at surgery. Such a situation could warrant the need of four or more units from the blood bank. This is just what the patient believes she is avoiding by autologous preoperative donations. Although the risk of contracting disease from donor blood is presumably lower than it has been in the past, it is still better to avoid all transfusions. The patient should be carefully counseled about these risks and the possible need for transfusion no matter how rare these occurrences may be.

Myomectomy approaches

Myomectomy is performed most commonly by the laparotomy route. Vaginal myomectomy, laparascopic myomectomy, as well as myomectomy by hysteroscopic resection are approached under special circumstances. For the present, abdominal myomectomy must be viewed as the gold standard. Many more data are needed to ensure that these alternative approaches are superior in every way. Prolapsed myomas should be approached vaginally. Laparoscopic approaches can be vexing in the removal of the myomas from the abdominal cavity. Moreover, it may not be possible to locate all the myomas. If the smaller ones are not removed, one can expect higher recurrence rates.

Abdominal myomectomy—the open surgical route

In carrying out the myomectomy, certain basic principles should be adhered to. Meticulous attention to hemostasis is essential. Most myomectomies can best be accomplished using Pfannenstiel's or a transverse incision in the abdomen, reserving a midline incision for the much larger myomas (e.g., arising above the umbilicus). The midline incision is less time consuming, but it is not as strong an incision as a transverse one. Moreover, it leaves the woman with a visible scar constantly reminding her of her surgery.

Good exposure, good assistance, and careful isolation of the tumor or tumors are essential to reduce blood loss. Moreover, meticulous hemostatic incision techniques help to defend against insidious blood loss. The use of the Shaw heated scalpel is strongly recommended. It justifies the time it takes to master its use because it does reduce the "insensible" blood loss incurred in opening the anterior abdominal wall. The dissection of the anterior sheath of the rectus should be made in a curvilinear manner as in the creation of a significant U-shaped flap. This should start from the initial midline transverse fascial incision and extend laterally with a cephalad course on each side to a level approaching that of the umbilicus (see Figs. 36-3, 36-4, 36-5 & 36-6). This U-shaped flap of the anterior sheath of the rectus affords an excellent exposure to the abdominal cavity after the recti have been retracted laterally. The peritoneum is then opened vertically in the midline. Occasionally, the lower pole of the peritoneal incision may need to be extended in a lateral direction, avoiding the bladder.

Of significance is excellent retraction. This can best be achieved by the use of the Iron Intern. It is ideally suited because it gives excellent exposure. It also has a gentle steady traction, which protects tissue from pressure points while also avoiding posterior pelvic compressions, which otherwise could lead to undesirable nerve and vessel trauma. The time taken to place these retractors is rewarded not only by the excellent exposure but also by the superior postoperative patient recovery. The retractor has a built-in safety clutch, which does not permit traumatic tissue pressures.

Hemostasis can be ensured with myometrial injection of vasoconstrictors such as dilute epinephrine, oxytocin (Pitocin), or vasopressin (Pitressin), as well as tourniquet application. Pitressin should be injected into the myometrium as a dilute solution (20 U in 40 to 50 ml normal saline). This can be used for small myomas or in conjunction with other techniques. Repeat use of dilute vasopressin may be needed. While some report a histamine reaction, it has never occurred in many hundreds of myomectomies over 30 years.[23]

The tourniquet technique is well-suited to large myomatous uteri with multiple intramural and submucous myomas. Reducing the intraoperative blood loss can be ensured by placing the tourniquet around the uterine mass. The tourniquet should be low enough to compress the infundibulopelvic ligaments and cervix, as well as to include the adnexa, which should be above the tourniquet to avoid being compressed. In this way, not only is the uterine blood supply to the uterus contained but also that by way of the ovarian anastomosis from the infundibulopelvic vessels. A simple piece of sterile rubber tubing or a catheter can serve as the tourniquet. The tourniquet is tightened in a stepwise fashion by alternately clamping with a Kelly

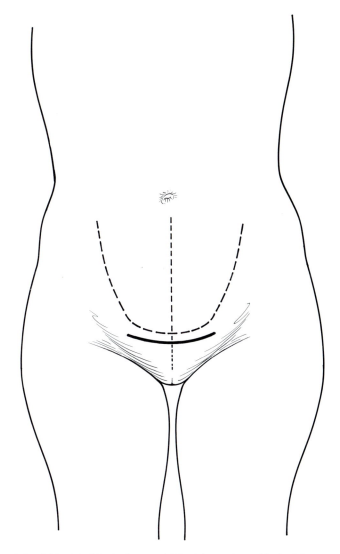

Fig. 36-3. Modified pfannenstiel incision: a low skin incision.

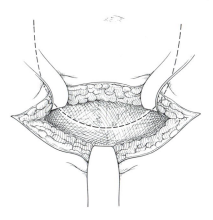

Fig. 36-4. Modified pfannstiel incision. Dissection exposing anterior sheath of the rectus. Tunneling of dissection at each angle follows dotted line.

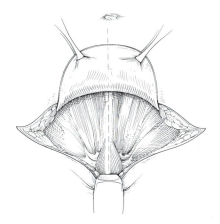

Fig. 36-5. Modified pfannenstiel incision. Shows flap of anterior sheath of rectus muscle that has been dissected free from the muscle bellies.

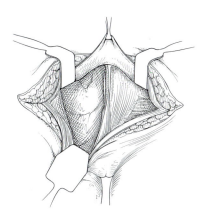

Fig. 36-6. Modified pfannenstiel incision. Right rectus muscle belly retracted, exposing the peritoneum prior to opening the celomic cavity.

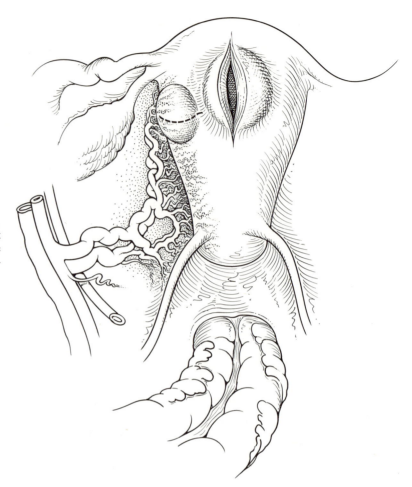

Figs. 36-7, 36-8, 36-9. Myomectomy incisions. The incisions should parallel the vasculature, except in the midline where the "avascularity" should be taken advantage of with a vertical or midline incision.

clamp, pulling on the tourniquet, and again clamping with another Kelly clamp. This repeated Kelly clamping and snugging of the tubing is continued until the compression is deemed adequate to constrict the blood flow. When Pitressin is injected into the myometrium before the application of the tourniquet, a vasoconstriction ensures reducing the blood volume within the organ. As a result, there is less bleeding on the initial uterine incision because the vasoconstriction has expressed the uterine blood into the peripheral circulation—a small autologous transfusion, as it were. This can be used for larger myomas as well as for smaller submucosal myomas.

Anoxia to the follicles causes them to become atretic during the current cycle; however, in the next cycle, a new crop of follicles develop from the primordial germ cells, which are resistant to the anoxia. This regeneration of follicles in the subsequent cycles has been consistent over the years even when the tourniquet has been in place some 5 hours. An alternate method of tourniquet application, suggested by Rubin[54a] in the 1930s, requires opening windows in the broad ligament through which the tourniquet is passed. This approach does not restrict the ovarian blood flow. It also has the disadvantage of creating broad ligament trauma.

The Shaw scalpel, electocautery, and laser[46,52] are useful tools for removing small myomas. Moreover, traction and compression are also helpful in reducing blood loss as

well as in the dissection of the myomas when tourniquets are not applied.

When approaching the uterus, the most important consideration is assessing the location and direction of the blood supply. A second consideration is to make as few incisions in the uterus as possible. The latter leads to a decreased chance of adhesion formation secondary to the effects of the uterine trauma. Posterior uterine wall incisions are of concern because of the potential of adhesions of bowel to these areas. Greater care in their repair is stressed.

Unless in the midline, the incision on the uterus should be made parallel with the course of the vascular bed of vessels. This is important when a more lateral uterine site is to be dissected. A vertical incision is preferable in the relatively avascular midline (Figs. 36-7, 36-8 & 36-9). Once through the serosa, the incision should be carried down through the myometrium into the pseudocapsule of the myoma. After the myoma has been exposed, it may be grasped with a towel clamp and traction can be applied. This traction reduces blood loss when a tourniquet has not been applied. The myoma is dissected free from the surrounding myometrium using a combination of sharp but principally blunt dissection (Fig. 36-10). The latter ensures remaining within the pseudocapsule. Strulli scissors and a periostial elevator are particularly well-suited to this purpose as are the surgeon's fingertips. Constant traction

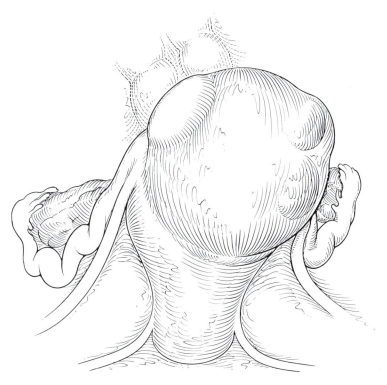

Fig. 36-8. For legend see opposite page.

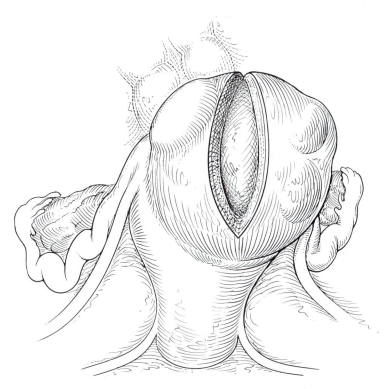

Fig. 36-9. For legend see opposite page.

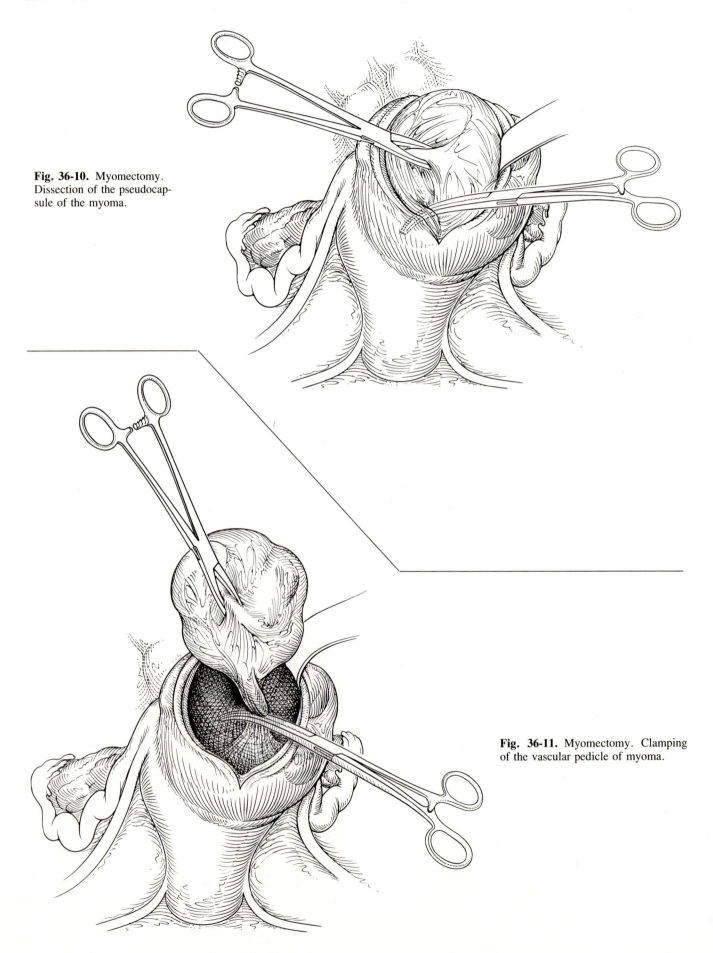

Fig. 36-10. Myomectomy. Dissection of the pseudocapsule of the myoma.

Fig. 36-11. Myomectomy. Clamping of the vascular pedicle of myoma.

on the myomas as well as a twisting motion are helpful. This dissection should not be difficult as long as the correct plane is maintained.

The dissection is carried down to the pedicle that contains the main blood supply to the myoma. The pedicle should be isolated, clamped, and ligated before the removal of the myoma as the first step in ensuring hemostasis (Figs. 36-11 & 36-12). Through the wall of the myometrial defect, other myomas are often detected and should also be dissected and excised. These surgically dissected uterine wall defects are repaired in a meticulous manner through the approximation of the tissues. This restores the anatomy previously distorted by the growing myomas. Several methods are suggested. The preferred approach uses a suture applied as a continuous concentric spiraling stitch, using vertically linear or radial bites. This closure is begun with a figure-of-eight stitch placed at the base of the operative defect. The important aspect of this stitch encompasses not only the anatomic reconstruction but also the securing of hemostasis. Both of these are achieved by closing all of the dead space (Fig. 36-13). It is most important to ensure continuous traction by snugging the stitch after each bite and maintaining constant tension on the suture as these stitches are being placed. Closing the defect is best accomplished by use of fine absorbable suture such as 3-0 or 4-0 Polyglactin (Vicryl). Catgut

should be avoided because of its inherent reactivity and lower tensile strength. The serosa is approximated using a baseball stitch that approximates the myometrium and inverts the serosa to minimize adhesion formation. For this approximation, 4-0 or 5-0 Vicryl sutures are used.

It is most important to identify all the myomas. If small myomas remain, the risk of them developing into larger myomas increases. This appears to be related to the high recurrence rates sometimes observed. Position and presence of myomas are determined by palpating the uterine wall carefully through the incision(s) and defects. Some myomas may be identified only by palpation through the defect created by the removal of the prior excised myomas. When palpated, it is preferable to remove the myoma through this existing incision. Incision techniques that also offer hemostasis, such as the Shaw scalpel, laser, and bipolar cautery, should be used. The removal of the myoma is accomplished by incising the myometrium overlying the myoma and removing the tumor as described above. Several myomas can be removed through the same incision in this manner. In doing so, care must be taken to identify blood supply ensuring hemostasis when closing all the defects that have been created. It is helpful to remove all myomas before closing defects so as not to confuse the digital palpation of sutured areas with remaining myomas.

With deep intramural or submucous myomas, the en-

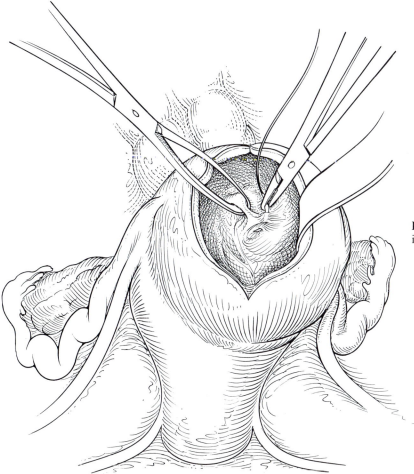

Fig. 36-12. Myomectomy. Suture ligature of pedicle of the base of the myoma.

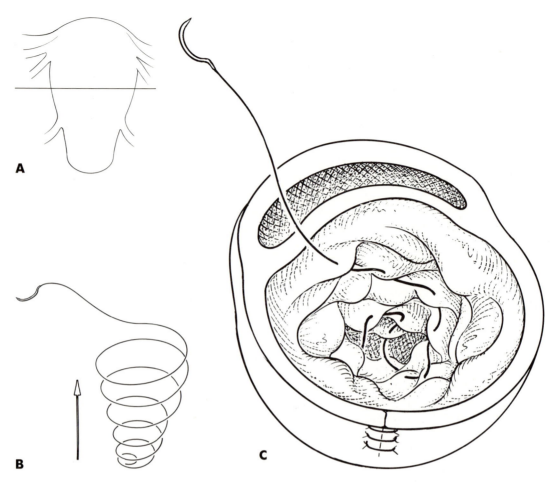

Fig. 36-13. A-D, Cross section of uterine cavity showing repair of myomectomy defect. A radial suture placement with a circumferential closure obliterates the dead space as well as providing hemostasis.   *Continued.*

dometrial cavity may be exposed or entered. It is best to avoid entry into the endometrial cavity because this could lead to adhesion formation (Asherman's syndrome). If the cavity is entered, care should be exercised in the repair. The cavity can be packed using one quarter inch iodoform gauze packing (Fig. 36-14). The endometrial cavity must be approximated using a fine running stitch with 5-0 or 6-0 Vicryl, taking care to ensure that the suture is free from the packing. The pack can be removed vaginally some 72 hours postoperatively.

Special care must be taken when myomas impinge on the oviducts. The course of the oviduct may be distorted by the myoma. Unless care is exercised, the oviducts may be injured or occluded during removal and repair. The pre-operative hysterosalpingography is useful in identifying variant anatomy. During surgery, a nylon stent of no. 1 monofilament nylon with a fine polished end may also be placed by way of the distal end of the tube to identify the oviduct by palpation during the resection. Microsurgical techniques are essential.

When a large myoma is removed, it is very tempting to use the approach that Bonney described as using the

monk's cowl type of closure[7] (Fig. 36-15). This approach should be reviewed as being of historical import. Such a repair is markedly anatomically unphysiologic in its context and should not be used. Reconstruction as outlined above produces a more physiologic anatomic restoration (Fig. 36-16).

Myomas, even when multiple and of sizes of 10 to 14 cm diameter, do not, per se, dictate hysterectomy. Meticulous conservational uterine surgery does allow for extirpation and reconstruction of large myomas while preserving the uterine function. With recurrent myomas, the technique of repeat myomectomy is similar to that described earlier when the myoma is initially dissected from the uterus.

Postoperatively, adhesion prophylaxis is recommended. dexamethasone/promethazine solution, high molecular dextron solution, and Ringer's lactated solution have all, in single or in combined manner, been instilled in the abdominal cavity before closure as an antiadhesions prophylaxis. Although Fayez[19] has reported no significant difference among the above techniques, the dexamethasone-promethazine regimen does have the advantage of accelerat-

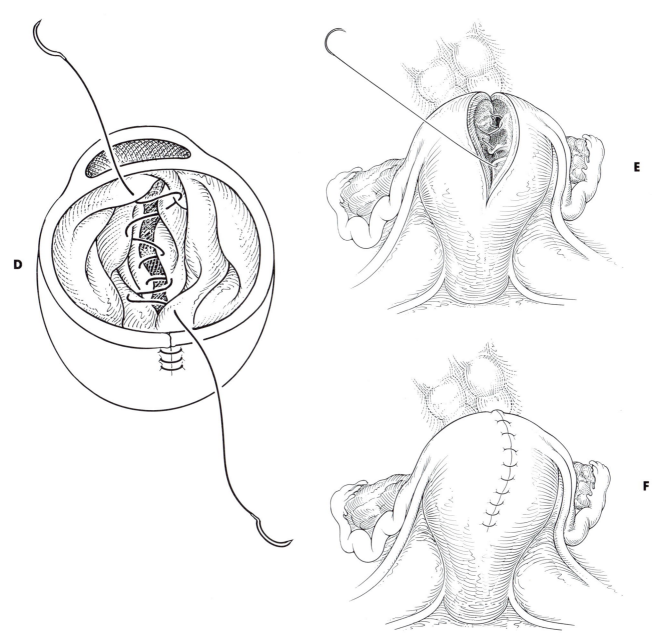

Fig. 36-13, cont'd. **E-F,** The superficial closure is achieved with a continuous simple approximation in layers.

ing the patient's postoperative recovery period with few if any side effects when used in a short, low-dose protocol.* Early ambulation and resumption of perfunctory activities are associated with that approach.

Intercede and Goretex have been advocated for adhesion prevention. Much work has to be done before using this routinely. Adhesions can occur with Intercede unless meticulous hemostasis is attained. Gortex needs a subse-

quent procedure for its removal. Prevention of adhesion formation or reformation is still best addressed by adhering to strict meticulous surgical principles. Constant irrigation using dilute solution of heparinized saline (5000 U/L) is helpful to prevent clot formation, which potentially can be viewed as a step in adhesion formation.

Laparoscopic myomectomy

Laparoscopic myomectomy is an appealing concept because major abdominal wall surgical trauma is avoided, which most frequently permits the woman to resume her normal physical activities sooner—often 12 to 24 hours after the procedure. The laparoscopic approach may well

*Low-dose protocol: 20 mg Dexamethasone and 25 mg Promethazine dissolved in 250 ml of n/s instilled into pelvis at end of procedure followed by 12.5 mg of Promethazine and 2 mg of Dexamethasone every 4 hours x 9 doses postoperatively.

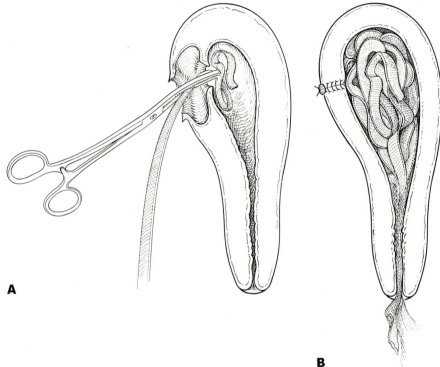

Fig. 36-14. A-B, Introduction of an intrauterine iodoform pack. This is done particularly when multiple entries to the cavity have occurred. Care must be exercised to prevent suturing the gauze in the closing of the defect.

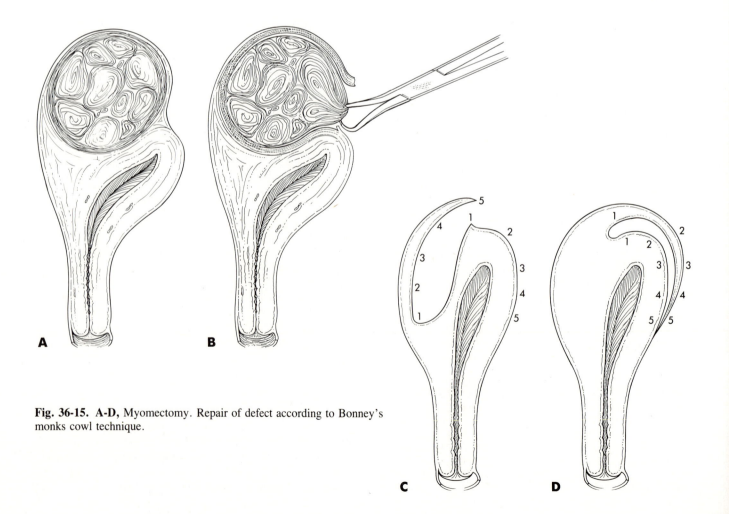

Fig. 36-15. A-D, Myomectomy. Repair of defect according to Bonney's monks cowl technique.

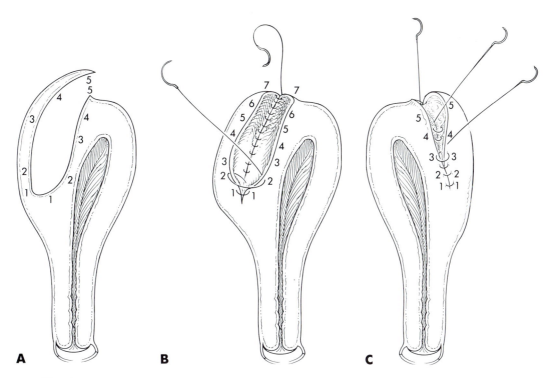

Fig. 36-16. A-C, Myomectomy cavity repair. Reconstruction of defect through repair approximating the anterior wall to the posterior wall in layers for a more anatomical reconstruction.

be suited to small superficial or pedunculated myomas. Limitations, however, occur with larger myomas, especially in intramural locations. The larger the myoma, the more significant the problems that can be encountered with this technique. Removing the myoma from the abdominal cavity after resection may require culdotomy or morcellation techniques. Other problems include adhesion formation seen with the laparoscopic suture material used in the repair.[49] Sutures cannot be applied as meticulously by laparoscopy as they can by laparotomy. Moreover, there are insufficient data to ensure that the uterine wall's strength is not weakened after such myomectomy approaches that could restrict the woman from carrying a gestation to term or viability. The use of laser drilling of myomas to destroy the blood supply of the tumor without removal of the myomas has been described to be followed by a reduction in the size of the myoma and, thus, uterine size and abatement of symptoms. Confirmatory safety studies are needed before these innovative promising techniques can be universally accepted as safe alternatives to laparotomy abdominal myomectomy.

Vaginal uterine myomectomy and hysteroscopic approaches

Often, women with submucosal myomas present with heavy vaginal bleeding (80% to 90%) and not necessarily with an enlarging uterus. Previously, the abdominal approach was the only method available for their removal. Vaginal myomectomy was reserved only for pedunculated myomas protruding through the cervix. However, with the technical advances in hysteroscopy, selected submucous myomas are being resected vaginally.

Prolapsed submucous myomas are relatively rare occurring in 2.5% of patients.[5] Patients present with menorrhagia, anemia, and foul vaginal drainage. These myomas can be necrotic and infected, causing systemic signs of infection in up to 13% of patients.[5,26] On examination, they can often have the appearance of a malignancy. Rarely, the patient can present with a complete uterine inversion caused by prolapsing of the myoma through the cervix.[31,53] The bladder and ureters are also exteriorized in this condition, and care is needed to avoid injury to these structures and to the uterine fundus during repair.[31] Vaginal myomectomy carries a lower morbidity than abdominal hysterectomy in these patients.[5,53] Prolapsed myomas are often attached to the cervical or endometrial cavity by a stalk. Removal of the tumors involves ligating the stalk or twisting the stalk to remove the myoma. Alternatively, a tonsil snare can greatly facilitate the removal.

Morcellation, hysterectomy, vaginal hysterectomy, and Dührssen's incisions have been used for large myomas.[15] A less traumatic approach using laminaria to dilate the cervix has facilitated exposure and removal of the myoma.[26] Myomas ranging from 10 to 180 g have been removed using this technique. Success rates of 90% to 94% have been reported.[5,26] Unfortunately, the early experiences of vaginal myomectomy have had some complications, which included uterine perforation (1%), excessive bleeding requiring insertion of Foley catheter as a tamponade (0 to 5%), febrile morbidity (1% to 6%), and cervical laceration with subsequent cervical incompetence (5%). Prophylactic antibiotics should be used. It should be pointed out that the incidence of malignancy in these tumors is similar to other myomas and reported as high as 2% to 3%.[26,53]

Submucous myomas that are nonprolapsing, if small, can sometimes be removed by sharp curettage. However, hysteroscopic removal first described by Norment in 1957[49a] is now a preferable alternative to abdominal myomectomy for the majority of submucous myomas. Hysteroscopic resection of myomas should be considered when there is definite evidence of submucous myomas proven by hysterosalpingogram, hysteroscopy, or MRI. However, before resection endometrial assessment should be performed to rule out a neoplastic cause of bleeding. It is probably preferable to limit hysteroscopic resection to myomas less than 4 cm, although larger myomas have been resected.[30] Sixty percent of the myoma should protrude into the endometrial cavity to allow safe resection with minimal bleeding and reduce risk of uterine perforation. Opposing wall myomas at the same level should be avoided because the dissected areas can and do grow together.

Transvaginal resection of intrauterine myomas

The technique with the operative hysteroscope or resectoscope involves shaving the protruding myoma to the level of the endometrium or, in the case of the laser, vaporizing out the myoma. The fragments of myoma can be removed at the time of the operative hysteroscopy. Some leave the fragments within the cavity to be expelled with menses. More experience is needed to assess the various approaches. The most popular approach uses laparoscopy. Complete resection of the myoma has not always been possible, and repeat hysteroscopic resection or definitive surgery has been required. The frequency with which this occurs has not always been reported. Some suggest the use of Gn-RH preoperatively with ablation of the endometrium and then resection of the submucous myomas. Neuwirth reported that, of 26 patients, 9 patients required further surgery after hysteroscopic resection of a myoma.[61] Other small series have reported no need for further surgery. Although the larger submucous myomas have been managed by repeated hysteroscopic resections on sequential procedures, not only is this approach fraught with risks but the pregnancy rates and safety have yet to be assessed. Certainly, great care needs to be taken that appropriate counseling of women be assigned prior to selecting these approaches in someone desirous of preserving reproductive function.

Hysteroscopic resection of submucosal myoma can be accomplished using the resectoscope at a power of 60 W

cutting current.[58] The applications of laser has favored the Nd-YAG laser at a power of 80 W.[16] CO_2 laser can only be used with a CO_2 distending medium. Gas-cooled fiber tips should never be used because several deaths have been attributed to gas embolism.[1]

Maintenance of adequate uterine distention and clarity of view have favored the use of a pump such as the electric Nezhat or the N_2 driven Davol disposable pump. When glycine is used as the distending medium, visualization of the cavity is quite good. However, hyponatremia has been reported with glycine.[64] Hyskon also allows a clear view of the uterine cavity because the pressure controls the bleeding that is present. High molecular weight Dextran, however, has been associated with pulmonary edema and disseminated intramuscular coagulation defects. These side effects are related to the length of the procedure and the volume of the distention medium used.

Donnez[16] described a technique for resection of myomas whose largest portion was located in the uterine wall.[22] He treated the patient preoperatively with Gn-RH agonist. Nd-YAG laser was then used to resect the myoma hysteroscopically. The remaining portion of the myoma was drilled with the laser to destroy the vascularity. After an additional 8 weeks of Gn-RH analogue therapy, repeat hysteroscopy revealed the residual portion of the myoma protruding, which could be readily resected. He reported 100% success and no complications. Most submucous resectionists advocate the preoperative use of Gn-RH agonist for submucous myomas because it reduces the size of the myoma by an average of 38%.[16] Moreover, the uterine myometrium is made atrophic and the vascularity is also reduced. Severe intractable hemorrhage has been reported when Gn-RH agonist therapy is used for submucous myomas.[22]

Endometrial ablation has also been used for treatment of hypermenorrhea and polymenorrhea.[6,32] This approach has been entertained in place of myomectomy or as an aid to reduce bleeding in the associated resection of myomas. Endometrial ablation is accomplished using the rollerball[6] followed by the use of the resectoscope[14,35] or the laser.[13,27,41,42] Concerns about using the endometrial ablation procedure include burying a nidus of endometrium. Reports of hematometria have been described after endometrial ablation[27] and support a concern about widespread use of endometrial ablation without stringent indications. Longer term follow-up is needed. We still do not know the extent of the problem secondary to burying endometrial niduses.

Myomectomy complications

Blood loss. Anemia is the most common complication after myomectomy. Strict adherence to a meticulous hemostatic technique as described above is essential to avoid this. Preoperative fluid loading is helpful to increase intravascular volume and promote hemodilution. Preoperatively, iron replacement and diet can be used to maximize hemoglobin in the case of an anemic patient. *Transfusions* *should be used only when the need is urgent!* Transfusions should not be given to the patient merely because she stored her own blood! This should be made clear to the patient before donation.

Hematoma formation. Seroma and hematoma formation can occur postoperatively. Meticulous closure of the defects in the myometrium avoids this. Patients may develop pain or fever when they occur. MRI and ultrasound are useful in making the diagnosis. Management involves conservative and supportive therapy and antibiotics. Surgical intervention is rarely necessary and preferably avoided.

Hysteroscopic complications. Complications of the hysteroscopic resection include hemorrhage and uterine perforation. The true incidence is not available because there are no well-controlled studies and the complications of these clinical experiences are sporadic. Concomitant use of laparoscopy is advocated to minimize risk of uterine perforation. It is apparent that the incidence decreases with experience but cannot but be lowest with those who are cautious. Hyponatremia and other electrolyte problems require careful vigilance with time and volume control.

Myoma recurrence after myomectomy. The recurrence rate of myomas after myomectomy is reported to be 5% to 30%.[9] Fedele found a 27% cumulative 10-year recurrence among 622 patients who underwent myomectomy between 1970 and 1984 at the University of Milan.[10] Garcia reported a 15% recurrence rate in 200 patients (unpublished data presented at the International Federation of Gynecology and Obstetrics). The recurrence rate reported depends on the skill and care of the surgeon in removing all of the myomas detected at the time of the initial surgery. If these small, seemingly insignificant myomas are ignored, with time they may develop into significant myomas.

Leiomyosarcoma

Leiomyosarcoma has been found in 0.1% to 0.7% of uterine myomas.[8,39] Occasionally, this diagnosis can be made preoperatively by D and C.[49] However, the majority may not be diagnosed until the intraoperative or postoperative period. Leiomyosarcoma is more frequent in solitary myomas and in tumors showing rapid growth, necrosis, hemorrhagic areas, and poor demarcation. The diagnosis is only confirmed after microscopic evaluation of the tissue sections reveal more than 10 mitoses per 10 higher powered field.[63]

Malignant transformation similar to leiomyosarcoma occurs in 0.1% to 0.7% of patients undergoing myomectomy.[8,39] This is most often associated with increased age of patient, abnormal uterine bleeding, rapid growth, and especially with solitary tumors.

Pregnancy after myomectomy

Appropriately performed myomectomy should improve the probability of pregnancy in those who would otherwise be fertile. Nonetheless, myomectomies can, on occasion, be resected from areas that may contribute to difficulties in either gamete tubal transport or implantation. With the techniques detailed above, the fertility appears enhanced or restored.

Generally speaking, there is less need for delay of attempted conception because the risk of potential immediate pregnancy is less after myomectomy than after other infertility procedures. By the time the earliest pregnancy occurs, which is not any sooner than 2 to 3 months after surgery and more often 6 months to 1 year, these patients experience no difficulty in safely carrying the pregnancy to term.

Mode of obstetric delivery is important. Cesarean section is advocated especially when intramural, submucosal, and large subserosal myomas have been removed. Small subserosal and some hysteroscopically removed submucosal myomas are not thought to represent a contraindication to trial of labor.

CONTROVERSIAL ISSUES

Despite the lack of approval by the FDA for the use of Gn-RH analogues in the management of myomas, it has been used for this purpose extensively. These medications are synthetic peptide analogues of gonadotropin-releasing hormone. Their effect is to down-regulate the pituitary, thereby creating a hypoestrogenic or menopausal state. Although the effects are believed to be reversed after discontinuing the medication, this is not universally the case.

Treatment with the Gn-RH agonists for 6 months has resulted in a shrinkage of the volume of myomas of 20% and shrinkage of total uterine volume in the range of 35% to 50%.[45,55,56] Initially, this was thought to be a significant advantage of this approach. However, several observations have been reported that may temper the initial enthusiasm for this therapy. First, the reduction in uterine volume has been shown to be greater than the reduction in myoma volume, 42.7% versus 30.4%, respectively, after 6 months of treatment.[55] This difference is explained by the fact that Gn-RH agonist results in shrinkage of myometrial cells but not fibrous or interstitial elements, which can make up a significant proportion of the myoma. Second, the reduction in size is transient. Myomas and uteri have been shown to return to pretreatment size within 4 months of completing the medication. Third, the return of ovarian function may be delayed.

Furthermore, the volume reduction observed can be misleading. Because the formula for calculating volume of a sphere or of a spheroid involves the cube of the radius, the reduction in volume in large myomas represents proportionately but a small reduction in the diameter. The volume reduction of 4% in a 10-cm myoma represents a 1.7 cm reduction in diameter. However, a similar percentage reduction in volume of a small myoma represents a greater proportionate reduction in diameter. Thus, the effect of the Gn-RH ovarian suppression on small seedlings is more significant because they may be reduced to an undetectable size, thereby making removal at time of myomectomy impossible. This has been proposed as the reason for the higher recurrence rates seen in postmyomectomy patients pretreated with Gn-RH agonists compared with those who have not. Fedele in a careful prospective well-designed study reported a 63% recurrence rate in patients treated preoperatively with Gn-RH versus 13% recurrence rate in those not treated.[20] Meticulous resection of all myomas without a menopausal state of estrogen suppression should provide a better long-term cure rate. Another advantage ascribed to the use of Gn-RH agonists has been a reported decrease in intraoperative myomectomy blood loss.[22a] More recent reports, however, have not reported such a conclusion.[20]

The most significant problem with the use of Gn-RH agonists has been their side effects. A 2% to 6% decrease in bone mineral density has been observed after the 6-month course.[36] The mean values approach normal in most patients 6 months after treatment. There is concern for those women who do not have a return to normal bone mineral content levels. Other effects include hot flashes (70% to 100%), vaginal dryness (30% to 60%), and the effects on lipids.[24,25,40,45,55] Because of these effects, those who are to use Gn-RH agonists should limit the course to a maximum of 6 months. Repeated courses of Gn-RH for reduction of uterine volume is not an acceptable approach. "Add on" progesterone therapies may or may not be acceptable and need more careful evaluation of efficacy and safety.

For these reasons, preoperative treatment with Gn-RH agonists has become a less favorable alternative. However, pretreatment with Gn-RH agonists appears to have a significant benefit in facilitating vaginal hysterectomy in those patients who would otherwise have required abdominal hysterectomy. Myomatous uteri the size of 14 to 18 weeks of gestation have successfully been removed vaginally after pretreatment with Gn-RH agonists.[12] Of course, morcellation could be used in those cases where the Gn-RH had been used and the potential problems of Gn-RH therapy can be avoided.

In a woman who has previously undergone myomectomy and has had a recurrent symptomatic myomatous uterus, the decision must be made to proceed with repeat myomectomy versus hysterectomy. The chance of successfully achieving pregnancy may be less favorable than with primary myomectomy. Although complications of myomectomy are infrequent, the overall risk is probably greater than hysterectomy. However, the effect of hysterectomy on the specific woman is difficult to quantify! Using a nondirective approach, one can usually guide the 40 to 45-year-old woman away from myomectomy. Supracervical hysterectomy is a reasonable alternative especially because preservation of the cervix is an acceptable alternative in those who feel strongly about preserving their organs from a sexuality standpoint. Pap smear and colposcopy have allowed for preservation of the healthy cervix with reasonable risk.

CONCLUSIONS

Myomectomy can be a difficult and often time-consuming procedure. However, with meticulous attention to technique, the procedure can be accomplished safely and effectively with relatively assured hemostasis. Myomectomy affords the option of preserving the uterus in those patients with symptomatic uterine myomas who desire to preserve their reproductive organs. However, careful assessment of the patient and counseling are essential. Hysteroscopic resection of submucous myomas has become the technique of choice in many cases. Abdominal myomectomy is the preferable technique for removal of intramural and subserosal myomas. Laparoscopic and hysteroscopic approaches must be viewed as being of very limited acceptability.

REFERENCES

1. Baggish MS, Daniell JF: Catastrophic injury secondary to the use of coaxial gas-cooled fibers and artificial sapphire tips for intrauterine surgery: a report of five cases, *Lasers Surg Med* 9:581, 1989.
2. Bakaknia A, Rock JA, Jones HW Jr: Pregnancy success following abdominal myomectomy for infertility, *Fertil Steril* 30(6):644, 1978.
3. Barter JF, Ízpak C, Creasman WT: Uterine leiomyomas with retroperitoneal lymph node involvement, *South Med J* 80(10):1320, 1987.
4. Beamis ELG et al: Ovarian functions after hysterectomy with conservation of the ovaries in premenopausal women, *J Obstet Gynecol Brit Commonwealth* 76:969, 1969.
5. Ben-Baruch G et al: Immediate and late outcome of vaginal myomectomy for prolapsed pedunculated submucous myoma, *Obstet Gynecol* 72(6):858, 1988.
6. Bent AE, Ostergaard DR: Endometrial ablation with the neodymium: YAG laser, *Obstet Gynecol* 75(6):923, 1990.
7. Bonney V: The technique and result of myomectomy, *Lancet*, January 24, 1931, p 171.
8. Buttram VC Jr: Uterine leiomyomata—aetiology, symptomatology and management. In: *Gonandotropin Down-Regulation in Gynecological Practice*, New York, 1986, Alan R. Liss.
9. Buttram VC Jr, Reiter RC: Uterine leiomyomata: etiology, symptomatology and management, *Fertil Steril* 36(4):433, 1981.
10. Candiani GB et al: Risk of recurrence after myomectomy, *Br J Obstet Gynecol* 98:385, 1991.
11. Centerwall BS: Premenopausal hysterectomy and cardiovascular disease, *Am J Obstet Gynecol* 139:58, 1981.
12. Damewood MD, Rock JA: Reproductive uterine surgery, *Obstet Gynecol Clin North Am* 14(4):1049, 1987.
13. Davis JA: Hysteroscopic endometrial ablation with the neodymium-YAG laser, *Br J Obstet Gynaecol* 96:928, 1989.
14. DeCherney AH et al: Endometrial ablation for intractable uterine bleeding: hysteroscopic resection, *Obstet Gynecol* 70(4):668, 1987.
15. Dicker D et al: The management of prolapsed submucous fibroids, *Aust N Z J Obstet Gynecol* 26:308, 1986.
16. Donnez J et al: Neodymium: YAG laser hyseroscopy in large submucous fibroids, *Fertil Steril* 54(6):999, 1990.
17. Dudiak CM et al: Uterine leiomyomas in the infertile patient: preoperative localization with MR imaging versus US and hysterosalpingography, *Radiology* 167(3):627, 1988.
18. Fan SX et al: Cytogenetic findings in nine leiomyomas of the uterus, *Cancer Genet Cytogenet (#74)* 47:179, 1990.
19. Fayez JA, Schneider PJ: Prevention of pelvic adhesions formation by different modalities of treatment, *Am J Obstet Gynecol* 157(5):1184, 1987.
20. Fedele L et al: Treatment of GnRH agonists before myomectomy and

the risk of short-term myoma recurrence, *Br J Obstet Gynecol* 97:393, 1990.

21. Ford JM et al: Metastasizing leiomyoma of the uterus, *Aust NZ J Obstet Gynecol* 28:154, 1988.

22. Friedman AJ: Vaginal hemorrhage associated with degenerating submucous leiomyomata during leuprolide acetate treatment, *Fertil Steril* 52(1):152, 1989.

22a. Friedman AJ et al: A randomized placebo-controlled, double-blind study evaluating the efficacy of leuprolide acetate depot in the treatment of uterine leiomyomata, *Fertil Steril* 51:251-255, 1989.

23. Garcia C-R, Tureck RW: Submucosal leiomyomas and infertility, *Fertil Steril* 42(1):16, 1984.

24. George M et al: Long-term use of LH-RH agonist in the management of uterine leiomyomas: a study of 17 cases, *Int J Fertil* 34(1):19, 1989.

25. Golan A et al: D-Trp-6 luteinizing hormone-releasing hormone microcapsules in the treatment of uterine leiomyomas, *Fertil Steril* 52(3):406, 1989.

26. Goldrath MH: Vaginal removal of the pedunculated submucous myoma: historical observations and development of a new procedure, *J Reprod Med* 35(10):921, 1990.

27. Goldrath MH, Fuller TGA, Segal S: Laser photovaporization of endometrium for the treatment of menorrhagia, *Am J Obstet Gynecol* 140(1):14, 1981.

28. Greenspoon JS et al: Pyomyoma associated with polymicrobial bacteremia and fatal septic shock: case report and review of the literature, *Obstet Gynecol Surv* 45(9):563, 1990.

29. Gross BH, Silver TM, Jaffe MH: Sonographic features of uterine leiomyomas: analysis of 41 proven cases, *J Ultrasound Med* 2:401, 1983.

30. Hallez JP, Perino A: Endoscopic intrauterine resection: principles and technique, *Acta Eur Fertil* 19(1):17, 1988.

31. Henderson PR: A large submucous fibroid polyp causing inversion of the uterus, *Aust NZ J Obstet Gynecol* 20:251, 1980.

32. Hill D, Maher P: Treatment of menorrhagia by endometrial ablation, *Med J Aust* 152:564, 1990.

33. Hofmann GE et al: Binding sites for epidermal growth factor in human uterine tissues and leiomyomas, *J Clin Endocrinol Metab* 58(5):880, 1984.

34. Honore LH: Parauterine leiomyomas in women: a clinicopathologic study of 22 cases, *Eur J Obstet Gynecol Reprod Biol* 11:273, 1981.

35. Indman PD, Soderstrom RM: Depth of endometrial coagulation with the urologic resectoscope, *J Reprod Med* 35(6):633, 1990.

36. Johanse JS et al: The effect of a gonadotropin-releasing hormone agonist analog (Nafarelin) on bone metabolism, *J Clin Endocrinol Metab* 67(4):701, 1988.

37. Jonas HS, Masterson BJ: Giant uterine tumor: case report and review of the literature, *Obstet Gynecol* 50(1 Suppl):2S, 1977.

38. Kulenthran A, Sivanesaratnam V: Recurrent uterine myomata in three sisters—an uncommon occurrence, *Int J Gynecol Obstet* 27:289, 1988.

39. Leibsohn S et al: Leiomyosarcoma in a series of hysterectomies performed for presumed uterine leiomyomas, *Am J Obstet Gynecol* 4:968, 1990.

40. Letterie GS et al: Efficacy of a gonadotropin-releasing hormone agonist in the treatment of uterine leiomyhomata: long-term follow-up, *Fertil Steril* 51(6):951, 1989.

41. Loffler FD: Laser ablation of the endometrium, *Obstet Gynecol Clin North Am* 15(1):77, 1988.

42. Lomano JM: Dragging technique versus blanching technique for endometrial ablation with the Nd:YAG laser in the treatment of chronic menorrhagia, *Am J Obstet Gynecol* 159(1):152, 1988.

43. Mark J et al: Cytogenetical observations in human benign leiomyomas, *Anticancer Res* 8:621, 1988.

44. Matamala MF et al: Leiomyomas of the ovary, *Int J Gynecol Pathol* 7(2):190, 1988.

45. Matta WHM, Shaw RW, Nye M: Long-term follow-up of patients with uterine fibroids after treatment with the LHRH agonist buserelin, *Br J Obstet Gynecol* 96:200, 1989.

46. McLaughlin DS: Metroplasty and myomectomy with the CO_2 laser for maximizing the preservation of normal tissue and minimizing bone loss, *J Reprod Med* 30(1):1, 1985.

47. Nelson WO: Endometrial and myometrial changes, including fibromyomatous nodules, induced in the uterus of the guinea pig by the prolonged administration of oestrogenic hormone, *Anat Rec* 68:99, 1937.

48. Neuwirth RS: Hysteroscopic management of symptomatic submucous fibroids, *Obstet Gynecol* 62(4):509, 1983.

49. Nezhat C et al: Laparoscopic myomectomy, *Int J Fertil* 36:175, 1991.

49a. Norment WB et al: Hysteroscopy, *Surg Clin North Am* 37:1377, 1957.

50. Puukka MJ et al: Oestrogen receptors in human myoma tissue, *Mol Cell Endocrinol* 6:35, 1976.

51. Rein MT et al: Cytogenetic abnormalities in uterine leiomyomata, *Obstet Gynecol* 77(6):923, 1991.

52. Reyniak JV, Corenthal L: Microsurgical laser technique for abdominal myomectomy, *Microsurgery* 8(2):92, 1987.

53. Riley P: Treatment of prolapsed submucous fibroids, *SA Med J* 62(3):22, 1982.

54. Rosenfeld DL: Abdominal myomectomy for otherwise unexplained infertility, *Fertil Steril* 46(2):328, 1986.

54a. Rubin I: Progress in myomectomy: Surgical measures and diagnostic aids favoring lower morbidity and mortality, *Am J Obstet Gynecol* 44:196, 1942.

55. Schlaff WD et al: A placebo-controlled trial of a depot gonadotropin-releasing hormone analogue (leuprolide) in the treatment of uterine leiomyomta, *Obstet Gynecol* 74(6):856, 1989.

56. Shaw RW: Mechanism of LHRH analogue action in uterine fibroids, *Horm Res* 32(Suppl 1):150, 1989.

57. Siddle N, Sarrel P, Whitehead M: The effect of hysterectomy on the age of ovarian failure, *Fertil Steril* 47(1):94, 1987.

58. Siegler AM: Therapeutic hysteroscopy, *Acta Europ Fertil* 17(6):467, 1986.

59. Singhabhandhu B et al: Giant leiomyoma of the uterus: report of a case and review of the literature, *Am Surg* p. 391, July, 1973.

60. Soules KMR, McCarty KS Jr: Leiomyomas: steroid receptor content: variation within normal menstrual cycles, *Am J Obstet Gynecol* 143(1):6, 1982.

61. Stovall TG et al: A randomized trial evaluating leuprolide acetate before hysterectomy as treatment for leiomyomas, *Am J Obstet Gynecol* 164(6):1420.

62. Tamaya T, Fujimoto J, Okada H: Comparison of cellular levels in steroid receptors in uterine leiomyoma and myometrium, *Acta Obstet Gynecol Scand* 64:307, 1985.

63. Townsend DE et al: Unicellular histogenesis of uterine leiomyomas as determined by electrophoresis of glucose-6-phosphate dehydrogenase, *Am J Obstet Gynecol* 107(8):1168, 1970.

64. Van Bove MJ et al: Dilutional hyponatremia associated with intrauterine endoscopic laser surgery, *Anesthesiology* 71:449, 1989.

65. Wilson EA, Yang F, Rees ED: Estradiol and progesterone binding in uterine leiomyomata and in normal uterine tissues, *Obstet Gynecol* 55(1):20, 1980.

66. Wong TC, Bard DS, Pearce LW: Unusual case of IUD-associated postabortal sepsis complicated by an infected necrotic leiomyoma, suppurative pelvic thrombophlebitis, ovarian vein thrombosis, hematoperitoneum and drug fever, *J Arkansas Med Soc* 83:138, 1986.

Chapter 37

PRESACRAL NEURECTOMY

L. Russell Malinak

Presacral neurectomy is the principal operation in modern gynecologic surgery performed for relief of severe central pelvic pain when preservation of uterine function is important. Secondary dysmenorrhea, deep dyspareunia, sacral backache with menses, perimenstrual pain of bowel or bladder origin, and chronic recurrent pain in the center of the pelvis constitute the type of pain relieved by this operation.

The operation was first described by Jaboulay[13] and Ruggi[25] in 1899. Its popularity increased in the mid 1920s when Cotte reported unusual success in the operative management of severe dysmenorrhea.[8] Since that time, many authors have documented the benefits of presacral neurectomy in the relief of central pelvic pain.*

INDICATIONS FOR PRESACRAL NEURECTOMY

The most common indication for presacral neurectomy is invasive endometriosis associated with significant central pelvic pain in patients who wish to preserve uterine function.[1,21,29] Lesions located in the uterosacral ligaments, the posterior and anterior cul-de-sacs, the proximal fallopian tubes and round ligaments, and myometrium trigger this type of pain. In addition, lesions in the region of the bladder and the rectosigmoid might promote major central pelvic pain. Few benign pelvic pathologic processes other than endometriosis promote the type of pelvic pain that is beneficially managed by presacral neurectomy.[9]

CONTRAINDICATIONS TO PRESACRAL NEURECTOMY

The general contraindications to any elective operation pertain to presacral neurectomy (i.e., if [1] the patient's general condition or vital signs are compromised, [2] pelvic infection or malignancy exists, or [3] adequate exposure cannot be obtained).

This operation is rarely indicated in the treatment of primary dysmenorrhea or in the absence of a demonstrable pelvic pathologic process. Typical of any operation in a patient with pelvic pain, the absence of disease contraindicates a surgical solution in most patients. A gynecologic surgeon is well advised to follow the old adage, "when you operate for pain, you get pain." Presacral neurectomy is not indicated in a patient who has had a hysterectomy or in the presence of malignancy. Furthermore, it is not indicated for the treatment of chronic pelvic inflammatory disease, which creates pain principally in the lateral pelvis. Also, I decline to attempt repeated presacral neurectomy because fibrosis and distorted anatomy render another attempt very difficult.

INNERVATION OF THE PELVIC VISCERA

Pain impulses from the cervix, the body of the uterus, the proximal portion of the fallopian tubes, and immediately adjacent tissues are transmitted through afferent fibers that accompany sympathetic nerves into the spinal cord at the level of T10, T11, T12, and L1.[3] These fibers pass through, and are component parts of, the uterine and cervical plexus, the pelvic plexus, the hypogastric nerve, the superior hypogastric plexus ("presacral nerve"), and the lumbar and lower thoracic sympathetic chain. The sensory nerves are special visceral afferents that course through the various plexus to higher levels and are functionally independent of the autonomic nervous system.[15]

The sensory fibers in the superior hypogastric plexus course upward from a lateral position near the sacral end of the uterosacral ligament. They are in close proximity to the lateral surface of the rectal ampulla in the pelvic plexus, sometimes known as Frankenhäuser's ganglion.[31]

The locations and relations of the superior hypogastric

*References 2, 9, 11, 14, 17, 20, 24, 27.

624

plexus are important. This plexus is present behind the peritoneum in a bed of loosely meshed areolar tissue that lies on the bodies of the fourth and fifth lumbar vertebrae. It is usually formed from two or three incompletely fused nerve trunks and is commonly present in more than one layer. In approximately 20% of cases, there is complete fusion with resultant formation of a single nerve.[29] In the midline, the middle sacral artery and vein lie between the nerve tissue and the periosteum of the vertebral bodies. Superior to the presacral nerve are the aorta and vena cava at their bifurcation and confluence, respectively. The common iliac artery and vein and the right ureter are at the right extension of the superior hypogastric plexus, and the inferior mesenteric vessels and the sigmoid mesocolon are at the left border. Inferiorly, the area occupied by the superior hypogastric plexus is bounded by the hollow of the sacrum, which contains a plexus of veins, interruption of which may cause troublesome bleeding during surgery.

Of importance in consideration of pelvic pain is that nerves from the ovaries, similar to their vascular supply, pass lateral and independent of the presacral nerve to the inferior mesenteric plexus, as do the sensory fibers from the lower bowel and distal fallopian tubes. The origin of the nerves that supply the ovary is the ovarian plexus, a meshwork of nerves that arise from the aortic and renal plexus and accompany the ovarian artery down its course. The ovarian plexus invests both the ovarian artery and vein and supplies fibers to the broad ligaments, the distal portion of the fallopian tube, and the ovary.

Technique

A Pfannenstiel incision (Fig. 37-1, *A*) provides adequate exposure for presacral neurectomy in most cases. If more room is needed, this incision may be easily converted into a Cherney incision,[9a] which provides adequate additional exposure. A transverse Maylard incision or a midline lower abdominal incision is also a reasonable choice. Some authors have recommended that a routine longitudinal incision be made in all cases.[1,29]

The sigmoid colon should be retracted and packed as far to the left as possible to accomplish maximum exposure of the sacral promontory.

At the anteriormost projection of the sacral promonotory, the posterior parietal peritoneum is lifted off the un-

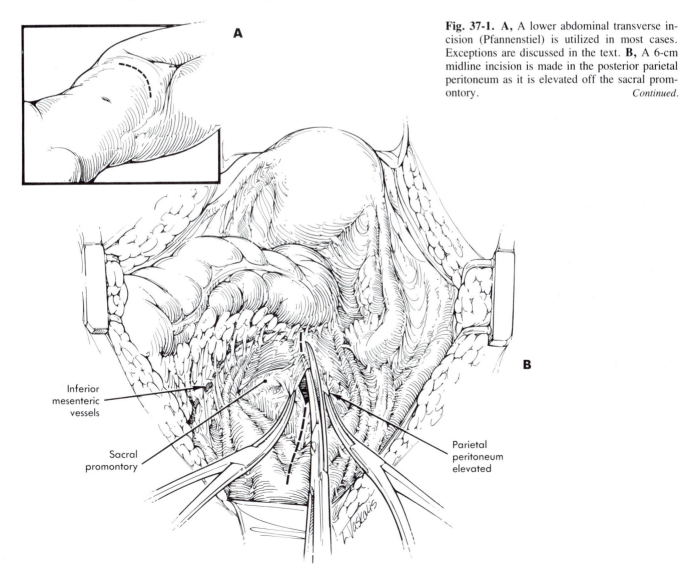

Fig. 37-1. A, A lower abdominal transverse incision (Pfannenstiel) is utilized in most cases. Exceptions are discussed in the text. **B,** A 6-cm midline incision is made in the posterior parietal peritoneum as it is elevated off the sacral promontory. *Continued.*

Inferior mesenteric vessels

Sacral promontory

Parietal peritoneum elevated

derlying tissue by the use of two long curved clamps, each placed just lateral to the midline. The promontory should be palpated as well as visualized before placement of these clamps so the location of the great vessels and their immediate branches can be better appreciated. In addition, the presence in the midline of other structures ordinarily in a more lateral position, such as the ureter, can be ruled out. An incision in the posterior parietal peritoneum is made in the midline between the two long clamps. This allows exposure of loose areolar tissue containing nerve fibers, as access to the retroperitoneal space is obtained. The incision is carried upward and downward to approximately 6 cm in length (Fig. 37-1, *B*) as the peritoneum is incised free of the underlying tissues. Stay sutures are placed on

each edge of the peritoneum to allow anterior traction, which provides exposure of the tissues overlying the sacral promontory.

After placement of these sutures, it is recommended that palpation of the promontory again be carried out, because the surgeon's perception of the location of the promontory might be slightly distorted by traction on the stay sutures.

Blunt dissection with fine pointed long clamps, right-angle clamps, or cotton pledgets at the right edge of the posterior peritoneal incision mobilizes the loose areolar tissue containing nerve fibers; this dissection is directed posterolaterally toward the promontory and proceeds immediately medial to the right ureter (Fig. 37-1, *C*). Occasion-

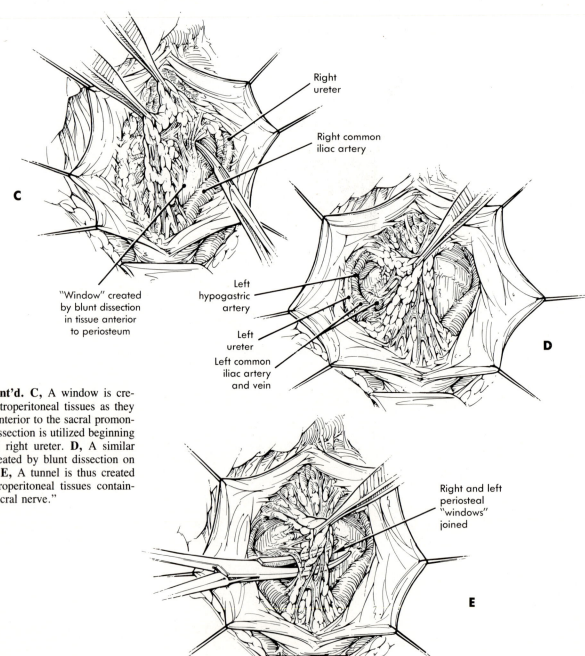

Right ureter

Right common iliac artery

"Window" created by blunt dissection in tissue anterior to periosteum

Left hypogastric artery

Left ureter

Left common iliac artery and vein

D

C

Right and left periosteal "windows" joined

E

Fig. 37-1, cont'd. C, A window is created in the retroperitoneal tissues as they are elevated anterior to the sacral promontory. Blunt dissection is utilized beginning medial to the right ureter. **D,** A similar window is created by blunt dissection on the left side. **E,** A tunnel is thus created under the retroperitoneal tissues containing the "presacral nerve."

ally, it is beneficial to initiate this blunt dissection sharply to liberate a few of the more tenacious fibers. Before this dissection, the right ureter should be clearly identified to avoid inclusion in the bundle of tissue being dissected off the posterior peritoneum. As the tissues are separated, they may be grasped in the midline to provide countertraction, so that dissection is simplified proceeding toward the promontory. When the periosteum comes into view, a small window is created to expose the white glistening tissue. At this point, dissection is initiated at the peritoneal edge of the left side and is carried down in a similar manner, medial to the base of the sigmoid mesocolon with its

contained inferior mesenteric artery and vein (Fig. 37-1, *D*). These structures constitute the left lateralmost extension of dissection in a majority of cases. It is ill-advised to dissect posterior to these structures. When the periosteum is reached, a similar small window is created by blunt dissection and is connected with the window previously formed on the right side (Fig. 37-1, *E*). Two long clamps may be placed across the bundle of nerve tissue that is resected and ligated (Fig. 37-1, *F*). Approximately 4 cm of this tissue are submitted for pathologic examination.

The severed ends of the nerve bundle are ligated with 0 silk suture, placed by suture carrier or "banjo" (Fig. 37-1,

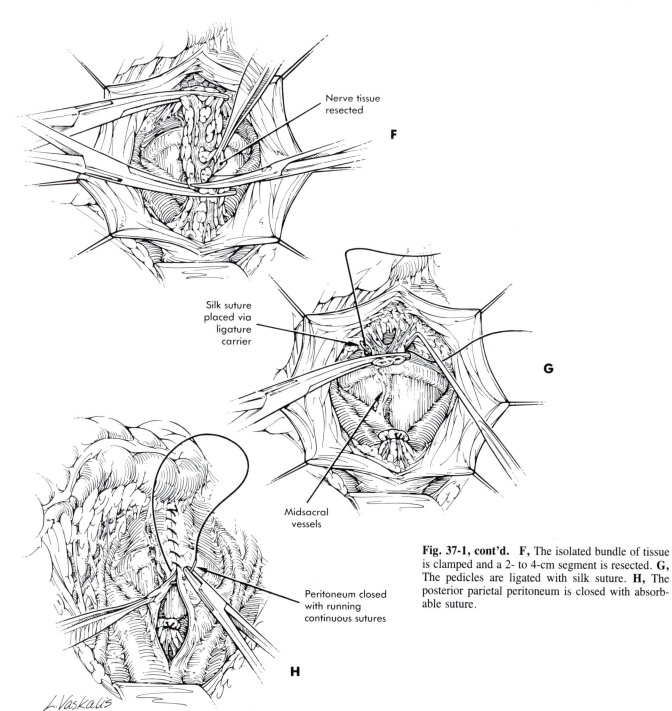

Nerve tissue resected

F

Silk suture placed via ligature carrier

G

Midsacral vessels

Peritoneum closed with running continuous sutures

H

L. Vaskalis

Fig. 37-1, cont'd. **F,** The isolated bundle of tissue is clamped and a 2- to 4-cm segment is resected. **G,** The pedicles are ligated with silk suture. **H,** The posterior parietal peritoneum is closed with absorbable suture.

G). Silk is chosen because its tensile strength is great and traction prevents slippage of the knot. There is no concern with peritoneal adhesion formation secondary to inflammatory reaction to silk, because the ligatures are present in the retroperitoneal space.

The superior hypogastric plexus at this level exists in more than one layer in approximately 80% of patients. After initial resection of the nerve tissue, the region of the promontory should be carefully examined. Clean, glistening periosteum indicates that complete resection has been accomplished. Any residual nerve tissue should be removed; loose areolar tissue without nerve present need not be resected.

The middle sacral artery and vein ordinarily overlie the promontory in the midline. These vessels may be ligated and divided if they are mobilized off the periosteum with the nerve tissue. If they are not included with the resected nerve, they may be left intact. If either vessel is disrupted, ligation is best accomplished with 3-0 suture anchored to the periosteum. Vascular clips may also be used for hemostasis.

The anatomy of the middle sacral vessels is quite variable, so careful identification before ligation is important.

Severe hemorrhage complicating this operation is unlikely if dissection is confined to the region immediately anterior to the promontory. The technique presented here minimizes the possibility of major intraoperative hemorrhage and postoperative bowel and bladder dysfunction, which might occur with more extensive dissection advocated by some surgeons.* Thus, dissection above the bifurcation of the aorta or into the hollow of the sacrum, where the rich venous plexus exists, is not necessary.[29] Dissection should not be carried out posterior to the aorta, vena cava, or the common iliac arteries or veins, because heavy bleeding will occur if a small vessel is avulsed from a great vessel or if direct injury occurs to a great vessel. Similarly, dissection should not extend into the sigmoid mesocolon, because injury to the inferior mesenteric artery or vein or a retroperitoneal hematoma might occur.

The retroperitoneal anatomy in this region is not constant. Large vessels ordinarily present in the lateral pelvis may course toward the midline. It is imperative to identify the origin and termination of such vessels before dissection. Occasionally, the ureter may course toward the midline rather than follow its usual lateral course. Thus, it is also important to note the position of the ureters before dissection.

After resection and ligation of the superior hypogastric plexus, it must be determined that hemostasis is adequate. Small bleeders may be cauterized using the needle-tip unipolar probe with extender or the bipolar instrument. Hemoclips or sutures, anchored to the periosteum if necessary, are indicated when heavier bleeding is present.

The posterior parietal peritoneum is then closed using 3-0 or 4-0 delayed absorbable suture (Fig. 37-1, *H*).

---

*References 5, 12, 18, 26, 28, 30.

COMPLICATIONS AND EFFECTS OF PRESACRAL NEURECTOMY

Complications of this operation are uncommon when performed by experienced surgeons.[17]

Because resected nerve tissue is in the midline, medial to the right ureter and sigmoid mesocolon, and because the autonomic nerves serving the bowel and bladder course lateral to the operative site, significant dysfunction in these viscera is rare. Corroboration of this site as effective for denervation to accomplish relief of deep, central pelvic pain has been demonstrated by an injection technique.[23] This new method is efficacious in relief of malignancy-related central pelvic pain. Other techniques of presacral neurectomy involve more extensive retroperitoneal dissection*; intraoperative complications and postoperative constipation or bladder dysfunction are more likely. I have found this operation to be quite harmless in its effect on function of the bowel and bladder. Other surgeons have reported similar results.[9,14,29] The only effect on menstruation I have observed has been a decrease in dysmenorrhea. Occasional hypermenorrhea has been limited to the first or second postoperative menses. There are no changes in sexual function except reduction in deep dyspareunia. There is usually partial reduction in discomfort in the first stage of labor.

LAPAROSCOPIC PRESACRAL NEURECTOMY

Presacral neurectomy has been performed by laparoscopy. There is insufficient published information to allow adequate appraisal of benefits, risks, results, and complications of this method.[22]

As with any operative procedure, knowledge of anatomy and the skill and experience of the surgeon are of paramount importance. The application of operative laparoscopic techniques in the retroperitoneal space, as in presacral neurectomy, should be undertaken only with great caution and after extensive practice in vitro and hands-on training with an experienced surgeon.

OTHER OPERATIONS FOR CENTRAL PELVIC PAIN
Uterosacral uterine denervation

Doyle[10] advocated transection of the uterosacral ligaments at their junction with the uterus at culdotomy or laparotomy to relieve pelvic pain. Because the afferent pain fibers from the uterus are present in and adjacent to these ligaments, some pain relief results. Limitations of the culdotomy approach include: (1) limited ability to detect extent of pelvic pathologic processes, and (2) difficulty in resection of significantly distorted ligaments. Modern indications for proximal uterosacral resection include: (1) presence of endometriosis or other lesions in and around the ligament, and (2) a contraindication to presacral neurectomy.

When uterosacral resection is carried out, reapproxima-

---

*References 5, 12, 18, 26, 28, 30.

tion of the distal segment to the posterior uterus should be accomplished, if possible.

Laparoscopic uterine denervation

Laparoscopic uterosacral ligament interruption by laser vaporization, electrosurgery, or transection is directed at relief of central pelvic pain. There is little documentation of indications, contraindications, results, and complications of this procedure. The available studies are largely uncontrolled,[6,7] involve small numbers of patients,[16,19] and have very brief duration of follow-up.[6,7,16] In addition, there is a high incidence of recurrence of pain.[19] Technique includes laser destruction to the depth of 3 to 4 mm[6] and 4 to 6 mm[7]; in most cases, such superficial incisions are unlikely to result in denervation. Until properly conducted clinical trials document efficacy and safety, this must be considered an experimental operation.

Another theoretical concern has been the potential loss of posterior-lateral support if the uterosacral ligament is transected and the distal end is not reattached to the uterus, as is customary at laparotomy. Because the depth of destruction reported to date is so superficial, it is unlikely that major loss of uterine support occurs. Nevertheless, the answer to this question awaits appropriate study. Anecdotally, some surgeons advocate round ligament uterine suspension by way of laparoscopy if uterosacral denervation is attempted. It seems unlikely this would provide significant long-term uterine support. If the round ligament suspension of a retroverted retroflexed uterus does not result in distortion of fallopian tube anatomy and can be accomplished in a atraumatic fashion, I see no contraindication. Patients with pelvic pain should be approached in the same manner whether the planned procedure(s) are accomplished at laparotomy or operative laparoscopy.

Ovarian denervation

Division of the infundibulopelvic ligaments, including blood vessels, or attempted division of nerves after isolation from blood vessels, has been recommended for control of pain thought to be of ovarian origin.[29,30] Neither of these techniques should be applied to the control of pelvic pain. Compromise of the ovarian blood supply is inevitable, and the relief of pain has not been substantiated.

REFERENCES

1. Behrman SJ: The surgical management of endometriosis: recent advances in endometriosis, *Excerpta Medica*, p. 62, 1976 (abstract).
2. Black WT: Use of presacral sympathectomy in the treatment of dysmenorrhea, *Am J Obstet Gynecol* 89:16, 1964.
3. Bonica JJ: *The management of pain*, Philadelphia, 1953, Lea & Febiger.
4. Browne OD: Survey of 113 cases of primary dysmenorrhea treated by neurectomy, *Am J Obstet Gynecol* 57:1053, 1949.
5. Campbell RM: The anatomy and histology of the sacrouterine ligaments, *Am J Obstet Gynecol* 59:1, 1950.
6. Corson SL et al: Treatment of endometriosis with Nd:YAG tissue contact laser probe via laparoscopy, *Int J Fertil* 34:284, 1989.
7. Corson SL et al: Laparoscopic laser treatment of endometriosis with the Nd:YAG sapphire probe, *Am J Obstet Gynecol* 160:718, 1989.
8. Cotte G: La sympathectomie hypogastrique a-t-ella sa place dana la therapeutique gynecologique? *Presse Med* 33:98, 1925.
9. Counseller VS, Winchell McKS: The treatment of dysmenorrhea by resection of the presacral sympathetic nerves: evaluation and end results, *Am J Obstet Gynecol* 28:61, 1934.
9a. Culp OS, DeWeerd JH: Advantages of the Cherney incision for urologic operations, *J Urol* 69:445, 1953.
10. Doyle JB: Paracervical uterine denervation by transection of the cervical plexus for the relief of dysmenorrhea, *Am J Obstet Gynecol* 70:1, 1955.
11. Garcia CR, David SS: Pelvic endometriosis: infertility and pelvic pain, *Am J Obstet Gynecol* 129:740, 1977.
12. Ingersoll F, Meigs JV: Presacral neurectomy for dysmenorrhea, *N Engl J Med* 238:357, 1948.
13. Jaboulay M: Le traitment de la nevralgie pelviene par la paralysie due sympathique sacre, *Lyon Med* 90:102, 1899.
14. Keene FE: The treatment of dysmenorrhea by presacral neurectomy, *Am J Obstet Gynecol* 30:534, 1935.
15. Kistner RW: *Nerve supply of the uterine corpus.* In *Gynecology: principals and practice,* ed 3, Chicago, 1979, Mosby–Year Book.
16. Kojima E et al: Nd:YAG laser laparoscopy for ovarian endometriomas, *J Reprod Med* 35:625, 1990.
17. Lee RB et al: Presacral neurectomy for chronic pelvic pain, *Obstet Gynecol* 68:517, 1986.
18. Leriche R: *Presse Med* 1:465, 1925.
19. Lichten EM, Bombard J: Surgical treatment of primary dysmenorrhea with laparoscopic uterine nerve ablation, *J Reprod Med* 32:37, 1987.
20. Mahfoud HK, Hewitt SR: A place for presacral neurectomy, *Ir Med J* 74:198, 1981.
21. Malinak LR: Management of endometriosis in the infertile female. In Givens JR, editor: *The infertile female,* Chicago, 1979, Mosby–Year Book.
22. Perez JJ: Laparoscopic presacral neurectomy: results of the first 25 cases, *J Reprod Med* 35:625, 1990.
23. Plancarte R et al: Superior hypogastric plexus block for pelvic cancer pain, *Anesthesiology* 73:236, 1990.
24. Polan ML, DeCherney A: Presacral neurectomy for pelvic pain in infertility, *Fertil Steril* 34:557, 1980.
25. Ruggi G: *La Simpathectomia abdominale utero-ovarica come mezzo di cura di alcune lesioni interne degli organi genitali della donna.* Bologna, Zanichelli, 1899
26. TeLinde RW: *Operative Gynecology,* ed 2, Philadelphia, 1953, JB Lippincott.
27. Tjaden B et al: The efficacy of presacral neurectomy for the relief of dysmenorrhea. *Obstet Gynecol* 76:89, 1990
28. Vara P: *Acta Obstet Gynecol Scand (suppl 5)* 30:1, 1950
29. Wharton LR: Presacral neurectomy. In Mattingly RF, editor: *Telinde's Operative Gynecology,* ed 5, Philadelphia, 1977, JB Lippincott.
30. White JC: Conduction of visceral pain. *N Engl J Med* 246:686, 1952
31. Woodruff JD, Pauerstein CJ: *Neuroanatomy of the fallopian tube.* In *The fallopian tube.* Baltimore, 1969, Williams & Wilkins.

Chapter 38

PELVIC INFECTION

Sebastian Faro

Pelvic infections that occur in the absence of an operative procedure can be divided anatomically into those of the lower and upper genital tract. Lower genital tract infections can be subdivided into those involving the vulva, the vestibule, and the vagina. Infections of the vulva are usually due to bacteria that inhabit the skin and cause diseases such as furunculosis, carbunculosis, pyodermatitis, erysipelas, and impetigo. These infections tend to be unimicrobial and are most frequently treated with topical or systemic antibiotics, depending upon the seriousness of the infection. Occasionally these infections will form abscesses, requiring incision and drainage. In contrast, hidradenitis suppurativa is a complex infection that may be polymicrobial and often does not respond to antimicrobial treatment.

Infections of the upper genital tract (i.e., the uterus and fallopian tubes) are usually more serious and often require the patient be hospitalized. These infections are treated with systemic antibiotics administered orally or parenterally. These infections can lead to infertility and damaged fallopian tubes, resulting in ectopic pregnancy, or abscess formation (e.g., pyosalpinx or tuboovarian abscess). Patients who develop abscesses often require surgical intervention to achieve a cure.

VAGINAL MICROFLORA

The bacterial microflora of the lower genital tract resembles the fecal flora except that the vagina is not as densely populated and usually does not contain abscessogenic bacteria (e.g., *Bacteroides fragilis* and the *B. fragilis* group). The endogenous vaginal bacterial population consists of gram-positive and gram-negative aerobic, facultative, and obligate anaerobes. In the healthy state the microflora of the vagina is dominated by the presence of commensal bacteria, which suppress the growth of the potentially pathogenic bacteria. There is a delicate balance between these two populations of bacteria (commensal versus pathogenic), which in turn must interact with environmental factors originating from the host and the exogenous environment. This dynamic but delicate equilibrium is tightly linked to the metabolic and hormonal activities of the host.[21,37] One crucial factor is the hydrogen ion concentration, which is dependent upon the metabolic activity of the bacterial community and the host. The normal hydrogen ion concentration of the vagina is between 3.8 and 4.2. The predominant bacteria at this hydrogen ion concentration are the commensals on the following list, *Lactobacillus* being the dominant genus.

Lactobacillus species
Diptheroids
Bacillus species
Nonhemolytic streptococci

Lactobacillus acidophilus is the dominant bacterium in the healthy vagina and is thought to suppress the growth of other bacteria, especially the pathogenic organisms, by production of lactic acid and hydrogen peroxide. The production of lactic acid aids in maintaining the pH between 3.8 and 4.2, which is unfavorable to the growth of many gram-positive and gram-negative bacteria. Hydrogen peroxide is toxic to the anaerobic bacteria.[13,23,24]

Many environmental factors, both exogenous and endogenous, can disturb the delicate equilibrium that exists in the healthy vagina. Once the pH is altered and the hydrogen ion concentration decreases, the pH rises, becoming more alkaline. A pH greater than 4.5 is more favorable to the growth of noncommensal, or pathogenic, endogenous bacteria. These coinhabitants of the healthy vagina are usually present in concentrations of less than 1,000 organisms per milliliter of vaginal fluid, but with a decrease in the acidity of the vagina they begin to reproduce more vigorously, and their numbers soon exceed 10,000 to

---

Endogenous microflora of the lower genital tract

Gram-positive	*Gram-negative*
Streptococcus agalactiae	*Escherichia coli*
Staphylococcus aureus	*Enterobacter agglomerans*
Staphylococcus epidermidis	*Enterobacter aerogenes*
Enterococcus faecalis	*Enterobacter cloacae*
	Klebsiella pneumoniae
Anaerobes	*Proteus mirabilis*
	Proteus vulgatus
Peptostreptococcus	
Bacteroides	
Fusobacterium	

100,000 organisms per milliliter of vaginal fluid. Eventually these potentially pathogenic bacteria dominate and essentially become the microflora of the vagina (box above).

Numerous studies have attempted to define the vaginal flora in healthy and unhealthy states. There is no doubt that the hydrogen ion concentration is a key factor in maintaining the vaginal ecosystem in a state of equilibrium that allows the commensal bacteria to dominate. The hydrogen ion concentration can influence the growth of all the various members of the endogenous microflora. There appear to be at least three distinct conditions that may exist with regard to the bacteriology of the vagina when the equilibrium is disrupted: (1) bacterial vaginitis, typified by the growth of various bacteria such as *Enterococcus faecalis, Streptococcus agalactiae,* and *Escherichia coli*[11]; (2) *Gardnerella vaginalis* vaginitis, characterized microscopically by the presence of clue cells (i.e., epithelial cells with adherent gram-negative rods that obscure the cytoplasmic membrane), aggregates or clumps of floating bacteria in the vaginal discharge, and the noticeable absence of white blood cells[12]; and (3) bacterial vaginosis, defined as an overgrowth of anaerobic bacteria and a decrease in the numbers of lactobacilli,[3] characterized microscopically by numerous individual free-floating bacteria, a noticeable absence of white blood cells, and the presence of clue cells.

Patients with abnormal vaginal bacterial flora typically have an altered hydrogen ion concentration (pH > 4.5). Bacterial vaginitis is not usually characterized by the presence of a large number of anaerobes, which typically produce amines that give the vaginal fluid a fishy odor, and therefore the KOH or amine test is negative. Microscopically, clue cells are not present, as is commonplace in the vaginal discharge of patients with *Gardnerella vaginalis* vaginitis and bacterial vaginosis, and the flora is dominated by an aerobic or facultative anaerobic bacteria. These patients usually complain of an increased amount of vaginal discharge, which may be dirty gray, greenish, or yellow in color and have a foul odor, and may state they have vaginal discomfort.[11] Individuals with *Gardnerella vaginalis* vaginitis complain of a homogenous liquid discharge, often foul-smelling, and may have a burning sen-

sation. The pH is usually > 4.5, and the KOH test is positive. Microscopic examination reveals the presence of clue cells and clumps of free-floating bacteria in the vaginal discharge. Typically the microflora is dominated by large numbers of *Gardnerella vaginalis* and the number of other bacteria is much smaller (e.g., > 100,000 versus 1000).[6] Bacterial vaginosis, in contrast to *Gardnerella vaginitis,* is characterized by an overgrowth of anaerobic bacteria, a decrease in lactobacilli, and *Gardnerella vaginalis* may or may not be present. The discharge is homogenous, dirty gray, runny, and usually gives off an amine odor when mixed with concentrated potassium hydroxide (KOH test). Microscopically there are large numbers of bacteria, which are free-floating and contain both gram-positive and gram-negative bacteria. Typically white blood cells are not present to any large degree in the vaginal discharge of patients with bacterial vaginosis, hence the suffix *-osis* to signify the absence of an inflammatory reaction.[16,17,34,44]

The endogenous bacterial vaginal flora apparently plays a role in infections of the female genital tract and is considered to be involved in vaginitis, cervicitis, endometritis, salpingitis, postpartum endometritis, and perhaps even pelvic abscesses, which may all be considered as stages in pelvic inflammatory disease. This is an important complex of infections since the end result may place the patient at risk for ectopic pregnancy, infertility, or perhaps castration.

LOWER GENITAL TRACT INFECTIONS
Hidradenitis suppurativa

This disease originates in the apocrine sweat glands and is initiated by closure of the duct or pore, which prevents egress of the gland contents. The gland also becomes colonized with bacteria that inhabit the skin and perhaps bacteria that are derived from the normal vaginal flora. The skin overlying the groin and labia is exposed to the vaginal discharge, which contains numerous gram-positive and gram-negative bacteria, both aerobic and anaerobic. Therefore hidradenitis of the vulva and groin has the potential to be a complex polymicrobial infection.[25,28,29] It is probable that closure of the duct or pore is initiated by bacteria colonizing the gland, inducing an inflammatory reaction in the cells lining and surrounding the duct. This results in swelling and closure of the duct. The gland becomes distended as it fills with mucus and bacteria, thus forming an abscess. Eventually the abscessed gland may rupture at the skin surface, resulting in the drainage of a foul-smelling purulent material that is characteristic of hidradenitis suppurativa. The abscessed gland may also rupture below the skin surface, infecting the surrounding tissue. Fistulae may form to other apocrine glands, which eventually become infected, thus resulting in a chronic infection as these glands abscess and rupture leading to infection of other apocrine glands. Typically, as the apocrine gland infection progresses to an abscess, nodules form on the skin surface. The area surrounding the infected gland becomes erythematous, swollen, and tender. The nodules suppurate and drain a thick, purulent, foul-smelling exudate. The recurrent formation of inflamed nodules that suppurate is a characteristic feature of this infection. Following rupture of an abscessed apocrine gland, fibrosis and hypertrophic scarring occur in the tissue overlying skin.

Hidradenitis suppurativa characteristically occurs in the axilla, groin, external genitalia, and perianal area. The recurrences or exacerbations typically occur at the time of menses, which coincides with an increase in gland activity. There is no antibiotic treatment currently available that will effectively cure this infection. Although antibiotic studies have not been conducted because it is difficult to obtain a significant number of patients, antibiotic regimens providing activity against anaerobes and facultative anaerobes appear to be most effective. The regimen should possess activity against bacteria such as *Propionibacterium, Peptostreptococcus, Staphylococcus,* and *Escherichia coli.* Two factors may be responsible for the inability to treat this infection successfully with antibiotics: (1) a lack in understanding the microbiological makeup, and (2) an inability to achieve adequate levels of the antibiotics in the inflamed and infected tissue. It may be that the fibrosis that accompanies the infection results in a decrease in vascular supply to the area, thereby preventing adequate tissue levels of antibiotic.

When antibiotic therapy fails, surgery is the only recourse. There are basically two operative approaches. One is to excise the infected tissue, including a margin of noninfected tissue and the underlying subcutaneous tissue but not the fascia. The incision can be closed primarily or allowed to heal by secondary intention. An alternative approach is to perform a skinning procedure and skin graft. The skinning procedure is preferred if large areas are involved, which if excised, would create large defects and leave behind unsightly scars. Whichever procedure is performed, it is extremely important that all infected tissue be removed. If infected tissue remains, the process will begin again within a period of less than 12 months.

Vulvovaginitis

Other microorganisms, such as viruses, play an important role in causing infections of the lower genital tract (e.g., molluscum contagiosum, condyloma acuminata, and herpes).[1,4,7] *Candida* is the most common fungus to cause lower genital tract infection and usually involves both the external genitalia and the vagina.[22] Vaginitis is probably the most common disease of the lower genital tract and is due to fungi, bacteria, viruses, parasites, and protozoans. These infections rarely lead to upper genital tract infections; however, they can often be responsible for chronic infections. Patients who have recurrent vaginal candidiasis should be examined for the presence of yeast in the oral cavity. If they complain of any symptoms that reflect possible infection of the gastrointestinal tract, this should be thoroughly investigated. Consideration should be given to screening the patient for HIV antibody, since esophageal candidiasis is often an indication of HIV infection.

Epidemiology

It is estimated that patients make approximately 1,000,000 outpatient visits to gynecologists per year for complaints of vaginitis. This indicates the immense amount of money that is spent on office visits and treatment regimens. The end result in some cases is that the physician is unable to correct the individual's problem and she is told that her condition is psychosomatic. Thus patients with recalcitrant vaginitis, be it yeast or bacterial, often avoid sexual activity or alter their sexual activity because of embarrassment. Thus this condition may be both a health and a social problem.

Attempts have been made to link bacterial vaginitis or vaginosis with more severe infections such as premature rupture of amniotic membranes, premature labor, postpartum endomyometritis, pelvic inflammatory disease, and postoperative pelvic cellulitis. The connection between bacterial vaginosis and upper genital tract infection is tenuous at best and is founded on the hypothesis that most of these infections are polymicrobial. The bacterial isolates from such sites as amniotic fluid, the endometrium, and the vaginal cuff in patients with pelvic cellulitis resemble the bacteriology of the lower genital tract. However, it must be emphasized that the bacterial isolates are often obtained not from the site of actual infection but from an area in close proximity, so this conclusion is based on an extrapolation from the available data.

UPPER GENITAL TRACT INFECTIONS

Upper genital tract infections include cervicitis, endometritis, salpingitis, and tuboovarian abscess. Other common infections that may occur in the pelvis, although not related to the female organs, are appendicitis and diverticulitis. Both of these infections are important because they are frequently confused with pelvic inflammatory disease and may cause damage to the fallopian tubes. Subsequently the patient may be infertile or, if pregnancy can be achieved, it may be located ectopically. The infections of the upper genital tract tend to be more serious and may give rise to systemic infection resulting in bacteremia, sepsis, and septic shock.

Therefore crucial to the successful treatment of any pelvic infection is an understanding of the microorganisms that are responsible for the disease. Female pelvic infections in general are derived from bacteria either introduced from the environment (most common are the sexually transmitted bacteria) or derived from the endogenous vaginal microflora. There has been great interest in the role of the endogenous microflora in upper genital tract infections. Although the specific role of the endogenous microflora in the production or development of upper genital tract infection has not been delineated, an association appears to exist between their presence in the lower genital tract and in upper genital tract infection.

PELVIC INFLAMMATORY DISEASE
Epidemiology

Pelvic inflammatory disease (PID) is predominant among sexually promiscuous women between the ages of 15 and 44 years old, with the peak incidence occurring in women between 18 and 25 years of age.[39,40] It is estimated that acute pelvic inflammatory disease may occur in 1% of sexually active women, and approximately 1.5% to 2% of the patients are sexually active teenagers between 15 and 19 years of age.

The relevance of these numbers of patients is manifested in the cost of treating pelvic inflammatory disease and its sequelae. It is estimated that 1,000,000 patient visits per year can be attributed to pelvic inflammatory disease. These generate between 200,000 and 300,000 hospitalizations per year, which in turn result in 110,000 operative procedures yearly. Several investigators have attempted to project the economic impact of this disease based on best estimates of the incidence of hospitalization and ambulatory patient visits to physicians. In the United States the estimated cost of treating pelvic inflammatory disease and its sequelae ranges from $300 million to $3 billion a year.[30,32,39] The sequelae may be not only physically traumatic but psychologically devastating as well. Approximately 25% of women who have had pelvic inflammatory disease will be left with chronic pelvic pain, infertility, or at risk for ectopic pregnancy.[14,38,42]

Individuals at risk for contracting pelvic inflammatory disease are primarily those with multiple sex partners or with a partner who has multiple sex partners. Patients exposed to gonorrhea are at risk for developing upper genital tract infection. Approximately 20% of women who contract cervical gonococcal infection, if left untreated or treated inappropriately, will develop pelvic inflammatory disease (i.e., endometritis or salpingitis).[33,42] Several factors have been found to be associated with the development of pelvic inflammatory disease:

1. Unmarried and sexually active
2. Sexually promiscuous
3. History of exposure to a sexually transmitted disease
4. Presence of an intrauterine device
5. Use of oral contraceptives
6. Adolescent

The patient who is known to have more than one sexual contact, directly or indirectly, regardless of age, should be evaluated for the presence of a sexually transmitted disease. If a sexually transmitted organism is found (e.g., *Trichomonas vaginalis, Herpes simplex, Neisseria gonorrhoeae, Chlamydia trachomatis,* human papilloma virus), specimens should be obtained for the detection of other sexually transmitted organisms.

Microbiology

The microbiologic makeup of pelvic inflammatory disease has not been completely elucidated. There is controversy over which organism—*Neisseria gonorrhoeae* or *Chlamydia trachomatis*—is most frequently responsible for pelvic inflammatory disease. The microbial causes of pelvic inflammatory disease are as follows:

1. *Neisseria gonorrhoeae*
2. *Chlamydia trachomatis*
3. Polymicrobial, nongonococcal, and nonchlamydial bacteria, ascending from lower genital tract
4. Iatrogenic placement of bacteria during diagnostic or therapeutic procedure

N. gonorrhoeae continues to be a leading isolate from patients diagnosed as having acute pelvic inflammatory disease. In studies conducted on the Baylor gynecologic service at the Ben Taub Hospital, which renders care for an indigent population, *N. gonorrhoeae* was recovered from 50% to 60% of the patients and *C. trachomatis* from 16% to 20% of the patients with acute pelvic inflammatory disease.[9,11,19] This is consistent with other isolation rates reported by other investigators[8,18,36,41] (e.g., 10% to 81% for *N. gonorrhoeae* and 5% to 20% for *C. trachomatis*). Sweet et al[36] reported a recovery rate of 48% for *N. gonorrhoeae* and 23% for *C. trachomatis* from patients with pelvic inflammatory disease. Sweet et al, in studying chlamydial and gonococcal colonization rates during the menstrual cycle, recovered *N. gonorrhoeae* from 40% of the patients and *Chlamydia* from 27%. Judson and Tavelli[18] reported in 1986 that *N. gonorrhoeae* was recovered from 27% of patients attending a sexually transmitted disease clinic, while 18% harbored *C. trachomatis,* and 16% had both organisms. Neither organism was found in 39% of the patients with symptoms suggestive of acute pelvic inflammatory disease. However, the experience in Sweden has been different. *C. trachomatis* has been isolated from 40% to 50% of the patients, and *N. gonorrhoeae* has been recovered from 10% to 15% of individuals with a diagnosis of pelvic inflammatory disease.[15,20,26,27] Kristensen et al reported a 13% isolation rate for *N. gonorrhoeae* and 24% for *C. trachomatis.*[25,35]

Although the U.S. data differs from the Scandinavian, empiric management of patients with acute salpingitis should include treatment for both organisms until definitive microbiologic data becomes available. Coinfections with *N. gonorrhoeae* and *C. trachomatis* have been reported to occur in 25% to 60% of women with gonorrhea who also have *Chlamydia.*[42,43]

Diagnosis

The initial infection begins with cervicitis, and all too often this goes unnoticed. Signs of cervicitis are as follows:

1. Endocervical purulent discharge
2. Cervical bleeding with minor trauma
3. Cervical pain with intercourse

It is uncommon for the patient to recognize that a cervical infection is present since it is usually asymptomatic. This is the major contributing factor to delay in establishing a diagnosis. However, the patient may relate that she has spotting after or pain during sexual intercourse. Frequently the physician will note the presence of endocervical pus when obtaining a Pap smear or, perhaps more commonly, note that the cervix bleeds easily while obtaining endocervical cells for a Pap smear with a cotton-tipped applicator. The physician may also note that the endocervical epithelium is hypertrophic. Any of these observations during the pelvic examination should lead the physician to ask questions relating to frequency of sexual intercourse, number of sexual partners, and if the patient has only one partner, whether she knows or suspects that other individuals may be involved with her partner and whether her consort has any symptoms that might suggest a genital tract infection. The patient's endocervix should be cultured for *N. gonorrhoeae,* and *C. trachomatis.* The urethra should be cultured for *Ureaplasma* and *Mycoplasma.* The vaginal discharge should be examined for the presence of *Trichomonas vaginalis.*

If gram reagents are readily available, then a gram stain of the endocervical specimen should be performed. If gram-negative intracellular diplococci are found, this can be taken as presumptive evidence for the presence of *N. gonorrhoeae.* If no bacteria are seen, rare squamous epithelial cells, but white blood cells are present and no detectable pathogen is found, then it is fair to suspect the presence of *C. trachomatis.* The patient should be treated with doxycycline (100 mg twice daily for 7 days) or other suitable antibiotic (Table 38-1).

The patient may progress from cervicitis to endometritis without developing symptoms that are easily recognized or considered to be significant. The most common symptoms of nongonococcal or chlamydial endometritis are vague lower abdominal pain, breakthrough vaginal bleeding if the individual is on the birth control pill, or intramenstrual spotting if not taking oral contraceptive pills. Patients who have an intrauterine device in place are at risk for developing or rapidly progressing to salpingitis if they develop cervicitis or endometritis. Patients with endometritis are best managed by obtaining an endometrial biopsy and culturing the specimen for *N. gonorrhoeae, C. trachomatis, Mycoplasma, Ureaplasma,* and aerobic and anaerobic bacteria. If an intrauterine device is present, it should be removed since it will serve as a nidus for infection. In addition, if the device becomes colonized, it will be difficult to rid it of bacteria with antibiotics administered systemically. The patient should be started on doxycycline—100

mg, administered orally twice a day for 7 days (box below). If the infection is thought or found to be due to aerobic and anaerobic bacteria then amoxicillin/clavulanic acid (Augmentin) or a combination of clindamycin plus a quinolone such as ciprofloxacin or ofloxacin (this agent will soon be available) should be used. The advantage of such a combination is that clindamycin provides activity against *Streptococcus agalactiae, Staphylococcus aureus,* anaerobes, and *C. trachomatis,* while the quinolone provides coverage against the Enterobacteriaceae, as well as *C. trachomatis.* The patient should be asked to return for the initial follow-up examination within 72 hours to determine if there is a response to the medication. If there is no evidence of improvement, then consideration must be given to the use of parenteral antibiotics, or perhaps the initial diagnosis was incorrect. If *N. gonorrhoeae* is isolated, it must be assayed for the production of penicillinase, especially if a penicillinlike agent is used. In addition, it is important epidemiologically to track the incidence of penicillinase-producing *N. gonorrhoeae* occurring within a community.

Patients hospitalized for the treatment of PID should receive intravenously administered antibiotics until all signs and symptoms of infection have resolved (box below). Therapy should be completed with doxycycline. The patient should be reevaluated within 7 to 10 days after being discharged from the hospital. Individuals who were positive for *N. gonorrhoeae* should be recultured on the day of discharge and within 7 to 10 days after release from the hospital. Patients who were positive for *C. trachomatis* should be recultured within 2 to 3 weeks of discharge from the hospital.

Critical to the management of pelvic inflammatory disease are early institution of antibiotic therapy, early surgical intervention if warranted, and early follow-up after the patient has been discharged from the hospital. The emphasis on early treatment is to prevent damage of the fallopian tubes, which if it occurs can result in ectopic pregnancy, infertility, pyosalpinx, hydrosalpinx, and tuboovarian ab-

Table 38-1. Antibiotics suitable for the treatment of *Chlamydia trachomatis* infection

Agent	Dosage
Doxycycline	100 mg, bid × 7 days
Erythromycin	500 mg, qid × 7 days
Clindamycin	150 to 300 mg, tid × 7 days

Antibiotic regimens for the treatment of pelvic inflammatory disease

Ambulatory

Ceftriaxone, 250 mg intramuscularly, and Doxycycline, 100 mg orally, twice daily for 7 days

Hospitalized Patients

Cefotetan, 2 g q 12 hr, or Ceftizoxime, 1 g q 8 hr, or Cefoxitin, 2 g q 8 hr, given intravenously, plus Doxycycline, 100 mg orally, twice daily for 7 days

Clindamycin, 900 mg q 8 hr, plus Gentamicin, 80 to 120 mg loading dose followed by 80 mg for the initial dose and subsequent doses based on serum peak and trough determination

scess. The tragedy of this disease is that it is primarily an infection of young women in the reproductive age group. Prevention of salpingitis is dependent upon recognition of the early signs of pelvic inflammatory disease.

Further, identification of the patient with cervicitis or endometritis represents the initial opportunity to prevent salpingitis in an individual who is at risk for upper genital tract infection. Once salpingitis has occurred, there is a risk that the patient will experience the sequelae of this tragic infection. It has been estimated that an individual who experiences a single episode of salpingitis has a 13% chance of being infertile, while if a second episode of salpingitis occurs the risk is approximately 33%, and if three episodes have occurred the risk is 75%.

ACUTE SALPINGITIS

Acute salpingitis is a difficult diagnosis to establish. There are no laboratory or physical findings that are pathognomic of pelvic inflammatory disease or acute salpingitis. Individuals who have fever, lower abdominal pain, purulent cervical discharge, tenderness or pain on motion of the cervix and uterus, and tenderness on gentle palpation of the adnexa are most likely to have acute salpingitis. However, these signs of infection are not always present. The accepted criteria for making a clinical diagnosis are as follows: (1) fever, (2) lower abdominal pain, (3) cervical motion and adnexal tenderness. In addition, the patient may have one or more of the following: an elevated white blood cell count, nausea and vomiting, evidence of pelvic peritonitis, a pelvic mass, and a purulent cervical discharge. The diagnosis must be differentiated from those clinical conditions that can easily mimic acute salpingitis (box below).

Patients with acute salpingitis should have specimens obtained from the endocervix for the isolation and identification of *N. gonorrhoeae* and *C. trachomatis*. There is no value in obtaining an endocervical specimen for the isolation and identification of aerobic and anaerobic bacteria. The cervical specimens will only reflect the vaginal flora. An endometrial biopsy should be obtained, preferably with a Pipelle. The tissue can easily be divided into two major portions, one for histologic evaluation and for the isolation of *N. gonorrhoeae*, *C. trachomatis*, *Mycoplasma*, *Ureaplasma*, and aerobic and anaerobic bacteria. The isolated aerobes and anaerobes should be identified, and antibiotic

sensitivities should be performed. Although almost all patients with acute salpingitis will respond to one of the recommended regimens of antibiotic therapy (box p. 634), it is the patient who fails or who progresses to advanced pelvic inflammatory disease that is of concern.

Complications

Pelvic inflammatory disease evolves into a complex infection when the large and small bowel become adherent to the adnexa, simulating an abscess. The bowel becomes inflamed, edematous, and densely adherent to the inflamed adnexa. The mucosal lining of the bowel becomes injured and develops microscopic breaks or leaks, permitting the transmigration of bacteria that are endogenous to the large bowel. These bacteria, many of which are abscessogenic and may interact synergistically with organisms already present in the infected tissue, form an abscess. Synergy can occur between bacteria such as *E. coli* and *B. fragilis*, perhaps between *E. faecalis* and *B. bivius*. The patient with acute salpingitis who does not have a pelvic mass should respond to antibiotic therapy within 48 to 72 hours. The patient should become afebrile, and the white blood cell count should be decreasing. If there were signs of peritonitis on admission, these should be abating, the patient's appetite should be returning, and a general sense of well-being should be present. However, if the patient continues to have spiking temperatures ($\geq 101°$ F), a persistent or elevated white blood cell count, and no change in the physical findings, it is imperative that a pelvic examination be repeated.

If a mass is detected, an ultrasonogram should be obtained, which may provide information concerning the number of masses, their size, whether they are unilocular or multilocular, and their location with respect to the uterus and bowel. The thickness of the wall of the mass can also be evaluated. This information may have a bearing on the treatment plan. A thick-walled multilocular mass is probably less likely to respond to antibiotic therapy than is a thin-walled, unilocular mass. The thick rind that is commonly found encasing a tuboovarian abscess is usually associated with thrombosed vessels that supply the abscess. This implies that blood flow is minimal at best, and the tissue may be necrotic. Antibiotics cannot be carried to the infected tissue in sufficient quantities, nor can they penetrate the thick wall of the abscess. Thus the effectiveness of the antibiotic will be limited to preventing bacteremia, and it will not eradicate the abscess. In addition, ultrasonography may assist in facilitating percutaneous drainage of the abscess. Specimens obtained should be cultured for the organisms mentioned thus far.

If a pelvic mass is present, a computed tomography (CT) scan will detail its location with respect to other structures, identify whether it is solid or cystic, and provide information about the nature of the fluid it contains (e.g., blood, pus, serous fluid). The CT scan is also of assistance in detecting and locating intraabdominal abscesses, including interloop bowel and subhepatic and sub-

---

Differential diagnosis for acute salpingitis

1. Ectopic pregnancy
2. Appendicitis
3. Ruptured appendix
4. Endometriosis
5. Torsion of an adnexa
6. Diverticulitis
7. Infection of Meckel's diverticulum
8. Abscess of Meckel's diverticulum

diaphragmatic abscesses. The location of the abscess is important because it will determine whether percutaneous drainage can be attempted or whether laparotomy is needed. The presence of gas in the abscess cavity indicates that anaerobic organisms are present. Gas in the tissue planes of the abscess suggests that a necrotizing infection is present (e.g., a clostridial or bacterial synergistic infection making surgical intervention imperative).

There are no specific clinical findings or laboratory tests that establish the presence of PID. Ideally laparoscopy should be performed to examine the pelvic cavity, but if this is not possible culdocentesis may prove helpful.

Before performing culdocentesis, a digital vaginal-rectal examination should be done to determine whether the cul-de-sac is clear. Combining this examination with ultrasonography will help make the culdocentesis successful. The fluid aspirated via culdocentesis can provide important clues for diagnostic evaluation and patient management. The presence of purulent fluid is suggestive of acute salpingitis. A ruptured tuboovarian abscess or pyosalpinx is unlikely unless the patient has signs of peritonitis or a mass on examination. Aspiration of nonclotting blood suggests an ectopic pregnancy, hemorrhagic corpus luteum, or retrograde menstruation. Aspiration of blood that clots suggests that the bleeding is recent or that a vessel has been injured. If serous fluid is aspirated, it should be gram stained and the fluid also tested for amylase. If numerous white blood cells are found, the patient may be suffering from acute salpingitis or another acute inflammatory process, such as appendicitis or pancreatitis.

Laparoscopy enables a more definitive examination of the fallopian tubes, ovaries, uterus, and cul-de-sac. Fluid from the cul-de-sac should be aspirated via the laparoscope and cultured for all aerobic and anaerobic bacteria associated with salpingitis. If a tissue biopsy is obtained from the fallopian tube or adhesive tissue is removed, it should also be cultured as directed earlier. If an abscess is found at the time of laparoscopy, it should be drained and a catheter left in place to allow continued drainage and permit lavaging of the abscess cavity. If the pelvic organs cannot be seen and evaluated, or the patient is believed to have right-sided salpingitis and the appendix cannot be examined, laparotomy should be performed.

An exploratory laparotomy is also indicated in patients with a surgical abdomen who are suspected of having a ruptured or leaking tuboovarian abscess. If the tubes are inflamed but not occluded, the pelvis and abdomen should be irrigated copiously with saline. If pyosalpinx is present unilaterally or bilaterally, salpingostomies should be performed. Fluid obtained should be gram stained and cultured. If tuboovarian abscesses are present, a bilateral salpingooophorectomy is indicated. In those infrequent instances in which only one adnexum is abscessed and the contralateral adnexum is normal, the involved adnexum should be removed.

Operative management of the tuboovarian abscess begins with thorough counseling of the patient. It is imperative that the patient understand that removal of her reproductive organs will place her in a postmenopausal state. She will require hormone replacement, which may not be entirely successful in relieving the vasomotor symptoms, and she may note a decrease in her desire for sexual activity. Injury to the bowel may necessitate a colostomy, and there is the risk that one or both ureters may be damaged.

Another approach to the operative management of tuboovarian abscess is incision and drainage. This approach is especially important to consider in the young nulliparous patient. The procedure may be accomplished via a percutaneous approach using ultrasonography, CT scan, laparoscopy, or laparotomy. Regardless of which method is used, a catheter should be left in place to allow for drainage and lavage with an antibiotic solution.

Time may not be sufficient to allow for preoperative bowel preparation, but high-dose antibiotics should be administered before commencing the operative procedure. Intravenous fluid should be administered, and the patient should be stable, in electrolyte balance, and euglycemic if possible. A ruptured tuboovarian abscess is to be considered life-threatening, and such patients are at risk for gram-negative sepsis. If aggressive management is not undertaken, they are likely to progress rapidly from sepsis to septic shock to adult respiratory distress syndrome. Therefore operative intervention should not be delayed.

The operative procedure begins with a generous vertical incision. The subdiaphragmatic, subhepatic, and subsplenic areas should also be thoroughly explored for abscesses. The appendix should be examined to determine whether it is ruptured. The appendix may be densely adherent to the tuboovarian abscess, making it difficult to determine its degree of involvement; in such a case, the appendix will have to be removed. Once the pelvic organs have been identified and isolated, a decision must be made as to whether they should be removed or drainage attempted.

If the patient is nulliparous or desires to retain her reproductive organs, it should be explained that drainage may be attempted but that this approach may be unsuccessful; the patient's condition may fail to improve or may deteriorate, necessitating a total hysterectomy with bilateral salpingoooophorectomy. If drainage is to be undertaken, the abscesses should be opened and all loculations disrupted. If necrotic or gangrenous tissue is present, the adnexa should be removed. Drains, preferably Jackson-Pratt or of similar large bore, should be placed into the cavities created and attached to a closed suction apparatus. The drains can also be used to lavage the cavities with antibiotic solution. Because tetracycline antibiotics (including doxycycline) will result in significant adhesion formation, they should not be used.

Management

The most difficult decision is whether or not a hysterectomy is necessary when the fallopian tubes and ovaries are abscessed (a tuboovarian abscess). If it is a unilateral condition, a unilateral salpingoooophorectomy can be performed with preservation of the contralateral adnexa. Often a pyosalpinx is present and the ovary is not involved. However, adhesions are usually present that involve the ovary, which often results in a salpingoooophorectomy. If the ovary appears normal and the capsule of the ovary has not been violated, there is no need to remove the ovary. Leaving one or both ovaries in place allows the patient the opportunity of in vitro fertilization and an endogenous supply of estrogen, progesterone, and androgens. If both tubes and ovaries are abscessed, the decision becomes more difficult. At the present time it is more common to perform a total hysterectomy with a bilateral salpingo-oophorectomy. However, consideration should be given to allowing the uterus to remain since it is not affected by the disease process. This will permit the patient to consider embryo transfer as a possibility for bearing children. Whatever the extent of the surgery, the procedure with its possible complications should be explained in detail to the patient and her family before the operation. The following complications are possible: damage to the bladder, ureters, and bowel; the possibility of a colostomy, hemorrhage, recurrent infection, or pulmonary embolus; and the possibility of additional operative procedures.

If at the time of laparotomy the abdomen and pelvis contain free pus, regardless of the amount, and the pelvic organs are inflamed, but no abscess is found, then no tissue or organ need be removed. Often the tube will appear to be markedly edematous if the fimbriae are not completely agglutinated and the tube is patent, but nothing need be done surgically. The edema and inflammation will resolve, and healing may occur with little residual scarring. The pelvis and abdomen should be irrigated with copious amounts of saline (3 to 6 L), and all fluid should be removed. Some individuals prefer to use an antibiotic-containing solution. I have not found this necessary or advantageous. When the abdomen is opened and subjected to the atmosphere, the oxygen present is toxic to the anaerobes, and the number of aerobic and facultative bacteria will be reduced to unimportant concentrations by the washing, leaving an inoculum too small to induce infection. Couple this with the fact that antibiotic serum and tissue levels will be maintained during, as well as after, the operative procedure, and continuation of the infection is unlikely. The remaining inoculum size will be too small to effectively reproduce in the presence of adequate antibiotic concentrations. If an inoculum is left behind in an area not adequately served by antibiotics, then a reinfection is likely, but since the bowel has not been injured, bacteria will not leak into the pelvic cavity, so infection is not likely to occur. It is imperative that if purulent fluid is found, upon entering the abdomen, an aliquot should be aspirated, placed in an anaerobic transport vial, and immediately taken to the laboratory. The specimen should be gram stained and processed for the isolation of aerobic, facultative, obligate, gram-positive, and gram-negative bacteria. The gram stain can be of great value in modifying antibi-

otic therapy. The patient is most likely to be on a cephalosporin (e.g., cefotetan, cefoxitin, ceftizoxime) or clindamycin plus gentamicin since these are the most commonly used antibiotics for the treatment of pelvic inflammatory disease. Doxycycline may or may not be given at this time. If the gram stain reveals the presence of gram-positive cocci, it is possible that streptococci or enterococci are present. All but the latter organism will be covered by any of the antibiotic regimens given above. Ampicillin should be added to the currently administered antibiotic regimen if enterococcus is suspected. There has been a great deal of concern over the significance of *Chlamydia,* whether it is isolated or not, it is recommended that the patient receive antibiotic therapy that is effective in eradicating this organism. It has not been our experience to frequently find *C. trachomatis* where advanced pelvic inflammatory disease is present. However, the patient receiving clindamycin plus gentamicin should be well covered. Clindamycin has been shown to have activity against *C. trachomatis.* The combination of clindamycin plus gentamicin has recently been shown to be synergistic in vitro against *C. trachomatis.*[31]

Once the patient's abdomen and pelvis have been completely and thoroughly washed, the bowel should be completely inspected, and if adhesions are found between loops of bowel, they should be taken down carefully. This may be done easily by sharp dissection. If blunt dissection is employed and resistance is encountered in attempting lysis of adhesions between loops of bowel, bowel and peritoneum, or bowel and another organ, this technique should be abandoned and sharp dissection used. It is important not to damage the serosa of the bowel since this will result in the formation of dense adhesions and may result in bowel obstruction. Since the bowel may be edematous, vigorous lysis of adhesions may result in evulsion of large amounts of serosa, thus exposing the subserosal surface. If the bowel is further traumatized or becomes greatly distended, spontaneous breaks in the mucosa can occur. This can result in leakage of bowel contents, carrying bacteria into the peritoneal cavity. Peritonitis and intraperitoneal abscesses can develop. This leads to a second exploratory laparotomy, which increases the risk for intraoperative complications, as well as for infection.

If the patient is found to have a pyosalpinx, unilaterally or bilaterally, and the ovaries are not involved in the infectious process, it is acceptable to perform a neosalpingostomy. The fallopian tubes should be copiously irrigated with sterile saline. A single stitch of permanent monofilament suture 4-0 gauge should be used to fix the ends of the incised fimbriae to the tubal serosa. The patient must be informed that this procedure was performed and that she is now at risk for ectopic pregnancy. If possible, a small tubal specimen from the end of the tube that was opened should be excised and cultured, especially for *N. gonorrhoeae* and *C. trachomatis.*

Parenteral antibiotic therapy should be continued until the patient has been afebrile for 48 hours, is tolerating oral

Table 38-2. Oral antibiotic regimens for posthospital treatment of PID

Antibiotic	Dosage (mg)	Duration (days)
Augmentin	500, tid	10
Metronidazole	500, tid	10
Ceftin or	500, bid	10
Ciprofloxacin	500, bid	10
Clindamycin	150, tid	10
Ceftin or	150, tid	10
Ciprofloxacin	150, tid	10

liquids and solid nourishment, and pulse and white blood cell count is normal. A pelvic examination should be performed to determine if the pelvic organs are normal. The patient will require antibiotic therapy for at least an additional 7 days. The choice should depend upon whether or not *Chlamydia* was present. If the organism was isolated, then the patient should receive doxycycline; if it was absent and the infection was polymicrobial, then perhaps amoxicillin/clavulanic acid (Augmentin) (500 mg orally three times a day for 10 days) (Table 38-2). Ideally the patient should be reexamined within 72 hours of being discharged from the hospital. This is to determine whether an exacerbation of the infection is occurring and whether the medication is being taken appropriately and to emphasize the serious nature of the infection. This education process is necessary and can only be accomplished by informing the patient that her infection could yet result in serious sequelae. The patient should also be placed on oral contraceptive pills to prevent pregnancy and possible abscess formation if the infection has not been eradicated. Her sex partner should be examined, and if she was found to harbor the gonococcus or *Chlamydia,* he should also be treated. It would be advisable for her to have complete pelvic rest for at least 3 to 6 weeks following discharge from the hospital. Patients who have undergone an exploratory laparotomy but have not had a hysterectomy should have a laparoscopic examination 6 weeks after they have recovered from their initial infection. This is necessary to assess the residual damage from the infection and surgery. At this time patency of the fallopian tubes can be assessed, lysis of adhesions can be performed, and a determination of the result of the initial infection can be established. Then a more definitive prognosis can be afforded the patient, as well as guidelines to follow if she desires pregnancy.

REFERENCES

1. Adam E et al: A prospective study of association of herpes simplex virus and human papillomavirus infection with cervical neoplasia in women exposed to diethylstilbestrol in utero, *Int J Cancer* 35:19, 1985.
2. Aly R, Britz MB, Marbach HI: Quantitative microbiology of human vulva, *Br J Dermatol* 101:445, 1979.
3. Amsel R et al: Nonspecific vaginitis: diagnostic criteria and microbial and epidemiologic association, *Am J Med* 74:14, 1983.
4. Becker TM et al: Trends of molluscum contagiosum in the United States 1966-83, *Sex Transm Dis* 13:88, 1986.
5. Bhatia NN, Bergman A, Broen EM: Advanced hidradenitis suppurativa of the vulva: a report of three cases, *J Reprod Med* 29:436, 1984.
6. Brown D Jr, Kaufman RH, Gardner HL: Gardnerella vaginalis vaginitis: the current opinion, *J Reprod Med* 29:300, 1984.
7. Corey L, Holmes KK: Genital herpes simplex virus infection: current concepts in diagnosis, therapy and prevention, *Ann Intern Med* 98:973, 1983.
8. Crombleholme WR et al: Ampicillin/sulbactam versus metronidazole-gentamicin in the treatment of soft tissue pelvic infections, *Am J Obstet Gynecol* 156:501, 1989.
9. Dodson MR, Faro S: The polymicrobial etiology of acute pelvic inflammatory disease and treatment regimen, *Rev Infect Dis* 7(4):S696, 1985.
10. Faro S, Phillips LE: Non-specific vaginitis or vaginitis of undetermined aetiology, *Int J Tissue React* 9(2):173, 1987.
11. Faro S et al: Ceftizoxime versus cefotaxime in the treatment of hospitalized patients with pelvic inflammatory disease, *Curr Therapeutic Res* 43:349, 1985.
12. Gardner HC, Dukes CD: Haemophilus vaginalis vaginitis: a newly defined specific infection previously classified "nonspecific" vaginitis, *Am J Obset Gynecol* 69:962, 1955.
13. Hammann R et al: Quantitative studies on the vaginal flora of asymptomatic women and patients with vaginitis and vaginosis, *Zentralbl Bakteriol Hyg* 265:451, 1987.
14. Hartford SL et al: Serologic evidence of prior chlamydial infection in patients with tubal ectopic pregnancy and contralateral tubal disease, *Fertil Steril* 47:118, 1987.
15. Henry-Suchet J et al: Microbiologic study of chronic inflammation associated with tubal factor infertility: role of *Chlamydia trachomatis, Fertil Steril* 47:274, 1987.
16. Hill LVH: Anaerobes and Gardnerella vaginalis in non-specific vaginitis, *Genitourin Med* 61:114, 1985.
17. Holst E et al: Bacterial vaginosis: microbiological and clinical findings, *Eur J Clin Microbiol* 6:536, 1987.
18. Judson FN, Tavelli BG: Comparison of clinical and epidemiological characteristics of pelvic inflammatory disease classified by endocervical cultures of *N. gonorrhoeae* and *Chlamydia trachomatis, Genitourin Med* 62:230, 1986.
19. Kirshon B et al: Correlation of ultrasonography and bacteriology of the endocervix and posterior cul-de-sac of patients with severe pelvic inflammatory disease, *Sex Transm Dis* 15:47, 1981.
20. Kristensen GB et al: Infections with *Neisseria gonorrhoeae* and *Chlamydia trachomatis* in women with acute salpingitis, *Genitourin Med* 61:179, 1985.
21. Larsen B, Galask RP: Vaginal microbial flora: composition and influences of host physiology, *Ann Intern Med* 96:926, 1982.
22. Leegaard M: The incidence of *Candida albicans* in the vagina of healthy young women, *Acta Obstet Gynecol Scand* 63:85, 1984.
23. Lidbeck A, Gustafsson J-A, Nord CE: Impact of *Lactobacillus acidophilus* supplement on human oropharyngeal and intestinal microflora, *Scand J Inf Dis* 19:531, 1987.
24. Lidbeck A et al: Impact of *Lactobacillus acidophilus* on the normal intestinal microflora after the administration of two antimicrobial agents, *Antimicrob Agents Inf* 16:329, 1988.
25. Lycke E et al: The risk of transmission of genital *Chlamydia trachomatis* infection is less than that of genital *Neisseria gonorrhoeae* infection, *Sex Transm Dis* 7:6, 1980.
26. Mardh P-A et al: Antibodies to *Chlamydia trachomatis, Mycoplasma hominis* and *Neisseria gonorrhoeae* in sera from patients with acute salpingitis, *Brit J Ven Dis* 57:125, 1981.
27. Moller BR et al: Infection with *Chlamydia trachomatis, Mycoplasma hominis,* and *Neisseria gonorrhoeae* in patients with acute pelvic inflammatory disease, *Sex Transm Dis* 8:198, 1981.
28. Mortimer PS: Mediation of hidradenitis suppurativa by androgens, *Br Med J* 292:245, 1986.

29. Mortimer PS et al: A double-blind controlled cross-over trial of cyproterone acetate in females with hidradenitis suppurativa, *Br J Dermatol* 115:263, 1986.

30. Nettleman MD, Jones RB: Cost-effectiveness of screening women at moderate risk for genital infections caused by *Chlamydia trachomatis,* JAMA 260:207, 1988.

31. Pearlman MD et al: *Chlamydia trachomatis* susceptibility testing: invitro synergy with clindamycin and aminoglycosides, *Antimicrob Chemother,* 34:1399, 1990.

32. Rice DP, Hodgson TA, Kopstein AN: The economic costs of illness: a replication and update, *Health Care Fin Rev* 7:61, 1985.

33. Spence MR: Epidemiology of sexually transmitted disease, *Obstet Gynecol Clin North Am* 16:453, 1989.

34. Spiegel CA, Amsel R, Holmes KK: Diagnosis of bacterial vaginosis by direct gram-stain of vaginal fluid, *J Clin Microbiol* 18:170, 1983.

35. Stamm WE et al: Effect of treatment regimens for *Neisseria gonorrhoeae* on simultaneous infection with *Chlamydia trachomatis, N Engl J Med* 310:545, 1984.

36. Sweet RL et al: The occurrence of chlamydial and gonococcal salpingitis during the menstrual cycle, *JAMA* 255:2062, 1986.

37. Tsai CC et al: Vaginal physiology in the postmenopausal woman: pH value, transvaginal electropotentiated difference and estimated blood flow, *South Med J* 80:986, 1987.

38. Walters MD et al: Antibodies to *Chlamydia trachomatis* and risk for tubal pregnancy, *Am J Obstet Gynecol* 159:942, 1988.

39. Washington AE, Arno PS, Brooks MA: Economic cost of pelvic inflammatory disease, *JAMA* 255:1735, 1986.

40. Washington AE, Johnson RE, Sanders LL: *Chlamydia trachomatis* infection in the United States: what are they costing us? *JAMA* 257:2070, 1987.

41. Westergaard L, Phillipsen T, Scheibel J: Significance of *Chlamydia trachomatis* infection in postabortal pelvic inflammatory disease, *Obstet Gynecol* 60:322, 1980.

42. Westrom L: Effect of acute pelvic inflammatory disease on fertility, *Am J Obstet Gynecol* 121:707, 1975.

43. Westrom L: Pelvic inflammatory disease: bacteriology and sequelae, *Contraception* 36:111, 1987.

44. Westrom L et al: Taxonomy of vaginosis: bacterial vaginosis—a definition, *Scand J Urol Nephrol* 86:259, 1984.

Chapter 39

METHODS OF FEMALE STERILIZATION

Jaroslav F. Hulka

Female sterilization is a popular method of maintaining family size in the United States. It is the leading method of family planning in married women over the age of 30, which is also the average age at which a woman in the United States undergoes sterilization. About 500,000 such operations are performed every year, about half of these at the time of delivery (postpartum sterilization) and about half in a nonpregnant state (interval). This chapter will review the techniques available and appropriate for these procedures.

GENERAL CONSIDERATIONS

Voluntary sterilization is legal in the United States and is funded by the federal government through Medicaid. Certain selection criteria should be kept in mind when offering sterilization to appropriate patients. The patient should be *mature,* with her decision based on solid emotional grounds. She should be *informed,* aware of the alternatives in contraception and of the risks of sterilization. Finally, she should be *unpressured,* not making this permanent decision under stress (e.g., during separation or divorce, at the time of delivery or abortion). Younger women (below 30) appear to have a greater risk for regret and a greater tendency to later request reversal[25]; for these women, a more reversible technique should be offered.

Involuntary sterilization for mentally retarded patients is an option in many states. North Carolina has model legislation for this process, involving presentation and documentation of the patient's condition by parents or guardians to a judge while the clerk of court acts on behalf of the patient. When the judge is convinced that sterilization is in the patient's and society's best interest, a court order is issued directing the surgeon to sterilize the patient.

STERILIZATION AT CESAREAN SECTION
Pomeroy technique

This procedure is probably the one most commonly performed worldwide and serves as the "gold standard" against which other techniques are measured. Although it was never published by Pomeroy, his associates published his technique in 1930.[3] A loop of tube is elevated by forceps or Babcock, an absorbable no. 1 plain catgut suture creates a loop of the tube, and the loop is excised for documentation by the pathology laboratory. Figure 39-1 illustrates this classic method.

Irving technique

In 1924, Irving[16] described a method that destroys no tube and achieves high success. The isthmus is divided, and the proximal stump is buried in myometrium, with the distal stump buried in the leaves of the broad ligament (Fig. 39-2). This technique has had no known failures but is associated with more morbidity than simple tubal ligation. Because no tube is destroyed, reversibility of this technique is high.

Fimbriectomy

It is easy to grasp the distal end of the tube, ligate, and excise the fimbria. This results in a permanent sterilization, since fimbriectomy reversal is seldom successful. Failures in this techniques have come from disregarding the fimbria ovarica, a strand of fimbria connecting the tube to the ovary. This structure will maintain patency and allow pregnancy if it is not identified and separately divided (Fig. 39-3).

POSTPARTUM STERILIZATION

After vaginal delivery, sterilization can be accomplished with ease through a minilaparotomy incision just

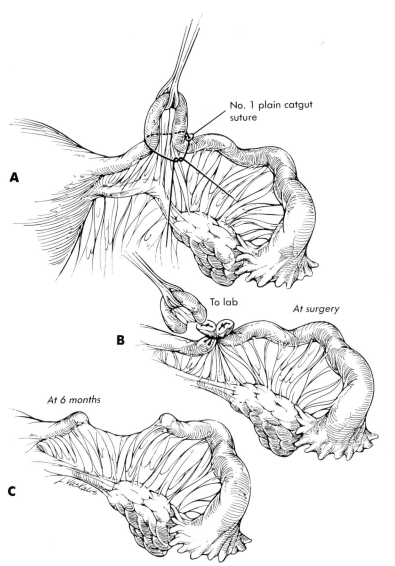

No. 1 plain catgut suture

A

To lab

At surgery

B

At 6 months

C

Fig. 39-1. Pomeroy technique. **A,** A Babcock clamp, scissors, and a length of no. 1 plain catgut are all the equipment necessary. **B,** A specimen confirms that tube and not round ligament was divided. **C,** Six months after division, the stumps have separated to about 3 cm apart. Elegantly simple and effective, this is the "gold standard" against which all other methods are compared.

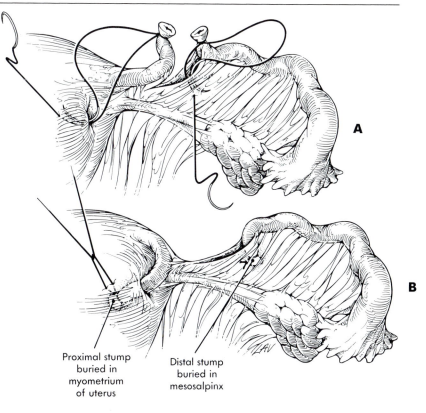

A

B

Fig. 39-2. Irving technique. **A,** The divided isthmic stumps are drawn underneath peritoneum to assure occlusion. **B,** The proximal stump is drawn under uterine, the distal stump under mesosalpingeal peritoneum. No failures with this method have been reported.

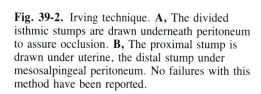

Proximal stump buried in myometrium of uterus

Distal stump buried in mesosalpinx

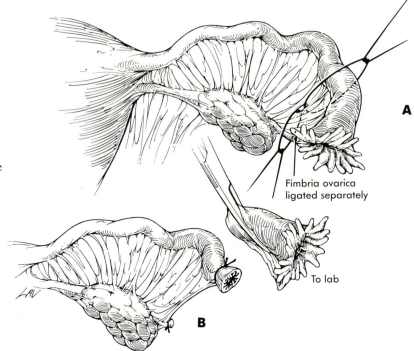

Fig. 39-3. Fimbriectomy. If a fimbrica ovarii is present **(A),** it should be separately divided to free the tubal fimbria for complete excision **(B).** This method is rarely reversed successfully.

Fimbria ovarica ligated separately

To lab

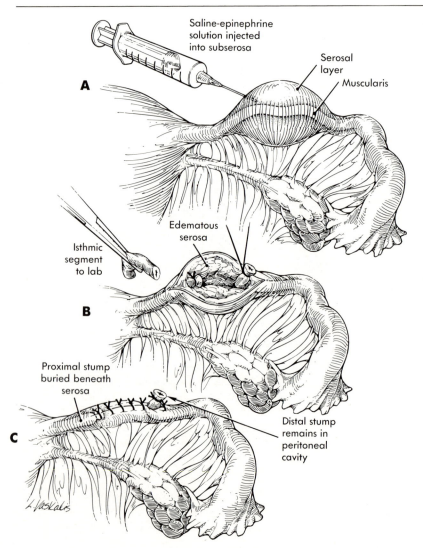

Saline-epinephrine solution injected into subserosa

Serosal layer

Muscularis

Isthmic segment to lab

Edematous serosa

Proximal stump buried beneath serosa

Distal stump remains in peritoneal cavity

Fig. 39-4. Uchida technique. **A,** Saline-epinephrine solution dissects the loose longitudinal musculature from the hard inner circular muscle of the isthmus. **B,** Uchida recommends stripping and excising this inner segment to minimize failures. **C,** The distal stump is drawn and tied outside the mesosalpinx.

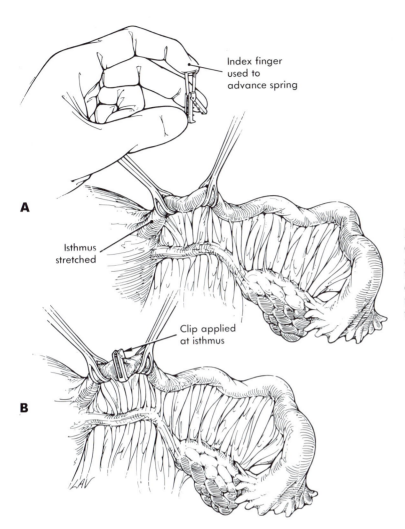

Index finger used to advance spring

A

Isthmus stretched

Clip applied at isthmus

B

Fig. 39-5. Clip at laparotomy. Two Babcocks, one close to the uterus, put a segment of isthmus on the stretch. **A,** A spring clip is held between thumb and third finger and placed on the stretched segment like a clothespin on a clothesline. **B,** The index finger pushes the metal spring over the plastic jaws to lock the clip on the isthmus.

below the umbilicus, where the uterus and its tubes lie postpartum. The tubal ligation is best delayed until it is certain that the newborn is healthy. This is the main reason that postpartum sterilization is often deferred till 6 weeks after delivery. If the child is obviously robust and healthy, a comfortable plan is to have the delivery accomplished with a epidural catheter, leaving the catheter indwelling until the operating room or labor room is available for this elective procedure.

Because there is limited access to the tube through the minilaparotomy, an Irving technique or a fimbriectomy may not be feasible. The Pomeroy technique is the one most universally used in this situation. Care must be taken to ensure that it is the tube, not the round ligament, that is operated on.

The Uchida technique[30] involves injection of saline-epinephrine solution into the tubal musculature to separate serosa from muscle layer. The edematous tube is incised, and the inner circular muscle of the tube can be identified and excised. The proximal stump is then buried beneath this edematous serosa, and the distal stump ligated outside the serosa (Fig. 39-4). The reversibility of this technique depends entirely on how much of the inner circular tubal lumen is excised for the pathology specimen.

Clip application

Although tantalum hemostatic clips do not work for tubal occlusion,[12] spring-loaded clips designed for laparoscopy can be placed by hand onto the postpartum tube.[18] The isthmus of the tube is held stretched between two Babcock clamps as the thumb and third finger close the jaws and the index finger pushes the spring into locked position (Fig. 39-5). The use of clips appears to produce lower morbidity compared to Pomeroy, with earlier recovery to full activity by the mother.

INTERVAL (NONPREGNANT) STERILIZATION

The introduction of laparoscopy in the 1970s was a major contributor to women's acceptance of sterilization as a method of family planning. The original unipolar electrocoagulation technique by Steptoe,[28] described in his textbook of laparoscopy, paved the way for worldwide use of the laparoscope and development of simpler and safer techniques.

Sterilization as an elective procedure not associated with pregnancy was infrequent before the acceptance of laparoscopy. Many vaginal surgeons were performing a vaginal fimbriectomy as described by Kroener (Fig. 39-3).[17] Other vaginal approaches incorporated the use of tantalum clips. Compared to laparoscopic approaches, however, the vaginal methods have been associated with a higher morbidity from postoperative infection, as well as higher pregnancy rates due to incomplete removal of the fimbria. Although a few good surgeons still recommend vaginal sterilization, this is no longer the trend in the United States.

Similarly, the concept of minilaparotomy has been introduced in developing countries as a means of avoiding the expensive equipment necessary for laparoscopy. In trained hands, and under general anesthesia, a minilaparotomy is an effective and comfortable method of accomplishing sterilization with the simple Pomeroy technique. Under local anesthesia, the abdominal invasion is usually sufficiently uncomfortable to make this procedure less acceptable by patients, particularly if laparoscopy is available as an alternative. For this reason, minilaparotomy has also been abandoned in the United States except by a few skilled practitioners.

Unipolar coagulation and division

This technique was the first used by gynecologists learning both laparoscopy and electrocoagulation techniques. The tube is grasped, and current is passed through the tube (and body) to a base plate (Fig. 39-6). The method produced considerable destruction of tube with electric current but was also associated with hemorrhage from incompletely coagulated vessels severed at the time of tubal division. Deaths were associated with unipolar coagulation,[20] perhaps as much because of complications of trocar entry as electrocoagulation of bowel. This method was abandoned by most laparoscopists in favor of the less destructive techniques described below.

Bipolar coagulation

This technique was developed independently in the early 1970s by Rioux in Canada, Kleppinger in the United States, and Hirsch in Germany. The Kleppinger technique emerged as the most popular method of laparoscopic sterilization in the United States. The bipolar technique is the simplest to perform technically and is the most common method of laparoscopic sterilization today. The poles of the forceps conduct the electricity between them, with no current flow beyond the forceps, so the patient is not part of the circuit (Fig. 39-7). Failures after bipolar coagulation have been due to incomplete coagulation, sometimes using inappropriate generators.[27] The end point of successful coagulation is indicated by a current flow meter on the ap-

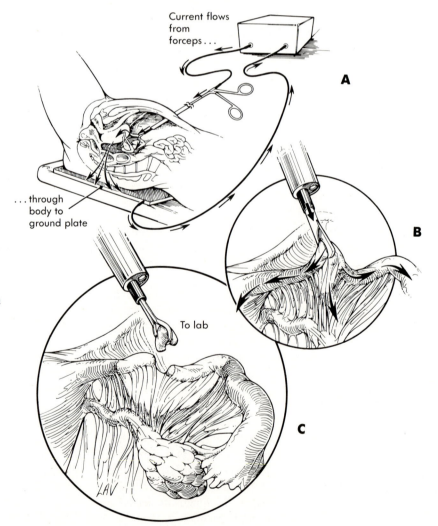

Fig. 39-6. Unipolar coagulation. Steptoe's original method involved grasping the tube **(A),** elevating it **(B),** and passing coagulating current through it until blanching occurred **(C).** Division with scissors sometimes resulted in bleeding from incompletely sealed mesosalpingeal vessels. Current running through the body caused skin and bowel burns.

propriate or matched generator. When the flow diminishes and ceases, the tubal tissue has been desiccated to the point that it no longer conducts electricity and the forceps can be moved to the next area for coagulation. Kleppinger stresses that three contiguous areas are to be coagulated. This results in at least 3 cm of tube being destroyed and prevents spontaneous recanalization, occurring as a result of the healing process bringing the two stumps closely together.[8] Recent reports of a high incidence of ectopic pregnancy following bipolar coagulation[19] may be the result of fistula formation between the uterus and peritoneum when the tube is destroyed too close to the uterus.[29] Sperm can travel through these uteroperitoneal fistulas, reach the egg in the distal tubal segment, and cause an ectopic pregnancy by this route (Fig. 39-8). This has led to the recommendation that the tube be grasped at least 2 to 3 cm away from the uterocornual junction at the time of sterilization so that a stump of isthmus remains to absorb the intrauterine fluid under pressure and minimize fistula formation.

Silastic band application

The Silastic band for sterilization was developed simultaneously by In Bae Yoon and Coy Lay in the early 1970s. Widely distributed by the U.S. Agency for International Development, the band was offered as a nonelectric (and therefore safer) method of tubal occlusion. The fallopian tube is drawn 1.5 cm into a 0.5-cm-diameter metal cylinder, destroying 3 cm of tube. A Silastic ring stretched on the outside of the cylinder is released to form an occlusion at the base of this knuckle (Fig. 39-9). Over time, about 3 cm of constricted tube undergoes necrosis and the tubes separate. Similar to the Pomeroy technique in theory, the laparoscopic application of band is associated with a 2.5% incidence of hemorrhage from stretching the vessels underneath the tube or tearing the tube itself. For this reason, Yoon and associates[34] have recommended that bipolar coagulation be available to manage this complication. Postoperatively, patients experience pain from hypoxic necrosis of the tube in the band. This subsides in 48 to 96 hours and can be diminished somewhat by topical application of anesthesia at the time of band application.

Spring clip application

Devised in the 1970s to offer a mechanical alternative to electrocoagulation, the spring clip occludes the isthmus of the tube by 2 plastic jaws, compressing the tube by a stainless steel spring pressing the jaws together.[13] Spring clip application by laparoscopy requires careful surgical technique to assure that the clip is completely across the isthmus of the tube (Fig. 39-10). Although the initial preg-

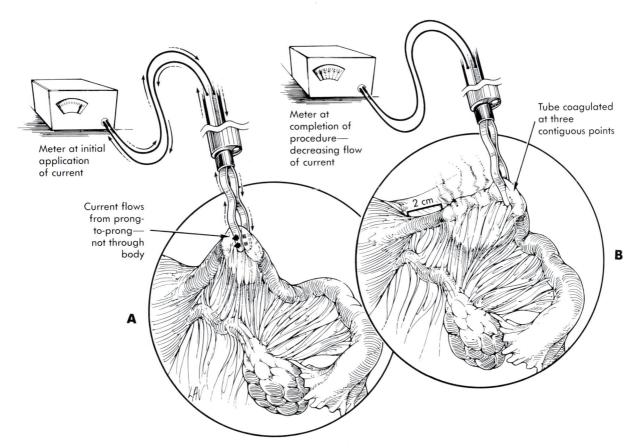

Fig. 39-7. Bipolar coagulation. **A,** Current passes only through the tube from prong to prong of the forceps. **B,** Three contiguous burns are needed to prevent spontaneous recanalization. The end point for coagulation is tissue desiccation, at which point current ceases to flow through the dry, nonconducting tube. A meter on the generator to monitor current flow is thus necessary.

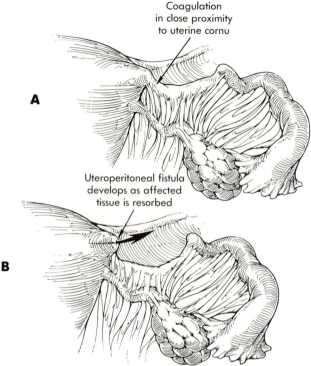

Fig. 39-8. Fistula formation. Destroying the isthmus too close to the uterus (**A**) may allow a uteroperitoneal fistula (**B**) to develop, through which sperm can get to the distal stump via the peritoneum. A fertilized ovum lodges as an ectopic pregnancy, a late serious complication of bipolar coagulation. Leaving a stump of isthmus should minimize this risk.

nancy rates were high as a result of misapplications, the current pregnancy rates for clip, coagulation, and band are comparable. The spring clip is the most reversible of the techniques[25] since less than 5 mm of tube is destroyed between the jaws of the clip. For this reason, it should be considered when one is selecting a method for a woman under 30.

Cautery techniques

True cautery is the direct application of heat to tissue, in contrast to electrocoagulation and desiccation, where electrical energy flows through tissue and heats it. In the United States, the Waters technique involves drawing the tube into a 10-mm insulated sheath with an electrode hook and applying current to the hook until the wire heats, cauterizes, and divides the tube in the sheath. The need for another 10-mm abdominal puncture has limited the appeal of this method. In Germany, the Semm Endotherm forceps is placed across the tube and one prong of the forceps is heated to 100° C, cauterizing the tube. The time (30 to 60 seconds) required for each cautery has limited the popularity of this method.

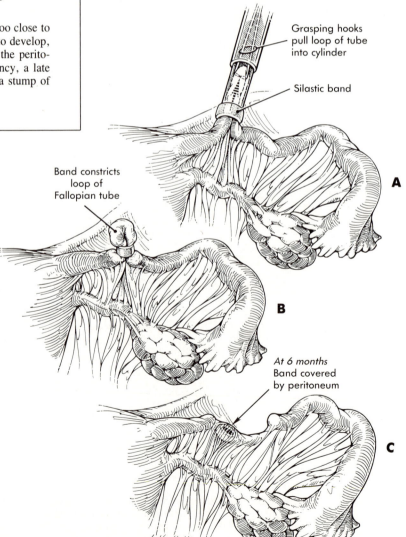

Fig. 39-9. Silastic band. **A,** About 3 cm of tube are drawn into a 5-mm cylinder over which a silastic band has been stretched. **B,** Releasing the band constricts the knuckle of tube with eventual necrosis. **C,** As with the Pomeroy, 6 months later the stumps are about 3 cm apart.

TECHNIQUES UNDER INVESTIGATION

The laser has been tried for tubal division at laparoscopy but offers no advantage over standard techniques. Burying the fimbria in a pouch of broad ligament peritoneum, and burying the ovary in an artificial plastic pouch, have been evaluated in animals but have not been used with humans because of the increased morbidity compared to standard techniques. Various other clips have been devised (Bleier clip, Filshie clip). The Bleier clip has been discontinued because of a high pregnancy rate due to the tube slipping into spaces within the jaws of the clip. The Filshie clip is undergoing extensive evaluation overseas but has not been approved by the FDA.

A number of hysteroscopic approaches have reached the human trial stage only to prove less cost-effective than standard laparoscopic techniques. In Europe, plastic tubal plugs developed by Steptoe in England and Hamou in France were abandoned after ectopic pregnancies developed. In the United States, the Silastic plug[7] was extensively evaluated[10] and found to be efficacious in about 85% to 90% of candidates, but technical failures persisted despite two or three hysteroscopic reapplications. The technique was intended to be reversible, but reversibility

has not been demonstrated. Other hysteroscopic approaches have included destroying the endometrium by freezing or coagulation, but these approaches have been abandoned or are still in preclinical evaluation stages. Similarly, the introduction of methylcyanoacrylate (crazy glue) into the tube has been clinically tested overseas but is not ready for clinical use. The Chinese have experimented with formalin injection into the tube, but reports of the efficacy and safety of this approach are incomplete. Although there are still active research projects concerning alternative sterilization techniques, the existing laparoscopic approaches of mechanical or electrocoagulation tubal occlusion remain the standard against which these alternatives must be measured in terms of cost, efficacy, and safety.

STERILIZATION FAILURES

To study the pregnancy rate following sterilization techniques, a large number of patients (over 1000) must be followed for a 2- to 3-year period with a high rate (over 85%) of follow-up. This enormously difficult task has been accomplished very few times: by Johns Hopkins University in the early days of electrocoagulation, and by the Univer-

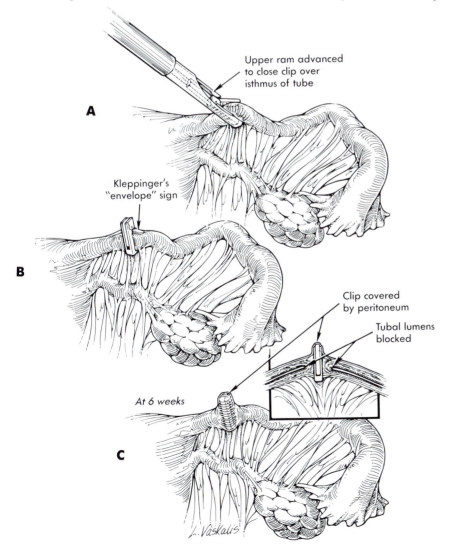

Upper ram advanced to close clip over isthmus of tube

A

Kleppinger's "envelope" sign

B

Clip covered by peritoneum

Tubal lumens blocked

At 6 weeks

C

L. Vaskalis

Fig. 39-10. Spring clip. **A,** The isthmic portion (first 2 to 3 cm of tube) is maneuvered into the open jaws of the clip until it is snug against the hinge. **B,** Closing the clip will create **C,** the "Kleppinger envelope sign," a fold of tubal peritoneum in the hinge of the clip. Failure to get the clip completely across the isthmus results in pregnancy. Some routinely use two clips close together on each tube.

Table 39-1. Risk of ectopic pregnancy following sterilization methods

Method	Number of pregnancies reported in 1979		Rate of ectopic to total pregnancies* (%)
	Intrauterine	Ectopic	
Pomeroy	657	145	18
Unipolar	168	133	45
Bipolar	197	98	41
Silastic ring	180	33	15
Spring clip	24	1	4

*As the amount of tubal destruction decreases, the rate of ectopic pregnancies among subsequent failures decreases.
From Phillips JM et al: American Association of Gynecologic Laparoscopists' 1979 membership survey, *J Reprod Med* 26:529, 1981.

sity of North Carolina in the development of the spring clip. Currently, the CREST study of the Centers for Disease Control (CDC) is following several thousand patients sterilized by a variety of techniques for a 5-year period. This ongoing national study is revealing a much higher pregnancy rate than was first appreciated for all methods of sterilization—approaching 0.8 per 100 pregnancies within 3 years. For these reasons, the latest education pamphlet on sterilization of the American College of Obstetricians and Gynecologists[1] states, "More than 99 out of every 100 women who have this procedure will not become pregnant, but you should be aware that the procedure does not guarantee sterility. Although the risk of failure is low, sometimes the procedure does not work."

Ectopic pregnancy is a rare but life-threatening form of pregnancy failure requiring early intervention for safe management. The CDC study has revealed that the late pregnancies after bipolar coagulation are mostly ectopic in nature. For this reason, we strongly recommend that a segment of isthmic tube next to the uterus be left when this technique is used, to minimize the risks of fistula formation.

Women with less tissue damage (from Pomeroy, band, and spring clip sterilization) have relatively less risk of ectopic pregnancy. Table 39-1 presents the comparative risks of ectopic pregnancy from different techniques.

COMPLICATIONS
Mortality

With widespread teaching of laparoscopic sterilization, major complication rates, defined as those requiring laparotomy for repair, have stayed below 2:1000 for the past decade. Mortality has not been reported since 1982.[15]

This makes the one-time risk of sterilization comparable to the annual risk of morbidity from oral contraceptives and probably explains why this method is so popular among U.S. women whose families are complete.

Posttubal syndrome

It is estimated that 6 million women in the United States have now undergone tubal sterilization. Many of these women's presenting symptoms are menometrorrhagia and pain, leading to the impression of a "posttubal syndrome" as a justification for hysterectomy. In an intensive analysis of this possibility, two prospective studies have recently been performed. Shain and co-workers[24] reported more initial menorrhagia, menstrual irregularity, and dysmenorrhea among women undergoing bipolar coagulation or Pomeroy ligation than among women undergoing mechanical tubal occlusion. Rulin and associates[23] reported a larger study showing only an increase in dysmenorrhea among sterilized women.

Endocrine changes

In a related issue, sterilization altering ovarian function has been observed independently by Radwanska and co-workers[22] and Donnez and co-workers.[6] In these studies, women who had undergone Pomeroy or coagulation sterilization had lower luteal progesterone levels (9 to 10 ng/ml) than normal controls or patients who had undergone clip sterilization (15 to 18 ng/ml). The authors postulated that extensive destruction of the vasculature with Pomeroy or coagulation caused interference in luteal function. However, other studies in both humans[2] and animals have failed to confirm these studies. After salpingectomy and hysterectomy, monkeys failed to reveal significant alterations in ovarian endocrine secretion.[4]

The conclusion to be drawn at the moment is that neither endocrine or symptomatic changes after sterilization have been consistently reported and that the posttubal syndrome remains to be documented.

Regret and reversibility

The permanent suspension of the reproductive function is not met with universal relief. Between 5% and 15% of women experience some form of regret over losing this function, but only 1% to 2% of sterilized women actually undergo reversal.[25] Since the average age of women requesting sterilization is 30, half of the requests are from women below this age. Recently, data from the United States[31] confirmed earlier findings among British[32] and Canadian[9] women that women sterilized below the age of 30 had a higher risk of requesting reversal later, usually after divorce and remarriage. The obstetrician-gynecologist thus faces a dilemma: whether to deny sterilization to hundreds of younger women who would benefit from the freedom from contraceptives and their risks in order to protect the reproductive ability of the few who may change their minds.

Recent experience with reversal has led to the insight, first proposed by Silber and Cohen,[26] that success of reversal sterilization is directly related to the length of tubal tissue remaining after sterilization. This was indirectly reported by Winston,[33] who found that anastomosis of isth-

Tubal Damage and Repair

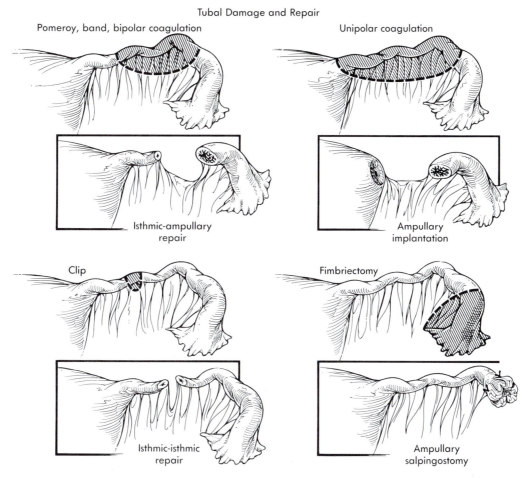

Fig. 39-11. Reversibility. Destroying a large portion of tube, particularly the junction of isthmus and ampulla, markedly diminishes the chance for a successful intrauterine pregnancy. (Adapted from Hulka JF, *Textbook of laparoscopy,* 1985, Grune & Stratton.)

mus to isthmus (after the least tubal damage) resulted in the highest success rates. A survey of microsurgeons who had performed reversal of clip sterilization[14] found an 87% intrauterine pregnancy rate. A review of the literature[25] revealed that unipolar coagulation, the most destructive method, had the lowest reversal rate, and the clip (least destructive) the highest. Figure 39-11 presents the nature of the repair necessary after different sterilization techniques.

Selection of the sterilization technique appropriate to a young patient should include preserving the option of reversal by choosing a minimally destructive method. It is important to stress that all sterilization procedures are *permanent,* requiring microsurgical procedures for reversal. In this context, if women are contemplating more pregnancies later in life, sterilization is not appropriate. However, patients and doctors make honest mistakes, and the younger patient is at greater risk for requesting reversal after divorce and remarriage. This is the single area in which the spring clip appears to offer a clear advantage over other methods.

COMPARISON OF TECHNIQUES

The trend in laparoscopic sterilization in the United States has been away from unipolar coagulation in favor of bipolar coagulation, band, and clip. Figure 39-12 presents the latest data, based on surveys of AAGL members.[15] A review of the literature concerning pregnancy failures and their management[11] revealed that the Irving procedure had no reported subsequent pregnancies. Interestingly, cornual resection (a sterilization technique no longer recommended) had a higher subsequent pregnancy rate than Pomeroy, and these pregnancies were interstitial or ectopic.

All laparoscopic sterilizations have a method failure of between 2 and 10 pregnancies per 1000 operations. The available studies cannot detect significant differences in failure rates among the various techniques. The largest comparative study,[2] based on 24,439 operations, showed no consistent differences among coagulation, band, and clip methods.

The *bipolar* method is the simplest to perform and the most popular method in the United States today but re-

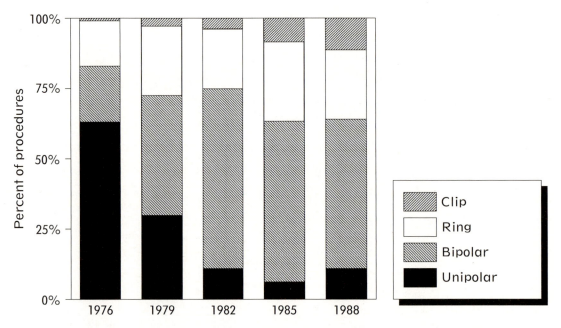

Fig. 39-12. Changing techniques in laparoscopic sterilization. Unipolar electrocoagulation has been displaced by bipolar coagulation as the leading method in the United States. (From Hulka JF et al: American Association of Gynecologic Laparoscopists' 1988 membership survey on laparoscopic sterilization, *J Reprod Med* 35(6):584, 1990.)

quires proper matched equipment (forceps and generator). Failures continue for years after the procedure and are often ectopic pregnancies, as recently reported from Scandinavia.[19] The cumulative bipolar failure rate in 6 years was 1.18%, all extrauterine. These authors urged the preservation of a 2-cm proximal isthmic stump to reduce the chance of subsequent fistula formation and ectopic pregnancies.

The *band* method is widely used and a good nonelectric method, though backup bipolar coagulation is recommended for occasional bleeding. Postoperative pain from the constricted tube is most severe with this technique.

The *clip* requires careful surgical technique to assure proper placement across the isthmus of the tube. Nonetheless, it is the least destructive technique, and therefore the most reversible, and should be offered to women below age 30 seeking sterilization. Pregnancies after clip applications appear to occur mostly within the first 2 years, with long-term follow-up studies showing few pregnancies afterwards. Thus, the long-term cumulative pregnancy rates with bipolar sterilization and the clip are similar.

Unipolar coagulation still has advocates among skilled practitioners, in whose hands patients will be well served, but this technique is not recommended for the younger patient who may later desire sterilization reversal.

Complication rates have been measured[5] for coagulation, band, and clip. All techniques had a similar rate of readmission for complications, but coagulation required a 10.5-day average stay (to rule out or manage bowel perforation); the band, 5.5 days (to rule out or manage pelvic

Table 39-2. Safety and efficacy: comparison of sterilization methods

	Coagulation	Band	Clip
Safety			
Days of readmission for complications	10.5	5.5	2.1
Late ectopic rate (%)	44	15	4
Reversibility			
Term pregnancies following reversal (%)	41	72	84
Efficacy			
1-year method failure range (rate per 1000)	1.9-2.6	3.3-4.7	1.8-5.9

Data from Chi IC et al,[5] Phillips JM et al,[21] and Siegler AM et al.[25]

infection); and the clip, 2.1 days, a statistically significant difference.

The comparative data available for safety and efficacy of different sterilization methods are summarized in Table 39-2.

I have consistently recommended that physicians choose the technique with which they are most comfortable and continue to provide this service to their patients until surgical misadventure or compelling reasons in the literature motivate a change of techniques.

REFERENCES

1. American College of Obstetricians and Gynecologists: *Sterilization for women and men,* AP011, April 1991.
2. Bhiwandiwala PP et al: A comparison of different laparoscopic sterilization occlusion techniques in 24,439 procedures, *Am J Obstet Gynecol* 144:319, 1982.
3. Bishop E, Nelms WF: A simple method of tubal sterilization, *N Y State J Med* 30:214, 1930.
4. Castracane VD et al: Ovarian function in hysterectomized Macaca Fascicularis, *Biol Reprod* 20:462, 1979.
5. Chi IC et al: Rare events associated with tubal sterilizations: an international experience, *Obstet Gynecol Surv* 41:7, 1986.
6. Donnez J et al: Luteal function after tubal sterilization, *Obstet Gynecol* 57:65, 1981.
7. Erb RA, Reed TP: Hysteroscopic oviductal blocking with formed-in-place silicone rubber plugs: method and apparatus, *J Reprod Med* 23:65, 1979.
8. Fishburne JI Jr, Hulka JF: Tubal healing following laparoscopic electrocoagulation, *J Reprod Med* 16:129, 1976.
9. Gomel V: Profile of women requesting reversal of sterilization, *Fertil Steril* 30:39, 1978.
10. Houck RM et al: Hysteroscopic tubal occlusion with formed-in-place silicone plugs: a clinical review, *Obstet Gynecol* 62:587, 1983.
11. Hulka JF, Mitchell L: *Resterilization after tubal sterilization failure.* In Nichols DH, editor: Reoperative gynecologic surgery, St Louis, 1991, Mosby–Year Book.
12. Hulka JF, Omran KF: Comparative tubal occlusion: rigid and spring-loaded clips, *Fertil Steril* 23:633, 1972.
13. Hulka JF et al: Spring clip sterilization: one-year follow-up of 1,079 cases, *Am J Obstet Gynecol* 125:1039, 1976.
14. Hulka JF et al: Reversibility of clip sterilizations, *Lancet* 2:927, 1982.
15. Hulka JF et al: American Association of Gynecologic Laparoscopists' 1988 membership survey on laparoscopic sterilization, *J Reprod Med* 35(6):584, 1990.
16. Irving FC: A new method of insuring sterility following cesarean section, *Am J Obstet Gynecol* 8:335, 1924.
17. Kroener WF Jr: Surgical sterilization by fimbriectomy, *Am J Obstet Gynecol* 104:247, 1969.
18. Lee SH, Jones JS: Postpartum tubal sterilization: a comparative study of Hulka clip application and the modified Pomeroy technique, *J Reprod Med,* in press.
19. Makar AP et al: Female sterilization failure after bipolar electrocoagulation: a 6 year retrospective study, *Eur J Obstet Gynecol Reprod Biol* 37:237, 1990.
20. Peterson HB et al: Deaths attributable to tubal sterilization in the United States, 1977 to 1981, *Am J Obstet Gynecol* 146:131, 1983.
21. Phillips JM et al: American Association of Gynecologic Laparoscopists' 1979 membership survey, *J Reprod Med* 26:529, 1981.
22. Radwanska E et al: Luteal deficiency among women with normal menstrual cycles, requesting reversal of tubal sterilization, *Obstet Gynecol* 54:189, 1979.
23. Rulin MC et al: Changes in menstrual symptoms among sterilized and comparison women: a prospective study, *Obstet Gynecol* 74:149, 1989.
24. Shain RN et al: Menstrual pattern change 1 year after sterilization: results of a controlled, prospective study, *Fertil Steril* 52:192, 1989.
25. Siegler AM et al: Reversibility of female sterilization, *Fertil Steril* 43:499, April 1985.
26. Silber SJ, Cohen R: Microsurgical reversal of female sterilization: the role of tubal length, *Fertil Steril* 33:598, 1980.
27. Soderstrom RM et al: Reducing bipolar sterilization failures, *Obstet Gynecol* 74:60, 1989.
28. Steptoe PC: *Laparoscopy in gynaecology,* Edinburgh, 1967, Livingstone.
29. Stock RJ: Histopathologic changes in tubal pregnancy, *J Reprod Med* 30:923, 1985.
30. Uchida H: Uchida tubal sterilization, *Am J Obstet Gynecol* 121:153, 1975.
31. Wilcox LS et al: Risk factors for regret after tubal sterilization: 5 years of follow-up in a prospective study, *Fertil Steril* 55:927, 1991.
32. Winston RML: Why 103 women asked for reversal of sterilisation, *Br Med J* 2(6082):305, 1977.
33. Winston RML: Microsurgery of the fallopian tube: from fantasy to reality, *Fertil Steril* 34:521, 1980.
34. Yoon IB et al: A two-year experience with the falope ring sterilization procedure, *Am J Obstet Gynecol* 127:109, 1977.

Chapter 40

ADNEXAL SURGERY FOR BENIGN DISEASE

James M. Wheeler

In 1809, McDowell removed a large benign ovary. Removal replaced the older practice of "tapping" a cyst, with its attendant risk of leaking the contents of the cyst into the peritoneal cavity—a facet of ovarian cyst removal that to this day is the subject of much debate. This chapter reviews aspects of surgical treatment of benign diseases of the ovary, tube, and adnexal appendages.

PREOPERATIVE DIAGNOSIS AND MANAGEMENT

Benign diseases of the adnexa usually present with the symptom of pain or the sign of palpable adnexal enlargement. A variety of preoperative evaluative techniques may aid the surgeon in the operating room. Although it is often true that "the only thing that separates us from the answer is the skin," most of us appreciate whatever hints we can ascertain preoperatively.

Serum markers—specifically CA-125—lack the sensitivity to be effective screening measures for benign *and* malignant adnexal disease and, if elevated, lack the specificity to distinguish benign *versus* malignant adnexal disease. If an elevated CA-125 drops significantly after the debulking of benign or malignant disease, it may be useful to check occasionally in follow-up to detect recurrent disease. Excellent work is underway in the development of monoclonal antibody techniques directed toward markers of malignant ovarian epithelial tumors; perhaps a marker will be developed to be a useful screening device as well as a differentiator between benign and malignant adnexal processes.

Ultrasonography can help a surgeon's clinical suspicion that an adnexal lesion is more likely benign than malignant.[1] The probability of a benign process increases with observation of a cystic rather than a solid lesion, unilocu-

lar rather than multilocular, localized rather than diffuse, and lack of ascites. Several benign processes are notoriously difficult to differentiate from more lethal disease on sonographic criteria, including teratomas and endometriomata. Doppler-aided sonography has been used to distinguish the normal architecture of vascular anatomy in benign disease from the aberrant vasculature associated with malignancies of the adnexa. Transvaginal sonography is preferred when the adnexal mass is confined to the true pelvis; otherwise, combined transvaginal/transabdominal scanning may offer the most accurate characterization of the mass. All surgeons performing sonography preoperatively are reminded that histology continues to be the gold standard of diagnosis of the adnexa. However, preoperative sonography may aid a surgeon in choosing a surgical approach (i.e., laparoscopy or laparotomy) or type of incision, as well as suggesting a benign or malignant process.

Computed tomography (CT) and magnetic resonance imaging (MRI) are generally less useful than sonography in studying adnexal masses. Perhaps with more experience, these more expensive techniques may have some demonstrable superiority, but the cystic/solid nature of adnexal disease is quite amenable to the less expensive evaluation by ultrasound.

For the large adnexal mass, knowledge of the course of the ureters may reduce the chances of operative trauma. Most commonly, an intravenous pyelogram (IVP) is ordered; the surgeon should designate in the request to the radiologist which portion of the ureter is particularly critical to be visualized and recorded on film. Often, a lateral view of the ureters on IVP supplements the visualization offered by the traditional anteroposterior view.

A preoperative mechanical bowel prep of some sort aids exposure in most adnexal cases. If the adnexa is particularly large, or immobile, or associated with ureteric compression or deflection on IVP, a full mechanical and antibiotic bowel prep is prudent.

Because of the possibilities of castration and sterility with adnexal surgery, full informed consent from the woman contemplating adnexal surgery is mandatory. Possibilities that must be addressed include removal of the ipsilateral ovary or tube, biopsy, and even removal of the contralateral adnexa. Whatever surgical option is recommended for the patient—laparoscopy or laparotomy, cystectomy or adnexectomy—*all* surgical and medical alternatives should be reviewed preoperatively. Written documentation of these critical points should be permanently represented in the medical record.

CHOOSING THE SURGICAL APPROACH

The sole goal of choosing a surgical approach is to optimize the likelihood of safe, effective treatment of the patient by the surgeon. Data and experience are insufficient to conclude that laparoscopy is always preferable to laparotomy (or vice versa) or that transvaginal ultrasound-guided aspiration is preferable to both.

Laparoscopic cystectomy and adnexectomy have been done for all types of benign conditions of all sorts and sizes; unfortunately, the superiority of endoscopic techniques has yet to be proven in randomized clinical trials compared directly to open techniques. Nevertheless, for certain adnexal processes, laparoscopic approaches are appropriate in most cases; these cases include simple ovarian cysts of fair size and small endometriomata. Again, there is no consensus as to what size a cyst should be to be handled laparoscopically, with experts suggesting ranges between 5 and 15 cm. Surgeons always vary where they "draw the line" in performing adnexal surgery by way of the laparoscope rather than laparotomy, but the decision should represent their own experience and skill as well as what has been demonstrated in the literature.[4] Most laparoscopic adnexectomies or cystectomies are best performed with a three puncture technique; a colpotomy incision is often useful in delivering larger masses from the peritoneal cavity. Retention bags have been marketed to aid retrieval of adnexal bits from the abdomen.

Regardless of the surgical approach taken, certain principles should be followed:

- *Minimal tissue handling.* When necessary, tissues should be handled gently with noncrushing instruments. Whenever possible, the tissue to be removed can be amply manipulated and undamaged, leaving the tissue preserved in better condition.
- *Constant irrigation.* Surgeons vary as to their favorite "magic solution," although heparinized (5000 U/L) lactated Ringer's solution seems most prevalent. Care must be taken not to sequester the fluid in the abdomen for a prolonged period of time because the heparin does gradually cross the peritoneum.
- *Minimal suturing.* When suturing is necessary, as

small a caliber a needle and the thinnest suture possible is chosen. Especially in the adnexa, sutures should be hidden as much as possible, and knots should be buried, to try to reduce de novo adhesion formation.
- *Complete hemostasis.* No adjunct to inhibit adhesion formation will work as well in the presence of even small amounts of blood.
- Whatever the energy sources used during the case, whether cautery or laser, whether endoscopic or open, the surgeon must have a thorough knowledge of the biophysics of the energy source (especially as applied to live tissue) to minimize the risk of damage to the repaired adnexa as well as the ureter and bowel.
- Careful inspection of the contralateral adnexum for disease, and appropriate biopsy and treatment.
- *Magnification when useful in suture placement or dissection.* Similar degrees of magnification (2.5 to 5×) are attainable at laparoscopy or laparotomy.

If there is any suspicion of malignancy, a frozen section is performed on the tissue. If the intraoperative histologic diagnosis is equivocal, peritoneal washings should be obtained, the contralateral ovary should be biopsied, and numerous peritoneal and omental biopsies should be taken in case the final histology suggests a lesion of indeterminate biologic activity, also known as a borderline tumor.[2,3]

Vascular surgical anatomy of the adnexum

The tube and ovary benefit from collateral circulation originating from two sources (Fig. 40-1). The distal tube and ovary derive most of their blood supply from the ovarian artery, whereas the proximal tube is largely supplied by a branch of the uterine artery. The blood vessels to the ovary are opposite those of the tube within the mesosalpinx; this area between the tube and ovary must be avoided, although sometimes it is difficult to determine where adhesions end and normal peritoneum begins. When bleeding is encountered, the most specific, least traumatic method of hemostasis must be applied—typically point ligature or bipolar cautery. As long as the hilar vessels are not overly traumatized, the adnexa are fairly resilient to some hemostatic measures. The adnexa should be removed only if there is no hope for blood supply to the ovary. If the tissue is still capable of oozing if nicked, there is a good chance that the tissue will be viable after healing. All consent forms should include the uncommon, but important, possibility of future adnexal removal if conserving the organ fails.

Besides blood vessels, the adnexal surgeon needs to keep manipulations, including incisions, away from the fimbria as much as possible if the adnexum is to be preserved. One favored technique is to make an ovarian incision on the underside of the ovary to keep the raw surface away from the fimbria; because this incision is at risk for adhering over the ureter, interposing an adjunct such as In-

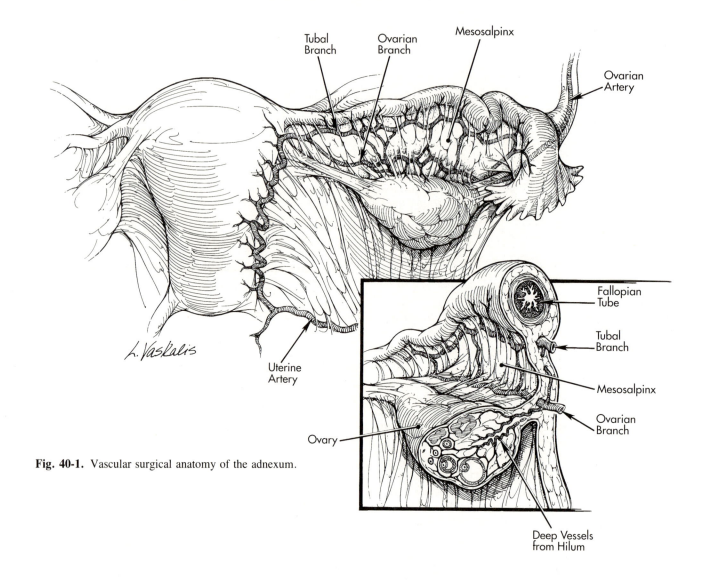

Fig. 40-1. Vascular surgical anatomy of the adnexum.

terceed TC-7 between the ovary and sidewall may be of use if hemostasis is complete.

Oophorectomy and oophorocystectomy

Similar techniques are used to remove the adnexa, regardless of the benign condition present (Fig. 40-2):

- *Identification of the ureter.* In the presence of obliterative benign conditions like endometriosis or severe adhesions, a retroperitoneal approach may be preferable.
- *Isolation of the blood supply.* The infundibulopelvic ligament should be occluded without damaging surrounding vital tissues including the ureter and iliac vessels. Ligature is preferred; experience with staplers suggests they are effective. If sufficiently small, the ovarian artery and vein may be bipolar or endocoagulated, remembering that adnexal enlargement often results in larger supplying vessels.
- *Complete removal of ovarian tissue.* Again, obliterative diseases such as endometriosis may mandate a retroperitoneal approach in which a significant patch

of peritoneum is removed from the ureter with the ovary to effect complete oophorectomy.

- *Retroperitonealization of knots and complete hemostasis to lessen adhesion risk.* Reperitonealization is counterproductive if the peritoneum is stretched or if sutures are too tight.

Ovarian follicular cysts. These cysts are the result of faulty ovulation and usually regress if given sufficient time. Typically presenting with pain, they are simple cysts on ultrasound of sizes varying from 1 to 7 cm, and sometimes larger. Multiple follicular cysts are not rare and especially follow the use of ovulation-inducing drugs. If the woman's pain can be conservatively managed, these cysts may simply be followed for 3 to 4 months; over 90% demonstrate shrinkage over this period of time and may simply be followed. The element of time seems to be more important than suppression of endogenous gonadotropin secretion with oral contraceptives.

Surgery is indicated if the pain is severe, or if rupture and bleeding are suspected, or more rarely, for torsion with its attendant acute abdomen. Follicular cysts are the

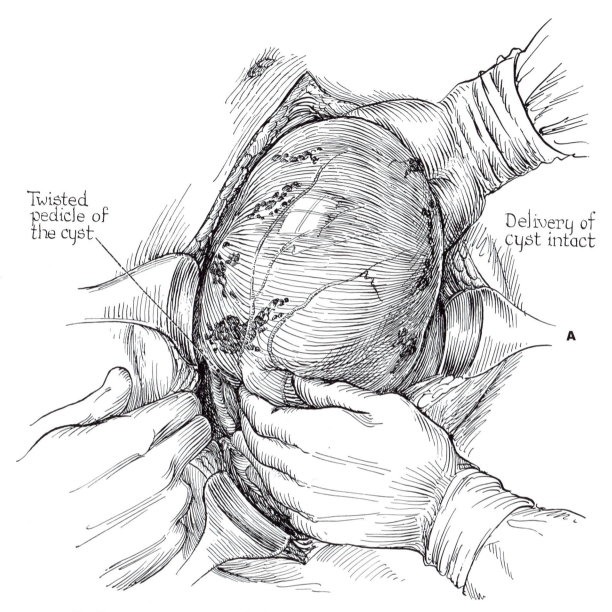

Twisted pedicle of the cyst

Delivery of cyst intact

A

Fig. 40-2. Oophorectomy. An incision believed to be adequate to deliver the cyst is made either in a longitudinal or a transverse direction. At times, this incision may extend from the symphysis to the xiphoid process. **A,** Delivery of a moderately large ovarian cyst with a twisted pedicle. The cyst was delivered intact and was not necrotic, although the circulation was impaired.

Continued.

type most amenable to transvaginal ultrasound-guided aspiration; laparoscopy just for aspiration is unwarranted. If the patient undergoes anesthesia for this cyst, it should be removed and sent for histologic confirmation of its benign nature. Many of these cysts are managed laparoscopically, although unusually large ones may require laparotomy. Oophorectomy is almost never required for these cysts.

The entire cyst should be removed or destroyed; bleeding is variable, but often minimal. Sutures or careful coagulation for hemostasis is usually all that is required; typically, the edges of the ovary oppose and may be returned safely to the pelvis.

Corpus luteum cysts. Similar to follicular cysts, corpus luteum cysts represent faulty ovulation. They tend to

be thicker, blood or clot filled, and more difficult to remove. However, also like follicular cysts, they resolve in most cases after 3 to 4 months should somatic symptoms not indicate quicker intervention. Sonographically, these cysts are echogenic and, with time, demonstrate lucency as hemolysis within the cyst occurs. Unfortunately, corpus luteum cysts are sonographically identical to endometriomata and even epithelial cancers of the ovary and must be followed closely.

If removal is necessary, frozen section is useful to address the possibility of malignancy. More bleeding occurs than with follicular cysts, but, often, waiting and point coagulation or ligature are all that is needed. More often than with similar-sized follicular cysts, persistent bleeding will

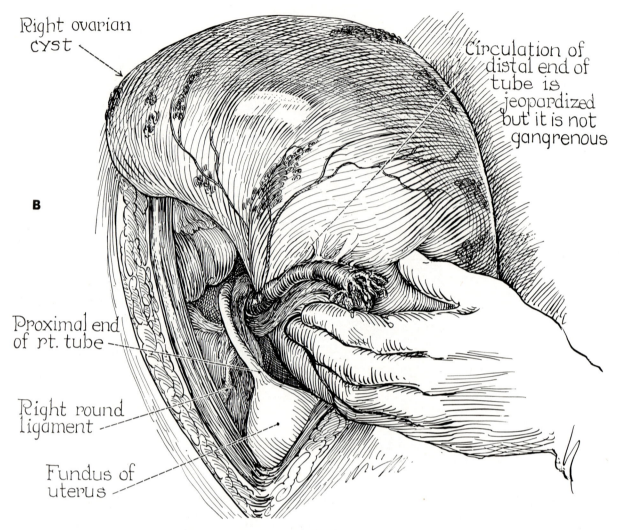

Right ovarian cyst

Circulation of distal end of tube is jeopardized but it is not gangrenous

B

Proximal end of rt. tube

Right round ligament

Fundus of uterus

Fig. 40-2, cont'd. B, Observation of the tube revealed the circulation to be adequate so that the tube could be preserved. No functional, normal ovarian tissue was observed. If even a fragment of normal ovarian tissue can be preserved, an oophorocystectomy, in a young patient with a benign lesion, is preferable to loss of the entire ovary.

indicate oophorectomy, again emphasizing the value of following these cysts for several months whenever possible.

Polycystic ovaries (also known as Stein-Leventhal syndrome, thecalutein cysts). Surgery is reserved in these women *only* if conservative medical treatment fails. The vast majority are managed by oral contraceptives or ovulation induction (if pregnancy is desired). Ovarian wedge resection is indicated only for progressive androgenization or anovulation refractory to medical treatment; the benefits of wedge resection are temporary, and the procedure is associated with a 50% risk of adhesion formation. If performed, the viability of the ovary must be maintained while a significant proportion of the ovarian stroma is removed. Again, minimal suturing is used: a few deep 4-0 absorbable sutures and a fine 6-0 to 8-0 polydioxanone subcortical suture are sufficient (Fig. 40-3).

Endometriomata. Women with endometriomata often

have dysmenorrhea or deep dyspareunia or are infertile. On ultrasound, these cysts are 1 to 6 cm in diameter (sometimes larger) and echo-filled. Contrary to corpus luteum cysts, their contents do not clear as a result of hemolysis. Sometimes, echo-dense areas including septa are seen within endometriomata, raising the possibility of benign teratoma.

Tiny endometriomata less than 1 cm are best vaporized, with care taken to ensure complete removal upon irrigation of the defect. Endometriomata larger than this are dissected free of the ovary, with care taken to ensure complete removal or destruction of the cyst wall. Spillage of cyst contents is inevitable with larger lesions; the "chocolate" fluid must be immediately and completely irrigated or aspirated because of the inflammation it causes.

These ovaries tend to be more contorted than those treated for a follicular or corpus luteum cyst. These cases have more inflammation and more adhesions, and are at

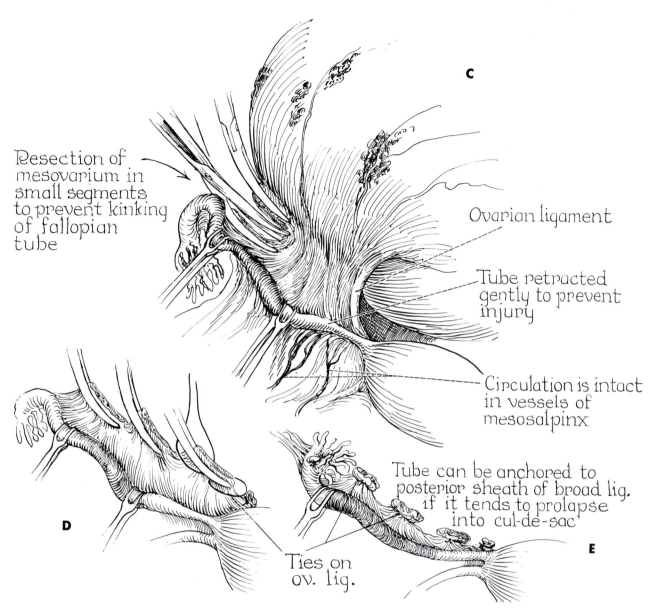

Resection of
mesovarium in
small segments
to prevent kinking
of fallopian
tube

Ovarian ligament

Tube retracted
gently to prevent
injury

Circulation is intact
in vessels of
mesosalpinx

Tube can be anchored to
posterior sheath of broad lig.
if it tends to prolapse
into cul-de-sac

Ties on
ov. lig.

C

D

E

Fig. 40-2, cont'd. C, The mesovarium is clamped, cut, and ligated in small segments to prevent kinking. Because this patient was desirous of having children, great care was exercised to prevent any injury to the tube, despite the fact that no ovarian tissue could be preserved. **D,** The ties on the mesovarium are of fine absorbable suture, which cause only a minimum of reaction. **E,** If the tube tends to prolapse into the cul-de-sac, it is anchored to the posterior sheath of the broad ligament so it remains near its normal position. (From Ball TL: *Gynecologic surgery and urology,* ed 2, St Louis, 1963, Mosby–Year Book.)

greater risk for postoperative adhesion formation. If the edges do not approximate, careful suturing is warranted with care taken to avoid devascularizing the ovary. Complete hemostasis is a must, but without destroying the ovary. Ample irrigation and the use of Interceed may help inhibit some adhesions; in the infertility patient, second-look laparoscopy should be discussed as a possibility, recognizing the lack of unequivocal proof of efficacy in terms of improved pregnancy rates.

Benign neoplasms of the ovary. The most common lesion in this category is the benign cystic teratoma; other

lesions include benign epithelial tumors, usually of the serous or mucinous type. Frozen section confirmation of the benign nature of these lesions is mandatory.

Even when the lesion is large, a cystectomy is usually possible. Although it seems that all that is left is a "shell" of ovary, it should be preserved if viable as a future source of oocytes, remembering oocytes are found in the cortex of the ovary rather than the stroma displaced by the tumor (Fig. 40-4). Often, the leaves of the ovaries oppose one another, with less inflammation than found with endometriomata.

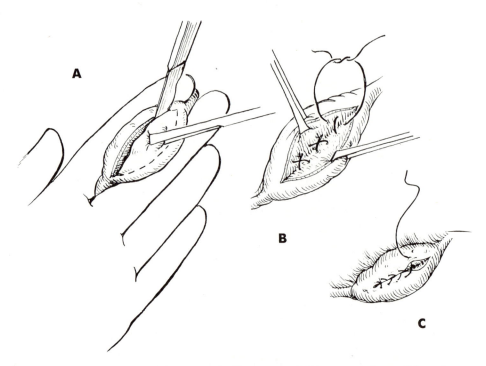

Fig. 40-3. Wedge resection of the ovary. **A,** The operator holds one ovarian pedicle and ovary between the index and middle fingers of the left hand. The broader inferior convexity of the ovary is grasped in an Allis clamp and approximately a third of the ovary is excised in wedge configuration by means of a scalpel down to the medulla. **B,** Allis' forceps are placed on the cut edges of the ovary and three or more figure-of-eight 4-0 absorbable sutures are used with the double intent of hemostasis as well as approximation of the two sides of the incision. **C,** The surface of the ovary is closed with an extremely fine, continuous nonabsorbable suture. (From Corson SL, Sedlacek TV, Hoffman JJ: *Greenhill's surgical gynecology,* ed 5, St Louis, 1986, Mosby–Year Book.)

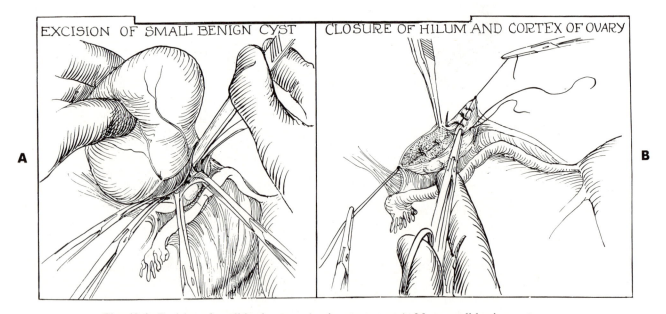

Fig. 40-4. Excision of small benign cysts (oophorocystectomy). Many small benign cysts are removed, with preservation of normal ovarian tissue. The surgical principles in this operation are shown in **A** and **B.** An incision is made along the base of the cyst between its wall and normal ovarian tissue. The cyst wall is carefully dissected from normal ovarian tissue. The contents of a dermoid cyst produce irritation if spilled in the peritoneal cavity, so the field of operation is protected with laparotomy pads. Bleeding points in the ovarian stroma are ligated, and the ovary is closed by interrupted sutures of fine suture. A minimum number of sutures consistent with adequate closure and hemostasis are employed. (From Ball TL: *Gynecologic surgery and urology,* ed 2, St Louis, 1963, Mosby–Year Book.)

The contralateral ovary must be carefully inspected and palpated due to the approximately 25% chance of it having a similar lesion. However, the ovary should not be incised if no palpable or visible defect is identified. Again, the possibility of future surgery for the condition should be covered during the informed consent procedure.

"Palpable post-menopausal ovary" (PMPO) syndrome. A special clinical circumstance is encountered in the menopausal woman with a small adnexal mass. These lesions are so frequently benign that some experts recommend expectant management. Unfortunately, few women today accept waiting and watching for signs of spreading of the lesion. This is one of the most useful aspects of laparoscopic evaluation and treatment, as long as any suspicion of malignancy is acted upon and laparotomy is performed appropriately. Adnexectomy is the usual course of treatment; some experts recommend the ovary be removed intact in these situations by way of a colpotomy incision. Again, extreme care must be taken to ensure the benign nature of these lesions so that traditional staging laparotomy would be performed otherwise.

Ovarian remnant syndrome. One of the dreaded complications of previous adnexal surgery is the ovarian remnant syndrome. Usually, these women present with pain, and, often, no identifiable gonad can be found by either palpation or sonography. At surgery, the best approach is retroperitoneal; once the ureter and hopefully the stump of the infundibulopelvic are identified, the entire peritoneal area that might contain ovarian tissue is dissected free.[5,6] The ureter may be obstructed or involved in adhesions; preoperative pyelography is mandatory in these cases. These are among the most challenging of benign adnexal operations. As such, an attempt at ovarian suppression with the oral contraceptive should be attempted if not contraindicated. In women with significant medical comorbidity, consideration can be given to radiation of the area, although this modality has its own attendant risks including bowel injury. When surgical extirpation has been selected because of persistent pain, and the ovarian tissue volume is small, the remnant may be easier to find at surgery if a preoperative course of clomiphene has been given.

Tubal and parovarian cysts

Sometimes, the supposed ovarian cyst proves to be tubal or, more appropriately termed, paratubal. (Operations pertaining to tubal function in fertility are discussed in Chapter 47.) Small paratubal cysts are rarely a problem, although they may undergo torsion and even more rarely require surgical removal. Larger hydatid cysts on the end of the fimbriae could potentially affect fertility and should be carefully removed. Some paratubal cysts may be 3 to 8 cm in size, typically simple on ultrasound, and somewhat challenging surgically as the tube is splayed over them. One useful technique is to make a small 2- to 3-cm incision on the end of the cyst farthest from the fimbria without breaking the cyst for as long as possible. Then, using a combination of sharp dissection and irrigator-assisted "hy-

dro-dissection," the surgeon separates the cyst from its attachments (Fig. 40-5). Bleeding is usually caused by the native tubal vessels, because these cysts are usually poorly vascularized. Once the cyst inevitably ruptures, the fluid is aspirated, and the entire cyst is dissected from its base. Point ligature or bipolar coagulation is used to achieve hemostasis; the small mesosalpingeal incision may be left open to heal.

Rarely, noncystic tubal benign disease is encountered and must be removed. Typically, women present with the presumed diagnosis of ovarian lesions. Most common among these entities are tubal leiomyomata; care must be taken in their removal because they may directly impinge on the tubal submucosa. All solid tumors must have a frozen section; localized fallopian tube carcinomas are usually incidental surgical findings.

Salpingo-oophorectomy and salpingectomy. When the ovary is being removed and the tube and its blood supply are badly damaged, salpingo-oophorectomy may be prudent. Careful attention to ligation of both the ovarian artery and the ascending branch of the uterine artery is necessary to ensure hemostasis. The technique is illustrated in Fig. 40-6. When only the tube is to be removed at laparotomy, the clamping and incision in the mesosalpinx are made as close to the tube as possible, preserving the blood supply of the ovary remaining.

Ovarian preservation at hysterectomy

A final adnexal operation is ovarian suspension after hysterectomy. If closure of the cuff or pelvic peritoneum affixes the ovaries to the cuff, placing the patient at risk for dyspareunia, the ovaries may be placed up on the sidewall to avoid this late complication. Attaching the utero-ovarian ligament and proximal tube to the round ligament is one useful technique that also allows burying of knots in the retroperitoneum. Care should be taken not to stretch the infundibulopelvic ligament or to leave the adnexum freely mobile, predisposing to torsion.

For the patient undergoing hysterectomy for malignancy, the ovaries may be marked with titanium clips so that they may be avoided if postoperative radiotherapy is required. Steel clips are more disruptive if CT or MRI scans are needed in the future.

SUMMARY

Many benign conditions of the ovary resolve with expectant management or hormonal suppression over 3 to 4 months. Because of the attendant risks of surgery and late complications of adhesion formation and infertility, ovarian lesions should be operated on only for severe pain or persistence after several months of sonographic follow-up. Once surgery is recommended, it is the obligation of each surgeon to recommend the best surgical approach to the problem, which always varies among physicians and specifics about the case. Adnexectomy is indicated if the ovary is destroyed or the woman is decidedly beyond childbearing; otherwise, most lesions may be removed

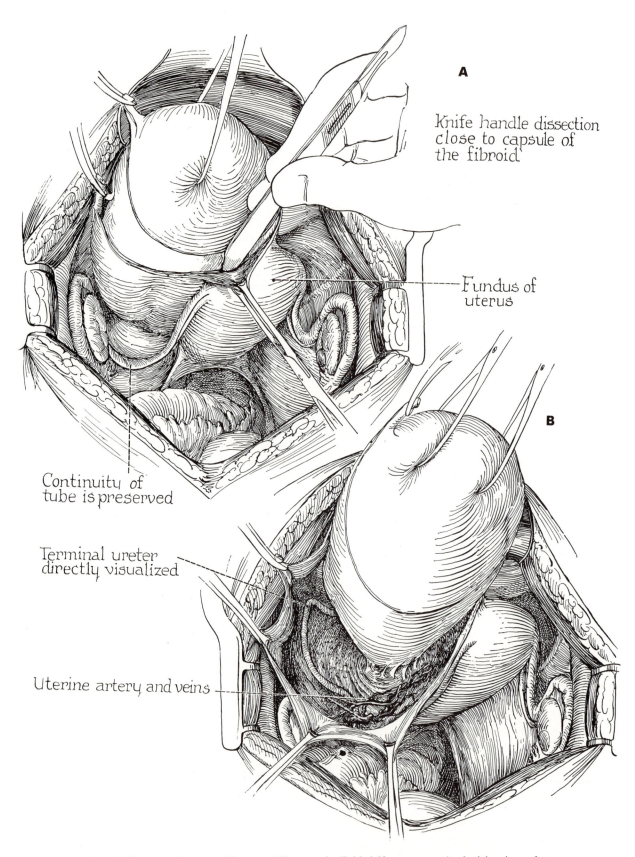

A

Knife handle dissection close to capsule of the fibroid

Fundus of uterus

B

Continuity of tube is preserved

Terminal ureter directly visualized

Uterine artery and veins

Fig. 40-5. Parovarian cyst. The round ligament is divided if necessary. An incision is made to remove the excess peritoneum over the tumor. By alternately using the finger, knife, and knife handle, the tumor is shelled from its bed. **A,** The dissection is done within the capsule, particularly near the tube, so as not to disturb the continuity of the latter. **B,** The intraligamentary lesion is almost removed from its bed. The dissection has now exposed the ureter and uterine artery and its accompanying veins.

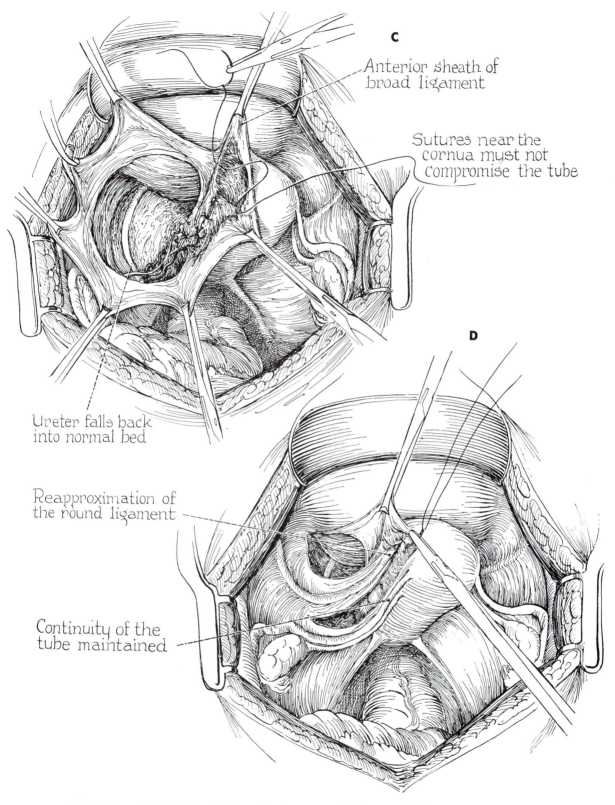

C

Anterior sheath of broad ligament

Sutures near the cornua must not compromise the tube

Ureter falls back into normal bed

D

Reapproximation of the round ligament

Continuity of the tube maintained

Fig. 40-5, cont'd. C, When the tumor has been removed, the ureter falls back into a normal bed. The round ligament is reapproximated by several interrupted sutures and the anterior sheath of the broad ligament is closed. **D,** The peritoneum is closed over the operative site, with care being exercised not to constrict or angulate the Fallopian tube. (From Ball TL: *Gynecologic surgery and urology,* ed 2, St Louis, 1963, Mosby–Year Book.)

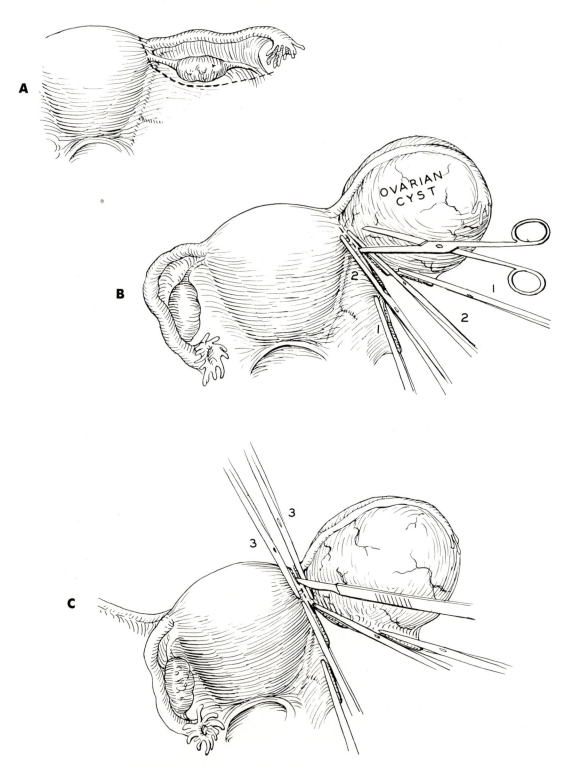

Fig. 40-6. Salpingo-oophorectomy. **A,** Relationship of a normal tube and ovary to the uterus. The dotted line shows the proposed line of incision for the removal of both tube and ovary. **B,** A large ovarian cyst is to be removed. Before a salpingo-oophorectomy is performed, one must be certain that both tube and ovary have been freed from the surrounding structures. Two clamps are placed high on the infundibulopelvic ligament about 1 cm apart to avoid the ureter, and the ligament is divided between them with a scissors. A second pair of clamps are placed in such a way that they take in not only the remainder of the broad ligament but also the ascending portion of the uterine artery. The tissue between these clamps is similarly divided. **C,** Two clamps are placed across the proximal isthmus of the fallopian tube. The tube is then bisected with a scissors. The proximal segment is trimmed with a fine scissors in such a way that the endosalpinx is not permitted to "pout." It is ligated with a 0 absorbable suture, as the clamp is removed.

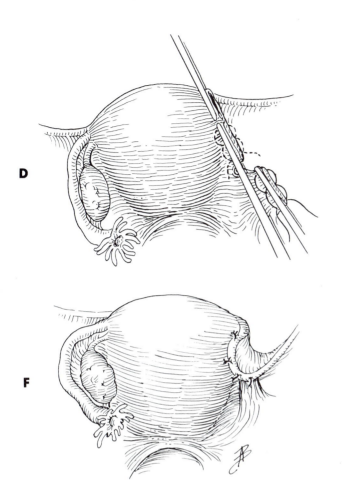

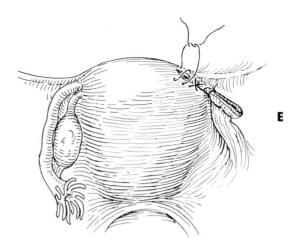

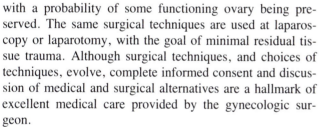

Fig. 40-6, cont'd. D, Two clamps remain. A figure-of-eight 0 absorbable suture is placed around the clamp on the infundibulopelvic ligament. A second similar suture placed around the second clamp takes in the remainder of the broad ligament as well as the ascending branch of the uterine artery. **E,** Before closing, it is advisable to observe the broad and infundibulopelvic ligaments for several minutes to be certain that there is not a hematoma forming between their leaves. If necessary, the infundibulopelvic ligament can be doubly ligated with a free tie of absorbable 0 suture material. **F,** The round ligament may be sutured over the raw area with absorbable suture. (From Corson SL, Sedlacek TV, Hoffman JJ: *Greenhill's surgical gynecology,* ed 5, St Louis, 1986, Mosby–Year Book.)

with a probability of some functioning ovary being preserved. The same surgical techniques are used at laparoscopy or laparotomy, with the goal of minimal residual tissue trauma. Although surgical techniques, and choices of techniques, evolve, complete informed consent and discussion of medical and surgical alternatives are a hallmark of excellent medical care provided by the gynecologic surgeon.

REFERENCES

1. American College of Obstetricians and Gynecologists: Benign ovarian cysts, *Precis* IV:202, 1991.
2. Chambers JT et al: Borderline ovarian tumors, *Am J Obstet Gynecol* 159(5):1088, 1988.
3. Lim-Tan SK, Cajigas HE, Scully RE: Ovarian cystectomy for serous borderline tumors: a follow-up study of 35 cases, *Obstet Gynecol* 72(5):775, 1988.
4. Perry CP, Upchurch JC: Pelviscopic adnexectomy, *Am J Obstet Gynecol* 162:79, 1990.
5. Pettit PD, Lee RA: Ovarian remnant syndrome: diagnostic dilemma and surgical challenge, *Obstet Gynecol* 71:580, 1988.
6. Steege JF: Ovarian remnant syndrome, *Obstet Gynecol* 70:64, 1987.

Chapter 41

SURGERY FOR CANCER OF THE OVARY

Stephen C. Rubin
John L. Lewis, Jr.

Ovarian cancer is the leading cause of death in women with gynecologic malignancies. Although it accounts for only approximately 27% of new gynecologic cancer cases each year in the United States, this deadly disease kills more U.S. women each year than all the other gynecologic malignancies combined. Because ovarian cancer is completely asymptomatic in its early stages and there is no effective screening test for early disease, early diagnosis is infrequent and generally serendipitous. The major advances that have been made in the chemotherapy of ovarian cancer over the last 15 years have tended to overshadow our enhanced understanding of the role of the gynecologic cancer surgeon in the management of this disease.

Surgery remains the cornerstone of the treatment of ovarian cancer, playing a critical part in diagnosis and staging, removal of tumor, assessment of response to chemotherapy, and palliation of symptoms including intestinal obstruction. Surgery plays three roles in the management of ovarian cancer:

1. Primary
   a. Establish diagnosis, histology, and grade of the cancer
   b. Define extent of the disease (staging)
   c. Resect tumor (primary cytoreduction)
2. Secondary
   a. Assess response to therapy (second-look laparotomy)
   b. Resect tumor (secondary cytoreduction)
3. Supportive and palliative
   a. Relieve intestinal obstruction
   b. Alleviate pleural effusion or ascites
   c. Intravenous access
   d. Intraperitoneal access

Despite the importance of surgery in the management of this disease, in most cases surgery alone is inadequate treatment for ovarian cancer and provides only a brief interruption in the inexorable progression of the disease. At the same time, both chemotherapy and radiotherapy depend heavily for their success on appropriate surgery. This true synergy among the therapeutic modalities highlights the fact that ovarian cancer, more than any of the other gynecologic malignancies, requires an interdisciplinary approach to treatment. This approach brings together the gynecologic surgeon, the medical and radiation oncologists, the pathologist, the nurse oncologist, and a number of supporting professionals including psychiatrists, nutritionists, geneticists, and social workers. Although this chapter deals only with the surgical management of ovarian cancer, one must remember that such surgery should be part of a comprehensive multimodality program for the management of the disease.

HISTOGENETIC CLASSIFICATION OF OVARIAN TUMORS

The ovary can give rise to a remarkable variety of neoplasms, both benign and malignant. A comprehensive classification of these tumors, adopted by the World Health Organization,[110] is based on currently accepted concepts of their histogenesis. Tumors may arise from any of the three main types of cells that make up the ovary: (1) the coelomic surface epithelium (actually mesothelium) that covers the ovary; (2) the cortical mesenchymal stroma and sex cords; and (3) the germ cells. The World Health Organization classification for the common epithelial tumors is given in the box on p. 665. Epithelial tumors comprise approximately 60% of all ovarian tumors and about 90% of malignant ovarian tumors. Although this chapter

---

World Health Organization Histologic classification of epithelial ovarian tumors

I. Common epithelial tumors
   A. Serous tumors
      1. Benign
         a. Cystadenoma and papillary cystadenoma
         b. Surface papilloma
         c. Adenofibroma and cystadenofibroma
      2. Of borderline malignancy (carcinoma of low malignant potential)
         a. Cystadenoma and papillary cystadenoma
         b. Surface papilloma
         c. Adenofibroma and cystadenofibroma
      3. Malignant
         a. Adenocarcinoma, papillary adenocarcinoma, and papillary cystadenocarcinoma
         b. Surface papillary carcinoma
         c. Malignant adenofibroma and cystadenofibroma
   B. Mucinous tumors
      1. Benign
         a. Cystadenoma
         b. Adenofibroma and cystadenofibroma
      2. Of borderline malignancy (carcinoma of low malignant potential)
         a. Cystadenoma
         b. Adenofibroma and cystadenofibroma
      3. Malignant
         a. Adenocarcinoma and cystadenocarcinoma
         b. Malignant adenofibroma and cystadenofibroma

   C. Endometrioid tumors
      1. Benign
         a. Adenoma and cystadenoma
         b. Adenofibroma and cystadenofibroma
      2. Of borderline malignancy (carcinoma of low malignant potential)
         a. Adenoma and cystadenoma
         b. Adenofibroma and cystadenofibroma
      3. Malignant
         a. Carcinoma
            i. Adenocarcinoma
            ii. Adenoacanthoma
            iii. Malignant adenofibroma
         b. Endometrioid stromal sarcomas
         c. Mesodermal (müllerian) mixed tumors, homologous, and heterologous
   D. Clear cell (mesonephroid) tumors
      1. Benign: adenofibroma
      2. Of borderline malignancy (carcinoma of low malignant potential)
      3. Malignant: carcinoma and adenocarcinoma
   E. Brenner tumors
      1. Benign
      2. Of borderline malignancy (proliferating)
      3. Malignant
   F. Mixed epithelial tumors
      1. Benign
      2. Of borderline malignancy
      3. Malignant
   G. Undifferentiated carcinoma
   H. Unclassified epithelial tumors

From Serou S, Scully R, Sobin L: Histological typing of ovarian tumors. In *International histological classification of tumors,* No. 9, pp. 17-18. Geneva, 1973, World Health Organization.

---

does not deal specifically with the surgical management of the less common stromal and germ cell malignancies of the ovary, for the most part the same principles and techniques apply.

The epithelial ovarian tumors are subdivided according to the predominant pattern of differentiation of the coelomic epithelial cell. These patterns tend to resemble the normally differentiated epithelium of the various areas of the female genital tract. The most common epithelial tumors are those of serous differentiation. The epithelium of these tumors contains a mixture of ciliated, goblet, and intercalated cells resembling those of the fallopian tube. Mucinous tumors contain endocervical type epithelium with tall columnar mucin-producing cells, or intestinal type epithelium with goblet cells. Other tumors, designated endometrioid, produce epithelium resembling that found in the endometrium. Related to the endometrioid group are the clear cell tumors, formerly misclassified as mesonephric. The so-called Brenner tumors produce epithelium resembling the transitional cells lining the urinary tract. Many ovarian tumors contain mixtures of the various types of epithelium, and some are so undifferentiated that they cannot be classified by this schema. Table 41-1, shows this classification of the differentiated epithelial tumors of the ovary.

EPIDEMIOLOGY OF EPITHELIAL OVARIAN CANCER

The epithelial cancers of the ovary most commonly occur in women in the early postmenopausal age range, with the average age at diagnosis about 54 years. Figure 41-1, based on data on over 8000 patients from the International Federation of Gynecology and Obstetrics (FIGO) 1988 Annual Report,[83] shows the distribution of cases by age. Epithelial ovarian cancer is rare in women under the age of 20, with a yearly incidence rate of less than 1 in 100,000 in this age group. This rate rises to about 33 per 100,000 at age 55. Although it is not generally appreciated, the incidence rate continues to rise thereafter, peaking at 52 cases per 100,000 women per year at age 78.[111]

Although the cause of epithelial ovarian cancer remains unknown and risk factors are poorly defined, some gener-

Table 41-1. Histogenetic classification of epithelial ovarian tumors

Differentiation	Benign tumor	Borderline tumor	Malignant tumor
Tubal	Serous cystadenoma	Borderline serous tumor	Serous carcinoma
Endocervical	Mucinous cystadenoma	Borderline mucinous tumor	Mucinous carcinoma
Endometrial	Endometrioid adenofibroma*	Borderline endometrioid tumor*	Endometrioid carcinoma
Clear cell	Clear cell adenofibroma*	Borderline clear cell tumor*	Clear cell carcinoma
Urothelial	Brenner tumor	Proliferating Brenner tumor*	Malignant Brenner tumor*

*Rare.

Modified from Gompel C, Silverberg S, and Zaloudek C: *The Ovary.* In Silverberg S and Zaloudek, C, editors: *Pathology in gynecology and obstetrics.* Philadelphia, 1985, JB Lippincott.

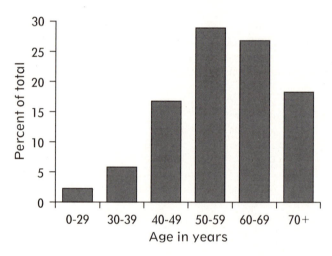

Figure 41-1. Age distribution of patients with epithelial ovarian cancer. Based on data from the International Federation of Gynecology and Obstetrical (FIGO) 1988 Annual Report.[83]

alizations can be made. The epidemiologic observation that incidence rates are highest in industrialized countries suggests that some as yet undefined environmental factors play a role in the etiology of the disease. A major exception to this observation is Japan, where recorded rates of ovarian cancer are among the lowest in the world. The risk of ovarian cancer is related to several aspects of reproductive and hormonal status. Young age at first pregnancy is recognized as protective,[48] whereas the risk is higher for women who have no or few children. Early menarche and late menopause have been associated with an increased risk.[30] The effect of obesity on the risk of developing ovarian cancer is controversial. In a large prospective study, Lew and Garfinkel found that women who were 40% or more overweight had an increased risk of dying from ovarian cancer compared to average-weight women.[51] Other studies have shown no relationship between body weight and risk.[124]

A number of studies have reported that the use of oral contraceptives decreases the risk of epithelial ovarian cancer. In a large case-control study published in 1987, the Centers for Disease Control reported that women who had used oral contraceptives had a risk of epithelial ovarian cancer of 0.6 compared with those who had never used them.[50] This protective effect was noted in women who had used oral contraceptives for as little as 3 to 6 months, and persisted for 15 years. This effect was independent of the specific type of oral contraceptive used. Rose and co-workers have found a relationship between high ovarian cancer mortality and high total intake of dietary fat, especially fats of animal origin.[99]

The known association of environmental carcinogens, specifically asbestos, with mesotheliomas, has led some to suggest a similar etiology for cancers of the ovarian epithelium, which shares a common embryologic origin with the peritoneal mesothelium. In a case-control study of ovarian cancer, Cramer and associates[22] noted that women with ovarian cancer were significantly more likely to report the regular use of talc as a dusting powder on the perineum or sanitary napkins, providing a possible route of direct ovarian exposure.

Some reports have suggested an association between viral infections and the development of ovarian cancer. McGowan and co-workers[70] found that patients with ovarian cancer had had rubella in their teens more often than a control group. A history of mumps has been suggested to increase the risk of ovarian cancer,[23] although others have suggested a protective effect.[121]

Although most cases of ovarian cancer are considered to be sporadic, with no discernable familial tendency, there are now a large number of recorded cases of familial ovarian carcinoma, defined as two or more cases among first-degree relatives.[59,60,90] These cancers tend to occur at an earlier age than the sporadic variety and are generally of the serous or undifferentiated cell types. The mode of transmission appears to be that of an autosomal dominant with variable penetrance. Lynch[58] has described three variants of familial ovarian cancer: (1) site-specific ovarian cancer; (2) ovarian cancer associated with colon and endometrial cancers; and (3) ovarian cancer associated with breast cancer. Management of women from families with a clear history of familial ovarian cancer is controversial. As yet no clear evidence shows that surveillance of such women with serum markers, sonography, laparoscopy, or frequent pelvic examinations is of any benefit, although some form of intensified surveillance and early intervention for adnexal enlargement or pelvic symptoms seems appropriate. Many would recommend prophylactic excision of the ovaries after age 35 if the woman has completed childbearing, recognizing that there have been reports of peritoneal carcinomatosis developing in women who previously had undergone prophylactic bilateral oophorectomy at which time normal ovaries were removed.[117] More difficult yet is the problem of women with a history of a single first-degree relative (mother, sister, daughter) with ovarian cancer, where there were no other female family members, or the family history is unknown.

NATURAL HISTORY AND PATTERNS OF SPREAD

Epithelial cancers of the ovary generally begin as cystic intraovarian growths, probably developing in invaginations of the normal ovarian surface epithelium. The tumors grow within the substance of the ovary for some time before dissemination begins by one of several routes. The rate of growth of early tumors and the length of time they remain confined to the ovary before spread are unknown. When spread does occur, two main routes are involved: exfoliation of cells into the peritoneal cavity, and spread by lymphatic dissemination. Occasionally, bloodborne spread to distant organs may be seen, but, in general, ovarian cancer remains confined to the peritoneal cavity and retroperitoneal lymphatics for most, if not all, of its natural history. In the past, spread of ovarian cancer by way of the lymphatics received little attention. Over the past 15 years, it has become clear that lymphatic spread is quite common in patients with advanced intraperitoneal ovarian cancer, and that even when the disease appears grossly confined to the ovaries, lymph nodes may already be involved.

The primary lymphatic drainage of the ovary follows the blood vessels in the infundibulopelvic ligament to terminate in aortic lymph nodes at approximately the level of the renal hilus.[91] Secondary channels traverse the broad ligament and terminate in the iliac lymph nodes. Spread may also occur by way of uterine cornual and tubal lymphatics along the path of the round ligament to terminate in the inguinal lymph nodes. While the clinical significance of lymphatic spread is uncertain in women with advanced intraperitoneal disease, in cases where the tumor appears grossly to be confined to the ovary, the detection of such spread is of critical importance. This topic is discussed further on pp. 668-672.

The intraperitoneal spread of ovarian cancer has appropriately received much greater attention than spread by way of the lymphatics. After growing for some time within the ovary itself, ovarian tumors eventually breach the capsule of the ovary where they may involve adjacent organs by direct extension or exfoliation. In its earliest form, intraperitoneal spread is clinically occult and must be actively searched for by the operating surgeon, or the patient may be understaged and then undertreated. In advanced cases, an amorphous mass of tumor may engulf the pelvic organs and obscure anatomic landmarks. Intraperitoneal spread by exfoliation of malignant cells from the surface of the ovary leads to viable tumor cells being carried throughout the peritoneal cavity by the normal clockwise circulation of the peritoneal fluid. Typically, tumor cells implant and grow as nodules on the parietal and visceral peritoneal surfaces, including the intestinal serosa, omentum, paracolic gutters, and undersurfaces of the diaphragm, particularly on the right. This initially produces the characteristic picture of miliary carcinomatosis so common in women with advanced ovarian cancer. Such metastatic implants can also become quite large. The specific surgical management of both occult and advanced intraperitoneal spread is discussed in subsequent sections.

Relatively late in the natural history of the disease, ovarian cancer can also spread beyond the peritoneal cavity to involve distant organs. Tumor cells may traverse the diaphragmatic lymphatics to involve the pleural space, producing malignant pleural effusions and pleural metastases. In one autopsy series of ovarian cancer patients, 36% had pleural metastases.[11] The disease may also spread by hematogenous dissemination to involve a variety of organs, most commonly the liver.

STAGING OF CANCER OF THE OVARY

The stage of a malignant tumor is determined by the extent of disease at the time of diagnosis. Once properly assigned, the stage does not change if the disease progresses or recurs. Unlike the staging systems for many malignancies, that used for cancer of the ovary is based on a surgical determination of the extent of disease. Because the stage of a patient's ovarian cancer correlates strongly with prognosis and is the basis for the selection of appropriate therapy, proper surgical staging is a critical element in the management of these patients. In 1985, the FIGO Cancer Committee[16] revised the surgical staging system for ovarian cancer to reflect not only the results of a thorough exploration of the areas at risk of spread but a more precise determination of the extent of such spread. This system is shown in the box on p. 668. Generally, early ovarian tumors are completely asymptomatic, although on occasion they may produce pain associated with rupture or torsion. Once the tumor has grown to considerable size, patients may complain of symptoms relating to pressure on the bladder or rectum such as urinary frequency, constipation, or tenesmus. With the development of ascites, they may notice abdominal bloating and an increase in the size of their waistline despite a loss of appetite. Because of the lack of specific symptoms early in the course of the disease, most patients with cancer of the ovary are not diagnosed until the malignancy has spread beyond the ovary. Table 41-2, taken from the FIGO 1988 annual report, shows the distribution by stage of more than 8000 patients with epithelial cancers of the ovary reported to FIGO from 95 participating institutions around the world.[83] Only about one quarter of these patients were diagnosed in stage

FIGO staging system for ovarian cancer

Stage I: Growth limited to the ovaries
   Ia: Growth limited to one ovary; no ascites; no tumor on the external surfaces; capsule intact
   Ib: Growth limited to both ovaries; no ascites; no tumor on the external surfaces; capsule intact
   Ic: Tumor either stage Ia or stage Ib but with tumor on the surface of one or both ovaries; or with capsule ruptured; or with ascites present containing malignant cells or with positive peritoneal washings
Stage II: Growth involving one or both ovaries with pelvic extension
   IIa: Extension and/or metastases to the uterus and/or tubes
   IIb: Extension to other pelvic tissues
   IIc: Tumor either stage IIa or IIb but with tumor on the surface of one or both ovaries; or with capsule(s) ruptured; or with ascites present containing malignant cells or with positive peritoneal washings

Stage III: Tumor involving one or both ovaries with peritoneal implants outside the pelvis and/or positive retroperitoneal or inguinal nodes; superficial liver metastases equals stage III; tumor is limited to the true pelvis but with histologically verified malignant extension to small bowel or omentum
   IIIa: Tumor grossly limited to the true pelvis with negative nodes but with histologically confirmed microscopic seeding of abdominal peritoneal surfaces
   IIIb: Tumor of one or both ovaries; histologically confirmed implants of abdominal peritoneal surfaces, none exceeding 2 cm in diameter; nodes negative
   IIIc: Abdominal implants greater than 2 cm in diameter and/or positive retroperitoneal or inguinal nodes
Stage IV: Growth involving one or both ovaries with distant metastases; if pleural effusion is present, there must be positive cytologic test results to allot a case to stage IV; parenchymal liver metastases equals stage IV

From Cancer Committee of FIGO: Staging announcement, *Gynecol Oncol* 25:383, 1986.

Table 41-2. Distribution by stage of ovarian cancer patients

	Patients	
Stage	**No.**	**%**
I	2230	26.1
II	1313	15.4
III	3339	39.1
IV	1391	16.3
Unstaged	268	3.1
TOTAL	8451	100.0

Data summarized from 1988 FIGO Annual Report.

I, and more than 50% were not diagnosed until stage III or IV disease was present.

PRIMARY SURGICAL MANAGEMENT OF APPARENT EARLY OVARIAN CANCER

Early ovarian cancers are most often detected at the time of exploration of a patient with an adnexal mass. Because the preoperative diagnosis of early ovarian cancer cannot be made definitively, nor the possibility excluded, the surgeon faced with a patient with an adnexal mass is well advised to form an opinion as to the likelihood of malignancy and to base the preoperative evaluation, discussion with the patient, and operative approach on this assessment.

With the ready availability of techniques such as sonography, computed tomography (CT), and magnetic resonance imaging (MRI), most patients with a persistent adnexal mass have some form of imaging of the mass performed preoperatively. Apart from confirming the presence of the mass, such tests may provide information about the precise size, composition, location, and origin of masses that may aid the clinician in refining the differential diagnosis. It should be remembered, however, that such techniques are not accurate in distinguishing benign from malignant masses because there is broad overlap in the imaging characteristics of each. Transvaginal color flow sonographic imaging to detect tumor neovascularization appears promising as a means of distinguishing benign from malignant ovarian tumors, but is currently not widely available.[10] Measurement of serum markers such as CA-125 is also often performed. If levels are elevated, suspicion should be increased, although CA-125 may be elevated in a variety of benign conditions including endometriosis and pelvic inflammatory disease[38,62] and may, in fact, be normal in many patients with early ovarian cancers.[82]

Laparoscopy has little place in the evaluation of persistent adnexal cystic masses, because benign cysts cannot be distinguished reliably from malignant ones on the basis of their appearance. The current trend toward laparoscopic removal of apparently benign ovarian masses has led to a marked increase in the number of patients referred to gynecologic oncologists after rupture of early ovarian cancers during laparoscopic surgery. Such rupture may increase the stage of the patient's malignancy and mandate the use of chemotherapy in patients who would otherwise be treated by surgery alone, thus worsening the chances for cure. Laparoscopy may occasionally be useful to distinguish an ovarian mass from other causes of apparent adnexal masses such as hydrosalpinx or pedunculated fibroid.

Before surgery for an adnexal mass, the experienced clinician forms an opinion as to the likelihood of malignancy based on the patient's age, the size and characteristics of the mass, and other factors. In all but the most clear-cut cases of benign disease, the physician should discuss the possibility of malignancy with the patient, review the surgical options if cancer is found, and ascertain the patient's wishes regarding these options. If the physician is not comfortable with this type of discussion, or if the suspicion of malignancy is high, consultation with a gynecologic oncologist should be obtained.

In the operating room, pelvic examination should be performed after the induction of anesthesia to allow a final assessment of the pelvic findings before exploration. If the adnexal mass is suspicious or other indications for evaluation of the endometrium exist, dilation and curettage (D and C) should be performed. The information obtained from this may aid in the decision-making process if an apparent early ovarian malignancy is found in a young woman who wishes to preserve fertility, because one is more comfortable leaving the uterus if the endometrium and uterine serosa are apparently free of disease. The choice of incision is determined by the surgeon's level of suspicion regarding malignancy. A low transverse incision, which does not allow the surgical exposure of the upper abdomen necessary for a proper ovarian cancer operation, should be avoided in favor of a vertical incision if there is a significant risk of cancer being found. If the patient insists on this as the initial incision, the possibility of her needing a second upper-abdominal incision if a malignancy is found should be discussed.

On entering the abdomen, cytologic washings should be taken from the pelvic cavity by saline lavage. If the ovaries are suspicious, washings should also be taken from both paracolic gutters and subdiaphragmatic areas before surgery in the pelvis. Manual exploration of the upper abdominal structures should be performed to identify any obvious abnormalities. The pelvic organs should be inspected, and the ovarian pathology should be identified. As the operation progresses, the surgeon should constantly be refining the estimate of the risk of malignancy based on inspection and palpation of the ovarian mass. The presence of ascites, bilateral ovarian involvement, surface excrescences, adherence to surrounding structures, or obvious solid areas in the ovarian tumor increase the chance of malignancy. The importance of such assessment lies in its effect on the operative management. In younger women with nonsuspicious masses, the surgeon may consider cystectomy with preservation of the remaining portion of the ovary. To the extent that cystectomy increases the risk of intraoperative rupture of an ovarian tumor, it should be avoided if that tumor might be malignant. Intraoperative rupture of a cystic ovarian cancer limited to the ovaries with resultant spillage of viable tumor cells into the peritoneal cavity worsens prognosis, as reflected in the official staging system.

After removal of the tumor, a frozen section should be studied. If malignancy is identified and there is no evidence of obvious metastatic disease, the role of further surgery is primarily diagnostic. Based on an understanding of the patterns of spread of ovarian cancer and of the patient's wishes for future fertility as determined in the preoperative discussion, a complete cancer staging operation should now be performed. This procedure should include a meticulous abdominal exploration, with special attention given to visualization and palpation of the serosal surfaces of the small and large intestine. The infracolic omentum is removed (Fig. 41-2) by serially clamping, transecting, and ligating the omental attachments to the transverse colon. Most gynecologic oncologists do not remove the gastrocolic portion of the omentum if it is grossly normal, because this adds little to the diagnostic accuracy of the omentectomy and increases the risk of damage to adjacent structures including the mesentery of the transverse colon and the vessels along the greater curvature of the stomach.

Aortic lymph nodes should be sampled, as should pelvic lymph nodes on the side of the primary tumor. The aortic lymph nodes can be approached by several routes. Either the ascending or the descending colon can be detached from its lateral peritoneal attachments and reflected medially to allow exposure of the aorta and vena cava. A somewhat simpler technique that usually provides adequate exposure for these purposes involves direct incision of the posterior parietal peritoneum overlying the right common iliac artery and the lower aorta. The small bowel must be packed above the operative field or displaced from the abdominal cavity. The retroperitoneal fat overlying the common iliac artery and the lower aorta is incised to expose the wall of the vessel and identify the proper plane of dissection. The right ureter should be carefully identified and retracted laterally. This procedure provides access to the fatty node-bearing tissue overlying the aorta and the vena cava, which is then carefully stripped from the vessels by blunt and sharp dissection, using stainless steel or titanium clips for hemostasis (Fig. 41-3). The dissection can be carried upward to approximately the level of the renal hilus. Through the same posterior parietal incision, the retroperitoneal space can be developed toward the left, elevating and mobilizing the mesentery of the descending colon and the inferior mesenteric artery and vein, and retracting them laterally to allow dissection of the nodes along the left common iliac artery and the left side of the aorta. This is particularly important if the primary tumor developed in the left ovary.

Pelvic lymph nodes on the same side as the primary tumor can be sampled by incising the peritoneum overlying the external iliac artery as far as the inguinal ligament. The ureter should be identified and retracted medially. The nodal tissue can be stripped from the external iliac artery and vein with care taken to avoid injury to the genitofemoral nerve, which lies along the psoas muscle just lateral to the vessels. If desired, nodal tissue can also be removed from the obturator fossa beneath the vessels. Although the yield is low, many gynecologic oncologists recommend

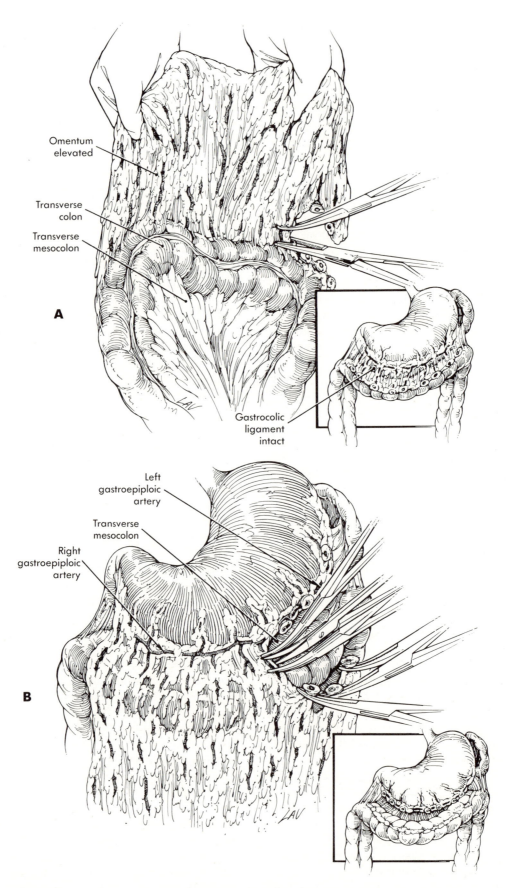

Figure 41-2. Infracolic omentectomy (**A**) is performed by removing the omentum near its attachments to the transverse colon. If there is gross involvement of the gastrocolic omentum this can also be resected (**B**).

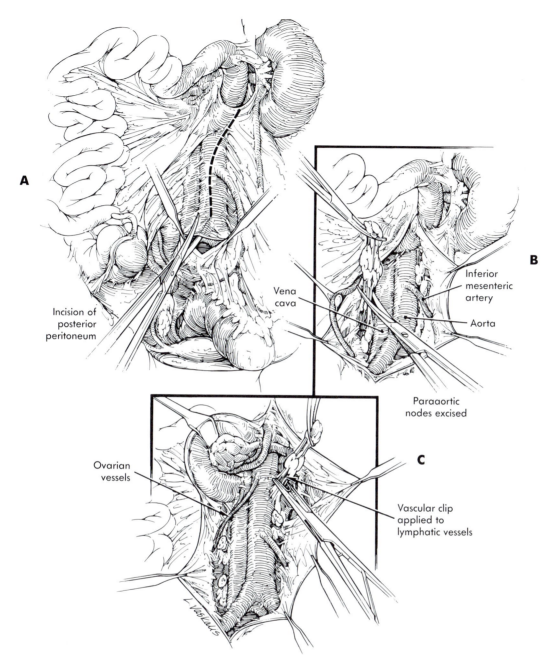

Incision of posterior peritoneum

Vena cava

Inferior mesenteric artery

Aorta

Paraaortic nodes excised

Ovarian vessels

Vascular clip applied to lymphatic vessels

Figure 41-3. Paraaortic node dissection for staging of apparent early ovarian cancer. The posterior parietal peritoneum overlying the aorta is incised (**A**), and the nodal tissue stripped from the vena cava (**B**) and the aorta (**C**) to the level of the left renal hilus.

taking random peritoneal biopsies from multiple sites in the pelvis, from the lateral paracolic gutters, and from the undersurfaces of both hemidiaphragms.

If the patient is not concerned about future childbearing, total hysterectomy and bilateral salpingoooophorectomy should be completed if malignancy is found. In younger women who wish to preserve fertility and who have no anatomic or functional barrier to successful pregnancy, it may be possible to preserve the uterus and the uninvolved tube and ovary. For this to be safe requires that there be no evidence of spread beyond the primary tumor as determined by complete surgical staging, including a

generous wedge biopsy of the contralateral ovary. The results of the preexploration D and C become important to rule out endometrial involvement. If the tumor is stage Ia and well-differentiated histologically, surgery alone should be curative in over 90% of cases. Women with stage I moderately or poorly differentiated tumors have a good likelihood of cure after adjuvant treatment with chemotherapy and may be able to retain fertility if the opposite ovary and uterus are left in place. Obviously, these issues must have been discussed with the patient preoperatively if the appropriate intraoperative decision is to be made. If they have not, it is generally best to perform the most conservative operative procedure possible and to subject the patient to reoperation if necessary. The same would apply if the frozen section diagnosis of malignancy is uncertain. The surgical approach to apparent early ovarian cancer is summarized as follows:

Vertical incision
Multiple cytologic washings
Intact tumor removal
Complete abdominal exploration
Removal of remaining ovary, uterus, tubes (May be preserved in selected patients.)
Omentectomy
Lymph node sampling
Random peritoneal biopsies, including diaphragm

The importance of a careful staging operation lies in the fact that a significant proportion of patients with ovarian cancers that appear grossly to be confined to a single ovary actually have microscopic spread detected by surgical staging. Table 41-3 shows the incidence of subclinical metastases in a relatively large group of women undergoing surgical staging for what appeared to be stage I ovarian cancer. Identification of these women with microscopic metastases will more accurately define their prognosis and allow them to receive potentially curative chemotherapy.

PRIMARY SURGICAL MANAGEMENT OF ADVANCED OVARIAN CANCER

Unfortunately, the typical ovarian cancer patient presents with advanced, rather than early, disease. Such patients may have obvious ascites and large pelvic and upper abdominal masses indicative of widespread malignancy. In such cases, the role of the surgery is primarily one of "debulking," or cytoreductive surgery. Unlike the experience in many other human solid tumors for which aggressive surgery is indicated only if all tumor can be resected, for ovarian cancer there is substantial theoretical and clinical evidence that debulking short of complete tumor removal is of benefit to the patient. Removal of bulky tumor masses with a resultant decrease in the formation of ascites may contribute to the patient's comfort and improve her ability to maintain adequate nutrition. Additionally, removal of large, poorly vascularized tumor masses with relatively low growth fractions may directly improve the response of remaining areas of tumor to chemotherapy by al-

Table 41-3. Subclinical metastases in apparent early ovarian cancer

Site	Patients	Involvement (%)
Peritoneal washings	79	33
Aortic nodes	58	10
Diaphragm	44	11
Omentum	27	3

From Piver MS, Barlow JJ, Lele SB: Incidence of subclinical metastasis in stage I and II ovarian carcinoma, *Obstet Gynecol* 52(1):100-104, 1978.

lowing more tumor cells to enter the active phase of the cell cycle, in which sensitivity to cytotoxic chemotherapy is greatest.[112] Because a given dose of chemotherapy will kill a constant fraction of the cancer cells present, regardless of the initial cell population,[113] cytoreduction should decrease the number of cycles of chemotherapy necessary, thus decreasing host toxicity and the development of spontaneous chemotherapy-resistant tumor cell populations.[33] Although mechanisms of acquired chemoresistance in ovarian cancer patients have not been clearly determined,[106] it is reasonable to assume that this might also be decreased by cytoreduction, which allows a decreased duration of exposure to chemotherapy.

Clinical studies supporting the concept of debulking in advanced ovarian cancer go back more than two decades.[29,74] Griffiths, in 1975, was able to quantify residual disease accurately after surgery in ovarian cancer patients, and showed a tripling of median survival time to 39 months in patients with no residual tumor who received melphalan.[35] More recently, reports of prospective clinical trials involving both non-platinum- and platinum-based combination chemotherapy regimens in ovarian cancer have supported the concept of primary cytoreductive surgery.[80,125] In general, studies examining the effect of cytoreductive surgery have reported an increase in the likelihood of a surgically documented complete response to chemotherapy (negative second-look),[100] an increase in median survival,[41] and a decrease in the risk of recurrence after negative second-look[107] for patients undergoing optimal primary cytoreduction. The definition of "optimal" primary cytoreduction has varied among reports and is generally defined as removal of all tumor masses greater than a certain maximum diameter in size, often 2 cm. This implies a "threshold" effect, in which cytoreduction of large tumor masses does not improve outcome unless they are reduced below a certain critical size. For this reason, most gynecologic oncologists feel that, unless optimal cytoreduction can be accomplished, aggressive surgery is unwarranted. For example, it would be inappropriate to do a major colon resection to debulk a pelvic tumor mass if there was a large volume of unresectable disease in the upper abdomen.

The preoperative evaluation of the patient with suspected advanced ovarian cancer must be tailored to the clinical situation. Imaging studies such as CT, sonography, or MRI may be performed to confirm the presence of a mass, and to look for ascites and evidence of metastatic disease. A barium enema should be considered to ascertain the extent of colonic involvement and to rule out a colonic primary tumor with metastases to the ovary. The preoperative discussion with the patient and her family should include a thorough review of the differential diagnosis, the risk of malignancy, and the surgical options that might be employed depending on the operative findings, including intestinal resection and possible colostomy. We generally use a regimen of oral antibiotics, cathartics, and enemas to cleanse the large intestine in case intestinal surgery is needed. We also routinely employ perioperative intravenous antibiotics and low-dose subcutaneous heparin prophylaxis. Intravenous fluid replacement is begun the evening before surgery because of the dehydration induced by the bowel preparation.

In the operating room, cystoscopy and proctoscopy may be performed under anesthesia to evaluate the bladder and lower colon. The abdomen should be entered through a vertical incision extending from the pubic symphysis into the upper abdomen. On entering the abdomen, ascites, if present, should be collected for cytologic evaluation. If none is present, saline washings can be taken, although in the presence of obvious intraperitoneal metastases, this may contribute little useful information.[101] A general exploration of the entire peritoneal cavity should be performed to assess the extent and resectability of both the pelvic and upper abdominal disease, and to identify any other pathology present. The aortic and pelvic lymph nodes should be palpated because these are often involved in advanced ovarian cancer.[123] Often, patients with advanced ovarian cancer present with extensive pelvic and upper abdominal disease and widespread abdominal carcinomatosis. Such situations can test the judgment of even the most experienced gynecologic cancer surgeon, who will have to determine the feasibility of optimal cytoreduction and weigh the benefits of such a procedure against the operative risks.

The surgical approach to the debulking of an extensive pelvic tumor is a retroperitoneal one. Even when the intraperitoneal pelvic anatomy is obliterated by massive tumor involvement, the retroperitoneal tissue planes are generally preserved and can be developed with relative ease. The infundibulopelvic ligament should be identified at the pelvic brim, and the parietal peritoneum lateral to it should be incised (Fig. 41-4). Retracting the infundibulopelvic ligament medially, the retroperitoneal space can be developed

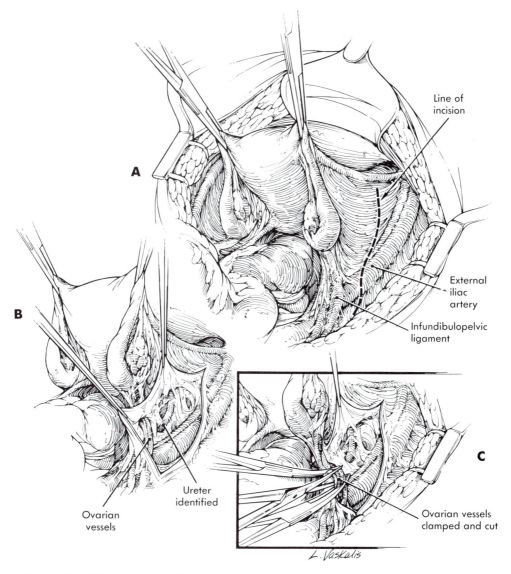

Figure 41-4. The retroperitoneal approach to the pelvis. The peritoneum in incised lateral to the infundibulopelvic ligament (**A**). Blunt development of the retroperitoneal space allows visualization of the ureter (**B**) prior to ligation of the ovarian vessels at the pelvic sidewall (**C**).

medially to identify the ureter and isolate the ovarian blood supply, which is then ligated and transected. By controlling the ovarian blood supply before any manipulation of the tumor, blood loss can be reduced. With the ureter under direct vision, a combination of blunt and sharp dissection can be used to free the tumor from the pelvic sidewall and cul-de-sac, stripping the peritoneum from these areas if necessary. In most patients, the uterus should be removed. Tumor nodules lateral or posterior to the uterus can often be removed in continuity with the uterine specimen by performing the type of dissection used in a modified radical hysterectomy, unroofing the ureter as it passes through the base of the broad ligament, and ligating the uterine vessels at this point. If removing the uterus will not contribute significantly to debulking the pelvic tumor, or if hysterectomy cannot easily be accomplished because of tumor encasement, the clinician may decide to leave the uterus in place or do a supracervical hysterectomy. In extreme cases where a bulky ovarian cancer involves the rectosigmoid colon, this can be resected together with the uterus by performing a procedure similar to posterior exenteration. The introduction of intestinal stapling devices has extended the ability to restore intestinal continuity in these patients by performing low colonic anastomoses. If this cannot be accomplished, colostomy is necessary. If a low colonic anastomosis is considered to be a possibility based on the preoperative findings, the patient's position on the operating table should allow direct access to the perineum to allow use of the stapling device through the anus. This can be accomplished by supporting the patient's legs in stirrups in a modified lithotomy position.

In the upper abdomen, omentectomy can be performed by dividing the omentum from its attachments to the transverse colon (Fig. 41-2). If the gastrocolic omentum is involved, the dissection can be continued upward to the greater curvature of the stomach (Fig. 41-2). In most patients, the omental tumor can be removed completely from the colon without intestinal resection. If it cannot, resection of the transverse colon should be performed if it contributes to an optimal debulking procedure. On occasion, extensive omental tumor may extend upward along the left side of the omentum to involve the spleen, necessitating splenectomy. Primary reanastomosis of the transverse colon can usually be accomplished after mobilization of the splenic or hepatic flexures. Bulky tumor involvement may require resection of other areas of the intestine, most commonly the terminal ileum, cecum, and ascending colon. Such aggressive cytoreductive procedures are justified only if they result in optimal tumor reduction or if there is evidence of obstruction.

The role of lymph node resection in advanced ovarian cancer remains unclear. The majority of patients with advanced ovarian cancer have involvement of retroperitoneal lymph nodes.[14,122] In a retrospective series, Burghardt et al reported an improved survival in patients with advanced ovarian cancer undergoing lymphadenectomy as compared to historical controls.[13] This same group also reported that the incidence of lymph node metastases after chemotherapy was approximately the same as that seen in newly diagnosed ovarian cancer patients, implying that chemotherapy may not be effective against retroperitonal disease. Although these data are interesting, they await confirmation. Lymphadenectomy is not considered a standard part of the surgical management of advanced ovarian cancer.

Ovarian cancer patients often have clinical features that increase the risk of incisional complications, including advanced age, obesity, medical complications, vomiting due to postoperative chemotherapy, and, perhaps most importantly, an advanced intraabdominal malignancy. In the past, surgeons often used retention suture closures in such patients. Recently, closure techniques similar to that commonly known as the Smead-Jones closure, first described in 1941,[44] have been used with great success in avoiding fascial dehiscense. These techniques, essentially internal retention sutures, incorporate large bites of fascia, rectus muscle, and peritoneum in a bulk closure that is extremely resistant to disruption. Several authors have reported good results using a bulk closure with a continuous monofilament nonabsorbable or delayed absorbable suture.[1,46]

SECOND-LOOK LAPAROTOMY

With regard to ovarian cancer, the term second-look laparotomy has been used with a variety of meanings. It has been used to describe all secondary operations including those performed for resection of known residual, progressive, or recurrent cancer, operations done for relief of symptoms such as intestinal obstruction, and operations to evaluate the response of tumor to treatment. In current usage, the term most commonly designates an exploratory operation performed in a patient who has completed a planned program of chemotherapy and has no clinical evidence of cancer. The primary goal of such an operation is to determine whether or not ovarian cancer is still present. A secondary goal may be to resect residual disease, if detected.

Second-look laparotomy has become a common part of the management of ovarian cancer for a number of reasons. Because ovarian cancer is a disease that generally remains confined to the peritoneal cavity and retroperitoneal lymph nodes for most or all of its natural history, it lends itself to reassessment by laparotomy. With the use of aggressive primary cytoreductive surgery and platinum-based combination chemotherapy, a large proportion of ovarian cancer patients have no clinically detectable tumor at the completion of their chemotherapy. No noninvasive method of reassessment of these patients that approaches the accuracy of surgical reexploration is available.

Laparoscopy has been investigated as a less invasive alternative to second-look laparotomy. Berek and others,[5] reporting on 119 laparoscopic examinations performed in ovarian cancer patients, observed a 14% incidence of major complications requiring laparotomy, most involving intestinal perforation. Ozols et al[81] have reported a false-negative rate of over 50% in ovarian cancer patients undergoing reassessment laparoscopy. In view of the high false-negative rate, the significant risk of complications, and the inability to resect residual disease by laparoscopy, this technique has little place in the reassessment of patients with ovarian cancer.

A number of authors have reported their results using imaging techniques such as CT, sonography, and MRI for detection of residual ovarian cancer after chemotherapy. Although these techniques may be useful in detecting large tumor masses, they are quite poor in detecting intraperitoneal tumor masses in the clinically important size range of less than 2 cm.[45,57,75] In one series, CT failed to detect large omental tumor cakes and abdominal and pelvic masses up to 3 cm in size.[12] Such techniques in no way approach the accuracy of surgical exploration in detecting residual disease.

Cytologic analysis of peritoneal fluid obtained by culdocentesis has been suggested as a means of detecting persistent cancer after treatment.[69] However, it has been demonstrated that the majority of women with biopsy-proven residual ovarian cancer in the peritoneal cavity have cytologically negative peritoneal washings. Rubin et al[101] reported on 96 women undergoing reexploration for ovarian cancer at Memorial Sloan-Kettering who had washings taken with the abdomen open at the time of laparotomy. Only 34% of patients with biopsy-proven gross intraperitoneal disease had positive washings.

The serial measurement of serum levels of CA-125 has been a significant advance in the management of ovarian cancer.[4] Such measurements correlate well with tumor response or nonresponse during chemotherapy. However, serum levels are often normal in patients with small amounts of tumor, and multiple studies have confirmed that many patients with normal CA-125 levels have tumor found on exploration. Rubin and associates[105] reported on CA-125 levels and surgical findings in 96 patients undergoing secondary operations for ovarian cancer. More than half the patients who had normal CA-125 levels had cancer documented at surgery. Similar findings have been reported by other authors.[8,71,79] Although an elevated CA-125 appears to be a reliable predictor of persistent tumor, it has been our practice to explore patients with elevated values to document the extent and location of tumor and attempt secondary cytoreduction[42] before the initiation of second-line chemotherapy protocols. To a large extent, the benefits of second-look laparotomy are related to the efficacy of second-line therapy for ovarian cancer. Given the encouraging results reported with second-line intraperitoneal chemotherapy in patients with small volume disease,[64,96] second-look laparotomy is likely to continue to play an important role in the management of ovarian cancer.

The surgical procedure is similar to that performed for the initial staging of apparently early stage ovarian cancer. The details of the patient's initial operation for ovarian cancer should be reviewed by the surgeon performing the second-look procedure, particularly with regard to the location and extent of areas of tumor left at the end of the initial surgery. The abdomen should be entered through a vertical incision adequate to allow full evaluation of the upper abdomen. If obvious tumor is identified, frozen section confirmation should be obtained, and involved areas should be resected if optimal cytoreduction appears possible. When no tumor is evident after initial exploration, the operation may actually become more difficult, because the surgeon must undertake a careful and thorough evaluation of the entire peritoneal cavity and selected retroperitoneal structures to detect areas of occult tumor. Washings for cytologic analysis should be obtained from multiple sites within the peritoneal cavity. Although these are not particularly sensitive in detecting residual disease, on occasion they may be the only positive finding. The upper abdomen should be carefully explored, including the undersurfaces of both hemidiaphragms. Some surgeons employ a sterile proctoscope or laparoscope to aid in visualization of the diaphragm. Suspicious areas should be biopsied. If there are none, random biopsies or scrapings for cytology should be obtained. Any remaining omentum should be removed. The intestines should be carefully examined. All adhesions should be lysed, and portions should be submitted for pathologic analysis. Biopsies are taken from both paracolic gutters. In the pelvis, biopsies should be taken from the peritoneal surfaces of the bladder, rectum, and pouch of Douglas. The surgical pedicles from the initial operation, particularly the stumps of the infundibulopelvic ligaments, should be identified and biopsied. Any remaining internal reproductive organs are generally removed. A thorough sampling of the para-aortic and pelvic lymph nodes should be performed. If no tumor is identified, a carefully performed second-look operation may take several hours and produce in excess of 20 individual histologic specimens.

Many reports on second-look laparotomy have appeared in the literature. We have compiled data from 27 reports comprising over 2000 patients.* Overall, about 55% of patients explored for second-look laparotomy had cancer detected. The likelihood of finding residual cancer at second-look laparotomy can be related to several clinical and histologic factors. These include stage, the amount of residual tumor left after the initial ovarian cancer operation, and perhaps the histologic grade of the tumor. Table 41-4 shows information compiled from the above cited references that relates these features to the probability of having no tumor found at the time of second-look laparotomy. Among the strongest predictors of findings at second-look laparotomy is the amount of tumor remaining after the initial operation for ovarian cancer, once again suggesting a benefit to aggressive primary cytoreduction.

The amount of tumor detected at second-look laparotomy has a clear effect on prognosis. In some reports, a

---

*References 2, 3, 7, 15, 17, 18, 20, 24, 25, 28, 31, 32, 39, 52, 56, 68, 72, 73, 86, 92, 93, 97, 98, 114, 116, 119, 120.

Table 41-4. Clinical correlates of second-look laparotomy

Feature	Percent Negative
Stage	
I	82
II	71
III	34
IV	33
Residual tumor after primary cytoreduction	
None	76
Optimal	46
Suboptimal	23
Histologic grade	
1	56
2	60
3	41

majority of patients with gross tumor detected were dead within 3 years.[93,109] More recent reports of salvage regimens for such patients portray a somewhat brighter picture, particularly in patients who are able to undergo optimal secondary cytoreduction, discussed below. Patients who have no visible disease found at second-look laparotomy but who have histologic or cytologic evidence of microscopic disease have a better outlook. Copeland and associates[21] reported a survival of 96% and 71% at 2 and 5 years, respectively, in a group of 50 patients with only microscopic disease found at second-look. Treatment of such patients with intraperitoneal chemotherapy regimens may improve survival.

Patients with no tumor detected at the time of second-look laparotomy have generally been felt to have a good prognosis, with recurrence rates reported in the range of 20% to 30%. Rubin and Lewis'[100] review of second-look laparotomy identified 12 studies published between 1980 and 1986 that provided information about recurrences after a negative exploration. In these combined series, the overall recurrence rate was 18%, with 26% of patients with stage III or IV disease having recurrence. All of these reports included patients treated with non-platinum containing chemotherapy. Subsequent studies by Rubin and co-workers[102,107] have demonstrated that the risk of recurrence in patients achieving a negative second-look laparotomy after platinum-based chemotherapy approximates 50%. Multivariate analysis showed that stage, histologic grade, and the amount of tumor remaining after primary cytoreduction were significant predictors of recurrence after negative second-look. At Memorial Sloan-Kettering, patients who have no tumor found at second-look laparotomy are offered participation in a prospective clinical trial of consolidation therapy to attempt to reduce their risk of recurrence. The success of this approach remains to be determined.

SECONDARY CYTOREDUCTION

Although the benefits of primary cytoreduction in ovarian cancer are well-established, the role of debulking surgery later in the course of the disease is considerably less clear. Because more than half of patients undergoing second-look laparotomy have tumor detected, and most of these have gross disease, many patients are potential candidates for secondary cytoreductive operations. Patients who experience tumor recurrence after a negative second-look operation, and patients who are reexplored after several cycles of chemotherapy to resect previously unresectable tumor (interval debulking) are examples of other situations in which secondary cytoreduction may be applied. The surgical principles and technical considerations are essentially the same as in primary debulking, except that the operation is likely to be more difficult because of prior surgery and the effects of treatment, particularly intraperitoneal therapy, on the condition of the abdominal contents. The reported rates of successful secondary cytoreduction vary from about 25% to 84%,* depending on the patient population, the surgeon's skill and aggressiveness, and the definition of "success" employed. Whether secondary cyto-reduction conveys a survival benefit is controversial. In relatively small series reported by Chambers and associates[18] and Luesley and co-workers,[55] there was no survival benefit associated with secondary cytoreduction. In a report from the Mayo Clinic, Podratz and co-workers described 116 patients with positive second-look laparotomy and found 4-year survival to be substantially greater in those with microscopic residual tumor as compared to those with larger disease.[94] In a recent report from Memorial Sloan-Kettering, Hoskins and co-workers found that patients whose tumors were reduced to microscopic residual at the time of a positive second-look procedure had a 5-year survival of 51%, as compared to less than 10% in patients left with gross disease.[42] Other authors have also reported an improved survival after optimal cytoreduction at the time of second-look laparotomy.[52] It seems quite likely that the value of secondary cytoreduction depends strongly on what therapy is employed after surgery. Promising second-line therapies based on increasing the exposure of tumor cells to cytoxic agents, such as intraperitoneal therapy or intensive intravenous therapy with autologous bone marrow support or colony-stimulating factors, will probably be most effective in patients with small residual disease.[66,67]

In patients with extensive tumor found at the time of diagnosis in whom primary optimal cytoreduction is not possible, reoperation after several cycles of chemotherapy may allow removal of previously unresectable masses. It has been shown both retrospectively[49] and in a prospective trial from Memorial Sloan-Kettering[78] that a high proportion of such patients can be optimally cytoreduced at the secondary procedure. Whether this will result in an im-

*References 6, 36, 55, 61, 95, 115.

proved outcome remains to be demonstrated, and probably depends in part on the type of therapy employed after the second operation. In one report, patients who underwent interval cytoreduction and then continued intravenous chemotherapy had no survival advantage over those who did not have interval cytoreduction.[77] On the other hand, Hakes and associates,[37] reporting on a subset of the Memorial Sloan-Kettering patients described by Ng and co-workers,[78] found that 47% of patients who underwent optimal interval cytoreduction followed by four courses of intraperitoneal platinum had a subsequent negative reexploration, a rate of complete pathologic response almost twice that usually reported for advanced ovarian cancer.

PALLIATIVE OPERATIONS

Despite the advances in our understanding of ovarian cancer that have accrued in the last decade, early diagnosis is still unusual, and the large majority of women diagnosed in the advanced stages die of the disease within 2 to 4 years. Because of the tendency of the disease to remain confined largely to the peritoneal cavity, many of these women eventually develop intestinal obstruction. In general, these patients are fully alert, in little or no pain, and might otherwise enjoy a reasonable quality of life, albeit for a limited time, were it not for the intestinal obstruction that necessitates gastric drainage and intravenous hydration. Although percutaneous endoscopic gastrostomy[40,63] and home intravenous therapy have been helpful in the management of intestinal obstruction, the question often arises as to whether an attempt at surgical relief of the obstruction would be appropriate. The physician making such a decision must weigh a number of factors, including the patient's overall medical condition, the extent of her cancer, prior therapeutic interventions, and the likelihood of a response to further cancer treatment. In addressing this issue, several authors have attempted to define factors that would predict a favorable outcome after exploration for intestinal obstruction in patients with advanced ovarian cancer. According to Krebs and Goplerud,[47] advanced age, poor nutritional status, palpable tumor masses, ascites, and prior irradiation are factors associated with a poor outcome. Clarke-Pearson and colleagues[19] reported that nutritional status and the amount of cancer remaining at the completion of the operation for intestinal obstruction were related to the duration of postoperative survival. On the other hand, in a report from Memorial Sloan-Kettering, Rubin and co-workers found no clinical features that were predictive of operability or duration of survival after surgery.[103] We do not believe it is possible to define firm criteria for deciding on surgery. Such decisions must be made on an individual basis after a frank discussion with the patient and her family.

If the patient is deemed an operative candidate, consideration should be given to the use of preoperative total parenteral nutrition because these patients are often in poor condition nutritionally, and therefore at increased risk for perioperative complications. A barium enema should be performed to determine if the obstruction involves the colon. In a report of 54 operations performed for intestinal obstruction on ovarian cancer patients, Rubin and associates[103] found that the site of obstruction was in the small intestine alone in 44%, the large intestine alone in 33%, and involved both small and large intestine in 22%. At the time of surgery, a definitive procedure for relief of obstruction was performed in 79% of the patients in this series. The remaining patients were felt to be inoperable at the time of exploration. Of the patients undergoing a definitive procedure, about 80% were discharged from the hospital eating a regular or low-residue diet. Their mean postoperative survival was 6.8 months. Other authors have reported similar findings.[47,89,118] Although survival is short, surgery may allow patients with intestinal obstruction to regain intestinal function and significantly improve the quality of their remaining months of life.

SURGICAL CONSIDERATIONS OF INTRAPERITONEAL THERAPY

Intraperitoneal therapy is one of a number of methods used to intensify the exposure of ovarian cancer cells to cytotoxic agents. The pharmacologic basis for intraperitoneal therapy has been well described by Dedrick and colleagues from the National Cancer Institute.[27] Multiple studies have documented the efficacy of this approach in selected patients with ovarian cancer[54,65]; some have documented responses in tumors that had been resistant to intravenous chemotherapy.[96]

The delivery of drugs into the peritoneal cavity has been accomplished using a variety of catheter systems.* Catheters that exit the skin (transcutaneous) require more maintenance and appear to have a substantially higher rate of infection than systems using a totally implanted port and catheter. The implanted systems consist of a stainless steel or titanium port with a Silastic septum. The port is attached with a locking collar to a Silastic tube with multiple side holes that is tunneled subcutaneously along the abdominal wall before entering the peritoneal cavity in the midabdomen. The technique of placement of the port and catheter has been well described by Lucas.[53] The port should be placed in a subcutaneous pocket and anchored to the fascia with permanent suture. Implantation of the port over the lower rib cage provides it with a firm support, which facilitates percutaneous puncture of the Silastic septum. These systems require no maintenance between uses.

The largest experience with totally implanted subcutaneous port and catheter systems has been reported from Memorial Sloan-Kettering by Rubin and associates[104] and Davidson and associates.[26] In the latter report, the authors described their experience with 227 patients receiving catheters for the first time for treatment on a variety of prospective intraperitoneal chemotherapy trials, most last-

*References 11, 43, 76, 84, 85, 87, 108.

ing from 5 to 6 months. These patients received a total of 1331 courses of chemotherapy during the study period. There were a total of 40 (17.6%) catheter-related complications noted, including an 8.8% rate of catheter blockage, generally caused by the formation of a fibrous sheath around the intraperitoneal portion of the catheter. An additional 8.8% of patients experienced catheter-associated infections. Included among these were eight patients with late erosion of the catheter into the intestinal lumen. The occurrence of profuse diarrhea shortly after chemotherapy infusion should alert the clinician to this possibility. Although the authors could not demonstrate a statistically significant increase in the rate of infection, they recommend against inserting catheters at the time of surgery on the large intestine.

The major technical problem associated with intraperitoneal chemotherapy is the formation of adhesions that limit the free distribution of the infusate within the peritoneal cavity, thus abrogating much of the advantage of direct drug delivery. These adhesions form as a result of the multiple insults suffered by the peritoneal contents: surgery, cancer, and the intraperitoneal treatment itself. There is no effective means of preventing the formation of adhesions, or of eliminating them once formed. If blockage of the catheter occurs, radiographic contrast studies should be used to determine if the blockage is caused by formation of a fibrous sheath around the catheter itself or to development of extensive adhesions within the peritoneal cavity. Repeat laparotomy for removal of a fibrous sheath may allow continued intraperitoneal chemotherapy. If the cause of catheter blockage is extensive intraperitoneal adhesions, repeat laparotomy with extensive lysis of adhesions usually does not result in a long-term reestablishment of catheter patency.

REFERENCES

1. Archie J, Feldtman R: Primary abdominal wound closure with permanent, continuous running monofilament sutures, *Surg Gynecol Obstet* 153:721, 1981.
2. Ballon SC et al: Second-look laparotomy in epithelial ovarian carcinoma: precise definition, sensitivity, and specificity of the operative procedure, *Gynecol Oncol* 17(2):154, 1984.
3. Barnhill DR et al: The second-look surgical reassessment for epithelial ovarian carcinoma, *Gynecol Oncol* 19(2):148, 1984.
4. Bast RJ et al: A radioimmunoassay using a monoclonal antibody to monitor the course of epithelial ovarian cancer, *N Engl J Med* 309:883, 1983.
5. Berek JS, Griffiths CT, Leventhal JM: Laparoscopy for second-look evaluation in ovarian cancer, *Obstet Gynecol* 58(2):192, 1981.
6. Berek JS et al: Survival of patients following secondary cytoreductive surgery in ovarian cancer, *Obstet Gynecol* 61(2):189, 1983.
7. Berek JS et al: Second-look laparotomy in stage III epithelial ovarian cancer: clinical variables associated with disease status, *Obstet Gynecol* 64(2):207, 1984.
8. Berek JS et al: CA 125 serum levels correlated with second-look operations among ovarian cancer patients, *Obstet Gynecol* 67(5):685, 1986.
9. Bergman F: Carcinoma of the ovary: a clinicopathological study of 86 autopsy cases with special reference to mode of spread, *Acta Obstet Gynecol Scand* 45:211, 1966.
10. Bourne T et al: Transvaginal colour flow imaging: a possible new screening technique for ovarian cancer, *Br Med J* 299(6712):1367, 1989.
11. Braly P, Doroshow J, Hoff S: Technical aspects of intraperitoneal chemotherapy in abdominal carcinomatosis, *Gynecol Oncol* 25(3):319, 1986.
12. Brenner DE et al: Abdominopelvic computed tomography: evaluation in patients undergoing second-look laparotomy for ovarian carcinoma, *Obstet Gynecol* 65(5):715, 1985.
13. Burghardt E, Lahousen M, Stettner H: The significance of pelvic and para-aortic lymphadenectomy in the operative treatment of ovarian cancer, *Baillieres Clin Obstet Gynaecol* 3(1):157, 1989.
14. Burghardt E et al: Pelvic lymphadenectomy in operative treatment of ovarian cancer, *Am J Obstet Gynecol* 155(2):315, 1986.
15. Cain J et al: A review of second-look laparotomy for ovarian cancer, *Gynecol Oncol* 23:14, 1986.
16. Cancer Committee of FIGO: Staging announcement, *Gynecol Oncol* 25:383, 1986.
17. Carmichael JA et al: A predictive index of cure versus no cure in advanced ovarian carcinoma patients—replacement of second-look laparotomy as a diagnostic test, *Gynecol Oncol* 27(3):269, 1987.
18. Chambers SK et al: Evaluation of the role of second-look surgery in ovarian cancer, *Obstet Gynecol* 72:404, 1988.
19. Clarke-Pearson D et al: Intestinal obstruction in patients with ovarian cancer. Variables associated with surgical complications and survival, *Arch Surg* 123(1):42, 1988.
20. Cohen CJ et al: Improved therapy with cisplatin regimens for patients with ovarian carcinoma (FIGO stages III and IV) as measured by surgical end-staging (second-look operation), *Am J Obstet Gynecol* 145(8):955, 1983.
21. Copeland LJ et al: Microscopic disease at second-look laparotomy in advanced ovarian cancer, *Cancer* 55(2):472, 1985.
22. Cramer D et al: Ovarian cancer and talc. A cost-control study, *Cancer* 50:372, 1982.
23. Cramer D et al: Mumps, menarche, menopause and ovarian cancer, *Am J Obstet Gynecol* 147:1, 1983.
24. Curry S et al: Second-look laparotomy for ovarian cancer, *Gynecol Oncol* 11:114, 1981.
25. Dauplat J et al: Second-look laparotomy in managing epithelial ovarian carcinoma, *Cancer* 57(8):1627, 1986.
26. Davidson SA et al: Intraperitoneal chemotherapy: analysis of complications with an implanted subcutaneous port and catheter system, *Gynecol Oncol* 1991.
27. Dedrick R et al: Pharmacologic rationale for peritoneal drug administration in the treatment of ovarian cancer, *Cancer Treat Rep* 62:1, 1978.
28. de Gramont A et al: Survival after second-look laparotomy in advanced ovarian epithelial cancer. Study of 86 patients, *Eur J Cancer Clin Oncol* 25(3):451, 1989.
29. Delclos L, Quinlan E: Malignant tumors of the ovary managed with post operative megavoltage irradiation, *Radiology* 93:659, 1969.
30. Franceschi S et al: Risk factors for epithelial ovarian cancer in Italy, *Am J Epidemiol* 115:714, 1982.
31. Gallup DG et al: Another look at the second-assessment procedure for ovarian epithelial carcinoma, *Am J Obstet Gynecol* 157(3):590, 1987.
32. Gershenson DM et al: Prognosis of surgically determined complete responders in advanced ovarian cancer, *Cancer* 55(5):1129, 1985.
33. Goldie JH, Coldman AJ: A mathematic model for relating the drug sensitivity of tumors to their spontaneous mutation rate, *Cancer Treat Rep* 63(11):1727, 1979.
34. Gompel C, Silverberg S, Zaloudek C: *The ovary*. In Silverberg S, Zaloudek C, editors: *Pathology in gynecology and obstetrics*, Philadelphia, 1985, JB Lippincott.
35. Griffiths CT: Surgical resection of tumor bulk in the primary treatment of ovarian carcinoma, *Natl Cancer Inst Monogr* 42(101):101, 1975.
36. Griffiths CT, Parker LM, Fuller AJ: Role of cytoreductive surgical

treatment in the management of advanced ovarian cancer, *Cancer Treat Rep* 63(2):235, 1979.

37. Hakes T et al: Pilot trial of high intensity intravenous cyclophosphamide/cisplatin and intraperitoneal cisplatin for advanced ovarian cancer: A preliminary report, *Proc ASCO* 8:152 (abstract #592), 1989.

38. Halila H, Stenman UH, Seppala M: Ovarian cancer antigen CA 125 levels in pelvic inflammatory disease and pregnancy, *Cancer* 57(7):1327, 1986.

39. Ho AG et al: A reassessment of the role of second-look laparotomy in advanced ovarian cancer, *J Clin Oncol* 5(9):1316, 1987.

40. Hopkins MP, Roberts JA, Morley GW: Outpatient management of small bowel obstruction in terminal ovarian cancer, *J Reprod Med* 32(11):827, 1987.

41. Hoskins WJ: The influence of cytoreductive surgery on progression-free interval and survival in epithelial ovarian cancer, *Baillieres Clin Obstet Gynaecol* 3(1):59, 1989.

42. Hoskins WJ et al: Influence of secondary cytoreduction at the time of second-look laparotomy on the survival of patients with epithelial ovarian carcinoma, *Gynecol Oncol* 34(3):365, 1989.

43. Jenkins J et al: Technical considerations in the use of intraperitoneal chemotherapy administered by Tenckhoff catheter, *Surg Gynecol Obstet* 154(6):858, 1982.

44. Jones T, Newell E, Brubaker R: The use of alloy steel wire in the closure of abdominal wounds, *Surg Gynecol Obstet* 72:1056, 1941.

45. Khan O et al: Ovarian carcinoma follow-up: US versus laparotomy, *Radiology* 159(1):111, 1986.

46. Knight C, Griffan F: Abdominal wound closure with a continuous monofilament polypropylene suture. Experience with 1,000 consecutive cases, *Arch Surg* 118:1305, 1983.

47. Krebs HB, Goplerud DR: Surgical management of bowel obstruction in advanced ovarian carcinoma, *Obstet Gynecol* 61(3):327, 1983.

48. La Vecchia C et al: Age at first birth and the risk of epithelial ovarian cancer, *J Natl Cancer Inst* 73:663, 1984.

49. Lawton FG et al: Neoadjuvant (cytoreductive) chemotherapy combined with intervention debulking surgery in advanced, unresected epithelial ovarian cancer, *Obstet Gynecol* 73(1):61, 1989.

50. Lee N et al: The reduction in risk of ovarian cancer associated with oral-contraceptive use, *N Engl J Med* 316:65, 1987.

51. Lew E, Garfinkel L: Variations in mortality by weight among 750,000 men and women, *J Chronic Dis* 32:563, 1979.

52. Lippman SM et al: Second-look laparotomy in epithelial ovarian carcinoma. Prognostic factors associated with survival duration, *Cancer* 61(12):2571, 1988.

53. Lucas W: *Surgical principles of intraperitoneal access and therapy.* In Howell S, editor: Intra-arterial and intracavitary cancer chemotherapy, pp. 53-60. Boston, 1984, Nijhoff.

54. Lucas WE, Markman M, Howell SB: Intraperitoneal chemotherapy for advanced ovarian cancer, *Am J Obstet Gynecol* 152(4):474, 1985.

55. Luesley DM et al: Second-look laparotomy in the management of epithelial ovarian carcinoma: an evaluation of fifty cases, *Obstet Gynecol* 64(3):421, 1984.

56. Lund B, Williamson P: Prognostic factors for outcome of and survival after second-look laparotomy in patients with advanced ovarian carcinoma, *Obstet Gynecol* 76:617, 1990.

57. Lund B et al: Correlation of abdominal ultrasound and computed tomography scans with second- or third-look laparotomy in patients with ovarian carcinoma, *Gynecol Oncol* 37(2):279, 1990.

58. Lynch HT, Bewtra C, Lynch JF: Familial ovarian carcinoma. Clinical nuances, *Am J Med* 81(6):1073, 1986.

59. Lynch HT et al: Familial association of carcinoma of the breast and ovary, *Surg Gynecol Obstet* 138(5):717, 1974.

60. Lynch HT et al: Familial excess of cancer of the ovary and other anatomic sites, *JAMA* 245(3):261, 1981.

61. Maggino T et al: Role of second look laparotomy in multidisciplinary treatment and in the follow up of advanced ovarian cancer, *Eur J Gynaecol Oncol* 4(1):26, 1983.

62. Malkasian GJ et al: CA 125 in gynecologic practice, *Am J Obstet Gynecol* 155(3):515, 1986.

63. Malone JJ et al: Palliation of small bowel obstruction by percutaneous gastrostomy in patients with progressive ovarian carcinoma, *Obstet Gynecol* 68(3):431, 1986.

64. Markman M et al: Intraperitoneal chemotherapy as treatment for ovarian carcinoma and gastrointestinal malignancies: the Memorial Sloan-Kettering Cancer Center experience, *Acta Med Austriaca* 16(3–4):65, 1989.

65. Markman M et al: Intraperitoneal therapy in the management of ovarian carcinoma, *Yale J Biol Med* 62(4):393, 1989.

66. Markman M et al: Responses to second-line cisplatin-based intraperitoneal therapy in ovarian cancer: influence of a prior response to systemic cisplatin. (Submitted).

67. Markman M et al: Second-line cisplatin therapy in patients with ovarian cancer previously treated with cisplatin, *J Clin Oncol* 9(3):389, 1991.

68. McCusker MC et al: The role of second-look laparotomy in treatment of epithelial ovarian cancer, *Gynecol Oncol* 28(1):83, 1987.

69. McGowan L, Bunnag B: The evaluation of therapy for ovarian cancer, *Gynecol Oncol* 4:375, 1976.

70. McGowan L et al: The woman at risk for developing ovarian cancer, *Gynecol Oncol* 7:325, 1979.

71. Meier W et al: Serum levels of CA 125 and histological findings at second-look laparotomy in ovarian carcinoma, *Gynecol Oncol* 35(1):44, 1989.

72. Miller DS et al: A critical reassessment of second-look laparotomy in epithelial ovarian carcinoma, *Cancer* 57(3):530, 1986.

73. Milsted R et al: Treatment of advanced ovarian cancer with combination chemotherapy using cyclophosphamide, adriamycin and cisplatinum, *Br J Obstet Gynaecol* 91(9):927, 1984.

74. Munnell E: The changing prognosis and treatment in cancer of the ovary, *Am J Obstet Gynecol* 100:790, 1968.

75. Murolo C et al: Ultrasound examination in ovarian cancer patients. A comparison with second look laparotomy, *J Ultrasound Med* 8(8):441, 1989.

76. Myers CE, Collins JM: Pharmacology of intraperitoneal chemotherapy, *Cancer Invest* 1(5):395, 1983.

77. Neijt J et al: Randomized trial comparing two combination chemotherapy regimens (CHAP-5 vs CP) in advanced ovarian carcinoma, *J Clin Oncol* 5:1157, 1987.

78. Ng LW et al: Aggressive chemosurgical debulking in patients with advanced ovarian cancer, *Gynecol Oncol* 38(3):358, 1990.

79. Niloff JM et al: Predictive value of CA 125 antigen levels in second-look procedures for ovarian cancer, *Am J Obstet Gynecol* 151(7):981, 1985.

80. Omura G et al: Randomized trial of cyclophosphamide plus cisplatin with or without doxorubicin in ovarian carcinoma: a Gynecologic Oncology Group study, *J Clin Oncol* 7:457, 1989.

81. Ozols RF et al: Peritoneoscopy in the management of ovarian cancer, *Am J Obstet Gynecol* 140(6):611, 1981.

82. Patsner B, Mann WJ: The value of preoperative serum CA 125 levels in patients with a pelvic mass, *Am J Obstet Gynecol* 159(4):873, 1988.

83. Pettersson F: Annual Report on the results of treatment in gynecological cancer, Stockholm: International Federation of Gynecology and Obstetrics, 1988.

84. Pfeiffer P et al: Intraperitoneal chemotherapy: introduction of a new "single use" delivery system—a preliminary report, *Gynecol Oncol* 35(1):47, 1989.

85. Pfeifle CE et al: Totally implantable system for peritoneal access, *J Clin Oncol* 2(11):1277, 1984.

86. Phibbs GD, Smith JP, Stanhope CR: Analysis of sites of persistent cancer at "second-look" laparotomy in patients with ovarian cancer, *Am J Obstet Gynecol* 147(6):611, 1983.

87. Piccart MJ et al: Intraperitoneal chemotherapy: technical experience at five institutions, *Semin Oncol* 90, 1985.

88. Piver MS, Barlow JJ, Lele SB: Incidence of subclinical metastasis in stage I and II ovarian carcinoma, *Obstet Gynecol* 52(1):100, 1978.

89. Piver MS et al: Survival after ovarian cancer induced intestinal obstruction, *Gynecol Oncol* 13(1):44, 1982.

90. Piver MS et al: Familial Ovarian Cancer Registry, *Obstet Gynecol* 64(2):195, 1984.

91. Plentyl A, Friedman E: *Lymphatic system of the female genitalia.* Philadelphia, 1971, WB Saunders.

92. Podczaski ES et al: Use of second-look laparotomy in the management of patients with ovarian epithelial malignancies, *Gynecol Oncol* 28(2):205, 1987.

93. Podratz KC et al: Second-look laparotomy in ovarian cancer: evaluation of pathologic variables, *Am J Obstet Gynecol* 152(2):230, 1985.

94. Podratz KC et al: Evaluation of treatment and survival after positive second-look laparotomy, *Gynecol Oncol* 31(1):9, 1988.

95. Raju KS et al: Second-look operations in the planned management of advanced ovarian carcinoma, *Am J Obstet Gynecol* 144(6):650, 1982.

96. Reichman B et al: Intraperitoneal cisplatin and etoposide in the treatment of refractory/recurrent ovarian carcinoma, *J Clin Oncol* 7(9):1327, 1989.

97. Roberts WS et al: Second-look laparotomy in the management of gynecologic malignancy, *Gynecol Oncol* 13(3):345, 1982.

98. Rocereto TF et al: The second-look celiotomy in ovarian cancer, *Gynecol Oncol* 19(1):34, 1984.

99. Rose D, Boyar A, Wynder E: International comparisons of mortality rates for cancer of the breast, ovary, prostate, and colon, and per capita food consumption, *Cancer* 58:2363, 1986.

100. Rubin SC, Lewis JJ: Second-look surgery in ovarian carcinoma, *Crit Rev Oncol Hematol* 8(1):75, 1988.

101. Rubin SC et al: Peritoneal cytology as an indicator of disease in patients with residual ovarian carcinoma [see comments], *Obstet Gynecol* 851, 1988.

102. Rubin SC et al: Recurrence after negative second-look laparotomy for ovarian cancer: analysis of risk factors, *Am J Obstet Gynecol* 159(5):109, 1988.

103. Rubin SC et al: Palliative surgery for intestinal obstruction in advanced ovarian cancer, *Gynecol Oncol* 34(1):16, 1989.

104. Rubin SC et al: Long-term access to the peritoneal cavity in ovarian cancer patients, *Gynecol Oncol* 33(1):46, 1989.

105. Rubin SC et al: Serum CA 125 levels and surgical findings in patients undergoing secondary operations for epithelial ovarian cancer, *Am J Obstet Gynecol* 160(3):667, 1989.

106. Rubin SC et al: Expression of P-glycoprotein in epithelial ovarian cancer: evaluation as a marker of multidrug resistance, *Am J Obstet Gynecol* 69, 1990.

107. Rubin S et al: Prognostic factors for recurrence following negative second-look laparotomy in ovarian cancer patients treated with platinum-based chemotherapy, *Gynecol Oncol* 1991.

108. Runowicz CD et al: Catheter complications associated with intraperitoneal chemotherapy, *Gynecol Oncol* 24(1):41, 1986.

109. Schwartz PE, Smith JP: Second-look operations in ovarian cancer, *Am J Obstet Gynecol* 138(8):1124, 1980.

110. Serov S, Scully R, Sobin L: *Histological typing of ovarian tumors.* In International histological classification of tumors. No. 9 (pp. 17–18). Geneva, 1973, World Health Organization.

111. Silverberg E: *Statistical and epidemiological information on gynecological cancer.* New York, 1986 American Cancer Society.

112. Skipper H: Thoughts on cancer chemotherapy and combination modality therapy, *JAMA* 230:1033, 1974.

113. Skipper H, Schabel FJ, Wilcox W: Experimental evaluation of potential anticancer agents XII: on the criteria and kinetics associated with "curability" of experimental leukemia, *Cancer Chem Rep* 35:1, 1964.

114. Smirz LR et al: Second-look laparotomy after chemotherapy in the management of ovarian malignancy, *Am J Obstet Gynecol* 661, 1985.

115. Smith JP, Delgado G, Rutledge F: Second-look operation in ovarian carcinoma: postchemotherapy, *Cancer* 38(3):1438, 1976.

116. Sonnendecker EW: Is routine second-look laparotomy for ovarian cancer justified? *Gynecol Oncol* 31(2):249, 1988.

117. Tobachman J, Tucker M, Kane R: Intraabdominal carcinomatosis after prophylactic oophorectomy in ovarian cancer-prone families, *Lancet* 2:795, 1982.

118. Tunca JC et al: The management of ovarian-cancer-caused bowel obstruction, *Gynecol Oncol* 186, 1981.

119. Webb MJ et al: Second-look laparotomy in ovarian cancer, *Gynecol Oncol* 14(3):285, 1982.

120. Webster KD, Ballard LJ: Ovarian carcinoma; second-look laparotomy postchemotherapy. Preliminary report, *Cleve Clin Q* 48(4):365, 1981.

121. West R: Epidemiologic study of malignancies of the ovaries, *Cancer* 19:1001, 1966.

122. Wu PC et al: Lymph node metastasis of ovarian cancer: a preliminary survey of 74 cases of lymphadenectomy, *Am J Obstet Gynecol* 155(5):1103, 1986.

123. Wu PC et al: Lymph node metastasis and retroperitoneal lymphadenectomy in ovarian cancer, *Baillieres Clin Obstet Gynaecol* 3(1):143, 1989.

124. Wynder E, Doko H, Barber H: Epidemiology of cancer of the ovary, *Cancer* 23:352, 1969.

125. Young R et al: Advanced ovarian adenocarcinoma: a prospective clinical trial of melphalan (L-PAM) versus combination chemotherapy, *N Engl J Med* 299:1261, 1978.

Chapter 42

PELVIC EXENTERATION

Hugh R.K. Barber
Jacqueline C. Johnson

HISTORICAL PERSPECTIVE

In December 1946, Brunschwig carried out an en bloc, one-stage excision of bladder, vagina, uterus, tubes and ovaries, lower ureters, and the rectosigmoid with a thorough bilateral pelvic lymph node dissection. The operation was designed to encompass and cure by a radical surgical approach pelvic cancer that could not be controlled or cured by any other modality of therapy. At that time, total pelvic exenteration was a viable option because radiation therapy had not achieved the sophistication that it has in the last decade.

At that time, any Department of Radiology included both diagnostic and therapeutic disciplines. The members of the department rotated through both sections, and it was not until the late 1950s into the mid 1960s that the disciplines were separated and the radiologist obtained special training in radiation therapy and devoted his or her energies to radiation therapy. As a result, the radiation therapist learned to control the local disease much better and it was in this group of patients that pelvic exenteration had its greatest application and impact.

In the late 1940s, chemotherapy was in its embryonic stages, and for certain select cancers the goal was to produce palliation. Now, more than 40 years later, chemotherapy too has advanced and is employed as a curative procedure, as well as for palliation. In the 1950s the Papanicolaou smear was introduced as a screening method to identify cancers of the cervix at an in situ or early invasive stage. These three advances, namely, improved radiation therapy, expanded use of chemotherapy, and lesions being identified at an earlier stage when they could be cured by a lesser procedure, markedly decreased the number of patients who qualified for pelvic exenteration.

Although Appleby[3] had carried out urinary and colonic diversions and at a later date excised pelvic organs, Brun-schwig is credited with doing the first en bloc, one-stage pelvic exenteration. Between 1935 and 1937, Brunschwig made a few desultory attempts to excise the bladder, prostate, and colon for advanced cancer of the colon by a three-stage operation (first, colostomy; second, cutaneous ureterostomies or nephrostomies; and third, excision of pelvic organs), but the results were disappointing and the technique was not pursued. However, his research identified that, although some cancers of the cervix metastasized out of the pelvis early, most remained within the pelvis for a long time. He felt that advanced or recurrent cancer of the cervix would be ideal for treatment by pelvic exenteration. In December 1946, he carried out the one-stage, en bloc total pelvic exenteration. Early in 1947, he did two more. In the fall of 1947, he was appointed chief of gynecology at Memorial Hospital in New York City and was given carte blanche to do radical surgery on both males and females. Brunschwig carried out the one-stage procedures as frequently as patients presented with the proper indications, and he published his first clinical report in 1948.[17] A less radical procedure, the anterior pelvic exenteration, was devised and reported in 1950. Brunschwig felt that the word *exenteration* was more appropriate for the operation than the original term *visceral evisceration*. He pointed out that exenteration was the surgical removal of the inner organs, commonly used to indicate radical excision of the contents of a body cavity as of the pelvis. Used in connection with the eye, it denotes removal of the entire contents of the orbit.

In the late 1940s and early 1950s, the total pelvic exenteration was referred to as the "all-American" operation. It is interesting to explore the reasons for this designation. Virginia K. Pierce, a fellow in oncology under Brunschwig and later an attending physician on the staff, was making rounds with the residents and fellows. They came to a patient who Pierce believed would require a pelvic exenteration to encompass the disease. It was the fall and the all-American football team was being chosen; in order not to upset the patient until she explained the type of operation to the residents outside the patient's room, she stated that the patient would need an all-American procedure. So, the term was born but did not meet with the approval of Brunschwig, who thought that it was not very scientific. Designating it the *total pelvic exenteration,* Pierce and the house staff began to call anterior pelvic exenteration, *the North American operation* and posterior exenteration, *the South American operation.* Because Brunschwig strongly disapproved of these terms, they were phased out and only the terms anterior, posterior, and total pelvic exenteration were used.

In the early part of the radical surgical approach to the control of locally advanced and recurrent carcinoma of the pelvis, there were no guidelines. As a result, the operation was attempted in any and all cases where the possibility existed that the disease could be cured or reasonable palliation could be achieved. The necessary surgical technique had to be established initially and then with greater experience had to be refined. The pitfalls of the operation were gradually elucidated, usually by bitter experience, but, in the end, Brunschwig and his staff learned how to do the operation so that the patient would have the maximum chance of survival and possible cure. The greatest number of cases were carried out by this group from 1947 through 1969.

GENERAL CONSIDERATIONS

Although other countries have many more advanced and recurrent cancers of the cervix than are found in the United States, pelvic exenteration is not commonly reported in these countries; most have been done within the United States. It is difficult to explain this because it has been proved that with limited selection of patients a very significant salvage rate (as high as 40%) can be achieved. This salvage rate cannot be achieved with radiation therapy or chemotherapy. Although central recurrence of cervical cancer represents the most suitable lesion for pelvic exenteration, the procedure can provide salvage cases of resectable primary or recurrent neoplasms of other types and origins. Brunschwig expanded his program and carried out pelvic exenteration for a variety of pelvic malignancies.

Pelvic exenteration is not as difficult an operation as a radical hysterectomy and pelvic lymph adenectomy that requires preservation of the bladder, ureters, and rectum, particularly if it is an extended radical hysterectomy.

Pelvic exenteration can be carried out with a mortality that is less than 5%. It is a taxing operation; the operator must be familiar with all pelvic structures and be able to expedite the operation. With the new hemoclips and stapling material, pelvic exenteration can be carried out in approximately 4 hours. Although the team approach of having a general surgeon, gynecologist, and urologist has been advocated, we believe that this is not in the best interest of the patient. It should be carried out by a gynecologic oncologist who has training in general surgery. Although cookbook protocols and stereotype programs have been advanced for the technique of the operation, the operator must be prepared to make adjustments, and because so many factors, including the patient and disease, enter into the operation, it is seldom possible to do the operation the same way repeatedly. The question of construction of a vagina is often raised, and whether this should be done at the time of the initial procedure depends on the difficulty in doing the primary operation, the age of the patient, the extent of the blood loss, and whether a perineal excision is necessary.

The "empty pelvis syndrome," in the early phase, may resemble a flulike illness with malaise, elevated temperature, and increased discharge from the perineal sinus that may continue for many years, particularly among those undergoing heavy irradiation. To avoid this syndrome, attempts have been made to cover the denuded pelvis. Numerous methods have been worked out. Brunschwig started using a pelvic pack that was removed on the second or third day; this has been followed by omental flaps and pedicles, peritoneal flaps, bovine pericardium grafts, collagen-filled small bowel mesentery leaf inserts, amnion chorion grafts, and synthetic pelvic floor slings. Although none of these has proved to be perfect, they have all decreased the postoperative morbidity by the management of the empty pelvic space.

INDICATIONS FOR PELVIC EXENTERATION AND CRITERIA FOR ESTIMATING PROGNOSIS

A quick review of the generally accepted 5-year salvage rates for cancer involving the different pelvic structures shows that about 30% to 40% of vulvar, 60% to 70% of vaginal, 40% to 60% of cervical, 30% of corpus, and 80% to 90% of ovarian cancers recur and need further treatment.[19]

The result of the treatment and the chances for long survival are difficult to predict. The operation is of considerable magnitude, and the patient has less resistance to any physical insult than has the nonexenterative patient, who is prone to develop infections. A high percentage of patients require additional surgery, usually for complications of the bowel or urinary tract. The success of treatment may be evaluated by the following:

At the time of operation, planes of dissection were developed with relative ease.

The recurrence was confined to the midline with minimal lateral spread.

There is relative certainty that all macroscopic disease was removed.

Technically, the urinary and bowel anastomoses were carried out with little trauma and no tension.

There was a reasonably uncomplicated postoperative course.

Hospital stay did not exceed 2½ to 3 weeks.

Postoperative pyelograms were within normal limits.

There were no attacks of pyelonephritis.

No fever occurred beyond the first 3 postoperative days.

There has been subjective improvement in association with a marked decrease in requirements of analgesic or narcotic drugs.

The clinical appearance correlates with the laboratory findings, indicating progressive improvement.

There has been a leveling off or reversal of the downward weight curve.

Performance status of the patient has improved.

There has been emotional adjustment to the operation.

Chemical and roentgen findings remain within normal limits.

All of the above are met and maintained for at least 1 year.

Absolute contraindications to surgery for cure[5]

Metastasis outside the pelvis (lung; supraclavicular, inguinal, or para-aortic nodes) and peritoneum (or positive cells in peritoneal fluid)

Visceral spread to the upper abdomen

"Skip" metastases to the bowel

Bilateral ureteral obstruction secondary to disease

Bilateral or multiple positive nodes in different lymph node chains

A triad of unilateral uropathy, unilateral leg edema, and sciatic pain

Relative contraindications to surgery for cure

Obesity

The patient over age 65

Doubt that all disease can be completely excised from the pelvis

Difficulty in mobilizing the specimen

Judgment decisions

Big, bulky, infected tumor

Localized abscess in pelvis

Lateral spread of tumor, especially in the posterior lateral part of the pelvis

Anaplastic tumor that has resisted initial treatment or recurs within 3 to 6 months of radiation therapy

Previously untreated cancer of the cervix

PREOPERATIVE EVALUATION TO DETERMINE OPERABILITY AND RESECTABILITY[20]
History

General health is important to the outcome in the management of patients with advanced cancer of the pelvis. Any metabolic or cardiopulmonary problem that would compromise the patient's chance for survival eliminates these patients as candidates for the pelvic exenteration. The patient should be mentally stable and come from a supportive family or have a support person available to them at all times.

Age of the patient at diagnosis is an important but highly variable factor. Although old age is listed as a contraindication in every series, none actually specifies an age beyond which exenteration is contraindicated. Old age is not a contraindication for radical surgery, with physiologic age being more important than chronologic age. However, in our series among patients receiving pelvic exenteration, morbidity and mortality rose significantly in patients older than 65. Therefore, the age of the patient must be considered when making the decision about whether to operate.

Other considerations include the time lapse from initial treatment to recurrence. If the interval is short, patients usually do poorly because of either the potency of the tumor or the decreased immunologic response of the patient. Weight loss over a short period of time is associated with a poor result, as are pain and swelling of the leg, especially when the pain radiates down the back of the leg.

Physical appearance

In general, the chronically ill, pale, emaciated patient who has difficulty in ambulating well or needs help in ambulation is a poor candidate for pelvic exenteration. The obese patient does poorly after surgery, particularly owing to cardiopulmonary complications. In addition, during the operation, obesity presents a difficult technical problem. Any evidence of extrapelvic spread is a contraindication to surgery. In general, a large lesion extending beyond the midline to the ischial spine and characterized by nodularity, fixed and with no spaces between the tumor and the pelvic side wall precludes the possibility of excision. A large cancer complicated by infection may be a contraindication to pelvic exenteration. Even with very potent broad-spectrum antibiotics, these patients are prone to develop further infection, and a higher number than would normally be anticipated develop sepsis.

Laboratory data

The usual metastatic work-up should be carried out. However, the backbone of the laboratory work-up consists of the blood count, urinalysis, blood chemistries, intravenous pyelogram, chest x-ray, and EKG. Various other scans and tests are optional. However, the best and the most accurate evaluation can be carried out at the time of exploratory surgery.

Preparation of the patient

When it has been decided that exenteration is a possibility after careful assessment of the patient, it is important to explain fully the magnitude of procedure to both the patient and her family. Before surgery the patient must be informed fully about her condition and the extent of the procedure. Ideally, she should meet the stomal therapist who must explain what responsibilities the patient will have in her own management.

It is also important to discuss with both the patient and her husband the full impact of the proposed operation, especially on sexual function and their perception of the alteration to body image. The possibility of producing a reconstructed vagina and the timing of this extra surgery must be discussed with the patient and her husband.

The anesthesiologist must assess the patient's ability to withstand the operation. Therefore the operating surgeon and the anesthesiologist must discuss this issue before surgery is undertaken.

Patient education

Crosson[21] has developed a patient teaching aid for the pelvic exenteration patient. She states that educational materials can greatly enhance patient teaching efforts when they meet the patient's information needs, are introduced at the appropriate times during the course of the disease, and are written at a level the patient understands.

The pamphlet is introduced to the patient after her discussion with the physician. The clinic nurse explains the pamphlet and encourages the patient and her family to read it before hospital admission. The nurse follows the teaching plan in a one-to-one teaching effort. Other members of the health care team refer to the educational booklet during their patient teaching sessions. Crosson's pamphlet is part of the patient education series at the University of Texas System Cancer Center, MD Anderson Hospital and Tumor Institute. It includes the description of the pelvic exenteration and the tests and preparation needed before the exenteration. It describes the procedure and the postoperative care. The discharge instructions are well presented and include important information for the patient in language that the patient can understand. It is also available in Spanish. A complimentary copy of the pamphlet can be obtained by writing to the Patient Education Program of the MD Anderson Hospital in Houston, Texas.

Parameters to be evaluated

Resectability. When it has been determined after a thorough work-up and evaluation that there is no contraindication to surgery, the patient is prepared to go to the operating room for exploratory laparotomy and the anticipated pelvic exenteration. Before any procedure the patient must be informed about all options, including the fact that if biopsies indicate that another modality of therapy should be chosen, the exenteration will not be carried out. This would apply in cases when the disease is beyond resection. Additionally, even though it has been determined preoperatively that no contraindication to surgery exists, resectability depends on the findings at exploratory laparotomy.

Positive peritoneal fluid or nodules on the peritoneum indicate lymphatic permeation; survival in this group of patients is brief indeed. Visceral and paraaortic involvement is also associated with a poor survival rate. However, in a few cases, the small bowel has dropped against the tumor and an area of serosal involvement can be resected en bloc including all of the tumor, or a small local encroachment of the tumor on the large bowel can be resected. These both have the potential for extended palliation or prolonged survival and are discussed in more detail later in the chapter.

Pelvic findings. If the tumor in the pelvis has extended to the pelvic side wall, either in the form of direct extension of the primary tumor or nodal metastasis, the prospects for cure are extremely small. Barber and Jones[12] showed that in a series of 671 patients receiving exenterative surgery for carcinoma of the cervix, there were 97 with involved pelvic nodes, only five of whom survived 5 years. They concluded that when pelvic nodes were involved, exenteration is contraindicated. The surgeon must, therefore, decide whether the procedure will materially improve the patient's quality of life and whether the short survival rate justifies the surgery.

Difficulty in establishing the planes of dissection often indicates extension of disease. These areas should be very carefully biopsied. It is important at the start of the pelvic exenteration to open up the planes along the pelvic wall and between the bladder and the obturator area as well as between the ureter and the hypogastric artery. This gives access to the pelvic side wall as well as the pelvic floor and helps determine operability rapidly.

The question is often raised whether pelvic bone excision has any place in the management of these patients. In patients where the bone is excised to obtain a wide margin, a small increase in survival may be anticipated, but in the presence of positive bone histology, excision should be abandoned.

Other considerations. When the triad of unilateral uropathy, unilateral leg edema, and sciatic pain occurs, the prospects for cure are extremely poor. This usually represents involvement of nerves and lymphatics of the pelvic side wall, which is not readily apparent using standard diagnostic techniques. The intravenous pyelogram has prognostic significance.[14] It has been observed that if the obstruction occurs at the ureterovesicle junction, the 5-year survival figures are similar to those of patients in whom normal bilateral visualization is recorded. However, the survival rate falls off progressively as the blockage occurs deeper in the pelvis, reaching practically zero when the obstruction is in the posterolateral aspect of the pelvis. Hydronephrosis is merely a stage in the progression to obstruction, and the amount of hydronephrosis is correlated with the extent of disease.

Failure to control the cancer after radiation or surgery is not very rewarding if the original treatment is simply continued. However, an increased complication rate usually occurs. The results obtained by pelvic exenteration after radiation therapy are comparable to those when pelvic exenteration is carried out after failure of initial radical hysterectomy surgery.[13] However, the difference lies in that very few patients are suitable for additional curative surgery after failure of primary radical surgery as opposed to those who fail to respond after radiation therapy.

Generally, exenterative surgery should not be used as a palliative method; very few series have advocated this approach. However, from time to time circumstances arise where exenteration offers a very much improved quality of life despite paraaortic metastases. These circumstances are limited to the presence of a fistula in the bladder or rectum accompanied by severe local pain and pelvic infection. Even here it may be argued that a bypass procedure will achieve a similar result with less trauma. Another consideration must be raised in evaluating the untreated advanced cervical cancer for pelvic exenteration. Despite the good survival rate after radical surgery in the treatment of cancer of the cervix stages III and IV, the loss of bladder or rectum with urinary or fecal diversion is a major complication and has decreased the enthusiasm for exenteration as a primary form of treatment. Million and associates[28] reported 28% survival of patients with bladder invasion managed only by radiation therapy. This survival was equivalent to survival after exenteration, and there were no fistulas in these patients. On the basis of this study, these authors preferred radiation therapy to primary exenteration in patients with advanced cervical cancer involving the bladder. In general, pelvic exenteration should be reserved for patients for whom there is no chance of cure by any other modality.

Inflammatory carcinoma is a recognized syndrome in the breast and is characterized by widespread lymphatic permeation. However, little attention has been given to this finding in the pelvis, possibly due to the fact that it is not as easily observed as in the breast. The pelvic peritoneum appears red and the vessels are dilated, a picture not too dissimilar from that seen in early peritonitis. The clinical findings are not secondary to infection but rather to extensive lymphatic permeation and carry a poor prognosis and high morbidity. It is important to rule out widespread disease. Usually in this clinical setting pelvic exenteration is not indicated.

The traditional philosophy has been to tailor the pelvic exenteration to fit the needs of the patient and the extent of disease. With limited disease, a procedure whose magnitude is less than that of total pelvic exenteration should achieve a significant 5-year survival, as borne out in patients undergoing anterior pelvic exenteration. Certain patients with vulvar, vaginal, and colon recurrence are candidates for treatment by limited pelvic exenteration such as the anterior or posterior exenteration. However, recurrent cervical cancer is probably best treated by total pelvic exenteration.

Cancer of the cervix spreading posteriorly quickly becomes adherent to the pelvic floor and also invades the venous plexus in this area. In treating recurrent cancer of the cervix, it is most important to excise the vagina, leaving behind denuded bladder and ureters in patients treated by posterior pelvic exenteration, which will slough from lack of support and blood supply. A high morbidity and mortality contraindicate posterior pelvic exenteration for the treatment of recurrent cancer of the cervix.

The question is raised whether pelvic exenteration should be carried out for palliation or only in the hope for a cure. It can be stated that pelvic exenteration should not be carried out if disease is left behind in the pelvis or even if it is thought that cancer may be left. There will be no

palliation and the brief survival will be accompanied by high morbidity. Only when all disease is removed, but where the clinical setting indicates an extended chance for long-term survival, can resection with the goal of palliation be justified. Among patients in whom disease was left after surgery was carried out for recurrent cervical cancer, the average survival rate is slightly over 3 months and there is little, if any, palliation. Commonly, patients in whom disease is left behind in the pelvis or in whom it is not recognized do poorly postoperatively and have a slow convalescence, characterized by ileus, low-grade fever, and lethargy without any other clinical cause for the poor postoperative course being determined.

McCullough and Nahhas[26] reported the futility of doing palliative pelvic exenteration. They stated that, "Following palliative exenteration, morbidity and mortality were high, survival was low and the quality of life was uniformly poor. With few exceptions, pelvic exenteration as a palliative procedure should not be performed."

Stanhope and Symmonds[34] reported on their experience at the Mayo Clinic. Eighteen percent of their surgeries were considered retrospectively to be palliative because of pelvic or aortic nodal metastases, pelvic peritoneal involvement, pelvic wall involvement, bone involvement or, in two cases, distant metastases. The survival statistics were 47% at 2 years and 17% at 5 years. When metastatic nodal disease was found after irradiated pelvic recurrence, the 2- and 5-year survivals were 46% and 23%, respectively. They stated that, although exenterative procedures are designed to be curative, the palliative benefits obtained in this group of patients appeared to be worthwhile and comparable to those achieved in advanced epithelial ovarian carcinoma for which aggressive surgical treatment is now strongly advocated.

It is obvious that there are cases in which all of the disease can be removed from the pelvis, eliminating the fistulas that are present, and, despite the presence of paraaortic disease, a significant survival rate can be achieved.

TECHNIQUE

The technique of pelvic exenteration has been described in great detail by several authors. However, there has been no significant advance since Brunschwig did the first pelvic en bloc, one-stage exenteration in 1946.

Essentially there are three types: anterior, posterior, and total pelvic exenteration. The total pelvic exenteration is a synthesis of three major procedures: (1) radical hysterectomy with bilateral pelvic lymph node dissection and bilateral salpingooophorectomy, (2) total cystectomy, and (3) combined abdominoperineal resection of the rectum.[6] Both anterior and posterior pelvic exenterations are less formidable procedures; although we will briefly outline their indications, the exact procedures will not be discussed separately.

Anterior pelvic exenteration is employed to encompass disease that is located in the region of the bladder. It is a fusion of radical cystectomy, radical hysterectomy, bilateral pelvic lymph node dissection, bilateral salpingooophorectomy, and partial vaginectomy. When the malignant disease arises in the posterior wall of the fornix and involves the rectovaginal septum and the rectum without encroaching anteriorly, a posterior pelvic exenteration may be indicated to excise the disease en bloc. In a posterior pelvic exenteration, which is merely an extended form of abdominoperineal resection, a radical excision of the lower bowel and rectum is carried out along with radical hysterectomy, bilateral pelvic lymph node dissection, bilateral salpingooophorectomy, and vaginectomy. Because the vagina must be excised, when pelvic exenteration is employed for management of cervical cancer, the floor of the bladder is denuded and left without support. This results in a very high incidence of bladder fistula and, as a result, there are few indications, if any, for posterior pelvic exenteration in the management of advanced or recurrent cancer of the cervix.

Total pelvic exenteration encompasses the bladder, rectum, uterus, tubes, ovaries and pelvic lymph nodes en mass. It is performed as follows[31]:

The abdomen is opened through a left pararectus incision that extends above the umbilicus as needed for better exposure. The abdomen and pelvis are carefully explored, with particular attention being given to the paraaortic area. Pelvic washings are obtained from the upper abdomen and the pelvis. The self-retaining retractor is set in place, and the intestines are carefully tacked out of the pelvis. In this operation, exposure is the keystone to success.

The paraaortic area may be evaluated on palpation alone or the peritoneum may be excised and lymph nodes removed for frozen section diagnosis.

The posterior peritoneum is picked up lateral to the infundibulopelvic ligament above the pelvic brim and is incised superficially, allowing the areolar tissue to fall away. The incision is carried to the round ligament. This ligament is clamped, cut, and ligated, and the incision in the peritoneum is carried to the inguinal area.

The ureter is dissected medially with finger dissection, care being taken to keep the ureter attached to the peritoneum. Then the common and external iliac vessels are freed from the pelvic wall by incising the tissue between the vessels and the pelvic wall. Using finger dissection, the tissue is separated from the pelvic wall down to the pelvic floor, thus exposing the lateral edge of the sacroiliac nerve plexus (sciatic nerve).

The tissue between the rectosigmoid and hypogastric artery is incised and a blunt dissection with the index finger is separated down to the pelvic floor. By identifying the distal portion of the obliterated vessels along the lateral edge of the bladder, another relatively avascular plane is located and the dissection is carried down to the pelvic floor. This facilitates identification and isolation of the obturator vessels and nerves.

The lymph nodes on the common and external iliac vessels are dissected starting at the origin of the common iliac artery and continuing along the external artery to the inguinal ligaments. At the distal segment of the external iliac vein, the pelvic tissue is dissected from the vein and removed from the obturator and levator ani muscles by finger dissection. This, in combination with the previous dissection, mobilizes the entire area.

The distal dissection is carried along the proximal part of the vein to the level of the hypogastric vessels. As the dissection is carried higher, care must be employed to prevent damage to the hypogastric vein as it joins the common iliac vein.

The obturator nerve is identified and protected from injury while the obturator vessels are clamped, cut, and ligated at the obturator foramen. The hypogastric artery is ligated either at its origin from the common iliac artery or wherever it can be mobilized easily, whereas the vein is ligated distally and then excised proximally, depending on whether a part of the vein or the entire vein is to be taken. If the hypogastric vein is taken, there is an increased amount of blood loss.

The vessels over the sacroiliac plexus are ligated individually. The entire side is mobilized, and a similar procedure is carried out on the contralateral side. The use of hemoclips during this dissection speeds up the operation.

The colon is mobilized at the pelvic brim, clamped, and transected, the inferior mesenteric artery and vein having been ligated. Then the rectosigmoid is freed from the posterior pelvis down to the coccyx; injury to the middle sacral veins must be avoided. The ureters are divided at a level below the pelvic brim. The bladder is mobilized readily from the posterior part of the pubis and is retracted backward. The mass of pelvic viscera is now freed from its attachments to the pelvic floor and the dissection is carried to the perineum, including the vulva. A pack may be placed in the pelvis.

Urinary diversion is carried out, using a segment of the ileum or sigmoid. The stapling method speeds up the operation.[16] A colostomy stoma is placed on the left at a different level from that of the ileal stoma (for urinary diversion); this is usually brought out to the skin surface in the right lower quadrant. A perineal phase may or may not be employed depending on the operator's preference.

The abdomen is closed in layers. New sutures, such as the Maxon no. 1, have cut down on the need for interrupted retention sutures.

RESULTS OF PELVIC EXENTERATION
Vulval cancer

The cure rate for primary treatment of vulval cancer by radical vulvectomy and lymph node dissection with or without radiation therapy is about 70%; therefore, 30% to 40% of the patients suffer a recurrence. However, because many of these patients are in the geriatric age group, the number dying from an intercurrent disease cuts down the number that presents finally for definitive treatment. In one series it was noted that, although all patients had a node dissection with the original radical vulvectomy, 33% of the patients with recurrent vulvar cancer had positive nodes at the time of pelvic exenteration. This indicates either that nodes were missed at the time of the original procedure or that regeneration of lymph channels had occurred.

Survival after treatment for cancer is related to the type of tumor and host resistance. There is no means of measuring either of these parameters. However, when considerable time has elapsed between initial treatment and recurrence, it may be assumed that either the tumor is of low virulence or the patient possesses a high degree of host resistance. A well-differentiated tumor usually remains localized for a longer period than an anaplastic cancer.

The lymphatics from the vulva course anteriorly, and the type of operation required to excise en bloc a recurrence of vulval cancer is directed toward eradication of the area drained by the lymphatics from the tumor. Failure after initial therapy probably results from small cancer emboli present in the lymphatics draining the cancer-bearing area. Most recurrent cancers of the vulva can be managed with an anterior exenteration. The complication rate is high among these patients, and the survival rate ranges from 15% to 20% at 5 years or more.

Morley[29] in a review of cancer of the vulva stated that the currently accepted treatment of invasive carcinoma of the vulva is radical vulvectomy and bilateral lymph node dissection. He states that no longer is pelvic lymph node dissection to be considered a routine part of the therapy but rather it is included only under specific circumstances. On rare occasions, a more radical procedure such as an anterior or posterior pelvic exenteration is considered appropriate therapy when the geographic location of the tumor requires this approach. The treatment of recurrent vulval cancer is influenced by its extent and location and must be tailored to the individual patient. In 1981, Morley reported on 14 cases of carcinoma of the vulva treated by pelvic exenteration. Three patients were treated with total pelvic exenteration, nine with posterior exenteration, and two with anterior pelvic exenteration. The overall 5-year survival was 66.6%. He stated that, if the lesion was geographically located so as to require only an anterior or posterior exenteration, he achieved an 80% 5-year survival on the 10 patients treated. As anticipated, total pelvic exenteration resulted in a much more dismal prognosis (see also Chapter 19).

Vaginal cancer[11]

Cancer of the vagina constitutes about 1% or 2% of the cancers of the female genital tract. It is less frequent than cancer of the vulva, but the number of reported cases is increasing, probably because of better diagnostic methods.

Carcinoma of the vagina is often well advanced when first diagnosed. The lesion may be concealed by the speculum unless the speculum is rotated to expose the entire vagina at the time of its removal and, therefore, the cancer is not detected until it has grown large or until signs and symptoms are quite evident. The vaginal lymphatics drain in three ways: the upper third of the vagina drains along

cervical lymphatics, the lower third along the vulval channels, and the middle third along either cervical or vulval channels.

The difference in the type of operation required to excise vaginal disease is of some interest. Most patients with advanced vulval cancer can be treated with an anterior pelvic exenteration, whereas most with advanced vaginal cancer require a total pelvic exenteration to encompass their disease. This could reflect either the location of the disease or possibly a more virulent cancer. If the cancer occurs in the anterior vaginal wall, particularly in the upper third, it is in close contact with the bladder. If it grows on the posterior wall, particularly in the middle third, it is very close to the rectum. In either of these situations, it is almost impossible to excise the cancer with an adequate margin without doing an exenterative procedure.

Talledo[36] reported on six cases of cancer of the vagina and vulvovaginal cancer and noted that there were two survivors. Rubin, Young, and Mikuta[33] reported that, in view of the satisfactory survival in stages I and II carcinoma of the vagina treated with radiotherapy, pelvic exenteration should be reserved for patients with central stage IV disease or with recurrences after radiotherapy. Patients in this series treated with exenteration did poorly, with only one of seven surviving 5 years. Phillips, Buchsbaum, and Lifshitz[32] reported on 16 pelvic exenterations performed for advanced and recurrent vulvovaginal cancer. Seven patients are alive and free of disease (six for more than 5 years and one for over 4 years). Three patients died free of disease, with an absolute 5-year survival rate of 54%.

Corpus cancer[9,22]

The survival rate for primary treatment of cancer of the endometrium is approximately 70%. Therefore, about 30% present with a recurrence. It has been reported that carcinoma of the cervix and carcinoma of the endometrium have similar natural histories or method of spread. However, this is now open to controversy. During an interval when several hundred exenterations were carried out for cancer of the cervix at Memorial Hospital, only 36 with advanced and recurrent corpus were found to be suitable for pelvic exenteration.

The finding of positive nodes at the time of treatment for carcinoma of the endometrium carries a very poor prognosis. Therefore, in patients with persistent or recurrent disease, positive nodes indicate an almost hopeless prognosis. Because there is an increased incidence of paraaortic node involvement in carcinoma of the endometrium a special effort must be made to rule out any possibility of paraaortic spread of disease before carrying out a pelvic exenteration.

Although there are fewer indications for pelvic exenteration in patients with carcinoma of the endometrium than in those with carcinoma of the cervix, there is a place for pelvic exenteration in the management of this malignancy. The number of patients qualifying for pelvic exenteration who present with carcinoma of the endometrium is small;

a survival rate of up to 20% can be anticipated. Falk and colleagues reported that pelvic exenteration has a place in the management of extensive, recurrent pelvic adenocarcinomas. It is of particular value in patients whose tumors can be completely removed, but it can also provide effective palliation of symptoms in selected patients with incurable disease.

Ovarian cancer[8]

At laparotomy, the characteristic finding in patients with advanced ovarian cancer is wide dissemination of tumor over the peritoneal surfaces of the pelvis, upper abdomen, and omentum, and frequent involvement of both ovaries either as spread from one primary malignancy or bilateral primary growths. Advanced and recurrent ovarian cancer is not amenable to surgical treatment except when a complication of the tumor, such as the relief of obstruction or drainage of an abscess, requires surgery.

Reports indicate that because the ovary and the entire peritoneal cavity are mesothelial structures, whatever is stimulating the ovary to form a malignancy is also stimulating other places in the peritoneal cavity. They conclude that the disease that has spread in the upper abdomen may represent multiple primary tumors rather than metastatic disease. This may account for the relatively few patients with ovarian cancer who are suitable for pelvic exenteration.

Theoretically, the natural history of ovarian cancer ordinarily contraindicates pelvic exenteration. However, in some instances recurrence is late and limited entirely to the pelvis, and a more radical procedure such as pelvic exenteration may be reasonable. Endometrioid ovarian cancer may lend itself to a radical surgical approach, because it has been shown that only 30% of cases are bilateral and 45% showed metastases to the upper abdomen. Endometrioid cancer of the ovary thus appears to be a less aggressive cancer than other ovarian cancers, especially in its potential for distant spread.

Patients with advanced recurrent ovarian cancer are an unfavorable group for pelvic exenteration, and, except in extremely rare instances, this surgical procedure is not indicated for the management of carcinoma of the ovary, particularly since the advent of combination chemotherapy, which is producing favorable 5-year survival rates. Less than a 10% 5-year survival can be anticipated when pelvic exenteration is carried out as a definitive procedure for carcinoma of the ovary.

Cervical cancer

About half of the patients with carcinoma of the cervix reported in the *Annual Report on the Results of Treatment in Gynecologic Cancer,* 20th volume, survive 5 years or more.[2] Therefore, almost half the patients treated for carcinoma of the cervix will have persistence or recurrence of their disease.

Surgical-pathologic classification. Meigs and Brunschwig established a classification for cases of cancer of the cervix[27] so that results could be compared objectively among different services. This classification of cervical cancer affords an opportunity for an accurate evaluation and serves to document the natural history of the tumor. The correlation of clinical and histopathologic findings permits a comparison of results among clinics carrying out a surgical program. This classification is not to be confused with the international classification. Classes of carcinoma of the cervix according to the surgical-pathologic classification are designated as follows:

A   Limited to the cervix
B   Involves vagina and/or corpus
C   Parametrial extension
CN   Parametrial node
D   Peripheral node and parametrial extension
E   Bladder and/or rectum
EN   Same as E, plus node involvement
F   Pelvic wall—beyond pelvis
FN   Same as F, plus node involvement
AO   After positive biopsy specimen of infiltrating carcinoma, no tumor in the cervix in the surgical specimen
PR   Preoperative irradiation
R   Curative radiation followed by failure
S   Surgical attempt at cure before recurrence
RS   Irradiation and surgery employed for cure but requires further surgery for persistence or recurrence of disease

Role of exenteration. Pelvic exenteration has its most important role in the management of persistent or recurrent cancer of the cervix.[25] In most instances, cancer of the cervix remains confined to the pelvis for a long time. These patients are suitable for further treatment of their cancer. Repeat irradiation therapy has little to offer in terms of cure and is accompanied by a high rate of complication and exacerbation of symptoms. The belief that if radiation has failed there is no further treatment affording cure is untenable today. The tendency for carcinoma of the cervix to remain localized to the pelvis provides an opportunity to encompass the disease by a surgical approach. The combination of surgery and multiple anticancer chemotherapy may add to the survival rate of these patients.

It is important to diagnose and treat recurrent cancer of the cervix soon after the recurrence is detected. The diagnosis of recurrence at an early stage is often difficult. In the early stages of recurrence the patient may have no symptoms and very few objective signs. A high index of suspicion is paramount in making the diagnosis. However, on pelvic examination, any change from previous examinations should indicate that more aggressive diagnostic procedures must be carried out. Intravenous pyelogram, ultrasound and/or computed tomography (CT) scans, and magnetic resonance imaging (MRI) contribute to making a diagnosis. A relatively new marker squamous cell cancer (SSC) has added another test, but, unfortunately, it is not very sensitive or specific. In cases of suspected recurrence, it is often possible to make a definitive diagnosis with the skinny needle biopsy. However, an exploratory laparotomy is usually required to make a definitive diagnosis.

At the time of exploration, the best results occur when the disease is confined to the central part of the pelvis. The survival rate drops as the disease moves toward the pelvic wall, and, if there is no free space between the recurrence and the pelvic wall, the chances for a 5-year survival are almost zero. In the favorable group of patients who have a central lesion of approximately 50% or higher, 5-year survival can be anticipated.[30] However, if there is lateral spread or the lesion is totally confined to the central pelvis, the survival rates range from 20% to over 50%.

The presence of positive pelvic lymph node involvement decreases the chance for survival. If more than one chain of nodes is involved, the results drop precipitiously, and when there is bilateral pelvic lymph node involvement, the survival rate is about zero. The overall results when pelvic lymph nodes are positive among patients with recurrent cancer are approximately 5% to 15%, although some series report a 0% 5-year survival. Symmonds and Webb[35] reported a 15% survival of patients with squamous cell carcinoma of the cervix with metastases to the lymph nodes.

Extensive radiation necrosis.[10] The management of radiation necrosis presents a real challenge. The clinical picture is complicated by severe pain, urinary or intestinal fistula, bleeding, copious foul discharge, and physical deterioration of the patient. It is difficult clinically to differentiate recurrent cancer from irradiation reaction and damage, but with proper selection of patients, pelvic exenteration is justified even though only radiation necrosis with fistula is found. Among patients treated for extensive radiation necrosis, a few will die of cancer despite the fact that cancer was not found at the time of pelvic exenteration. This confirms the natural history of cervical cancer and also reinforces the observation that it is difficult to differentiate clinically between persistent cancer and radiation necrosis even in the presence of a negative biopsy. Patients treated by pelvic exenteration for visceral necrosis are labile, and constant supervision is essential. Many develop complications, most of which are small bowel fistulas. The results achieved in terms of physical well-being appear to justify the operation, because before surgery existence is just bearable in most instances.

It appears that pelvic exenterations are indicated in selected patients for radiation necrosis and other damage-producing severe symptoms. However, before pelvic exenteration, the patient should be evaluated to see if diversion of the urinary and fecal streams could possibly provide palliation. If in the judgment of the surgeon this can be achieved, there is a great deal less morbidity and practically no mortality as opposed to those receiving pelvic exenteration. However, this method of management by merely diverting the urinary and fecal stream may not control the bleeding, foul discharge, or pain that accompanies visceral necrosis.

Exenteration for other cancers

Pelvic exenteration has been carried out for approximately 20 different disease entities. Aside from those already discussed, exenteration has been employed to control cancer of the rectum, embryonal cancer of the vagina, sarcoma of the uterus, cancer of the bladder, mixed mesodermal tumor of the uterus, granular cell myoblastoma, cancer of the urethra, adenocarcinoma of the tubes, cancer of the perineum, lymphosarcoma, leiomyosarcoma of the bladder, leiomyosarcoma of the cervix, sarcoma of the prostate, fibrosarcoma, and reticulum cell sarcoma of the cervix.

Symmonds and Webb[35] have also reported on a variety of tumors and organ systems treated with pelvic exenteration. They stated that the physician should consider pelvic exenteration when indicated regardless of the origin or cell type of the tumor. Averette and co-workers[4] carried out pelvic exenteration for 12 different organ systems.

DISCHARGE FROM THE HOSPITAL[7]

Criteria have been established for discharge from the hospital. The patient:

Feels well physically and mentally
Tolerates a normal diet
Has no fever for at least 5 days
Walks without difficulty
Shows interest in being discharged from the hospital
Starts to resume interest in her previous work or hobbies
Demonstrates that she can take care of herself at home
Has skill and confidence in managing her "ostomies"
Has stable or increasing weight
Has minimal drug requirements
Understands the labile nature of her condition and accepts her responsibility for reporting any complications immediately
Understands the importance of continued follow-up examinations
Has immediate family members who understand the nature of the problem
Can return to home surroundings where the problems presented by the patient are accepted
Has, in the judgment of the responsible physician, been rehabilitated to the point where she can be discharged

PSYCHOSEXUAL ADJUSTMENT AND REHABILITATION[37]

The rehabilitation of the patient who has had a pelvic exenteration should be well-structured. There are several excellent articles in the literature on this subject.[23,24]

It has been stated that patients who have survived for some time after pelvic exenteration are happy. Happiness probably means that they have become well-adjusted to the operation that they received. After a period of time, the patient realizes that the cancer is controlled. The patient's partner often can play a significant role in the rehabilitation of the patient. It is important to have a careful sexual history in the preoperative period and to explain to the patient that it is possible to make a psychosexual adjustment after pelvic exenteration.

Sexual functioning, particularly under age 65, continues as the area of greatest disruption for these patients. It is important to construct a vagina to restore confidence to the patient and help in her rehabilitation. If a perineal phase is not required to encompass the entire disease, the vulva and clitoris can be left in place. This provides a psychological uplift for the patient, particularly when she realizes that a functioning vagina can be constructed. These women are able to recapture some of their previous sexual activity and, although it may not be as complete and satisfying as before the exenteration, it is usually acceptable and satisfying for both the patient and her partner. Patients who have a fairly strong sex drive before the pelvic exenteration do better than those who have a low sex drive.

Berek and colleagues[15] reported on 28 patients who underwent vaginal reconstruction simultaneously with pelvic exenteration performed for recurrent pelvic malignancy. A satisfactory neovagina was created in 86% of the patients. When vaginal reconstruction can be performed simultaneously with pelvic exenteration, it is in the best interest of the patient.

It is important to provide continuing support and regular counseling to the patient who has had a pelvic exenteration. Every gynecologic oncologist should have one or two patients who have had a pelvic exenteration and made a satisfactory physical, psychological, and sexual rehabilitation available to meet with the patient who is about to undergo a pelvic exenteration. In my experience, this has provided an important support mechanism, particularly when the patient who has survived a pelvic exenteration for a long time is available at any time to talk to the patient who is about to have an exenteration or who has recently recovered from a pelvic exenteration. These patients should be encouraged to return to productive activity as soon as possible. They must be instructed and advised to engage in all of their previous social functions, including golf, horseback riding, or whatever activities they enjoyed. The aim is to bring about total rehabilitation and a satisfactory adjustment to the loss of bladder, rectum, and vagina. The quality of life is almost as important as the quantity of life. Andersen and Hacker[1] reported on 15 pelvic exenteration patients they studied and found that after the patients were asymptomatic and clinically free of disease that they still appear mildly depressed and distressed. However, these women report active and satisfactory levels of social and leisure activities. Sexual functioning continues as the area of greatest disruption for these patients, and, as a group, they resemble severely sexually dysfunctional healthy women. Anderson and Hacker also reported that there was a reduction in the frequency of sexual activity, both sexual arousal and satisfaction, and disruption of sexual competence and body image. These difficulties appear to be more or less distressing to a patient, depending on the availability of a sexual partner and the patient's own desire for the continuation of her sexual life.

SUMMARY

Pelvic exenteration continues to play a role in the treatment of recurrent or persistent gynecologic malignancy confined to the central pelvis. It is most frequently employed in cases of recurrent or persistent cervical cancer, but is also well-suited for recurrent vaginal and vulvar lesions.

A survey of the literature over a 40-year period suggests that exenteration operations have not been widely accepted or perhaps not commonly reported except in the United States. Even in the United States, the series reported are usually very small. The reasons for this are difficult to explain except that the most widely indicated reason for the operation is carcinoma of the cervix and this has been decreasing in incidence as far as the more advanced stages and recurrences are concerned. Cancer of the cervix is being diagnosed at earlier stages with a greater chance for cure without recurrence.

Since 1946, there have been very few significant changes in the approach for carrying out a pelvic exenteration. There have been some refinements in the technique, and the use of hemoclips and stapling apparatus has significantly cut down on the time required to do an exenteration. New techniques have been introduced to manage the denuded pelvis.

Endometrial and ovarian cancer have been on the increase, with endometrial cancer being diagnosed early with excellent results. Ovarian cancer, which is diagnosed most commonly in stages III and IV, does not lend itself readily to exenterative surgery. The pelvic exenteration has a limited role as primary therapy and as treatment for recurrent or persistent endometrial and ovarian cancer. It has been stated that ovarian cancer only lends itself to management by pelvic exenteration when it violates its natural history, that is, it remains in the pelvis and does not spread to the upper abdomen or there is a late recurrence from the original treatment to the time that the exenteration is to be carried out.

In cases where pelvic exenteration is indicated (and these are highly selected patients), there is no other equally curative form of therapy that exists for the distressing problem of recurrent pelvic cancer.

With the new stapling techniques and use of clips along the pelvic wall to control bleeding from the blood vessels in that area, it is possible to do a pelvic exenteration with little blood loss and in considerably less time than previously. The improved methods of monitoring these patients with the Swan-Ganz catheter and a better understanding of the metabolic and physiologic processes has reduced the mortality to less than 5%. The new, very potent broad-spectrum antibiotics given in combination have significantly decreased the morbidity associated with pelvic exenteration. The adjuvant use of anticancer chemotherapy has added another dimension to the management of these patients.

Having given these patients a quantity of life, it is important to give them a quality of life. These patients should be rehabilitated and, if indicated, a new vagina should be constructed and the patient should be encouraged to lead a normal life. In constructing the new vagina, it is important to elevate the vagina so that during intercourse there will be adequate contact with the clitoris.

Perhaps these patients cannot be described as happy patients but at least they have been given a second chance for life; they can become well-adjusted and make significant contributions to their family and the community. Many of these patients are at the height of their social and economic productivity and must receive strong support from their family, physician, nurses, social workers, counselors, and clergy.

The improved methods of treating patients with radiation therapy and combination therapy, such as radiation, surgery, chemotherapy, immunotherapy, and hyperthermia, have reduced the number of patients who require pelvic exenteration. However, rather than relegating patients with recurrent malignancy to the scrapheap of repeated irradiation and chemotherapy, which are rarely curative, the responsible physician should consider pelvic exenteration, regardless of the origin or cell type of the tumor.

Acknowledgments. The author wishes to thank Ruzena Danek, Marcia Miller, and Shirley Dansker, Chief Librarian, for their assistance in the preparation of this chapter.

REFERENCES

1. Andersen BL, Hacker NF: Psychosocial adjustment following pelvic exenteration, *Obstet Gynecol* 61(3):331, 1983.
2. Annual Report on the Results of Treatment of Gynecological Cancer. Vol. 20. *Statement of results obtained in 1976 to 1978 inclusive,* Stockholm, 1988, International Federation of Gynecology and Obstetrics.
3. Appleby LH: Proctocystectomy: the management of colostomy with ureteral transplants, *Am J Surg* 79:57, 1950.
4. Averette HE et al: Pelvic exenteration: a 15 year experience in a general metropolitan hospital, *Am J Obstet Gynecol* 150:179, 1984.
5. Barber HRK: Relative prognostic significance of preoperative and operative findings in pelvic exenteration, *Surg Clin North Am* 49:431, 1969.
6. Barber HRK: *Exenteration procedures in pelvic malignancy.* In *Davis' Gynecology and Obstetrics,* vol 3, chap 63, Hagerstown, 1977, Harper and Row.
7. Barber HRK: Pelvic exenteration, *Cancer Invest* 5(4):331, 1987.
8. Barber HRK, Brunschwig A: Pelvic exenteration for advanced and recurrent ovarian cancer, *Surgery* 58:935, 1965.
9. Barber HRK, Brunschwig A: Treatment and results of recurrent cancer of corpus uteri in patients receiving anterior and total exenteration 1947-1963, *Cancer* 22:949, 1968.
10. Barber HRK, Brunschwig A: Definitive treatment of radiation necrosis. Five year results in 77 patients, *Obstet Gynecol* 35:344, 1970.
11. Barber HRK, Brunschwig A, Mangioni C: Advanced cancer of the vulva and vagina treated by anterior and total pelvic exenteration 1947-1962 at the Memorial-James Ewing Hospital. Estratto dalla Rivista, *Annali di Ostetrica e Gynecologica,* 1968.
12. Barber HRK and Jones W: Lymphadenectomy in pelvic exenteration for recurrent cervix cancer, *JAMA* 215:1945, 1971.
13. Barber HRK, O'Neil W: Recurrent cervical cancer after treatment by a primary surgical program, *Obstet Gynecol* 37(2):165, 1971.
14. Barber HRK, Roberts S, Brunschwig A: Prognostic significance of the preoperative nonvisualizing kidney in patients receiving pelvic exenteration, *Cancer* 16:1614, 1963.
15. Berek JS, Hacker NF, Lagasse LD: Vaginal reconstruction performed simultaneously with pelvic exenteration, *Obstet Gynecol* 63:318, 1984.
16. Bricker EM: *The technique of ileal segment bladder substitution.* In Meigs JA, editor: *Progress in gynecology,* vol 3, New York, 1957, Grune & Stratton.
17. Brunschwig A: Complete excision of pelvic viscera for abdominal carcinoma, *Cancer* 1:177, 1948.
18. Brunschwig A: What are the indications and results of pelvic exenteration? *JAMA* 194:274, 1965.
19. *Cancer Facts and Figures 1992.* New York, 1990, American Cancer Society.
20. Creasman WT, Rutledge FN: Preoperative evaluation of patients with recurrent carcinoma of the cervix, *Gynecol Oncol* 1:111, 1972.
21. Crosson K: A patient teaching aid for the pelvic exenteration patient, *Oncology Nursing Forum* 8(4):53, 1981.
22. Falk RE et al: Pelvic exenteration for advanced primary and recurrent adenocarcinoma, *Can J Surg* 28(6):539, 1985.
23. Lagasse LD et al: *The gynecologic oncology patient: restoration of function and prevention of disability.* In McGowan L, editor: *Gynecologic oncology,* New York, 1978, Appleton-Century-Crofts.
24. Lamont JA, DePetrillo AD, Sargeant EJ: Psychosocial rehabilitation of exenterative surgery, *Gynecol Oncol* 6:236, 1978.
25. Lawhead RA Jr. et al: Pelvic exenteration for recurrent or persistent gynecologic malignancies: a ten-year review of the Memorial-Sloan Kettering Cancer Center experience (1972-1981), *Gynecol Oncol* 33:279, 1989.
26. McCullough WN, Nahhas WA: Palliative pelvic exenteration—futility revisited, *Gynecol Oncol* 27:97, 1987.
27. Meigs JV, Brunschwig A: Proposed classification for cases of cancer of the cervix treated by surgery, *Am J Obstet Gynecol* 64:413, 1952.
28. Million RR, Rutledge F, Fletcher GH: Stage IV carcinoma of the cervix with bladder invasion, *Am J Obstet Gynecol* 113:239, 1972.
29. Morley GW: Infiltrative carcinoma of the vulva: results of surgical treatment, *Am J Obstet Gynecol* 124:874, 1976.
30. Morley GW, Lindenauer SM: Pelvic exenterative therapy for gynecologic malignancy: an analysis of 70 cases, *Cancer* 38:581, 1976.
31. Parsons L, Ulfelder H: *An atlas of pelvic operations,* ed 2, Philadelphia, 1968, WB Saunders Co.
32. Phillips B, Buchsbaum HJ, Lifshitz S: Pelvic exenteration for vulvovaginal carcinoma, *Am J Obstet Gynecol* 141(8):1038, 1981.
33. Rubin SC, Young J, Mikuta JJ: Squamous carcinoma of the vagina: treatment, complications and long-term follow-up, *Gynecol Oncol* 20:346, 1985.
34. Stanhope CR, Symmonds RE: Palliative exenteration—What, when and why? *American J Obstet Gynecol* 151:12, 1985.
35. Symmonds RE, Webb MJ: *Pelvic exenteration.* In Coppleson M, editor: *Gynecologic oncology. Fundamental principles and clinical practice,* New York, 1981, Churchill Livingstone.
36. Talledo OE: Pelvic exenteration—Medical College of Georgia experience, *Gynecol Oncol* 22:181, 1985.
37. Wabrek AJ, Gunn JL: Sexual and psychological implications of gynecologic malignancy, *J Obstet Gynecol Neonatal Nurs* Nov/Dec: p 371, 1984.

Chapter 43

CHEMOTHERAPY AND TUMOR MARKERS OF GYNECOLOGIC CANCER

Robert C. Park
John D. Nash

Generally the clinical value of a tumor marker depends on its ability to reflect the extent of disease and its usefulness in monitoring efficacy of treatment. Certain gynecologic cancers respond quite well to various chemotherapeutic regimens, and in some of these cancers, tumor markers reflect treatment response earlier than clinical observation. Because of this interaction, it is pertinent to discuss tumor markers and the chemotherapy of gynecologic malignancies together.

TUMOR MARKERS

A tumor marker may be considered as any biologic aberration that indicates the presence of tumor. Ideally, a tumor marker should have several characteristics to be clinically useful. It should be expressed by all tumor cells and released within a body compartment. It must be easily determinable, reflect the presence and amount of tumor, and distinguish between benign and malignant tissue. In addition, the more specific the marker is for the tumor type, the more useful it is, especially if it is related to tumor growth and development. Also, the earlier the marker is detectable, the earlier a diagnosis can be made.

In that context, a number of tumor markers are available to patients with preinvasive and invasive gynecologic malignancies. These include cytologic screening (Pap smear) in cervical cancer and the presence of postmenopausal bleeding in endometrial cancers. However, what will be discussed in this chapter are those tumor markers that are present only in serum, particularly those that have efficacy in monitoring response for patients undergoing chemotherapy.

Serum tumor markers can be divided into several categories: oncofetal antigens, hormones, enzymes, proteins, metabolic products, and cell surface antigens. Although no tumor-specific markers have as yet been defined in the human, monoclonal antibody technology (MABS) has allowed the identification of a large number of tumor-associated markers. Generally the clinical value of a tumor marker depends on its sensitivity, specificity, ability to reflect the extent of disease (early diagnosis), and usefulness in monitoring the efficacy of treatment or the progression of disease. The appearance of a nonspecific tumor marker, be it produced early or late in tumor development, does not preclude its use in the management of the cancer patient.[16] Following is a discussion of those serum markers of clinical use with the gynecologic oncology patient.

Human chorionic gonadotropin

Possibly the most dramatic and successful application of a serum tumor marker has been that of human chorionic gonadotropin (HCG) in the management of patients with gestational trophoblastic disease (GTD). HCG is normally produced by the syncytiotrophoblast cells of the placenta and reaches a maximum value by about 10 weeks of normal pregnancy.[86] HCG is a hormonal glycoprotein with a molecular weight of approximately 37,000 daltons and a serum half-life of 36 hours.[127] The molecule is composed of two subunits—alpha and beta. The alpha subunit is shared with luteinizing hormone (LH), follicular-stimulating hormone (FSH), and thyroid-stimulating hormone (TSH). The beta subunit is unique to the HCG molecule, although it is similar to the beta subunit of LH. A specific radioimmunoassay for HCG based on the immunologic properties of the beta subunit was developed by Vaitukaitis, Braunstein, and Ross[126] in 1972. The normal nonpregnant value for HCG is less than 5 mlU/ml.

Marked elevation of serum HCG levels in the absence of pregnancy is highly specific for GTD. Serial HCG levels accurately reflect the clinical course of disease, and the presence of as few as 1000 tumor cells is sufficient to maintain a significant elevation of serum levels.[3] Since GTD is exquisitely sensitive to chemotherapy, HCG levels can be used in the clinical setting to determine the optimum intensity and duration of therapy.[50]

In addition to conditions of pregnancy, HCG can be mildly elevated in a number of benign diseases, including fibrocystic hyperplasia of the breast, and nongynecologic malignancies.[23] These causes of HCG elevation are rarely confused with GTD, which is associated with HCG elevations that are several orders of magnitude higher. More commonly the differential diagnosis of an elevated HCG involves the distinction between GTD and either intrauterine or ectopic pregnancy, conditions where diagnostic ultrasound is frequently helpful.

Measurement of serum beta HCG levels has four major clinical applications in the management of GTD: (1) postevacuation monitoring of molar pregnancy to detect development of persistence, (2) establishing prognosis in patients with metastases, (3) monitoring response to treatment, and (4) surveillance of patients who are treated and have achieved remission. Measurement of this marker can allow detection of persistent or recurrent disease long before clinical manifestations become apparent. Because of the relatively long half-life of HCG, regression to normal may require 8 to 12 weeks.[27]

Nongestational ovarian choriocarcinoma is a rare ovarian germ cell malignancy that secretes low levels of HCG.[128] However, the more common postgestation form of choriocarcinoma should be ruled out in each instance. Also, dysgerminoma, the most common ovarian germ cell malignancy, occasionally (in 3% of cases) contains multinucleated syncytiotrophoblastic cells, which produce low levels of HCG. In addition, the rare embryonal ovarian germ cell tumor frequently produces HCG.[65]

Alpha-fetoprotein

Alpha-fetoprotein (AFP) is a glycoprotein with a molecular weight of approximately 70,000 daltons and a serum half-life of 4 to 6 days. It was first described in the serum of mice by Abelev[1] in 1963 and has structural and physical characteristics similar to those of human albumin.[99] AFP was one of the first oncofetal proteins studied in relation to germ cell tumors and normal pregnancy. In the fetus, AFP is produced by parenchymal cells of the yolk sac, liver, and, to a lesser extent, by the upper gastrointestinal tract.[30] Its serum level peaks at 13 weeks gestation, when it approaches 3 mg/ml.[117] Shortly after birth, levels decrease rapidly to those observed in healthy adults (20 to 25 ng/ml). The function of AFP is not known, but in normal pregnancy it may facilitate down regulation of maternal immunity.

In the clinical setting, serum AFP levels are useful in the diagnosis and management of patients with ovarian endodermal sinus tumor (EST) and embryonal carcinoma (EC).[29,65] The production of AFP by these tumors is consistent with their histologic appearance, which resembles that of fetal yolk sac.[103,119] Endodermal sinus tumor is the second most common ovarian germ cell malignancy, while EC is quite rare, arising much more frequently in the testes than the ovary. As reported by Kurman and Norris[64,65] in 1976, EST contains only AFP, while EC produces both AFP and HCG. Although not all patients with EST and EC have elevated serum AFP levels, AFP, when present, has proven to be a reliable serum marker by which to monitor the status of disease.[26,118,132] In general, it has been noted that in patients who initially have elevated serum AFP levels, failure of the AFP to return to normal following treatment is associated with persistent disease. The converse is not always true, since a normal serum AFP level following treatment does not rule out persistence of elements other than EST or EC in the case of mixed germ cell tumors. Also, EST has been present at second look when the serum AFP levels are normal.[58] However, rising levels of AFP in patients who appear to be cured is predictive of recurrence.[58,135]

CA-125

The first clinically useful tumor marker for epithelial ovarian cancer was CA-125. The CA-125 assay, described by Bast and associates[5,6] in 1981, uses the monoclonal antibody OC-125, which reacts with an antigenic determinant common to most nonmucinous ovarian carcinoma. CA-125 has been found on a high molecular weight glycoprotein and has a serum half-life of 4.5 days. The specific epitope recognized by OC-125 is composed of carbohydrate and amino acids. Multiple epitopes exist on the CA-125 molecule, which have facilitated the development of a double determinant immunoradiometric assay, the test available today. With this test less than 1% of nonpregnant individuals have circulating CA-125 levels greater than 35 U/ml, while approximately 83% of individuals with epithelial ovarian cancer have elevated serum levels at the time of diagnosis.[59]

Unfortunately, CA-125 is not specific for ovarian cancer, so it has minimal utility as a screening test. Immunohistochemical studies have revealed that CA-125 is present on the cell surface of amnion and fetal tissues derived from coelomic epithelium. In the adult, CA-125 is found on the surface of epithelial cells of the fallopian tube, endometrium, endocervix, peritoneum, pleura, pericardium, and bronchus. Interestingly, normal ovarian epithelium does not express CA-125, although it is seen in inclusion cysts and benign papillary excrescences of the ovary.[51] In addition to epithelial ovarian cancer, CA-125 is elevated in association with other malignancies such as those of breast, colon, lung, and pancreas.[6,38] Also CA-125 is elevated in a number of benign conditions that include endometriosis, pregnancy, pelvic inflammatory disease, leiomyomata uteri, adenomyosis, cystadenomas, peritonitis, liver disease, pancreatitis, and renal failure.[10,37,40,129]

Since false-positive testing can occur in a number of conditions, CA-125 is most useful in two settings involving epithelial ovarian cancer patients: (1) the workup of an adnexal mass and (2) monitoring the course of therapy in patients with known disease.

A number of studies have confirmed the utility of CA-125 during the workup of a pelvic mass, especially in the postmenopausal age group.[111,129] Malkasian and co-workers[73] reported 158 patients who underwent exploratory laparotomy for an adnexal mass. In this group a CA-125 level greater than 65 U/ml predicted malignancy with a sensitivity of 91% for nonmucinous carcinomas. In the postmenopausal group, the positive predictive value was 98% and the negative predictive value was 72%. In the premenopausal patients, these values were 49% and 93% respectively. The specificity in the premenopausal group was notably lower because of the higher incidence of benign conditions associated with an elevated CA-125.

The use of CA-125 testing in patients with known disease has been well established. Serum CA-125 can describe the status of disease and response to therapy in over 90% of patients who have elevated CA-125 at the time of diagnosis.[51] With some degree of certainty, the knowledge of CA-125 trends will help identify those patients who are not responding to initial therapy or who will have evidence of disease after completion of primary therapy.[100] Numerous studies have shown that consistently elevated CA-125 levels correlate with the discovery of persistent disease at the time of second look exploration.[9,76] Also, 20% of patients with no clinical evidence of disease after the completion of primary cytotoxic therapy will have an elevated CA-125, of which 95% will have a positive second-look. Therefore, a diagnostic second look may not be required in this group of patients because of the high probability of persistent disease.[86] Unfortunately, a negative CA-125 does not guarantee the absence of disease, since 40% to 50% of these patients will have a positive second-look.[80] Lavin et al[67] demonstrated that those who have a negative CA-125 within 3 months of primary cytoreductive surgery after beginning cytotoxic therapy will have a negative second look laparotomy. The ability of CA-125 to predict recurrence is of interest. A rising CA-125 during the follow-up period after completion of primary therapy can predict recurrence of disease before clinical manifestation in up to 94% of patients.[86] This observation, however, has not translated into improved patient survival, since at the present time effective salvage therapy does not exist.

The stage or extent of disease at the time of diagnosis is the most important prognostic factor in patients with epithelial ovarian cancer. Early-stage disease is clearly associated with better prognosis. Therefore, the detection of patients with early-stage disease improves overall survival since disease confined to the ovary at the time of diagnosis

is associated with an 85% cure rate. The use of a single CA-125 determination to screen for early-stage disease, however, is plagued by its low sensitivity. In an often quoted study of screening with CA-125, 915 nonhospitalized patients were evaluated.[141] If the upper limit of normal CA-125 is defined as 65 U/ml, only 0.51% of women older than age 50 had elevated levels. None of the patients in the study with elevated CA-125 were found to have ovarian cancer, however, and only one patient in the study had cancer (metastatic breast cancer). In other investigations, CA-125 determinations were falsely elevated secondary to a variety of benign conditions.

On the basis of these initial studies, it would appear that mass screening of asymptomatic women for the presence of clinically undetectable ovarian cancer with a single CA-125 assay is not cost-effective because of the high false-positive rate relative to the low incidence of the disease. Serial CA-125 determinations might provide higher predictive value. At present, new approaches are being used to develop monoclonal antibodies that will complement CA-125 and these may allow development of monoclonal antibody panels with both high sensitivity and specificity.[7,62,101] Also, studies combining CA-125 and pelvic ultrasonography as screening procedures in the postmenopause age group are ongoing.

Serum CA-125 levels are elevated in most patients with metastatic endometrial cancer. A study of 81 patients with endometrial cancer clinically confined to the uterus showed that 95% of those with an elevated serum CA-125 had occult extrauterine disease at laparotomy.[92] Conversely, only one patient with a normal serum CA-125 had occult extrauterine disease. Other studies have shown similar results.[8,84] Serum CA-125 may play a role in planning the extent of surgical staging in patients with apparent early-stage disease.

Serum CA-125 has been shown to be elevated in 73% of patients with adenocarcinoma of the cervix and to a lesser degree in patients with squamous cell carcinoma of the cervix.[33,68] The data suggest that patients with initially elevated CA-125 levels that return to normal after therapy have a favorable prognosis. Persistent elevation of CA-125 levels during and after therapy in patients with carcinoma of the cervix was associated with a poor prognosis. However, to draw firm conclusions concerning CA-125 in cervix cancer patients requires further study.

Miscellaneous tumor markers

There are a number of tumor markers, new and old, that have limited value for gynecologic oncology patients. Undoubtedly, there will be many additional markers in the future, particularly with the further development of monoclonal antibody technology.

Carcinoembryonic antigen (CEA). Carcinoembryonic antigen is a heavily glycosylated protein with a molecular weight of approximately 180,000 daltons. It was first detected in 1965 in colon carcinoma, and its primary site of origin in both the fetus and adult is the gastrointestinal tract.[31,32] CEA is nonspecific and has been described in a wide variety of human cancers, including colon and pancreas, as well as in benign liver disease and in smokers free of malignant disease.[13] Although CEA can be found in most gynecologic cancers, serum levels usually are not sufficiently elevated to be useful for diagnosis or monitoring the clinical course of disease.[21,22]

In squamous cell cervix cancers, advanced-stage disease is often accompanied by elevated CEA, while early-stage disease is not.[21] This fact may be of some use. In epithelial ovarian cancer, elevations of CEA are most frequently associated with advanced stage, poor tumor differentiation, and mucinous histology.[43,128] Since serum CA-125 levels are most often low in patients with mucinous ovarian cancers, it has been thought that CEA and CA-125 together might yield higher sensitivity and specificity than CA-125 alone. In one study, however, this approach was not superior, although the proportion of mucinous tumors in the study was low.[7] For CEA to become a useful gynecologic tumor marker, more studies and data are necessary.

Placental alkaline phosphatase (PLAP). Placental alkaline phosphatase is an oncofetal protein that normally is expressed by the placenta. Elevated serum levels of PLAP have been reported in a variety of tumors, including cervical and ovarian cancers.[113] However, serum levels are elevated in only 30% to 60% of patients, making the usefulness of this marker suspect.

Inhibin. Inhibin is a peptide hormone produced by the granulosa cell. Under normal circumstances, it provides regulatory feedback to the hypothalamus, causing decrease in follicle-stimulating hormone release. Recently six patients with granulosa cell tumors were described in whom markedly elevated levels of inhibin were noted.[66] Inhibin levels became normal after treatment but reappeared at 5 and 20 months in two women who eventually showed clinical evidence of recurrence. When the assay becomes commercially available, inhibin may prove to be useful in diagnosis of recurrent disease and monitoring of therapy in patients with granulosal cell tumors.

Lactic dehydrogenase (LDH). Lactic dehydrogenase is a glycolytic enzyme that may be elevated in any of the ovarian germ cell malignancies, and in many other solid tumors. More consistently the two fast fractions LDH-1 and LDH-2 are increased with dysgerminoma where it seems to parallel response to therapy.[28] LDH would appear to be a useful marker in diagnosis and monitoring of patients with ovarian dysgerminoma.

Lipid-associated sialic acid (LSA). Lipid-associated sialic acid has been shown to be elevated in the serum of patients with gynecologic cancers.[101] In those patients with clinical evidence of disease, LSA is elevated in 70% with ovarian cancer, 63% with cervical cancer, and 43% with endometrial cancer. The addition of LSA to CA-125 resulted in only a slight improvement in the sensitivity and specificity of CA-125 alone in the diagnosis of ovarian cancer.[93,114] Further studies are needed to define a clinical role for LSA in the monitoring of patients with gynecologic cancers.

Squamous cell carcinoma antigen (SCC). Squamous cell carcinoma antigen is one of 14 subfractions of tumor-associated antigen (TA-4) discovered by Kato and Torigoe[53] in 1977. Available data on serum SCC antigen in normal healthy controls indicates SCC levels below 2 ng/ml.[102] In squamous cell carcinoma of the cervix, the frequency of elevation above 2 ng/ml increases with stage of disease from 34% in stage I to 85% in stage IV. In general, good agreement has been found between SCC antigen values and regression, progression, or recurrence in patients with squamous cell carcinoma of the cervix.[55] However, the test is not suitable as a screening tool since elevated SCC antigen levels may be found in patients with cervical intraepithelial neoplasia, and values less than 2 ng/ml can be found in patients with invasive squamous carcinoma.[54] Elevated levels of SCC antigen have been found in 42% of patients with squamous cell carcinoma of the vulva and 17% of patients with squamous cell carcinoma of the vagina.[78] However, the reported series are small and further evaluation is necessary to determine if SCC has clinical potential in these diseases.

Other antigens defined by monoclonal antibodies. NB-70K is a relatively new tumor-associated antigen that shows some promise. NB-70K is elevated in all types of epithelial adenocarcinomas, including mucinous cell types.[61] Combining this antigen with CA-125 may increase the diagnostic ability to determine epithelial ovarian cancers. Studies are in progress. CA-72, CA-15-3, and CA-19-9 are other antigens defined by monoclonal antibodies.[86,101,111] All of these are found in epithelial ovarian cancers and are presently under study to determine if they might complement CA-125, allowing development of monoclonal antibody panels with both high sensitivity and specificity.

Current use of serum tumor markers

There are several gynecologic neoplasms in which serum tumor markers are useful in diagnosis and monitoring of therapy. Also, there may be some use for CA-125 in the evaluation of undiagnosed pelvic masses.

Hydatidiform mole. All patients with a diagnosis of hydatidiform mole should have serial HCG determinations. Human chorionic gonadotrophin is a highly sensitive and specific tumor marker for gestational trophoblastic neoplasia (GTN). It accurately reflects volume of tumor, as well as the clinical course of disease. If there is post-evacuation titer plateau or rise, evaluation and treatment for persistent GTN can be instituted. During therapy serial HCG determinations should be continued since it is extremely accurate in reflecting tumor response. After cure, GTN patients should continue HCG monitoring for 6 to 12 months for evidence of recurrence.

Germ cell malignancies. In women with endodermal sinus tumors and embryonal carcinomas, alpha-fetoprotein is usually a reliable marker. In addition, AFP accurately predicts the presence of yolk sac elements in mixed germ cell tumors. Patients with embryonal cancer and nongestational choriocarcinoma will usually show HCG presence as well. Patients with dysgerminoma often show elevation of lactic dehydrogenase. All or any of these markers, when initially elevated, should be followed as indicators of response to treatment. Immature ovarian teratoma, in its pure form, has no described tumor marker.

Epithelial ovarian cancer. Any patient with a diagnosis of epithelial ovarian carcinoma may benefit from CA-125 determinations. When positive, CA-125 levels can predict tumor response to therapy with reasonable accuracy, often eliminating the necessity for a second look operative procedure.

Undiagnosed pelvic mass. The diagnostic utility of HCG and AFP in patients suspect for ovarian germ cell tumors is obvious. Levels should be determined in young patients with rapidly growing adnexal masses. Any patient with an undiagnosed adnexal mass, particularly those who are postmenopausal, may benefit from CA-125 determination. Most of these patients will require diagnostic laparotomy regardless of the CA-125 level, but in those whose CA-125 is elevated the chance of finding a malignancy is high. These patients may then be better prepared for a cancer operation.

Screening for ovarian cancer. At the present time there is no good marker for generalized screening of patients for ovarian cancer. In certain high-risk situations, such as a family history of ovarian cancer, serial CA-125 levels may facilitate diagnosis of occult early-stage disease. However, mass screening with CA-125 is not practical because of its low sensitivity. Monoclonal antibody panels with both high sensitivity and specificity are under study. These or other markers may become useful for screening in the future.

CHEMOTHERAPY

Chemotherapy plays a variety of roles in the management of patients with gynecologic malignancies. On one end of the spectrum, essentially all patients with gestational trophoblastic neoplasias are cured with cytotoxic agents as the exclusive therapeutic modality. Similarly, modern chemotherapy now enables a substantial majority of patients with ovarian germ cell tumors to survive their disease. In the middle of the spectrum, advances in chemotherapy over the past two decades have improved response and complete remission rates in patients with advanced epithelial ovarian cancer. However, cure rates have not improved, and few of these patients survive their disease. At the other end of the spectrum, the role of chemotherapy in the management of other gynecologic malignancies, such as squamous cancers of the cervix, adenocarcinomas of the endometrium, and sarcomas of the uterus, is limited to those patients with advanced or recurrent disease. Although sometimes palliative in these patients, rarely does chemotherapy promote cure. Continued treatment trials, increased knowledge of tumor biology, and in-

creased understanding of the mechanisms associated with the development of drug resistance, will undoubtedly lead to additional curative treatments in the future.

Ovarian epithelial malignancies

The 20,700 cases of ovarian cancer estimated to have occurred in the United States in 1991 place it second to uterine corpus as the most frequent site of malignancy in the female genital tract, but the 12,500 deaths estimated for the same year make ovarian cancer the most lethal female pelvic malignancy.[104] Following the introduction of alkylating agents as treatment for this disease in the late 1950s, a number of cytotoxic agents, alone and in combination, have produced significant improvement in tumor response and progression-free interval of disease.[91,123] However, in spite of improved quality of life for ovarian cancer patients, use of chemotherapy has unfortunately had little impact on long-term survival, with approximately 70% of patients eventually succumbing to their disease. The search for new active chemotherapeutic agents, and other treatment modalities must continue.

Early-stage disease. Despite the fact that most patients with epithelial ovarian cancer are first seen with advanced disease, 20% to 25% are found to have the tumor localized to the ovary or ovaries at the time of staging laparotomy. It is important to identify these early-stage patients because they have a much higher potential for cure than those in whom the tumor has spread away from the ovary. The necessity of a thorough, meticulous staging procedure cannot be overemphasized.[139] Accurate determination of disease spread not only has important prognostic implications but is essential to the selection of appropriate adjuvant therapy as well. Early-stage, low-risk disease is curable by surgery alone in better than 90% of patients.

Well-designed prospective, randomized clinical trials conducted by the Ovarian Cancer Study Group and the Gynecologic Oncology Group stratified patients into favorable and nonfavorable prognosis groups.[140] Subjects included in the favorable prognosis group had FIGO stage Ia or Ib disease with either well (grade 1) or moderately well (grade 2) differentiated tumors. All patients were randomized postoperatively to receive either melphalan (0.2 mg/kg per day for 5 days repeated every 4 to 6 weeks for up to 12 cycles) or no further therapy. After a median follow-up of more than 6 years, there was no significant difference in 5-year survival between the two groups (94% versus 98%, p = 0.43). The unfavorable prognosis group comprised patients with FIGO stage IaG3, Ic, IIa, IIb, or IIc tumors. These patients were treated with either melphalan (the same dosage schedule as the favorable prognosis group) or a single dose of 15 mCi radioactive chromic phosphate (P-32) administered intraperitoneally. The overall 5-year survival for each group was not significantly different (81% for the melphalan treated patients versus 78% for those receiving P-32, p = 0.48). These clinical trials clearly establish that patients with localized disease (FIGO stages I and II) comprise two groups, the first a group at low risk for recurrence in whom surgery alone is adequate treatment and the second a group at high risk for recurrence in whom adjuvant therapy is essential.

Since either an alkylating agent or intraperitoneal P-32 achieve identical results (80% survival), P-32 has become the standard therapy because of its limited toxicity and ease of administration. Alkeran, although effective, has the added risk of producing a secondary malignancy associated with chemotherapy.[52] Optimal therapy for this group of higher risk early-stage patients has not yet been established. Accordingly, trials are ongoing in which a short course of cisplatin-based combination chemotherapy is being tested against the standard control of intraperitoneal P-32 in an attempt to further improve long-term outcome.

Advanced-stage disease. The management of patients with advanced stage epithelial ovarian cancer involves a multimodal approach. The maximal removal of bulk tumor at the time of staging laparotomy is well established as the initial cornerstone of management.[45] The volume of residual disease is clearly an important prognostic indicator.[39] Reduction in tumor burden dramatically affects patient comfort and improves the ability to maintain nutritional status. Also, tumor removal results in a recruitment of additional tumor cells into the active, more chemosensitive phase of the cell cycle, whereas large residual tumor masses with their inherently poor blood supply are likely to receive inadequate doses of chemotherapy. Finally, the reduction in tumor volume results in a substantial log kill. It has been shown that the reduction of 1 kg of tumor to 1 g of residual disease reduces the number of tumor cells from 10^{12} to 10^{9}.[34] Theoretically, fewer courses of chemotherapy would then be required to eliminate the last tumor cell, lessening the opportunity for the tumor to become resistant to therapy.

Alkylating drugs were the original agents used as adjuvant management in patients with advanced epithelial ovarian cancer following surgical cytoreduction. Single-agent trials using a variety of alkylators in over 1000 patients yield response rates of 33% to 65%.[91,138] However, the 5-year survival of the patients reported in these series is only 9%. As new active drugs were identified, many of which differed in both mechanism of action and toxicity profile from the alkylating agents, combinations of drugs were tested in clinical trials. In 1978 the results of the first randomized, prospective trial testing the combination of the four-drug regimen HexaCAF (hexamethylmelamine, cyclophosphamide, methotrexate, 5-fluorouracil) against melphalan, an alkylating agent, were published.[137] Those patients treated with HexaCAF achieved a significantly increased overall response rate (75% versus 54%, p<0.05) and a significantly longer median survival (29 months versus 17 months, p<0.02) than those treated with melphalan. Multiple published series subsequently confirmed the superiority of combination regimens over single-agent therapy.[18,87,125]

The basis for the modern management of ovarian cancer

was established shortly after cisplatin became available for clinical use some 15 years ago. The superiority of cisplatin-based combination chemotherapy regimens over combinations not including cisplatin has been demonstrated. In a large prospective clinical trial conducted by the Gynecologic Oncology Group (GOG), patients were randomized to receive cyclophosphamide (50 mg/m^2) and doxorubicin (50 mg/m^2) with or without cisplatin (50 mg/m^2) every 3 weeks for 8 cycles.[88] Although there were no significant differences in survival between the two treatment arms, the cisplatin-containing combination yielded a significantly better progression-free interval and pathologic response rate than the combination without cisplatin. These results have been confirmed in reports by other investigators.[17,82]

More recently, in an effort to reduce toxicity, the role of doxorubicin has been rigorously explored in several well-designed clinical trials. In one of these trials, the GOG compared the combination of cisplatin (50 mg/m^2) plus cyclophosphamide (1000 mg/m^2) against cisplatin (50 mg/m^2), doxorubicin (50 mg/m^2), and cyclophosphamide (500 mg/m^2), both regimens administered every 3 weeks for 8 cycles.[89] The pathologic complete remission rate and the progression-free survival interval were the same in both treatment arms, indicating that the addition of doxorubicin to a regimen containing an alkylating agent and cisplatin does not improve response rate or survival. Similar results have been reported from other well-designed trials, establishing cisplatin and cyclophosphamide as the treatment of choice for patients with advanced-stage epithelial ovarian carcinoma.[11,83] However, despite the emergence of cisplatin and cyclophosphamide as the preferred regimen, optimal dosage schedules remain undefined. Results from clinical trials in which high-dose platinum compounds achieved significant responses in previously platinum-refractory patients, and retrospective meta-analyses of published trials of ovarian cancer support the concept of maximizing dose intensity.[48,69,90] Whether dose intensity will achieve more sustained complete remission from disease awaits confirmation from ongoing randomized, prospective clinical trials.

Since higher doses of cisplatin are associated with severe renal and neurologic toxicity, the less toxic platinum analog carboplatin has recently been tested in clinical trials.[2,25,74,120] These preliminary reports indicate that carboplatin has similar activity to cisplatin but is less toxic. Similarly, the results of carboplatin-containing combination regimens versus cisplatin-containing combination regimens indicate an improved therapeutic index for carboplatin. In spite of these encouraging preliminary results, more confirmatory data are necessary to make carboplatin the drug of choice in patients with epithelial ovarian cancer.

Salvage therapy remains unsatisfactory, although remarkable responses in heavily pretreated, platinum-resistant patients with a new agent, Taxol, are promising.[75] Taxol is a natural product, isolated from the Western yew tree, with a unique antimicrotubule mechanism of action.

Because its toxicities are manageable and do not overlap those of cisplatin, phase III trials with Taxol in combination with cisplatin as primary therapy are currently ongoing.

Ovarian cancer frequently remains confined to the peritoneal cavity throughout most of its course. The delivery of cytotoxic agents directly into the peritoneal cavity permits high intraperitoneal concentrations of drug with relative sparing of systemic toxicity. Studies using intraperitoneal chemotherapy, principally cisplatin or cisplatin-based combinations, with or without systemic toxicity protectors, have shown responses in patients who have not responded to other therapy, particularly those with minimal residual disease.[36,46] However, definitive conclusions regarding the efficacy of the intraperitoneal approach await the results of ongoing multi-institutional randomized, prospective clinical trials.

Ovarian germ cell malignancies

Malignant ovarian germ cell tumors (GCT) account for 5% to 8% of all ovarian malignancies. These tumors most frequently occur in young women with a mean age of 22 at diagnosis. The ovarian malignant germ cell tumors, in order of frequency, are dysgerminoma, endodermal sinus, immature teratoma, mixed cell types, embryonal, and choriocarcinoma. Before the use of combination chemotherapy, first reported in 1975, the prognosis of nondysgerminomatous tumors was dismal, even in patients with disease confined to an ovary.[9,73,85,108] Endodermal sinus tumors had a 2-year survival rate of 10% following surgical removal with or without adjuvant irradiation and single-agent chemotherapy.[117] Successful use of postoperative combination chemotherapy was first reported by Smith and Rutledge in 1975.[108] Although there have been no randomized clinical trials for this disease, advances in chemotherapy now enable a substantial majority of these patients to survive.

Once a diagnosis of malignant GCT is established, often aided by elevation of serum AFP, HCG, or LDH (described previously), the patient should undergo surgery as described in Chapter 41. Fortunately, ovarian germ cell malignancies, other than those containing dysgerminoma, do not have bilateral ovarian involvement. Since most of these patients are young, this allows sparing of the uterus and the uninvolved ovary, regardless of tumor spread, thus preserving fertility.[136]

Surgical cures can be anticipated in patients with dysgerminoma, since 5-year survival rates of 85% for all stages and 10-year survival rates of 90% for stage I disease are reported. Recurrences are well treated by irradiation, since these are among the most radiosensitive tumors in the human. Cytotoxic chemotherapy may be useful in advanced disease and recurrent situations, but its role to date remains experimental. FIGO stage Ia grade 1 immature teratomas are also adequately treated by surgery alone, with reported cure rates of greater than 90%. All the other

malignant germ cell tumors, regardless of disease spread, including all stages of grade 2 and 3 immature teratomas, benefit from postoperative chemotherapy.[106]

Patients with FIGO stage Ia grade 2 and 3 and all stage II and III immature teratomas without residual tumor and those with any other stage I, II, or III nondysgerminomatous germ cell malignancy that has been totally resected are best treated with vincristine, actinomycin-D, and cyclophosphamide (VAC). Vincristine is given weekly (1.5 mg/m² IV) for 8 to 12 weeks, while actinomycin-D (350 μg/m² IV) and cyclophosphamide (150 mg/m² IV) are given daily for 5 days every 4 weeks for a minimum of 10 weeks. With this treatment regimen, cure rates of 84% for patients with immature teratomas and 73% for all other cell types have been reported.[106] Toxicity must be closely monitored; 30% of patients will require dose modification because of severe bone marrow and/or neuromuscular toxicities.

All patients with FIGO stage II, III, and IV germ cell malignancies with residual, unresected tumor, and any with recurrences after previous treatment are well served by cisplatin-containing regimens. The standard is treatment with vinblastine, bleomycin, and cisplatin (VBP): vinblastine (12 mg/m² IV every 3 weeks), bleomycin (20 U/m² IV weekly), and cisplatin (20 mg/m² IV daily for 5 days every 3 weeks). Drug courses should be continued for 9 to 12 weeks. Two-year survival rates of 71% are reported.[118,133] As with the VAC regimen, toxicity with VBP can be substantial, and frequently only three courses of therapy (9 weeks) can be delivered.

Recent studies in male patients with disseminated germ cell tumors and females with recurrent GCT have substituted Etoposide for vinblastine (PEB) in the VBP regimen.[132,135] This regimen appears to have substantially less neuromuscular toxicity, and in patients with high tumor volume, better efficacy. Whether this observation can be used to improve first-line therapy is being studied by the GOG. Patients with advanced and recurrent disease are given PEB followed by "consolidation" with VAC. Another study by the GOG involves the use of PEB as a surgical adjuvant in completely resected early-stage patients. Although these regimens appear promising, they cannot be recommended as first-line treatment until clear superiority over VBP has been demonstrated. In addition, ifosfamide has shown activity in testes tumors and is also undergoing clinical trials as salvage therapy for patients with refractory ovarian GCT.[77] Its use as a front-line agent must await results of clinical trials.

Gestational trophoblastic neoplasms

Gestational trophoblastic neoplasms (GTN) are relatively rare malignant tumors arising from the trophoblast of human pregnancy. They invariably secrete human chorionic gonadotropin (HCG), a hormone described in some detail earlier in this chapter. The production of HCG is directly related to the number of viable tumor cells present, which makes it an excellent marker for diagnosis and monitoring response to therapy in patients with GTN. Before the introduction of chemotherapy by Li, Hertz, and Spencer[71] in 1956, the survival rate for patients with trophoblastic malignancies was universally poor. However, at the present time, with proper monitoring and chemotherapy, essentially all patients can be cured. Gestational trophoblastic neoplasms include hydatidiform mole, invasive mole (chorioadenoma destruens), and choriocarcinoma. All these tumors secrete HCG; therefore specific histologic diagnosis is not necessary.

Hydatidiform mole occurs in the United States in approximately 1 in 1200 pregnancies.[14] Following diagnosis, which is facilitated by ultrasonography, evacuation is indicated by means of suction curettage. Within 6 to 8 weeks following evacuation, 80% to 85% of patients achieve remission without further treatment, but 15% to 20% of patients persist as cases of invasive mole or choriocarcinoma, conditions that require treatment. All cases of invasive mole follow hydatidiform mole, while about one half of the choriocarcinoma cases follow mole and the other half follow term gestation, abortion, or ectopic pregnancies. The incidence of choriocarcinoma is approximately 1 in 40,000 episodes of pregnancy. Diagnosis of persistence is made by finding an elevated HCG titer at 6 to 8 weeks following any of the above conditions in the absence of an intervening pregnancy. In addition, diagnosis can be made by finding metastatic disease or by finding tissue diagnostic of chorioadenoma destruens or choriocarcinoma.

Once the diagnosis of malignant GTN has been established, using clinical staging studies, the disease status must be rapidly categorized into nonmetastatic or metastatic. Metastatic disease should be further identified as good prognosis (good risk) or poor prognosis (poor risk). Nonmetastatic GTN is defined as disease confined to the uterus without evidence of metastatic lesions. Usually the diagnosis is made during follow-up of a patient after molar pregnancy. However, in approximately 25% of patients a diagnosis is made following other conditions of pregnancy.[41] Metastatic GTN is defined as any presence of lesions outside the uterus. In good prognosis metastatic neoplasia, the disease has been present for a short time (4 months or less following the event of pregnancy), the pretreatment HCG titer is low (less than 42,000 mlU/ml), no brain or liver metastases are present, and there has been no prior significant use of chemotherapy for the current diagnosis. In poor prognosis metastatic disease, the neoplasia has been present longer than 4 months, the pretreatment HCG titer is greater than 42,000 mlU/ml, brain or liver metastases are present, the preceding event of pregnancy has resulted in a term infant, or significant chemotherapy has been given and the disease has failed to respond.[4,42]

Treatment should begin as soon as possible following diagnosis and evaluation for prognostic factors (usually within 24 hours). Nonmetastatic disease and good prognosis metastatic disease respond well to single-agent chemo-

therapy, and cure rates approaching 100% should be anticipated.[42,98] The traditional agents methotrexate (0.2–0.4 mg/kg IM) or actinomycin-D (10–13 mcg/kg IV), each given daily for 5 days, are equally effective, with remission rates of 72% to 98%.[41,42] The between-course interval with either drug is 7 to 10 days, depending on toxicity. Drug courses should be continued until the HCG, which should be monitored weekly, is normal (less than 5 mlU/ml). If toxicity has not been excessive, it is probably wise to give one course of therapy after the first normal HCG titer has been obtained. Remission is diagnosed when three consecutive HCG determinations are normal. A switch to the alternate drug is indicated if the HCG titer rises or plateaus at an elevated level for 3 weeks or longer. A drug change is also indicated if new metastatic lesions appear during therapy. Those who fail to respond to initial single-agent therapy respond to the alternate drug regimen in almost 100% of cases.[42]

One effective alternate drug regimen for nonmetastatic disease is actinomycin-D (1.25 mg/m^2 IV every 2 weeks until remission). A GOG study of 30 patients showed response in 28, with the remaining 2 responding after a change to traditional chemotherapy.[94] Advantages of this regimen include ease of administration, patient convenience, and cost-effectiveness. Also effective is methotrexate (30 mg/m^2 IM weekly until remission). Another GOG study showed an 81% complete response rate with a 100% salvage by traditional 5-day actinomycin-D for the 19% nonresponders.[44]

Poor prognosis metastatic disease is well treated by the three-drug regimen of methotrexate (7 mg/m^2 IM), actinomycin-D (350 mcg/m^2 IV), and chlorambucil (5 mg/m^2 po) (MAC). Each drug is given daily for 5 days and courses are reported every 14 to 21 days depending on toxicity, which may be severe. Drug courses are continued until HCG assays are normal for 2 to 3 recordings. Remission rates of 70% to 90% can be expected with this regimen.[42] The addition of 2000 to 3000 cGy of whole brain radiation when brain metastases are present enhances cure since it appears to decrease intracranial bleeding early in the treatment process.[130] The addition of radiation to the liver in light of metastases to that organ remains controversial. Some investigators have substituted cytoxan for chlorambucil with results being equal to the more traditional MAC therapy.[49] Drugs that appear to be active when the MAC regimen fails include etoposide, Velban, bleomycin, and cisplatin. Patients with prolonged duration of disease and nonmolar antecedent gestation are at high risk for failure to respond to the MAC regimen (40% failed in a recent publication).[110] Therefore, new combinations using the above active drugs and others as they become available need to be continually evaluated. Use of the Bagshawe EMA/CO regimen in high-risk GTN patients is controversial. A nonrandomized study by Bolis et al[12] showed it to be superior to MAC therapy. However, a head-on comparison by the Gynecologic Oncology Group showed the MAC regimen to be more effective and less toxic than a modified Bagshawe.[15] Until additional studies show greater efficacy for the Bagshawe treatment, MAC therapy remains the gold standard in patients with poor risk disease.

Uterine corpus malignancies

The most common invasive neoplasms of the female genital tract involve the uterine corpus. Of these lesions, the most frequent are endometrial carcinoma and uterine sarcoma, two neoplasms that accounted for an estimated 34,000 new cases and 6000 deaths in the United States in 1991 due to malignancy in the female.[104]

Endometrial cancer. Carcinoma of the endometrium is the most common invasive neoplasm of the female genital tract.[104] Since the disease process produces bleeding at a relatively early point in its development, most are diagnosed while the lesion is still limited to the uterine corpus (FIGO stage I). As a result, surgical excision, with or without postoperative radiation, leads to a high cure rate. Because the overall 5-year survival rate approaches 70%, the potential role of chemotherapy has been minimized. However, chemotherapy has proven useful in certain situations.

Progestational agents have been found valuable in patients with recurrence.[56,63,95,97] Hydroxyprogesterone caproate (Delalutin), medroxyprogesterone acetate (Provera), and megestrol acetate (Megace) have been used in varying dose forms, giving an overall response rate of 25%. The specific progestin dose and route of administration do not appear to be related to response. The overall survival for all progestin treated patients is approximately 1 year.[95,97,121] However, in one series, 15% of patients were alive 4½ years after the beginning of treatment.[97] A long disease interval (exceeding 2 or 3 years),[60,95] well-differentiated histologic type,[96] and positive estrogen and/or progesterone receptor status have all been related to an increased frequency of response.[24,105,116] Receptor-positive patients have a 70% response rate to therapy compared to a 16% response rate in receptor-negative patients. Tamoxifen has been tried as salvage therapy in several studies. Results have varied, but in general response rates are minimal in untreated patients. Currently tamoxifen cannot be recommended as treatment.

Although some cytotoxics are capable of inducing objective remission, all treatment with these agents for advanced and recurrent disease is palliative, and chances of response and survival remain small.[19] Active agents include doxorubicin, cisplatin, cytembena, and carboplatin. Clinical trials to ascertain the effectiveness of these and other cytotoxic agents continue.

For patients with recurrent endometrial cancer, progestin treatment remains the cornerstone of therapy, and anyone with metastases who is not eligible for clinical trials should be given a progestin. Those with long disease-free intervals, well-differentiated tumors, or receptor-positive malignancy will respond best to such treatment. Delalutin

(1 to 3 g IM per week), Provera (200 mg to 1 g IM per week or 200 mg to 1 g orally each day), or Megace (160 to 320 mg daily) are equally effective. Regardless of the agent used, treatment should continue for as long as remission is evident. As previously discussed, the tumor marker CA-125, when positive, may be helpful in monitoring response.

Chemotherapy as an adjuvant in the treatment of patients with endometrial carcinoma is an evolving discipline. Several clinical trials have been reported using hormonal and cytotoxic therapies as adjuvants in the early disease setting. However, to date none of these trials have increased survival over the traditional surgical/radiation approach.[70,79]

Uterine sarcoma. Sarcoma of the uterus includes a variety of histologic types. The two most common, accounting for 90% of all cases, are mixed mesodermal sarcoma (both homologous and heterologous) and leiomyosarcoma. Because these lesions are considerably less common than endometrial carcinoma, clinical studies with cytotoxic agents have been few.

Available evidence on the activity of single agents in advanced or recurrent sarcoma of the uterus comes almost entirely from GOG trials.[81,107,115,122] Although not absolutely conclusive, these data suggest that the two major histologic types respond differently to chemotherapy and must be studied as separate groups. In mixed mesodermal sarcoma, Ifosfamide and cisplatin as single agents demonstrate strong activity with overall response rates of 20% to 30%. In leiomyosarcoma, doxorubicin appears to be the most active agent, showing a 25% partial and complete response rate. Ifosfamide also exhibits modest activity, but cisplatin produces only a minimal response rate. In addition, there is some evidence of modest effectiveness for Etoposide (VP-16). The only randomized (phase III) trial in both histologic types showed no difference between doxorubicin alone and doxorubicin plus DTIC.

Despite the obvious need for effective adjuvant therapy in uterine sarcomas, only one study has been conducted, of patients with stages I and II uterine sarcoma randomized to receive no further therapy or adjuvant doxorubicin.[122] There was no significant difference between the two arms of the study. Current and future efforts should be directed to the identification of additional active drugs (phase I and II trials) and identification of effective combination chemotherapy.

Uterine cervix malignancies

Although the incidence of cancers of the uterine cervix has declined in the past 30 years, there were still an estimated 13,000 new cases diagnosed in the United States in 1991. In addition, the 4,500 deaths predicted for the same year rank cervical cancer as the ninth most frequent cause of death due to malignancy in females.[104] Most invasive cases are first seen as squamous cell carcinoma confined grossly to the pelvis, and the principal approach to management consists of surgery, radiotherapy, or both. Before mid-1970 there was little interest or information available on the role of systemic therapy.[20] In the past 15 years the GOG and other investigators have initiated a concerted effort to evaluate the efficacy of cytotoxic therapy in advanced and recurrent cervical cancer. However, the role of systemic cytotoxic therapy has not as yet been clearly defined in cervical cancer patients.

The only proven effective use for chemotherapy in cervix cancer involves the administration of hydroxyurea in combination with radiotherapy for patients with locoregionally advanced disease (FIGO stages IIb through IVa). In a GOG trial comparing radiotherapy plus either hydroxyurea or placebo, patients receiving hydroxyurea demonstrated significantly better response, progression-free interval, and survival than patients receiving placebo.[47] The current standard of care indicates that all patients stage IIb and greater receiving radiotherapy as primary treatment should also receive hydroxyurea (80 mg/kg 2 times each week) as an effective radiosensitizer.

A number of cytotoxic agents alone and in combination have been evaluated in advanced and recurrent disease. Cisplatin and dibromodulcitol show moderate overall response rates in the 20% to 30% range, with cisplatin showing a 6% to 10% complete response rate in both squamous and nonsquamous tumors.[112,133,124] Carboplatin appears to exhibit response rates similar to cisplatin's.[131] To date no other single drugs or combinations show a superior response rate to cisplatin alone. Single-agent and combination clinical trials, as well as neoadjuvant use in poor risk early-stage patients, need to be continued.

REFERENCES

1. Abelev GI: Study of antigenic structure of tumors, *Acta Intern Cancer* 19:80, 1963.
2. Alberts D et al: Improved efficacy of carboplatin plus cyclophosphamide versus cisplatin plus cyclophosphamide: preliminary report by the Southwest Oncology Group of a phase III randomized trial in stages III & IV suboptimal ovarian cancer, *Proc Am Soc Clin Oncol* 8:151, 1989.
3. Bagshawe KD: Treatment of trophoblastic tumors, *Ann Acad Med* 5:273, 1976.
4. Bagshawe KD: Risk and prognostic factors in trophoblastic neoplasia, *Cancer* 38:1373, 1976.
5. Bast RC Jr et al: Reactivity of a monoclonal antibody with human ovarian carcinoma, *J Clin Invest* 68:1331, 1981.
6. Bast RC Jr et al: A radioimmunoassay using a monoclonal antibody to monitor the course of epithelial ovarian cancer, *N Engl J Med* 309:883, 1983.
7. Bast RC Jr et al: Monitoring human ovarian carcinoma with a combination of CA-125, CA 19-9 and carcinoembryonic antigen, *Am J Obstet Gynecol* 149:553, 1984.
8. Berchuck A et al: Immunohistochemical expression of CA-125 in endometrial adenocarcinoma: correlation of antigen expression with metastatic potential, *Cancer Res* 49:2091, 1989.
9. Berek JS et al: CA-125 levels correlated with second-look operations among ovarian cancer patients, *Obstet Gynecol* 67:685, 1986.
10. Bergman J-F et al: Elevation of CA-125 patients with benign and malignant ascites, *Cancer* 59:213, 1987.
11. Bertelsen K et al: A randomized study of cyclophosphamide and cis-platinum with or without doxorubicin in advanced ovarian cancer, *Gynecol Oncol* 28:161, 1987.
12. Bolis G et al: EMA/CO regimen in high-risk gestational trophoblastic tumor (GTT), *Gynecol Oncol* 31:439, 1988.
13. Costanza ME et al: Carcinoembryonic antigens: report of a screening study, *Cancer* 33:583, 1974.
14. Curry S et al: Hydatidiform mole: diagnosis, management and long-term followup of 347 patients, *Obstet Gynecol* 45:1, 1975.
15. Curry S et al: A prospective randomized comparison of methotrexate, dactinomycin, chlorambucil vs methotrexate, dactinomycin, cyclophosphamide, doxorubicin, meythalan, hydroxyurea and vincristine in "poor prognosis" metastatic gestational trophoblastic disease, *Obstet Gynecol* 73:357, 1989.
16. Daunter B: Review—tumor markers in gynecologic oncology, *Gynecol Oncol* 39:1, 1990.
17. Decker DG et al: Cyclophosphamide plus cisplatin in combination: treatment program for stage III or IV ovarian carcinoma, *Obstet Gynecol* 60:481, 1982.
18. Delgado G et al: L-PAM vs cyclophosphamide, hexamethylmelamine and 5-fluorouracil (CHF) for advanced ovarian cancer, *Proc Am Assoc Cancer Res* 20:434, 1979.
19. Deppe G: *Chemotherapy for endometrial cancer.* In Deppe G, editor: *Chemotherapy for gynecologic cancer,* New York, 1990, Alan R Liss.
20. DeVita V Jr, Wasserman T, Young R: Perspectives and research in gynecologic oncology, *Cancer* 38:509, 1976.
21. DiSaia PJ et al: Carcinoembryonic antigen in patients with gynecologic malignancies, *Am J Obstet Gynecol* 121:159, 1975.
22. Donaldson ES et al: Multiple biochemical markers in patients with gynecologic malignancies, *Cancer* 45:948, 1980.
23. Dosogne-Guerin M, Stolarczyk A, Borkowski A: Prospective study of the alpha and beta subunits of human chorionic gonadotropin in the blood of patients with various benign and malignant conditions, *Eur J Cancer* 14:525, 1978.
24. Edmonson JH et al: Ineffectiveness of tamoxifen in advanced endometrial carcinoma after failure of progestin treatment, *Cancer Treat Rep* 70:1019, 1986.
25. Edmonson JH et al: Cyclophosphamide-cisplatin versus cyclophosphamide-carboplatin in stage III-IV ovarian carcinoma: a comparison of equally myelosuppressive regimens, *J Natl Cancer Inst* 81:1500, 1989.
26. Forney JP, DiSaia PF, Morrow CP: Endodermal sinus tumor: a report of two sustained remissions treated postoperatively with a combination of actinomycin-D, 5-fluorouracil and cyclophosphamide, *Obstet Gynecol* 95:186, 1975.
27. Franke HR et al: Plasma human chorionic gonadotropin disappearance in hydatidiform mole: a central registry report from the Netherlands, *Obstet Gynecol* 62:467, 1983.
28. Fujii S et al: Analysis of serum lactice dehydrogenese levels and its isoenzymes in ovarian dysgerminoma, *Gynecol Oncol* 22:65, 1985.
29. Gallion H et al: Therapy for endodermal sinus tumor of the ovary, *Am J Obstet Gynecol* 135:447, 1979.
30. Gitlin D, Perricelli A, Gitlin GM: Synthesis of alpha-fetoprotein by liver, yolk sac and gastrointestinal tract of the human conceptus, *Cancer Res* 32:979, 1972.
31. Gold P, Freedman SO: Demonstration of tumor specific antigens in human colonic carcinomata by immunological tolerance and absorption techniques, *J Exp Med* 121:439, 1965.
32. Gold P, Freedman SO: Specific carcinoembryonic antigens of the human digestive system, *J Exp Med* 122:567, 1965.
33. Goldberg GL et al: CA-125: a potential prognostic indicator in patients with cervical cancer, *Gynecol Oncol* 40:22, 1991.
34. Griswold DR Jr et al: Success and failure in the treatment of solid tumors. 1. effects of cyclophosphamide on primary and metastatic plasmacytoma in the hamster, *Cancer Chemother Rep* 52:345, 1968.
35. Gurpide E: Hormone receptors in endometrial cancer (review), *Cancer* 48:638, 1981.
36. Hacker NF, Berek JS, Pretorious RG: Intraperitoneal cis-platinum as salvage therapy for refractory epithelial ovarian cancer, *Obstet Gynecol* 70:759, 1987.
37. Haga Y et al: Clinical significance of serum CA-125 values in pa-

tients with cancers of the digestive system, *Am J Med Sci* 292:30, 1986.

38. Haglund C: Tumor marker antigen CA-125 in pancreatic cancer: a comparison with CA-19-9 and CEA, *Br J Cancer* 54:897, 1986.

39. Hainsworth JD et al: Advanced ovarian cancer: long term results of treatment with intensive cisplatin-based chemotherapy of brief duration, *Ann Intern Med* 108:165, 1988.

40. Halila H, Stenman U, Seppala M: Ovarian cancer antigen CA-125 levels in pelvic inflammatory disease and pregnancy, *Cancer* 57:1327, 1986.

41. Hammond C et al: Primary chemotherapy for nonmetastatic gestational trophoblastic neoplasms, *Am J Obstet Gynecol* 98:71, 1967.

42. Hammond C et al: Treatment of metastatic trophoblastic disease: good and poor prognosis, *Am J Obstet Gynecol* 115:4, 1973.

43. Heald J, Buckley CH, Fox H: An immunohistochemical study of the distribution of CEA in epithelial tumors of the ovary, *J Clin Pathol* 32:918, 1979.

44. Homesley H, Blessing J, Schlaerth J: Rapid escalation of weekly intramuscular methotrexate for nonmetastatic gestational trophoblastic disease: a Gynecologic Oncology Group study, *Gynecol Oncol* 39:305, 1990.

45. Hoskins W: The influence of cytoreductive surgery on progression-free interval and survival in epithelial ovarian cancer, *Baillieres Clin Obstet Gynaecol* 3:59, 1989.

46. Howell SB et al: Long term survival of advanced refractory ovarian carcinoma patients with small volume disease treated with intraperitoneal chemotherapy, *J Clin Oncol* 5:1607, 1987.

47. Hreshchyshyn M et al: Hydroxyurea or placebo combined with radiation to treat stages IIIB and IVA cervical cancer confined to the pelvis, *Int J Radiat Oncol Biol Phys* 5:317, 1979.

48. Jacobs AJ et al: Therapy of ovarian carcinoma: the relationship of dose level and treatment intensity to survival, *Gynecol Oncol* 33:23, 1988.

49. Jones WB: Treatment of chorionic tumors, *Clin Obstet Gynecol* 18:247, 1975.

50. Jones WB, Lewis JL, Lehr M: Monitor of chemotherapy in gestational trophoblastic neoplasm by radioimmunoassay of the beta subunit of human chorionic gonadotropin, *Am J Obstet Gynecol* 121:669, 1975.

51. Kabawat SE et al: Tissue distribution of coelomic-epithelium related antigen recognized by the monoclonal antibody OC-125, *Int J Gynecol Pathol* 2:275, 1983.

52. Kaldor JM et al: Leukemia following chemotherapy for ovarian cancer, *N Engl J Med* 322:1, 1990.

53. Kato H, Torigoe T: Radioimmunoassay for tumor antigen of human cervical squamous cell carcinoma, *Cancer* 40:1621, 1977.

54. Kato H et al: Value of tumor-antigen (TA-4) of squamous cell carcinoma in predicting the extent of cervical cancer, *Cancer* 50:1294, 1982.

55. Kato H et al: Prognostic significance of the tumor antigen TA-4 in squamous cell carcinoma of the uterine cervix, *Am J Obstet Gynecol* 145:350, 1983.

56. Kauppila A: Progestin therapy of endometrial, breast and ovarian carcinoma: a review of clinical observations (review), *Acta Obstet E Gynecol Scand* 63:441, 1984.

57. Kauppila A: Estrogen and progestin receptors as prognostic indicators in endometrial cancer: a review of the literature (review), *Acta Oncol* 28:561, 1989.

58. Kawai M et al: α-fetoprotein in malignant germ cell tumors of the ovary, *Gynecol Oncol* 39:160, 1990.

59. Kenemans P et al: Mucins and mucin-like antigens as serum tumor markers, *Cancer Rev* 4:1, 1988.

60. Kistner RW, Griffiths CT: Use of progestational agents in the management of metastatic carcinoma of the endometrium (review), *Clin Obstet Gynecol* 11:439, 1968.

61. Knauf S: Clinical evaluation of ovarian tumour antigen NB/70K: monoclonal antibody assays for distinguishing ovarian cancer from other gynecologic disease, *Am J Obstet Gynecol* 158:1067, 1988.

62. Knauf S et al: A study of the NB-70K and CA-125 monoclonal antibody radioimmunoassays for measuring serum antigen levels in ovarian cancer patients, *Am J Obstet Gynecol* 152:911, 1985.

63. Kohorn EI: Gestagens and endometrial carcinoma, *Gynecol Oncol* 4:398, 1975.

64. Kurman RJ, Norris HJ: Endodermal sinus tumor of the ovary, *Cancer* 38:2404, 1976.

65. Kurman RJ, Norris HJ: Embryonal carcinoma of the ovary: a clinicopathological entity distinct from endodermal sinus tumor resembling embryonal carcinoma of the adult testes, *Cancer* 38:2420, 1976.

66. Lappohn RE et al: Inhibin as a marker for granulosa-cell tumors, *N Engl J Med* 321:790, 1989.

67. Lavin PT et al: CA-125 for the monitoring of ovarian carcinoma during primary therapy, *Obstet Gynecol* 69:223, 1987.

68. Leminen A: Tumor markers CA-125, carcinoembryonic antigen and tumor associated trypsin inhibitor in patients with cervical adenocarcinoma, *Gynecol Oncol* 39:358, 1990.

69. Levin L, Hryniuk WM: Dose intensity analysis of chemotherapy regimens in ovarian carcinoma, *J Clin Oncol* 5:756, 1987.

70. Lewis GC Jr et al: Adjuvant progestogen therapy in the primary definitive treatment of endometrial cancer, *Gynecol Oncol* 2:368, 1974.

71. Li MC, Hertz R, Spencer DB: Effects of methotrexate therapy upon choriocarcinoma and chorioadenoma destruens, *Proc Soc Exp Biol Med* 93:361, 1956.

72. Li MC et al: Effects of combined drug therapy on metastatic cancer of the testis, *JAMA* 174:145, 1960.

73. Malkasian GD et al: Preoperative evaluation of serum CA-125 levels in premenopausal and postmenopausal patients with pelvic masses: discrimination of benign from malignant disease, *Am J Obstet Gynecol* 159:341, 1988.

74. Mangioni C et al: Randomized trial in advanced ovarian cancer comparing cisplatin and carboplatin, *J Natl Cancer Inst* 81:1464, 1989.

75. McGuire WP et al: Taxol: a unique antineoplastic agent with significant activity in advanced ovarian epithelial neoplasms, *Ann Int Med* 111:273, 1989.

76. Meier W et al: Serum levels of CA-125 and histological findings at second-look laparotomy in ovarian carcinoma, *Gynecol Oncol* 35:44, 1989.

77. Metzer R et al: The role of ifosfamide plus cisplatin-based chemotherapy as salvage therapy for patients with refractory germ cell tumors, *Cancer* 66:2476, 1990.

78. Montag T: Tumor markers in gynecologic oncology, *Obstet Gynecol Surv* 45:94, 1990.

79. Morrow C et al: Doxorubicin as an adjuvant following surgery and radiation therapy in patients with high-risk endometrial carcinoma, stage I and occult stage II: a Gynecologic Oncology Group study, *Gynecol Oncol* 36:166, 1990.

80. Moskovic E et al: Monitoring patients with ovarian carcinoma: the relationship of serum CA-125 levels to CT scanning, *Int J Gynecol Cancer* 1:125, 1991.

81. Muss H et al: Mitoxantrone in the treatment of advanced uterine sarcoma, *Am J Clin Oncol* 13:32, 1990.

82. Neijt JP et al: Randomized trial comparing two combination chemotherapy regimens (HexaCAF vs CHAP-5) in advanced ovarian carcinoma, *Lancet* 2:594, 1984.

83. Neijt JP et al: Randomized trial comparing two combination chemotherapy regimens (CHAP-5 vs CP) in advanced ovarian carcinoma, *J Clin Oncol* 5:1157, 1987.

84. Niloff JM et al: Elevation of serum CA-125 in carcinomas of the fallopian tube, endometrium and endocervix, *Am J Obstet Gynecol* 148:11057, 1984.

85. Norris H, Zirkin H, Benson W: Immature (malignant) teratoma of the ovary, *Cancer* 36:669, 1975.

86. Olt G, Berchuck A, Bast RC: The role of tumor markers in gynecologic oncology, *Obstet Gynecol Surv* 45:570, 1990.

87. Omura GA et al: Randomized comparison of melphalan vs melphalan plus hexamethylmelamine vs adriamycin plus cyclophosphamide in ovarian carcinoma, *Cancer* 51:783, 1983.

88. Omura G et al: A randomized trial of cyclophosphamide and doxorubicin with or without cisplatin in advanced ovarian carcinoma: a Gynecologic Oncology Group study, *Cancer* 57:1725, 1986.

89. Omura GA et al: Randomized trial of cyclophosphamide plus cisplatin with or without doxorubicin in ovarian carcinoma: a Gynecologic Oncology Group study, *J Clin Oncol* 7:457, 1989.

90. Ozols R et al: High dose (HD) cisplatin (P) (40 mg/m² qd × 5) and HD carboplatin (CBDCA) (400 mg/m² qd × 2) in refractory ovarian cancer: active salvage drugs with different toxicities, *Proc Am Soc Clin Oncol* 4:119, 1985.

91. Park RC et al: Treatment of women with disseminated or recurrent ovarian carcinoma, *Cancer* 45:2529, 1980.

92. Patsner B et al: Predictive value of preoperative serum CA-125 levels in clinically localized and advanced endometrial carcinoma, *Am J Obstet Gynecol* 158:399, 1988.

93. Patsner B et al: Comparison of serum CA-125 and lipid-associated sialic acid (LASA-P) in monitoring patients with invasive ovarian adenocarcinoma, *Gynecol Oncol* 30:98, 1988.

94. Petrilli E et al: Single dose actinomycin-D treatment for nonmetastatic gestational trophoblastic disease: a prospective phase II trial of the Gynecologic Oncology Group, *Cancer* 60:2173, 1987.

95. Piver MS et al: Medroxyprogesterone acetate (Depo-Provera) vs hydroxyprogesterone caproate (Delalutin) in women with metastatic endometrial adenocarcinoma, *Cancer* 45:258, 1980.

96. Podratz KC et al: Effects of progestional agents in treatment of endometrial carcinoma, *Obstet Gynecol* 66:106, 1985.

97. Reifenstein EC Jr: The treatment of advanced endometrial cancer with hydroxyprogesterone caproate (review), *Gynecol Oncol* 2:377, 1974.

98. Ross G et al: Sequential use of methotrexate and actinomycin-D in treatment of metastatic choriocarcinoma and related trophoblastic diseases in women, *Am J Obstet Gynecol* 93:223, 1965.

99. Ruoslahti E, Hirai H: Alpha fetoprotein, *Scand J Immunol* 8(suppl):3, 1978.

100. Rustin GJS et al: Use of CA-125 to predict survival of patients with ovarian carcinoma, *J Clin Oncol* 7:1667, 1889.

101. Schwartz PE et al: Circulating tumor markers in the monitoring of gynecologic malignancies, *Cancer* 60:353, 1987.

102. Senikjian EK et al: An evaluation of squamous cell carcinoma antigen in patients with cervical squamous cell carcinoma, *Am J Obstet Gynecol* 157:433, 1987.

103. Shirai T et al: Immunofluorescent demonstration of alpha-fetoprotein and other plasma proteins in yolk sac tumor, *Cancer* 38:1661, 1976.

104. Silverberg E, Boring CC, Squires BA: Cancer statistics 1991, *CA* 41:29, 1991.

105. Slavik M et al: Phase II clinical study of tamoxifen in advanced endometrial adenocarcinoma: a Gynecologic Oncology Group study, *Cancer Treat Rep* 68:809, 1984.

106. Slayton RE et al: Vincristine, dactinomycin and cyclophosphamide in the treatment of malignant germ cell tumors of the ovary, *Cancer* 56:243, 1985.

107. Slayton RE et al: Phase II trial of etoposide in the management of advanced or recurrent mixed mesodermal sarcomas of the uterus: a Gynecologic Oncology Group study, *Cancer Treat Rep* 71:661, 1987.

108. Smith J, Rutledge F: Advances in chemotherapy for gynecologic cancer, *Cancer* 36:669, 1975.

109. Soper J, Christensen CW: Steroid receptors and endometrial cancer, *Clin Obstet Gynecol* 13:825, 1986.

110. Soper J et al: Metastatic gestational trophoblastic disease: prognostic factors in previously untreated patients, *Obstet Gynecol* 71:338, 1988.

111. Soper JT et al: Preoperative serum tumor-associated antigen levels in women with pelvic masses, *Obstet Gynecol* 75:249, 1990.

112. Stehman FB et al: A phase II evaluation of mitolactol in patients with advanced squamous cell carcinoma of the cervix: a Gynecologic Oncology Group study, *J Clin Oncol* 7:1892, 1989.

113. Stigbrand T et al: On the value of placental alkaline phosphatase as a marker for gynecological malignancy, *Acta Obstet Gynecol Scand* 64:99, 1985.

114. Stratton JAS et al: Relationship of serum CA-125 and lipid-associated sialic acid tumor associated antigen levels to the disease status of patients with gynecologic malignancies, *Obstet Gynecol* 71:20, 1988.

115. Sutton G et al: Phase II trial of ifosfamide and mesna in mixed mesodermal tumors of the uterus: a Gynecologic Oncology Group study, *Am J Obstet Gynecol* 161:309, 1989.

116. Swenerton KD: Treatment of advanced endometrial adenocarcinoma with tamoxifen, *Cancer Treat Rep* 64:805, 1980.

117. Talerman A, Haije WB: Alpha-fetoprotein and germ cell tumors: a possible role of yolk sac tumor in production of alpha-fetoprotein, *Cancer* 34:1722, 1974.

118. Taylor MH, DePetrillo AD, Turner AR: Vinblastine, bleomycin and cisplatin in malignant germ cell tumors of the ovary, *Cancer* 56:1341, 1985.

119. Teilum G, Albrechtsen R, Norgaard-Pedersen B: Immunofluorescent localization of alpha-fetoprotein synthesis in endodermal sinus tumor (yolk sac tumor), *Acta Pathol Microbiol Scand* 82A:586, 1974.

120. ten Bokkel Huiniuk WW et al: Carboplatin in combination chemotherapy for ovarian cancer, *Cancer Treat Rev* 15(suppl B):9, 1989.

121. Thigpen J, Blessing J, DiSaia P: *Oral medroxyprogesterone acetate in advanced or recurrent endometrial carcinoma: results of therapy and correlation with estrogen and progesterone levels: the gynecologic oncology experience.* In Baulieu EE, Slacobelli S, McGuire WL, editors: *Endocrinology of malignancy,* 1986.

122. Thigpen J et al: Chemotherapy for advanced or recurrent gynecologic cancer, *Cancer* 60:2104, 1987.

123. Thigpen J et al: Chemotherapy in ovarian carcinoma: present role and future prospects, *Semin Onco* 16:58, 1989.

124. Thigpen J et al: A randomized comparison of a rapid versus prolonged (24 hr) infusion of cisplatin in therapy of squamous cell carcinoma of the uterine cervix: a Gynecologic Oncology Group study, *Gynecol Oncol* 32:198, 1989.

125. Trope C: A prospective and randomized trial comparison of melphalan vs adriamycin-melphalan in advanced ovarian carcinoma, *Proc Am Soc Clin Oncol* 22:469, 1981.

126. Vaitukaitis JL, Braunstein GP, Ross GT: A radioimmunoassay which specifically measures human chorionic gonadotropin in the presence of human luteinizing hormone, *Am J Obstet Gynecol* 113:751, 1972.

127. Vaitukaitis JL et al: Gonadotropins and their subunits: basic and clinical studies, *Recent Prog Horm Res* 32:289, 1974.

128. van Nagell JR et al: Biochemical markers in the plasma and tumors of patients with gynecologic malignancies, *Cancer* 48:495, 1981.

129. Vasilev SA et al: Serum CA-125 levels in preoperative evaluation of pelvic masses, *Obstet Gynecol* 71:751, 1988.

130. Weed JC Jr, Hammond CB: Cerebral metastatic choriocarcinoma: intensive therapy and prognosis, *Obstet Gynecol* 55:89, 1980.

131. Weiss G, Green S, Hannigan E: A phase II trial of carboplatin for recurrent or metastatic squamous carcinoma of the uterine cervix: a Southwest Oncology Group study, *Gynecol Oncol* 39:323, 1990.

132. Wilkinson EJ, Friedrich EG, Hosty TA: Alpha-fetoprotein and endodermal sinus tumor of the ovary, *Am J Obstet Gynecol* 116:711, 1973.

133. Williams S et al: Treatment of disseminated germ-cell tumors with cisplatin, bleomycin and either vinblastine or etoposide, *N Engl J Med* 316:1435, 1987.

134. Williams SD et al: Cisplatin, vinblastine, and bleomycin in advanced and recurrent ovarian germ cell tumors, *Ann Intern Med* 111:22, 1989.

135. Wong LC et al: Etoposide combination chemotherapy in refractory ovarian malignant germ cell tumors, *Gynecol Oncol* 39:123, 1990.

136. Wu P et al: Treatment of malignant ovarian germ cell tumors with preservation of fertility: a report of 28 cases, *Gynecol Oncol* 40:2, 1991.

137. Young RC, Chabner BA, Hubbard SP: Prospective trial of melphalan (L-PAM) versus combination chemotherapy in ovarian adenocarcinoma, *N Engl J Med* 299:1261, 1978.

138. Young RC, Hubbard SP, DeVita VT: The chemotherapy of ovarian carcinoma, *Cancer Treat Rev* 1:99, 1974.

139. Young RC et al: Staging laparotomy in early ovarian cancer, *JAMA* 250:3072, 1983.

140. Young RC et al: Adjuvant therapy in stage I and II epithelial ovarian cancer, *N Engl J Med* 322:1021, 1990.

141. Zurawski VR Jr et al: Serum CA-125 levels in a group of non-hospitalized women: relevance for the early detection of ovarian cancer, *Obstet Gynecol* 69:606, 1987.

Chapter 44

RADIATION AND ISOTOPE THERAPY IN GYNECOLOGIC CANCER

Ronald E. Hempling
M. Steven Piver

Nearly a century has passed since Roentgen described the x-ray and was awarded the first Nobel Prize in physics for his discovery.[77] The possible medical implications of this discovery were recognized in 1903 when Cleaves first treated a cervical cancer with radiation.[13] Since that time, substantial progress has been made in the use of radiation therapy in malignant diseases of the female pelvis.

This chapter reviews the nature of radiation and its cellular and biologic effects and outlines its use in gynecologic cancers.

THE NATURE OF RADIATION

Radiation is a descriptive term that encompasses an entire spectrum of potential sources of energy. Some of these are beneficial, indeed perhaps essential, to the continued existence of life on this planet, whereas others may result in cellular death. The selective exposure of cells to specific wavelengths of radiation energy forms the basis of radiation therapy.

The band in the electromagnetic spectrum that most concerns this discussion is composed of x-rays and gamma rays. These electromagnetic radiations encompass wavelengths of 10^{-7} to 10^{-10} cm or 10^{-3}Å.

Crucial to an understanding of radiation energy is a basic knowledge of atomic structure, because atomic interaction is the source of electromagnetic radiation.

Atoms, which are the smallest unit of matter, are described as a central core or nucleus around which are various numbers of electrons in orbit. The nucleus of an atom contains neutrons, which are uncharged particles, and protons, which are positively charged particles. Electrons are negatively charged and are arrayed in various orbits around the nucleus. The number of electrons is the signature of a given atom or its atomic number Z. In a neutral atom, the number of electrons and the number of protons are equal. The atomic mass, conventionally denoted by a symbol A, represents the total number of protons and neutrons in the nucleus of a given atom.

Electromagnetic radiation is created when an atom is in an unstable condition. This instability may arise either in the nucleus or in the electron cloud that orbits it. Nuclear instability arises in atoms whose atomic number (number of protons) is the same as a parent compound, but whose atomic weight (number of neutrons) is different from its parent compound. Such atoms are referred to as *isotopes*. These atoms are unstable and seek to achieve equilibrium by ejecting nuclear particles. The energy released in this process frequently takes the form of ionizing radiation. The particulate radiation generated in this process takes the form of alpha particles, which are positively charged helium nuclei composed of two neutrons and two protons; beta particles, which are electrons; and gamma rays, which are high-frequency electromagnetic waves comprised of discrete energy bundles called photons.

Electromagnetic radiation also results from extranuclear or electron–electron interactions. Electrons are held in their orbits around the nucleus by a *binding energy*, which is proportional to their proximity to the nucleus and its size. When an incident, high-energy electron interacts with the orbiting electrons of a target atom, an inner shell electron may be ejected. An outer shell electron moves centrally to fill its place and, in the process, releases a photon

Table 44-1. Isotopes commonly used in radiation therapy

Isotope	Energy (meV)	Half-life
^{137}Cs	0.662	30 years
^{60}Co	1.173, 1.332	5.3 years
^{125}I	0.027-0.035	60 days
^{192}Ir	0.47	74 days
^{226}Ra	0.8	1620 years
^{222}Rn	0.8	3.83 days
^{182}Ta	1.18	115 days

^{226}Ra, ^{137}Cs, ^{192}Ir, and ^{182}Ta are suitable for temporary implants; ^{222}Rn is suitable for permanent implants that remain in the patient; ^{60}Co has some uses in intracavitary therapy.
Reprinted with permission from DiSaia PJ: *Radiation therapy in gynecology.* In Scott JR et al, editors: *Danforth's obstetrics and gynecology,* p 1130, Philadelphia, 1988, JB Lippincott.

Table 44-2. Modalities of external radiation

Modality	Voltage	Source
Low voltage (superficial)	85-150 kV	X-ray
Medium voltage (orthovoltage)	180-400 kV	X-ray
Supervoltage	500 kV-8 mV	X-ray ^{60}Co ^{137}Cs ^{226}Ra
Megavoltage	Above supervoltage energy	Betatron Synchrotron Linear accelerator

Reprinted with permission from DiSaia PJ: *Radiation therapy in gynecology.* In Scott JB et al, editors: *Danforth's obstetrics and gynecology,* p 1122, Philadelphia, 1988, JB Lippincott.

of energy equal to the difference in the binding energies between the inner and outer shell electrons. Such quanta of energy, or photons, are x-rays.

In summary, electromagnetic radiation capable of ionization results from nuclear decay, or isotopes, in which case the radiation is referred to as *gamma radiation,* or electron–electron interactions, in which case it is referred to as *x-radiation.*

Isotopes and generators

X-rays and *gamma rays* are both terms used to describe ionizing radiation. As previously mentioned, gamma rays are spontaneously emitted from unstable radionuclides and x-rays result from electron–electron interactions.

The most frequently employed sources of gamma radiation are listed on Table 44-1. The half-life of each isotope is also listed. The half-life denotes the time in which the radioactivity originally associated with a sample of isotope will be reduced by one half through radioactive decay.

X-rays are generated whenever fast-moving electrons strike a suitable target. Such targets have high atomic numbers. The incident electron interacts with the electron cloud of the atoms in the target material, resulting in energy expenditure in the form of heat and characteristic x-ray production. The energies produced by these interactions depend on the speed of the incident electron as well as the target medium. A simple diagnostic x-ray machine produces accelerated electrons as a result of a difference in the electrical potential between the target and the heated filament that produces the electrons. Electrons may also be accelerated in a straight line by high-frequency microwaves. Such a system produces photons of energy and is called a *linear accelerator.*

When electrons are accelerated through a circular core by a changing of magnetic fields, yet higher energy photons may be produced. Such a system is referred to as a *betatron.*

The energies of the photons (x-rays or gamma rays) produced by various radiation sources are all measured in

electron volts. An electron volt (eV) is the energy required to move an electron through an electrical potential of 1 V and is equivalent to 1.6×10^{-12} ergs. The abbreviation meV is equivalent to 1 million electron volts, and the abbreviation keV is equivalent to 1000 electron volts. As can be seen from Table 44-2, these ranges of energy are classified into low-voltage, orthovoltage, supervoltage, and megavoltage, and have important therapeutic implications.

INTERACTIONS OF RADIATION WITH MATTER
The concept of ionization

The object of exposing living tissue to high-energy photons is the selective destruction of unwanted cells. This object is achieved by the formation of electrically charged entities and free hydroxyl radicals within the target, hence the term *ionizing radiation.* The ionizing effects of high-energy photons may be the result of direct action on the target medium in which the charged particles effect atomic destabilization by direct collision, or indirect action by interaction with atoms other than the target medium and secondary production of free radicals that diffuse for some distance to damage critical targets.

In either case, direct or indirect action, the interaction of ionizing radiation with water and resultant formation of free radicals and peroxides are crucial in understanding the molecular effects of photons and tissue. These interactions result in the disruption of water molecules with the production of hydrogen ions and hydroxyl radicals (Fig. 44-1). About one half of the hydrogen atoms encounter hydroxyl radicals and form H_2O_2. In the presence of sufficient quantities of oxygen, HO_2 radicals are also formed and subsequently H_2O_2.

In addition to peroxide formation, degradation of large molecules and cross-linking can result when the excited species interact with cellular constituents. Such interactions, if unrepaired, cripple the cell and lead to a loss of component integrity and eventual cell death.

The interactions of ionizing radiation with matter take place in three mechanisms depending on the energy of the

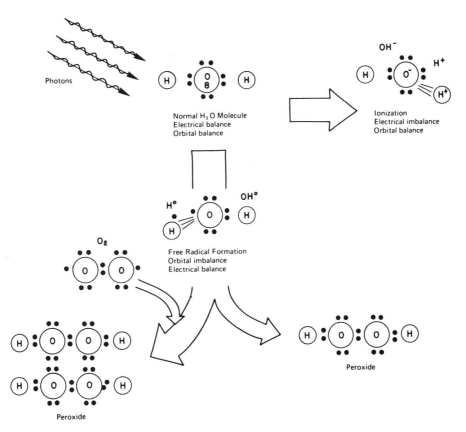

Fig. 44-1. Effects of radiation on water. Ionizing radiation produces water ions and, possibly, free radical formation, yielding peroxide. Latter process is enhanced by addition of pure oxygen. (Reprinted with permission from DiSaia PJ: *Radiation therapy in gynecology.* In Scott JR et al, editors: *Danforth's obstetrics and gynecology,* Philadelphia, 1988, JB Lippincott.)

incident photon and the target material. These three mechanisms are the photoelectric effect, the compton effect, and pair production.

The photoelectric effect

The interactions described by the term *photoelectric effect* are ones in which all, or nearly all, of the energy of the incident photon is transferred to an inner shell electron of an atom in the target tissue. The target atom electron is ejected with a kinetic energy equal to the difference between the energy of the incident photon and the binding energy of the ejected electron. The loss of the inner shell electron results in an inner shell vacancy, which is filled by movement of an outer shell electron. This shift from inner to outer shell results in energy emission in the form of characteristic x-rays. The ejected electron dissipates its energy by collision interactions in the medium.

The photoelectric effect is a characteristic interaction of low-energy photons (0.05 meV). The likelihood of this type of interaction also depends on the target medium and is directly proportional to Z^3. Accordingly, osseous media with a higher Z than soft tissue can more effectively attenuate low-energy photons. This difference forms the physical basis for the use of low-energy x-rays in diagnostic radiology.

Compton effect

Higher energy photons (0.1 meV to 5 meV) more readily interact with outer shell electrons in the target medium. These interactions are described by the Compton effect. In such collisions, the incident photon interacts with a loosely bound outer orbiting electron. A portion of the energy in the incident photon is transferred to the electron, which is then ejected from its orbit. The ejected electron, also called the Compton electron or recoil electron, is ejected in a "forward" direction, as is the energy-reduced photon, also called the scatter photon. Both proceed to further interactions within the target medium, either by Compton scattering or photoelectric effect, until their energy is dissipated. Unlike the photoelectric effect, the probability of a Compton interaction is nearly independent of the atomic number of the target tissue. This property provides a therapeutic advantage because the presence of higher atomic number media do not significantly change the dose of radiation delivered to target tissues within the patient.

Pair production

Photon interactions with nuclear components of the atoms in the target tissue are described by the process of pair production and occur with incident photon energies greater

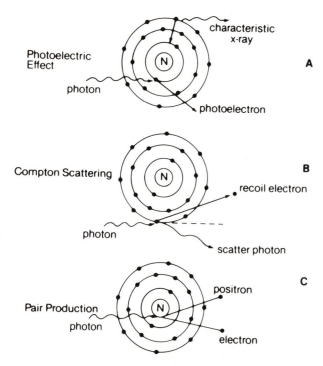

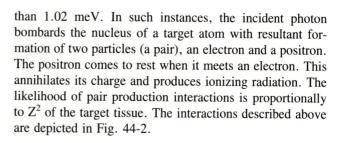

Fig. 44-2. The three main photon interaction processes in matter. **A,** Photoelectric effect: an incident photon interacts with an atom to eject an electron from the K shell, producing a photoelectron. An outer-shell electron fills this vacancy, and the excess energy is emitted as characteristic x-rays. **B,** Compton scattering: an incident photon is scattered by an outer-shell electron. Part of the incident photon energy is transferred to the recoil electron, and the rest is carried by the scatter photon. **C,** Pair production: an incident photon interacts with the nucleus of the atom, and a positron-electron is produced. (Reprinted with permission from Chin LM, Bloomer WD: *The practice of radiotherapy.* In Knapp RC, Berkowitz RS, editors: *Gynecologic oncology,* New York, 1986, Macmillan.)

than 1.02 meV. In such instances, the incident photon bombards the nucleus of a target atom with resultant formation of two particles (a pair), an electron and a positron. The positron comes to rest when it meets an electron. This annihilates its charge and produces ionizing radiation. The likelihood of pair production interactions is proportionally to Z^2 of the target tissue. The interactions described above are depicted in Fig. 44-2.

BIOLOGIC EFFECTIVENESS OF IONIZING RADIATION

The therapeutic effectiveness of ionizing radiation depends on the energy of incident photons and the atomic number of the target material. However, living tissues are in a constant flux, and ongoing biologic changes with any living system also affect the therapeutic index of any treatment modality. Photon radiation is no exception (Fig. 44-3).

The effect of the cell cycle

Evaluations of mammalian cell population by sophisticated molecular techniques demonstrate that various subpopulations are in different phases of reproduction at any given time. These phases have been characterized as the various compartments of the cell cycle (Fig. 44-4). These compartments have been designated as G_1, S, G_2, and M. They represent the presynthetic phase, DNA synthesis, the postsynthetic phase, and mitoses, respectively.

Histochemical staining techniques have allowed identification of the proportion of cells undergoing mitoses. The ratio of this number of cells to the entire cell population is called the *mitotic index.* In most mammalian cell populations, the mitotic index approximates 2% to 7%. Approximately 50% to 60% of an exponentially growing mamma-

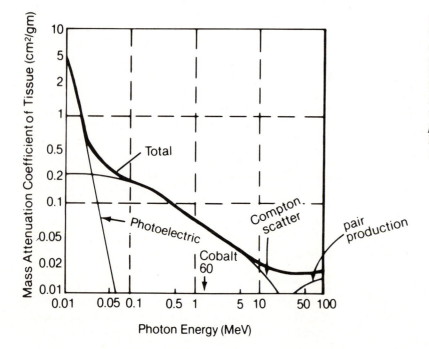

Fig. 44-3. The mass attenuation coefficient of soft tissue as a function of photon energy. The relative components of the three photon interaction processes are plotted. Most of the high-energy linear accelerators operate at an effective energy between 1 and 5 meV. Therefore, most of the interactions are Compton scattering. (Reprinted with permission from Chin LM, Bloomer WD: *The practice of radiotherapy.* In Knapp RC, Berkowitz RS, editors: *Gynecologic oncology,* New York, 1986, Macmillan.)

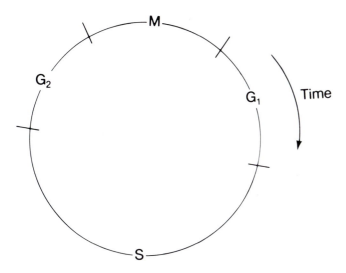

Fig. 44-4. The cell cycle. M = mitosis; G_1 = presynthetic; S = DNA synthesis; G_2 = postsynthetic. (Reprinted with permission from Chin LM, Bloomer WD: *The practice of radiotherapy*. In Knapp RC, Berkowitz RS, editors: *Gynecologic oncology*, New York, 1986, Macmillan.)

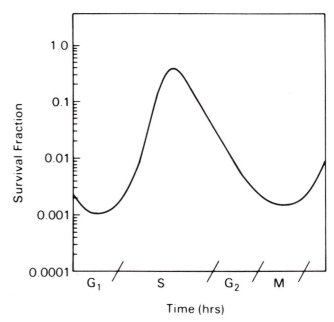

Fig. 44-5. Variation in survival relative to radiation can be considered a function of the cell-cycle phase. Middle and late S constitute a resistant phase, and G_2 and M are sensitive phases. G_1 may be sensitive or resistant, depending on its length. (Reprinted with permission from Chin LM, Bloomer WD: *The practice of radiotherapy*. In Knapp RC, Berkowitz RS, editors: *Gynecologic oncology*, New York, 1986, Macmillan.)

lian cell population are in the synthetic phase (DNA synthesis) of the cycle. Additionally, the proportion of cells in exponentially growing populations found in the four compartments remains constant, and the proportion of cells in each compartment is roughly proportional to the time required to complete that particular activity.

Terasima and Tolmach[84] synchronized cells in mitoses and were able to demonstrate different survival properties as cells passed through each component of the cell cycle. The following general conclusions may be drawn from their work:

1. When cells are in the process of DNA synthesis—S phase—they are the most resistant to ionizing radiation.
2. Cells in the G_2 or M phase are the most radiation-sensitive cells in a population.
3. Cells in the G_1 compartment may be sensitive if the time in the compartment is short but demonstrate increased resistance as the compartment occupies an increasing proportion of the time in the cell cycle.

These findings are depicted in Fig. 44-5. In summary, it may be stated that radiation therapy represents a classic cell cycle specific antineoplastic agent.

The oxygen effect

Among the multitude of factors that may affect the ability of ionizing radiation to achieve therapeutic cell kill, the presence or absence of oxygen must be considered among the most significant.

The survival fraction of hypoxic cells is larger after a single dose of radiation than is the survival fraction of oxic cells (Fig. 44-6). These results indicate that oxygen enhances cell kill for a given dose of radiation. The differ-

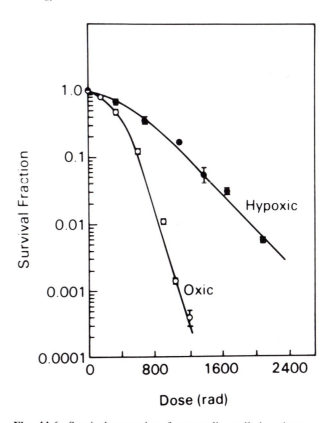

Fig. 44-6. Survival properties of mammalian cells in culture under oxic or hypoxic conditions. The ratio of the final slopes is the oxygen enhancement ratio (OER), usually 2.5 to 3.5. (Reprinted with permission from Chin LM, Bloomer WD: *The practice of radiotherapy*. In Knapp RC, Berkowitz RS, editors: *Gynecologic oncology*, New York, 1986, Macmillan.)

ence between the final slope of these two curves is called the *oxygen enhancement ratio*. For most human cells, this ratio ranges from 2.5 to 3.5.

The relative radiation sensitivity of cells in the presence or absence of oxygen reaches its maximum effect at oxygen tensions that are lower than normal venous blood (Fig. 44-7). However, the diffusion distance for oxygen is only 150 μm. Thomlinson and Gray[85] demonstrated that hypoxic areas ($Po_2 < 20$ mm Hg) in tumors may exist when cells are < 100 μm from a capillary.

The exact mechanism by which oxygen serves as a radiation sensitizer (i.e. enhances the cell-killing ability of a given dose of photons) remains occult. It is generally believed that its presence enhances injury by combining with an unpaired electron in an outer shell of a free radical to form a peroxide. Peroxides are more unstable and toxic than simple free radicals.

In summary, oxygen serves as an important radiation sensitizer in therapeutic radiation systems. Hypoxic cells are 2.5 to 3.5 times more resistant to radiotherapy than are oxic systems. This finding is of clinical significance in the treatment of large and bulky tumors of the female pelvis, which not infrequently contain areas of hypoxic cells.

CELLULAR DAMAGE

It should be clear that cell death resulting from radiation therapy is not an all or none phenomenon. The stage of the cell cycle, availability of oxygen, and host tolerances,

among other factors, virtually preclude this from happening. However, for a given dose of radiation, a constant fraction of cells is destroyed.

The level of damage imparted to exponentially growing mammalian, malignant cells has been classified with respect to its effect on the population. This classification rates damage as lethal, sublethal, and potentially lethal.

Lethal damage describes the situation in which a given dose of radiation results in irreparable cell damage, suspension of unlimited division, and cell death.

Cells that suffer sublethal damage may effect repairs of altered mechanisms and proceed to division. However, if a second insult ensues, the additive effects of both doses result in a lower survival fraction. If repairs are effected and sublethally damaged cells progress from a relative radioresistant phase of the cell cycle to a more radiosensitive one, a second dose of radiation also effects a greater cell kill. This finding serves as one of the major bases for the fractionization of radiation therapy.

Potentially lethal damage may be reparable to a nonlethal state if favorable postradiation conditions are present. For example, potentially lethal damage is repaired in cells incubated in balanced salt solution for several hours after radiation, as opposed to those incubated in full-grown medium.

In summary, whereas some members of a cell population may be destroyed by a given dose of radiotherapy, others suffer damage that is reparable. The repair of such damage may allow for progression into a more radiosensitive phase of the cell cycle where lethal damage may be effected by a subsequent dose of radiation.

DOSE–RESPONSE RELATIONSHIPS

Although early researchers realized that the total dose of radiation given in one exposure rarely eradicated a given tumor, the role played by tumor size and response to radiation was not clarified until the 1970s. Fletcher[23] codified principles that are crucial to the treatment of malignant neoplasms by ionizing radiation. Although a detailed discussion of this work is beyond the scope of this chapter, several vital points should be recognized.

Control of gross disease

Employing data from collected series of tumors of the head and neck, Fletcher demonstrated that there are differences in response among various stages of the same tumor and various tumors of the same stage. These differences he ascribed to differences in cell composition, as well as the existence of anoxic areas within the tumor. Fletcher also demonstrated that some control for small (T_1) lesions could be achieved with all doses of radiation, and that increasing doses effected increased control for moderate sized lesions (T_2, T_3). However, although larger lesions (T_4) show some control at all doses of radiation, this control increases only minimally with increasing doses. Similar findings are seen in grossly positive metastatic lymph nodes.

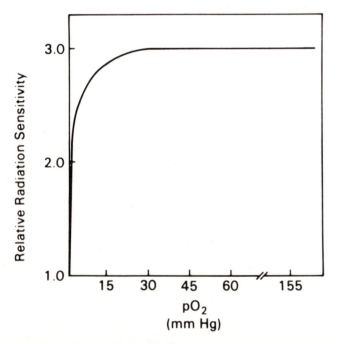

Fig. 44-7. Relationship between relative radiation sensitivity and Po_2. Relative radiation sensitivity increases rapidly with small increases in oxygen tension and reaches a maximum below the Po_2 of venous blood. (Reprinted with permission from Chin LM, Bloomer WD: *The practice of radiotherapy.* In Knapp RC, Berkowitz RS, editors: *Gynecologic oncology,* New York, 1986, Macmillan.)

Control of subclinical disease

Arguably the most significant information from Fletcher's work deals with the treatment of subclinical disease. In series of patients with carcinomas of the breast and squamous cancers of the upper respiratory tract and digestion system, in each case less than 90% control of subclinical disease was achieved if less than 5000 cGy were delivered (Table 44-3).

TOLERANCE OF PELVIC ORGANS

The tolerance of pelvic organs to ionizing radiation varies from patient to patient and from disease to disease depending on factors such as volume of tissue treated, dose of radiation given, fractionization of radiation, and the energy of photons employed as well as the technique of administration. Some general guidelines of organ tolerance are outlined in Table 44-4.

As indicated in Fig. 44-8, uncomplicated cures are the desired outcome. At dose A, there are virtually no complications, but there are no cures either. At dose C, there are substantial numbers of cures, but the numbers of complications are prohibitive. The ideal situation is that of dose B where the optimum number of cures and the lowest number of complications are encountered. However, one must be prepared to accept an increase in complication to

Table 44-3. Percentage of control of subclinical disease in function of dose*

	Adenocarcinoma of the breast		Squamous cell carcinoma of the upper respiratory and digestive tracts	
3000-3500 rads (89 patients)		60%-70%	3000-1000 rads (50 patients)	60%-70%
4000 rads (121 patients)		80%-90%	5000 rads (356 patients)	>90%
5000 rads (273 patients)		>90%	6000 rads (65 patients)	>90%

*1000 rads/week—five days a week.
Reprinted with permission from Fletcher GH: Clinical dose response curves of human malignant epithelial tumors, *Br J Radiol* 46:1, 1973.

Table 44-4. Approximate tolerance of tissues to radiation therapy

Tissue	Approximate tolerance dose (rads)
Bladder	6,000–7,000
Rectum	6,000–7,000
Vaginal mucosa	7,000
Bowel	6,000
Cervix	>12,000
Kidney	2,000–2,300
Liver	2,500–3,500

Reprinted with permission from Droegenmueller W et al: *Principles of radiation therapy and chemotherapy in gynecologic cancer.* In *Comprehensive gynecology,* p 719, St Louis, 1987, The Mosby–Year Book.

achieve a cure. Although most patients suffer some acute side effects of pelvic radiotherapy, these effects are frequently minor and often manageable by conservative techniques.

Perez and Thomas[62] have demonstrated that late com-

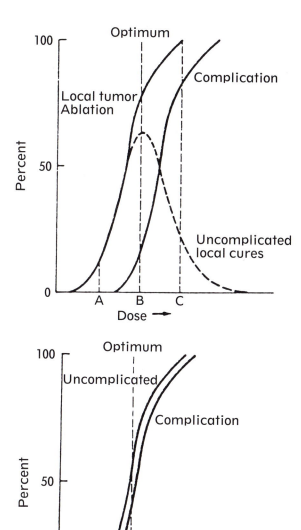

Fig. 44-8. Treatment outcomes. Uncomplicated cures *(dashed line)* are the desired result of treatment. This is illustrated as a function of the therapeutic ratio. That is, the greater the separation between the tumor control curve and the normal tissue complication curve, the greater number of uncomplicated cures will result. The letters *A, B,* and *C* represent three different dose levels that, if chosen, would lead to three different outcomes: *A* would result in few tumor cures but no complications; *C* would lead to complete cure in many cases, but virtually all patients would suffer complications. The optimal choice in this group of dose levels is *B,* which would result in the greatest number of cured patients without complications. (Reprinted with permission from Perez CA, Brady LW, editors: *Principles and practices of radiation oncology,* Philadelphia, 1987, JB Lippincott.)

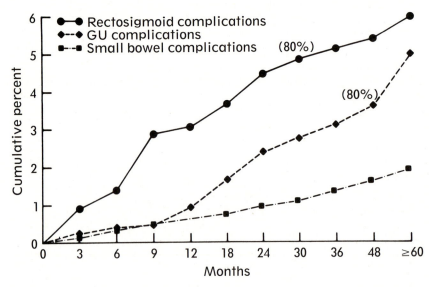

Fig. 44-9. Time to appearance of complications in the rectosigmoid, bladder or ureter, and the small intestines in patients treated with radiation alone for carcinoma of the uterine cervix. (Reprinted with permission from Perez CA and Brady LW, editors: *Principles and practices of radiation oncology,* Philadelphia, 1987, JB Lippincott.)

plications may occur up to 60 months after therapy (Fig. 44-9). Such chronic side effects, however, occur only in between 5% and 10% of treated patients.

ADMINISTRATION OF RADIATION THERAPY

Therapeutic ionizing radiation is delivered to patients by two primary methods. These are external therapy, in which the source of photon radiation is at a distance from the patient, and local radiation or brachytherapy, in which the sources of radiant energy are in direct contact with the tumor.

Three concepts are important in understanding the nature of these differences.

1. *Radiation dose*—The absorbed dose of radiation is the mean energy imparted by radiation to the target material per unit of mass. The unit of measurement employed is the *rad*. The rad represents absorption of 100 ergs of energy per gram of tissue. Recently, by international convention, the gray has been accepted as the unit of radiation dose. One gray = 1 J/kg = 100 rad; 1 rad = 1 centigray (cGy).

2. *Linear energy transfer (LET)* refers to the amount of energy deposited per unit length of the tract of the radiation beam. It is expressed in kiloelectron volts (keV). LET values depend on factors other than radiant energy, and the concept is one of a measure of radiation quality. Low values are calculated for x-rays, and high values are calculated for heavy particle radiation.

3. *Relative biologic effectiveness* is the ratio of the dose of 250 kV x-rays to that of another kind of radiation to produce the same biologic effect. The 250-kV x-rays were chosen because the biologic effect of this radiation is well-known. The value is not absolute and depends on many factors. Some of these factors are radiation quality and the biologic end point evaluated.

TELETHERAPY

Teletherapy or external therapy is the term given to techniques of delivering ionizing radiation in which the source of photons is remote from the target. As mentioned earlier, photons used in this technique may be derived from radionuclides (Co^{60} is the most common) or from accelerated electrons. Figure 44-10 demonstrates schematically two photon generating systems. One employs electrons, and the other employs gamma rays. In each case, a source of photons and a columnator, or beam limiting device, are present. The latter directs the photons to a given target area and reduces the lateral scatter (penumbra).

The energy of the photons generated from teletherapy machines varies with the sources of these photons and has been nosologically divided depending on these energies. In general, it is well to remember that the higher the energy generated, the deeper the penetrating ability of the incident photons (see Table 44-2).

Orthovoltage therapy refers to x-rays generated with potentials of 150 to 500 kV. Although they were used for the treatment of deep-seated tumors early in the history of radiation therapy, use of teletherapy devices has declined as higher energy generators have been invented.

Supervoltage/megavoltage therapy refers to the generation of photons (x-ray or electrons) with potentials of as much as 40 meV. This type of generator includes the linear accelerator, which is the most common source of photons employed in modern teletherapy.

The difference in the energies of photons is of vital clinical importance. It should be recalled that photons dissipate their energy after contact with the target and that this energy is dissipated over various lengths depending on the energy of the incident photon (the concept of LET). The higher the energy of the incident photon, the greater will be the depth at which the maximum ionization occurs. This concept is embodied in the principle of *percent depth dose* (Fig. 44-11). Note that in Fig. 44-11, the maximal ionization takes place close to the surface of the target for

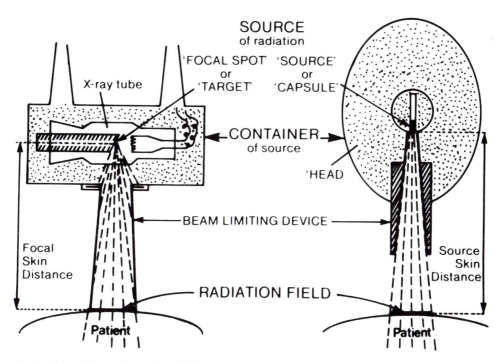

Fig. 44-10. Comparison of two devices used to produce ionizing electromagnetic radiation. (Reprinted with permission from DiSaia PJ: *Radiation therapy in gynecology.* In Scott JR et al, editors: *Danforth's obstetrics and gynecology,* Philadelphia, 1988, JB Lippincott.)

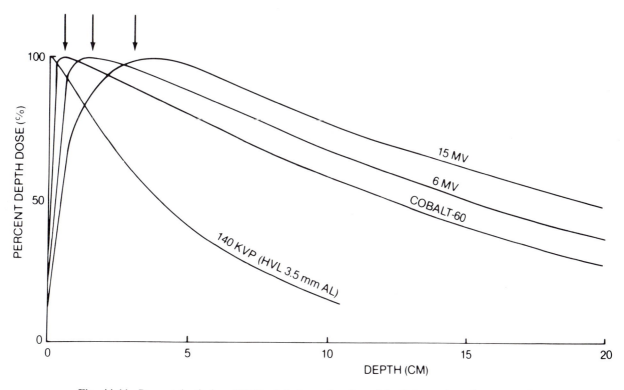

Fig. 44-11. Percent depth dose (PDD) plotted as a function of depth for various photon energies. The depth of maximum buildup for each energy is indicated by the arrow of each curve. (Reprinted with permission from Chin LM, Bloomer WD: *The practice of radiotherapy.* In Knapp RC, Berkowitz RS, editors: *Gynecologic oncology,* New York, 1986, Macmillan.)

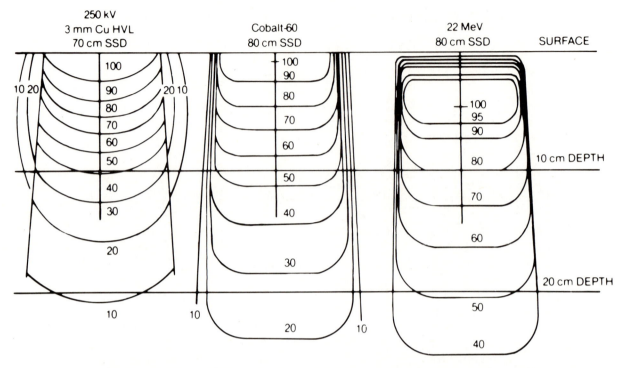

Fig. 44-12. Comparison of isodose distribution for 250-kV, cobalt-60, and 22-mV linear accelerator beams. The field size is 10 × 10 cm at the surface for all beams; respective SSDs (source to surface distance) are indicated. (Reprinted with permission from Chin LM, Bloomer WD: *The practice of radiotherapy.* In Knapp RC, Berkowitz RS, editors: *Gynecologic oncology,* New York, 1986, Macmillan.)

lower energy photons; for higher energy photons, maximal ionization takes place at progressively deeper levels. Another method of evaluating this phenomenon is the isodose curve (Fig. 44-12). This two-dimensional concept is one that depicts a line that connects the points in a target tissue that receive equivalent doses of radiation.

Note that in each case, lower energy photons (140 and 250 kV) have maximal ionization close to or at the surface of the target, whereas the higher energy photons deliver maximal ionization at deeper levels.

This advantage of photons in the supervoltage or megavoltage range is of clinical significance in the treatment of tumors located deep to the surface. In such cases, the introduction of a sufficiently high dose of orthovoltage radiation is not practical.

BRACHYTHERAPY

Local therapy or brachytherapy refers to the placement of radioactive sources in body tissues or in natural cavities in close proximity to a given tumor. This technique permits the delivery of high doses of radiation to a small volume of tissue. The most commonly employed radiation sources for brachytherapy are listed in Table 44-5. The primary advantage of brachytherapy is that it allows for the delivery of a high dose of radiation to a given area with low or acceptable dose exposure to surrounding normal tissues.

Table 44-5. Radionuclides used for brachytherapy

Radionuclide	Half-life ($T_{1/2}$)	Photon energy (meV)
Radium (^{226}Ra)	1600 years	0.83 (avg)
Radon (^{222}Rn)	3.83 days	0.83 (avg)
Cobalt (^{60}Co)	5.26 years	1.17, 1.33
Cesium (^{137}Cs)	30 years	0.662
Iridium (^{192}Ir)	74.2 days	0.38 (avg)
Iodine (^{125}I)	60.2 days	0.028 (avg)

Reprinted with permission from Piver MS, editor: *Manual of gynecological oncologic/gynecology,* Boston, 1989, Little, Brown.

Devices used to deliver such radiation are designed for placement in natural body cavities (e.g., Fletcher Suit after loading appliance; Heyman capsules; Delclos vaginal cylinders) or for interstitial placement (e.g., radium needles or seeds; Fig. 44-13).

The dose of radiation absorbed by brachytherapy applications is governed in large part by the inverse square law. This law states that for radiation emitted by a point source, the dose rate varies inversely as the distance from the source squared.

$$\text{Dose proportional to } \frac{1}{d^2}$$

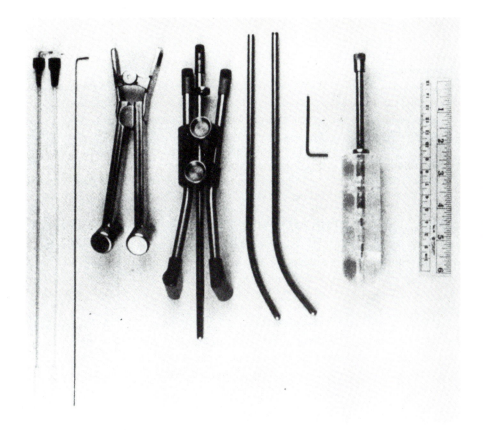

Fig. 44-13. Common applicators used for intracavitary irradiation of gynecologic tumors. *Right to left,* Simon's capsules, Fletcher colpostats, Delclos colpostats, and a tandem combination (two tandems and a vaginal cylinder). (Reprinted with permission from Khalil M: *Principles of radiation therapy.* In Piver MS, editor: *Manual of gynecologic oncology and gynecology,* Boston, 1989, Little, Brown.)

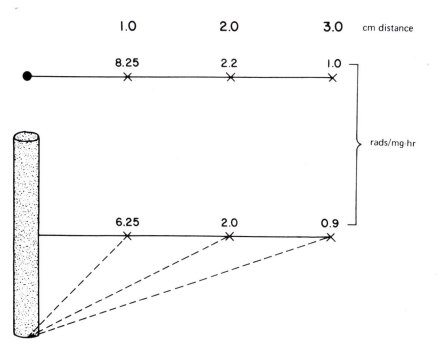

Fig. 44-14. Radiation effects at various distances from 1-mg point source of radium and 1-mg, 2-cm long tubular source of radium. (Reprinted with permission from DiSaia PJ: *Radiation therapy in gynecology.* In Scott JR et al, editors: *Danforth's obstetrics and gynecology,* Philadelphia, 1988, JB Lippincott.)

Therefore, for example, if the dose at a point 1 cm from a source is 100 cGy/hr, the dose at 2 cm from the source is 25 cGy/hr, and at 3 cm the dose is 11.1 cGy/hr (Fig. 44-14).

TREATMENT PLANNING

The compilation of clinical, surgical, and radiographic data is used to generate a plan that defines the total volume of tissue to be treated, the dose to be received, and the time over which treatment is to take place. The use of computers has aided remarkably in creating individualized treatment plans, and their use is nearly routine.

The dose of radiation required to eradicate a tumor is usually given in small increments over periods of days or weeks. The dose given daily is called a *fraction.* The rationale for fractionation is determined by four factors that contribute to the difference in dose response between normal and neoplastic tissues. These four factors are regeneration, repair of cellular damage, reoxygenation, and redistribution within the cell cycle. Conventional treatment regimens have been determined because they optimize normal tissue repair of sublethal damage and increase efficient cell kill in malignant neoplasms by allowing for reoxygenation of hypoxic tumors and redistribution of cells to more sensitive phases of the cell cycle.

The response of normal tissue to ionizing radiation may be divided with respect to the promptness with which the effects of radiation are seen. Early or acutely responding tissues include epithelial surfaces or membranes and the hematopoietic system. These organs contain a population of rapidly dividing cells, and radiation produces acute effects such as ulceration and desquamation. Late responding or chronic responding tissues contain slowly dividing cells and constitute the dose-limiting factors in most clinical situations. Examples of chronic responding tissues are the spinal cord and kidney.

Conventional radiation fractions range between 180 and 200 cGy. Increasing the dose per fraction increases the severity of injury. This phenomenon is more readily observed in late responding than in early responding tissues. Modifications of dose fractionation patterns in clinical practice include:

1. *Hyperfractionation:* Treatments are divided into smaller than conventional doses per fraction without changing the overall treatment duration.
2. *Accelerated fractionation:* The overall regimen is shortened, but conventional dose fractions are employed.
3. *Hypofractionation:* Larger treatment fractions are used over the same period of time.

THE CONCEPT OF WHOLE PELVIS RADIATION

The clinical application of radiotherapy in gynecologic malignancy most frequently revolves around the delivery of tumoricidal radiation to cancers involving the pelvic viscera and lymph nodes. Accordingly, the term *whole pelvis radiation* is frequently employed.

The field of therapy described by this term extends from the lower border of the obturator foramena to the L4–5 interspace. The lateral extent of the field is a point 1 to 2 cm lateral to the pelvic brim (Fig. 44-15).

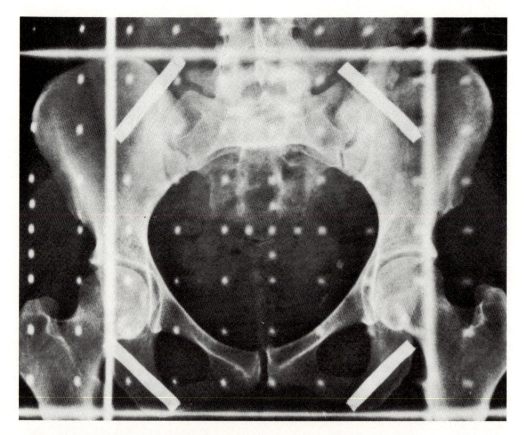

Fig. 44-15. Whole pelvis irradiation for cervical cancer extending to involve upper part of vagina. Lower margin of 18 × 18 cm field is well below pubic symphysis. Lead tapes (white strips) show technique of excluding corners of a square field, thus reducing volume irradiated by roughly 10%. (Reprinted with permission from DiSaia PJ: *Radiation therapy in gynecology.* In Scott JR et al, editors: *Danforth's obstetrics and gynecology,* Philadelphia, 1988, JB Lippincott.)

The usual dose delivered to this target volume for the eradication of microscopic disease is 5040 cGy. This dose may be delivered in a number of ways, the most common of which are depicted in Fig. 44-16. Each technique, parallel opposing beams, the "box technique," and rotational therapy, has advantages in given patient situations, and the treatment plan must reflect such individualization.

The dose of radiotherapy delivered to specific areas in the pelvis may be altered with the use of lead shielding or by limiting the size of the beam at its source. This technique is referred to as the "shrinking field technique" and allows for the delivery of higher doses (up to 7000 cGy) of radiotherapy to specific areas in the pelvis (Fig. 44-17).

CLINICAL APPLICATIONS
Vulvar cancer

Vulvar carcinoma represents a relatively rare gynecologic malignancy and accounts for 3% to 4% of all gynecologic cancers in the United States. The majority of lesions are diagnosed in relatively early stages, and radical surgery or, in selected cases, more conservative surgery result in cure rates that exceed 90%. However, the presence of inguinal pelvic lymph node metastasis significantly worsens prognosis. Curry and co-workers[15] reported on

191 patients, 57 (30%) of whom were found to have lymph node metastasis. The overall survival for the entire group was 73%, but patients with positive nodes demonstrated a survival of 38%. Moreover, there were no survivors among patients with three or more positive inguinal lymph nodes. Positive pelvic lymph nodes were found in one half of the patients who had more than four ipsilateral positive nodes and in one quarter of the patients with bilateral inguinal nodes.

Hacker et al[31] also demonstrated a substantial difference in survival for patients with inguinal lymph node metastasis. The corrected actuarial survival for patients with negative nodes in his series was 96%. For patients who had one positive lymph node, the 5-year actuarial survival was 94%, and patients who had two positive lymph nodes had a 5-year actuarial survival of 80%. Patients with three or more positive nodes had a 5-year actuarial survival of 12%. Additionally, no patient who had less than three positive inguinal lymph nodes had positive pelvic lymph nodes.

The treatment of patients with positive inguinal lymph nodes and pelvic lymph nodes with groin and whole pelvic radiotherapy has demonstrated a salutary effect on local tumor control and survival. Malfetano and Piver[50a] reported

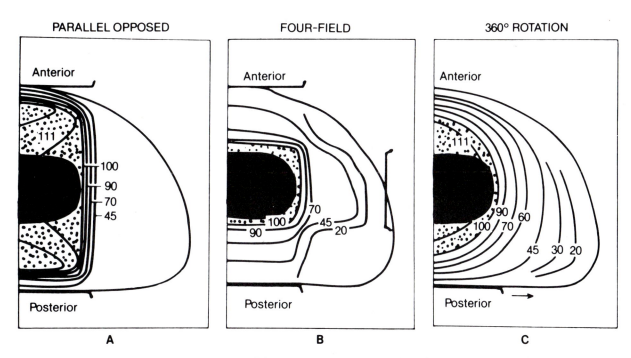

Fig. 44-16. Comparison of three high-energy photon treatment plans for a target volume with an elliptical cross section. The plans were normalized so that the target receives 100% of the prescribed dose. Plan A is clearly not optimal, because a large volume of normal tissue (stippled area) outside the target (blackened area) also receives a dose higher than 100%. By simply adding a pair of opposed lateral beams to plan A, the 100% isodose conforms well to the target volume, and the transit doses through normal tissue are relatively low (plan B). Plan C is a 360-degree rotation and is not optimal to cover an elliptical target, because the field width must be larger than the longer axis of the ellipse. A 360-degree rotation is better suited for circular target volumes. (Reprinted with permission from Chin LM, Bloomer WD: *The practice of radiotherapy.* In Knapp RC, Berkowitz RS, editors: *Gynecologic oncology,* New York, 1986, Macmillan.)

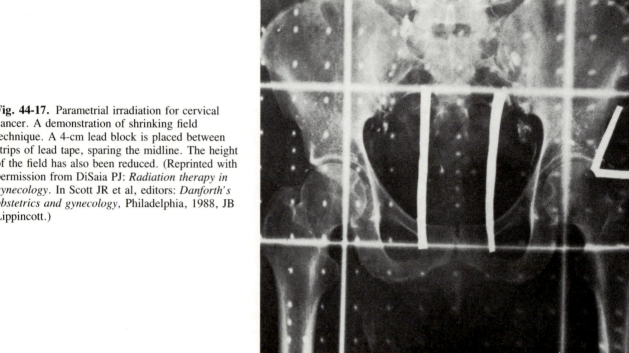

Fig. 44-17. Parametrial irradiation for cervical cancer. A demonstration of shrinking field technique. A 4-cm lead block is placed between strips of lead tape, sparing the midline. The height of the field has also been reduced. (Reprinted with permission from DiSaia PJ: *Radiation therapy in gynecology.* In Scott JR et al, editors: *Danforth's obstetrics and gynecology,* Philadelphia, 1988, JB Lippincott.)

only one recurrence in the treated field among eight patients with advanced disease and histologically positive regional lymph nodes.

Homesley and coworkers[35] demonstrated significant advantages for patients with positive lymph nodes treated with radiotherapy as opposed to those treated with pelvic lymphadenectomy. The 2-year progression-free survival for patients with positive lymph nodes was 68% when treated with radiotherapy, whereas those who had undergone pelvic lymphadenectomy demonstrated a 2-year progression-free survival of 51%. This difference was statistically significant.

In light of these findings, it is recommended that patients with three or more positive inguinal lymph nodes or bilateral metastasis to the groin nodes undergo inguinal and pelvic radiotherapy after primary surgery.

Electron beam radiation lends itself particularly well to the treatment of inguinal lymph nodes. As can be seen from Fig. 44-18, electrons with energies of 6 meV deliver nearly 100% of their dose at depths most likely to harbor occult metastasis. Accordingly, treatment plans for the patient in need of radiotherapy for nodal disease arising from vulval cancer should include higher energy photons for the pelvis, but should include electrons with energies of 6 meV or less for eradication of subclinical disease in the inguinal lymph nodes.

The treatment of locally advanced vulval cancer that involves the anus or urethra may require exenterative surgery to effect tumor-free margins. In an attempt to obviate the need for such surgery, several authors have proposed the use of preoperative radiotherapy. Boronow[2] reported on the treatment of 26 patients with locally advanced vulvar cancers. Vaginal radium with or without teletherapy was employed, followed by surgery. Eight patients developed major complications, and the survival for the group was 65% at between 1 and 11 years. Hacker[32] and Rotmensch et al,[79] have reported on smaller series that have demonstrated survival rates approximating those achieved by exenterative surgery in advanced disease.

The combination of preoperative chemotherapy and radiotherapy in patients with advanced disease used in hopes of averting the need for exenterative surgery has also been reported.[37,39,40] Several small series demonstrate promising results, and further exploration of this modality appears to be warranted.

Vaginal cancer

Carcinoma of the vagina is rare, representing a little more than 1% of all gynecologic malignancies. The overwhelming majority are squamous cancers and occur primarily in patients of advanced years.

Although lesion size and depth of invasion play significant roles in the treatment of vaginal cancer, lesion location is of crucial importance (Fig. 44-19). Lymphatic drainage of the upper two thirds of the vagina is directed to the pelvic lymph nodes; the lower one third drains to the inguinal lymph nodes.

The treatment of vaginal cancer has varied in the last

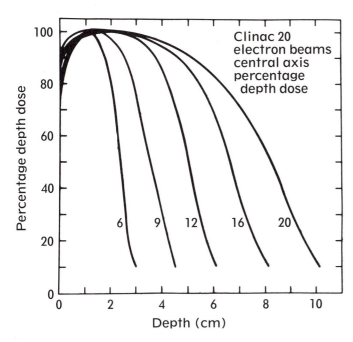

Fig. 44-18. Electron beam central axis isodose curves for a 10 × 10 cm field at 100-cm SSD. These data are from the Varian Clinac 20 at Mallinckrodt Institute of Radiology in St Louis. (Reprinted with permission from Glasgow GP, Sampiere VA, Purdy JA: *External beam dosimetry and treatment planning.* In Perez CA, Brady LW, editors: *Principles and practice of radiation oncology,* ed 2, Philadelphia, 1992, JB Lippincott.)

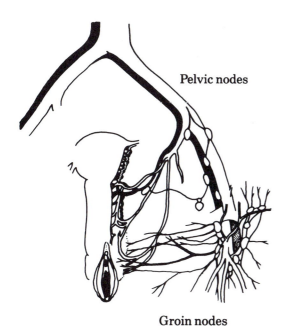

Fig. 44-19. Lymphatic drainage of the upper and lower vagina. The upper two thirds of the vagina drains directly to the pelvic lymph nodes, and the lower one third drains to groin lymph nodes. (Reprinted with permission from Karlen J: *Cancer of the vagina.* In Piver MS, editor: *Manual of gynecologic oncology and gynecology,* Boston, 1989, Little, Brown.)

half century from exclusively surgical methods to methods employing only radiation therapy. Many authors have employed a combination of therapies. By the early 1970s, surgery had become the preferred treatment modality for patients with vaginal cancer. The two primary reasons for this trend were the high complication rate of orthovoltage radiation used in the precedent 45 years, and the lack of uniformity in staging among authors reporting results. Additionally, a convincing treatise by Herbst[33] demonstrated a significant survival advantage for patients treated by radical surgery. In this study, 32 patients were treated with radical surgery and 36 were treated by radiation therapy. The 5-year survival for the surgically treated group was 48%, and for those treated with radiation therapy was 21.1%. The study, however, failed to consider patient selection. Patients with more advanced lesions more frequently received radiation therapy as opposed to surgery.

In 1971, Brown and coworkers[6] reported their experience using a primary radiotherapeutic approach to vaginal cancer. This report of 76 patients with stages I to IV vaginal cancer demonstrated an overall 5-year survival of 70%, a low complication rate, and retention of sexual function in most patients. The report demonstrated the efficacy of modern radiotherapy techniques in the treatment of vaginal cancer and shifted the emphasis in therapy from surgery to radiation.

The literature is replete with techniques for the treatment of vaginal cancer. Most combine teletherapy and brachytherapy. The teletherapy portion of the regimen usually involves delivery of 4000 to 6000 cGy of fractionated radiation to the whole pelvis. When the lesion is located in the lower two thirds of the vagina, inguinal node radiation is also included. The lesser dose is usually administered to stage I or stage II lesions with increasing amounts given to larger lesions. When brachytherapy is not feasible, the dose of external radiation therapy may be increased to 7000 cGy with appropriate shielding and shrinking field techniques.

Local radiotherapy techniques also play a significant role in the treatment of vaginal cancer. Several authors have demonstrated excellent survival in patients with stage I disease using local therapy alone. Perez,[60,61,63] in a series of three studies spanning 11 years, demonstrated an 81% 5-year survival among 22 patients treated with local therapy. Similar survival data were reported by Dancuart.[15a] The choice of brachytherapy technique is determined in large measure by tumor thickness. Tumors that measure less than 0.5 cm in width lend themselves well to intracavitary therapy, because the dosimetry offered by colpostat or vaginal cylinders, as determined by the inverse square law, allows for delivery of tumoricidal radiation to the cancer and to a depth great enough to treat subvaginal tissues at risk. However, tumors of greater than 0.5 cm in thickness preclude the delivery of such doses and demand the use of interstitial therapy. Radium or iridium-192 needles are usually used for this technique. They are placed in a manner that gives an adequate

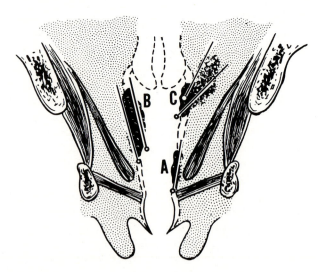

Fig. 44-20. Interstitial radium implants for tumors of different depths on the lateral vaginal wall. (Reprinted with permission from Fletcher GH, editor: *Vagina and female urethra. Textbook of radiotherapy,* Philadelphia, 1966, Lea & Febiger.)

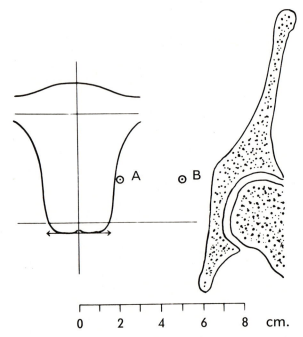

Fig. 44-21. Technique for determining radiation dose to various areas of pelvis. Point *A* is 2 cm lateral to cervical canal and 2 cm superior to lateral vaginal vault. Point *B* is 3 cm lateral to point *A.* Calculation of radiation dose to point *A* indicates radiation delivered to paracervical structures that may be involved in cervical cancer; calculation of radiation dose at point *B* indicates radiation delivered to pelvic lymph glands draining cervix. (Reprinted with permission from DiSaia PJ: *Radiation therapy in gynecology.* In Scott JR et al, editors: *Danforth's obstetrics and gynecology,* Philadelphia, 1988, JB Lippincott.)

homogeneous radiation dose to the entire tumor, but avoids "hot spots," which could cause necrosis and fistula formation (Fig. 44-20).

Brachytherapy techniques, similar to those described above, are also used in conjunction with teletherapy for larger and more advanced lesions. Their purpose is the destruction of residual disease. Criteria for the choice of treatment modality are similar to those outlined above.

Cervical cancer

Nearly a century has passed since the first reported cure of cervical cancer using radiation therapy. While during that time advances in surgical technique, anesthesia, and antibiotics have made surgery a viable option for selected patients, radiation therapy has emerged as the treatment of choice for most patients with locally advanced cervical cancer.

Although the reasons for this statement include an improved knowledge of the pathologic spread pattern of the disease, newer radiation modalities, improved supportive care, and the use of radiation sensitizers, the most important factors that have led to this conclusion are the accessibility of the tumor and the fact that it lies in a relatively radioresistant bed of tissue. Although the tolerance of surrounding organs may be a limiting factor in some cases, the careful planning of therapy allows for the delivery of 15,000 to 20,000 cGy of ionizing radiation to the cervix and upper vagina. These tissues tolerate such high doses without significant difficulty, thereby allowing eradication of the neoplasm.

In all but a few cases, teletherapy and brachytherapy are combined to deliver tumoricidal radiation to carcinomas of the cervix.

Teletherapy. Teletherapy is usually employed first. A dose of 5040 cGy in approximately 28 fractions is deliv-

ered to the whole pelvis. Supervoltage or megavoltage photons are used. Shrinking field techniques and the use of midline blocks allow doses to the parametria to be raised to 7000 cGy in selected cases. The purpose of teletherapy is the delivery of tumoricidal radiation to node-bearing tissues in the pelvis and the reduction of cervical tumor bulk. The latter affords the restoration of normal cervical and intravaginal anatomy and allows for more efficacious placement of brachytherapy devices.

Brachytherapy. Radium has traditionally been the source of photons for the overwhelming majority of brachytherapy applications in gynecologic oncology. It has been more recently supplanted by cesium 137, which offers the advantages of monoenergetic emission, a shorter half-life, and improved shielding ability.

The standardization of the dose of radiation delivered by brachytherapy presented some difficulties and, until recently, had been described in terms of two imaginary points in the pelvis: A and B. These points, originally proposed by the developers of the Manchester System (see below), serve as guidelines from which doses delivered to the parametria and the lymph nodes in the pelvis may be calculated. Point A is defined as being 2 cm superior to the mucosa of the vaginal fornix and 2 cm lateral to the cervical os. Point B is 3 cm lateral to point A (Fig. 44-21). It was suggested that control of squamous cell carcinoma of

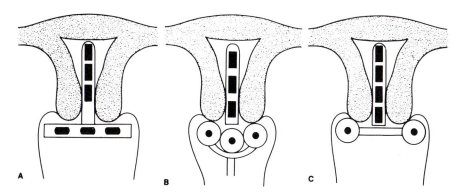

Fig. 44-22. Application of radium in treatment of cervical cancer. **A,** Stockholm technique. **B,** Paris technique. **C,** Manchester technique. (Reprinted with permission from DiSaia PJ: *Radiation therapy in gynecology.* In Scott JR et al, editors: *Danforth's obstetrics and gynecology,* Philadelphia, 1988, JB Lippincott.)

the cervix required a tumor dose of 7000 to 8000 cGy. Accordingly, most followers of the Manchester System attempted to deliver 7000 cGy to point A. Although computer simulation has all but obviated the need for these somewhat arbitrary mathematical constructs, they are still frequently used in discussing delivered doses.

Three primary systems have been developed. All three employ an intrauterine tandem, a long hollow tube that is inserted into the uterus and projects from the vagina, and colpostats or ovoids in which sources are placed to allow close proximity to the cervix.

The Stockholm technique. The Stockholm technique of brachytherapy employs high doses of radiation over two separate insertions separated by 2 to 3 weeks (Fig. 44-22, *A*). The intrauterine tandem is loaded with 50 to 75 mg of radium in its distal aspect, whereas the proximal, intracervical portion is loaded with a dummy source. The vaginal portion of the application consists of two to four rows of boxes or small cylinders containing 60 to 80 mg of radium. The average treatment time approximates 24 hours and delivers slightly less than 6000 cGy to point A and 2000 cGy to point B in two applications. Although the Stockholm technique offers good doses, it has the disadvantage of being a live loaded technique (i.e., the unshielded sources are placed in the operating room).

The Paris technique. The Paris technique employs lower doses of radium administered over a longer period of time (Fig. 44-22, *B*). The uterine tandem contains three sources. The two cephalad sources are 13-mg sources, and the intracervical source is a 6-mg source. Three cork cylinders, each containing a 13- or 13-mg source, are placed in close proximity to the cervix, one in each fornix and one near the external os. Again, point A receives slightly less than 6000 cGy. Each treatment lasts between 96 and 200 hours.

The Manchester technique. The Manchester technique, a variation of the Paris technique, has gained wide popularity (Fig. 44-22, *C*). With the advent of afterloading hardware, the Fletcher-Suit system, this technique offers

Table 44-6. Survival rates for squamous cell carcinoma of the cervix treated by radiation only, September 1954 through December 1967, MD Anderson Hospital and Tumor Institute

Stage	5-Year survival rate* (%)	10-Year survival rate* (%)
Cervical carcinoma, intact uterus (1705 patients)†		
Ib	91.5	90.0
IIa	83.5	79.0
IIb	66.5	57.0
IIIa	45.0	39.0
IIIb	36.0	30.0
IV	14.0	14.0
Carcinoma of cervical stump (189 patients)		
Ib	97.0	97.0
IIa	93.0	89.0
IIb	67.0	67.0
IIIa	61.0	61.0
IIIb	32.0	32.0
IV	0	0

*Modified life table method. Patients dying of intercurrent disease are excluded.
†Includes patients treated incompletely or for palliation.
Reprinted with permission from DiSaia PJ: *Radiation therapy in gynecology.* In Scott JR et al, editors: *Danforth's obstetrics and gynecology,* p 1137, Philadelphia, 1988, JB Lippincott.

homogeneity of dose and safety (Fig. 44-23). Isodose curves for the Manchester technique are demonstrated in Fig. 44-24. In each case, dose is calculated as 100% at point A. Other numbers demonstrate the percentage of this dose at various depths. Note that the doses at points A and B are considerably improved by the use of larger ovoids.

Excellent results for early stage disease are achieved with radiation therapy (Table 44-6). Results for more advanced disease are less encouraging, but several studies indicate that these may be improved with radiation sensitizers (see below).

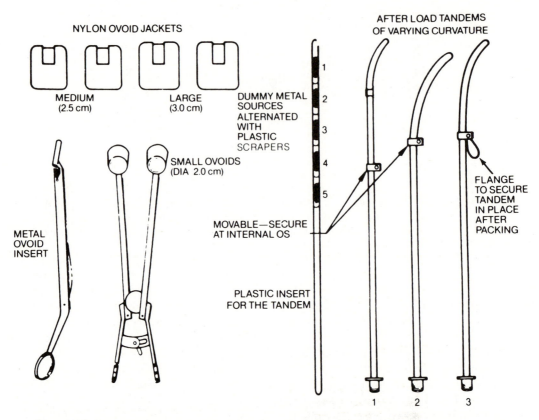

Fig. 44-23. Fletcher-Suit afterloading applicators. Different sizes and shapes of tandems and ovoids are shown. (Reprinted with permission from Chin LM, Bloomer WD: *The practice of radiotherapy.* In Knapp RC, Berkowitz RS, editors: *Gynecologic oncology,* New York, 1986, Macmillan.)

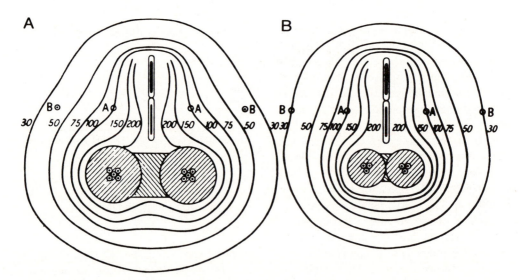

Fig. 44-24. Isodose curves showing dose delivered by Manchester technique to different depths in two cases in which differing amounts of radium could be used. In each, dose is calculated as 100% at point *A*, or *x* number of centigrays. Other numbers show percentage of this dose delivered at other depths. **A,** Standard applicators for large vagina. **B,** Standard applicators for small vagina. *Note:* The dose at points *A* and *B* is considerably improved by using larger vaginal ovoids. Thus, with the larger ovoids, the same maximal normal tissue tolerance of the bladder, rectum, and vaginal mucosa is arrived at, with more radiation being delivered to the parametria as represented by point *A* and point *B*. (Reprinted with permission from DiSaia PJ: *Radiation therapy in gynecology.* In Scott JR et al, editors: *Danforth's obstetrics and gynecology,* Philadelphia, 1988, JB Lippincott.)

CARCINOMA OF THE ENDOMETRIUM

Adenocarcinoma of the endometrium is the most common of all gynecologic malignancies. The mainstay of therapy for all but rare cases remains surgical. Although the use of radiotherapy in more advanced stages of the disease is clearly beneficial, its use in stage I disease remained, until recently, controversial.

Stage I disease

The use of radiation therapy in stage I endometrial cancer varies from institution to institution. The difficulty in demonstrating its efficacy lies in the fact that a clear understanding of the surgicopathologic spread pattern of the disease was not available until the last quarter century. Although Ng and Reagan[57] clearly demonstrated that patients with deeply invasive or poorly differentiated endometrial cancer had a worse prognosis than patients with well differentiated or superficially invasive tumors, the reason for this finding remained unknown until Lewis and Stallworthy,[47] Creasman,[14] Boronow,[4] and Piver,[72] among others, demonstrated the importance of the depth of invasion and grade of tumor as regards the potential for pelvic and paraaortic lymph node metastasis. The risk for pelvic lymph node metastasis in well differentiated tumors and superficially invasive tumors is approximately 7%, whereas one quarter to one half of deeply invasive or poorly differentiated tumors demonstrate pelvic lymph node metastasis (Tables 44-7 and 44-8). Of perhaps greater significance was the finding that one quarter to one half of patients with deeply invasive or poorly differentiated tumors had metastasis to paraaortic lymph nodes (Tables 44-9 and 44-10). These metastasis lay outside the standard treatment fields for adjuvant whole pelvis radiation, and patients with metastasis to these nodes had no hope of being cured with such therapy. With these findings

in mind, a series of studies have been carried out that allow for individualization of adjuvant therapy in stage I corpus cancer and maximization of its efficacy.

Vaginal vault radiation. Studies indicate that between 2% and 14% of patients with stage I endometrial cancer will suffer vaginal cuff recurrence if untreated with vaginal vault radiation. The question of when and how to apply such radiation has remained a matter of controversy. Early reports extolled the virtues of preoperative brachytherapy. This method of vaginal vault radiation supposedly served the twofold purpose of "sterilizing the uterus" and delivering tumoricidal radiation to microscopic nests of disease in the subvaginal lymphatics. Such brachytherapy was followed traditionally by hysterectomy some 6 weeks later. Although efficacious in diminishing cuff recurrence, this methodology suffers from three significant detractors. First, the use of intracavitary radium/cesium and remote hysterectomy destroyed the architecture of the tumor and the depth of invasion, which is now known to be a vital prognostic indicator. Second, sterilization of the uterus was shown to be of little, if any, therapeutic value. Third, two anesthetics are required: one for the placement of the brachytherapy hardware and one for hysterectomy. Additionally, statistical support for the contention that preoperative brachytherapy offers treatment to the paravaginal tissues and improved dosimetry is lacking. A solution to two of these problems was found when studies demonstrated that preoperative brachytherapy followed by immediate (48 hours) hysterectomy preserved uterine architecture and was accompanied by no increase in postoperative infectious morbidity. The question of a second anesthetic in frequently elderly, obese, hypertensive, glucose-intolerant patients, however, remains unanswered. Several studies have demonstrated that the use of postoperative intravaginal radium or cesium is equally effective as preoperative,

Table 44-7. Pelvic lymph node metastases in FIGO stage I endometrial cancer

		Metastases	
	No. patients	No.	(%)
Grade			
1 (well differentiated)	36	2	(5.5)
2 (moderately differentiated)	50	5	(10.0)
3 (poorly differentiated)	19	5	(26.0)
Not known	2	—	
TOTAL	107	12	
Myometrial invasion			
None	16	0	(0.0)
Superficial	41	0	(0.0)
Intermediate	28	4	(14.3)
Deep	22	8	(36.2)
TOTAL	107	12	

Reprinted with permission from Piver MS: Uterine cancer. New thoughts on postoperative therapy, *Contemp Obstet Gynecol* 28:45, 1986.

Table 44-8. Pelvic lymph node metastases in surgical stage I endometrial cancer

		Metastases	
	Patients	No.	(%)
Grade			
1	85	1	(1.2)
2	74	4	(5.4)
3	35	9	(25.7)
TOTAL	194	14	
Myometrial invasion			
Endometrial	87	0	(0.0)
Superficial	73	4	(5.5)
Intermediate	13	3	(23.1)
Deep	21	7	(33.3)
TOTAL	194	14	

Reprinted with permission from Piver MS: Uterine cancer. New thoughts on postoperative therapy, *Contemp Obstet Gynecol* 28:45, 1986.

Table 44-9. Paraaortic lymph node metastases in surgical stage I

		Metastases	
	Patients	No.	(%)
Grade			
1	64	0	(0.0)
2	44	2	(4.5)
3	27	7	(25.9)
TOTAL	135	9	
Myometrial invasion			
Endometrial	63	0	(0.0)
Superficial	48	4	(8.3)
Intermediate	8	1	(12.5)
Deep	16	4	(25.0)
TOTAL	135	9	

Reprinted with permission from Piver MS: Uterine Cancer. New thoughts on postoperative therapy, *Contemp Obstet Gynecol* 28:45, 1986.

Table 44-10. Paraaortic lymph node metastases in FIGO stage I

		Metastases	
	Patients	No.	(%)
Grade			
1	11	0	(0.0)
2	22	3	(13.6)
3	8	3	(37.5)
TOTAL	41	6	
Myometrial invasion			
Endometrial	8	0	(0.0)
Superficial	22	1	(4.5)
Deep	11	5	(45.5)
TOTAL	41	6	

Reprinted with permission from Piver MS: Uterine cancer. New thoughts on postoperative therapy. *Contemp Obstet Gynecol* 28:45, 1986.

and the technique obviates the need for a second anesthetic.

In 1979, Piver and co-workers,[73] expanding on earlier seminal work by Graham,[27] reported a series of 189 patients with stage I endometrial cancer treated either by surgery alone, surgery plus preoperative vaginal radium, or surgery plus postoperative vaginal radium. All patients were followed for a minimum of 10 years or until death. The actuarial cancer-free 5- and 10-year survival rates, respectively, were 90.5% and 88.0% for patients treated with hysterectomy alone, 91.4% and 91.4% for patients treated with hysterectomy and preoperative brachytherapy, and 95.7% and 93.4% for patients treated with hysterectomy and postoperative brachytherapy. Not only was the survival somewhat better for those treated with hysterectomy and postoperative brachytherapy, but not one of the patients so treated developed a vaginal recurrence. In contrast, 7.5% of those treated with surgery alone and 4% of those treated with preoperative intravaginal radium or cesium developed vaginal cuff recurrence. Two studies from the Roswell Park Cancer Institute have also demonstrated the efficacy of postoperative vaginal cesium in preventing vaginal recurrence. Between 1975 and 1982, 68 patients with stage I disease at low risk for pelvic or paraaortic lymph node metastasis (grade 1 or 2 lesions with less than 50% myometrial invasion) were treated with postoperative vaginal cylinders that delivered 6000 cGy to the vaginal mucosa and 3000 cGy to 0.5 cm below the surface of the vaginal mucosa. Not one of these patients suffered a vaginal cuff recurrence during a median follow-up of 4.8 years.[51] Interestingly, during that same 7 years, 19 patients with similar pathology treated with surgery only who suffered vaginal cuff recurrence were referred to Roswell Park Cancer Institute for further therapy. Their 5-year survival was 21.1%. Most recently, Piver and Hempling[66] reported 92 surgically staged patients with adenocarcinoma

of the endometrium. These patients were all at low risk for nodal metastasis (i.e., grade 1 or 2 with less than 50% myometrial invasion). All received vaginal vault radiation postoperatively within 8 to 10 days of surgery. A Delclos vaginal cylinder was used that delivered 6000 cGy to the vaginal surface and 3000 cGy at a depth of 0.5 cm. All patients have been followed for 2 to 10 years or until death. The estimated 5-year disease-free survival for this group was 99%, and there have been no vaginal cuff recurrences. Only one patient suffered a complication of radiation therapy. This was a radiation proctitis that was managed conservatively to a successful conclusion. In short, the use of postoperative vaginal cesium/radium in appropriately selected patients offers the advantages of maintaining uterine architecture, eliminating the need for two anesthetics, and, most importantly, virtually eliminating vaginal cuff recurrence.

Postoperative teletherapy. Postoperative pelvic teletherapy has been widely prescribed for patients with endometrial cancer. However, a clear benefit ascribable to the therapy, vis-a-vis survival, has been difficult to establish. This difficulty arose, no doubt, from the treatment of patients who did not need or could not benefit from the therapy.

Recent work has more clearly defined a subgroup of patients with stage I disease most likely to benefit from adjuvant pelvic radiotherapy. These patients have deeply invasive (greater than 50% of the myometrium) tumors of any grade or poorly differentiated tumors of any invasive depth. Studies previously cited demonstrate that 25% to 45% of these patients have metastasis to the pelvic lymph nodes. Accordingly, adjuvant therapy with tumoricidal radiation to the whole pelvis is warranted. However, if this therapy is to be effective, pathologic confirmation of the absence of disease in the next highest lymph node chain, the paraaortic nodes, is mandatory. Work by Creasman,[14]

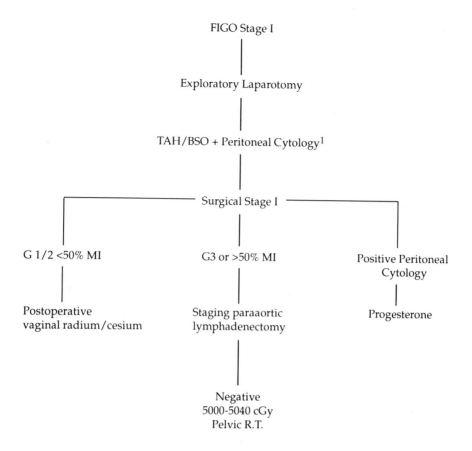

FIGO Stage I

Exploratory Laparotomy

TAH/BSO + Peritoneal Cytology[1]

Surgical Stage I

G 1/2 <50% MI

G3 or >50% MI

Positive Peritoneal Cytology

Postoperative vaginal radium/cesium

Staging paraaortic lymphadenectomy

Progesterone

Negative
5000-5040 cGy
Pelvic R.T.

[1] Added in 1982.
TAH/BSO = total abdominal hysterectomy and bilateral salpingo-oophorectomy.
MI = myometrial invasion.
RT = radiation therapy.

Fig. 44-25. Protocol—Surgical stage I endometrial adenocarcinoma. (Reprinted with permission from Piver MS, Hempling RE: A prospective trial of postoperative vaginal radium/cesium for grade 1 to 2 less than 50% myometrial invasion and pelvic radiation for grade 3 or deep myometrial invasion in surgical stage I endometrial adenocarcinoma, *Cancer* 66:1133, 1990.)

Piver,[72] and Boronow[4] has confirmed that deeply invasive or poorly differentiated tumors carry a 25% to 45% risk of paraaortic lymph node metastasis (Table 44-10).

The use of adjuvant teletherapy in surgically staged patients is rarely reported. Piver and Hempling[66] reported 41 patients with stage I disease who demonstrated deep myometrial invasion or grade 3 histology. All underwent paraaortic lymph node dissection, and all had histologically negative nodes. This group was subsequently treated with 5000 to 5040 cGy whole pelvis radiation over 5 to 5½ weeks. The estimated 5-year disease-free survival for this group was 88%. Four recurrences were noted (9.7%), and only one of these (2.4%) was inside the treated field. Four significant complications were reported (9.7%), including three small bowel obstructions and one large bowel obstruction. Although these results are gratifying, the finding of distant metastasis in the face of tumoricidal pelvic radiotherapy and histologically negative paraaortic lymph nodes is of concern and may lend some support to

the contention that other routes of metastasis, principally vascular, may play a role in the spread of disease.

Treatment recommendations. Based on the findings cited above, the treatment recommendations for patients with stage I adenocarcinoma of the endometrium are outlined in the algorithm depicted in Fig. 44-25. All patients should undergo exploratory laparotomy, peritoneal cytologic sampling, total abdominal hysterectomy, and bilateral salpingo-oophorectomy. Frozen section evaluation of the specimen should be carried out to determine tumor grade and depth of invasion. Patients who demonstrate grade 3 differentiation or deep myometrial invasion (greater than 50%) should undergo paraaortic lymph node dissection. Patients who demonstrate grade 1 or 2 tumors with superficial (less than 50%) myometrial invasion should receive postoperative brachytherapy by vaginal cylinder. Such an application should deliver 5000 to 6000 cGy to the vaginal mucosa and 3000 cGy to a depth of 0.5 cm. Patients who demonstrate poorly differentiated or deeply invasive tumors with histologically negative paraaortic lymph nodes should undergo 5040 cGy whole pelvic radiation delivered in 5 to 5½ weeks.

Stage II disease

Although extensive research has permitted the development of a rational and effective treatment plan for patients with stage I endometrial cancer, the same cannot be said for patients with stage II (cervical stromal involvement) disease. This finding is due to the small number of cases, staging errors, and an incomplete knowledge of the surgicopathologic spread pattern of disease, vis-a-vis pelvic and paraaortic lymph nodes.

Five-year survival for patients treated with combined radiation therapy and surgery varies between 59.5% and 85%.* Patients treated with radiotherapy alone demonstrate survivals ranging between 42% and 77%. Most radiotherapy regimens for stage II adenocarcinoma of the endometrium are very similar to those employed for treating cervical cancer. These involve the administration of preoperative brachytherapy and teletherapy, but vary widely from institution to institution. The choice of the optimal treatment regimen, therefore, becomes difficult. It would appear that combined therapy (radiation plus surgery) offers some advantage over radiation alone. Because total abdominal hysterectomy and bilateral salpingo-oophorectomy followed by radiation therapy do not appear to compromise survival, surgical staging for patients with endocervical involvement followed by radiotherapy is recommended. In the absence of paraaortic lymph node metastasis, 5040 cGy whole pelvis radiation should improve survival over hysterectomy alone.

Stage III disease

Stage III endometrial cancer encompasses a wide variety of pathologic findings and accounts for about 10% of all cases. Although survival for patients with parametrial extension, vaginal or nodal metastasis remains poor, patients with isolated adnexal metastasis or those in whom all disease is removed and adjuvant radiotherapy is administered appeared to enjoy improved survival. Again, however, it must be recalled that these studies are relatively small and suffer from a lack of complete surgical staging as well as a lack of uniformity in treatment modality.

Although the overall survival for stage III endometrial cancer approximates 30%, the range is wide and depends on the site of metastasis as well as the extent of surgery. Bruckman,[8] Mackillop,[50] and Genest[25] reported small series of patients in whom isolated adnexal metastasis was treated with complete resection and adjuvant whole pelvic radiation. Five-year survivals between 70% and 82.3% were reported, and the majority of failures occurred outside the treated field. In contrast, patients who demonstrated parametrial extension, vaginal metastasis, or multiple intraperitoneal masses did not fare nearly so well.

*References 3, 7, 9, 20, 29, 30, 41, 43, 44, 58, 59, 80, 86.

Among such patients treated with radiation therapy alone or radiation therapy in combination with surgery in which all disease was not removed, 5-year survival ranged between 8% and 40% with the majority of studies reporting survivals that approximate 12%.

Ideally, if patients are discovered to have extrauterine disease at the time of initial surgery, a complete staging procedure should be performed. Adjuvant therapy should be tailored to pathologic findings. In the absence of extrapelvic disease, whole pelvis radiation should prove efficacious. Extended field radiation for paraaortic lymph node involvement should be given strong consideration when such lymph nodes demonstrate microscopic metastasis.

Medically inoperable patients

The 5-year survival for patients whose medical condition precludes surgery and who are treated by radiation only is decreased by 20% to 30% (Table 44-11). In light of the fact that depth of invasion, cervical involvement, or adnexal metastasis cannot be determined, all such patients should be treated with 5040 cGy whole pelvic radiation plus intracavitary brachytherapy.

OVARIAN CANCER

The mainstay of therapy for patients with ovarian cancer, regardless of its origin, remains surgical. Adjuvant therapy, when indicated, has centered around cisplatin-based chemotherapy protocols. Nevertheless, two modalities, intraperitoneal radioactive colloids and pelvic and whole abdominal radiotherapy, have been used in the treatment of this disease.

Radiocolloids

Ovarian malignancy, particularly cancers of epithelial origin, which comprise some 80% of all ovarian cancers,

Table 44-11. Five-year survival after radiation therapy alone for stage I and II endometrial adenocarcinoma

Study	No.	Stage	5-Year survival (%)
Roswell Park	285	I	63
University of Maryland	42	I	72
		II	40
Tufts-New England	50	I	78*
		II	
University of Michigan	64	I	65
		II	
MD Anderson	124	IA	75†
		IB	71†
		II	59†
University of North Carolina	73	I	57‡
		II	26‡

*Three-year actuarial.
†Estimated.
‡Disease-free.
Reprinted with permission from Piver MS, editor: *Manual of gynecologic oncology/gynecology*, p 97, Boston, 1989, Little, Brown.

remains confined, for the majority of its course, to the peritoneal cavity. Accordingly, the use of a therapeutic modality that delivers tumoricidal radiotherapy to this area with minimal side effects is particularly appealing. Suspensions of radiocolloids offer such a modality.

Whereas earlier workers reported the use of intraperitoneal radioactive colloidal gold for the treatment of various malignancies, radiocolloidal phosphorus is now the most widely used agent. The popularity of ^{32}P is the result of several advantages it offers over gold. These advantages are outlined in Table 44-12.

Physical properties of ^{32}P (Table 44-13). Commercially available chromic phosphate is a colloidal suspension in a solution of 30% glucose and 2% benzyl alcohol. It is made by neutron bombardment of $_{16}S^{32}$, which forms $_{16}S^{33}$, which then decays to ^{32}P. The fact that neutron bombardment is required adds an extra step to the process; this makes ^{32}P more expensive than ^{198}Au.

The radiation emitted by ^{32}P is in the form of electrons. The nucleus of this atom acts as a negatron (electron) emitter. The decay process results in the formation of sulfur and a beta particle with an energy emission up to 1.7 meV. The average energy of the electrons is 0.69 meV. The beta particle interacts with other subatomic particles primarily by the Compton effect. As the particle slows, the amount of energy increases dramatically and, eventually, the beta particle comes to rest by entering an atomic orbit.

In theory, the administration of 15 mCi of ^{32}P to the peritoneal cavity delivers 5000 cGy to a depth dose of 3 to 4 mm with tumoricidal effects. Nevertheless, this dose has been arrived at empirically and its distribution (dosimetry) has never been actually calculated.

Catheter placement and pretherapy evaluation of distribution. A polyethylene or Silastic catheter may be left in the peritoneal cavity at the time of surgery. If not placed at that time, then approximately 1 week postoperatively a 14-gauge intravenous catheter is inserted into the peritoneal cavity under local anesthesia. Even distribution of fluid may be ensured by either instillation or water-soluble contrast and conventional x-ray (peritoneogram) or by the use of scanning with ^{99m}Tc. The primary contraindica-tion to the administration of intraperitoneal therapy would be the presence of adhesions that preclude adequate distribution of the isotope. Such an uneven distribution results not only in suboptimally treated areas of the peritoneal cavity, but an increase in complications.

Rosenshein et al,[78] using female adult rhesus monkeys, demonstrated that the use of small volumes of fluid to instill radioactive isotopes into the peritoneal cavity resulted in an inadequate distribution. Accordingly, the use of large volumes of fluid is essential to ensure even distribution and to take advantage of the "peritoneal circulation" in aiding the distribution of ^{32}P throughout the peritoneal cavity.

Approximately 1000 ml of normal saline are injected into the peritoneal cavity followed by a bolus injection of 15 mCi of ^{32}P. An additional 60 ml of saline are injected intraperitoneally to clear the injection material of residual radiocolloid. The injection site is secured with a suture to prevent leakage.

The patient is turned every 15 minutes for approximately 2 hours in five different positions: head down supine, right side, prone, left side, head elevated. To evaluate the distribution of ^{32}P, an abdominal scan is performed 24 hours after administration. Although ^{32}P is a beta emitter, bremsstrahlung x-rays (less than 1% of total energy) are emitted and allow for the production of adequate scans. Although the risk of complication associated with the administration of ^{32}P is small, it can be associated with significant life-threatening gastrointestinal complications if given concomitantly with pelvic radiotherapy.

Radiocolloids in early staged ovarian cancer

Before the advent of surgical staging in ovarian cancer, three small series reported an overall survival of 92.7% using intraperitoneal ^{32}P in presumed stage I ovarian cancer patients.[12,34,65] Subsequently, Piver[75] reported 25 evaluable patients with FIGO stage I ovarian cancer treated with adjuvant intraperitoneal ^{32}P. All patients had undergone total abdominal hysterectomy with (28%) or without (72%) omentectomy. Patients were restaged by laparoscopy with inspection of the diaphragm, abdomen, and pel-

Table 44-12. Comparison of ^{198}Au and ^{32}P

	Gold	Chromic Phosphate
	^{198}Au	$Cr^{32}P^4O$
Physical characteristic	Colloid	Suspension
Emission	Beta 90%	Beta 100%
	Gamma 10%	
Energy (kV)	1700	960
Half-life (days)	2.7	14.5
Usual dose (MiC)	150	10-20

Reprinted with permission from Buchsbaum HJ, Keetel WC, Latovrette HB: Radioisotopes as adjunct therapy of localized ovarian cancer, *Semin Oncol* 2:248, 1975.

Table 44-13. Physical properties—^{32}P

Chemistry	Colloidal Suspension
pH	3-5
Particle size	0.5-1.5 μm
Physical half-life	14.3 days
Average beta energy	.69 meV
Maximum beta energy	1.7 meV
Average tissue range	1.4 to 3 mm
Maximum tissue range	8 mm
Color	Blue-green

Reprinted with permission from Rosenshein et al: Radiocolloids in the treatment of ovarian cancer, *Obstet Gynecol Surv* 34:713, 1979.

vis, biopsies of suspicious lesions, and peritoneal cytology. The estimated 5-year recurrence-free rate was 84%, but was only 75% at 10 years.

Most recently, Young et al[91] reported the results of a randomized trial of patients with early ovarian cancer who underwent surgical staging. These stage I grade 3, stage Iaii, stage Ibii, stage Ic, IIa, b, and c patients received either adjuvant chemotherapy with melphalan or adjuvant intraperitoneal ^{32}P at a dose of 15 mCi. With a median follow-up of 6 years, the 5-year disease-free rate for each arm was identical at 80%.

Several studies have been reported in which ^{32}P has been used as adjuvant therapy for patients with minimal residual disease at second-look surgery or as consolidation therapy for those with negative restaging operations.[10,82,83] Varia et al[87] reported on 43 patients who were treated after negative second-look operation with 15 mCi of intraperitoneal ^{32}P. The 4-year disease-free survival for this group after second-look operation was 89%. Fifteen patients with no evidence of disease at second-look received no further therapy. The 4-year post-second look disease-free survival for the latter group was 67%. These differences were hopeful but failed to achieve statistical significance. The same study also reported the use of intraperitoneal ^{32}P in patients with minimal residual disease at second-look operation. Among 29 such patients, 7 were treated with ^{32}P only, 10 were treated with ^{32}P plus adjuvant chemotherapy, and 12 were treated with chemotherapy alone. The 4-year survival for those who received ^{32}P was 59% as opposed to 22% for those who did not. Again, these data failed to achieve statistical significance but were indicative of some benefit. A prospective study evaluating the efficacy of intraperitoneal ^{32}P as consolidation after chemotherapy or for patients with minimal residual disease is ongoing.

Whole abdominal radiation

Whole abdominal radiation has been employed at several institutions as adjuvant therapy for patients with epithelial ovarian cancers. When whole abdominal radiation is used, only 2250 to 3000 cGy can be delivered to the whole abdomen and 4500 to 5000 cGy can be delivered to the pelvis. These doses represent the maximum doses tolerated by intraperitoneal structures. Fletcher[23] has demonstrated that a dose of at least 5000 cGy of external therapy is needed to cure 90% of subclinical disease.

In hopes of overcoming this difficulty, workers at the MD Anderson Hospital developed the moving strip technique for delivering radiation to the peritoneal cavity.[16] Small areas (2.5-cm strips at a time) are radiated over a shorter period to lessen intestinal reaction and obtain a larger biologic effect. Each 2.5-cm strip is radiated anteriorly and posteriorly for a total dose of about 2250 to 2500 cGy in eight treatments over 10 calendar days. Open field techniques, also used in delivering whole abdominal radiation, deliver comparable doses over 8 weeks. In a randomized trial comparing moving strip to open field techniques

in patients with ovarian cancer, Dembo et al[19] were unable to demonstrate a clear advantage for either technique. A significant increase in bowel complications, however, was reported among those treated with moving strip techniques.

The efficacy of whole abdominal radiation in the treatment of epithelial ovarian cancer remains controversial. Dembo[18] reported a 73% disease-free survival among 79 patients with stage I disease who were treated with whole abdominal radiation. The advent of surgical staging has demonstrated, however, that not all patients with stage I ovarian cancer are in need of adjuvant therapy. Furthermore, excellent survival in those patients at risk for recurrence can be achieved with adjuvant chemotherapy, obviating the risk of complication with whole abdominal radiation.

Macbeth and co-workers[49] employed whole abdominal radiation techniques described by Dembo et al[19] to deliver 2500 cGy in surgically staged patients. A 5-year estimated disease-free survival of 65% was reported in 28 stage I patients, and a 5-year estimated disease-free survival of 39% was reported in 25 stage II patients. The authors conclude that these data do not seem to support the idea of a curative role for postoperative radiotherapy in such patients.

The efficacy of whole abdominal radiation in patients with advanced disease as compared to multiagent cisplatin-based chemotherapy regimens has not been evaluated.

RADIATION ENHANCEMENT

The ability to generate photons that produce a tumoricidal effect is not a limiting factor in the delivery of efficacious radiotherapy. Indeed, it is the biology of the tumor and the tolerance of normal surrounding tissues that have restricted radiation doses. Accordingly, attempts have been made to enhance the cell-killing ability of ionizing radiation.

Experimental designs to decrease hypoxic areas in tumors by increasing ambient oxygen tension (hyperbaric oxygen)* and techniques to raise the temperature of a tumor or the core temperature of patients (hyperthermia)[42,81] have met with limited success.

The nitroimidazoles have been explored as hypoxic cell sensitizers. Theoretically, these compounds mimic the effect of oxygen in tumors by forming free radicals and have the advantage of not being as rapidly metabolized as oxygen. Among the nitroimidazoles, the compound most extensively studied is misonidazole. Three randomized trials carried out in patients with stage IIb through IVa cervical cancer have not demonstrated a statistically significant benefit to the use of the drug.[22,45,56]

Hydroxyurea is an S-phase cell cycle specific inhibitor of DNA synthesis (inhibits ribonucleotide reductase) that reportedly acts as a radiation potentiator by three separate mechanisms:

*References 5, 21, 24, 28, 38, 89, 90.

1. Destroying cells in the relatively radioresistant S phase of the cell cycle.
2. Collecting the surviving cells at the G_1/S interphase, a relatively radiosensitive portion of the cell cycle.
3. Inhibiting the repair of tumor cells that have suffered only sublethal damage as a result of prior radiation and that are capable of repair if uninhibited by the continued presence of hydroxyurea after the completion of radiation therapy.

Seven prospective randomized trials and one nonrandomized trial have been conducted using hydroxyurea in locally advanced cervical cancer. Piver et al[67,71,74] performed six prospective trials—five randomized trials comparing hydroxyurea and radiation to placebo and radiation and one nonrandomized trial using hydroxyurea and radiation. In addition, the Gynecologic Oncology Group (GOG)[67,71,74] reported two prospective trials—one comparing hydroxyurea and radiation to placebo and radiation and one comparing hydroxyurea and radiation to misonidazole and radiation (Table 44-14).

Hreshchyshyn et al[36] reported on 104 stage IIIb and IVa, clinically staged patients who had significantly improved progression-free survival when treated with hydroxyurea plus radiation therapy compared to placebo plus radiation therapy ($p < 0.05$). Stehman et al[83a] (GOG) compared hydroxyurea as the standard to misonidazole in a group of 296 surgically staged patients with stage IIb, III, and IVa cervical cancer. Hydroxyurea and misonidazole were administered twice weekly during external radiotherapy only. Patients received a median of 5 days of hydroxyurea (1 to 8) and a median of 5 days of misonidazole (1 to 10) and did not receive either after completing external radiation. The median progression-free survival was 43 months for hydroxyurea and 40 months for misonidazole.

In studies by Piver et al,[67–71,74] patients received hydroxyurea or placebo during radiation for a total of 28 courses of hydroxyurea or placebo over 12 weeks. The last 4 to 5 weeks' doses of hydroxyurea or placebo were administered after the completion of radiotherapy. This administration is based on the mechanism of action of hy-

Table 44-14. Randomized hydroxyurea trials in cervical cancer

Author	No. of Patients	Stage	Staging	Drug therapy	Control	Survival
Hreshchyshyn et al (GOG)	104	IIIb, IVa	Clinical	HU: 80 mg/kg every 3 days	Placebo	Median 14 months (HU) versus 8 months (placebo) ($p < 0.05$)
Stehman et al (GOG)	296	IIb, III, IVa	Surgical	Miso: 1 g/m^2 twice weekly	HU: 80 mg/kg twice weekly	Median 43 months (HU) versus 40 months (miso) ($p = 0.08$)
Piver et al	37	IIb, IIIb	Clinical	HU: 80 mg/kg every 3 days	Placebo	2 yr PFS HU: 67% Placebo: 32% ($p < 0.0014$)
Piver et al	130	IIb, IIIb	Surgical (66 pts.) Clinical (64 pts.)	HU: 80 mg/kg every 3 days	Placebo	2 yr stage IIb HU: 74% Placebo: 44% ($p = 0.01$) Stage IIIb HU: 52% Placebo: 33% ($p = 0.22$)
Piver et al	40	IIb	Surgical	80 mg/kg every 3 days	Placebo	5 yr actuarial survival: HU: 94% Placebo: 53% ($p = 0.006$)
Piver et al	45	IIIb	Surgical	HU: 80 mg/kg every 3 days	Placebo	5 yr PFS HU: 91% Placebo: 60% (continuous radiation therapy) ($p < 0.06$)
Piver et al	25	IIIb	Clinical	HU: 80 mg/kg every 3 days	Placebo	5 yr actuarial survival: HU: 54% Placebo: 18%

HU: hydroxyurea; miso: misonidazole; PFS: progression-free survival.
Reprinted with permission from Piver MS, Hempling R, and Craig KA: *Neoplasms of the cervix.* In Bast RC, editor: *Cancer medicine 1992,* in press.

droxyurea, which prevents repair of sublethally damaged cells. In the first of these trials in which clinically staged IIb and IIIb cervical cancer patients were treated, the 2-year progression-free survival rate was 67% for hydroxyurea and 32% for placebo ($p < 0.001$). In the next trial, the same group combined clinically and surgically staged patients. The 2-year survival rate was 74% for stage IIB patients treated with radiotherapy plus hydroxyurea and 44% for those treated with radiotherapy plus placebo ($p < 0.01$). A trend toward improvement was noted in stage IIIB patients (52% for hydroxyurea and 33% for placebo). In the subsequent trial of surgically staged IIB patients, the 5-year actuarial survival for hydroxyurea was 94% compared to 53% for placebo ($p < 0.06$). For surgically staged IIIB patients who received continuous pelvic radiation (rather than split course), the 5-year actuarial survival was 91% for hydroxyurea and 60% for placebo. The 5-year actuarial survival was 54% for hydroxyurea and 18% for placebo among stage IIIB cervical cancer patients who were not candidates for, or who refused, surgical staging. In a nonrandomized trial of stage IIB patients in which no evidence of paraaortic lymph node metastasis could be demonstrated by pretherapy lymphangiography rather than paraaortic lymphadenectomy and all patients received pelvic radiotherapy plus hydroxyurea, the 5-year actuarial survival rate was 92%.

In a review of concomitant chemotherapy and radiation therapy in patients with solid tumors, Vokes and Weichselbaum concluded that "while each of these studies (above quoted studies) by itself is open to some criticism, taken as an entity, they do suggest a role for hydroxyurea with radiotherapy as standard therapy for patients with cervix cancer."[88]

NEW RADIATION TECHNIQUES

In addition to modalities that sensitize cells to standard photon therapy, those that produce ionizing radiation less dependent on oxygen for its effect have been explored. Among these techniques are those that employ fast neutrons. Studies have demonstrated that these nuclear particles offer several theoretical advantages over standard photon radiation, including diminished dependency on oxygen, an effect in relatively radioresistant phases of the cell cycle, and a diminished capacity for cells exposed to fast neutrons to repair sublethal damage.

Among the three studies[54,55,64] that have evaluated the use of neutron teletherapy in patients with advanced cervical cancer, a slight advantage was observed in patients treated with mixed beam (neutrons plus photons) therapy in terms of local control. However, no advantage in complication rate or survival was reported.

Californium 252 serves as a source of fast neutrons employed in brachytherapy. Small clinical trials have attempted to explore its use in patients with far advanced cervical cancer. However, patient compliance and small numbers have precluded deriving meaningful conclusions from these studies.[53,54]

INTRAOPERATIVE RADIOTHERAPY

The use of intraoperative radiotherapy dates back at least to the 1930s when it was described in patients with incompletely resected bladder cancers.[11] Research in Japan in the mid 1960s demonstrated that delivery of 2000 to 4000 cGy of teletherapy as a single intraoperative dose was biologically as effective as 6000 cGy given over 5 to 6 weeks.[1]

Electron beam generators deliver electron energy over well-defined fields and shallow depths. This technique is particularly appealing in treating patients with gynecologic malignancy in the pelvis who have suffered metastasis to the paraaortic lymph nodes. Intraoperative radiotherapy, if effective, would obviate the morbidity of extended field radiotherapy.

Physically, the technique involves the isolation of the area to be treated with packs and thin lead shielding followed by the delivery of approximately 2000 cGy using 6-meV electrons delivered over several minutes.

Goldson et al[26] and Delgado et al[17] have reported on two small series of patients with paraaortic lymph node metastasis treated with intraoperative radiotherapy. The results of these studies were disappointing. Of 11 patients with positive paraaortic nodes, 7 died of disease. However, the sites of failure were unspecified and may represent persistence outside the treated field. No complications directly attributable to the technique were reported.

PHOTODYNAMIC THERAPY

Photodynamic action is a biologic process in which the combined effects of visible light, a photosensitizing substance, and oxygen produce cellular destruction. The photosensitizing material, hematoporphyrin derivative (HPD), is injected intravenously 24 to 48 hours before therapy and localizes preferentially in skin, muscle, and neoplastic tissues. The exposure of sensitized tissue to light of 630-nm wavelengths produces a cytotoxic effect. Monochromatic red light generated by a laser is the most frequently employed source.

The putative mechanism of action of photodynamic therapy is the generation of molecular oxygen from the light-sensitizing material and subsequent cellular destruction primarily at the cell membrane. The primary side effect of photodynamic therapy is sensitivity to light. This effect lasts for approximately 4 weeks. Prior cytotoxic therapy with ionizing radiation or drugs has not proved to be a contraindication to the employment of photodynamic therapy.

Several researchers have used photodynamic therapy in gynecologic malignancies with some success. Four of seven sites of local recurrence of endometrial and cervical cancers treated by Rettenmaier et al[76] responded to therapy. One was a complete response. Lobracio et al[48] treated 45 sites in seven patients and demonstrated a 76% complete response rate and an 18% partial response rate.

Recently, researchers at the Roswell Park Cancer Institute reported their experience with the use of photodynamic therapy among 21 patients with recurrent gynecologic cancers.[46] Seven patients with cutaneous lesions were complete responders, and four patients with cervical or vaginal recurrence also responded. Of the four vaginal/cervical responders, two were complete responders and remained disease free at 40+ and 58+ months after therapy. The use of photodynamic therapy in patients with intraperitoneal malignancy is under study, and preliminary findings are encouraging.

REFERENCES

1. Abe M, Takahisi M: Intraoperative radiotherapy; the Japanese experience, *Int J Radiat Oncol Biol Phys* 7:863, 1981.
2. Boronow RC: Combined therapy as an alternative to exenteration for locally advanced vulvovaginal cancer, *Cancer,* 49:1085, 1982.
3. Boronow RC: Advances in diagnosis, staging, and management of cervical and endometrial cancer stages I and II, *Cancer* 65:648, 1990.
4. Boronow RC et al: Surgical staging in endometrial cancer: clinical-pathologic findings of a prospective study, *Obstet Gynecol* 63:825, 1984.
5. Brady LW et al. Hyperbaric oxygen for carcinoma of the cervix stages IIB, IIIA, IIIB, IVA—Results of a randomized study by the Radiation Therapy Oncology Group, *Int J Radiat Oncol Biol Phys* 7:991, 1981.
6. Brown GR, Fletcher GH, Rutledge FN: Irradiation of in situ and invasive squamous cell carcinoma of the vagina, *Cancer* 28:1278, 1971.
7. Bruckman JE et al: Combined irradiation and surgery in the treatment of stage II carcinoma of the endometrium, *Cancer* 42:1146, 1978.
8. Bruckman JE et al: Stage III adenocarcinoma of the endometrium: two prognostic groups, *Gynecol Oncol* 9:12, 1980.
9. Burman ML et al: Risk factors and prognosis in stage II endometrial cancer, *Gynecol Oncol* 14:49, 1982.
10. Carlson JA et al: Hexamethylmelamine, methotrexate and 5-fluorouracil (HMF) for progression of ovarian carcinoma during therapy with cisplatin, cyclophosphamide ± doxorubicin, *Gynecol Oncol* 22:189, 1985.
11. Chaoul H: Weiter Beitrag zur Rontgennahbestrahlung des Karzinomas, Strahlentherapie 50:446, 1934.
12. Clark DG et al: The role of radiation therapy (including isotopes) in the treatment of cancer of the ovary. Results of 614 patients treated at Memorial Hospital in New York, NY, *Prog Clin Cancer* 5:227, 1973.
13. Cleaves M: Radium therapy, *Med Rec NY* 64:601, 1903.
14. Creasman WT et al: Adenocarcinoma of the endometrium: its metastatic lymph node potential, *Gynecol Oncol* 4:239, 1976.
15. Curry SL, Wharton JT, Rutledge F: Positive lymph nodes in vulvar squamous carcinoma, *Gynecol Oncol* 9:63, 1980.
15a. Dancuarte F et al: Primary squamous cell carcinoma of the vagina treated by radiotherapy: a failure analysis. The MD Anderson Hospital experience 1955-1982, *Int J Radiat Oncol Biol Phys* 14:745-769, 1988.
16. Delclos L, Quinlan EJ: Malignant tumors of the ovary managed with postoperative megavoltage radiotherapy, *Radiology* 93:659, 1969.
17. Delgado G et al: Intraoperative radiation in the treatment of advanced cervical cancer, *Obstet Gynecol* 63:246, 1984.
18. Dembo AJ: Abdominal radiotherapy in ovarian cancer. Ten year experience, *Cancer* 55:2285, 1985.
19. Dembo AJ et al: A randomized clinical trial of moving strip versus open field whole abdominal radiation in patients with invasive epithelial cancer of the ovary, *Proc Am Soc Clin Oncol* 2:146, 1983.
20. DePalo G et al: A retrospective analysis of 53 patients with pathologic stage II and III endometrial carcinoma, *Tumori* 68:341, 1982.
21. Dische S: The hyperbaric oxygen chamber in the radiotherapy of carcinoma of the uterine cervix, *Br J Radiol* 47:99, 1974.
22. Dische S: *Clinical trials with hypoxic cell sensitizers—The European experience.* In Mirand EA, Hutchinson WB, Mihich E, editors: *13th International Cancer Congress. Part D. Research and treatment,* 1983, Alan R Liss, New York.
23. Fletcher GH: Clinical dose-response curves of human malignant epithelial tumors, *Br J Radiol* 46:1–12, 1973.
24. Fletcher GH et al: Hyperbaric oxygen as a radiotherapeutic adjuvant in advanced cancer of the uterine cervix. Presented at the American Radium Society, May 1975, *Cancer* 39:617, 1977.
25. Genest P et al: Stage III carcinoma of the endometrium. A review of 41 cases, *Gynecol Oncol* 26:77, 1987.
26. Goldson AL et al: Intraoperative radiation of the paraaortic lymph nodes in cancer of the uterine cervix, *Obstet Gynecol* 52(6):713, 1978.
27. Graham J: The value of preoperative and postoperative treatment by radium for carcinoma of the uterine body, *Surg Gynecol Obstet* 132:855, 1971.
28. Gray LA et al: The concentration of oxygen dissolved in the tissues at the time of irradiation as a factor in radiotherapy, *Br J Radiol* 26:638, 1953.
29. Greenberg SB et al: Management of carcinoma of the uterus stage II, *Cancer Clin Trials* 4:183, 1981.
30. Grigsby PW et al: Stage II carcinoma of the endometrium: results of therapy and prognostic factors, *Int J Radiat Oncol Biol Phys* 11:1915, 1985.
31. Hacker NF et al: Management of regional lymph nodes and their prognostic influence in vulvar cancer, *Obstet Gynecol* 61:408, 1983.
32. Hacker NF et al: Preoperative radiation for locally advanced vulvar cancer, *Cancer* 54:2056, 1984.
33. Herbst AL, Green TH, Ulfelder H: Primary carcinoma of the vagina. An analysis of 68 cases, *Am J Obstet Gynecol* 106:210, 1970.
34. Hester LL, White L: Radioactive colloidal chromic phosphate in the treatment of ovarian malignancies, *Am J Obstet Gynecol* 103:911, 1969.
35. Homesley HD et al: Radiation therapy versus pelvic node resection for carcinoma of the vulva with positive groin nodes, *Obstet Gynecol* 68:733, 1986.
36. Hreshchyshyn MM et al: Hydroxyurea or placebo combined with radiation to treat stages IIIB and IVA cervical cancer confined to the pelvis, *Int J Radiat Oncol Biol Phys* 5:317, 1979.
37. Iverson T: Irradiation and bleomycin in the treatment of inoperative vulvar carcinoma, *Acta Obstet Gynecol Scand* 61:195, 1982.
38. Johnson RJR, Walton RJ: Sequential study on the effect of the addition of hyperbaric oxygen on the five year survival rates of carcinoma of the cervix treated with conventional fractional radiation, *Am J Roentgenol* 120:111, 1974.
39. Kalra JK et al: Preoperative chemoradiotherapy for carcinoma of the vulva, *Gynecol Oncol* 12:256, 1981.
40. Kelly J: Malignant diseases of the vulva, *J Obstet Gynecol Br Commonw* 79:265, 1972.
41. Kinsella TJ et al: Stage II endometrial carcinoma: 10 year follow-up of combined radiation and surgical treatment, *Gynecol Oncol* 10:290, 1980.
42. Kong JS et al: *Hyperthermia in the treatment of gynecologic cancers.* In Rutledge FN, Freeman RS, Gershenson DM, editors: *Gynecologic cancer diagnosis and treatment strategies,* Austin, 1987, University of Texas Press.
43. Landgren RC et al: Irradiation of endometrial cancer in patients with medical contraindications to surgery or with unresectable lesions, *Am J Roentgenol* 126:148, 1976.
44. Larson DM et al: Stage II endometrial carcinoma: results and complications of a combined radiotherapeutic-surgical approach, *Cancer* 61:1528, 1988.
45. Leibel S et al: Radiotherapy with or without misonidazole for patients with stage IIIB or IVA squamous carcinoma of the uterine cervix: a Radiation Therapy Oncology Group randomized trial, Abstract No 94, *Int J Radiat Oncol Biol Phys* 11:1439, 1985.

46. Lele SB et al: Photodynamic therapy in gynecologic malignancies, *Gynecol Oncol* 34:350, 1989.

47. Lewis BU, Stallworthy JA, Cowdell R: Adenocarcinoma of the body of the uterus, *J Obstet Gynecol Br Commonw* 77:343, 1970.

48. Lobraico RV et al: Photodynamic therapy for cancer of the lower female genital tract, *Colposc Gynecol Laser Surg* 2:185, 1986.

49. Macbeth PR, MacDonald H, Williams CJ: Total abdominal and pelvic radiotherapy in the management of early stage ovarian carcinoma, *Int J Radiat Oncol Biol Phys* 15:353, 1988.

50. Mackillop WJ, Pringle JF: Stage III endometrial cancer: a review of 90 cases, *Cancer* 56:2519, 1985.

50a. Malfetana JH, Piver MS, Tsukada Y: Stage III and IV carcinoma of the vulva, *Gynecol Oncol* 23:192, 1986.

51. Marchetti D et al: Prevention of vaginal recurrence of stage I endometrial adenocarcinoma with postoperative vaginal radiation, *Obstet Gynecol* 67:399, 1986.

52. Maruyama Y: CF-252 neutron brachytherapy. An advance for bulky localized cancer therapy, *Nucl Sci Appl* 1:677, 1984.

53. Maruyama Y et al: Feasibility study of californium 252 for the therapy of stage IV cervical cancer, *Cancer* 61:2448, 1988.

54. Morales P et al: Preliminary report of the MD Anderson Hospital randomized trial of neutron and photon irradiation for locally advanced carcinoma of the uterine cervix, *Int J Radiat Oncol Biol Phys* 7:1533, 1981.

55. Morita S et al: Clinical experience of fast neutron therapy for carcinoma of the cervix, *Int J Radiat Oncol Biol Phys* 11:1439, 1985.

56. MRC Working Party on Misonidazole for Cancer of the Cervix: The Medical Research Council trial of misonidazole in carcinoma of the uterine cervix, *Br J Radiol* 57:491, 1984.

57. Ng AB, Reagan JW: Incidence and prognosis of endometrial carcinoma by histologic grade and extent, *Obstet Gynecol* 35:437, 1970.

58. Nori D et al: Combined surgery and radiation in endometrial carcinoma: an analysis of prognostic factors, *Int J Radiat Oncol Biol Phys* 13:489, 1987.

59. Onsrud M et al: Endometrial carcinoma with cervical involvement (stage II) prognostic factors and value of combined radiological-surgical treatment, *Gynecol Oncol* 13:76, 1982.

60. Perez CA, Camel HM: Long term follow-up of radiation therapy of carcinoma of the vagina, *Cancer* 49:1308, 1982.

61. Perez CA, Kobra A, Subhash S: Dosimetric considerations in irradiation of carcinoma of the vagina, *Int J Radiat Oncol Biol Phys* 3:639, 1977.

62. Perez CA, Thomas PRM: *Radiation therapy: basic concepts and clinical implications.* In Sutow WW, Fernbach DJ, and Vietti TJ, editors: *Clinical pediatric oncology,* 3, St Louis, 1984, Mosby–Year Book.

63. Perez CA et al: Definitive irradiation in carcinoma of the vagina: long term evaluation of results, *Int J Radiat Oncol Biol Phys* 15:1283, 1988.

64. Peters LJ et al: *Second preliminary report of the MD Anderson study of neutron therapy for locally advanced gynecologic tumors.* In Barendsen GW, Broerse JT, Breur K, editors: *High-LET radiation in clinical radiotherapy,* Proceedings of the 3rd Meeting on Fundamental and Practical Aspects of the Application of Fast Neutrons and Other High LET Particles in Clinical Radiotherapy, The Hague, The Netherlands, September 13–15, 1978, Eur J Cancer Suppl 3:15, 1979.

65. Piver MS: Radioactive colloids in the treatment of stage IA ovarian cancer, *Obstet Gynecol* 40:42, 1972.

66. Piver MS, Hempling RE: A prospective trial of postoperative vaginal radium/cesium for grade 1-2 less than 50% myometrial invasion and pelvic radiation therapy for grade 3 or deep myometrial invasion in surgical stage I endometrial adenocarcinoma, *Cancer* 66:1133, 1990.

67. Piver MS, Khalil M, Emrich LJ: Hydroxyurea plus pelvic radiation versus placebo plus irradiation in non-surgically staged stage IIIB cervical cancer, *J Surg Oncol* 42:120, 1989.

68. Piver MS, Krishnamsetty RM, Emrich LJ: Survival of non-surgically staged patients with negative lymphangiograms who had stage IIB carcinoma of the cervix treated by pelvic radiation plus hydroxyurea, *Am J Obstet Gynecol* 151:1006, 1985.

69. Piver MS, Vongtama V, Emrich LJ: Hydroxyurea plus pelvic radiation versus placebo plus radiation in surgically staged IIIB cervical cancer, *J Surg Oncol* 35:129, 1987.

70. Piver MS et al: Hydroxyurea and radiation therapy in advanced cervical cancer, *Am J Obstet Gynecol* 120:969, 1974.

71. Piver MS et al: Hydroxyurea as a radiation sensitizer in women with carcinoma of the uterine cervix, *Am J Obstet Gynecol* 129:379, 1977.

72. Piver MS: Paraaortic node biopsy in staging women with cervical ovarian and endometrial carcinoma: a review, *J Surg Oncol* 12:365, 1979.

73. Piver MS et al: A prospective trial of comparing hysterectomy, hysterectomy plus vaginal radium and uterine radium plus hysterectomy in stage I endometrial carcinoma, *Obstet Gynecol* 54:85, 1979.

74. Piver MS et al: Hydroxyurea: a radiation potentiator in carcinoma of the uterine cervix, *Am J Obstet Gynecol* 147:803, 1983.

75. Piver MS et al: Five and ten year estimated survival and disease free survival rates after intraperitoneal chromic phosphate; Stage I ovarian adenocarcinoma, *Am J Clin Oncol* 11:515, 1988.

76. Rettenmaier MA et al: Photoradiation therapy of gynecologic malignancies, *Gynecol Oncol* 17:200, 1984.

77. Roentgen WC: On a new kind of rays (preliminary communication). Translation of a paper before Physikalische-Medicinischen Gesellschaft of Wurzburg on 12/28/85, *Br J Radiol* 4:32, 1931.

78. Rosenshein N et al: The effect of volume on the distribution of substances into the peritoneal cavity, *Gynecol Oncol* 6:106, 1978.

79. Rotmensch J et al: Preoperative radiotherapy followed by radical vulvectomy with inguinal lymphadenectomy for far advanced vulvar carcinomas, *Gynecol Oncol* 36:181, 1990.

80. Rustowski T, Kupsc W: Factors influencing the results of radiotherapy in cases of inoperable endometrial cancer, *Gynecol Oncol* 14:185, 1982.

81. Scott RS et al: Local hyperthermia in combination with definitive radiotherapy: increased tumor clearance, reduced recurrence rate in extended follow-up, *Int J Radiat Oncol Biol Phys* 10:2119, 1984.

82. Smirz LR et al: Second look laparotomy after chemotherapy in the management of ovarian malignancy, *Am J Obstet Gynecol* 152:661, 1985.

83. Soper JT et al: Intraperitoneal chromic phosphate P^{32} as salvage therapy for persistent carcinoma of the ovary after surgical restaging, *Am J Obstet Gynecol* 156:1153, 1987.

83a. Stehman FB et al: A randomized trial of hydroxyurea versus misonidazole adjunct to radiation therapy in carcinoma of the cervix, *Am J Obstet Gynecol* 159:87, 1988.

84. Terasima R, Tolmach LJ: X-ray sensitivity and DNA synthesis in synchronous populations of HeLa cells, *Science* 140:490, 1963.

85. Thomlinson RH, Gray LH: The histological structure of some human lung cancers and the possible implications for radiotherapy, *Br J Cancer,* 9:539, 1955.

86. Trimble EL, Jones HW III: Management of stage II endometrial adenocarcinoma, *Obstet Gynecol* 71:323, 1988.

87. Varia M et al: Intraperitoneal chromic phosphate therapy after second look laparotomy for ovarian cancer, *Cancer* 61:919, 1988.

88. Vokes EE, Weichselbaum RR: Concomitant chemoradiotherapy: rationale and clinical experience in patients with solid tumors, *J Clin Oncol* 8:911, 1990.

89. Watson ER et al: Hyperbaric oxygen and radiotherapy: a medical research clinical trial in carcinoma of the cervix, *Br J Radiol* 51:879, 1978.

90. Watson TA et al: Clinical experience with hyperbaric oxygen in radiotherapy, *J Can Assoc Radiol* 20:132, 1969.

91. Young RC et al: Adjuvant therapy in stage I and II epithelial ovarian cancer: results of two prospective randomized trials, *N Engl J Med* 322:1021, 1990.

Part VI

OPERATIONS FOR RESTORATION OF FERTILITY

Chapter 45

LAPAROSCOPY

Dan C. Martin

Laparoscopy is useful for diagnosis and treatment of infertility patients. The diversity of uses is reflected in the many names applied to this technique; operative laparoscopy,[30,62,67] therapeutic laparoscopy,[57] pelviscopy,[89] videolaseroscopy[69] and laser laparoscopy[54] are but a few of the names applied. Although a distinction is often made between diagnostic and therapeutic procedures, there is therapeutic benefit to having a proper diagnosis.

Published material on diagnostic and sterilization aspects of laparoscopy include the techniques, complications, and avoidance of complications.* This chapter does not cover sterilizations but covers complications as they pertain to the material of this chapter.

TISSUE EFFECTS

An important concept is the tissue effect produced by the various types of equipment. Three terms are generally used to describe these effects: coagulation, vaporization, and excision.[30,62,63] Coagulation is a term whose meaning encompasses heating, desiccation, cautery, denaturation, and tissue death. This is generally the result of heat produced by conversion of laser light to heat, conversion of electricity to heat, conduction of heat from a heat probe, and conduction of heat from the heated tissue. Vaporization is produced by high-power density energy laser or electricity.[60,61] The power density must be above a vaporization threshold so that there is instantaneous conversion of tissue water into a vapor. Excision is performed with various types of equipment. At the most basic form, scissors are used to excise the tissue and hemostasis is obtained with coagulation. Although more precise dissections have been accomplished with the CO_2 laser, this level of precision may not be biologically important in the long-term care of the patient.

*References 6, 14, 44, 77, 78, 92, and see Chapter 39.

EQUIPMENT

Equipment is generally broken into four categories: mechanical, electrosurgical, thermal, and laser. Although each of these technologies has its own originating proponents, most of them use multiple modalities in an attempt to individualize the approach to the problem. Coagulators and mechanical devices appear to be the most useful for hemostasis and are easy to use, whereas lasers appear to add more precision.

Mechanical instruments

The basic mechanical instruments for all endoscopic procedures are atraumatic blunt probes, irrigators, aspirators, scissors, and graspers. The probes used to manipulate and push equipment are smooth so as to avoid inadvertently pulling tissue into the hinges of grasping forceps or scissors. These generally have centimeter markings for measuring structures in the pelvis and may be roughened or blackened for use with lasers. A hinge is at about 2 cm from the end so that the probe can be angled. This angling increases the ability to manipulate structures and to measure tissue tangential to the viewing angle.

Irrigation and aspiration systems change constantly. High-pressure irrigation systems may be needed for dissection techniques. Nezhat[70] has used this type of dissection to place water barriers between targeted endometriosis and the underlying structures. Reich[81,82] has used these techniques to dissect organs.

In addition to specifically designed systems, standard blood pressure cuffs can be used to pressurize irrigation solution. Straight suction to the wall can be used. When the aspiration system is also used for laser plume, protective filters are placed in the line to prevent the hydrocarbons in the plume from depositing in the wall pipes. If this material accumulates in the pipes, these can occlude and require major repair.

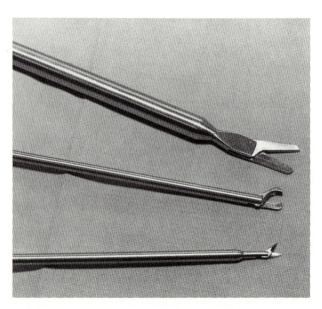

Fig. 45-1. Scissors range from microscissors with delicate tips to heavy scissors designed to go through an 11-mm trocar.

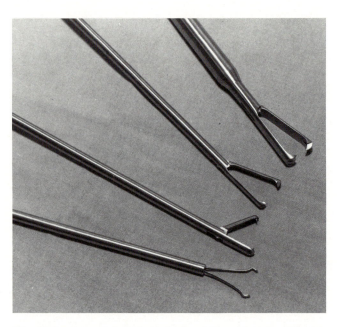

Fig. 45-2. Graspers have been designed for work on various pelvic organs.

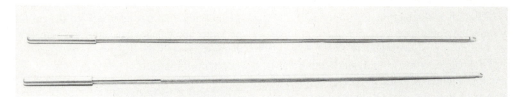

Fig. 45-3. Suturing technique can be aided by extracorporeal ties with the knot pushed by ligating devices such as the Clarke-Reich ligators (Marlow Surgical Technologies, Inc.).

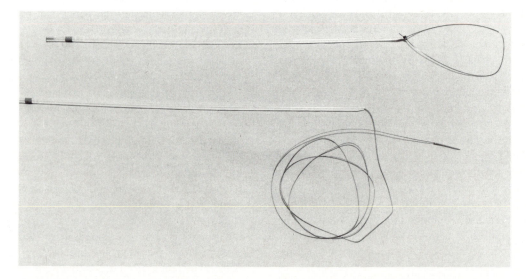

Fig. 45-4. Endoloops and Endoknots (Ethicon, Inc.) have been very easy to place and use at laparoscopy.

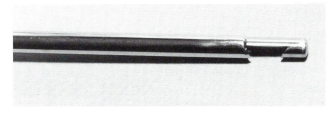

Fig. 45-5. The tissue morcellator (WISAP, Inc.) is used to remove large fragments of tissue by slowly fragmenting the tissue using the jaws and loading it into the barrel of the morcellator.

Scissors and grasping forceps are made in sizes designed for procedures from delicate lysis of peritubal adhesions to gross morcellation of large tissue. Although one set of scissors and graspers may be used for all procedures, a combination of two or more sizes appears more useful (Figs. 45-1 and 45-2).

The development of suturing techniques and loops by Clarke[10] (Marlow Surgical Technologies) and the subsequent adaptation of the Roeder loop by Semm[90] preceded the development of other mechanical occlusive devices (Figs. 45-3 and 45-4). Semm subsequently developed a series of instruments, such as morcellators, to fragment and remove large tissue masses (Fig. 45-5). Although gut was the only suture available for some time, a large line of sutures is now available including Vicryl and PDS (Ethicon, Inc.). The ability to tie and place knots is a useful skill.[53] In addition, small and modified needles have been developed for ease in placement at laparoscopy (Ethicon, Inc.; Fig. 45-6). Dissolvable clips are in development (Fig. 45-7), and a gastrointestinal anastomosis (GIA) stapling device (U.S. Surgical Corporation; Fig. 45-8) has been used for a laparoscopically assisted vaginal hysterectomy.[71] Other GIA devices have been used for laparoscopic appendectomy, laparoscopic bowel resection, and thoracoscopic segmental pneumonectomy.

Transabdominal suturing of the specimen may be helpful in holding specimens toward the anterior wall for better visualization. A 3-0 Vicryl suture (Ethicon, Inc.) on a Keith needle is passed into the abdomen, being careful to avoid vessels. The end is held out of the abdomen. This is used to suture the specimen, and the needle is reversed and pushed out of the abdomen and cut off. The tension on the sutures is controlled by clamping the two free ends at the abdominal surface. The suture is pulled through at the end of the case.

Biopsy forceps are available that produce small areas of tissue for analysis. However, excision and excisional biopsies have been more accurate in diagnosis.[65,66]

Rectal, vaginal, and other probes are used to mobilize the various areas of the pelvis. A sponge on ring forceps for the vagina, an 81 Fr rectal probe, and a no. 4 Sim's blunt curette have been suggested.[82]

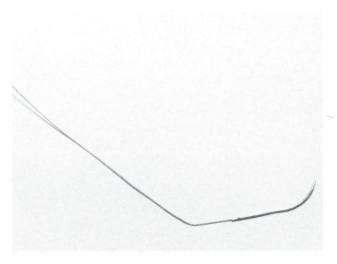

Fig. 45-6. Sutures specifically designed for use at laparoscopy are available. The skislope needle (Ethicon Inc.) is designed so that the straight portion can be grasped with the laparoscopic needle holder while maintaining a curved tip.

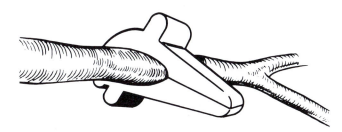

Fig. 45-7. Polydioxanon absorbable clips (Ethicon, Inc.) can be used by surgeons who wish to avoid permanent devices.

Electrosurgical equipment

Electrosurgical equipment includes unipolar (Fig. 45-9) and bipolar (Fig. 45-10) modes of delivery.[45,84] For both of these, the tissue effect is produced by converting electrical energy into heat. At low power, this desiccates, denatures, coagulates, and destroys tissue while leaving it in place. This is generally referred to as coagulation. If the current is continued until the tissue is sufficiently heated, thermal spread by conduction occurs and the instrument acts like a cautery tip. Coagulation and cautery are the general effects of bipolar electrosurgical units. Most hospitals have bipolar electrosurgical units designed for sterilization; newer units have smaller jaws for more precise use (Fig. 45-11). Sterilization units are broad and have a wider area than the smaller bipolar units developed for operative procedures.

The wave form has a significant influence on the tissue effect. If the peak power and the delivery unit are constant, a damped wave form has less electrical driving force and appears better for coagulation. On the other hand, an undamped wave form has more electrical driving force and is better for vaporization (cutting) or fulguration. Although these concepts are useful for unipolar units, they do not always apply to bipolar units. A bipolar system generally works better with an undamped driving wave form to ensure rapid and adequate coagulation of the tissue between the jaws.[45,84]

Unipolar delivery can be of low or high power. At low power, these unipolar units behave in a fashion similar to bipolar coagulation but with penetration determined by the amount of energy delivered. This is different from bipolar coagulation in which the energy transfer is between the jaws of the coagulator.[45] On the other hand, at high power, the electrosurgical units are capable of vaporization of tissue in a fashion very similar to that of lasers. At power densities of approximately 60,000 W/cm^2, the ther-

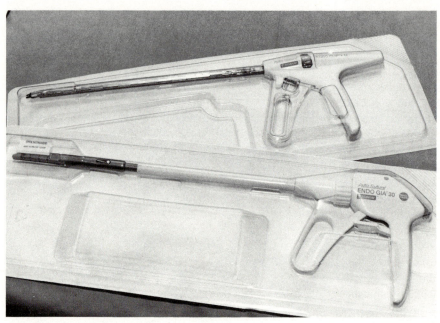

Fig. 45-8. A complete line of Endo GIA and Endo Clip (US Surgical) instruments has been designed to aid in the removal of larger structures.

Fig. 45-9. Unipolar techniques use a single pole instrument with the action at the interaction level of a grounded patient. At high-power density, this produces vaporization, and, at low-power density, this produces coagulation.

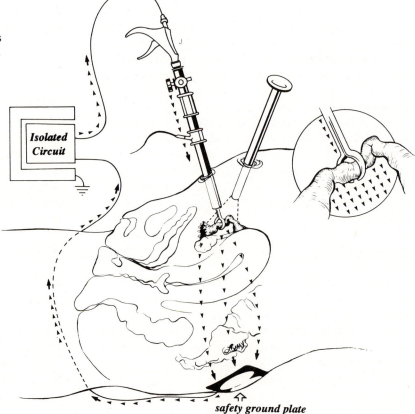

safety ground plate

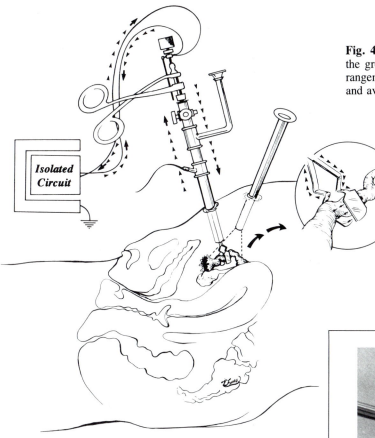

Fig. 45-10. Bipolar coagulation places both the active pole and the grounding pole on the same piece of equipment. In this arrangement, electrical flow is between the poles of the equipment and avoids deeper electrical damage to the patient.

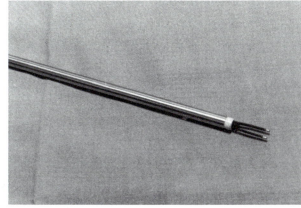

Fig. 45-11. Small bipolar electrical tips are available for discrete bipolar coagulation (WISAP, Inc.).

mal damage from an electrosurgical unit approximates that of a CO_2 laser unit.[48,49,60,61]

Dangers of electrosurgical burn. There is concern about the danger of any equipment. Unipolar electrosurgery burns have been attributed to the equipment itself and to misuse by surgeons.[4,46,92,102] In six cases, deep and extensive bowel burns were possibly related to electrical sparking,[102] but the same areas of the bowel were banded with the Falope ring when this equipment was used to replace electrosurgery.[40] In addition, of the 11 cases reported by Thompson and Wheeless, one was recognized as traumatic and five were direct bowel burns recognized at the time of surgery. The remaining five may have been from the needle, the trocar, direct contact, or sparking.[96] Borten states that the blind spot in single puncture technique may be responsible for unseen accidents.[6] All equipment can be dangerous when used in an unsafe fashion; unipolar electrosurgery is safe when used in an appropriate fashion.

One of the most difficult parts about diagnosing these burns is that they may not be seen when they occur. This is similar to cutting the bowel with scissors or lasers when doing adhesiolysis. Laparotomy may be necessary to determine if the bowel has actually been cut with scissors. Determining whether a burn has resulted from electrosurgery can be more difficult because the exact extent of burn

may not show up until after necrosis has taken place.[102] A patient who has progressive abdominal pain, distention, and peritoneal signs should be evaluated for the possibility of bowel perforation. This is true for all trocar insertion techniques and all types of equipment. Bowel perforation has been noted with all equipment and techniques.

The majority of such complications at laparoscopy appear clustered in the early learning experience. This increase in the early phase of learning techniques has been documented by American Association of Gynecologic Laparoscopists (AAGL) safety surveys[76] and, more recently, by the Southern Surgeons Club (SSC) in studying cholecystectomy.[93] The AAGL showed the highest incidence in the first 25 cases with a significant decline after the first 250 cases. The SSC study demonstrated that 71% of their bile duct injuries occurred in the first 13 cases. This resulted in an overall incidence of 2.2% in the first 13 cases and 0.1% thereafter.

Endocoagulation

Endocoagulation (Fig. 45-12) is one of the hallmarks of pelviscopy[90] and is used to avoid electrosurgery and the potential for electrosurgical burns. Although it is possible to produce a thermal burn inadvertently, this should be a rare clinical occurrence due to the slow mechanism of action when compared with electrosurgical or laser techniques. Although thermal units have grasping forceps, which would imply spread from both grasping jaws, the equipment frequently produces a thermal effect from one jaw only. This is used to great advantage with the thermal wedge (Fig. 45-13). This wedge can be placed behind myomas to coagulate the vessels before shelling the myomas out of the uterus. On the other hand, thermal coagulation is a slow technique that can increase the operating time. In addition, coagulation distorts tissue and may obscure disease and result in incomplete treatment.

Lasers

The four lasers (Fig. 45-14) most commonly used in gynecology are the carbon dioxide (CO_2), argon, potassium-tantinyl-phosphate (KTP), and neodymium: yttrium-aluminum-garnet (Nd:YAG).[32,63] The CO_2 laser produces the most predictable effect. In addition, nontouch techniques and avoiding blind spots with single puncture make this a very useful and safe laser. However, mirror alignment and smoke plume can be difficult to control. This is the most commonly used laser for both external and internal gynecologic use.

Although the thermal damage from a CO_2 laser can be limited to 100 to 500 μm, this is adequate for hemostasis in most infertility surgery. Although the fine coagulation line created with this laser is helpful in identifying tissue planes, coagulation and occlusive devices are needed for some vessels.

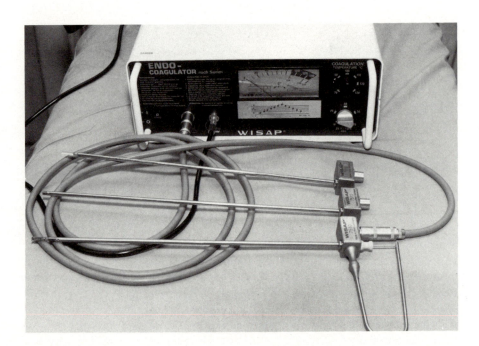

Fig. 45-12. The Endocoagulor (WISAP, Inc.) developed by Semm is a hallmark of pelviscopy.

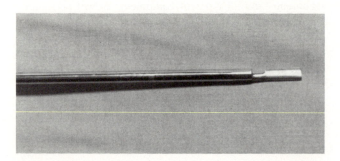

Fig. 45-13. The myoma enucleator is used to provide hemostasis at the depth of a myoma even when this cannot be seen during surgery. This helps avoid inappropriate tearing and hemorrhage from vessels coagulating them before they are seen.

Laser wavelengths		
Carbon dioxide	Infrared	10,600 nm
Nd:YAG	Infrared	1,064 nm
Helium neon	Red	632 nm
KTP	Green	532 nm
Argon	Green	515 nm
	Blue	488 nm
KrCl Excimer	Ultraviolet	222 nm

Fig. 45-14. The lasers used in gynecology are the argon with a wavelength of 488 to 514 nm, the KTP with a wavelength of 532 nm, the Nd:YAG with a wavelength of 1064 nm and the carbon dioxide with a wavelength of 10,600 nm.

Argon, KTP, and Nd:YAG lasers can be directed down quartz fibers. These lasers have a greater intrinsic depth of penetration than the CO_2 laser; the Nd:YAG laser has the greatest penetration. However, this depth of penetration is most apparent at the low-power densities used for coagulation. On the other hand, high-power densities are created with small fibers and artificial tips. These higher power densities are associated with decreased thermal coagulation. Very small tips and high-power density can create a thermal coagulation zone similar to that of the CO_2 laser.[36,37,91]

Like any equipment or technique that is closely monitored, lasers have been associated with complications. These include hypothermia, emphysema, hemorrhage, transfusion, laparotomy, colostomy, urinary leak, and death.[62] The rate of these appears to be less than occurs at laparotomy. Furthermore, many of these occurred in the initial learning phase as was discussed for bowel burns earlier in this chapter.

One logistical problem that arises with the use of lasers is the variation in electrical and water requirements. Different types of equipment require a range of 110 to 240 V, 5 to 50 A, and up to 4 gal/min of water at 60 psi.[8] The specific requirements must be known before setting up a laser in an operating room. The specific equipment requirements for water and for 220-V single phase current may require changes in many operating rooms.

ENDOMETRIOSIS

The approach to endometriosis depends on the indications for surgery. When the primary indication for the surgery is infertility with little pain or tenderness, intentionally limiting therapy may be associated with fewer adhesions and improved pregnancy rates when compared to extensive dissection and suturing.[26,57] This may be accomplished as readily with coagulation as with vaporization. On the other hand, focal tenderness frequently persists after coagulation or superficial vaporization. For these lesions, deep vaporization or excision (Fig. 45-15) is more likely to result in relief of pain and tenderness.*

*References 13, 17, 56, 57, 62, 64.

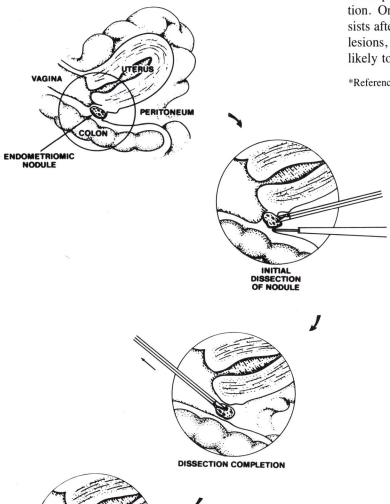

Fig. 45-15. Peritoneal nodules require dissection and careful palpation for removal. These may include full thickness resection to the vagina.

Although it is frequently difficult to distinguish superficial disease from deep disease, the white fibrotic scarring of deep infiltration more commonly causes tissues distortion (Fig. 45-16). At the same time, this white infiltrating lesion can be more difficult to distinguish from the underlying tissue, particularly when it is in the area of the uterosacral or other ligaments. Superficial lesions generally move without resulting in motion of the underlying tissue whereas the entire area appears to move when there is deep infiltration. These superficial lesions are generally

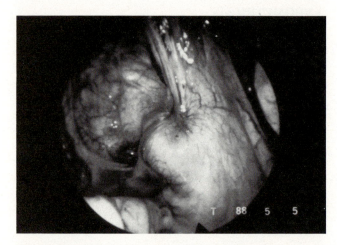

Fig. 45-16. Fibrotic infiltration of the peritoneum and bowel causes distortion. This picture is an example of deep involvement of the rectosigmoid with the rectosigmoid pulled up into the right uterosacral ligament. With this level of distortion, lesions are most commonly full thickness through the muscularis. See Color Plate 8, facing p. 754.

easily destroyed with either coagulation or superficial vaporization. From the studies on the depth of penetration,[13,56,64] it is extrapolated that 70% to 85% of all lesions first diagnosed at laparoscopy can be adequately treated with techniques designed for surface lesions.[57]

An additional 5% to 10% of lesions are too deep for surface coagulation but can be vaporized or excised at laparoscopy. Excision can be performed with scissors, high-power density unipolar electrosurgery, or laser. An additional advantage to excision is that tissue diagnosis is more commonly obtained.

However, some lesions of endometriosis are more palpable than visible. This includes retroperitoneal lesions (Fig. 45-17) as well as deep bowel involvement (Fig. 45-16). Although many of these are palpable at preoperative office examination, they can be missed at laparoscopy and found only on careful palpation at laparotomy. This type of lesion appears to be present in 5% to 15% of patients.[13,57,64]

Deep involvement is of greatest concern around the ureters, bladder, and bowel. Although lesions on the surface of any of these can be vaporized or coagulated, deep involvement into the muscularis may not be noted except at laparotomy. For these lesions, an initial attempt is made to lift the serosa or peritoneum away from the organ. When these can be lifted off and loose connective tissue is noted, complete dissection is feasible. However, when the organ does not push away easily, deep infiltration is suspected and this type of dissection is avoided unless the patient is ready for bowel resection, ureteral reimplantation, or bladder repair.

Fig. 45-17. This schematic diagram shows infiltrating endometriosis in the rectovaginal septum extending from the peritoneum. When a dissection plane can be found between the lesion and the sigmoid colon, these can be performed by a combined laparoscopic and vaginal approach. If there is muscularis involvement in the bowel, a surgeon familiar with deep rectal anastomosis and surgery is needed.

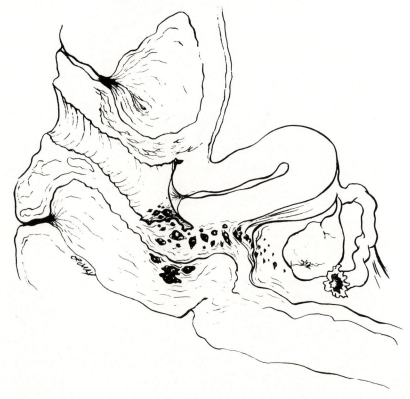

The pregnancy rate for a collective series of 754 patients was 68%.[57] This was relatively independent of stage with 65% pregnancy in severe and extensive disease and 74% in minimal and mild disease. These results followed CO_2 laser laparoscopy. When these studies were analyzed by life table analysis, the success rates were the same as or greater than those from previous laparotomy series.[1,69,74] Many of the patients with deep lesions or bowel lesions had superficial treatment of deep disease. This suggests that intentionally limiting therapy may be advantageous in correcting infertility. However, complete excision appears needed when a patient experiences pelvic pain and tenderness.

CHOCOLATE CYSTS OF THE OVARY

Chocolate cysts of the ovary can be endometrioma, residual of a hemorrhagic corpus luteum, or nonspecific on histology. When these are opened and examined, the general appearance of an endometrioma is a mottled lining with red or brown areas on a white fibrotic base. Corpus lutea tend to have a smoother, more uniformly brown or yellow-brown lining. Biopsies for confirmation of endometriosis are best taken from the red streaks of tissue coming off the base. Biopsies of the brown areas frequently show hemosiderin resulting from either old corpus lutea or endometriomas. The chance that a biopsy will miss a cancer is small,[75] but the consequences are significant.[52,86] Preoperative sonography and serologic markers may aid in clinical decisions regarding specific patients.[28,87]

Stripping techniques can be used to remove the entire capsule for complete histologic analysis. However, these stripping techniques are more difficult and may not be more effective for endometriosis than biopsy followed by coagulation. In addition, stripping removes not only the pseudocapsule but also a thin rim of healthy ovary immediately adjacent to the capsule. With large endometriomas, this small rim may have adequate volume to compromise the overall function of the ovary.

Chocolate cysts of less than 5 mm have little or no fibrotic reaction and tend to be irregular in their infiltration (Fig. 45-18). These are generally biopsied and then coagulated or vaporized. When cysts measure from 5 to 20 mm, various techniques are used, determined by the appearance as the procedure progresses. When the cysts are greater than 2 cm, the fibrotic reaction is prominent and stripping of the pseudocapsule is accomplished in a slow fashion. Stripping also removes a rim of healthy ovary (Fig. 45-19). Two grasping forceps are usually all that is needed. However, as the cysts exceed 4 cm, a third grasping forcep or a transabdominal suture to hold the tissue to the anterior abdominal wall frequently increases visualization.

As the stripping approaches the hilum, special attention and care are taken to avoid the hilar vessels. When stripping is difficult in this area, the capsule is generally amputated above the hilar vessels and the remnant base is coagulated. When these cysts have been greater than 5 cm, laparoscopies have taken up to 5 hours.[57,62] Treating these large chocolate cysts by biopsy and coagulation followed by examinations and sonograms may help preserve healthy ovarian tissue. However, this increases the risk of missing an ovarian cancer.[75]

In the management of these chocolate cysts, an incision is made at the most dependent portion so that the walls tend to collapse back together at the end of the procedure. Sutures are generally avoided because suturing techniques have been shown to increase adhesions in both peritoneum[23-25,73] and in ovaries.* Furthermore, the highest pregnancy rate reported with ovarian cystectomy at laparoscopy was 92% by Reich[83] when no other factors were present. This is similar to Martin's report of an 80% pregnancy rate after treatment of severe endometriosis using laser and no sutures.[55] When ovarian suturing is needed, laparotomy with true intracapsular closure is preferred.[11,12] The use of fibrin glue has been suggested to avoid the ischemic sequelae of suturing.[2,21] This glue is not yet commercially available in the United States.

*References 3, 9, 16, 18, 59, 79.

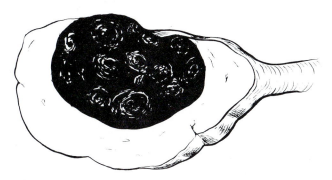

Fig. 45-19. When endometriomas exceed 2 cm, they are more likely to be flattened and have a regular round configuration. Old blood and debris are inside of these. There is a thin lining at the inner wall, which may have glands and stroma, a nonspecific hemosiderin containing lining, or a nonspecific flat lining. When these are greater than 2 cm, the glands and stroma have not infiltrated more than 1.5 mm into the fibrotic capsule. On the outside of the fibrotic capsule is a rim of healthy ovary which is removed in the process of stripping the ovaries.

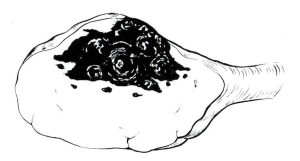

Fig. 45-18. Small ovarian endometriomas of up to 20 mm may be irregular in their infiltration and frequently have little or no fibrotic reaction.

OTHER CYSTS

In treating cysts, the chance of opening an ovarian cancer is of major concern.[52,75,86] Preoperative assessment by ultrasonography,[28] magnetic resonance imaging[88] or tumor markers such as CA-125, α-fetoprotein, and human chorionic gonadotropin (HCG)[87] may be useful.

Oophorectomy may be more reasonable than ovarian cystectomy.[38] If a dermoid is spilled while doing a cystectomy, the patient and table must be reversed to put the head in an up position to keep the fluid in the pelvis. The pelvic volume is approximately 20 to 80 ml, and spill into the upper abdomen can occur rapidly with irrigation.[59]

ADHESIONS
Adhesion prevention

Laparoscopic techniques result in fewer new adhesions than laparotomy techniques.[20,50,51] In addition, many studies have suggested or denied that multiple agents help in adhesions prevention. Of the agents suggested, two are FDA approved: Interceed (TC7) (Johnson & Johnson)[19] and Gore-Tex (WL Gore and Associates).[7] The advantage of Interceed is that it can be cut into small pieces and laid into the pelvis through a laparoscope. Gore-Tex requires suturing and is not absorbable, and, when used in infertility patients, a second operation is required for removal to allow egg transit. Comparative studies between Interceed and Gore-Tex are needed.

Needle and trocar insertion

In treating patients with known pelvic or abdominal adhesions, the insertion techniques are very important.[33,35,39,41] Increased preparation of the patient for the possibility of bowel damage includes informed consent and bowel prep. Although minilaparotomy, open trocar insertion, and safety trocars have proponents who claim a

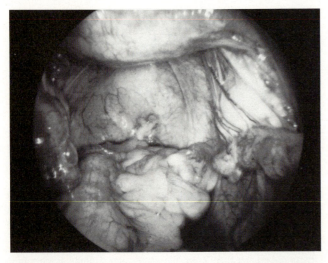

Fig. 45-20. Filmy adhesions are easy to lyse with any equipment. Blunt lysis is avoided because this increases bleeding and petechial hemorrhage. See Color Plate 9, facing p. 755.

decreased chance of complications, this has not been the general observation in clinical use. One specific advantage of these techniques is that, if the bowel is entered, it will be noted as the front wall is opened. When closed techniques are used, it is possible to penetrate both the front and back wall of bowel.

Techniques of insertion include percussing the gas in the stomach with use of nasogastric tubes for decompression when needed, percussing liver dullness, using intraabdominal negative pressure to pull saline through the hub, and injecting 10 ml of saline through the needle followed by aspiration to check for contents.

Before surgery, informed consent and preparation for patients with histories of pelvic and abdominal adhesions and previous abdominal surgery must include the possibility of laparotomy for bowel repair. Many general surgeons consider bowel prep to be essential in these patients.

Filmy adhesions

Filmy adhesions (Fig. 45-20) can be lysed using several techniques.* Although blunt dissection and lysis has been renounced, there is worry that the abraded surfaces with their oozing and biochemical activity may adhere more readily than surfaces that are cleanly cut and hemostatic. Data suggest that adhesions are more common with ischemic tissue than dead tissue.[23-25,62]

Scissors and coagulation are very useful for upper abdominal incisions from the omentum and epiploic fat to the anterior abdominal wall. These are progressively cut, and coagulation is used when bleeding occurs. Many of these adhesions are avascular. A significant area of concern is that the adhesions that are seen through the laparoscope can sometimes hide bowel on the other side. Care is taken to identify both sides of the adhesions when possible. This sometimes includes placing the laparoscope through a lower port to get a view from the other side. Furthermore, while trying to avoid bowel, dissections have been kept so far anterior that the bladder has been entered. This has required minilaparotomy, repair of the bladder, and indwelling catheterization.

Lasers and electrosurgery can be used to cut the adhesions under direct visualization. The electrosurgical knife and fiber-equipped lasers disperse rapidly in space and need no backstop. On the other hand, the CO_2 laser will continue in space until tissue is hit. This can be dangerous, or it can be used to advantage by using the adherent tissue as its own backstop. A pulsed CO_2 laser technique is sometimes helpful in controlling this possibility.

Dense adhesions

Dense adhesions are more difficult to control with scissors and coagulation, and there is an increased chance that bowel is hidden in these. Slow dissection with electrosurgical knife or with lasers is generally performed.[15,72,95]

*References 30, 62, 67, 70, 95.

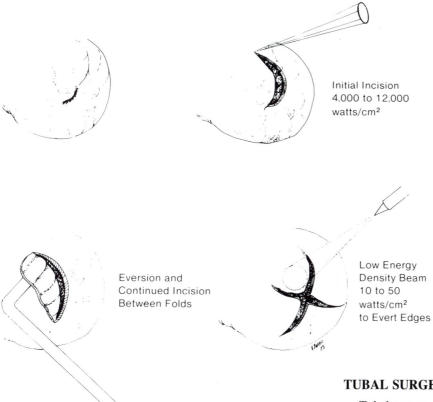

Initial Incision
4,000 to 12,000
watts/cm²

Eversion and
Continued Incision
Between Folds

Low Energy
Density Beam
10 to 50
watts/cm²
to Evert Edges

Fig. 45-21. A cuff salpingostomy can be performed with several types of equipment. The Bruhat technique using a carbon dioxide laser is performed by making an incision into the tube at high-power density (>4000 W/cm²) and then coagulating the serosal surface to turn back the tube using low-power density beam (<50 W/cm²).

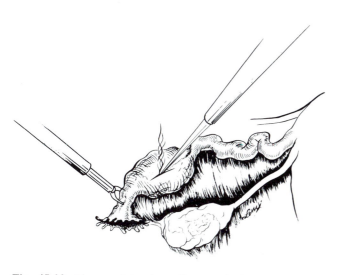

Fig. 45-22. Linear salpingotomy for an ectopic pregnancy can be performed with a laser, unipolar cautery, or scissors. Pitressin injection is used to decrease bleeding, and bipolar coagulation may be helpful in obtaining hemostasis.

TUBAL SURGERY

Tubal surgery at laparoscopy includes adhesiolysis, cuff salpingostomy for hydrosalpinx (Fig. 45-21), salpingotomy for tubal gestation, and anastomosis.[98] Laparoscopic results have generally been compatible with microsurgical results. However, these have not been corrected for stage for adequate comparison. Boer-Meisel noted significant differences in term and ectopic pregnancy rates in the various stages. She reported a 59% term rate, 18% abortion rate, and 4% ectopic rate in class I tubes as opposed to a 3% term pregnancy rate and 16% tubal pregnancy rate in class III tubes. The largest group in her series was a class II tube that had a 17% term pregnancy rate, a 5% abortion rate, and a 27% tubal pregnancy rate.[5]

Laparoscopic techniques have included the use of scissors to open up the tube followed by coagulation of any bleeders.[31] Other surgeons use a Bruhat or modified Bruhat procedure.[62] This includes opening the tube along radial scarred lines in the tube. A probe inside the tube helps in the identification of the folds and can serve as a backstop for the CO_2 laser when used. The tube is opened using high-power density laser or electrosurgical techniques. This is turned back using a defocused technique of the laser with low-power density or by using a coagulator as a heat source. This can be accomplished by coagulating saline in the jaws and keeping those near the serosa of the tube. However, direct application of electrical current to the serosa of the tube can coagulate the deep vasculature and destroy the tube. If electrosurgery is used, care is taken to avoid excess tubal damage.

Ectopic pregnancies are treated at laparoscopy just as they are treated at laparotomy. Linear salpingostomy[97] (Fig. 45-22) is used in patients who want to preserve fertility. Vasopressin can be injected along the antimesenteric border of the tube to aid in hemostasis. A dilute solution of 1 mU Pitressin (0.1 ml of a 10-mU ampule) in 50 ml of normal saline can be used. This is injected using a spinal needle placed directly through the abdominal wall. After the antimesenteric incision is made, the products of conception are removed from the tube. These may spontaneously extrude but more often require general teasing of the trophoblastic tissue from the bed. When multiple clots are in the tube, the distal and proximal margins of the incision are closely observed to ensure that the trophoblastic tissue is not at the margin and hidden by the clots. Sutures do not appear to be beneficial.[99] Persistent ectopic pregnancy has been a problem in 5% of patients treated by this technique.[68,80] All patients having conservative surgery should undergo follow-up HCG titers to ensure that these are declining. Depending on the speed of decline, these titers can be anywhere from every 3 days to every 2 weeks. It is not uncommon for the titers to be positive for up to 24 days.[97]

Salpingectomy is a technically easier procedure and is useful in patients who do not desire to preserve fertility and in patients who have significant tubal damage from rupture.[100] This technique can be performed using bipolar coagulation for hemostasis and scissors for the excision, and loops for hemostasis followed by excision or other devices such as the GIA. In all of these techniques, the tube is removed intact through a minilaparotomy or colpotomy incision. Morcellating the tube may fragment and spread the ectopic, resulting in persistence.

Laparoscopic techniques have also been adequate for the care of both unruptured[34] and ruptured[85] interstitial pregnancies. With experience, indications for laparoscopic surgery increase and the contraindications are few and resolve around hemodynamic status of the patient, the medical status of the patient, and the surgical history. Patients who are hemodynamically unstable, who have a history of diaphragmatic hernia, or who have known extensive pelvic adhesions appear to be best treated at laparotomy.

The results of anastomosis have generally been poor with a few tubal pregnancies and very uncommon intrauterine pregnancies. True microsurgical anastomosis at laparotomy or minilaparotomy is still preferable. Minilaparotomy microsurgical anastomoses are performed on an outpatient basis at several centers.

STEIN-LEVENTHAL SYNDROME

Stein-Leventhal syndrome has been treated at laparoscopy by microcyst puncture, biopsy of the multiple microcystic areas, furrowing of the ovary, and true wedge resection.* The change in hormones after this shows a decrease in testosterone and luteinizing hormone.[3,94] Pregnancy rates after this treatment have been from 52% to 57%.[3,16,94]

*References 3, 16, 29, 30, 42, 62, 67, 94.

LAPAROSCOPIC UTERINE NERVE ABLATION

The concept of uterine nerve ablation or uterosacral transection was developed at laparotomy by Doyle[22] and adapted to laparoscopy by Feste.[27] Lichten[47] subsequently performed a randomized prospective study showing that 81% of patients had relief at 3 months and 45% had relief at 12 months after this procedure. Lichten renamed this procedure the laparoscopic uterine nerve ablation (LUNA). Although this procedure is advocated by some as a primary therapy for dysmenorrhea, the more common use is as an ancillary procedure at the time of laparoscopy.

However, many surgeons are worried about hemorrhage from the vaginal branch of the uterine artery, ureteral transection, and uterine prolapse as a delayed effect. Bilateral ureteral transection has occurred; care in the area of delicate organs is important.

UTERINE SUSPENSION

Although indications for uterine suspension are hard to define, this can be performed in patients who appear to have symptomatic retroversion or in patients where there is extensive posterior dissection and the surgeon wishes to attempt to keep the uterine fundus out of the pelvis during healing. Simple techniques include placing a loop ligature or a Falope ring around the round ligament to shorten this. Other surgeons have pulled the round ligament directly anterior and tacked this to the fascia. This technique can produce open areas lateral to the suspension and the possibility of internal herniation.

A technique similar to the Gilliam suspension can be performed. Lateral incisions are made, and the external oblique fascia is identified. Pressure is placed to ensure that the site is above the insertion of the round ligament. An Allis clamp is placed through the fascia at this level and worked retroperitoneally down the round ligament under direct visualization through the laparoscope. This is taken one third to one half the length of the round ligament and then pushed through the peritoneum into the peritoneal cavity. The round ligament is grasped at this point and pulled back upon itself to the fascia. Two Tevdek sutures are used to anchor this to the external oblique fascia. This is performed on both sides, and the incision is closed. Because these are outpatient surgeries, a Marcaine and morphine block of this area is generally performed.

MARCAINE-MORPHINE BLOCKS

As outpatient procedures become increasing complex with multiple incisions at laparoscopy and with minilaparotomy being used, deadening of incisional pain increases the ability of postoperative patients to be comfortable at home. A solution of 2 mg of morphine in 10 ml of 0.25% Marcaine is injected into the incision. The total amount used is generally 2 to 6 mg in 10 to 30 ml. This is very similar to the Marcaine blocks used by anesthesiologists in long-term pain therapy.[58]

ECONOMIC IMPACT

Levine has documented a savings of $1007 to $1581 when laparoscopy was used instead of laparotomy for removal of adnexa, lysis of adhesions, fulguration of endometriosis, and salpingostomy. He reported an average reduction of 49% in overall hospital costs. In addition, he pointed out that women who normally waited 4 to 6 weeks to return to full activity were fully recovered at 7 to 10 days.[43]

One other area of concern and cost is the increased use of disposable equipment. Although it may be argued that it is economical to replace permanent equipment with disposables, until this happens, hospitals will still place both the permanent and disposable equipment on the table. The net effect at cholecystectomy is an increase of $425 when compared to nondisposable equipment. When this was added to the use of a laser, and the routine use of cholangiography, there was an increase of $1271 per case when compared with using electrosurgery, permanent sutures, and selective cholangiography.[101]

CONCLUSION

Bipolar coagulators, unipolar electrosurgery, thermal cautery, and lasers can be used to coagulate, vaporize, or excise tissue. Combining these techniques is better than concentrating on any one of them. Changes in the use of this equipment have been very rapid; attending update courses appears essential to develop and maintain optimal techniques.

REFERENCES

1. Adamson GD, Lu J, Subak LL: Laparoscopic CO_2 laser vaporization of endometriosis compared with traditional treatments, *Fertil Steril* 50:704, 1988.
2. Adamyan LV, Myinbayev OA, Kulakov VI: Use of fibrin glue in obstetrics and gynecology: a review of the literature, *Int J Fertil* 36:76, 1991.
3. Armar NA et al: Laparoscopic ovarian diathermy in the management of anovulatory infertility in women with polycystic ovaries: endocrine changes and clinical outcome, *Fertil Steril* 53:45, 1990.
4. Baumann H, Jaeger P, Huch A: Ureteral injury after laparoscopic tubal sterilization by bipolar electrocoagulation, *Obstet Gynecol* 71:483, 1988.
5. Boer-Meisel ME et al: Predicting the pregnancy outcome in patients treated for hydrosalpinx: a prospective study, *Fertil Steril* 45:23, 1986.
6. Borten M, editor: *Laparoscopic complications*, Philadelphia, 1986, BC Decker.
7. Boyers S, Diamond M, DeCherney A: Reduction of postoperative pelvic adhesions in the rabbit with Gore-Tex surgical membrane, *Fertil Steril* 49:1066, 1988.
8. Boyers SP: Operating room setup and instrumentation, *Clin Obstet Gynecol* 34:373, 1991.
9. Brumsted JR et al: Postoperative adhesion formation after ovarian wedge resection with and without ovarian reconstruction in the rabbit, *Fertil Steril* 53:723, 1990.
10. Clarke HC: Laparoscopy—new instruments for suturing and ligation, *Fertil Steril* 23:274, 1972.
11. Cohen BM: *Surgery of the ovary including anatomic derangements of the fimbrial-gonadal ovum-capture mechanism*. In Hunt RB, editor: *Atlas of female infertility surgery*, Chicago, 1986, Mosby–Year Book.
12. Cook AS, Rock JA: The role of laparoscopy in the treatment of endometriosis, *Fertil Steril* 55:663, 1991.
13. Cornillie FJ et al: Deeply infiltrating pelvic endometriosis: histology and clinical significance, *Fertil Steril* 53:978, 1990.
14. Corson SL, Soderstrom RM, Levy BS: *Emergencies and laparoscopy*. In Martin DC, editor: *Manual of endoscopy*, Santa Fe Springs, 1990, American Association of Gynecologic Laparoscopists.
15. Daniell JF: Laparoscopic enterolysis for chronic abdominal pain, *J Gynecol Surg* 5:61, 1989.
16. Daniell JF, Miller W: Polycystic ovaries treated by laparoscopic laser vaporization, *Fertil Steril* 51:232, 1989.
17. Davis GD, Hruby PH: Transabdominal laser colpotomy, *J Reprod Med* 34:438, 1989.
18. De Leon FD, Edwards M, Heine MW: A comparison of microsurgery and laser surgery for ovarian wedge resections, *Int J Fertil* 35:177, 1990.
19. Diamond MP et al: Adhesion reformation: reduction by the use of Interceed (TC7) plus heparin, *J Gynecol Surg* 7:1, 1991.
20. Diamond MP et al: Postoperative adhesion development after operative laparoscopy: evaluation at early second-look procedures, *Fertil Steril* 55:700, 1991.
21. Donnez J et al: CO_2 laser laparoscopy in peritoneal endometriosis and in ovarian endometrial cyst, *J Gynecol Surg* 5:361, 1989.
22. Doyle JB: Paracervical uterine denervation by transection of the cervical plexus for the relief of dysmenorrhea, *Am J Obstet Gynecol* 70:1, 1955.
23. Elkins TE et al: A histologic evaluation of peritoneal injury and repair: implications for adhesion formation, *Obstet Gynecol* 70:225, 1987.
24. Ellis H: The cause and prevention of postoperative intraperitoneal adhesions, *Surg Gynecol Obstet* 1333:497, 1971.
25. Ellis H: Internal overhealing: the problem of intraperitoneal adhesions, *World J Surg* 4:303, 1980.
26. Fayez JA: An assessment of the role of operative laparoscopy in tuboplasty, *Fertil Steril* 39:476, 1983.
27. Feste JR: Laser laparoscopy: a new modality, *J Reprod Med* 30:413, 1985.
28. Fleischer AC: Transabdominal and transvaginal sonography of ovarian masses, *Clin Obstet Gynecol* 34:433, 1991.
29. Gadir AA et al: Ovarian electrocautery versus human menopausal gonadotrophins and pure follicle-stimulating hormone therapy in the treatment of patients with polycystic ovarian disease, *Clin Endocrinol* 33:585, 1990.
30. Gomel V: Operative laparoscopy: time for acceptance, *Fertil Steril* 52:1, 1989.
31. Gomel V, Urman CB: Laparoscopic surgery, *Curr Opin Obstet Gynecol* 2:303, 1990.
32. Harris DM, Werkhaven JA: Biophysics and applications of medical lasers, *Arch Otolaryngol Head Neck Surg* 3:91, 1989.
33. Hasson HM: *Open techniques for equipment insertion*. In Martin DC, editor: *Manual of endoscopy*, Santa Fe Springs, 1990, American Association of Gynecologic Laparoscopists.
34. Hill GA, Segas JH, Herbert CM: Laparoscopic management of interstitial pregnancy, *J Gynecol Surg* 5:209, 1989.
35. Jarrett JC: Laparoscopy: direct trocar insertion without pneumoperitoneum, *Obstet Gynecol* 75:725, 1990.
36. Joffe SN et al: Resection of the liver with the Nd:YAG laser, *Surg Gynecol Obstet* 163:437, 1986.
37. Joffe SN et al: Splenic resection with the contact Nd:YAG laser system, *J Pediatr Surg* 23:829, 1988.
38. Johns A: Laparoscopic oophorectomy/oophorocystectomy, *Clin Obstet Gynecol* 34:460, 1991.
39. Kaali SG, Bartfai G: Direct insertion of the laparoscopic trocar after an earlier laparotomy, *J Reprod Med* 33:739, 1988.
40. King TM: Personal communication, November 20, 1986.

41. Kleppinger RK: *Closed techniques for equipment insertion.* In Martin DC, editor: *Manual of endoscopy,* Santa Fe Springs, 1990, American Association of Gynecologic Laparoscopists.

42. Kojima E et al: Ovarian wedge resection with contact Nd:YAG laser irradiation used laparoscopically, *J Reprod Med* 34:444, 1989.

43. Levine RL: Economic impact of pelviscopic surgery, *J Reprod Med* 30:655, 1985.

44. Levinson CJ, Wattiez A: *Complications and safety of laparoscopy.* In Martin DC, editor: *Manual of endoscopy,* Santa Fe Springs, 1990, American Association of Gynecologic Laparoscopists.

45. Levy BS, Soderstrom RM: *Electrical techniques of sterilization.* In Martin DC, editor: *Manual of endoscopy,* Santa Fe Springs, 1990, American Association of Gynecologic Laparoscopists.

46. Levy BS, Soderstrom RM, Dail DH: Bowel injuries during laparoscopy, *J Reprod Med* 30:168, 1985.

47. Lichten EM, Bombard J: Surgical treatment of primary dysmenorrhea with laparoscopic uterine nerve ablation, *J Reprod Med* 32:37, 1987.

48. Luciano AA: *Effects of electrosurgery and lasers on tissue.* In Martin DC, editor: *Lasers in endoscopy,* Santa Fe Springs, 1990, Resurge Press and American Association of Gynecologic Laparoscopists.

49. Luciano AA et al: A comparison of thermal injury, healing patterns, and postoperative adhesion formation following CO_2 laser and electromicrosurgery, *Fertil Steril* 48:1025, 1987.

50. Luciano AA et al: A comparative study of postoperative adhesions following laser surgery by laparoscopy versus laparotomy in the rabbit model, Obstet Gynecol 74:220, 1989.

51. Lundorff P et al: Adhesion formation after laparoscopic surgery in tubal pregnancy: a randomized trial versus laparotomy, *Fertil Steril* 55:911, 1991.

52. Maiman M, Seltzer V, Boyce J: Laparoscopic excision of ovarian neoplasms subsequently found to be malignant, *Obstet Gynecol* 77:563, 1991.

53. Marrero MA, Corfman RS: Laparoscopic use of sutures, *Clin Obstet Gynecol* 34:387, 1991.

54. Martin DC: Avoid laparotomy by using laser laparoscopy, *Contemp OB/GYN: Update on Surgery* 25:101, 1985.

55. Martin DC: CO_2 laser laparoscopy for endometriosis associated with infertility, *J Reprod Med* 31:1089, 1986.

56. Martin DC: Laparoscopic and vaginal colpotomy for the excision of infiltrating cul-de-sac endometriosis, *J Reprod Med* 33:806, 1988.

57. Martin DC: *Therapeutic laparoscopy.* In Martin DC, editor: *Laparoscopic appearance of endometriosis,* ed 2, vol I, Memphis, 1990, Resurge Press.

58. Martin DC, editor: *Laparoscopic appearance of endometriosis,* Memphis, 1990, Resurge Press.

59. Martin DC: Laparoscopic treatment of ovarian endometriosis, *Clin Obstet Gynecol* 34:452, 1991.

60. Martin DC: Tissue effects of lasers, *Semin Reprod Endocrinol* 9(2):127, 1991.

61. Martin DC: Tissue effects of lasers and electrosurgery. In Sanfilippo J, Vitale G, Perissat J, editors: *Atlas of laparoscopic general surgery,* Philadelphia, JB Lippincott, in press.

62. Martin DC, Diamond MP: Operative laparoscopy: comparison of lasers with other techniques, *Curr Probl Obstet Gynecol Fertil* 9:563, 1986.

63. Martin DC, Diamond MP, Yussman MA: *Laser laparoscopy for infertility surgery.* In Sanfilippo JS, Levine RL, editors: *Operative gynecologic endoscopy,* New York, 1989, Springer-Verlag.

64. Martin DC, Hubert GD, Levy BS: Depth of infiltration of endometriosis, *J Gynecol Surg* 5:55, 1989.

65. Martin DC, Vander Zwaag R: Excisional techniques for endometriosis with the CO_2 laser laparoscope, *J Reprod Med* 32:753, 1987.

66. Martin DC et al: Laparoscopic appearances of peritoneal endometriosis, *Fertil Steril* 51:63, 1989.

67. Murphy AA: Operative laparoscopy, *Fertil Steril* 47:1, 1987.

68. Nager CW, Murphy AA: Ectopic pregnancy, *Clin Obstet Gynecol* 34:403, 1991.

69. Nezhat C, Crowgey SR, Nezhat F: Videolaseroscopy for the treatment of endometriosis associated with infertility, *Fertil Steril* 51:237, 1989.

70. Nezhat C, Nezhat FR: Safe laser endoscopic excision or vaporization of peritoneal endometriosis, *Fertil Steril* 52:149, 1989.

71. Nezhat C, Nezhat F, Silfen SL: Laparoscopic hysterectomy and bilateral salpingo-oophorectomy using multifire GIA surgical stapler, *J Gynecol Surg* 6:287, 1990.

72. Nezhat C et al: Endoscopic infertility surgery, *J Reprod Med* 34:127, 1989.

73. Nezhat CR et al: Adhesion reformation after reproductive surgery by videolaseroscopy, *Fertil Steril* 53:1008, 1990.

74. Olive DC, Martin DC: Treatment of endometriosis-associated infertility with CD_2 laser laparoscopy: the use of one- and two-parameter exponential models, *Fertil Steril* 48:18, 1987.

75. Parker WH, Berek JS: Management of selected cystic adnexal masses in postmenopausal women by operative laparoscopy: a pilot study, *Am J Obstet Gynecol* 163:1574, 1990.

76. Phillips JM: Complications in laparoscopy, *Int J Gynaecol Obstet* 15:157, 1977.

77. Phillips JM, editor: *Endoscopy in gynecology,* Downey, CA, 1977, American Association of Gynecologic Laparoscopists.

78. Phillips JM, editor: *Laparoscopy,* Baltimore, 1977, Williams & Wilkins.

79. Portuondo JA et al: Periovarian adhesions following ovarian wedge resection or laparoscopic biopsy, *Endoscopy* 16:143, 1984.

80. Pouly JL et al: Conservative laparoscopic treatment of 321 ectopic pregnancies, *Fertil Steril* 46:1093, 1986.

81. Reich H: Laparoscopic treatment of extensive pelvic adhesions, including hydrosalpinx, *J Reprod Med* 32:736, 1987.

82. Reich H: Pelvic sidewall dissection, *Clin Obstet Gynecol* 34:412, 1991.

83. Reich H, McGlynn F: Treatment of ovarian endometriomas using laparoscopic surgical techniques, *J Reprod Med* 31:577, 1986.

84. Reich H, Vancaillie TG, Soderstrom RM: *Electrical techniques.* In Martin DC, editor: *Manual of endoscopy,* Santa Fe Springs, 1990, American Association of Gynecologic Laparoscopists.

85. Reich H et al: Laparoscopic treatment of ruptured interstitial pregnancy, *J Gynecol Surg* 6:135, 1990.

86. Schwartz PE: An oncologic view of when to do endoscopic surgery, *Clin Obstet Gynecol* 34:467, 1991.

87. Schwartz PE: Ovarian masses: serologic markers, *Clin Obstet Gynecol* 34:423, 1991.

88. Scoutt LM, McCarthy SM: Imaging of ovarian masses: magnetic resonance imaging, *Clin Obstet Gynecol* 34:443, 1991.

89. Semm K: Advances in pelviscopic surgery, *Curr Probl Obstet Gynecol Fertil* 5(10):1, 1982.

90. Semm K, Friedrich ER, editors: *Operative manual for endoscopic abdominal surgery,* Chicago, 1987, Mosby–Year Book.

91. Shirk GJ: Use of the Nd:YAG laser for the treatment of endometriosis, *Am J Obstet Gynecol* 160:1344, 1989.

92. Soderstrom RM, Levy BS: *Medical and legal aspects of laparoscopy.* In Martin DC, editor: *Manual of endoscopy,* Santa Fe Springs, 1990, American Association of Gynecologic Laparoscopists.

93. The Southern Surgeons Club: A prospective analysis of 1518 laparoscopic cholecystectomies, *N Engl J Med* 324:1073, 1991.

94. Sumioki H et al: The effect of laparoscopic multiple punch resection of the ovary on hypothalamo-pituitary axis in polycystic ovary syndrome, *Obstet Gynecol Surv* 44:208, 1989.

95. Sutton C, MacDonald R: Laser laparoscopic adhesiolysis, *J Gynecol Surg* 6:155, 1990.

96. Thompson BH, Wheeless DR: Gastrointestinal complications of laparoscopy sterilization, *Obstet Gynecol* 41:669, 1973.

97. Thornton KL, Diamond MP, DeCherney AH: Linear salpingostomy for ectopic pregnancy, *Obstet Gynecol Clin North Am* 18(1):95, 1991.

98. Tulandi T: Reconstructive tubal surgery by laparoscopy, *Obstet Gynecol Surv* 42:193, 1987.

99. Tulandi T, Guralnick M: Treatment of tubal ectopic pregnancy by salpingotomy with or without tubal suturing and salpingectomy, *Fertil Steril* 55:53, 1991.

100. Vancaillie TG: Salpingectomy, *Obstet Gynecol Clin North Am* 18(1):111, 1991.

101. Voyles CR et al: A practical approach to laparoscopic cholecystectomy, Am J Surg 161:365, 1991.

102. Wheeless CR: *Thermal gastrointestinal injuries.* In Phillips JM, editor: *Laparoscopy,* Baltimore, 1977, Williams & Wilkins.

Chapter 46

HYSTEROSCOPY

Charles M. March

The exact incidence of infertility and pregnancy wastage caused by structural uterine abnormalities is unknown. However, such pathology has been implicated in 5% to 10% of infertile couples and in up to one third of those with recurrent pregnancy loss. Although intrauterine defects have been found in 13% of asymptomatic patients undergoing surgical sterilization, up to 62% of patients who are infertile have been reported to have lesions.[9,67] Losses in the second trimester and early in the third trimester are likely to be caused by congenital anomalies and submucosal myomas.

Before the advent of hysteroscopy, gynecologists could investigate the uterine cavity only indirectly. Although members of other surgical specialties such as orthopedics and urology have considered endoscopy to be one of their indispensable diagnostic and therapeutic tools, gynecologists have not embraced hysteroscopy with the same enthusiasm. Table 46-1 demonstrates the differences between the urinary bladder and the uterus with respect to endoscopy and highlights the limitations that uterine anatomy places upon gynecologists. Thus for many decades we used only hysterosalpingography, curettage, and the limited palpatory sensations afforded by the tip of a uterine sound to detect intrauterine pathology. Although the deficiencies of these different approaches have been known, difficulties with adequate illumination and the lack of suit-

able uterine distending media hindered acceptance of hysteroscopy, a procedure described in 1869 by Panteleoni.[52]

Cold-light fiberoptics solved the problem with illumination. However, only after Edstrom and Fernstrom[18] demonstrated the feasibility of using a highly viscous dextran solution to provide both uterine distention and a clear view even in the presence of blood and cellular debris did hysteroscopy emerge as a valuable procedure with many applications.[18]

Hysteroscopy not only permits the nature of a lesion suggested by hysterography to be confirmed but also allows the surgeon to plan therapy and to assess the defect's proximity to tubal ostia or the internal cervical os. A comparison of hysterosalpingography (HSG) and hysteroscopy is shown in Table 46-2. These two studies should be considered complementary rather than competing or mutually exclusive. The advantages of hysteroscopy make it the first choice for patients who are likely to have uterine pathology. However, as a screening procedure the HSG is preferred for those physicians who do not have office hysteroscopy available. In addition, for infertile patients the additional information about the fallopian tubes that can only be obtained by the HSG makes this procedure an important one.

Table 46-1. Endoscopy of the uterus and urinary bladder

Uterus	Urinary bladder
Virtual cavity, thick muscle	Thin muscle
Distended by high pressure	Distended by gravity only
Fragile lining, bleeds easily	No lining
Cyclic epithelial changes	None
Communicates with peritoneal cavity	No communication

Table 46-2. Comparison of hysterosalpingography and hysteroscopy

Hysterosalpingography	Hysteroscopy
Outlined by contrast	Direct view of cavity
Presumptive diagnosis	Definitive diagnosis
Localization difficult	Lesion location mapped
No surgery possible	Surgery possible
Tubal study also required	Uterine evaluation possible
Low cost	Moderate cost

INDICATIONS
Sterilization

The first widespread application of hysteroscopy was in transcervical sterilization under direct visualization (see box). Although this application remains investigational and therefore is outside the scope of this chapter, a brief summary is warranted. Fulguration of the tubal ostia was adopted as a rapid, simple method of achieving tubal closure.[54] However, this technique has a high failure rate and is associated with many ectopic pregnancies, especially intramural ectopics.[13] Excessive thermal damage to the intramural portion of the tube has been postulated as the cause of this complication.[43] A variety of plugs, implants, and sclerosing agents have had an unacceptably low rate of success.[19,59] Formed-in-place silicone plugs have been approved in some European countries but await further study in the United States.[41,55]

Reproductive failure

Unexplained infertility and recurrent abortion continue to frustrate gynecologists and their patients. Although it was believed that direct inspection of the uterine cavity in women with normal hysterograms would provide important information about the preimplantation phase of the endometrium and thus provide clues to diagnosis and treatment, this hope was not realized. Although the correlation between the presumptive diagnosis of a uterine abnormality detected by hysterosalpingography and the definitive diagnosis established by hysteroscopy is excellent, discrepancies do occur.[60,63] If the properly performed hysterogram is normal, hysteroscopy is not necessary.[21] However, if any the necessary elements of that radiographic study are absent (long axis of the uterus parallel to the film plate, view of endocervical canal, view of uterus during the early filling phase, absence of uterine contractions that obscure the upper fundus), or if a cavity defect is present, hysteroscopy is a mandatory step in the evaluation of the infertile woman, the patient with recurrent abortion, and

---

Indications for hysteroscopy

A. Sterilization
B. Reproductive failure
  1. Unexplained infertility
  2. Recurrent abortion
C. Intrauterine pathology
  1. Confirm abnormal HSG
  2. Intrauterine adhesion
  3. Congenital anomalies
  4. Embedded IUDs
  5. Abnormal bleeding
    a. Polyps
    b. Myomas
    c. Carcinoma
    d. Ablation
  6. Proximal tubal obstruction

---

the patient with only one second trimester loss. Obviously the iodine contrast media for hysterography should not be introduced via a balloon catheter, which would obscure the uterine contour.

Intrauterine pathology

Hysteroscopy is used to establish the presence of intrauterine pathology in the following conditions:

1. Intrauterine adhesions can be diagnosed definitively and their extent classified. Synechiae can be lysed completely and safely under direct vision. The success of treatment can be evaluated by repeat hysteroscopy (or HSG) at a later date.

2. The nature and extent of congenital uterine anomalies can be defined if hysteroscopy is combined with laparoscopy. A treatment plan can then be formulated. The septate uterus can be unified and the results assessed by a follow-up hysteroscopy or hysterosalpingography.

3. Submucous leiomyomas can be differentiated from polyps, their extent evaluated, and they can be biopsied or resected. If pedunculated, the lesion can be excised completely.

4. Endometrial polyps can be differentiated from submucous leiomyomas, which is not always possible by HSG. The polyps should be excised under direct vision and then their bases should be curetted or fulgurated to reduce the risk of recurrence.

5. In cases of abnormal bleeding, structural abnormalities of the uterine cavity can be detected and classified so that appropriate medical or surgical treatment can be employed. Malignancies occasionally missed by curettage can be diagnosed. Endometrial carcinoma can be staged more accurately than by fractional curettage. Endometrial ablation can be performed.

6. Embedded IUDs can be visualized and removed under direct vision, thereby minimizing endometrial trauma.

7. In some patients with proximal tubal obstruction, only a small portion of the intramural segment of tube is occluded, and the placement of a series of wires and catheters in a coaxial fashion under hysteroscopic and laparoscopic guidance may achieve patency.

INSTRUMENTATION
Hysteroscopes

Hysteroscopes are of three types: rigid panoramic, rigid contact, and "flexible" panoramic. Most panoramic hysteroscopes are modified cystoscopes. The telescope may have an outer diameter of 2.7 to 4.0 mm. The telescope may have a 0° viewing angle and thus provide a straight-on view or may have a foreoblique lens that is offset from the horizontal by 12°, 15°, 25°, or 30°. Some telescopes have a focusing knob that allows them to be used as a contact device. Others allow magnification. The

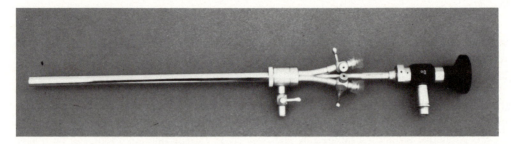

Fig. 46-1. Double channel hysteroscope.

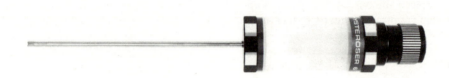

Fig. 46-2. Contact hysteroscope.

sheaths for panoramic hysteroscopes may be 3.3 to 4.5 mm in diameter and are only for diagnostic use. These are ideally suited for office work without anesthesia or after a paracervical block has been introduced. For operative hysteroscopy, 7- or 8-mm sheaths are available to permit the placement of one or two accessory instruments. The newest hysteroscope (Fig. 46-1) has two accessory channels. In its sheath the four channels (telescope, medium, two accessory) are completely isolated from one another; therefore this is the only panoramic hysteroscope that can provide true continuous flow. Special luer-lock nipples fit over the operating instrument ports to prevent leakage of medium. Some sheaths have a modification at their distal end, the Albarran bridge, which allows the accessory instrument to be deflected toward a lesion. This modification is especially valuable for patients whose tubal ostia are eccentrically placed and who wish to have transcervical tubal surgery–sterilization or relief of proximal tubal obstruction.

The microcolpohysteroscope provides a magnified view of the endocervix and uterine cavity and may be useful in evaluating patients with CIN lesions that extend into the canal.[29] If the full extent of the lesion can be seen, directed biopsy may reduce the need for conization. Another operating panoramic hysteroscope has an offset eyepiece and accepts rigid accessory instruments.

The contact hysteroscope (Fig. 46-2) is an office instrument that is valuable for diagnosing all types of intrauterine pathology, but not for therapy.[2] The hallmark of contact hysteroscopy is simplicity. Neither a light source nor distending medium is necessary. Two instruments are available: one with a 6-mm diameter and one of 8 mm.

The former is favored because it requires less cervical dilatation. Biopsy/grasping forceps that fit over the 6-mm endoscope can be used to remove embedded IUDs. A focusing device that increases the depth of field is a mandatory attachment.

Because the contact hysteroscope does not provide a panoramic view of the cavity, most physicians find it more difficult to master than the panoramic hysteroscope. Achieving complete inspection of the cavity requires discipline and patience. However, its simplicity of use and maintenance makes the contact hysteroscope a valuable and convenient diagnostic tool.

"Flexible" hysteroscopes (Fig. 46-3) are not truly flexible but rather steerable.[38] The outer diameter varies between 3.5 and 4.8 mm and the distal end can be deflected over an arc of 130° to 160°. By rotating the entire instrument it is possible to view the entire cavity. The 1-mm media channel can be used to deliver either CO_2 or 5% glucose in water. The larger flexible hysteroscope can be used for surgery and has a 2-mm operating channel for biopsy forceps and microscissors. The view afforded by flexible hysteroscopes is inferior to that obtained by a rigid telescope, but because the leading edge can be maneuvered around lesions and because it can provide a parallel view of even the most eccentrically placed ostium, this instrument can help to cannulate tubes and to deliver a balloon to relieve obstruction or a plug or chemical to cause sterilization.

The choice of hysteroscope depends upon the goals of the user and the needs of the patient. All instruments have a role, and the "complete" hysteroscopist will be able to use all types well.

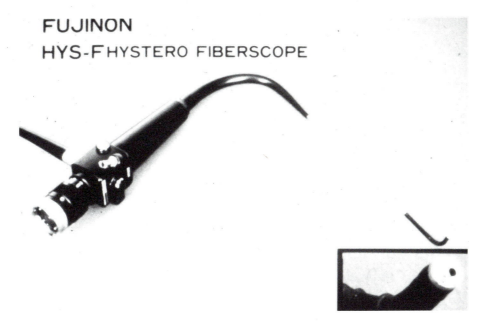

Fig. 46-3. "Flexible" hysteroscope.

Ancillary equipment

The ancillary equipment available includes an aspirating cannula, biopsy forceps, scissors, alligator-jaw grasping forceps, and a fulgurating electrode. The aspirating cannula and fulgurating electrode are both flexible and are either 6 or 7 f. The aspirating cannula is really an essential instrument rather than an accessory one. Because blood and cellular debris may be present before beginning the hysteroscopy or as a consequence of intrauterine surgery, a method of maintaining a clear view is important. Even though dextran media are not miscible with blood, and continuous flow instruments can irrigate the cavity well, an aspirating catheter permits pinpoint clearing of certain regions, especially the cornual recesses.

Scissors can be used to incise a septum, to lyse adhesions, or to excise a polyp or pedunculated submucosal myoma. Biopsy forceps should be used to document the histology of any lesion that is not excised. Alligator-jaw grasping forceps can retrieve retained intrauterine devices or other foreign bodies. All of these instruments can be flexible, semirigid, or rigid depending upon the sheath used. Rigid instruments are the most durable. They can be used with an offset eyepiece hysteroscope or can be attached to the sheath. If the latter, they remain a fixed distance in front of the telescope and cannot be moved. Because depth of field is poor with monocular instruments, this class of instrument may be associated with an increased risk of uterine perforation and a relative inability to approach eccentrically placed lesions.

Coagulation can be obtained via a flexible electrode or a fiber to deliver laser energy from an Argon or Nd:YAG source. The latter can use a bare 600-mm fiber or one with a sapphire tip. If the latter is used, the tip *cannot* be cooled with gas.

A four-pronged "cervical-sealing" tenaculum, which reduces the leakage of medium through a patulous cervix, is well designed and permits the telescope to be passed through its prongs.[24] At the base of each prong is a broad base, which reduces the depth of penetration of the prong and exerts pressure against any vessel that may have been punctured. A simple bivalve speculum with only one attachment between both blades permits it to be removed easily following insertion of the instruments, thereby reducing patient discomfort.

Resectoscope

The resectoscope, an essential tool for the urologist, has been modified for use by the gynecologist. This instrument has inner and outer sheaths to provide continuous flow of the medium. Although this instrument can be used with only the inner sheath, which has an insulated tip, most gynecologic surgeons prefer the continuous flow instrument because of its ability to clear the operative field of blood and cellular debris. Commercially available resectoscopes have two outer sheath sizes, a 25 or a 27 Fr. The medium is instilled via the inner sheath into the uterus and then flows out via perforations in the outer sheath. Either gravity or suction can be used to withdraw the medium. Most instrument companies have now modified the outflow sheath to place the outflow holes around the entire sheath.

The working element. The electrodes extend a maximum of 4 cm beyond the end of the outer sheath. Two types of working elements are available to extend and retract the electrodes over that distance—two-handed and one-handed mechanisms. The two-handed mechanism, exemplified by the Stern-McCarty unit, works on a rack and pinion lever. Two types of one-handed models are the Baumrucker and Iglesias mechanisms, both of which use a spring mechanism.

The most common electrodes used in gynecologic surgery are the roller ball and the cutting loop. A number of variations of the roller ball are available ranging in diameter from 2 mm upwards. The cutting loops available are generally between 6 and 8 mm in outer diameter. Another electrode with application in gynecology is the knife, useful in cutting septa and synechiae.

Conversion to operating hysteroscope. The Circon/ACMI resectoscope allows the outflow sheath mechanism to be converted to use as an operating hysteroscope by use of a bridge. This bridge allows the surgeon to use a 7-Fr operating channel for insertion of semirigid instruments or a laser fiber.

TECHNIQUE

Hysteroscopy may be performed at any time during the menstrual cycle except during menses. However, visualization is best within 2 to 3 days after the cessation of menstrual flow. The endometrium is thin early in the cycle, but later the tubal ostia may become obscured by endometrial growth. In addition, the endometrium is less friable in the early proliferative phase. If hysteroscopy is performed during the secretory phase, it is necessary for the couple to be using adequate contraception.

Hysteroscopy may be performed in the office. No special preoperative instructions or tests are necessary. For patients with a history of pelvic infection, a cervical culture should be obtained before surgery. Pelvic tenderness should be considered possible evidence of infection and may dictate postponing the procedure. For most patients prophylactic antibiotics are not necessary. For brief procedures, premedication with 600 mg of ibuprofen is sufficient. If a longer or more difficult hysteroscopy is anticipated, sedation consisting of meperidine, midazolam, or diazepam should be given IV. The use of these drugs mandates that the patient leave the office in the care of another. If general or regional anesthesia is necessary, an outpatient surgical unit provides an adequate setting, and the patient may be discharged in a few hours.

Following introduction of a paracervical block with 10 ml of 1% lidocaine without epinephrine into each uterosacral ligament, the uterine cavity is sounded. The cervix is then dilated to between 4 and 7 mm, and the hysteroscope is engaged in the external os and advanced into the uterine cavity only if a clear view is available. A 4.5-mm sheath is used if the procedure is to be diagnostic only, and a 7- or 8-mm sheath for operative procedures. Because the anterior and posterior uterine walls are in apposition, the cavity must be distended by one of three different types of media (described below) to ensure proper visualization. After inspection of the endocervical canal and lower uter-

ine segment, the hysteroscope is advanced into the cavity, and the lateral walls, upper fundus, both cornual recesses, and both tubal ostia are inspected in a systematic fashion. If necessary, scissors may be introduced through the operating channel of the hysteroscope for lysis of synechiae. In addition, polyps may be excised and embedded IUDs removed. Resection of myomas or lysis of moderate or severe adhesions requires general or regional anesthesia. If a uterine division is found, simultaneous laparoscopy is necessary to differentiate the bicornuate from the septate anomaly. If the anomaly proves to be septate, the laparoscopist will guide the hysteroscopist in treating the defect and preventing uterine perforation.

MEDIA
Low viscosity

An inexpensive medium is 5% glucose in water. It is introduced via an IV infusion bag. The rate of flow is controlled by gravity or by increasing the infusion pressure by a hand pump or a blood pressure cuff. The high-volume, high-flow-rate system of delivery increases uterine cramping and thus hinders the use of this medium for office procedures. Another disadvantage of this type of medium is that it mixes with blood, thus obscuring vision. Normal saline, Ringer's lactate, 3.3% sorbitol, or 1.5% glycine may also be used for hysteroscopy and have the same attributes and limitations as glucose in water.[30] Electrolyte-containing media cannot be used if any electrosurgical procedure is planned. More recently special pumps have been developed to control the pressure under which low-viscosity media are delivered.

Carbon dioxide

A special insufflator is required (the CO_2 insufflator used to create the pneumoperitoneum for laparoscopy *must not* be used).[40] CO_2 is instilled at a flow rate of 25 to 100 ml/min at a maximum pressure of 200 mmHg. Because the refractile index of CO_2 is 1.00, the appearance of the tissue is more "true to life" than with other media.[39] There is less magnification than with other media because of the lower index of refraction of CO_2. A patulous cervix limits the ability to maintain adequate uterine distention. During prolonged procedures, up to 500 ml of CO_2 may be needed to compensate for both absorption and spill into the peritoneal cavity. Intraperitoneal CO_2 will cause shoulder pain when the patient resumes an erect position. This medium is perfectly suited for office diagnostic procedures.

High viscosity

Dextran, being immiscible with blood, provides excellent visualization. It is instilled via a 50-ml syringe attached to large-diameter (5-mm) infusion tubing. An alternative is instillation via a CO_2-driven pump with special infusion tubing. Intermittent delivery of 5- to 10-ml volumes to enhance visualization results in less uterine cramping. This medium is very difficult to remove from instruments; thus, instruments *must* be rinsed immediately

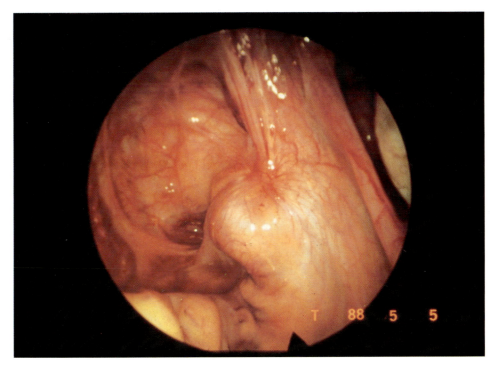

Color Plate 8. Fibrotic infiltration of the peritoneum and bowel causes distortion. This picture is an example of deep involvement of the rectosigmoid with the rectosigmoid pulled up into the right uterosacral ligament. With this level of distortion, lesions are most commonly full thickness through the muscularis.

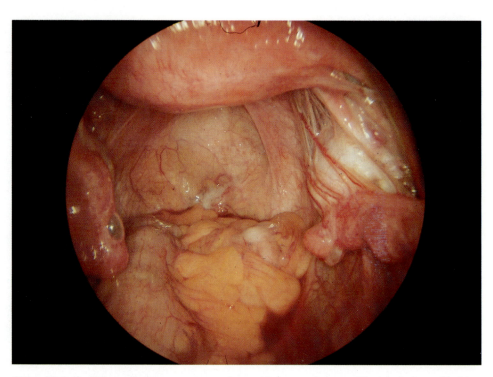

Color Plate 9. Filmy adhesions are easy to lyse with any equipment. Blunt lysis is avoided because this increases bleeding and petechial hemorrhage.

after the procedure with copious amounts of hot water. Two forms of dextran have been used for hysteroscopy. The first, Rheomacrodex, is a 10% dextran solution with a molecular weight of 40,000 in 5% glucose in water. The second, Hyskon Hysteroscopy Fluid, is a 32% dextran solution with a molecular weight of 70,000 in 10% glucose in water. This medium was developed specifically for use in hysteroscopy.[18] The excellent clarity and minimal equipment needed make Hyskon the medium of choice for operative hysteroscopy. Almost all examinations can be completed using one 100-ml bottle. For difficult operative procedures, much larger volumes may be necessary, but the total amount infused should not exceed 500 ml. Hyskon is delivered via wide-diameter tubing, which facilitates the introduction of this very viscous medium.

CONTRAINDICATIONS

The only absolute contraindication to hysteroscopy is acute pelvic infection. Active uterine bleeding, pregnancy, a recent uterine perforation, and uterine cancer are relative contraindications. If Hyskon is used to distend the uterine cavity, a satisfactory examination can usually be accomplished even if the patient is bleeding heavily. If the low-viscosity media are used in a continuous flow system, similar results can be obtained because the blood and cellular debris will be flushed from the cavity. The contact hysteroscope may also be used in patients with a recent uterine perforation. Although hysteroscopy may be used to diagnose and stage cancer, the potential for tumor dissemination has prevented its widespread use. This theoretical objection does not apply if contact hysteroscopy is performed or if CO_2 is used for panoramic hysteroscopy.

SPECIFIC PROCEDURES
Intrauterine adhesions (IUA)

Lysis of adhesions under direct vision is safer and more complete than blind curettage or hysterotomy. Before beginning adhesiolysis, the extent of the disease is classified (Table 46-3).[1,47] Under hysteroscopic guidance, it is pos-

Table 46-3. Classification of IUA by hysteroscopic findings

Class	Findings
Severe	More than three fourths of uterine cavity involved; agglutination of walls or thick bands; ostial areas and upper cavity occluded
Moderate	One fourth to three fourths of uterine cavity involved; no agglutination of walls, adhesions only; ostial areas and upper fundus only partially occluded
Minimal	Less than one fourth of uterine cavity involved; thin or filmy adhesions; ostial areas and upper fundus minimally involved or clear

From March CM, Israel R, March AD: Hysteroscopic management of intrauterine adhesions, *Am J Obstet Gynecol* 130:653, 1978.

sible to cut only scar tissue, thereby sparing adjacent normal endometrium and permitting it to be a source for endometrial regrowth over the freshly dissected surfaces. Each adhesive band is identified and divided with miniature scissors (Fig. 46-4). Restoration of normal uterine architecture can be achieved even in women with complete uterine obliteration. However, patients who have very extensive disease should undergo simultaneous laparoscopy. The laparoscopist will guide the hysteroscopist in order to reduce the risk of uterine perforation. If the intensity of the light source for the laparoscope is reduced markedly, the laparoscopist will more readily detect dissection into the myometrium because the light of the hysteroscope will begin to shine through the uterine serosa at a single point. In contrast, after the cavity's configuration has been restored, the uterus will have a uniform glow. Following adhesiolysis, as large a loop IUD as possible is placed in the cavity and retained for 2 months. Postoperative use of an IUD may reduce the chances that the raw dissected surfaces

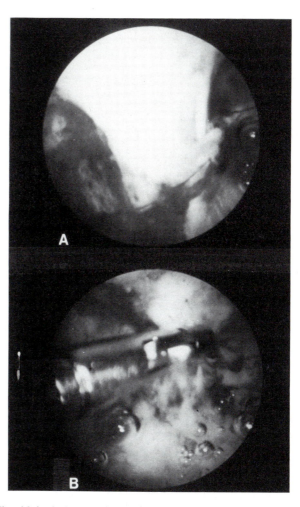

Fig. 46-4. A, Intrauterine scar as seen through the hysteroscope. **B,** Division of scar using miniature scissors. (From March CM: *Hysteroscopy and the uterine factor in infertility.* In Mishell DR Jr, Davajan V, Lobo RA, editors: *Infertility, contraception and reproductive endocrinology,* ed 3, Cambridge, Mass, 1991, by permission of Blackwell Scientific Publications.)

will readhere.[44] Copper-bearing IUDs and the Progestasert IUD may have too small a surface area to prevent adhesion reformation, and copper may induce an excessive inflammatory reaction. Therefore their use is not advised. If a loop IUD is not available, an 8 Fr Foley catheter with a 3-ml balloon can be used. The balloon is inflated, the catheter remains for 1 week, and a broad-spectrum antibiotic is prescribed during that time period. Special Silastic uterine splints are also available to maintain separation of the uterine walls.

Conjugated equine estrogens (5 mg daily) are given to all patients for 60 days, and medroxyprogesterone acetate (10 mg) is added during the last 5 days of estrogen thera-

py.[44] High-dose sequential estrogen-progestin therapy maximally stimulates the endometrium so that the previously scarred surfaces are reepithelialized. The adequacy of therapy should be assessed accurately by repeat hysteroscopy or by HSG following the steroid-induced withdrawal bleeding. If the HSG is normal, complete resolution may be presumed. An abnormal HSG, however, does not definitively indicate persistent adhesions and the hysteroscopy should be repeated.

The results of this approach to our first 175 patients with IUA are summarized in Table 46-4. Of the 105 patients who originally had symptoms of secondary amenorrhea, 100 have cyclic, spontaneous, painless menses of normal flow and duration, 4 have hypomenorrhea, and 1 has remained amenorrheic. Of the 28 who had hypomenorrhea before therapy, all have normal menses. After one hysteroscopic treatment, 90% of our patients have had a normal follow-up hysteroscopy or HSG. Although most of the others have needed a second procedure only to restore normal uterine architecture, a few women have needed three to six operations. Therefore, our approach to patients with IUA is a four-pronged one (Table 46-5). The importance of a postoperative study to verify normalcy of the cavity before permitting conception cannot be overemphasized. Severe obstetric complications have been reported in patients who conceived before postoperative studies were performed to document complete resolution of the adhesions.[22] It is likely that these women had persistent disease, causing the subsequent obstetrical problems.

The pregnancy results of the approach are excellent and surpass those with other types of therapy[34,45] (Table 46-6). Of these 175 patients, 69 wished to conceive and had no other known infertility factors. Of the 69, 52 (75%) conceived 62 times, and 54 (87%) of the 62 pregnancies have gone to term. Two patients have had placenta previa and two required manual removal of the placenta. One patient had retained placental fragments, which were detected when a curettage was performed to stop hemorrhage 3 weeks after delivery. Her follow-up HSG had been abnormal but she conceived before another hysteroscopic procedure was performed. These results are superior to those achieved by outdated treatment modalities such as blind disruption of adhesions by a sound or curette.

Table 46-4. Results of lysis of IUA using hysteroscope

Before		After	
Findings	No. of patients	Findings	No. of patients
Amenorrhea	105	Normal menses	100
		Hypomenorrhea	4
		Amenorrhea	1
Hypomenorrhea	28	Normal menses	28
Infertile	69	Delivered or currently pregnant	54

Table 46-5. Principles of treating intrauterine adhesions

Goal	Method
Restore normal uterine architecture	Hysteroscopic lysis
Prevent readherence	Splint
Promote endometrial overgrowth	High-dose estrogen
Verify uterine normalcy	Follow-up HSG or hysteroscopy

Table 46-6. Gestational outcome after treatment for IUA*

Method	No. of pregnancies	First or second trimester losses no. (%)	Term no. (%)
Traditional*	369	104 (28)	147 (40)
USC†	62	8 (13)	54 (87)

*Includes blind disruption of adhesions; data gathered from the literature.
†University of Southern California data have been corrected to eliminate losses from known causes (e.g., elective abortion, cervical incompetence).
From Jewelwicz R et al: Obstetric complications after treatment of intrauterine synechiae (Asherman's syndrome), *Obstet Gynecol* 47:701, 1976. Reprinted with permission from The American College of Obstetricians and Gynecologists.

Congenital anomalies

Uterine anomalies are found in 1% to 2% of all women, in 4% of infertile women, and in 10% to 15% of women with recurrent abortion.[5]

Congenital uterine anomalies may be classified as follows:

1. Unicornuate: complete developmental arrest of one müllerian duct.
2. Didelphic: a complete lack of fusion, with duplication of corpus and cervix. The duplication may extend into the vagina. This anomaly is associated with premature delivery and abnormal presentations.

3. Bicornuate: partial lack of fusion or associated with a single or septate cervix. The defect is manifested externally and internally. This is the most common anomaly and is associated with malpresentations and premature delivery.
4. Septate: a partial lack of resorption of the midline septum. In some, the upper cavity is normal.[64] This defect is manifested internally only. It may be associated with a septate cervix. This is the anomaly most often associated with recurrent first trimester abortions.[57]
5. Arcuate: a very mild, asymptomatic form of septate uterus. It is a hysterographic or hysteroscopic diagnosis only and has no reproductive consequences.
6. Rudimentary horn: incomplete development of one horn. The horn may be either communicating or noncommunicating. The latter is more common. Rudimentary horns may or may not have functioning endometrium.

Abortion and obstetrical problems such as premature labor and abnormal fetal presentations are the most common symptoms in patients with uterine anomalies.[61] Uterine defects have not been proven to cause primary infertility. Although two thirds of pregnancies in women with uterine duplications progress to term, abortion has been reported to occur in as many as 30% of pregnancies in women with septate uteri.[31] If the endometrium present in a noncommunicating rudimentary horn is functional, recurrent abdominal pain, hematometra, and even rupture simulating an ectopic pregnancy may occur. Longitudinal vaginal septa, which are usually asymptomatic, may be found alone or combined with other müllerian anomalies, especially uterus didelphys. Some patients with a septate vagina have one side obstructed, thus the outflow of one uterus is restricted to a variable degree, causing a mass due to hydrocolpos or hematocolpos to form.

HSG and hysteroscopy (Fig. 46-5) can be used to delineate uterine defects and serve as a baseline prior to treatment. The HSG also provides information regarding tubal patency. Before metroplasty a complete investigation is mandatory so that other infertility factors and other causes of recurrent abortion can be ruled out.

Only the anomalies related to in utero diethylstilbestrol (DES) exposure and the septate uterus are definitely associated with early reproductive failure. A uterine septum is not usually an indication for surgery in infertile patients, because this defect has not been reported to cause infertility. Laparotomy with uterine unification and incision or excision of the septum was formerly the procedure of choice for women with this anomaly and a history of recurrent abortion. The procedures advocated by Tompkins and by Jones were the most popular.[56] Hysteroscopic treatment of septa has relegated these procedures to antiquity.

Hysteroscopy is used not only to assess the size and extent of the septum but also to treat the anomaly.[12] Simultaneous laparoscopy is needed to verify that the uterus is unified externally and also to provide guidance for the hys-

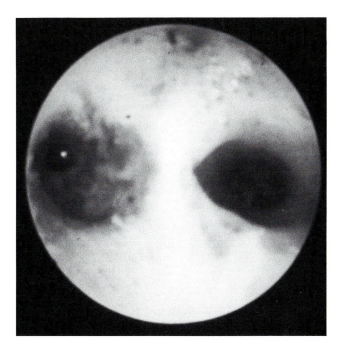

Fig. 46-5. Hysteroscopic view of uterine septum. (From March CM: *Hysteroscopy and the uterine factor in infertility.* In Mishell DR Jr, Davajan V, Lobo RA, editors: *Infertility, contraception and reproductive endocrinology,* ed 3, Cambridge, Mass, 1991, by permission of Blackwell Scientific Publications.)

teroscopist. Flexible scissors are passed through the operating channel of the hysteroscope, and the central portion of the anteroposterior column of the septum is incised. If the septum is 3 cm or less wide at the top of the fundus, the incision is carried cephalad from the most inferior point of the septum and directed laterally as the most superior aspect of the uterus is approached. The fibroelastic band of tissue retracts immediately and does not bleed. The dissection is continued until the septum is incised completely and the uterine architecture is normalized.[32,46] Broader septa are treated differently. The incision is begun at the most inferior portion of the septum, and the scissors are directed superiorly along one lateral margin of the septum up to 0.5 cm from the junction with normal myometrium (Fig. 46-6). Next the other lateral margin is incised up to the same level, and subsequently each new lateral aspect is incised alternatively until only a short broad notch (Fig. 46-6, *E*) between the tubal ostia remains. Finally this notch is incised beginning from one cornual recess and progressing to the other. This approach is used because minimal bleeding usually occurs at the interface between myometrium and septum and if treatment of this portion is delayed until the end of the procedure, blood loss is minimized and excellent visualization ensured. The dissection is complete when both tubal ostia can be visualized simultaneously even when the hysteroscope is high in the cavity, when the hysteroscope can move freely from one cornual recess to another, and/or when the laparoscopist observes that the entire uterus glows uniformly, even

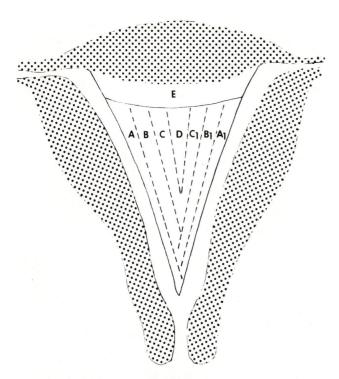

Fig. 46-6. Diagram of surgical approach to wide uterine septum. Sequential incisions are made through all of area A, then A_1, B, B_1, C, C_1, and D. Finally, the residual notch E is incised. (From March CM, Israel R: Hysteroscopic management of recurrent abortion caused by septate uterus, *Am J Obstet Gynecol* 156:834, 1987.)

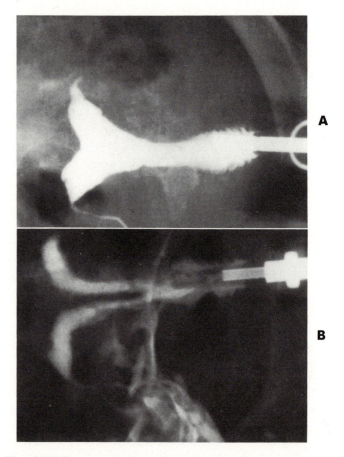

Fig. 46-7. Preoperative **(A)** and postoperative **(B)** hysterogram of patient with septate uterus who underwent hysteroscopic treatment.

when the distal end of the hysteroscope is located in one cornual recess.

If the cervix is septate also, it is not incised, because this area is very vascular, because cervical incompetence may ensue, and because the cervical portion of the septum will not hinder labor. The hysteroscope is placed in one horn and a uterine sound in the other. The sound is used to deflect the septum toward the hysteroscope and the scissors that incise it just above the internal os. After a small communication has been made between the two horns, the remaining upper portion of the septum is treated as described above.

Some have used a laser (Nd:YAG, KTP, or Argon) or even a resectoscope to incise the septum. These instruments offer no advantage over scissor incision and cause more tissue damage.[7] In addition, anatomic results are worse when a resectoscope is used.[16] There is no need to place an intrauterine splint.

The patient may be discharged from the surgery unit a few hours after the procedure is finished. To epithelialize the area over the incised septum, conjugated estrogens (1.25 mg daily) are prescribed for 25 days. Medroxyprogesterone acetate (10 mg daily) is given during the last 5 days of the estrogen treatment. Office CO_2 hysteroscopy or an HSG should be performed after the withdrawal

menses. If normal, the patient may attempt to conceive immediately thereafter.

Preoperative and postoperative HSGs of a patient treated by hysteroscopic incision are shown in Fig. 46-7. Outcomes have been excellent in four series of hysteroscopic treatment of patients with uterine septa and histories of recurrent abortion.[11,16,46,53] The rates of abortion were reduced from 95% (pretreatment) to less than 15% (posttreatment) (Table 46-7).[46] These results equal those of abdominal metroplasty.[58] A comparison of transfundal and transcervical techniques for incision of the septate uterus is shown in Table 46-8. These differences were demonstrated most clearly in a report by a single surgeon who compared his personal results.[20] The multiple advantages of hysteroscopic therapy make it the method of choice for treating uterine septa. In fact, because this method of treatment is so easy and safe, it may permit us to expand the indications for treating patients with uterine septa. For example, it should be used before in-vitro fertilization or gamete intrafallopian transfer (GIFT) and may be used before complex therapy such as ovulation induction with gonadotropins, or even for patients with unexplained infertility. The

Table 46-7. Reproductive outcome before and after hysteroscopic metroplasty

	Preoperatively (N = 240)	Postoperatively (N = 63)
Term, survived	7	51
Premature, survived	5	4
Premature, neonatal death or stillbirth	16	—
Spontaneous abortion	212	8
Successful	12 (5%)	55 (87%)

Table 46-8. Comparison of hysteroscopic and abdominal metroplasty

Hysteroscopic	Abdominal
Minor surgery	Major surgery
Outpatient	Inpatient
½-hour operating time	2-hour operating time
Contraception for 1 month	Contraception for 3 months
Vaginal delivery	Cesarean section needed
Postoperative HSG	Postoperative HSG

value of hysteroscopic treatment of uterine septa for these expanded indications remains uncertain. However, its value for those with reproductive failure is unquestioned. This operation has made abdominal metroplasty for the septate uterus obsolete.

Currently, the most common müllerian anomaly is that following in utero exposure to DES. Typical radiographic findings include a T shape with cornual constriction bands and pretubal bulges, lower uterine segment dilatation, and small cavities with irregular borders resembling intrauterine adhesions. These findings occur in over 80% of women who have typical DES changes in the cervix or vagina. These anomalies may be confirmed by hysteroscopy, but this technique adds little and surgical correction is not possible.

Excessive bleeding

Curettage and hysterectomy are often used as methods of controlling abnormal bleeding. A dilatation and curettage (D and C) is usually required if the patient has evidence of endometrial hyperplasia or if the biopsy is inadequate to exclude malignancy and in cases of profuse bleeding, hypovolemia, recurrent bleeding, and failed medical therapy. Curettage has no place in the long-term management of DUB. There are recurrences of excessive bleeding in more than 68% of patients with DUB treated by curettage alone. If the patient is anovulatory, intermittent progestational therapy will prevent recurrences in most patients. In one study of those with ovulatory menorrhagia, menstrual blood loss was unchanged 2 or more months after D and C.[50] Hysteroscopic examination of the endometrial cavity at the time of D and C helps to rule out the presence of a polyp or submucosal myomas. Among 113 patients who had abnormal bleeding that was investigated by both curettage and hysteroscopy, either a polyp or a submucosal myoma was found in 58 (85%) of the 68 whose excessive bleeding persisted for 6 months or more; 26 (84%) of the 31 women who had secretory endometrium had a cavity defect; of the 78 whose abnormal bleeding recurred despite having had one or two curettages in the previous 6 months, 58 (78%) had a polyp and 18 (23%) had a myoma; and of the 33 with minimal uterine enlargement, 24 (73%) had a submucosal myoma.

Among 342 patients who underwent both hysteroscopy and curettage, uterine inspection and directed biopsy were six times more likely to demonstrate more advanced pathology than did curettage in the group of 71 women whose histologic findings were not in agreement.[25] If the patient is bleeding heavily, a clear view can be obtained if patience is combined with a high-viscosity medium such as Hyskon or one of the low-viscosity media together with a continuous flow instrument. Hysterectomy, the last resort for the treatment of abnormal bleeding, is indicated when all other modalities fail or when there is associated pelvic pathology.

Endometrial carcinoma

Although the standard method of differentiating stage I endometrial carcinoma from stage II disease is the fractional curettage, errors in staging occur 10% to 15% of the time. For those physicians who treat all women in both stages with primary surgery of the same type and who use intraoperative findings or the final pathology report as a guide to selection of further surgery or adjunctive therapy, this distinction is not critical. However, contact hysteroscopy or panoramic hysteroscopy with CO_2 is a safe and accurate method of differentiating between these two stages and of providing important information about the progression of the disease.[62]

Endometrial polyps

Endometrial polyps (Fig. 46-8) are frequently a cause of menometrorrhagia and often cannot be removed completely with polyp forceps and/or a curette.[4] However, hysteroscopic excision by means of scissors or a loop electrode is an easy procedure. If scissors are used to excise the polyp, its base should be fulgurated or curetted to reduce the risk of recurrence. If curettage rather than excision under hysteroscopic control is employed for removal, the hysteroscope must be reinserted to verify that no polyps or fragments thereof remain.

Leiomyomata uteri

Leiomyomas of the uterus are the most common solid pelvic tumor and occur in 20% of women 35 years of age or older.[48] Despite their frequency, their cause and patho-

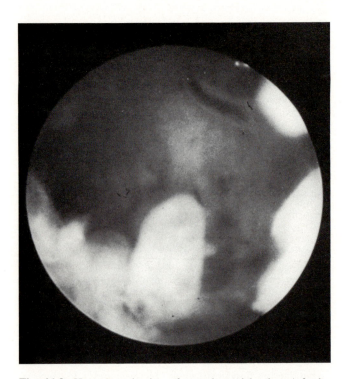

Fig. 46-8. Hysteroscopic view of an endometrial polyp. A feathery appearance and transillumination distinguish a polyp from a myoma. (From March CM: *Hysteroscopy and the uterine factor in infertility*. In Mishell DR Jr, Davajan V, and Lobo RA, editors: *Infertility, contraception and reproductive endocrinology,* ed 3, Cambridge, Mass, 1991, by permission of Blackwell Scientific Publications, Inc.)

physiology remain unclear, although they appear to be unicellular in origin.[66] Myomas arise most often during the third and fourth decades and therefore have an important impact upon reproductive performance. Because first pregnancies are delayed beyond age 35 more commonly today, the relative incidence of myomas in women attempting to conceive is rising. Myomas tend to be multiple and to grow slowly. Most patients are asymptomatic but have firm nodular masses that distort the uterine contour. Infertility, abortion (during either the first or second trimester), premature labor, and abnormal presentations have all been associated with the presence of submucous myomas.[6]

Intramural and submucous myomas have the greatest impact upon reproductive capability. Submucous myomas may hinder endometrial nutrition and afford a poor implantation site (resulting in abortion or infertility). Large intramural myomas may cause enlargement of the endometrial cavity (possibly resulting in poor sperm transport) and may, on occasion, occlude the intramural portion of the tube(s). Both types, but particularly the submucous variety, may not allow normal uterine enlargement during pregnancy and thus lead to abortion and premature labor.

The diagnosis of intramural myomas is usually made at the time of bimanual examination. The presence of submucous tumors may be suspected during curettage, but an HSG or hysteroscopy is necessary for confirmation. Smooth, circular, or crescent-shaped defects persisting after the entire cavity is filled suggest submucous myomas (Fig. 46-9). Occasionally it is impossible to differentiate the defect caused by a myoma from that of an endometrial polyp or a gestational sac. The HSG also gives prognostic information, because marked tubal disease would contraindicate conservative surgery unless the patient is interested in in-vitro fertilization. An HSG may also demonstrate the

Fig. 46-9. Hysterogram of patient with submucous myoma. (From March CM: *Hysteroscopy and the uterine factor in infertility*. In Mishell DR Jr, Davajan V, Lobo RA, editors: *Infertility, contraception and reproductive endocrinology,* ed 3, Cambridge, Mass, 1991, by permission of Blackwell Scientific Publications, Inc.)

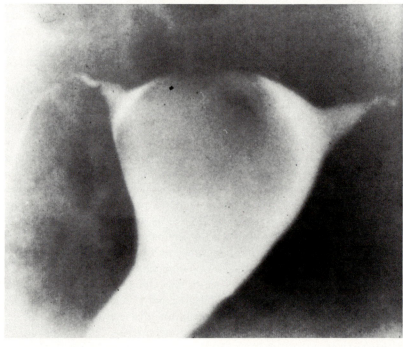

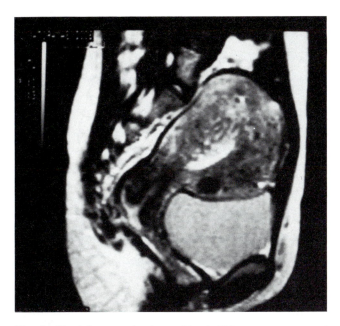

Fig. 46-10. Adenomyosis. (From March CM: *Hysteroscopy and the uterine factor in infertility*. In Mishell DR Jr, Davajan V, and Lobo RA, editors: *Infertility, contraception and reproductive endocrinology,* ed 3, Cambridge, Mass, 1991, by permission of Blackwell Scientific Publications, Inc.)

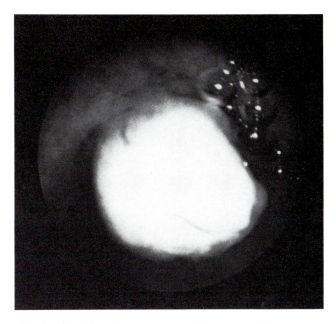

Fig. 46-11. Pedunculated submucous leiomyoma visualized with the hysteroscope. Myomas appear white and glistening. (From March CM: *Hysteroscopy and the uterine factor in infertility*. In Mishell DR Jr, Davajan V, Lobo RA, editors: *Infertility, contraception and reproductive endocrinology,* ed 3, Cambridge, Mass, 1991, by permission of Blackwell Scientific Publications, Inc.)

filling of multiple channels in the tumor mass that communicate with the endometrial cavity, and thus the diagnosis of adenomyosis can be made (Fig. 46-10).

The definitive diagnosis of a submucosal myoma is made by hysteroscopy. Direct visualization can establish the nature of the defect(s) more accurately and pinpoint the location, size, and relation to the tubal ostia and internal os (Fig. 46-11).

Because myomas develop and enlarge during the reproductive years and especially during pregnancy but tend to involute after delivery and following menopause, all medical methods of treatment have been directed toward inducing estrogen deficiency. The response to progestins has been variable, but high-dose medrogestone acetate has been shown to induce marked degeneration, fibrosis, and hyalinization.[27] The response to danazol has been variable.[14] Recently, a significant reduction in myomas has been demonstrated with gestrinone, an antiestrogen, antiprogesterone, when administered orally or vaginally.[10] Preoperative treatment with a potent gonadotropin-releasing hormone (GnRH) agonist such as nafarelin or leuprolide causes cellular myomas to shrink markedly and thus facilitates surgery.[37] Maximal tumor shrinkage occurs after 3 months of therapy.[23] Before surgery anemic patients should be treated with a GnRH agonist and iron until their iron stores have been replenished. The medical management of myomas cannot replace surgery for the symptomatic infertile woman or one with recurrent abortion, because ovarian function is restored promptly after the agonist is discontinued, and myomas usually return to their original size within 3 months. Calcified myomas and those that are fibrous and avascular do not respond to medical treatment.

Indications for myomectomy are (1) to conserve the uterus in a woman with large or symptomatic myomas and (2) to improve reproductive potential. Before performing a myomectomy to improve reproductive potential, a complete infertility investigation must be carried out to place the role of the myoma(s) in proper perspective. Additional infertility factor(s) should be corrected, if possible, before surgery. Subsequent pregnancy rates are reduced if myomectomy is performed in patients with multifactorial infertility. Smaller myomas (less than 7 cm) may be resected or, if pedunculated, may be excised under hysteroscopic control.

Three types of instruments have been used. A standard operating hysteroscope with scissors has been used to resect submucosal myomas. The line of resection follows that of the adjacent normal endometrial surface. This technique is most suitable for myomas in the center of the endometrial cavity and has been used to resect solitary or multiple myomas of up to 5 cm in diameter. After resection, the mass must be morcellated to permit removal via the cervical os.

Another approach involves using a resectoscope (Fig. 46-12) and "shaving" the myoma gradually to a point even with the normal endometrial surface[28,49] (see box). This technique may be used for larger myomas and for those more eccentrically placed (Fig. 46-13). If multiple submucosal myomas are present and if these myomas occupy

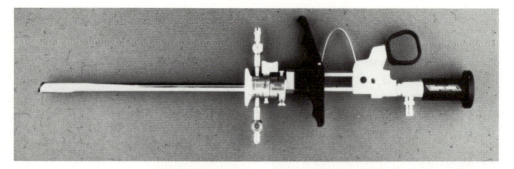

Fig. 46-12. Continuous flow rectoscope.

Steps in hysteroscopic myomectomy

Inspection of cavity
Coagulation of surface vessels
Resection
Coagulation of cut vessels
Evacuation of chips
Reinspection
Doxycycline (100 mg BID × 5 days)
Conjugated equine estrogens (CEE), (1.25 mg daily × 21)
Medroxy progesterone acetate (10 mg daily, d 16–21 of CEE)

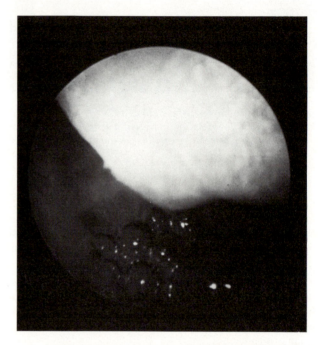

Fig. 46-13. Large myoma via hysteroscope.

most of the endometrial surface and/or oppose one another, endoscopic resection is not advised. Much of the endometrial surface will be damaged by resection, and the risk of synechiae formation is high. An alternative for moderate-sized opposing wall myomas is a two-stage procedure; that is, resecting the myomas at 2-month intervals so that only one uterine surface is raw at one time.

Following the induction of anesthesia and a pelvic examination, the uterine cavity is sounded and the cervix is dilated to 9 mm. The resectoscope and all tubing are filled with medium, the instrument is introduced into the endocervical canal, and systematic inspection of the cavity is performed (see box above). The technique of resecting a myoma involves the systematic shaving of the intracavitary portion of the tumor. If the depth of myometrial involvement is thought to be great, a preoperative magnetic resonance imaging (MRI) should be performed. This study will identify myomas that have an intramural component so large that transuterine resection would be of little value if only the intracavitary component were excised or dangerous if the resection were carried far into the uterine wall. Any large surface vessels are coagulated before beginning the resection. The resection is carried out beginning with the portion of the myoma that bulges most into the uterine cavity. The electrosurgical unit is set initially at 30 W, but more power is often needed, especially for tumors that are more fibrous. Cutting current only is used. The resecting loop is passed superior to the myoma and

withdrawn back toward the insulated sheath. As the loop passes the tumor, it is activated and a piece of the myoma is excised. The loop should only be activated when it is completely in view and not in contact with adjacent normal endometrium or a tubal ostium. As fragments are resected, they should be pushed superior to the myoma in order to maintain a clear view. If the view becomes obscured the fragments should be rinsed out of the cavity or retrieved with polyp forceps. All of the resected tumors should be sent to the laboratory for examination (see Fig. 46-13).

As the resection progresses, some of the tumor that had been intramural is commonly extruded into the cavity and becomes available to the resecting electrode. The resection may be continued to a point even with the normal adjacent endometrium or even to just below this level *but no further*. If the resection is continued into the underlying muscle, marked hemorrhage may occur and the risk of uterine perforation is a real one. Moreover, deep dissection is usually not necessary. If a small intramural component is left

Table 46-9. Results of hysteroscopic resection
of myomas

Number	60
Follow-up	½– 10 yr
Largest	
Pedunculated	8 cm
Sessile	6 × 4 cm
Recurrence (6)	
Abdominal myomectomy	3
Hysterectomy	2
Repeat resection	1

in situ, uterine contractions over the ensuing weeks often cause that fragment to be extruded into the uterine cavity and subsequently aborted. This mechanism probably explains the high rate of success even if a portion of the myoma remains. Myomas that are located on the most superior aspect of the uterus are more difficult to resect because access to them is limited. Newer loops and other cautery elements are being designed to permit excision of these masses. At present, the easiest access to these myomas is with a quartz fiber transmitting energy from an Nd:YAG laser and delivered via a panoramic hysteroscope.

Operator caution is critical to endoscopic resection of submucosal myomas. Tumors that are attached to the region of the internal cervical os are more vascular, and injury to large vessels may occur. Abdominal removal should be considered. Myomas that have a large intramural component (more than one half of the uterine wall) may be resected, but these tend to cause recurrent symptoms shortly after surgery. If the MRI demonstrates that the submucosal myoma extends close to the uterine serosa, an abdominal approach should be used. The same approach is needed in patients who have bothersome symptoms related to other myomas that are intramural or subserosal. A combined approach of resection of myomas and endometrial ablation may be used in women with multiple or solitary submucosal myomas who do not wish to conserve fertility. Pretreatment with a GnRH agonist, danazol, or a progestin should be used before ablation to induce endometrial atrophy.

Since Neuwirth[49] reported resecting of submucosal myomata with a resectoscope, the value of this technique has been proven by other investigators. The largest published experience is that of Hallez, Netter, and Cartin.[28] Ninety percent of my patients have had no recurrence of bleeding over 1 to 10 years of follow-up (Table 46-9). Similar results have been reported by others.[68]

Recently the Nd:YAG laser has been used to resect a submucosal myoma.[17] Most investigators were experienced hysteroscopists before undertaking resection of submucosal myomas via a resectoscope or laser. A thorough preoperative investigation and correction of anemia will reduce the risk of complications. Although simultaneous laparoscopy has not been used at the USC center, it may be helpful, especially during a surgeon's early experience

with this valuable approach to the symptomatic submucosal leiomyoma. In contrast to abdominal myomectomy, patients may attempt to conceive 1 month after surgery and may deliver vaginally. If a GnRH agonist is used before myomectomy, estrogen therapy should be used immediately after surgery to reduce the risk of adhesion formation. An HSG or repeat hysteroscopy should be performed before conception.

Endometrial ablation

Laser photovaporization of the endometrium has been investigated for treatment of menorrhagia.[26] A neodymiun-YAG laser was used under hysteroscopic visualization. Before the procedure, all patients were given danazol (800 mg/day) for 2 to 3 weeks. An additional 2 weeks of danazol treatment followed the laser procedure. This regimen cured 203 of 210 patients, including many with organic lesions such as submucosal myomas. Similar results have been reported by Loffer,[42] using a "nontouch" technique to destroy the endometrium. Photovaporization causes varying degrees of uterine contraction, scarring, and adhesion formation, as follow-up HSGs and hysteroscopy showed. DeCherney et al,[15] Townsend et al,[65] and Vancaille[69] have used a standard urologic resectoscope or a modified one that permits continuous flow of the distending medium (and therefore reduced fluid absorption) to destroy the endometrium with cautery. The instruments employed are different but the techniques of endometrial destruction are similar. Preoperative endometrial sampling is mandatory to rule out the presence of any endometrial atypicalities. If the patient has more than minimal uterine enlargement or other symptoms related to leiomyomata, this procedure will not relieve all her complaints. The use of a drug to cause endometrial atrophy before surgery will facilitate ablation and increase efficacy. USC uses leuprolide acetate for 2 months before surgery.

Surgery is performed on an outpatient basis under general or regional anesthesia. The results of endometrial ablation are similar irrespective of whether a resectoscope or a laser is used. I prefer to use the former: the instrument is readily available, is less costly, and the procedure can be performed more rapidly. A 2.5-mm roller electrode is used to coagulate the endometrium. The electrosurgical unit is set at 50 W, but occasionally 70 W or more are needed. The end point is a series of overlapping yellow-brown furrows. It is important that the thermal injury be conducted down to the basalis so that the endometrium will not regenerate. Although a loop electrode may be used to resect the endometrium, the depth of resection is more difficult to control and therefore damage to uterine muscle may occur with resultant hemorrhage and increased absorption of medium. A continuous flow resectoscope is used. Sorbital, glycine, and Hyskon all provide a clear view. The ablation is begun in the cornual regions and carried inferiorly to just above the level of the internal os. Ablation below this point increases the risk of damage to large blood vessels. Medroxyprogesterone acetate (150 mg) is given intramuscularly on the day of the procedure to maintain hypoestrogenism and therefore facilitate adhesion formation. During the 2 months after surgery the uterine cavity is sounded intermittently in order to disrupt adhesions in the lower segment so that the process of endometrial obliteration proceeds from above downward. Thereby the chance of developing hematometra is reduced.

Endometrial ablation is an alternative to hysterectomy when other modalities have failed, are contraindicated, or are undesirable. The goal of endometrial ablation is relief of hypermenorrhea, and thus hypomenorrhea or normal menses should be considered successful outcomes. Only about two thirds of patients develop amenorrhea. The rest have hypomenorrhea, and there is a 5% to 10% failure rate. Therefore any patient who demands amenorrhea might be served better by hysterectomy.

All patients must be willing to accept sterilization as a consequence of the surgery, and although the risk of subsequent pregnancy is small, some have advocated simultaneous tubal sterilization. If the patient is at risk for pregnancy, a barrier method should be employed until long-term amenorrhea has been documented. When postmenopausal hormone replacement therapy is given to these patients, a progestin should be added to the estrogen to protect any remaining islands of endometrium from unopposed estrogen stimulation.

Tubal obstruction

The cause of proximal tubal obstruction remains obscure. In many cases the presumptive diagnosis, made by hysterosalpingography, is proven incorrect when laparoscopy with transcervical hydrochromoperturbation is performed. Most of these patients have spasm at the proximal uterotubal junction during the HSG. Others have anatomic damage at both the proximal and distal tubal regions or at only the proximal segments. Those with bipolar disease should probably undergo in-vitro fertilization because the results of microsurgery remain poor. Those with salpingitis isthmica nodosa usually have a poor prognosis because the disease tends to be extensive and progressive and produces a predisposition to ectopic pregnancy. Until recently, tubal reimplantation or microsurgical tubocornual anastomosis was the only method of treating patients who had occlusion of the proximal fallopian tube. Although transcervical balloon tuboplasty (TBT) under fluoroscopic control is probably efficacious, treatment via hysteroscopy offers advantages.[51] Most TBT protocols require that patients have normal distal tubes. Therefore, laparoscopy is usually a prerequisite to TBT. During that laparoscopy, coaxial dilatation of the proximal fallopian tube under hysteroscopic guidance is a convenient alternative to TBT because treatment is carried out at the same time, thereby speeding treatment and reducing cost and discomfort.

As an adjunct to salpingography and to assess the tubal surface anatomy after relief of proximal obstruction and/or before salpingostomy, falloposcopy has emerged as a tool of the future. Although falloposcopy has been performed

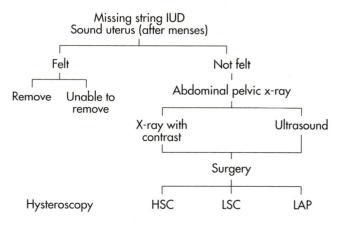

Fig. 46-14. Algorhythm for locating and removing an IUD whose filaments cannot be identified.

from the peritoneal side, more recently these have been passed into the tube after being guided up to the tubal ostium via a flexible hysteroscope.[35]

Foreign bodies

The combination of ultrasound and alligator-jaw grasping forceps can remove most "lost" or embedded IUDs. This approach is safer than the use of an IUD hook. Rather than subjecting all patients to hysteroscopy, USC uses a simple flow chart (Fig. 46-14). The first step is to provide a second method of contraception as soon as the possibility of an expelled or extrauterine device is encountered. Following the next menstrual period, an attempt is made to retrieve the filaments from the endocervical canal. If they are not detected, the cavity is sounded in order to "palpate" the device. If the device is felt, it is retrieved via an alligator-jaw grasping forceps or hysteroscopy. If it cannot be felt, one or more imaging procedures should be used to localize the device, which is then removed by the appropriate surgical procedure. However, for those who have the capability of office hysteroscopy, it can readily be performed before the imaging studies outlined on the right side of Fig. 46-14. If an embedded device is partially intracavitary, the base is grasped with forceps and the device, forceps, and hysteroscope are withdrawn as a single unit. If only a small portion of the device is visible, it may be partially extrauterine and may have involved the bowel. In these instances simultaneous laparoscopy is advised.

POSTOPERATIVE CARE

Little care is needed after hysteroscopy. Those who have had only local anesthesia may leave the office after a brief rest period. If a parenteral narcotic or tranquilizer has been administered, the patient may leave in the care of another after an hour. If general anesthesia has been used, standard guidelines of the hospital or day surgery unit are followed. Bleeding, usually light, should be expected for a few to 10 days. Mild cramping should persist for less than 1 day. Coitus may be resumed in 1 week, and if the patient wishes to conceive she may attempt to do so after 1 month provided all adjunctive therapy has been completed and if any necessary postoperative inspection of the cavity proves it to be normal.

COMPLICATIONS AND MANAGEMENT

Complications have been infrequent and most have been mild in the more than 3000 hysteroscopies performed at USC. The frequency of complications can be reduced if strict guidelines are followed:

Careful history and physical

Follicular phase

Advance telescope only in a clear field

Do not overdilate

Monitor media volume

Use cautery and laser with care

Liberal use of laparoscopy

Pain is usually mild to moderate during hysteroscopy. Most brief hysteroscopies can be performed on an outpatient basis using a paracervical block. Meperidine, midazolam, diazepam, or a prostaglandin synthetase inhibitor may be used to supplement the paracervical block. Cramps increase substantially if operating time exceeds 20 to 30 minutes. Following hysteroscopy, mild cramping may persist for a few hours and is easily controlled with a mild analgesic.

Bleeding

In the USC series of more than 3000 procedures, bleeding has occurred in 12 patients, usually secondary to a laceration at the site of tenaculum placement. In 2 women, a branch of the uterine artery was severed, and tamponade using an intrauterine balloon successfully arrested the bleeding. In another patient, heavy bleeding necessitating transfusion occurred after IUD placement following incision of a uterine septum (splints are no longer used after hysteroplasty). Bleeding may also occur following extensive dissection of synechiae or resection of polyps or a submucous myoma. Almost all bleeding is caused by myometrial injury, not incision of a septum, scar, polyp, or myoma.

Infection

Only 2 of the USC patients have developed pelvic infection following hysteroscopy. Both had histories of salpingitis and 1 was found to have a positive cervical culture for *Neisseria gonorrhoeae* when she was admitted for IV antibiotic therapy. Broad-spectrum antibiotic therapy, including an agent effective against anaerobic organisms, such as clindamycin or chloramphenicol, should be instituted immediately if symptoms of infection develop. Prophylactic antibiotic therapy for hysteroscopy is not necessary.

Uterine perforation

This is a rare complication of hysteroscopy and usually occurs only in the most severe cases of IUA. If the dissec-

tion proves to be extremely difficult, general anesthesia should be administered and laparoscopy performed simultaneously to reduce the chance of uterine perforation. Central perforations may be managed by observation only. Antibiotics are not used and hospitalization is unnecessary.

The use of electrocautery and lasers inside the uterus increases the potential sequelae of uterine perforation because bowel or bladder injury may occur or damage to large blood vessels. The surgeon can only activate the electrosurgical electrode or fire the laser when the view is clear and all of the electrode or laser fiber can be seen. If a resectoscope is used, the electrode should only be activated when it is being withdrawn toward the sheath, never going away. For patients undergoing endometrial ablation, the endocervical canal and internal os should not be treated because of the risk of damage to large blood vessels.

Endometrial dislocation

The subsequent development of endometriosis is probably only a theoretical complication. Avoidance of hysteroscopy during menses further reduces the risk.

Anesthetic accidents

The rare anesthetic complications are related to the agents used rather than to the hysteroscopic procedure itself.

Complications related to the medium

Allergic reactions to dextran occur rarely. If a large amount of dextran enters the venous circulation, circulatory overload is possible.[36,70] A symptom complex consisting of acute noncardiogenic pulmonary edema and disseminated intravascular coagulation has occurred in 12 of the USC patients.[33] All received large volumes (600 to 800 ml) of Hyskon and had extensive dissection of their endometrial surfaces. In order to avoid this serious complications, it is advisable to limit the total amount of Hyskon used to 500 ml or less, even if this means that the procedure must be terminated prematurely and completed at a later date. Hyskon enters the vascular system and can draw almost 10 ml of fluid from the extravascular space for each ml of Hyskon absorbed. After approximately 200 ml of Hyskon is absorbed, platelet dysfunction will result.

Acute fluid overload has also been reported when large volumes of glucose in water, saline, or sorbital have been used. If large volumes of glucose in water have been absorbed, hyperglycemia and hyponatremia may develop.[8] This same complication can occur if large amounts of sorbital or glycine are absorbed. If low-viscosity media are used, intake and output must be recorded accurately at 15-minute intervals. Only rarely should fluid absorption exceed 3000 ml. The use of warm low-viscosity media will reduce the occurrence of hypothermia. In some patients, potent diuretics have been used prophylactically. If fluid overload or pulmonary edema occur, treatment is identical to that used when these events are not preceded by intrauterine surgery.

CO_2 acidosis and arrhythmias are probably only theoretical complications if the proper insufflator is used. However, deaths have occurred when the sheathed fiber used to deliver Nd:YAG energy had a sapphire tip that was cooled by gas delivered at a high rate of flow.[3] These tips should be cooled by the liquid medium being used to distend the cavity. If CO_2 is used as the uterine distending medium, a bare fiber should deliver the laser energy.

LEARNING HYSTEROSCOPY

Although hysteroscopy is easier to learn than laparoscopy, a disciplined approach and patience are necessary. Books, postgraduate courses, and a preceptorship serve to get the novice ready to perform diagnostic hysteroscopy, first under supervision and then independently. After the physician becomes adept at recognizing normal and abnormal structures, excision of polyps and small pedunculated myomas and lysis of minimal adhesions may be undertaken. Incision of septa and more extensive adhesions and the management of larger myomas are procedures of moderate difficulty and risk. If all the cavity is obliterated by scar tissue or if a laser or resectoscope is to be used inside the uterus, an accomplished hysteroscopist should be in charge of the procedure.

REFERENCES

1. American Fertility Society: The American Fertility Society classification of adnexal adhesions, distal tubal occlusion, tubal occlusion secondary to tubal ligation, tubal pregnancies, Mullerian anomalies and intrauterine adhesions, *Fertil Steril* 49:944, 1988.
2. Baggish MS: Contact hysteroscopy: a new technique to explore the uterine cavity, *Obstet Gynecol* 59:350, 1979.
3. Baggish MS, Daniell MS: Death caused by air embolism associated with neodymium: yttrium-aluminum-garnet laser surgery and artificial sapphire tips, *Am J Obstet Gynecol* 161:877, 1989.
4. Burnett JE: Hysteroscopy-controlled curettage for endometrial polyps, *Obstet Gynecol* 24:621, 1964.
5. Buttram VC, Gibbons WE: Mullerian anomalies: a proposed classification (an analysis of 144 cases), *Fertil Steril* 32:40, 1979.
6. Buttram VC, Reiter RC: Uterine leiomyomata: etiology, symptomatology and management, *Fertil Steril* 36:433, 1981.
7. Candiani GB et al: Argon laser versus microscissors for hysteroscopic incision of uterine septa, *Am J Obstet Gynecol* 164:87, 1991.
8. Carson SA et al: Hyperglycemia and hyponatremia during operative hysteroscopy with 5% dextrose in water distention, *Fertil Steril* 51:341, 1989.
9. Cooper JM, Houck RM, Rigberg HS: The incidence of intrauterine abnormalities found at hysteroscopy in patients undergoing elective hysteroscopic sterilization, *J Reprod Med* 10:659, 1983.
10. Coutinho EM, Goncalves MT: Long-term treatment of leiomyomas with gestrinone, *Fertil Steril* 51:939, 1989.
11. Daly DC, Maier D, Soto-Albors C: Hysteroscopic metroplasty: six years experience, *Obstet Gynecol* 73:201, 1989.
12. Daly DC et al: Hysteroscopic metroplasty: surgical technique and obstetric outcome, *Fertil Steril* 39:623, 1983.
13. Darabi KF, Roy K, Richart RM: *Collaborative study on hysteroscopic sterilization procedures: final report.* In Sciarra JJ, Zatuchni GL, Speidel JJ, editors: *Risks, benefits and controversies in fertility control,* Hagerstown, Md, 1978. Harper & Row.
14. DeCherney AH, Maheux R, Polan ML: A medical treatment for myomata uteri, *Fertil Steril* 39:429, 1983.
15. DeCherney AH et al: Endometrial ablation for intractable uterine bleeding: hysteroscopic resection, *Obstet Gynecol* 70:668, 1977.
16. DeCherney AH et al: Resectoscopic management of mullerian fusion defects, *Fertil Steril* 45:726, 1986.
17. Donnez J et al: Treatment of uterine fibroids with implants of gonadotropin-releasing hormone agonist: assessment by hysterography, *Fertil Steril* 51:947, 1989.
18. Edstrom K, Fernstrom I: The diagnostic possibilities of a modified hysteroscopic technique, *Acta Obstet Gynecol Scand* 49:327, 1970.
19. Falb RD et al: *Transcervical fallopian tube blockage with gelatin-resorcinol-formaldehyde (GRF).* In Sciarra JJ, Droegemuller W, Speidel JJ, editors: *Advances in female sterilization techniques,* Hagerstown, Md, 1976, Harper & Row.
20. Fayez JA: Comparison between abdominal and hysteroscopic metroplasty, *Obstet Gynecol* 68:399, 1986.
21. Fayez JA, Mutie G, Schneider PJ: The diagnostic value of hysterosalpingography and hysteroscopy in infertility investigation, *Am J Obstet Gynecol* 156:558, 1987.
22. Friedman A, DeFazio S, DeCherney A: Severe obstetric complications after aggressive treatment of Asherman syndrome, *Obstet Gynecol* 67:864, 1986.
23. Friedman AJ et al: A randomized, placebo-controlled, double-blind study evaluating the efficacy of leuprolide acetate depot in the treatment of uterine leiomyomata, *Fertil Steril* 51:251, 1989.
24. Gimpelson R: Preventing cervical reflux of the distention medium during panoramic hysteroscopy, *J Reprod Med* 31:7, 1986.
25. Gimpleson RJ, Rappold HO: A comparative study between panoramic hysteroscopy with directed biopsies and dilatation and curettage, *Am J Obstet Gynecol* 158:489, 1988.
26. Goldrath MH, Fuller TA, Segal S: Laser photovaporization of endometrium for the treatment of menorrhagia, *Am J Obstet Gynecol* 140:14, 1981.
27. Goldzieher JW et al: Induction of degenerative changes in uterine myomas by high-dose progestin therapy, *Am J Obstet Gynecol* 96:1078, 1966.
28. Hallez JP, Netter A, Cartin R: Methodical intrauterine resection, *Am J Obstet Gynecol* 156:1080, 1987.
29. Hamou J: Microhysteroscopy, *J Reprod Med* 26:375, 1981.
30. Haning RV Jr, Harkins PG, Uehling DT: Preservation of fertility by transcervical resection of a benign mesodermal uterine tumor with a resectoscope and glycine distending medium, *Fertil Steril* 33:209, 1980.
31. Heinonen PK, Saarikoski S, Pystynen P: Reproductive performance of women with uterine anomalies, *Acta Obstet Gynecol Scand* 61:157, 1982.
32. Israel R, March CM: Hysteroscopic incision of the septate uterus, *Am J Obstet Gynecol* 149:66, 1984.
33. Jederkin R, Olsfanger D, Kessler I: Disseminated intravascular coagulopathy and adult respiratory distress syndrome: life threatening complications of hysteroscopy, *Am J Obstet Gynecol* 162:44, 1990.
34. Jewelwicz R et al: Obstetric complications after treatment of intrauterine synechiae (Asherman's syndrome), *Obstet Gynecol* 47:701, 1976.
35. Kerin J et al: Falloposcopy: a microendoscopic technique for visual exploration of the human fallopian tube from the uterotubal ostium to the fimbria using a transvaginal approach, *Fertil Steril* 54:390, 1990.
36. Leake JF, Murphy AA, Zacur HA: Noncardiogenic pulmonary edema: a complication of operative hysteroscopy, *Fertil Steril* 48:497, 1987.
37. Letterie GS et al: Efficacy of a gonadotropin-releasing hormone agonist in the treatment of uterine leiomyomata: long-term follow-up, *Fertil Steril* 51:951, 1989.
38. Lin BL et al: Flexible hysterofiberscope: the development of a new flexible hysterofiberscope and its clinical application, *Acta Obstet Gynecol Jap* 39:649, 1987.
39. Lindermann H-J: The use of CO_2 in the uterine cavity for hysteroscopy, *Int J Fertil* 17:221, 1972.
40. Lindemann H-J, Siegler AM, Mohr J: The hysteroflator 1000s, *J Reprod Med* 16:145, 1976.

41. Loffer FD: Hysteroscopic sterilization with the use of formed-in-place silicone plugs, *Am J Obstet Gynecol* 149:261, 1984.

42. Loffer FD: Hysteroscopic endometrial ablation with the Nd:YAG laser using a nontouch technique, *Obstet Gynecol* 69:679, 1987.

43. March CM, Israel R: A critical appraisal of hysteroscopic tubal fulguration for sterilization, *Contraception* 11:261, 1975.

44. March CM, Israel R: Intrauterine adhesions secondary to elective abortion: hysteroscopic diagnosis and management, *Obstet Gynecol* 48:422, 1976.

45. March CM, Israel R: Gestational outcome following hysteroscopic lysis of adhesions, *Fertil Steril* 36:455, 1981.

46. March CM, Israel R: Hysteroscopic management of recurrent abortion caused by septate uterus, *Am J Obstet Gynecol* 156:834, 1987.

47. March CM, Israel R, March AD: Hysteroscopic management of intrauterine adhesions, *Am J Obstet Gynecol* 130:653, 1978.

48. Miller NF, Ludovici PP: On the origin and development of uterine fibroids, *Am J Obstet Gynecol* 70:720, 1955.

49. Neuwirth RS: A new technique for and additional experience with hysteroscopic resection of submucous fibroids, *Am J Obstet Gynecol* 131:91, 1978.

50. Nilsson L, Rybo G: Treatment of menorrhagia, *Am J Obstet Gynecol* 110:713, 1971.

51. Novy MJ et al: Diagnosis of cornual obstruction by transcervical fallopian tube cannulation, *Fertil Steril* 50:434, 1988.

52. Pantaleoni DC: On endoscopic examination of the cavity of the womb, *Med Press Circ* 8:26, 1869.

53. Perino A et al: Hysteroscopy for incision of uterine septa: report of 24 cases, *Fertil Steril* 48:321, 1987.

54. Quinones RG, Aznar RR, Duran HA: Tubal electrocauterization under hysteroscopic control, *Contraception* 7:195, 1973.

55. Reed TP III, Erb R: Hysteroscopic tubal occlusion with silicone rubber, *Obstet Gynecol* 61:388, 1983.

56. Rock JA, Jones HW Jr: The clinical management of the double uterus, *Fertil Steril* 28:798, 1977.

57. Rock JA, Schlaff WD: The obstetrical consequences of utero-vaginal anomalies, *Fertil Steril* 43:681, 1985.

58. Rock JA, Zacur HA: The clinical management of repeated early pregnancy wastage, *Fertil Steril* 39:123, 1983.

59. Sciarra JJ: *Hysteroscopic approaches for tubal closure.* In Zatuchni GL, Lablock MH, Sciarra JJ, editors: *Research frontiers in fertility regulation,* Hagerstown, Md, 1980, Harper & Row.

60. Siegler AM: Hysterography and hysteroscopy in the infertile patient, *J Reprod Med* 18:143, 1977.

61. Stein AL, March CM: The outcome of pregnancy in women with Müllerian duct anomalies, *J Reprod Med* 35:411, 1990.

62. Sugimoto O: Hysteroscopic diagnosis of endometrial carcinoma, *Am J Obstet Gynecol,* 105, 1975.

63. Taylor PJ: Correlations in infertility: symptomatology, hysterosalpingography, laparoscopy and hysteroscopy, *J Reprod Med* 18:339, 1977.

64. Toaff ME, Lew-Toaff AS, Toaff R: Communicating uteri: Review and classification with introduction of two previously unreported types, *Fertil Steril* 41:661, 1984.

65. Townsend D et al: "Rollerball" coagulation of the endometrium, *Obstet Gynecol* 76:310, 1990.

66. Townsend DE et al: Unicellular histogenesis of uterine leiomyomas as determined by electrophoresis of glucose-6-phosphate dehydrogenase, *Am J Obstet Gynecol* 107:1168, 1970.

67. Valle RF: Hysteroscopy in the evaluation of female infertility, *Am J Obstet Gynecol* 137:425, 1980.

68. Valle RF: Hysteroscopic removal of submucous leiomyomas, *J Gynecol Surg* 6:89, 1990.

69. Vancaille T: Electrocoagulation of the endometrium with the ball-end resectoscope, *Obstet Gynecol* 74:425, 1989.

70. Zbella EA, Moise J, Carson SA: Noncardiogenic pulmonary edema secondary to intrauterine instillation of 32% dextran 70, *Fertil Steril* 43:479, 1985.

Chapter 47

RESTORATION OF TUBAL PATENCY

Robert B. Hunt

Tubal surgery is a valuable option for the infertile female with tubal obstruction. The viable pregnancy rates after correction of most tubal conditions compare favorably with those obtained with assisted reproductive technologies.

PRELIMINARY EVALUATION
Fertility testing

Although they vary from couple to couple, fertility tests usually include (1) *Mycoplasma* and *Chlamydia* culture or antibody level; (2) blood studies such as complete blood count and sedimentation rate, thyroid stimulating hormone, prolactin, follicle-stimulating hormone, luteinizing hormone, and midluteal phase progesterone levels; (3) postcoital test and semen analysis; (4) basal body temperature chart and timed endometrial biopsy; (5) hysterosalpingogram or hysteroscopy; and (6) laparoscopy.

Counseling

When the possibility of tubal surgery is being discussed with a couple, the proposed plans of the operation are explained with emphasis on the chances of a viable pregnancy. Complications of the procedure, including ectopic pregnancy, are discussed, as well as the availability and applicability of other options such as advanced reproductive technologies. The couple is given ample time to ask and receive answers to all their questions.

After the consultation is completed, a letter is sent to them restating all the important information relative to the proposed procedure. A copy is sent to the referring physician, and one is retained in the patient's office record. When the couple calls to schedule the operation, the appropriate informed consent documents are mailed to them. These are returned before surgery with each page initialed and the final page signed and witnessed. This methodical approach to the consent process results in a well-informed couple, provides an opportunity for the staff to detect any omissions in the evaluation, builds layers of legal protection, and is superb public relations.

BASIC PROCEDURE
Magnification

Some advocate the use of the operating microscope in tubal surgery; others believe magnification is not necessary for most procedures.* Having used the operating microscope for virtually all tubal operations in the past, I find it most valuable in tubal anastomosis. The ×2.5 operating loupe augmented with a bright headlamp is perfectly satisfactory for adhesiolysis, fimbrioplasty, and salpingostomy.

Anesthesia

General, epidural, or spinal anesthesia may be chosen for these operations, unless an assessment laparoscopy is required at the time of laparotomy. Under those circumstances, a general anesthetic is preferable.

Incision

If the patient has had a previous low midline incision, I generally use the same one. With rare exception, I use the Hunt-Acuna version, consisting of a low transverse skin incision with a vertical fascial and peritoneal opening.[16] This provides ample exposure, prevents damage to the ilioinguinal nerves, and appears to cause less postoperative discomfort than Pfannenstiel's incision.

Pelvic preparation

With the patient appropriately anesthesized, a pelvic examination is performed. An intrauterine catheter connected

*References 4, 9, 13, 23, 27, 30, 38.

768

to a syringe of indigo carmine is inserted into the uterine cavity. A portion of Kerlix gauze soaked in lactated Ringer's solution is inserted into the vagina to elevate the uterus and support the catheter. A Foley catheter is inserted into the urinary bladder, and, if the patient is under general anesthesia, an orogastric tube is placed in the stomach. The vaginal pack, intrauterine catheter, and orogastric tube are removed at the conclusion of the operation.

Once the abdomen is draped and opened and the abdominal exploration is completed, the patient is placed in Trendelenburg's position. A Kirschner retractor is positioned over a wound protector, the bowel is displaced, and the posterior cul-de-sac is packed with a single Kerlix gauze placed over a sump drain. The drain is connected to continuous suction to remove excess fluids. A silicone mat is inserted to provide an unencumbered background on which to work (Fig. 47-1).

Microsutures

Several studies have compared the synthetic absorbable and nonabsorbable sutures available. Some minor differences among them have been shown in animal studies, but not enough to affect patency or pregnancy rates.* Nylon and polybutester (Sharpoint and Davis and Geck, respectively) are excellent choices because of their color contrast, tensile strength, and memory, and the availability of tapered needles with cutting tips.

Irrigant

Based on animal research by Blandau, I use warm, lactated Ringer's solution for irrigation. Heparin, 5000 U, is added to each 1-L bottle of irrigant to prevent blood clotting on peritoneal surfaces.[2]

Antibiotics

Although their value in preventing adhesions and infections after reproductive surgery is unclear, I administer antibiotics intravenously before beginning surgery and continue them postoperatively while the patient is hospitalized. My choice is 100 mg doxycycline given in an antecubital vein (to prevent phlebitis) and switching to 100

*References 12, 18, 19, 25, 32.

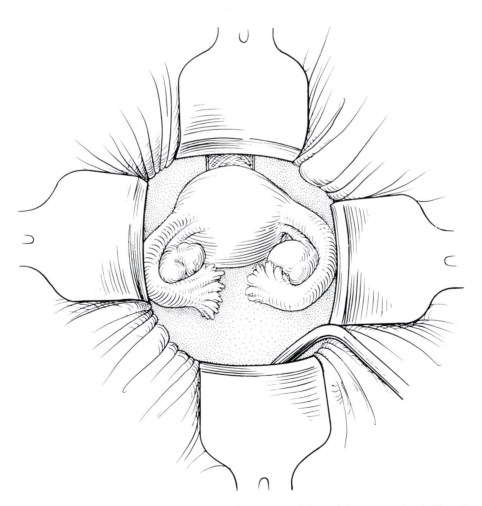

Fig. 47-1. Placement of Kirshner retractor and exposure of the pelvis are completed. Note the wound protector and sump drain. (From Hunt RB, Acuna HA: *Pelvic preparation and choice of incision.* In Hunt RB, editor: *Atlas of female infertility surgery,* ed 2, St Louis, 1992, Mosby– Year Book.)

mg orally when appropriate. Sometimes the choice of antibiotic is determined by other medical indications, such as mitral valve prolapse.

Tubal cannulation and danazol

Tubal cannulation to relieve cornual obstruction has been successful in a significant percentage of patients.[31] Unless the proximal tube is obviously involved in severe disease, such as salpingitis isthmica nodosa, I attempt to relieve the obstruction by passing a catheter into the proximal tube, either by hysteroscopy or by fluoroscopy. The fallopian tube is irrigated thoroughly with either dilute indigo carmine (hysteroscopy) or water-soluble contrast medium (fluoroscopy).

Some advocate the use of danazol to correct pathologic cornual occlusion. One group found 5 of 12 patients achieved patency and 1 of 12 conceived after danazol treatment.[3]

TUBAL IMPLANTATION

Although implantation has been largely replaced by tubal cannulation and cornual anastomosis, it is still indicated occasionally. An example of its appropriate application would be in the patient with total destruction of the intramural portion of the fallopian tube, perhaps having had a previous cornual resection for an ectopic gestation. The technique has many variations; I prefer the one advocated by Levinson.[20]

After pelvic preparation is completed and pelvic exposure is obtained, the tubes are checked for patency with dilute indigo carmine, by either transcervical or transuterine lavage. If hysteroscopy or past surgical history indicates the intramural portion of the tube is unsatisfactory for anastomosis, the surgeon may go directly to implantation. Otherwise, the tube is transected approximately 1 cm from the cornu and the proximal segment is serially sectioned

into the wall of the uterus, with continual checks for patency (Figs. 47-2 and 47-3). Once it is determined that implantation is indicated, the dissection into the uterine wall is terminated, the defect is closed, and the procedure is begun.

Attention is turned to the lateral tubal segment. The operating microscope is used for this portion of the operation. The tube and ovary are kept moist at all times. The tube is dissected from the mesosalpinx, preserving the longitudinal nutrient vessels coursing just beneath and parallel to it, until patency and relatively normal-appearing tissue is reached, as determined by probing or retrograde lavage and inspection (Figs. 47-4 and 47-5).

The tube is divided into mesenteric and antimesenteric halves with microscissors, resulting in a fishmouth configuration. An additional 1 cm is liberated from the mesentery (Figs. 47-6 and 47-7). A 2-0 or 3-0 absorbable suture is placed through each half of the fishmouth (Fig. 47-8). Substantial amounts of tissue are incorporated into the sutures to prevent the sutures from cutting through as they are pulled into the uterine cavity. The respective needles are removed, and the sutures are secured with fine hemostats and set aside. If the contralateral tube is to be implanted, it is prepared at this time.

Loupes replace the microscope as attention is focused on the uterus. The uterus is anteverted, sometimes requiring a Buxton uterine clamp. Approximately 2 to 3 ml dilute vasopressin (20 U in 50 ml lactated Ringer's solution) is injected into the posterior uterine wall with a 25-gauge needle at the level of the uteroovarian ligament (Fig. 47-9). If the contralateral tube is to be implanted also, a similar quantity of vasopressin is injected into the uterine wall in the vicinity of the contralateral uteroovarian ligament. A 1-cm cork bore is placed against the uterine wall just medial to the insertion of the uteroovarian ligament. The bore is angled slightly medially and, with the uterus elevated

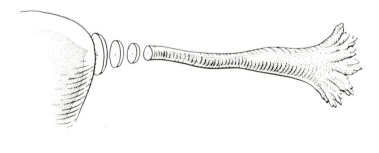

Fig. 47-2. Progressive incisions are made toward the uterus to determine patency proximally. (From Levinson CJ, Lam F: *Tubal implantation.* In Hunt RB, editor: *Atlas of female infertility surgery,* ed 2, St Louis, 1992, Mosby–Year Book.)

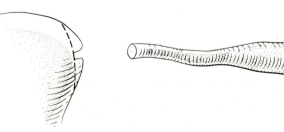

Fig. 47-3. Occlusion persists well into the uterine wall. (From Levinson CJ, Lam F: *Tubal implantation.* In Hunt RB, editor: *Atlas of female infertility surgery,* ed 2, St Louis, 1992, Mosby–Year Book.)

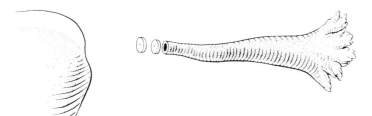

Fig. 47-4. Segments of tube are excised until patency is achieved. (From Levinson CJ, Lam F: *Tubal implantation.* In Hunt RB, editor: *Atlas of female infertility surgery,* ed 2, St Louis, 1992, Mosby–Year Book.)

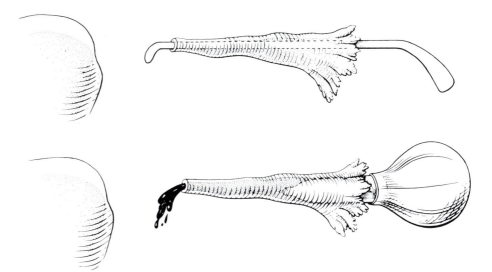

Fig. 47-5. Patency is ascertained by passage of a small probe or by retrograde lavage. (From Levinson CJ, Lam F: *Tubal implantation.* In Hunt RB, editor: *Atlas of female infertility surgery,* ed 2, St Louis, 1992, Mosby–Year Book.)

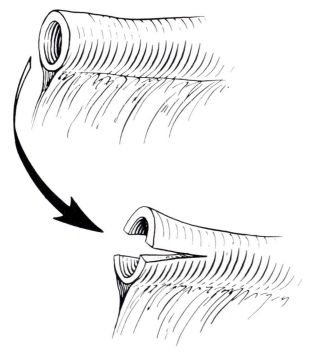

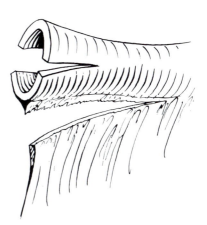

Fig. 47-6. By dividing the tube into mesenteric and antimesenteric halves, a fishmouth is formed. (From Levinson CJ, Lam F: *Tubal implantation.* In Hunt RB, editor: *Atlas of female infertility surgery,* ed 2, St Louis, 1992, Mosby–Year Book.)

Fig. 47-7. The tube is dissected from the mesosalpinx for an additional 1 cm. (From Levinson CJ, Lam F: *Tubal implantation.* In Hunt RB, editor: *Atlas of female infertility surgery,* ed 2, St Louis, 1992, Mosby–Year Book.)

and anteverted by the opposite hand or Buxton clamp, it is rotated, applying firm pressure that results in its traversing the uterine wall. Entry into the uterine cavity is facilitated by distending the cavity with indigo carmine and is determined by a sudden reduction of resistance on the bore and the appearance of indigo carmine in the defect. The core of tissue is removed (Fig. 47-10). The intrauterine catheter or transuterine needle used for lavage is removed from the uterus. If the contralateral tube is to be implanted, a similar opening is made on the opposite side of the uterus.

The proximal end of the tube is positioned so that the suture on the mesenteric side of the fishmouth is facing inferiorly and that on the antimesenteric side is facing superiorly (Fig. 47-11). The mesenteric half is dealt with first. A no. 4 Mayo needle is threaded on one end of the suture and positioned in a standard needle carrier so that the end near the tip is grasped. The blunt end of the needle with its

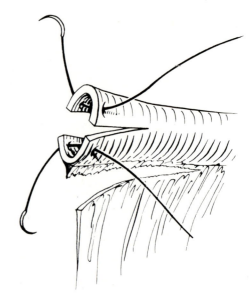

Fig. 47-8. A synthetic absorbable suture is placed through each half of the fishmouth. (From Levinson CJ, Lam F: *Tubal implantation.* In Hunt RB, editor: *Atlas of female infertility surgery,* ed 2, St Louis, 1992, Mosby–Year Book.)

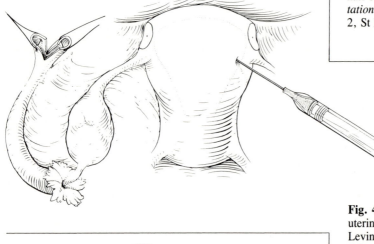

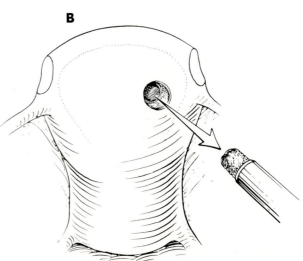

Fig. 47-9. Vasopressin is injected on both sides of the posterior uterine wall at the level of the uteroovarian ligament. (From Levinson CJ, Lam F: *Tubal implantation.* In Hunt RB, editor: *Atlas of female infertility surgery,* ed 2, St Louis, 1992, Mosby–Year Book.)

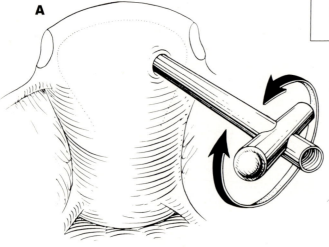

A

B

Fig. 47-10. A, The borer is inserted into the serosa. **B,** The borer is removed together with the core containing serosa, myometrium, and endometrium. (From Levinson CJ, Lam F: *Tubal implantation.* In Hunt RB, editor: *Atlas of female infertility surgery,* ed 2, St Louis, 1992, Mosby–Year Book.)

When retrograde lavage with a cannula inserted through the fimbriae does not exhibit satisfactory flow through the transected end, additional tube must be excised. The medial portion of this lateral segment is grasped with heavy-toothed forceps, the peritoneum is incised on either side of the mesosalpinx and the connective tissue beneath it, and the tube is dissected away from the underlying nutrient vessels (Fig. 47-25). Bipolar coagulation is performed as necessary.

When the tube seems normal by appearance and palpation, a peritoneal tract is created with the aid of ring forceps and a dissecting rod (Fig. 47-26). The tube is transected with iris scissors, taking care to avoid cutting the underlying vessels (Fig. 47-27). Hemostasis is achieved, and patency is determined by retrograde lavage. The mucosa should appear pink and well perfused, and the muscularis should be devoid of scar. If the cut end does not meet these criteria, additional tube should be removed. Often the tube becomes normal in appearance at the ampullary-isthmic junction, which is fortunate because it avoids excessive luminal disparity. Figure 47-28 depicts a patent distal segment after dissection and transection of the proximal end.

At this point in the operation, both proximal and distal segments are prepared for anastomosis. Stay sutures of 6-0 material on a tapered needle are placed (Fig. 47-29). Failure to place them accurately results in misalignment of the lumina and possible failure of the anastomosis. The stay sutures are secured with fine hemostats.

If tension exists at the site of anastomosis, additional dissection must be done to reduce it. This may be accom-

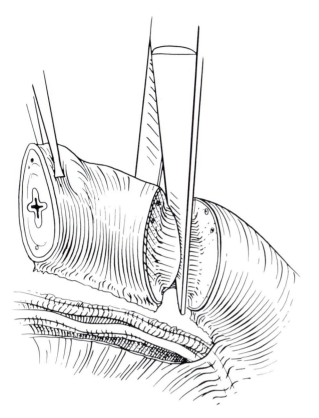

Fig. 47-27. The tubal segment is excised with iris scissors. (From Hunt RB, Diaz DG: *Tubal anastomosis.* In Hunt RB, editor: *Atlas of female infertility surgery,* ed 2, St Louis, 1992, Mosby–Year Book.)

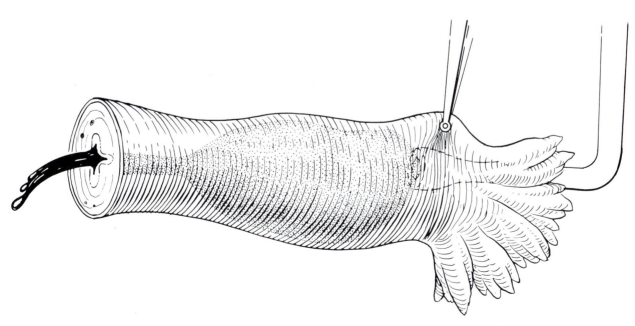

Fig. 47-28. Retrograde lavage confirms patency. (From Hunt RB, Diaz DG: *Tubal anastomosis.* In Hunt RB, editor: *Atlas of female infertility surgery,* ed 2, St Louis, 1992, Mosby–Year Book.)

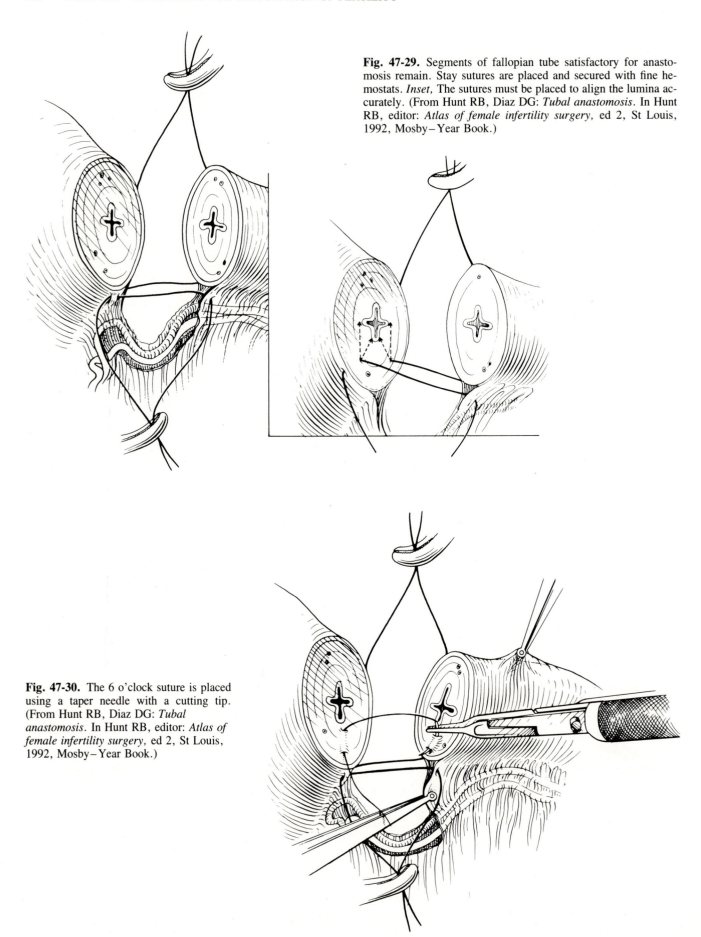

Fig. 47-29. Segments of fallopian tube satisfactory for anastomosis remain. Stay sutures are placed and secured with fine hemostats. *Inset,* The sutures must be placed to align the lumina accurately. (From Hunt RB, Diaz DG: *Tubal anastomosis.* In Hunt RB, editor: *Atlas of female infertility surgery,* ed 2, St Louis, 1992, Mosby–Year Book.)

Fig. 47-30. The 6 o'clock suture is placed using a taper needle with a cutting tip. (From Hunt RB, Diaz DG: *Tubal anastomosis.* In Hunt RB, editor: *Atlas of female infertility surgery,* ed 2, St Louis, 1992, Mosby–Year Book.)

plished by one or a combination of several maneuvers. First, the peritoneum on either side of the mesosalpinx may be incised widely. Second, a moist sponge may be placed lateral to the uterus on the contralateral side and lateral to the adnexa on the ipsilateral side. Third, if the proximal tubal segment is positioned superior to the distal segment, some vaginal packing may be removed to place the two segments into the same horizontal axis.

With the microscope properly centered and focused, the anastomosis begins. An 8-0 or 9-0 suture is placed extramucosally at the 6 o'clock position with the knot outside the tubal lumen (Fig. 47-30). If the distal segment consists of ampulla at the site of anastomosis, a tiny bit of mucosa may be incorporated. The knot is tied and cut. Stay sutures may be tied at this time or later (Fig. 47-31).

The first of two lateral sutures is placed but not tied, followed by placement of the second (Figs. 47-32 and 47-33). The 12 o'clock suture is placed, and all sutures are tied, including stay sutures (Figs. 47-34 and 47-35). Patency is tested by transcervical or transuterine lavage. If the myometrial defect is large, it is partially closed (Fig. 47-36). The serosal layer is approximated (Fig. 47-37). Additional sutures that are required to close the mesosalpinx are placed at this time. Only the anterior mesosalpinx is closed. The overall tubal length is determined and recorded for statistical purposes. The completed anastomosis is shown in Fig. 47-38.

Leakage at the anastomosis site occurs often and is acceptable provided that there is no tension at the anastomosis site and that flow of indigo carmine out of the distal tube is adequate. What is not acceptable is leakage at the

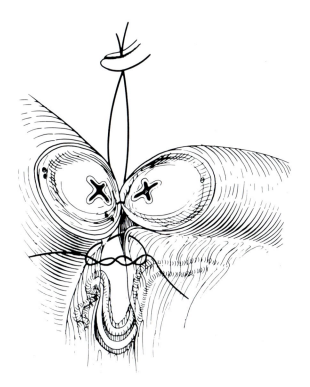

Fig. 47-31. The 6 o'clock suture is tied. The stay sutures may be tied now or later. (From Hunt RB, Diaz DG: *Tubal anastomosis.* In Hunt RB, editor: *Atlas of female infertility surgery,* ed 2, St Louis, 1992, Mosby–Year Book.)

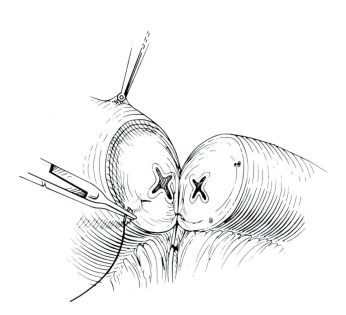

Fig. 47-32. The first lateral suture is positioned. (From Hunt RB, Diaz DG: *Tubal anastomosis.* In Hunt RB, editor: *Atlas of female infertility surgery,* ed 2, St Louis, 1992, Mosby–Year Book.)

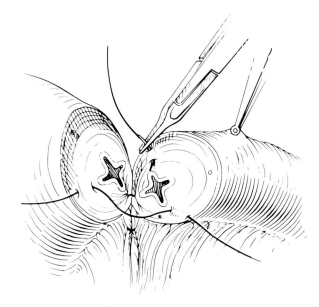

Fig. 47-33. The second lateral suture is placed. Both lateral sutures may be tied now or later. (From Hunt RB, Diaz DG: *Tubal anastomosis.* In Hunt RB, editor: *Atlas of female infertility surgery,* ed 2, St Louis, 1992, Mosby–Year Book.)

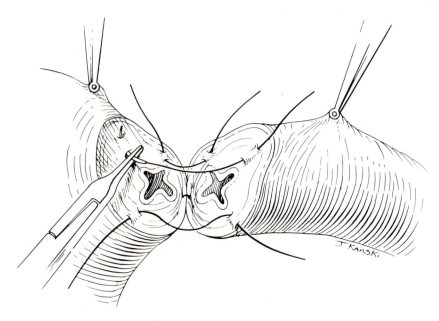

Fig. 47-34. The 12 o'clock suture is placed. (From Hunt RB, Diaz DG: *Tubal anastomosis*. In Hunt RB, editor: *Atlas of female infertility surgery*, ed 2, St Louis, 1992, Mosby–Year Book.)

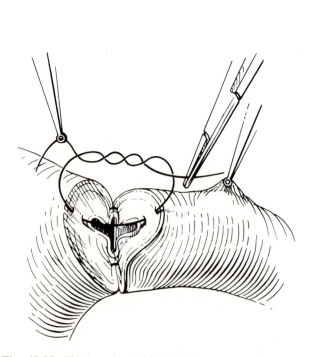

Fig. 47-35. The lateral and 12 o'clock sutures are tied. (From Hunt RB, Diaz DG: *Tubal anastomosis*. In Hunt RB, editor: *Atlas of female infertility surgery*, ed 2, St Louis, 1992, Mosby–Year Book.)

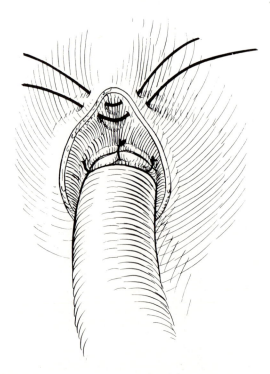

Fig. 47-36. The superior portion of the uterine defect is closed with 6-0 or 8-0 suture. (From Hunt RB, Diaz DG: *Tubal anastomosis*. In Hunt RB, editor: *Atlas of female infertility surgery*, ed 2, St Louis, 1992, Mosby–Year Book.)

anastomosis site with no spillage of dye. If it appears that dye fails to flow into the proximal tube, and the uterus is not expanding as dye is injected, the intrauterine catheter should be removed and transuterine lavage carried out with an 18-gauge needle. If the uterus expands with the injection of indigo carmine and the proximal tubal segment still does not fill, the surgeon may gently massage the myometrium in the vicinity of the cornu, which sometimes results in satisfactory dye flow. If these maneuvers are not successful, but if the surgeon is confident the anastomosis is technically satisfactory, and ample flow of dye out of the proximal segment was observed when the segment was prepared, the anastomosis need not be taken down.

Tubotubal anastomosis

Because most patients with conditions applicable to tubotubal anastomosis have had previous tubal sterilization procedures, they are the focus of this discussion. The same techniques may be used to reestablish patency in patients with localized obstruction from such problems as a previously treated isthmic or ampullary pregnancy, or that caused by localized tubal endometriosis.

Figure 47-40 depicts the appearance of the fallopian tube after ligation with a Falope ring. The anastomosis technique varies little whether coagulation, partial salpingectomy, clip, or ring was used for the sterilization.

The operation begins with removal of the Falope ring. It is grasped with heavy-toothed forceps and excised (Fig. 47-39). A fibrous band of tissue connects the proximal and distal segments of fallopian tube. This band is grasped and lifted superiorly, and is dissected from the mesosalpinx until the proximal segment is reached (Fig. 47-40). Excis-

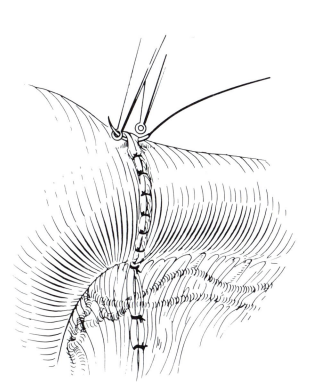

Fig. 47-37. Serosal sutures are placed. A technique to facilitate grasping the needle tip is illustrated. (From Hunt RB, Diaz DG: *Tubal anastomosis*. In Hunt RB, editor: *Atlas of female infertility surgery,* ed 2, St Louis, 1992, Mosby–Year Book.)

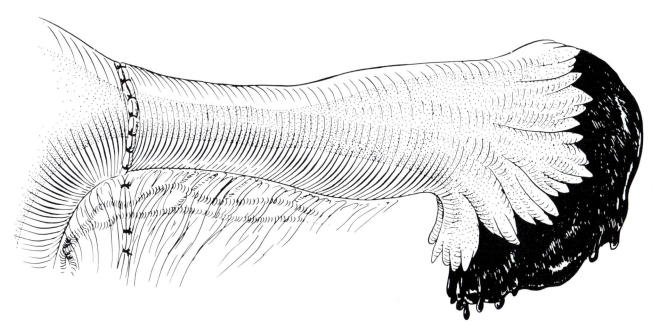

Fig. 47-38. Indigo carmine exits from the fimbriae. Optimally, this is done before serosal closure. (From Hunt RB, Diaz DG: *Tubal anastomosis*. In Hunt RB, editor: *Atlas of female infertility surgery,* ed 2, St Louis, 1992, Mosby–Year Book.)

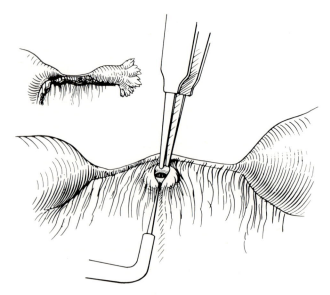

Fig. 47-39. The fallopian tube after Falope ring ligation. The ring is removed. (From Hunt RB, Diaz DG: *Tubal anastomosis.* In Hunt RB, editor: *Atlas of female infertility surgery,* ed 2, St Louis, 1992, Mosby–Year Book.)

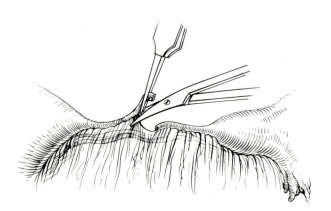

Fig. 47-40. The fibrous band joining the tubal segments is divided and dissected toward the proximal tube.

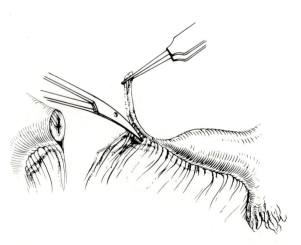

Fig. 47-41. The fibrous band is dissected toward the distal tubal segment.

ing a portion of the band and using the remaining section attached to the proximal segment, the surgeon prepares the proximal segment for anastomosis (Fig. 47-41). The surgeon will have to excise 0.5 to 1.0 cm of tube at the site of previous sterilization, because this section is usually diseased.[6,29,34,35] Because this is an isthmic-to-ampullary anastomosis, the tube is transected at approximately a 30-degree angle. Care must be taken to avoid damaging the underlying vascular tree.

Attention is turned to the lateral segment. The fibrous band attached to it is lifted and dissected to the medial portion of the lateral segment, in this case, ampulla (Fig. 47-41). Using the band as traction, a cap of serosa is excised from the proximal ampulla (Fig. 47-42). None of the muscularis is excised, and the tubal mucosa is not exposed. When dissection of the ampulla is performed, the microelectrode is avoided to lessen thermal damage to the mucosa through this very thin muscle layer.

Applying retrograde lavage or advancing the lavage cannula will identify the most medial portion of the ampullary lumen. This portion is grasped with ring forceps, and a tiny bit is excised, exposing the mucosa (Fig. 47-43). Patency is documented by retrograde lavage. Stay sutures of 6-0 material are placed to align the tubal lumina and to relieve tension (Fig. 47-44). Four sutures of 9-0 material are placed, avoiding the isthmic mucosa but incorporating a tiny bit of ampullary mucosa with the ampullary muscularis. All sutures are tied (Fig. 47-45). After patency is confirmed, serosal sutures of 8-0 material are placed and tied, and additional sutures are placed in the serosa of the mesosalpinx as required.

When placing the inner layer of sutures, visibility may be hampered by ampullary mucosa draping over the surgical site. The mucosa may be brushed back into the ampullary lumen with the needle tip or ring forceps as each su-

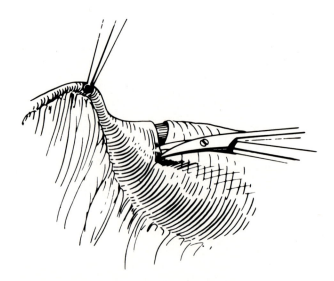

Fig. 47-42. A serosal cap is excised with microscissors. (From Hunt RB, Diaz DG: *Tubal anastomosis.* In Hunt RB, editor: *Atlas of female infertility surgery,* ed 2, St Louis, 1992, Mosby–Year Book.)

ture is placed. Another aid is to lift the 3 o'clock and 9 o'clock sutures superiorly and return the mucosa to the ampullary lumen by irrigation or ring forceps.

Occasionally, a large luminal disparity exists between tubal segments. Two steps lessen this problem. First, the proximal stump is cut at an approximately 30-degree angle. Second, two or three sutures of 9-0 material are placed transversely in the distal segment and tied. The standard anastomosis is then performed (Figs. 47-46 through 47-48). Ampullary obstruction is associated with such conditions as tubal ligation and salpingotomy for ectopic pregnancy (Fig. 47-49). To correct it, the fibrous band or narrowed tube connecting the ampullary segments is divided and dissected away from the underlying vessels

(Fig. 47-50). A peritoneal tract is made over the proximal segment with microscissors, and the tube is transected. Again, care must be taken to avoid damaging the longitudinal vessels (Fig. 47-51). Because there is no luminal disparity, the cut is perpendicular to the long axis of the tube. A similar procedure is performed on the distal segment (Fig. 47-52). A standard anastomosis is carried out (Figs. 47-53 and 47-54), usually requiring approximately six sutures on the inner layer. Patency is documented.

If at least 2 cm of distal ampulla with healthy fimbriae remain and the proximal tube is deciliated or otherwise damaged, the surgeon should consider resecting the proximal ampulla and performing an isthmic-ampullary anastomosis.

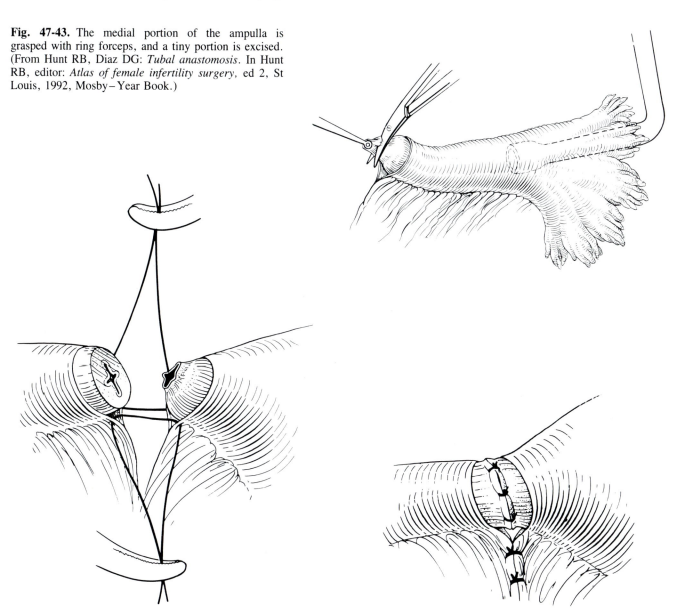

Fig. 47-43. The medial portion of the ampulla is grasped with ring forceps, and a tiny portion is excised. (From Hunt RB, Diaz DG: *Tubal anastomosis.* In Hunt RB, editor: *Atlas of female infertility surgery,* ed 2, St Louis, 1992, Mosby–Year Book.)

Fig. 47-44. The proximal tube has been cut at a 30-degree angle. The luminal disparity is acceptable. (From Hunt RB, Diaz DG: *Tubal anastomosis.* In Hunt RB, editor: *Atlas of female infertility surgery,* ed 2, St Louis, 1992, Mosby–Year Book.)

Fig. 47-45. The inner layer of sutures of 9-0 material has been placed and tied. Serosal and additional mesosalpinx sutures complete the anastomosis. (From Hunt RB, Diaz DG: *Tubal anastomosis.* In Hunt RB, editor: *Atlas of female infertility surgery,* ed 2, St Louis, 1992, Mosby–Year Book.)

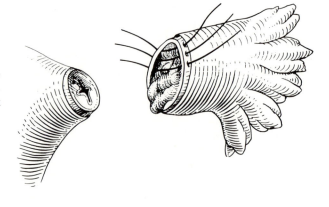

Fig. 47-46. Transverse sutures are placed to correct a luminal disparity unacceptable for anastomosis. (From Hunt RB, Diaz DG: *Tubal anastomosis*. In Hunt RB, editor: *Atlas of female infertility surgery*, ed 2, St Louis, 1992, Mosby–Year Book.)

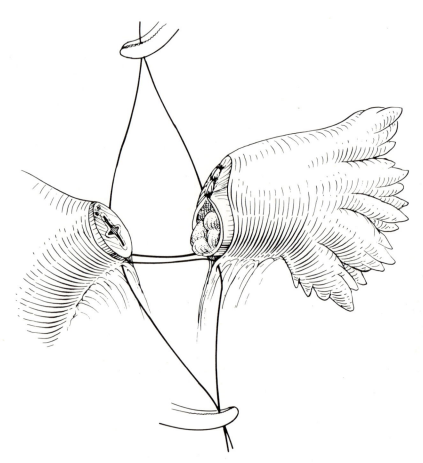

Fig. 47-47. The anastomosis is begun with placement of stay sutures. (From Hunt RB, Diaz DG: *Tubal anastomosis*. In Hunt RB, editor: *Atlas of female infertility surgery*, ed 2, St Louis, 1992, Mosby–Year Book.)

Fig. 47-48. The inner layer of the anastomosis is complete, and stay sutures are tied. The serosal sutures are placed next. (From Hunt RB, Diaz DG: *Tubal anastomosis*. In Hunt RB, editor: *Atlas of female infertility surgery*, ed 2, St Louis, 1992, Mosby–Year Book.)

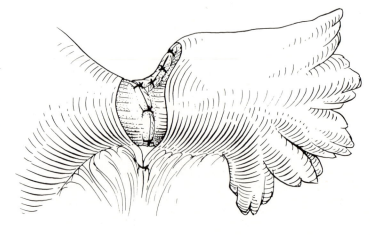

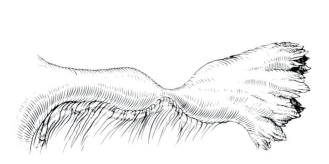

Fig. 47-49. Ampullary obstruction.

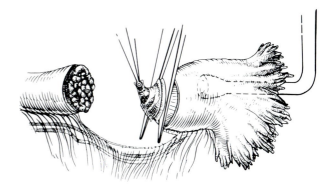

Fig. 47-52. The distal segment is prepared similarly.

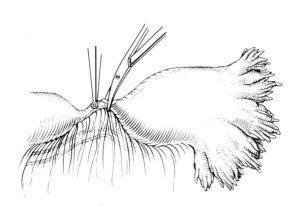

Fig. 47-50. The fibrous band is divided.

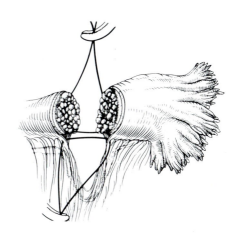

Fig. 47-53. Stay sutures are placed and secured.

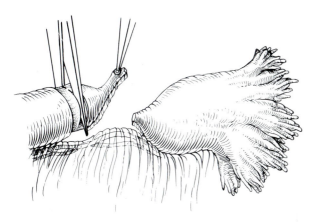

Fig. 47-51. The proximal tube is cut vertically.

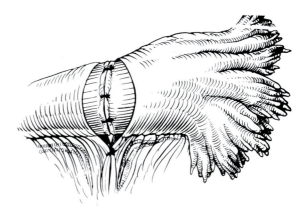

Fig. 47-54. The inner layer of 9-0 sutures is placed and tied. Serosal approximation with 8-0 sutures completes the anastomosis.

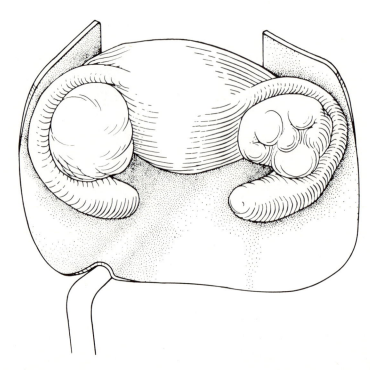

Fig. 47-55. Adhesiolysis has been completed, and exposure is obtained. (From Hunt RB, Verhoeven HC, Schlosser HLS: *Adhesiolysis, fimbrioplasty, and salpingostomy*. In Hunt RB, editor: *Atlas of female infertility surgery*, ed 2, St Louis, 1992, Mosby–Year Book.)

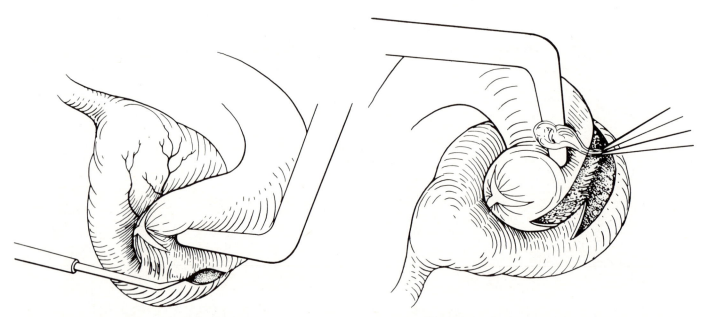

Fig. 47-56. The distal tube is mobilized from the ovary by microscissors, microelectrode, or laser. (From Hunt RB, Verhoeven HC, Schlosser HLS: *Adhesiolysis, fimbrioplasty, and salpingostomy*. In Hunt RB, editor: *Atlas of female infertility surgery*, ed 2, St Louis, 1992, Mosby–Year Book.)

Fig. 47-57. Hemostasis is obtained with bipolar coagulation. (From Hunt RB, Verhoeven HC, Schlosser HLS: *Adhesiolysis, fimbrioplasty, and salpingostomy*. In Hunt RB, editor: *Atlas of female infertility surgery*, ed 2, St Louis, 1992, Mosby–Year Book.)

SALPINGOSTOMY

After adhesiolysis has been accomplished, the surgeon focuses on the distal end of the tube. This is frequently tightly adherent to the ovary and should be released (Figs. 47-55 through 47-57).

I prefer the technique of salpingostomy developed by Kosasa.[17] The distal end of the tube is stabilized with a Babcock forceps and distended with indigo carmine. The distal tube is incised with a microelectrode, and the opening is enlarged with a fine hemostat (Figs. 47-58 and 47-59). Microscissors or laser may also be used. The edges created by the incision are grasped with fine hemostats and rotated outward, providing marked mucosal eversion (Fig. 47-60). If mucosal bridges are encountered, they should be divided. The mucosa is fixed to the serosa with 6-0 sutures (Fig. 47-61). The eversion and suturing processes are repeated until all mucosa has been everted (Figs. 47-62 through 47-64). Tubal and ovarian defects are repaired (Fig. 47-65). After the salpingostomy is completed, the in-

terior of the tube should be inspected with a tuboscope, which provides valuable prognostic information.

In spite of laparoscopic screening, a thick-walled hydrosalpinx is sometimes encountered, requiring modification of the technique. The serosa and tubal muscularis are incised but not through the mucosa (Fig. 47-66). The fibrotic and thickened ampullary serosa and musculature are excised distally (Fig. 47-67). Approximately four incisions are made in the mucosa, and the flaps are sutured to the corresponding serosal sites (Figs. 47-68 and 47-69).

An alternative technique is to excise the very distal end of this thickened tube (Fig. 47-70). Approximately four incisions are made through the full thickness, and the edges are everted and fixed with fine sutures (Fig. 47-71).

To avoid adherence of the adnexae to the lateral pelvic sidewall, the surgeon may develop peritoneal platforms (Fig. 47-72). This is accomplished by placing a 3-0 suture just beneath the lateral one third of the ovary. Several passes are made through the tissue inferior to the ovary,

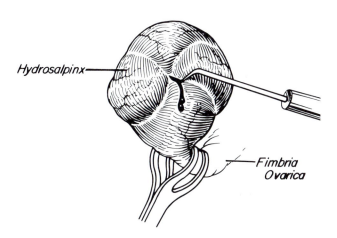

Fig. 47-58. The fimbria ovarica is stabilized with a Babcock forceps, and the distal tube is opened with a microelectrode.

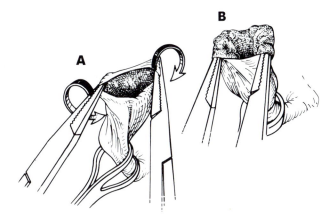

Fig. 47-60. A, The mucosal flaps are grasped with fine hemostats and, **B,** everted by rotation.

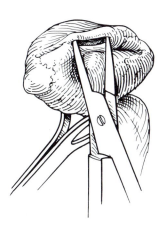

Fig. 47-59. The tubal opening is enlarged with a fine hemostat.

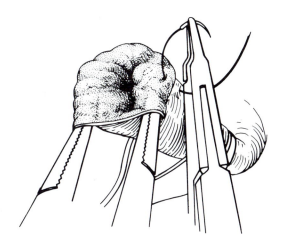

Fig. 47-61. The mucosa is fixed to serosa by interrupted 6-0 sutures.

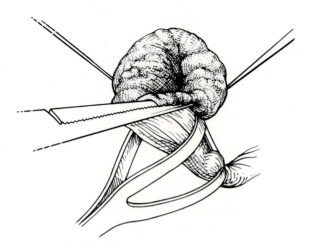

Fig. 47-62. The inferior portion of the mucosal flap is grasped with a fine hemostat.

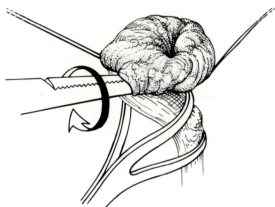

Fig. 47-63. The mucosa is everted by rotation of the hemostat.

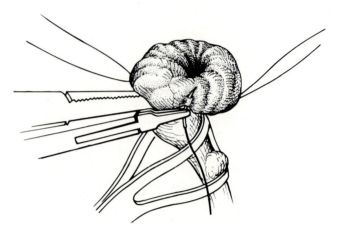

Fig. 47-64. The process is continued until all mucosa is everted and fixed with sutures.

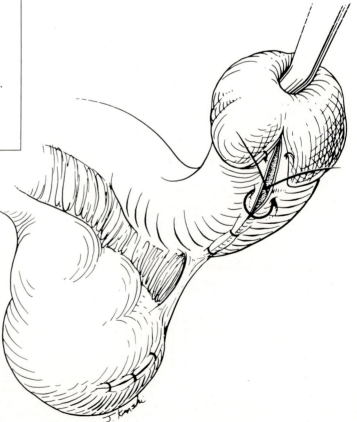

Fig. 47-65. Tubal and ovarian defects are closed as necessary. (From Verhoeven HC et al: *Surgical treatment of distal tubal occlusion, J Reprod Med* 28:293, 1983.)

advancing toward the uterus. The suture is anchored just inferior to the insertion of the uteroovarian ligament into the uterus and tied. The ureter must be kept free of this suture.

To avoid cul-de-sac adhesions, the surgeon may elect to triplicate the round ligaments (Fig. 47-73).

POSTOPERATIVE FOLLOW-UP

I monitor patients carefully, either personally or with the referring physician. At 1 month, patients return for their postoperative checkup. Anastomosis patients are encouraged to attempt conception at that time, but implantation patients are asked to wait for 3 months. At 4 months, a hysterosalpingogram is performed unless contraindicated. The patients are seen every 2 months from then on, with indicated studies and observations to maximize their chances of conceiving. A second-look laparoscopy is considered at 12 to 18 months if conception has not occurred. In addition to detecting reproductive problems, this follow-up gives the patients valuable emotional support.

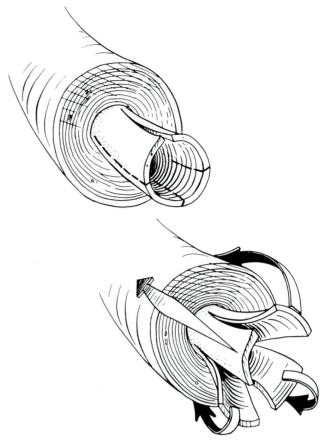

Fig. 47-68. Four incisions are made in the mucosa of the tube. (From Verhoeven HC et al: *Surgical treatment of distal tubal occlusion, J Reprod Med* 28:293, 1983.)

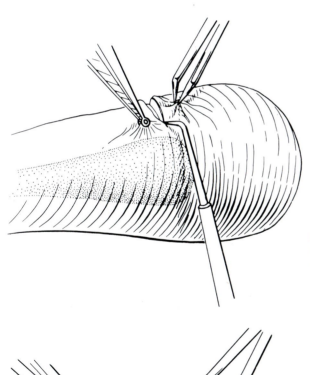

Fig. 47-66. Tubal serosa and muscularis are incised in this thick-walled hydrosalpinx. (From Verhoeven HC et al: *Surgical treatment of distal tubal occlusion, J Reprod Med* 28:293, 1983.)

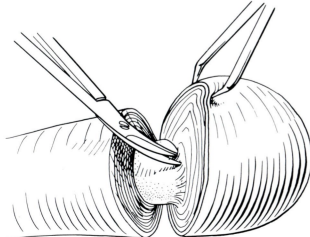

Fig. 47-67. Seromuscular layers of the distal tube are excised. (From Verhoeven HC et al: *Surgical treatment of distal tubal occlusion, J Reprod Med* 28:293, 1983.)

PREGNANCY RESULTS
Tubal implantation

The success of tubal implantation depends on the disease process. When performed to reverse tubal sterilization, the procedure has an excellent prognosis. Of 38 patients in whom sterilization was reversed using the posterior wall implantation technique, 26 (68.4%) had a viable pregnancy. Of 30 patients with pathologic cornual occlusion, 11 (36.7%) achieved a viable pregnancy. In the total series of 68 patients, 4 (5.9%) suffered an ectopic pregnancy.[20]

A series of 60 patients underwent posterior wall implantation either to reverse sterilization or to correct pathologic cornual occlusion. In this group, 45% achieved a pregnancy.[24]

Using a slightly different technique, one author reported pregnancy in 8 of 16 patients. In a brief report 8 years later, the same author described much poorer results and

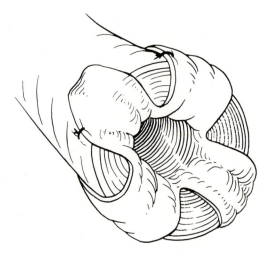

Fig. 47-69. Mucosal flaps are sutured to tubal serosa with fine sutures. (From Verhoeven HC et al: *Surgical treatment of distal tubal occlusion, J Reprod Med* 28:293, 1983.)

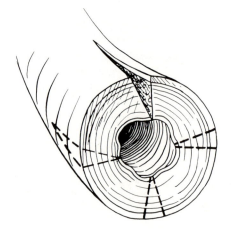

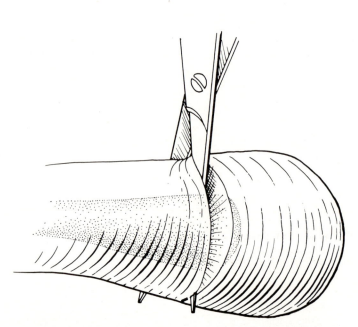

Fig. 47-70. The distal tube is excised in this thick-walled hydrosalpinx. (From Verhoeven HC et al: *Surgical treatment of distal tubal occlusion, J Reprod Med* 28:293, 1983.)

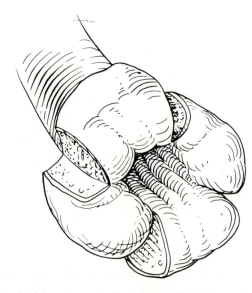

Fig. 47-71. Four incisions are made through the full thickness of the tube, and the flaps are everted and sutured to tubal serosa with fine sutures. (From Verhoeven HC et al: *Surgical treatment of distal tubal occlusion, J Reprod Med* 28:293, 1983.)

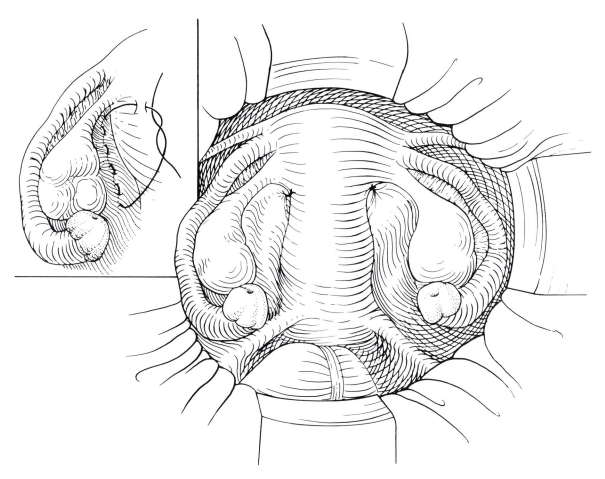

Fig. 47-72. Peritoneal platforms *(inset)* are created to prevent the ovaries from adhering to pelvic sidewalls and posterior broad ligaments. (From Hunt RB, Verhoeven HC, Schlosser HLS: *Adhesiolysis, fimbrioplasty, and salpingostomy*. In Hunt RB, editor: *Atlas of female infertility surgery*, ed 2, St Louis, 1992, Mosby–Year Book.)

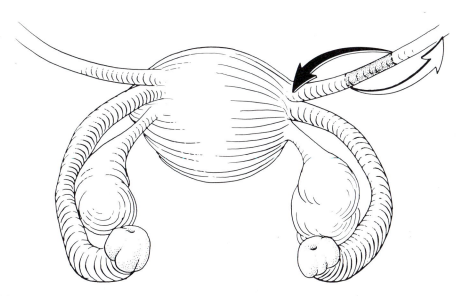

Fig. 47-73. Round ligament triplication. (From Hunt RB, Verhoeven HC, Schlosser HLS: *Adhesiolysis, fimbrioplasty, and salpingostomy*. In Hunt RB, editor: *Atlas of female infertility surgery*, ed 2, St Louis, 1992, Mosby–Year Book.)

concluded that posterior wall tubal implantation has a limited role in the management of cornual occlusion.[28]

Cornual anastomosis

Cornual anastomosis has yielded excellent results. Of 43 patients undergoing the procedure to reverse sterilization, 26 (61%) achieved a pregnancy; 1 had an ectopic gestation.[39] Eighteen (64.3%) of 28 patients had a term pregnancy after cornual anastomosis for mixed indications.[4]

The viable pregnancy rates for correction of pathologic cornual occlusion have also been excellent. In one series, 27 (56.2%) of 48 patients had a term pregnancy, and 3 (6.2%) had an ectopic pregnancy.[10] Of 27 patients in whom this condition was treated by microsurgical anastomosis, 53.2% had a viable pregnancy and 11% had an ectopic gestation.[26] Term pregnancies in three series were 15 (57.7%) of 26 patients,[22] 27 (56.2%) of 48 patients,[11] and 36 (44%) of 82 patients.[5] The ectopic pregnancy rates were 15.4%, 6.2%, and 7%, respectively. A collected series of 506 patients undergoing cornual anastomosis for proximal occlusion revealed 274 (54%) intrauterine pregnancies and 18 (3.6%) ectopic pregnancies.[33]

Tubotubal anastomosis

Reversal of sterilization by tubal anastomosis has produced many reports of superb pregnancy results. Of 118 patients, 93 (78.8%) achieved a term pregnancy; 2 (1.7%) experienced an ectopic pregnancy.[11] The figures in a collected series of 1803 patients were 1149 (63.7%) intrauterine pregnancies and 68 (3.8%) ectopic gestations.[33]

One author reported a 61.1% pregnancy rate after reversal of sterilization when the only or the longer oviduct was 4 cm or less. The mean time for conception to occur was 19.1 months.[38] Another study was not so encouraging. When the longer tube was greater than 7 cm, the delivery rate was 75%; if the longer tube was shorter than 7 cm, it fell to 16%.[15] Significant improvement was reported when the longer oviduct was greater than 4 cm in length.[29] Although the minimal tubal length, particularly ampullary length, required for humans to conceive after reversal of sterilization has not been determined, I proceed with the reversal if there is at least 2 cm ampulla with healthy fimbriae on the longer tube.

Salpingostomy

To determine accurately the intrauterine and ectopic pregnancy rates after salpingostomy, experience has shown the need for prolonged follow-up. A minimum of 5 years is necessary.[1]

The outcomes for 143 patients undergoing distal salpingostomy in one clinic were as follows: 19.6% term pregnancies, 4.2% abortions, and 2.1% ectopic pregnancies.[36] A collected series of 692 patients undergoing microsurgical salpingostomy in seven centers revealed term pregnancy rates between 18% and 31% (median 24%) and ectopic pregnancy rates between 0% and 18% (median 10%).[1]

A collected series taken from 14 centers and including 1275 patients undergoing salpingostomy revealed a term pregnancy rate of 21% and an ectopic pregnancy rate of 8%. Patients with a favorable prognosis had a term pregnancy rate of 59%, compared to 4% in those judged to have a poor prognosis. The ectopic pregnancy rate rose predictably, from 4% to 16%, respectively. The authors concluded that patients with poor prognosis should be encouraged to have in-vitro fertilization (IVF) instead of surgery, whereas surgery seemed most reasonable in patients with either a favorable or an intermediate prognosis. The authors based this recommendation on a collected series from 22 IVF centers reporting 7713 cycles in which ova were retrieved, resulting in an overall pregnancy rate of 12%.[21]

The Mayo Clinic experience revealed a term pregnancy rate of 29% for 71 patients undergoing salpingostomy. The rate was 39% in patients with moderate adhesions compared with 27% in those with severe adhesions.[37] This is consistent with the findings of a direct correlation between the extent and type of adhesions and successful pregnancy outcome reported elsewhere.[14]

In a collected series of 135 patients undergoing repeat salpingostomy reported by five centers, term pregnancy rates varied from 8.4% to 33% (median 10%).[1]

SUMMARY

Surgical management of most tubal obstructions yields positive results; however, continued research and honest reporting of surgical results are essential. Seldom are corrective surgery and assisted reproductive technologies mutually exclusive, and they should not be considered competitive.

REFERENCES

1. Bateman BG, Nunley WC Jr, Kitchin JD III: Surgical management of distal tubal obstruction—are we making progress? *Fertil Steril* 48:523, 1987.
2. Blandau RJ: Comparative aspects of tubal anatomy and physiology as they relate to reconstructive procedures, *J Reprod Med* 21:7, 1978.
3. Claman P et al: Danazol therapy for proximal obstruction of the oviduct, *J Reprod Med* 31:687, 1986.
4. Diamond E: A comparison of gross and microsurgical techniques for repair of cornual occlusion in infertility: a retrospective study, 1968-1978, *Fertil Steril* 32:370, 1979.
5. Donnez J, Casanas-Roux F: Prognostic factors influencing the pregnancy rate after microsurgical cornual anastomosis, *Fertil Steril* 46:1089, 1986.
6. Donnez J et al: Tubal polyps, epithelial inclusions, and endometriosis after tubal sterilization, *Fertil Steril* 41:564, 1984.
7. Ehrler P: Anastomose intramurale de la trompe, *Bull Fed Soc Gynecol Obstet* 17:866, 1965.
8. Fortier KJ, Haney AF: Pathologic spectrum of uterotubal junction obstruction, *Obstet Gynecol* 65:93, 1985.
9. Gomel V: Microsurgical reversal of female sterilization: a reappraisal, *Fertil Steril* 33:587, 1980.
10. Gomel V: An odyssey through the oviduct, *Fertil Steril* 39:144, 1983.

11. Gomel V: *Microsurgery in female infertility,* Boston, 1983, Little, Brown.

12. Gomel V, McComb P, Boer-Meisel M: Histologic reactions to polyglactin-910, polyethylene, and nylon microsuture, *J Reprod Med* 25:56, 1980.

13. Hedon B, Wineman M, Winston RML: Loupes or microscope for tubal anasomosis? An experimental study, *Fertil Steril* 34:264, 1980.

14. Hulka JF: Adnexal adhesions: a prognostic staging and classification system based on a five-year survey of fertility surgery results at Chapel Hill, North Carolina, *Am J Obstet Gynecol* 144:141, 1982.

15. Hulka JF, Halme J: Sterilization reversal; results of 101 attempts, *Am J Obstet Gynecol* 159:769, 1988.

16. Hunt RB, Acuna HA: *Pelvic preparation and choice of incision.* In Hunt RB, editor: *Atlas of female infertility surgery,* Chicago, 1986, Mosby–Year Book.

17. Kosasa TS, Hale RW: Treatment of hydrosalpinx using a single incision eversion procedure, *Int J Fertil* 33:319, 1988.

18. Laufer N et al: Macroscopic and histologic tissue reaction to polydioxanone, a new, synthetic, monofilament microsuture, *J Reprod Med* 29:307, 1984.

19. Leader A et al: Histologic reaction to a new microsurgical suture in rabbit reproductive tissue, *Fertil Steril* 40:815, 1983.

20. Levinson CJ, Lam F: *Tubal implantation.* In Hunt RB, editor: *Atlas of female infertility surgery,* Chicago, 1986, Mosby–Year Book.

21. Marana R, Quagliarello J: Distal tubal oclusion: microsurgery versus in vitro fertilization; a review, *Int J Fertil* 33:107, 1988.

22. McComb P: Microsurgical tubocornual anastomosis for occlusive cornual disease: reproducible results without the need for tubouterine implantation, *Fertil Steril* 46:571, 1986.

23. McCormick WG, Torres J: A method of Pomeroy tubal ligation reanastomosis. *Obstet Gynecol* 47:623, 1976.

24. Musich JR, Behrman SJ: Surgical management of tubal obstruction at the uterotubal junction, *Fertil Steril* 40:423, 1983.

25. Neff MR, Holtz GL, Betsill WL Jr: Adhesion formation and histologic reaction with polydioxanone and polyglactin suture. *Am J Obstet Gynecol* 151:20, 1985.

26. Patton PE, Williams TJ, Coulam CB: Microsurgical reconstruction of the proximal oviduct, *Fertil Steril* 47:35, 1987.

27. Pauerstein CJ: Why has not man a microscopic eye? *Fertil Steril* 34:289, 1980.

28. Peterson EP: Uterotubal implantation—a reappraisal, *Fertil Steril* 39:401, 1983.

29. Rock JA et al: Tubal anastomosis following unipolar cautery, *Fertil Steril* 37:613, 1982.

30. Rock JA et al: Comparison of the operating microscope and loupe for microsurgical tubal anastomosis: a randomized clinical trial, *Fertil Steril* 41:229, 1984.

31. Rosch J et al: Selective transcervical fallopian tube catheterization: technique update, *Radiology* 168:1, 1988.

32. Sojo D, Pardo JD, Nistal M: Histology and fertility after microsurgical anastomosis of the rabbit fallopian tube with nylon and polyglactin sutures, *Fertil Steril* 39:707, 1983.

33. Sotrel G: *Tubal reconstructive surgery,* Philadelphia, 1990, Lea & Febiger.

34. Stock RJ: Postsalpingectomy endometriosis: a reassessment, *Obstet Gynecol* 60:560, 1982.

35. Vasquez G et al: Tubal lesions subsequent to sterilization and their relation to fertility after attempts at reversal, *Am J Obstet Gynecol* 138:86, 1980.

36. Verhoeven HC et al: Surgical treatment for distal tubal occlusion, *J Reprod Med* 28:293, 1983.

37. Williams TJ: Surgical procedures for inflammatory tubal disease, *Obstet Gynecol Clin North Am* 14:1037, 1987.

38. Winston RML: The future of microsurgery in infertility, *Clin Obstet Gynecol* 5:607, 1978.

39. Winston RML: Reversal of tubal sterilization, *Clin Obstet Gynecol* 23:1261, 1980.

Chapter 48

SURGERY TO REPAIR DISORDERS OF DEVELOPMENT

Sir John Dewhurst

The variety of genital tract malformations is infinite. Some, to be sure, fall into regular patterns and are the ones most commonly seen; even among these, minor differences are to be found that need to be taken into account if correct treatment is to be undertaken.

Fusion defects of the uterine body are a good example of the variations to be found within a single group of malformations. The uterus may be of normal outline with a septate cavity, or its external appearance may be clearly bicornuate. If septate the septum may be thick or thin and may be complete down to the internal os or may stop at any point between there and the fundus. If bicornuate the horns may be equal in size or one may be poorly developed or rudimentary and with or without a patent orifice.

Similar differences are to be found within other more commonly encountered groups such as that in which there is vaginal obstruction by a membrane, which is usually close to the hymen but may be much higher in the vagina. Variations such as these, and many that are rarer and more bizarre, clearly show how important it is to consider each individual malformation on its own merits and to determine precisely what the state of affairs may be so that appropriate treatment can be chosen.

A question that gynecologists often ask themselves when confronted with an unusual malformation is "How can we explain this in terms of normal development?" The answer is that one cannot explain bizarre malformations in terms of what normally occurs. Malformations are, by definition, abnormal, and many cannot be explained as simple variations of the normal. More importantly, if one assumes some variation of the normal when confronted by an abnormality, errors of diagnosis and management are likely to be made.

Most of the malformations to be discussed in this chapter are development errors, the reasons for which are un-

known. Those concerning intersexuality fall into a different category since their causes can generally be determined.

ABSENCE OF THE VAGINA

When the vagina is absent, the uterus is absent too in all but the rarest cases. This section will consider the more common abnormality of congenital absence of vagina and uterus; the problem presented by the absent vagina and functioning uterus will be dealt with later under the heading of Genital Tract Obstruction.

Diagnosis

The diagnosis of congenital absence of the vagina is not usually difficult. The patient, who displays normal secondary sexual development, has primary amenorrhea but—and this is a most important feature—no symptoms suggesting that blood is collecting in the pelvis. Examination reveals a normal vulva apart from an imperforate vaginal orifice (Fig 48-1) but without the bulging often seen in patients with hematocolpos. A rectal examination discloses no pelvic mass of retained blood.

Investigations need not be elaborate. An ultrasound scan[7] will show no pelvic collection of blood, such as that shown in Fig. 48-18, and the uterus will not be seen. At the same time the renal area should be scanned since in a significant percentage of cases renal anomalies coexist with vaginal ones. If the scan shows two normally situated kidneys, an intravenous pyelogram (IVP) may be omitted, but if an anomaly is suspected it is best to proceed to the IVP to identify precisely the abnormality in question: a kidney may be absent (Fig. 48-2) and the remaining one normal or abnormal in appearance and position. Magnetic resonance imaging (MRI)[76] may well have a place in these investigations in the future. Laparoscopy, although fre-

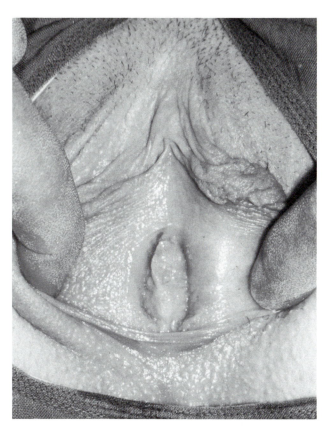

Fig. 48-1. The vulva in a patient with congenital absence of the vagina. Note that apart from absence of the vaginal opening, the vulva is of normal appearance. (From Dewhurst J: *Female puberty and its abnormalities,* Edinburgh, 1984, Churchill Livingstone.)

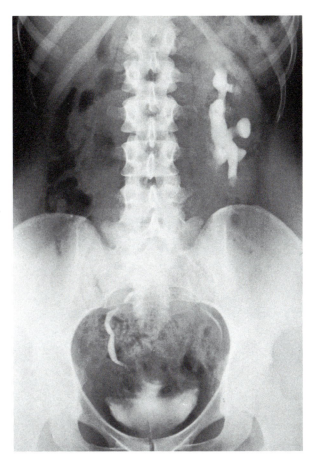

Fig. 48-2. An IVP showing a single abnormal kidney and ureter in a patient with congenital absence of the vagina.

quently employed to confirm the absence of the uterus and the presence of normal ovaries, is generally unnecessary since all this information can be obtained from the above observations and studies. If the operation is employed, the presence of a pelvic kidney should be eliminated first for fear of injury. When viewing the pelvis through the laparoscope, it must be remembered that the ovaries are often placed more laterally than usual and may escape detection unless the instrument is directed toward the pelvic side walls.

In differential diagnosis in the adolescent the condition to be remembered is androgen insensitivity,[19] with presenting symptoms of primary amenorrhea in a 46XY phenotypic female patient with a short blind vagina and absent pubic hair. This sparsity of pubic hair is the important physical sign, which calls for chromosomal analysis to reveal the 46XY karyotype.

The diagnosis of congenital absence of the vagina in the infant or child is not easy. Since, except in cases of hydrocolpos, mentioned later, there is no retained fluid in the pelvis, the distinction cannot easily be drawn between vaginal absence and an imperforate membrane. An ultrasound scan[50] can again be helpful here. If a uterus can be seen on the scan, the likelihood is that the diagnosis is an imperforate membrane; if there is no uterus or upper vagina to be seen, the diagnosis is probably congenital absence of the vagina.

A condition often mistaken for congenital absence of the vagina in a young child is labial adhesions.[15,18] Here the labia minora stick together in the midline, obscuring the normal vaginal orifice (Fig. 48-3). If it is remembered that in a patient with an absent vagina, the vulva is otherwise normal, the distinction between this condition and the grossly abnormal vulva of a girl with labial adhesions can easily be drawn.

Management

The management of an adolescent with congenital absence of the vagina calls, first and foremost, for a gentle, sympathetic approach in which the problem is explained to the girl in simple terms and she is made to understand what can be done for her. The realization that, suitably treated, she can live a normal sexual life can transform a depressed, withdrawn teenager into an optimistic, cooperative young lady. Time spent with such a patient, outlining what can be done and how it might be achieved, is invaluable to the ultimate result, as a number of earlier writers have stressed[28,41,65]; Edmonds[22] gives an excellent ac-

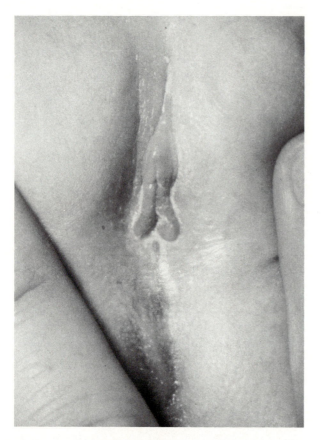

Fig. 48-3. Labial adhesions completely obscuring the vaginal introitus. The condition is often mistakenly diagnosed as congenital absence of the vagina. Compare with Fig. 48-1.

count of the correct approach to these sensitive young women, and Poland and Evans[61] look at the problem in detail.

Whatever form of treatment is employed the girl's wholehearted cooperation is required, and in order to give this kind of cooperation to the full, there needs to be a degree of emotional maturity, which the younger adolescent may not yet have. The timing of the discussions and of the start of treatment must be carefully decided after an assessment of the patient's attitude and maturity. A rapport must be established between patient and therapist, and there is much to be said for involving a young female physician or knowledgeable nurse in these discussions at an early stage so that this kind of helpful relationship can come about between two people of the same sex and similar age.

The most difficult point to manage is the inevitable infertility of the affected patient. To help her accept this, very gentle, sympathetic handling indeed is necessary.

Several choices of treatment are available[71]; this may be surgical or nonsurgical. If an operation is to be performed, various techniques can be employed.

Nonsurgical treatment. Nonsurgical techniques should be explored first since, in a considerable proportion of cases, success may be achieved without operation. The ba-

sis of this approach is the graduated dilatation method of Frank.[34]

Where the vagina should be, there is loose connective tissue, which can be indented to quite an extent by the examining finger (Fig. 48-4, *A*) or a dilator or, in rare cases, a penis. Many senior gynecologists have encountered a patient without a vagina who was unaware of it—and so was her husband since his repeated attempts at coitus gradually created a large vaginal indentation (Fig. 48-4, *B*).

The patient should be made aware that, with her cooperation—and only with her cooperation—a vagina can be made by this form of graduated dilatation. Dilators, similar to that shown in Fig. 48-5, *A*,, are placed against the fourchette, and firm pressure is kept up for, say, 15 minutes twice a day or more often if this is possible. Slowly, over several months, the dilator will go farther and farther in until a full-length vagina can be achieved (Fig 48-5, *B*). In my own unit, a few years ago, 50% of patients with congenital absence of the vagina were treated successfully in this way.[24] More recently, under my colleague and successor, D.K. Edmonds, a success rate of 80% has been achieved.[22]

One matter that sometimes limits the value of this approach is that the hand holding the dilator gets tired. Ingram[42] tried to avoid this by the ingenious method of using dilators graduated for length and circumference and worn inside a panty belt; almost continual dilatation was achieved by having the girl sit on a bicycle seat mounted as a stool, the ridge of the seat giving a firm upward thrust to the dilator.

It must be emphasized that, whatever approach is employed, the patient's enthusiasm will inevitably flag from time to time and must be reinforced by the attendant supervising her case.

Surgical techniques. A number of ingenious methods have been devised for the surgical creation of an artificial vagina. Some, although enjoying success in the hands of their originator, have not been widely adopted and will not be described in this chapter; these include the Vecchietti[79] and Davydov[13,68] procedures. Three methods will principally be considered here: the Abbe-McIndoe-Read procedure, in which the new vagina is lined by a split skin graft; a similar operation in which human amnion is used instead of skin; and the Williams vulvovaginoplasty. On rare occasions one will encounter an anteriorly placed anus in association with absence of the vagina. A mold cannot be used in this circumstance, and the perineum is too short for a vulvovaginoplasty. A new vagina can be made using cecum with success, but the procedure is a surgical tour de force.

The use of split skin grafts. In this procedure, described first by Abbe,[1] then by McIndoe and Banister,[52,53] but modified since by a number of authors,* a space is created, largely by blunt dissection, between rectum and bladder. An incision is first made across the region of the

---

*References 10, 30, 33, 36, 40, 44, 65, 66, 70.

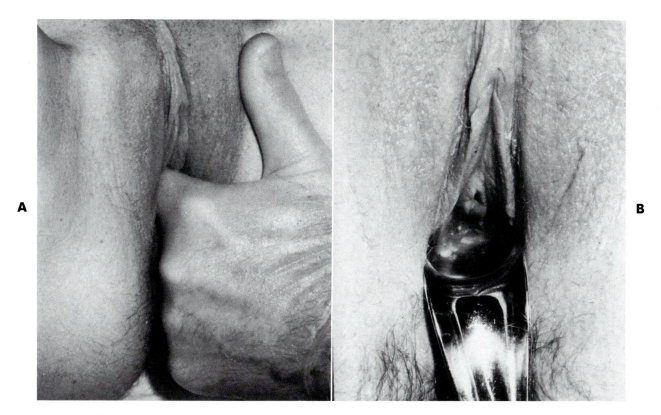

Fig. 48-4. A, A finger indenting the loose tissue in the space that the vagina, which is here congenitally absent, should occupy. **B,** A Sims speculum passed for its full length into a "vagina" created by coitus.

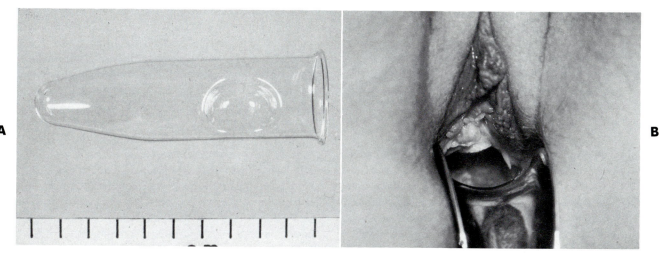

Fig. 48-5. A, A type of dilator used in the graduated dilatation method of vaginal construction. **B,** A vagina created by Frank's graduated dilatation method.

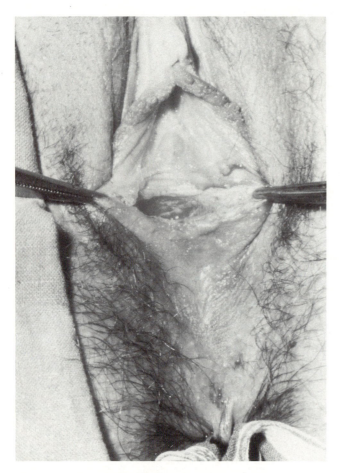

Fig. 48-6. The initial transverse incision across the fourchette prior to blunt finger dissection to dissect the space for the new vagina.

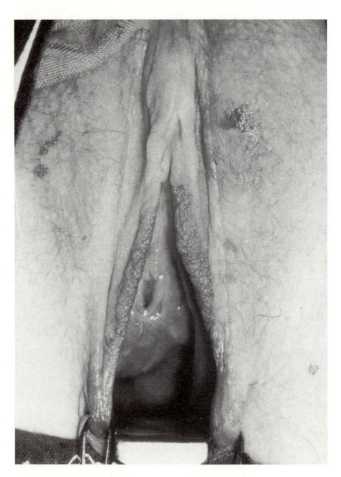

Fig. 48-7. Following the incision shown in Fig. 48-6 the space for the new vagina has been easily constructed by finger dissection. The cavity is clean and dry and ready for grafting.

fourchette (Fig. 48-6) and deepened to about 0.5 cm. The knife is then put aside and, by blunt finger dissection, a space some 10 to 12 cm in length can be achieved in 10 minutes or so (Fig. 48-7). The finger pressure must be exerted laterally and not posteriorly or the rectum may be entered. Gauze pressure or temporary packing is usually sufficient to achieve hemostasis. A variation of this method of creating the space was described by Sheares,[33,70] in which ordinary Hegar dilators are used to stretch up the region of the paramesonephric ducts on each side of a midline septum between them, which is then divided by scissors.

This space is then lined by a split skin graft taken from the buttock, thigh, or suprapubic region (Fig. 48-8). The gynecologist may do this if he or she feels able, or a plastic surgeon may be asked to undertake this part of the procedure. The graft is then sewn onto a suitable mold so as to enshroud it completely, with, of course, the deep surface of the graft facing outward so that it will be in contact with the newly created vaginal walls. The molds originally used were rigid ones of dental stent or other material, but a more malleable form made from folded foam rubber packed firmly into a condom is now preferred (Fig. 48-9). It should be of sufficient length and bulk to fit snugly into the new cavity for a distance of some 10 cm or slightly

more; it should not be so large as to bring undue pressure on the rectum, urethra, or bladder, lest pressure necrosis lead to a fistula. The labia are then approximated with silk sutures to hold the mold in place.

Variations concern mainly the postoperative management. For example, McIndoe[52,53] originally left the mold in place for 3 months, and when it was removed, a glass one of similar size was worn every night for 6 weeks. Jackson[44] removed the original rigid mold after 2 weeks, washed out the cavity, and inserted a sponge rubber one covered with a condom, closing the perineum over it once more and leaving it in the patient for 4 to 5 months. Sheares[70] removed the mold for the first time after 21 days, thereafter teaching the patient to insert and remove it, although it was to be left in situ most of the time for 2 months. At the opposite extreme, Farber and Mitchell[30] left the mold in for only 1 week, after which it was inserted 3 times a day until full coital activity was established.

It will be apparent that these and other minor differences are aimed at the avoidance of contraction of the new vagina, which will inevitably result unless prevented by the prolonged wearing of a mold, repeatedly passing it, or by the practice of frequent regular coitus. Undoubtedly the

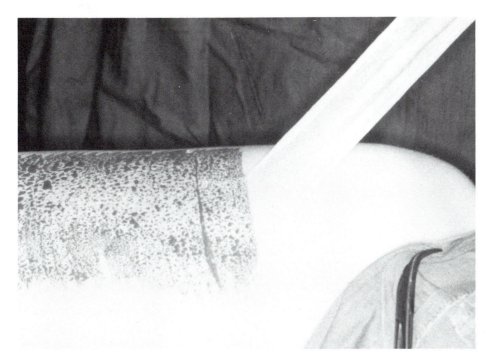

Fig. 48-8. Split skin graft being taken from the thigh.

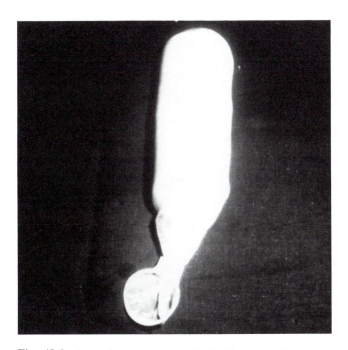

Fig. 48-9. A condom has been packed with foam rubber onto which skin or amnion will be applied.

prolonged suturing together of the labia is uncomfortable and distressing, so that removal of the mold after, say, 2 weeks, followed by repeated insertions of it, accompanied whenever possible by wearing it at night, recommends itself most.

There can be no doubt that in the hands of experienced, capable operators results can be excellent. Jackson,[44] reviewing 128 vaginoplasties, for example, showed a satis-

factory anatomic result in 109 (85%), and Rock et al[66] reported satisfactory coitus in all of 79 patients, although in 7 (9%) the anatomic result was judged imperfect.

Nevertheless, the operation is not without its complications. Fistula formation[32] is the most serious, and if this occurs during the course of the operation the procedure should be abandoned and treatment to close the fistula employed first before reoperation on the vagina is considered. It is these reoperations that carry the greatest danger of fistula formation since the dissection through tough fibrous tissue is much more difficult than that through the loose, soft tissues at the first operation.

The donor site from which the graft has been taken is often painful during the postoperative period and unsightly thereafter. For this reason my preference is for the use of human amnion as a graft instead of split skin.

The use of amnion. When human amnion is to be used, the entire surgical procedure, up to the point of coating the mold, is the same as that just described.[3,56] Amnion is then used instead of skin.

The amnion is obtained, within a day or two of the vaginal procedure if possible, from the placenta of a parturient who has been tested and found negative for acquired immunodeficiency syndrome (AIDS). It may be taken at elective cesarean section, emergency section with membranes ruptured for less than 12 hours, or even at uncomplicated vaginal delivery. The following steps are then taken.

1. Careful washing of the membranes in sterile saline
2. Separation of the chorion from the amnion, leaving a tiny piece attached to identify which surface of the amnion is which

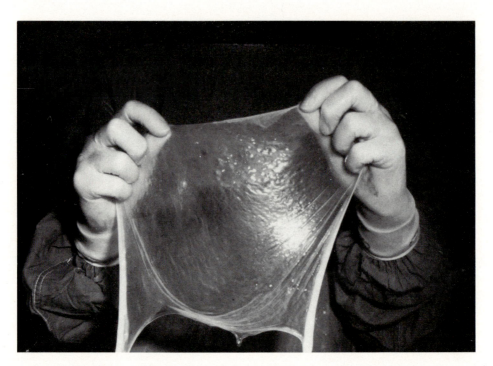

Fig. 48-10. A suitable piece of human amnion cleaned and ready for use.

3. Storage at 4° C in an ordinary refrigerator in sterile saline containing 100,000 U of penicillin per 100 ml, to which solution hydrogen peroxide has been added

In the operating room the amnion is again washed well (Fig. 48-10) and draped around the mold, as described above, with its deep—or mesothelial—surface outward; the mold is then inserted as above and the labia approximated. After 1 week the mold is removed, the cavity of the new vagina—which now appears lined with a glistening white membrane—is irrigated with hydrogen peroxide, and the mold is then coated with a second piece of amnion, reinserted, and left for a second week. Management thereafter is as above. As with the Abbe-McIndoe procedure, there are variations of this procedure. Dhall[20,21] does not make a second application of amnion but, after 1 week, allow the patient to remove and reinsert the mold herself and to wear it as often as possible.

The results of constructing an artificial vagina using this method appear at least as good as when a skin graft is employed; indeed the quality of the vaginal epithelialization may be superior. It has been reported that in 20 patients managed in this way all were successful provided that coitus began 6 to 8 weeks after the operation.[1] My own experience of over 30 cases confirms this. Nevertheless, the risk of contraction of the new vagina is as great as when skin is used, and efforts to prevent this are mandatory until regular coitus is practiced.

The main advantage of amnion over skin is that there is no painful or unsightly donor site on the patient's leg or buttock. The disadvantage is the theoretical risk of transmitting AIDS to the recipient. Time alone will tell whether this risk is a real one and if preliminary treatment of the amnion with hydrogen peroxide,[23] which has been reported to render it safe in this respect, can be relied upon. Certainly the capacity of the amnion to stimulate epithelialization appears not to be adversely affected by hydrogen peroxide treatment.[37]

The Williams vulvovaginoplasty. This procedure[31,81] has several advantages over the other two methods.[1] It is simple to perform and takes only some 20 to 25 minutes; no molds are needed, and the new canal has no tendency to contract even though the vagina is neither dilated nor used for natural coitus for some time after the operation.

The technique is as follows. An indwelling catheter is first inserted into the bladder; if this step is forgotten, insertion of the catheter later may be very difficult since the urethral orifice is covered by the skin of the new vagina. A U-shaped incision is then made in the vulva 4 cm lateral to the midline and passing anterior to the urethral orifice for a similar distance (Fig. 48-11, *A*); the base of this U passes across the region of the fourchette in a gentle curve. The incision is deepened to go through the superficial tissues, but a really deep incision is not required. The edges are freed by gentle undercutting and careful separation of the tissues with scissors to render them loose. The internal skin edges on each side are then brought together in the midline with fine catgut (Fig. 48-11, *B*); there may be some advantage in placing these stitches so that the knots lie within the new vagina. This inner layer complete, the outer skin edges are brought together over it, closing the original incision in such a way that a cavity or pouch is constructed between the outer skin and that of the region of the vaginal introitus and urethral orifice (Fig. 48-11, *C*).

If any deep suturing is undertaken, it should be limited

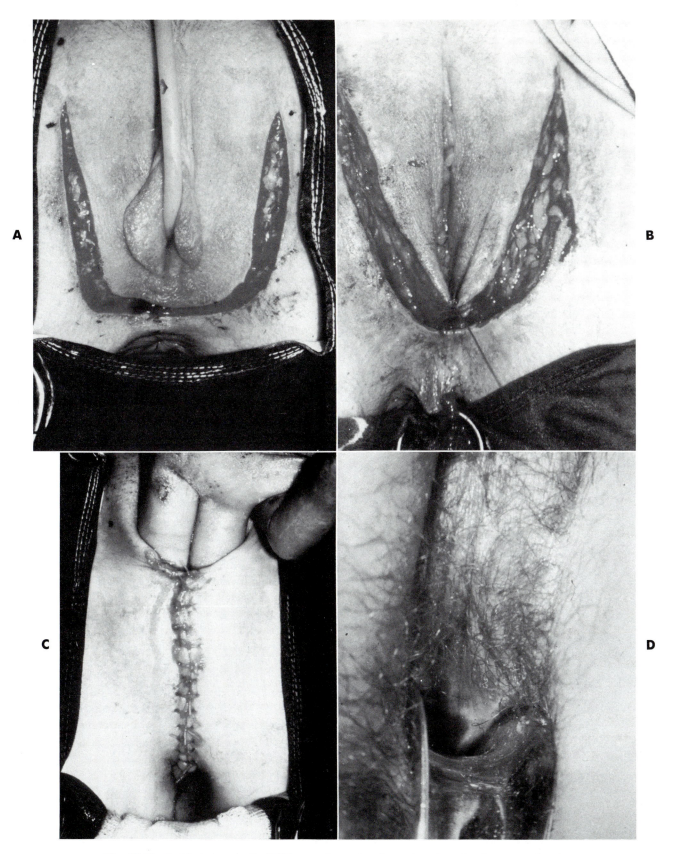

Fig. 48-11. A, First steps in the Williams vulvovaginoplasty. A catheter has been passed and a U-shaped incision made. **B,** The incision has been deepened, and the inner layer is being sutured; the cavity of the new vagina can be seen. **C,** Both layers have been sutured, and the site of the new vagina is shown. **D,** A Sims speculum inserted for its full length into the vagina constructed by the Williams method.

to, at the most, one or two stitches to bring loose tissues together in the posterior part of the area; if several deep sutures are put firmly in place, they will effectively constrict the cavity that is to form the new vagina. The pouch so formed should be some 10 cm long and capable of receiving one and a half to two fingers at the conclusion of the operation (Fig. 48-11, *D*).

The urethral catheter should stay in place for 5 or 6 days and may then be removed. While in place it should be strapped upward onto the abdomen or it may drag posteriorly onto the anterior stitches of the incision and break them down.

Several advantages of this operation have already been enumerated, to which must be added good coital results with orgasm, perhaps because the angle of the new vagina allows maximum clitoral stimulation during penile insertion. It is worthwhile remembering, too, that should the new vagina prove unsatisfactory later, for any reason, the original status quo can easily be restored and another vagina made by either of the methods described above (Fig. 48-12).

Disadvantages are minor and include the unusual angle of the new vagina, minor urinary difficulties, calling perhaps for manual squeezing out from the vagina of the last few drops of urine at the end of micturition, and the occasional turning in of hair-bearing skin. These disadvantages tend to become less evident in time. The angle of the vagina changes as repeated intercourse depresses the superficial part of the new vagina while indenting the deepest parts farther into the region of the introitus; this improves any earlier urinary problems there may have been. The turning in of hair-bearing skin is a theoretical concern that I have never found to be a problem, since such hair becomes thin.

An interesting modification of this operation was reported by Capraro and Capraro.[9] Realizing that the success of the procedure depended to some extent on the penile tip indenting the region of the introitus—in a similar fashion to the graduated dilatation procedure described above—they constructed a shorter vagina that did not obscure the vaginal introitus; good results have been reported from both the original technique and this modification.[12,32]

The Williams vulvovaginoplasty is applicable to most patients with congenital absence of the vagina. Exceptions are where the perineum is very shallow, the vulval tissues unusually rigid, or the labia minora large and fleshy; in this latter instance, because these labia fill the newly constructed vagina and cause problems, they may be removed beforehand.

Other procedures. Exceptionally, patients are seen with congenital absence of the vagina who are not suitable for any of these procedures. These include, principally, the rare patient in whom the anus is displaced so far forward that a mold placed into a newly created cavity would inevitably exert great pressure on the rectum and anus with fistula formation. In these uncommon cases cecum has been satisfactorily used in a technique devised by Richard Turner-Warwick at the Middlesex Hospital, London.[55] A full-length abdominal incision is required, and the omentum is mobilized from the greater curve of the stomach on a pedicle from the right gastroepiploic artery. Cecum is mobilized on a vascular pedicle, and end-to-end ileocolic anastomosis restores bowel continuity. A dissection is then made between bladder and bowel down to the introitus, and into this is led the cecum wrapped in omentum for protection and additional blood supply. The technique can give excellent results when little else will do but is a formidable one only to be attempted by surgeons of excellence. Burger et al[8] report a similar procedure.

GENITAL TRACT OBSTRUCTION

The genital tract may be obstructed by any degree of failure of canalization, from absence of the whole vagina and cervix, at one extreme, to persistence of a thin imperforate membrane. Clinical features vary depending upon the position and extent of the obstruction; treatment may be extremely simple or incredibly difficult.

Obstruction by a membrane

The most common condition to result from the presence of an imperforate membrane in the vagina is hematocolpos

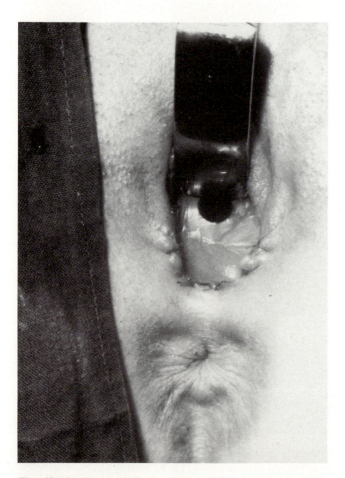

Fig. 48-12. Construction of a new vagina by the McIndoe technique after a Williams vulvovaginoplasty has been taken down. Skin has not yet been applied to the mold.

beginning at puberty; much less commonly, clinical features become evident in the newborn in the condition of hydrocolpos.

Uncomplicated hematocolpos is usually seen in a 13- to 16-year-old girl who has never menstruated and who complains of intermittent lower abdominal pain, which may or may not be at more or less monthly intervals. If nothing is done, more and more blood collects in the vagina, causing difficulty in emptying the bladder and culminating in acute retention of urine (Fig. 48-13).

Examination of such a patient will show her to have normal secondary sexual development, a substantial lower abdominal swelling—the overfull bladder perched on top of a vagina full of blood, a tense membrane just deep to the hymen, and, on rectal examination, a cystic swelling in front of the examining finger. If the membrane—often called an imperforate hymen, although the hymen can frequently be distinguished from it (Fig. 48-14)—is very thin it may appear blueish and bulge markedly; if thicker there may be neither bulging nor discoloration.

The condition constitutes an acute emergency, in view of the retention of urine. Treatment consists of simple incision of the membrane, which will release a quantity of dark, thickish blood. The redundant portions of the membrane may then be snipped away until an adequate opening has been made for drainage and subsequent coitus. Nothing more need be done—indeed nothing more should be done, since to explore the vagina further or to attempt to douch out the blood may introduce infection. It is rare for any further treatment to be required; usually normal menstruation follows and subsequent fertility is unaffected. Any concern there may be that blood has been retained in one or other tube—a rare event indeed—can be dispelled by an ultrasound scan, which will display normal internal pelvic organs.

Histologic examination of the excised membrane is not without interest. The external and internal aspects of it will usually show stratified squamous epithelium, but on occasion the deep surface may show columnar epithelium.[25]

The higher the membrane in the vagina, the more likely it is that its deep surface will have a columnar lining (Fig. 48-15).

When the obstructing membrane is at a higher level in the vagina, a condition that is rarer but that may occasionally be seen, the retained blood will in all probability be above the level of the bladder neck, and urinary obstruction will not be a feature; other aspects of the case are similar, however, as is treatment. It is of particular interest that sometimes—and especially when the obstruction is higher in the vagina—the proximal vaginal segment shows the presence of vaginal adenosis when it is inspected after the obstruction is relieved.[2,20]

The condition corresponding to hematocolpos in the newborn child is hydrocolpos (Fig. 48-16).[15,22] Here the retained fluid is milky white in color and, presumably, represents the combined secretions of the cervix and vagina. These are usually small in amount and, even if there is obstruction, cause no clinical features until their volume is added to at puberty by menstrual flow. Occasionally these neonatal secretions are sufficient in amount to produce a large abdominal swelling, a bulging introital membrane, and urinary retention. So large may the abdominal

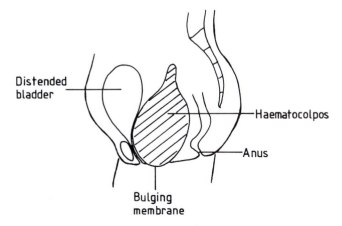

Fig. 48-13. Diagrammatic representation of hematocolpos. (From Dewhurst J: *Female puberty and its abnormalities,* Edinburgh, 1984, Churchill Livingstone.)

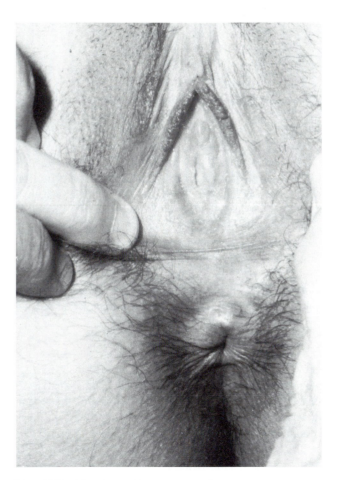

Fig. 48-14. The obstructing membrane in a case of hematocolpos. The hymen can easily be distinguished from the imperforate membrane.

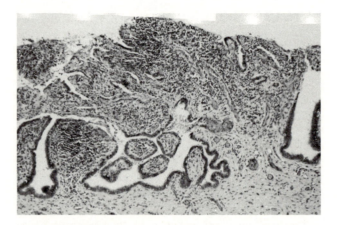

Fig. 48-15. Vaginal adenosis deep to the obstructing membrane in a case of hematocolpos.

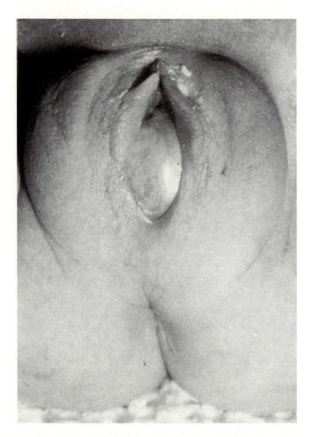

Fig. 48-16. Vulval appearance in a newborn child with hydrocolpos.

swelling be that it has many times been mistaken for an ovarian tumor and the tumor and the abdomen opened—even with fatal results.

Proper treatment is very simple; the membrane should be incised and the retained milky fluid released.

In any of these forms of obstruction, an ultrasound scan of the kidneys should be undertaken at some convenient time.[3] If both appear normal, well and good; if not, an IVP should be undertaken.

Complicated hematocolpos

Under this heading[17] will be discussed all forms of genital tract obstruction due to more than a simple membrane. The least rare forms of these abnormalities are those in which the vagina is absent in part and those in which the genital tract is double and one half is obstructed.

Absence of part of the vagina shows some clinical features that are similar to those of ordinary hematocolpos but others that are different. The patient is of similar age, with primary amenorrhea and good secondary development. There is cyclic, but not necessarily regular, abdominal pain. There is no retention of urine, however, since the obstruction is at a higher level than the bladder base (Fig. 48-17); nor is there a bulging swelling at the introitus, although this is imperforate. The mass of retained blood is palpable at a higher level on rectal examination and is less easy to identify clearly.

The most helpful investigation by far in this group of cases is an ultrasound scan (Fig. 48-18).[6,49] This not only demonstrates the presence of retained blood but also gives some indication of the height at which the blood is retained. Therefore an estimate can be made of the amount of vagina that is absent, which is far from easy to do on examination. If a hematosalpinx is also present, this should be evident.

The management of these cases can be comparatively easy but tends to show increasing difficulty the more vagina is absent. If it is thought that only some 2 to 3 cm of vagina are absent, a dissection can be undertaken from be-

low with every expectation that the lower pole of the retained blood will be easily found and drained (Fig. 48-19). If more than this is absent a dissection may be started from below, but if difficulty is experienced in finding the blood—and such difficulty is commonplace—it is prudent to open the abdomen so that palpation from above and below can direct the dissection into the retained blood and not into the rectum or bladder; injury to either will seriously complicate an already difficult problem. If, at the outset, it is thought that only a small amount of vagina is patent close to the cervix, it is wise to open the abdomen first to establish precisely what the state of affairs is and to guide the dissection from below.

By this type of approach it is usually possible to locate the collection of blood and let it out. This is only half the battle, however, and the easy half at that. The difficult part is keeping the vagina open thereafter. The procedure of vaginal advancement[45] is helpful in those patients in whom a relatively short segment of vagina is missing. After draining the blood, the stretched vaginal skin of the upper portion is brought down to line the new lower part and stitched to the region of the introitus (Fig. 48-20). This maneuver can work well, but there is a tendency for the upper portion to retract, and a ring of constriction may develop later at the point where the upper skin was fixed to

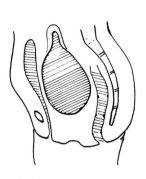
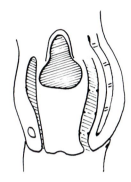

Fig. 48-17. Two diagrams showing retained blood at a higher level in cases of partial vaginal atresia. (Courtesy of Longman Group, Ltd.)

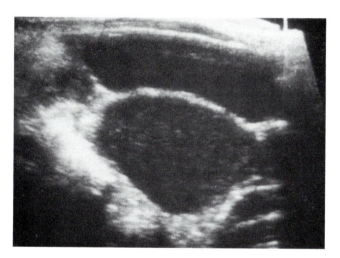

Fig. 48-18. Appearance on ultrasound scan in a case of hematocolpos due to absence of the lower part of the vagina. (From Dewhurst J: *Female puberty and its abnormalities,* Edinburgh, 1984, Churchill Livingstone.)

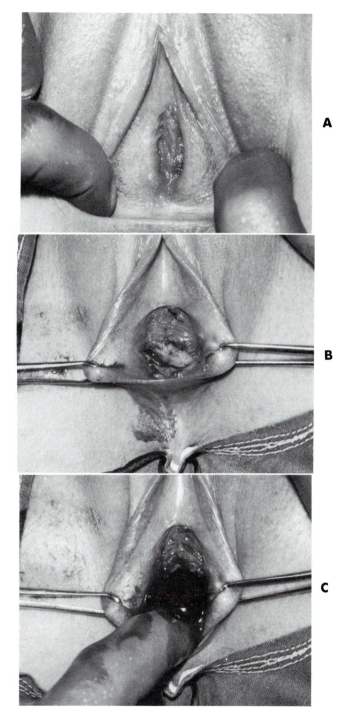

Fig. 48-19. A, Absence of lower 2 cm of the vagina in a case of hematocolpos; appearance before surgery. **B,** Dissection is in progress, and retained blood can just be seen. **C,** Blood is released.

the introitus, which has now retracted back up the vagina; this may need division later.

If the vagina is absent for more than half its length, this procedure of vaginal advancement will probably not suffice. When all the retained blood has drained away, which takes only a few days as a rule, the patient can begin taking a combined oral contraceptive continuously to prevent further endometrial breakdown, and the new portion of the vagina can be grafted with amnion or skin. This has the same tendency to contract as in the construction of an entire new vagina, so regular passage of a dilator of suitable size, which may be worn also at night, is essential. The problem is that since the emergency nature of the case may necessitate operating on a younger, and therefore less mature, adolescent, the patient cooperation so essential to success may be less than wholehearted. If the patient is young both in years and emotionally, there is much to be said for postponing the operation for several years, keeping her symptom-free meanwhile by a 2-monthly injection

of Depo-Provera or by the continuous use of a combined oral contraceptive.

Brief mention must be made of those well-nigh impossible cases in which the vagina and cervix are both absent and blood is retained within the uterine body and tubes.[29,62,82] Symptoms are similar to those described

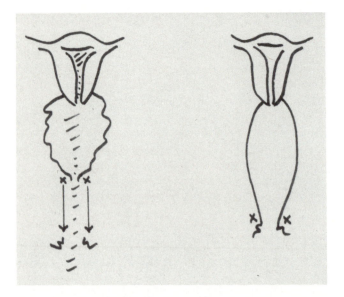

Fig. 48-20. Diagrammatic representation of the operation of vaginal advancement. The stretched vaginal skin lining the upper vagina (seen on the left) is brought down to line the new lower vaginal canal. (From Dewhurst J: *Female puberty and its abnormalities,* Edinburgh, 1984, Churchill Livingstone.)

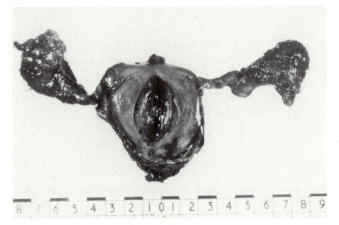

Fig. 48-21. Specimen removed from an adolescent girl with hematometra due to absence of the vagina and cervix. Pelvic adhesions were widespread and both tubes badly damaged, necessitating radical treatment.

above, but determination of the exact state of affairs by clinical examination is far more difficult. Precise diagnosis rests first upon the appearance of the ultrasound scan and ultimately on the findings at laparotomy.

The theoretical management of such serious cases consists of constructing a vagina by the use of a split skin graft or human amnion and artificially canalizing the cervix to drain the retained blood. A hollow tube of some kind must then be left through the cervix for some weeks or even months to keep this artificial canal open. The success rate of such procedures is woefully small, and the risk of pelvic sepsis from the presence of the intrauterine drain is high. Because of these two factors the gynecologist must seriously question whether an attempt at cervical canalization is reasonable or not. This depends to some extent upon the condition of the other pelvic organs. If both tubes are distended with blood and blocked, as they are very likely to be, and there are, in addition, widespread pelvic adhesions, serious thought must be given to hysterectomy, despite the youth of the patient (Fig. 48-21). If the condition of the other pelvic organs is more favorable and the cervical block can be overcome, this must be tried first and consideration of hysterectomy left until the response to conservative treatment has been determined.

Endometriosis,[67,69] usually in the ovaries but sometimes on the pelvic peritoneum also, is almost always seen whenever there is high genital tract obstruction. Relief of the obstruction is generally sufficient to permit these endometriotic lesions to regress, but a short course of danazol, or similar therapy, may occasionally be considered wise.

The clinical problems produced by a double genital tract are discussed below under the heading of Fusion Defects. Mention must be made here, however, of those cases in which one half of a double tract is blocked (Fig. 48-22).

Cyclical, if not necessarily regular, lower abdominal pain in an adolescent with good secondary sexual development is again the presenting symptom. The main difference from those cases of hematocolpos already discussed is that, since the other half of the genital tract is normal and functioning, there is no symptom of primary amenorrhea. The cyclical pain nevertheless calls for investigation, and a cystic swelling extending well down the patent vagina will be detected on either rectal or vaginal examination. An ultrasound scan,[6,49] either conventional or with a rectal or vaginal probe, will clarify the picture. A renal scan will show absence of the kidney on the side of the obstruction in most instances.

Management of the obstruction is not difficult once a correct diagnosis has been made. The septum between the patent and the imperforate vaginas should be opened widely and the blocked vagina drained into the patent one. The only minor surgical problem that these cases present is due to the emerging blood obscuring the field and preventing a really large opening being made in the septum. If this should occur, it is wise to reexamine the patient under anesthesia a few days later when all the blood has drained away so that the opening can, if necessary, be enlarged. If only a tiny hole is made, this may be inadequate for proper drainage and may close later, causing reappearance of symptoms. As in the case of a high obstructing membrane, the proximal section of the blocked vagina may show evidence of vaginal adenosis.[2,25]

Should the retained blood be in a rudimentary horn that has no connection with the other uterus or with the vagina, diagnosis is much more difficult. Examination may reveal a unilateral swelling, which ultrasound will help to identify. Removal of the rudimentary horn is almost always

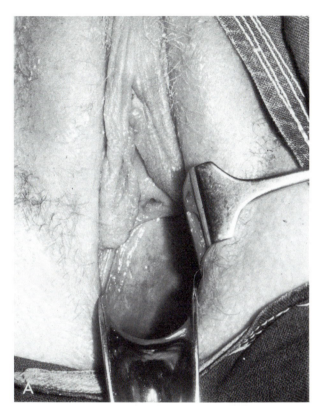

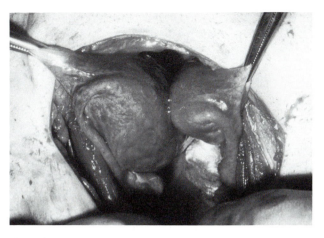

Fig. 48-23. Retained blood in the left horn of a bicornuate uterus. The horn had no connection with the vagina, and its cervix was absent, necessitating hysterectomy on the left side.

Fig. 48-22. Unilateral hematocolpos. The speculum has been inserted into the patent vagina revealing the bulging mass of blood in the blocked vagina before incision to release it. (From Dewhurst J: *Female puberty and its abnormalities,* Edinburgh, 1984, Churchill Livingstone.)

necessary (Fig. 48-23). Even should it be possible to establish a permanent drainage hole to the outside, a pregnancy in such a poorly developed horn would be likely to lead to uterine rupture long before viability.[57]

FUSION DEFECTS

The uterus and most of the vagina develop from the fusion in the midline of bilateral paramesonephric ducts. This fusion is sometimes less than complete, and a variety of fusion faults result. The main examples of these are as follows (Fig. 48-24).

1. The arcuate uterus where a small fundal depression is the only departure from the normal. Such a uterus is without clinical significance.
2. The uterus bicornis unicollis (bicornuate uterus), which has two distinct horns and a single cervix.
3. The septate uterus, which has a normal external outline but a cavity that is divided in part or in whole by a septum. This form of abnormality, and the bicornuate uterus above, constitute lesions of clinical significance.
4. The rudimentary uterine horn, which represents a considerable hazard should a pregnancy implant in it.
5. The uterus didelphys, in which there are two uterine

cavities with or without a septate vagina. Only the septate vagina, if present, is likely to require surgical treatment unless, as already discussed, one half of the double tract is blocked.
6. A septate vagina with no fault at a higher level. This is a simple abnormality easily corrected.

Other bizarre forms of fault are very rarely seen. The unicornuate uterus is not, strictly speaking, a fusion defect, and since it is not susceptible to surgical correction it will not be described further.

In the absence of obstruction to part of a double tract, these abnormalities come to light clinically only after coitus or conception.

Dyspareunia may result from the presence of a vaginal septum, but many patients with a small septum remain unaware of it until it is noticed during a vaginal examination (Fig. 48-25).

Infertility is not usually the result of a fusion abnormality and, if present in a patient with such an abnormality, is likely to be explained by some other fault.

Recurrent reproductive failure, such as abortion or premature labor, is the most common symptom of the bicornuate or septate uterus,[7] and it is this feature that may call for surgical treatment. The uterus didelphys may be associated with premature labor or, less commonly, with recurrent abortion at an earlier stage in pregnancy but is not an indication for surgical unification attempts. The rudimentary horn may cause cyclical pain if there is obstruction to menstrual outflow or may rupture during pregnancy[57] when the poor uterine development can no longer contain the enlarging fetus; I have recently encountered two such examples with profuse intra-abdominal bleeding around 4 months of pregnancy.

Reproductive failure

This feature is classically associated with the bicornuate or septate uterus. However, a patient becoming pregnant

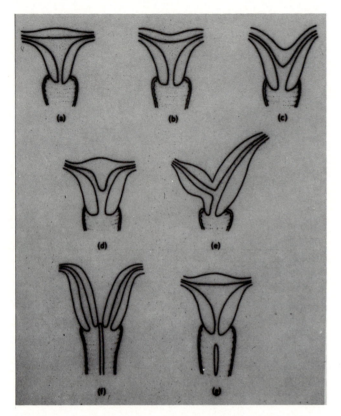

Fig. 48-24. Diagrammatic representation of the various forms of fusion defect of the uterus and vagina. **A,** Normal. **B,** Arcuate fundus of no clinical significance. **C,** Uterus bicornis unicollis. **D,** Septate uterus. **E,** Rudimentary horn. **F,** Uterus didelphys. **G,** Normal uterus with septate vagina.

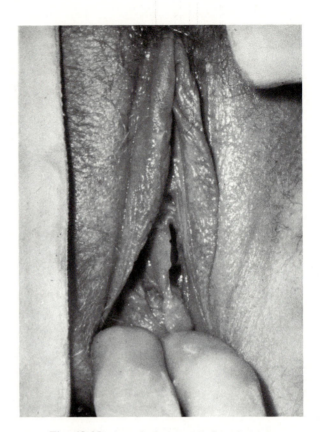

Fig. 48-25. A vaginal septum before division.

with either abnormality is more likely to have a successful than an unsuccessful pregnancy; approximately 60% of pregnancies in patients with these fusion faults can be expected to have a live child, although this may be born somewhat prematurely. Nonetheless, a considerable number of women remain whose pregnancies may not reach viability and who may be considered candidates for a surgical procedure to unify the endometrial cavity.

Such cases must be carefully selected for surgery. Should a bicornuate or septate uterus be discovered in a patient with a history of recurrent pregnancy loss, a metroplasty operation is not automatically the answer. It is important to eliminate any other possible cause first,[47] such as, for example, cervical incompetence or husband-wife histocompatibility. If these and other causes can be excluded, good results attend various metroplasty procedures. An abdominal operation is necessary in the case of the bicornuate uterus, but for a septate uterus, a hysteroscopic approach now seems a simpler and more realistic one.

In attempting to determine the precise abnormality present, hysterography, hysteroscopy, and laparoscopy are all necessary (Fig. 48-26). Ultrasound examination may be

of some help[31,59] but is unlikely to be as useful as in other types of cases already discussed.

For the management of the bicornuate uterus, the Strassmann[74,75] operation or some modification of it is preferred (Fig. 48-27). The technique I have employed is first to instill 1 ml of methylene blue into the uterine cavity through the cervix. This outlines the cavity well and facilitates opening it when the uterus is incised. The abdomen is then opened, and a transverse incision is made across the fundus of the two horns, beginning a little anterior and medial to the insertions of the fallopian tubes, care being taken not to approach too near to them. The incision is deepened into the cavity of the uterus for its whole length. Bleeding can be quite brisk at this point unless a Bonney's myomectomy clamp or a tight rubber catheter has been placed around the cervix at the level of the internal os to occlude the uterine arteries temporarily. The transverse incision is then sewn up anteroposteriorly in three layers: a deep layer taking half the thickness of the muscle but not encroaching on the endometrium, a second layer taking most of the remainder of the uterine muscle, leaving a narrow subserous zone into which a subcuticular stitch can be placed.

The operation is not difficult to perform, and its success depends not so much on the surgical skill of the operator as on the care with which the cases for surgery have been selected.

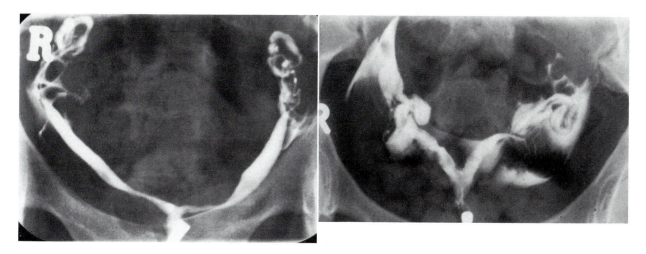

Fig. 48-26. Two examples of bicornuate uteri outlined by hysterography.

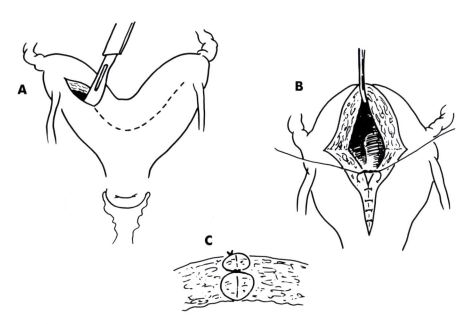

Fig. 48-27. Strassmann operation. **A,** Transverse incision across the bicornuate fundus. **B,** Incision is sewn up anteroposteriorly. **C,** Two layers of sutures are used as shown or three as described in text.

For the abdominal approach to the septate uterus, the technique of Tompkins[77] is advised (Fig. 48-28). The preliminaries are similar to those already described until the abdomen is open and the Bonney clamp in place. The uterus is then incised vertically through its midline, and the incision is carried as far toward the cervix as is necessary to enter the cavity. The uterine body will then be almost in two halves, and the septum of each half can be slit upward toward the cornua so that the right and left cavities of the endometrium are exposed. Any thickened portion of the septum that remains can be excised as appropriate, although this is seldom needed, followed by anteroposterior suturing, which is carried out as before. An alternative to this operation, although one with less appeal, is the Jones procedure,[47] in which a wedge of tissue containing the septum is excised and the organ then reconstituted.

The results of these operations in properly selected cases can be excellent, success rates of 80% or more for subsequent pregnancies being commonly reported; Craig[11] even achieved a 94% success rate.

Admirable though some of these results are, hysteroscopic methods[14,43,59,78] seem likely to replace abdominal ones for the septate uterus in most cases. The procedure has generally been undertaken during the proliferative

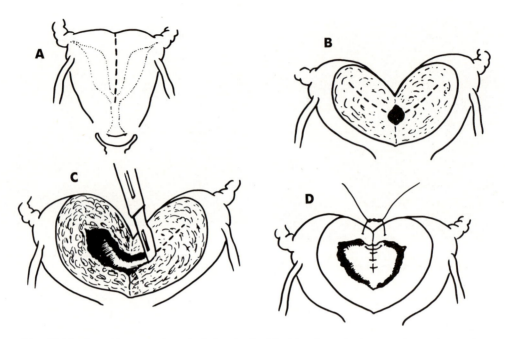

Fig. 48-28. Tompkins operation. **A,** A longitudinal incision is made down to the uterine cavity. **B,** The uterus is almost bisected. **C,** The uterus is incised laterally into the cavity. **D,** Reconstruction is commenced posteroanteriorly.

phase of the cycle and with minimal or no cervical dilatation. Miniaturized semirigid scissors are used, and the relatively avascular septum is snipped upward from below until bleeding is encountered; division is then halted. By this time, in favorable cases, a smooth fundal appearance will be seen and both tubal ostia should be visible. Simultaneous laparoscopy is employed as a precaution against penetration of the uterine wall. Postoperative management involves insertion of an intrauterine device and a period of 1 to 2 months of estrogen therapy. Toward the end of this time a progestogen is given for 5 days to ensure good withdrawal bleeding when these hormones are stopped. The IUD is then removed.

Results appear to be at least as good as those following the Tompkins operation, and there are several advantages to this hysteroscopic technique: short hospital stay, avoidance of an abdominal procedure and a uterine incision, and every chance of a vaginal delivery in a subsequent pregnancy as a result.

Vaginal septum

If a longitudinal vaginal septum is discovered, which has already given rise to dyspareunia or seems likely to do so, its division should be undertaken. This presents no serious surgical problem other than the control of a few bleeding points, and it can be undertaken at any convenient time.

Such a septum is occasionally encountered during pregnancy, when division is recommended. This can safely be undertaken during the second trimester and is indicated to avoid the risk of serious tearing during delivery, which might otherwise occur.

OTHER ANOMALIES

Some reference must now be made to a variety of other malformations that, rare though they be, might be encountered at any time by a gynecologist. A detailed account of these is not appropriate, but some guidance on an approach to management will be provided.

Bladder exstrophy

The problem of bladder exstrophy in the newborn is one for the pediatric surgeon, but because of the vulval deformities that accompany it, a gynecological consultation is sometimes requested.[16,22,47,72]

The most important of the gynecological aspects is an extreme narrowing of the introitus, which may be so marked as to make identification of the opening extremely difficult (Fig. 48-29, *A*). If such difficulty is encountered, an examination under anesthesia while the patient is menstruating is of real help. It seems evident that the labial folds come together in the midline in a manner similar to that seen in cases of congenital adrenal hyperplasia (discussed below). This reduces the size of the vaginal opening to a variable extent.

It is important to realize that deep to these fused folds there is a vagina of normal capacity, which will permit normal intercourse when the opening has been enlarged (Fig. 48-29, *B*). Treatment is simple, a posterior incision exposing the vagina quite easily. Care should be taken not to make this incision too large, however, because of the risk that genital prolapse might follow. The normal supports of the genital organs are greatly attenuated in bladder exstrophy since there is a large bony defect in the fore pelvis and the levator ani muscles are much reduced or ab-

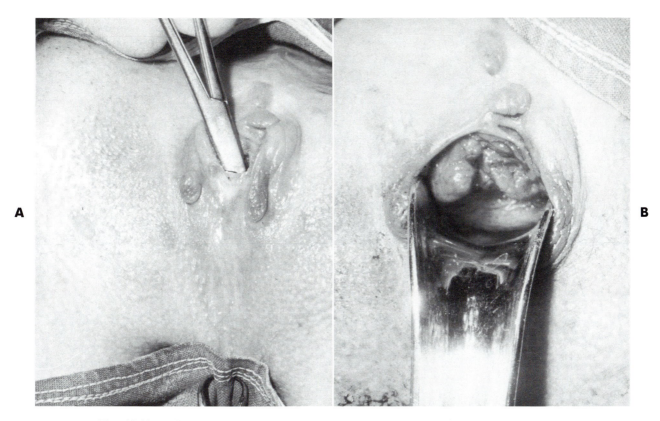

Fig. 48-29. Vulval appearance in an adolescent girl whose bladder exstrophy was managed by urinary diversion in childhood. **A,** Constricted vaginal opening. **B,** A normal vagina exposed after incision of the excessively fused labial folds.

sent. The shelf provided by the fused labial folds has previously prevented genital prolapse from being apparent, but, when incised, a cystocele and vault prolapse may soon follow, even in the early teenage years. For this reason the incision in the folds must be taken no farther back than is essential to allow intercourse.

Should prolapse occur it cannot be satisfactorily repaired by conventional means and some form of sacral fixation procedure is likely to be required.

The deformity of the vulva that arises from the presence of a bifid clitoris, even after the bladder problem has been treated, is an ugly one, and some type of plastic reconstruction may be needed to overcome the feelings of sexual inferiority to which this gives rise. Consideration of the accounts given by earlier authors on this subject[15,26] may prove helpful if confronted by this rare anomaly.

Ectopic anus

During the normal process of development of the anus it migrates posteriorly from a position immediately adjacent to the vagina, which it initially occupies. This posterior migration may either not occur at all, leaving the external bowel opening at the fourchette or even just within the vagina (Fig. 48-30), or may be arrested, with the anus left much further on the perineum than is usual. The actual anal opening in these cases is generally markedly contracted, which interferes with the normal process of defecation.

The abnormality may be managed in a variety of ways by the pediatric surgeon, who often prefers some kind of pull-through procedure. However, one form of treatment is to leave the anal opening where it is, near to that of the vagina, but to incise the contracted anus by a cutback procedure (Fig. 48-31).[22] Anal continence is usually good in patients managed in this way. Moreover, vaginal soiling with fecal matter is uncommon, and intercourse is often possible despite the proximity of the bowel. In earlier years[15] I sometimes attempted a type of perineorrhaphy procedure to achieve greater separation of the two organs, but this approach was later abandoned since little was achieved, the risk of disturbing anal continence was ever-present, and the procedure was, in any event, unnecessary. The maintenance of bowel continence is paramount here, and nothing must be done that might possibly interfere with it. When the patient becomes pregnant, delivery by cesarean section is usually wise.

Cloacal and other gross faults

A gynecologist may occasionally be consulted about a child with an extremely gross genital tract fault such as a high rectovaginal fistula, a complete cloaca, or a reduplicated urethra. Solutions to the most immediate problems in these cases lie with the pediatric surgeons, but if the infant survives childhood, difficult gynecological problems may arise later.

Both cloacal and high rectovaginal fistula cases require

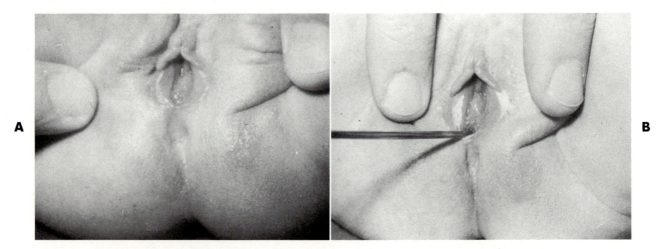

Fig. 48-30. A, Ectopic anus in newborn; anus is absent from its usual site. **B,** Ectopic opening is indicated with a probe.

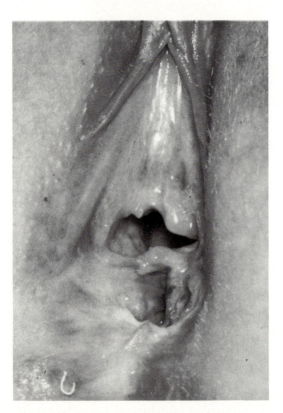

Fig. 48-31. Ectopic anus that has been enlarged by a cutback procedure. It functioned well and did not give rise to vaginal contamination.

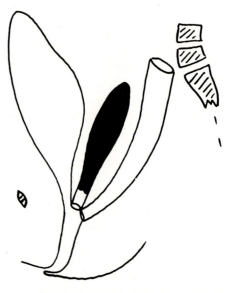

Fig. 48-32. Diagrammatic representation of a child with a cloaca, seen some years ago. Note the sacral agenesis.

an early colostomy after which some assessment of the possibilities of later treatment may be undertaken.* Considerable ingenuity is required to assist those few patients who survive childhood. The coexistence of sacral agenesis in some of these cases is a further complication (Fig. 48-32).

A group of bizarre cases in which a child is born with a

narrow clitoral urethra and a second urethra that opens into the lower vagina has occasionally been reported (Fig. 48-33). The enlargement of the clitoris gives rise initially to doubts about the sex of the child. Whatever the explanation of the clitoral enlargement may be, it appears not to be one of the common ones considered in the section entitled "Intersexual Surgery," which follows. An account such as this can do little more than draw the attention of the reader to the existence of such abnormalities. The variations that have been encountered over the years[4,5,15,37,41] have been so great that these accounts should be consulted for guidance should the need arise. The account by Stephens[73] has always seemed particularly helpful.

*References 15, 27, 25, 39, 58, 80.

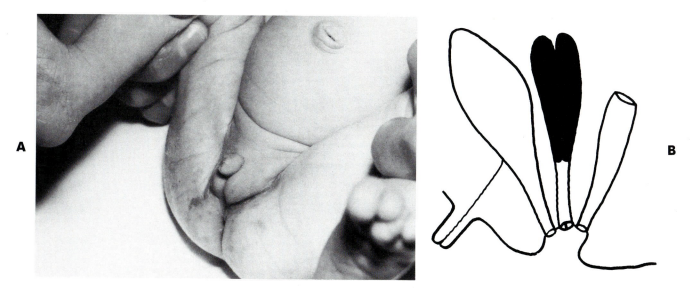

Fig. 48-33. A, A female child with a prominent phallus. **B,** Diagrammatic representation of the findings in this child. There was a cloaca, a double uterus, and a second filiform urethra passing down the enlarged phallus.

INTERSEXUAL SURGERY

The gynecologist may be called upon for several surgical procedures associated with intersexual states, and some account of these is appropriate. The investigations that must be performed before the correct diagnosis is established, and the choice of the more suitable gender role, are complex and require cooperation between specialists in several disciplines: endocrinologists, pediatricians, gynecologists, and others. Diagnosis must be confirmed and a firm decision made on the sex of rearing before any definitive surgery is carried out. Details of the investigations necessary in the various intersexual states will not be included here, but consideration will now be given to the more common forms of surgical operation needed in these intersexual individuals (Fig. 48-34).

Reduction in phallic size

When an intersexual patient is to be brought up in the female role and the phallus is sufficiently enlarged to be or to become a source of sexual embarrassment, reduction in its size should be undertaken. Most of the patients with this kind of large phallus will be infant girls with congenital adrenal hyperplasia (CAH), although a few subjects with this disease may not be seen until puberty. Phallic reduction may also be necessary in true hermaphrodites or in males with such poor external genital masculinization that normal sexual life in the male role will never be possible.

When the patient is an infant with CAH the optimum time for surgery to the clitoris is during the neonatal period soon after birth and before discharge from the hospital. To operate then has two supreme advantages: the infant will almost certainly be under excellent pediatric control of the

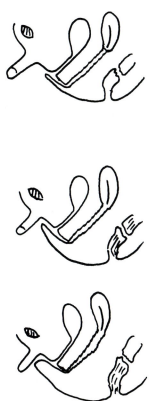

Fig. 48-34. Diagram showing the appearance of patients with congenital adrenal hyperplasia. The clitoris is enlarged in all. In the upper drawing the fused labial folds are thin and barely obscure the urethra; in the middle one the folds are thicker and extend further forward; in the lower drawing the folds are very thick and not only narrow the vagina but extend some distance along the shaft of the clitoris.

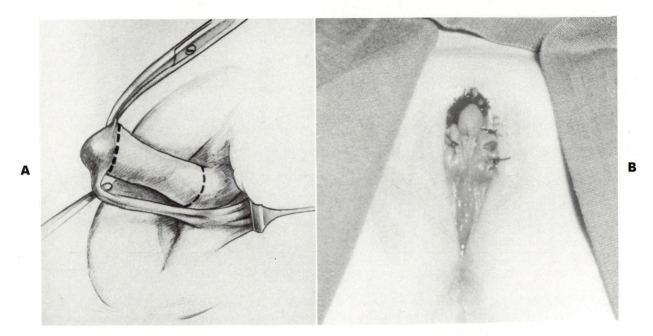

Fig. 48-35. A, Diagram indicates portion of the corpora cavernosa to be excised after preservation of nerve and blood supply. **B,** The preserved glans has been stitched back into place.

adrenal hyperplasia, and the parents can take their daughter home without any external evidence of maleness.

The preferred operation is excision of the corpora cavernosa with preservation of the sensitive glans with its blood and nerve supply (Fig. 48-35). The technique was devised by Dr. Hugh Allen of London, Ontario.[22] Vessels and nerves reach the glans closely applied to the sheath of the corpora on the dorsal surface of the clitoris; an additional blood supply comes from the ventral surface. An incision along the dorsum of the organ allows the skin and subcutaneous tissues to be reflected laterally without difficulty; nerves and blood vessels can be identified and displaced in the same way, leaving the corpora themselves completely isolated. They are then excised, taking the division, at a deep level, toward the region of the fusion of the two crura, although it is not necessary to go quite as deep as this point. The cut ends are firmly ligated and the glans stitched back in its normal place. Redundant skin may be trimmed if required and then closed; a good cosmetic result is easily obtained. Local edema is often evident during the early postoperative period but subsides quickly in most cases.

The same approach to clitoral reduction is used in older patients and is equally applicable whether they are females with congenital adrenal hyperplasia, true hermaphrodites, or 46XY males to be reared as females.

This is easily the most successful surgical procedure I have adopted, and it avoids the need for total amputation, the idea of which distresses parents. Procedures that bend the clitoris ventrally and bury it beneath the skin are not recommended, since discomfort or pain is common later during the erections that accompany sexual excitement.

Exposure of the vagina

In CAH, masculinization due to androgenic drugs, and in true hermaphrodites, excessive fusion of genital folds usually occurs in utero. These folds come together in the midline in front of the vagina and urethra, leaving only a single external opening on the perineum. Surgical division of these fused folds is generally necessary to expose the two orifices satisfactorily. If the folds are thin the division can be performed at virtually any time; if they are thick, and especially if there is narrowing of the lower vagina as well, the division is much more difficult and it is recommended that surgery be postponed until puberty or after (Fig. 48-34).

A simple posterior division of thin folds will easily expose the urethra and vagina. A few stitches are now used to unite the cut edges of the incision, and no more need be done (Figs. 48-36 and 48-37). Even the simplest procedure, however, is best not undertaken on the newborn subject at the same time as clitoral reduction. Bleeding, which is external and easily controlled during the clitoral part of the procedure, is now within the cavity of the infant's tiny, narrow vagina where control is much more difficult. Moreover, a satisfactory result is not always obtained, and I have often been called upon to reoperate after puberty on patients whose original operation had been carried out at a very early age.

With thicker folds it is even more important to postpone this operation until the time of puberty. Simple division may still be sufficient, but if there is narrowing of the lower vagina—and, in extreme cases, the upper vagina as well—extra tissue must be brought into the introital ring. This can be achieved by employing some type of flap procedure (Fig. 48-38).[22]

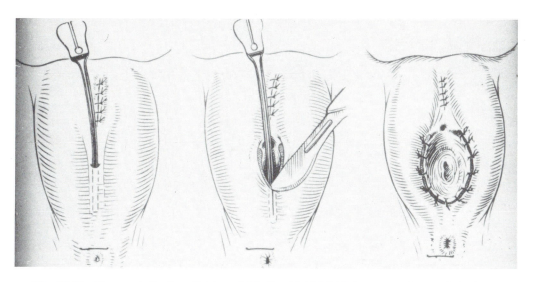

Fig. 48-36. Diagram indicating division of thin fused labial folds in a case of congenital adrenal hyperplasia.

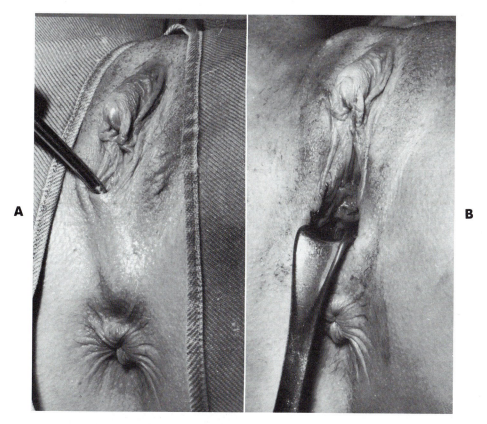

Fig. 48-37. A, Adolescent with fused labial folds due to congenital adrenal hyperplasia. **B,** The folds have been divided exposing a normal vagina.

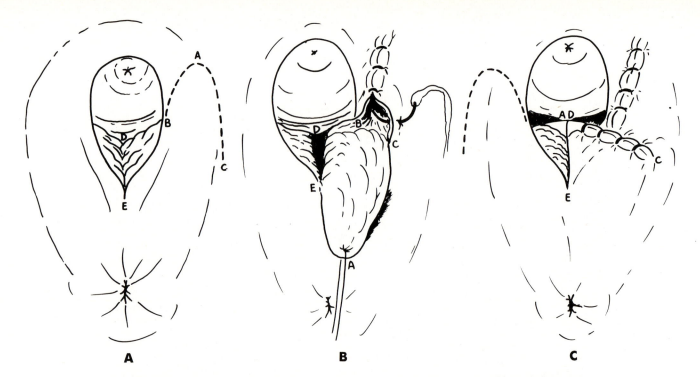

Fig. 48-38. One type of flap operation for enlarging the introitus. **A,** A longitudinal incision is made along the length of the contracted segment of the vagina, and a flap is outlined in which the height from the base to A is not more than $1\frac{1}{2}$ times the length of the base from B to C. **B,** The flap has been turned down and the donor site is closed. **C,** The flap is folded into half the vaginal defect, point A being taken to point D. The procedure is then repeated on the opposite side.

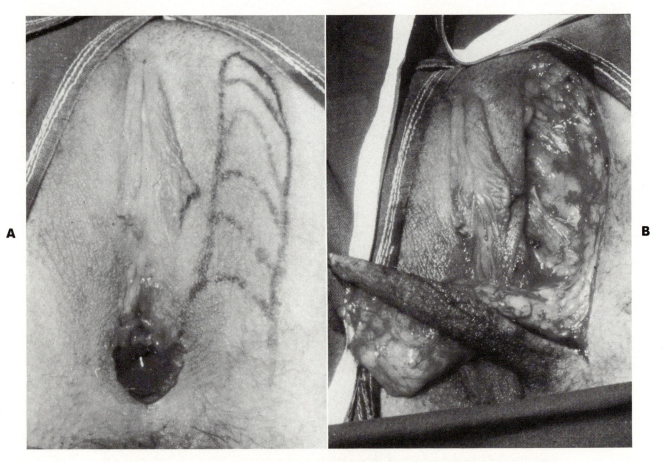

Fig. 48-39. Taking a fasciocutaneous flap. **A,** The vagina has been divided in the midline throughout its narrowed portion, and the area of the proposed flap is outlined. **B,** The flap has been turned down; the amount of bulbocavernosus tissue and fat attached to it can be seen.

The vagina is first divided longitudinally in the midline, carrying the incision completely through the narrowed portion. An inverted V-shaped flap of skin with a little subcutaneous tissue attached is then raised on each side of the vulva, the triangle being so shaped that its vertical height from base to apex does not exceed $1\frac{1}{2}$ times the length of its base, in order to preserve the blood supply. The donor site is then closed, the triangle of skin is folded into the incised portion of the vagina from each side, and the triangles are sutured together. Flaps made in this fashion will probably suffice if the contracted part does not extend more than halfway up the vagina. If it does, such flaps will probably be too short, and longer fasciocutaneous ones will be needed (Fig. 48-39).[54]

A longer flap may now be outlined by skin pencil until its length and width, compared with the extent of the contracted portion of the vagina, seem appropriate. Only one flap need be outlined first since this may be sufficient without a contribution from the other side. The incision is taken right down to the deep fascia so that all the subcutaneous tissues contained within the sides of the flap, including fat and bulbocavernus muscle, are left attached to it, thus ensuring maintenance of its blood supply. The donor site is then closed as before and the flap folded into the narrowed portion of the vagina.

A technique that may be a useful adjunct to any form of flap procedure, and therefore useful in cases such as these where extra tissue is needed in the vagina, is the tissue expansion method reported by Lilford, Sharpe, and Thomas.[51] Inflatable tissue expanders are inserted beneath the labia and the incision through which they were put in place closed. The expanders are then gradually distended with fluid over the next few weeks, so greatly increasing the area of labial skin without interference with blood supply—a useful technique to have up one's sleeve when confronted with a difficult situation for which the usual methods do not appear to offer a satisfactory solution.

Other procedures

Removal of testes is necessary in most 46XY patients being brought up in the female role. Where it is feared that testicular activity at puberty may produce masculinization, which would be greatly distressing to a patient who had lived to that age as a female, the operation should be carried out at any convenient time during childhood. If the removal of the gonads is to be undertaken because of their cancer potential in girls with androgen insensitivity (testicular feminization) who will feminize at puberty, it is better to await the breast development that accompanies this syndrome and to remove the organs once this is complete; their removal in childhood followed by the administration of estrogens seldom achieves comparable breast growth.

The actual removal of the gonads can easily be accomplished by excision and ligation of vessels (Fig. 48-40). When they are retained within the peritoneal cavity they are likely to be located on the lateral pelvic walls, which is where they should be sought. Often they can be seen and palpated in the groins when their removal is even simpler.

Hysterectomy, perhaps of a unicornuate uterus, may be necessary in a true hermaphrodite being brought up in the male role. In such cases identification of the cervix during the operation may be less easy than usual and care should be taken to avoid bladder injury.

Construction of an artificial vagina, or elongation of a very short one, will be needed in genetic males who are to live as females. In androgen insensitivity there is always at least a small dimple present, which should allow elongation by graduated dilatation if the patient is cooperative. If a new vagina is to be constructed, the principles described earlier in this chapter apply. The management of such

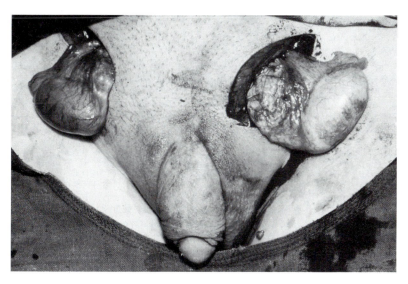

Fig. 48-40. Exposure of the testes in the groins in an intersex individual before their removal.

cases has been the subject of an excellent report by Rock and Jones.[65]

REFERENCES

1. Abbe R: New method of creating a vagina in a case of congenital absence, *Med Rec* 56:836, 1898.
2. Amortegui AJ, Kanbour AI: Diffuse vaginal adenosis with imperforate hymen, *Obstet Gynecol* 53:760, 1979.
3. Ashworth MF et al: Vaginoplasty using amnion, *Obstet Gynecol* 67:443, 1986.
4. Belis JA, Hrabovsky EE: Idiopathic female intersex with clitoromegaly and urethral duplication, *J Urol* 122:805, 1979.
5. Bellinger MF, Duckett JW: Accessory phallic urethra in the female patient, *J Urol* 127:1159, 1982.
6. Bennett MJ: In Bennett MJ, Edmonds DK, editors: *Spontaneous and recurrent abortion,* Oxford, 1987, Blackwell Scientific Publications.
7. Bennett MJ, Dewhurst Sir John: The use of ultrasound in the management of vaginal atresia, *Ped Adol Gynecol* 1:25, 1983.
8. Burger RA et al: Ileocecal vaginal reconstruction, *Am J Obstet Gynecol* 161:162, 1989.
9. Capraro VJ, Capraro EJ: Creation of a neovagina, *Obstet Gynecol* 39:544, 1972.
10. Counsellor VS, Flor FS: Congenital absence of the vagina, *Surg Clin North Am* 25:1107, 1957.
11. Craig CJT: Congenital abnormalities of the uterus and fetal wastage, *South Afr Med J* 47:2000, 1973.
12. Creatsas G, Loutradis D: Our experience of the Williams vaginoplasty, *Ped Adol Gynecol* 2:43, 1984.
13. Davydov SN: Colpoiesis from the peritoneum of the urorectal space, *Obstet Gynecol* (Moscow) 12:55, Dec 1969.
14. DeCherney AH et al: Rectoscopic management of mullerian fusion defects, *Am J Obstet Gynecol* 149:66, 1984.
15. Dewhurst CJ: *Gynaecological disorders of infants and children,* London, 1963, Cassell.
16. Dewhurst Sir John: *Congenital malformation of the lower urinary tract.* In Stanton SL, editor: *Clinics in Obstetrics and Gynaecology: Gynaecological Urology,* vol 5, Eastbourne, 1978, WB Saunders.
17. Dewhurst Sir John: Complicated haematocolpos and haematometra, *Gynecologie* 31:19, 1980.
18. Dewhurst Sir John: *Practical pediatric and adolescent gynecology,* New York, 1980, Marcel Decker, Inc.
19. Dewhurst Sir John, Spence JEH: The XY female, *Br J Hosp Med* 17:498, 1977.
20. Dhall K: Amnion graft for treatment of congenital absence of the vagina, *Br J Obstet Gynaecol* 91:279, 1984.
21. Dhall K: Congenital absence of the vagina; simple surgical procedure for its relief, *Aust NZ J Obstet Gynaecol* 27:240, 1987.
22. Edmonds DK: *Dewhurst's practical paediatric and adolescent gynaecology,* ed 2, London, 1989, Butterworth.
23. Edmonds DK: Personal communication, 1990.
24. Ellis C, Dewhurst Sir John: A simplified approach to management of congenital absence of the vagina and uterus, *Ped Adol Gynecol* 2:25, 1984.
25. Ellis C, Pryse Davies J, Dewhurst Sir John: Vaginal adenosis in the vaginal septum of a double genital tract, *Ped Adol Gynecol* 1:197, 1983.
26. Erich JB: Repair of deformity in bladder exstrophy, Proceedings of the Staff Meetings of the Mayo Clinic 34:235, 1959.
27. Escobar LF et al: Urorectal septum malformation sequence, *Am J Dis Child* 141:1021, 1987.
28. Evans T, Poland ML, Boving RL: Vaginal malformations, *Am J Obstet Gynecol* 141:910, 1981.
29. Farber M: Congenital atresia of the uterine cervix, *Semin Reprod Endocrinol* 4:33, 1986.
30. Farber M, Mitchell GW: Surgery for congenital absence of the vagina, *Obstet Gynecol* 51:365, 1978.
31. Fedele L et al: Ultrasonography in the differential diagnosis of "double" uteri, *Fertil Steril* 50:361, 1988.
32. Feroze RM, Dewhurst CJ, Welply G: Vaginoplasty at Chelsea Hospital for Women: a comparison of two techniques, *Br J Obstet Gynaecol* 82:536, 1975.
33. Fleigner JR: Congenital atresia of the vagina, *Surg Gynecol Obstet* 165:387, 1987.
34. Frank RT: The formation of an artificial vagina without operation, *Am J Obstet Gynecol* 35:1053, 1938.
35. Gale DH, Stocker JT: Cloacal dysgenesis with urethral, vaginal outlet, anal agenesis and functioning internal genito-urinary excretion, *Pediatr Pathol* 7:457, 1987.
36. Garcia J, Jones HW: The split thickness graft technique for vaginal agenesis, *Obstet Gynecol* 49:328, 1976.
37. Gau G: Personal communication,
38. Hansen K, Egholm M: Diffuse vaginal adenosis, *Acta Obstet Gynecol Scand* 54:287, 1975.
39. Hendren WH: Urogenital sinus and anorectal malformation: experience of 22 cases, *J Pediatr Surg* 15:628, 1980.
40. Howkins J, Hudson CN, editors: *Shaw's textbook of operative gynaecology,* ed 5, Edinburgh, 1983, Churchill Livingstone, Inc.
41. Hurwitz RS, Fitzpatrick TJ: Vaginal urethra, clitoral hypertrophy and accessary phallic urethra: a rare syndrome of female pseudohermaphroditism, *J Urol* 127:1165, 1982.
42. Ingram J: The bicycle seat stool in the treatment of vaginal agenesis, *Am J Obstet Gynecol* 140:867, 1981.
43. Israel R, March CM: Hysteroscopic incision of the septate uterus, *Am J Obstet Gynecol* 149:66, 1984.
44. Jackson I: The artificial vagina, *J Obstet Gynaecol Br Commonwealth* 72:336, 1965.
45. Jeffcoate TNA: Advancement of the upper vagina in the treatment of haematocolpos and haematometra caused by vaginal atresia: pregnancy following construction of an artificial vagina, *J Obstet Gynaecol Br Commonwealth* 76:961, 1969.
46. Jones HW: An anomaly of the external genitalia in female patients with exstrophy of the bladder, *Am J Obstet Gynecol* 117:748, 1973.
47. Jones HW, Jones GES: Double uterus as an etiological factor of repeated abortion; indications for surgical repair, *Am J Obstet Gynecol* 65:325, 1956.
48. Kounami T et al: Vaginal and phallic urethra with prominent clitoris in female pseudohermaphroditism, *J Urol* 136:915, 1986.
49. Lange AP et al: Uterus didelphys with obstructed hemivagina diagnosed by transrectal ultrasound scanning, *Ped Adol Gynecol* 1:19, 1983.
50. Lilford RJ, Morton K, Dewhurst Sir John: The diagnosis and management of the imperforate vaginal membrane in the pre-pubertal child, *Ped Adol Gynecol* 1:115, 1983.
51. Lilford RJ, Sharpe DT, Thomas DFM: The use of tissue expansion techniques to create skin flaps for vaginoplasty, *Br J Obstet Gynaecol* 95:402, 1988.
52. McIndoe AH: Treatment of congenital absence and obliterative conditions of the vagina, *Br J Plast Surg* 2:254, 1950.
53. McIndoe AH, Banister JB: An operation for the cure of congenital absence of the vagina, *J Obstet Gynaecol Br Empire* 45:490, 1938.
54. Morton K, Davies D, Dewhurst Sir John: The use of fascio-cutaneous flaps in vaginal reconstruction, *Br J Obstet Gynaecol* 93:970, 1986.
55. Morton K, Dewhurst Sir John: The use of bowel to create a vagina: a follow up study, *Ped Adol Gynecol* 2:51, 1984.
56. Morton K, Dewhurst Sir John: Human amnion in the treatment of vaginal malformations, *Br J Obstet Gynaecol* 93:50, 1986.
57. Muram D, Spence JEH: Rupture of a pregnant rudimentary horn in an adolescent girl followed by a successful pregnancy, *Ped Adol Gynecol* 1:53, 1982.
58. Nakayama DK et al: Posterior sagittal exposure for reconstructive surgery for cloacal abnormalities, *J Pediatr Surg* 22:588, 1987.
59. Perino A et al: Hysteroscopy for metroplasty of uterine septa: report of 24 cases, *Fertil Steril* 48:321, 1987.
60. Perino A et al: Hysteroscopic metroplasty: the role of ultrasound in the diagnosis of patients with uterine septa, *Acta Eur Fertil* 18:349, 1987.

61. Poland ML, Evans TN: Psychological aspects of vaginal agenesis, *J Reprod Med* 30:340, 1985.
62. Regan L, Dewhurst Sir John: Atresia of the cervix, *Ped Adol Gynecol* 3:83, 1985.
63. Rock JA: Diagnosing and repairing uterine anomalies, *Contemp Obstet Gynecol* 17:43, 1981.
64. Rock JA, Jones HW: The clinical management of the double uterus, *Fertil Steril* 28:798, 1977.
65. Rock JA, Jones HW: Construction of a neovagina for patients with a flat perineum, *Am J Obstet Gynecol* 160:845, 1989.
66. Rock JA et al: Success following vaginal creation for Mullerian agenesis, *Fertil Steril* 39:809, 1983.
67. Rodeck C, Craft IL, Dewhurst CJ: Genital tract obstruction and endometriosis, *Int J Gynaecol Obstet* 13:197, 1975.
68. Rothman D: The use of peritoneum in the construction of a vagina, *Obstet Gynecol* 40:835, 1972.
69. Sanfilippo JS et al: Endometriosis in association with uterine anomaly, *Am J Obstet Gynecol* 154:39, 1986.
70. Sheares BH: Congenital atresia of the vagina; a new technique for tunnelling the space between bladder and rectum and construction of a new vagina by a modified Wharton technique, *J Obstet Gynaecol Br Empire* 67:24, 1960.
71. Smith MR: Vaginal aplasia; therapeutic options, *Am J Obstet Gynecol* 146:488, 1983.
72. Stanton SC: Gynecological complications of epispadias and bladder exstrophy, *Am J Obstet Gynecol* 119:749, 1974.
73. Stephens FD: *Congenital malformations of the rectum, anus and genital tracts,* Edinburgh, 1963, Churchill Livingstone, Inc.
74. Strassmann EO: Plastic unification of a double uterus; a study of 123 collected and five personal cases, *Am J Obstet Gynecol* 64:25, 1952.
75. Strassmann EO: Fertility and unification of double uterus, *Fertil Steril* 17:163, 1966.
76. Togashi K et al: Vaginal agenesis: classification by magnetic resonance imaging, *Radiology* 162:675, 1987.
77. Tompkins P: Comments on bicornuate uterus and twinning, *Surg Clin North Am* 42:1049, 1962.
78. Valle RF, Sciarra JJ: Hysteroscopic treatment of the septate uterus, *Obstet Gynecol* 67:253, 1986.
79. Vecchietti RF: Neovagina nella sindrome di Rokitansky-Kuster-Hauser, *Attual Ost Gin* 11:131, 1957.
80. Waters EG: Cloacal dysgenesis; related anomalies and pregnancies, *Obstet Gynecol* 59:398, 1982.
81. Williams EA: Congenital absence of the vagina; a simple operation for its relief, *J Obstet Gynaecol Br Commonwealth* 71:511, 1964.
82. Zarou GS, Esposito V, Zarou DM: Pregnancy following the surgical correction of congenital absence of the cervix, *Int J Gynaecol Obstet* 11:143, 1973.

Part VII

OPERATIONS UPON THE URINARY TRACT

Chapter 49

THE REPAIR OF URETHRAL INJURIES, DIVERTICULA, AND FISTULA

Raymond A. Lee

The female urethra is well-protected and rarely involved in injury except during childbirth or operation. Occasionally, usually as a result of a motor vehicle accident, a woman may experience an avulsion of the urethra, generally in the area of the bladder neck. Less commonly, women may experience a penetrating wound as a result of being impaled while fence climbing or being struck by farming tools; such injuries frequently result in hematoma of the vulva and laceration of the urethra. Occasionally, injuries to the vagina, rectum, and urethra result from a disproportion between the size of the penis and that of the vagina. These usually result in disruption of the posterior vaginal wall and the anal sphincter rather than trauma to the urethra and the base of the bladder.

Any injury to the urethra and anterior vaginal wall usually consists of a longitudinal laceration of the vaginal wall extending into the lateral vaginal fornix, but rarely is the urethra itself disrupted. We have seen several patients who were unaware that they had agenesis of the vagina and were attempting or experiencing intercourse in the urethra. Early in her experience, such a patient generally will have pain with few other symptoms. With sufficient time, the urethra dilates to accommodate a normal penis, and this process eventually results in significant urinary incontinence because of the stretched urethra and bladder neck but not because of laceration. Bleeding is not a frequent problem.

An appropriate diagnosis can generally be made on careful inspection of the area, but anesthesia may be required to ensure an accurate assessment of the urethra. This examination in combination with a cystourethroscopic examination assists in determining the integrity of the urethra, the bladder neck, and the base of the bladder. If they are found to be intact, depending on the degree of trauma, a urethral catheter may be required for a short time to ensure adequate drainage of the bladder during recovery. If a defect is noted in the urethra and if the tissues can be assessed accurately, immediate operative repair may be accomplished by reconstructing the urethra, its supporting tissues, and the anterior vaginal wall with interrupted 4-0 delayed absorbable sutures. This reconstruction is an attempt to restore the urethra and the anterior vaginal wall to their normal anatomy and to avoid the potential of later fistula formation. Space does not permit detailing the approach of disruption of the urethra and the abdominal repair that is frequently associated with disruption of the symphysis and other pelvic fractures.

URETHROVAGINAL FISTULA
Etiology

Prolonged labor continues to be a common cause of destruction of the urethra and base of the bladder in medically deprived countries,[5,11,14] whereas elective urethral and vaginal operation is the leading cause of these low-lying fistulas in the United States.[4,13] The excision of a friable, infected urethral diverticulum can be tedious and inexact.[8] Despite meticulous efforts to reconstruct the urethral floor accurately, infection and edema may lead to imperfect healing and fistula formation. In addition, over-zealous plication of the urethra or the inadvertent intramural placement of a suture (vaginal or retropubic

Portions of this chapter were previously published in Lee RA: *Surgical management of genitourinary fistulas*. In WG Hurt, editor: *Urogynecological surgery,* Gaithersburg, Md, 1991, Aspen Publishers, Inc. By permission of the publisher.

needle suspension) may produce a fistula of the urethra or, a greater calamity, actual slough of the entire floor and the bladder neck.[13]

Clinical symptoms

Patients who experience trauma to the urethra from forceps delivery or automobile accident have leakage immediately or within the first 24 hours after damage. If a urethral catheter is in place, either after delivery or trauma, removal of the catheter is generally followed promptly by leakage of urine. Patients who have undergone an operation generally have a catheter in place for 2 to 7 days. Some patients who have had an operation may have an unrecognized suture through the wall of the urethra; this generally results in necrosis of the tissue, possibly associated with hematoma formation or some degree of infection, the combination of which results in leakage of urine. The patient may initially be continent only to experience leakage 1 to 2 weeks postoperatively. Patients who have had irradiation generally note the leakage some time after the treatment, generally within 2 to 4 weeks after therapy.

Simple urethrovaginal fistula, depending on its location relative to the bladder neck, may not produce urinary incontinence and may not require operative repair. A fistula located near the bladder neck may be technically more difficult to repair, and urinary continence cannot be ensured. Even after what appears to be a successful repair, the patient may experience urinary stress incontinence due to fibrosis, fixation, and poor contractility of the urethral musculature. A more complex problem is presented by patients who have had a major slough resulting in a linear loss of the floor of the urethra and frequently involving the bladder neck and the base of the bladder.

Operative repair

The basic phases of operative reconstruction consist of a linear incision, much like that for an anterior colporrhaphy, and mobilization of the vaginal mucosa laterally off the underlying cervicopubic fascia. This procedure must be accomplished in the proper bloodless tissue plane sufficiently lateral (to establish mobility) so that a tension-free closure of the urethra can be accomplished.

Once the fistula is completely mobilized and the scar tissue (fistula tract) is removed, the fistula is closed with fine 4-0 delayed absorbable sutures placed extramucosally, and the tissue edges are approximated free of tension and with excellent hemostasis. The presence of a small-caliber catheter within the urethra frequently assists in accurate placement of the sutures to close the fistulous tract. This initial suture line is imbricated with a second set of sutures, the most distal suture being just distal to the original suture line. Snug plication of the bladder neck by approximation, under the urethra, of the tissue (cervicopubic fascia) lateral to the urethra to create a tension-free second layer of sutures is mandatory for a successful repair. A tension-free closure of the vaginal wall as a third layer, or

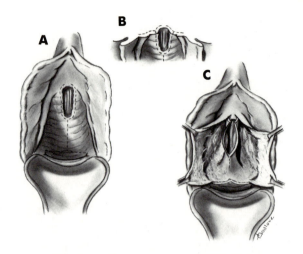

Fig. 49-1. Mobilization of tissue. **A,** Proposed midline incision about defect. **B,** Proposed line of dissection about urethra through mucosa of vagina. **C,** Wide mobilization of vaginal mucosa off cervicopubic fascia. (From Symmonds RE: Loss of the urethral floor with total urinary incontinence: a technique for urethral reconstruction, *Am J Obstet Gynecol* 103:665, 1969.)

when necessary for the obliteration of dead space and actual replacement of the anterior vaginal wall with a pedicled-skin, fibrofatty labial graft, may be indicated.

A "second-stage" retropubic urethral vesical suspension for patients who have a good anatomic result with an apparently intact urethra but who nevertheless remain incontinent (intact urethra with stress incontinence) may be necessary at a later date. This result cannot be predicted at the time of closure of the urethral fistula.

Loss of the floor of the urethra

One of the most challenging forms of genitourinary fistula is the fistula that involves the loss of a major portion of the proximal urethra and bladder neck. Several operative techniques can correct the anatomic defect (urethrovaginal fistula), but urinary continence rather than the anatomic result is a far better criterion of a successful operation. Regardless of the operative technique selected, the surgeon cannot anticipate successful restoration of urinary continence in all patients who have loss of the urethra. Symmonds and Hill[13] reported on 50 Mayo Clinic patients with loss of the urethra. The etiologic factors are the same as those that result in simple urethrovaginal fistula—anterior colporrhaphy and repair of urethral diverticulum.

Operative repair. A midline incision is made in the anterior vaginal wall and extended up and around the margins of the urethral defect (Fig. 49-1). The dissection is carried laterally to the descending pubic ramus much like that carried out for an anterior colporrhaphy (Fig. 49-1). With appropriate traction on the edges of the urethral wall, the urethra is mobilized sufficiently that a tension-free closure can be constructed. All palpable bands of scar tissue that distort the urethra and the bladder neck must be dissected and released. In patients who have loss of a major

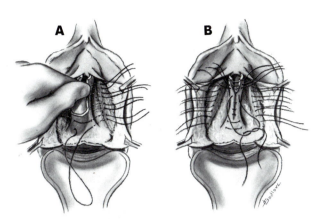

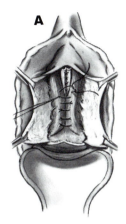

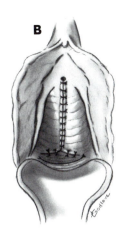

Fig. 49-2. Closure of urethra. **A,** A finger through the bladder neck assists the placement of bladder neck and proximal urethral sutures. **B,** Reconstructed urethral tube with fine extramucosal sutures. (From Symmonds RE: Loss of the urethral floor with total urinary incontinence: a technique for urethral reconstruction, *Am J Obstet Gynecol* 103:665, 1969.)

Fig. 49-3. Bladder neck and urethral plication and vaginal closure. **A,** Placement of second layer; reconstruction sutures inverting initial suture line of newly reconstructed urethra. **B,** Tension-free closure of anterior vaginal wall. (From Symmonds RE: Loss of the urethral floor with total urinary incontinence: a technique for urethral reconstruction, *Am J Obstet Gynecol* 103:665, 1969.)

portion of the proximal urethra and the bladder neck, it may be preferable to insert what will be the second row of interrupted sutures before reconstructing the urethra. If this procedure is done in this sequence, one can be assured that the suture is not within the lumen of the bladder or proximal urethra; thus, the maximal amount of all available tissue can be used in attempting to reconstruct the urethra, and a satisfactory continence mechanism will result. A finger inserted through the defect (Fig. 49-2, *A*) into the bladder aids in identifying the bladder wall and the ureters (previously placed ureteral stents), and the suture can be accurately placed. This initial layer of sutures (2-0 delayed absorbable) is tagged and held laterally. The urethral reconstruction is accomplished over a small catheter (8 to 12 Fr) with the use of interrupted 3-0 delayed absorbable sutures. These sutures are placed in a manner that accurately inverts and approximates the epithelial edges without entering the urethra. On completion of the first layer (Fig. 49-2, *B*), the sutures are tied in the order in which they were placed. The bladder can be tested by passing 200 ml of sterile evaporated milk solution or infant formula through the previously placed urethral catheter to ensure that the closure of the floor of the bladder, the proximal urethra, and the bladder neck is watertight.

After the urethral floor and the bladder neck have been constructed, the initially placed second row of sutures is tied to create a broad approximation of tissue that reinforces the initial suture line and the newly reconstructed urethra (Fig. 49-3). The sutures that act as plicating sutures to the bladder neck are tied and usually consist of 2-0 monofilament delayed absorbable sutures.

In this "much-operated" group of patients, occasionally a complete second layer of sutures cannot be obtained throughout the entire length of the urethra. In this circumstance, one needs to rely on the single set of sutures of the

more distal portion of the urethra. Not infrequently, once the vaginal wall is incised and the dissection is performed, it is impossible to reapproximate the vaginal wall without undue tension. In this circumstance, we prefer to use a labial pad with an anterior pedicle (Fig. 49-4). The flap should be of sufficient width and length to replace the defect in the anterior vaginal wall. The flap is rotated into the vagina, filling the defect, where it is fixed with fine interrupted (4-0) delayed absorbable sutures in an accurate and meticulous fashion. The blood supply of the labial flaps has always proved to be adequate, regardless of whether the pedicle is based anteriorly or posteriorly. Once the repair is accomplished, a small vaginal pack is inserted to compress the pedicle and aid in obliterating any underlying dead space or venous oozing. The transurethral catheter is removed, and a suprapubic catheter is placed.

Postoperative management. For patients in whom approximation of vaginal wall would result in tension on the suture line, we prefer to use a Martius-type (bulbocavernosus) muscle flap to obliterate the dead space and interpose a living tissue layer between the urethral and vaginal suture lines. When much of the lower anterior vaginal wall is absent or is the site of excessive scar, the wall should be completely replaced with a labial skin flap.

Postoperatively, the patient receives appropriate antibiotic coverage. The suprapubic catheter is clamped on the tenth postoperative day, when voiding may be undertaken. Almost always, the patient is voiding within the first week that the catheter is clamped, and only 1 of our last 25 patients has required suprapubic drainage for more than 20 days.

Despite adequate vesical neck plication and satisfactory elevation of the support of the urethra and even though an anatomically sound–appearing urethra has been obtained by the operation, some persistent urinary incontinence

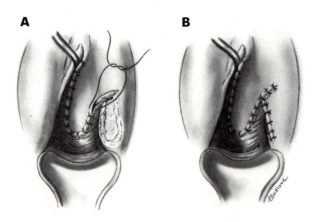

Fig. 49-4. A, Mobilization of labial skin-fibrofatty flap. Placement of pedicled fibrofatty labial flap replacing defect in anterior vaginal wall. **B,** Vaginal wall reconstruction. Individual sutures fixing labial flap in place and closing defect in the labia majora. (From Symmonds RE: Loss of the urethral floor with total urinary incontinence: a technique for urethral reconstruction, *Am J Obstet Gynecol* 103:665, 1969.)

eventually may be noted. In this case, a second-stage retropubic suspension of the neourethra may be necessary at a later date. Obviously, the goal of surgical correction is to construct a urethra that provides sufficient resistance to ensure good urinary continence; regrettably, a neourethra that appears to be anatomically sound, perfectly supported, and in excellent position does not guarantee good urethral function and urinary control. A scarred, fixed, noncontractile urethra does not provide good urinary control regardless of the urethral angles or support.

In some instances, perhaps when there has been significant destruction of the proximal urethra and the smooth muscle of the bladder neck, a second-stage retropubic suspension may be necessary to increase urethral support and resistance and provide better urinary control. Certainly, use of some type of labial flap to replace a deficient anterior vaginal wall or to reduce tension on the suture line frequently will improve the chance for successful repair. The type of vaginal closure required depends on the anatomic relationships noted after urethral bladder neck reconstruction. As our experience has increased, it has become apparent that approximately 70% of patients will not require a second-stage retropubic procedure. We have been reluctant to perform a concomitant suspension because it might produce undesirable stress or pull on the suburethral suture line, promoting disruption of the urethral repair. The caliber of the new urethra is, of necessity, small. Although this was an initial concern of ours, urethral dilation is rarely required.

DIVERTICULUM OF THE URETHRA

Diverticulum of the female urethra causes untold misery in the patient and frequently is well-disguised, resulting in a prolonged period of symptoms before diagnosis. Numerous investigative studies have been undertaken to clarify

its cause and its clinical presentation. Various innovative techniques have been suggested to improve the accuracy of diagnosis of this elusive condition because attempts at surgical correction may be technically difficult and occasionally result in serious complications. New operations and modifications of old procedures continue to be recommended.

Etiology

Several theories have been advanced to explain the pathogenesis of urethral diverticulum. Evidence for a congenital origin is based on case reports of children and neonates. The reports by Glassman et al[3] of a diverticulum in a 6-hour-old female infant reinforced this concept. They suggested that the exact cause of their patient's diverticulum could be a collecting system duplication, now obliterated except for a tiny ectopic ureterocele. We have had no evidence to support the congenital origin of diverticulum of the urethra. Huffman[6] aptly likened the urethra to a tree from the base of which arise numerous stunted branches—the periurethral ducts and glands. In some patients, they form a labyrinthine mass encircling the urethra on all sides with ducts opening into the lateral, dorsal, and a few ventral urethral walls. Most investigators agree with Routh,[10] who postulated that infection and obstruction of the periurethral glands result in the formation of retention cysts that when infected rupture into the lumen and give rise to a diverticulum. Urethral trauma from catheterization and childbirth has also been suggested as contributing to the formation of a diverticulum. Because 20% of our patients were nulliparous,[8] a finding also reported by Davis and TeLinde,[2] we do not support childbirth as an important etiologic factor. Rather, it appears that there are several different etiologic factors, any one of which may result in the formation of a diverticulum of the female urethra.

Clinical presentation

Although the complaints of patients vary, most patients experience urgency, frequency, dysuria, and dyspareunia. A history of recurrent urinary tract infection is common; hematuria, dribbling after voiding, and urinary stress incontinence are infrequently mentioned. A palpable, tender, suburethral mass is found in approximately 60% of patients; actual protrusion of a diverticulum from the vaginal introitus is rare.

Diagnosis

The diagnosis initially must be suspected but is customarily confirmed by cystourethroscopy or voiding cystourethrography. Double-balloon urethrography, while theoretically appealing, has not proved very efficacious in our experience. Vaginal ultrasonography has recently been proved to be an extremely effective diagnostic tool and may become the standard method.

Huffman[6] found that most openings to the periurethral glands ended in the distal (external) third of the urethra; however, there is marked individual variation with open-

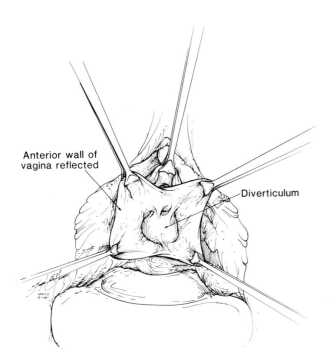

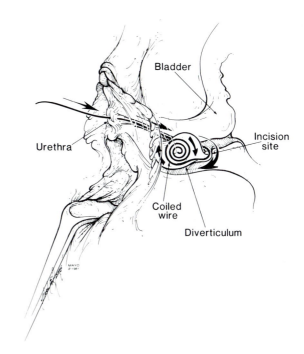

Fig. 49-5. Diverticulum exposed, with vaginal lining and endopelvic fascia retracted. (From Lee RA: Diverticulum of the female urethra: postoperative complications and results, *Obstet Gynecol* 61:52, 1983. By permission of The Mayo Foundation.)

Fig. 49-6. Coiled ureteral catheter distends diverticulum and aids in its identification and dissection. (From Lee RA: Diverticulum of the female urethra: postoperative complications and results, *Obstet Gynecol* 61:52, 1983. By permission of The Mayo Foundation.)

ings extending throughout the entire length and involving the bladder neck. These findings correlate well with the site of origin of most diverticula of the urethra and further support a direct relationship between the periurethral ducts and the formation of diverticula.

Menville and Mitchell[9] reported that 85% of diverticula were located in the distal two thirds of the urethra. Cook and Pool[1] stated that the orifices were located more often in the middle of the urethra. In our experience, 65% of the diverticula are located in the proximal two thirds of the urethra and the bladder neck area, and an additional 20% of the diverticula have multiple sites of origin, most of which are in the midurethra with a second opening in the inner or outer segment. Only 15% are in the distal (external) third of the urethra. When cystourethroscopy is used in combination with urethrography, the size, ramifications, and number of diverticula usually can be determined. Occasionally, a saddlebag diverticulum or even multiple diverticula can be demonstrated with voiding cystourethrography when only a single orifice can be seen on urethroscopic examination.

Operative technique

A vertical incision is made in the anterior vaginal wall, the underlying pubocervical fascia is exposed, and the lateral vaginal wall flaps are mobilized to the descending pubic ramus. A similar incision is made in the fascia, which is mobilized laterally to expose the underlying diverticulum (Fig. 49-5). The wall of the diverticulum is recognized as a smooth, shiny, thin-walled structure. The dissection must be sharp, accurate, and meticulous. The pre-

operative placement (coiling) of a ureteral catheter within the diverticulum to distend its walls when this can be accomplished may enhance the identification and dissection of the diverticulum (Fig. 49-6). Not infrequently, the diverticulum is in immediate apposition or even perforating the pubocervical fascia, and it can be easily identified (perhaps even inadvertently entered) during the dissection. If the diverticulum is entered, the surgeon simply may introduce the tip of the left index finger into the diverticulum and, with appropriate traction with a broad Allis forceps on the edge of the diverticulum, further dissect it from the surrounding cervicopubic fascia (Fig. 49-7). Rarely, a linear incision is made through the full thickness of the urethra to expose the urethral floor and permit the passage of a probe through the ostium to aid in the identification of the diverticulum. Depending on the size of the diverticulum, it may present with loculations containing various amounts of urine, purulent material, necrotic debris, and even gravel; such loculations or septae should be incised. The use of Allis forceps on the rim of the diverticulum permits gentle traction on the wall of the diverticulum and aids in the dissection with Metzenbaum scissors to ensure total excision.

Occasionally, the sac of the diverticulum extends laterally and upward around the urethra. Rarely, it may extend into the retropubic space, or the urethral orifice of the diverticulum may be located laterally or may even enter the roof of the diverticulum. In the latter instance, the dissection is continued as far superiorly as possible, at which point the neck of the diverticulum is simply transected and permitted to retract; no attempt is made to close the defect

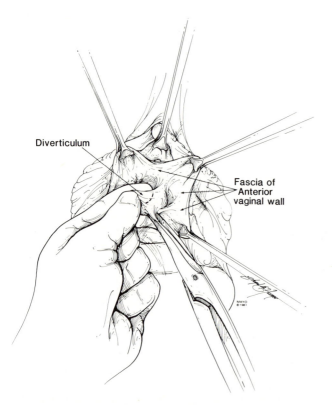

Fig. 49-7. Finger within diverticulum permits traction, which aids in dissection and identification of ostium. (From Lee RA: Diverticulum of the female urethra: postoperative complications and results, *Obstet Gynecol* 61:52, 1983. By permission of The Mayo Foundation.)

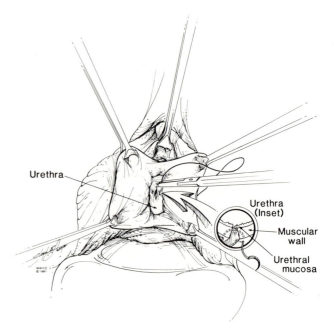

Fig. 49-8. After complete resection of the diverticulum, the urethra is closed with fine interrupted extramucosal chromic sutures. (From Lee RA: Diverticulum of the female urethra: postoperative complications and results, *Obstet Gynecol* 61:52, 1983. By permission of The Mayo Foundation.)

in the urethra. In some patients, the diverticulum is saddle-shaped around the entire urethra or bladder neck; thus, extensive dissection of the lower trigone or a major portion of the urethral floor is required.

The urethra is closed in a linear direction over a urethral catheter (the size varies depending on the size of the urethra and the size and shape of the defect in the urethra) with interrupted 4-0 delayed absorbable sutures (Fig. 49-8). Rarely, the tissues can be most appropriately approximated in a transverse direction to prevent tension on the suture line. After the urethral defect is repaired, the pubocervical fascia is imbricated in a side-to-side (vest-over-pants) fashion with 3-0 delayed absorbable sutures (Fig. 49-9). By providing two additional supporting layers and avoiding a superimposed suture line, this method appears to diminish the possibility of fistula formation. In addition, it provides good support for the proximal urethra and the bladder neck. Before closure of the vaginal wall, complete hemostasis must be accomplished with use of fine interrupted absorbable sutures and meticulous electrocoagulation; the vaginal wall is closed with 3-0 delayed absorbable suture material. A urethral retention catheter is inserted; generally, this remains in place until the sixth postoperative day. In individual cases, the complexity of the repair may require that the catheter be retained for a longer time.

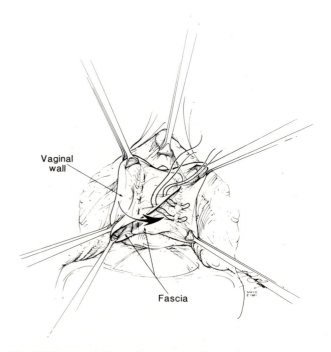

Fig. 49-9. Overlapping of paraurethral fascia in vest-over-pants fashion further supports repair and reduces opportunity for formation of fistulas. (From Lee RA: Diverticulum of the female urethra: postoperative complications and results, *Obstet Gynecol* 61:52, 1983. By permission of The Mayo Foundation.)

Most repairs of diverticula are tedious and difficult and are associated with more loss of blood than one would expect from such a small incision. The potential for development of a serious complication depends on the size and the number of the diverticula, the degree of inflammation, and the friability of the tissues and the position of the ostium in relation to the floor of the urethra and the bladder neck. The resection of multiple, large, multiloculated or saddle-shaped diverticula can require extensive dissection about the floor of the urethra, the bladder neck, and the lower trigone. In these conditions, the placement of ureteral catheters before the operation can facilitate identification of the ureters and actually reduce the risk of damage during the dissection. Actual or potential destruction or fixation of the smooth muscle of the urethra and the bladder neck produced by both the expanding inflammatory mass and the trauma associated with this excision can result in a urethral fistula or stress incontinence. Accurate reconstruction of the urethra and its supporting structures in combination with good hemostasis and routine antibiotic therapy for control of the infectious process significantly reduces the frequency of these potentially disabling complications.

Other surgical management applicable to individual situations should be considered. Lapides[7] reported a technique of transurethral marsupialization or resection of the roof of the diverticulum by use of a transurethral knife electrode. This technique involves enlarging the orifice of the diverticulum by incising the roof linearly. The result is an internal marsupialization or saucerization of the diverticulum. This procedure, for certain complicated or recurrent diverticula depending on their size and the location of the urethra, deserves further consideration.

Another operative approach reported by Spence and Duckett[12] is applicable to patients with the ostium of the diverticulum distal (external) to the peak urethral closure pressure. The operative approach consists of a transvaginal marsupialization of the diverticulum with one blade of the scissors in the urethra and the other blade in the vagina. With the exception of lesions involving the distal third of the urethra, it is conceivable that with menopausal atrophy of pelvic supports and resulting loss of tone of the remaining smooth muscle, a significant incidence of urinary incontinence may result some years after what appeared to be a successful marsupialization procedure.

Complications and results

Prompt, complete, and long-lasting relief of symptoms is usually obtained after successful diverticulectomy.[8] Urethroscopic examination demonstrates either a normal urethra or a shallow depression or a dimple at the operative site. We have seen no evidence of a urethral stricture in patients undergoing diverticulectomy. More than 80% of patients remain asymptomatic and have not required postoperative medical or surgical management. A small number of patients may have persistent pain, dyspareunia, or recurrent urinary tract infection. In this group, cystourethroscopy, cystourethrography, and appropriate cultures of

the urine should be reevaluated. Rarely, there may be a recurrence of a diverticulum of the urethra, either in the same location or presumably a second diverticulum at another location. If it occurs in the same location, the original diverticulum may have been incompletely excised. Recurrence of a diverticulum elsewhere in the urethra may be a diverticulum that was overlooked at the original operative procedure or may represent the development of a second diverticulum. Whatever the cause, the frequency of recurrent diverticular disease after diverticulectomy emphasizes the difficulties associated with the surgical treatment of this disease. Of 85 of our patients who underwent diverticulectomy, a urethrovaginal fistula developed in 1.[8] This followed the use of anticoagulant therapy necessary for the management of a myocardial infarction. A hematoma developed in the suture line, and a fistula developed later.

We continue to favor transvaginal excision of the diverticulum, even though it is a more complex and tedious operation. Resection of the diverticulum has provided a relatively good long-term rate of cure with an extremely low incidence of fistula and other serious complications.

Injury to the urethra, whether by trauma, childbirth, or operation, can result in disabling complications for the patient. The operative area is relatively small, the supporting tissues are of variable quality, and the wall of the urethra is thick. Given sufficient blood supply, laceration, fistula, loss of the floor, or diverticulum of the urethra can be reconstructed to form an intact tube. However, the functional result—a contractile, continent urethra—is more difficult to predict and cannot be ensured, even when the anatomic result appears satisfactory.

REFERENCES

1. Cook EN, Pool TL: Urethral diverticulum in the female, *J Urol* 62:495, 1949.
2. Davis HJ, TeLinde RW: Urethral diverticula: an assay of 121 cases, *J Urol* 80:34, 1958.
3. Glassman TA, Weinerth JL, Glenn JF: Neonatal female urethral diverticulum, *Urology* 5:249, 1975.
4. Gray LA: Urethrovaginal fistulas, *Am J Obstet Gynecol* 101:28, 1968.
5. Hamlin RHJ, Nicholson EC: Reconstruction of urethra totally destroyed in labour, *Br Med J* 2:147, 1969.
6. Huffman JW: The detailed anatomy of the paraurethral ducts in the adult human female, *Am J Obstet Gynecol* 55:86, 1948.
7. Lapides J: Transurethral treatment of urethral diverticula in women, *Trans Am Assoc Genitourin Surg* 70:135, 1978.
8. Lee RA: Diverticulum of the female urethra: postoperative complications and results, *Obstet Gynecol* 61:52, 1983.
9. Menville JG, Mitchell JD Jr: Diverticulum of the female urethra, *J Urol* 51:411, 1944.
10. Routh A: Urethral diverticula, *Br Med J* 1:361, 1890.
11. Shigui F, Qinge S: Operative treatment of female urinary fistulas: report of 405 cases, *Chin Med J* 92:263, 1979.
12. Spence HM, Duckett JW Jr: Diverticulum of the female urethra: clinical aspects and presentation of a simple operative technique for cure, *J Urol* 104:432, 1970.
13. Symmonds RE, Hill LM: Loss of the urethra: a report on 50 patients, *Am J Obstet Gynecol* 130:130, 1978.
14. Vanderputte SR: Obstetric vesicovaginal fistulae: experience with 89 cases, *Ann Soc Belg Med Trop* 65:303, 1985.

Chapter 50

SURGERY FOR URINARY STRESS INCONTINENCE

Neil D. Jackson

SCOPE

The aim of every gynecologic surgeon involved in surgical therapy for urinary incontinence is to make every wet patient dry. A noble aim, indeed, with a conservative estimation that in the United States over 10 million patients suffer from urinary incontinence and three quarters of them are women.[30,58,72] The Surgeon General of the United States estimates that Americans spend in excess of $10 billion per year in continence control, nursing care, materials, and supplies.[22,39] To be in control of one's life in all aspects is precious to every person. More specifically, to always be in control of one's own bodily functions is a life-long expectation. When this is not so, it grates harshly at one's self-image and threatens to jeopardize one's self-confidence, interpersonal relationships, careers, and ignites a morass of fears, anxieties, and depression. Progressive separation and reclusive behavior often supervene. Patients suffering from this debilitating malady all too frequently are unaware that help is available.

In recent years, an increase in media advertising of products for incontinence control has served as evidence that the problem is commonplace and help is available. Patients who previously hid their problem are reaching out to the medical community for assistance. The receptive, empathic, and sensitive gynecologic surgeon has the greatest opportunity for curative success. The key to that success is a comprehensive diagnosis.

HISTORY AND PHYSICAL EXAMINATION

A careful history of circumstances surrounding the episodes of incontinence can provide general clues to the diagnosis.[33,73] Urgency and frequency may be associated with uninhibited detrusor activity, which, in turn, may be related to infection, stones, or tumor. But spontaneous, inappropriate detrusor contractile activity may occur in the absence of these—a condition referred to as *detrusor instability*.[5] Urinary loss may occur during instances of increased intraabdominal pressure with coughing, sneezing, lifting, and exercise. Classically, these occasions of urinary loss have been termed *stress incontinence*.[6] Stress incontinence has been identified with anatomic displacement conditions of the urethra and bladder. The term *anatomic stress urinary incontinence* is more descriptive and in the standard nomenclature of the International Continence Society (ICS) is referred to as type I incontinence, more recently termed *genuine stress incontinence*.[1] It is quite clear from careful objective analysis of bladder function correlated with presenting symptoms that there is a great overlap of presenting symptomatology and discreet diagnostic entities. The presenting patient's symptomatology, therefore, is only suggestive but by no means diagnostic. Too much diagnostic emphasis on presenting symptoms without detailed functional analysis of the urinary tract is misleading. Diagnosis and therapy based on such hasty conclusions have led to misdiagnosis and misapplication of surgical therapy, doubtless contributing heavily to the perception that antiincontinent surgery frequently fails. Such a view is held by the lay community and a substantial portion of the medical community as well.

A detailed history must include a list of the patient's medications and caffeine intake.[59] Many medications prescribed for treatment of disorders of other organ systems have an indirect bearing on the physiology of the lower urinary tract. Particular note in the patient's history should be made of any prior incontinence or past pelvic surgery. If prior pelvic surgery has been performed, an exact copy of the operative report is most helpful in determining the specifics of the procedure done and of the suture material used on that occasion.

A comprehensive physical examination including a neurologic examination with attention to evaluation of the S_2-S_4 nerve distribution is fundamental. Particular attention to discover all aspects of pelvic pathology prepares the therapist with the needs to be addressed and by what route at the time of anticipated surgery. Is there a cystocele, rectocele, enterocele, vaginal vault eversion, or paravaginal sulcus detachment? All of these pelvic prolapse conditions would direct one to vaginal surgical repair. Are there large uterine leiomyomata, ovarian neoplasms, endometriosis, or other pelvic disorders, which may dictate an abdominal approach?

URODYNAMIC EVALUATION

The International Continence Society has defined clinically significant incontinence as voluntary loss of urine that is a social or hygienic problem and can be *objectively* demonstrated. During the filling phase of the lower urinary tract function, disturbance of the bladder acting as a proper reservoir, or disturbance of the urethral outflow resistance as a proper sphincter, can lead to an incontinent state. The International Continence Society has classified these diagnostic entities as shown below. These entities can occur as solitary conditions, or in any combination. When causes are multiple, the conditions are often synergistic.

Types of incontinence
Type I -Genuine stress incontinence
Type II -Detrusor instability
Type III-Low pressure urethra
Type IV-Unstable urethra

The role of the urodynamics laboratory is to identify the particular contribution of the bladder and of the urethra during the filling and emptying phases of lower urinary tract function. The bladder and urethral sphincter normally work in reciprocal accord under control of the autonomic nervous system.

Water or gas cystometry measures the pressure in the bladder while it is filling. Under sympathetic autonomic control, rich in β-adrenergic smooth muscle relaxing receptors,[4,82] the bladder fills by dynamic relaxation of the detrusor wall creating low intravesical pressure. At the same time, changes in intraabdominal pressure engendered by Valsalva's maneuver, coughing, or straining transmitted to the bladder can be demonstrated.[28,31] Not only failure of the bladder to relax but also involuntary contraction of the bladder during filling generates an uninhibited contraction and is diagnostic of detrusor instability. Turner-Warwick[81] and McGuire[54] have found some degree of detrusor instability in about 10% of the population, most of whom have sufficient urethral closing pressure to remain continent. In very specific terms, detrusor instability is a cystometric diagnosis and comprises about 15% to 30% of patients with clinically significant incontinence. Therapy

for this problem is medical rather than surgical, employing anticholinergics, estrogen replacement therapy, dietary caffeine restriction, supplemented with exercise, timed voiding, and biofeedback.* Many patients with detrusor instability describe urgency and frequency as their presenting complaint. However, detrusor instability can masquerade as stress incontinence, hence the same stressful conditions of coughing, sneezing, and lifting can precipitate an uninhibited detrusor contraction. The incautious surgeon unequipped with urodynamic analysis and with the wrong diagnosis may schedule this patient for unhelpful surgery—a proposal fraught with failure from the outset (Fig. 50-1).

During cystometry, the bladder is filled through a small catheter (8 Fr) containing two pressure-sensitive microtransducers 6 cm apart (Fig. 50-2). During cystometric testing, the transducer at the tip remains in the bladder and records intravesical pressure while the proximal transducer simultaneously measures intraurethral pressure.[19]

Urethral profilometry is conducted through the measurement of pressure present within the urethra throughout its course as recorded by the second transducer, drawn by a catheter puller from the vesicourethral neck to the external meatus. This outlet resistive pressure is a quantification of urethral sphincter activity. During the filling phase of bladder function, pressure present within the urethra must exceed the pressure present within the bladder to ensure a continent state. The value of urethral pressure in excess of bladder pressure is termed *urethral closing pressure* and normally is greater than 20 cm of water. Values less than 20 cm of water are termed *low urethral pressure* and often lead to incontinence.

Maximum urethral closing pressure is derived by subtracting detrusor pressure from urethral pressure:

$$\begin{array}{ccc} \text{Maximum urethral} \\ \text{closing pressure} \\ \text{MUCP} \end{array} = \begin{array}{c} \text{Urethral} \\ \text{pressure} \\ \text{UP} \end{array} - \begin{array}{c} \text{Bladder} \\ \text{pressure} \\ \text{BP} \end{array}$$

Urethral pressure is a composite summation of smooth muscle tone within the wall of the urethra, surface adhesive activity of the urethral mucosa, striated muscle tone of the external sphincter, vascularity, and an abundance of supporting connective tissue elements—collagen, elastin, and ground substance.[24,25,31] All of these components in the female urethra are estrogen-dependent.[40,84] Deficiency of estrogen can contribute to a reduction in sustained urethral pressure and, in turn, can lower the effective urethral closing pressure.

The vesicourethral junction is positioned normally in a high retropubic location (Fig. 50-3). The most important portion of the urethra in respect to outlet resistance is the proximal half. It rests above the pelvic and urogenital diaphragms and is, therefore, under the influence of increased intraabdominal pressure.[9,67] Increases in intraabdominal pressure occur coincident with stress (e.g., coughing,

*References 7,8,12,41,45,78,80.

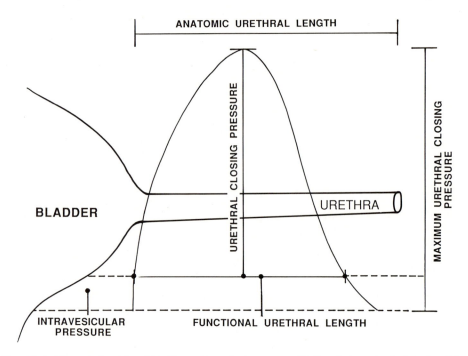

Fig. 50-1. The relationship of bladder and urethral pressure. Notice that anatomic length of the urethra is greater than the functional length and that the urethral closing pressure, identified by the curved line, is greatest at the midpoint of the functional urethral length.

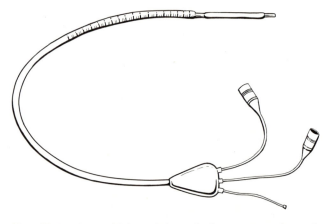

Fig. 50-2. The multichanneled urethral pressure catheter is shown. There is a pressure transducer at the catheter tip and a second transducer 6 cm down the shaft.

sneezing, and lifting). When the bladder and proximal urethra are in their normal position, they are both equally affected by increased intraabdominal pressure and the equation given above is unaffected.

The additional pressure within the bladder and the urethra caused by intraabdominal distribution is the transmission pressure. The relationship of the extent that abdominal pressure affects the bladder and urethra is the transmission pressure ratio.[10,20] It is obvious that if additional pressure is transmitted only to the bladder and not to the urethra, there would be a reduction in maximum urethral closing pressure. If this reduction is great enough (i.e., in-

travesicular pressure exceeds intraurethral pressure), incontinence will occur.

Failure to maintain normal urethral position is termed *urethral hypermobility* and is caused by a failure of supportive connective tissues or striated muscle tone within and about the urethra. Hypermobility can be measured in the laboratory by the Q-tip test (Fig. 50-4).[14,23,83] It can also be seen with the aid of the urethroscope.[70] With the urethroscope in midurethra and the patient straining down with Valsalva's maneuver while the observer keeps the bladder neck in view, the angle inscribed by the inclination of the Q-tip or urethroscope is usually parallel to the floor. With straining, there is an elevation of 30 degrees or less in the patient with normal urethral support. When hypermobility of the proximal urethra is present, there is elevation of the urethroscope or Q-tip greater than 30 degrees caused by abnormal descent of the proximal urethra. The external meatus acts as a fulcrum and is a relatively fixed structure. The elevation seen on the examiner's side is a direct and opposite reflection of urethral hypermobility. Hypermobility and descent of the proximal urethra displaces it below the pelvic diaphragm, removing it from the influence of intraabdominal pressure and, thus, effectively reducing urethral closing pressure.

Urethral hypermobility can also be measured by cystourethrography.[29,34] This had been the gold standard for years. However, it involves the disadvantage of ionizing radiation and in most centers cannot be conducted concurrent with other urodynamic investigation.

With the development of vaginal and rectal probes,

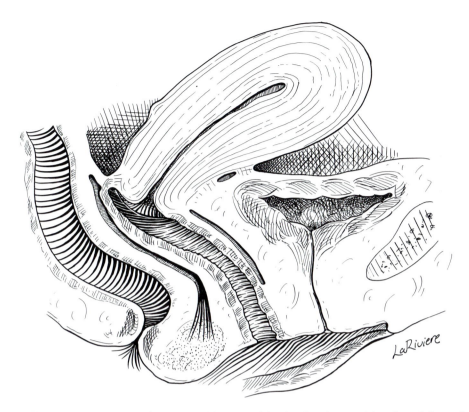

Fig. 50-3. Vaginal drawing of the normal female pelvis showing the usual location of the vesicourethral position at about the junction of the lower third with the upper two thirds of the back of the pubis.

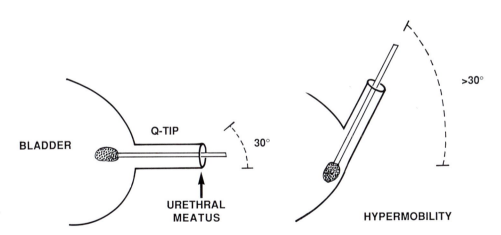

Fig. 50-4. Demonstration of how the angle of urethral hypermobility may be measured. Patient at rest is shown on left. Effect of Valsalva's maneuver in patient with urethral hypermobility is shown at right.

real-time display with linear array, and sector scanning techniques, the bladder and urethra can be visualized and mobility can be measured by ultrasound.[11,15,16,18,42] Anatomic visualization by ultrasound with simultaneous physiologic assessment by multi-channel urodynamics provides a comprehensive documentation of the lower urinary tract.

When incontinence is a consequence of normal urethral closing pressure at rest, a stable bladder, hypermobility of the urethra and on effortful activity, loss of effective urethral closing pressure secondary to reduction of transmitted abdominal pressure to the otherwise normally functioning urethra, the condition is given the ICS preferred designation—genuine stress incontinence. Other designations in the literature for this condition are anatomic stress urinary incontinence or type I incontinence.

This comprises 65% to 70% of all patients with incontinence and is the group of patients to which antiincontinence surgery is properly directed.

Analysis of the urethral pressure profile can disclose the patient with low urethral pressure (i.e., urethral closing pressures of less than 20 cm of water).[72] It may be seen de novo or may follow prior injury or surgery.[17] Patients with a denervated, defunctionalized "drainpipe" urethra also fall into this category. Patients with low urethral pressure are sometimes referred to having as type III incontinence.

A fourth and much smaller group of patients are those with an unstable urethra. The unstable urethra is defined by the ICS as a sudden drop in urethral pressure measurable during urethral profilometry, resulting in urinary incontinence in the absence of provocative maneuvers such as detrusor contraction, coughing, or Valsalva's maneuver. It is often only apparent when performing the urethral profile study on the patient in the erect rather than the supine position. Variations in urethral pressures of 10 to 20 cm of water have been reported.[50,71] This disorder has been termed type IV incontinence.

From a therapeutic standpoint, the patient with low urethral pressure or an unstable urethra needs early identification. The usual surgical procedures associated with correction of genuine stress incontinence are ineffective in addressing the needs of this special group of patients. Surgical procedures engineered to replace the proximal urethra to a high retropubic position in patients with low urethral pressure are fraught with failure. In the not so distant past, such surgical elections may have contributed significantly to the popular notion that antiincontinence surgery may benefit only temporarily and frequently may fail altogether. When the preoperative urodynamic evaluations identify a single cause of urinary incontinence, therapeutic planning can be straightforward. However, frequently, the patient presenting with incontinence, on close evaluation, represents a combination of etiologic entities of varying severity.[36] Urodynamic evaluation can identify these components and serve as a means to weigh the contribution that each is making to the overall problem.[43] Often this leads to a combination of therapeutic procedures including medication, exercise, biofeedback, and surgery to address appropriately all the contributing diagnostic elements.

GENERAL PRINCIPLES

Successful therapy for patients suffering from urinary incontinence clearly demands precise diagnosis supported by laboratory confirmation. When the diagnosis indicates medical management to be the prime focus, then medical management should be pursued. If, however, there is a combination of entities indicating medical management for one and surgery for the other, then the less traumatic medical management should be maximized first. The results and conditions are then reassessed before embarking on invasive surgical therapy.

In most instances of urinary incontinence, pubococcygeal perineal resistive exercises of Kegel's type are helpful. The contractions of at least 3 seconds' duration

each should be employed with sufficient frequency (five sets of fifteen per day) for many months, both preoperatively and postoperatively. The patient may be standing, sitting or, reclining. It is of extreme importance that the patient employ the correct muscle group. She should be tightening the voluntary muscles around the introitus and not bearing down. (Bearing down or straining as in Valsalva's maneuver increases intraabdominal pressure.) The physician/therapist should not rely solely on a verbal description of the exercise to the patient. In the examining situation with a finger in the vagina, the therapist can feel and estimate the strength of the increased perineal tension produced by the correct maneuver. At the same time, the patient can be encouraged to monitor the degree of tension produced when at home with her own fingers placed vaginally. This is a very simple but effective and inexpensive home biofeedback exercise. Many investigators have reported the increased benefits of biofeedback in training patients to use the correct muscles, and a positive program will improve the effectiveness of surgery.

Patients who are deficient in estrogen should be encouraged to use it locally as long as there is no contraindication to estrogen therapy. Because so many elements in the continence mechanism of the lower urinary tract contain estrogen receptors and are estrogen-dependent for maximum physiologic performance, it seems axiomatic that direct therapy with local estrogen cream would be helpful. One gram of local estrogen cream instilled into the vagina at bedtime twice weekly for an initial 2-month period followed by maintenance of 1 g once a week for a very long time may be all that is necessary for effective supplementation.

SURGERY FOR GENUINE STRESS INCONTINENCE

The literature contains the descriptions of more than 100 surgical procedures for urinary incontinence. The objective of surgical correction for genuine stress incontinence, or type I, is to replace the hypermobile proximal urethra to a high retropubic position to improve transmission of abdominal pressure changes to the urethra. Some of these procedures involve a retropubic approach through an abdominal incision and still others are carried out from a vaginal approach, and others a combination of the two. Either way, the objective is the same—reestablishment of a normal position of the urethra into a high retropubic location.

Each approach, vaginal or abdominal-retropubic, has its champions.[75,83,85] Much appears in the literature to support the thesis of each proponent that their's is the best operation with the best results, ease of procedure, shortest recovery time, and long-term prognosis. In the hands of each proponent, it is certainly reasonable that it may very well be a very successful procedure. Unfortunately, far too much argument is devoted to the deprecation of one procedure to the support of another.[61] What is needed is a large prospective study containing randomly selected patients, matched for severity of anatomic defect, total body weight, age, general physical condition, history of prior surgery, and urodynamic functional profile. These groups must be followed and objectively evaluated during the postoperative follow-up period (3 to 5 years). Although such studies are planned and underway, only preliminary, inconclusive results are available.[13]

Patients suffering from urinary incontinence may have concurrent pathologic difficulties. There may be cystocele, rectocele, uterine prolapse, lateral vaginal sulcus detachment, eversion of the vaginal vault, or enterocele. Each of these conditions may require coincident vaginal surgery, and the therapist should consider one of the vaginal surgical procedures to correct the patient's genuine stress incontinence. Correcting all of the accompanying defects by this single-approach manner is quite possible and appears most reasonable.

Transabdominal procedures

Patients with type I genuine stress incontinence may have coincident pelvic pathology that may require a transabdominal operation. Among such disorders are large uterine leiomyomata, ovarian neoplasms, endometriosis, chronic pelvic pain of old adhesive pelvic inflammatory disease. When using a transabdominal approach to solve these problems, the surgeon could employ a retropubic antiincontinence operation of the Marshall-Marchetti-Krantz, Burch, or paravaginal sulcus fixation type. Coexistent pelvic conditions contribute to a decision as to which surgical approach to take.

In an abdominal procedure, one needs to access the retropubic space of Retzius. The bladder and urethra are separated from the posterior surface of the symphysis pubis by gentle blunt dissection of the loose connective tissue with the fingers. A Foley catheter placed in the bladder at the beginning of the operation can serve to define the urethrovesical junction. Often there is considerable fat overlying the bladder, urethra, and paraurethral tissues. Time taken to dissect away this fat tissue reveals the white-appearing stronger submucosal endopelvic "fascia." Care should be taken to avoid the paraurethral veins in this area to diminish the possibility of intraoperative bleeding. Frequently, a branch of the obturator vein is encountered, which courses diagonally through this space. Removing

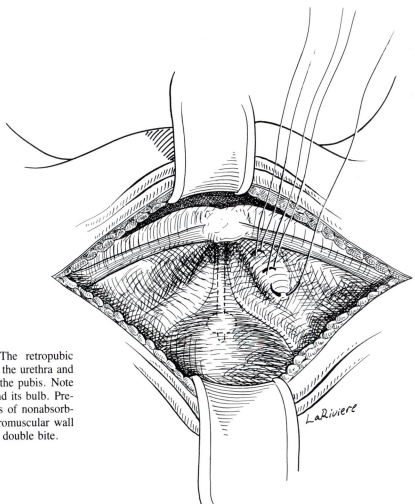

Fig. 50-5. The Burch-type colposuspension. The retropubic space of Retzius has been entered as shown, and the urethra and bladder are carefully dissected from the back of the pubis. Note the position of the transurethral Foley catheter and its bulb. Prevesical fat has been dissected away, and a series of nonabsorbable synthetic sutures are placed through the fibromuscular wall of the vagina lateral to the urethra, each taking a double bite.

the fat helps to ensure accurate placement of paraurethral sutures into tissue with substantial tensile strength and scarification potential for permanent support.

A double-gloved hand in the vagina with the patient prepped and draped in the "frog-leg" position allows the surgeon to feel the depth of the placement of the sutures to incorporate all but the vaginal mucosa in these paraurethral supporting stitches. After the first pass of the needle, slight traction on the suture elevates the bite of tissue, facilitating a second pass of each suture. Three or four sutures are placed on each side of the urethra with particular attention to the urethrovesical junction (Fig. 50-5). The sutures are held with consecutively numbered hemostats.

In the Marshall-Marchetti-Krantz operation,[52] the paraurethral supporting sutures are secured to the periosteum of the posterior symphysis pubis. The more distal sutures are first tied on each side and then sequentially followed until all are secured to the pubic periosteum, pulling the urethra and bladder neck ventrally. The vaginal examining hand will feel the course of the Foley catheter (i.e., the urethra applied to the posterior surface of the symphysis with a concavity on each side, earmarking the anchoring supporting sutures). In the Burch variation[21] of this retropubic fixation procedure, the supporting sutures are secured to the conjoined tendon (Cooper's ligament) rather than the pubic periosteum (Fig. 50-6). The sutures are placed lateral to one another, creating a supporting hammock of anterior wall elevating the urethra (Fig. 50-7). At times, the surgeon cannot fully approximate the paraure-thral tissues to Cooper's ligament without avoiding excessive tension. Deliberate suture bridges of nonabsorbable suture material may be created. During healing, scarification bridges the gap. Either permanent nonabsorbable plastic synthetic suture, slowly absorbable synthetic polyglycolic acid-type suture can be used for paraurethral support.

Drainage of the retropubic space is rarely necessary and depends on how "wet" the operative site appears, paying due heed to hemostasis. Although it has been suggested that the space of Retzius should always be drained, experience dictates that it is seldom desirable or necessary to drain this area. When it is, a Jackson-Pratt drain led through a separate incision serves the purpose well.

Cystoscopic visualization of the interior of the bladder can be done with the cystoscope positioned transurethrally by the operator (with appropriate change of gown and gloves) or it can be done by an assistant; or at the operative site, the surgeon can insert the cystoscope through a small incision in the bladder fundus, first placing a purse-string suture around the incision site. This suture allows introduction of the scope with a liquid seal for bladder filling and serves as a primary closure at the end of the procedure. The fundus of the bladder heals quite promptly. An incision here represents no greater potential for complication than a suprapubic cystotomy.

Cystoscopy serves two purposes. Visualization of the operative results from the vesical side can confirm satisfactory elevation of the bladder neck, and, if any sutures are present within the bladder, they can be identified, removed, and replaced.

Some surgeons prefer to open the bladder at the time of suspension to visualize the bladder neck directly correct any funneling that may be present, and guide the placement of the suspensory sutures. Direct visualization also

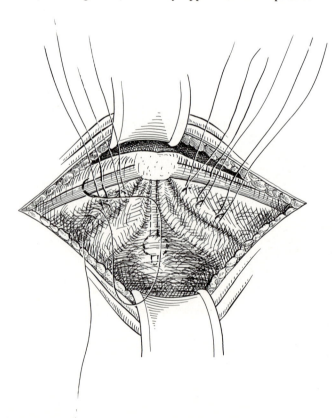

Fig. 50-6. Each suture is placed through the conjoined tendon.

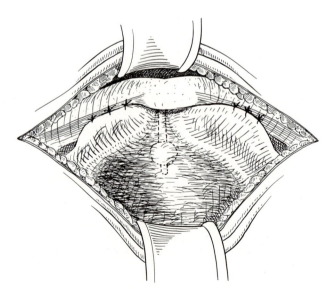

Fig. 50-7. When all stitches have been placed, they are tied. To avoid excess tension, deliberate suture bridges may be employed if nonabsorbable suture is used.

helps to prevent obstruction or injury to the ureters. Because the fundus of the bladder has such an abundant blood supply and is not a dependent area of the bladder, any incision in the fundus will heal well when properly closed.[27,47]

Transvaginal procedures

Over 30 years ago, Armand J. Pereyra first introduced the concept of suspension of the urethra and bladder neck with the use of a single needle passed through the retropubic space. There have been a number of modifications to that procedure.[61,62] Stamey was the first to suggest direct visualization of the bladder neck with the cystoscope to ensure adequate elevation and to detect the presence of any sutures in the bladder.[76] The procedure was further modified by Raz and others.[46,69] The advantage of the modified Pereyra procedure is its vaginal approach, permitting the operator concurrently to address additional pelvic prolapse.[64,66]

First, a longitudinal full-thickness incision is made in the anterior vaginal wall exposing the bladder base, bladder neck, and proximal urethra (Figs. 50-8 and 50-9). With sharp and blunt dissection, the vaginal flaps are raised laterally, with care taken to remain close to the undersurface of the pubic ramus, pushing the bladder neck medially. Pelvic prolapse is often accompanied by the development of extensive periurethral venous dilatations secondary to prolonged venous congestion. Chemical hemostasis can be aided by prior injection of a dilute solution

(1:200,000) of epinephrine under the vaginal epithelium. Lateral to the urethrovesical junction, demarcated by the Foley catheter, the periurethral supporting tissues are sutured in a helical fashion incorporating the overlying full-thickness vaginal flap excluding only the superficial epithelium. At least three helical loops are made on each side (Fig. 50-10). The suture used is nonabsorbable 0 polypropylene. If there is insufficient flexibility of the bladder neck and urethra as a result of prior operative scarring, dissection of the surrounding scar tissue to free this constraint is carried out to permit satisfactory elevation of the bladder neck without tension.

A short transverse incision is made suprapubically two finger-breadths above the symphysis pubis. This is carried down to the rectus abdominis fascia with care to clear the fascia of overlying fat (Fig. 50-11). With the aid of the Pereyra ligature carrier, the rectus fascia is perforated and the needle is advanced through the space of Retzius closely applied to the posterior surface of the symphysis to avoid entering the bladder. The bladder must be empty. With the operator's index finger under the dissected vaginal flap beneath the pubic ramus, the needle is guided into the region of the helical suture. Both ends of the suture are threaded onto the needle, and the needle is withdrawn, bringing the ends of the polypropylene suture above the rectus fascia. The same procedure is repeated on the opposite side.

Before proceeding, the Foley catheter is removed and the patient is examined with a cystoscope. We use both a 30-degree and 70-degree lens to visualize all surfaces of the bladder and proximal urethra. If a cystoscope is unavailable, a laparoscope or hysteroscope or even an arthro-

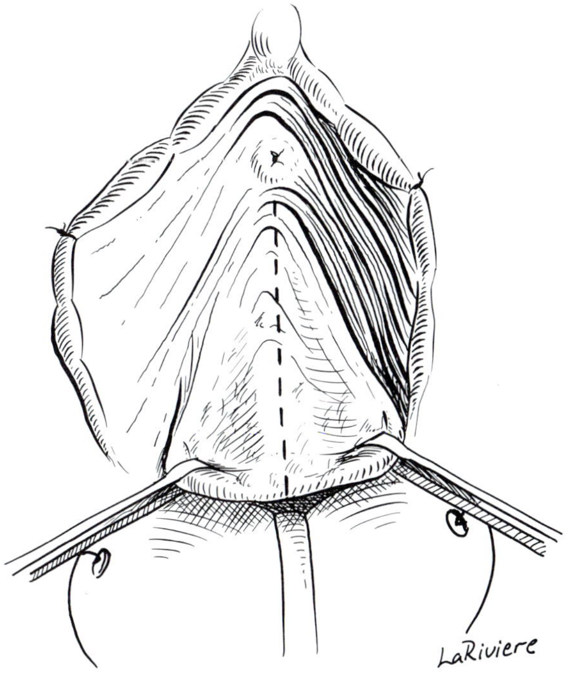

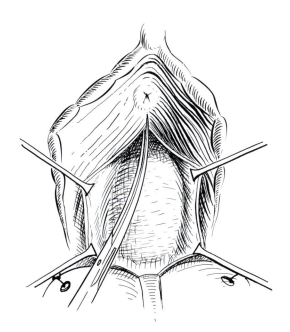

Fig. 50-8. Needle suspension of the vesicourethral junction. The anterior vaginal wall beneath the bladder is grasped between Allis clamps, and a longitudinal full-thickness incision is made along the path shown by the dashed line.

Fig. 50-9. The incision is carried to within 1 cm of the external urethral meatus, and the vaginal flaps are dissected carefully from the underlying bladder.

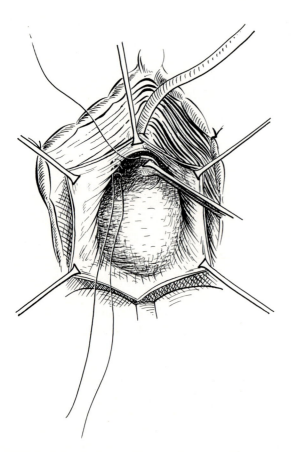

Fig. 50-10. The periurethral supporting tissues on the patient's right have been sutured in a helical fashion, incorporating the full fibromuscular thickness of the vaginal wall excluding only the superficial epithelium. At least three loops are made on each side.

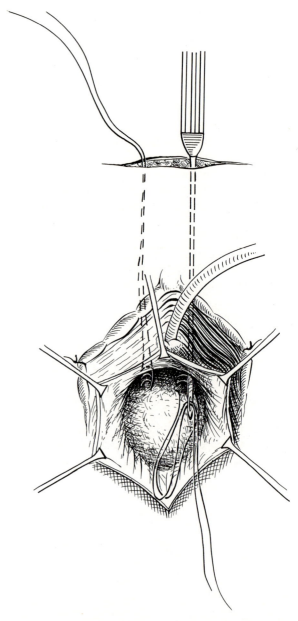

Fig. 50-11. Through a short transverse suprapubic incision, a Pereyra ligature carrier is introduced as shown, perforating the rectus aponeurosis and muscle, progressing through the space of Retzius, to appear in the vaginal wound lateral to the vesicourethral junction. The previously mentioned helical stitches are threaded into the tip of the ligature carrier as shown on the right, and the ligature carrier is withdrawn, bringing the sutures through the space of Retzius into the abdominal wound as shown to the left of the drawing.

scope can be substituted. Intravenously injected indigocarmine will be seen 5 to 10 minutes later pulsating from the unobstructed ureteral orifices. If there has been a penetration of the bladder by suture material, the suture can easily be withdrawn and rerouted through the space of Retzius. Once the surgeon is satisfied with the suture placement, traction on the sutures (with the cystoscope in mid-urethra) will reveal satisfactory elevation of the urethra and closure of the bladder neck.

At the completion of the cystoscopy, the Foley catheter is replaced in the bladder. The posterior pubourethral ligaments are brought together under the proximal urethra with a figure-eight suture of slowly absorbable polyglycolic type suture (Maxon or PDS; Fig. 50-12). Any attendant cystocele can now be reduced in the standard fashion using the subvaginal fascia. Redundant vagina is excised. After closure of the vaginal wall, the elevating sutures are pulled up with the same tension and visual elevation of the bladder neck as was seen with the cystoscopy. The sutures are either tied across the rectus fascia to one another or one end on each side is brought back through the fascia with a Mayo needle and tied to the other end of the same suture (Figs. 50-13 and 50-14).

The Foley catheter is left in place for approximately 48 hours. The author likes to remove the catheter at bedtime with a simple, offhand instruction that if the patient remembers we would like to measure the amount voided when she does so in the morning. But if she forgets to collect it for measurement, we will measure the next voiding. This casual, expectant, positive approach defuses the patient's anxiety and often on first arising she will void with-

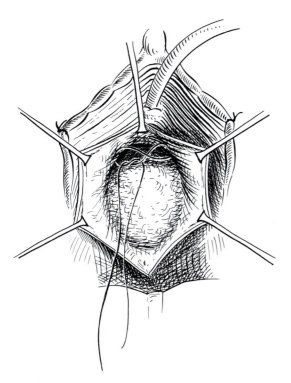

Fig. 50-12. The posterior pubourethral ligaments are plicated beneath the proximal urethra with a figure-eight stitch.

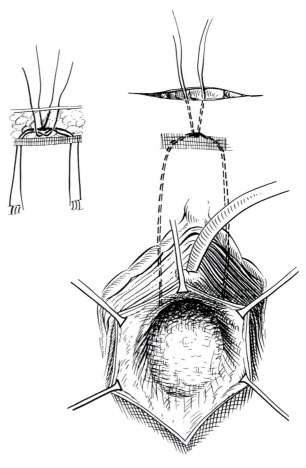

Fig. 50-13. After proper traction to this suture has been made, the sutures are tied.

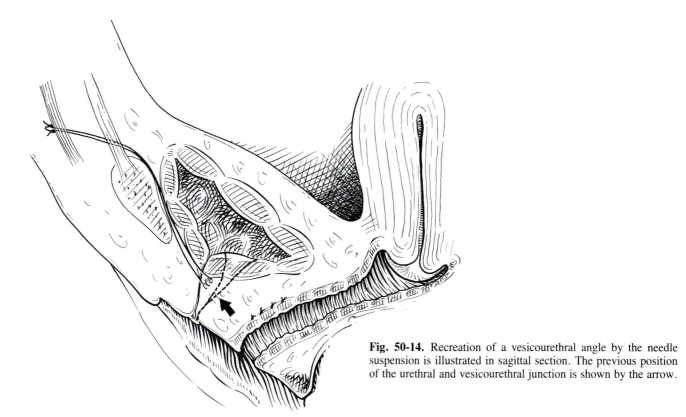

Fig. 50-14. Recreation of a vesicourethral angle by the needle suspension is illustrated in sagittal section. The previous position of the urethral and vesicourethral junction is shown by the arrow.

out giving it much thought. After due course, if postoperative bladder hypotonia persists, the patient is instructed in self-catherization, preferably using the Mentor flexible plastic catheter for the female. This procedure will not be entirely foreign to the patient because the possibility has been discussed with her preoperatively in the office.

There have been several variations of this operative procedure. Stamey proposed a loop of suture on each side with a pledget of synthetic material at the loop to buttress the paraurethral tissues.[77] The pledget, in effect, replaces the helical suture loops. The author's experience with this procedure has not been favorable. On a number of occasions, the pledget has required removal because of a foreign body reaction. A simplified loop of suture led through two suprapubic incisions down through the vagina and returned without any attempt to bury it beneath the vaginal mucosa has been proposed by Gittes and Loughlin.[32,48,49] They find that the suture is soon covered by vaginal mucosa as a matter of course. This procedure can be done under local anesthesia in a surgical day care setting. Although the long-term results are disheartening, this procedure may be a consideration for an elderly person with compromising medical problems for which a limited procedure may be desirable.

Anterior colporrhaphy as a treatment for genuine stress incontinence is discussed in Chapter 21.

Suburethral sling procedures

Recurrent and socially disabling incontinence is devastating not only for the patient but also for her physician. Before embarking on any additional therapy, it is of utmost importance to restudy the patient from the beginning with a fresh history, drug history, examination, and urodynamic evaluation as outlined earlier in this chapter.

Patients who fail usual antiincontinence surgery have frequently been successfully treated with a suburethral sling operation.[53,58] A special subset of incontinent patients have been identified with low urethral pressure. These patients fail standard antiincontinence surgery in an extraordinarily high percentage.[70] Experience has shown that these patients with low urethral pressure (closure pressure less than 20 cm of water) are more predictably cured by a suburethral sling procedure.

The patients who are more likely to have low urethral pressure have had prior surgery with fibrosis and fixation of the urethra. Robertson has described patients with an inflexible fixed "drainpipe" urethra. Additionally, patients with long-standing diabetes, those with neurologic injuries to the pelvic floor for whatever reason, patients with chronic obstructive lung disease, as well as patients over the age of 65, are more likely to have low urethral pressure resistance.

Since sling procedures were first introduced, a number of different materials have been used, including rectus fascia,[55] dura mater, round ligament,[37] fascia lata,[62] as well as synthetic materials such as Mersilene,[57,58] Gore-Tex,[38] Marlex,[26] and the Silastic sling,[44] to mention a few. Each

material has its proponent, but the basic purpose is the same—to elevate the bladder neck, support and compress the base, thereby increasing outlet resistance.

There have been two basic approaches to this operation. The first is to accomplish it entirely through an abdominal incision, making a tunnel under the urethra and bladder neck through which the supporting material is passed, as in the Millin sling procedure.[56] This approach has the disadvantage of increasing the likelihood of bladder and urethral injury and potential fistula formation. In the second approach, a combined abdominovaginal route allows direct visualization of the undersurface of the bladder neck through an open dissection of anterior vaginal wall, minimizing the possibility of urologic injury.

We prefer the abdominovaginal approach and generally use Mersilene mesh for support,[58] although a strap of fascia lata may be alternately used. With the patient in a modified lithotomy position using either standard lithotomy hanging leg supports or the Allen universal supports, the abdomen and perineum are prepared and draped. Two short lower abdominal transverse incisions are made two fingerbreadths above and two fingerbreadths lateral to the pubic tubercle. The incisions are carried down to the rectus fascia, which is cleared of fat. The rectus fascia on each side is incised in the direction of its fibers. With scissor tips followed by finger dissection, the rectus muscle is penetrated near its medial border, and the dissection is carried through the transversalis fascia down behind the pubis into the space of Retzius to the level of the obturator for amen.

Next, the surgeon moves to the transvaginal approach and opens the anterior vaginal wall longitudinally, exposing the bladder neck and proximal urethra. The urogenital diaphragm is penetrated on each side lateral to the urethra and opening into the space of Retzius from below, and a pilot suture is introduced on each side from below up using a Bozeman uterine packing forceps (Fig. 50-15). Alternately, as in the modified Pereyra procedure, the Pereyra needle may be passed abdominally through the rectus incision and brought out into the vaginal incision at the urethrovesical junction. A strip of single-thickness Mersilene gauze mesh cut in the direction of least stretch and trimmed to allow a midsegment of at least an inch in width, is placed over the bladder neck and urethra. The Mersilene mesh is sutured in place with 000 slowly absorbed synthetic suture, preventing wrinkling. The vaginal end of the pilot suture is tied to each end of the Mersilene and serves the purpose of retropubic retrieval. Traction to the abdominal ends of the pilot sutures brings the ends of the Mersilene gauze retropubically up into the abdominal incisions (Fig. 50-16).

At this point, the Foley catheter is removed and the bladder is viewed cystoscopically to ensure that there has not been a bladder or urethral penetration and to see that satisfactory elevation is obtained. If foreign material is present in the bladder, it is retrieved and replaced more satisfactorily. Intravenous indigo-carmine facilitates recog-

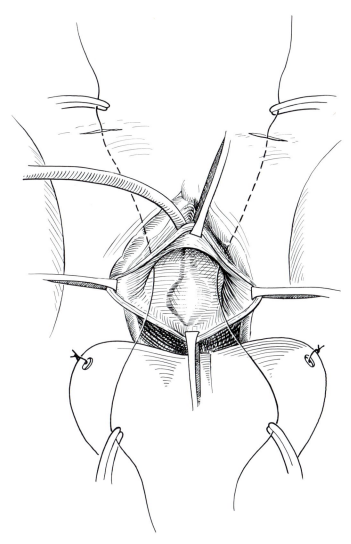

Fig. 50-15. The vesicourethral sling procedure. Incisions have been made in each groin and in the anterior vaginal wall. The latter is separated from the vesicourethral junction by sharp dissection. A pilot stitch has been introduced into the space of Retzius on each side, and the ends are clamped.

nition of the ureteral orifices and ensures their patency. At the completion of the cystoscopy, the Foley catheter is replaced.

Any necessary anterior or posterior colporrhaphy is accomplished. The vaginal incision is closed in two layers to protect against an erosion of the synthetic material into the vagina. The vaginal canal is packed with iodoform or Betadine-impregnated gauze packing. This elevates the bladder base and urethra to a normal retropubic position (Fig. 50-17).

After changing gloves, the surgical team returns to the abdominal incisions and sutures the ends of the Mersilene mesh to the rectus sheath after gently pulling out any wrinkling redundancy. Without further traction, the tail of the sling is sewn to the rectus aponeurosis or fascia at the point where each end of the sling crosses through the apo-

neurosis. This helps to reduce undue strain on the supports and to guard against over-correction. After closure of the rectus fascia, the skin edges are approximated in the usual fashion. Perioperative antibiotics are given to reduce the possibility of cross-contamination of the vaginal to abdominal wound areas.

Postoperatively, the catheter is removed as described earlier. There is a greater potential for postoperative bladder hypotonia after a sling procedure, and this must be part of preoperative counseling. Clean self-catheterization can be taught and practiced until voiding function returns. Even when this is required for lengthy periods of time, one rarely encounters an incontinent patient who would not prefer to self-catheterize and be dry. One should be very cautious in considering a sling procedure for the uncommon patient with impaired and hypoactive detrusor function. Increased outlet resistance engendered by the sling may permanently prevent satisfactory emptying.

Raz has proposed a sling procedure using a sheath of rectus fascia under the bladder neck elevated by four sutures at the four corners of the sheath. The elevating sutures are led through the retropubic space by a needle and then secured to the rectus fascia.[69] This is essentially a transvaginal approach.

Postoperative detrusor instability is more common after a sling operation. If there is detrusor instability present before surgery, it may be intensified postoperatively. In most instances, instability can be satisfactorily controlled by musculotropic agents such as oxybutynin in conjunction with timed voiding. In time, most detrusor instability will modify or regress completely.

A simpler procedure for patients with deficient outlet resistance is the submucosal injection of biodegradable glutaraldehyde cross-linked collagen (Gax) beneath the urethral mucosa at the bladder neck.[2] This procedure has particular appeal for patients with limiting medical conditions because the surgery is very short and can be done with local anesthesia in an outpatient setting.[3] Early results are promising. It works by effectively increasing periurethral outlet resistance. Biodegradable Gax collagen has an advantage over nonbiodegradable polytetrafluoroethylene (Teflon), which has been shown to migrate after injection.[51,68]

SUMMARY

The surgery for urinary incontinence has many varied techniques and methods of approach. The breadth of variety is a direct reflection of the complexity of urinary incontinence and its individual patient expression. The key to success resides in a clear understanding of this individual expression in each patient through complete evaluation before surgery. With this information in hand, the surgeon can pick and choose from the surgical armamentarium and tailor it to meet the specific needs of that person.

Despite the level of our present understanding and the scope of therapeutic applications available, therapy is not always successful. Current expectations for long-term suc-

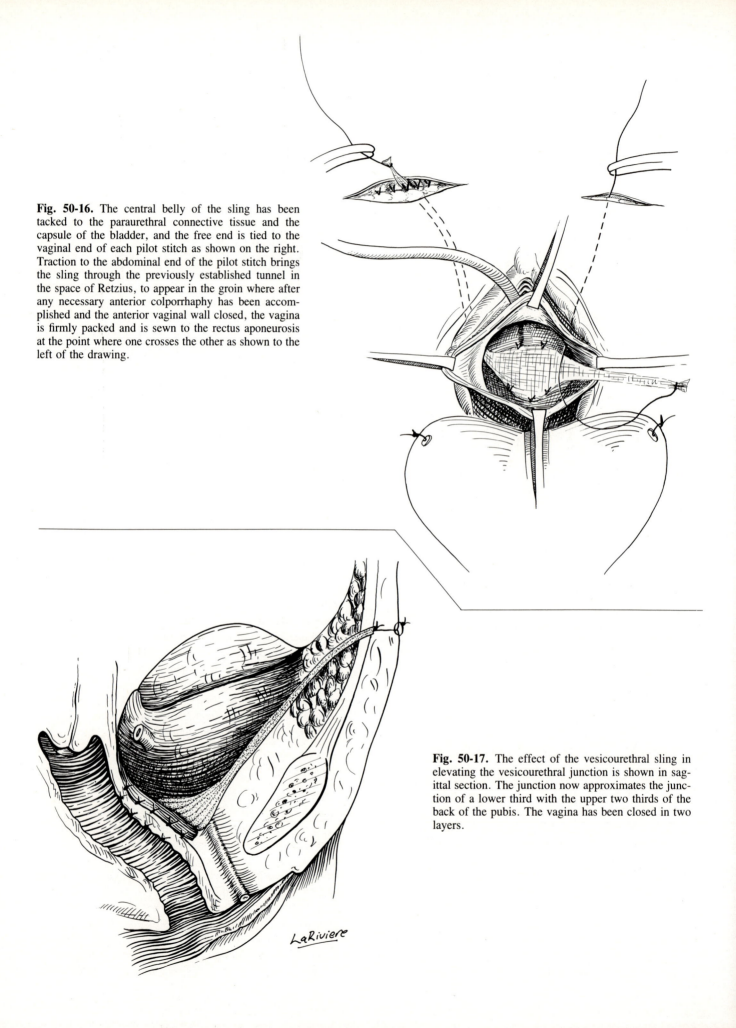

Fig. 50-16. The central belly of the sling has been tacked to the paraurethral connective tissue and the capsule of the bladder, and the free end is tied to the vaginal end of each pilot stitch as shown on the right. Traction to the abdominal end of the pilot stitch brings the sling through the previously established tunnel in the space of Retzius, to appear in the groin where after any necessary anterior colporrhaphy has been accomplished and the anterior vaginal wall closed, the vagina is firmly packed and is sewn to the rectus aponeurosis at the point where one crosses the other as shown to the left of the drawing.

Fig. 50-17. The effect of the vesicourethral sling in elevating the vesicourethral junction is shown in sagittal section. The junction now approximates the junction of a lower third with the upper two thirds of the back of the pubis. The vagina has been closed in two layers.

LaRiviere

cess range between 75% and 85%. There is much work to be done in refining diagnosis and therapy. The need is great but the rewards are profound when a physician assists in removing an enormous burden of incontinence from a patient.

REFERENCES

1. Abrams P et al: Sixth report on the standardization of terminology of the lower urinary tract function. Procedures related to neurophysiological investigations. Electromyography, nerve conduction studies, reflex latencies, evoked potentials and sensory testing, *World J Urol* 4:2, 1986; *Scand J Urol Nephrol* 20:162, 1986.
2. Appell RA: Injectables for urethral incompetence, *World J Urol* 8:208, 1990.
3. Appell RA et al: Multi-center study of periurethral and transurethral injection of GAX-collagen in female urinary incontinence, *Int Urogynecol J* (sample issue): 41, 1990.
4. Awad SA et al: Distribution of alpha and beta receptors in the human urinary bladder, *Br J Pharmacol* 50:525, 1974.
5. Bates P et al: Fourth report on the standardization of terminology of the lower urinary tract function, *Br J Urol* 53:333, 1981.
6. Bates P et al: First and second reports of the standardization of terminology of lower urinary tract function, *Am J Obstet Gynecol* 59:269, 1982.
7. Beck RP: Detrusor instability: Diagnosis and therapy, *Current Opinion Obstet Gynecol* 2:591, 1990.
8. Beck RP, Arnush D, King C: Results in treating 210 patients with detrusor overactivity incontinence of urine, *Am J Obstet Gynecol* 125:593, 1976.
9. Beck RP, McCormick S: Treatment of urinary incontinence with anterior colporrhaphy, *Obstet Gynecol* 59:369, 1982.
10. Beck RP, McCormick S, Nordstrom L: Intraurethral-intravesical cough-pressure spike differences in 267 patients cured of stress incontinence of urine, *Obstet Gynecol* 72:302, 1988.
11. Benson JT, Sumners JE: Ultrasound evaluation of female urinary incontinence, *Int Urogynecol J* 1:7, 1990.
12. Bent A: Concurrent genuine stress incontinence and detrusor instability, *Int Urogynecol J* 1:124, 1990.
13. Bergman A, Ballard CA, Koonings PP: Comparison of three different surgical procedures for genuine stress incontinence: Prospective randomized study, *Am J Obstet Gynecol* 160:1102, 1989.
14. Bergman A et al: Role of the Q-tip test in the evaluation of stress urinary incontinence, *J Reprod Med* 32:273, 1987.
15. Bergman A et al: Ultrasonic prediction of stress urinary incontinence development in surgery for severe pelvic relaxation, *Gynecol Obstet Invest* 26:66, 1988.
16. Bhatia N: *Ultrasound in gynecologic urology.* In Ostergard DR, editor: *Gynecologic urology and urodynamics,* ed 2, p 219, Baltimore, 1985, Williams & Wilkins.
17. Bowen LW et al: Unsuccessful Burch retropubic urethropexy: A case-controlled urodynamic study, *Am J Obstet Gynecol* 160:452, 1989.
18. Brown MC et al: Potential use of ultrasound in place of x-ray fluoroscopy in urodynamics, *Br J Urol* 57:88, 1985.
19. Bump RD: The urodynamic laboratory, *Obstet Gynecol Clin North Am* 16:795, 1989.
20. Bump RC, Fantl JA, Hurt WG: The mechanism of urinary continence in women with severe uterovaginal prolapse: Results of Barrier studies, *Obstet Gynecol* 72:291, 1988.
21. Burch JC: Urethrovaginal fixation to Cooper's ligament for correction of stress incontinence, cystocele and prolapse, *Am J Obstet Gynecol* 81:281, 1961.
22. Consensus Development Conference. National Institutes of Health, October 3, 1988.
23. Crystle CD, Charme LS, Copeland WE: Q-tip test in stress urinary incontinence, *Obstet Gynecol* 38:313, 1971.
24. DeLancy JOL: Correlative study of paraurethral anatomy, *Obstet Gynecol* 68:91, 1986.
25. DeLancy JOL: Structural aspects of the extrinsic continence mechanism, *Obstet Gynecol* 72:296, 1988.
26. Drutz HP et al: Clinical and urodynamic re-evaluation of combined abdomino-vaginal Marlex sling operations for recurrent stress urinary incontinence, *Int Urogynecol J* 1:70, 1990.
27. Duthoy EJ et al: Suprapubic urethropexy: Management with a transvesical exposure. *J Urol* 137:225, 1987.
28. Enhorning G: Simultaneous recording of intravesical and intraurethral pressure, *Acta Chir Scand* 276(suppl):10, 1961.
29. Fantl JA et al: Bead-chain cystourethrogram: An evaluation, *Obstet Gynecol* 58:237, 1981.
30. Garnell JWG, St. Leger AS: The prevalence, severity and factors associated with urinary incontinence in the elderly, *Age Ageing* 8:81, 1979.
31. Gilpin SA et al: The pathogenesis of genitourinary prolapse and stress incontinence of urine: A histological and histochemical study, *Br J Obstet Gynecol* 96:15, 1989.
32. Gittes RF, Loughlin KR: No-incision pubovaginal suspension for stress incontinence, *J Urol* 138:568, 1987.
33. Glezerman M et al: Evaluation of the reliability of history in women complaining of urinary stress incontinence, *Eur J Obstet Gynecol Reprod Biol* 21:159, 1986.
34. Green TH: Urinary stress incontinence: Differential diagnosis, pathophysiology and management, *Am J Obstet Gynecol* 122:368, 1975.
35. Hadley HR et al: Transvaginal needle bladder neck suspension, *Clin Obstet Gynaecol* 12:497, 1985.
36. Hodgkinson CP: Recurrent stress urinary incontinence, *Am J Obstet Gynecol* 132:844, 1978.
37. Hodgkinson CP, Kelly WT: Stress urinary incontinence in the female. Round ligament technique for retropubic suspension of the urethra, *Obstet Gynecol* 10:493, 1957.
38. Horbach NS et al: A suburethral sling procedure with PTFE for the treatment of genuine stress incontinence in patients with low urethral closure pressure, *Obstet Gynecol* 71:648, 1988.
39. Hu TW: Economic impact of urinary incontinence, *Clin Geriatr Med* 1:673, 1986.
40. Iosif S et al: Estrogen receptors in the human female lower urinary tract, *Am J Obstet Gynecol* 141:817, 1981.
41. Jorgenson L, Lose G, Molsted-Pederson L: Vaginal repair in female motor urge incontinence, *Eur Urol* 13:382, 1987.
42. Kohorn EI et al: Ultrasound cystomethrography by perineal scanning of the assessment of female urinary incontinence, *Obstet Gynecol* 68:269, 1986.
43. Koonings P, Bergman A, Ballard CA: Combined detrusor instability and stress urinary incontinence: Where is the primary pathology? *Gynecol Obstet Invest* 26:250, 1988.
44. Korda A, Peat B, Hunter P: Silastic slings for female incontinence, *Int Urogynecol J* 1:66, 1990.
45. Langer R et al: Detrusor instability following colposuspension for urinary stress incontinence, *Br J Obstet Gynecol* 95:607, 1988.
46. Leach GE, Raz S: Modified Pereyra bladder neck suspension after previously failed anti-incontinence surgery, *Urology* 23:359, 1984.
47. Lee RA: Abdominal operations for urinary incontinence. In Sciarra JL et al, editors: *Gynecology and Obstetrics,* vol 1, Ch 86, 1980.
48. Loughlin KR et al: The comparative medical costs of two major procedures available for the treatment of stress urinary incontinence, *J Urol* 127:436, 1982.
49. Loughlin KR et al: Review of an 8 year experience with modifications of endoscopic suspension of the bladder neck for female stress incontinence, *J Urol* 143:44, 1990.
50. Low JA, Armstrong JB, Mauger GM: The unstable urethra in the female, *Obstet Gynecol* 74:69, 1989.
51. Malizia AA et al: Migration and granulomatous reaction after periurethral injection of Polytef (Teflon), *JAMA* 251:3277, 1984.
52. Marshall VF, Marchetti AA, Krantz KE: The correction of stress in-

continence by simple vesicourethral suspension, *Surg Gynecol Obstet* 88:509, 1949.

53. McGuire EJ, Lytton B: Pubovaginal sling procedure for stress incontinence, *J Urol* 119:82, 1978.

54. McGuire EJ, Savastano JA: Stress urinary incontinence and detrusor instability/urge incontinence, *Neurol Urodyn* 4:313, 1985.

55. McLaren AG: Late results from sling operations, *Obstet Gynaecol Br Commonw* 75:10, 1968.

56. Millin T, Reed CD: Stress incontinence of urine in the female, *Postgrad Med J* 24:51, 1948.

57. Moir JC: The gauze hammock operation, *J Obstet Gynaecol Br Commonw* 75:1, 1968.

58. Nichols DH: *The sling operations.* In Cantor EB, editor: *Female stress incontinence,* Springfield, Ill, 1979, Charles C Thomas.

59. Ostergard DR: The effect of drugs on the lower urinary tract, *Obstet Gynecol Surv* 34:424, 1979.

60. Ouslander JG, Kane RL, Abrams GB: Urinary incontinence in elderly nursing home patients, *JAMA* 248:1194, 1982.

61. Park GS, Miller EJ: Surgical treatment of stress urinary incontinence: A comparison of the Kelly plication, Marshall-Marchetti-Krantz and Pereyra procedures, *Obstet Gynecol* 71:575, 1988.

62. Parker RT, Addison WA, Wilson CJ: Fascia lata uterovesical suspension for recurrent stress urinary incontinence, *Am J Obstet Gynecol* 135:843, 1979.

63. Pereyra AJ: A simplified surgical procedure for the correction of stress incontinence in women, *West J Surg Obstet Gynecol* 67:223, 1959.

64. Pereyra AJ: *Revised Pereyra procedure using colligated pubourethral supports.* In Slate WG, editor: *Disorders of the female urethra and urinary incontinence,* Baltimore, 1978, Williams & Wilkins.

65. Pereyra AJ, Lebherz TB: Combined urethrovesical suspension and vaginourethroplasty for correction of stress incontinence, *Obstet Gynecol* 30:537, 1967.

66. Pereyra AJ et al: Pubourethral supports in perspective: Modified Pereyra procedure for urinary incontinence, *Obstet Gynecol* 59:643, 1982.

67. Peters WA, Thornton WN: Selection of the primary procedure for stress urinary incontinence, *Am J Obstet Gynecol* 137:923, 1980.

68. Politano VA: Periurethral Teflon injection for incontinence, *Urol Clin North Am* 5:415, 1978.

69. Raz S: Modified bladder neck suspension for female stress incontinence, *Urology* 18:82, 1981.

70. Robertson JR: Gynecologic urethroscopy, *Am J Obstet Gynecol* 115:986, 1973.

71. Sand PK, Bowen LW, Ostergard DR: Uninhibited urethral relaxation in unusual cause of incontinence, *Obstet Gynecol* 68:645, 1986.

72. Sand PK et al: The low pressure urethra as a factor in failed retropubic urethropexy, *Obstet Gynecol* 69:399, 1987.

73. Sand P, Hill RC, Ostergard DR: Incontinence history as a predictor of detrusor instability, *Obstet Gynecol* 71:257, 1988.

74. Sier H, Ouslander J, Orzeck S: Urinary incontinence among geriatric patients in an acute care hospital, *JAMA* 257:1767, 1987.

75. Spencer JR, O'Connor VJ, Schaeffer AJ: A comparison of endoscopic suspension of the vesical neck with suprapubic vesicourethropexy for treatment of stress urinary incontinence, *J Urol* 137:411, 1987.

76. Stamey TA: Endoscopic suspension of the vesical neck for urinary incontinence, *Surg Gynecol Obstet* 136:547, 1973.

77. Stamey TA: Endoscopic suspension of the vesical neck for urinary incontinence, *Surg Gynecol Obstet* 192:465, 1980.

78. Susset J, Galea G, Read L: Biofeedback therapy for female incontinence due to low urethral resistance, *J Urol* 143:1205, 1990.

79. Tanagho EA: The way we do it, *J Urol* 116:751, 1976.

80. Tries J: Kegel exercises enhanced by biofeedback, *J Enterostom Ther* 17:67, 1990.

81. Turner-Warwick R: Some clinical aspects of detrusor dysfunction, *J Urol* 113:539, 1975.

82. vanGeelen H: Drug action on the bladder and urethra, *Int Urogynecol J* 1:19, 1990.

83. vanGeelen JM et al: The clinical and urodynamic effects of anterior vaginal repair and Burch colposuspension, *Am J Obstet Gynecol* 159:137, 1988.

84. Walter S et al: Stress urinary incontinence in postmenopausal women treated with oral estrogen (estriol) and an alpha-adrenergic stimulating agent (phenylpropanolamine): A random double-blind placebo-controlled study, *Int J Urogynecol* 1:74, 1990.

85. Wheelahan JB: Long-term results of colposuspension, *Br J Urol* 65:329, 1990.

Chapter 51

TRANSVAGINAL REPAIR OF BLADDER INJURIES AND OF UROGENITAL VESICOVAGINAL FISTULA

David H. Nichols

SURGICAL PRINCIPLES IN BLADDER FISTULA SURGERY

The late Tom Ball[3] described the following surgical principles that are universally applicable to the successful closure of genitourinary fistulas.

1. Surfaces are to be opposed that will require all the factors concerned with the union of tissues to be as near normal as possible. Evaluate the patient's general health and nutrition. Postpone operation until any nutritional deficiencies are corrected by diet and supplementary therapy. Investigate the patient's blood chemistry with attention to the plasma proteins, blood sugar, and electrolytes. Latent diabetes should be suspected and a sugar tolerance test performed in patients who have experienced multiple failures. The most skillful closure may fail when the essential conditions for proper wound healing are neglected.

2. Infection and the deposition of urinary salts about the edges of the fistula compromise healing. Upper urinary tract disease should be eliminated by appropriate study and treatment and the bladder freed of infection by urinary antiseptics. An intravenous pyelogram, cystoscopy, and retrograde studies as indicated should precede the operation. Urine cultures and sensitivity tests—so you know you have one or more agents effective against any organism identified—guide your choice of antibiotics and other urinary antiseptics. The importance of confirming the presence of healthy edges by cystoscopic observation will be apparent to those who attempt a closure only to find themselves inverting tissue into an encrusted bladder mucosa. The preoperative preparation of the fistulous tract requires attention to bladder irrigations and vaginal douches. The solutions should be mildly acid since the deposition of urinary encrustations is most frequent in an alkaline urine. Water intake should be forced despite the discomfort attendant upon the increased output.

3. Study the accessibility of a fistula and the means by which the position on the operating table (lithotomy, Sims, knee-chest) may help to bring it into the field. As Kelly said regarding accessibility, "Either the operator must go up to the fistula or the fistula must be brought down to the operator; or a combination of both may be necessary for success."

4. Regardless of how distant the tract may seem from the vaginal aspect, it is not, with few exceptions, so far away as it is through a large abdominal panniculus, deep pelvis, and across the bladder through a suprapubic cystotomy. In short, everything favors the vaginal approach to all but a few fistulas. *From the abdomen you operate in the dark so far as the vaginal wall is concerned and at the bottom of a chasm on the bladder wall; from the vagina you see the vaginal wall directly, and the mucosa of the bladder can be visualized as frequently as necessary by the simplest of endoscopes!*

5. Remember that fistulas in the lateral sulci are accessible only with some risk of damage to the ureter unless this structure is positively identified. Place a catheter in the ureter, if possible, on the side of the fistula, and remove it only when all sutures in the fistula closure have been placed and tied. A small catheter can be left in place as a splint if the particular fistula involves the intramural ureter. If the catheter is removed, the ureteral orifice should be visualized with a simple observation endoscope to note the efflux of urine and whether it contains blood.

6. Schuchardt's incision, correctly performed, makes a high fistula readily accessible.

7. Vesicovaginal fistulas recognized on the delivery table are closed immediately only if the edges of the tear are clean, not edematous or necrotic, and the patient's condition is good. The frantic closure of a fistula after a long labor, edema and ischemia of the edges, and contamination of the field by repeated examinations and instrumentation will most surely result in complete

breakdown of the wound and complicate future closure. Exercise restraint since the fistula may close spontaneously or be a simple procedure in a few months.

8. Develop the patience to study before and during a fistula repair the direction, density, and firmness of the scar tissue adjacent to the fistula, not only in all directions, but also along its course directly to the bladder or through other structures. Master gynecologic surgeons—renowned for dexterity and speed—have the wisdom to proceed painstakenly and deliberately in performing a fistula repair. Remember that you can observe the pliability of the bladder wall through a cystoscope while manipulating the vaginal aspect of the fistulous tract and add to your information regarding the direction of forces that may disrupt your repair.

9. Midline vesicovaginal fistulas are best approached by a vertical (in axis of vagina) incision that circumscribes the vaginal orifice of the fistula. After the separation and mobilization of the vaginal and bladder walls, the bladder is closed transversely and the vaginal wall vertically. By this method the ultimate strain on the suture lines is minimized and the blood supply left intact to both layers.

10. Lateral sulcus fistulas of small dimensions are best approached with a transverse vaginal incision since the blood supply to the vagina originates from that direction. A long vertical incision in the lateral vaginal wall, while leaving the lateral vaginal flap of the closure with an intact blood supply, may compromise the medial flap since it would have to receive vessels from above or across the midline.

11. Adequate mobilization of the bladder frequently requires a total hysterectomy, either vaginal or abdominal. This is necessary to remove a uterus to which the bladder is adherent by dense scar tissue that would cause retraction of the edges of the fistula closure if left behind.

12. Fistulas not infrequently course through a cervical stump when they are the result of an emergency Porro section or other surgery to stem bleeding. Elimination of the entire fistula is best accomplished by excision of the cervical stump, which effects an adequate mobilization of the bladder at the same time.

13. *Study the cause of a fistula and you will learn where to expect its edges to be scarred and retracted!* An example of this is a vault fistula following a total abdominal hysterectomy. The posterior edge of such a fistula is farthest from the introitus and coincides with the transverse scar of the vaginal vault. *This, then, is the segment of the opening that must be carefully mobilized!* In an obliteration type of procedure (Latzko) this must be appreciated so that an adequate denudation is done posteriorly to cover the opening that anatomically lies in the anterior vaginal wall just as it is reflected anteriorly from the scar of the closed vaginal vault.

14. Recognize a situation in which the blood supply adjacent to the fistula is so impaired as to require some type of transplant as an artificial means of providing nourishment to the flaps used in the closure. The gracilis muscle or a Martius graft (bulbocavernosus and vestibular bulb) is a source of providing a new blood supply.

15. Will the patient have gross urinary stress incontinence from an incompetent bladder neck after a successful fistula closure and thus be little better off than before? Studies of the position of the bladder neck before surgery by urethroscopy and urethrography may anticipate this complication, permitting the surgeon to incorporate some type of bladder neck plication for restoration of the posterior urethrovesical angle and a competent bladder neck in his fistula repair.

16. The principles of bladder fistula surgery that permit approximation of the edges without strangulation or tension are put into effect the moment tissue is touched. Use traction sutures to gain exposure or fix tissues for dissection wherever this is possible.

17. Crushing instruments must not be used, and *all tissues are delicately handled and as little as possible!*

18. Aim for the approximation of broad, raw, healthy surfaces.

19. When a suture has to be tied under tension, the dissection has been inadequate, and this suture should be removed. It will only cause a sloughing of the immediate area and may doom the entire procedure to failure.

20. The availability of strong, small caliber, and atraumatic suture material has outmoded nonabsorbable material such as silkworm gut and silver or steel wire. Use small, round-body, atraumatic needles and interrupted sutures throughout. Pursestring, figure-of-eight, and other fancy variations are tissue stranglers and have no place in fistula surgery.

21. Characteristic of the anastomosis in most hollow structures (bowel, ureterovesical and ureterointestinal transplants, vascular surgery), the success of the closure depends, to a great extent, upon the approximation of the internal lining of the structure. Strive to approximate mucosa to mucosa, with your sutures passing in the submucosa in the closure of a bladder fistula.

22. Close the bladder and vaginal walls in different planes so that as little as possible of one suture line is superimposed on the other. The exception to this principle is a situation where such a closure would cause undue tension. The direction of retraction of the edges of the fistula may necessitate closure in the same plane to avoid tension, and this is more important than superimposition of the suture lines.

23. Do not neglect the use of the cystourethroscope during the course of an operation. It is invaluable in determining the proper eversion of healthy tissue and mucosa-to-mucosa approximation within the bladder.

24. A urethral catheter is satisfactory for fistulas in the base, provided it does not lay on the suture line. A suprapubic cystotomy is used after an abdominal approach to some fistulas or a combined approach.

25. Postoperatively the urinary tract is kept free of infection by the use of an effective urinary antiseptic or a combination of drugs. The patient's nutrition is important, and appropriate electrolyte studies are done as indicated. Patients should be mobilized immediately and careful attention paid to the avoidance of straining at stool, coughing, or sneezing. Complete immobilization of the patient would seem to add little to the chance of successful closure since the patients still have to strain to evacuate their bowels.

In younger patients with a history of urinary loss, particularly in those with evidence of congenital malformation of the genitalia, the surgeon must thoroughly inspect both the urinary tract and the genital tract. Intravenous pyelography may be the only way to determine whether the patient has an aberrant or third ureter opening into the vagina. It is equally important to confirm that the patient with a urinary fistula has two patent, normally placed ureters. Should the patient have only a single kidney and ureter, the operator should certainly be aware of this fact before planning and undertaking the repair of the fistula. The

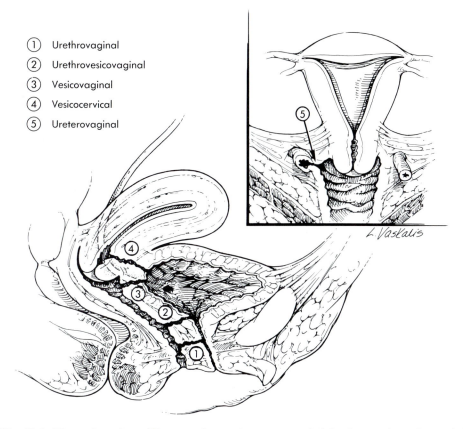

1. Urethrovaginal
2. Urethrovesicovaginal
3. Vesicovaginal
4. Vesicocervical
5. Ureterovaginal

L. Vaskalis

Fig. 51-1. The various sites of the more frequently seen urogenital fistulas are shown in saggital section. A combination of fistulas is possible, and the tracts may course through several structures. Vesicouterine, vesicocervicovaginal, urethrovesicovaginal, and ureterovaginal fistulas are indicated. One or more fistulas may exist at the same time.

operator should also determine the relationship of the fistula to the ureteral orifices, bladder neck, and trigone by means of preoperative cystoscopy.

Trauma, necrosis secondary to invasion by neoplastic growth, or rarely the reaction to certain types of necrotizing inflammation may lead to fistulae involving the female urinary tract and genitalia. Genital tract trauma is by far the most common cause.

Some possible locations of urinary fistula are shown in Fig. 51-1. The cause, diagnosis and treatment of each is sufficiently distinctive that the surgeon must be familiar with each one, bearing in mind that a patient may have more than one at a given time.

ACCIDENTAL INJURY TO ADJACENT STRUCTURES

Because unrecognized or unrepaired full-thickness trauma in the urinary or intestinal system usually results in the formation of a fistula, it is essential for the surgeon who is performing any gynecologic operation or obstetric procedure to recognize immediately any penetration of a neighboring viscus. The presence of a *small* amount of urine in the bladder is desirable at the time of vaginal hysterectomy or anterior colporrhaphy because its appearance in the operative field alerts the surgeon to a penetrating in-

jury. Any suspicion of such an injury must be investigated thoroughly and an appropriate repair accomplished without delay. Although the incidence of accidental penetration is small and becomes smaller as the experience of the operator increases, unexpected relationships may occasionally lead to accidental injuries no matter how often a surgeon operates.

Preoperatively, the surgeon should consider all sites of possible accidental trauma, such as an undesirable laceration, avulsion, or unwanted incision of nearby pelvic organs.

It is essential that any suspected injury be evaluated and treated promptly. A problem that is neglected intraoperatively may eventually necessitate one or more secondary surgical procedures, which can be as damaging to the surgeon's reputation as to the patient's health. There is no room for procrastination in the hope that the suspected damage did not occur or will resolve itself. Therefore, as soon as any injury is recognized, the operator should mobilize the tissues sufficiently to accomplish the repair under direct vision. The remainder of the operation can then proceed as planned. The effective management of such problems requires candor, scientific objectivity, and confident surgical technique.

One indication of a possible bladder injury during the

course of surgery is the escape of a recognizable urinelike fluid into the vagina. For this reason, it is desirable that some urine remains in the bladder during surgery. Patients about to undergo vaginal surgery should be asked to void shortly before they come to the operating suite and then should be catheterized at the beginning of surgery only if bimanual examination reveals bladder overdistention.

It is best to repair a visceral injury with two or three layers of fine absorbable suture (e.g., 3-0 polydiaxanone, polygluconate, polyglycolic-acid type, or chromic catgut). In the repair of injuries to the bladder or ureter, however, knots should be extraluminal in order to reduce the risk of calculus formation at the site of the suture. Accurate approximation of the submucosal muscular layers must provide the primary support in these cases; although mucosal sutures are hemostatic, they supply minimal support. A layer of watertight running horizontal mattress sutures in the muscular layer inverts the previous stitches, and another layer of interrupted reinforcing mattress stitches may be added, if desired, to reduce the tension on the deeper layer (Fig. 51-2). The operator must always be careful to avoid tying mattress sutures so tightly as to strangulate the tissues involved.

After repairing a recognized penetration in the bladder wall, the operator may test the repair for watertightness by instilling a methylene blue solution, an indigo carmine solution, or sterile milk (e.g., evaporated milk, canned condensed milk, or infant formula milk from the nursery) and checking for leakage. (Sterile milk has the obvious advantage over dyes in that the leakage of milk does not cause prolonged staining of adjacent tissues.) If there is evidence of leakage after the initial repair, the operator should place additional reinforcing sutures and again test the repair for leakage. Should the wall of the bladder be penetrated near its attachment to the cervix, the adjacent peritoneum can be mobilized and sewn over the site of the repair after the defect in the musculature has been repaired; such a peritoneal flap provides support and increases the blood supply to the area.

If the ureteral orifices are near or part of an accidental laceration, the operator should insert ureteral catheters. Ureteroneocystostomy is advisable if it is not possible to ensure the integrity of the ureters.

If the ureter is transected, as may occur quite inadvertently when the patient has an undiagnosed duplication of the ureter on one or both sides, the severed ureter can be successfully reimplanted under direct vision. Postoperative splinting with both ureteral and urethral catheters is desirable for 2 weeks.

A fistula that follows an obstetric laceration should be repaired within 24 hours of the injury. If a fistula develops after hysterectomy or if the first attempt to repair a fistula fails, however, the surgeon should allow an interval of 3 to 6 months to pass so that adequate lymphatic drainage can return to the tissue and the infection, swelling, and edema of surgery can subside. If necrosis and edema subside earlier, successful nondelayed repair has been reported.[21,22,23] If the fistula results from necrosis after irradiation, the vagina should be given local estrogen supplementation by transvaginal instillation of estrogen cream (1 to

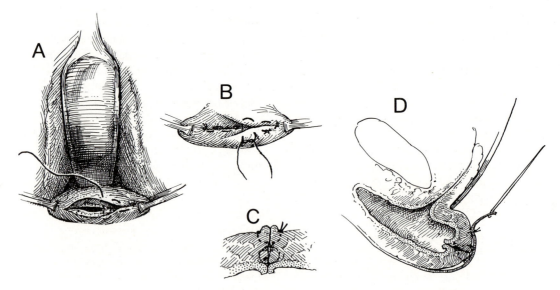

Fig. 51-2. Closure of accidental cystotomy is depicted. The defect has been identified and widely mobilized. A suture tagging the peritoneum is noted on the right side of **D.** If no mucosal stitch is used, a running mattress suture in the muscularis, starting and finishing lateral to the defect, may be placed as shown in **A.** This may be covered by a second layer of interrupted mattress sutures **(B)**, establishing full-thickness reapproximation of the muscularis as seen in cross-section **(C).** An anterior peritoneal flap has been excised from the anterior surface of the uterus as shown **(D)** and tacked in place over the operative repair, providing the security of an additional fresh tissue layer. (From Nichols DH, Randall CL: *Vaginal surgery,* ed 3, Baltimore, 1989, Williams & Wilkins, p 428.)

2 g at bedtime, two or three times weekly) and the repair postponed for at least a year to permit the progression of the causative endarteritis obliterans to cease.[24]

While awaiting the appropriate time for the repair of a fistula, the patient can obtain some temporary but welcome relief by wearing an intravaginal contraceptive diaphragm[4,5,31] the center of which has been perforated by a 3-mm hole through which the tip of a Foley catheter has been inserted. The balloon is inflated with 5 to 10 ml of air and the base of the balloon cemented by a cyanoacrylate watertight glue on cement to the inside of the diaphragm creating a watertight seal. After the adhesive has dried for 15 minutes, the diaphragm can be inserted into the vagina and connected to a urinary leg bag. It has been recommended that application of an estrogen cream be applied to the edges of the diaphragm each time it is inserted, to minimize trauma, and that the diaphragm be removed for several hours every few day, either at night or during the day, to avoid vaginal ulceration. The resulting improvement makes it easier for the patient to wait until the condition of the tissues is optimal for surgical repair. Although some authorities recommend cortisone treatment to accelerate tissue preparation for surgery, it seems preferable to wait the length of time required for inflammation and edema to subside, and not compromise wound healing by coincident steroid use, which may precipitate premature absorption of sutures.

Thompson[21,22,23] has described a technique of transvaginal repair of the distal ureter (i.e., along its lowest 3 cm). Ureteral catheters are inserted transurethrally, if possible. Palpation of the tip of this catheter identifies the area where operative exposure must be obtained. The proximal ureter is identified (if necessary, by the passage of urine made blue by an injection of intravenous indigo carmine) and dissected free. If the stump of a transsected ureter is long enough to permit ureteroureteral anastomosis without tension, a series of four 4-0 PGA sutures are placed through the muscularis (stent in place) (Fig. 51-3) and tied, establishing a ureteroureteral anastomosis. If the vesical stump of ureter is too short to be used safely, it is ligated and a ureteroneocystostomy performed.

Technique of transvaginal ureteroneocystostomy

A small cystotomy is made of a size sufficient to permit retrieval of the vesical end of the ureteral catheter (or infant-sized plastic feeding tube as a substitute for the ureteral catheter), which has been introduced into the bladder through the urethra. The internal tip is brought out through the cystotomy wound and inserted into the lumen of the cut end of the proximal ureter. The stent is advanced along the ureteral lumen for several centimeters. The tip of the proximal ureter is spatulated or fish-mouthed for about 1 cm on each side, and a 3-0 or 4-0 PGA suture is placed through the full thickness of the ureteral wall (Fig. 51-4). Both ends of each suture are sewn through the full thickness of the bladder mucosa and muscularis, one set on each side of the cystotomy, and gentle traction is applied to them, drawing the spatulated end of the ureter into the bladder (Fig. 51-5). The transmural sutures are tied, fixing the ureter in place. Tension on the anastomosis is reduced by placing several circumferential interrupted PGA sutures that fix the external surface of the implanted ureter to the bladder muscularis. (A "psoas hitch" to the bladder to achieve this is not possible with this transvaginal operative exposure.) If the site of ureteral repair or anastomosis cannot be covered by the flap of anterior vaginal wall, a Martius graft (see Figure 51-13, *F, G*) can be readily obtained and transposed into place.

The vagina is packed, and the ureteral stent taped to a transurethral Foley catheter. A postoperative intravenous

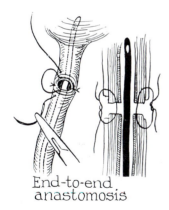

End-to-end anastomosis

Fig. 51-3. Ureteroureterostomy. Damage may be treated by ureteroureterostomy if there are unmistakably viable segments above and below the injury and the ureter can be anastomosed without tension. The ends are brought together with interrupted sutures of 0000 PGA on chromic catgut on atraumatic needles. The sutures should not pass into the lumen and should accurately approximate mucosa to mucosa. The anastomosis may also be done side to side or end to side. An end-to-end anastomosis restores the normal course of the ureter—a surgical principle that is observed whenever possible. A small splinting catheter is left in place. (From Ball TL: *Gynecologic surgery and urology,* ed 2, St Louis, 1963, Mosby–Year Book, p 542.)

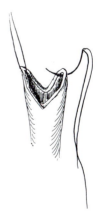

Fig. 51-4. Ureteroneocystostomy. A fish-mouth incision is made in the terminal ureter, and traction sutures of 4-0 PGA or chromic catgut are placed in the edge of each flap. (From Ball TL: *Gynecologic surgery and urology,* ed 2, St Louis, 1963, Mosby–Year Book, p 542.)

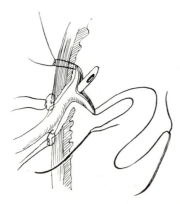

Fig. 51-5. The ureter is drawn into the bladder and the traction sutures are threaded on fine needles and passed through the adjacent bladder wall to anchor the flaps. These are tied on the outside to just approximate the tissues without strangulation. A few sutures are used to anchor the ureter at the point of entrance into the bladder wall. They should be placed in the adventitia of the ureter and into the bladder wall without constricting the anastomosis. (From Ball TL: *Gynecologic surgery and urology,* ed 2, St Louis, 1963, Mosby–Year Book, p 542.)

pyelogram is obtained, and another ordered following removal of the stent on an outpatient basis 2 to 3 weeks later. The pyelogram may be repeated periodically for several years in an attempt to ensure the integrity of the anastomosis and absence of progressive hydroureter-hydronephrosis that would suggest ureteral stricture.

With an absorbant tampon in place within the vagina, 100 cc of dilute Congo red solution may be instilled into the bladder through a transurethral catheter. The catheter is removed, and the patient is instructed to stand and move around. After half an hour, the vaginal tampon is removed and inspected. If the tip of the tampon is stained red, the dye will be presumed to have come from the Congo red, and the presence of a vesicovaginal fistula is likely. If the tampon is unstained, a fresh one is inserted into the vagina and the patient is given a 5-cc ampule of indigo-carmine intravenously. The second tampon is removed after half an hour and inspected. If the tip of the second tampon is stained blue, the dye will have come from the intravenous indigo-carmine, and the presence of a vesicovaginal fistula should be suspected.

VESICOVAGINAL FISTULA

A history of low cervical cesarean section is a factor predisposing to the development of a vesicovaginal fistula following hysterectomy because cesarean section may alter tissue relationships between the bladder and the cervix, thus increasing the risk of inadvertent injury during hysterectomy. When a patient with a history of cesarean section must undergo hysterectomy, it is helpful to instill 60 ml of indigo carmine or methylene blue solution into the bladder preoperatively. Not only can the violet-stained bladder mucosa sometimes be seen before the bladder may be opened, but violet-stained urine in the operative field is a priori evidence of unwanted penetration. Gynecologic sur-

geons must remember that approximately 20% of the present generation of parous women who will require hysterectomy in the future will have such a history.

When a vesicovaginal fistula develops after a hysterectomy, it is likely to be at the very apex of the vagina if the vaginal cuff was not closed or just anterior to the suture line if the vaginal cuff was closed. Vesicovaginal fistula in the lower vagina is more likely to occur after colporrhaphy.

A fistula first recognized after hysterectomy is usually the result of an unrecognized penetration or laceration at the time of the primary operative procedure; the result of trauma recognized but inadequately repaired; or, sometimes, the result of postoperative necrosis of a small area of bladder epithelium secondary to an infected hematoma or to devascularization by a suture placed into or immediately adjacent to the lumen of the bladder. Carelessly placed hemostatic mattress sutures in the bladder wall near the cut edge of the vagina may devitalize the spot of tissue in which they have been placed. In addition, incomplete surgical separation from the vaginal cuff during hysterectomy places the bladder at risk.

The presence of hematuria after the initial operative procedure should alert the operator to the possibility of a subsequent fistula, particularly if the bloody urine persists for longer than 48 postoperative hours. When this occurs, inspection by cystoscopy is advisable, and catheter drainage should usually continue for a number of days beyond the usual period. When a fistulous tract, even a small one, is relatively short, the patient is usually incontinent. When the fistulous tract is longer, especially if it is tortuous, the patient is likely to be incontinent only intermittently because the flow of urine through the tract may be inversely proportional to the amount of urine within the bladder. Patients with this type of fistula are frequently prone to infection and calculus formation along the tract, however. The presence of an intermittent spontaneous bloody urethral or urinary discharge is ominous, requiring evaluation and biopsy to rule out the presence of malignant disease, which may be coexisting with the fistulous tract.

Preoperative considerations

The gynecologic surgeon must always consider the possibility of multiple fistulas when investigating a recognized fistula. Obviously, the surgical correction of the recognized fistula will not eliminate incontinence resulting from an unrecognized and thus unrepaired coexistent fistula. Both operator and patient may believe that the treatment failed when the apparent failure may be due to the inadequacy of the preoperative study and appraisal. Careful review of the history and circumstances preceding the recognition of a fistula is essential.

Differentiation between a vesicovaginal and a ureterovaginal fistula is of primary importance. In making this distinction, many surgeons find that the tampon test is helpful.[9] A rather long menstrual tampon is inserted into the vagina and 6 to 8 ounces of strongly colored methylene blue or indigo carmine solution are then injected into the bladder. The patient is instructed to walk around for 10 or 15 minutes, after which the tampon is examined. If only the lowest part is wet and blue, the patient presumably suffers from urinary stress incontinence or detrusor instability; if the upper thirds are wet and blue, the patient probably has a vesicovaginal fistula; if the upper third is wet but not blue, the diagnosis is a damaged ureter.

General principles of repair

Several excellent techniques are available for the repair of a vesicovaginal fistula, and they are adaptable to a variety of clinical circumstances. There are certain general principles that a surgeon should consistently adhere to in performing a urinary fistula repair, however. The operator should:

1. Supplement or replace estrogen preoperatively and postoperatively if the patient is postmenopausal.
2. Postpone the repair until infection and inflammation have subsided and healthy granulation tissue may be present.
3. Dissect, mobilize, and excise the epithelialized tract and adjacent scar tissue until healthy, normal tissue is reached, thus converting the lesion to a fresh wound. As a rule, a fresh wound of bladder or rectum heals promptly and primarily if the initial repair is adequate and appropriate. It should be closed without tension.
4. Make lateral vaginal relaxing incisions if the repair has been closed under tension.
5. Try to interrupt the continuity of the fistulous tract so that the orifice of repair in one viscus no longer overlies or underlies its counterpart in the other.

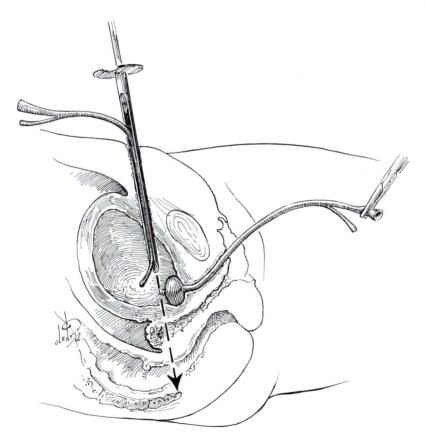

Fig. 51-6. Suprapubic cystostomy. The bladder has been distended by 400 ml of sterile saline solution instilled through a transurethral Foley catheter, shown in place and clamped. At a midline point two fingerbreadths above the superior border of the pubis, a no. 22 spinal needle was introduced through the anterior abdominal and bladder wall and pointed toward the coccyx. When a free flow of clear urine has been observed, the needle is immediately removed and a 1.5-cm transverse incision through the skin only is made using a no. 12 scalpel blade at the site of the needle puncture. The operator, having noted the approximate depth at which the spinal needle entered the bladder, bluntly introduces the Campbell trochar in the same direction until the characteristic "give" is noted. The sharply pointed obturator of the trochar is withdrawn about an inch, the blunt end of the sleeve is inserted an additional inch or two, and the obturator is removed. There is prompt escape of urine and saline, and immediately a no. 16 Foley catheter is inserted through the trochar into the bladder as shown. The 5-ml bulb is inflated, the trochar is removed, and a brief tug on the catheter until resistance is encountered brings the now inflated bulb to the undersurface of the fresh cystostomy. (Reproduced with permission from Nichols DH, Milley PS: A simplified technique for suprapubic cystostomy, *Ob/Gyn Digest* 12:30-35, 1970.)

6. Approximate anatomically strong layers or flaps and, when available, interpose between the previous fistulous orifices a strong tissue layer that has an independent blood supply.

7. When infection or abscess formation is likely, provide adequate drainage of the low pressure side of the previous tract.

8. Catheterize the ureter at the time of the repair if it is adjacent to or incorporated in the fistula to avoid unintentional operative ureteral stricture. If the repair seems likely to compromise the ureter, a ureteroneocystostomy may be desirable.

9. Decompress the bladder by catheter postoperatively. If the inflated bulb of a transurethral Foley catheter would touch the bladder side of the fistula, possibly interfering with the healing process, the catheter may be placed suprapubically (Fig. 51-6).

A few special instruments can be very helpful at the time of fistula repair, such as a pair of fine dissecting scissors, right-angled scissors, Sims hooks, and Sims or Breisky retractors. A small suction tip is desirable. A variety of scalpel blades and handles should also be available to the operator, particularly the no. 11- and no. 15-type blades and the no. 7-type scalpel handle. It is also extremely helpful to have a flexible operative schedule that allows the operator as much surgical time as necessary for the particular reconstruction because the length of time required for an adequate operation is not always predictable.

Adequate exposure of the fistula is of paramount importance. If for any reason the exaggerated lithotomy position does not provide adequate exposure, as when it is found to be fibrosed to the symphysis pubis, it may be necessary to use the knee-chest position or even the jackknife or Kraske position, in which the patient is face down with the hips well flexed, the table bent at this point, and extra padding supplied under the hips[14,18] (Fig. 51-7). This enables the operator to look down on the fistula. Adequate, well-focused lighting is equally important; at times the operator may find it advantageous to wear a forehead fiberoptic light to concentrate illumination and reduce annoying shadows.

The gynecologic surgeon should examine both sides of the fistulous tract in choosing the appropriate procedure for the repair of a genital fistula. This examination will reveal the size of each aperture and will afford the surgeon a better opportunity to appraise scarring, fibrosis, and the possibility of multiple openings.

When biopsy of any suspicious area in the margin of the postirradiation fistula has excluded active malignancy, successful repair generally requires not only the delicate handling and approximation of tissue but also the introduction of a new layer of tissue that will provide a new blood supply to the organs involved. If the labia are fleshy, it may be possible to obtain from them a bulbocavernosus fat pad for this new layer.[6] If the labial tissues are atrophic, a nonirradiated graft of omentum, with its blood supply intact, may be brought down and sutured in place to provide the new blood supply and the necessary insulation[24] (see Chapter 53).

Techniques of repair

Electrosurgical or chemical cautery of a very small fistulous opening may destroy the epithelial lining of the tract

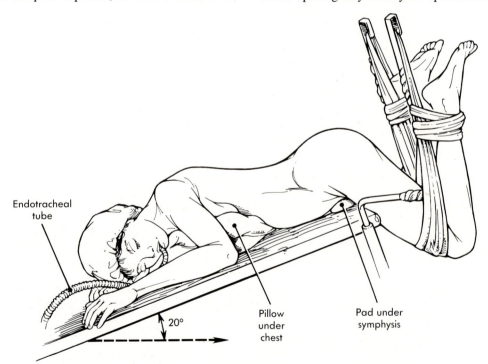

Fig. 51-7. Lawson's[14] prone position to improve the surgeon's view of the operative field when a vesicovaginal fistula is adherent to the pubic symphysis.

and permit spontaneous healing in a small percentage of tiny fistulae.[7] Coagulation must be followed by immediate decompression of the bladder and constant drainage for 2 to 3 weeks. This technique is most likely to be effective when the fistula is only 1 or 2 mm in diameter; follows an oblique course; and has thick, healthy bladder wall around it, as may be seen after the inadvertent placement of a stitch through the bladder wall.

The insertion of a small or pediatric Foley catheter (no. 8, 9, or 10) into the bladder through the fistula itself may facilitate the mobilization of a fistulous tract. When the bulb on the Foley is inflated, the catheter not only serves as an identifying handle but also makes it possible to apply traction on the fistula in all directions.[11] If the fistulous opening is not big enough to permit the entry of a small Foley catheter, the operator can gently enlarge the opening by spreading the tips of a small hemostat or inserting a small Hegar dilator. Infiltration of the area with dilute epinephrine-lidocaine solution has a hemostatic effect; in addition, the local hemostatic effect of using small sponges (e.g., wisps, pushers, or "peanuts") soaked in an epinephrine solution often improves visibility, especially when the surgeon is dissecting and mobilizing the healthy mucosal tissue. There may be considerable oozing, but few vessels are large enough to require clamping and tying.

Most experienced gynecologic surgeons repair vesicovaginal fistulae by a transvaginal approach,[13,16,27] reserving the transabdominal route for very unusual situations in which mobility is limited, the ureter is involved, earlier repeated attempts at repair have failed, or the fistula has developed in tissues previously irradiated.[16,19,23] (See Chapter 53.)

As Moir[16] has written, ". . . the vaginal operation is, from the patient's point of view, relatively simple; and, if need should arise, it can be repeated without much ado. This last argument can be epitomized by the cynical and doubtless exaggerated comments: 'The surgeon who chooses to operate on a vesico-vaginal fistula through the abdominal wall is the surgeon who would remove a child's tonsils by dissecting through the side of the neck.' "

Rarely a transvaginal fistula repair will be chosen for a patient previously irradiated, after persistent or recurrent malignancy as a cause for the fistula has been excluded. Generous and frequent applications of intravaginal estrogen cream should be given to such a patient for a month preoperatively to thicken the vagina, and postoperatively to promote healing. However, generally, the surgeon will wish to insulate the fistula repair during the prolonged healing time by either a Martius bulbocavernosus fat pad transplant (if the patient has fleshy and thick labia majora)[6] or a gracilis muscle transplant as practiced by Ingelman-Sundberg and described by Ball.[3,10]

Latzko technique. If the patient has a deep vagina and a posthysterectomy fistula at the very apex of the vagina, the simplest and most effective operative repair is often the Latzko colpocleisis.[15,18,19] This technique is also useful for a small residual vault fistula that remains after the closure of a larger fistula. If there is any problem in exposure of the fistula, a preliminary episiotomy or Schuchardt-type incision (Fig. 51-8, *A*) is strongly recommended to improve accessibility and ensure visibility of the fistula.

It is not necessary or even desirable to excise the fistulous tract into the bladder as the edges will be coapted in a linear fashion when the supporting tissues in the fibromuscular vaginal wall have been placed and tied. Furthermore, the location of this fistula following hysterectomy is such that it will be near the bladder trigone, and not in the area of bladder that would expand and contract with normal bladder function. The ureters are not generally a part of the fistula, and the repair is in the fibromuscular wall of the vagina, well removed from the ureters, so that ureteral catheterization is superfluous. By the same token, all vesicovaginal fistula repairs benefit from immediate postoperative inspection of the bladder by cystoscopy following injection of intravenous indigo-carmine and waiting for it to appear at the ureteral orifice on each side, guaranteeing ureteral patency.

In this technique (Fig. 51-8, *B*), the operator excises a 1.5- to 2-cm disk—of only the superficial layers of the vaginal epithelium—from around the fistulous opening which denudes but does not remove the vaginal epithelium. (Were the *full* thickness of both epithelium and fibromuscular layer of the vaginal wall removed, the remaining soft muscular wall of the bladder muscle around the fistula might be too fragile to support the deeper layers of suture to be placed and the repair might fail.) When approximated by suture, the disk effectively closes the area turned into the bladder lumen where it will be subsequently covered by a process of vesical epithelialization. It is essential for the operator to excise outward from the line of the initial incision a disk of the superficial layers of the vaginal membrane wide enough to ensure that the deeper fibromuscular tissue layer (i.e., vaginal wall denuded of superficial epithelium by excision of the epithelial disk) can be brought together as a thickened supporting layer beneath the segment of vaginal membrane that is being invaginated into the bladder lumen (Fig. 51-8, *C*). The excised disk of vaginal epithelium should be ovoid rather than round, usually with the long axis of the ovoid transverse across the vault so that the infolding of a portion of the vaginal wall does not constrict the vaginal caliber. When the depth of the vagina is likely to be more critical than the diameter, the long axis and repair of the denuded ovoid of connective tissue that surrounds the invaginated segment of vaginal membrane can parallel the length rather than the width of the vagina.

The sutures of the first layer should be placed to bring together the narrow margins of preserved vaginal membrane around the fistula in what should effectively serve as a subcuticular closure of the denuded segment of vaginal wall, precluding a postoperative bladder diverticulum. Results are best if (1) mobilization is sufficient to permit approximation of the supporting connective tissue layer with no tension and with no irregular buckling of the surfaces

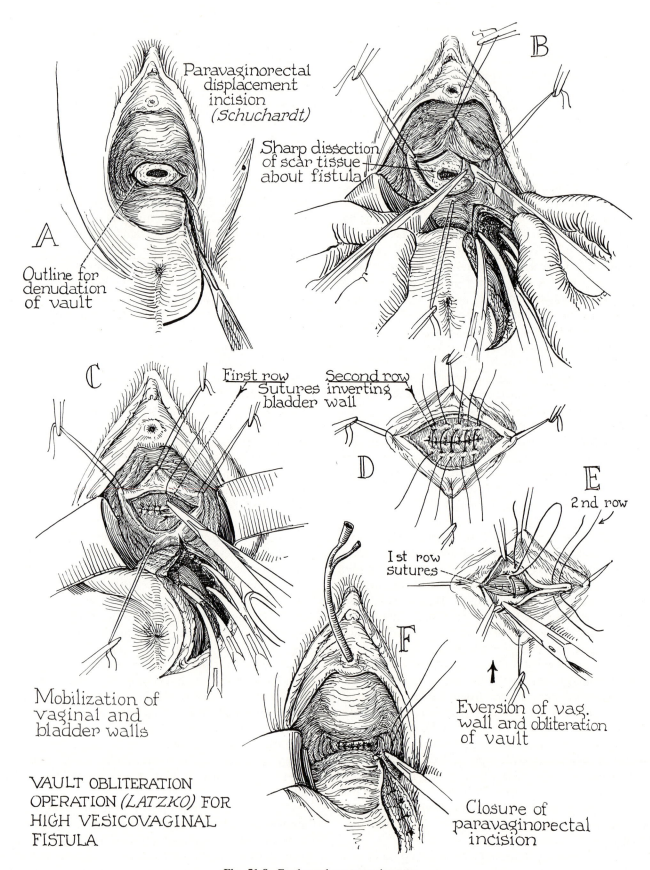

A

Paravaginorectal
displacement
incision
(Schuchardt)

Outline for
denudation
of vault

B

Sharp dissection
of scar tissue
about fistula

C

First row   Second row
Sutures inverting
bladder wall

D

E

2nd row

1st row
sutures

Mobilization of
vaginal and
bladder walls

F

Eversion of vag.
wall and obliteration
of vault

VAULT OBLITERATION
OPERATION *(LATZKO)* FOR
HIGH VESICOVAGINAL
FISTULA

Closure of
paravaginorectal
incision

Fig. 51-8. For legend see opposite page.

as they are brought together, obliterating the angle at each side of the vault, and (2) no suture material goes into the lumen of the urinary tract or through both bladder and vaginal walls into the lumen of the vagina.

If the bladder opening is too large to close from side to side without unusual tension, the operator may transpose a flap of vaginal wall to cover the defect (Figs. 51-9 and 51-10).[25] The instillation of sterile milk or infant formula into the bladder makes it possible to determine the watertightness of the repair because any presence of milk in the operative area indicates a leak; the operator must correct any leakage promptly. To avoid tangling the sutures that have been placed but not yet tied, the operator may clamp the free end pairs in small hemostats and then place each handle over the free tip of a long hemostat whose handle has been clamped to the drape by two towel clips.

The operator should place one or more additional layers of interrupted stitches (Fig. 51-8, *D*), coapting the denuded vesical musculature, and should close the vaginal wall with interrupted sutures (Fig. 51-8, *E* and *F*). If the closure is not watertight at the conclusion of the operation, the operator should remove the stitches and reapproximate the wound as part of the same operation. When it is desirable not to overlap the vaginal closure over the vesical suture line, as in the repair of a recurrent fistula, the modification of Hurd[5] (Fig. 51-11) is effective. Because it requires some undermining of the vaginal wall, however, it further shortens the vagina.

Bladder decompression by catheter drainage usually continues postoperatively for 10 to 14 days, but the patient should ambulate the day after surgery. The patient should take stool softeners so as to evacuate the bowel without straining. A 6% failure rate may be expected; if there is a failure, which is usually recognized promptly after surgery, and the patient wishes rerepair, the operator can take the repair down and repeat the procedure 6 or 8 weeks later when epithelization is complete, paying special attention to dissecting and repairing the lateral tissues of the wound.

When employed at the apex of the vagina, the Latzko technique may shorten the vagina by as much as an inch. Should the shortened vagina constitute a marital problem, the operator can create a distal additional depth by using a Williams vulvovaginoplasty. As with any type of fistula repair, no coitus should be permitted for 2 months postoperatively.

Layered closure technique. Moir[16] reintroduced a modification of the standard Sims vaginal operation for the repair of vesicovaginal fistulae, particularly those distal to the vaginal apex. This operation, which has been popular for many years, does not shorten the vagina as does the Latzo "colpoclesis." Moir[16] went on to say:

The treatment of vesico-vaginal fistula has a fascination of its own. No branch of surgery calls for greater resource, never is patience so sorely tried, and never is success more dependent on

---

Fig. 51-8. Paravaginorectal displacement incision (Schuchardt). This technique of making the upper vagina accessible for fistula closure or radical surgery has been poorly understood. Many surgeons make a superficial cut in the perineum to permit the introduction of a larger retractor and describe this as the operation originally described by Schuchardt. Correctly performed, a paravaginorectal incision displaces the vagina and rectum to the left (for right-handed operators) and changes the vagina from a tubular structure to a wide-open field of operation. This incision provides wide exposure of the operative field from the introitus to a point a few centimeters distal to the fistula. It extends posteriorly and laterally along the extensions of the obturator fascia on the levator ani. It is impossible not to cut some of the fibers of the levator muscles that pass posteriorly.

The tissues to be incised may be infiltrated by no more than 50 cc of 0.5% lidocaine in 1:200,000 epinephrine—the "liquid tourniquet"—to reduce blood loss.

Make an incision in the left lateral sulcus of the vagina about 6 cm. above the introitus and carry it down through the full thickness of the vaginal wall. Continue this to the vulva, curving more laterally after the edge of the puborectalis is passed.

At the mucocutaneous junction the incision is continued in a half circle about the anus to the midline posteriorly. It should clear the anus by at least 3 cm. in order to avoid any fibers of the external sphincter ani muscle (**A**).

The incision is now carried deeper along the lateral wall of the rectum. Bleeding points from the inferior and middle hemorrhoidal vessels will be numerous and require ligation. The extension of the incision to the deeper layers in the perineum will cut the superficial and deep layers of the urogenital diaphragm, and the anal, deep and superficial transverse perineal branches of the pudendal artery, vein, and nerve.

Retractors are placed on either side to further expose the vaginal vault. The rectum and vagina tend to fall caudad from loss of support and in this way bring the vaginal vault closer to the operator (**C**).

The incision (after completion of the fistual repair) is closed in layers, using 00 chromic catgut (**F**). Dead space is avoided particularly where the incision has opened up the ischiorectal fossa.

Vault obliteration operation *(Latzko)*. **A** shows the outline for denudation of the vault about the area of the fistula.

The scar tissue about the fistula is completely excised from both the vaginal and bladder walls. This excision should be carried a sufficient distance from the edges of the fistula to ensure removal of all the scar tissue even though it is anticipated that the vault will be shortened (**B**).

The vaginal and bladder walls are mobilized for some distance from the fistula. The bladder wall is then inverted toward the interior of the bladder by two rows of sutures of 0000 PGA or chromic catgut on atraumatic needles (**C** and **D**).

The vaginal vault is partially obliterated by eversion of the vaginal wall toward the vaginal aspect. This is accomplished by two rows of sutures as shown in **E**. These sutures are placed so that broad, healthy surfaces oppose each other as the incision heals.

The paravaginorectal incision is closed in layers (**F**). (From Ball TL: *Gynecologic surgery and urology,* ed 2, St Louis, 1963, Mosby–Year Book, p 232.)

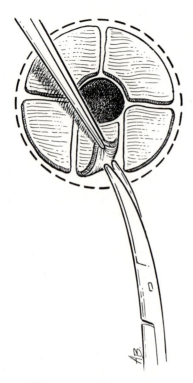

Fig. 51-9. Ueda's[25] alternate method of closing a large fistula.[14] Vaginal wall around fistula is divided into five sections as shown. Four are removed, but the fifth, the width of the fistula, is developed as a flap. (From Nichols DH, Randall CL: *Vaginal surgery,* ed 3, Baltimore, 1989, Williams & Wilkins.)

the exercise of constant care both during operation and, even more perhaps, during the anxious days of convalescence. But never is reward greater. Nothing can equal the gratitude of the woman who, wearied from constant pain, depressed by an ever-growing sense of the humiliating nature of her infirmity, and desperate with the realization that her very presence is an offence to others, finds suddenly that she is restored to full health and able to resume a rightful place in the family—who finds, as it were, that life has been given anew and that she has again become a citizen of the world. To J. Marion Sims, more than to any man, is due the honour for this transformation. And if in these days a moment can be spared for sentimental reverie, look again, I beg, at the curious speculum and, gazing through the confused reflections from its bright curves, catch a fleeting glimpse of an old hut in Alabama and seven negro women who suffered, and endured, and had rich reward.

After obtaining suitable exposure, the operator injects or infiltrates the margins of the fistulous tract, which are often quite vascular, with a few cubic centimeters of 0.5% lidocaine in 1:200,000 epinephrine solution. A small Foley catheter maybe inserted through the fistula (enlarged, if necessary, by the tip of a small hemostat) into the bladder, and the bulb is inflated. Traction on the catheter will stabilize the position of the fistula and bring it closer to the operator. Alternatively, guide sutures may be placed for traction (Fig. 51-12, *A*).

The operator circumscribes the circumference of the fistula with the point of the scalpel blade 0.5 cm from the edge of the fistula. After making a circular incision

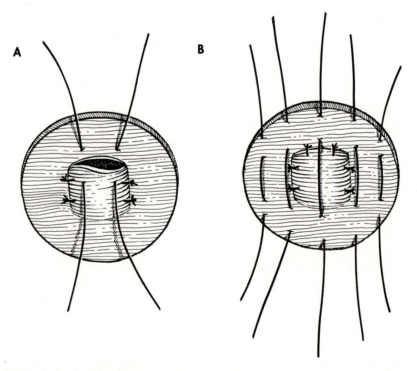

Fig. 51-10. A, Vaginal flap has been turned to cover fistula and sewn in place by several interrupted sutures, sufficient to make closure watertight. **B,** A second layer of sutures approximates exposed tissues, and when these have been tied, cut edges of vagina are approximated by interrupted through-and-through sutures. (From Nichols DH, Randall CL: *Vaginal surgery,* ed 3, Baltimore, 1989, Williams & Wilkins.)

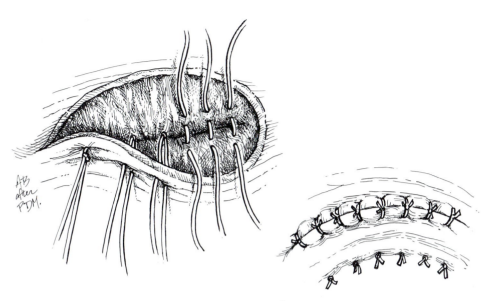

Fig. 51-11. Hurd's alternate method of closing vault,[5] useful for a recurrent fistula. Posterior vaginal wall margin has been undermined for 1½ cm, and ends of final reinforcing layer of stitches approximating bladder wall have been tied, reinserted through full thickness of vaginal wall as shown, and tied again to avoid overlapping of bladder closure with that of vagina. Vaginal incision is closed by a separate layer. (From Nichols DH, Randall CL: *Vaginal surgery,* ed 3, Baltimore, 1989, Williams & Wilkins.)

through the full thickness of the bladder wall (Fig. 51-8, *B*), the operator removes the fistulous tract. Any remaining fibrous tissue is carefully excised to a point where tissue vascularity is normal; it is desirable to remove as much scar and fibrous tissue as possible in order to convert the edges of the defect to a fresh operative wound. Then, with a no. 11 taper-pointed Bard-Parker blade, the operator makes a sagittal incision completely through the vaginal wall (but not into the bladder muscularis or cavity) for a distance of 1 cm superior and inferior to the fistula. The vaginal wall is undercut approximately 1 cm along each side of the fistulous tract (Fig. 51-8, *C*). Undercutting is continued until the bladder adjacent to the fistulous tract is mobilized sufficiently to facilitate closure without tension.

If necessary for hemostasis, the operator may close the bladder mucosa with a layer of running 3-0 polyglycolic or chromic suture, using a subcuticular stitch that inverts any exposed bladder mucosa into the lumen of the bladder. The bladder muscularis is closed with interrupted sutures of 3-0 or 4-0 PGA suture (Fig. 51-12, *D*).

As with the Latzko technique, the watertightness of the closure may be tested by examining the area for leakage after the instillation of sterile milk or infant formula into the bladder; additional sutures may be inserted as a second layer, if necessary. The bladder neck may be plicated prophylactically if desired (Fig. 51-12, *E*). If there is any question about the viability of the tissues, either a Martius bulbocavernosus graft[6] (Fig. 51-13) or a gracilis muscle transplant[3,10] (Figs. 51-14 and 51-15).

Gracilis interposition operation. Frequently, the decision to use a new source of blood supply at the site of the fistula will be

determined at the time of operation. The operator will have excised the fistulous tract. He then begins to mobilize layers to approximate viable tissue to viable tissue but finds that he is cutting through avascular scar tissue that cuts like plaster board and bleeds little. The patient should have signed an informed operative permit since the leg incision to mobilize the gracilis is the length of the thigh. This should have been explained in detail. The patient should also be told that, if in the judgment of the surgeon the closure shows a good chance for success without a transplant, the muscle will not be used.

Surgical anatomy of the gracilis muscle. The gracilis is a long, flat muscle that is the most medial of the adductors of the thigh. The fact that its upper portion is wide and flat, with an abundant blood supply, together with its proximity to the vagina, make it ideal for inclusion in plastic procedures for the cure of fistulas. It arises from the medial margin of the body and ramus of the pubis by a thin, broad tendon about 6 cm in width. It becomes more round in the lower thigh and terminates in a round tendon, which passes behind the medial condyle of the femur, over the internal lateral ligament of the knee joint, and between the tendons of the semitendinosus and sartorius, to be inserted into the proximal part of the medial aspect of the shaft of the tibia below the medial tuberosity. The long saphenous nerve passes between the tendons of the gracilis and sartorius. Loss of the gracilis as an adductor of the thigh and flexor of the knee is of no importance, since the remaining muscles of the adductor group are more than adequate.

The general principles of fistula surgery—viable, fresh edges for approximation, liberal dissection to avoid tension of the suture lines, and the use of fine, atraumatic, catgut—apply here in every particular. Since the interposition of the muscle is done to supply blood to tissue with an inadequate supply, it is important to excise every fragment of scar tissue from the edges of the fistulous tract. Excision of scar tissue may enlarge the opening, but, if it removes scarred edges, the size of the fistula is unimportant.[3]

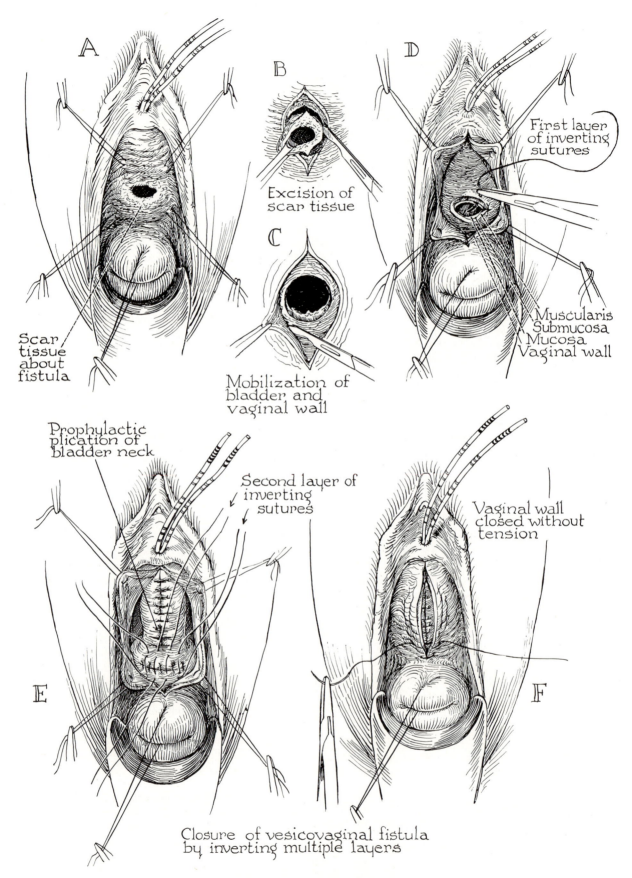

A

B

Excision of scar tissue

C

Mobilization of bladder and vaginal wall

D

First layer of inverting sutures

Muscularis
Submucosa
Mucosa
Vaginal wall

Scar tissue about fistula

Prophylactic plication of bladder neck

Second layer of inverting sutures

E

Vaginal wall closed without tension

F

Closure of vesicovaginal fistula by inverting multiple layers

Fig. 51-12. For legend see opposite page.

Fig. 51-12. Multiple-layer closure of vesicovaginal fistula. **A,** shows a vesicovaginal fistula in the bladder base that is readily accessible. The ureters may be catheterized to identify them in the event that the dissection is extended near the intramural ureter. Four traction sutures are placed about the fistulous tract, and the tissue is grasped by instruments only when absolutely necessary. The scar tissue about the fistulous tract is studied, and the direction of any retraction caused by this tissue is noted.

The scar tissue about the fistula is completely excised **(B),** including that which has formed in the bladder musculature as well as the vaginal wall.

By sharp dissection the plane of cleavage between the bladder and vaginal wall is located. Flaps, free of scar tissue, are mobilized for some distance from the fistula **(C).** The mobilization of healthy tissue extends far enough away from the fistulous tract to ensure approximation without tension.

The bladder mucosa is inverted toward the interior of the bladder by interrupted sutures of 0000 PGA or chromic catgut on ataumatic needles **(D).** This suture passes through the muscularis of the bladder down to, but not including, the mucosa **(D).**

In **E,** a second layer of inverting sutures has been placed in the bladder, and when the sutures are tied, the bladder mucosa in the area of the former fistula will be precisely inverted toward the interior.

If the fistula is in the bladder base and preoperative studies have indicated that the patient, after successful closure of the fistula, would have ordinary stress incontinence, a prophylactic plication of the bladder neck is done **(E).**

The vaginal wall is closed with interrupted sutures in the opposite (longitudinal) direction to the closure of the bladder wall **(F).**

The ureteral catheters are replaced by a silicone coated 16 Fr transurethral Foley catheter. (From Ball TL: *Gynecologic surgery and urology* ed 2, St Louis, 1963, Mosby–Year Book, p 234.)

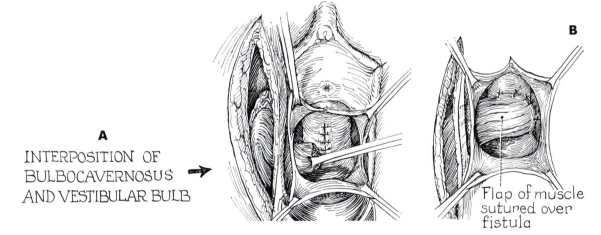

A

INTERPOSITION OF BULBOCAVERNOSUS AND VESTIBULAR BULB

B

Flap of muscle sutured over fistula

Fig. 51-13. Interposition of bulbocavernosus in a fistula repair. A lateral incision over the labia majora is made, and the bulbocavernosus and part of the vestibular bulb are mobilized, with care being exercised not to disturb the blood supply of the bulbocavernosus, which comes from the deep perineal brance of the external pudendal artery. This approaches the muscle near its point of origin, so care should be exercised not to disturb the major vessels. The vaginal wall is mobilized further on the lateral edge of the incision, and finally the anterolateral wall is dissected free along the upper portion of the descending pubic rami. A canal is formed behind the labia majora and vaginal wall, through which the bulbocavernosus can be drawn **(A).**

The bulbocavernosus is detached anteriorly and the free edge observed for viability. The muscle is sutured across the area of the fistula or to the periosteum of the opposite pubic ramus **(B).**

The full thickness of the vaginal wall is closed by interrupted sutures. The incision in the labia majora is likewise closed, and the skin edges are everted by interrupted sutures. (From Ball TL: *Gynecologic surgery and urology,* ed 2, St Louis, 1963, Mosby–Year Book, p 234.)

Fig. 51-14. Gracilis muscle interposition operation. The medial aspect of either the right or left leg is prepared and draped from the genitocrural fold to the region of the medial epicondyle of the knee. The vagina and vulva are prepared and draped. The preparation of the vaginal flaps about the fistula may be done in the knee-chest position and the patient turned around for the gracilis transplant. It is awkward to attempt to mobilize the gracilis in the knee-chest position. If exposure is adequate, the entire procedure is better done in the dorsal lithotomy position. The sketches accompanying this description were drawn in the dorsal lithotomy position, and the right gracilis was transplanted.

The edges of the fistula are denuded of all scar tissue, and the natural line of cleavage between the bladder and anterior vaginal wall is entered when reasonably normal tissue is found some distance from the fistula. Continue the dissection farther until the bladder is freely mobilized and until the edges of the fistula will come together without tension. With large fistulas this may not be possible, and the transplanted muscle will be used to fill the gap. If the edges will come together, they are loosely approximated with interrupted sutures of 0000 atraumatic, chromic catgut. No attempt should be made to close the fistula in several layers, which adds a lot of suture material in the wound. The area of the fistula is then avoided and protected from trauma and pressure during the rest of the operation **(A).**

If the fistula is at the bladder neck, trigone, or adjacent bladder base, the patient should be drained by a vaginal cystotomy as illustrated in **A.** A fistula in the bladder base may be drained by an indwelling catheter as long as it does not cause pressure on the edges of the wound or muscle transplant. A suprapubic cystotomy is preferable to an indwelling urethral catheter and can be done as a preliminary operation or at the time of the gracilis transplant procedure.

The medial epicondyle of the femur is then palpated and an incision made through the skin and subcutaneous tela from here to point on the descending ramus of the pubis and 2 cm. below the inferior border of the symphysis **(B).** The fascia lata is then split along the course of the incision to within a few centimeters of the knee where it thickens and sends fibers into the joint capsule. The fascia lata is then dissected laterally and medially, exposing the gracilis, adductor longus, and medial to the gracilis, the edge of the adductor magnus.

The success of the transplant depends on the next maneuver. Retract the fascia lata laterally about 12 cm. distal from the origin of the gracilis muscle. Gently lift up its lateral edge and look for the anterior branch of the obturator artery, vein, and nerve. It will be seen entering the lateral edge of the muscle together with some connective tissue extensions of the muscle sheath. In some patients the vessels are located by retracting the lateral edge of the gracilis medially. This is best done with a vein retractor, and once the bundle of vessels and nerve are located, the area must be carefully protected.

To protect the blood and nerve supply, a rubber dam is sutured across the point of entrance of the vessels and attached to skin or adjacent muscle. During the ensuing phase of the operation, the blood and nerve supply can be compromised as the surgeon draws the muscle through the obturator foramen and under the bladder. The rubber dam serves as a landmark and prevents traction on the vessels **(C).**

The gracilis is now dissected free from the other muscles of the adductor group to a point where its tendon is overlapped by the tendon of the sartorius. This portion of tendon is useful in passing the muscle through the obturator space but is later resected almost down to the belly of the muscle since the latter is the part that has an abundant blood supply. The distal portion of the muscle is bathed in wet gauze while the path for its transplantation between bladder and vaginal wall is being prepared.

The index finger is now inserted between the medial edge of the gracilis and the medial edge of the adductor magnus that lies behind and at a deeper level. Direct the dissecting finger posteriorly between the adductor magnus and the adductor brevis, which is anterior to the adductor magnus. This may avoid injuring the posterior branches of the obturator artery, vein, and nerve. The index finger of the other hand is then inserted between the bladder and vaginal wall and directed laterally until the most caudad edge of the obturator membrane is felt. The finger dissecting from the thigh then separates some of the fibers of the obturator externus to meet the vaginal finger, with the obturator membrane interposed between them. The finger in the vagina will rupture some of the fibers of the levator ani and obturator internus in this dissection.

A long, curved Kelly clamp is then passed along the index finger, dissecting from the thigh until the tip reaches the most caudad part of the obturator membrane. The clamp is then forced through the membrane and opened to make a passageway of sufficient size to admit the belly of the gracilis. It is important to make the opening adequate so the edges do not necrose the muscle or constrict its blood supply.

A silk traction suture is then inserted in the tendon of the gracilis. A large curved clamp or large aneurysm needle is passed from the vaginal aspect, through the rent in the obturator membrane, and between the muscles, to emerge medial to the gracilis and a few centimeters from its origin. (From Ball TL: *Gynecologic surgery and urology,* ed 2, St Louis, 1963, Mosby–Year Book, p 240.)

If the cut edge of the vaginal incision appears ragged, torn, or suspiciously thin, the operator may trim the edge. The full thickness of the vaginal membrane is closed from side to side with vertical mattress sutures of 2-0 PGA or polydiaxonone (PDS) or polyglyconate (Maxon) (Fig. 51-12, *F*). These additional layers of closure relieve much of the tension on the stitches of the first layer. The operator should place and hold all these interrupted stitches before tying them; when the stitches are tied, the operator should be certain to incorporate a double turn on the first cast of each knot, followed by four additional casts of the suture, to prevent postoperative slipping. As Moir correctly emphasized, these sutures should be only tight enough to approximate the tissue securely—not so tight as to strangu-late the tissue. The ends of any *nonabsorbable* sutures should be left long to facilitate their removal on approximately the 21st postoperative day.

If necessary, the operator may make full-thickness lateral relaxing incisions in the vagina to relieve any tension on the suture line. The vagina should then be loosely packed with iodoform gauze for 24 hours and an in-dwelling catheter inserted to ensure bladder contraction for 10 days. If the patient is postmenopausal, both local and systemic estrogen should be administered through the postoperative period.

Vaginal lapping. For the larger vesicovaginal fistula, it is particularly important to ensure that the dissection of the vaginal wall from the bladder wall is sufficiently exten-

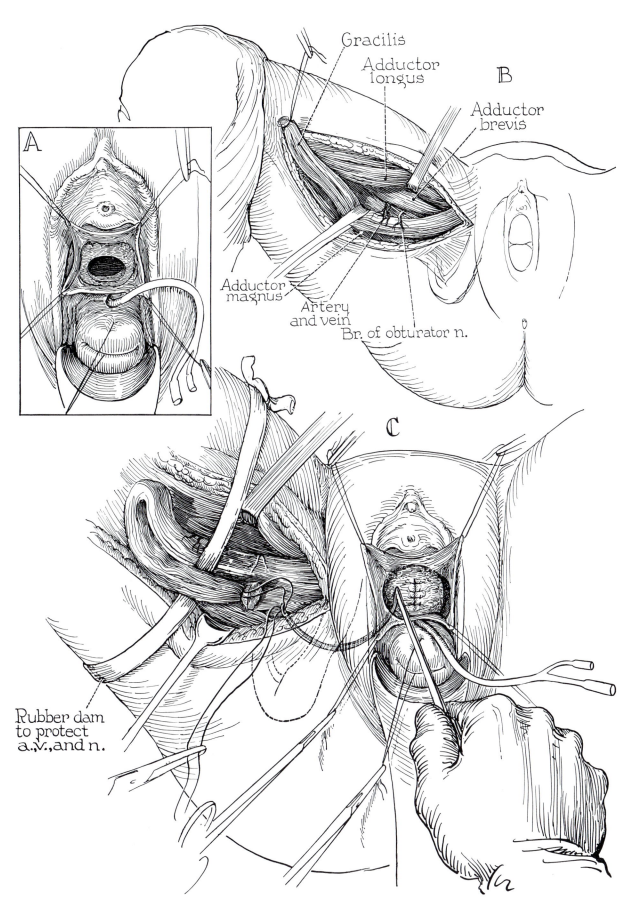

Fig. 51-14. For legend see opposite page.

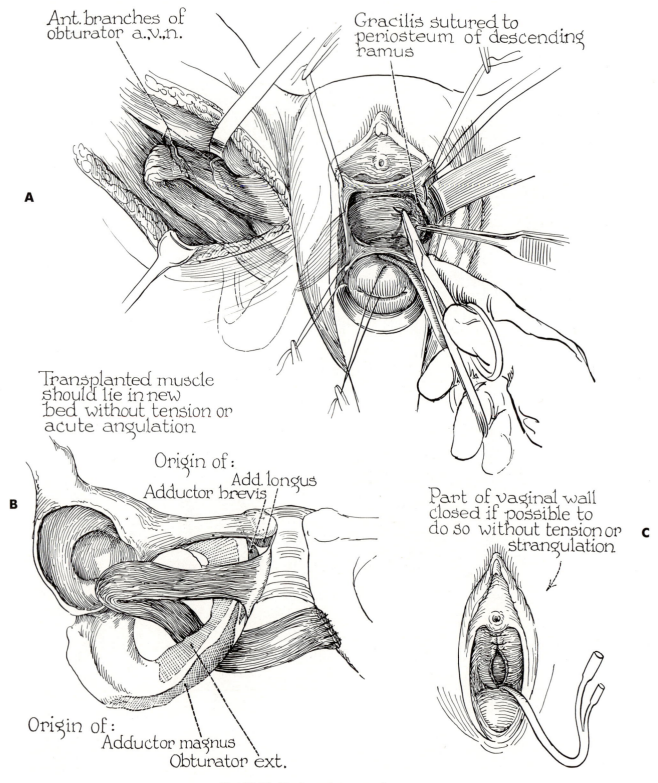

Ant. branches of
obturator a.,v.,n.

Gracilis sutured to
periosteum of descending
ramus

A

Transplanted muscle
should lie in new
bed without tension or
acute angulation

Origin of:
Adductor brevis   Add. longus

B

Part of vaginal wall
closed if possible to
do so without tension or
strangulation

C

Origin of:
Adductor magnus
Obturator ext.

Fig. 51-15. For legend see opposite page.

Fig. 51-15. The traction suture is drawn through this pathway and out the vagina. A clamp then grasps the tendon of the gracilis, and by a combination of pushing with the clamp and traction on the suture, the muscle is inserted through the obturator fossa and between the bladder and vaginal wall to the opposite descending ramus of the pubis **(A).** This must be accomplished without tension or angulation of the blood and nerve supply of the muscle **(B).** Since the detached distal end of the muscle retracts, it frequently seems that there is not enough muscle to reach across the vagina. This is not the case, and one finds ample length to span even the widest pubic arch.

The viable ends of the muscle or tendon that have not been disturbed by traction suture or clamp are then sutured to the inner aspect of the opposite descending ramus of the pubis. These sutures pass through the remains of the attachment of the levator ani and the extensions of the obturator fascia that once formed the inferior layer of the urogenital diaphragm that in these patients has long since lost its identity. The muscle should now lie between the bladder and vaginal wall without tension and should cover the fistula. With large fistulas the muscle will present into the interior of the bladder and with a successful transplant soon become covered with bladder mucosa **(C).**

If the vaginal wall can be closed without tension, this is done with interrupted sutures of 00 PGA or chromic catgut, tied to provide approximation without strangulation. Should the anterior vaginal wall be so deficient that approximation is not feasible without tension, the edges should be sutured to the muscle graft in a few places to eliminate dead space, but again the sutures should be few and far between and not tied tightly **(C).** The vagina should not be packed, nor should petroleum jelly gauze or other foreign bodies be placed against the suture lines to impede vascularization and healing.

The leg incision is closed in layers with fine and medium silk sutures.

There is no contraindication to early mobilization of the patient. (From Ball TL: *Gynecologic surgery and urology*, ed 2, St Louis, 1963, Mosby–Year Book, p 240.)

---

sive to permit the mobilization and interposition of a large layer of subcutaneous tissue between the sutures that close the bladder and those that close the defect in the vagina. When the vaginal wall is suitably redundant, the vaginal lapping technique[1,12] may provide insulation and reinforcement for these suture layers.

The underlying fibromuscular layer of the right vaginal flap is split from the vaginal epithelium to the lateral margins of the vesicovaginal space (Fig. 51-16). Dissection along this line of cleavage should separate the musculoelastic layer of the vaginal wall from the overlying layer of vaginal epithelium. The vaginal flap of the left side is not similarly split, however; all connective tissue should remain attached to the epithelial layer of the left flap of the vagina in order to preserve as much of its blood supply as possible. Leaving the vaginal muscularis attached to the

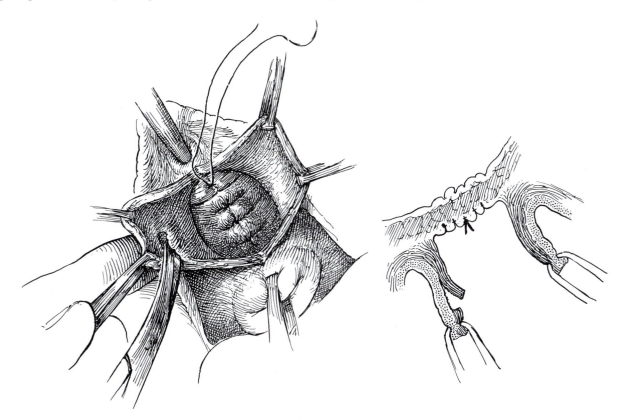

Fig. 51-16. The vaginal lapping operation. Fibromuscular layer of right vaginal flap is dissected from superficial vaginal skin. (From Nichols DH, Randall CL: *Vaginal surgery*, ed 3, Baltimore, 1989, Williams & Wilkins.)

epithelium on one side also effectively doubles the thickness of the connective tissue layer supporting the anterior vaginal wall.

Using a series of interrupted sutures of 2-0 polyglycolic suture), the operator sews the medial edge of the right inner vaginal or fibromuscular flap to the undersurface of the unsplit full-thickness flap of the left vaginal wall, along the lateral extent of the vesicovaginal space. Each untied suture is held loosely until all have been placed; then all are tied (Fig. 51-17).

At this point, trimming an appropriate amount of the right epithelial covering layer of vaginal flap along the left lateral margin of the vesicovaginal space brings the edges of the vaginal membrane together again, making them

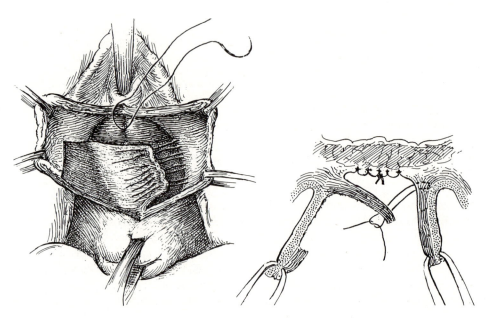

Fig. 51-17. Fibromuscular layer of right vaginal flap is sewn to undersurface of unsplit left vaginal wall. The excess of the split right vaginal flap is trimmed. (From Nichols DH, Randall CL: *Vaginal surgery,* ed 3, Baltimore, 1989, Williams & Wilkins.)

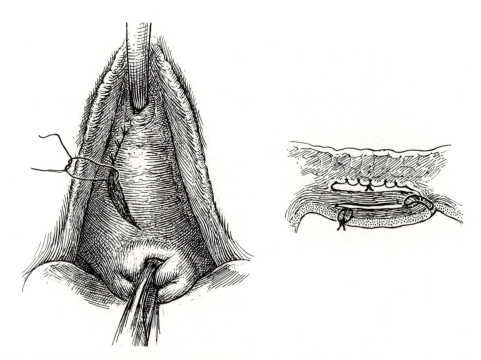

Fig. 51-18. Full thickness of left flap is sewn to right. (From Nichols DH, Randall CL: *Vaginal surgery,* ed 3, Baltimore, 1989, Williams & Wilkins.)

roughly parallel over the now doubled fibromuscular tissue layers. Finally, the operator attaches the full thickness of the unsplit left vaginal flap to the cut edge of the right flap by a series of interrupted sutures of 2-0 polyglycolic suture (Fig. 51-18). Any noticeable damage to or relaxation of the posterior vaginal wall and perineum could be repaired at this time.

Under rare circumstances, when the anterior vaginal wall is unusually thin and it is desirable to preserve the full vaginal depth and width, the Ocejo modification of the Watkins-Wertheim[28,29,30] interposition operation may be useful in patients who still have their uterus. In this modification, which Gallo[4] advocated, the operator amputates the cervix and excises the endometrium through a longitudinal incision in the anterior wall of the uterus, safely removing this potential source of future endometrial trouble or symptoms. The uterine fundus is interposed as a separate tissue layer between the bladder and the vagina and sewn into position as shown (Fig. 51-19).

Postoperative care

Although the bladder of a patient who has been totally incontinent as a result of a vesicovaginal fistula is usually capable of physiologic regeneration and function within a few weeks, even when the incontinence has persisted for a number of years, the capacity of the bladder is likely to be relatively small immediately after the repair. The surgeon should warn the patient to expect a certain amount of urgency and should advise the patient of the need to empty her bladder frequently for the first few postoperative weeks, even during the night. It may be suggested that she

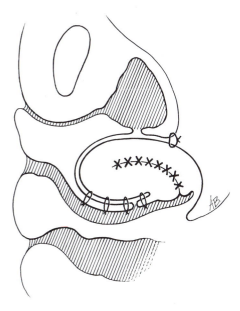

Fig. 51-19. Uterine corpus may be transposed between bladder and vagina in certain cases of vesicovaginal fistula when blood supply is poor. In Acejo's modification,[8] endometrium has been removed by sharp dissection and cavity obliterated by sutures as shown. An elongated cervix will have been amputated. (From Nichols DH, Randall CL: *Vaginal surgery,* ed 3, Baltimore, 1989, Williams & Wilkins.)

set an alarm clock to arouse her for this purpose in order to avoid nocturnal distention. Because primary healing is so important, the patient should be maintained on urinary antisepsis for several weeks after the surgery. For postmenopausal patients, it is sometimes advisable to prescribe estrogen to improve vascularity and wound healing in these estrogen-sensitive tissues.

Any element of postoperative detrusor instability giving rise to precipitancy or incontinence must be sought and, if found, promptly treated, usually by a program of dietary caffeine restriction and bladder drill (voiding every 2 hours during the waking hours) supplemented by anticholinergic medication as necessary; "closure of the fistula does not always mean success. Urinary continence must be restored."[27]

VESICOUTERINE AND VESICOCERVICAL FISTULA

If the escape of urine through the external cervical os is not identified, a standing lateral cystogram or hysterogram using a short-tipped canula will supply the confirmation. "Menouria," which may consist of cyclic hematuria, a vesicouterine-fistula above the level of the internal cervical os, and apparent amenorrhea in the presence of a patent cervix but without coincident urinary incontinence has come to be known as *Youssef's syndrome.*[20,32]

Vesicouterine or vesicocervical fistula, with its accompanying incontinence, is almost invariably the aftermath of a cesarean section at which a suture used in the repair of the uterine incision compromised the integrity of the bladder. Occasionally such a fistula develops after uterine rupture as a result of precipitate labor.[2] Surgery involves the anatomic dissection and separation of the bladder from the uterus at the site of the fistula, freshening of the edges, and separate repair of each organ with absorbable suture. Catheter decompression of the bladder for a period of not less than 10 days postoperatively is desirable.

Such a fistula may be repaired either transvaginally or abdominally, and the option of coincidental hysterectomy determined according to the patient's wishes for future reproduction. Normal subsequent pregnancy and delivery have been reported in cases in which the uterus was retained.

Urinary incontinence does not always occur with vesicocervical fistula; the sole symptom is sometimes menstrual hematuria, erroneously suggesting endometriosis of the bladder. In such instances, some valvelike structure has developed within a fistulous tract, creating a flap effect that permits fluid to pass from the uterus to the bladder but not in the reverse direction. Vesical endometriosis should have been excluded by careful cystoscopy.

URETEROVAGINAL FISTULA

Although freshly damaged or transected ureters may be transvaginally reimplanted into the bladder at the time of the initial injury—if the operator is familiar with the technique of repair[21,22]—the postoperative ureterovaginal fistula is most often approached through a transabdominal route, either for reconstruction or reimplantation.

Urinary diversion

Permanent diversion of the patient's urine to a biologic reservoir appropriated from another system within the body may be required rarely. This subject is considered in Chapter 54.

REFERENCES

1. Aldridge AH: Modern treatment for vesicovaginal fistula, *J Obstet Gynaecol Br Emp* 60:1, 1953.
2. Al-Juburi A, Aloosi I, Khundra S: Unusual vesicocervical fistulas, *J Obstet Gynaecol* 4:264, 1984.
3. Ball TL: *Gynecologic surgery and urology,* ed 2, St Louis, 1963, Mosby–Year Book.
4. Banfield PJ, Scott G, Roberts HR: A modified contraceptive diaphragm for relief of utero-vaginal fistula: a case report, *Br J Obstet Gynaecol* 98:101, 1991.
5. Dotters DJ, Droegemueller W: Diaphragm catheters for vesicovaginal fistula management, *Contemp Obstet-Gynecol* Technology 1992 (special issue), 45-46, 1992.
6. Elkins TE, De Lancey JOL, McGuire EJ: The use of modified Martius graft as an adjunctive technique in vesicovaginal and rectovaginal fistula repair, *Obstet Gynecol* 75:727-733, 1990.
7. Falk HC, Orkin LA: Nonsurgical closure of vesicovaginal fistulas, *Obstet Gynecol* 9:538, 1957.
8. Gallo D: *Ocejo modification of interposition operation.* In *Urologica Ginecologica,* Guadalajara, 1969, Gallo.
9. Hurd JK: *Vaginal repair of vesicovaginal fistula.* In Libertino JA, Zinman L, editors: *Reconstructive urologic surgery,* Baltimore, 1977, Williams & Wilkins.
10. Ingelman-Sundberg A: Repair of vesicovaginal and rectovaginal fistula following fulguration of recurrent cancer of the cervix after radiation. In Meigs JV, editor: *Surgical treatment of cancer of the cervix,* New York, 1954, Grune & Stratton.
11. Janisch H, Palmrich AH, Pecherstorfer M: *Selected urologic operations in gynecology,* Berlin, 1979, Walter de Gruyter.
12. Judd GE, Marshall JR: Repair of urethral diverticulum or vesicovaginal fistula by vaginal flap technique, *Obstet Gynecol* 47:627, 1976.
13. Keettel WC et al: Surgical management of urethrovaginal and vesicovaginal fistulas, *Am J Obstet Gynecol* 131:425-431, 1978.
14. Lawson JB, Stewart DB: *Obstetrics and gynaecology in the tropics,* London, 1967, Arnold.
15. Latzko W: Postoperative vesicovaginal fistulas, *Am J Surg* 58:211, 1942.
16. Moir JC: *The vesicovaginal fistula,* London, 1967, Balliere, Tindall & Cassell.
17. O'Connor VJ Jr: Repair of vesicovaginal fistula with associated urethral loss, *Surg Gynecol Obstet* 146:251, 1978.
18. Robertson JR: *Vesicovaginal fistulas.* In Slate WG, editor: *Disorders of the female urethra and urinary incontinence,* Baltimore, 1982, Williams & Wilkins.
19. Tancer L: Personal communication, 1985.
20. Tancer ML: Vesicouterine fistula—a review, *Obstet Gynecol Survey* 41:743-753, 1986.
21. Thompson JD: *Transvaginal ureteral transection with vaginal hysterectomy and anterior colporrhaphy.* In Nichols DH, editor: *Clinical problems, injuries and complications of gynecologic surgery,* ed 2, Baltimore, 1988, Williams & Wilkins.
22. Thompson JD, Benigno BB: Vaginal repair of ureteral injuries, *Am J Obstet Gynecol* 3:601, 1971.
23. Thompson JD, Rock JA, editors: *TeLinde's operative gynecology,* ed 7, Philadelphia, 1992, JB Lippincott.
24. Turner-Warwick R: The use of pedicle grafts in the repair of urinary tract fistulae, *Br J Urol* 44:644, 1972.
25. Ueda T et al: Closure of a vesicovaginal fistula using a vaginal flap, *J Urol* 119:742, 1978.
26. Wang Y, Hadley HR: Nondelayed transvaginal repair of high lying vesicovaginal fistula, *J Urol* 144:34-36, 1990.
27. Ward A: Personal communication, 1980.
28. Watkins TJ: The treatment of cystocele and uterine prolapse after the menopause, *Am Gynaec Obstet J* 15:420-423, 1899.
29. Watkins TJ: Treatment of cases of extensive cystocele and uterine prolapse, *Surg Gynecol Obstet* 2:659-667, 1906.
30. Wertheim E: Zur plastichen Verwendung des Uterus bei Prolapsen, *Centralbl f Gynäk* 23:369-372, 1899.
31. Wolff HD, Gililand NA: Vaginal diaphragm catheters, *J Urol* 78:681, 1957.
32. Youssef AF: Menouria following lower segment cesarean section, *Am J Obstet Gynecol* 73:759-767, 1957.

Chapter 52

MASSIVE VESICOVAGINAL FISTULA

Reginald Hamlin
Catherine Nicholson
Robert Zacharin

The incidence of massive vesicovaginal fistula, considered worldwide, makes it the most common major gynecologic surgical problem existing today. Although it is extremely rare in communities with access to expert medical help, in many countries such care is minimal or nonexistent and the problem very common. The tragedy, of course, is that such fistulas are entirely preventable.

CAUSES

Urinary fistula in the Western world usually results from pelvic surgery or pelvic malignancy and its treatment. Obstructed labor leading to fistula formation should not occur. In third world countries there is a clear relationship between such fistulas and poor or absent obstetric care, associated with a wide range of contributing social conditions. The prime factor is unrelieved obstructed labor, leading to pressure necrosis. The duration of obstruction and the level at which descent of the presenting part is arrested determine the extent of tissue damage. Not only the bladder but commonly the urethra and ureters together with the rectum and cervix may be involved in the sloughing process. Associated medical factors include disproportion due to large babies or contracted pelvis, delay in diagnosis, and added difficulties of a traumatic delivery either by forceps, cesarean section, or destructive procedure. Social factors with an important impact include poor diet and associated systemic diseases (e.g., malaria) that stunt growth, poor or absent medical care, obstruction to quick transport from villages to hospitals by distance or rugged terrain, and use of traditional remedies including deliberate genital tract injury and mutilation.

PATHOLOGY

Fistula site and extent are determined by the level of obstruction, the tissues passing through various phases from discoloration to eventual sloughing. The bladder wall is subjected to both mechanical pressure from the impacted presenting part and hydrostatic pressure from unrelieved retention of urine. Usually the bladder neck and trigone area bear the brunt, but often the urethra and ureters are included in the tissue loss. For some weeks after damage, necrotic debris continues to be discharged (Fig. 52-1), and healing follows by secondary intention. This process leads to gross scarring, adhesion to the ischiopubic rami, and cross-union between bladder and vaginal epithelial linings. Such a healing phase requires a period of 10 to 12 weeks for completion. This healing process presents several important clinical features to be appreciated when later surgical correction is being considered. Scar tissue is maximal at or near the fistula track but nevertheless extends, although diminished, into tissues well removed from the fistula. Scar tissue must be divided to allow access into the vagina and also to free the fistula from its attachment to pelvic bones. Only following satisfactory mobilization of bladder and vagina will the true extent of the tissue deficit become apparent.

CLASSIFICATION

Site and size of the fistula determine what reparative measures will be necessary. There have been many proposals for classification, but most are too complex, attempting to consider every variant and failing to appreciate that there are no clearcut divisions between these described

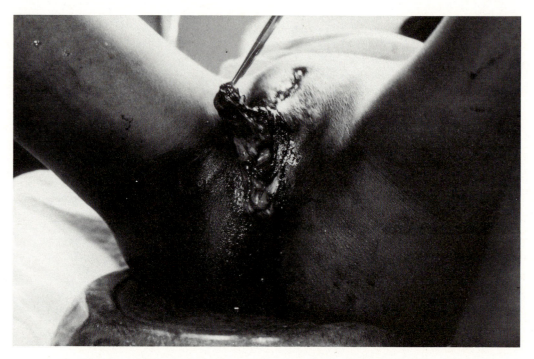

Fig. 52-1. Necrotic tissues discharged through the vulva some weeks following obstructed labor. (From Zacharin RF: *Obstetric fistula,* New York, 1987, Springer.)

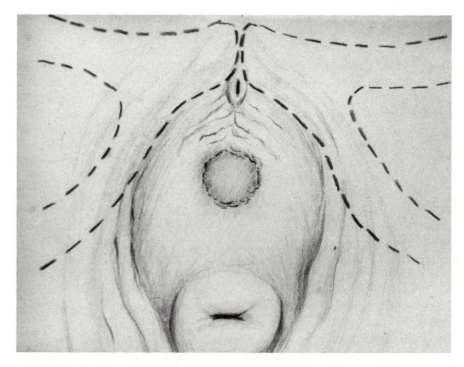

Fig. 52-2. Line drawing of a small fistula: central situation, minimal tissue deficit, and scarring without bony adhesion. (From Zacharin RF: *Obstetric fistula,* New York, 1987, Springer.)

varieties. In a clinical setting, important features are (1) the anatomic site of damage, (2) the size of the defect, and (3) the degree of associated scarring.

Fistula site

The clinical grouping of fistulas involving the urinary system is as follows:

1. Vesicovaginal fistula without urethral involvement
2. Vesicovaginal fistula with partial or complete urethral destruction
3. Vesicocervicovaginal fistula

Fistula size

The following simplification into small, medium, and large is based on realities of surgical correction.

Small fistula. Although small compared to other obstetric fistulas, it is not to be compared with a small posthysterectomy fistula. It lies in the anterior vaginal wall, does not involve bladder neck or urethra, is not fixed to bone, and has minimal tissue deficit (Fig. 52-2).

Middle-sized fistula. A large area of the anterior vaginal wall and urethrovesical junction, including part of the proximal urethra, is lost. Bony adhesion is usual, and one

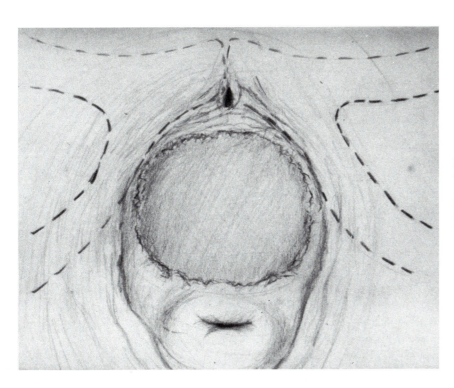

Fig. 52-3. Line drawing of a middle-sized fistula: increased tissue deficit with scarring and the likelihood of ureteral involvement together with moderate bony adhesion. (From Zacharin RF: *Obstetric fistula,* New York, 1987, Springer.)

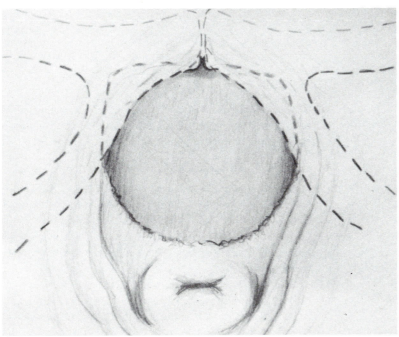

Fig. 52-4. Line drawing of a large fistula: massive tissue loss, scarring, bony adhesion, and the ureteral orifices may lie near to the fistula edge or even outside it. (From Zacharin RF: *Obstetric fistula,* New York, 1987, Springer.)

or both ureteral orifices may be near the fistula edge and, on occasion, even outside (Fig. 52-3).

Large fistula. A large amount of bladder floor, urethrovesical junction, and often the whole urethra are affected, with the anterior vaginal wall replaced by massive scarring. The ureteral orifices are always displaced near to the fistula margin or outside it. There are dense adhesions between bladder remnant and pelvic bones (Fig. 52-4).

DIAGNOSIS AND INVESTIGATION

It is always wise to assume that there is something unusual about each patient and to conduct a thorough and thoughtful examination.[15] Accuracy with physical signs is essential and usually straightforward, but suspicious granulating areas separate from the major defect must be investigated carefully with probe, dye, or vaginal swab test. Ureterovaginal fistula, which may occur in association with vesicovaginal fistula, must be excluded or confirmed by complete urological assessment. An especially difficult diagnostic problem is a ureterovaginal fistula occurring at the lower end of the ureter, right against the bladder wall. Following are the important details in diagnosis.

Anatomic facts

1. Site and size of the fistula into the vagina, its relation to cervix, bladder, urethrovesical junction, and urethra; cervix involvement, identification of external os.
2. Number of fistulas.
3. Patency of the urethra.
4. Relationship of ureteral orifices to the fistula and their proximity to the fistula edge. In larger fistulas, one or both orifices can lie outside the fistula edge, and this possibility must be clarified with certainty early on during reparative surgery.

Pathologic features

All these features are compounded by previous attempts at surgical correction. The more attempts have been made, the more obvious are these changes.

1. Amount of tissue deficit.
2. Extent of scarring at the fistula edge and degree of associated vaginal fixity and stenosis.
3. Adhesion of the fistula to the ischiopubic rami and pubic bones.
4. Bladder inversion through the defect.
5. Presence of bladder calculi.
6. Progress of epithelial healing in the bladder and vagina as gauged by a return of normal epithelial appearance. After frequent attempts at surgical repair, return to normal is much delayed. Assessment of normality is made by periodic vaginal inspections and cystoscopic examination of the bladder. Major indexes of normality are as follows:
   a. Loss of tissue edema and return of normal epithelial color.
   b. Softening and return of tissue mobility.

c. Decrease in inflammatory reaction shown by diminution in blanching test: compression of vaginal epithelium with the tip of a uterine sound produces marked blanching in inflamed tissues, diminishing as healing progresses.

Additional considerations

Finally, there must be an assessment of renal function, restoration of vulval and vaginal cleanliness before any surgery, and a general examination, excluding common associated problems of malaria, anemia, bilharzia, and various parasites.

Consideration of all these factors enables planning to commence, for both general and local preparation, and a decision to be made about an appropriate time for surgical intervention. General diseases, especially bilharzia and malaria, must be treated and local vaginal cleanliness achieved by simple hygiene, especially mechanical scrubbing and washing and intravaginal douches. With long-standing fistulae, calculi must be sought and removed. Urinary tract infection is not a problem before surgery because of free urinary drainage but requires appropriate prophylaxis after fistula closure with the need for prolonged catheter drainage.

SURGICAL CORRECTION
Prophylaxis

Hamlin[8] succinctly described the causes of obstetric fistula as obstructed labor and obstructed transport. Therefore, prophylaxis should be directed to these major problems. According to Lister[12]:

The real answer as to what can be done in decreasing the incidence of fistula comes within the wide term of education of the patient, husband, relatives and influential people at the village level, and they should be made to realize that all women should be brought to hospital when undelivered after 24 hours, and also that certain women are high risk, i.e., short young girls, elderly primagravidae, grand multiparity, patients with still-births and those who have had operative deliveries in the past or a repaired vesicovaginal fistula. If all these women came to hospital early in labor or even attended an antenatal clinic, fistulae in many countries would become things of the past.

Should bladder injury occur during cesarean section, it demands prompt recognition and careful management to avoid cervicovesicovaginal fistula.

Difficulties associated with urinary fistulas

Sir Reginald Watson-Jones, emphasizing the importance of controlled treatment of fractures, remarked, "Bones are filled not with red marrow; but with black ingratitude." Similar words might be used to underline the meticulous care necessary for successful fistula management.

The nature of the injury that caused the fistula and the type of fistula and its location are the main factors determining the result of attempted repair.[3] Two most important factors that can militate against a successful outcome are the amount of tissue deficit and dense fibrosis with adhesion to the rami and body of the pubic bones. The ability to mobilize grossly scarred tissues adequately without destroying blood supply and then to close them carefully in layers without tension is vital for successful repair. Associated vaginal stenosis can usually be overcome by adequate incision. Concurrent rectal lesions complicate the problem of bladder fistula, and in general the rectal defect should not be attempted until the bladder has been closed, although we have stated that our usual practice in Addis Ababa is to close both fistulas at the one operation.[8] Scarring produced by repeated operations, particularly near the bladder neck, may result in a rigid patulous internal urinary meatus densely adherent to bone, further resulting in severe incontinence even if successful closure is achieved.

Methods available for surgical correction

Vaginal surgery. Hamlin and Nicholson[8] have operated upon all their fistula patients with the patient in the lithotomy position. In their experience with 12,000 vaginal fistulas, they have never found it necessary to employ the knee-chest position, the left pateral position, or the abdominal approach. The vaginal approach embodies two techniques: the first, saucerization, was popularized by Sims but has been largely replaced by the alternative method of layered repair attributed to Mackenrodt. This second technique is also known as flap-splitting or dedoublement.

Ureteric transplantation. This procedure is usually unnecessary and in third world countries with limited or absent medical care may in fact be lethal. Lawson[11] performed the procedure 30 times in 377 patients, but with increasing experience the technique was required much less often.

Principles of vaginal closure

Fistula surgery is difficult and demanding, and success will be gained only by meticulous attention to detail, for the tissues are scarred, with a poor blood supply leading to slow healing, and tissue loss of greater or lesser degree. Accordingly, the best chance of surgical success is at the first attempt, so everything possible related to the surgery must be as right as conditions permit. The accepted time for all inflammatory changes and scar contraction to have subsided is 10 to 12 weeks, and surgical intervention during this time is considered most unwise. Despite the increased risk of failure with early intervention, attempts to speed up healing using cortisone have been advocated. Similarly, selective intervention for surgically produced fistulas is suggested by some, believing the tissue reaction to be much less than that following obstetric trauma. Failure means a great emotional letdown and prolonged delay before a second attempt can be made, however. A more reliable result will follow thorough observance of the principles laid down long ago, but despite the best care, failures will still occur, for the nature of the tissues precludes 100% success.

Immediate preoperative requirements

Intervention should be well away from the menstrual period, when the tissues become unduly vascular and engorged, making dissection more difficult. Similarly, oral contraceptives should cease several weeks before surgery. Blood group and hemoglobin should be known, and blood should be available for replacement in patients requiring extensive surgery with gracilis muscle grafting. Following are additional considerations:

1. Anesthesia. Depending on availability, either low spinal or general is suitable.
2. Position on the operating table. Throughout their experience over the past 33 years, Hamlin and Nicholson have emloyed the exaggerated lithotomy position for every vaginal fistula operation.
3. Lighting. A properly focussed, adequately bright theater light is essential.
4. Vaginal access. A variety of specula are necessary depending upon the degree of stenosis. Access can be improved by episiotomy, but with gross degrees of scarring, a modified Schuchardt incision could be required.
5. Suturing. The labia are stitched with no. 00 silk. When feasible the fistula should be drawn toward the vaginal introitus using four guy sutures of no. 00 chromic catgut inserted about its periphery, but in many large obstetric fistulas scarring and adhesion inhibit vaginal mobility in varying degrees.
6. Proper instruments. Essentials include a range of sharp-pointed scissors and fine-toothed dissecting forceps of adequate length so the surgeon's hand does not obscure the field. A long-handled Bard-Parker scalpel with No. 11 blades, fine Allis forceps and skin hooks, a small neurosurgical sucker, and a range of fine needleholders together with no. 00 chromic catgut and no. 00 nylon sutures on small curved strong needles are necessary.

Assessment under anesthesia

All preoperative impressions should be confirmed and, if necessary, ureteral catheters passed.

Mobilization

The primary object of mobilization is to free the bladder from the vaginal wall, and flap-splitting is the standard procedure. First, the fistula is steadied, with guy sutures, Allis forceps, or transfixion with the point of the no. 11 scalpel blade. Next, the junctional zone between bladder and vagina is incised, beginning where access is easiest (Fig. 52-5). The freed vaginal skin edge is held by Allis or long-toothed forceps, and incision of the junctional zone continues until the circular incision is complete. Then extensions of 1 to 2 cm are made anterior and posterior at the 6 o'clock and 12 o'clock positions through the full thickness of the vaginal wall. Judicious use of suction enhances speed and accuracy, and progressive undercutting to free

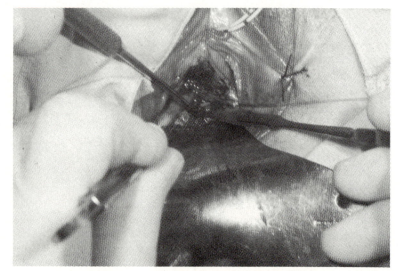

Fig. 52-5. Mobilization begins, using fine-toothed dissectors, a no. 11 blade, and a neurosurgical sucker. The traction suture can be seen on the right. (From Zacharin RF: *Obstetric fistula*, New York, 1987, Springer.)

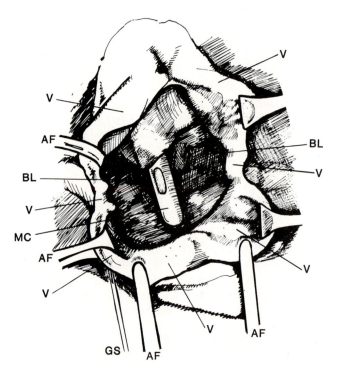

Fig. 52-6. Mobilization completed with a small fistula. V = vagina; AF = Allis forceps; BL = bladder; MC = metal catheter. (From Zacharin RF: *Obstetric fistula*, New York, 1987, Springer.)

the bladder from the vagina is achieved using the no. 11 blade and sharp scissors. Ultimately, mobilization must be sufficient to allow bladder closure without tension, for tension means failure. Therefore, the larger the defect, the more extensive the necessary mobilization (Fig. 52-6). Special attention must be directed to lateral extensions of the fistula, particularly bony adhesion to the ischiopubic rami. All such attachments must be freed using sharp scissors aided by palpation and finger pressure between bladder and vagina. The finger detects ridges of scar tissue and

areas of adhesion that need division so that the next tissue cut can be directed with accuracy.

Excision of scar tissue

This is a separate heading to emphasize the point that scar excision is never—repeat never—necessary. This step, emphasized in many textbooks, has been copied, it would seem, from one publication to another but never by the pen of an experienced fistula surgeon. Excision of bladder scar tissue not only makes the present tissue deficit even greater, leading to a more difficult and more hazardous closure, but also creates unnecessary bleeding, which hinders closure and allows the bladder to fill with blood. One need only review the pathologic processes in the healing of a fistula to appreciate that the bladder wall for some distance around is infiltrated heavily with scar tissue.

Care of the ureters

With massive fistulas the likelihood of ureteral involvement at or near the fistula edge, or even outside it, must be presumed in each case until disproven. Early in dissection the orifices must be identified and catheterized so that mobilization proceeds superiorly, laterally, and centrally, carefully avoiding the lateral angles of the defect near the cervix (Fig. 52-7). It is most important that the bladder be mobilized centrally from the cervix. Pockets of freedom produced by this preliminary mobilization aid eventual ureteral orifice identification by freeing the bladder, but with larger fistulas identification often can be made before any attempt at mobilization begins.

Methods of ureteral orifice identification

1. After preliminary mobilization has been completed, the terminal ureter and orifice may be palpable. Eversion of the lateral angles of the fistula might enable the orifice to be seen, allowing the passage of a fine probe gently through the orifice, particularly if the probe lies flat on the bladder mucosa and is

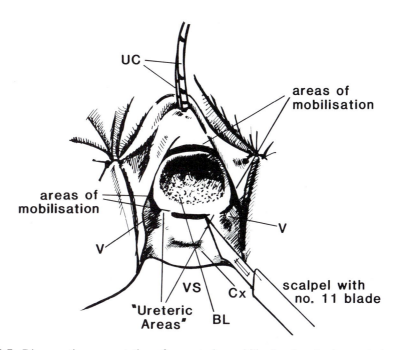

Fig. 52-7. Diagramatic representation of areas to be mobilized and ureteral areas to be avoided until the ureters have been identified and catheterized. UC = ureteric catheter; V = vagina; VS = vaginal speculum; BL = bladder; Cx = cervix. (From Zacharin RF: *Obstetric fistula*, New York, 1987, Springer.)

passed carefully in several areas in the anticipated line of the distal ureter (Fig. 52-8).

2. With a very large fistula, or when probing is unrewarded, 5 ml of 0.5% indigo carmine injected intravenously will produce telltale blue dye within 5 minutes and identify the orifices.

3. Should dye investigation fail, a second indigo carmine injection or even a double dose together with 10 mg of intravenous Lasix will usually complete identification. When the ureters have been catheterized and the catheters drawn through the urethra by artery forceps, then bladder mobilization can proceed and be safely completed (Fig. 52-9).

Bladder wall closure

Although there are no fixed rules to be followed, the bladder is usually closed with interrupted sutures of no. 00 chromic catgut (W565 Ethicon is recommended) while the surgeon observes the following principles:

1. The limits of the fistula are defined and the bladder mucosa inverted with interrupted sutures passing through muscle and submucosal layers only, avoiding the bladder lumen. Wide bites will prevent tearing out, and sutures should ensure apposition without strangulation. Never should the surgeon forget that these tissues have been subjected to excessive trauma. Even though they appear nearly normal, they are far from it. Healing will be slow, for blood supply is much less than usual, and tight suturing is unnecessary and dangerous.

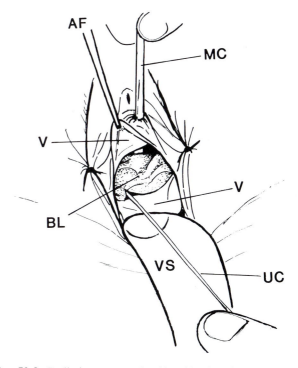

Fig. 52-8. Preliminary ureteral orifice identification, then passage of a ureteral catheter. AF = Allis forceps; V = vagina; BL = bladder; VS = vaginal speculum; UC = ureteric catheter; MC = metal catheter. (From Zacharin RF: *Obstetric fistula*, New York, 1987, Springer.)

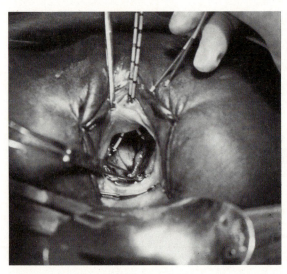

Fig. 52-9. When both ureteral catheters are in place, bladder mobilization can proceed. AF = Allis forceps; V = vagina; UC = ureteric catheter; VS = vaginal speculum; BL = bladder. (From Zacharin RF: *Obstetric fistula*, New York, 1987, Springer.)

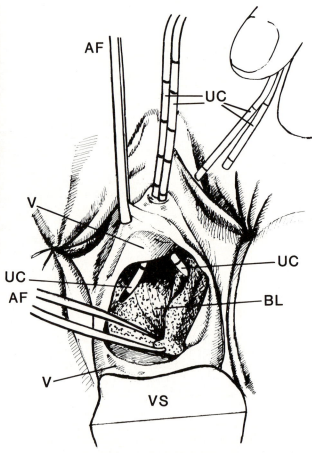

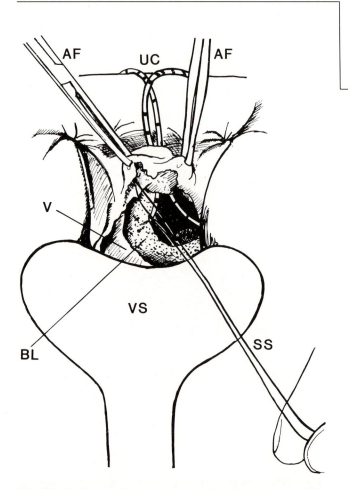

Fig. 52-10. The stabilizing suture is tied, anchoring the bladder to the pubic symphysis. AF = Allis forceps; V = vagina; BL = bladder; VS = vaginal speculum; SS = stabilizing suture. (From Zacharin RF: *Obstetric fistula*, New York, 1987, Springer.)

2. Before beginning closure of larger fistulas, the lateral edges of the bladder defect are identified on either side and the bladder wall immediately lateral to this fixed to the periosteum of the ischiopubic ramus on that side. This important and key step stabilizes the bladder against the rami, minimizing postoperative movements of the recent bladder suture line (Fig. 52-10).

3. Bladder wall closure begins laterally and moves centrally either in the natural transverse direction or in the anteroposterior direction should this seem more appropriate. Occasionally, a combination of transversely placed sutures laterally with centrally sited anteroposterior sutures can be the best method for closing a large defect. The important principle to be remembered and reemphasized is that *there must never be any tension on this suture line*.

4. Usually it is possible to insert a double layer of sutures, the outer overlapping the inner.

5. Following fistula closure the patency of the suture line must always be tested by injecting dye into the bladder through the catheter. Moderate pressure may be applied to the bladder, and any leaks detected will require extra sutures (Fig. 52-11).

Grafting

Historically, the placing of a graft between bladder and vagina is a relatively recent innovation, yet it ranks

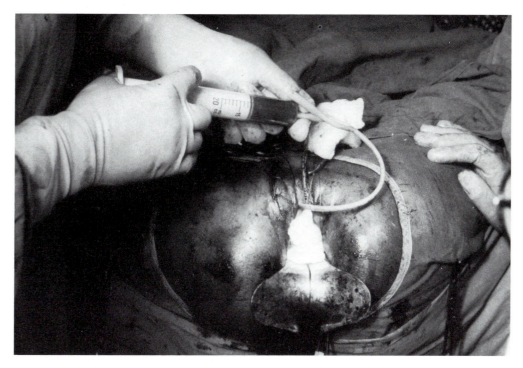

Fig. 52-11. Injecting methylene blue into the bladder to confirm a watertight closure. (From Zacharin RF: *Obstetric fistula,* New York, 1987, Springer.)

equally in importance with other principles of fistula closure. Some form of grafting should be employed during the closure of every fistula, for there is no point in saving this technique for future surgical attempts. Undoubtedly a graft enhances the quality of fistula closure and makes a successful outcome more likely. The two grafting techniques employed are the Martius graft and the gracilis muscle graft.

Martius graft. This graft should be employed with most fistulas, excluding the very small and the very large with urethral loss when it would be inadequate. Key points in the technique in taking this graft and placing it in position are that the fat pedicle must be mobilized back to the inferior margin of the ischiopubic ramus without disturbing the blood supply of the graft, and the tunnel for the graft must lie in close apposition to the inferior margin of the ramus to avoid undue bleeding. The tunnel should allow easy passage of the little finger to avoid strangulation, and the fat pedicle should be fixed in position over the closed fistula with anchor sutures, avoiding undue tension.

Gracilis graft. Described originally by Garlock[5] and embellished by Ingelman-Sundberg,[9] this graft was simplified by Hamlin and Nicholson,[7] making it similar in principle to a Martius graft in being transferred from the donor site subcutaneously into the vagina. It is required in correcting some large fistulas, especially those involving urethral reconstruction. The vaginal wound is closed with no. 00 monofilament nylon inserted as vertical mattress sutures, incorporating the underlying graft to help eliminate dead space. Just enough tension is applied to bring the

skin edges into apposition without strangulation. Should there be a deficit of vaginal skin, a labial skin flap can be raised from the lesser labium of one or the other side and laid over the muscle or fat graft as a full-thickness skin graft.

Vaginal pack

The vagina is packed gently but firmly with gauze soaked in paraffin. This pack remains for 48 hours, a step that encourages the various layers to adhere and minimizes dead space and hematoma formation.

Postoperative management

Immediately following surgery, urine should be draining from all catheters. If not, intravenous Lasix will start a flushing action. Bladder washout should be avoided. Two important principles must be observed:

1. The bladder must be kept empty during the healing phase.
2. Antibiotics are required to prevent urinary tract infection so long as the catheter is required.

A nurse should be present until the patient is fully recovered from the anesthesia, a precaution that minimizes any risk of interference with catheter drainage. Suction is never employed, for it has inherent problems. The patient is instructed to watch catheter drainage and to notify the nursing staff should there be any concern about adequacy of drainage. If there is any doubt, the catheter should be changed immediately without question. Depending upon

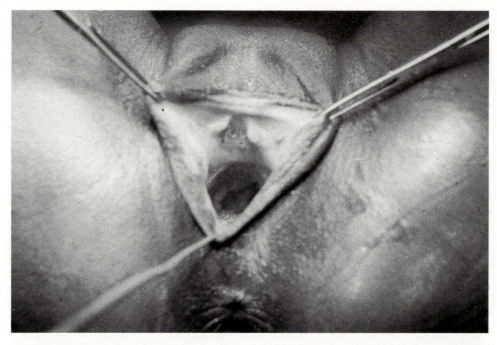

Fig. 52-12. The residual fistula after some months of healing: "the urethra has vanished and the examiner looks straight into the bladder." (From Zacharin RF: *Obstetric fistula*, New York, 1987, Springer.)

the size of the bladder defect, catheter drainage is required for a minimum of 10 days and up to 14 days for larger defects. Ureteral catheters remain in situ for 8 to 10 days to allow meatal edema to subside. Following catheter removal, there is usually no difficulty voiding, but the patient must be observed carefully and catheterized at 4- to 6-hour intervals, depending on fluid intake, if unable to void. In practice, voiding usually occurs easily, and providing that volumes are 200 ml or more, no checks are necessary. The patient remains under supervision for a further 24 hours, a specimen of urine is checked for infection, and antibiotics are stopped. The patient is instructed to avoid sexual intercourse until the postoperative visit in 1 month, when the nylon sutures are removed.

Complications

The addition of partial or complete urethral destruction to a vesicovaginal fistula has been regarded as a serious complicating factor difficult to correct. Many procedures have been designed to correct the situation. Hamlin and Nicholson,[7] drawing on an extensive experience with difficult fistulas, have described their technique for reconstructing a urethra totally destroyed in labor, a detailed procedure that includes contributions from earlier publications by Martius, Chassar Moir, and Ingleman-Sundberg. Principles of repair are as follows:

1. Lithotomy with steep Trendelenburg tilt is the procedure to be used.
2. Posterolateral introital incision opens the stenosed vagina.

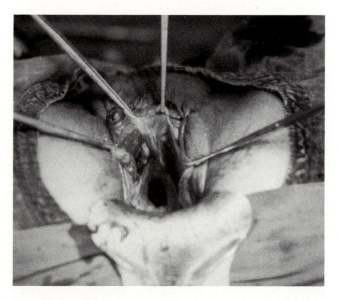

Fig. 52-13. Paraurethral incision outlining the new urethra. (From Zacharin RF: *Obstetric fistula*, New York, 1987, Springer.)

3. The vesical defect in these patients is such that usually ureteral orifices can be identified and catheterized. However, if not then, along with mobilization of tissues to be used in reconstructing the new urethra, bladder mobilization begins laterally and centrally, avoiding the ureteral areas. Then the ureters are identified and catheterized.
4. Remains of the external urethral meatus can be

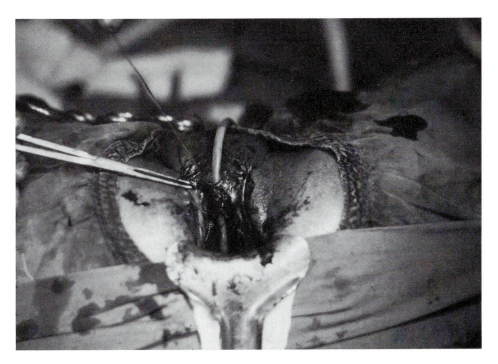

Fig. 52-14. Urethral reconstruction. (From Zacharin RF: *Obstetric fistula,* New York, 1987, Springer.)

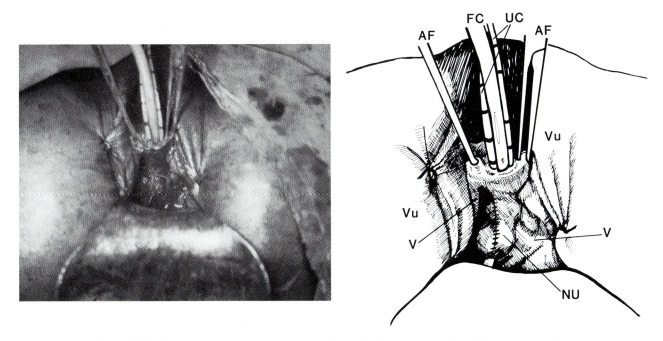

Fig. 52-15. Completion of urethral reconstruction, bladder closure and stabilizing sutures in place. (From Zacharin RF: *Obstetric fistula,* New York, 1987, Springer.)

seen as two small epithelial elevations adherent anterior to the pubic bone, while the site of the absent urethra is marked by tough scar tissue joining urethral remnants to the ischiopubic rami and anterior edge of the bladder defect (Fig. 52-12).

5. Deep paraurethral incisions are made, demarcating tissue to be used in forming the new urethra. Ex-

tending the incisions deeply allows mobilization of this tissue, which is then rolled over a Foley 12 catheter to form the new urethra (Figs. 52-13 and 52-14).

6. The bladder is mobilized widely with special attention given to bony adhesion.

7. Before beginning urethral closure, the Foley and

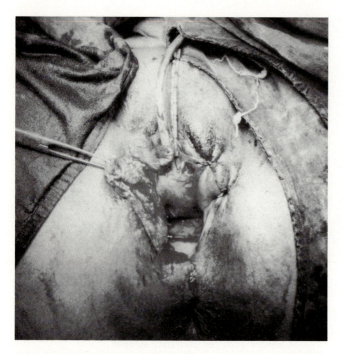

Fig. 52-16. Labial graft prepared to cover the gracilis graft. (From Zacharin RF: *Obstetric fistula*, New York, 1987, Springer.)

two ureteral catheters are held in place against the new urethral roof while the first inverting suture of no. 00 chromic catgut is placed. Then the urethral tube transmitting the three catheters is completed down to the bladder defect with a series of mattress sutures, not too many and not too tight. During urethral reconstruction, the danger point at the urethrovesical junction is reinforced with extra sutures, drawing bladder muscle over this junctional zone to invert the join and minimize the risk of later stress incontinence.

8. The bladder is closed, rolling in the mucosa with the contained ureteral orifices and catheters. Often the bladder defect, because of its size, is closed transversely. It is important to insert anchor sutures to stabilize the bladder wall laterally against the ischiopubic rami (Fig. 52-15). Following closure, a dye test is performed.

9. The repair is reinforced with a gracilis muscle graft, and in some cases a Martius fat graft is also used.

10. The anterior vaginal wall is closed, if necessary, using a labial fat graft (Fig. 52-16).

REFERENCES

1. Bardescu N: Ein neues Verfahren für die Operation der tiefen Blasen-Uterus-Scheidenfisteln, *Zentralbl Gynakol* 24:170, 1900.
2. Blaikley JB: Colpocleisis for difficult vesicovaginal and rectovaginal fistulas, *Am J Obstet Gynecol* 91:589, 1965.
3. Carter B et al: Vesicovaginal fistulas, *Am J Obstet Gynecol* 63:479, 1952.
4. Counsellor VS, Haigler FH: Management of urinary vaginal fistula in 253 cases, *Am J Obstet Gynecol* 72:367, 1956.
5. Garlock JH: The cure of an intractable vesicovaginal fistula by the use of a pedicled muscle graft, *Surg Gynecol Obstet* 47:255, 1928.
6. Greenslade NF: Vesico-vaginal fistula: a method of repair, *Aust N Z J Surg* 38:283, 1969.
7. Hamlin RHJ, Nicholson EC: Reconstruction of urethra totally destroyed in labour, *Br Med J* 2:147, 1969.
8. Hamlin RHJ, Nicholson EC: Personal communication, 1986.
9. Ingelman-Sundberg A: *Pathogenesis and operative treatment of urinary fistula in irradiated tissue.* In Youssef AF, editor: *Gynaecological urology,* Springfield, Ill, 1960, Charles C Thomas.
10. Kiricuta I, Goldstein AMB: The repair of extensive vesicovaginal fistulas with pedicled omentum: a review of 27 cases, *J Urol* 108:724, 1972.
11. Lawson JB: *Vesico-vaginal fistulae.* In Proceedings of the 1st International Conference of the Faculty of Gynaecology and Obstetrics, Ibadan, Nigeria, 1977.
12. Lister U: Personal communication, 1986.
13. O'Connor VJ et al: Suprapubic closure of vesico-vaginal fistula, *J Urol* 109:51, 1973.
14. Roen PR: Combined vaginal and transvesical approach in successful repair of vesicovaginal fistula, *Arch Surg* 80:628, 1960.
15. Russell CS: The vesical fistula high in the vagina, *Proc R Soc Med* 59:1022, 1966.
16. Simon G: *Fälle von Operation bei Urinfisteln am Weibe, Beobachtung einer Harnleiter-Scheidenfistel,* 1856. Cited by Latzko WA.
17. Su CT: A flap technique for repair of vesicovaginal fistula, *J Urol* 102:56, 1969.
18. von Dittel (1893) from Latzko W: *Postoperative vesicovaginal fistulas: genesis and therapy, Am J Surg* 58:211, 1942.
19. Weyrauch HM, Rous SN: Transvaginal-transvesical approach for surgical repair of vesicovaginal fistula, *Surg Gynecol Obstet* 123:121, 1966.
20. Zacharin RF: Grafting as a principle in the surgical management of vesicovaginal and rectovaginal fistulae, *Aust N Z Obstet Gynaecol* 20:10, 1980.
21. Zacharin RF: *Obstetric fistula,* New York, 1988, Springer-Verlag New York, Inc.

Chapter 53

THE ABDOMINAL-APPROACH REPAIR OF SIMPLE AND COMPLEX VESICOVAGINAL FISTULAS

Richard Turner-Warwick

It is almost always possible to close urinary vaginal fistulas. Meticulous technique is naturally essential, but reliable success with the more complicated problems depends on the ability of the surgeon to select the procedure best suited to the particular clinical situation and, furthermore, to vary it according to the findings in the course of the operation on the basis of a wide personal experience.

Because urinary fistulas in women are commonly the result of gynecologic and obstetric complications, in addition to the most unpleasant inconvenience for the patient, they often present a medico-legal aspect. The essential of treatment is, therefore, to resolve the situation without delay and without any complications. Failure should be a rare event.

The basic surgical option for the repair of a vesical fistula lies between a vaginal-approach procedure and an abdominal-approach procedure. Many surgeons have an instinctive personal preference for one of these, but this is not as it should be. Although many simple vesicovaginal fistulas can be closed by a vaginal repair procedure, the access that this provides is relatively restricted and any significant incidence of failure after this suggests under-usage of the abdominal approach. Similarly, a significant incidence of failure after a simple abdominal-approach layer-closure can be resolved by a formal omental-interposition procedure, because, in the absence of active tumor or infection, this procedure should be almost invariably successful.[2,15] Thus, the most reliable fistula-closure procedure must be the "three option" (vaginal-abdominal-omen-tal) progression-approach (TOPA) procedure,[10,11] and almost the only indication for urinary diversion after a fistula operation is urinary incontinence due to irremediable sphincter damage.

Thus, ideally, the closure of even an apparently simple vesicovaginal fistula should be regarded as a specialist gynecourologic or urogynecologic procedure and the surgeon who created the fistula is not always the best person to undertake its repair.

THE TIMING OF REPAIR

Even the smaller vesicovaginal fistulas rarely respond to conservative treatment by simple catheter drainage of the bladder. A definitive closure is almost invariably required.

Traditionally, a delayed repair has been advocated for the treatment of urinary fistulas to ensure that the local tissue reaction has settled. The major change in the management of postoperative vesical and ureteric fistulas in recent years has been an immediate repair procedure, in preference to a delayed one. However, this does not generally apply to urethrovaginal fistulas because these are invariably associated with damage to the all-important intrinsic urethral sphincter mechanism on which continence depends. The appropriate procedure for these is usually a delayed definitive reconstructive sphincteroplasty (see p. 882).

Early diagnosis and immediate specialist referral are important because, after about 2 weeks, the local healing reaction tends to make a repair more difficult and precarious so it may then be advisable to defer it for 2 to 3 months or more to ensure that this has settled. However, when an omental interposition procedure is used, the success of the closure is less dependent on the perfect healing of a simple layer-closure. Thus, the timing of a repair must be carefully considered in each particular case.

THE MANAGEMENT OF FISTULOUS INCONTINENCE

When it is necessary to delay the repair of a vesicovaginal or urethrovaginal fistula for a few months, the collection of incontinent urine becomes a major problem in the patient's life. All too often, there is no alternative to simple absorbent pads. However, once the decision for a delayed repair has been made, the deferment should be carried through with fortitude until the most appropriate time because disasters can lurk in premature closure endeavors.

The urine leakage from a small vesicovaginal fistula can sometimes be reduced by indwelling urethral catheter drainage. However, this is usually ineffective when the fistula is large. When the caliber of the vaginal introitus is narrow enough to retain a 40- to 50-ml balloon catheter, vaginal catheter drainage is an effective and underused technique, both for vesicovaginal and ureterovaginal fistulas.

FISTULOUS INJURIES

Unrecognized or inadequate or ineffectively repaired injuries to the urinary tract during gynecologic surgery and complicated childbirth generally result in fistulation into the vagina from the ureter, the bladder, or the urethra. Each of these presents an entirely different surgical problem involving quite separate considerations. However, a vesicovaginal fistula may be associated with a terminal ureterovaginal fistula or a proximal urethrovaginal fistula. Occasionally, the rectum may also be involved.

Gynecologic injuries

Because of their proximity, the ureter and the bladder are particularly vulnerable during both abdominal and vaginal gynecologic surgery for benign and for malignant conditions.

The ureters are particularly at risk during the course of a difficult dissection and ligation of the lateral pedicles that contain the uterine, vaginal, or ovarian vessels; the ureters may be divided, windowed, or simply included in the ligature.

Often, however, the development of a simple vesicovaginal fistula is not the direct result of a surgical misadventure. These are commonly large and located in the midline above the trigone. Frequently, they are not immediately identifiable, the vaginal leakage starting a few days postoperatively. This type of fistula can result from a patch of ischemia that develops after the separation of a particularly thin-walled bladder from the anterior aspect of the uterus and cervix. Even the most experienced surgeons are not immune from this fortuitous complication.

The surgical significance of infrequent voiding

It is important that gynecologic surgeons should recognize that patients who void infrequently have a characteristically thin-walled bladder and that this predisposes to the development of an ischemic supratrigonal vesicovaginal fistula. Thus, it is generally advisable to monitor carefully the postoperative voiding efficiency of patients with thin-walled bladders, using a temporary prophylactic suprapubic catheter to avoid overdistention or retention that can predispose to the development of necrosis of the ischemic patch and consequent fistulation.

Patients who void infrequently (at intervals of 4 to 6 hours or more) are prone to develop voiding difficulties after simple pelvic surgery and, incidentally, they are also prone to late-onset urine infection.[3,4,13] Having identified this situation from the history preoperatively, it is wise to forewarn the patient that socially convenient infrequent voiding can be associated with a somewhat precarious degree of voiding dysfunction and cause voiding difficulties postoperatively. If, in spite of extra care, such a patient does, nevertheless, develop a fistula, such a forewarning may help them understand that it was their particularly thin-walled bladder that was the underlying cause of their vesicovaginal fistula, not simply a surgical misadventure.

Obstetric injuries

Injuries to the urinary tract during natural delivery are unusual in obstetrically developed countries. However, bladder-base injury caused by ischemic pressure necrosis due to fetal-head compression against the pubis during uncontrolled prolonged labor is by far the most common cause of vaginal fistulas, worldwide. The proximal urethra is commonly involved in such injuries, and, if the damage to this is circumferential, the irremediable sphincter deficiency is naturally a disaster.

The bladder is also vulnerable during cesarean section and, occasionally, one or even both ureters may be involved. Rupture of the uterus resulting from a trial of labor after a previous cesarean section is particularly likely to involve the bladder as a result of secondary adhesions between its posterior surface and the lower segment hysterotomy scar. The consequent vesical disruption is often severe and may extend distally into the urethra, causing potentially critical sphincter damage.

Unfortunately, the early repair of an obstetric fistula is often contraindicated for a critical period by the postpartum involution, so a delayed repair may be advisable.

FISTULA REPAIR PROCEDURE OPTIONS

Even the smaller vesicovaginal fistulas rarely respond to conservative treatment by simple catheter drainage of the bladder. Immediate procedure to a definitive closure is generally advisable.

From the patient's, the medical, and the legal viewpoints, it is important to ensure that a postoperative fistula is repaired both expeditiously and successfully at the first attempt, preferably without an additional skin incision as a

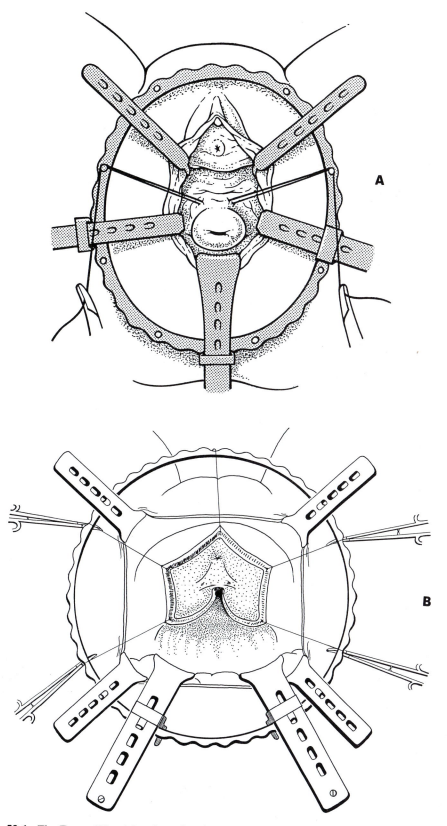

Fig. 53-1. The Turner-Warwick universal perineoabdominal ring retractor and abdominal ring retractor. **A,** The perineal ring retractor with stay-suture guide knobs and malleable copper vaginal blades. **B,** The Turner-Warwick abdominal ring retractor and the particular advantages of elevating traction stay sutures retained by ring-margin hemostats for fistula repairs. (© 1970, Institute of Urology.)

lasting reminder of the complication even if additional omental mobilization is required in the more complicated situations to ensure success.

Vaginal-approach repair procedures

Vaginal-approach repair procedures are discussed in Chapter 51.

The traditional "exaggerated lithotomy" operating position is widely used for repair of vaginal fistulas. The disadvantage of this is that it does not provide the facility of immediate extension to a synchronous abdominal procedure if necessary. Consequently, the exaggerated position is only appropriate when the surgeon is certain that a vaginal approach will be both sufficient and successful—a conviction that sometimes proves questionable. Thus, the author invariably uses the open-option perineoabdominal progression approach (PAPA) operating position for vaginal surgery (see p. 891) because it facilitates the TOPA procedure.

A synchronous vaginal approach is essential for an abdominal omental-interposition repair (see p. 891). Appropriate instrumentation greatly facilitates vaginal surgery. The perineal element of the Turner-Warwick (TW) universal perineoabdominal ring retractor system has malleable copper blades for vaginal retraction posteriorly and posterolaterally (Fig. 53-1); its guide knobs maintain the direction of traction stay-sutures that can be used to draw a fistula down toward the introitus, and this greatly improves surgical access to it. Thus, ring retraction provides more efficient vaginal retraction than the traditional weighted Auvard retractor, and it also obviates the need for a retracting surgical assistant, for whom there is little room during the perineal component of a synchronous perineoabdominal repair procedure.

Abdominal-approach repair procedures

Preoperative urographic proof that the upper tracts are draining freely into the bladder is naturally essential before any repair of a vesicovaginal fistula. It is generally helpful to insert temporary catheters into the ureters as an immediate preliminary to a repair because this facilitates their extravesical identification, especially during an abdominal procedure after a previous surgical failure or irradiation.

Even if a preoperative decision has been made to use an abdominal-approach repair procedure, there is considerable advantage in the PAPA operating position (see p. 891) because a guiding finger in the vagina greatly facilitates the separation and the development of the tissue layers around a vesicovaginal fistula (see below).

Abdominal access to the pelvis is also greatly increased by ring retraction (Fig. 53-1). A particular advantage of this is that multiple stay-sutures, retained by the tips of hemostats tucked under the margin of the ring, can be used to elevate the bladder and the vaginal vault: this greatly improves the exposure and facilitates the repair of a fistula. Thus, combined with the circumferential disposition of appropriately shaped blades, it eliminates the misuse of an assistant as a retractor.

Transperitoneal supravesical approach repair procedures

The traditional anterior transvesical approach, which provides only relatively restricted exposure for a simple layer-closure of a fistula, is no longer advocated and should be abandoned.

The transperitoneal supravesical approach provides the best exposure for the abdominal repair of vesicovaginal fistulas (Fig. 53-2).

1. It facilitates separation of the vagina from the back of the bladder and the urethra.
2. It enables the separation of the vagina to be extended into an effectively wide abdominoperineal tunnel for omental interposition, should this be indicated (see p. 891).
3. It facilitates a reflux-preventing reimplantation of the ureter when one or both of these are involved in the fistulous margin (see below).
4. It facilitates a synchronous perineoabdominal urethral sphincteroplasty when a vesical fistula extends downward through the bladder neck creating an additional urethral defect (see below).

The incision in the posterior bladder wall should be laterally curved whenever the tissues are somewhat rigid as a result of irradiation or inflammatory fibrosis because this enables the bladder to be closed by rotation of the conse-

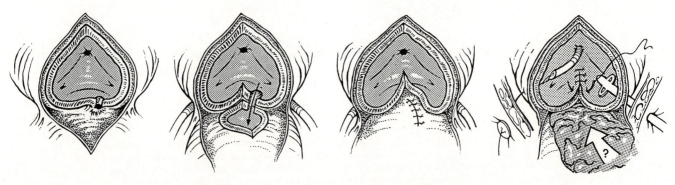

Fig. 53-2. The transperitoneal supravesical approach for the abdominal repair of vesicovaginal fistulas. (© 1970, Institute of Urology.)

quently eccentric flap of its posterior wall. After irradiation, a vertical midline incision in the bladder can prove impossible to close side-to-side.

The synchronous PAPA operating position is a great advantage for this procedure; in particular, a guiding finger in the vagina facilitates the development of the plane of separation and hemostasis.

Principles of layer closure of a fistula

The basic principles of the layer-closure of a fistula are well-established, but there are many technical options.

After appropriate separation of the vagina and bladder, facilitated by a guiding finger in the vagina, the abnormal tissue at the margin of the fistula is resected. The author always uses polyglycolic acid (PGA) sutures—never catgut—and ties the knots on the lumen whenever possible. The technique of suturing and the duration of catheter drainage are discussed below. The vagina is usually closed with a single layer of inverting interrupted sutures. If the tissue quality and the closure of the bladder are deemed sufficiently good for a simple layer-closure procedure, the bladder is closed with two layers of sutures. However, if there is any doubt about the success of this procedure, a single layer of carefully placed, interrupted, inverting sutures is used in combination with omental support.

Supporting the closure of complex fistulas by interposition grafts

When the healing potential of the tissue around a fistula is compromised by fibrotic scar tissue resulting from infection, from the failure of previous repairs, or from irradiation, the reliability of a simple layer-closure procedure diminishes abruptly unless an additional well-vascularized transposition graft is interposed. The advisability of interposition support generally becomes obvious in the course of an operation so that, in general, surgeons should regard the recurrence of a fistula after a simple layer-closure procedure as an avoidable complication, even though it may be fortuitously inevitable on occasion.

A sizeable flap of parapelvic peritoneum sometimes provides sufficient additional interposition support for a layer-closure, but this is generally inappropriate when it is also involved in the local pathology, especially irradiation. Pedicled muscle flaps, such as gracilis, can be used as a simple tissue-bulk interposition; however, skeletal muscle is ill-adapted to resist infection and to resolve inflammation so it contributes little to the local healing reaction. Its vascular response-potential is primarily exercise-related, and, ultimately, inactivity results in disuse atrophy and fibrosis.

Surgical value of omental redeployment support

The omentum is unique in that it is the only body tissue specifically developed for the purpose of resolving inflammation. This function is partly due to its vascularization, which is capable of rapid augmentation in response to inflammation. However, the "magic" of the omentum is fundamentally dependent on its abundant lymphatic drainage, which is so good it can rapidly reabsorb macromolecular inflammatory exudates, the accumulation of which can create purulent collections that compromise the healing of a repair. Thus, the omentum acts as a physiologic drain that generally prevents the formation of pus in the peritoneal cavity except in locations it does not normally reach, such as the pelvis and the subdiaphragmatic areas.

Surgically, the omentum is invaluable for the support of the more precarious urinary tract reconstructions.[15] Furthermore, unlike the retroperitoneal and retropubic fat, the omentum always regains its suppleness after an inflammatory response has settled. Thus, the omentum provides a unique urodynamic quality of support that is fundamentally important to the reliable success of functional reconstructions, especially sphincteroplasty, because it ensures the freedom of its subsequent functional movements.[2,10,11]

Appropriately used, the omentum can virtually guarantee the closure of a vesicovaginal fistula (Fig. 53-3) or a complex vesicovaginorectal fistula (Fig. 53-4) provided an adequate bulk of it is appropriately mobilized and interposed between PGA-sutured closure lines of the vagina

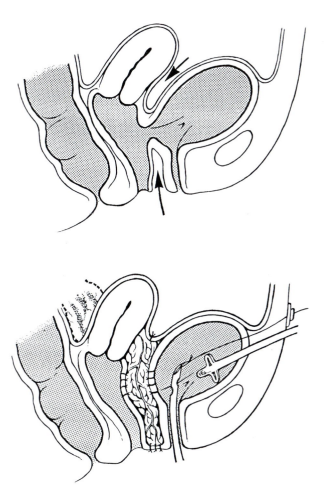

Fig. 53-3. Omental interposition for a recurrent vesicovaginal fistula after the creation of a wide intervening abdominoperineal tunnel. (© 1966, Institute of Urology.)

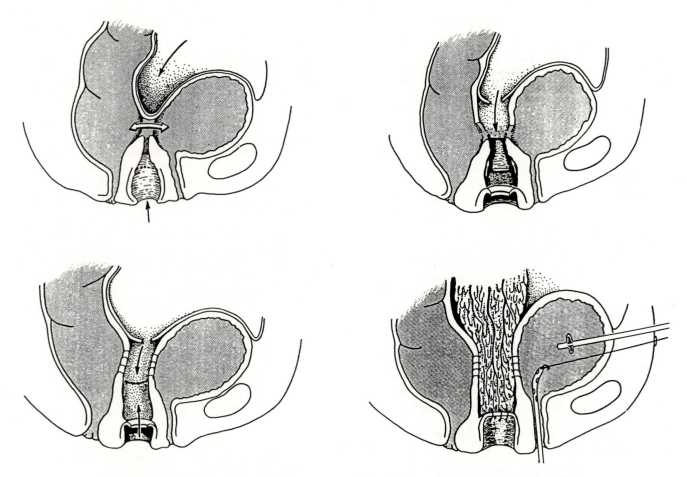

Fig. 53-4. The closure of a complex hysterectomy + irradiation vesicovaginal fistula achieved by excising the stenotic vault of the irradiated vagina to create a wide abdominoperineal tunnel for omental interpositioning. (© 1966, Institute of Urology.)

and the bladder/urethra. This interpositioning procedure requires the synchronous abdominoperineal exposure provided by the PAPA operating position (see p. 891).

The omentum should completely fill an interposition abdominoperineal tunnel that is properly developed laterally to admit three or four fingers so that a good tissue-overlap is ensured. It should not be regarded simply as an "omental plug." The lower margin of the interposed omentum is anchored by including it in the perineal sutures used to close the vaginal wall opening, just proximal to the introitus, at the lower end of the abdominoperineal interposition tunnel.

Anatomical basis of omental mobilization

The "magic" of the omentum depends on the "pulsating efficiency" of its vascularization, and this must be preserved during its mobilization: the preservation of this depends on an accurate knowledge of its anatomical features, and these are detailed elsewhere.[2,6,10,11]

The blood supply of the omentum is derived from the right gastroepiploic branch of the gastroduodenal vessels and the left gastroepiploic branch of the splenic vessels (Fig. 53-5). The right gastroepiploic vascular pedicle is considerably larger than that on the left, and it directly supplies the major part of the omental apron. Within the omental apron, the collateral anastomoses between the vertical branches of the gastroepiploic arcade are relatively minor and somewhat unreliable.

In about 30% of patients, the omentum reaches the perineum without any mobilization of its vascular pedicles (Fig. 53-5). Even so, when it is surgically redeployed to support reconstructive procedures in the pelvis, it is generally advisable to separate its natural adhesion to the transverse colon and the mesocolon to avoid its distraction by gaseous distention of the bowel postoperatively.

Simple mobilization by division of its relatively minor left gastroepiploic vascular pedicle enables a further 30% of omental aprons to reach the perineum, and, normally, this does not significantly reduce its blood supply.

In about 40% of patients (more in children whose apron is often relatively short), meticulous full-length mobilization of the right gastroepiploic vascular arcade from the stomach is required to enable it to be effectively redeployed in the pelvis. Because the bulk of a fully mobilized

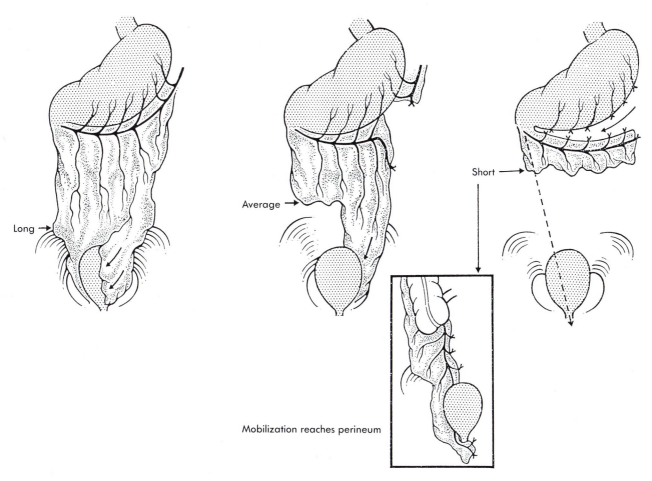

Long

Average

Short

Mobilization reaches perineum

Fig. 53-5. In 30% of cases, the omental apron is long enough to reach the perineum after its simple separation from the transverse colon and mesocolon. In another 30%, an additional division of its left gastroepiploic pedicle is required. Formal mobilization of the whole length of its right gastroepiploic pedicle from the stomach is required in 40%. In such cases, the pedicle should be protected by positioning it behind the mobilized right colon, and a prophylatic appendicectomy is generally advisable. (© 1987, Institute of Urology.)

omentum is based on its slender vascular pedicle, this should be protected by mobilizing the right colon so that it can lie retroperitoneally behind this. Failure to do this can result in the division of the all-important pedicle during a subsequent laparotomy for obstruction, a complication we have seen during several retrievoplasty procedures.

Thus, even when its apron is underdeveloped, as it often is in children, a normal omentum can always be redeployed into the pelvis.

Unfortunately, some surgical and gynecologic texts advocate basing the mobilization of the omentum on its relatively minor vascular pedicle on the left; others even elongate the apron by a simple horizontal incision that transects its vertical vessels and this inevitably reduces its pulsating efficiency. Furthermore, in about 10% of patients, there is no anastomotic junction between the right and the left gastroepiploic vessels that usually form a complete gastroepiploic arcade on the greater curvature of the stomach (Fig. 53-6).

Operative procedure for full-length mobilization of the right gastroepiploic pedicle

A midline abdominal wall incision must always be used whenever there is any possibility that a reconstruction in the pelvis may require omental support; this is essential to enable the incision to be extended upward to provide appropriate surgical access to the stomach for the meticulous mobilization of its pedicle vessels. The need for an extended mobilization cannot be predicted preoperatively.

It is fundamentally important to remember that there is only one omentum and that damage to its blood supply by inappropriate mobilization of its vascular pedicle not only compromises the success of the procedure, but also the success of a subsequent retrievoplasty.

The individual ligation of the 20 to 30 short gastric branches involves meticulous vascular technique to avoid damage to the main gastroepiploic pedicle vessels (Fig. 53-7); this takes time.

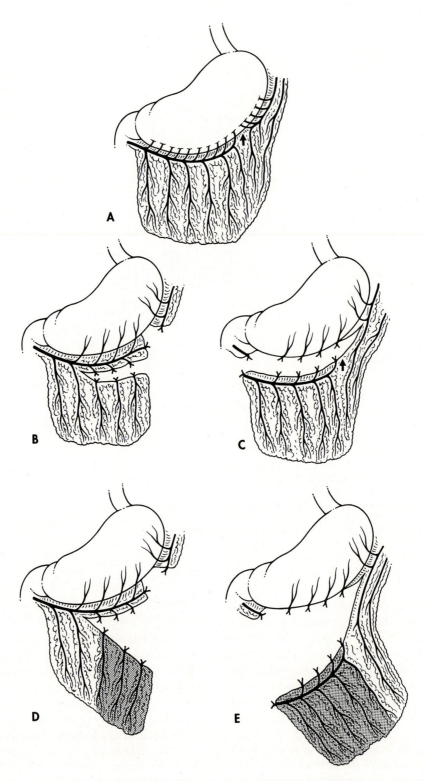

Fig. 53-6. A, In 10% of patients, the right and left gastroepiploic vessels do not anastomose to form an "arch." **B** and **C,** The omentum should not be mobilized by a horizontal incision across the apron below the gastroepiploic arch because this divides the vertical branches and the distal collateral communications between these are poor. **D** and **E,** The right gastroepiploic vessels vascularize more than two thirds of the omental apron. Mobilization of the omentum on the basis of the left gastroepiploic pedicle may result in ischemia if the gastroepiploic arch is incomplete. (© 1977, Institute of Urology.)

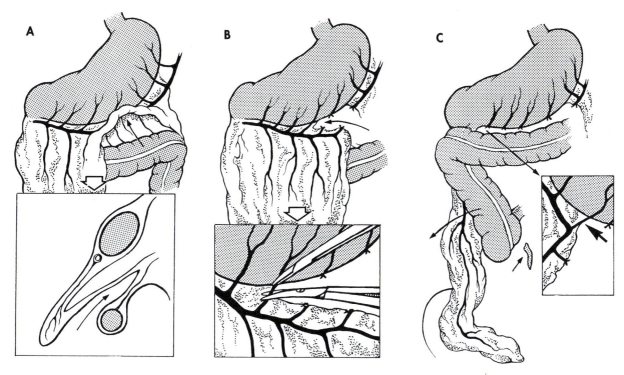

Fig. 53-7. Mobilization of the right gastroepiploic pedicle of the omentum requires meticulous vascular technique. **A,** Separation from the transverse mesocolon by development of the avascular plane is always advisable to prevent postoperative displacement of the redeployed omentum by gaseous bowel distention. **B,** Ligation-in-continuity reduces the risk of developing an interstitial hematoma. Ligation between hemostats risks vessel escape. Nonabsorbable ligature material should always be used. **C,** Once started, mobilization of the right gastroepiploic vessels from the stomach should be extended to their gastroduodenal origin; otherwise, tension on the pedicle at the point of the last undivided branch may rupture it. (© 1977, Institute of Urology.)

1. Bunch ligation of vessels foreshortens the pedicle and increases the risk that they may escape and bleed.
2. Absorbable ligatures should be used for mobilization of the omental pedicle vessels. Nonabsorbable sutures and ligaclips can come to lie exposed within a fistulous area and can result in stone formation.
3. The technique of the division of the short gastric vessels must be meticulous to avoid damage to the parent gastroepiploic vessels. The proximal end of these branches should be ligated in continuity, before division, not between hemostats. This is because their inadvertent escape can result in the immediate development of an interstitial hematoma in the omentum, and even greater care is then necessary to retrieve it for secure religation without damaging the main pedicle vessels. Hemostat ligation can be used for the gastric end because this is easy to retrieve if it slips off.
4. Once started, mobilization of the right gastroepiploic arch from the greater curvature of the stomach should be completed to its gastroduodenal origin; otherwise, there is a risk that traction on the pedicle might rupture the last undivided branch or "window" the main pedicle vessel.
5. The slender pedicle vessels at the root of a fully mobilized right omental pedicle should be protected by relo-

cating them behind the mobilized ascending colon. A prophylactic appendectomy avoids incidental surgical damage to the pedicle during a subsequent acute appendectomy immediately adjacent to it.

Avoidable causes of failure of omental interposition repairs

Failure of an omental interposition repair can almost always be prevented by ensuring
1. An adequate size of the abdominoperineal interposition tunnel to provide a sufficient tissue overlap laterally. The tunnel should be three to four fingerbreadths wide.
2. Mobilization of a sufficient bulk of omentum to fill the appropriately sized interposition tunnel.
3. Appropriate mobilization procedure and meticulous vascular technique to avoid impairment of the "pulsating efficiency" of the mobilized omentum.
4. Protection of the pedicle of a fully mobilized right gastroepiploic pedicle behind the mobilized ascending colon to protect it from subsequent surgery (see above).

In our experience of secondary and tertiary repairs, the previous failure of an omental interposition procedure was almost always attributable to one or more of these; however, despite meticulous care, the occasional fortuitous loss of a fully mobilized omental flap is inevitable.

SOME PRINCIPLES OF RECONSTRUCTIVE SURGERY

The basic essential for the avoidance of postoperative complications is to anticipate and to prevent them. An essential feature of this is the surgeon's inclination and ability to adapt a procedure according to the actual findings at the time of operation, many of which cannot be anticipated, however detailed the preoperative evaluation: hence, the basic principles of the TITBAPIT (Take It To Bits And Put It Together) and the PAPA procedures (see below).[2,6,7,10,11]

Technique and tissue handling

Successful reconstructive surgery is all about technique and tissue handling. Almost all surgeons regard their surgical technique as "meticulous and immaculate," however, some are more "tissue-sensitive" than others. For instance, tissue forceps applied to tissue that will remain in situ should be gentle enough to apply to a fold of one's finger skin. Would-be reconstructive surgeons who use Allis forceps for handling tissue might do well to take a course in microsurgery to improve their technique and "tissue-understanding."

Sutures

Dexon and Vicryl sutures cause much less tissue reaction than catgut and are consequently much more suitable for urinary tract reconstruction. The author thankfully abandoned catgut for all urinary tract operations in 1970 when Davis and Geck pioneered the production of PGA sutures. Size for size, these are much stronger than catgut, enabling smaller sizes to be used, and they retain their tensile strength longer. The 30- to 40-day survival of the tensile strength of 3/0 and 4/0 PGA sutures is generally appropriate for urinary tract reconstruction. Catgut causes a severe tissue reaction, which is generally unacceptable for meticulous reconstructive surgery (except for certain special purposes when this excessive reaction is unimportant or even a particular advantage).

The knots of bladder and urethral sutures are tied on the lumen, as far as possible, because the relative bulk of the knot is naturally the point of maximum tissue reaction to any suture and, located here, it falls off and is voided when PGA loses its tensile strength during the fifth or sixth week. In the course of many thousand urinary tract reconstructions over the 20 years since they were introduced, the author has not yet encountered significant encrustation or stone formation on an in situ PGA suture. Although PGA causes a relatively mild tissue reaction in the course of their dissolution (which is primarily the result of passive hydrolysis rather than an active foreign-body tissue reaction), an excessive tissue reaction can be generated by the mass ligation of an oversize pedicle that strangulates a large cuff of tissue.

Interrupted sutures allow the best possible vascularization of the tissue intervening between the suture bites and are generally preferable when the vascularization is relatively precarious. If interrupted runs of a continuous suture are used, it is most important that they be snugged down lightly so they gently approximate the tissue without strangulating it. Consequently, assistants should be dissuaded from their natural instinct to use a continuous suture as an elevating retractor.

Postoperative urine drainage

Suprapubic catheter drainage of the urine is strongly advocated after all vesical fistula repairs; it is efficient, reliable, and less uncomfortable than a urethral catheter. Furthermore, at the conclusion of the drainage period, it is easy to verify the restoration of voiding efficiency by clamping the suprapubic drainage and checking the postvoiding residual urine volumes before removing it. This compares favorably with the emotionally charged situation that can arise when only a urethral catheter is used so that it has to be reinserted repeatedly for the management of a voiding difficulty—the "yo-yo catheter."[3,4,13]

An additional urethral catheter is an insurance against early postoperative bladder distention that can occasionally arise as a result of obstruction of suprapubic catheter drainage. However, the use of a Foley balloon catheter is most inadvisable because inadvertent traction on this can disastrously disrupt the bladder-base closure; a urethral catheter is best retained by a sling suture, button-fixed on the abdominal surface.

Unobstructed catheter drainage is all that a fistula repair requires, hence the added safety of using an additional urethral catheter for the first week or so. Suction urinary drainage systems are unnecessary. Unfortunately, however, the caliber of the connecting tubes of many standard urologic drainage bag systems is so large that they have a tendency to retain air and the consequent fluid levels in a hanging loop at the bedside can create a positive hydrostatic resistance to the flow of urine. If the internal diameter of the connecting tube does not much exceed the lumen of the catheter that it is draining, it remains bubble free so that, hanging by the bedside, it naturally creates a syphonic-suction negative pressure.

The duration of catheter drainage after a fistula repair should relate to the quality of the tissue healing of the particular patient; drainage should be maintained until it has served its intended function. This depends on the surgeon's judgment, and, on the principle that there should be no brave surgeons, just brave patients, the author maintains catheter drainage until he does not have to feel brave when deciding to discontinue it—in other words, at least 2 weeks after a simple fistula closure. Naturally, when the quality of the tissue healing is relatively poor after infection, the failure of previous surgery or irradiation, a longer period is advisable, say 3 weeks, with a preliminary check on the watertightness of the suture line by suprapubic cystography.

Wound drains and antibiotics

The use of wound drains is a matter of personal surgical preference. In general, the reliability of suture-line healing is enhanced when it is immediately surrounded by well-vascularized tissue; it is diminished by adjacent accumulations of inert hematoma and tissue fluid, especially if these become infected, as they tend to, in the pelvis. Consequently the author always uses an appropriate wound drain for as long as he feels it is fulfilling its intended purpose. Suction drainage may be relatively inefficient when positioned within folds of omentum because this tends to get sucked into the fenestrations of the tubing and occlude them. A soft Penrose drain may be more efficient.

The use of prophylactic antibiotics is optional—but preferable. The problem is that a precarious suture line may occasionally separate as a result of infection before this is clinically identifiable. There is good evidence that the incidence of postoperative hip-prosthesis infection is significantly reduced by the use of prophylactic antibiotics.

Perineoabdominal progression-approach (PAPA) operating position and procedures

The PAPA operating position, with the perineum and abdomen prepped and draped in a single sterile operating field, is strongly advocated for the repair of *all* urinary fistulas in the pelvis. It provides good access for both perineal and abdominopelvic surgery (Fig. 53-8).

The patient is placed on the operating table in a flat, slightly head-down position, and the legs are widely abducted with only moderate hip flexion. For a vaginal-approach procedure, the surgeon is seated, the instrument table is immediately to the right (or left if left-handed), and the scrub nurse is also seated. The bundle of suction tube, fiberlight, and diathermy cables is arranged over the patient's leg on the side opposite the scrub nurse. If the vaginal approach proves difficult or inappropriate, the surgeon simply walks round to the abdominal-approach position and the scrub nurse repositions the instrument table between the patient's legs. It is rarely necessary to have two

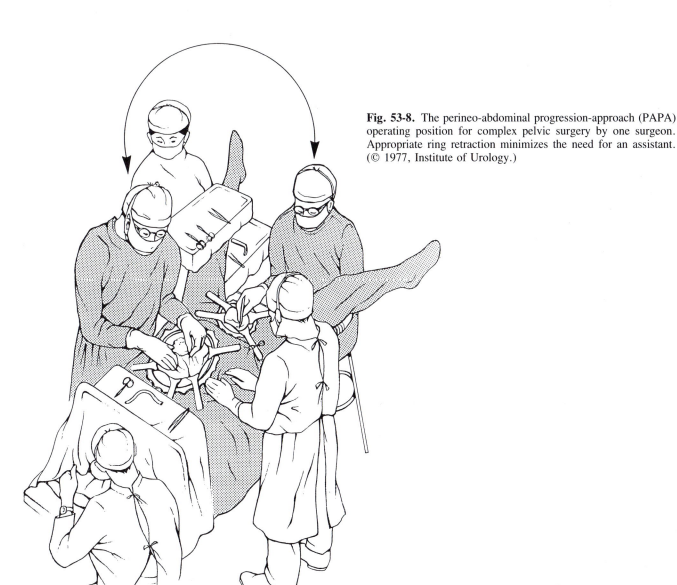

Fig. 53-8. The perineo-abdominal progression-approach (PAPA) operating position for complex pelvic surgery by one surgeon. Appropriate ring retraction minimizes the need for an assistant. (© 1977, Institute of Urology.)

surgeons for a synchronous approach because the perineo-abdominal interchange is so simple. Furthermore, if appropriate ring retraction is used (both perineal and abdominal), one assistant is more than enough. Certainly no assistant should intervene between the surgeon and the instrument table/scrub nurse.

If a foot control is used to operate the diathermy (as it has to be if the TW combination of insulated diathermy knife/forceps/scissors is used), the cable should be tracked around the head end of the operating table pedestal and back to the surgeon's right foot so that minimal movement of it enables it to be operated with the same foot when the surgeon moves back and forth from the perineal to the abdominal approach position.

When the PAPA position is used for an intended vaginal-approach repair, the option of its extension to a synchronous perineoabdominal procedure is immediately available with minimal rearrangement. However, a synchronous approach is, of course, essential for the proper development and distal perineal closure of the abdominoperineal tunnel required for the omental interposition repair procedure.

During a definitive abdominal approach, the advantage of the synchronous vaginal access provided by the PAPA position is that it facilitates urethral catheter manipulation and it also enables a finger in the vagina to guide the separation of the fused tissue layers around the fistula. Any bleeding that develops during the lateral development of an abdominoperineal interposition tunnel can be immediately controlled by vaginal finger-pressure until hemostasis is secured.

However, the PAPA operating position is so convenient for the surgeon, for the scrub nurse, and for the instrumentation that the author invariably uses it for all major abdominopelvic surgery, even when there is no expectation of need for a synchronous perineal approach.

Incisions for the abdominal approach

The traditional Pfannenstiel incision provides an avoidably restricted surgical access to the pelvis. It was designed for gynecologic procedures for which neither the proximal nor the retropubic extent of the procedure is usually critical. Most urologic procedures are more demanding in terms of access. Pfannenstiel incision is not advisable for a pelvic operation that could become unexpectedly complex because the exposure that it provides cannot be extended without a radical revision-incision. Gynecologic surgeons in general, and those in training in particular, could find that their routine pelvic surgical procedures are considerably simplified by the improved access provided by the simple "suprapubic V" modification of Pfannenstiel incision.

The "suprapubic V" incision

The suprapubic V procedure uses a skin incision identical to that of Pfannenstiel procedure, but it makes better use of the local anatomy to provide a greatly improved surgical exposure, not only of the pelvis but also of the lower abdomen.

Many surgeons modify the straight horizontal Pfannenstiel incision in the rectus sheath into one that is somewhat curved. However, a definitive V-shaped incision into it has distinct advantages (Fig. 53-9).[10,11,16]

1. An initial 4 cm horizontal incision is made into the rectus sheath 2 cm *below* the upper margin of the pubis. This is possible because of the anatomical extent of the distal aponeurotic origin of the rectus abdominis (see below).
2. Laterally, the V-shaped incision in the sheath is sharply angled upward so the width of the consequent flap remains within the width of the rectus muscle. It does not encroach beyond it, into the lateral abdominal muscles, unless a definitive upward extension is required.
3. The distal extent of the incision provides a wide exposure of the upper border of the pubis, and, of course, the distal margin of the rectus sheath is prepubic so it does not require retraction to provide good access to the retropubic space.
4. An unextended V incision provides good proximal access as far as the midureter, above the iliac vessels. It is a general-purpose incision for all lower abdominal and pelvic surgery, including a reflux-preventing reimplantation of the midureter into the bladder, above the iliac vessels, using the bladder elongation psoas hitch (BEPH) procedure (see p. 895).
5. The V incision can be extended upward and laterally into a supracostal incision for a synchronous nephrectomy; however, this proximal extension does not provide good access to the stomach, in the midline, for the mobilization of the omentum.

Midline abdominal wall incision and the "suprapubic cross incision"

A midline incision in the abdominal wall is essential to provide access for the radical mobilization of the vascular pedicle of the omentum when necessary, the mobilization of which may be fundamental to the success of the closure of a difficult fistula repair. The need for the mobilization of the pedicle of a short omental apron from the stomach cannot be predicted preoperatively, but, in fact, a subumbilical midline abdominal wall incision is sufficient to achieve its effective transposition in more than half the cases in which this is necessary.

The traditional transverse Pfannenstiel incision cannot be simply extended for an extensive mobilization of the omental pedicle. However, many of the patients presenting with a vesicovaginal fistula have already had a Pfannenstiel-approach procedure, and the routine use of an additional vertical midline skin incision for a fistula repair results in a scar, which is a lasting reminder of the complication and may contribute to the initiation of medico-legal proceedings.

The "suprapubic cross incision" was developed to en-

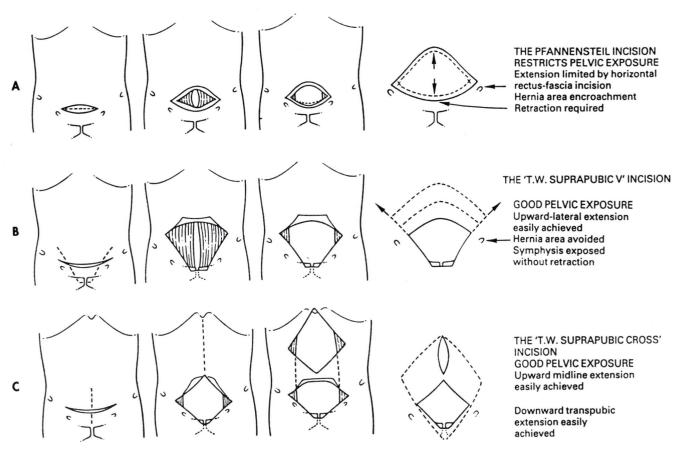

Fig. 53-9. A, The traditional Pfannenstiel incision provides a relatively restricted surgical access to the pelvis. The lateral extent of its horizontal incision in the rectus sheath is limited by the inguinal canal area and the lower margin of the rectus sheath requires retraction. **B,** The TW suprapubic V incision uses the same horizontal skin incision, but the access to the pelvis and the lower abdomen is greatly improved by the V-shaped incision in the rectus sheath, which can be extended upward and laterally, if necessary, to provide a good exposure of the upper urinary tract without division of the rectus muscle **C,** The TW suprapubic cross incision also uses the same horizontal skin incision, but its subumbilical midline incision in the abdominal wall can be extended upward to provide supraumbilical upper abdominal access for mobilization of the right gastroepiploic pedicle of the omentum from the stomach by using an additional vertical epigastric midline skin incision. (© 1974, Institute of Urology.)

able the majority of abdominal-approach fistula repairs to be completed through the original Pfannenstiel skin incision (Fig. 53-9).[7,10,11] After only a minor lateral extension of this horizontal skin incision, the upper and lower skin/ subcutaneous tissue flaps are separated from the rectus fascia to enable a midline abdominal wall incision to be made up to the level of the umbilicus, leaving the original horizontal Pfannenstiel rectus sheath closure intact (with suture reinforcement if necessary).

In the event that upper abdominal access is required to mobilize the vascular pedicle of a short-apron omentum (30% to 40% of cases), this can be achieved by a relatively small additional midline epigastric skin incision and a supraumbilical extension of the midline incision in the abdominal wall under the wide skin bridge. Thus, a secondary midline skin incision is avoided in the majority of patients who require a postoperative fistula-repair proce-

dure without compromising the option of a safeguarding omental-interposition procedure in the event of need for this.

Increasing the midline incisional access to the retropubic space

Simple application of surgical anatomy can greatly improve the midline incisional access to the retropubic space. Although traditional anatomical texts often describe a pubic attachment of the rectus abdominis aponeurosis to the pubic crest, in reality it spreads down, over the anterior surface of the pubis, to its inferior margin. After a distal prepubic extension of the midline incision into the prepubic aponeurosis, it can be reflected off the surface of the pubic bone by sharp dissection (Fig. 53-10).[9,15] This creates a remarkably effective exposure of the whole width of the upper border of the pubis. This access to the retropubic

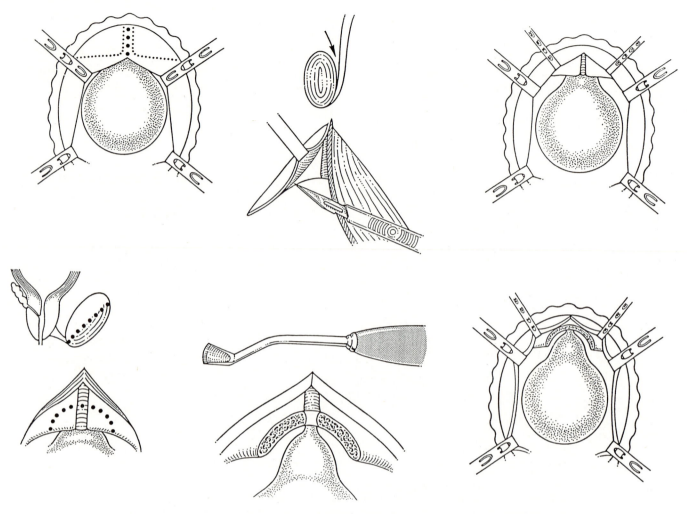

Fig. 53-10. Simple procedures for increasing the retropubic exposure of the subprostatic area. The insertion/origin of the rectus abdominis tendon is not confined to the pubic crests but extends down the anterior pubis. The width of a retropubic exposure can be greatly increased by a prepubic extension of the midline incision and sharp dissection separation of its margins from the bone. *Bottom,* Exposure of the urethra can be further increased, if necessary, by partial removal of the pubic bone with a Capener bone gouge. (© 1987, Institute of Urology.)

space can be increased still further by a partial resection of the pubic bone, but this is rarely necessary in women.

Instrumentation

In addition to the TW universal perineoabdominal ring retractor system that maximizes the access provided by any incision (Fig. 53-1), two instruments in particular facilitate complex pelvic reconstructive surgery in general and fistula closure in particular (Fig. 53-11).

1. The TW needle holders are gently curved to keep the hand out of the line of sight of the needle. This is particularly helpful for accurate suturing when surgical access to a delicate reconstruction deep in the pelvis is unavoidably restricted.

2. The fiberlight sucker provides an invaluable combination of "suck and see" in deep dark places. It is also appropriately curved.

COMPLEX VESICOVAGINAL FISTULAS

A fistula that is "complex" as a result of impaired local tissue healing due to infection, to previous surgery, or to irradiation may be further complicated by the additional involvement of the terminal ureter on one or both sides, by a urethral sphincter deficiency, by a coincident rectal fistula, by a vaginal abnormality, or by a "frozen pelvis" due to extensive radiation fibrosis. These naturally make an already difficult repair procedure even more difficult. However, almost all are nevertheless synchronously remediable by an appropriate variation of the available procedures.

Operative injury to the ureter and ureterovaginal fistulas

Gynecologic surgical injuries to the ureter are generally located in its terminal third. If the injury is identified at the time of surgery, naturally it should be repaired at that

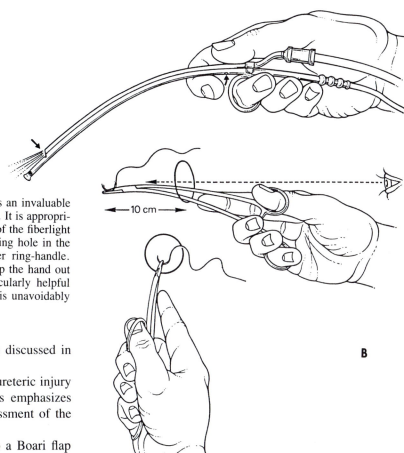

Fig. 53-11. A, The TW fiberlight sucker provides an invaluable combination of "suck and see" in deep dark places. It is appropriately curved, with a suction hole at the distal end of the fiberlight to keep it blood-free and a suction-pressure-reducing hole in the "trigger-finger" position beyond the middle-finger ring-handle. **B,** The TW needle holder is gently curved to keep the hand out of the line of sight of the needle. This is particularly helpful when surgical access to a delicate reconstruction is unavoidably restricted. (© 1977, Institute of Urology.)

time. The management of ureteral fistulae is discussed in Chapter 49.

However, not infrequently, an associated ureteric injury complicates a vesical fistula repair, and this emphasizes the importance of appropriate prerepair assessment of the upper urinary tracts.

A BEPH procedure is much preferable to a Boari flap procedure or a transureteroureterostomy for the resolution of lower ureteric injuries (Fig. 53-12). Its advantages are discussed elsewhere.[8,10,14] The particular advantage of the BEPH procedure is that the simple bladder elongation, achieved by the vertical closure of an initial horizontal hemicircumferential incision in the equator-line of the bladder, greatly facilitates the reflux-preventing reimplantation of the normal middle third of the ureter into normal, relocated, neofundus of the bladder, well away from the local healing reaction at the site of the original ureteric injury in the pelvis. A single BEPH procedure can also be used for reimplantation of both ureters.

Urethrovaginal fistulas

The resolution of urethrovaginal fistulas is discussed in Chapter 49. The essential factor to bear in mind is that urinary incontinence depends entirely on the function of the intrinsic urethral sphincter musculature within the thickness of the wall of the urethra. The urethra is located in the capacious urogenital hiatus of the pelvic floor in front of the relatively large vagina. There is no intervening pubourethral "muscle sling" mechanism, and, consequently, contraction of the pelvic floor levator muscles cannot possibly directly occlude the urethra in multiparous women.[10,11]

If a bladder-base injury extends down into the urethra to form a vesicourethrovaginal fistula, it creates a traumatic defect in the posterior sector of the urethral sphincter mechanism—just as a urethral diverticulum is associ-

ated with a congenital midposterior sector defect. Naturally, therefore, the appropriate procedure for the resolution of such a fistula is the extension of the vesical fistula repair to include a definitive repair of the sphincter (Fig. 53-13). This involves a synchronous combination of a perineal prevaginal reduction sphincteroplasty with an abdominal transvesical reconstruction of the bladder neck and mobilization of an omental support to ensure that its functional occlusive movement is not subsequently impaired by secondary periurethral fibrotic tethering.[5,10,11] Without such a definitive extension of the reconstruction procedure, the risk of impaired urinary control is considerable.

Neovaginoplasty fistulas

The creation of a neovagina involves the development of a neovaginal space between the bladder and the urethra anteriorly and the anorectum posteriorly. The development of this plane is relatively easy in simple congenital vaginal atresia. In gender-reassignment procedures, it is complicated by the dense adhesion of the male rectourethral ligament. Postirradiation fistulas are naturally associated with extensive adhesions, which increase both the risk of injury and the difficulty of the reconstruction.

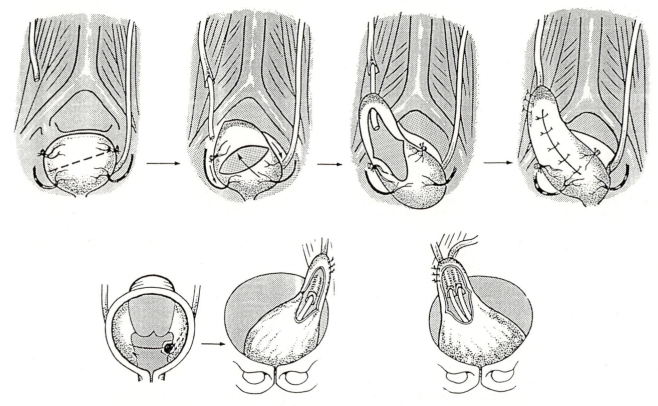

Fig. 53-12. The BEPH procedure for replacement of the lower ureter. The particular advantage of the BEPH procedure is that the simple bladder elongation procedure achieved by the vertical closure of a horizontal hemicircumferential incision in the equator of the bladder facilitates a reflux preventing reimplantation of the normal middle third of the ureter into the normal relocated fundus of the bladder, well away from the local healing reaction at the site of the original ureteral injury in the pelvis. A single BEPH procedure can also be used for reimplantation of both ureters. (© 1972, Institute of Urology.)

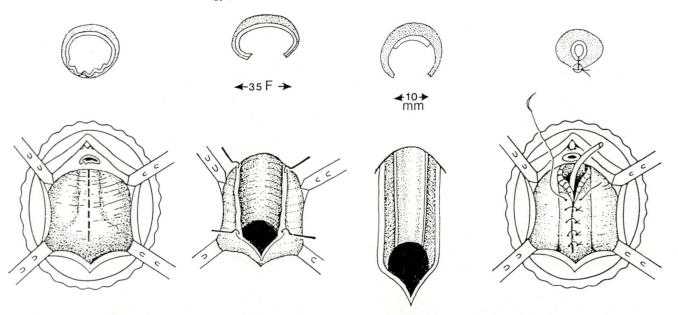

Fig. 53-13. Reduction sphincteroplasty. The urethra is exposed through a hemicircumferential introital prevaginal approach: it is opened posteriorly in the midline, the incision extending through the bladder neck into the trigone. The 3-cm width of the opened urethral uroepithelial lining is reduced to a 1-cm anterior strip, and the urethral sphincter mechanism is overclosed around a 10 Fr stenting catheter, suture-slung through the abdominal wall. An accurate functional reconstruction of the bladder neck mechanism generally requires a synchronous transvesical approach to achieve an appropriate trigonal reduction. (© 1982, Institute of Urology.)

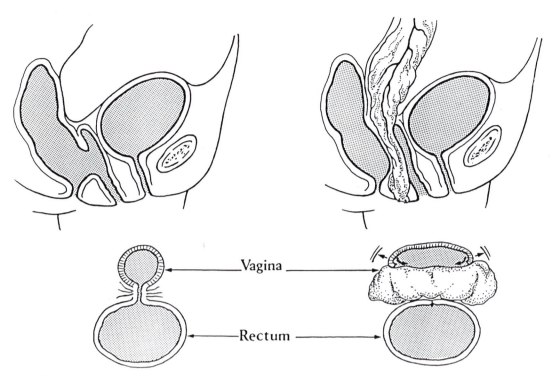

Fig. 53-14. A complex neovaginal-rectal fistula after a skin-graft vaginoplasty for atresia, closed by separation and lateral fixation of the neovaginal skin strip. The surface of the interpositioned omentum opposed to the skin strip epithelializes, greatly increasing the vaginal capacity. (© 1973, Institute of Urology.)

Various surgical options are available for the creation of a neovaginal lining. Split-skin and amnion can be satisfactory substitutes, but both have the disadvantage that the wall of the neovagina is not only very thin but its capacity is relatively small and tends to contract. Thus, its size has to be maintained by regular intercourse or by the passage of dilators, which can occasionally result in neovaginal rupture and the development of a fistula into the rectum or the bladder. The resolution of neovaginal fistulas presents particular problems and an omentoneovaginoplasty can be a useful reconstructive procedure (Fig. 53-14).[7,10,11]

In general, cecolovaginoplasty[1,12] offers particular advantages, not only for the primary creation of a vagina but also for the resolution of neovaginal fistulas. The result is not only relatively robust but it does not tend to contract so that regular use or dilation is not required to maintain an adequate capacity (Fig. 53-15).

Postirradiation "frozen pelvis"

Inevitably, the effective treatment of carcinoma of the cervix by radiotherapy results in a degree of irradiation tissue damage to the bladder and to the rectum. It is important to recognize that the extent of irradiation damage is not always directly related to the dose—there is considerable variation in the particular tissue response of the individual. Thus, a given depth dose that causes a moderate reaction in one patient may cause extensive radiation fibrosis in another.

Severe radiation injury can result in incarceration of the rectum and ureters by radiation fibrosis and the development of a vesicovaginal fistula, occasionally associated with a radionecrotic cavity in the vaginal vault area. Traditionally, such a "frozen pelvis" has been treated by a urostomy and colostomy, but even this does not always relieve the unfortunate patient of an offensive purulent discharge from a radionecrotic cavity.

Although the fibrotic reaction in such cases is extensive, the anal canal, its sphincter mechanism, and the lower segment of the vagina are rarely severely damaged (Fig. 53-15). Consequently, it is often possible to exenterate the fibrosis and to restore bowel continuity by anastomosis of the mobilized unirradiated descending colon to the partially irradiated anal canal. Naturally, this anastomosis is potentially precarious, but, if it is meticulous and it is wrapped with a well-vascularized omental flap, it is often successful.[7,10,11]

The functional result of reconstructing a small-capacity irradiated bladder by a bowel-substitution cystoplasty depends primarily on whether the residual urethral sphincter mechanism is capable of maintaining continence. The cystoplasty/bladder-base anastomosis is potentially precarious, but, again, this is generally successful if a good omental wrap can be achieved. The anastomosis of the unirradiated proximal ureters to the relatively unirradiated bowel cystoplasty rarely presents difficulties.

The main additional problem involving the exenteration

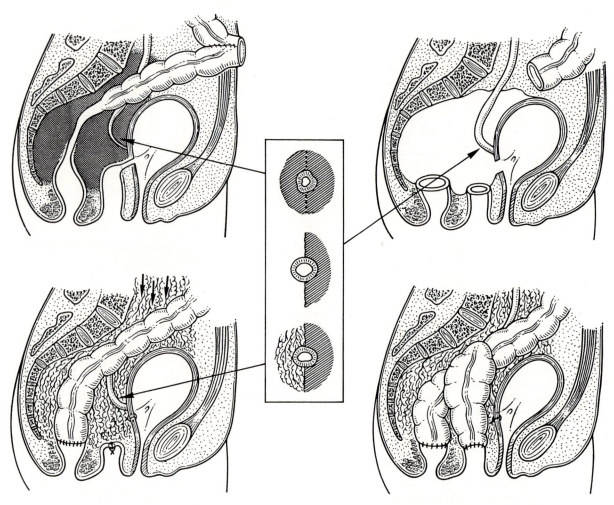

Fig. 53-15. Extensive resection of the radiation fibrosis of a "frozen pelvis" results in a rigid-walled cavity. Restoration of bowel continuity by coloanal anastomosis is usually possible and "hemi-liberation" of obstructive ureteral incasement avoids the risk of necrosis resulting from circumferential mobilization. The pelvic "deadspace" is best filled by mobilized omentum when sufficient is available, otherwise the cecum can be used as a space-occupying procedure. (© 1975, Institute of Urology.)

of a large mass of radiation fibrosis is the obliteration of the consequently large "dead space" cavity in the pelvis. Sometimes, redeployment of the whole omental apron, on the basis of a full-length mobilization of its right gastroepiploic vascular pedicle from the greater curvature of the stomach (Fig. 53-5), provides a sufficient bulk to fill this cavity. However, these patients are often thin so that even the fully mobilized omental apron is only sufficient to provide the critical vascular support for the actual suture line.

In such cases, the well-vascularized inverted colocecal segment of the large bowel provides a satisfactory "space-filling vaginoplasty" that effectively relines the margins of the exenteration cavity, the irradiation ischemia of which prevents natural healing by proliferation of vascular granulation tissue.[7,10,11] The mucosal lining of such a "neovaginal colocavity" naturally produces some mucous discharge, but this is minimal, inoffensive, and easily controllable.

There is always a possibility of residual tumor cells in the fibrosis associated with an irradiation fistula, even when preoperative biopsy proves negative and even if the treatment was concluded 10 or more years previously. It is clearly inappropriate to attempt to close a fistula when the bulk of the pelvic induration associated with it is active, recurrent macroscopic tumor. However, when a patient develops a postirradiation vesicovaginal fistula and a representative preliminary biopsy shows only a few residual cells in extensive irradiation fibrosis, the local tumor may be relatively quiescent. Under these circumstances, because the prognosis is very poor, it is all the more important to resolve the incapacitating incontinence as swiftly and as efficiently as possible. Closure of such a fistula by omental interposition is not only a simpler procedure than a ureteroileal surface conduit but it offers the patient a good chance of normal voiding and urinary control for their few short remaining months.[7,10,11]

Prevention of vesicovaginal fistulas

A discussion of the treatment of vesicovaginal fistulas should naturally include some consideration of their prevention.[11]

The confines of the pelvis naturally restrict the access for gynecological surgery; however, the operation notes of procedures that have resulted in fistulas, particularly ureteral injuries, often relate difficulties with hemostasis that might have been avoided if better surgical access had been obtained. The adoption of the much-improved access provided by the suprapubic V modification of the traditional Pfannenstiel incision (Fig. 53-9), combined with the much improved retraction provided by the ring-retractor system (Fig. 53-1), simplifies the more difficult abdominopelvic and gynecologic procedures and could reduce the incidence of complications. The routine preliminary passage of relatively large ureteric catheters (6-7 Ch) for the duration of the operation is the best way of protecting the ureters during potentially difficult pelvic wall dissections.

The curved TW fiberlight sucker provides an invaluable combination of "suck and see" in deep dark places, and similarly the curved TW needle holders that keep the hand out of the line of sight of the needle facilitate the accurate insertion of sutures when the surgical access in unavoidably restricted (Fig. 53-11).

CONCLUSION

It has long been recognized that the boundaries between some traditional areas of surgical specialization are inappropriate to the proper development and improvement of our care of patients; this is reflected in the evolution of a number of regional surgical specialities such as head and neck surgery, hand surgery, and so forth.

The proximity of the genital and the lower urinary tracts naturally results in a degree of structural and functional interdependence. Consequently, some incidence of urinary tract complications is inevitable during childbirth and gynecologic operations.

Within the traditional confines of gynecology and of urology, we have to recognize the need for cross-boundary training and sub-specialization by the development of specialist interests in urogynecologic and in gynecourologic functional reconstruction. The natural progress of this must surely be the development of a small number of referral units with special expertise in a "horizontal speciality" of "pelvic surgery" to avoid the shortcoming of "committee surgery" in the pelvis for the treatment of complex congenital, trauma, incontinence, and oncologic gynecourologic problems. Proper training in pelvic surgery should also involve an appropriate experience of reconstructive colorectal surgery.

Successful functional reconstruction should be primarily based on a particular aptitude for meticulous surgical minutiae and, furthermore, an instinctive inclination to adopt and to adapt procedures according to the findings at the time of operation. Thus, in addition to a training in general gynecourology or urogynecology, a surgeon undertaking reconstructive procedures should have an additional period of training in plastic surgical techniques and tissue handling.

Furthermore, because all parts of the urinary tract are specifically developed to subserve a particular function, appropriate functional reconstruction requires not only an accurate understanding of the local anatomical structure but also a personal hands-on experience of videourodynamic assessment, for which there is no substitute.

Finally, it is essential to appreciate that any operative procedure that fails, however well-intentioned and however well-performed, inevitably complicates a subsequent retrievoplasty—"having a go" cannot be in the best interests of one's patients.

The Turner-Warwick range of instruments is supplied by Baxter V. Mueller, Chicago; by Leibinger, Germany; by Downs and by Thackray, UK.

REFERENCES

1. Kirby RS, Turner-Warwick R: Reconstruction of the vagina by caecolo-vaginoplasty, *Surg Gynecol Obstet* 170:132, 1990.
2. Turner-Warwick R: The use of the omental pedicle graft in urinary tract reconstruction, *J Urol* 116:341, 1976.
3. Turner-Warwick R: Impaired voiding efficiency and retention in the female, *Clin Obstet Gynecol* 5:193, 1978.
4. Turner-Warwick R: Clinical urodynamics, *Urol Clin North Am* 6:13, 1979.
5. Turner-Warwick R: *Female sphincter mechanisms and their relation to incontinence surgery.* In Dubruyne FMJ, Van Karrenbrock PEUA, editors: *Practical aspects of urinary incontinence,* 1986, Martinns Nijoff.
6. Turner-Warwick R: *Urinary fistula in the female.* In *Campbell's urology,* Philadelphia, 1986, Saunders.
7. Turner-Warwick R: *Vesico-vaginal fistula: the resolution of the 'frozen pelvis' by caeco-vaginoplasty.* In Robb C, Smith R, editors: *Operative Surgery,* 1986, Butterworth.
8. Turner-Warwick R: The Turner-Warwick bladder elongation psoas hitch BEPH procedure for substitution ureteroplasty. In Abrams P, Gingell JC, editors: *Controversies and innovations in urological surgery,* 1988, Springer Verlag.
9. Turner-Warwick R: *Improving the access to retropubic space, Br J Urol* 1990.
10. Turner-Warwick R: *The functional anatomy of the urethra.* In Droller MJ, editor: *The surgical management of urologic disease,* St Louis, 1992, Mosby–Year Book.
11. Turner-Warwick R: *Obstetric and gynaecological injuries of the urinary tract—their prevention and management.* In Bonnar J, editor: *Recent advances in obstetrics and gynaecology 18,* London, Churchill Livingstone (in press).
12. Turner-Warwick R, Handley Ashken M: The functional results of cystoplasty with special reference to caecocystoplasty (and mention of caeco-vaginoplasty), *Br J Urol* 39:3,
13. Turner-Warwick R, Kirby RS: *Urodynamic studies and their effect upon management.* In Chisholm GD, Fair WR, editors: *Scientific foundations of urology,* ed 3, 1991, Heineman.
14. Turner-Warwick R, Worth PHL: The psoas-hitch procedure for the replacement of the lower third of the urethra, *Br J Urol* 41:701, 1969.
15. Turner-Warwick R, Wynne EJC, Handley Ashken M: The use of the omentum in the repair and reconstruction of the urinary tract, *Br J Surg* 54:849, 1967.
16. Turner-Warwick R et al: The 'supra-pubic V' incision, *Br J Urol* 46:39, 1974.

Chapter 54

INTRAOPERATIVE URETERAL INJURIES AND URINARY DIVERSION

W. Glenn Hurt
Charles M. Jones III

The close anatomic relationship that exists between the lower urinary tract and the internal genitalia predisposes the distal ureter to involvement by gynecologic disorders and places it at risk for injury during pelvic surgery and radiation therapy. Intraoperative repair of ureteral injuries is successful in over 90% of cases. Patients whose ureteral injuries are missed during the operation in which they occur are much more likely to have a poor result following a subsequent attempt at repair.[7]

Unrecognized ureteral injuries or unsuccessful ureteral repairs may cause oliguria or anuria, fever, chills, and flank pain. If there is intraperitoneal or retroperitoneal leakage of urine, it may cause abdominal distention, ileus, and urinoma formation. Ultimately, a urinary fistula may develop or there may be ureteral obstruction with loss of renal function.

INCIDENCE OF URETERAL INJURY

Operative injuries to the ureter are most commonly associated with gynecologic or urologic surgery, rectosigmoid resections, and repeat surgical procedures within the pelvis and retroperitoneum. The surgical literature attributes between 50% and 90% of all ureteral injuries to gynecologic procedures. Although, the true incidence of ureteral injuries at the time of major gynecologic surgery is unknown, studies suggest an incidence of 0.5% to 2.5%.[3,5,15,23,25]

Ureteral injury is much more likely to occur at the time of an abdominal hysterectomy than at the time of a vaginal hysterectomy.[25] There appears to be a slight increase in the number of ureteral injuries associated with periaortic

node dissections and with obstetric procedures (e.g., cesarean sections and cesarean or postpartum hysterectomies).

Pelvic surgery will never be free of ureteral injuries. It should, however, be possible to minimize the risk of ureteral injury by identifying the course of the pelvic ureters and keeping them out of harm's way. Unfortunately, most surgical injuries to the ureter are not recognized at the time they occur. Therefore, to reduce the postoperative morbidity associated with ureteral injuries, it is important, whenever the ureter is jeopardized by a disease process or a surgical procedure, for the surgeon to demonstrate the integrity of the ureter by surgical dissection or intraoperative testing.

Some pelvic conditions that distort the anatomy, infiltrate the tissues, affect the blood supply, and predispose to ureteral injury are listed in the box at right. Yet, Symmonds reminds us that it is not the complicated surgical procedure that is responsible for the majority of ureteral injuries; it is the "simple" abdominal hysterectomy performed for a benign indication (i.e., abnormal uterine bleeding, cervical intraepithelial neoplasia, and so forth) that is most often associated with a ureteral injury.[25] If this is true, it should be possible to prevent the majority of ureteral injuries.

PREVENTION OF URETERAL INJURY

Preoperatively, the history and physical examination, urinalysis, urine culture, and blood chemistries may give a clue to the condition of the urinary tract and its potential involvement by pathologic conditions. Preoperative intravenous urograms assist in detecting congenital anomalies

```
┌─────────────────────────────────────────────┐
│   Conditions associated with ureteral injury │
│                                              │
│   Large pelvic tumors                        │
│   Cervical leiomyomas                        │
│   Endometriosis                              │
│   Ovarian remnants                           │
│   Pelvic inflammatory disease                │
│   Pelvic malignancies                        │
│   Pelvic hematomas and lymphocysts           │
│   Pelvic organ prolapse                      │
│   Diverticulosis                             │
│   Congenital anomalies                       │
│   Pregnancy                                  │
│                                              │
│   Prior pelvic surgery                       │
│   Prior radiation therapy                    │
└─────────────────────────────────────────────┘
```

of the urinary tract and in documenting involvement by pelvic tumors, pelvic inflammatory disease, or invasive processes such as endometriosis or cancer. Routine preoperative urograms have not been shown to lower the overall incidence of operative ureteral injuries.[18] Ultrasound examinations, computed tomography (CT) scans, and radionucleotide scans can document the preoperative integrity and function of the urinary tract but do not facilitate ureteral identification during pelvic surgery nor obviate the surgeon's obligation to identify the ureters.[2,13,25]

Preoperative placement of ureteral catheters to assist in the identification and dissection of the ureters at the time of surgery is not always practical or desirable. Ureteral catheterization cannot be expected to reduce the overall incidence of ureteral injuries, most of which occur in patients for whom there is no indication that their use is needed. When pelvic findings suggest the need for preoperative ureteral catheterization because of fixation of the tissues or malignancy, the catheters often are difficult to palpate within the ureter. It has been suggested that during dissection of a ureter, an unyielding ureteral catheter may, in fact, cause mucosal injury or predispose the ureter to devascularization or laceration.[25] If ureteral catheterization is needed during a difficult pelvic dissection, it can be easily performed by linear ureterotomy, suprapubic cystotomy, or cystoscopy. Most pelvic surgeons find this preferable to preoperative ureteral catheter placement.

Intraoperatively, the principles that contribute to the safety of all pelvic procedures include: adequate exposure of the surgical field; adequate light within the surgical field; restoration of anatomic relationships; traction and countertraction to expose adjacent structures; dissection along tissue planes; appropriate dissection of extraperitoneal spaces; clamping, cutting, and suturing under direct vision; and the avoidance of mass ligation of tissues. These surgical principles help protect all vital organs. The most effective way to prevent ureteral injury during pelvic laparotomy is to identify the ureters as they enter the pelvis over the bifurcations of the common iliac arteries[13] and

to trace the pelvic course of each ureter during dissection of the retroperitoneal spaces. In demonstrating the course of the ureter, its attachment to the pelvic peritoneum should be preserved. Every effort should be made to protect the blood supply to each ureter and the longitudinal network of the microvasculature within its adventitial sheath.

COMMON SITES OF URETERAL INJURY

Most ureteral injuries that are the result of gynecologic surgery occur in the lower third of the ureter. The three most common sites of ureteral injury at the time of hysterectomy are: (1) at the pelvic brim where the ureters lie beneath the insertions of the infundibulopelvic ligaments and over the bifurcations of the common iliac arteries; (2) lateral to the cervix where the ureters pass under the uterine arteries; and (3) lateral to the vaginal fornices where the ureters course about the cervix and upper vagina to enter the bladder.

Ureteral angulation, perforation, or ligation may occur during reperitonealization of the pelvis, posterior culdeplasty, colporrhaphy, or as a result of retropubic urethropexy/vaginopexy. Dissecting the ureter within a pathologic process and "tunneling" the ureter near the bladder may result in devascularization or laceration.

In the obstetric patient, ureteral injury most often occurs as a result of extension of the uterine incision, suturing of the incision, or an effort to control hemorrhage within one of the broad ligaments.[6] Cesarean and postpartum hysterectomies may be associated with ureteral injuries because of the increased vascularity of the pelvis, the distortion of the anatomy, the loss of tissue turgor that maintains the shape of the pelvic organs during traction and countertraction, and the effacement and dilation of the cervix.

Ureteral injury as a result of pelvic radiation therapy for cervical cancer is uncommon (less than 0.5%). The immediate effect of radiation therapy is an inflammatory response; over time, it causes devascularization and fibrosis of the tissues and places the ureter at risk for injury during subsequent surgical procedures.

DETECTION OF URETERAL INJURY

During surgery, if there is reason to suspect that ureteral injury has occurred, a number of procedures can be used to determine the location and extent of the injury. They include the following:

Ureteral dye injection. Indigo carmine is injected through a 22-gauge needle into the ureter above the suspected site of injury. Resistance to the injection suggests ureteral obstruction, leakage of dye into the operative field below the injection site indicates ureteral injury, and excretion of dye in the urine suggests ureteral patency.

Intravenous dye injection. Injection of intravenous indigo carmine (5 ml) should be followed in 5 to 10 minutes by the excretion of blue urine. Complete bilateral ureteral obstruction prevents urine from reaching the bladder. Unilateral ureteral obstruction cannot be detected by the intravenous administration of indigo carmine unless ureteral excretion is observed by cystotomy or cystoscopy (suprapubic or transurethral). Leakage of blue urine through an injured ureter into the operative site identifies an area of ureteral injury.

Intraoperative ureteral catheterization. The ureter(s) may be catheterized during surgery by ureterostomy, cystotomy, or cystoscopy. A linear ureterotomy above the site of suspected injury permits catheter passage down the ureter and into the bladder. A cystotomy may be performed in the anterior wall of the bladder to visualize the ureteral orifices and to pass ureteral catheters. During an abdominal procedure, transurethral cystoscopy is a somewhat cumbersome method of ureteral catheter placement.

Intravenous excretory urography. Constant infusion intraoperative intravenous urography may be performed during surgery to evaluate the integrity of the urinary tract.

Dissection of the ureter. When there is concern about the integrity of a ureter, there is no substitute for dissecting the pararectal space and visualizing repetitive vermiculation of the ureter throughout its course.

SURGICAL ANATOMY

The ureters are bilateral tubular structures, 25 to 30 cm in length, that serve as urinary conduits between the kidneys and bladder. The ureters originate rather indistinctly from the renal pelves lateral to the transverse processes of the first lumbar vertebra. They descend, retroperitoneally, lateral to the transverse processes of the vertebrae, over the anterior surface of the psoas muscles to pass posterior to the ovarian vessels and then cross the pelvic brim and enter the true pelvis. Within the pelvis, they descend over the bifurcations of the common iliac vessels, forming the posterior boundary of the ovarian fossae. They then pass under the uterine arteries and turn anteriorly, medial to the obturator vessels and nerve, to pass about the cervix and upper vagina to enter 1.5- to 2.0-cm intramural tunnels within the base of the bladder. The ureters open into the bladder on either end of the interureteral ridge (Mercier's bar) that forms the base of the trigone of the bladder.

In descent, the right ureter is crossed by the right colic and ileocolic vessels and the left ureter is crossed by the left colic vessels. The ureters are slightly constricted and more firmly attached by their adventitial layer to adjacent structures at the ureteropelvic junction, as they cross over the iliac vessels, and at the ureterovesical junction. The pelvic portion of the ureter is more intimately attached to the overlying parietal peritoneum than is the abdominal portion.

Congenital anomalies of the ureter are common. A bifed or Y-shaped ureter may connect anywhere between the ureteropelvic junction and the bladder. When there is ureteral duplication, the two ureters commonly cross within the retroperitoneal spaces and enter the bladder wall through the same ureteral tunnel but open into the bladder in a predictable relationship in which the upper ureteral or-

ifice drains the lower pole and the lower ureteral orifice drains the upper pole of the kidney (Weigert-Meyer rule). The rare ectopic ureter may have its distal opening into the lower urinary tract anywhere between its normal location within the bladder and the external urethral meatus, or it may open into the vagina or vestibule.

The arterial supply of a ureter is unpredictable. The upper ureter usually receives a branch of the renal artery that descends within the adventitial sheath. The ureter may receive additional branches from the aorta and the ovarian, iliac, uterine, middle hemorrhoidal, superior vesical, and/or vaginal arteries. When there is no single artery that runs the length of the ureter, there is usually a longitudinal anastomosis of branches of some or all of the arteries mentioned. In both cases, arteries within the adventitial layer of the ureter give off arterioles and capillaries that penetrate and supply its muscular and submucosal layers (Fig. 54-1).[9,10] The fact that the arterial blood supply to the ureter is unpredictable and may depend on only one or two vessels within the adventitial layer makes it important to handle the ureter with care and, whenever possible, to perform all dissection outside of the adventitial sheath.

The venous drainage of the ureter arises within its submucosal and muscular layers and forms a network within the adventitial layer that closely parallels its arterial blood supply. The ureteral lymphatics arise in its muscular layer and drain from the upper ureter to the lumbar nodes along the aorta and inferior vena cava or from the lower ureter to the internal iliac nodes.

The nerve supply to the upper ureter comes from the celiac and aorticorenal plexus and to the lower ureter from the superior and inferior hypogastric plexus. Its sympathetic supply arises in the T11, T12, and L1 spinal segments. The parasympathetic supply to the upper ureter arises from the celiac plexus and to the lower ureter from S2, S3, and S4 sacral segments. The ureter receives primarily visceral sensory, not visceral motor, fibers. When

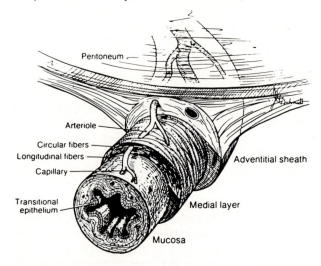

Fig. 54-1. Arterial supply and microvasculature of ureter. (Reprinted with permission from Guerriero WG: *AUA Update Series,* lesson 22, vol II, p 1, Bellaire, TX, 1983, AUA Office of Education.)

the extrinsic nerve supply to the ureter is cut, there is relief of ureteric pain, but no loss of normal peristaltic activity.

The wall of the ureter has three layers: an outer adventitial (Waldeyer's sheath) layer of connective tissue containing collagen, elastic, and nonmyelinated nerve fibers and blood vessels; a middle layer of smooth muscle fibers that interdigitate in a longitudinal, circular, and spiral fashion; and an inner mucosal layer of transitional epithelium resting on a basement membrane or lamnia propria.

Animal experiments have shown that, after ureterotomy, mucosal healing is complete at 3 weeks and smooth muscle bridging is complete at 6 weeks. Conduction of peristalsis across the anastomosis is not seen until 28 days after surgery. Ureters with extensive fibrosis, angulation, or poor smooth muscle regeneration may fail to regain their peristaltic activity. An oblique or spatulated end-to-end anastomosis heals faster and regains its peristaltic activity faster than a circular anastomosis.[20]

REPAIR OF URETERAL INJURY

Common types of ureteral injury are listed in the box at right. Any significant angulation of the ureter should be released to prevent obstruction. Minor devascularization and crush injuries may not require additional treatment. Stenting the injured ureter may be beneficial.[22] A ligated ureter should have the suture removed and should be treated as if it were a crush injury. Partial lacerations of the ureter may be closed with several interrupted 4-0 absorbable sutures over a ureteral stent. The treatment of ureteral transection and the loss of a segment of ureter depend on the location of the injury. Figure 54-2 shows treatment options for major ureteral injuries, and the box on p. 904 lists surgical principles that favor successful ureteral repair.

Unfortunately, most ureteral injuries that occur as a result of surgery are not recognized during the course of the surgical procedure. As a rule, when ureteral injuries that require definitive repair are recognized, it is best not to delay the repair,[26] unless it would be complicated by the presence of a pelvic infection or a history of recent pelvic radiation therapy.

URETERONEOCYSTOSTOMY

Ureteroneocystostomy, or ureteral reimplantation, is recommended for the repair of significant injuries to the lower 4 to 5 cm of either ureter. It is easier to perform and more likely to be successful than ureteroureterostomy. Most injuries that are the result of gynecologic surgery or

---

Types of ureteral injury
Angulation
Devascularization
Crushing
Ligation
Penetration
Laceration, partial or complete
Loss of segment

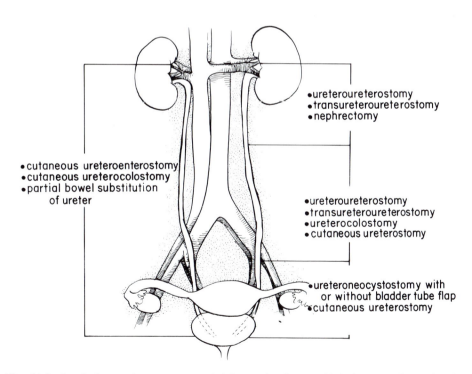

Fig. 54-2. Surgical procedures recommended for repair of ureteral injuries according to involved ureteral segment. (Reprinted with permission from Hurt WG, Dunn LJ: *Complications of gynecologic surgery and trauma.* In Greenfield LJ, editor: *Complications in surgery and trauma,* ed 2, Philadelphia, 1990, JB Lippincott.)

- ureteroureterostomy
- transureteroureterostomy
- nephrectomy

- cutaneous ureteroenterostomy
- cutaneous ureterocolostomy
- partial bowel substitution of ureter

- ureteroureterostomy
- transureteroureterostomy
- ureterocolostomy
- cutaneous ureterostomy

- ureteroneocystostomy with or without bladder tube flap
- cutaneous ureterostomy

Principles for successful ureteral repair

1. Perform meticulous ureteral dissection using atraumatic instruments
2. Preserve ureteral blood supply and microvasculature by leaving peritoneal attachment and dissecting outside adventitial sheath
3. Perform a tension-free anastomosis
4. Use the minimal amount of smallest absorbable suture needed to obtain watertight anastomosis
5. Surround anastomosis with retroperitoneal fat or omentum to assist healing
6. Drain retroperitoneal anastomotic site to prevent accumulation of urine
7. Consider prominal urinary diversion, with or without stenting

---

Modified from Schlossberg SM: Ureteral healing, *Semin Urol* 5:198, 1987.

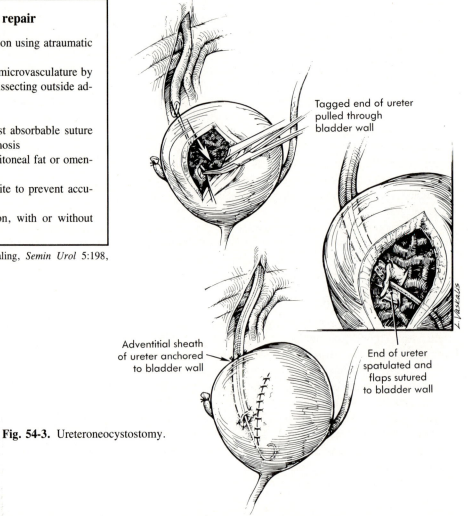

Tagged end of ureter pulled through bladder wall

Adventitial sheath of ureter anchored to bladder wall

End of ureter spatulated and flaps sutured to bladder wall

Fig. 54-3. Ureteroneocystostomy.

pelvic radiation therapy involve this portion of the ureter and can be repaired by ureteroneocystostomy.[14]

The pelvic peritoneum is incised anterolateral to the ureter as it crosses the bifurcation of the common iliac artery, and continued caudally to the bladder. The distal ureter is meticulously dissected to prevent damage to its adventitial sheath and blood supply.

The ureter is ligated with permanent suture at the ureterovesical junction. Any damaged ureteral segment is excised. A 3-0 suture affixed to an atraumatic tapered needle is passed through the diameter of the distal ureter about 0.5 cm from its end. The needle is removed, and the ends of the untied suture are tagged with a small forceps.

An extraperitoneal vertical cystotomy is performed in the dome of the bladder, and the ureteral orifices are identified. A finger is placed inside the fundus of the bladder, which is displaced toward the cut end of the ureter to determine the best site for a tension-free reimplantation. If direct reimplantation is to be performed, the entire thickness of the bladder wall is perforated with a right-angled forceps from within the bladder at the site of reimplantation. The tips of the forceps are opened about 1 cm to enlarge the hole in the bladder wall and to grasp the tagged end of the ureter, which is gently drawn through the blad-

der wall and into the bladder a distance of 1.0 cm. The end of the ureter is spatulated about 0.5 cm on opposite sides of its circumference, and the tagging suture is removed. Four 3-0 absorbable sutures are placed to secure the distal ureteral flaps to the inside of the bladder wall (Fig. 54-3).

Several 3-0 delayed absorbable sutures are used to anchor the adventitial sheath of the ureter to the outside of the bladder wall. If a peritoneal flap was left attached to the ureter, it may be secured to the outside of the bladder wall with 3-0 or 4-0 delayed absorbable sutures.[8,25]

In adults with normal kidney function, no bladder outlet obstruction, and no history of significant urinary tract infections, direct reimplantation of the ureter is satisfactory. Hydrodynamically, the female bladder is a low-pressure organ; and because bladder outlet obstruction in uncommon, vesicoureteral reflux is a rare cause of upper urinary tract damage. If, however, there is physiologic compromise of the upper urinary tract, a submucosal tunnel may be created within the wall of the bladder to prevent vesicoureteral reflux. A submucosal tunnel requires 2.0 cm of the length of the ureter. Therefore, it is important to determine that, as a result of the placement of 2.0 cm of the ureter in the tunnel, there will be no undue tension on the reimplantation site. The submucosal tunnel (modified Paquin,[17] Politano-Leadbetter,[19] and so forth) may be created by passing closed Metzenbaum scissors or small tapered forceps (i.e., Adson tonsil forceps) obliquely through the outer visceral peritoneum and the muscular layer of the bladder. The distal three quarters or half of the tunnel should be submucosal before its final entry into a predetermined site for the new ureteral orifice within the bladder. The size of the tunnel may be increased by opening the scissors or forceps slightly as they are removed. An Adson tonsil forceps may be used to traverse the tunnel within the bladder wall to grasp the suture tag on the distal end of the ureter and to draw the tagging suture and distal ureter through the tunnel. The ureter may be fed into the tunnel as gentle traction is applied to the tagging suture. The distal ureter is secured to the mucosal and muscular layers of the bladder by several 4-0 absorbable sutures, and the tagging suture is removed. The adventitial sheath of the ureter may be anchored to the outer bladder wall by several 3-0 delayed absorbable sutures.

It is usually not necessary to stent a ureter when performing an open, direct ureteroneocystostomy. It is recommended that a ureteral stent (8 Fr double J ureteral catheter or polyethylene or polyurethane drainage tube) be placed if a submucosal tunnel is used.[22] It is necessary to provide extraperitoneal drainage of the reimplantation site, preferably with a silicone suction drainage system. After placement of the drain, the opening in the peritoneum about the reimplanted ureter may be closed. A suprapubic or transurethral bladder drainage system is placed, and a two-layer closure of the cystotomy incision is performed using 3-0 absorbable or delayed absorbable suture. The bladder drainage system is usually discontinued after 7 to 10 days unless there is reason to keep the bladder drained longer. The drain from the reimplantation site is removed when there is no drainage or evidence of leaking urine.

URETEROURETEROSTOMY

Ureteroureterostomy is recommended for significant injuries above and just below the pelvic brim. It is often difficult to perform an end-to-end anastomosis on the lower 4 to 5 cm of either ureter; when it is attempted, it is likely to be unsuccessful.

The cut ends of a ureter may be joined when there will be no tension on the anastomosis. This is usually possible if there is loss of less than 2 cm of ureteral length. The damaged portion of the ureter is excised, and each end is dissected free of the peritoneum. One end of the ureter is spatulated anteriorly, and the opposite end is spatulated posteriorly to help prevent stenosis at the site of the anastomosis.[8] A vertical extraperitoneal cystotomy is performed in the dome of the bladder, and a ureteral catheter (8 Fr double J ureteral catheter or polyurethrane or polyethylene drainage tube) is passed through the ureteral orifice up the distal ureteral segment and then up the proximal ureter into the renal pelvis as a stent for the anastomosis and to drain urine from the renal pelvis. The cut ends

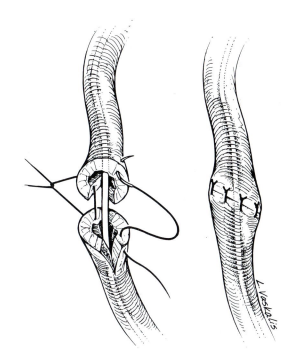

Fig. 54-4. Ureteroureterostomy.

of the ureter are approximated with four or five interrupted 4-0 absorbable sutures that pass through the adventitial and muscular coats of the ureteral wall. The anastomosis should be watertight but not ischemic (Fig. 54-4). The distal end of the ureteral catheter may be brought out through the anterior bladder and abdominal wall and secured to the abdominal wall or through the urethra and secured to a transurethral Foley catheter. An extraperitoneal suction drain should be placed adjacent to, but not touching, the ureteroureteral anastomosis. The catheters may usually be removed after 10 days. The suction drain is removed 24 hours later, if there is no evidence of urinary leakage.

BLADDER EXTENSION AND MOBILIZATION

When performing a ureteroneocystostomy or ureteroureterostomy, it is essential that the ureteral anastomosis be tension-free. This may require mobilization of the bladder by severance of the attachments to its anterior wall. A vesicopsoas hitch may be performed to elongate the bladder in the direction of the proposed anastomosis. Bladder flaps of the Boari-Ockerblad[1,16] or Demel[4] type have been recommended for further extension of the bladder fundus toward the site of a ureteral anastomosis, but they may be technically difficult to perform and may be a source of postoperative complications (e.g., ureteral reflux or stenosis).

The upward mobility of the bladder may be increased to a moderate degree by dissecting the retropubic space (of Retzius) and freeing the dome of the bladder from its loose attachments to the retrosymphysis. This procedure often provides enough mobility of the bladder to relieve minor degrees of tension that may be placed on a ureteral anastomosis or reimplantation site.

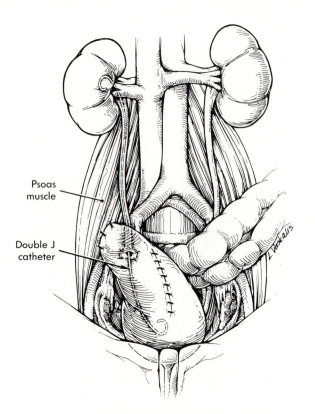

Psoas
muscle

Double J
catheter

Fig. 54-5. Vesicopsoas hitch.

Vesicopsoas hitch

If there is any question as to whether there will be tension on the reimplantation or anastomotic site after mobilization of the bladder, a vesicopsoas hitch may be performed to ensure that the reimplantation site is protected. The vesicopsoas hitch should be performed before reimplantation or reanastomosis of the ureter.

To perform a vesicopsoas hitch, one or two fingers are placed through an anterior vertical extraperitoneal cystotomy in the dome of the bladder, which is displaced toward the end of the ureter that is to be reimplanted. The leading point of the outer wall and muscular layer of the bladder is sutured to the psoas major fascia with several interrupted 2-0 or 1-0 delayed absorbable sutures. The bladder must be anchored to the psoas major fascia without undue tension to prevent pressure necrosis about the sutures and premature detachment of the bladder (Fig. 54-5).[8]

Boari-Ockerblad bladder flap

The bladder is fully mobilized by lysis of all attachments to its anterior wall. A vesicopsoas hitch is performed on the side of the reimplantation. A full-thickness, wide-based flap with adequate blood supply is cut out of the anterior bladder wall as shown in Fig. 54-6.[1,16] The

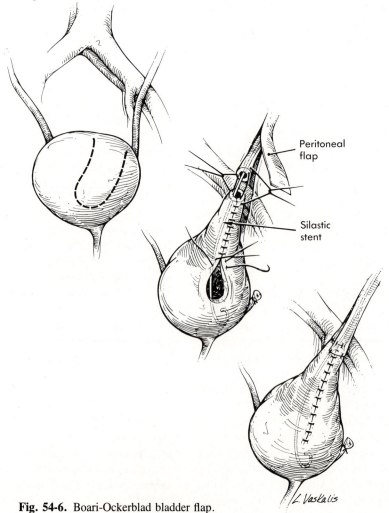

Peritoneal
flap

Silastic
stent

Fig. 54-6. Boari-Ockerblad bladder flap.

distal ureter is reimplanted directly or by way of a submucosal tunnel into the upper end of the bladder flap with 4-0 interrupted absorbable or delayed absorbable sutures. The cut edges of the flap are approximated with one layer of interrupted 4-0 or 3-0 absorbable or delayed absorbable sutures.

Demel bladder flap

The bladder is fully mobilized by lysis of all attachments to its anterior wall. A vesicopsoas hitch is performed on the side of the reimplantation. A curved incision is made about the anterolateral wall of the bladder on the side of the ureteral reimplantation as shown in Fig. 54-7.[4] The distal end of the ureter is reimplanted directly or by way of a submucosal tunnel into the upper end of the bladder flap with 4-0 interrupted absorbable or delayed absorbable sutures. The incision in the bladder is closed with interrupted 4-0 or 3-0 absorbable or delayed absorbable sutures.

TRANSURETEROURETEROSTOMY

Transureteroureterostomy may be performed when there is loss of a significant portion of one of the lower ureters.

The distal end of the ureter is tied with a permanent suture at its ureterovesical junction. The proximal ureter is mobilized and carried retroperitoneally below the inferior mesenteric artery and in front of the great vessels to meet the opposite ureter. The recipient ureter is longitudinally incised, and an end-to-side anastomosis is performed using interrupted 4-0 absorbable sutures placed through the adventitial and muscular layers of both ureters. The anastomosis should be watertight, but not ischemic (Fig. 54-8).[8] The anastomotic site should be drained by an extraperitoneal suction drain. Stenting catheters are usually not necessary. The suction catheter is not removed until there is no drainage from the anastomotic site.

CUTANEOUS URETEROSTOMY

This is the least complicated and also the least permanent of all ureteral diversions. The distal end of the ureter is tied with permanent suture. The cut end of the ureter is brought out retroperitoneally, and a ureteral skin anastomosis is performed.[8] Stenting is usually not necessary. Cutaneous ureterostomies, which are not considered permanent procedures, may be performed in patients whose chances of survival are expected to be limited or in cases in which the surgeon is not prepared to perform a definitive repair.

FOLLOW-UP OF URETERAL ANASTOMOSES

Prophylactic antibiotics (e.g., a cephalosporin) are recommended until all stents and drains are removed. The extravasation of urine into tissues often leads to infection, impaired healing, and fibrosis and can contribute to ureteral stenosis and loss of kidney function. Intravenous

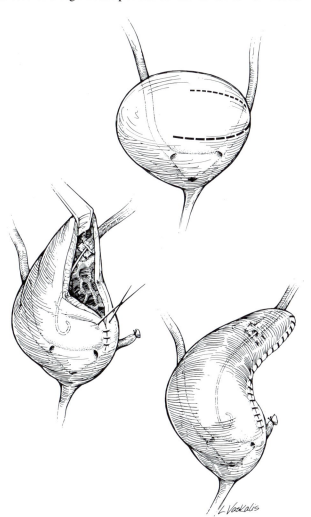

Fig. 54-7. Demel bladder flap.

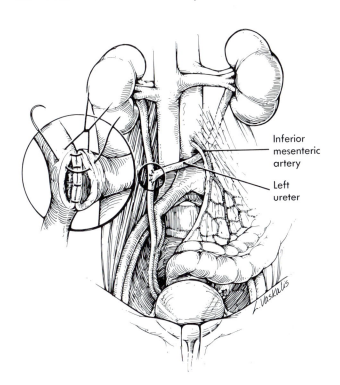

Inferior mesenteric artery

Left ureter

Fig. 54-8. Transureteroureterostomy.

urography should be performed after the repair of ureteral injuries to detect ureteral stenosis and to evaluate kidney function.

URINARY DIVERSIONS

In gynecology, urinary diversions have become an integral part of the management of patients with pelvic disease that obstructs and ultimately destroys the lower urinary tracts. Urinary diversions are performed primarily during treatment of advanced gynecologic malignancies, exenterative procedures, and to treat complications of cancer therapy (i.e., radiation-induced urinary fistulas). Less commonly, urinary diversion may be indicated for refractory cystitis and irreparable urinary fistulas due to "benign" disease processes. Regardless of the indication, urinary diversions are major surgical procedures, requiring advanced surgical training, and are associated with a significant potential for morbidity and mortality.

Methods of urinary diversion have evolved as a result of advances in surgical techniques and a better understanding of the effects of urinary diversion on renal physiology. The reduction in operative and postoperative morbidity and mortality makes urinary diversion an option for patients who were previously considered not suitable for such a procedure.

Percutaneous nephrostomy, image-directed insertion of a small urinary drainage catheter through the skin into the renal pelvis, is an excellent means of urinary diversion in patients with an injured or obstructed lower urinary tract. This procedure is used primarily as a palliative measure in patients with progressive pelvic malignancies, but it may be used to alleviate obstructive symptoms in patients who are being prepared to undergo corrective surgery or urinary diversion.

In gynecologic patients, the pathologic processes requiring urinary diversion dictate a supravesical surgical approach and a ureterocutaneous or ureteroenteric diversion of urinary flow. Advances in the construction of intestinal conduits make ureteroenteric diversion preferable to ureterocutaneous diversion, which has frequent stomal complications. Although the ileal conduit, as popularized by Bricker in 1950,[11] is the most frequently performed technique of ureteroenteric diversion, attention also has been directed to the use of transverse colon conduits in an effort to avoid complications inherent in operating on previously irradiated bowel.[21] Efforts to minimize stomal complications associated with incontinent conduits have resulted in the introduction of the "continent conduit." Since being introduced by Kock, there have been numerous modifications of high-volume/low-pressure reservoirs using terminal ileum and proximal colon.[12] The role of the continent conduit in gynecologic disease is being defined. Therefore, the ileal conduit is described with the understanding that only minor alterations in surgical technique are required to construct conduits using the large intestine.

The preoperative evaluation must focus on the patient's physical and psychologic suitability for urinary diversion.

She should be counseled regarding the required care and the possible complications of permanent urinary diversion. An enterostomal therapist can assist in choosing potential stomal sites and provide information regarding necessary supplies and stomal care. Preoperative medical evaluation should include an evaluation of the cardiac and respiratory systems and provide baseline hematologic and metabolic data. Imaging studies should include an intravenous urogram to define renal function and the location and extent of lower urinary tract involvement. Depending on which segment of bowel is to be used for the conduit, an upper gastrointestinal series with small bowel follow-through or a barium enema is indicated to document the condition of the alimentary tract.

Beginning 2 to 3 days before surgery, the patient should be placed on a liquid diet. Twenty-four hours before surgery, she should begin mechanical bowel preparation by drinking a purgative (Golytely, Braintree Laboratories, Inc., Braintree, Mass, 4 L ingested at a rate of 8 oz every 10 to 15 minutes on morning prior to surgery), and initiate antibiotic bowel preparation using erythromycin, neomycin, or one of the cephalosporins that have been shown to be effective in reducing postoperative infections caused by intestinal and urinary tract pathogens. The patient should take nothing by mouth, except oral medications, for 6 hours before her surgical procedure. Perioperative low-dose heparin (5000 units subcutaneously every 12 hours) and intermittent pneumatic compression stockings are recommended as prophylaxis against thromboembolic disorders.

ILEAL CONDUIT

The patient is placed on the operating table in the supine position, and general anesthesia is administered. The abdomen is prepared and draped in the usual manner. A midline abdominal incision is made. The entire abdomen is explored to determine if there is evidence of malignant disease. If malignant disease is present, a decision must be made about performing the urinary diversion. Once the decision has been made to perform an ileal conduit, an appropriate segment of ileum is chosen for the urinary reservoir. The bowel must be well-vascularized, mobile, and free of injury due to prior irradiation therapy, and so forth. If such a segment of ileum is not available, a transverse colon or sigmoid conduit should be considered (Fig. 54-9).

In performing an ileal conduit, the ureters next to but not involved in disease are isolated by meticulous sharp dissection to minimize damage to the microvasculature and to preserve the peritoneal attachments. The ends of the ureters, next to the diseased tissues, are ligated with permanent suture, and the healthy ureters are transected proximal to the ligating sutures. The ureters and their peritoneal attachments are mobilized up to the bifurcation of the common iliac arteries, ensuring adequate length to reach, without tension, a midline intestinal conduit. The distal ureters are spatulated and a Silastic stent, either an 8 Fr double J catheter or polyurethrane or polyethylene drainage tube, is passed proximally through the ureters and into

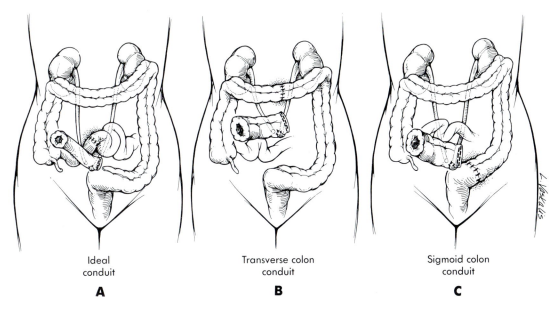

Fig. 54-9. Conduits. **A,** Ileal. **B,** Sigmoid. **C,** Transverse colon.

the renal pelves. A 4-0 absorbable suture is passed through the ureter and stent to prevent stent dislodgement. Urinary output by way of the stenting catheter is monitored. If the postoperative course is uncomplicated, the stents are removed after the tenth postoperative day.

A portion of ileum 20 to 30 cm from the ileocecal valve is isolated and delivered into the surgical incision. A segment 15 to 20 cm in length, with adequate vasculature from the superior mesenteric or ileocolic arteries, is chosen to cross the abdominal wall and extend 4 cm beyond the proposed stomal site. The mesentery of this portion of ileum is divided, and attention is given to protecting its blood supply. The mesenteric dissection is carried 3 to 4 cm beyond the proximal dissection to provide additional mobility for the development of the stoma. The isolated portion of ileum is removed from the rest of the small intestine using standard surgical techniques and intestinal staplers. Intestinal staplers reduce operating time, protect the blood supply, minimize wound contamination and trauma, and appear to facilitate the return of bowel function. Once the ileal segment has been isolated, the continuity of the small bowel is reestablished using bowel staplers, and defects in the mesentery are sutured to prevent intestinal herniation.

The distal end of the intestinal segment that is to be used for the conduit is opened, and the segment is irrigated with normal saline. The left ureter is tunneled retroperitoneally, deep to the inferior mesenteric vessels to reach without tension the proximal end of the conduit. Similarly, the right ureter is brought to the proximal end of the conduit. Two 0.5-cm incisions are made 2 to 4 cm from the proximal end of the conduit on opposite sides midway between its mesenteric and antimesenteric edges. The ureteral stents are threaded through these incisions and out through the distal end of the conduit. The ureteroenteric anastomosis is made using interrupted 4-0 absorbable su-

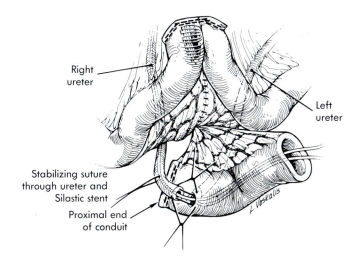

Fig. 54-10. Ureteral implantation into intestinal conduit.

ture with the knots placed on the serosal side of the anastomosis (Fig. 54-10). The anastomosis should be watertight but not ischemic. It may be protected and strengthened by approximating the periureteral peritoneum to the conduit. The integrity of the anastomosis should be tested by filling the conduit with sterile saline and testing for leakage.

Patients who have an incontinent conduit do not require an antireflux ureteroenteric anastomosis. On the other hand, patients having continent conduits may benefit from an antireflux anastomosis.

The distal end of the ileal conduit is passed through the stoma site and matured in the standard fashion. The serosa of the conduit should be sutured to the parietal peritoneum and the abdominal wall fascia to prevent herniation. The proximal end of the conduit is sutured to the sacral promontory or the medial peritoneal surface of the sigmoid mesentery to stabilize the conduit and reduce any tension on the ureteroenteric anastomosis.

Perioperative complications associated with ileal conduits may be significant. Early postoperative complications include hemorrhage, infection, bowel obstruction, herniation or volvulus, anastomotic leaks or disruption, fistula formation, stomal necrosis, and so forth. Late complications include stomal stenosis, parastomal herniation, peristomal dermatitis, and so forth.[24] Metabolic complications include hyperchloremic metabolic acidosis secondary to the reabsorption of urinary chloride by the conduit's mucosa and renal failure resulting from either the acidosis or stomal or ureteroenteric obstruction. Periodic assessment of renal function and of blood urea nitrogen and creatinine are recommended. Elevations in these parameters may indicate a need for renal scans or intravenous urograms to determine renal function.

REFERENCES

1. Boari A: Contributo sperimentale alla plastica dell' uretere, *Atti Acad Sci Med Nat Ferrara* 68:149, 1894.
2. Cruikshank SH: Surgical method of identifying the ureters during total vaginal hysterectomy, *Obstet Gynecol* 67:277, 1986.
3. Daly JW, Higgins KA: Injury to the ureter during gynecologic surgical procedures, *Surg Gynecol Obstet* 167:19, 1988.
4. Demel R: Ersatz des Ureters durch eine Plastik aus der Harnblase (Vorlaufige Mitteilung), *Zentralbl Chir* 51:2008, 1924.
5. Dowling RA, Corriere JN Jr, Sandler CM: Iatrogenic ureteral injury, *J Urol* 135:912, 1986.
6. Eisenkop SM et al: Urinary tract injury during cesarean section, *Obstet Gynecol* 60:591, 1982.
7. Fry DE, Milholen L, Harbrecht PJ: Iatrogenic ureteral injury, *Arch Surg* 118:454, 1983.
8. Greenstein A, Koontz WW Jr, Smith MJV: *Surgery of the ureter.* In Walsh PC et al, editors: *Campbell's urology,* ed 6, Philadelphia, 1991, WB Saunders.
9. Guerriero WG: *Ureteral trauma.* In Guerriero WG, editor: *Management of acute and chronic urologic injury,* Norwalk, 1984, Appleton-Century-Crofts.
10. Guerriero WG: Ureteral injury, *Urol Clin North Am* 16:237, 1989.
11. Jaffee BM, Bricker EM: Bladder substitution after pelvic evisceration, *Surg Clin North Am* 30:151, 1950.
12. Kock NG et al: Urinary diversion via a continent ileal reservoir: clinical results in 12 patients, *J Urol* 128:469, 1982.
13. Manetta A: Surgical maneuver for the prevention of ureteral injuries, *J Gynecol Surg* 5:291, 1989.
14. Mann WJ et al: Ureteral injuries in obstetrics and gynecology training program: etiology and management, *Obstet Gynecol* 72:82, 1988.
15. Miyazawa K: Urological injuries in gynecological surgery, *Hawaii Med J* 39:11, 1980.
16. Ockerblad NF: Reimplantation of the ureter into the bladder by a flap method, *J Urol* 57:845, 1947.
17. Paquin AJ Jr: Ureterovesical anastomosis: the description and evaluation of a technique, *J Urol* 82:573, 1959.
18. Piscitelli JT, Simel DL, Addison WA: Who should have intravenous pyelograms before hysterectomy for benign disease? *Obstet Gynecol* 69:541, 1987.
19. Politano VA, Leadbetter WF: An operative technique for correction of vesicoureteral reflux, *J Urol* 79:932, 1958.
20. Schlossberg SM: Ureteral healing, *Semin Urol* 5:197, 1987.
21. Schmidt JD, Buchcharm HJ, Jacoby EC: Transverse colon conduit for supravesical urinary diversion, *Urology* 8:542, 1976.
22. Shore ND, Bragg KJ, Sosa RE: Indwelling ureteral stents, *Semin Urol* 5:200, 1987.
23. Solomons E et al: A pyelographic study of injuries sustained during hysterectomy for benign conditions, *Surg Gynecol Obstet* 111:41, 1960.
24. Sullivan JW, Grabstald H, Whitmore WF: Complications of ureteroileal conduit with radical cystectomy: review of 336 cases, *J Urol* 124:797, 1980.
25. Symmonds RE: Ureteral injuries associated with gynecologic surgery: prevention and management, *Clin Obstet Gynecol* 19:623, 1976.
26. Witters S, Cornelissen M, Vereecken R: Iatrogenic ureteral injury: aggressive or conservative treatment, *Am J Obstet Gynecol* 155:582, 1986.

Part VIII

OPERATIONS UPON THE ALIMENTARY TRACT

Chapter 55

THE APPENDIX

David H. Nichols

Primary appendectomy is but rarely within the province of the gynecologic surgeon, but considerations concerning secondary appendectomy arise regularly.

ELECTIVE APPENDECTOMY

Although generally not a formidable procedure, appendectomy must be viewed strategically within the context of what is best for the patient (i.e., a very thoughtful consideration of the risk-benefit ratio for each particular person, which is indirectly the risk of future development of appendicitis). The hazards of elective appendectomy, although uncommon, must be considered and are concentrated on postoperative infection, which may involve abscess formation, either intraperitoneal or extraperitoneal, wound infection, or even peritonitis. Infection of the incisional wound is certainly more common in patients who have sustained appendectomy and may involve colonic anaerobes; wound infection may not only disturb wound healing, but may weaken the abdominal scar leading to an increased risk of postoperative wound weakness including that of the scar with the possibility of evisceration and of wound hernia.

The patient's views concerning retention or removal of her appendix should be solicited preoperatively, and, if elective appendectomy is a consideration, the surgeon should outline his or her position and recommendation to the patient and her consent must be obtained.

Although the patient may express gratitude to the surgeon post-operatively for her unexpected appendectomy, in the absence of her informed consent to appendectomy, the surgeon is fully liable for any unexpected misfortune that may develop postoperatively as a consequence to appendectomy (e.g., bowel obstruction or abscess formation from contamination or peritonitis as may develop from a tie that has slipped from around the appendiceal stump). An almost indefensible charge against the surgeon in such a situation is that of assault and battery for having under-

taken an elective procedure without the patient's knowledge and consent. The extent of liability will be proportionate to the pain, suffering, and damage produced. That a "routine appendectomy" may be the surgeon's "custom" would be of scant comfort to the surgeon and his or her legal defense during litigation. One simple preoperative statement by the surgeon may save a great deal of trouble if the patient has given a positive response to the surgeon's question, "In the event that during the course of your operation it appears, in my judgment, that removal of your appendix is in your best interest, may I have your permission to do so?"

The location of the appendix should always be visualized as part of a laparotomy (Fig. 55-1), the peritoneal surface should be inspected for inflammation, and the lumen should be palpated to detect any fecalith(s) present, which are thought by most to be precursors of appendicitis and by their very presence may constitute an indication for appendectomy. There are certain circumstances in which it is felt that elective appendectomy should be strongly considered:

1. When the surgeon has discovered a retrocecal location of the appendix, appendectomy may be warranted for two reasons—a retrocecal location of the appendix may confuse and delay the diagnosis of a future appendicitis, promoting an increased risk of appendiceal abscess and peritonitis. Future appendectomy or an inflamed retrocecal appendix is invariably more difficult than when appendectomy is performed electively on the uninflamed appendix.
2. Palpation of one or more fecaliths within the lumen of the appendix (thought to be a precursor of appendicitis)
3. Carcinoid of the appendix, if easily resectable, as the lesion is usually of a low grade of malignancy
4. Gross involvement of the appendix by endometrio-

sis. This may predispose to future symptomatology or mechanical obstruction

5. Benefit from appendectomy is less certain during exploratory laparotomy in a patient with chronic or repeated episodes of right lower quadrant pain, in whom at laparotomy there is no explanation for the pain. A misdiagnosis of chronic pelvic inflammatory disease, unsubstantiated by preliminary laparoscopy, may be evident. More likely, there may be follicle cysts of the patient's possibly dominant right ovary, although they generally should not be disturbed

6. With laparotomy performed to remove a mucinous tumor of the ovary

7. During staging operations for ovarian malignancy, because metastases are not uncommon[14]

8. Upon the patient's request for appendectomy

Appendectomy at this time eliminates consideration of the procedure in a future, different clinical situation and location often at the hands of a different practitioner.

Contraindications to elective appendectomy of a grossly normal, freely movable appendix are especially noteworthy in the patient who wishes to preserve her future fertility. These include:

1. Surgical treatment of a coincident ectopic pregnancy

2. Coincident pelvic operations to restore or enhance fertility (e.g., myomectomy, tubal reanastamosis, adhesiolysis, and fimbrioplasty, especially where there may be postoperative oozing of the surgical site)

3. Cesarean section, in a patient with uterine infection

4. The patient having expressly forbidden the procedure

5. A strong suspicion of Crohn's disease in the patient (e.g., weight loss, frequent bowel movements, and chronic crampy lower abdominal pains), because appendectomy in the face of active Crohn's disease is an invitation for postoperative enterocutaneous fistula

Relative contraindications to elective appendectomy include:

1. Preoperative failure to have obtained the patient's informed consent

2. The patient is already at greater than average medical risk for surgery

3. The risk of prolonging the total operative time

4. The operator's lack of experience with the technical steps of the procedure and management of its possible complications

It appears that the incidence of subsequent colon cancer, lymphomas, and leukemias is slightly increased in later years among women who had appendectomy in their youth. This is, of course, difficult to explain, but it has been suggested that the removal of lymphoid tissue from the younger patient might deprive the patient of some protective influences.[4,10]

At times, when one has determined that appendectomy may be in the patient's best interest, as, for example, in the patient with a retrocecal appendix, there may be difficulty in initial exposure of the base of the appendix, and it may be removed in a retrograde fashion starting at the ap-

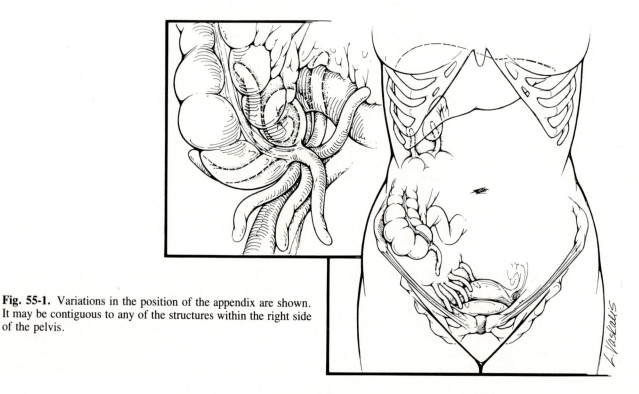

Fig. 55-1. Variations in the position of the appendix are shown. It may be contiguous to any of the structures within the right side of the pelvis.

pendiceal tip, and with the ligation and transection of the base being the final step of the appendectomy.

Occasionally after transvaginal colpotomy or vaginal hysterectomy, the appendix may appear in the operative field. Although it can be easily removed at this time using the same techniques as one might employ abdominally, the surgeon must be assured that to do so is in the patient's best interest and that the procedure meets with her approval. The surgeon must be certain to inform the patient in such a circumstance that her appendix has been removed, lest a future development of right lower-quadrant pain might be interpreted by another examiner as indication for appendectomy, unaware due to the presence of an unscarred abdomen that the appendix had been previously removed.

A history of previous appendectomy does not guarantee

against the development of appendicitis, because the latter may be seen in an appendiceal stump residual after subtotal appendectomy.

An uncommon observation may be that of a "hunter's appendix," in which, during the course of a barium enema or IVP, a "bag" full of buckshot may be seen at the site of the appendix in the patient who is accustomed to consuming freshly shot game from which all the buckshot had not been removed before cooking.

CARCINOID OF THE APPENDIX

The appendix should always be examined at laparoscopy, and the presence or absence of adhesions should be noted as well as any signs of inflammation or tumors. Carcinoma of the appendix is quite rare, the vast majority of which will be carcinoid, although a small number may

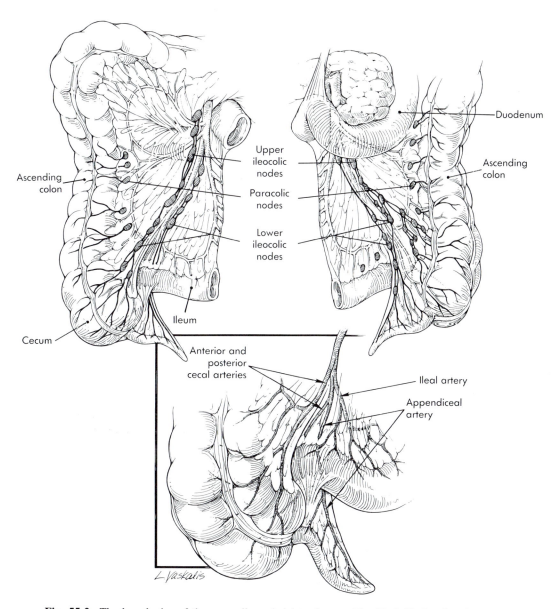

Fig. 55-2. The lymphatics of the appendix and right colon are identified. Notice that the appendiceal artery arises as a branch of the posterior cecal artery and enters the mesoappendix several millimeters away from the base of the appendix.

harbor adenocarcinoma. The diagnosis is established by frozen section and, if positive for carcinoid, the rest of the bowel must be inspected for other areas of carcinoid, and palpation of any lymph nodes should be undertaken of the right colon and mesoappendix (Fig. 55-2). If any nodes are positive, or if adenocarcinoma is found, right hemicolectomy is indicated. The characteristic appearance of carcinoid is a firm nodule at the tip of the appendix, which in cross section appears as a yellow submucous ring encircling the appendix. Microscopically, there are masses of polyhedral cells with granulated or vacuolated cytoplasms. The tumor is yellow because the cells are rich in lipid material. These tumors are chromaffinomas, or tumors of the endocrine system arising from Kulchitsky's cells of the intestinal mucosa, which are found between the columnar cells of the crypts of Lieberkühn and belong to the chromaffin system.[5] Intestinal carcinoid, in contrast, is primarily a tumor of the ileum where it may form a yellow mass partly encircling the bowel and projecting into the lumen and is best treated by resection, although there may be secondary carcinoid growths in the liver which may produce serotonin in the carcinoid syndrome.

SYMPTOMS AND PATHOGENESIS OF APPENDICITIS

Appendicitis is the consequence of obstruction to the lumen. In most instances, this is the consequence of submucosal lymphoid follicle hyperplasia secondary to infection anywhere in the body, although the second most common cause of obstruction may be from a fecalith, and far more rarely tumor or foreign bodies.

This obstruction may give rise to abscess formation within the lumen of the appendix, which, as it progresses, may cause local circulatory embarrassment and edema, and as the vessels become obstructed, gangrene may develop. Perforation and peritonitis may evolve as a consequence. Periappendicitis is less ominous because it may involve infection from without rather than within the appendix, as might be secondary to an episode of pelvic inflammatory disease. As the inflammatory disease resolves, the periappendicitis may tend to resolve as well, without necessarily passing through a stage of luminal obstruction.

The symptoms of appendicitis generally begin with epigastric pain, which is followed by anorexia and may be followed later by nausea and vomiting. As the area of inflammation comes in contact with the parietal peritoneum, the pain may seem to migrate to the right lower quadrant, where tenderness on deep palpation and rebound tenderness may be found. Fever may or may not be present before perforation, and it is important to differentiate appendicitis from acute pyelonephritis, and a careful urinalysis should always be obtained. With pyelonephritis, the temperature tends to be higher than with appendicitis. Chills are more common with pyelonephritis, but leukocytosis is more common with appendicitis. Confusion may be generated when a retrocecal appendix overlies the patient's ure-

ter, because appendiceal inflammation here may generate ureteral inflammation and pyuria as well (Fig. 55-1).

Differential diagnosis of appendicitis must include pyelonephritis, mesenteric adenitis, Crohn's disease, pelvic inflammatory disease (although the latter is usually bilateral), and adnexal torsion or hemorrhage.

THE DIAGNOSIS OF APPENDICITIS

Anorexia, right lower-quadrant pain, leukocytosis, and fever are characteristic of acute appendicitis, although occasional periappendicitis will be seen unexpectedly during laparotomy for some other reason. The significance of the latter is unclear, but its presence should be recorded. In the patient with recurrent episodes of right lower-quadrant pain that has subsided and is now recurrent, with borderline leukocytosis, further diagnostic study is indicated. Barium enema may be useful, because an inflamed appendix will not fill and presence of a visualized appendiceal filling tends to exclude appendicitis. There appears to be no hazard to barium enema, even in the patient with appendicitis, providing that perforation has not occurred before the procedure.

To avoid unnecessary exposure to ionizing radiation, ultrasound examination may demonstrate a mass.

Diagnostic laparoscopy may be useful in inspecting the appendix directly.

APPENDICITIS IN PREGNANCY

Although appendicitis during pregnancy is not common, it is very real, and the surgeon evaluating symptoms of possible appendicitis in a prenatal patient must be cognitive of the changes of the location in the site of the appendix coincident with the advancing state of pregnancy, because it is displaced further toward the right upper quadrant. Although it is possible for appendicitis during pregnancy to have been undiagnosed and, therefore, untreated, an appendiceal abscess may have formed. Labor in the presence of an appendiceal abscess can be deadly, because the excursions of uterine contraction and later involution may rupture the wall of an appendiceal abscess, promoting a disseminated peritonitis.

Acute appendicitis is more common in women under 25 than those over 25, and because this is the age group of most reproduction, the incidence during pregnancy, 1 in 5000, will be that of the population as a whole. It may occur at any time during pregnancy, although it is perhaps a slight bit more common in the first and second trimester. The location of the appendix is altered considerably by displacement from the enlarging uterus, because the appendix is pushed laterally and cranially[2,13,16] (Fig. 55-3). At times, the diagnosis may be difficult to establish, but Alders' sign[1,3] may be helpful in which, after the right-sided tenderness has been localized in the supine position, the patient is turned on her left side, and, if the tenderness or pain shifts to the left along with the pelvic organs, it is thought to be of gynecologic origin unassociated with ap-

Fig. 55-3. Location of the appendix in relation to the McBurney's point as pregnancy advances (mo, months; pp, postpartum). (Modified from Baer JL, Reis RA, Arens RA: Appendicitis in pregnancy with changes in position and axis of a normal appendix in pregnancy, *JAMA* 98:1359, 1932.)

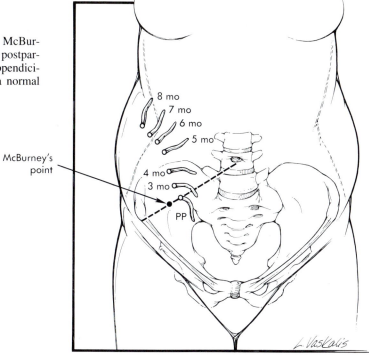

pendicitis. Because the white blood count is generally elevated during the course of pregnancy, a mild leukocytosis is not pathognomonic, but a distinct left shift should be expected in the presence of appendicitis, particularly if the count is over 18,000 cells/cm^3.

Removal of the unruptured appendix during pregnancy carries little risk to the fetus, but rupture with abscess formation has a grave significance because, should there be onset of labor, the walls of the abscessed cavity are likely to be disturbed considerably by the movement of the uterus, risking purulent dissemination of the abscess contents producing a generalized peritonitis. The toxins from the latter may be fatal for the baby, as well as the mother. When appendiceal abscess is encountered, the cavity should be entered and cultures taken, but loculations should be broken up without disturbing the walls of the abscessed cavity or surrounding adhesions, lest the infection be disseminated. The appendix should be removed only if it is easy to do. The abscessed cavity should be emptied and irrigated, and closed drainage through a separate stab wound should be instituted. Appropriate antibiotics should be used. For the fetus younger than 33 weeks gestation, concurrent cesarean section usually should not be performed because the risks of prematurity outweigh the risks of possible infection to the fetus; beyond the 33rd week, concurrent section should be seriously considered if there is evidence of fetal compromise.[11]

Incidental appendectomy at the time of cesarean section is generally safe, although not widely practiced, because there is a very small risk of infection of the peritoneal cavity. If the surgeon contemplates incidental appendectomy, it would be wise to obtain the patient's permission preoperatively.[12]

TECHNIQUE OF APPENDECTOMY

It is easy to remove an appendix if the cecum can be brought out of the abdomen and there are no complications. If the appendix is badly infected, bound down by adhesions or if retrocecal, its removal can be a very difficult operation. "The inexpert will use numerous packs, retract forcefully, use sponge sticks on the intestine, injure the peritoneum and even tear the mesentary with the results of the postoperative course being marked by distention, often dangerous peritonitis and many later adhesions and even death. The worse the appendix and the more difficulty exposing, the greater the demands for gentleness and the more dangerous the gauze pack."[7]

There should be adequate preliminary operative exposure, making the organ accessible. If there is any peritoneal exudate, it should be cultured and, as the appendix and cecum are visualized, moist packs should isolate this area from the rest of the abdominal cavity, often permitting the site for surgery to be delivered into the wound.[15]

The mesoappendix at the tip of the appendix is grasped with the hemostat and gently elevated while traction is applied caudally and medially to the cecum[9] (Fig. 55-4). The mesoappendix is clamped perpendicular to the appendiceal axis (Fig. 55-5), and the clamp is replaced by transfixion ligature. The appendiceal artery may be several millimeters from the base of the appendix (Fig. 55-1). In the event

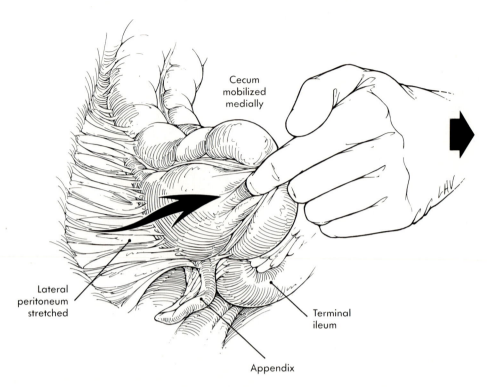

Cecum
mobilized
medially

Lateral
peritoneum
stretched

Terminal
ileum

Appendix

Fig. 55-4. Cecum is mobilized by traction medially, exposing the appendix and the lateral peritoneum. The latter may require incision if necessary to mobilize the appendix further.

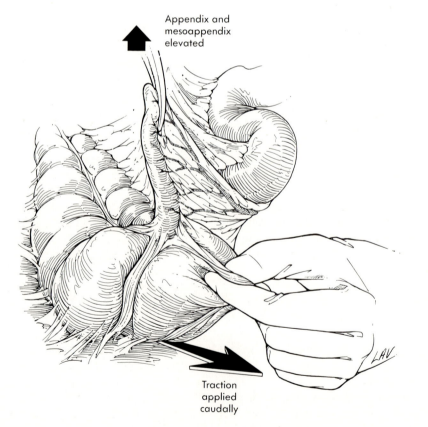

Appendix and
mesoappendix
elevated

Traction
applied
caudally

Fig. 55-5. The mesoappendix is grasped near the appendiceal tip, while traction in a caudal direction brings the cecum into the wound.

of infection and inflammation, the peritoneum overlying the mesoappendix should be incised on each side[9] (Fig. 55-6), the edematous fat should be removed, and the appendiceal artery should be clamped, cut, and ligated. The base of the appendix is ligated with an absorbable suture, the ends are held with the hemostat just beyond the knot and cut, and a second tie is placed a few millimeters distal to the first. A hemostat is placed across the body of the appendix and closed but not locked, stripping the appendiceal contents toward the distal tip, and, when about 1 cm away from the tie, the hemostat is locked and the appendix (doubly tied at its base) is gently severed with the scalpel. Both appendix and scalpel are handed off the table.

An alternate method of handling the stump is that it be inverted and the seromuscular layer closed by a series of interrupted mattress sutures, but there seems to be no advantage to separate ligation followed by inversion of the stump, because this would lead to postoperative intramural abscess formation, which would probably rupture into the intestinal lumen. If it was the surgeon's desire to employ this combined treatment of the stump, it would be desirable to tie the stump off first with an absorbable suture in the area crushed by hemostat and then invert this with a pursestring suture placed in the seromuscular layer of the bowel[17] (Fig. 55-7).

If the appendix is gangrenous and the latter extends to its base, there may be considerable induration and edema

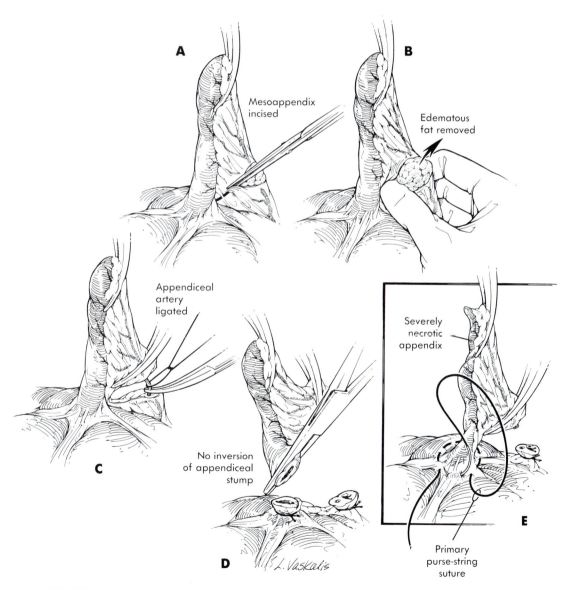

Fig. 55-6. A, When the appendix is acutely inflamed, the tip is elevated and the mesoappendix is incised along either side. **B,** Edematous fat is squeezed out. **C,** The appendiceal artery is clamped, cut, and ligated. **D,** The base is ligated; the appendix is transected and removed. **E,** When the appendix is necrotic, it may be better to place a primary pursestring suture in the seromuscular layer, which will be tied after the appendix has been amputated.

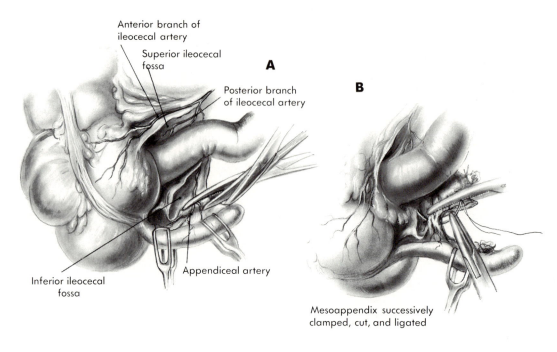

Anterior branch of ileocecal artery

Superior ileocecal fossa

A

B

Posterior branch of ileocecal artery

Inferior ileocecal fossa

Appendiceal artery

Mesoappendix successively clamped, cut, and ligated

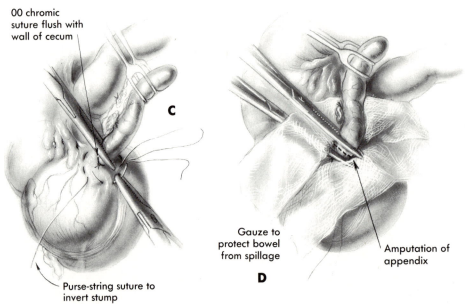

00 chromic suture flush with wall of cecum

C

Purse-string suture to invert stump

Gauze to protect bowel from spillage

Amputation of appendix

D

Fig. 55-7. A technique for appendectomy. **A,** Some of the anatomy of the appendix and cecum and the first step in the excision of an appendix that lies at or near the pelvic brim. Kelly clamps are successively placed along the mesoappendix, and the mesoappendix is cut. With each successive bite of the Kelly clamps, the mesoappendix is ligated with fine sutures. The appendiceal artery, which arises from the posterior cecal branch of the ileocecal artery, is usually located at or near the junction of the terminal ileum with the cecum. **B,** Technique of ligating the appendiceal artery is shown. Although some operators prefer to ligate the appendiceal artery at the beginning of the appendectomy, with ligation of the mesoappendix by one large tie, the method of successively clamping, cutting, and ligating the mesoappendix allows for every variation in the length of the appendix and position of the mesoappendix. A pursestring suture is placed around the base of the appendix with the ends left long. **C,** A straight hemostat is used to crush the appendix at its junction with the cecum, the clamp is moved a few millimeters toward the distal end of the appendix, and an absorbable ligature is placed flush with the wall of the cecum. A straight clamp is used to grasp the ligature placed at the base of the appendix, and the other straight clamp is moved further distally on the appendix preparatory to amputation. Several gauze sponges are placed around the base of the appendix to protect adjacent bowel from the caustic phenol solution used later. **D,** The appendix and all the instruments that have touched the organ are placed in a separate basin from the rest of the operative field.

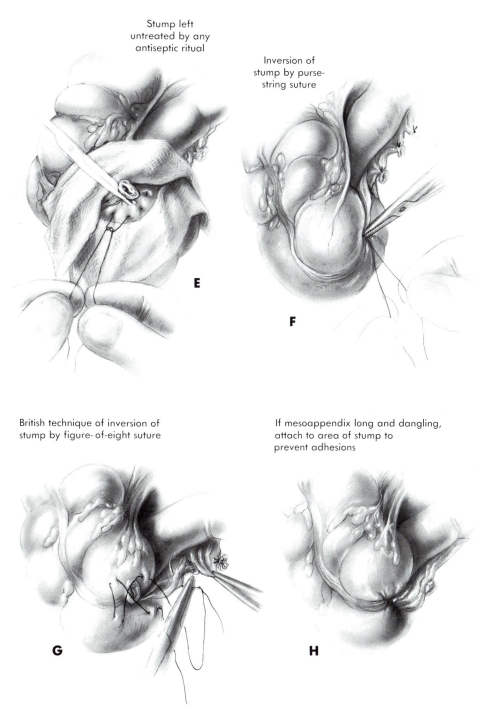

Stump left
untreated by any
antiseptic ritual

Inversion of
stump by purse-
string suture

E

F

British technique of inversion of
stump by figure-of-eight suture

If mesoappendix long and dangling,
attach to area of stump to
prevent adhesions

G

H

Fig. 55-7, cont'd. E, The stump of the appendix may be wiped successively by an applicator tip saturated with povidone-iodine. **F,** The stump of the appendix is grasped with a straight hemostat and is inverted as the pursestring suture is tied. **G,** An alternate method of inverting the appendiceal stump is shown. This consists of passing a double figure-of-eight mattress suture about the stump of the appendix and also into the adjacent segment of the mesoappendix. This is a faster method and effectively inverts the stump and sutures the mesoappendix over the area of operation. **H,** The final appearance of the inverted stump by the alternate method is shown. The area about the inverted stump and all of the ligated points on the mesoappendix are inspected for any bleeding before the abdomen is closed.

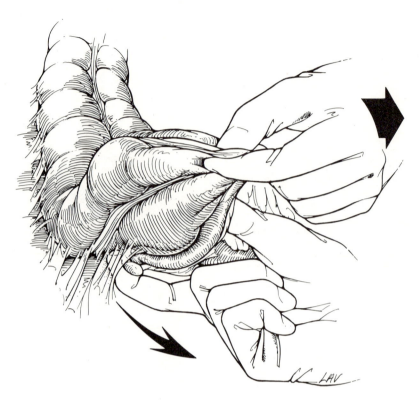

Fig. 55-8. The retrocecal appendix must be mobilized by traction of the cecum to the patient's left, combined with digital identification of the fibrous band at the tip of the retrocecal appendix.

of the cecum, making it desirable to reinforce the site of amputation of the stump with a series of interrupted mattress stitches. If the appendix has a retrocecal location, the cecum will have to be mobilized. Often, there is a small avascular band running from the tip of the appendix ending close to the lower pole of the right kidney. This will have to be divided, care being taken to divide the band and not the tip of the appendix[15] (Fig. 55-8).

Occasionally, a retrocecal appendix must be removed in a retrograde fashion starting with the base of the appendix, the stump now ligated, and it may be possible to demonstrate the ill-defined mesoappendix; by blunt dissection the mesoappendix is clipped and cut until it has been removed.

Dewhurst[6] has described an interesting alternative to inversion appendectomy that does not risk peritonitis. The appendix is cleaned of its mesentery and attached fatty tissue, and, by pressure with a blunt-ended probe at the tip of the organ, the appendix is inverted into the cecum. When this is complete, the appendix lies "inside out" in the lumen of the cecum and its site is marked only by a dimple in the cecal wall, which is closed with a single catgut suture. The appendix sloughs off and is "digested" in the course of its passage through the colon. The surgeon must be careful to determine that a fibrous appendix with obliteration of its lumen is not present if this treatment is to be possible.

MECKEL'S DIVERTICULUM

If a Meckel's diverticulum is encountered, it may be removed because about half of such diverticula contain ectopic gastric mucosa, which occasionally may be the site of future gastrointestinal bleeding, perforation, or obstruction. It has its own mesentery, the mesenteriolum, which should be be separately clamped, cut, and tied. The base is clamped in an axis at a right angle to that of the small intestine, and the diverticulum is excised. In most instances, the Meckel's diverticulum will be 25 to 50 cm from the ileocecal valve. Clamping must be done at right angles to the long axis of the small bowel. It may be done by a gastrointestinal (GI) stapler at right angles to the intestine (Fig. 55-9) or between two Kocher clamps, the wound in the bowel closed by a running absorbable nonlocking suture over the clamp, or a running back and forth absorbable suture beneath the clamp, both areas reinforced with a synthetic nonabsorbable suture, much as one might close a laceration into the intestinal lumen.[9]

APPENDICEAL ABSCESS

A small percentage of patients demonstrate the presence of a right lower-quadrant mass, and it is important to determine whether this represents a localized inflammation with edema or has progressed to abscess formation; the latter invariably requires drainage because it has no effective circulation and it is difficult to deliver systemic antibiotics to

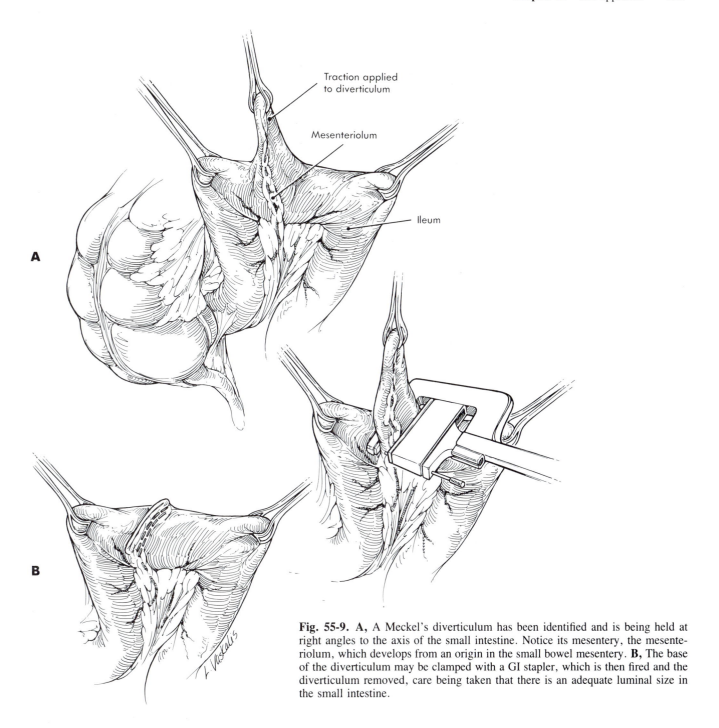

Fig. 55-9. A, A Meckel's diverticulum has been identified and is being held at right angles to the axis of the small intestine. Notice its mesentery, the mesenteriolum, which develops from an origin in the small bowel mesentery. **B,** The base of the diverticulum may be clamped with a GI stapler, which is then fired and the diverticulum removed, care being taken that there is an adequate luminal size in the small intestine.

the center of the abscessed cavity.[16] Although some would favor bedrest with intravenous hydration and antibiotics (a cephalosporin and metronidazole, or a gentamicin and clindamycin combination), it is important that the presence of abscess formation be identified, because the latter must be surgically drained. Following clinical improvement after 7 to 10 days of drainage and antibiotic administration, consideration should be given to interval appendectomy in 3 to 4 months because appendicitis will recur in about 10% of such patients, usually within the year.[16]

This lower-quadrant abscess must be differentiated from that of diverticulitis, which may be more common in the patient over 60, although the latter may be more common on the left side with left lower-quadrant pain, often cramplike with diarrhea alternating with constipation and the presence of a palpable mass. If, however, the diverticulosis is present also in the right side of the pelvis and diverticulitis should develop in this area, the symptoms may be on the right side. There are several options for treatment of a diverticular abscess, the latter often having been diagnosed by computed tomography (CT) scan. If the lesion is well-circumscribed and less than 3 cm in diameter, excision of the involved segment and removal of the abscess can be undertaken.[15] If the abscess if larger that 5 cm, CT-guided percutaneous drainage may be instituted with delayed primary resection and reanastamosis. An alternate is for the surgeon to excise the involved segment at the time of the initial operation, bringing the proximal segment of the colon out in an end colostomy, the distal remaining segment oversewn as a Hartmann pouch. Some 6 to 12 weeks later, when the acute phase has passed and clinical resolution of the inflammation is evident, reanastomosis may be accomplished and the colostomy taken down.[16]

DIVERTICULAR ABSCESS

The abscessed cavity should be opened with care and a stab wound should be brought down to the site. The opening of the perforation is usually invisible, so no attempt should be made to close it. Transverse colostomy is not altogether satisfactory because there is probably a column of feces in the splenic flexure and descending colon and the source of sepsis and fecal contamination will remain; for this reason, excision of the affected loop with an end colostomy and Hartmann's pouch may be favored.

Percutaneous drainage of diverticular abscess and subsequent one-stage resection and anastomosis are as effective as surgical drainage of intraabdominal abscesses including those that communicate with the lumen of the intestine, with lower mortality.[8]

When surgery demonstrates an appendiceal abscess, it should always be drained through a separate stab wound, and manipulation should be kept to a minimum. Interval appendectomy may be considered at some future date, usually 6 months or more beyond the original surgery, but the likelihood of subsequent appendicitis in such a patient is estimated to be at around 10%, and subsequent appendectomy is, therefore, not mandatory. Future appendicitis will make itself known by recurrence of inflammatory symptoms.

REFERENCES

1. Alders N: A sign for differentiating uterine from extrauterine complications of pregnancy, *Br Med J* 2:1194, 1951.
2. Baer JL, Reis RA, Arens RA: Appendicitis in pregnancy with changes in position and axis of a normal appendix in pregnancy, *JAMA* 98:1359, 1932.
3. Bey M, Pastorek J: Appendicitis complicating pregnancy, *Clin Adv in Treatment of Infections* 3:1, 1989.
4. Bierman H: Human appendix and neoplasia, *Cancer* 21:109, 1968.
5. Boyd W: *A textbook of pathology*. Philadelphia, 1961, Lea & Febiger.
6. Dewhurst J: *Integrated obstetrics and gynaecology for post-graduates*. London, 1981, Blackwell.
7. Dudley G: The surgical assistant, *Surg Gynecol Obstet* 115:245, 1962.
8. Hemming A, Davis NL, Robins RE: Surgical vs. percutaneous drainage of intra-abdominal abscesses, *Am J Surg* 161:593, 1991.
9. Lee PL, Mariner DR: Appendectomy. In Sanz LE, editor: *Gynecologic surgery*, 1988, Medical Economics Books.
10. McVay, Jr: The appendix in relation to neoplastic disease, *Cancer* 17:929, 1964.
11. Newton M, Newton E: *Surgical problems in pregnancy*. In Dilts PV, Sciarra JJ, editors: *Gynecology and obstetrics*, vol 2, Philadelphia, 1991, JB Lippincott.
12. Parsons AK et al: Appendectomy at cesarean section: A prospective study, *Obstet Gynecol* 68:479, 1986.
13. Pritchard JA, MacDonald PG, Gant NF: Medical and surgical illness during pregnancy and the puerperium. In *Williams Obstetrics*, ed 17, Norwalk, CT, 1985, Appleton-Century-Crofts.
14. Rose PG et al: Appendectomy in primary and secondary staging operations for ovarian malignancy, *Obstet Gynecol* 77:116, 1991.
15. Simmons SC, Luck RJ: *General surgery in gynaecological practice*, Oxford, 1971, Blackwell.
16. Triedman L, Adler LM: Differentiation of subtle GI pathology from common gynecologic conditions, *Obstetrics and Gynecology Forum* 5 (4):2, 1991.
17. Weingold AB: Appendicitis in pregnancy, *Clin Obstet Gynecol* 26:801, 1983.

Chapter 56

SMALL INTESTINAL SURGERY INCIDENTAL TO GYNECOLOGIC PROCEDURES

Seymour I. Schwartz

MANAGEMENT OF OPERATIVE COMPLICATIONS

Traumatic perforation during laparoscopy

The diagnosis can be confirmed by direct visualization during the procedure or may be suggested postoperatively by accentuation of the signs of peritonitis. A laceration of the small intestine mandates celiotomy, and repair closure of the intestinal wound can be achieved by a two-layer technique, the first layer through mucosa, muscularis, and serosa (Fig. 56-1), and the second layer placed seromuscularly in a Lembert fashion. A single layer of sutures is equally effective (Fig. 56-2). There is no indication to irrigate or drain the peritoneal cavity. A 3-day regimen of cephalosporin and metronidazole is reasonable.

Postoperative ileus

Following an abdominal operation, small bowel motility usually returns within 24 hours and gastric motility within 48 hours, while colon inertia may persist for 3 to 5 days.[5] Nasogastric decompression of the stomach is usually sufficient. In the unusual case of prolonged ileus (i.e., greater than a week), a long tube can be passed into the duodenum under radiologic control and allowed to progress distally. Most cases of ileus resolve spontaneously.

Postoperative mechanical obstruction

This may be caused by an adhesion, volvulus, or internal herniation. The diagnosis is usually suggested by abdominal distention and intensified by radiologic findings of distended bowel with air/fluid levels. There is no conclu-sive method of differentiating between simple and strangulated obstruction preoperatively.

With few exceptions, mechanical obstruction requires urgent surgical intervention. Preoperative nasogastric suction should be instituted; fluid replacement and antibiotic should be administered. The abdomen is best explored through a generous midline incision that will provide access to the pelvis. The decompressed distal ileum is isolated first, and the bowel is "run" proximally until a distended segment is identified. If an adhesion is noted, it is transected; if a volvulus is noted, it is detorted; if an internal hernia is the cause, generally the herniated bowel is reduced and the defect closed. The bowel is adequately assessed by inspection. In rare cases, the injection of fluorescein intravenously and viewing the bowel with a Wood's lamp illumination will define nonperfused areas. In most instances closure of the abdominal wall can be achieved in the face of distention. If this is not feasible, a Baker tube can be inserted perorally or through an enterostomy, and suction applied as the tube is advanced will effect adequate decompression and permit closure. If an enterostomy was performed, it is closed after the tube is removed before closure.[1]

INTRAOPERATIVE CONSIDERATIONS

In the course of gynecologic operations several affections or lesions of the small intestine may be encountered.

Adhesions

The most common circumstance confronting the gynecologic surgeon is adhesions resulting from previous ce-

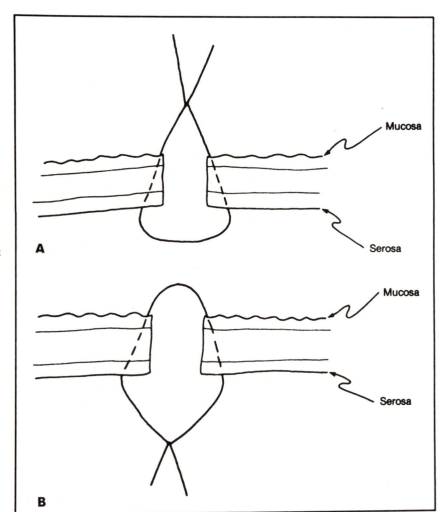

Fig. 56-1. A, Demonstration of angle of penetration of suture through posterior row. **B,** Demonstration of angle of penetration of suture through anterior row. (From Schwartz SI: *Intestinal resection and anastomosis.* In Schwartz SI, Ellis H, editors: *Maingot's abdominal operations,* ed 9, vol 1, East Norwalk, Conn, 1989, Appleton & Lange, with permission.)

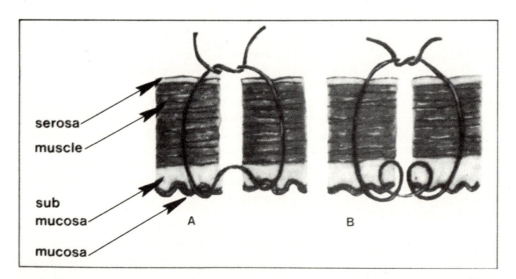

Fig. 56-2. Two methods of intestinal suture. **A,** Conventional two-layer inverting technique. **B,** Gambee single-layer technique designed to end-on apposition of the cut edges of bowel without puckering of the mucosa. (From Schwartz SI: *Intestinal resection and anastomosis.* In Schwartz SI, Ellis H, editors: *Maingot's abdominal operations,* ed 9, vol 1, East Norwalk, Conn, 1989, Appleton & Lange.)

liotomy. The vast majority of adhesions are harmless; the presence of adhesions per se does not constitute an indication for lysis. It is tempting to divide all the filmy adhesions encountered as the small intestine is "run." Not only is this procedure not indicated, but it may be contraindicated because the adhesions may play a protective role, and lysis may result in denudation of areas of serosa and consequently increase the risk of postoperative ileus or subsequent obstruction. Indications for lysis of adhesions during gynecologic operations are: (1) to facilitate exposure when adhesions between the small intestine and pelvic peritoneum or pelvic organs interfere with dissection and (2) when there is evidence of partial or complete intestinal obstruction, manifest by dilatation of the intestine proximal to the point of obstruction and distal collapse. Lysis of adhesions should be performed by sharp dissection. Denuded areas of the muscularis of the intestine should be oversewn with interrupted sutures placed in a Lembert fashion to invaginate the muscularis beneath the reapproximated serosa. Enterotomy performed during dissection should be closed with interrupted sutures.

Acute ileitis

In some patients explored for acute abdominal signs and symptoms, a beefy-red edematous terminal ileum with thickened mesentery and enlarged lymph nodes is encountered. This condition is self-limiting and usually does not progress to Crohn's disease. The cause is unknown, but some cases are due to *Yersinia* or *Campylobacter* infections. The ileum involved in the process of acute ileitis should *not* be removed. A regional node should be excised for pathologic evaluation and culture, including a specified culture for *Yersinia* and *Campylobacter*. The normal appendix should be removed to reduce confusion in diagnosis of subsequent episodes of abdominal pain.

Crohn's disease

This is a chronic granulomatous disease characterized by spontaneous remissions and acute exacerbations. Grossly, there are thickened, matted loops of intestine with fat wrapping of the individual loops and a thickened and shortened mesentery. Areas of involved bowel are separated by areas of grossly normal bowel. The diseased terminal ileum may become adherent to the pelvic wall or its contents, and a fistula may extend from the ileum to the vagina or rectum. The National Cooperative Crohn's Disease Study indicates that although 75% of patients require at least one surgical procedure within 20 years of onset, surgical resection is rarely curative and operations should be reserved to treat specific complications.[7]

A segment or segments of small intestine involved with Crohn's disease encountered during a gynecologic procedure should usually be noted and avoided. If there is evidence of obstruction and/or internal fistulization, and resection is believed to be indicated, the resection should be limited to the grossly involved adjacent intestine. Frozen section for definition of microscopic disease is not indi-

cated, because the amount of bowel removed should be minimized and microscopic involvement does not impact on the healing of an anastomosis. Ileosigmoid fistulas do not require resection of the sigmoid, because the disease is generally confined to the small intestine.

In selected patients with obstruction caused by single or multiple strictures, stricturoplasty may be appropriate. This is accomplished by longitudinal incision down to pouting submucosa, extending 1 cm proximal and distal to the stricture. The longitudinal incision is then closed transversely. Bypass procedures are rarely indicated in patients with Crohn's disease and are applicable only when resection would endanger adjacent structures.

Meckel's diverticulum and diverticulosis of the small intestine

Meckel's diverticulum is the most common congenital abnormality of the gastrointestinal tract and results from persistence of the vitelline duct that connected the intestinal tract to the yolk sac. This antimesenteric outpouching occurs in approximately 2% of the population, is usually located within 2 feet of the ileocecal valve, and may contain two types of aberrant lining cells, gastric and/or pancreatic tissue. Some surgeons would advise removal of an asymptomatic Meckel's diverticulum when found incidently in children or young adults. Leijonmarck et al[3] have recently provided evidence that in the adult, a wide-mouth diverticulum should not be resected. Resection is indicated if there has been evidence of bleeding, usually manifest by passage of bloody, maroon, or tarry stools, or if there is inflammation or an umbilical fistula, or if the Meckel's diverticulum has caused obstruction by a band, torsion, or intussusception.

Solitary or multiple diverticula may be found incidentally in the jejunum and less commonly in the ileum.[2] They are usually located on the mesenteric border, are symptomless in most cases, and should not be removed. Hemorrhage, perforation, and obstruction are specific indications for resection.

Meckel's and other small intestinal antimesenteric diverticula are excised by clamping the base in the transverse axis of the ileum (Fig. 56-3) to avoid narrowing the lumen when the defect is closed. Closure can be accomplished by two layers of Dexon or Vicryl, the first layer placed as a through-and-through suture and the second layer as an inverting Connell suture. Closure can also be accomplished with silk, using a single-layer or double-layer interrupted technique. Resection of a segment of adjacent intestine is reserved for cases in which the base is involved with inflammation or ulceration. In the unusual circumstance in which jejunal or ileal diverticula demand removal because of their location within the mesentery, an incision is made in the mesentery overlying the diverticulum and the diverticulum is dissected to its base, taking care to avoid the adjacent vasa recti. The diverticulum is then excised, and the defect is closed as described above. In some instances single or multiple diverticula are best

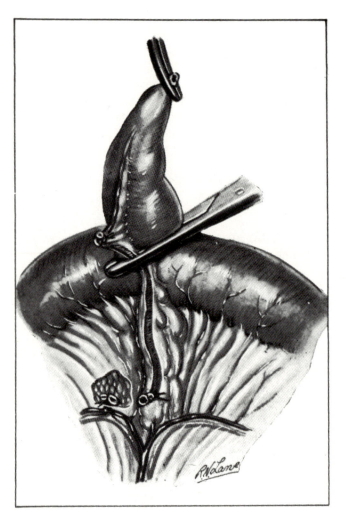

Fig. 56-3. Excision of a Meckel's diverticulum. (From Ellis H: *Meckel's diverticula, diverticulosis, umbilical fistulae and tumours.* In Schwartz SI, Ellis H, editors: *Maingot's abdominal operations,* ed 9, vol 1, East Norwalk, Conn, 1989, Appleton & Lange.)

managed by resection of the involved segment of small intestine.

Tumors of the small intestine

These are uncommon lesions. Primary benign tumors of the small intestine include adenomas, leiomyomas, lipomas, hemangiomas, and adenomatous polyps. The most common malignant tumor is an adenocarcinoma. Carcinoids usually are present in the ileum within 2 to 3 feet of the ileocecal valve, and they extend into the mestenteric nodes. Primary intestinal lymphomas also occur most frequently in the ileum. The most common intestinal sarcoma is the leiomyosarcoma. Treatment of an incidentally encountered tumor of the small intestine is generally effected by resection and immediate reconstruction of intestinal continuity.

RESECTION OF SMALL INTESTINE
General principles

Currently almost all anastomoses are carried out openly. Closed anastomoses are essentially of historical interest only. The amount of spillage into the peritoneal cavity can be controlled by atraumatic clamps or by occlusive tapes placed proximally and distally to the resection. The extent of resection is determined by the nature and size of the lesion. In the case of benign lesions, resection of the intestine 1 cm proximally and distally to the lesion is sufficient. In the case of malignant tumors, a 5- to 6-cm segment of normal intestine should be resected on either side of the grossly involved segment. The extent of resection may also be dependent on the lymphatic drainage; all grossly enlarged nodes should be removed. In the case of Crohn's disease, the resection is carried out just beyond the limits of grossly involved intestine. Healthy segments of intestine with adequate blood supply should be anastomosed. The anastomosis should be watertight, with an adequate stoma, and the suture line should be free from any tension. Transecting the intestine in an oblique fashion so that a greater portion is removed from the antimesenteric side ensures adequate vascularization of the anastomosis.

Types of anastomoses

End-to-end anastomosis. This is usually readily applied and can be established by suture or staple technique. The disparity between the two stomas can be compensated for by enlarging the smaller lumen, either by cutting the limb with a smaller lumen in an oblique fashion or by dividing the intestine longitudinally along the antimesenteric border (Fig. 56-4).[4] In the case of disparate lumena, a functional end-to-end anastomosis may be accomplished by closing the two ends of the intestine and performing a side-to-side anastomosis in immediate proximity to the closed ends. This may be performed by a suture technique (Fig. 56-5) or by using staples to close the two ends and creating the anastomosis with the GIA stapler (see below).

Side-to-side anastomosis. This technique is used to bypass an obstructed segment to the intestine, leaving that segment in place. The anastomosis should be carried out in the antimesenteric portion using either a suture technique or the GIA stapler.

In the side-to-side or functional end-to-end anastomosis, the anastomosis is carried out with the proximal segment transected. It is important that no more than 1.5 cm of proximal segment be allowed to extend beyond the anastomosis, because the pouch may enlarge or balloon and produce a "blind-loop syndrome."

Techniques of anastomoses

The major holding power of an intestinal anastomosis is found in the submucosa. The consensus opinion is that it is important to achieve serosal apposition. This is most readily accomplished by using an inner layer of sutures

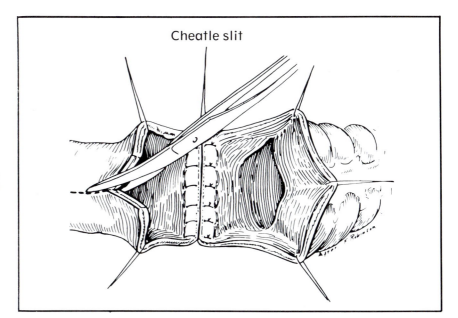

Fig. 56-4. Ileocolostomy; the Cheatle slit. (From Schwartz SI: *Intestinal resection and anastomosis*. In Schwartz SI, Ellis H, editors: *Maingot's abdominal operations,* ed 9, vol 1, East Norwalk, Conn, 1989, Appleton & Lange, with permission.)

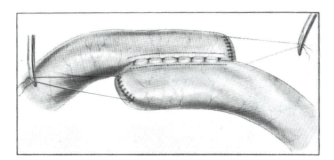

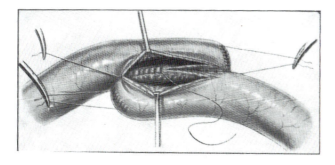

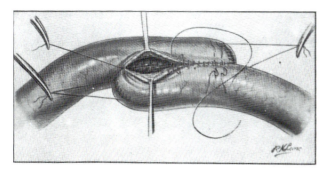

Fig. 56-5. Lateral, or side-to-side, anastomosis. (From Schwartz SI: *Intestinal resection and anastomosis*. In Schwartz SI, Ellis H, editors: *Maingot's abdominal operations,* ed 9, vol 1, East Norwalk, Conn, 1989, Appleton & Lange.)

made with absorbable material and an outer layer of nonabsorbable sutures placed in the seromuscular layer in an inverting Lembert fashion. Initially, the posterior row of seromuscular sutures is placed (Fig. 56-6), followed by a through-and-through continous suture placed in a locked fashion and continued anteriorly as an inverting Connell suture (Fig. 56-7). This layer is then covered with interrupted Lembert sutures (Fig. 56-8).

The suture material for intestinal anastomoses is determined by individual preference. It has been suggested that polyglycolic or polyglactin is superior to catgut for the inner layer of a conventional two-layer anastomosis. A technique using interrupted single-layer sutures has been associated with acceptable, and in some hands equivalent, results.

The techniques for staple anastomosis of the small intestine have been well defined by Steichen and Ravitch,[6] most frequently performed as a functional end-to-end anastomosis in which the GIA stapler is inserted into the two limbs of small intestine to be joined. After the stapler has been fired, laying down two rows of staples and cutting between, the open end is closed with a TA-55 instrument (Fig. 56-9). The staple line should be reinforced with several silk sutures. A functional end-to-end anastomosis can also be performed by initially clamping the two ends with a TA stapler and then either removing a segment of the staple line or making two small openings proximal to the staple line, inserting a GIA stapler, and establishing a stoma. The opening into which the GIA stapler has been inserted can then be closed either with sutures or with a TA stapler (Fig. 56-10). An end-to-end anastomosis can be made in the colon or the small intestine using an EEA stapler (Fig. 56-11).

Enteroenterostomy is achieved initially by securing two stay-sutures along the line of anastomosis and then insert-

Text continued on p. 934.

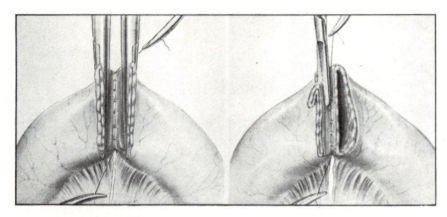

Fig. 56-6. Enterectomy followed by end-to-end anastomosis. (From Schwartz SI: *Intestinal resection and anastomosis*. In Schwartz SI, Ellis H, editors: *Maingot's abdominal operations,* ed 9, vol 1, East Norwalk, Conn, 1989, Appleton & Lange.)

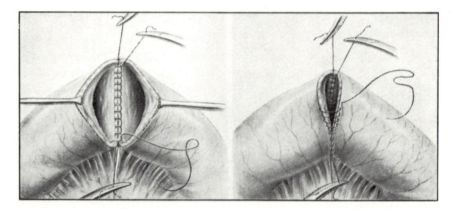

Fig. 56-7. Enterectomy followed by end-to-end anastomosis. (From Schwartz SI: *Intestinal resection and anastomosis*. In Schwartz SI, Ellis H, editors: *Maingot's abdominal operations,* ed 9, vol 1, East Norwalk, Conn, 1989, Appleton & Lange.)

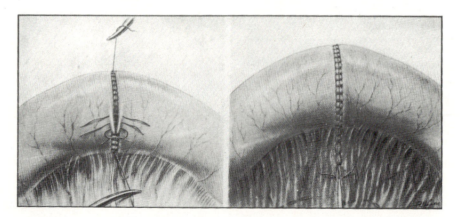

Fig. 56-8. Enterectomy with end-to-end anastomosis. Operation was completed by closing the defect in the mesentery. (From Schwartz SI: *Intestinal resection and anastomosis*. In Schwartz SI, Ellis H, editors: *Maingot's abdominal operations,* ed 9, vol 1, East Norwalk, Conn, 1989, Appleton & Lange.)

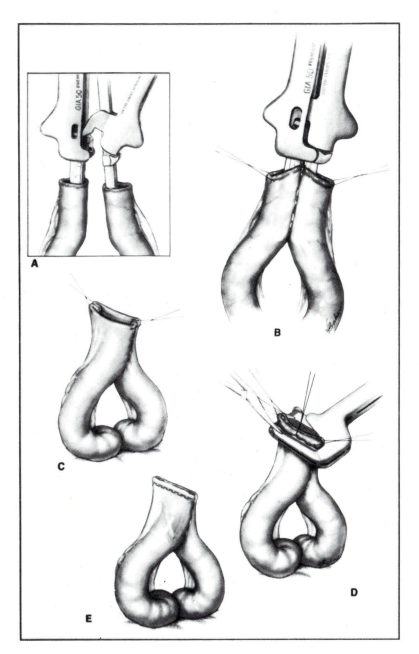

Fig. 56-9. Functional end-to-end anastomosis—wide V-mode. See text. (From Steichen FM, Ravitch MM: *Staplers in gastrointestinal surgery.* In Schwartz SI, Ellis H, editors: *Maingot's abdominal operations,* ed 9, vol 1, East Norwalk, Conn, 1989, Appleton & Lange.)

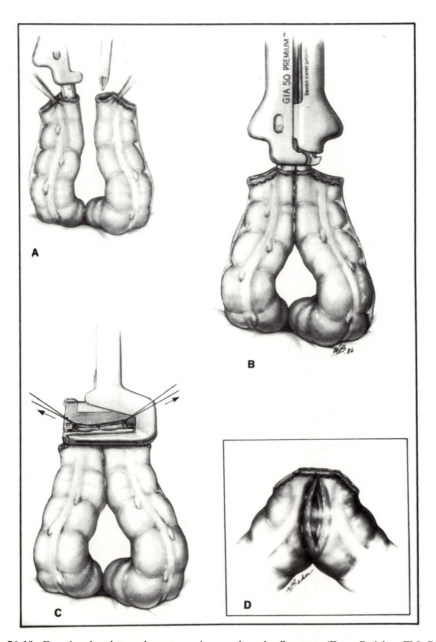

Fig. 56-10. Functional end-to-end anastomosis—oval mode. See text. (From Steichen FM, Ravitch MM: *Staplers in gastrointestinal surgery*. In Schwartz SI, Ellis H, editors: *Maingot's abdominal operations,* ed 9, vol 1, East Norwalk, Conn, 1989, Appleton & Lange.)

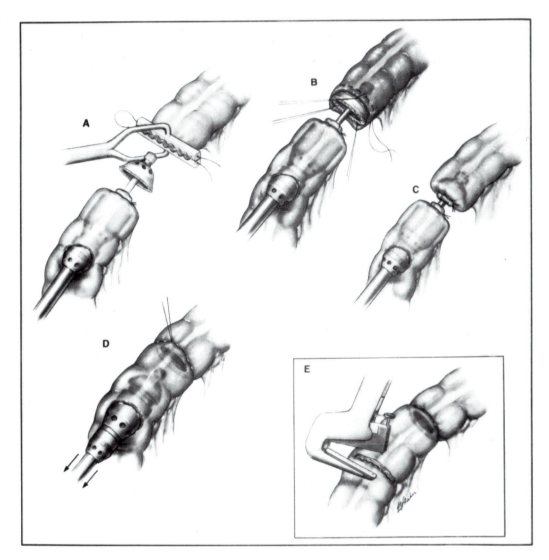

Fig. 56-11. End-to-end colocolostomy. See text. (From Steichen FM, Ravitch MM: *Staplers in gastrointestinal surgery.* In Schwartz SI, Ellis H, editors: *Maingot's abdominal operations,* ed 9, vol 1, East Norwalk, Conn, 1989, Appleton & Lange.)

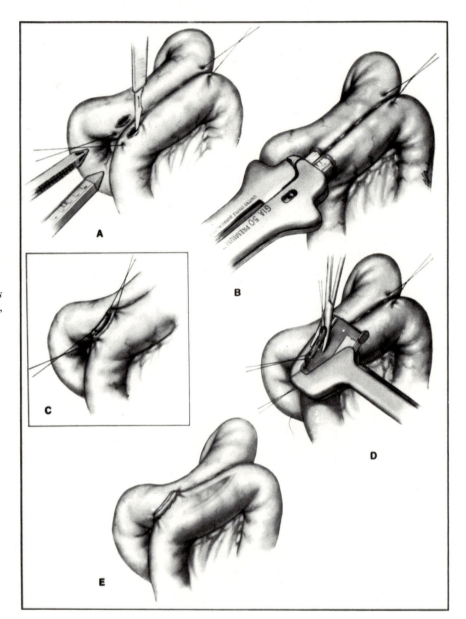

Fig. 56-12. Enteroenterostomy. See text. (From Steichen FM, Ravitch MM: *Staplers in gastrointestinal surgery.* In Schwartz SI, Ellis H, editors: *Maingot's abdominal operations,* ed 9, vol 1, East Norwalk, Conn, 1989, Appleton & Lange.)

ing the GIA stapler to achieve the anastomosis and closing the GIA stab wounds with a TA staple (Fig. 56-12).

After the creation of an anastomosis, using sutures or staples, a good lumen should be demonstrated by invaginating the two limbs of the intestine between thumb and index finger to define the large stoma. Following anastomosis, if there is a rent in the mesentery, it should be closed to obviate development of a internal hernia.

REFERENCES

1. Ellis H: *Acute intestinal obstruction.* In Schwartz SI, Ellis H, editors: *Maingot's abdominal operations,* ed 9, vol 1, East Norwalk, Conn, 1989, Appleton & Lange.
2. Ellis H: *Meckel's diverticulum, diverticulosis of the small intestine, umbilical fistulae and tumours.* In Schwartz SI, Ellis H, editors: *Maingot's abdominal operations,* ed 9, vol 1, East Norwalk, Conn, 1989, Appleton & Lange.
3. Leijonmarck CE et al: Meckel's diverticulum in the adult, *Br J Surg* 73:146, 1986.
4. Schwartz SI: *Intestinal resection and anastomosis,* In Schwartz SI, Ellis H, editors: *Maingot's abdominal operations,* ed 9, vol 1, East Norwalk, Conn, 1989, Appleton & Lange.
5. Schwartz SI: *Manifestations of gastrointestinal disease.* In Schwartz SI, Shires GT, Spencer F, editors: *Principles of surgery,* ed 5, New York, 1989, McGraw-Hill Publishing Co.
6. Steichen FM, Ravitch MM: *Stapling in surgery,* Chicago, 1984, Mosby–Year Book.
7. Townsend CM, Thompson JC: *Small intestine.* In Schwartz SI, Shires GT, Spencer F, editors: *Principles of surgery* ed 5, New York, 1989, McGraw-Hill Publishing Co.

Chapter 57

SURGERY OF THE COLON, INCIDENTAL TO GYNECOLOGIC SURGERY

Seymour I. Schwartz

PREOPERATIVE BOWEL PREPARATION

Unlike the small intestine, the colon contents have sufficient bacterial colonization that spillage is associated with a higher rate of intraperitoneal and wound infections. The colon and rectum cannot be sterilized, but the bacterial count can be sufficiently decreased to reduce the incidence of infection by a mechanical cleansing. The time-honored regimen of a 3-day course of a clear liquid diet, purgatives, and enemas generally has been replaced by whole gut lavage with polyethylene-glycol solution (Golytely or Colyte). The patient either drinks the solution or has it administered by way of a nasogastric tube at a rate of 250 ml every 10 minutes until the rectal effluent is clear. Because this process may take 3 to 10 hours, the regimen should be started the afternoon before the operation. Prophylactic antibiotics also have been shown to reduce the incidence of infection. Either a second-generation cephalosporin or the combination of metronidazole and a first-generation cephalosporin is equally effective. If the colonic lumen has not been traversed, there is no need to continue the medication postoperatively. If the lumen has been entered, a 3-day course of postoperative medicine is sufficient; a longer course increases the incidence of superinfection with *Clostridium difficile*.

COLONIC OBSTRUCTION
Mechanical obstruction

The mechanically obstructed colon cannot be prepared preoperatively. If obstruction of the descending or sigmoid colon is encountered intraoperatively, a colostomy should be created proximal to the point of obstruction and brought out through a separate incision. The obstructing lesion can be resected, and the colon distal to the lesion can be closed with a TA stapler and dropped back into the pelvis (Hartmann's procedure). Dudley and Phillips have advocated converting the distended colon into a nondistended state by intraoperative lavage. A catheter is inserted into the cecum, and, after the colon is transected proximal to the obstruction, warm Hartmann's solution is instilled by way of the catheter to cleanse the colon by allowing the effluent to be evacuated through a large tube tied into the end of transected end of the colon.

Colonic obstruction encountered intraoperatively by a gynecologist is most frequently related to diverticulitis or carcinoma. Endometriosis rarely causes complete colonic obstruction. The preferable management of any of these lesions is resection with proximal colostomy and creation of a Hartmann's pouch. If resection cannot be safely achieved because of the extent of the lesion or because of a surrounding inflammatory process that precludes identification of the major blood vessels in the area and the ureter, it is preferable to perform a double-barrel transverse colostomy as an initial procedure and plan to carry out a second operation weeks later at which time the offending lesion can be safely resected.

Ileus of the colon

Rarely, after a pelvic operation, marked distention has been noted, confined largely to the colon, without evidence of mechanical obstruction or vascular compromise. X-ray examination reveals dilation of the entire large bowel; the cecum shows the most pronounced dilation. If the cecum distends to the extent of compromising its vascular supply, perforation occurs. Barium enema defining the absence of mechanical obstruction establishes the diagnosis. The treatment is colonoscopy to decompress the colon. If this is not feasible and critical distention of the cecum evolves, cecostomy may be required.

IATROGENIC INJURY OF THE COLON

Penetrating wounds of the colon may occur during celiotomy procedures or during pelvic dissections. Seromuscular injuries without entrance into the lumen should be closed with an interrupted suture. Small primary wounds located on the antimesenteric border, in which there is minimal tissue destruction and peritoneal soilage, including those of the left colon, should be closed in two layers with interrupted sutures; antibiotic therapy should be initiated and maintained for 3 to 5 days. If there is significant tissue loss, devascularization, contamination, hypotension, or delay of treatment, simple closure is contraindicated. The therapeutic alternatives are proximal colostomy and drainage, primary repair and proximal colostomy, resection and colostomy with a mucous fistula, or creation of a Hartmann's pouch in the distal segment. Major wounds of the right colon can be managed, even in the unprepared bowel, by resection and ileotransverse colostomy.

COLONIC LESIONS DETECTED INTRAOPERATIVELY

Diverticular disease, ulcerative colitis, granulomatous colitis, or ischemic colitis might be unanticipated findings during a gynecologic procedure.

Diverticular disease

Diverticula of the colon are pulsion type in which there is herniation of the mucosa and the muscularis mucosa through the colonic muscle wall leaving outpouchings covered by serosa. Diverticulosis implies the presence of diverticula without inflammation. The condition is present in one third of people over 60 years old. Diverticula encountered during an operation should be noted, and the patient should be placed on a high-residue diet to avoid the complications of diverticular disease.

If an inspissated fecal plug obstructs the neck of a diverticulum, continued secretion of mucus and proliferation of bacteria can result in an inflammatory process known as diverticulitis. The initial spread is into the pericolic fat, resulting in a thickened segment of colon and mesocolon. If this is encountered intraoperatively in a patient with an unprepared colon, no surgical treatment should be performed. The patient should be placed on metronidazole and a first-generation cephalosporin for 3 to 5 days postoperatively. The inflammatory process might subside as a result of the conservative therapy, but a barium enema should be carried out after the patient has recovered. If the phlegmonous mass persists, elective resection of the involved segment with immediate anastomosis of the two ends to reestablish intestinal continuity is preferable.

The most common complication of diverticulitis is perforation. The following classification has been proposed for perforated diverticulitis:

1. *Stage I:* The abscess is confined by the mesocolon.
2. *Stage II:* There is a localized pelvic abscess that has extended beyond the colon and mesocolon. It may be walled off by the colon, mesocolon, omentum, small intestine, pelvic organs, and peritoneum.
3. *Stage III:* Generalized peritonitis due to rupture of the pericolonic abscess without gross communication between the peritoneal cavity and the lumen of the colon.
4. *Stage IV:* Fecal peritonitis with escape of feces from the colon into the free peritoneal cavity.

If stage I or II disease is encountered, the patient might respond to antibiotics and definitive operation postponed for 6 weeks at which time resection and anastomosis of prepared bowel can be performed. If the patient fails to improve, computed tomography (CT) guided percutaneous drainage of the abscess can be performed. Low pelvic abscesses may be drained transrectally by way of the cul-de-sac. One-stage elective resection can be carried out at a later date.

If the abscess cavity has been entered intraoperatively or if diffuse peritonitis with or without fecal contamination is encountered, the abscess should be drained and options for managing the offending segment of colon are available. If the inflammatory process is so extensive that it precludes safe dissection, a proximal transverse colostomy should be performed preemptive to an anticipated resection of the diseased colon about 8 weeks later. The transverse colostomy is closed at a third operation in the so-called three-stage approach. If, during the gynecologic operation, the offending colon is deemed resectable, resection should be carried out and preferably an end-to-end anastomosis performed; this should be protected by a proximal (transverse) colostomy, which is closed at a second procedure. An alternative is to resect the offending segment of colon and not anastomose the two ends but rather bring out an end-descending colostomy and close the distal segment (Hartmann's pouch; two stage approach).

The most common internal fistula associated with diverticular disease is the colovesical type. In women, it occurs less frequently because of the interposed uterus. This fistula may be manifested by urinary tract infection, pneumaturia, or fecaluria. Cystoscopy and barium enema might fail to reveal the fistula. Treatment consists of removal of the involved segment of sigmoid colon and closure of the opening into the bladder. Coloenteric fistulas generally require resection of the involved colon and segment of small intestine. The small intestinal continuity should be restored at the operation, and the options for management of the colon are the same as those presented for the management of diverticular perforation.

In all circumstances in which colonic resection is performed for diverticular disease, the extent of resection should be limited to the involved segment and about 5 cm proximal and distal to the inflammation. The distal resection often extends below the pelvic peritoneum because the rectum contains no diverticula. Uninflamed colon bearing diverticula proximally should not be resected. Diverticulitis rarely recurs in these proximal segments.

Ulcerative colitis and granulomatous colitis

Inflammation in ulcerative colitis is usually confined to the mucosa and submucosa. The serosal surface of the colon does not appear inflamed, but the wall may feel thickened and the bowel is foreshortened in long-standing cases. Ulcerative colitis encountered during a gynecologic operation should not be addressed intraoperatively. Similarly, granulomatous (Crohn's) colitis should not be resected in the course of a gynecologic procedure. The typical gross finding of granulomatous colitis is manifestation of its transmural involvement. The bowel wall may demonstrate skip areas of involvement; the regional lymph nodes are enlarged, and there is creeping of mesenteric fat around the bowel wall.

Ischemic colitis

Ischemic colitis occurs with or without major vascular occlusion. Most patients with ischemic colitis are in the older age group and have associated cardiovascular disease. If a vascularly compromised or ischemic segment of colon is encountered during gynecologic exploration for an acute abdomen, the entire segment of ischemic colon plus a generous margin of normal colon proximal and distal to the involvement should be resected. An end colostomy should be brought out through a separate incision, and the distal limb should be closed and positioned in the pelvis as a Hartmann's pouch.

TECHNIQUES

The colon can be anastomosed using suture or staple techniques. Colonic continuity can be established using two layers of suture (Fig. 57-1) or one layer (Fig. 57-2). Using staples, a functional end-to-end anastomosis can be performed using the TA and GIA devices. In the case of low colorectal anastomosis, the EEA stapler passed transanally can be used (Fig. 57-3).

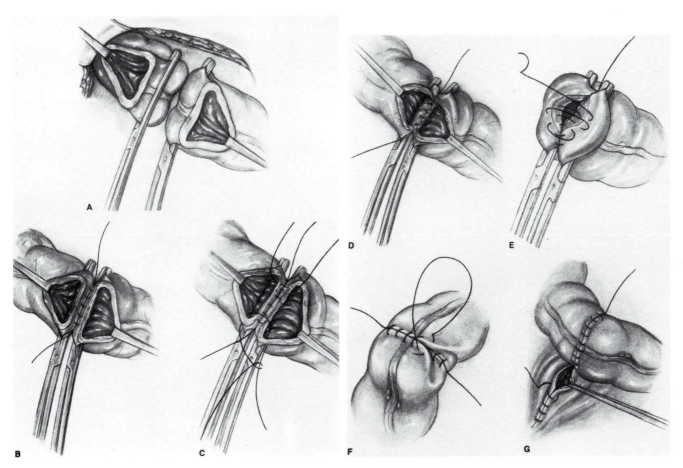

Fig. 57-1. Colectomy: the steps in the two-layer anastomosis. **A,** Mobilized bowel ends apposed in noncrushing clamps. **B,** Posterior serosal continuous layer. **C,** Posterior all-coats continuous layer. **D,** Corner is turned by means of a loop on the mucosa suture, and the anterior all-coats continuous layer is begun. **E,** Anterior layer is inserted. **F,** Anterior serosal layer is completed. **G,** Mesocolic defect is repaired. (From Ellis H: *Resection of the colon.* In Schwartz SI, Ellis H, editors: *Maingot's abdominal operations,* ed 9, East Norwalk, 1989, Appleton Lange.)

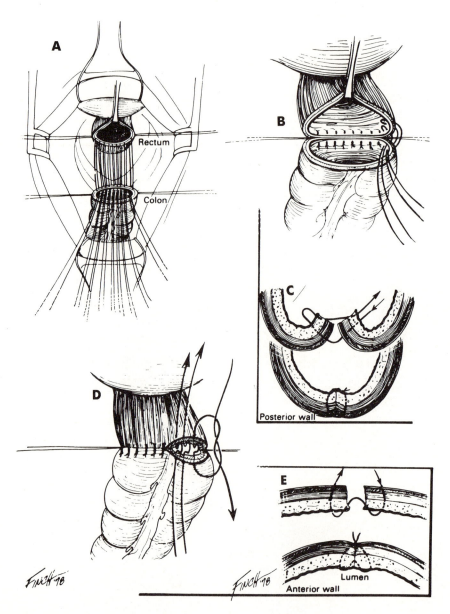

Fig. 57-2. Technique of handsewn one-layer anastomosis. **A,** Horizontal mattress sutures of 4-0 PDS placed in the posterior row. **B,** Sutures tied. **C,** Detail of suture placement in posterior row. **D,** Gambee's stitches in anterior row. **E,** Detail of suture placement in anterior row. (From Goldberg SM, Nivatvongs S, Rotherberger DA: *Colon, rectum, and anus.* In Schwartz SI, Shires GT, Spencer FC, editors: *Principles of surgery,* ed 5, New York, 1989, McGraw-Hill.)

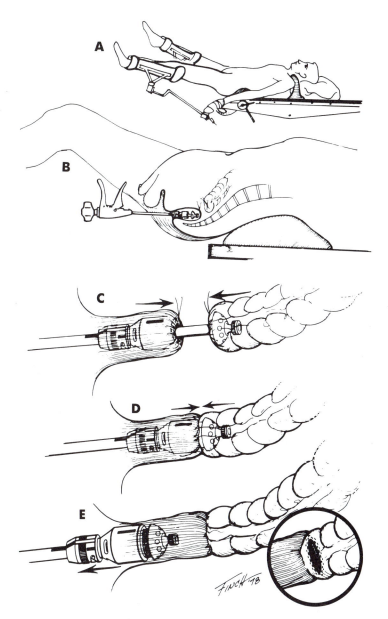

Fig. 57-3. Technique of anastomosis using EEA stapler. **A,** Patient's legs put in stirrups for exposure of perineum. **B,** Insertion of EEA stapler into rectal stump. **C,** Purse-string suture of 2-0 prolene on rectum tied over cartridge on the shaft. Purse-string suture on the colon tied over the anvil. **D,** Anvil brought down to meet cartridge. **E,** Staple gun fired and withdrawn. (From Goldberg SM, Nivatvongs S, Rothenberger DA: *Colon, rectum, and anus.* In Schwartz SI, Shires GT, Spencer FC, editors: *Principles of surgery,* ed 5, New York, 1989, McGraw-Hill.)

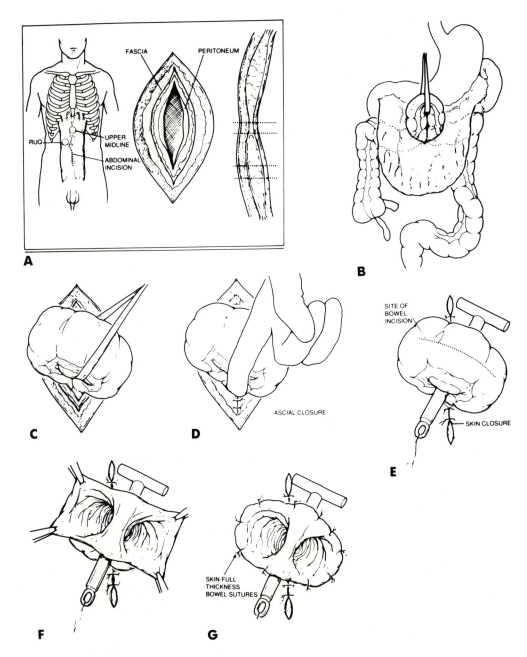

Fig. 57-4. Construction of a loop-transverse colostomy. **A,** Choice of stoma's location. **B,C,** Tracheostomy tape is used to pull the loop of colon through the incision. **D,** The fascia is closed tightly around the loop of intestine. **E-G,** The loop of colon is opened over a supporting rod and is sutured to the skin of the abdominal wall. (From Kodner IJ, Fleshman JW, Fry RD: *Intestinal stomas.* In Schwartz SI, Ellis H, editors: *Maingot's abdominal operations,* ed 9, East Norwalk, 1989, Appleton Lange.)

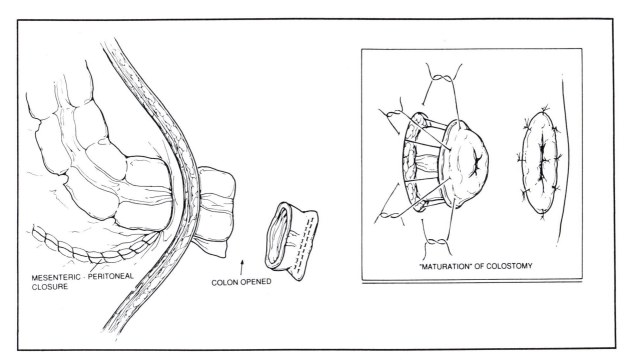

Fig. 57-5. Final stages of constructing a "mature" end colostomy. (From Kodner IJ, Fleshman JW, Fry RD: *Intestinal stomas*. In Schwartz SI, Ellis H, editors: *Maingot's abdominal operations*, ed 9, East Norwalk, 1989, Appleton Lange.)

For the first part of the three-stage procedure for an obstructing or nonresectable descending colon lesion, a loop transverse colostomy can be performed rapidly (Fig. 57-4). The end-descending colostomy should be brought out through a separate incision (Fig. 57-5) planned to permit convenient application of a colostomy bag.

APPENDIX
Normal appendix

The appendix can occupy various positions (Fig. 57-6). It is readily located by tracing the teniae of the colon to their termination. It is generally believed that a normal appendix should not be removed during the course of a pelvic procedure because there is an increased potential for intraperitoneal contamination.

Acute appendicitis

Acute appendicitis should be considered in the differential diagnosis of all patients with abdominal pain, particularly caudad to the level of the umbilicus. The pain is classically located at McBurney's point, but may be to the left of the midline if there is congenital lack of fixation of the ascending colon. The location of pain and point tenderness changes during pregnancy (Fig. 57-7).

If an acutely inflamed appendix is encountered, it should be removed by the purse-string method (Fig. 57-8) or simply by ligating the crushed area of the stump. If an inflammatory mass is encountered in the region of the ap-

pendix, it usually represents a walled-off perforation. The appendix should be removed, if possible. If an abscess is entered, an attempt should be made to remove the appendix, and the abscess should be drained through a stab wound. If the appendix cannot be readily located, drainage should be established, and an interval appendectomy should be performed 2 months later. A short course of metronidazole and a first-generation cephalosporin should be instituted intraoperatively.

Tumors

Carcinoid tumors are the most common tumor of the appendix. They are typically less than 1 cm in diameter, firm, circumscribed, and yellowish-brown. Three quarters of appendiceal carcinoid tumors occur in the distal third. Simple appendectomy with excision of the mesoappendix is adequate treatment unless invasion beyond the line of resection or nodal metastases is noted, in which case, right colectomy and ileotransverse colostomy are indicated. Adenocarcinoma of the appendix is also indication for a right colectomy. Mucocele of the appendix is a cystic dilatation containing mucoid material. Most mucoceles are benign, but there is a rare malignant lesion, mucous papillary carcinoma, which can be difficult to distinguish grossly. Appendectomy is indicated, and care should be taken to avoid rupture because of the potential consequence of pseudomyxoma peritonei. Some of the surgical aspects of appendectomy are considered and discussed more fully in Chapter 55.

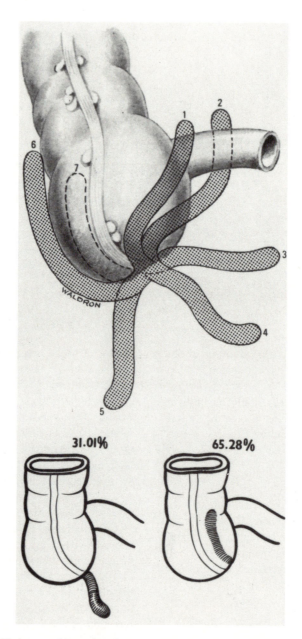

Fig. 57-6. *Top:* Various positions that the appendix can occupy: (1) preileal; (2) postileal; (3) promontoric; (4) pelvic; (5) subcecal; (6) paracolic or prececal; (7) retrocecal. *Bottom left:* Location of the appendix in Wakelely's series of 10,000 cases (pelvic or descending position). *Bottom right:* Location of the appendix in Wakeley's series of 10,000 cases (postcecal and retrocecal). (From Ellis H: *Appendix.* In Schwartz SI, Ellis H, editors: *Maingot's abdominal operations*, ed 9, East Norwalk, 1989, Appleton Lange.)

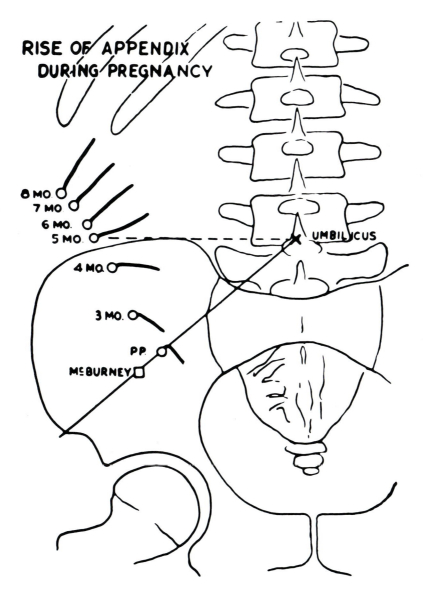

Fig. 57-7. Changes in position and direction of appendix during pregnancy. (From Schwartz SI: *Appendix.* In Schwartz SI, Shires GT, Spencer FC, editors: *Principles of surgery,* ed 5, New York, 1989, McGraw-Hill.)

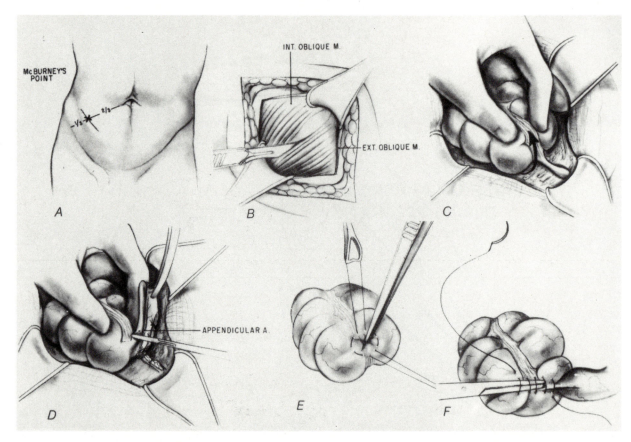

Fig. 57-8. Appendectomy. (From Schwartz SI: *Appendix*. In Schwartz SI, Shires GT, Spencer FC, editors: *Principles of surgery*, ed 5, New York, 1989, McGraw-Hill.)

BIBLIOGRAPHY
Colon

Dudley H, Phillips R: *Intra-operative techniques in large bowel obstruction: methods of management with bowel resection.* In Fielding LP, Welch J, editors: *Intestinal obstruction,* Edinburgh, 1987, Churchill Livingstone.

Ellis H: *Resection of the colon.* In Schwartz SI, Ellis H, editors: *Maingot's abdominal operations,* ed 9, East Norwalk, 1989, Appleton Lange.

Morton JH, Schwartz SI: Ileus of the colon: a complication in obstetrics and gynecology, *Prog Gynecol* 4:637, 1963.

Parks TG: *Diverticular disease of the colon.* In Schwartz SI, Ellis H, editors: *Maingot's abdominal operations,* ed 9, East Norwalk, 1989, Appleton Lange.

Slater G, Aufses AH Jr: *Granulomatous colitis and ulcerative colitis.* In Schwartz SI, Ellis H, editors: *Maingot's abdominal operations,* ed 9, East Norwalk, 1989, Appleton Lange.

Steichen FM, Ravitch MM: *Stapling in surgery.* Chicago, 1984, Mosby–Year Book.

Appendix

Anderson JR, Wilson BG: Carcinoid tumours of the appendix, *Br J Surg* 72:545, 1985.

Bower RJ, Bell MJ, Ternberg JL: Controversial aspects of appendicitis management in children, *Arch Surg* 116:885, 1981.

Doberneck RC: Appendectomy during pregnancy, *Am Surg* 51:265, 1985.

Engstrom L, Fenyo G: Appendicectomy: assessment of stump invagination versus simple ligation—a prospective randomized study, *Br J Surg* 72:971, 1985.

Svendsen LB, Bulor S: Carcinoid tumours of the appendix in young patients, *Acta Chir Scand* 146:137, 1980.

Schwartz SI: *Appendix.* In Schwartz SI, Shires GT, Spencer FC, editors: *Principles of surgery,* ed 5, New York, 1989, McGraw-Hill.

Wakeley CP: The position of the vermiform appendix as ascertained by an analysis of 10,000 cases, *J Anat* 67:277, 1933.

Part IX

OPERATIONS UPON THE BREAST

Chapter 58

BREAST BIOPSY

Douglas J. Marchant

There has been a dramatic change in the role of the obstetrician/gynecologist in the diagnosis and treatment of breast diseases. In 1985, the American Board of Obstetrics and Gynecology indicated that a knowledge of breast disease would be required for certification, and, in May 1986, a Consensus Meeting was held in Chicago to discuss the implications of this new position.[2] As a result of this meeting, the American Board recommended that the obstetrician/gynecologist have a knowledge of the embryology, anatomy, and physiology of the breast and be able to provide adequate information concerning screening and to perform simple diagnostic studies including aspiration of cysts, fine needle aspiration (FNA), and appropriate follow-up for patients treated for breast cancer. Because open biopsy often becomes part of the treatment for breast cancer, the Board stopped short of recommending that *every* obstetrician/gynecologist perform this procedure. It is anticipated that as training programs are established and the parameters for conservative treatment are more clearly defined, appropriately trained gynecologists may participate in the treatment of breast cancer. This will require additional surgical training and close collaboration with the cytopathologist, radiotherapist, and medical oncologist.

The American College of Obstetricians and Gynecologists has published a number of position papers dealing with breast disease and breast cancer, and, in the fall of 1990, the Jacob's Institute, a nonprofit organization founded by the American College, released the results of a study that evaluated the use of mammography in the United States.[7] This survey showed that 64% of women age 40 and older had at least one mammogram—an increase from 37% noted in 1987. However, only 31% of American women followed the recommended guidelines for mammograms beginning at age 40. Nearly three quarters of all women who obtained mammograms did so because their doctors recommended it, but almost half (45%) of the women who had never had a mammogram said that

their doctor had not recommended it. Additional statistics on women's attitudes concerning mammography revealed that:

1. Forty percent of women who had never had a mammogram stated that no one in their family had breast cancer—in spite of the fact that it has been noted by the American Cancer Society that 80% of women who get breast cancer have none of the usual risk factors.
2. One third of women who had only one mammogram did not *believe* that it was necessary to have a second mammogram if the first one was negative. Clearly, it is important that a mammogram be obtained on a regular basis as determined by physical examination and the recommended guidelines.
3. Women 65 years of age and older are the least likely to get mammograms. Only 24% follow the published guidelines.

As a result of this survey, a workshop was held by the American College of Obstetricians and Gynecologists in September 1990, and a number of recommendations were suggested.

1. The only proven tool to reduce mortality from breast cancer is periodic screening mammography.
2. Mammography is the only method of detecting lesions that are not palpable at a time when curability is over 90%.
3. Mammography is safe and effective with a highly favorable risk/benefit ratio.

It was also suggested that organizations representing primary care providers, particularly obstetricians and gynecologists, remind their membership of the current screening guidelines and disseminate information to back up these guidelines. This should include review articles in their professional journals. Special attention should be focused on the increased rate of breast cancer and the higher mortality among black women, particularly those under the age of 50. It was also suggested that the American College of Radiology (ACR) clarify the standard definition of a *screening* mammogram as distinguished from the diagnostic examination.

As a follow-up, it was suggested that the Jacob's Institute formally request the National Institutes of Health (NIH) Office of Women's Health to make breast cancer a high priority, especially emphasizing the importance of screening mammography. In addition to publishing the proceedings of this workshop, it was recommended that the Jacob's Institute submit an article or an editorial to the *Journal of the American Medical Association* (JAMA) for wider dissemination of this information.

On October 18, 1990, a special meeting of the American College of Obstetricians and Gynecologists Committee on Gynecologic Practice was held to address the lack of national standards to evaluate training in breast surgery.

At the request of the College, I prepared a statement concerning the role of the obstetrician/gynecologist in the diagnosis of breast disease and the training required to perform breast surgery. One of my concerns continues to be the definition of "adequate training for breast surgery." My comments presented to the Committee are as follows:

I am concerned about who should be eligible for this training and under what conditions the obstetrician/gynecologist be permitted to practice surgery related to the breast.

There is no question that the breast is an organ of reproduction and that the diagnosis and treatment of breast disease is within the responsibility of gynecologic practice as noted both by the American Board and the American College of Obstetricians and Gynecologists. The American Board has deliberately stopped short of recommending or suggesting training for major surgical procedures involving the breast because it was felt by a number of observers that the obstetrician/gynecologist should become involved in the diagnosis and treatment of breast disease in a stepwise fashion. As this concept is developed, consideration should be given to structuring residency programs to include such training and eventually outlining the surgical training required both for breast biopsy and the contemporary treatment of breast cancer.

To immediately announce to our colleagues in general surgery, and radiation and medical oncology that the obstetrician/gynecologist should manage breast cancer including the surgical treatment seemed inappropriate. It was realized, however, that at some point, steps should be taken to outline surgical training and the conditions for which such surgical training and practice would be appropriate. There are several issues involved, not the least of which is the multifaceted nature of the current practice of obstetrics and gynecology. In my opinion, while the proper examination of the breast is essential to the practice of good obstetrics and gynecology, and a knowledge of breast disease including breast cancer is necessary to advise patients and request appropriate referral, I do not believe that *every* obstetrician/gynecologist should proceed beyond simple diagnostic studies including breast examination, aspiration of cysts or fine needle aspiration when appropriate cytologic evaluation is available.

In 1965, I first began discussing these issues with the American College of Obstetricians and Gynecologists. At this time the management of breast cancer was a simple matter. Mammography had not yet been introduced, at least not on a widescale basis and there was only one treatment for breast cancer and that was radical mastectomy. Now, the situation is quite different. Mammography as a screening procedure is performed on a regular basis, frequently with the discovery of the occult lesion, and alternative treatments for breast cancer are available. Breast cancer is no longer a simple surgical problem. Appropriate treatment requires a multidisciplinary approach including the expertise not only of the surgical specialist but the medical oncologist, the radiation oncologist and, in many cases, the services of a well trained plastic surgeon. It must be understood that open biopsy often becomes part of the definitive treatment for breast cancer. In the past, a biopsy performed in any area of the breast and even one associated with local complications did not compromise the total treatment of breast cancer since the entire breast would be removed.

There is no lesion that is obviously benign, and every biopsy must be considered to be a cancer and appropriately handled by the pathologist. This means requesting immediate frozen section to determine whether cancer is present and, if so, the determination of estrogen and progesterone receptor values and the appropriate marking of the margins to facilitate discussion concerning conservative versus radical treatment.

Breast biopsy must be considered a plastic procedure, and the surgeon must be appropriately trained in tissue handling and the requirements of cosmetic surgery. The procedure is not difficult, but it must be practiced repetitively to produce satisfactory results. In terms of the definitive surgical procedures for breast cancer, the same philosophy applies. The radical mastectomy is no longer appropriate, and, in my opinion, the modified radical mastectomy is a more difficult procedure since there is less exposure when performing the lymph node dissection. Conservative management is even more difficult. The incisions must be carefully chosen and the surgery meticulously performed in accordance with the recommendations of the radiation therapist.

The position of the Board could be interpreted to indicate that *every* obstetrician/gynecologist should proceed with an open biopsy and surgical treatment, the only requirement being "approved surgical training." This is not the position of the Board nor the College, furthermore, in the average practice, breast cancer would occur so infrequently that the value of special training and skill so acquired soon would be lost. In dealing with this disease on a daily basis, it is my firm belief that the patient is best served by obtaining treatment from a multidisciplinary center with a sufficient volume to maintain a high level of surgical skill and appropriate interaction among the various disciplines associated with the treatment. This means that those obstetricians and gynecologists who wish to devote a significant amount of their practice to the diagnosis and treatment of breast disease should avail themselves of an approved training program and join their surgical colleagues as part of the multidisciplinary team in the diagnosis and treatment of this disease.

Since January of 1991, screening mammography subject to frequency limitations, quality standards, and special payment rules, is covered by Medicare, so a number of these recommendations are of interest to the primary care physician.[3] It is clear from a review of these rules that the Health Care Financing Administration (HCFA) is interested in quality control. Quality control as described in these rules concerns equipment and personnel. The equipment must be specifically designed for mammography. The rules also deal extensively with the training of the personnel who administer the procedure, the precautions to be taken for safety, and the qualifications and training of the personnel interpreting the mammogram. It is understood that the person interpreting the mammogram will be a *radiologist,* and the rules go into some detail to describe the training and qualifications of these individuals. It has also been noted by HCFA that

Medicare entitled women might not have a mammogram because they were unwilling to take the time or because the service was not readily available on site during their medical visit, i.e., a gynecologic examination. Of potential concern in this context is the use of primary care physicians as suppliers of mammographic services. For example, taking the x-ray, attendant to manual examination of the breast or during a gynecologic examination with the use of a radiologic technician who may not have received formal education meeting the standards which have been approved.

The implications of these HCFA rules and the findings of the Jacob's Institute-National Cancer Institute (NCI) survey will significantly affect the practice of obstetrics and gynecology. There will be increasing pressure to provide free-standing mammographic units, and an increase in screening will ultimately result in the diagnosis of more occult lesions. This chapter discusses diagnostic procedures that may be appropriately performed by the obstetrician/gynecologist.

MAKING THE DIAGNOSIS

The diagnosis begins with a careful history and physical examination. It is important that the physician note the chief complaint including the date of onset. A thorough physical examination should be performed with the patient in both the sitting and the supine positions. Regrettably, a number of the current textbooks still discuss breast findings in terms of a mass, ulceration, erythema, edema, retraction, and other signs that indicate advanced disease. It should be remembered that a cancer 1 cm in size, with the average doubling time, has been present for at least 7 or 8 years, ample time for the establishment of metastases. Therefore, we must search for subtle changes that suggest smaller or (earlier) cancers for which conservative treatment may be appropriate. The most important feature of the physical examination of the breast is the time spent during the examination, not the examination technique.

If a dominant mass is felt, it must be resolved within a reasonable time frame. There is no lesion that is obviously benign. Resolution includes reexamination during the menstrual cycle, appropriate additional diagnostic studies, or referral.

In my opinion, an attempt should be made to aspirate every dominant mass, the single exception being the obvious cancer for which fine needle aspiration (FNA), as discussed in the following pages, is the appropriate proce-

dure. It is a mistake to assume that because a mass is firm, mobile, and nontender it represents a fibroadenoma. I have seen a number of macrocysts from 5 mm to 2 cm in diameter that had all the hallmarks of a solid lesion. They were firm, they were nontender, and they were quite mobile, but all were cysts.

Aspiration is a simple procedure that does not require special equipment—only a plastic 10-ml syringe and a 23-gauge needle. The mass is stabilized as shown in Fig. 58-1, *A* through *C,* and the area over the mass is wiped with an alcohol sponge. Without the use of local anesthesia, the needle is quickly plunged into the mass. It is important to attempt to gauge the size of the mass so the needle actually penetrates the cyst but does not pass through the opposite wall. This is particularly true in very small masses. The fluid is withdrawn until the mass has completely disappeared (Fig. 58-1, *D, E*). An adhesive bandage is placed over the site.

It is important to note the exact location and size of the cyst and the date the aspiration was performed. With rare exceptions, the patient should be requested to return in 1 month to reevaluate this area. If the mass returns, one must be suspicious of a carcinoma and open biopsy is recommended. There are exceptions to this rule. It is almost impossible to aspirate completely a large (3 to 4 cm) cyst. The wall becomes quite flaccid, and, inevitably, a few milliliters remain. Reexamination in a month often reveals a mass that can be completely emptied, and follow-up can again be recommended in 1 month.

Not every macrocyst requires aspiration. Often a mammogram reveals asymmetric densities that on ultrasound prove to be multiple macrocysts. Many of these are nonpalpable. All that is required is a repeat mammogram or ultrasound to assess the stability of these lesions.

Should the aspirated fluid be sent to cytology? From a practical standpoint, no. The incidence of intracystic cancer is approximately one in 100,000. However, if the fluid is bloody or if the patient is in her late reproductive years without a longtitudinal history, it is probably wise to submit the fluid for cytologic evaluation.

FINE NEEDLE ASPIRATION

Fine needle aspiration (FNA) is not difficult, although certain precautions must be taken.[7] First, there must be a dominant mass. It is important for the surgeon to determine if there is a cytopathologist available to interpret the aspirate. The material obtained, in essence, is "tissue juice," and it is a cytologic not a tissue diagnosis. Even the best aspiration technique is useless unless the cytopathologist is capable of providing an accurate diagnosis.

In my opinion, special equipment is not required. It is important that the needle be of a small calibre, 23 to 25 gauge. It is a mistake to use a larger needle because the negative pressure available becomes much less and the specimen is often inadequate. Occasionally, the uninformed physician confuses FNA with a "core" needle biopsy in which a large diameter needle is employed and a

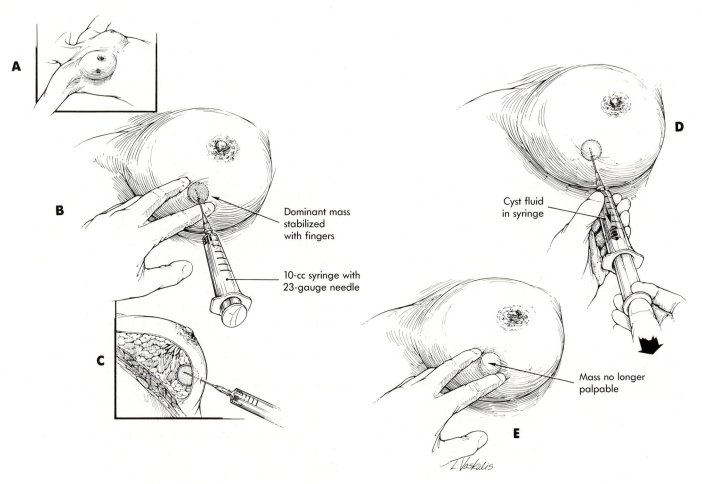

Fig. 58-1. Aspiration of cyst. **A,** Mass palpated and skin wiped with alcohol sponge. **B** and **C,** Needle penetrates cyst without passing through opposite wall. (No local anesthesia is necessary.) **D** and **E,** Fluid is withdrawn until mass disappears.

tissue sample is obtained. This type of biopsy is discouraged because often it is associated with hematoma formation, which may interfere with additional diagnostic studies and the conservative approach to treatment for breast cancer.

Because multiple "passes" must be made with the needle, it is wise to employ local anesthesia. We use 1% lidocaine without adrenaline. A small wheal is made, and the mass is immobilized with the fingers as shown in Fig. 58-2, *A* through *C*. A 10-ml syringe with a 25-gauge needle is used. It is important to test the needle before it is inserted into the breast. The needle is inserted into the breast, and suction is applied as the needle is withdrawn and replaced in a repetitive manner to cover a defined area of the lesion (Fig. 58-2, *D, E*). It is very important that the "tissue juice" not enter the syringe. It should remain in the needle. As the needle is withdrawn, the suction is released, and the material is spread on a slide and processed according to the recommendations of the cytopathologist (Fig. 58-3). In our Breast Health Center, the pathologist is present and immediately determines whether enough material has been obtained. If not, additional samples are re-

quested. As many as three or four samples may be required. In some cases, syringes are rinsed with saline and processed later using a millipore filter to obtain additional cellular detail.

Consultation between the physician and the pathologist is essential. Can the surgeon rely on FNA to proceed with definitive treatment? If an unequivocal diagnosis of carcinoma is made, the surgeon may, in my opinion, proceed directly with the definitive surgical procedure. If there is any question, an open biopsy should be obtained as part of the surgical management. This requires consultation with the pathologist and a review of the slides. FNA, in my opinion, is useful only if positive. A negative result, because of the high percentage of false negatives, is suspect.

OPEN BIOPSY

Open biopsy often becomes part of the definitive treatment for breast cancer. In the past, the choice of the incision was unimportant because, if cancer was diagnosed, a radical mastectomy would be performed. With the advent of conservative management, the placement of the incision is crucial, and the appearance of the wound may influence

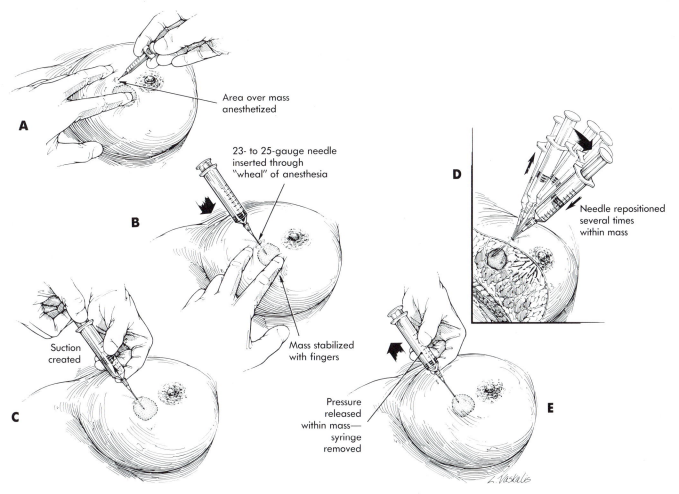

Fig. 58-2. Fine needle aspiration (FNA). **A,** Mass located. Local anesthesia (1% xylocaine without adrenalin) applied. **B,** Mass stabilized and needle inserted. **C,** Suction created as needle is withdrawn. **D,** Needle repositioned several times. **E,** Suction released as needle is withdrawn.

the timing and even the feasibility of conservative treatment.

Once the decision has been made to perform an open biopsy, the surgeon should discuss with the patient the type of anesthesia to be used and the immediate outcome of the biopsy procedure. With rare exception, almost all breast biopsies can be performed under local anesthesia. I have three exceptions. First, a teenager often is terrified with the operating room setting and the use of any type of needle. In this situation, we proceed with an open biopsy on a day surgery basis under general anesthesia. In some cases, local anesthesia is no problem, but this should be discussed both with the patient and her parents. Second, patients with a language barrier are not ideally suited for local anesthesia. It is a frightening experience to be unable to understand the conversation in the operating room and, for these patients, unless an interpreter is available, we proceed on a day surgery basis with general anesthesia. The final group of patients who are best operated on under general anesthesia are those with very large breasts and le-

sions deep within the breast for which extensive exposure is required to reach the lesion.

It is essential that breast biopsy be performed in an operating room setting with nurses familiar with the technique. Conversation must be kept to a minimum and appropriate to the procedure being performed. In our Day Surgery Center, the draping is such that the patient is unable to watch the procedure (although, if the patient looks directly at the reflection in the operating room light, a portion of the procedure can be seen).

It is important to examine the patient immediately before she is brought into the operating room. Occasionally, a mass that had been noted is no longer present, and, of course, in this situation, the procedure is canceled.

I mark my incisions with the patient in the sitting position. The patient is brought into the operating room and placed in the supine position with the arm extended. The breast is carefully prepared. We use a Betadine preparation, but almost any standard operating room preparation can be used. It is important to include the nipple in the

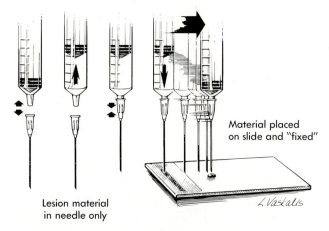

Material placed
on slide and "fixed"

Lesion material
in needle only

L. Vaslalis

Fig. 58-3. FNA being readied for processing. Note "tissue juice" remains in needle and does not enter syringe.

Equipment required for open biopsy procedure	
Equipment	**Sutures**
Mayo stand	3-0, 4-0 plain ties
Prep table	3-0, 4-0 chromic ties
2 arm boards	4-0 plain sutures
Bovie	4-0, 5-0 Nylon sutures
Drapes	
Chux	**Instruments**
Sponges	Small snaps—curved
"Fluffs"	and straight
Telfa	2 Allis clamps
6-in Ace bandage	2 small rake retractors
2-in silk tape	2 skin hooks
Specimen cup	1 curved Mayo scissors
1% lidocaine without	1 small Metzenbaum
adrenaline	scissors
0.25% bupivacaine with-	Knife handle and #15
out adrenaline	blades
Marking pencil and ruler	Small right-angle retrac-
Suction (poole or plas-	tors
tic)	

draped area for orientation. When the draping is complete, the Mayo tray with the appropriate instruments is brought over to the patient. The instruments most commonly used are listed in the box at right.

It is important to explain to the patient that she will be told what is going to happen during the procedure, not in technical terms, but, for example, before the breast is touched or the needle for local anesthesia is inserted into the skin. For local anesthesia, we use 1% lidocaine without adrenaline. I believe it is important to identify any bleeding immediately, and, because I do not use a drain, the wound must be absolutely dry before closure. The previously marked incision is infiltrated, noting the amount of anesthesia used (Fig. 58-4, *A, B*). While the local anesthesia is diffusing into the tissue, this is a good time to prepare the sutures and be certain that the Mayo tray contains all of the instruments required for the procedure. This delay has another practical application. For small lesions, the introduction of the local anesthesia often obscures the anatomy and the lesion no longer can be palpated.

The incision is made (Fig. 58-4, *C*). I use a #15 blade. Bleeding is controlled with fine 4-0 plain catgut ligatures. I do not use the actual cautery near the surface nor during the excision of the specimen, but this is a matter of personal preference. Bleeding is controlled during the dissection with appropriate hemostats and fine catgut ligatures (Fig. 58-4, *D*). Retraction is provided using either skin hooks or very small rake retractors. Every effort should be made not to damage the skin edges. To provide appropriate exposure, an assistant is essential. This may be a nurse or another physician.

The patient is instructed to indicate if she has any discomfort during the procedure. It is essential that a minimal amount of normal tissue be removed. Most of the lesions are benign, and, if a cancer is present, in most cases, this will be obvious. It is inappropriate to insert large Allis clamps to elevate tissue into the incision and blindly excise the breast tissue. Instead, the lesion should be directly identified. At this point, a suture of plain or chromic cat-

gut can be placed into the lesion, and the lesion can be elevated into the incision (Fig. 58-4, *E*). The lesion is easily excised by sharp dissection, and the bleeding points are clamped and ligated. The lesion is passed to the nurse and submitted to pathology for frozen section analysis. This is important because even the most benign-appearing lesion may contain cancer for which estrogen and progesterone receptors and the marking of margins are essential in the treatment planning process.

Once the lesion has been removed, the wound is inspected for hemostasis. It is at this point, particularly in the young patient with very dense breast tissue, that use of the actual cautery is appropriate. Small bleeding points can be cauterized. The major vessels, however, are ligated with fine plain catgut. When the wound is dry, the breast tissue is *loosely* reapproximated with 4-0 plain catgut (Fig. 58-4, *F*). No attempt is made to obliterate the cavity completely. The skin is closed with vertical mattress sutures of fine nylon (Fig. 58-4, *G*). No drain is employed. A close-up view of the skin closure is shown in Fig. 58-4, *H*. It is important that the sutures are placed evenly along the incision line and that the most superficial suture barely grasps the dermis. In this way, a cosmetic closure is achieved. The sutures should be removed in 5 to 7 days.

The most important part of this procedure is the placement of the pressure dressing. Once the skin has been closed, additional lidocaine without adrenaline is injected into the incision, and Telfa and a pressure dressing are applied directly over the incision and secured with a 6-inch Ace bandage for 48 hours (Fig. 58-4, *I, J*). The use of the pressure dressing immobilizes the breast, reduces discom-

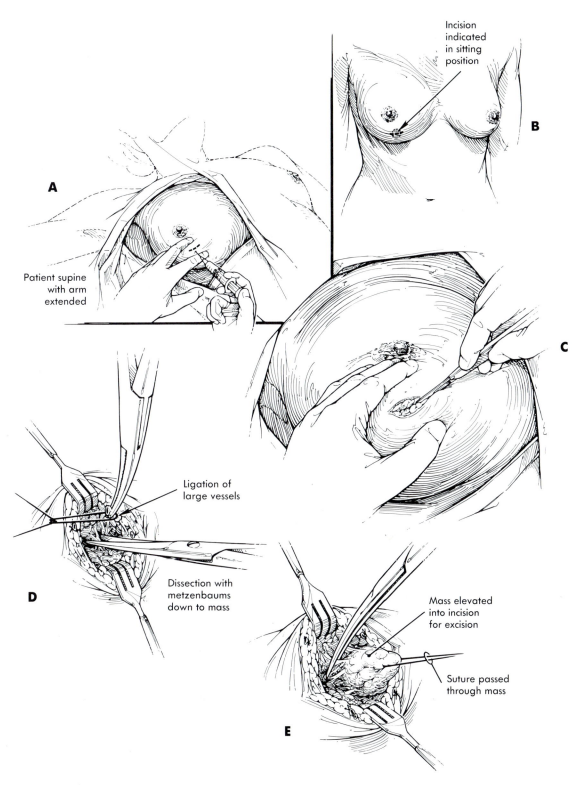

Fig. 58-4. Open breast biopsy. **A,** Incision marked while patient in sitting position. **B,** Patient now in supine position. Breast has been prepared and local anesthesia (1% xylocaine without adrenalin) administered. **C,** Incision made. **D,** Large vessels ligated and dissection proceeds. **E,** Suture placed into lesion and mass elevated into incision for excision.

Continued.

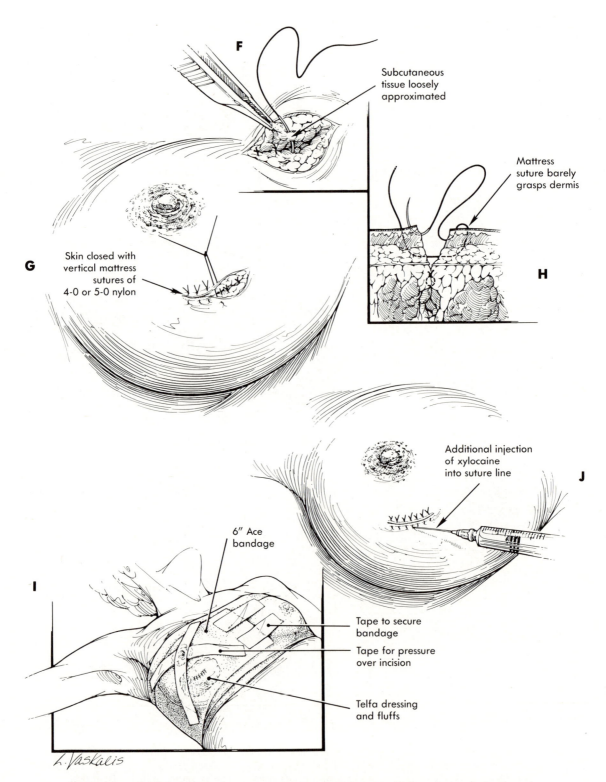

F

Subcutaneous
tissue loosely
approximated

Mattress
suture barely
grasps dermis

G

Skin closed with
vertical mattress
sutures of
4-0 or 5-0 nylon

H

Additional injection
of xylocaine
into suture line

J

I

6" Ace
bandage

Tape to secure
bandage

Tape for pressure
over incision

Telfa dressing
and fluffs

L. Vaskalis

Fig. 58-4, cont'd. F, Breast tissue loosely reapproximated. **G** and **H,** Skin closed with vertical mattress sutures. **I** and **J,** Additional local anesthesia injected and pressure dressing applied.

fort, and prevents ecchymosis and induration. The latter is essential if reexcision is required at a later date as part of the definitive surgical procedure for breast cancer.

Using this technique, we have not found it necessary to administer narcotics. The patient is simply told to take Tylenol and to begin normal activities once the dressing has been removed. We do not use prophylactic antibiotics.

LOCALIZATION AND BIOPSY

With the introduction of screening mammography, the discovery of an occult lesion is an increasing possibility. These include microcalcifications and the asymmetric density. The decision to perform a biopsy is the responsibility of the radiologist.[4-6,8] These patients have no symptomatology, and the physical examination is entirely negative. In my opinion, the handling of the occult lesion is one of the most difficult aspects of the diagnosis and treatment of breast disease. A number of patients have been referred to our Breast Health Center with an "abnormal" mammogram, and this has resulted in considerable anxiety for the patient and her family. When we have received the films, in many cases, the lesion is of no consequence and follow-up films to assess stability are all that are required.

When we see a patient with an abnormal mammogram (i.e., microcalcifications or an asymmetric density), there are three possibilities.

1. Additional studies are required to clarify the situation. This may include an additional mammogram with special views or an ultrasound.
2. Follow-up films in 4 to 6 months to assess stability
3. Localization and biopsy

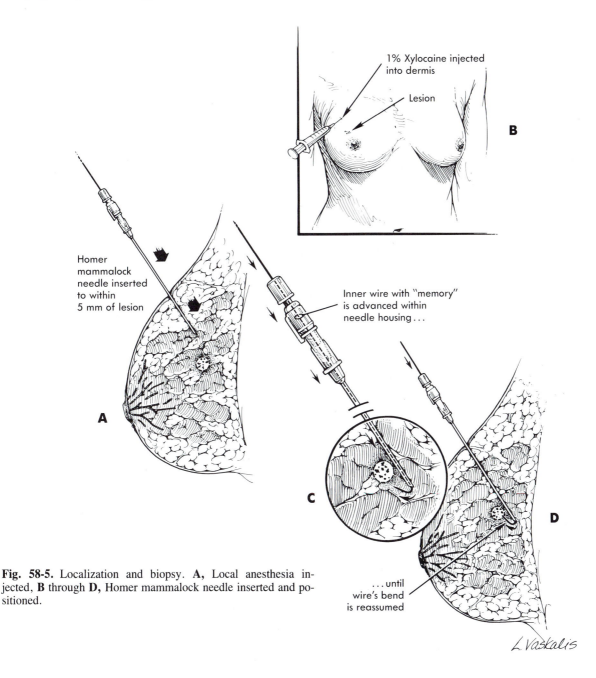

Fig. 58-5. Localization and biopsy. **A,** Local anesthesia injected, **B** through **D,** Homer mammalock needle inserted and positioned.

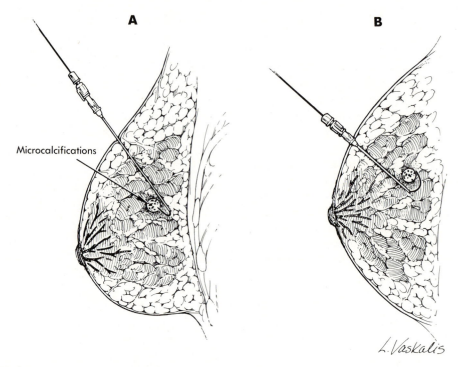

Fig. 58-6. Needle in mediolateral and craniocaudal positions. **A,** Mediolateral view; **B,** craniocaudad view.

It is very helpful to show the patient the films and point out the lesion. I have found that patients are reassured by this procedure, and it also helps to explain the localization process. The patient is shown where and how the needle will be inserted.

On the day of localization, the patient reports to the radiology suite. No premedication is employed because the films must be taken in the sitting position. The radiologist, noting the position of the lesion on the original films, places a small amount of lidocaine in the dermis (Fig. 58-5, *A*). We use a Homer mammalock needle as shown in Figs. 58-5, *B* through *D*, and 58-6. The illustrations show the technique of insertion of the needle and the final position of the needle relative to the occult lesion. The needle is inserted, and additional films are taken (Fig. 58-6). If the needle is not within 5 mm of the lesion, it is withdrawn and reinserted to obtain the final position.

The films are reviewed by the radiologist and the surgeon, and the patient is taken to day surgery for open biopsy. The films are brought to the operating room for review during the procedure. We use local anesthesia for this procedure as in the routine open biopsy. We have found this to be quite satisfactory. Our figures indicate that we obtain the lesion 96% of the time on the first operation and the other 4% in a second operation if this is required. We have had no significant complications using this technique, and, because there is an appreciable amount of "down time" waiting for specimen radiography, we feel that the patient should be awake rather than subjected to the risk of general anesthesia.

The patient is placed in the supine position on the oper-

ating room table with the arm extended. In this case, a decision must be made where to make the incision. Should the incision be made at the entrance of the needle or should the needle be intercepted (Fig. 58-7, *A, B*)? This decision is based largely on the probability of the lesion being a cancer and the need for additional surgery. An improperly placed incision may make a modified mastectomy difficult. A circumareolar incision is seldom used unless the lesion is directly beneath the incision.

The x-ray films are reviewed, and measurements are taken to locate the needle relative to the skin surface. This is helpful in deciding where to make the incision. The location of the occult lesion relative to the needle also is noted. Is it superior or inferior? Is it toward the mid line or the axilla? The incision is chosen and marked. The 1% lidocaine without adrenaline is injected, and the incision is made as in the open biopsy. If, however, the incision is made adjacent to the needle, it is essential to leave a small portion of dermis attached to the needle to provide stability during the dissection.

Using the films as a guide, sharp dissection is continued toward the lesion using appropriate retraction as in the open biopsy (Fig. 58-7, *C, D*). Care must be taken not to disturb the needle. When the proper distance has been reached, the needle is freed from the dermis and the tissue is stabilized with a single Allis clamp. Using the films as a guide, the area in question is removed by sharp dissection (Fig. 58-7, *E*). A fresh number 15 blade is useful for this procedure, but appropriate scissors can be used as well. This is not an easy procedure, and it requires experience to know exactly when to stabilize the lesion and begin exci-

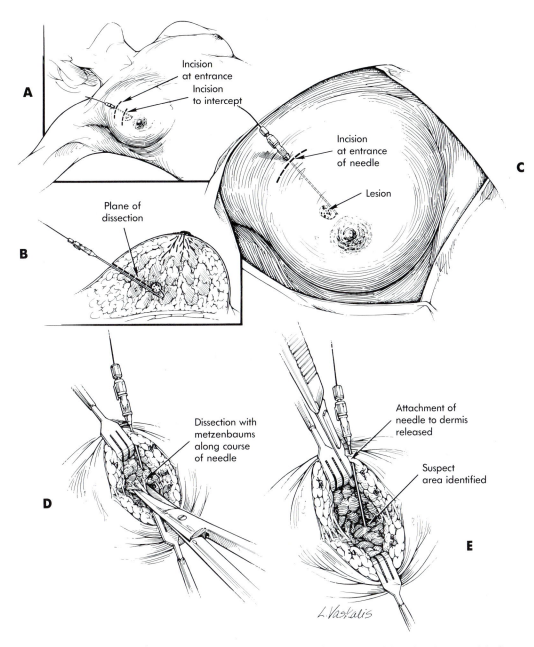

Fig. 58-7. Localization and biopsy, operative procedure. **A** and **B,** Incision site chosen and incision made. **C** and **D,** Sharp dissection continues along needle toward lesion. **E,** Needle freed from dermis.

sion of the specimen. It must be remembered that the needle is placed with the patient in the *sitting* position and the operation is performed with the patient in the *supine* position, therefore, there is displacement of the lesion, which must be considered during the dissection. In the very firm breast, there is little movement. However, in a pendulous or fatty breast, the breast tissue may roll away from the midline and make identification of the lesion difficult.

If the incision is made midway between the needle and the nipple, once the dissection has reached the area in question, the needle is stabilized and withdrawn into the incision (Fig. 58-8, *A* through *E*). To perform this maneuver, the outer or larger needle is removed, leaving the

wire, which is withdrawn through the incision and stabilized with the Allis clamp.

Once the lesion has been removed, preferably with the needle, it is placed on an appropriate tray with wet sponges and delivered with the films to the radiologist for specimen radiography (Fig. 58-8, *F* through *H*). In most cases, the wound is not closed until it has been confirmed that the lesion has been removed. No attempt should be made to use the actual cautery because, if additional tissue is removed, the cautery may obscure the histology and make the definitive diagnosis difficult if not impossible.

If the lesion is not present, additional tissue can be removed. We do not proceed beyond a second attempt be-

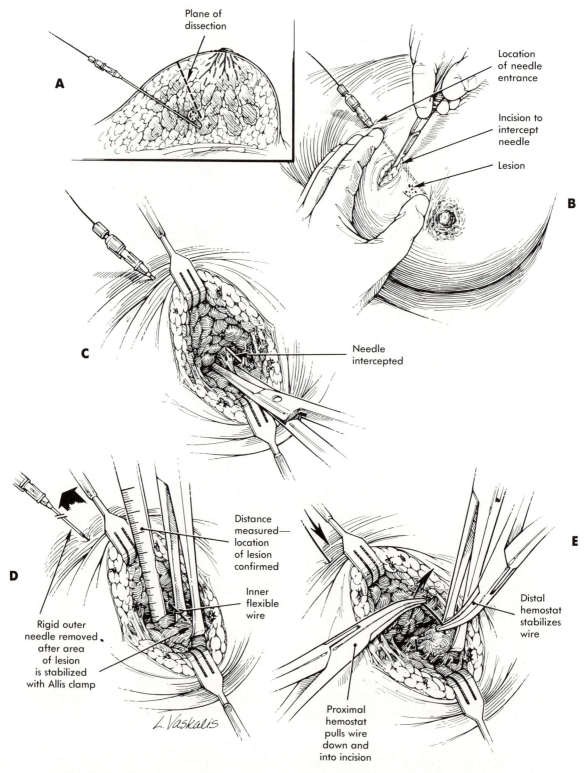

Plane of
dissection

A

Location
of needle
entrance

Incision to
intercept
needle

Lesion

B

Needle
intercepted

C

Distance
measured—
location
of lesion
confirmed

Inner
flexible
wire

E

D

Rigid outer
needle removed
after area
of lesion
is stabilized
with Allis clamp

Distal
hemostat
stabilizes
wire

Proximal
hemostat
pulls wire
down and
into incision

L. Vaskalis

Fig. 58-8. Localization and biopsy. Needle is intercepted. **A,** Plane of dissection midway between needle and nipple. **B** and **C,** Incision and dissection made to intercept needle. **D** and **E,** Needle stabilized and withdrawn into incision.

Continued.

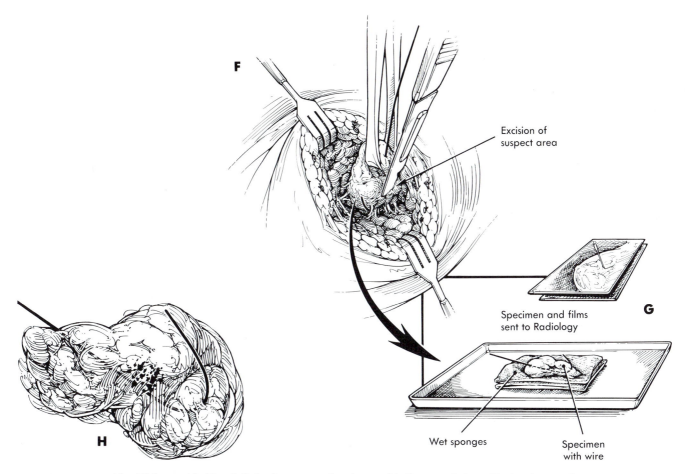

Fig. 58-8, cont'd. F and **G,** Lesion removed and sent with film to radiology. **H,** Specimen radiography showing microcalcifications.

cause the landmarks are no longer available and successful removal is unlikely.

Once it has been determined that the lesion is present in the specimen, bleeding is controlled with the actual cautery or ligatures of fine plain catgut. Again, no drain is employed. The breast tissue is loosely reconstructed, and the skin is closed with vertical mattress sutures of 5-0 nylon as in the open biopsy. Additional lidocaine without adrenaline is injected into the incision, and the pressure dressing is applied and left in place for 48 hours.

Successful removal of an occult lesion is not an easy procedure, particularly when using local anesthesia. It should only be performed in a setting in which there is communication between an experienced radiologist and a skillful surgeon. In our institution, once a specimen radiography has confirmed the presence of the lesion, the pathologist is called to the radiology suite and takes over responsibility for processing the specimen. In most cases, a rapid section is not performed because of the small size of the lesion. The margins are marked to assist in treatment planning. In most cases, receptor analysis is not possible because of the small size of the specimen, however, this can be determined by immunocytochemical techniques. In some cases, localization and biopsy may constitute a wide

local excision and definitive treatment of the cancer. Obviously, this depends on the site and size of the lesion and the experience of the operating surgeon. In most cases, re-excision is required, and often this is performed at the time of the axillary dissection.

REFERENCES

1. Adye B, Jolly PC, Bauermeister DE: The role of fine needle aspiration and the management of solid breast masses. *Arch Surg* 123:37, 1988.
2. The American Board of Obstetrics and Gynecology: *Conference proceedings: conference on breast disease—an initiative for curriculum development and residency education,* Chicago, 1986.
3. Department of Health and Human Services Health Care Financing Administration Medicare Program: Medicare coverage of screening mammography. *Federal Register* 55:53510, 1990.
4. Feig SA: Decreased breast cancer mortality through mammographic screening: results of clinical trials. Radiology 167:659, 1988.
5. Homer MJ: Nonpalpable breast lesion localization using a curved-end retractable wire. *Radiology* 157:259, 1985.
6. Homer MJ, Marchant DJ, Smith TJ: The geographic cluster of breast microcalcifications—is it really intramammary? *Surg Gynecol Obstet* 161:532, 1985.
7. Marchant DJ, Sutton SM: Use of mammography—United States, 1990. *MMWR* 39:621, 1990.
8. Moskowitz M: Predictive value, sensitivity and specificity in breast cancer screening. *Radiology* 167:576, 1988.

Chapter 59

TREATMENT OPTIONS FOR BREAST CANCER

Douglas J. Marchant

The American Cancer Society has predicted that, for 1993, breast cancer will represent 32% of the cancer incidence and 18% of the deaths. Lung cancer now surpasses breast cancer as the leading cause of cancer in women. It is also predicted that, for 1993, there will be 182,000 new cases and 46,000 deaths.[1] This is an increase of 2,000 new cases predicted from 1990. The reason for this increase is not clear. It may be due to a combination of an aging population and increased screening.

HISTORY

Surgical removal of the breast was described in the first and second centuries AD. The lesions observed were far advanced, and the treatment was unsuccessful. Later refinements in surgical technique resulted in a lower operative mortality, but, again, cures were infrequent. In 1867, Z.H. Moore[11] suggested that the entire breast be removed with a wide margin of skin. Halsted's mastectomy was first mentioned in 1891, and, by 1894, he had performed 50 "complete mastectomies."[5] This radical mastectomy, as the operation came to be known, was enthusiastically adopted in the United States and abroad. Because the lesions for which the Halsted procedure was designed were far advanced, the operation was not associated with an increase in cure, although there was a dramatic decrease in chest wall recurrences. During the next several decades, the results of the radical mastectomy improved principally because of earlier diagnosis and more selective use of the operation. Because the radical mastectomy did not include resection of the internal mammary lymph nodes, it was suggested that the classic operation be extended to include resection of the internal mammary nodes and the chest wall. In 1951, Urban[17] described the extended radical mastectomy that included an en bloc dissection of the chest wall.

It is widely accepted that cancer of the breast is a systemic disease and that some patients will not be cured even with the most extensive local treatment. This has resulted in a more conservative approach and participation of the patient in treatment planning. Lesser surgical procedures have largely replaced the classic Halsted radical mastectomy.

EVALUATION OF THE PATIENT

Treatment planning for breast cancer includes a multidisciplinary approach. Alternatives in treatment require the expertise not only of the surgeon but of the radiotherapist and the medical oncologist.

Once the diagnosis of breast cancer has been established, a number of preoperative studies should be obtained. Mammography is essential even in the most obvious case. Synchronous cancer is present in 5% of patients, and multicentric disease may be discovered in the involved breast. This may preclude wide local excision and radiation therapy. Patients should have a pretreatment chest radiograph, routine blood studies, and liver function tests. For invasive lesions, many surgeons recommend a bone scan, however, the yield is very low for T_1 lesions. Because many patients are placed on protocol studies, bone scan may be required as part of the staging procedure for these studies. Clinical staging using the tumor, node, metastasis (TNM) system is recommended, although most students of breast disease recognize that this system does not adequately segregate patients nor does it help to select appropriate patients for surgical treatment (Table 59-1). The TNM system was designed so that patients could be categorized, thereby enabling centers to group patients similarly for intercenter comparison. It is well known that the clinical nodal status of the patient may be incorrect. In addition, it is difficult to obtain an accurate tumor size ei-

Table 59-1. The staging of cancer: Staging for breast carcinoma

Definitions:

Primary tumor (T)

TX   Primary tumor cannot be assessed

T0   No evidence of primary tumor

Tis   Carcinoma in situ: Intraductal carcinoma, lobular carcinoma in situ, or Paget's disease of the nipple with no tumor

T1   Tumor 2 cm or less in greatest dimension
 T1a 0.5 cm or less in greatest dimension
 T1b More than 0.5 cm, but not more than 1 cm in greatest dimension
 T1c More than 1 cm, but not more than 2 cm in greatest dimension

T2   Tumor more than 2 cm, but not more than 5 cm in greatest dimension

T3   Tumor more than 5 cm in greatest dimension

T4   Tumor of any size with direct extension to chest wall or skin
 T4a Extension to chest wall
 T4b Edema (including peau d'orange) or ulceration of the skin of breast or satellite skin nodules confined to same breast
 T4c Both T4a and T4b
 T4d Inflammatory carcinoma

Regional lymph nodes (N)

NX   Regional lymph nodes cannot be assessed (e.g., previously removed or not removed for pathologic study)

N0   No regional lymph node metastasis

N1   Metastasis to movable ipsilateral axillary lymph node(s)
 N1a Only micrometastasis (none larger than 0.2 cm)
 N1b Metastasis to lymph node(s), any larger than 0.2 cm
  N1bi Metastasis in 1 to 3 lymph nodes, any more than 0.2 cm and all less than 2 cm in greatest dimension

  N1bii Metastasis to 4 or more lymph nodes, any more than 0.2 cm and all less than 2 cm in greatest dimension

  N1biii Extension of tumor beyond the capsule of a lymph node metastasis less than 2 cm in greatest dimension

  N1biv Metastasis to a lymph node 2 cm or more in greatest dimension

N2   Metastasis to ipsilateral axillary lymph nodes that are fixed to one another or to other structures

N3   Metastasis to ipsilateral internal mammary lymph node(s)

Distant metastasis (M)

MX   Presence of distant metastasis cannot be assessed

M0   No distant metastasis

M1   Distant metastasis (includes metastasis to ipsilateral supraclavicular lymph node(s)

AJCC/UICC stage grouping

Stage 0	Tis	N0	M0
Stage I	T1	N0	M0
Stage IIA	T0	N1	M0
	T1	N1	M0
	T2	N0	M0
Stage IIB	T2	N1	M0
	T3	N0	M0
Stage IIIA	T0	N2	M0
	T1	N2	M0
	T2	N2	M0
	T3	N1	M0
	T3	N2	M0
Stage IIIB	T4	Any N	M0
	Any T	N3	M0
Stage IV	Any T	Any N	M1

ther from the pathologist or from the surgeon. However, the TNM system is the best available and it does have some value in that it makes the physician record the patient and tumor information. Clearly, the future rests with some form of biologic staging.

Appropriate treatment planning requires formal consultation with a radiotherapist and a medical oncologist. This should not be presented to the patient as a competition among the specialties. This concept of pretreatment evaluation inevitably results in some delay in the treatment, but there is no evidence that a delay of 2 to 3 weeks or more between diagnosis and definitive treatment affects prognosis.

SURGICAL OPTIONS FOR LOCAL TREATMENT

A number of factors influence the definitive surgical treatment for breast cancer. Important considerations include the size and histology of the lesion, the skill and experience of the multidisciplinary team, and the wishes of the patient. Treatments discussed include:

1. Radical mastectomy
2. Modified radical mastectomy
3. Simple mastectomy
4. Subcutaneous mastectomy
5. Conservative treatment including quadrantectomy or wide local excision with or without axillary dissection

There is no doubt that the conservative approach appeals to many patients, however, statistics clearly indicate that most patients are treated with the modified radical mastectomy. This operation has replaced the Halsted procedure. However, for completeness, the radical operation is described.

Radical mastectomy

There are few indications today for the classic radical mastectomy. This operation assumed that cancer spread locally involving the deeper structures of the breast and the pectoral muscles and then, in a predictable manner, the regional nodes (Figs. 59-1 and 59-2). The operation required a vertical incision with removal of sufficient skin to include the primary tumor and the nipple areolar complex (Figs. 59-3, *A*). In this operation, relatively thin skin flaps are developed medially and laterally or, if the incision is

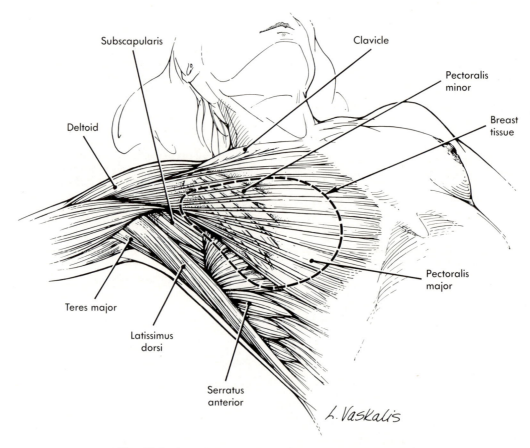

Fig. 59-1. Anatomy and musculature of chest wall and axilla.

more oblique or transverse, superiorly and inferiorly. The pectoralis major muscle is identified and removed leaving the clavicular head. It is divided at its humeral and sternal attachments (Fig. 59-3, *B*). The dissection is carried laterally toward the latissimus dorsi until the pectoralis minor is encountered. This is divided at the coracoid process, and the axillary dissection is performed (Fig. 59-3, *C* through *E*).

This operation is a more standardized procedure than are the many operations often described as the "modified radical mastectomy."

Even if patients present with large lesions, these are probably best treated with external radiation therapy and removed. Lesions that involve the pectoral fascia can be excised with a portion of this muscle, and the area can be treated with postoperative radiation therapy.

Four complications of radical mastectomy have been described.

1. Infection
2. Necrosis of the skin
3. Seroma
4. Edema of the arm

Infection is rare and occurs in fewer than 10% of cases. It is more common in older patients with prolonged suc-

tion drainage. Treatment with appropriate antibiotics resolves the problem.

Skin necrosis is not unusual because very thin flaps are the exception rather than the rule. It is rare for these areas to require additional treatment, and healing usually takes place by secondary intention (Fig. 59-3, *F*).

A seroma may develop if the drains are removed prematurely. This complication requires continued aspiration, which may result in secondary infection. This complication can be avoided by continued drainage until the skin flap is securely attached to the underlying tissues.

Lymphedema is unusual in the early postoperative period, but the later development of this complication is a distressing problem for the patient. Usually it results from a low-grade infection in the hand or arm with ascending lymphangitis. The patient must be instructed to avoid trauma to the hand or arm, and, if infection does occur, appropriate antibiotics must be promptly administered.

Modified radical mastectomy (simple mastectomy with axillary dissection)

This operation, as the name implies, is, in essence, a total mastectomy (simple) and axillary node dissection with preservation of the pectoral muscles. There have been a number of modifications of this operation including re-

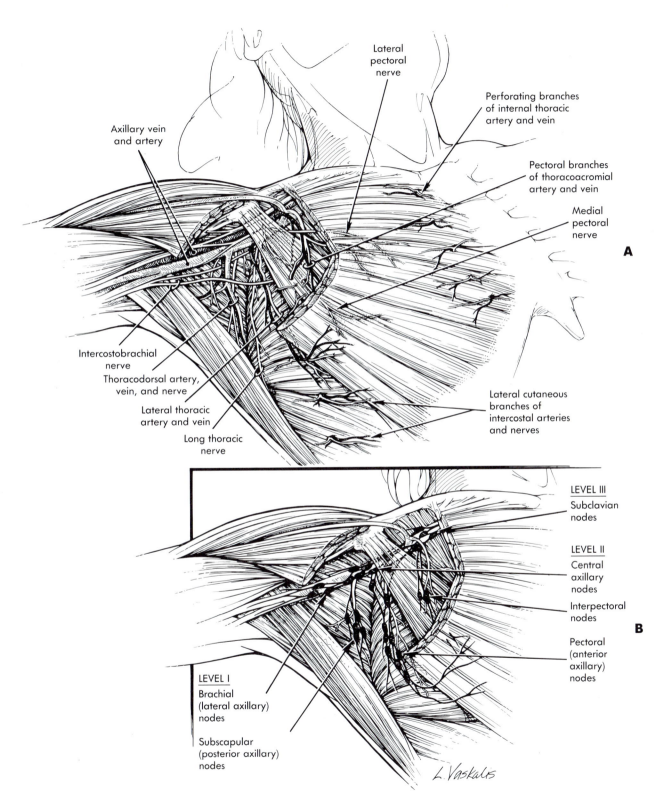

Lateral
pectoral
nerve

Perforating branches
of internal thoracic
artery and vein

Axillary vein
and artery

Pectoral branches
of thoracoacromial
artery and vein

Medial
pectoral
nerve

A

Intercostobrachial
nerve

Thoracodorsal artery,
vein, and nerve

Lateral thoracic
artery and vein

Long thoracic
nerve

Lateral cutaneous
branches of
intercostal arteries
and nerves

LEVEL III
Subclavian
nodes

LEVEL II
Central
axillary
nodes

Interpectoral
nodes

B

Pectoral
(anterior
axillary)
nodes

LEVEL I
Brachial
(lateral axillary)
nodes

Subscapular
(posterior axillary)
nodes

L. Vaskalis

Fig. 59-2. Anatomy. **A,** Vasculature and nerves of chest wall and axilla. **B,** Lymphatics. Level I, II, and III lymph nodes.

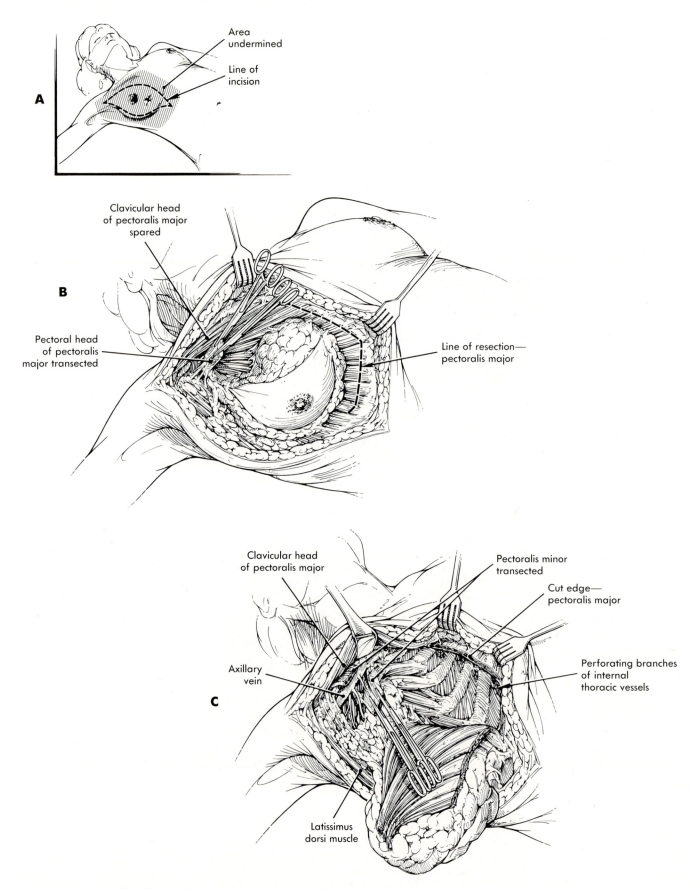

Area
undermined

Line of
incision

A

Clavicular head
of pectoralis major
spared

B

Pectoral head
of pectoralis
major transected

Line of resection—
pectoralis major

Clavicular head
of pectoralis major

Pectoralis minor
transected

Cut edge—
pectoralis major

Axillary
vein

Perforating branches
of internal
thoracic vessels

C

Latissimus
dorsi muscle

Fig. 59-3. Radical mastectomy. **A,** Line of incision and area to be included in the dissection. **B,** Extent of muscular resection, pectoralis major and minor. **C,** Pectoralis major and minor resected. Exposure of axillary contents and anterior chest wall.

Continued.

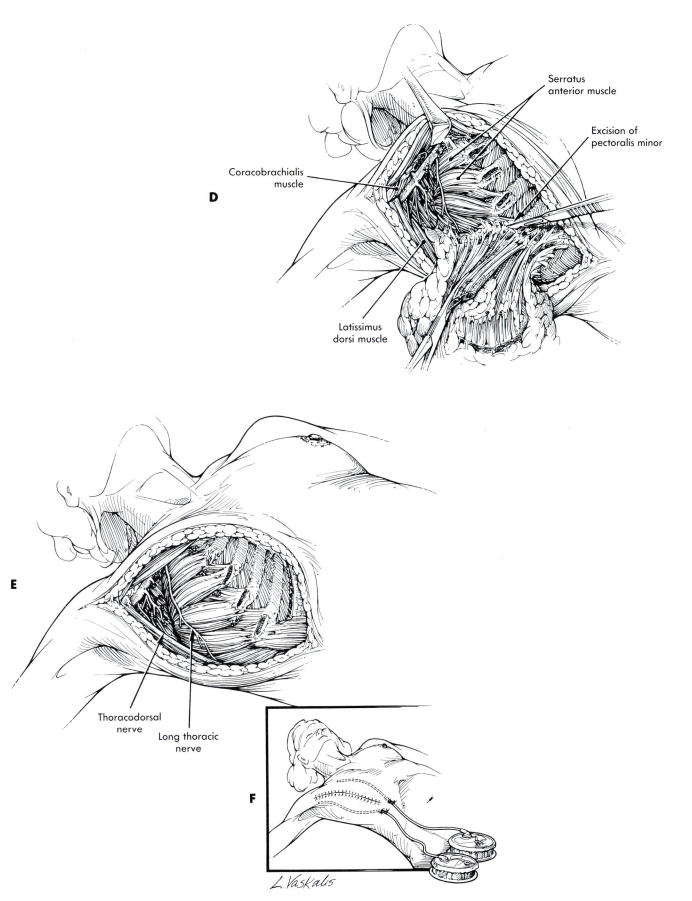

Serratus
anterior muscle

Excision of
pectoralis minor

Coracobrachialis
muscle

D

Latissimus
dorsi muscle

E

Thoracodorsal
nerve

Long thoracic
nerve

F

L. Vaskalis

Fig. 59-3, cont'd. D, Extent of axillary dissection. **E,** Completed dissection. Note position of thoracodorsal and long thoracic nerves. **F,** Closure with suction drainage.

moval of the pectoralis minor muscle. Most contemporary surgeons agree, however, that the operation today is best performed with preservation of both the pectoralis major and minor muscles.

The modified mastectomy is the procedure of choice for large operable lesions, for patients with smaller lesions in relatively small breasts, and for patients who refuse conservative treatment. It is also the procedure of choice for large lesions demonstrated by mammography and proven by biopsy.

For most patients, this operation is performed on an "admit after surgery basis." Therefore, the work-up, as previously described, is obtained on an outpatient basis. It is important that the operating surgeon supervise this evaluation to avoid cancellation of the procedure on the day of surgery because of an incomplete work-up.

The procedure is performed using appropriate endotrachial anesthesia. I usually request a muscle relaxant, although some surgeons prefer no paralysis so that the nerves in the axilla can be stimulated if necessary during dissection. A transverse incision is ideal because it makes later reconstruction more cosmetic. However, the actual line of incision depends on the site of the primary tumor. A number of maneuvers can be used that result in a transverse incision. These include an S-shaped incision that includes not only the lesion but the nipple areolar complex as well. In some cases, the lesion is in the midline, high in the breast tissue or in the inframammary fold. In these cases, the tissue can be mobilized so that a vertical incision is avoided. In all cases, the nipple areolar complex must be included in the incision. An alternative to mobilizing large flaps is to proceed directly with a transverse incision including the nipple areolar complex and leave the biopsy incision in situ. Because relatively thin flaps are obtained, there is little danger of local recurrence in this area.

To relax the pectoral muscles, I prefer to elevate the arm on a crossbar (Fig. 59-4, *A*). It is secured with an Ace bandage and, after axillary dissection, is placed at the patient's side to complete the skin closure.

After the marking of the incision and the positioning of the arm, the chest, the upper arm and the upper portion of the abdomen are carefully prepared and the area is draped. The incision is made, and the skin flaps are developed. This is accomplished by placing small Allis clamps in the subcutaneous tissue, not in the skin, and elevating these under slight tension as the flaps are developed by sharp dissection (Fig. 59-4, *B*). Bleeding is controlled on the skin side with fine absorbable ligatures and on the breast side with the actual cautery (Fig. 59-4, *C*). The dissection is carried to the chest wall superiorly, inferiorly, and medially (Fig. 59-4, *D* and *E*). The breast is removed by sharp dissection from the sternum toward the latissimus dorsi muscle. As this is being accomplished, the perforating vessels appear. These are clamped and suture ligated with 3-0 chromic catgut or similar suture material (Fig. 59-4, *F*). These vessels should be very carefully ligated

because, if they retract, it is almost impossible to secure adequate hemostasis.

The dissection is carried to the latissimus dorsi muscle laterally, being careful not to proceed beneath the muscle. Bleeding points are clamped and ligated with fine chromic catgut. As this dissection proceeds, the lateral edge of the pectoralis major muscle is identified. The fascia of the muscle has been removed with the specimen, and, with dissection toward the axilla, the pectoralis minor muscle also comes into view (Fig. 59-4, *F* and *G*).

At this point, the breast is wrapped in a moist towel and attention is turned to the axilla. The costocoracoid fascia is now visible and is incised with Metzenbaum scissors. The axillary fat is distinct from the adipose tissue noted during the breast dissection. It has a much lighter color and is obvious when one has entered the axilla. A small right-angle retractor is placed beneath the pectoralis major muscle. The axillary vein is identified, and the tissue immediately beneath and inferior to the vein is removed by sharp dissection (Fig. 59-4, *H*). The intercostal brachial nerves may be sacrificed; however, if possible, at least some of the branches are spared to avoid lack of sensation on the medial surface of the upper arm. As the dissection proceeds, the thoracodorsal vessels and nerve become apparent at the floor of the axilla, and often the long thoracic nerve is visible along the chest wall, although, with the modified radical mastectomy, this is not always apparent (Fig. 59-4, *I* and *J*). Bleeding in the axilla is controlled by using right-angle clamps and fine silk ligatures. As the dissection proceeds, an attempt should be made to remove at least some of the interpectoral (Rotter's) nodes. With the modified radical mastectomy, level 1 and 2 nodes can be removed, but, by definition, level 3 nodes are not routinely removed.

With proper exposure and sharp dissection, a minimum of 12 to 15 axillary nodes will be recovered. The number of nodes actually removed depends on the thoroughness of the surgeon and the diligence of the pathologist at the surgical desk. Repeated recovery of but one to two nodes suggests either that the surgeon is not performing a true modified radical mastectomy or that the pathologist is careless in locating the lymph nodes in the specimen.

Because of the extensive elevation of the flaps, suction drainage is required (Fig. 59-4, *K*); although, for some very thin patients, I have simply closed the incision and wrapped the patient in a pressure dressing using a 6-inch Ace bandage. If suction drainage is employed, care must be taken in the placement of the drains. Some patients require external radiation therapy, and, if the exit incision is beyond the projected field of radiation, these patients may require extension of the radiation field to avoid local recurrence. The suction catheters are secured with a pursestring suture of silk (Fig. 59-4, *L*).

The wound is inspected for bleeding. The axilla is irrigated with normal saline, and additional bleeding points are ligated. The bleeding points on the muscle may be cauterized with the actual cautery, and those in the subcutane-

Text continued on p. 970.

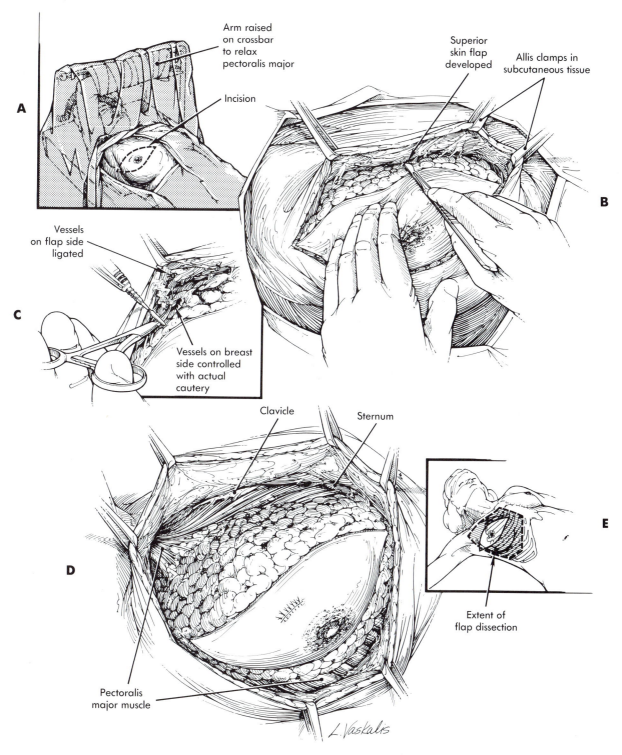

Fig. 59-4. Modified radical mastectomy. **A,** Position of patient and extent of incision. Note position of the arm to relax pectoralis major muscle. **B,** Development of skin flap. Allis clamps on subcutaneous tissue, not skin. **C,** Control of bleeding. Vessels on flap ligated; vessels on specimen cauterized. **D,** Beginning removal of the breast. **E,** Extent of dissection.   *Continued.*

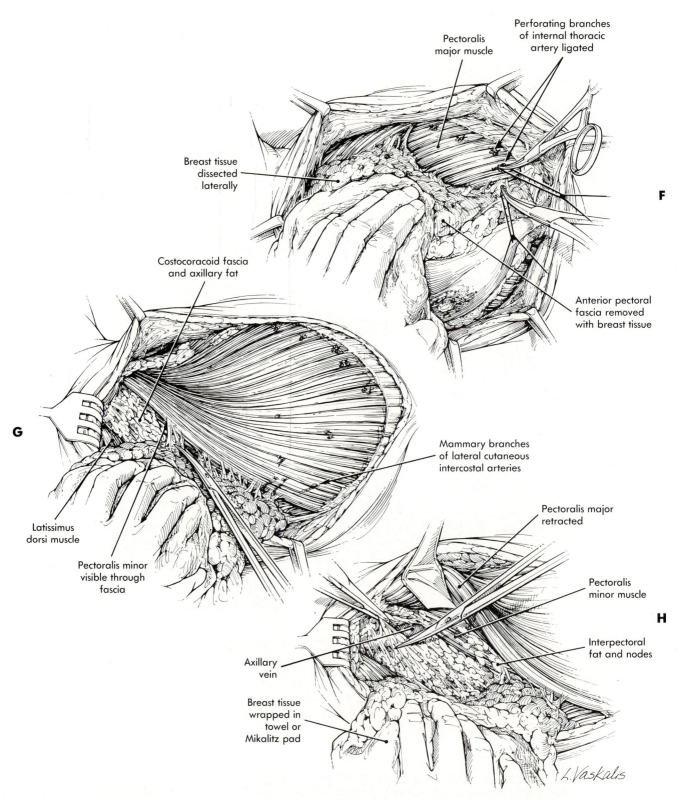

Fig. 59-4, cont'd. F, Using sharp dissection, breast removed toward latissimus dorsi muscle. Perforating vessels ligated. **G,** Costocoracoid fascia exposed. **H,** Pectoralis major muscle retracted medially, and axillary dissection begins.

Continued.

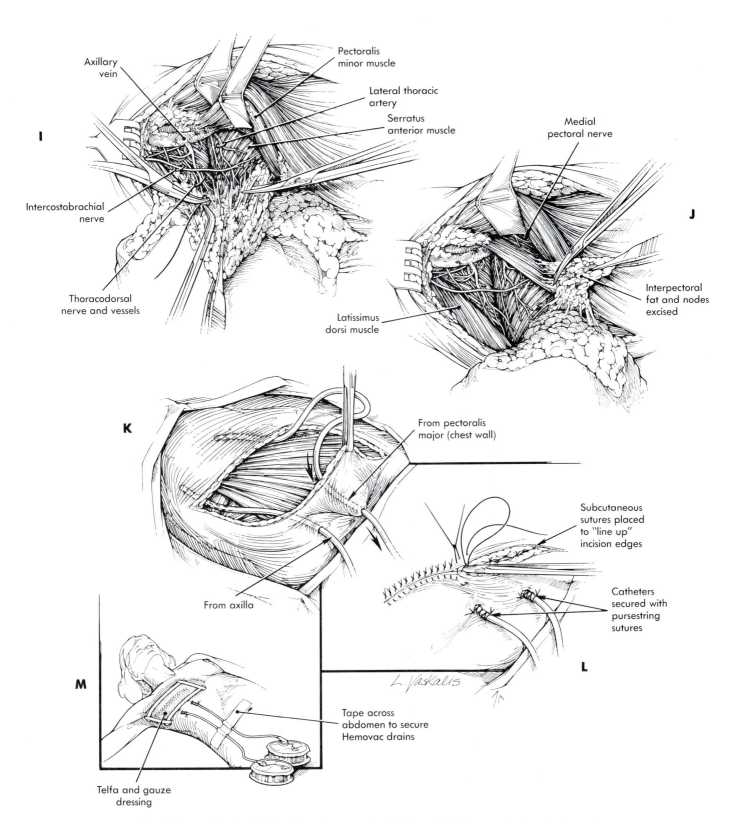

Axillary
vein

Pectoralis
minor muscle

Lateral thoracic
artery

Serratus
anterior muscle

Intercostobrachial
nerve

Thoracodorsal
nerve and vessels

Latissimus
dorsi muscle

Medial
pectoral nerve

Interpectoral
fat and nodes
excised

From pectoralis
major (chest wall)

Subcutaneous
sutures placed
to "line up"
incision edges

Catheters
secured with
pursestring
sutures

From axilla

L. Vaskalis

Tape across
abdomen to secure
Hemovac drains

Telfa and gauze
dressing

Fig. 59-4, cont'd. I, Axillary dissection completed. Note similarity to radical mastectomy. **J,** Pectoralis minor exposed and interpectorial nodes excised. **K,** Suction drainage placed on axilla and over pectoral muscles. **L,** Skin closure with vertical mattress sutures of 4-0 nylon (staple closure optional). Note that drains are secured by pursestring sutures. **M,** Completed closure and small dressing applied to cover incision. Note that suction drainage is secured to point with tape.

ous tissue are ligated with fine absorbable suture material. When the wound is dry, the arm is brought to the patient's side and any redundant skin is excised.

The closure, in my opinion, is best achieved with a few sutures of absorbable catgut in the subcutaneous tissues to "line up" the skin edges. The skin is closed with vertical mattress sutures of fine nylon, although some surgeons prefer to use staples. I think a more cosmetic closure can be achieved with interrupted sutures, but this is a matter of personal preference (Fig. 59-4, *L*).

A simple dressing is applied (Fig. 59-4, *M*). No pressure dressing is required, and the hemovacs are secured with additional tape across the abdomen to prevent their inadvertent removal. The usual operating time is 2 to 3 hours. The blood loss depends, to some extent, on the size of the breast and the age of the patient. In older patients with very fatty breasts, often there is very little bleeding; however, in younger patients, the breast is definitely a functional organ and well supplied with vessels that require time-consuming hemostasis.

Most patients can be mobilized soon after the surgical procedure, and usually there is little discomfort, which can be controlled with analgesics. The suction drainage should be recorded, and the drains, in my opinion, should not be removed until the drainage is less than 10 to 15 ml per 24 hours through each catheter. Premature removal invites seroma formation and the necessity for repeated aspiration. Orders should be written to have the patient seen by a physiotherapist so that arm and chest wall exercises can be established early in the postoperative period.

The length of hospital stay varies with the surgeon and the requirements of the patient; it is usually no more than 4 or 5 days. Some surgeons send patients home with their drains. This may or may not be appropriate depending on the home situation.

Total (simple) mastectomy

This operation is the same as described for the modified radical mastectomy. It differs in that the axillary dissection is omitted, although level 1 nodes often are removed. The entire breast, including the nipple areolar complex and the fascia of the pectoralis major muscle, is removed (Fig. 59-5, *A* and *B*).

There are a number of indications for this procedure.

1. Extensive ductal carcinoma in situ or lobular carcinoma in situ (DCIS or LCIS)
2. Recurrence after partial mastectomy or wide local excision with axillary dissection followed by radiation (i.e., conservative treatment)
3. Bulky or ulcerated lesions or in patients with distant metastases when local control will improve quality of life
4. Elderly patients or those who are a poor operative risk and in whom there is no palpable axillary adenopathy and no evidence of distant disease
5. Selected cases when prophylactic removal of the opposite breast is recommended

It must be stated that there is considerable debate concerning the best treatment for patients with documented DCIS. The standard treatment continues to be total mastectomy; however, in selected cases, conservative surgery (i.e., wide local excision with or without radiation therapy) may be considered.[3,8–10,12,13,15,16]

Local recurrence after modified or simple mastectomy is unusual, occurring in less than 10% of cases. Lymphedema, which may occur in 30% of patients with the radical mastectomy, is unusual with the modified procedure.

Variations in surgical technique and length of hospital stay are the rule rather than the exception depending on the type of third-party reimbursement and the home situation of the patient. Some surgeons recommend prophylactic antibiotics and anticoagulation, but I have not used this in my own practice. One surgeon of my acquaintance has suggested that the modified mastectomy can be performed on a "day surgery" basis and has actually discharged patients immediately after the operation. My conversations with some of these patients indicate less than total satisfaction with this arrangement.

Subcutaneous (prophylactic) mastectomy

Total mastectomy is the operation of choice. It is the only operation that completely removes all of the breast tissue. Subcutaneous mastectomy is inadequate. Studies have indicated that even with the most carefully performed subcutaneous procedure, breast tissue remains under the areola and is found in other locations in 80% of cases.[4,7] Thus, it is not a prophylactic procedure; however, there are no studies indicating whether removal of 80% of the breast tissue would yield an equivalent reduction in risk. In addition, the subcutaneous mastectomy may result in a less than satisfactory cosmetic result. A number of complications are associated with this operation including hematoma and subsequent scarring and fibrosis.

Breast preservation (conservative) procedures

A number of consensus development conferences have dealt with the treatment of primary breast cancer in an effort to determine treatment recommendations that provide the best chance for disease-free survival. These conferences have dealt with the question whether conservative treatment including dissection of the axillary lymph nodes followed by irradiation to the breast is as effective as the modified mastectomy.

Although the concept of conservative treatment has gained favor, there has been continued controversy concerning the technical details of the surgery and the radiation therapy. Several definitions dealing with these issues were proposed at a consensus conference in New York in 1985.[6]

1. Conservative surgery implies wide local excision and resection of the tumor with 1 or 2 cm of adjacent breast tissue designed to provide clear margins.
2. Quadrantectomy implies the resection of the tumor with the involved quadrant of the breast including the over-

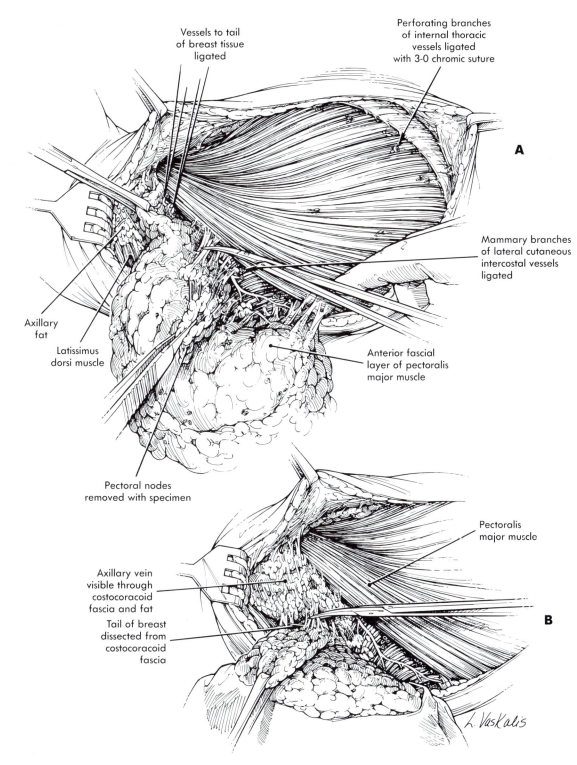

Vessels to tail
of breast tissue
ligated

Perforating branches
of internal thoracic
vessels ligated
with 3-0 chromic suture

A

Mammary branches
of lateral cutaneous
intercostal vessels
ligated

Axillary
fat

Latissimus
dorsi muscle

Anterior fascial
layer of pectoralis
major muscle

Pectoral nodes
removed with specimen

Pectoralis
major muscle

Axillary vein
visible through
costocoracoid
fascia and fat

Tail of breast
dissected from
costocoracoid
fascia

B

L. Vaskalis

Fig. 59-5. Total (simple) mastectomy. **A,** Extent of dissection. Costocoracoid fascia not excised. **B,** Breast is removed, including fascia and pectoralis major muscle. Exposure of axillary contents and lateral chest wall.

lying skin. The terms *lumpectomy* and *segmental mastectomy* are imprecise, and their use is discouraged.

3. Axillary dissection implies the removal of the axillary contents from the tail of the breast to the latissimus dorsi, the axillary vein superiorly, and the lateral border of the pectoralis minor medially. The use of the term *axillary sampling* is discouraged because it is not a precise definition concerning the extent of the surgical procedure.

The use of breast conservation procedures involves four important criteria:

1. Patient selection
2. Surgery of the primary tumor
3. Surgery of the axilla
4. Radiotherapy to the retained breast

The principal advantage of conservative treatment is cosmetic. There are no data to indicate that the conservative approach provides improved survival compared to the radical procedure. Thus, the surgeon must select patients for whom an adequate resection results in an acceptable cosmesis. Patients who are poor candidates include those with widely separated tumors in the same breast, patients whose mammograms reveal diffuse disease in many quadrants, and patients with large tumors in relatively small breasts. Patients with central lesions involving the nipple areolar complex can be treated by resection of the nipple with careful attention to the final cosmetic result. Reconstruction of the nipple has been accomplished after radiation therapy. Advanced age is not a contraindication. Patients in their middle seventies often request conservative treatment for cosmetic reasons, and younger patients may request not only total mastectomy but prophylactic mastectomy "to avoid concern about recurrence of cancer in the treated breast and the development of new cancer in the opposite breast."

Adequate surgical resection implies grossly clear margins. The surgeon marks the specimen for orientation by the pathologist. The pathologist then "inks" the margins to assist in the examination of the permanent sections. The tissue is submitted for estrogen and progesterone receptor analysis without disturbing the resected margins.

We consider the margins positive if there is microscopic involvement within 2 mm of the margin. A 5-mm margin is adequate and does not require additional boost radiation therapy or reexcision.

A cosmetic incision is important. These incisions are marked with the patient in the sitting or the standing position. Often, a fold can be noted in the axilla and used for the axillary incision. Cosmetic skin lines in the breast are best observed in the sitting or the standing positions, and these should be marked immediately before the operative procedure (Fig. 59-6, *A*).

If no axillary dissection is contemplated, wide local excision can be performed under local anesthesia. However, in most cases, this is combined with an axillary dissection, and general anesthesia is required. Again, these patients fall under the category of "admit after" and must be carefully evaluated on outpatient basis before the surgical procedure.

Once the incisions have been marked, the patient is taken to the operating room suite and endotracheal anesthesia is administered. Again, the arm is placed on a crossbar to relax the pectoralis muscles and facilitate exposure (Fig. 59-6, *B*). The breast, upper arm, and upper abdomen are carefully prepared and draped as in the modified mastectomy. I usually perform the axillary dissection first, and the breast is covered with a drape. The previously marked incision is used, and bleeding is controlled with ligatures of fine absorbable catgut. The dissection is carried to the pectoralis major muscle, which is easily identified in the superior portion of the incision (Fig. 59-6, *C* and *D*). It is not necessary to carry the incision beyond the muscle toward the midline. The costocoracoid fascia is identified as in the modified radical procedure and incised with Metzenbaum scissors. The axillary dissection is exactly the same as that performed with the modified radical mastectomy. The pectoral muscles are retracted by the assistant, and the tissue below the axillary vein, lateral to the pectoralis muscle and medial to the latissimus dorsi muscle, is removed (Fig. 59-6, *E*). Bleeding is controlled with ligatures of fine silk. The same number of nodes should be recovered in this procedure as in the modified radical mastectomy. The elevation of the arm on a crossbar facilitates relaxation of the muscle and provides improved exposure for the axillary dissection. Once the dissection has been completed, the axilla is irrigated and inspected for hemostasis. If the wound is dry, I do not employ any type of drainage. The subcutaneous tissue is simply closed with fine absorbable catgut, and the skin is closed with vertical mattress sutures of 4-0 or 5-0 nylon (Fig. 59-6, *F*). A temporary pressure dressing is placed over the incision, and the arm is brought to the patient's side.

New instruments, drapes, and gloves are employed, and the wide local excision is performed. It is helpful to have the original mammogram in the operating room because many of these cases represent an occult lesion. The wide local excision may be a "reexcision." It is important to know exactly where the original lesion was located so that grossly clear margins can be obtained. The previous incision is removed, and flaps are developed very similar to the modified radical mastectomy (Fig. 59-7, *A* and *B*). The subcutaneous tissues are grasped with the Allis clamp, and, using sharp dissection, superior and inferior flaps are developed on either side of the previous incision (Fig. 59-7, *C*). With the mammogram as a guide, the dissection is carried to the chest wall, and all indurated tissue is removed (Fig. 59-7, *D* and *E*). Bleeding is controlled with ligatures of fine absorbable catgut or the actual cautery. It is best to proceed quickly with the removal of the specimen so the anatomy is not distorted by repeated attempts to ligate vessels and reposition the retractors. Once the specimen has been removed, hemostasis can be achieved

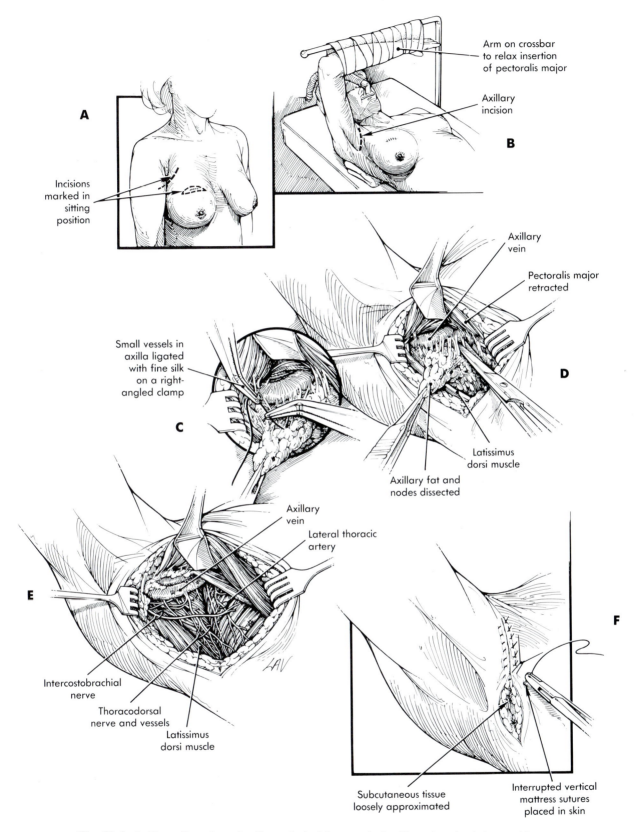

Fig. 59-6. Axillary dissection. **A,** Cosmetic incisions marked with patient in sitting position. Note that axillary incision can be placed in "skin fold." **B,** Position of patient before draping. Note that arm is elevated on a crossbar to relax pectoralis major muscle. **C,** Costocoracoid fascia is entered, and dissection is begun. **D,** Axillary vein and tributaries exposed. Vessels are ligated with 3-0 silk (hemoclips optional). **E,** Axillary dissection is completed. Note similarity to modified radical mastectomy dissection. **F,** Skin closure with 4 or 5-0 nylon. No drain is employed.

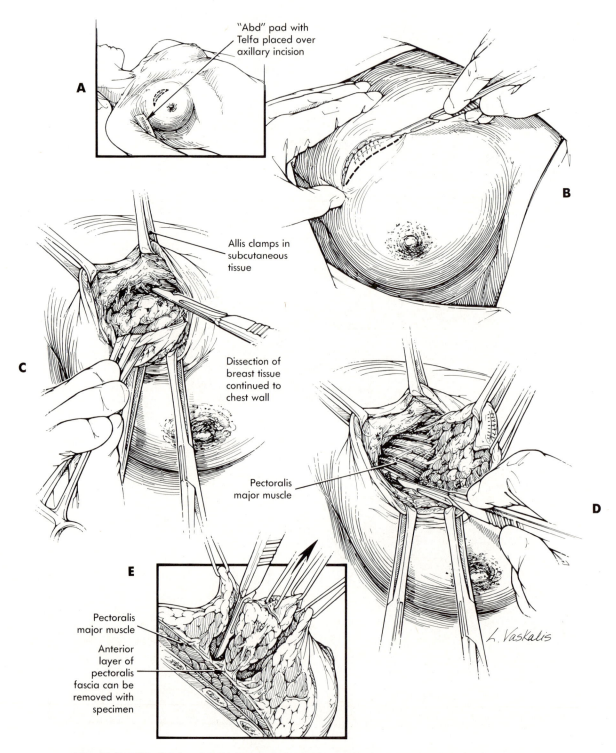

"Abd" pad with
Telfa placed over
axillary incision

A

B

Allis clamps in
subcutaneous
tissue

Dissection of
breast tissue
continued to
chest wall

C

D

Pectoralis
major muscle

E

Pectoralis
major muscle

Anterior
layer of
pectoralis
fascia can be
removed with
specimen

L. Vaskalis

Fig. 59-7. Wide local excision. **A,** Arm is brought to patient's side and covered with temporary
pressure dressing. **B,** Incision is made, removing small amount of skin, including previous incision. **C,** Skin flaps are developed by sharp dissection. **D,** Dissection continues to anterior chest
wall. **E,** Sagittal view showing extent of dissection.

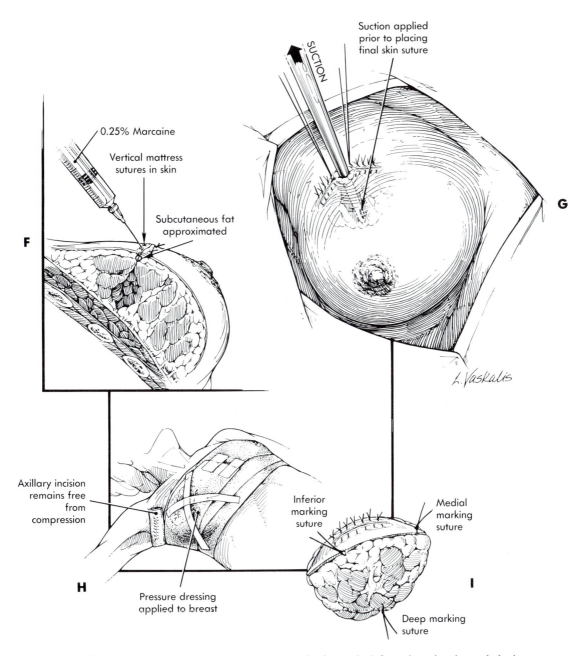

Fig. 59-7, cont'd. F, Final specimen is appropriately marked for orientation by pathologist. **G,** 0.25% Marcaine injected. No attempt is made to obliterate cavity. Only subcutaneous fat is approximated. **H,** Wound is partially closed with vertical mattress sutures of fine nylon. One suture is left "long" to permit suction before closure is completed. **I,** Pressure dressing with "fluffs" and 6-inch Ace bandage applied. Depending on location of axillary incision, this may or may not be included in dressing.

either with the actual cautery or ligatures of absorbable catgut.

The specimen is carefully marked usually before removal at least for the medial and inferior margins. I prefer to do this with a variety of sutures, for example, silk sutures for the medial margin, chromic catgut sutures for the inferior margin, and plain catgut for the deep margin (Fig. 59-7, *F*). It is absolutely essential that some type of marking system be employed and recorded on the pathology requisition. In most cases, the specimens are sent in a

fresh condition to the pathologist. This provides additional material for estrogen and progesterone receptor analysis.

Once hemostasis has been achieved, no attempt should be made to obliterate completely the dead space in the central portion of the excision. The subcutaneous tissues are closed with fine absorbable catgut, and the skin is closed with vertical mattress sutures of 4-0 or 5-0 nylon. A few milliliters of 0.5% Marcaine without adrenaline are injected into the incision (Fig. 59-7, *G*). Before tying the last suture, I usually insert the suction to remove any fresh bleeding, and then an immediate pressure dressing is applied (Fig. 59-7, *H*). I do not employ suction drainage, which inevitably results in retraction of the skin and a less than perfect cosmetic result. With the use of a pressure dressing, the breast is "molded" into its normal configuration. When the dressing is applied, compression of the axillary incision should be avoided (Fig. 59-7, *I*).

Most of these patients can be discharged within 24 to 48 hours. I leave the pressure dressing on for a full 48 hours. When this is removed, there is seldom any ecchymosis and a relatively normal contour of the breast is achieved. Occasionally, there is some minor ecchymosis in the region of the axillary dissection as a result of the pressure dressing. Before discharge, the patient should be instructed in arm and chest exercises. This is important because of the fibrosis that may be associated with the subsequent radiation therapy.

These patients are treated over a 4- or 5-week period by the department of radiotherapy receiving 180 to 200 cGy per day for a total of 45 to 50 Gy. Doses in excess of 50 Gy result in fibrosis and retraction and an unacceptable cosmetic result. This is particularly true for patients who require "boost" therapy. If possible, we prefer to reexcise the area to avoid this cosmetic complication.[14] There is controversy concerning the technique for supplemental radiation. It can be delivered by insertion of radioactive nucleotides or an electron beam. Whichever technique is employed, it should not diminish the cosmetic result.

There are advantages and disadvantages associated with the conservative and radical approaches. In terms of the surgical procedure performed, wide local excision and axillary dissection require as much time as the modified mastectomy and, in my opinion, is a more difficult operation if a satisfactory cosmetic result is achieved. Obviously, the main advantage of the conservative approach is the preservation of the breast. However, the price to be paid is the extended radiation treatments and the real concern of some patients that future symptomatology in the retained breast may be associated with recurrent tumor. In the more radical approach, the treatment is accomplished in a few days and, obviously, the cancer cannot recur in the removed breast.

RECONSTRUCTIVE SURGERY

Although this subject will be covered in detail in Chapter 60, it is important for the surgeon to be aware of the possibility or reconstruction and discuss this with the patient as part of the pretreatment planning. The American Cancer Society[2] at a recent consensus meeting recognized that there are few, if any, contraindications to immediate reconstruction. Adjuvant chemotherapy can be given to patients undergoing reconstruction, and many radiation therapists note few adverse sequelae after reconstructive surgery and radiation. In my opinion, this discussion is an important part of treatment planning, and consultation with the plastic surgeon should be obtained early in this process.

REFERENCES

1. American Cancer Society: *Cancer facts and figures,* 1993.
2. American Cancer Society: Workshop on Breast Reconstruction: Prospects/Problems supplement. *Cancer* 68:1143, 1991.
3. Fisher ER et al: Pathologic findings from the National Surgical Adjuvant Breast Project (protocol 6). 1. Intraductal carcinoma (DCIS), *Cancer* 57:197, 1986.
4. Goldman LD, Goldwyn RM: Some anatomical considerations of subcutaneous mastectomy, *Plast Reconstr Surg* 51:501, 1973.
5. Halsted WS: The results of operations for the cure of cancer of the breast performed at the Johns Hopkins Hospital. 4:297, 1894-1895.
6. Harris JR, Hellman S, Kinne DW: Limited surgery and radiotherapy for early breast cancer, *N Engl J Med* 313:1365, 1985.
7. Humphrey LJ: Subcutaneous mastectomy is not a prophylaxis against carcinoma of the breast: opinion or knowledge?, *Am J Surg* 145:311, 1983.
8. Hutter RVP: The management of patients with lobular carcinoma in situ of the breast, *Cancer* 53:798, 1984.
9. Lagios MD et al: Duct carcinoma in situ: relationship of extent of noninvasive disease to the frequency of occult invasion, multicentricity, lymph node metastases, and short term treatment failures, *Cancer* 50:1309, 1982.
10. Lagios MD et al: Mammographically detected duct cancer in situ, *Cancer* 63:618, 1989.
11. Moore ZH: On the influence of inadequate operations on the theory of cancer, *R Med Chir Soc (Lond)* 1:245, 1867.
12. Robert NJ et al: In situ breast cancer: a multidisciplinary approach, *Hosp Pract* 169:185, 1989.
13. Rosen PP, Braun DW, Kinne DE: The clinical significance of preinvasive breast carcinoma, *Cancer* 46:919, 1980.
14. Schmidt-Ullrich R et al: Tumor margin assessment as a guide to optimal conservation surgery and irradiation in early stage breast carcinoma, *Int J Radiat Oncol Biol Phys* 17:733, 1989.
15. Schnitt SJ et al: Ductal carcinoma in situ (intraductal carcinoma) of the breast, *N Engl J Med* 318:898, 1988.
16. Silverstein MJ et al: Axillary lymph node dissection for intraductal breast carcinoma—is it indicated? *Cancer* 59:1819, 1987.
17. Urban JA, Marjani MA: Significance of internal mammary lymph node metastases in breast cancer, *AJR* 111:130, 1971.

Chapter 60

BREAST PLASTIC SURGERY AND RECONSTRUCTION

Sumner A. Slavin
Robert M. Goldwyn

A large segment of the average plastic surgeon's practice in the United States concerns the female breast. We shall describe the most common conditions for which women seek plastic and reconstructive surgery.

BREAST AUGMENTATION

Augmentation mammaplasty seems to satisfy the psychologic and anatomic needs of women who are concerned about the small size of their breasts.[13] In North America, it is a very popular procedure despite its technical limitations and consumer alerts against the supposed dangers of silicone implants. At the outset, it should be stated that no study has demonstrated an increased incidence of cancer in women who have had breast augmentation with silicone prostheses. What is true, however, is that women who have had breast enlargement with implants present a slightly greater difficulty in examination to some of their physicians as well as to mammographers who, nevertheless, have developed newer techniques for a more accurate depiction.

Patients for augmentation mammaplasty (Fig. 60-1) have usually one thing in common: a preoccupation with what they consider to be their inadequately developed breast. They commonly feel poor self-esteem despite the fact that they may be very attractive and extremely accomplished. They may complain of the difficulty in purchasing the clothes they wish. Psychologically, they are usually not abnormal although they may have a greater than normal concern with their bust size. During the initial consultation, the plastic surgeon must be certain that the patient is undertaking the operation for herself and is not doing it to please a partner or possibly to save a marriage. In those instances, the patient would be better served by a psychotherapist than by a plastic surgeon.

In determining a woman's suitability for this procedure, it is important to inquire about the family history, especially whether a close relative—mother or sister—has had premenopausal breast cancer. It is also important to know whether the patient has had biopsies in the past or a history of breast masses that require frequent aspiration. Under those conditions, the presence of a foreign body, such as a silicone implant, would be unwise. One cannot emphasize enough the need for a careful, thorough breast examination to rule out the presence of a malignancy. In patients 30 or older, mammography is mandatory. In some instances, it may be indicated with a younger patient.

The plastic surgeon must inform the patient that no matter what technique is used, the presence of a foreign body may induce an abnormal appearance and firmness to the breast, which results from the capsular and spherical contracture that occurs in a certain percentage of women having this procedure. If the patient expects that her breasts will be absolutely normal to inspection and examination, then she is liable to be seriously disappointed. The fact that there are literally scores of different implants of various textures and sizes attests more to the inadequacy of the procedure than to the imagination of the manufacturer. Implants that may have an original tear drop shape and a soft texture may become round and hard after operation.

Most plastic surgeons favor inserting a silicone gel implant under the muscle rather than immediately under the breast to lessen the incidence of capsular contracture. Another popular alternative is to use a polyurethane or silicone textured implant (the so-called rough implant) rather than the smooth silicone gel implant with or without a saline component to obtain a more natural appearing breast and one that has less tendency to form a distorting, firm capsule. Implants may be inserted through the axilla, through or

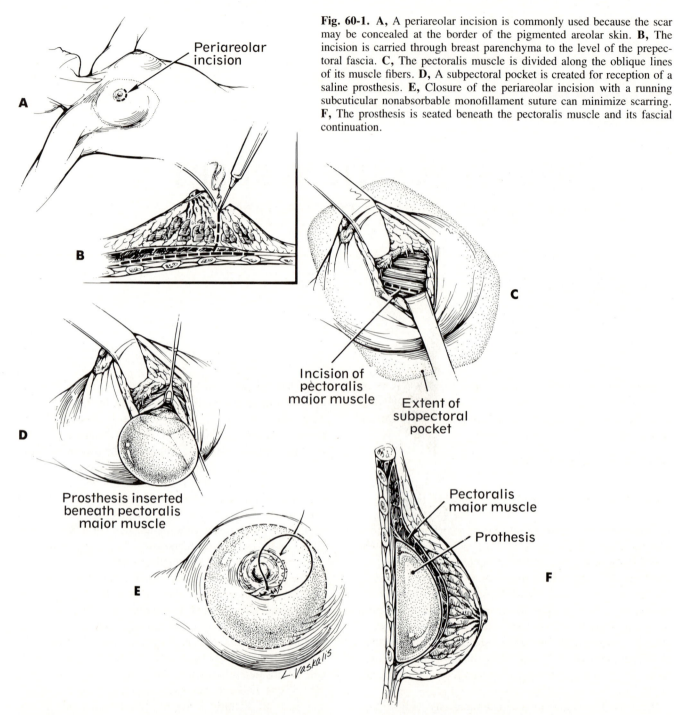

Fig. 60-1. A, A periareolar incision is commonly used because the scar may be concealed at the border of the pigmented areolar skin. **B,** The incision is carried through breast parenchyma to the level of the prepectoral fascia. **C,** The pectoralis muscle is divided along the oblique lines of its muscle fibers. **D,** A subpectoral pocket is created for reception of a saline prosthesis. **E,** Closure of the periareolar incision with a running subcuticular nonabsorbable monofilament suture can minimize scarring. **F,** The prosthesis is seated beneath the pectoralis muscle and its fascial continuation.

Periareolar incision

Incision of pectoralis major muscle

Extent of subpectoral pocket

Prosthesis inserted beneath pectoralis major muscle

Pectoralis major muscle

Prothesis

L. Vaskalis

around the areola, or by way of an inframammary incision. The decision concerning what type of implant to use and how and where to insert it depends on the needs of the patient, the preferences of the patient and the surgeon, and the ruling of the Federal Drug Agency, which has determined that silicone-covered, saline-filled implants can now be used only for patients desiring augmentation.

Before the operation, the plastic surgeon and the patient must decide on the eventual size of the breast. Most patients do not want their breasts to be excessively large; if so desired, the plastic surgeon should warn the patient that the chance of getting abnormal firmness is greater if the pocket created for the implant can barely contain it.

The operation is generally performed on an ambulatory basis, either under local anesthesia with intravenous sedation or under general anesthesia.

The patient should be aware not only of the possibility of abnormal firmness on one or both sides but also of the possibility of postoperative bleeding (less than one percent) and infection (less than one percent). Altered or decreased sensation in the nipple and areola may occur, but it is infrequent (less than ten percent).

In the immediate postoperative phase, patients are instructed not to lift more than ten pounds for two weeks, usually are asked not to drive for five days, but may return to work a week or ten days after operation. By four weeks,

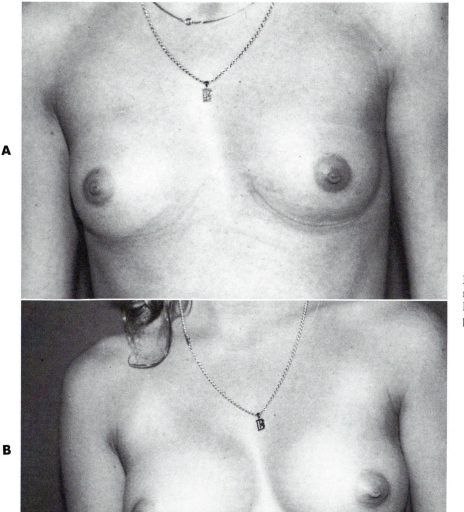

Fig. 60-2. A, A 32-year-old woman with mammary hypoplasia. **B,** Result after bilateral subpectoral augmentation mammoplasties.

they are able to resume almost all activities, including the use of a Nautilus.

It is important that patients having had augmentation mammaplasty continue their periodic follow-up with their physician who should continue to do careful breast examination and order mammograms on a regular basis, depending on the age of the patient and other conditions intrinsic to the breast. In surveys of women who have had augmentation mammaplasty, satisfaction with the result is extremely high, about 96%, even in the presence of abnormal firmness and shape secondary to capsular contracture. This incidence varies from 3% to 10% with silicone implants placed below the pectoral muscle to 30% if silicone implants (not rough textured) are placed immediately below the mammary gland. The incidence of abnormal firmness in patients having the polyurethane implant or the silicone textured implant is less than 8%; however, long-term follow-up of patients with these implants is lacking.

The following case is typical of the kind of patient, the type of operation, and the outcome that one can usually, but not always expect.

Case report. A 32-year-old married woman complained of bilateral mammary hypoplasia (Fig. 60-2, *A*). She described herself as having a breast size of approximately an A cup bra and requested enlargement to a size B cup bra. There was no family history of breast cancer. The patient described her marital relationship as stable. Her primary reason for requesting the procedure was a self-motivated desire to improve body image, which was supported by her husband.

A preoperative mammogram, the patient's first, disclosed no abnormalities. Bilateral subpectoral augmentation mammoplasties were performed under general anesthesia on an outpatient basis using 200-ml gel implants. Postoperatively (Fig. 60-2, *B*), she noted some diminution of sensation medially on each breast, but nipple areolar sensory function was unchanged. She has been followed for 3 years and has maintained a satisfactory breast form and natural softness.

BREAST PTOSIS

Ptosis is literally sagging of the breast. Although ptosis can occur in women who have very large breasts, pure ptosis is a condition in which the elastic envelope of the breast has been stretched. Ptosis may be either incipient, mild, moderate, or severe. Treatment may include correcting the ptosis and also augmenting the breast. This therapy would be for a women whose breasts are not only sagging but, when elevated, are too small for her liking. Although the operation of correction of breast ptosis seems technically not difficult, it is not an easy procedure in terms of long-term results because the condition can recur as a result of the passage of time and the effect of gravity.[13] Patients whose ptosis has been corrected by excision of the skin and elevation of the breast on the chest wall (Fig. 60-3) present a less complicated problem than do those who have had augmentation as well. Quite often, these women's breasts tend to sag again, their breasts going downward over the implant, which by now has become fixed to the chest wall. This possibility must be completely and clearly explained to the patient. The correction of breast ptosis requires incisions; in some procedures, the incision goes only around the areola; in others, additional incisions are made from the areola to the inframammary fold and then along the inframammary crease. Patients who have ptosis usually, but not always, heal without thick scars. Perhaps that is evidence of the cause, still unexplained, of why their breast skin has stretched. Patients frequently complain that their breast ptosis and perhaps atrophy have occurred after childbirth, particularly after

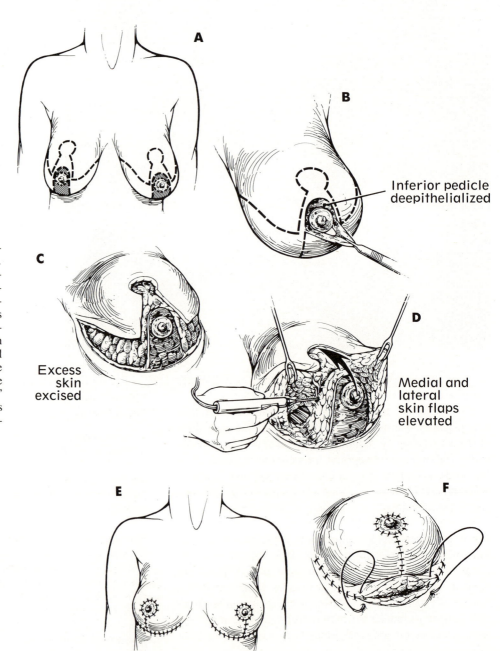

Fig. 60-3. A, Preoperative marking of excess skin to be removed. The nipple is sited at a more superior location. **B,** Deepithelialization of the inferior pedicle is commenced. Deeper blood vessels supplying the nipple are preserved. **C,** Excess skin has been resected. **D,** Medial and lateral flaps are elevated to facilitate wound closure. **E, F,** Wounds are closed to create an inverted "T" appearance. Most plastic surgeons prefer a subcuticular type of suture closure.

Inferior pedicle deepithelialized

Excess skin excised

Medial and lateral skin flaps elevated

nursing. In some women, it happens without pregnancy and quite often is a family trait.

The correction of breast ptosis with or without augmentation is usually done on an outpatient basis, under local or general anesthesia. Patients are given approximately the same instructions for their postoperative activities as they are after augmentation mammaplasty even when no implant has been used. These patients with ptosis should be advised to wear a bra as much as possible after operation and for years to come. Whether or not the bra decreases the chance of ptosis recurring is only conjecture. In this procedure, as in breast augmentation, infection and bleeding are possible, and, if an implant has been used, unfavorable results or complications associated with the implant, particularly abnormal firmness, can also occur.

Case report. A 39-year-old woman complained of bilateral mammary ptosis (Fig. 60-4), which became more noticeable after

the birth of her second child. Formerly, her breasts had a youthful form with a full shape of approximately size C cup bra. She had nursed both children for approximately 6 months each, noting loss of skin tone and atrophy of breast mass. Her breasts became increasingly ptotic, and she felt restricted in her choice of clothing. There was no family history of breast cancer. She had undergone a prior removal of a fibroadenoma at age 26.

Mastopexy was reviewed with the patient, emphasizing the location of incisions and the anticipated scarring. She requested concomitant breast augmentation to restore her former breast size. Under general anesthesia, bilateral mastopexies were performed along with subpectoral augmentation mammaplasties using 160-ml gel implants. She was discharged that same day. Results at 6 months after operation are shown in Fig. 60-5.

BREAST ASYMMETRY OR AGENESIS

Unilateral or bilateral agenesis of the breast or marked asymmetry can understandably distress a woman. Many

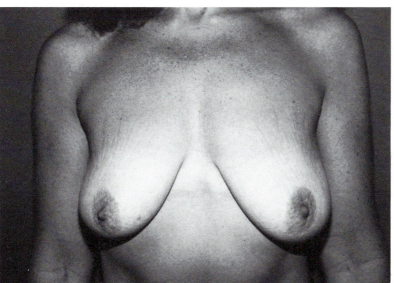

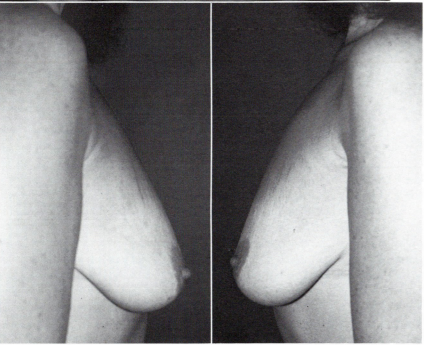

Fig. 60-4. A 39-year-old woman with bilateral mammary ptosis developing after the births of her two children.

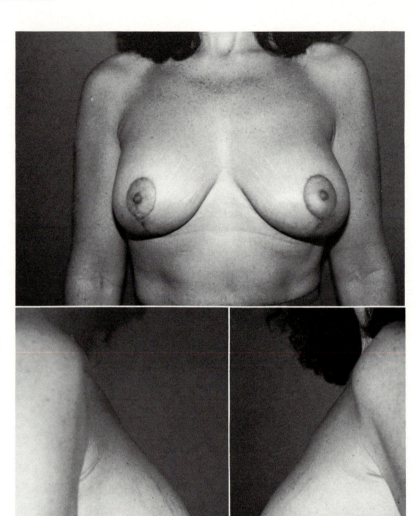

Fig. 60-5. Appearance of the patient 6 months after bilateral mastopexies with concomitant subpectoral augmentation mammoplasties.

are so ashamed of the condition that they have kept it a secret even from their parents, as well as their siblings and friends. Some adolescent girls have described the problem to their mother but have never allowed a parent to see it.

Because those who seek plastic surgery have obviously not adjusted to their abnormality, they may not be representative of all those who have this problem.[13] Some teenage girls engage in promiscuous sexual activity almost to prove to themselves that they can still be women despite their abnormality. One of our patients stated that she wanted to get pregnant to be able to see whether she could nurse.

Like the husbands of patients for augmentation, reduction, or correction of ptosis, the partners of many women

with mammary agenesis or asymmetry do not believe that their wife has to undergo the operation because the man has obviously adapted to it—at least to the degree that he has married that woman.

In taking a history, it is important to elicit from the patient whether she prefers that the breast that is large be reduced or whether she wishes the one that is smaller to be enlarged. It is easier, technically, to reduce the larger breast to match the opposite but only if that breast is of normal development. Frequently the situation involves a breast that is excessively large and one that is abnormally small. One may have to operate on both to get some kind of symmetry.

On physical examination, one must look carefully for

abnormalities of the chest wall, pectoral muscles, and spinal column, such as scoliosis.

Informing the patient depends on what has to be done: reduce or augment, one breast or both; whether to use inflatable or gel prostheses or an expander or whether to make a moulage of the chest and breast and insert something that will not only augment the breast but restore the chest wall to relative normalcy. It is almost impossible in a significant case of asymmetry to obtain perfection; perfection, as a matter of fact, in plastic surgery is more often the ideal than the reality. One should stress to the patient and to the parents, if the patient is a teenager, that the operation hopefully will give improvement but only seldom, if ever, perfection. As with augmentation mammaplasty, the patient and family must understand the possibility of infection, hematoma, abnormal contour and firmness if, indeed, the small breast is to be enlarged. Those patients require general anesthesia, possibly an overnight stay in the hospital, and then a postoperative recovery period similar to that of the patient undergoing augmentation mammaplasty or reduction mammaplasty, if one breast has been reduced. The patient should be wearing a bra for the initial few weeks after operation.

If an expander is to be used, the patient is informed of the necessity for serial injections of fluid after the insertion of the implant and eventual replacement of the inflatable expander with a permanent implant. There are expanders that are permanent, but these have not yet been developed without problems.

REDUCTION MAMMAPLASTY

Reduction mammaplasty, which is being performed increasingly, combines features of both aesthetic and nonaesthetic surgery (Fig. 60-6).[13,14] Although there may be controversy about how to classify reduction mammaplasty, there is little argument that most patients are pleased with the results. Indeed, the more severe the problem, the happier the patient is postoperatively unless a complication has occurred. The age of patients wanting this operation ranges from adolescent to postmenopausal. Most women with very large breasts consider their condition a deformity.[6] They feel conspicuous and resent being singled out for this aspect alone. They complain that men fixate on their breasts to the exclusion of their personality or intellect. Buying clothes is frustrating and expensive. Bras also are extremely costly. Commonly, women avoid athletics or going to the beach. Many dread the summer. Some adolescent patients give a history of avoiding male contact, of overeating, of encouraging in themselves obesity almost so that their large breasts are in proportion to their overweight body. This is one of the few situations in which the plastic surgeon would be advised not to have the patient lose weight before he or she operates; weight loss usually follows reduction because the patient is more pleased with herself and has already reached a goal that can be further maximized.

Not uncommonly, the father or husband opposes the operation. Many men like women with large breasts, despite the fact that the women suffer from this encumbrance. Patients commonly complain of pain in their neck and upper back and pain in pulling over the shoulders in the bra strap line.

The surgeon who treats the female breast not only for this condition but for others must be aware that the patient could have cancer, and every means must be taken to rule out its presence—careful physical examination as well as history, and mammography if the patient is 30 or older, or even younger if the patient has a strong family history of breast cancer.

The patient and the family, if the patient is a teenager, must be informed that the operation inevitably produces scars and can sometimes alter or decrease nipple-areola sensation. In addition, there is the possibility of bleeding and infection, for which antibiotics are usually given perioperatively. Surgery can interfere with the blood supply to the nipple and areola. This is obviously true if the nipple-areola are taken as a graft, a procedure less frequently done today unless the breasts are gigantic. Even with transposing the nipple and areola on a pedicle, it is possible that the blood supply will be compromised. This is more likely to happen in a patient who is a smoker and women who are should be enjoined to terminate that habit, at least 3 weeks before the operation and hopefully forever. Breast reduction decreases the likelihood of nursing from about 98% to approximately 70%. It is impossible to predict which patient will nurse and whether it will be from one or both breasts.

The surgeon should show patients examples of what is considered excellent, good, and poor scarring. It must be emphasized that scars do not disappear, although they usually become less prominent. The patient should also be told that this operation with its scars should be discussed between her and her partner. Occasionally, a husband adamantly opposes the operation, and that puts the plastic surgeon "in the middle." Although the patient obviously has the right to have the operation, the plastic surgeon might be wise not to perform it until the dissension can be worked out between the husband and the wife, perhaps through the intervention of a psychotherapist. If this is not done, the patient and her husband may unite in condemning the plastic surgeon for having performed an operation that has caused them marital problems, when, in fact, those problems have always existed and merely have been intensified by the operation.

In our practice, we almost never need to give a transfusion, but if it is a possibility, the patient should donate the blood herself (autotransfusion) so it can be used later at the time of surgery.

Insurance coverage must be discussed with patients. Insurance plans have differing criteria, usually based on weight of tissue removed per breast. In Massachusetts, for example, Blue Cross/Blue Shield honors both the hospitalization and the surgeon's fee (without balance billing) if a weight of 300 g is removed per side. The patient and her

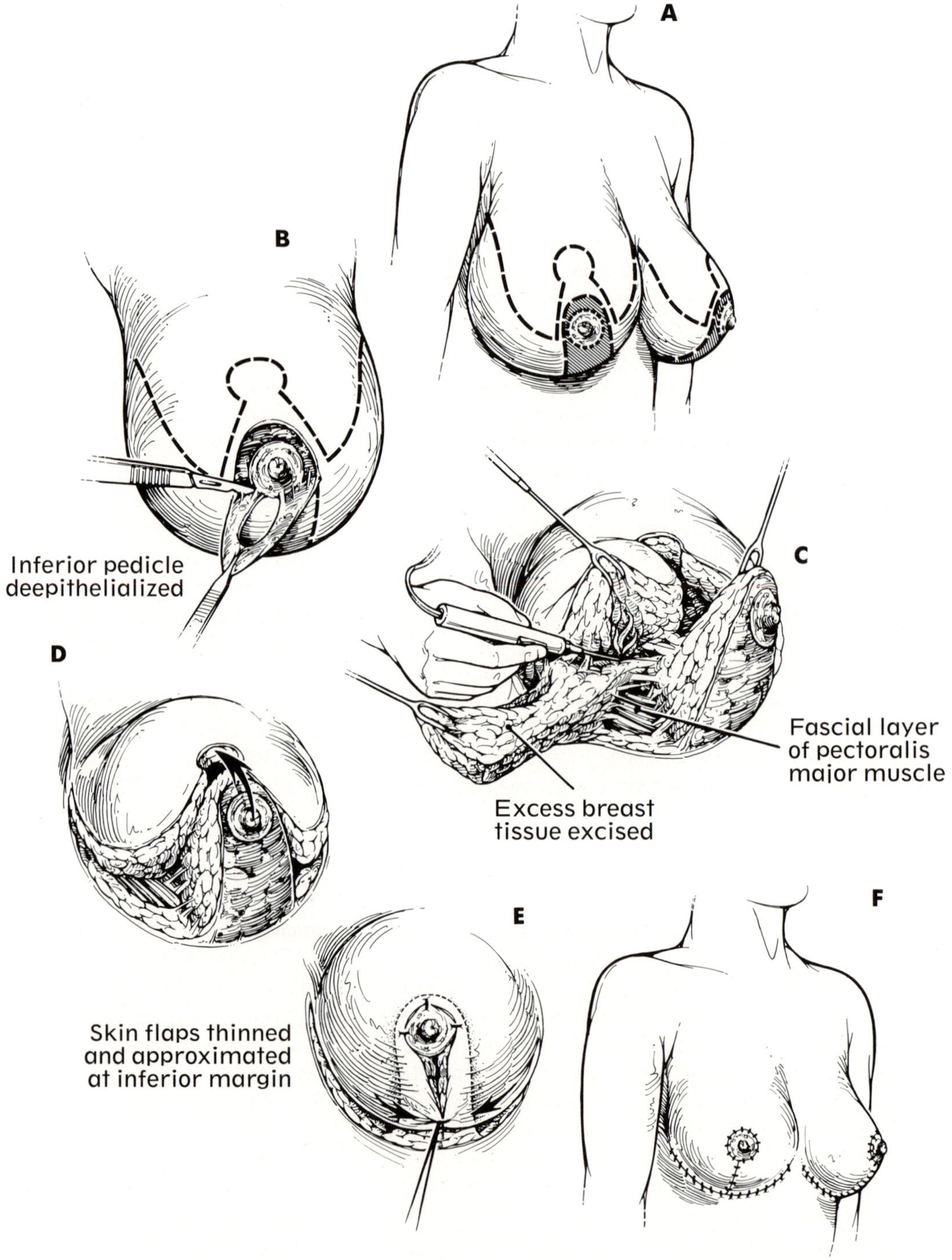

Fig. 60-6. A, Preoperative markings are similar to the technique for mastopexy. **B,** Deepithelialization of the inferior pedicle is performed. **C,** Excision of breast parenchyma from medial, lateral, and superior poles of the breast. Perforating vessels penetrating the inferior pedicle toward the nipple areolar complex are carefully preserved to maintain nipple vascularity. **D,** Reapproximation of the breast commences with elevation of the nipple to a more cephalad location. **E,** Excess skin is trimmed and contoured. **F,** Result demonstrates smaller size and improved contour following breast reduction.

Inferior pedicle
deepithelialized

Fascial layer
of pectoralis
major muscle

Excess breast
tissue excised

Skin flaps thinned
and approximated
at inferior margin

family must find out and the surgeon also should know whether or not the procedure and hospitalization will be covered. This can be a source of major disruption in the patient–doctor relationship.

The operation is almost always done under general anesthesia with a day or two in the hospital. There is pressure on the surgeon as well as the patient to have the procedure done on an ambulatory basis. This is difficult for the patient, who needs careful watching postoperatively as well as medication to relieve pain. The operation generally lasts 3 to 4 hours.

Although most patients who have reduction mamma-

plasty are ultimately satisfied with the results, not every woman is joyful immediately after operation. Despite their complaints about the large size of their breasts, some women experience transitory depression as the result of having their "badge" (though unwelcomed) of femininity removed. Many patients say they do not want to look at their incisions when their dressing is changed for the first time, but most eventually do. The reluctance to view their operative site is not only because of the presence of blood and stitches but also because of their need to accommodate to a new body image. In most patients, this takes just a few weeks.

Before operation, the surgeon must know approximately what size the patient wants her breasts to be. No guaranteed size should be given, but one should hopefully achieve a size that pleases the patient. When in doubt, the surgeon should take less rather than more because it is always easier to take out more afterwards than it is to enlarge the breast if one has been too zealous in performing the reduction.

Postoperatively, patients usually return to work in 2 weeks, although they are usually asked not to drive for a week and not to lift heavy bundles for 2 weeks. They are usually asked not to resume physical activity for 3 to 5 weeks, depending on what they wish to do and the surgeon's preferences.

If a woman develops a mass after operation, the surgeon or any physician who sees the patient must evaluate it carefully. It may be scar tissue or fat necrosis or reaction to a suture that has absorbed or is absorbing. A persistent lump, however, even in the presence of histologically normal tissue, may move during operation and requires a bi-

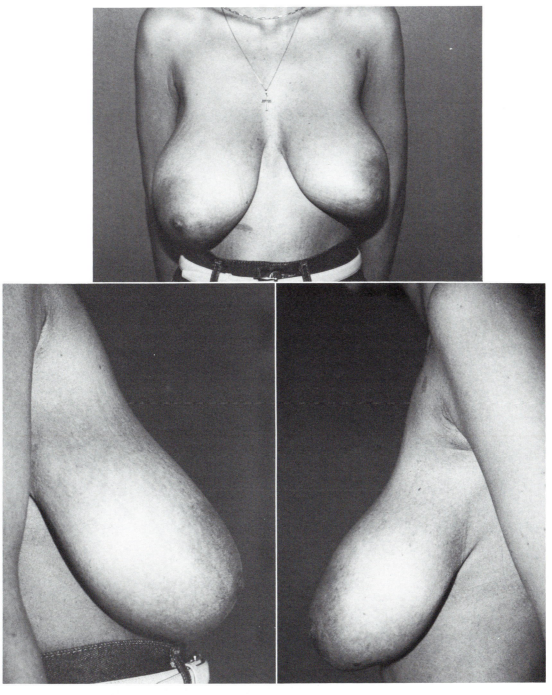

Fig. 60-7. Preoperative appearance of a 26-year-old woman with severe mammary hyperplasia, ptosis, and asymmetry.

opsy, particularly if the mass makes its appearance a few months later. Although mammograms are helpful, only the pathologist can provide the precise diagnosis.

Case report. A 26-year-old unmarried woman with bilateral mammary hyperplasia was evaluated for reduction mammoplasty. She complained of neck, shoulder, and back pain in association with her extremely hyperplastic breasts. The patient confided that she was embarrassed by her appearance, lacked self-esteem, and generally avoided social interaction with men.

Her preoperative mammograms demonstrated dense glandular tissue but no abnormalities. On physical examination (Fig. 60-7), she was noted to have marked mammary hyperplasia, ptosis, and asymmetry. Her breast size was severely disproportionate for her slender frame of 5 feet 3 inches tall and 103 lb. Bilateral reduc-

tion mammoplasties were performed with correction of the ptosis and asymmetry deformities. A final breast size of approximately a bra cup size B, as had been discussed with the patient preoperatively, was achieved (Fig. 60-8). Her satisfaction with the surgical result has been accompanied by psychologic benefits of improved body image and social adaptation.

SELECTING A MASTECTOMY INCISION

Optimal selection of an incision for mastectomy, whether it be simple or modified radical, requires close cooperation and careful planning by the surgeon performing the mastectomy and the plastic surgeon. Whenever possible, most plastic surgeons prefer a low transverse or oblique incision, which preserves the integrity of the infra-

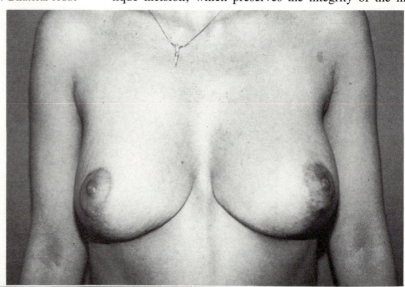

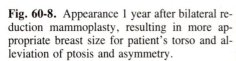
Fig. 60-8. Appearance 1 year after bilateral reduction mammoplasty, resulting in more appropriate breast size for patient's torso and alleviation of ptosis and asymmetry.

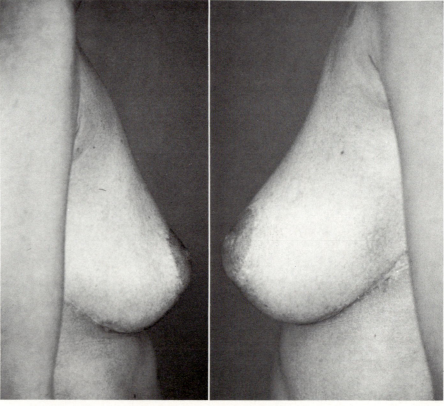

clavicular, medial, and superior native breast skin flaps. Because these areas are the most socially conspicuous portions of the breast, their preservation is critical. The oblique incision, in particular, facilitates the creation of a new breast that mimics the teardrop characteristics of normal breast anatomy. In those situations where a myocutaneous flap of tissue harvested from the back or abdomen is needed, inferiorly placed transverse or oblique incisions allow the flap to be shaped into a breastlike configuration with appropriate lateral, medial, and inferior pole curvature. Recreation of the breast's natural ptosis is also enhanced by these lower incisions. Any suture closure technique that leaves obtrusive suture marks on both borders of the incision should be avoided. In our experience, the best technique has been a subcuticular, running nonabsorbable suture, usually of Prolene because of its tissue sliding properties, which can be removed in its entirety approximately 10 to 14 days later. Layered closures, which approximate the dermis with fine absorbable suture material (5-0 Vicryl, for example), may enhance final scar appearance.

A number of factors can adversely affect incision placement. Breast lesions present along the medial, superior, or superolateral borders of the breast are the least favorable situations. When tumor persists along the edges of wide excisional biopsies, encompassment of these incisions within the mastectomy incisional lines may result in a significant alteration of the anticipated scar. Extension of the incision medially onto parasternal or even sternal skin surface invites the formation of hypertrophic and keloidlike scar appearances. If possible, these types of incisional designs should be avoided. Similarly, incisions that extend superiorly to the axilla or infraclavicular hollow pose major aesthetic problems during breast reconstruction. Often, the prosthesis or flap appears displaced and unnatural. Because the efficacy of mastectomy in controlling or curing breast cancer supercedes all aesthetic considerations, unfavorably located incisions may accompany the removal of any lesion located outside of the lower pole or periareolar locations. The patient should be appraised of these possibilities preoperatively so that she can anticipate a less than optimal scar placement or configuration.

Patients should also be informed of other local factors that can negatively influence the aesthetic result. The actual performance of the mastectomy may be associated with significant contour irregularities such as dimpling, retraction, thinning, atrophy, or inadvertent perforation of the cutaneous surface of the chest wall. In such instances, the reconstruction can appear flawed. Postoperatively, skin necrosis and local wound infections contribute to widened scars healed by secondary intention, or skin surfaces discolored by partial thickness loss.

BREAST RECONSTRUCTION

Although the goal of breast reconstruction is to restore the patient to a more normal physical appearance, no procedure ever recreates the unique aesthetic qualities and characteristics of a natural breast. However, the benefits of breast reconstruction far exceed considerations of anatomic form. Psychologic benefits,[12,38] including improved self-image, have been documented by many authors. Most women describe a sense of well-being and self-confidence after undergoing such procedures. A diminished fear of the mutilation of mastectomy has been shown to encourage patients to seek earlier diagnosis and treatment for breast lesions. As breast reconstructive procedures have improved and the number of available techniques has increased accordingly, it seems likely that more women will choose from these reconstructive options.

Immediate versus delayed reconstruction

Until the last decade, most breast cancer patients were advised to forego breast reconstruction until some mandatory period of cancer surveillance had been completed. This philosophy of delaying the reconstructive procedure for some period of time, usually in the order of 5 years, was based not only out of concern that a combined mastectomy and reconstructive procedure was too formidable and stressful a surgical undertaking, but also out of fear that cancer recurrence might be concealed by the presence of the reconstructed breast. Fortunately, these fears have receded as evidence has emerged that recurrences can be expeditiously detected in the presence of the reconstructed breast. Although not all physicians are completely convinced, most oncologists support breast reconstruction undertaken immediately after completion of the mastectomy or delayed some period of months thereafter. The actual period of delay may be influenced by issues of wound healing or the necessity for adjuvant chemotherapy or radiation therapy. The leukopenia and thrombocytopenia of most chemotherapy regimens require waiting until normal cell levels have been achieved. Radiation therapy, now being given less commonly on a postoperative basis, significantly influences the selection of a reconstructive procedure and is reviewed elsewhere in this chapter.

The two-stage procedure—mastectomy followed by delayed reconstruction—remains popular with many plastic surgeons who cite the greater control over local wound conditions and the enhanced results they can obtain. Immediate reconstruction may be associated with increased wound complications, such as skin necrosis, infection, hematoma, and exposure or extrusion of a prosthetic device. Nevertheless, immediate reconstruction has evolved to a point of proven safety.[10,26] It does require strenuous efforts by both the cancer surgeon and the plastic surgeon to plan and coordinate the two procedures. As the option of immediate breast reconstruction becomes more available to patients confronted by mastectomy, the trend toward choosing immediate reconstruction, observed in our practice for the past 10 years, will probably continue.

Neither term—immediate or delayed reconstruction—denotes a specific reconstructive technique. All procedures, including implants, inflatable expanders, and myocutaneous and microvascular flaps, can be performed on either basis. Although plastic surgeons initially preferred the simplest technique, insertion of a silicone implant beneath the pectoralis muscle for immediate breast reconstruction, improved inflatable expanders and complex flap procedures have been reported as successful choices for immediate reconstruction.[7] Availability of skin and soft tissues on the chest wall, more than any other factor, determines technique selection. The anatomy of the contralateral breast, if such exists, may also be a prime factor. In most patients, more than one breast reconstruction technique is appropriate for the patient's needs. The plastic surgeon who is most familiar with all of the available surgical options can customize the technique to the patient's unique reconstructive requirements.

Breast reconstruction techniques

Silicone implants. The modern era of breast reconstruction began with the introduction of silicone implants made of medical grade dimethyl polysiloxane approximately 30 years ago. Although the silicone implant has undergone considerable modification over this period and now includes an array of products that may or may not contain separate additional chambers for insertion of saline, the basic product has a silicone outer shell and liquid silicone fill. Recently, concern has focused on the issue of carcinogenicity, but no proven relationship exists between these products and breast cancer.

Originally placed subcutaneously, implants are now routinely located in a subpectoral location.[9,39] Added coverage from the adjacent serratus anterior muscle and rectus fascia permits total enclosure in a myofascial envelope. When these elements of the chest wall are absent, or the remaining chest wall skin at the mastectomy site is excessively tight and scarred, placement of the implant may be contraindicated. Ideal candidates for a silicone implant are women with a smaller breast size and healthy skin and soft tissues and no previous history of radiation therapy to the operative site.

Unlike augmentation mammoplasty, which can be performed under local or general anesthesia, dissection of the chest wall musculature almost always requires a general anesthetic. Given the relative paucity of soft tissues that characterizes most postmastectomy deformities, the procedure may be subject to complications of wound healing caused by skin necrosis, wound infection, exposure of the prosthesis, and ultimately extrusion. When compelled by local wound factors to remove the device, most plastic surgeons choose a different technique for subsequent reconstructive attempts. From an aesthetic point of view, silicone implants yield breasts that are small, rounded, and sometimes lacking definition in the area of the inframammary crease. The natural ptotic qualities of a normal breast may be absent. The simplicity of the technique is appealing to both patient and plastic surgeon, and the quality of the match for a woman with smaller breasts is usually satisfactory to excellent.

The major problem encountered with silicone implants is encapsulation, a process marked by deposition of fibrous

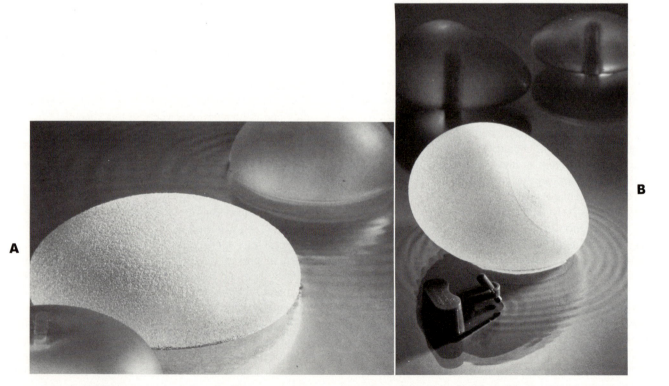

Fig. 60-9. A, Newer style of silicone implant has a roughened or textured surface designed to promote ingrowth of fibroblasts and decrease encapsulation. **B,** Inflatable expander with textured surface.

tissue in a circumferential manner about the implant. A number of factors have been identified in the causation of this process, including migration of molecules of silicone across the outer membrane of the prosthesis, but surface characteristics of the prosthesis and its interaction with surrounding local tissues appear to predominate.[2,5,17] Research directed at the surface kinetics and histology of the fibrous capsule suggests, but certainly does not confirm, that alteration of the implant's outer envelope may reduce the incidence of encapsulation. Newer products (Fig. 60-9) designed to counteract the process of fibrous deposition contain roughened surfaces of textured silicone or are coated with a polyurethane foam to permit ingrowth of fibroblasts. Proof of the efficacy of such products remains elusive.

Inflatable expanders. Recognition of the elastic and expandible qualities of skin and application of these concepts to the field of breast reconstruction were pioneered by a number of investigators during the past decade.[1,11,27] Specifically, the development of a hollow silicone device that could be injected percutaneously with saline in a stepwise manner (usually by weekly injections) represented a watershed breakthrough for the postmastectomy patient with tight skin and inadequate chest wall soft tissues. The device is inserted in a retropectoral position, just as is done for placement of a single implant (Fig. 60-10). As with all breast reconstruction techniques, inflatable expanders can be used on an immediate or delayed basis. The technique, known as skin-expansion breast reconstruction, stretches the available cutaneous and muscular layers through weekly injections of saline in volumes averaging 50 to 75 ml. A process of skin expansion encompassing 12 weeks of injection, followed by a sustained period of full inflation for 1 to 3 months, is the most common regimen. During the time of serial weekly injections of saline into a defined port valve located within or adjacent to the actual expander reservoir, the patient observes a full panorama of breast sizes evolving. The technique not only allows the patient to visualize these different sizes on the chest wall and select an optimal configuration based on this preview, but also deliberately overexpands the skin and its underlying layers. After full saline expansion has been performed, a second operation involving removal of the expander and placement of the permanent implant completes the breast reconstruction. Because the final silicone implant is smaller than the maximal volume of saline used for expansion, an excess of skin and underlying muscle results. Unlike the original tissues at the commencement of the process, the final tissues have an augmented microcirculation. The expansion process is believed to inhibit capsule formation and provide durable and supple soft tissue coverage for the prosthesis. This technique appears to be appropriate for women requiring a breast of virtually any size; it has been particularly well-suited for women in the mid to full breast size (bra size B or C) range. Some authors have achieved the creation of extremely large breasts through filling of inflatable expander reservoirs up to volumes of 1000 ml or higher. Numerous modifications of the original inflatable expander design have occurred, including the addition of a textured surface, a self-enclosed valvular mechanism, preferential lower pole directional expansion, and a device that can be permanently left in place without silicone implant substitution.[3]

Despite its purported advantages, the inflatable expander has had its limitations. In general, it has not been proven suitable for placement in an irradiated field. These tissues not only lack the requisite vascularity for adequate wound healing over the device but also develop a fibrotic rigidity, which resists stretching. Nonradiated wounds have not been immune to complications. In some series, an overall complication rate of approximately 40% has been reported, with skin necrosis, infection, hematoma, seroma, and extrusion predominating.[22,25] Some patients require removal of the inflatable expander from an infected field and replacement after secondary wound healing is completed. Under these circumstances, the aggregate number of procedures needed for the breast reconstruction may approach three (instead of two) in some instances.[32] Most plastic surgeons choose to reconstruct the nipple-areolar complex as a separate operation rather than add it to the final stage of the skin expansion breast reconstruction. General anesthesia is routinely used at each stage of the process, but hospitalization can usually be brief, involving a 1- or 2-day stay.

Case report. A 46-year-old woman was evaluated for bilateral breast reconstruction (Fig. 60-11, *A*). Three years earlier, she had undergone a left mastectomy for lobular carcinoma. A mirror biopsy on the right side was initially negative, but a subsequent excision also revealed lobular carcinoma, necessitating a right mastectomy. Her nodes were negative on both sides, and no additional therapy was recommended. At the time of her consultation, she had bilateral postmastectomy defects characterized by tight skin. Her former breast size had been a bra size C, and she requested breast reconstructions of similar size. The first stage of the reconstruction was accomplished by placement of a 700-ml inflatable expander under bilateral pectoralis major-serratus anterior muscle flaps. A 3-month course of weekly saline percutaneous injections of 60 ml into each expander reservoir was followed by the second-stage procedure. The expanders were removed, and 360-ml gel implants were inserted. One month after placement of gel implants, bilateral nipple-areolar complex reconstructions were performed as the third and final procedure (Fig. 60-11, *B*).

From an aesthetic point of view, the result achieved with an inflatable expander is deemed superior to simple insertion (one stage) of a breast implant. Nevertheless, defects in breast contour may be notable, including a deficient inframammary crease, inadequate lower pole contour, and excess upper pole fullness. Breast ptosis, while surpassing that of an implant, may be modest. To improve breast symmetry, many plastic surgeons have found it necessary to alter the contralateral breast by means of an improving procedure, either an augmentation, reduction, or mastopexy, in more than half of their patients. Inflatable

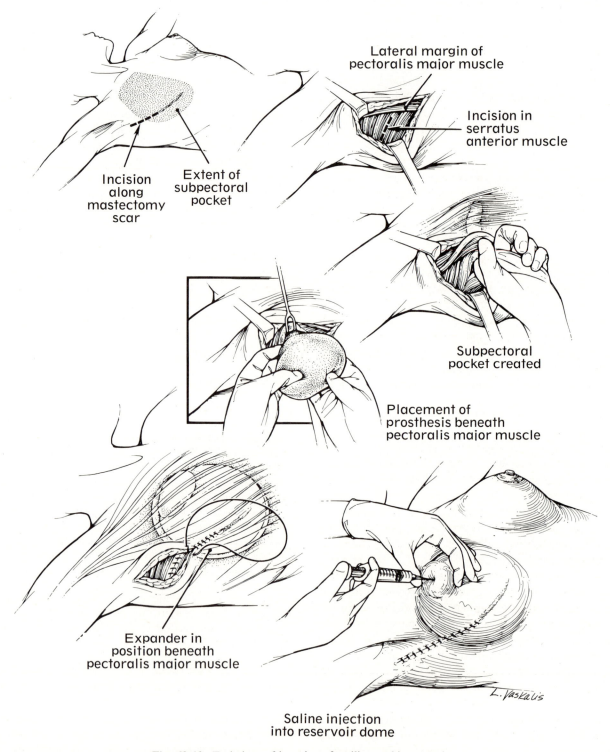

Fig. 60-10. Technique of insertion of a silicone skin expander.

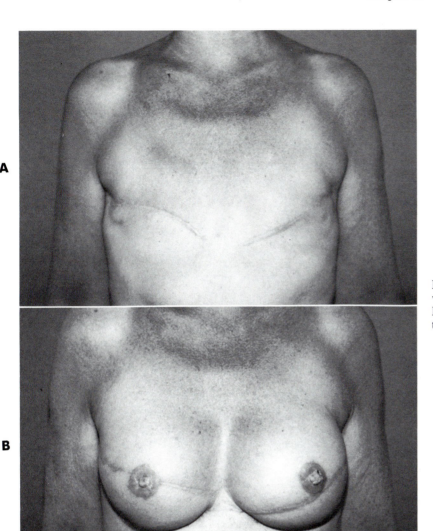

Fig. 60-11. A, A 46-year-old woman who underwent bilateral mastectomies for lobular carcinoma. **B,** Appearance of the patient after completion of a two-stage procedure using inflatable expanders.

expanders, unlike flaps, preserve other areas of the body from use as potential donor sites, thereby reducing the total amount of scarring incurred by a breast reconstruction patient. Encapsulation and its attendant deformity of breast shape appear lessened. The procedure has achieved its most satisfying results when bilateral breast reconstructions are necessary and the complex problems of symmetry with the contralateral breast do not exist.

Myocutaneous flaps. Myocutaneous flaps are composites of skin, subcutaneous fat, and muscle supplied by one or more dominant vascular pedicles. Although every muscle is potentially a flap donor site, not all are suitable for transfer. Depending on the specific donor site selected, myocutaneous flaps can consist of varying amounts of skin, fat, fascia, muscle, and bone. Some of the more common units were recognized for centuries, but the ability to transfer them with an intact blood supply was developed in the 1970s. Mobilization of these flaps requires careful preservation and dissection of the vascular pedicle to prevent any interruption of flow. Despite the abundance of myocutaneous flaps described for reconstruction of areas injured by neoplasm, infection, trauma, and radiation, two units—the latissimus and the rectus myocutaneous flaps—deserve special recognition.

Latissimus dorsi myocutaneous flap. Considered the workhorse favorite of myocutaneous flaps, the latissimus dorsi flap (Fig. 60-12) is preferred for its proven safety, ample size, and superb vascularity.[4,23] Although recognized as the body's largest motor unit, the latissimus dorsi muscle is actually an expendable mass of soft tissue. Despite its location on the back, the muscle functions as a shoulder rotator. The extensive cutaneous surface overlying the muscle is vascularized by a multitude of direct perforating vessels that traverse the subcutaneous fat superficial to the muscle to enter the skin above. A dominant vascular pedicle, the thoracodorsal artery and vein, enter the hilum of the muscle in association with its motor innervation, the thoracodorsal nerve.

During the transfer of the flap, or "transposition" as it is customarily designated, the latissimus dorsi muscle is ele-

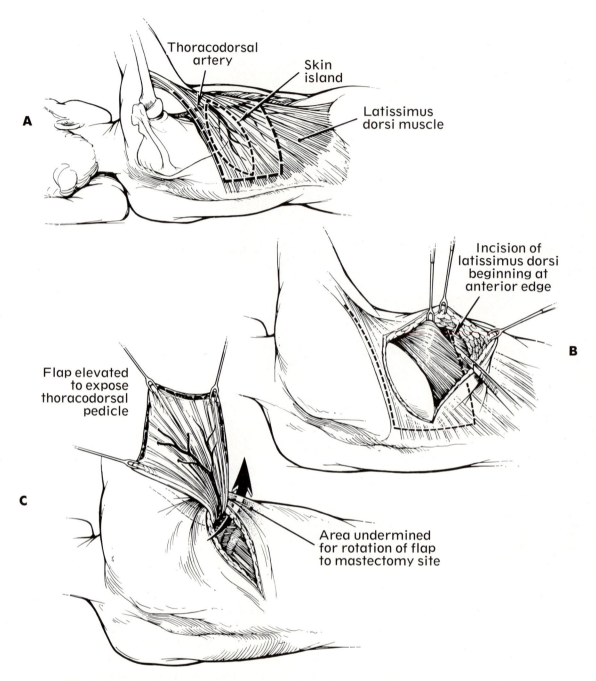

Fig. 60-12. A, Latissimus dorsi myocutaneous flap outlined on back prior to elevation. **B,** Borders of the latissimus dorsi muscle are elevated off the posterior chest wall by sharp dissection. **C,** The entire myocutaneous flap has been elevated. It will be transposed to the anterior chest wall by passing it subcutaneously beneath intact lateral chest wall skin.   *Continued.*

vated off the posterior chest wall by dividing most, but not necessarily all, of its attachments to structures of origin and insertion. Its vascular pedicle is identified and carefully preserved throughout the procedure. Depending on the extent of dissection of the pedicle, and its actual length, the muscle can be mobilized with portions of the overlying fat and skin. The cutaneous attachment is usually designed as an ellipse of varying dimensions; those patients with redundant skin of the back will permit transfers of cutaneous islands large enough to resurface exten-

sive wounds. Closure of the elliptical skin defect creates a linear scar that tends to be located transversely in the area of the bra strap (Fig. 60-12, *E*). Virtually any part of the ipsilateral hemithorax is accessible with this flap as are defects involving sternum and proximal portions of the contralateral chest.

The latissimus dorsi myocutaneous flap has proven to be particularly useful for the majority of postmastectomy defects. Its large expanse of muscle recreates the natural fullness and contour of the pectoralis major muscle and an-

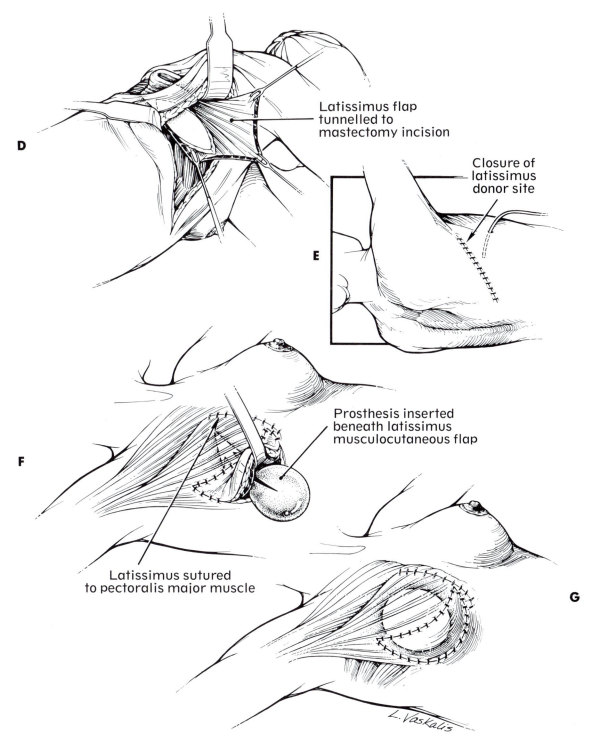

Latissimus flap
tunnelled to
mastectomy incision

Closure of
latissimus
donor site

Prosthesis inserted
beneath latissimus
musculocutaneous flap

Latissimus sutured
to pectoralis major muscle

L. Vaskalis

Fig. 60-12, cont'd. D, Latissimus dorsi transposed anteriorly and sutured to anterior chest wall.
E, Back donor site is closed after placement of suction catheters. **F,** An appropriately sized saline
prosthesis is inserted beneath the flap but anterior to the pectoralis muscle. **G,** Flap is shaped to
approximate the contralateral breast.

terior axillary fold when these structures are absent, while
simultaneously providing a soft tissue complement to areas
of deficiency in the infraclavicular hollow and the anterior
axilla. Even the most formidable defect, such as the wash-
board chest deformity of a radical mastectomy, can be satisfactorily reconstructed with this technique. Placement of

a silicone implant beneath the muscle enhances the breastlike contour of the flap unit while simultaneously facilitating the creation of a breast of any desired size. Patients
with radiated wounds and with extreme soft tissue loss are
excellent candidates for reconstruction with this technique.[19] Loss of the latissimus muscle as a functioning

motor unit is easily compensated by the remaining shoulder rotators. Most importantly, this myocutaneous flap has been distinguished by the reliability of its blood supply and a low incidence of either complete or partial necrosis. It is appropriate for use in any wound with diminished vascularity.

The addition of new skin, imported from the back and transferred by means of the cutaneous island of the flap, permits reconstruction of chest wall areas severely constricted by scarring after mastectomy. Latissimus flaps create a reconstructed breast with distinctly visible qualities of ptosis. For women who require a larger breast form, the latissimus reconstruction provides an excellence of symmetry and ptosis that matches the pendulousness of a generously proportioned remaining breast.

This versatile myocutaneous flap has proven to be equally applicable for breast reconstruction undertaken on an immediate or delayed basis. The patient scheduled for immediate reconstruction must be alternately shifted from the supine position of mastectomy to a lateral decubitus position for the latissimus flap. The donor site is closed, and the patient is returned to a supine position. Some plastic surgeons prefer delayed reconstruction because it allows them to situate the flap in a precise and optimal manner on the chest wall. When a large amount of skin or portions of the pectoralis muscle have been resected, the latissimus flap amply supplies the requisite tissues.

A major disadvantage of this technique is the encapsulation around the submuscular silicone prosthesis that normally accompanies the flap procedure. Although the exact incidence of this problem has not been determined, it occurs with enough frequency to compromise the result achieved.[24] Encapsulation may develop within months or years after the procedure, causing the reconstructed breast to be unnaturally firm in its consistency and distorted in contour. This process has been observed around different types of breast prostheses, including a new model group with a roughened or textured surface. The hardened breast is characterized by pain, superior pole prominence, and retraction of the entire reconstruction to a more cephalad position on the chest wall. Removal of the prosthesis, surgical incision of the fibrous capsule (or excision), and replacement with a different type of prosthesis sometimes can alleviate this unfavorable result.

Other objections to the latissimus flap point to differences in color tone and consistency between back and chest wall skin. Back skin tends to be slightly darker in tone and thicker than its anterior counterpart.

Complications. Seroma is, by far, the most common complication observed after latissimus dorsi breast reconstruction, developing in 20% or more cases.[30] The serous fluid accumulates in dependent portions of the back donor site wound and can cause pain or contribute to wound dehiscence. There is no agreement as to the optimal management of this problem, but many plastic surgeons aspirate large collections as an office procedure; smaller volumes of fluid gradually and spontaneously resorb. Infections appear to be infrequent problems, attesting to the superb vascularity of the flap and its elimination of scar and skin tension at the recipient site. Likewise, hematomas are most unusual after this procedure. Care must be taken, however, to ensure that vessels along the border and undersurface of the latissimus muscle have been properly controlled. Dehiscence of the back donor site wound is unusual, but lesser degrees of wound separation are more common and tend to heal uneventfully. As mentioned, complete necrosis or even partial necrosis of the flap is rarely encountered.

Case report. A 41-year-old woman underwent a left mastectomy for infiltrating ductal carcinoma. Two nodes were positive, and a course of chemotherapy was commenced after the mastectomy. Two years after mastectomy, she was evaluated for left breast reconstruction. During the consultation, the patient requested that the opposite breast be lifted but its size (bra size C) maintained. On physical examination, she was noted to have a significant left chest depression deformity characterized by an absence of skin and subcutaneous tissues (Fig. 60-13, *A*). Flexion of the pectoralis muscles revealed that the entire lower half of the left pectoralis either had been removed or was scarred and atrophic (Fig. 60-13, *B*). Based on this finding, she was considered an unsatisfactory candidate for placement of a subpectoral implant or expander. Despite a slim body habitus and scarcity of abdominal soft tissues, she had adequate laxity of the skin overlying the left latissimus dorsi muscle. A latissimus dorsi myocutaneous flap breast reconstruction was performed with insertion of a 260-ml gel implant beneath the myocutaneous flap complex. Three months later, a right mastopexy was done in conjunction with a left nipple areolar reconstruction (Fig. 60-13, *C*).

Transverse rectus abdominis myocutaneous flap (TRAM flap). The transverse rectus abdominis myocutaneous flap (Fig. 60-14) consists of a cutaneous island of abdominal skin attached to an underlying rectus abdominis muscle.[8,16] Usually, the cutaneous island is oriented transversely as an ellipse of varying sizes. It can incorporate upper, mid, or lower abdominal skin and extends as far laterally as the anterior superior iliac spine. Mobilization of this complex flap requires elevation of a rectus muscle with careful inclusion of the deep epigastric arterial pedicle located on its undersurface. A large subcutaneous tunnel is dissected between the abdominal donor site and the chest wall wound, which allows transposition of the flap to its new site. The flaps blood supply is derived from the internal mammary artery and its continuation beyond costal margin as the superior deep epigastric artery. Any encroachment of the internal mammary artery, either by surgical interruption or radiation injury, compromises the vascularity of the flap. In the absence of such factors, the TRAM flap is noteworthy for providing a large and well-vascularized mass of soft tissue. Abdominal fat included with the cutaneous island is strongly similar in consistency to breast tissue.

Because this particular myocutaneous flap provides such an abundance of tissue borrowed from the abdomen, it concomitantly creates a formidable defect at the donor site. After transposition of the flap, it is necessary to ap-

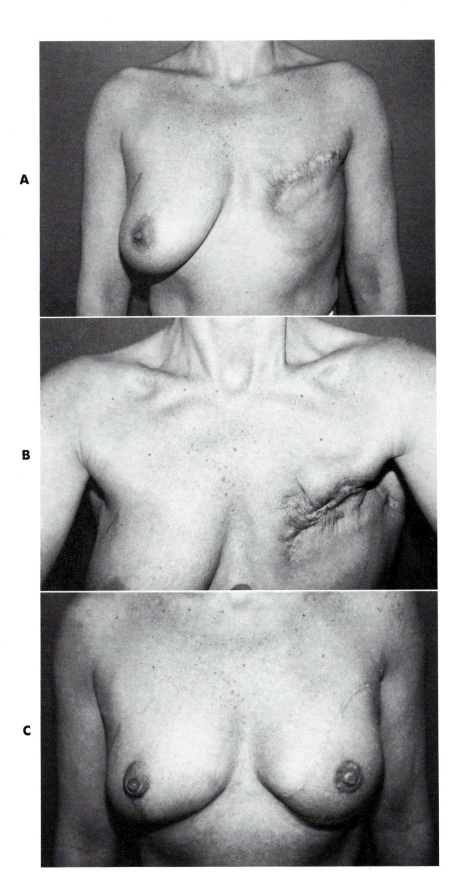

Fig. 60-13. A, A 41-year-old woman 2 years after left mastectomy for stage I breast cancer. **B,** During active contraction of the left pectoralis muscle, the lower pole of the muscle is noted to be absent. When significant portions of the pectoralis have been removed with the breast, the remaining muscle may provide inadequate soft tissue coverage for an implant or expander. **C,** Appearance of the patient after left breast reconstruction using a latissimus flap and placement of an implant beneath the flap. A right mastopexy was also performed as was left nipple areolar reconstruction.

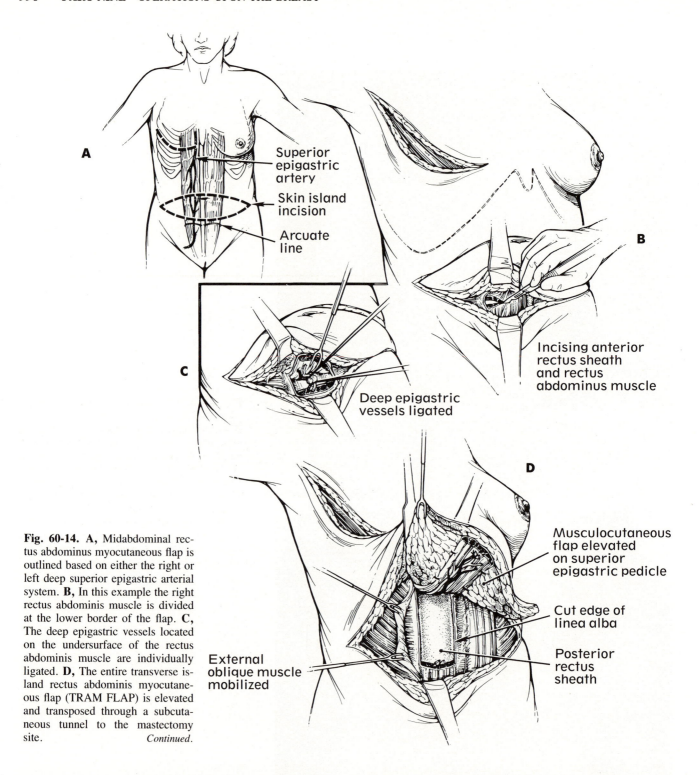

A, Superior epigastric artery
Skin island incision
Arcuate line

B, Incising anterior rectus sheath and rectus abdominus muscle

C, Deep epigastric vessels ligated

D, Musculocutaneous flap elevated on superior epigastric pedicle
Cut edge of linea alba
Posterior rectus sheath

External oblique muscle mobilized

Fig. 60-14. **A,** Midabdominal rectus abdominus myocutaneous flap is outlined based on either the right or left deep superior epigastric arterial system. **B,** In this example the right rectus abdominis muscle is divided at the lower border of the flap. **C,** The deep epigastric vessels located on the undersurface of the rectus abdominis muscle are individually ligated. **D,** The entire transverse island rectus abdominis myocutaneous flap (TRAM FLAP) is elevated and transposed through a subcutaneous tunnel to the mastectomy site. *Continued.*

proximate residual fascial layers of anterior and posterior rectus sheath to avoid subsequent hernia formation. Additional buttressing of the abdominal closure has been achieved by placement of a sheet of synthetic mesh or by mobilization of adjacent flaps of external oblique muscle. The entire operation may be lengthy and difficult.

Despite such obstacles of execution, the rectus abdominis myocutaneous flap is appropriate for reconstruction of most postmastectomy deformities. For extensive wounds of the chest wall characterized by osteomyelitis and radia-

tion injuries, the rectus flap supplies a vast surface area of skin. The underpinning of this flap—the rectus muscle—is well-suited to healing complex wounds injured by tumor, infection, or radiation. The entire procedure is performed with the patient in a supine position, an advantage for both immediate and delayed breast reconstruction. Like the latissimus flap, the rectus flap is also well-suited for reconstruction of a radical mastectomy defect. Some plastic surgeons consider it to be a superior choice, based primarily on its abundant soft tissues and ease of filling areas of

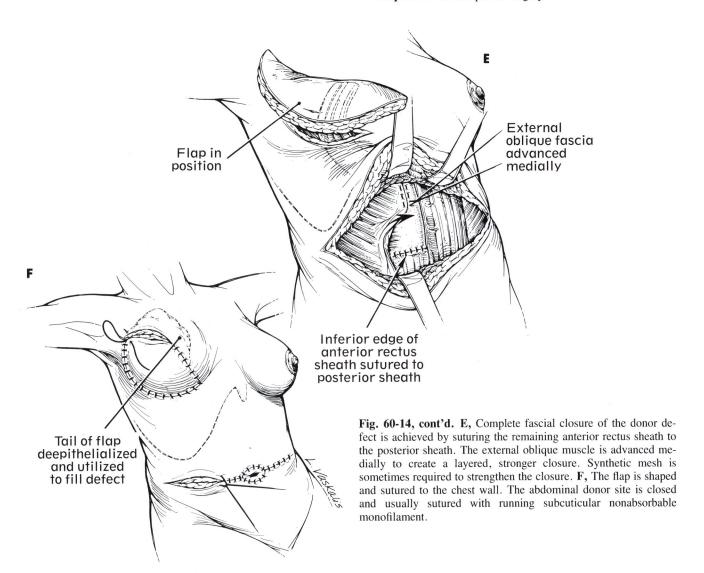

Fig. 60-14, cont'd. **E,** Complete fascial closure of the donor defect is achieved by suturing the remaining anterior rectus sheath to the posterior sheath. The external oblique muscle is advanced medially to create a layered, stronger closure. Synthetic mesh is sometimes required to strengthen the closure. **F,** The flap is shaped and sutured to the chest wall. The abdominal donor site is closed and usually sutured with running subcuticular nonabsorbable monofilament.

axillary and infraclavicular hollowing. The rectus flap is routinely used for total and modified radical mastectomy defects that require a moderate or large breast reconstruction for matching the contralateral side.[33] Elimination of the need for a breast implant, with its associated problems of encapsulation, is considered a major advantage of the technique.

Although a single pedicled rectus flap is sufficient for most problems in breast reconstruction, augmentation of the flap and its blood supply has been accomplished by inclusion of the other rectus muscle. These double-pedicled rectus flaps are designed with a single overlying elliptical skin island.[18] They are most appropriate for salvage mastectomy in patients suffering from osteoradionecrosis of ribs and sternum with large associated skin deficiencies.

Complications. Given the complexity of this procedure, it is not surprising that an array of complications have been reported. Flap loss constitutes the most serious complication, followed by varying degrees of partial loss. The exact incidence of this complication is unknown, but it occurs with enough frequency to warrant significant con-

cern. Some plastic surgeons have attempted to select out patients who are deemed to be high risk, but it is not clear precisely which patients are poor candidates. Obese patients, diabetics, and smokers have all been implicated. Pretreatment of these patients using exercise regimens or corticosteroids has not been proven to be effective. Why some flaps develop complete or partial necrosis is not well understood, but vasospasm, venous obstruction, and microcirculatory failure have all been attributed. Strengthening of the pedicle by inclusion of the opposite rectus muscle does appear to create a flap of improved vascularity. In addition to double-pedicled vascular augmentation, microsurgical techniques have been tried that connect the inferior deep epigastric artery to a separate source of blood supply on the lateral chest wall. This particular method, known as turbocharging the flap, results in a rectus flap with dual blood supply through the superior and inferior deep epigastric arteries.[15] Although successful for selected cases, it exposes the patient to a significantly lengthened operating room time and to the perils of a failed microvascular anastomosis.

Major problems of abdominal wall competence have occurred after rectus flap breast reconstruction. Mobilization of the rectus muscle with its anterior fascial sheath exposes the underlying posterior rectus to the forces of intraabdominal pressure. Although intact, this posterior fascial layer may become so severely attenuated in some middle-aged and older patients that a transitional zone of progressive fascial thinning extending from the level of the umbilicus to the arcuate line is observed. Extremely atrophied fascia is often located just cephalad to the arcuate line. This area of the abdomen, previously occupied by the muscle and its vigorous anterior sheath, constitutes a definite zone of vulnerability for subsequent hernia formation. Postoperative hernia incidence has ranged from 1% to 20%; concomitant loss of abdominal wall strength is another expected sequel of the procedure.[35] Patients need to be advised that the important spinal flexion function served by the paired rectus muscles is impaired by removal of either or both motor units. Postoperatively, they may experience a decreased ability to elevate the head while lying supine, or difficulty getting up from a sitting or lying position. Many patients spontaneously develop a number of compensatory mechanisms, such as grasping of a knee with both hands or rolling onto a side, to expedite rising from a reclining position. All patients should be examined carefully for signs of abdominal wall laxity or incompetence, which can predispose them to worsened abdominal wall function, or outright herniation, after operation. In particular, patients with an established history of low back pain who have required medical or surgical intervention for treatment may be unsuitable candidates for a rectus flap procedure. Finally, women of childbearing age should be informed of the paucity of information available regarding any increased risk during pregnancy or labor resulting from loss of portions of the rectus musculature. A recent case report[15] documented successful labor and delivery in one patient who had undergone previous rectus flap breast reconstruction, but more detailed information is lacking. Despite that apparently favorable outcome, some plastic surgeons are reluctant to recommend this procedure for women of childbearing age.

Other complications occurring after rectus flaps are fat necrosis, infection, hematoma, seroma, wound healing complications, and umbilical necrosis. When the flap is elevated on a single muscular pedicle, the contralateral portion of the transverse skin ellipse must derive its blood supply through a series of crossover myocutaneous perforators. For this reason, the ipsilateral hemiellipse of skin has a superiority of blood flow as compared to the marginal vascularity of the more distal (contralateral) skin segments. The contralateral skin can be discarded when ipsilateral sections are sufficient; when it is retained for the breast reconstruction, it may undergo necrosis and, ultimately, calcification. These calcifications may cause confusion and an inaccurate diagnosis if an inadvertent mammogram of the reconstructed breast is performed.

Given the diminished intrinsic blood supply of the lower abdominal skin and subcutaneous fat, delayed wound healing and skin dehiscence are not rare events. Most of these wounds heal secondarily, but leave obtrusive scars that are permanently thickened. Whether located on mid or lower parts of the abdomen, donor site scars tend to be coarse and discolored in many patients. Hematomas are uncommonly reported in most series, but may require operative intervention when the bleeding originates from the deep epigastric arterial pedicle. Seromas, however, do occur frequently despite suction drainage. Most seromas resolve spontaneously, but some necessitate aspiration for reasons of patient comfort. Uncommonly, some seromas coalesce in the epigastrium, developing a fibrinous wall, which gradually forms a pseudocyst.[34] These established masses continue to grow unless they are drained and their anterior walls are excised.

Umbilical necrosis occurs when its blood supply is compromised during flap elevation. Because the embryologically derived umbilical blood vessels are obliterated in most adults, it is important to maintain a cuff of periumbilical fat for purposes of umbilical vascularity. Overzealous skeletonization of the umbilicus will risk its devascularization, and, although functionally insignificant, the umbilicus exerts enough symbolic importance to many people to warrant its preservation.

Case report. A 54-year-old woman had undergone a left modified radical mastectomy for stage II breast cancer 6 years earlier. Her opposite breast was hyperplastic and pendulous—physical features that had not disturbed her before the mastectomy. Over the past 2 years, she had noticed progressive neck and shoulder pain, which both she and an orthopedic surgeon attributed to the unilateral pendulousness of the right breast. She requested right breast reduction and left breast reconstruction (Fig. 60-15, *A*). On physical examination, she had a large abdominal panniculus, which was considered optimal for a rectus abdominis myocutaneous flap breast reconstruction. After preoperative consultation with the patient, a left breast reconstruction of approximately a bra size C-D was determined to be aesthetically appropriate for her body habitus and consistent with her desire for the full-breasted appearance to which she was accustomed. The left breast reconstruction with a left rectus flap was performed as the first part of an anticipated two-stage procedure. Three months later, right breast reduction was accomplished in conjunction with left nipple areolar reconstruction (Fig. 60-15, *B* and *C*).

Microvascular free flap breast reconstruction. For most mastectomy defects, adequate breast reconstruction can be achieved with the use of synthetic devices such as silicone implants and expanders or with autogenous tissue borrowed from the back or abdomen. The simplicity of using synthetic material is sometimes belied by complications of firmness, encapsulation, and extrusion. Autogenous techniques, exemplified by the latissimus dorsi and rectus abdominis myocutaneous, supply soft tissues of suitable bulk and warmth, which can be sculpted into a breast of virtually any size or contour. In certain situations, previous abdominal surgery may render that site unavailable for a rectus flap procedure, or the thoracodorsal

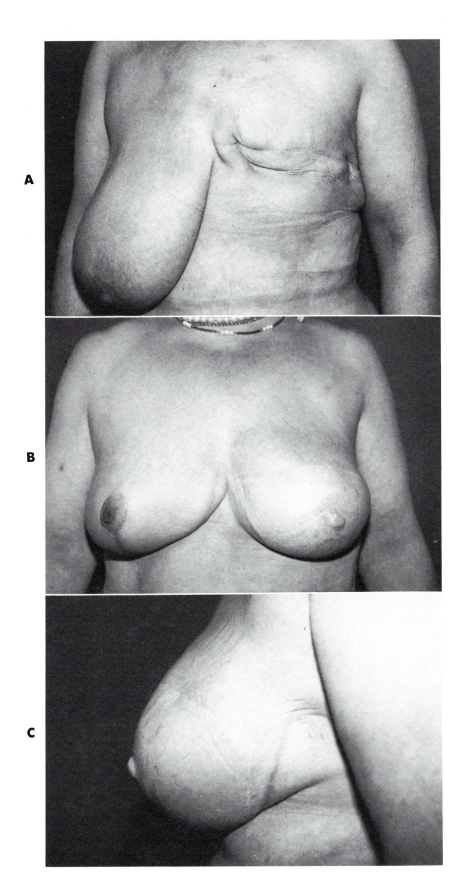

Fig. 60-15. A, A 54-year-old woman who had undergone previous left modified radical mastectomy. She complained of neck pain, which she and her orthopedist related to the right breast hyperplasia. **B,** Appearance of the patient after a left rectus flap breast reconstruction was performed as the initial procedure, followed by right breast reduction and left nipple-areolar reconstruction 3 months later. (Anterior view.) **C,** Lateral view of same patient.

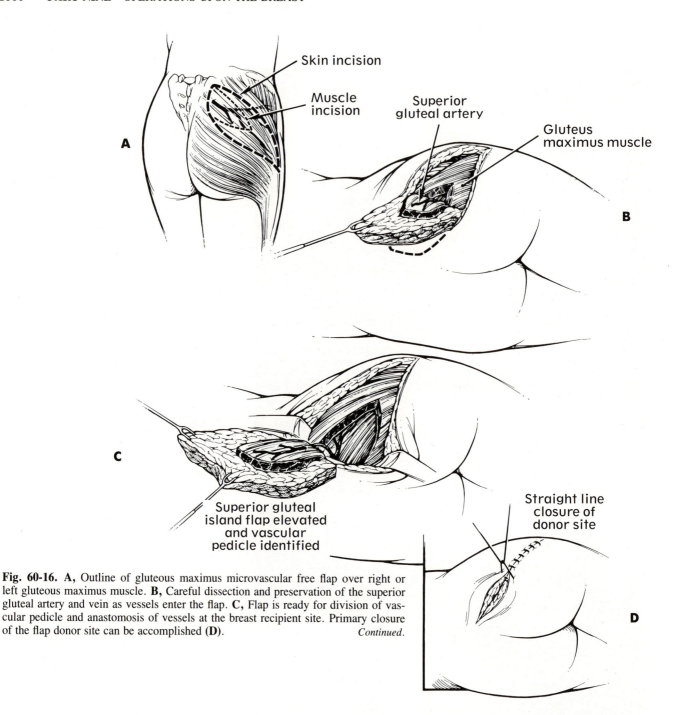

Fig. 60-16. A, Outline of gluteous maximus microvascular free flap over right or left gluteous maximus muscle. **B,** Careful dissection and preservation of the superior gluteal artery and vein as vessels enter the flap. **C,** Flap is ready for division of vascular pedicle and anastomosis of vessels at the breast recipient site. Primary closure of the flap donor site can be accomplished (**D**). *Continued.*

arterial pedicle may have been previously ligated (during the course of a radical mastectomy) or heavily radiated, obviating use of a latissimus flap. Microvascular free flaps comprised of abdominal or buttock skin, fat, and muscle were developed to remedy such situations. These exceedingly complex and challenging operations differ fundamentally from pedicled myocutaneous flaps. In free flap procedures, the donor tissues and their attendant nourishing vessels are dissected and divided. A recipient vessel on the chest wall is selected and prepared for the microvascular reanastomosis, which reestablishes flow into the donor flap. The donor site is closed primarily, just as is done for myocutaneous flaps. After successful reanastomosis, the

microvascular flap is shaped and contoured to create the desired breast reconstruction.

The superior gluteal flap (Fig. 60-16). This flap of the upper portion of the gluteus maximus muscle, subcutaneous fat, and skin derives its blood supply from the superior gluteal artery.[28] Most patients have adequate or even generous amounts of tissue available for transfer from this site. The flap leaves an inconspicuous donor site scar on the upper portion of the buttock and little, if any, functional deficit. Inferior gluteal contributions to gait controlled by the inferior gluteal neurovascular bundle remain largely intact.

Like all microvascular free flaps, the tissue must be re-

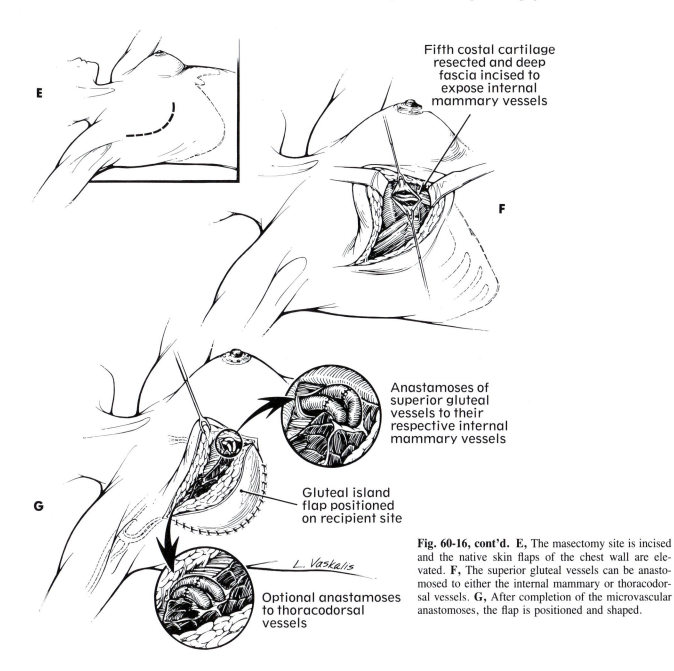

Fifth costal cartilage resected and deep fascia incised to expose internal mammary vessels

Anastamoses of superior gluteal vessels to their respective internal mammary vessels

Gluteal island flap positioned on recipient site

L. Vaskalis

Optional anastamoses to thoracodorsal vessels

Fig. 60-16, cont'd. **E,** The masectomy site is incised and the native skin flaps of the chest wall are elevated. **F,** The superior gluteal vessels can be anastomosed to either the internal mammary or thoracodorsal vessels. **G,** After completion of the microvascular anastomoses, the flap is positioned and shaped.

attached to a suitable vessel in the vicinity of the breast reconstruction. Internal mammary, thoracodorsal, lateral thoracic, and external jugular vessels have been preferred for that purpose. Constraints created by the limited length of the donor vessels, or unsuitability of the recipient ones, have restricted the placement or contouring of the flap into a breast mound. The relatively short vascular pedicle of the superior gluteal flap abetted the search for other free flap donor sites, as did the difficulty of the donor site dissection.

Transverse rectus abdominis myocutaneous free flap.
As a result of the extensive experience gained from pedicled TRAM flaps, this site became the next logical source of free flap donor tissue.[15] Unlike the superior gluteal flap, the TRAM flap contains donor vessels of superior caliber and length—the inferior deep epigastric artery and vein.

The longer vascular leash obtained has eliminated problems of tethering of the breast reconstruction and has greatly reduced episodes of microvascular thrombosis and flap loss. Another advantage of the rectus free flap, the use of the supine position for the entirety of the procedure, contrasts with the need for alternate positioning of the patient from lateral decubitus to supine when the superior gluteal procedure is performed. Also, in a free TRAM flap, less muscle and fascia need to be taken, thereby facilitating closure of the abdominal wall and lessening the chance of subsequent hernia. Finally, the free TRAM flap supplies generous portions of abdominal skin and subcutaneous fat, which may exceed the availability of soft tissue in the upper buttock.

From an aesthetic point of view, microvascular free flaps harvested from the abdomen may provide a greater versatility of reconstruction than is usually possible with its gluteal counterpart. Like all microsurgical transfers, the free TRAM flap is vulnerable to major complications of thrombosis of the microvascular anastomosis and ultimate necrosis of the donor tissues. The possibility of complete loss of the breast reconstruction can be emotionally devastating to this group of patients who have already lost a breast to cancer. Although some microsurgeons have reported a 95% success rate of free tissue transfer, others indicate an overall complication rate, including reexploration for vascular problems, of 25% to 30%. Many plastic surgeons and their patients are daunted by these formidable statistics.

NIPPLE-AREOLAR RECONSTRUCTION

Reconstruction of the nipple-areolar complex is usually performed weeks or months after completion of the breast reconstruction.[21] This period of delay allows time for healing and descent of the reconstructed breast. In addition to issues of size and symmetry, a reconstructed nipple should match the color, texture, and configuration of the existing contralateral structure, assuming such exists. When needed, bilateral nipple areolar reconstructions optimize the opportunity for matching.

A variety of donor sites have been identified, including the opposite breast, medial thigh and labial skin, inguinal and buttock creases, ear, and toe. Most plastic surgeons

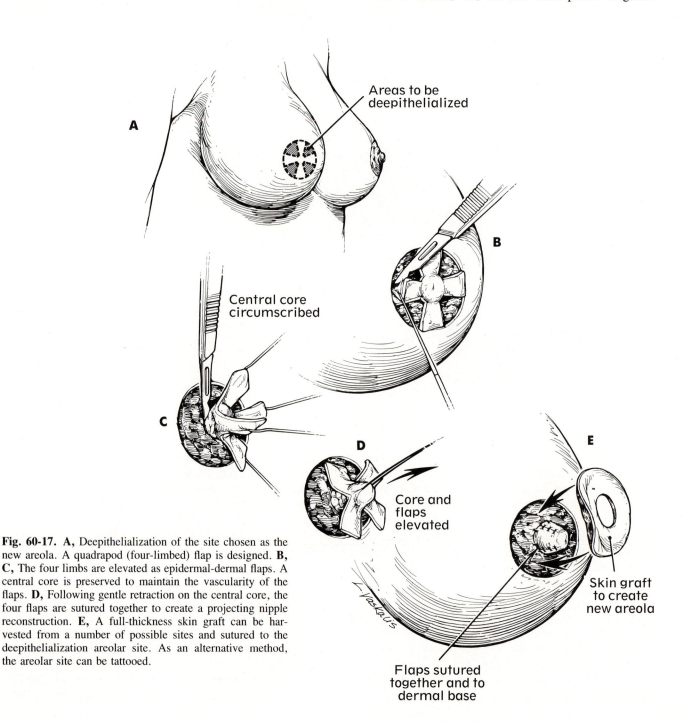

Fig. 60-17. A, Deepithelialization of the site chosen as the new areola. A quadrapod (four-limbed) flap is designed. **B, C,** The four limbs are elevated as epidermal-dermal flaps. A central core is preserved to maintain the vascularity of the flaps. **D,** Following gentle retraction on the central core, the four flaps are sutured together to create a projecting nipple reconstruction. **E,** A full-thickness skin graft can be harvested from a number of possible sites and sutured to the deepithelialization areolar site. As an alternative method, the areolar site can be tattooed.

prefer to harvest a full-thickness skin graft from the medial thigh because the increased pigmentation of this area creates a natural contrast of tone with the surrounding skin of the breast reconstruction. The tendency of a full-thickness skin graft to darken its color varies from patient to patient, but, in most cases, the match is satisfactory. In those situations where significant tonal contrasts are necessary, intradermal tattooing with medical grade pigment is an excellent remedy.[37]

Creation of a projecting central nipple of approximately the same diameter and height as the other side can pose a significant challenge. Most techniques involve elevation of local flaps of skin and subcutaneous fat from the surface of a myocutaneous flap or from the residual native skin present after mastectomy and reconstruction with implants or expanders.[20] Depending on the particular design on the surface of the breast reconstruction site, these flaps have been dubbed quadrapod (Fig. 60-17), skate, pin wheel, or other descriptive terms. Each design involves sculpting of skin flaps based on the vascularity of the subdermal plexus.

Application of a wide variety of techniques has resulted in the creation of aesthetically pleasing nipples that reasonably match the contralateral form. All of the techniques can be performed under local anesthesia and on an outpatient surgery basis, adding minimal morbidity for the patient. Major complications occurring after nipple reconstruction have consisted of partial or complete necrosis of the central nipple, combined with varying degrees of loss of the areolar graft. Fortunately, complete necrosis of the nipple has been a most unusual complication. Donor site complications have involved wound separation, delayed healing, and infection. It is unclear what percentage of patients return for this final stage of breast reconstruction, but those who do express a high degree of satisfaction with the results achieved.

SENSATION AFTER BREAST RECONSTRUCTION

Most patients fail to inquire about sensation after breast reconstruction, either because it may not have been discussed with the plastic surgeon or because they mistakenly assume there will be a complete absence of feeling. The normal surface sensuality of the breast is always diminished after mastectomy, a result of the removal of breast parenchyma and its associated sensory innervation. Among the intercostal nerves that penetrate the breast substance from the lateral pectoral border, the fourth intercostal directly innervates the nipple-areolar complex and underlying tissues. Unfortunately, this important sensory nerve, along with other cutaneous contributors, is routinely removed during mastectomy. Skin sensation is, however, preserved in the superior and inferior native flaps, which are approximated at the conclusion of the procedure. Breast reconstruction procedures that recreate the breast mound by stretching the available chest wall skin tend to retain some qualities of light touch and pressure, but normal sensation is never present. When myocutane-

ous flaps are used from the back (latissimus dorsi) or abdomen (rectus abdominis), the transferred tissues lack sensory innervation. These flaps do contain their respective motor nerves—thoracodorsal for the latissimus flap and intercostal for the rectus flap—but the cutaneous component of each flap has no sensory trunk. Although they will gradually note some ingrowth of sensory branches around the periphery of the cutaneous island, usually appearing about a year later, patients should be advised that the flap reconstruction is generally devoid of sensation. Chest wall recipient sites that have been previously irradiated or require postoperative radiation therapy may not develop even a rudimentary level of sensory innervation. Similarly, the nipple-areolar complex reconstruction, usually sited centrally on the myocutaneous flap or the native skin flaps, will lack any appreciable surface sensory function.

BREAST RECONSTRUCTION AND RADIATION

The increasing popularity of conservative surgery and radiotherapy poses unique reconstructive challenges for the plastic surgeon. As the technique of lumpectomy and radiation has gained international recognition, more patients with radiation changes of the skin and soft tissues of the chest wall and residual breast parenchyma are requiring additional procedures. Two important groups are involved: patients who have undergone lumpectomy or quadrantectomy and radiation therapy, and those who have failed conservative therapy because of cancer recurrence in the irradiated breast. In both situations, the reconstructive surgeon must understand the effects of radiation therapy on breast tissue.[31]

Physical findings after radiation consist of breast edema, retraction, fibrosis, induration, skin discoloration, and telangiectasia formation. Vascularity of the breast is significantly reduced by radiation, resulting in ischemic tissues prone to wound healing complications. Previously radiated chest wall skin is characterized by a leathery induration that is rigid and unyielding when subjected to stretching by an inflatable expander. Cutaneous sensory function is significantly reduced. Even the minimally increased skin tension occurring when a subpectoral implant is placed may abet skin necrosis and ultimate extrusion of the prosthetic device. Such patients are, in general, poor candidates for techniques using foreign body placement and must instead rely on the independent vascularity provided by a myocutaneous flap. In more extreme situations characterized by cancer recurrence in the irradiated breast, or in the presence of ulceration and osteoradionecrosis, a myocutaneous flap is always necessary. Patients with these life-threatening problems become candidates for salvage mastectomy with immediate reconstruction using a myocutaneous flap.

Radiation therapy may create a zone of injury that encompasses skin and soft tissues extending from clavicle to costal margin and lateral chest wall to sternum. Microvascular free flap transfers can be especially hazardous in this group of patients due to radiation-induced injury of the intended recipient vessels and the increased probability of thrombosis. For this reason, most plastic surgeons select a latissimus or rectus myocutaneous flap, based on availability of the particular unit and the requirements of the wound defect. If neither flap is available, a microvascular free flap procedure may have to be undertaken.

RECURRENCE AFTER BREAST RECONSTRUCTION

Breast cancer surveillance after mastectomy and reconstruction is an issue of critical importance for the patient and the physicians involved in her care. Earlier concerns that implants would impede the detection of breast cancer recurrence have not materialized. Gradually, the imposition of a mandatory waiting period for commencement of the reconstruction was replaced by the concept of immediate breast reconstruction. A number of studies have demonstrated that immediate breast reconstruction with implants or expanders does not affect cancer recurrence rates or survival rates in clinical stage I and II patients. Locoregional recurrences, usually manifested by visible and palpable cutaneous or subcutaneous tumor aggregates, are readily diagnosed by simple physical examination and can be treated by excision, radiation, or chemotherapy. Optimal cancer detection and management are not compromised.

When myocutaneous flaps were introduced for both delayed and immediate breast reconstruction, there was renewed concern that transfer of large masses of autogenous soft tissue could obscure a recurrence and lead to a delay in diagnosis. It was theorized that tumor cells would proliferate beneath the flap, escaping detection. Fortunately, a large review of this potential problem showed that breast cancer recurrences invariably developed on the native skin surface bordering the myocutaneous flap.[36] Again, all of the locoregional recurrences were detectable by physical examination and no instances of occult recurrent cancer cells beneath the flap have been documented. These findings suggest that the use of myocutaneous flaps for immediate breast reconstruction does not interfere with the detection or treatment of a local recurrence. Furthermore, 90% of patients with local recurrence, whose incidence is about 9%, have systemic disease.

MANAGEMENT OF THE OPPOSITE BREAST

The basic premise of breast reconstruction is the achievement of symmetry with the remaining breast. In those situations where the opposite breast is aesthetically acceptable, all efforts are directed at creating a new breast of approximately the same size, shape, and configuration. Not uncommonly, the opposite breast can be altered by one or more of the techniques described earlier in this chapter—augmentation, mastopexy, or reduction. Some patients perceive in the plan to reconstruct the postmastectomy defect an opportunity to improve their opposite breast, which they might have spurned under other circumstances. The belief that they might look better than they did before mastectomy provides considerable psychologic comfort.

Women who were not satisfied with a small breast size may choose to augment the opposite breast. After consultation with the patient's oncologist, it is usually permissible to place the breast implant in a subpectoral location that impedes to a lesser degree the mammographic or physical evaluation of the patient.

Similarly, patients with hyperplastic and pendulous breasts often choose either a reduction mammoplasty and mastopexy technique of breast correction, or may prefer a breast reconstruction that attempts to match the opposite breast. Loss of a breast can lead to a protective stance in regard to any proposed surgical intervention for the other side. Scarring after breast reduction does not appear to interfere with the performance of an accurate physical examination.

In the most extreme situations, prophylactic mastectomy may be recommended for optimal management of high-risk patients. For those patients whose breast pathology indicates a likelihood of bilaterality, total mastectomy is preferred to subcutaneous mastectomy. Total mastectomy achieves a more complete removal of breast parenchyma, leaving only residual microscopic foci of breast tissues at the limits of the dissection. The resulting bilateral mastectomy defects lend themselves to placement of implants or expanders because of the ease in attaining symmetry.

REFERENCES

1. Argenta LC: Reconstruction of the breast by tissue expansion, *Clin Plast Surg* 11:247, 1984.
2. Asplund O: Capsule contracture in silicone gel and saline filled breast implants after reconstruction, *Plast Reconstr Surg* 73:270, 1984.
3. Becker H: The expandable mammary implant, *Plast Reconstr Surg* 79:631, 1987.
4. Bostwick J III, and Scheflan M: The latissimus dorsi myocutaneous flap: one stage breast reconstruction, *Clin Plast Surg* 7:71, 1980.
5. Caffee HH: The influence of silicone bleed on capsule contracture, *Ann Plast Surg* 17:284, 1986.
6. Cline CJ: Psychological aspects of breast reduction surgery. In Goldwyn RM, editor: *Reduction mammaplasty,* Boston, 1990, Little, Brown.
7. Cohen IK, Turner D: Immediate breast reconstruction with tissue expanders, *Clin Plast Surg* 14:491, 1987.
8. Dinner MI, Labandter HP, Dowden RV: The role of the rectus abdominis myocutaneous flap in breast reconstruction, *Plast Reconstr Surg* 69:209, 1982.
9. Dowden RV, Dinner MI: Breast reconstruction without skin flaps, *Clin Plast Surg* 11:265, 1984.
10. Georgiade GS et al: Long-term clinical outcome of immediate reconstruction after mastectomy, *Plast Reconstr Surg* 76:415, 1985.
11. Gibney J: The long-term results of tissue expansion for breast reconstruction, *Clin Plast Surg* 14:509, 1987.
12. Goin MK, Goin JM: Psychological reactions to prophylactic mastectomy synchronous with contralateral breast reconstruction, *Plast Reconstr Surg* 69:632, 1982.
13. Goldwyn RM: *The patient and the plastic surgeon,* Boston, Little, Brown.
14. Goldwyn RM, Courtiss EH: *Inferior pedical technique*. In Goldwyn RM, editor: Reduction mammaplasty, pp 255-266, Boston, 1990, Little, Brown.

15. Grotting JC et al: Conventional TRAM flap versus free microsurgical TRAM flap for immediate breast reconstruction, *Plast Reconstr Surg* 83:828, 1989.

16. Hartrampf CR, Scheflan M, Black PW: Breast reconstruction with a transverse abdominal island flap, *Plast Reconstr Surg* 69:216, 1982.

17. Hester TR Jr: *Augmentation mammoplasty: polyurethane covered mammary implant*. In Marsh JL, editor: *Current therapy in plastic and reconstructive surgery,* Toronto, 1989, BC Decker.

18. Ishii CH et al: Double-pedicle transverse rectus abdominis myocutaneous flap for unilateral breast and chest-wall reconstruction, *Plast Reconstr Surg* 76:901, 1985.

19. Larson DL, McMurtrey MJ: Musculocutaneous flap reconstruction of chest wall defects: an experience with 50 patients. *Plast Reconstr Surg* 73:734, 1984.

20. Little JW: Nipple reconstruction by quadrapod flap (letter), *Plast Reconstr Surg* 72:422, 1983.

21. Little JW: Nipple-areolar reconstruction, *Clin Plast Surg* 11:351, 1984.

22. Manders EK et al: Soft-tissue expansion: concepts and complications, *Plast Reconstr Surg* 74:493, 1984.

23. Maxwell GP: Latissimus dorsi breast reconstruction: an aesthetic assessment, *Clin Plast Surg* 8:373, 1981.

24. Maxwell GP: Selection of secondary breast reconstruction procedures, *Clin Plast Surg* 11:253, 1984.

25. McCraw JB et al: An early appraisal of the methods of tissue expansion and the transverse rectus abdominis musculocutaneous flap in reconstruction of the breast following mastectomy, *Ann Plast Surg* 18:93, 1987.

26. Noone RB et al: A 6-year experience with immediate reconstruction after mastectomy for cancer, *Plast Reconstr Surg* 76:258, 1985.

27. Radovan C: Tissue expansion in soft-tissue reconstruction, *Plast Reconstr Surg* 74:482, 1984.

28. Shaw WW: Breast reconstruction by superior gluteal microvascular free flaps without silicone implants, *Plast Reconstr Surg* 73:490, 1983.

29. Shaw WW: Microvascular free flap breast reconstruction, *Clin Plast Surg* 11:333, 1984.

30. Slavin SA: Drainage of seromas after latissimus dorsi myocutaneous flap breast reconstruction. Letter to the editor, *Plast Reconstr Surg* 83:925, 1989.

31. Slavin SA: *Salvage mastectomy and reconstruction*. In Noone RB, editor: *Plastic and reconstructive breast surgery,* Toronto, 1991, BC Decker.

32. Slavin SA, Colen SR: Sixty consecutive breast reconstructions with the inflatable expander: a critical appraisal, *Plast Reconstr Surg* 74:493, 1990.

33. Slavin SA, Goldwyn RM: The midabdominal rectus abdominis myocutaneous flap: review of 236 flaps, *Plast Reconstr Surg* 81:89, 1988.

34. Slavin SA, Howrigan P, Goldwyn RM: Pseudocyst formation following rectus flap breast reconstruction: diagnosis and treatment, *Plast Reconstr Surg* 83:670, 1989.

35. Slavin SA et al: Abdominal wall function after rectus flap breast reconstruction. Presented at the 55th Annual Scientific Meeting of the American Society of Plastic and Reconstructive Surgeons, Plastic Surgery Educational Foundation, American Society of Maxillofacial Surgeons, Los Angeles, Calif, Oct 27, 1986.

36. Slavin SA, Love SM, Goldwyn RM: Breast cancer recurrence and detection following immediate breast reconstruction with myocutaneous flaps. Presented at the 59th Annual Scientific Meeting of the American Society of Plastic and Reconstructive Surgeons, Boston, Mass, Oct. 23, 1990.

37. Spear SL: *Intradermal tattooing*. In Marsh J, editor: *Current therapy in plastic and reconstructive surgery,* Toronto, 1989, BC Decker.

38. Stevens LA et al: The psychological impact of immediate breast reconstruction for women with early breast cancer, *Plast Reconstr Surg* 73:619, 1984.

39. Woods JE, Irons GB, and Arnold PG: The case for submuscular implantation of prostheses in reconstructive surgery, *Ann Plast Surg* 5:115, 1980.

Part X

OBSTETRIC OPERATIONS

Chapter 61

INVASIVE FETAL DIAGNOSTIC PROCEDURES

Devereux N. Saller, Jr.
Marshall W. Carpenter

The availability and techniques of invasive prenatal diagnosis of congenital malformations have changed dramatically in recent years. These advances are particularly striking when one recalls that chromosome analysisis has only become widely available within the last 30 years. Additional laboratory advances (including biochemical and microenzyme assay and the most recent molecular techniques) have focused increasing attention on the development of safe clinical techniques of obtaining appropriate specimens for laboratory analysis. This chapter will describe the development of these clinical techniques, their indications, and their risks.

AMNIOCENTESIS
Historical perspectives

The use of amniocentesis was first described in the treatment of polyhydramnios as early as the 1880s.[27] These early interventions were unaided by any visualization of the internal anatomy. In the early 1900s, with the availability of ionizing radiation, Menees, Miller, and Holly[36] employed amniocentesis to evaluate fetal anatomy and to localize the placenta by injecting contrast media into the amniotic cavity. It was not until the 1950s that broad clinical application of this technique became possible. At that time amniocentesis was reported in the evaluation of erythroblastosis fetalis. It was then noted that spectrophotometric analysis of amniotic fluid for bilirubin correlated with the severity of fetal anemia and the prognosis for the fetus in at-risk pregnancies.[4,29,55]

Amniocentesis was first used for prenatal diagnosis of congenital malformations in the late 1950s. Before the availability of chromosome analysis, the ability to identify the inactivated X chromosome (or Barr body) in amniotic fluid cells (and thereby to identify fetal sex) was reported.[15a,22,34,46] With the advent of cytogenetic studies of cultured cells from various tissues in the late 1950s and early 1960s, chromosome analysis from cultured amniotic fluid cells became possible. Successful karyotyping of amniocytes was first reported by Steele and Breg[50] and quickly became commonly available.

Utility

Amniocentesis provides the substrate for three types of laboratory studies. First, after centrifugation the supranatent fluid may be studied directly by biochemical assay. The relative amounts of amniotic fluid alpha-fetoprotein and acetylcholinesterase, for example, may be valuable in the prenatal diagnosis of open neural tube defects.[48] Second, the cells in the pellet may be analyzed directly in biochemical studies (such as microenzyme assays for the diagnosis of certain inborn errors of metabolism) or molecular deoxyribonucleic acid (DNA) studies. Third, the cells may be cultured to provide material for similar biochemical or DNA studies, or they may be cultured for chromosomal analysis. At later gestations, amniotic fluid may be cultured for bacterial infection or may be used for biochemical studies such as fetal lung maturity studies or for spectrophotometric analysis (for bilirubin, in the evaluation of erythroblastosis fetalis).

Currently the most common indication for genetic amniocentesis is increased risk of a chromosomally abnormal fetus. Women of relatively advanced age[43] and women with a known balanced chromosomal rearrangement (in either parent of the fetus) or with a history of a previous child with a chromosomal abnormality are at increased risk for chromosomal abnormalities. Genetic amniocentesis may also be indicated in the evaluation of fetuses at risk for open neural tube defects[48] or for metabolic or other biochemical defects in which either the gene or gene product has been identified and can be quantitated.[37] Genetic amniocentesis is also indicated when a gross anatomic malformation that is associated with karyotypically abnormal pregnancies is prenatally diagnosed.

Technique

The technique of amniocentesis (Fig. 61-1) involves the percutaneous insertion of a needle into the amniotic cavity and the aspiration of amniotic fluid. As with any other percutaneous biopsy procedure, care must be taken to assure asepsis. Additionally, there is evidence that sonographically monitored procedures result in 5.7% fewer "dry" or unsuccessful needle insertions (7.7% in the guided group compared to 2% in the monitored group) and 4% fewer "bloody" specimens (5.2% in the guided group compared to 1.2% in the monitored group).[42] With the current availability of ultrasound, all amniocentesis should be performed with ultrasound guidance.

Several methods of insertion have been described. Jeanty et al[23] have described needle insertion immediately adjacent to the side of a linear array transducer at a slight angle. The tip of the needle is kept within the ultrasound beam and is thereby visualized throughout the insertion, but the entire length of the needle cannot be visualized.

Benacerraff[1] suggested inserting the amniocentesis needle at one end of a sector probe (or more recently, a curvilinear array transducer). With this method, the entire needle is within the ultrasound beam and can be visualized throughout the procedure, thereby enhancing the operator's spatial orientation. However, this technique may require an assistant to hold the ultrasound transducer adjacent to the sterile field. Although this technique does not require that the transducer be placed within a sterile sheath, it does depend upon successful coordination of the sonographer and the operator.

Amniocentesis may be performed in the second or third trimesters (after 14 to 16 weeks of gestation). The technical aspects of the procedure and laboratory evaluations are the same in either trimester. Amniocentesis in the first 20 weeks, however, provides the option for termination of pregnancy.

The safety and feasibility of amniocentesis as early as 10 weeks have been more recently investigated.[18,14,24] These procedures remove a relatively larger volume of amniotic fluid and may change the size of the amniotic cavity to a greater extent than second trimester amniocentesis because the total amniotic fluid volume at early in gestation is less than it is later. These changes in intrauterine volume may theoretically impact on uterine contractility, placental perfusion, or embryologic development. Although none of the early studies suggest a significant increase in the risk of amniocentesis before 14 weeks compared to second trimester amniocentesis, relatively small numbers of procedures have been reported and most are at 13 or 14 weeks. Conclusions regarding the safety of first trimester amniocentesis await further study.

Risks

The maternal risks of amniocentesis include chorioamnionitis, hemorrhage, injury to abdominal viscera, and blood group isoimmunization. Fetal risks include premature rupture of membranes, abortion or preterm labor, abruptio placentae, injury from needle trauma, orthopedic deformities, and possibly respiratory difficulties.

Several investigators[31,51,52] have addressed the precise risks of second trimester amniocentesis. A prospective American study[31] of over 2000 pregnancies was coordinated by the National Institute of Child Health and Human Development. Ultrasound "was used in only about one-third of the taps." Of the 1040 pregnancies undergoing amniocentesis, 950 (91.3%) were performed for cytogenetic analysis, while 90 (8.7%) were to evaluate the possibility of an inherited metabolic disorder (such as Tay-Sachs disease). This study reported that immediate complications (including bleeding and amniotic fluid leakage) were noted in 2.4% of patients, and 3.5% of the pregnancies were lost following amniocentesis compared to 3.2% lost in the control group. No other physical problems were noted more commonly following amniocentesis. A report of the Canadian collaborative group[35] suggested similar complication rates in a study of 1020 pregnancies but did not have a control group.

A collaborative British study[52] of over 4800 pregnancies was reported in 1978. The use of ultrasound in conjunction with the amniocentesis was considered optional. Of 3131 patients undergoing amniocentesis, 1632 (52.1%)

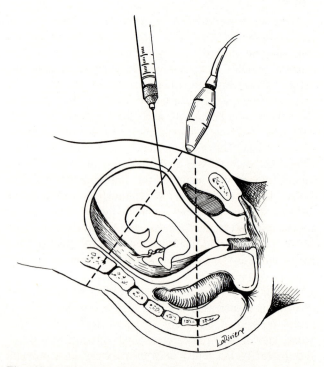

Fig. 61-1. Schematic representation of amniocentesis under ultrasonic guidance.

were having it for chromosomal analysis and 1282 (40.9%) for an increased risk of neural tube defects. This study suggested that the risks of midtrimester abortion following amniocentesis was on the order of 2.6% compared to 1.1% in the control group. Additionally, approximately 1.2% of newborns in the amniocentesis group were reported to have nonfatal respiratory difficulties compared to 0.4% in matched controls, and orthopedic postural deformities (including talipes equinovarus and congenital hip dislocations) were noted in 1.4% of newborns in the amniocentesis group and in none of the matched controls. The rate of orthopedic defects in the control group was unexpectedly low, however. It is also noteworthy that there were significant differences between the amniocentesis group and the control group in maternal age. In addition, this study included a large number of patients (30%) for whom the indication for amniocentesis was elevated maternal serum alpha-fetoprotein, which in the absence of open fetal defects has been associated with poor pregnancy outcome.[16] Whether these factors account for the differences between this study and the American and Canadian studies is unclear.

A more recent randomized, controlled Danish study of 4606 pregnancies[51] reported a pregnancy loss rate in the amniocentesis patients of 1.7%, while the control group had a loss rate of 0.7%. Respiratory distress and pneumonia were also more common in neonates from the amniocentesis group. No differences were noted in orthopedic problems, however. Although all of the amniocentesis procedures in this study were done with ultrasound guidance, an 18-gauge needle was used to aspirate the fluid. In other reports, a 20- or a 22-gauge needle was usually used for the amniocentesis.

With these data in mind, although the precise risks of amniocentesis remain unclear, it may be considered a generally safe procedure with attributable risks of under 1% and probably under 0.5%. Its use, however, must be weighed in each case against the need and value of the information to be gained and the risk of an unexpected or abnormal result (such as a chromosomal abnormality).

CHORIONIC VILLUS SAMPLING
Historical perspectives

Although investigations into placental biopsy for prenatal diagnosis date back to the late 1960s,[17] until recently prenatal diagnosis for chromosomal abnormalities was mainly carried out through amniocentesis. This preference was primarily based on assumptions about the safety and technical ease of amniocentesis compared to that of chorionic villus sampling at a time when high-resolution ultrasound was unavailable. By the early 1980s, high-resolution ultrasound was able to adequately image the developing placental tissue and provide guidance for a biopsy catheter or needle.[26] This, as well as technical cytogenetic laboratory advances, made chorionic villus sampling (CVS) a potential alternative to amniocentesis for genetic prenatal diagnosis.

Utility

Chorionic villus sampling provides tissue for prenatal diagnosis of a wide variety of indications. After careful cleaning, the tissue may be analyzed directly, in a manner similar to amniocytes, in biochemical studies (such as microenzyme assays for the diagnosis of certain inborn errors of metabolism) or molecular DNA studies. Additionally, since the cells in the developing placenta (chorion) are rapidly dividing, the cells may be directly analyzed for karyotype[47] with results available within 72 hours. The cells are also placed into culture to provide material for similar biochemical or DNA studies or for chromosomal analysis. The directly analyzed cells offer the advantage of less maternal cell contamination, while the cultured cells show fewer incorrect predictions of fetal cytogenetic status.[28] The combination of both methods is considered optimal and resulted in no incorrect predictions of fetal status in a large collaborative trial.[28] Karyotypic results from such cultures are generally available within 10 to 12 days.

A major advantage of chorionic villus sampling over amniocentesis is the earlier gestational age at which this procedure can be performed. CVS appears to have a lower attributable risk when performed between 9 and 11 weeks of gestation.[20] This earlier gestational age may be an important advantage to patients at increased risk for specific types of genetic abnormalities, since the results of this diagnostic test allow for termination of pregnancy before 14 weeks of gestation. Termination of pregnancy at this early stage offers a lower risk of hemorrhage and uterine or cervical trauma than later terminations. There may also be social and emotional advantages to earlier prenatal diagnosis for certain patients, relating to the fact that a first trimester pregnancy is not obvious to social contacts and therefore may remain a private matter. Additionally, awareness of fetal movement has not occurred in the first trimester, and such awareness following second trimester amniocentesis may make decisions regarding pregnancy termination more difficult.

Chorionic villus sampling may be employed for any prenatal diagnostic indication for which amniocentesis is used except for the diagnosis of neural tube defects (in which the biochemical evaluation of amniotic fluid is advantageous).[48] Since chorionic villus sampling is usually performed between 9 and 11 weeks of gestation, it is of less use in the evaluation of most second or third trimester pregnancies. Currently, chorionic villus sampling is most commonly used for karyotypic evaluation of pregnancies at risk for chromosomal abnormalities (usually related to the increasing risk of nondisjunction with advancing maternal age).

Technique

Chorionic villus sampling involves a biopsy of the chorionic villi, which are the fetal aspect of the developing placenta. CVS is usually performed either by a transabdominal route (Fig. 61-2) using percutaneous needle biopsy of the placenta[6,39] or by transcervical passage of a catheter (Fig. 61-3) into the chorion or developing placenta.[20]

The performance of second or third trimester chorionic villus biopsy by the percutaneous transabdominal approach has been described by several authors.[21,41,53] Although late chorionic villus sampling has been shown to be feasible, its safety in comparison to amniocentesis has not yet been reported. Nevertheless, in selected cases when a high index of suspicion for a chromosomal abnormality exists and when amniocentesis is deemed difficult or impossible, late chorionic villus sampling is currently a viable alternative.

Risks

Risks related to CVS have been categorized as maternal or fetal risks. The maternal risks of chorionic villus sampling are rare but mainly involve intrauterine infection presenting as acute chorioamnionitis.[20] Fetal risks mainly involve oligohydramnios, with or without a clear history of amniotic fluid leakage[20] and fetal loss. Recently, several cases of limb abnormalities have been reported in pregnancies that underwent CVS.[14a] Neither these, nor any other anomalies, have been noted more frequently in the large collaborative trials of CVS.[41a,56a] Both the transabdominal and transcervical techniques have achieved clinical acceptance and are felt to be equal in safety.[5,33]

The results of two large collaborative trials are now available. The Canadian Collaborative Trial[56a] was a multicenter trial of 2787 women aged 35 or more, randomized to CVS or amniocentesis. Of these, 396 women were excluded after randomization because of a nonviable fetus, multiple gestation, infection, or incorrect gestational age. The report suggested that the excess risk of pregnancy loss in patients undergoing chorionic villus sampling (compared to patients undergoing amniocentesis) was 0.6% (7.6% in the CVS group compared to 7% in the amniocentesis group). This difference, however, was not statistically significant (the 95% confidence interval for the total pregnancy loss rate for chorionic villus sampling was 6.2% to 9.3%, while the 95% confidence interval for the amniocentesis group was 5.6% to 8.6%).

A similar collaborative multicenter trial from the United States[41a] reported on 2278 pregnancies undergoing CVS.

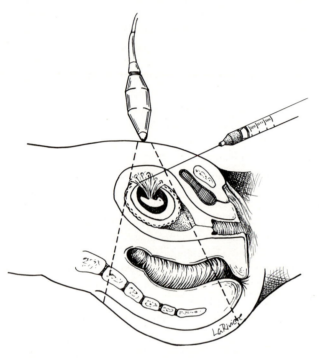

Fig. 61-2. Schematic representation of transabdominal chorionic villus sampling.

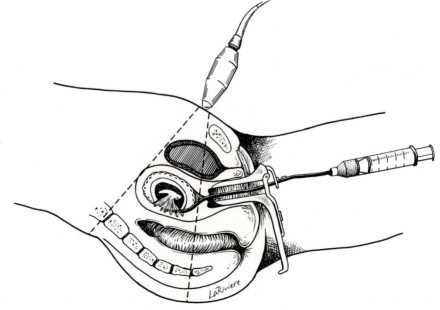

Fig. 61-3. Schematic representation of transcervical chorionic villus sampling.

This report suggested that the total loss rate for women undergoing chorionic villus sampling was 0.8% greater than for those undergoing amniocentesis, after adjustment for slight differences in maternal and gestational age at enrollment. Again, there was a higher loss rate following CVS, but this was not statistically significant (the 80% confidence interval for the excess total loss in the CVS group was −0.6% to 2.2%).

FETAL BLOOD SAMPLING
Historical perspectives

Another source of fetal cells for prenatal diagnosis is fetal blood. This has been described since the early 1970s.[54] Early reports described sampling using fetoscopy, which required percutaneous and transuterine insertion of a 1.7-mm or greater fiberoptic scope and involved significant risk of fetal morbidity and mortality.[3,49] This limited its application to only a few centers and to a limited number of diagnoses. As with the development of CVS, high-resolution ultrasound has allowed accurate real time localization of fetal umbilical vasculature. Percutaneous umbilical blood sampling (PUBS) was first reported by Daffos, Capella-Pavlovsky, and Forestier[9] in 1983. In this report, 66 samples were taken from 63 pregnancies. Although no long-term complications were reported, 35 pregnancies were ongoing at the time of the report and in 17 cases a therapeutic abortion was induced between 2 and 10 days after the PUBS. PUBS (with ultrasound guidance) has now become the preferred technique of fetal blood sampling.

Utility

Percutaneous umbilical blood sampling, or PUBS, may be useful in any diagnostic situation in which fetal blood provides the best-quality information for management of a disorder. Common indications for this technique include possible fetal anemia due to isoimmunization[40] or possible fetal thrombocytopenia due to autoimmune thrombocytopenia.[12] The lymphocytes in fetal blood provide an attractive alternative to amniocentesis or CVS for fetal karyotype when rapid chromosome results (48 to 72 hours) are desired. This may occur when an anatomic malformation is identified on ultrasound late in the previable period (to allow the option of pregnancy termination) or in the third trimester (when delivery is anticipated) to aid in the management of the perinate.[38] PUBS has also been employed for the evaluation of fetal infections and has been used extensively in Europe for the evaluation of patients at risk for toxoplasmosis.[11] In the latter instance, 746 such pregnancies were evaluated with PUBS, and if the fetus was demonstrated to be infected, the mother either terminated the pregnancy or was treated with additional antimicrobial agents.

Technique

The technique of umbilical blood sampling (Fig. 61-4) involves the insertion of a needle into the umbilical vein, preferably near the placental insertion site, under high-res-

olution ultrasound.[8,10,19,56] In previable gestations, the procedure may be done in a location remote from an operating room, usually in an ultrasound room. In later gestations, the procedure should be performed in close proximity to an operating room allowing for immediate cesarean delivery in the event of fetal compromise. Local anesthesia alone is usually sufficient for patient comfort. In cases of maternal obesity, difficult access to the cord insertion site, or when performing PUBS transfusions, maternal sedation with small doses of a narcotic may be considered. In cases where the fetus is quite active or for transfusions, transient fetal paralysis may be accomplished by fetal intramuscular or intravenous injections of d-tubocurare or pancuronium bromide.[45]

Possible contamination of the fetal blood specimen by amniotic fluid or maternal blood can be detected by hematologic studies of the specimen.[15] The fetal red blood cell, which is larger than the adult red blood cell, can be distinguished from the latter by measuring the mean corpuscular volume (MCV). The presence of nucleated red cells in fetal blood (on smear) and differences in the hemoglobin molecule may also be employed (as in the Kleihauer-betke test).

PUBS can be performed as early as at 18 weeks of gestation and becomes technically easier as gestation advances. Because of these gestational age limitations and the procedure-related risks (which are significantly greater than with amniocentesis or chorionic villus sampling), umbilical blood sampling is a technique of prenatal diagnosis generally limited to the later half of pregnancy.

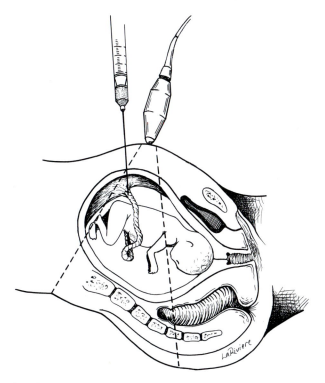

Fig. 61-4. Schematic representation of percutaneous umbilical blood sampling.

Risks

The maternal complications of percutaneous umbilical blood sampling include chorioamnionitis, hemorrhage, injury to abdominal viscera, and blood group isoimmunization. Fetal complications include fetal bleeding,[8,32] fetal infection,[8,32] and fetal bradycardia.[2,8,32] Rarely, persistent bradycardia at advanced gestations may require emergent cesarean section. The induction or augmentation of blood group isoimmunization by the introduction of even small volumes of fetal blood into the maternal circulation has not been well studied.

The risks of percutaneous umbilical blood sampling appear to be low in the hands of experienced operators. Daffos reported an in-utero fetal death rate of 1.1%, an abortion rate of 0.8%, and a premature delivery rate of 5% among 606 consecutive PUBS.[10] More recent data on over 2000 PUBS (including the 606 previously reported cases) suggest that the combined risk of abortion and fetal death in experienced hands is between 0.5% and 1%.[8] These risks are also being measured in pregnancies that are complicated or otherwise at high risk (they all have an indication for an invasive procedure). This may result in increased a priori risk in these pregnancies and thus an increased reported complication rate of the procedure.

CONCLUSIONS
Risk-benefit analysis

Diagnostic procedures in pregnancy, whether invasive or not, require consideration of the value of the information to be obtained versus the possible risks of the procedure. Not only must the physician consider the risks and benefits, but these must be clearly explained to the patient and documented. The availability of a variety of techniques (amniocentesis, chorionic villus sampling, and fetal blood sampling) now allows a choice of which fetal tissue might be most appropriate to make a given diagnosis. Other considerations in the choice of procedure include the gestational age at the time of procedure and the risk of a given procedure in relation to the risk of a suspected diagnosis.

Since these procedures are employed at differing gestational ages, it is important to consider (and to discuss with the patient) the background risks of spontaneous pregnancy loss, to which the procedure-related risks are added. It is also true that the prevalence of chromosomal abnormalities decreases with advancing gestational age. Therefore the risk of finding aneuploidy increases as earlier prenatal diagnosis is employed.

The future

These invasive diagnostic procedures have dramatically changed the practice of obstetrics. Future developments, which are certain to continue this process, are likely to include less invasive and less risky diagnostic procedures for prenatal diagnosis. For example, there is renewed interest in isolating fetal cells directly from the maternal circulation.[57] If this becomes possible, only a maternal venipuncture would be required to obtain fetal DNA for diagnostic purposes. However, the technical feasibility of fetal lymphocyte isolation remains to be demonstrated. Additionally, the use of newer laboratory techniques such as fluorescent in-situ hybridization[25] may allow the diagnosis of certain cytogenetic abnormalities, within hours, from any fetal tissue (including amniotic fluid cells).

In-utero therapy, other than transfusion, may also soon be available.[30] Recent attempts at open fetal surgery with the return of the fetus to the womb and the prolongation of the pregnancy have met with limited success and must be considered investigational.[18a] These interventions require appropriate candidates to be diagnosed early in pregnancy so as to allow the attempts at therapy to occur at appropriate gestational ages for optimal outcome. Investigations into fetal surgery are only beginning, but already the ethical implications of such interventions are raising great concern.[30] The financial and social implications of these advances must also be considered.[7]

REFERENCES

1. Benacerraff BR, Frigoletto FD: Amniocentesis under continuous ultrasound guidance: a series of 232 cases, *Obstet Gynecol* 62:760, 1983.
2. Benacerraf BR et al: Acute fetal distress associated with percutaneous umbilical blood sampling, *Am J Obstet Gynecol* 156:1218, 1987.
3. Benzie R et al: Fetoscopy and fetal tissue sampling, *Prenat Diagn* 1(suppl):29 (special issue), 1980.
4. Bevis DCA: The antenatal prediction of haemolytic disease of the newborn, *Lancet* 1:395, 1952.
5. Bovicelli L et al: Transabdominal versus transcervical routes for chorionic villus sampling, *Lancet* 2:290, 1986.
6. Brambati B, Oldrini A, Lanzani A: Transabdominal chorionic villus sampling: a freehand ultrasound-guided technique, *Am J Obstet Gynecol* 157:134, 1987.
7. Cook-Deegan RM: Social and ethical implications of advances in human genetics, *South Med J* 83:879, 1990.
8. Daffos F: Fetal blood sampling, *Ann Rev Med* 40:319, 1989.
9. Daffos F, Capella-Pavlovsky M, Forestier F: Fetal blood sampling via the umbilical cord using a needle guided by ultrasound: report of 66 cases, *Prenat Diagn* 3:271, 1983.
10. Daffos F, Capella-Pavlovsky M, Forestier F: Fetal blood sampling during pregnancy with use of a needle guided by ultrasound: a study of 606 consecutive cases, *Am J Obstet Gynecol* 153:655, 1985.
11. Daffos F et al: Prenatal management of 746 pregnancies at risk for congenital toxoplasmosis, *N Engl J Med* 318:271, 1988.
12. Daffos F et al: Prenatal diagnosis and management of bleeding disorders with fetal blood sampling, *Am J Obstet Gynecol* 158:939, 1988.
13. Deleted in proof.
14. Evans MI et al: Early genetic amniocentesis and chorionic villus sampling: expanding the opportunities for early prenatal diagnosis, *J Reprod Med* 33:450, 1988.
14a. Firth HV et al: Severe limb abnormalities after chorion villus sampling at 56-66 days' gestation, *Lancet* 337:762, 1991.
15. Forestier F et al: The assessment of fetal blood samples, *Am J Obstet Gynecol* 158:1184, 1988.
15a. Fuchs F, Riis P: Antenatal sex determination, *Nature* 117:330, 1956.
16. Haddow JE et al: Data from an alphafetoprotein screening program in Maine, *Obstet Gynecol* 62:556, 1983.
17. Hahnemann N, Mohr J: Genetic diagnosis in the embryo by means of biopsy from extraembryonic membranes, *Bull Eur Soc Hum Genet* 2:23, 1968.

18. Hanson FW et al: Amniocentesis before 15 weeks gestation: outcome risks and technical problems, *Am J Obstet Gynecol* 156:1524, 1987.

18a. Harrison MR et al: Successful repair in utero of a fetal diaphragmatic hernia after removal of herniated viscera from the left thorax, *N Engl J Med* 332:1582, 1990.

19. Hobbins JC et al: Percutaneous umbilical blood sampling, *Am J Obstet Gynecol* 152:1, 1985.

20. Hogge WA, Schonberg SA, Golbus MS: Chorionic villus sampling: experience of the first 1000 cases, *Am J Obstet Gynecol* 154:1249, 1986.

21. Holzgreve W et al: Safety of placental biopsy in the second and third trimester, *N Engl J Med* 317:1159, 1987.

22. James F: Sexing foetuses by examination of amniotic fluid, *Lancet* 1:202, 1956.

23. Jeanty P et al: How to improve your amniocentesis technique, *Am J Obstet Gynecol* 146:593, 1983.

24. Johnson A, Godmilow L: Genetic amniocentesis at 14 weeks or less, *Clin Obstet Gynecol* 31:345, 1988.

25. Julien C et al: Rapid prenatal diagnosis of Down's syndrome with in-situ hybridisation of fluorescent DNA probes, *Lancet* 863, 1986.

26. Kazy S, Stigar AM, Bakharev VA: Chorionic biopsy under immediate real-time (ultrasound) control, *Orv Hetil* 121:2765, 1980.

27. Lambl D: Ein seltener Fall von Hydramnios, *Zentralbl Gynakol* 5:329, 1881.

28. Ledbetter DH et al: Cytogenetic results of chorionic villus sampling: high success rate and diagnostic accuracy in the United States collaborative study, *Am J Obstet Gynecol* 162:495, 1990.

29. Liley AW: Liquor amnii analysis in the management of the pregnancy complicated by rhesus sensitization, *Am J Obstet Gynecol* 82:1359, 1961.

30. Longaker MT et al: Maternal outcome after open fetal surgery: a review of the first 17 human cases, *JAMA* 265:737, 1991.

31. Lowe CU et al: *The NICHD amniocentesis registry: the safety and accuracy of mid-trimester amniocentesis,* DHEW Pub. no. (NIH) 78-190. U.S. Department of Health, Education, and Welfare, Washington, D.C., 1978.

32. Ludomirsky A et al: Percutaneous fetal umbilical blood sampling: procedure safety and normal fetal hematologic indices, *Am J Perinatol* 5:264, 1988.

33. MacKenzie W, Holmes D, Newton J: A study comparing transcervical with transabdominal chorionic villus sampling (CVS), *Br J Obstet Gynaecol* 95:75, 1988.

34. Makowski EL, Prem K, Kaiser IH: Detection of sex of fetuses by the incidence of sex chromatin body in nuclei of cells in amniotic fluid, *Science* 123:542, 1956.

35. Medical Research Council: *Diagnosis of genetic disease by amniocentesis during the second trimester of pregnancy,* Rep no 5, Ottawa, Canada, 1977.

36. Menees TO, Miller JD, Holly LE: Amniography: preliminary report, *Am J Roentgenol Radium Ther* 24:363, 1930.

37. Nadler HL, Gerbie AB: Role of amniocentesis in the intrauterine detection of genetic disorders, *N Engl J Med* 282:596, 1970.

38. Nicolaides KH, Rodeck CH, Gosden GM: Rapid karyotyping in non-lethal fetal malformations, *Lancet* 5:283, 1986.

39. Nicolaides KH, Soothill PW, Rosevear S: Transabdominal placental biopsy, *Lancet* 2:855, 1987.

40. Nicolaides KH et al: Have Liley charts outlived their usefulness? *Am J Obstet Gynecol* 155:90, 1986.

41. Nicolaides KH et al: Why confine chorionic villus (placental) biopsy to the first trimester? *Lancet* 1:543, 1986.

41a. Rhoads GG et al: The safety and efficacy of chorionic villus sampling for early prenatal diagnosis of cytogenetic abnormalities, *N Engl J Med* 320:609, 1989.

42. Romero R et al: Sonographically monitered amniocentesis to decrease intraoperative complications, *Obstet Gynecol* 65:426, 1985.

43. Schreinemachers DM, Cross PK, Hook EB: Rates of trisomy 21, 18, 13, and other chromosome abnormalities in about 20,000 prenatal studies compared with estimated rates in live births, *Hum Genet* 61:318, 1982.

44. Second report of the UK collaborative study on alpha-fetoprotein in relation to neural tube defects: amniotic fluid alpha-fetoprotein measurement in antenatal diagnosis of anencephaly and open spina bifida in early pregnancies, *Lancet* 2:652, 1979.

45. Seeds JW, Corke BC, Speilman FL: Prevention of fetal movement during invasive procedures with pancuronium bromide, *Am J Obstet Gynecol* 155:818, 1986.

46. Shettles LB: Nuclear morphology of cells in human amniotic fluid in relation to sex of infant, *Am J Obstet Gynecol* 71:834, 1956.

47. Simoni G et al: Efficient direct chromosome analyses and enzyme determinations from chorionic villi samples in the first trimester of pregnancy, *Hum Genet* 63:349, 1983.

48. Smith AD et al: Amniotic fluid acetylcholinesterase as a possible diagnostic test for neural tube defects in early pregnancy, *Lancet* 1:685, 1979.

49. Special Report: The status of fetoscopy and fetal tissue sampling, *Prenat Diagn* 4:79, 1984.

50. Steele MW, Breg WR Jr: Chromosome analysis of human amniotic fluid cells, *Lancet* 1:383, 1966.

51. Tabor A et al: Randomized controlled trial of genetic amniocentesis in 4606 low risk women, *Lancet* 1:1287, 1986.

52. Turnbull AC et al: Report to the Medical Research Council: an assessment of the hazards of amniocentesis, *Br J Obstet Gynaecol* 85:1, 1978.

53. Vachon F et al: Second trimester placental biopsy versus amniocentesis for prenatal diagnosis of β-thalassemia, *N Engl J Med* 322:60, 1990.

54. Valenti C: Antenatal detection of hemoglobinopathies, *Am J Obstet Gynecol* 115:851, 1973.

55. Walker A: Liquor amnii studies in the prediction of haemolytic disease of the newborn, *Br Med J* 2:376, 1957.

56. Weiner CP: Cordocentesis for diagnostic indications: two years' experience, *Obstet Gynecol* 70:664, 1987.

56a. Wilson D et al: Multicentre randomised clinical trial of chorionic villus sampling and amniocentesis, *Lancet* 1:1, 1989.

57. Yeoh SC et al: Detection of fetal cells in maternal blood, *Prenat Diagn* 11:117, 1991.

Chapter 62

FIRST AND SECOND TRIMESTER ABORTION

Phillip G. Stubblefield

Abortion is a common procedure, yet most abortions are performed in free-standing clinics, out of the mainstream. Physicians in training may not understand the central role safe, legal abortion plays in the health of women. Before considering the technology for abortion, we think it important to describe something of the social and medical background of pregnancy termination.

Pregnancy carries a risk of illness and death. The U.S. maternal mortality rate is about 9 per 100,000 live births.[40] The death rate for first trimester abortion is far less: 1 per 100,000.[11] Young mothers are especially in need of abortion because fertility is greater and intercourse without contraception more common than for older people.[18] For women 15 to 19 the abortion rate, 43.8 per 1000 women in 1985, was only a little less than the birth rate, 51.3 per 1000.[25,26] Without legal abortion, births to teenaged mothers would double. For all age groups, contraception fails more often than medical personnel usually realize. For this reason and because of fear of side effects, sterilization is the most common method of contraception among U.S. couples.[39] Deaths from complications of illegal abortion were a major cause of maternal mortality until the 1960s. With the increasing availability of legal abortion, the number of these deaths fell. In 1980 there were only 6 deaths from spontaneous abortion, 8 from legal abortion, and 1 from illegal abortion (abortion induced by a nonphysician) in the United States.[11]

The problems of fertility control and health are far worse in the third world. Maternal mortality rates are markedly higher, typically 300 to 500 per 100,000 births; access to contraception is poor; and illegal abortion is widely practiced. In many countries half or more of pregnancy-related deaths are from complications of illegal abortions. However, safe abortion services can be provided at low cost and reduce maternal mortality.[2]

Risk of death from abortion increases with gestational age and after 16 weeks is no safer than continuing pregnancy (Table 62-1). For individual women with high-risk conditions, even late abortion is undoubtedly safer. More than 90% of U.S. abortions are performed in the first trimester when they are safest.

FIRST TRIMESTER ABORTION
Surgical techniques

Virtually all first trimester abortions in the United States are performed by vacuum curettage. The technique was first reported in China in 1954.[62] It spread to Eastern Europe and was then introduced into England in the 1960s. It was introduced into the United States through the efforts of Laylor Burdick. Standard vacuum curettage uses rigid

Table 62-1. Death-to-case rate for legal abortions by weeks of gestation, United States, 1972-1980

Weeks of gestation	Deaths*	Abortions†	Rate‡	Relative risk§
> 8	19	4,073,472	0.5	1.0
9-10	31	2,382,516	1.3	2.6
11-12	25	1,197,915	2.1	4.2
13-15	20	419,767	4.8	9.6
16-20	55	430,907	12.8	25.6
> 21	14	91,343	15.3	30.6
Total	164	8,595,920	1.9	

*Excludes deaths from ectopic pregnancy.
†Based on distribution of 6,108,658 abortions (71.1%).
‡Deaths per 100,000 abortions.
§Based on index rate of < 8 menstrual weeks' gestation of 0.5 deaths per 100,000 abortions.
From Centers for Disease Control: Abortion surveillance 1979-80, Jan 1983, Atlanta, CDC. By permission.

plastic cannula, 8 to 12 mm in diameter, with an electric pump. A more recent innovation is the menstrual regulation, or minisuction, technique with smaller, flexible cannula, often used with only a modified 50-cc syringe as vacuum source.[34]

Standard vacuum curettage. A medical history is taken and a physical exam is performed to rule out complicating factors. There are no absolute contraindications to first trimester vacuum curettage performed under local anesthesia, but some conditions will dictate additional consultation and preparation or referral. The patient deserves the opportunity to discuss her decision with a nonjudgmental person and to have full information about her options and time to make an informed choice.[50] However, since complications increase with gestational age, providing abortion services should be regarded as urgent, once the patient has reached a decision.

Pelvic exam. A bimanual examination is performed, noting uterine size, position, tenderness, and the presence of adnexal masses. Suspicion of abnormality or size-date discrepancy calls for an ultrasound examination. A speculum is inserted and specimens taken for cervical cytology,

gonorrhea culture, and *Chlamydia* antigen test. For local anesthesia procedures the familiar weighted speculum is uncomfortable, and the short, Moore modification of the Graves speculum is preferred. It requires some experience to easily expose the cervix with this speculum, but once in place and the cervix grasped with a tenaculum, it is easy to draw the cervix down to the introitus, facilitating safe introduction of instruments through the cervical canal (Fig. 62-1).

Next the cervix is cleansed with a germicide such as povidone iodine. Full sterile technique is not necessary. Most U.S. abortions are carried out following the "no touch technique." The surgeon wears sterile gloves and works from a small sterile instrument kit, but sterile drapes and gowns are not used.[9] The surgeon takes care never to touch that portion of an instrument that will enter the uterus.

Paracervical block. We use a 1% lidocaine solution containing 0.5 mg of atropine in 20 cc. Atropine is added to prevent "cervical shock," a form of vasovagal syncope that can be seen with cervical dilatation. Some have advocated use of epinephrine-containing solutions, but these

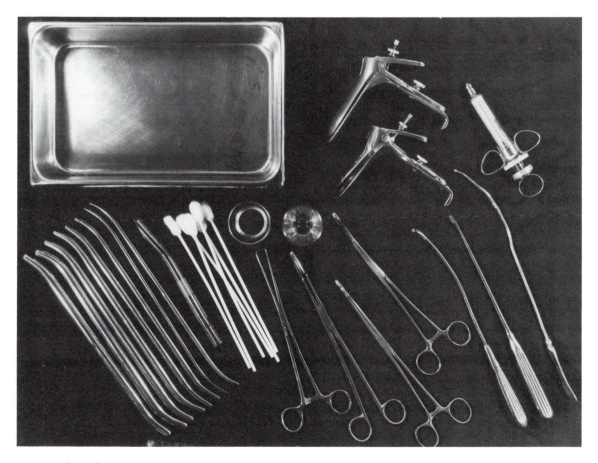

Fig. 62-1. Instrument kit for vacuum curettage abortion. *Left to right:* sterile tray, Graves speculum, Moore speculum, control syringe, uterine sound, no. 1 curette, no. 3 curette, curved Foerester forceps, straight Foerester forceps, Moore ovum forceps, single tooth tenaculum, medicine glasses, cotton swabs, plastic vacurette, Pratt cervical dilators. (From Stubblefield PG: *Surgical techniques for first trimester abortion.* In Sciarra JJ, Zatuchni GI, Daly MJ, editors: *Gynecology and obstetrics,* vol 6, Hagerstown, Md, 1982, Harper and Row.)

can cause cardiac arrhythmias even at concentrations as low as 1:200,000, and in asthmatic patients the metabilsulfite preservative in all epinephrine solutions can cause fatal anaphylaxis.[55] There are several variations in technique for the block. In the past we used the superficial technique, where the local anesthetic is injected submucosally. We are convinced that the combination of superficial and deep technique introduced by Glick[20] is superior. Wiebe[59] has confirmed this in a comparative study. We use a modification of Glick's technique, injecting at three sites rather than the multiple locations he described. The cervix is infiltrated superficially with 2 to 3 cc at the 12 o'clock position, and the needle is then advanced through the anesthetized area for approximately 3 cm to reach the junction of the cervix and lower uterine segment, where an additional 2 cc are injected. This allows for painless placement of the tenaculum. The procedure is repeated at the 4 and 8 o'clock positions, injecting 2 to 3 cc superficially and then advancing the needle 3 cm to infiltrate the lower uterine segment on each side with 4 to 5 cc. Care is taken to aspirate before each injection to avoid intravascular injection. This is important. Deaths have been reported with paracervical block. A 22-gauge 3½-inch spinal needle or a needle extender with a 1½-inch needle is used (Fig. 62-2). We use a total of 20 cc of 1% lidocaine (200 mg) in patients who weigh 100 lbs or more. One should not exceed 2 cc/lb as an initial dose, so the amount is reduced in smaller patients.[22] Occasionally the block is less effective on one side. If this occurs, an additional 5 to 6 cc of 1% lidocaine are injected deeply into the junction of cervix and lower uterine segment on that side.

Tenaculum placement. We use a single-tooth, square-jaw tenaculum, placed vertically with one branch inside the cervical canal. Placement of the tenaculum in this fashion, grasping the cervix about 2 cm proximal to the external os, provides traction near the internal os, the region of greatest resistance. Outward traction with the tenaculum then serves to reduce the angle between the cervical canal and the uterine cavity, making it easier to insert dilators in the proper direction to avoid perforation (Fig. 62-3).

Sounding and dilatation. When forcible dilatation will be performed, we favor sounding the uterus in the conventional fashion. Some view the sound as a "perforator" and do not use it. We believe that the additional information gained regarding uterine size and position is worth the small risk, and that if perforation were to occur, it would be far less serious from the small, blunt tip of the sound than from a dilator or curette. With the uterine sound, as with any instrument inserted through the cervical canal, it is important to avoid excessive force. The rule to follow is "If it isn't easy, something isn't right." Do not push harder. Check that the cervical opening has been correctly identified, that the tenaculum is properly placed, and that the cervix is pulled well down toward the introitus. Bend the sound to a gentle curve, then slowly rotate it around its

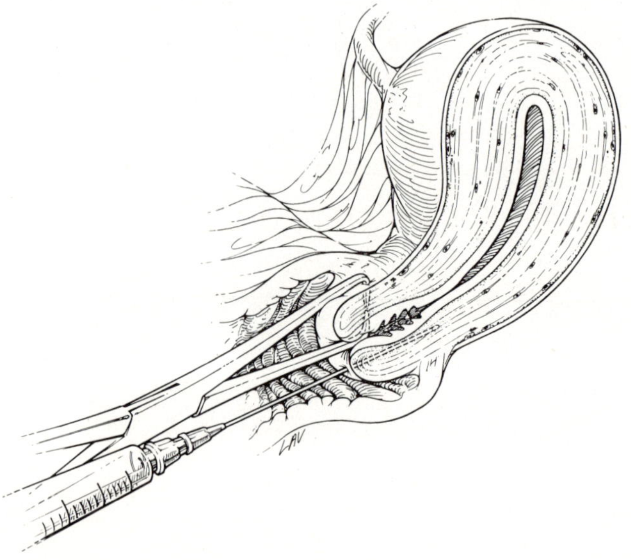

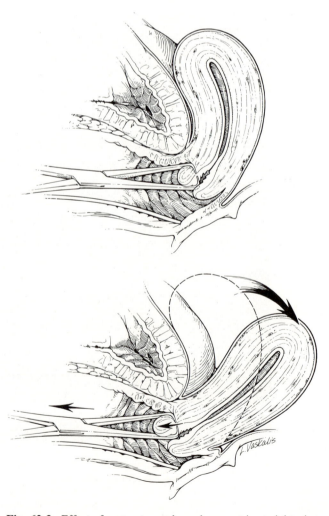

Fig. 62-2. Deep technique for paracervical block. Infiltrating the lower uterine segment at the 4 o'clock position.

Fig. 62-3. Effect of proper tenaculum placement in straightening the angle between the cervix and the uterus by traction.

axis while pressing it gently through the canal. This allows the sound to find the true passage. Especially in the young nulligravida, and especially in early pregnancy, the cervix can be tortuous and firm. Caution is required. Dilatation is accomplished with gently tapered dilators; Pratt's or Denniston's plastic modification of the Pratt dilator is recommended (Fig. 62-4). Full-sized Hegar dilators should not be used, because their blunt design requires excessive force. Half-sized Hegars, with increases of only 0.5 mm between dilators, are an excellent choice, though rarely seen in U.S. operating rooms. Each dilator is inserted slowly and carefully, keeping in mind that the dilator tip must negotiate a curve where cervix and uterus join. With an anteflexed uterus the operator's hand must follow a downward curve to properly direct the dilator (Fig. 62-5).

The direction is reversed when the uterus is retroverted. Failure to incorporate these simple concepts can lead to perforation. Sometimes placement of the tenaculum on the posterior lip of the cervix is helpful if the uterus is markedly retroverted.

If much resistance is encountered during dilatation, one should stop, reassess the position of tenaculum and cervix, and redirect the dilator along the proper curve. If there is still excessive resistance, remove the dilator and insert the next smallest dilator to that previously used to confirm the correct angle. Insert this smaller dilator so that its widest portion traverses the internal os and leave it in place for a minute or two before proceeding to the next larger. There may come a point where continued dilatation will require considerable force. At this point the operator should con-

Fig. 62-4. Denniston dilators. (Photo courtesy of International Projects Assistance, Chapel Hill, NC.)

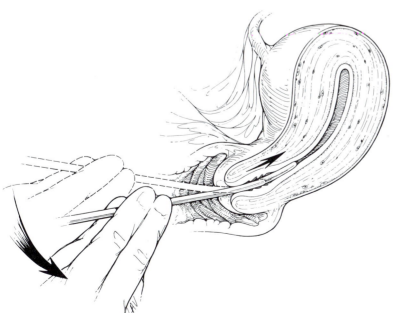

Fig. 62-5. Inserting the dilator along the proper curved path to avoid perforation. The tenaculum is omitted.

sider whether the abortion can be successfully completed with a smaller vacuum cannula than originally intended. Ordinarily we use a cannula that is 1 mm smaller than the gestational age in menstrual weeks (i.e., 9 mm for 10 weeks). However, the 6-mm flexible Karman cannula used for minisuction (see below) works for pregnancies of 8 and 9 weeks, though the aspiration takes longer and more cannula action is required. At times use of the flexible cannula allows safe evacuation of the pregnancy from a markedly anteverted or retroverted uterus where the rigid cannula cannot negotiate the curve from cervical canal into uterine cavity. An 8-mm cannula can evacuate 10-week pregnancies, and a 9-mm rigid cannula will suffice through 12 weeks, though the procedure takes longer and requires more of the operator in order to avoid an incomplete procedure than would a larger cannula. Angulated cannula are used in first trimester procedures. After 12 weeks we prefer straight cannulas because the uterine size is large relative to the cannula and the curve of the angulated cannula just gets in the way.

Uterine evacuation. After insertion of the selected cannula, vacuum is established. An electric vacuum pump is used at its maximum setting. Initially the cannula is rotated vigorously around its long axis. This usually ruptures the membranes and begins the aspiration of amniotic fluid and tissue. After 30 seconds or so, tissue may block the cannula. At this point an in and out motion is combined with rotation. As the cannula is pulled back almost to the internal os, the lower uterine segment serves as a funnel, linearizing the tissue into the cannula orifice and helping to shear off pieces of placenta and membranes so they can be evacuated. Depending on cannula size relative to gestational size, uterine evacuation is essentially complete in 1 to 2 minutes. When all tissue has been aspirated, the operator sees only a pink foam entering the cannula and the gritty feel of the cannula passing over the endometrial surface becomes apparent. The vacuum cannula is removed and a light curettage is performed, using the curette as one would use a finger, to palpate and confirm that the cavity is empty. Forceful curettage should be avoided because it is not necessary. Pregnancy tissue is only lightly adherent to the uterine wall. If tissue has been retained, it is best to continue evacuation with the vacuum cannula. After the check with the sharp curette, reinsert the vacuum cannula for a final few seconds. The tenaculum is then removed and the tenaculum site observed for bleeding. Such bleeding will stop with pressure. Sometimes it is necessary to compress the full thickness of the cervix with the ring forceps for 2 to 3 minutes to stop tenaculum site bleeding. Rarely, the tenaculum will have slipped off during the procedure and lacerated the cervical mucosa. If so, the laceration should be inspected to make sure it does not extend into the lower uterine segment and should be immediately repaired with a figure-eight suture of an absorbable material.

Tissue examination. Next, the operator must carefully examine the aspirated tissue to be sure complete abortion has been performed and rule out ectopic or molar pregnancy.[10] The tissue is placed in a strainer, rinsed with normal saline, and then poured into a clear glass or plastic dish with a small amount of saline. Inspection over a light source facilitates identification of chorionic villi. From 8 weeks onward, fetal parts are also identified, and for later first trimester procedures (11 to 12 weeks), care must be taken to identify the calvarium, the axial skeleton, and extremities. Routine pathologic examination is not necessary, provided the surgeon rigorously performs and documents the fresh inspection. Pathologic consultation is mandatory when the gestational sac is not identified, when tissue is scant for gestational age, or where abnormality is suspected.

Rhesus-negative patients not already sensitized are given Rh immune globulin immediately after the procedure.

Prophylactic antibiotics. Perioperative antibiotics are widely used in U.S. clinics. Whether this is necessary has not been resolved. Two large nonrandomized studies showed benefit.[29,47] Others found the benefit limited to patients with a history of previous pelvic inflammatory disease.[49] A recent randomized study found that most of the benefit accrued to patients colonized with *Chlamydia,* but *Chlamydia*-negative patients also benefited.[37] On the other hand, antibiotics were not routinely used in Hakim-Elahi, Tovell, and Burnhill's[24] large series, yet serious infection was rare. Tetracycline, doxycycline, or minocycline have been most used. When patients can be conveniently cultured for gonorrhea and *Chlamydia* in advance, routine antibiotics probably offer little advantage. If cultures and procedure will be performed the same day, and the rate of colonization of these organisms is known to be significant in the community served, an argument can be made in favor of short courses of prophylactic doxycycline.

Alternative means for cervical dilatation. Osmotic dilators can be used instead of forcible dilatation. Presently three types are available: laminaria tents, magnesium sulfate sponges (Lamicel), and synthetic tents of polyacrilonitrile (Dilapan). Laminaria is a genus of seaweed. When inserted into the cervical canal, laminaria take up water from the cervix, causing it to swell and exert gentle pressure that produces dilatation (Fig. 62-6). Only tents of *L. japonicum* should be used. The other medical laminaria, *L. digitata,* become too soft when wet and easily fragment with removal. Two or more small tents should be used rather than a single larger tent. A single tent may swell above a resistant internal cervical os and be difficult to remove.

Early studies found that use of laminaria reduced cervical laceration[46] and perforation[21] without increasing risk of postabortal infection. In current U.S. practice, rates of cervical laceration and perforation are very low for experienced surgeons using conventional forcible dilatation with Pratt dilators.[24] In our own practice the main use of osmotic dilators is for the midtrimester. The main drawback of laminaria is that several hours are needed for dilation to

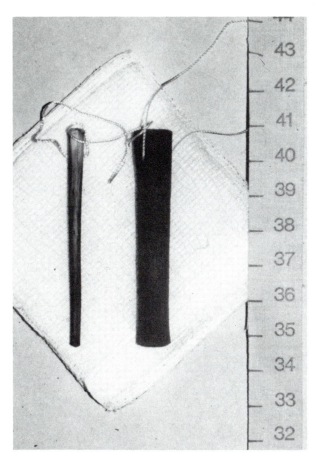

Fig. 62-6. Tents of *Laminaria japonicum*. Dry tent *(left)* as it would be just before insertion. Wet tent *(right)* as it would be after several hours exposed to water. (Photo courtesy of Mildred Hanson, M.D.)

be accomplished. Lamicel acts more quickly to pull water from the cervix and produce softening but exerts little force. Dilapan swells rapidly and exerts more force than natural laminaria. Analogues of prostaglandin produce useful dilatation within 2 to 3 hours, but gastrointestinal side effects and pain are common. In a three-way trial, Dilapan produced more dilatation than laminaria, while a prostaglandin analog produced less dilatation and had more side effects of vomiting and pain.[15]

Minisuction. In U.S. practice the minisuction technique is not used beyond 7 weeks. The procedure begins with a careful bimanual exam, and as with standard vacuum curettage, the cervix is exposed with a speculum, grasped with a tenaculum placed vertically, and then infiltrated with 20 cc of 1% lidocaine containing 0.5 mg of atropine. Flexible Karman cannulas of 4 and 5 mm are passed through the cervical canal as dilators and used to sound the uterus. Then a 6-mm cannula is inserted and attached to the evacuated 50-ml syringe to establish suction. The 4- and 5-mm cannulas are too small to dependably evacuate the uterus in pregnancy but are very useful in treatment of anovulatory bleeding. The 6-mm cannula is rotated and pushed in and out with gentle strokes. The

cannula must not be rotated when it is pushed against the fundus, because the flexible tip can be twisted off. When no more tissue comes through, the cannula is withdrawn, its tip cleared in a sterile fashion, and vacuum reestablished to prove the uterus empty. Optionally, a small sharp curette can also be used to check, as with standard vacuum curettage. Fresh exam of the aspirated tissue is even more important with these early procedures, because ectopic pregnancy is seen more often before 8 weeks than after and failed abortion is more likely as well. To prevent failed abortion, it is not enough to identify a few chorionic villi. The gestational sac must be seen.[17] Figure 62-7 shows the appearance of an early pregnancy.

In the third world, minisuction instrumentation may be the only modern technology available. In some countries physicians have modified the procedure so as to successfully terminate pregnancy throughout the first trimester. Rigid dilators are used, usually half-sized Hegars, to dilate the cervix to 8 to 9 mm. The 6-mm Karman cannula is advanced to the fundus and back to just above the internal os several times to begin shearing the gestational sac off the uterine wall. Then the syringe plunger is withdrawn to create vacuum, rupture the sac, and aspirate the amniotic fluid. When the cannula tip plugs with tissue, cannula and tissue are withdrawn together without breaking the vacuum. Some of the pregnancy tissue will pass through the lumen of the cannula, but larger portions are removed in this fashion, held in the cannula tip by the vacuum. A small, sharp curette is used as well, alternating with the vacuum. When the syringe is partially full, vacuum becomes reduced. The syringe is emptied and reevacuated to again establish vacuum. This is repeated until the cavity feels empty. A 12-week procedure done in this fashion may take 10 to 15 minutes, much longer than is needed with an 11-mm rigid cannula and electric pump as is standard in U.S. practice. Nevertheless, an experienced operator can provide abortion services successfully and safely under field conditions with only the simple instruments described: 6-mm flexible cannula and syringe, dilators, and a small steel curette. With the addition of a slender ovum forceps, early midtrimester dilatation and evacuation (D and E) procedures can be performed as well.[56]

Medical abortion. Prostaglandins are effective abortifacients at any gestational age, and two forms are available in the United States that could be used in the first trimester: vaginal suppositories of prostaglandin E_2 (PGE_2) and carboprost tromethamine, the 15-methyl analog of prostaglandin F_{2a} (Hemabate)* given by intramuscular injection. These agents have frequent side effects and, because of the widespread availability of surgical abortion, are not often used in the first trimester. The first practical medical abortifacient is mifepristone (RU486), an analog of the progestin norethindrone. Mifepristone is an antagonist to progesterone, acting at the level of progesterone receptors in the nucleus of steroid-sensitive tissues. A single oral dose

*Upjohn Co, Kalamazoo, Mich.

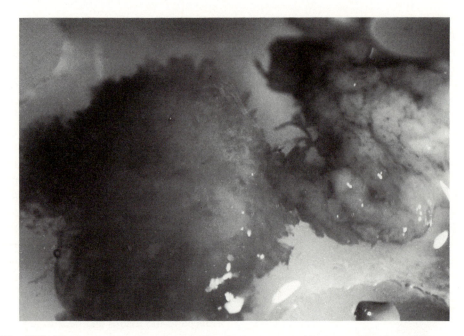

Fig. 62-7. Tissue specimen from 6-week pregnancy, as seen without magnification. The conceptus is on the left. To the right is the decidual lining of the uterus. (From Stubblefield PG; *Surgical techniques for first trimester abortion*. In Sciarra JJ, Zatuchni GI, and Daly MJ, editors: *Gynecology and obstetrics,* vol 6, Hagerstown, Md, 1982, Harper and Row.)

given to women in early pregnancy produces complete abortion in about 85% of cases. The addition of a single small dose of prostaglandin markedly improves efficacy. In a large French experience, 2115 women at or before 49 days of amenorrhea were given 600 mg of mifepristone as a single dose on day 1.[48] On day 3 they were treated with a prostaglandin, either 1 mg of gemeprost given vaginally or intramuscular sulprostone (0.25 to 0.5 mg). Altogether, 96% aborted completely; 1% required urgent vacuum curettage for heavy bleeding, but only 1 of the 2115 patients had to be transfused; 2% aborted incompletely and required a later curettage; 1% failed to abort and needed vacuum curettage. Later in pregnancy the drug becomes less effective and there is a greater chance of incomplete abortion that will require curettage. Mifepristone can also be used to trigger cervical softening and dilatation before surgical abortion.[36] The drug is approved in France and England, but extremists in the United States have thus far prevented its study outside of clinical trials in one institution.

Reduction of multifetal pregnancies

Extreme prematurity and perinatal loss are likely with multifetal pregnancy. In recent years there has been considerable interest in reduction of multifetal pregnancies and in selective termination of twin gestations where one fetus has major anomalies. The most often used technique is ultrasound-guided intracardiac injection of potassium chloride. Using high-resolution ultrasound, a 22-gauge spinal needle is advanced through the abdominal and uterine walls toward the cardiac echo. A 2-mmol solution of

KCl is used. In the first trimester, 0.2 to 0.4 ml are injected at a time until cardiac asystole is observed. In the series reported by Wapner et al,[57] 0.2 to 1.8 ml total volume was required. Visualization is continued until 2 minutes of asystole have been observed. The needle is then withdrawn and redirected into another gestational sac as needed. Usually two gestations are left intact, because the morbidity of diamniotic twins is not unacceptably greater than that of singletons. For second trimester procedures, 0.5 ml is injected at a time and total doses of 0.5 to 3 ml are required. In Wapner's series, 2 of 42 first trimester cases and 1 of 4 second trimester cases showed resumed cardiac activity 30 minutes later despite 2 minutes observation of asystole. These were successfully reinjected the same day. In Berkowitz's initial series[6] of 12 patients treated, 4 went on to abort the entire pregnancy, 7 delivered twins and 1 delivered a singleton at term. All were healthy.[6] Wapner and colleagues treated 46 pregnancies. Of 80 fetuses remaining after reduction, 75 (94%) survived. They caution that monoamniotic twins should not be treated, because this usually results in death of the remaining normal fetus. Similarly treatment of twin-twin transfusion syndrome by selective termination of one fetus has been troublesome, with infarctions resulting from embolism of tissue from the dead fetus through the shared circulation. Serum maternal alpha-fetoprotein is elevated after selective termination. Maternal coagulation defects were not seen, but most of the patients were treated in the first trimester when risk for this phenomenon is very low. Maternal coagulation surveillance is warranted after second trimester procedures.

Complications of first trimester abortion

Postabortal triad. The syndrome of pain, bleeding, and low-grade fever is the most frequent complication of first trimester abortion. The symptoms may respond to treatment with ergot preparations and oral antibiotics; however, in most cases the symptoms indicate some amount of retained tissue or blood clot in the uterine cavity. Repeat evacuation is readily accomplished under local anesthesia without need for the operating room and usually resolves the problems quickly. Since some amount of endometritis is usually present, we use a 7- to 10-day course of oral antibiotics after reevacuation.

Hematometra. In this syndrome, a type of uterine atony, the patient experiences increasing lower abdominal pain soon after the abortion.[45] The symptoms can be quite dramatic, with severe lower midline pain, diaphoresis, and tachycardia. On exam the uterus is enlarged, tense, and tender. This could be mistaken for perforation with a broad ligament hematoma except that the mass is midline. Immediate reevacuation is the treatment of choice. In Hakim-Elahi, Tovell, and Burnhill's large series,[24] 1 in 500 experienced this complication, and were managed with reaspiration of the uterus in the clinic the same day. It has been suggested that perioperative use of an intramuscular ergot preparation will reduce the incidence.[45] The same syndrome can develop more slowly with symptoms of pain and bleeding a few days after the abortion.

Hemorrhage. Excessive bleeding with vacuum curettage may be caused by uterine atony, perforation, or a pregnancy of more advanced gestational age than anticipated. Rare causes are low-lying implantation or cervical pregnancy and disseminated intravascular coagulopathy. General anesthesia leads to additional concerns because all of the potent anesthetic gases will relax the uterus in proportion to the inhaled concentration. Management of excess bleeding requires a rapid reassessment of gestational age by examination of the fetal parts already extracted and gentle exploration of the uterine cavity with curette or forceps to confirm that there is no perforation. Intravenous oxytocin is administered and the abortion completed. The uterus is massaged between two hands to ensure contraction. Intracervical administration of 10 U of vasopressin diluted to 10 cc and intracervical or intramuscular administration of 250 mcg of carboprost tromethamine are helpful. If these measures fail, the patient should be transferred immediately to the hospital with intravenous fluids running. Continued brisk bleeding from atony persisting after complete evacuation is very uncommon, as is coagulopathy with first trimester procedures. If bleeding persists, coagulopathy is ruled out and the patient prepared for laparoscopy and repeat curettage. Cervical pregnancy and cervical perforation (described below) are special cases, best managed by arteriography and selective embolization of the bleeding vessels. Selection of this form of treatment requires prompt and accurate assessment to rule out other causes, and volume support for the patient while arrangements are made for the radiologic procedure.

Perforation. The rate of perforation was 0.9 per 1000 in a multicenter study of 67,175 abortions.[23] Risk of perforation was greater for patients at more advanced gestational ages and for parous women than for women with no previous delivery. Use of laminaria reduced risk, as did operator skill. Resident physicians were more likely to perforate than were attending physicians. A much lower rate, only 1 per 10,000 was reported in the series of 170,000 procedures through 14 weeks from the Planned Parenthood Clinic of New York City where all procedures were performed by a small number of experienced physicians.[24] In that series dilatation was by Pratt dilators. Laminaria were not used.

In our own experience with patients hospitalized for perforation, the perforations were lateral and usually occurred either at the junction of the cervix and lower uterine segment or were perforations of the cervix itself (Fig. 62-8).[4] These lateral perforations produced different clinical syndromes depending on the anatomic location of the injury. Lateral perforations at the junction of the cervix and lower uterine segment can lacerate the ascending branch of the uterine artery within the broad ligament, causing severe pain, a broad ligament hematoma, and intraabdominal bleeding. This type of injury is usually recognized immediately. Laparoscopy is required to confirm the injury, with laparotomy to ligate the severed uterine artery and repair the uterine injury. Hysterectomy should not be required and may not stop the bleeding should the operator fail to perceive that the vascular injury is lateral to the site where the vessels are ligated in standard hysterectomy technique. Low cervical perforations, on the other hand, may injure the descending branch of the uterine artery within the dense collagenous substance of the cardinal ligaments. In this case there is only external bleeding through the cervical canal and no broad ligament hematoma will form. Bleeding from this injury will cease as the arteries go into spasm, but it recurs. Deaths have occurred when a low cervical perforation was not appreciated and bled again several hours later when the patient was at home. Hysterectomy has usually been required for management, but there are other options if the injury is suspected. Freiman[19] has described a case managed by laparotomy and placement of sutures through the cardinal ligaments after downward mobilization of the bladder and identification of the ureter. We have proposed that arteriography and selected embolization of the injured vessel should be attempted. Both types of injuries undoubtedly occur during dilation. Midline and fundal perforations generally do not cause heavy bleeding, but if they are not recognized and curettage is continued, extensive damage to the bowel or bladder may result. Management requires laparoscopy to assess the extent of injury, and then laparoscopic-guided completion of evacuation and coagulation of the bleeding site on the uterus. Antibiotics are administered and the patient observed overnight in the hospital.

Bowel injury. When bowel injury is suspected, as when the bowel has been drawn into the perforation, it is

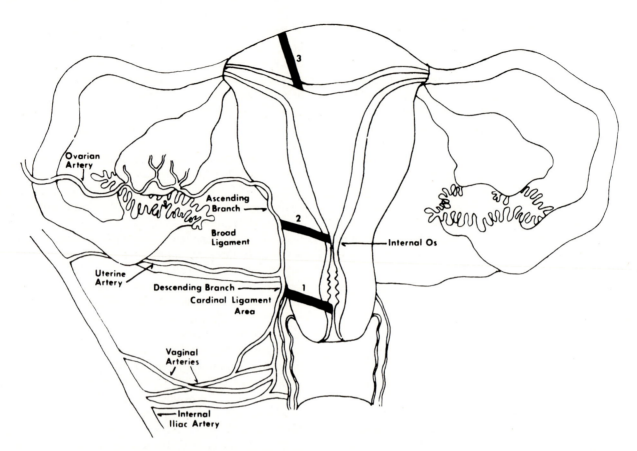

Fig. 62-8. Possible sites of uterine perforation at abortion. *1,* Low cervical perforation with laceration of descending branches of uterine artery. *2,* Perforation at junction of cervix and lower uterine segment with laceration of ascending branch of uterine artery. *3,* Fundal perforation. (From Berek JS, Stubblefield PG: Anatomical and clinical correlations of uterine perforations, *Am J Obstet Gynecol* 135:181, 1979.)

essential to completely visualize the affected area. Often this can be accomplished at laparoscopy by an experienced operator, but if there is difficulty in visualizing the site of injury, laparotomy is indicated. Failure to recognize and adequately treat a bowel injury can be fatal. If there is full-thickness injury or the mesentery has been stripped, segmental resection and anastomosis are required. Small areas of injury can be managed successfully by oversewing the lesion, irrigating the peritoneal cavity, and leaving a large intraabdominal drain. High-dose antibiotics are given prophylactically. Larger injuries to the colon require a diverting colostomy after resection and anastomosis.

Bladder injury. Anterior perforations can lacerate the bladder trigone. Part of the evaluation of a major perforation is bladder catheterization to look for gross hematuria. The injury is confirmed at laparoscopy, but laparotomy is needed for management. Direct repair should not be attempted for injury to the trigone. An ample cystotomy incision is made on the dome, the ureters are catheterized, and the rent then repaired in two layers with absorbable suture. It is important to obtain the best possible operative consultation with a general surgeon or urologist for man-

agement of these more extensive injuries. Inadequate initial management of major injury adds markedly to the patient's problems and may jeopardize survival.

Failed abortion, continued pregnancy, and ectopic pregnancy. Failure to interrupt the pregnancy is more often a problem with very early abortions. For this reason, many U.S. clinics refuse to accept patients before 8 menstrual weeks. In contrast, abortion services in the third world, having only equipment for minisuction procedures, prefer operating at 6 or 7 weeks. With early procedures the gestational sac must be identified with a fresh exam of the tissue.[17] When no chorionic villi are found in the fresh exam, the patient is at risk for ectopic pregnancy. Patients are considered either high-risk or low-risk for ectopic pregnancy based on symptoms and physical findings. High-risk patients should have immediate laparoscopy. Low-risk patients are followed with serial quantitative assays for beta chorionic gonadotropin with frequent contact until the problem is resolved.[10] Vaginal probe ultrasound is often helpful.

Incomplete and septic abortion. Preexisting colonization with pathogenic bacteria and retained tissue are the principal causes of postabortal sepsis. If there is bleeding and the uterus is enlarged, repeat curettage is indicated. When the uterus is larger than 12 weeks, a preoperative ultrasound is advised. Where fever is present, a cervical gram stain and appropriate cultures are taken. Then high-dose intravenous antibiotic therapy is begun and curettage performed shortly thereafter. Delay of several hours is unnecessary and adds risk for the patient. Fever, pelvic pain, minimal bleeding, and a small firm uterus suggest endometritis-myometritis without retained tissue. When there is question, ultrasound is useful in making the decision whether to perform curettage or to treat with antibiotics alone.

Rarely, clostridial sepsis is seen as a complication of legal abortion. This should be suspected from the presence of large gram-positive rods on gram stain of the cervical secretions or curetted tissue, or when tachycardia seems out of proportion to the fever. Hematuria, shock, and severe adult respiratory distress syndrome can develop rapidly. Initial treatment requires high-dose intravenous penicillin, curettage, and fluid management. A superficial clostridial infection will respond to these measures. If hemolysis is present, indicating systemic release of clostridial toxins, prompt hysterectomy is probably necessary if the patient is to survive.[30]

SECOND TRIMESTER OR MIDTRIMESTER ABORTION
Dilatation and evacuation (D and E)

Surgical evacuation is the most common method for midtrimester abortion in the United States through 20 weeks[11]; hence, this procedure will be described in detail.

Technique. After adequate counseling, complete medical history, and physical examination, laminaria tents are placed in the cervical canal and held in place with two 4 × 4 gauze sponges tucked into the fornices. At 13 to 15 weeks, 2 small tents will suffice, but at 16 to 20 weeks 4 or more small tents are inserted, and after 20 weeks, 8 to 10 small tents. Paracervical anesthesia is produced with 10 cc of 1% lidocaine for the insertion. To avoid syncope, the patient is kept lying on her side for a few minutes after insertion and then goes home. If the membranes are ruptured during insertion, the abortion is performed as scheduled the next day. We leave the tents in place for 12 to 24 hours. Dilapan tents provide about the same dilatation as 2 medium *L. japonicum* tents and can be used instead of or in combination with laminaria. An analgesic is prescribed because some patients will experience moderate abdominal discomfort through the night. We routinely give doxycycline, 100 mg after insertion, 100 mg at bedtime, and then 100 mg twice a day for 2 days after the procedure. Tests for gonorrhea and chlamydia are performed before or at laminaria insertion. Results are rarely available until after the procedure. Patients are then treated following current guidelines of the Centers for Disease Control.

Ultrasound examination is advised if there is a discrepancy between menstrual dates and uterine size or if there is an abnormality on bimanual examination and for all cases 20 weeks and beyond. Operative ultrasound guidance is helpful for the more advanced cases.[14]

Uterine evacuation is performed as follows.[1] An intravenous line is established. The anesthetic of choice is begun. The patient is placed in lithotomy position, and the previously placed vaginal sponges and laminaria are removed. The vagina and cervix are cleansed with a germicide. Paracervical block is administered with 20 cc of 1% lidocaine containing 10 U of vasopressin.[13] When a general anesthetic is used, the lidocaine is omitted but the same dose of vasopressin is given in 10 cc of saline at the 4 and 8 o'clock positions deep into the cervical stroma to reach the junction of cervix and lower uterine segment. Great caution is exercised to avoid intravascular injection. Two single-tooth tenaculums are placed vertically side by side, each with one branch inside the cervical canal. A large dilator is gently inserted to confirm dilatation. Intravenous oxytocin is started, 40 U per 1000 cc solution, at 150 to 200 cc/hr. The vacuum cannula is then inserted and vacuum established briefly to rupture the membranes and drain amniotic fluid. The 12- or 14-mm cannulas are used for 13 to 15 week procedures; the 16-mm system is used for more advanced cases.* The cannula is then removed and evacuation begun with the ovum forceps. A Foerrester forceps is adequate for 13 to 15 weeks. Beyond this, the small Sopher forceps and the Kelly placental forceps are used for most procedures (Fig. 62-9). If there is difficulty in locating fetal parts, the uterine cavity is explored with the Kelly placental forceps, preferred for its rounded contour and light feel to the heavier Sopher instrument. When the fetal parts are located, they may be extracted with the Kelly forceps, but more often the Sopher or Bierer forceps will be needed. Fetal parts are extracted slowly and carefully, rotating the instrument as they are brought through the cervical canal to avoid lacerating the cervix. The Bierer forceps are used for larger gestations. The vacuum cannula is reinserted as needed to pull tissue downward where it can be grasped with the forceps. When the procedure feels complete, the vacurette is gently inserted all the way to the fundus and slowly rotated for 1 to 2 minutes, then a large sharp curette is used to explore the cavity. If any additional tissue is encountered, the forceps or cannula are reinserted to remove it. After the procedure the operator carefully examines the fetal parts to be sure all have been evacuated. On occasion the fetal calvarium is retained in the uterus. If exploration with the Kelly placental forceps does not locate it, the vacuum cannula is inserted and slowly rotated as described above, producing a strong uterine contraction that may push the retained parts down where they can be grasped with the forceps. If these attempts are not successful, it is best to stop, administer an oxytocin infusion for 2 hours, and then try again. By then the remaining fetal parts will be pushed down to the inter-

---

*16-mm vacuum systems are available from Rocket of London, Inc, Branford, Conn.

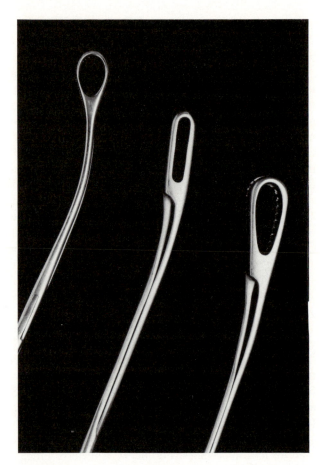

Fig. 62-9. Instruments for D and E. Kelly placental forceps, Sopher forceps, and Bierer forceps.

nal os where they can be easily extracted. Hern's monograph[27] provides a more detailed description of the procedure.

Attempting evacuation of a pregnancy beyond the operators's skill and experience poses serious risk and mandates liberal use of preoperative ultrasound. If the cervix has been widely dilated by multiple laminaria tents, the experienced surgeon can satisfactorily extract a pregnancy up to 20 or 21 weeks. Beyond this we feel the procedure should be abandoned unless the surgeon regularly performs more advanced procedures. Intravenous oxytocin or systemic prostaglandins can be used instead.

Modifications of technique are often used to facilitate D and E in the late midtrimester. Hern[28] has described a combination method. After multistage laminaria treatment over 2 days, urea is injected into the amniotic sac to produce fetal demise and initiate labor. When expulsion begins, an assisted delivery is performed under local anesthesia. Wright[61] practices another approach. Multiple laminaria or four Dilapan tents are inserted into the cervix, and under ultrasound guidance, a fetal intracardiac injection of 1.5 mg of digoxin is given. The D and E is carried out under brief general anesthesia the following day. Oxytocin is administered as 50 to 100 U per 1000 cc during the procedure. As noted below, digoxin has been used to produce

fetal death prior to prostaglandin abortion. Wright has described 2400 cases at 19 to 23 weeks with no perforations.

Anesthesia. With good psychological support from trained counselors, midtrimester D & E can be performed under paracervical block with low-dose intravenous sedation. This may be difficult to provide in the operating rooms of a busy general hospital, oriented towards major anesthetics. In a multicenter study, general anesthesia increased the risk for cervical laceration and hemorrhage with D and E.[38] On the other hand, large series have been reported in which very low rates of uterine injury occurred with general anesthesia.[33,61] When general anesthesia is used, it is all the more critical to have adequate preparation of the cervix with laminaria or Dilapan tents. Suitable regimens for intravenous sedation are diazepam (5 mg) followed by fentanyl (0.05 mg), repeated after several minutes if needed. Alternatively, midazolam (2 to 4 mg) is given 1 mg at a time, followed with 200-mcg doses of alfentanyl given at 3- to 4-minute intervals during the procedure. A pulse oximeter is advisable with these regimens because all of these agents depress respiration and when combined have the potential for greater respiratory depression.[3] If general anesthesia is used, full compliance with current standards for monitoring tissue oxygen levels, end expiratory CO_2, and frequent vital signs are mandatory.[16] When these procedures take place out of hospital, more stringent patient selection is required. Combinations of short-acting barbiturates, nitrous oxide, and oxygen are preferred. Potent inhalant agents are avoided altogether or used in very low concentrations. Close observation during recovery is essential. Use of IV sedation or general anesthesia requires personnel trained in cardiorespiratory support.

Labor induction methods

Hypertonic saline. Hypertonic saline is still widely used after 20 weeks. There are hazards unique to this method: cardiovascular collapse, pulmonary and cerebral edema, and renal failure occur if there is intravascular injection, and disseminated intravascular coagulopathy is a risk for all. Intravascular injection is avoided by careful amniocentesis and instillation of the saline through a catheter placed in the amniotic sac. Given alone, hypertonic saline produces mean times to abortion of 33 to 35 hours.[5,35] Addition of oxytocin at 17 to 67 mU per minute reduces the mean time to 25 to 26 hours; thus there are fewer failed abortions, fewer retained placentas, less blood loss, and less risk of infection.[5] Addition of the oxytocin increases the rate of occurrence of disseminated intravascular coagulation (DIC) and requires caution to avoid water intoxication.

Intraamniotic urea. Urea is safer than saline because inadvertent intravascular injection of small amounts is harmless. Urea requires augmentation to avoid prolonged intervals from injection to abortion. The combination of 80 g of urea plus 5 mg of prostaglandin F_{2a} instilled into the amniotic sac produces abortion in a mean time of 17.5

hours, with 80% aborting within 24 hours. The urea-prostaglandin combination offers a shorter injection to abortion interval than hypertonic saline and has fewer serious complications.[7]

Intrauterine prostaglandins. Prostaglandin F_{2a} was the first prostaglandin approved by the U.S. Food and Drug Administration. Initial problems were the need for a second injection in many cases, transient fetal survival in some cases, failure of the primary technique, incomplete abortion and, in the primigravida, risk for cervical rupture. Overnight treatment with laminaria tents reduces the mean times to abortion from 29 to 14 hours, reduces the risk for cervical injury, and reduces the need for a second dose.[52] Routine exploration of the uterine cavity with forceps and vacuum curette reduces postabortal hemorrhage and injection from retained products.

Prostaglandin F_{2a} is no longer available in the United States. An alternative is the 15-methyl analog of PGF_{2a}, carboprost tromethamine (Hemabate). For intraamniotic injection, 2 mg of this drug replace 40 mg of PGF_{2a}, and 0.250 mg replaces the 5-mg dose of PGF_{2a} used to augment intraamniotic urea. Osathanondh[39] has described an extensive experience with intraamniotic carboprost in a combination method. Patients are treated overnight with multiple laminaria tents packed around one Lamicel tent. The following morning, the tents are removed and an intraamniotic injection of 2 mg of carboprost is given in combination with 64 cc of 23.4% sodium chloride. After 4 hours the membranes are artificially ruptured, and unless the cervix is already well dilated, a 20-mg prostaglandin E_2 (Prostin E_2) suppository is placed into the cervical canal on the end of a Dilapan tent. Subsequently, PGE_2 vaginal suppositories are given at 3-hour intervals until abortion. All patients have a brief exploration of the uterine cavity and curettage under low-dose sedation after expulsion of the placenta. If the patient has not aborted by 14 hours, a D & E procedure is performed. A mean time from instillation to abortion of 8 hours was reported, and neither cervical laceration nor uterine rupture occurred in more than 4000 consecutive cases following this protocol.

Systemic prostaglandins. PGE_2 vaginal suppositories and intramuscular carboprost are available in the United States. Both are highly effective. With vaginal PGE_2 (20 mg every 3 hours), the mean time to abort is 13.4 hours, and 90% of patients abort within 24 hours.[54] Mean times to abort are 15 to 17 hours with carboprost given as 0.25 mg IM injections at 2-hour intervals and 80% abort within 24 hours.[43] Vomiting and diarrhea are frequent with both, usually more frequent with carboprost. PGE_2 produces temperature elevation of $1°$ C or more in about one third of patients. Overnight treatment with laminaria shortens the length of prostaglandin treatment, reduces the dose of drug required, and hence reduces prostaglandin-related side effects.[53] Transient fetal survival is a problem with all prostaglandin methods. One group has reported ultrasound-guided intracardiac injection of digoxin to ensure fetal death.[58]

Oxytocin. Oxytocin is used to augment other methods but is generally considered to be poorly effective by itself. In fact, oxytocin can be a primary method for abortion in the midtrimester, but very high infusion rates are required. Winkler et al[60] compared a high-dose oxytocin protocol to vaginal PGE_2 suppositories at 17 to 24 weeks and found the oxytocin just as effective and with fewer side effects. Their protocol was as follows: Fifty units of oxytocin is given in 500 ml of 5% dextrose and normal saline over 3 hours (approximately 278 mU/min), followed by a 1-hour rest period off oxytocin. Then 100 U in 500 ml are given over 3 hours, followed by a 1-hour rest, and repeated, adding 50 U of oxytocin to each infusion until the patient aborts or a final solution of 300 U in 500 ml (1667 mV/min) is reached. Of 59 patients in the PGE_2 group, 2 experienced severe bronchospasm. No signs of water intoxication were seen with the oxytocin. This report is instructive and offers more options for managing late abortion, fetal death, and premature rupture of the membranes. However, the lessons we have learned from high-dose oxytocin used to augment saline or prostaglandin must be remembered. Uterine rupture, cervical-vaginal fistula, and annular detachment of the cervix can be seen when the uterus is overstimulated without adequate cervical preparation.

Midtrimester complications

Failed abortion. Labor induction methods share the common problem that not all patients abort from the primary method within a reasonable period of time and so become at increasing risk for bleeding and infection. For these methods, a graph showing cumulative percentage of patients aborted versus time shows a plateau (Fig. 62-10). At this point a second method is indicated. High-dose intravenous oxytocin can be used, but caution is required to avoid uterine rupture in multigravida[42] and cervical rupture in primigravida. A better alternative is to change to a different prostaglandin or a different route of administration (i.e., if the primary method was intraamniotic carboprost, change to vaginal suppositories of PGE_2). If the second prostaglandin is unsuccessful after a defined period of time, a D and E is performed.[8] Since failure of a second prostaglandin is uncommon and may indicate a uterine anomaly, it is wise to consider an ultrasound exam before surgical intervention if this was not already done.

Disseminated intravascular coagulopathy (DIC). Disseminated intravascular coagulopathy (DIC) is very rare after first trimester vacuum curettage, occurring in approximately 8 cases per 100,000 procedures, but the incidence is higher after midtrimester D and E (191 per 100,000) and highest for saline instillation (658 per 100,000).[31] DIC must be considered whenever postabortal hemorrhage is seen and, if present, requires aggressive management with cryoprecipitate, fresh frozen plasma, and packed red cells. Heparin therapy is not helpful in these cases.

Others. Perforation with midtrimester D and E is more

likely to result in major visceral injury than in the first trimester and usually requires laparotomy for management. Inexperienced operators may confuse maternal small intestine for late midtrimester fetal bowel, although the diameters are different, and fail to appreciate a perforation until considerable harm has resulted. The labor induction methods can lead to fetal expulsion through a rent in the cervix above the external os, a cervicovaginal fistula. These are repaired by debridement of the avascular edges and primary closure of the defect. Uterine rupture can occur when saline, urea, or prostaglandin is augmented with high-dose oxytocin. Uterine rupture is suspected because of severe pain followed by falling blood pressure and rising pulse from intraabdominal bleeding. Management requires blood replacement and laparotomy with repair of the uterine laceration.

Choice of midtrimester procedure

The mortality risk for different methods is shown in Table 62-2. Early midtrimester D and E is the safest. Labor induction methods and D and E are comparable in the later midtrimester, and both are much safer than hysterotomy or hysterectomy for abortion. The labor induction methods all involve overnight hospitalization, which in the United States greatly increases expense and limits accessability. The D and E technique can be safely provided on an outpatient basis and in well-equipped free-standing clinics at much reduced cost. Also, the psychological impact on the patient is much less than with labor induction techniques.[33] In the early midtrimester, D and E has fewer complications than labor induction.[32] Several skilled surgeons offer D and E to 24 weeks. Indeed, the lowest reported rate of complications for any late abortion technique is that of Hern[28] for his combination method of laminaria, intraamniotic urea, and D and E. For the occasional operator faced with the need to provide midtrimester abortion, we would suggest ultrasound-guided fetal intracardiac injection of 1.5 mg of digoxin, and intracervical laminaria, followed the next day by vaginal suppositories of PGE_2. If abortion is prolonged beyond 24 hours, carboprost injections of 0.25 mg at 2-hour intervals would be substituted.

Fetal death in utero. Fetal death in utero can be managed as abortion of an intact pregnancy, with either D and E techniques, vaginal PGE_2, or IM carboprost. The intraamniotic route is not advised, as increased permeability of the membranes and the greater difficulty of amniocentesis may result in systemic reaction to saline or prostaglandin. The response of the uterus to prostaglandin is quicker

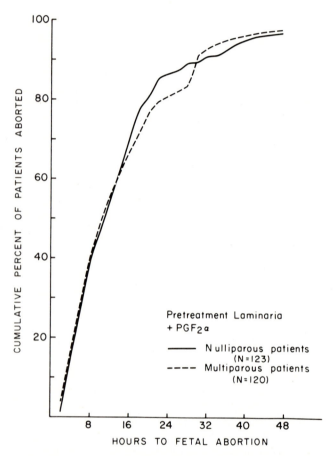

Fig. 62-10. Curve showing the cumulative percentage of patients aborted as a function of time since start of prostaglandin therapy. (From Stubblefield PG et al: Combination therapy for midtrimester abortion: laminaria and analogues of prostaglandin, *Contraception* 13:723, 1976, by permission.)

Table 62-2. Death-to-case rate* and deaths (in parentheses) for legal abortions by type of procedure and weeks of gestation, United States 1972-1980

Type of procedure	Weeks of gestation					
	≥8	9–10	11–12	13–15	16–20	≥21
Curettage	0.4(18)	1.2(29)	2.1(24)	0.0(0)	0.0(0)	0.0(0)
D and E	0.0(0)	0.0(0)	0.0(0)	3.6(10)	10.7(9)	15.0(2)
Saline or prostaglandin instillation	0.0(0)	0.0(0)	0.0(0)	1.9(1)	16.2(34)	15.1(7)
Other instillation	0.0(0)	0.0(0)	0.0(0)	14.1(4)	6.6(7)	16.0(3)
Hysterotomy/hysterectomy						
Total	0.5(18)	1.3(31)	2.2(25)	5.4(18)	3.6(53)	17.7(13)

*Deaths per 100,000 abortions, excluding deaths associated with ectopic pregnancy. Centers for Disease Control: Abortion surveillance 1979-80. Jan. 1983, Atlanta, CDC. By permission.

after fetal death. With PGE$_2$ suppositories, the mean time to abortion is about 10 hours. Special caution is required for use of prostaglandins after 28 weeks. The full dose of 20 mg of PGE$_2$ is too much and has produced fatal uterine rupture on occasion. Our protocol, used successfully for many years, is to cut the suppository into quarters and administer one quarter of the full dose (approximately 5 mg of PGE$_2$) at 1- to 2-hour intervals, titrating uterine activity to avoid hyperstimulation. This also markedly reduces gastrointestinal side effects and fever. In patients with ruptured membranes or much vaginal bleeding, vaginal PGE$_2$ may be poorly effective because dilution by blood or amniotic fluid may limit absorption. IM carboprost (0.25 mg every 2 to 3 hours) is a better choice in these cases. Patients who will receive prostaglandins are given antiemetics and antidiarrheal agents on a routine basis to reduce vomiting and diarrhea. Acetaminophen suppositories are given at 4-hour intervals to block the febrile response to PGE$_2$.

When laminaria are used to prepare the cervix after fetal death, labor can sometimes be triggered by the laminaria alone. This is not a problem if the patient knows it may happen and has been instructed to return to the hospital. DIC is more common with D and E for fetal death than with the same procedure and an intact pregnancy and can also be triggered by the labor induction methods. Preoperative evaluation of the clotting system is advised before intervention for fetal death. Excessive postabortal bleeding is immediately evaluated with clotting studies so that DIC, if present, can be treated early.

ABORTION IN THE THIRD TRIMESTER

Viability is the limit for abortion based on the decision of the woman in most U.S. jurisdictions, following the Supreme Court's decision in *Roe v. Wade*.[44] Viability is a legal concept, usually meaning the ability to survive indefinitely, with or without medical support. Fetuses with major malformations incompatible with life thus could be considered as previable at any gestational age, and intervention to induce labor could be considered in order to spare the woman the prolongation of a pregnancy that will have no fetal benefit. Chervenak et al[12] have explored the ethical dimensions of the issue and conclude that third trimester abortion is ethical, provided two conditions are met: (1) the fetus has a condition with no prospect for prolonged survival after birth, and (2) there exists a completely accurate way to diagnose this condition. Anencephaly is one such condition.

REFERENCES

1. Altman A et al: Midtrimester abortion by laminaria and evacuation (L & E) on a teaching service: a review of 789 cases, *Adv Plan Parent* 16:1, 1981.
2. Begum SF, Jalil K: *Problems of septic abortion in Bangladesh and the need for menstrual regulation*. In Landy U, Ratnam SS, editors: *Prevention and treatment of contraceptive failure*, New York, 1986, Plenum Press.
3. Bell GP et al: A comparison of diazepam and midazolam as endos-copy premedication: assessing changes in ventilation and oxygen saturation, *Br J Clin Pharmacol* 26:595, 1988.
4. Berek JS, Stubblefield PG: Anatomical and clinical correlations of uterine perforations, *Am J Obstet Gynecol* 135:181, 1979.
5. Berger GS, Edelman DA: Oxytocin administration, instillation to abortion time, and morbidity associated with saline instillation, *Am J Obstet Gynecol* 121:941, 1975.
6. Berkowitz, RL et al: Selective reduction of multifetal pregnancies in the first trimester, *N Engl J Med* 318:1043, 1988.
7. Binkin NJ et al: Urea-prostaglandin versus hypertonic saline for instillation abortion, *Am J Obstet Gynecol* 146:947, 1983.
8. Burkeman RT et al: The management of midtrimester abortion failures by vaginal evacuation, *Obstet Gynecol* 49:233, 1977.
9. Burnhill M: *Physician's manual: standard medical procedures,* ed 3, Newton, Mass, 1975, Preterm Institute.
10. Burnhill MS, Armstead JW: Reducing the morbidity of vacuum aspiration abortion, *Int J Gynaecol Obstet* 16:204, 1978.
11. Centers for Disease Control: *Abortion surveillance* 1979-80, Jan 1983, CDC.
12. Chervenak FA et al: When is termination of pregnancy during the third trimester morally justifiable? *N Engl J Med* 310:501, 1984.
13. Christensen D: Use of vasopressin to reduce D & E blood loss. Paper presented at the 8th Annual Meeting of the National Abortion Federation, Los Angeles, May 14, 1984.
14. Darney PD: Midtrimester abortion under ultrasound guidance. Postgraduate course presented by the National Abortion Federation, Tampa, Fla, Jan 31, 1983.
15. Darney PD, Dorward K: Cervical dilatation before first-trimester elective abortion: a controlled comparison of meteneprost, laminaria and hypan, *Obstet Gynecol* 70:397, 1987.
16. Eichhorn JH et al: Standards for patient monitoring during anesthesia at Harvard Medical School, *JAMA* 256:1017, 1986.
17. Fielding WL et al: Continued pregnancy after failed first trimester abortion, *Obstet Gynecol* 63:421, 1984.
18. Forrest JD, Henshaw SK: What U.S. women think and do about contraception, *Fam Plann Perspect* 15:157, 1983.
19. Freiman M: Personal communication, April 2, 1982.
20. Glick E: Paracervical and lower uterine field block anesthesia for therapeutic abortion and office D & C. Paper presented at the 11th Annual Convention of the National Abortion Federation, Salt Lake City, Utah, May 18, 1987.
21. Gold J et al: *The safety of laminaria and rigid dilators for cervical dilatation prior to suction curettage for first trimester abortion: a comparative analysis.* In Naftolin F, Stubblefield PG, editors: *Dilatation of the uterine cervix: connective tissue biology and clinical management,* New York, 1980, Raven Press.
22. Grimes DA, Cates W: Deaths from paracervical anesthesia used for first trimester abortion, 1972–1975, *N Engl J Med* 295:1397, 1976.
23. Grimes DA, Schulz KF, Cates WJ: Prevention of uterine perforation during curettage abortion, *JAMA* 251:2108, 1984.
24. Hakim-Elahi E, Tovell HMM, Burnhill MS: Complications of first trimester abortion: a report of 170,000 cases, *Obstet Gynecol* 76:129, 1990.
25. Henshaw SK, Silverman J: The characteristics and prior contraceptive use of U.S. abortion patients, *Fam Plann Perspect* 20:158, 1988.
26. Henshaw SK, Van Vort J: Teenage abortion, birth and pregnancy statistics: an update, *Fam Plann Perspect* 21:85, 1989.
27. Hern WM: *Abortion practice,* Philadelphia, 1984, JB Lippincott.
28. Hern WM: Serial multiple laminaria and adjunctive urea in late outpatient dilatation and evacuation abortion, *Obstet Gynecol* 63:543, 1984.
29. Hodgson JE et al: Prophylactic use of tetracycline for first trimester abortions, *Obstet Gynecol* 45:574, 1975.
30. Hoyme UB, Eschenback DA: *Postoperative infections.* In Iffy L, Charles D, editors: *Operative perinatology,* New York, 1984, Macmillan.
31. Kafrissen ME et al: Coagulopathy and induced abortion methods: rates and relative risks, *Am J Obstet Gynecol* 147:344, 1983.

32. Kafrissen ME et al: A comparison of intraamniotic instillation of hyperosmolar urea and prostaglandin F$_{2a}$ vs dilatation and evacuation for midtrimester abortion, *JAMA* 253:916, 1984.

33. Kaltreider NB, Goldsmith S, Margolis AJ: The impact of midtrimester abortion techniques on patients and staff, *Am J Obstet Gynecol* 135:235, 1979.

34. Karman H, Potts M: Very early abortion using syringe as vacuum source, *Lancet* 1:7759, 1972.

35. Kerenyi TD, Mandelaman N, Sherman DH: Five thousand consecutive saline abortions, *Am J Obstet Gynecol* 116:593, 1973.

36. LeFebre Y et al: The effects of RU38486 on cervical ripening, *Am J Obstet Gynecol* 162:61, 1990.

37. Levallois P, Rioux JE: Prophylactic antibiotics for suction curettage abortion: results of a clinical controlled trial, *Am J Obstet Gynecol* 158:100, 1988.

38. MacKay HT, Schulz KR, Grimes DA: The safety of local versus general anesthesia for second trimester dilatation and evacuation abortion, *Obstet Gynecol* 66:661, 1985.

39. Mosher WD: Fertility and family planning in the United States: insights from the national survey of family growth, *Fam Plann Perspect* 20:207, 1988.

40. National Center for Health Statistics: *Monthly vital statistics report* 39(suppl 11):7, 1990.

41. Osathanondh R: *Conception control.* In Ryan KJ, Barbieri R, Berkowitz RS: *Kistner's gynecology,* ed 5, St Louis, 1990, Mosby–Year Book.

42. Propping D, Stubblefield PG, Golub J: Uterine rupture following midtrimester abortion by laminaria, prostaglandin F$_{2a}$ and oxytocin: report of two cases, *Am J Obstet.*

43. Robins J, Mann LI: Second generation prostaglandins: midtrimester pregnancy termination by intramuscular injection of a 15 methyl analog of prostaglandin F$_{2a}$, *Fertil Steril* 27:104, 1976.

44. *Roe v. Wade,* 410 U.S. 113, 1973.

45. Sands RX, Burnhill MS, Hakim-Elahi E: Post-abortal uterine atony, *Obstet Gynecol* 43:595, 1974.

46. Schulz KF, Grimes DA, Cates W Jr: Measures to prevent cervical injury during suction curettage abortion, *Lancet* 1:1182, 1983.

47. Schulz KF et al: Prophylactic antibiotics to prevent febrile complications of curettage abortion. Paper presented at 8th Annual Meeting of the National Abortion Federation, Los Angeles, May 15, 1984.

48. Silvestre L et al: Voluntary interruption of pregnancy with mifepristone (RU486) and a prostaglandin analogue: a large scale French experience, *N Engl J Med* 322:645, 1990.

49. Sonne Holme S et al: Prophylactic antibiotics in first trimester abortion: a clinical controlled trial, *Am J Obstet Gynecol* 139:693, 1981.

50. Stubblefield PG: *Induced abortion: indications, counseling, and services.* In Sciarra JJ, Zatuchni GI, Daly MJ editors: *Gynecology and obstetrics,* Philadelphia, 1982, Harper and Row.

51. Stubblefield PG, Altman AM, Goldstein SP: Randomized trial of one versus two days of laminaria treatment prior to late midtrimester abortion by uterine evacuation: a pilot study, *Am J Obstet Gynecol* 143:481, 1982.

52. Stubblefield PG et al: Laminaria augmentation of intraamniotic PGF$_{2a}$ for midtrimester pregnancy termination, *Prostaglandins* 10:413, 1975.

53. Stubblefield PG et al: Combination therapy for midtrimester abortion: laminaria and analogues of prostaglandin, *Contraception* 13:723, 1976.

54. Surrago EJ, Robins J: Midtrimester pregnancy termination by intravaginal administration of prostaglandin E$_2$, *Contraception* 26:285, 1982.

55. U.S. Food and Drug Administration: Warning for prescription drugs containing sulfite, *Drug Bull* 17:2, 1987.

56. VanLith DAF et al: *Aspirotomy.* In Berger GS, Brenner WE, Keith LG, editors: *Second trimester abortion: perspectives after a decade of experience,* Boston, 1981, John Wright PSG.

57. Wapner RJ et al: Selective reduction of multifetal pregnancies, *Lancet* 335:90, 1990.

58. Waters JL, Pitts-Hames M: Digoxin induction abortion. Paper presented at 8th annual meeting of the National Abortion Federation, Los Angeles, May 14, 1984.

59. Weibe ER: Comparison of the efficacy of different local anesthetic techniques in therapeutic abortions. Paper presented at Annual Meeting of Canadian College of Family Physicians, Vancouver, BC, Nov 24, 1990.

60. Winkler CL et al: Mid second trimester labor induction: concentrated oxytocin compared with prostaglandin E$_2$ vaginal suppositories, *Obstet Gynecol* 77:297, 1991.

61. Wright PC: Late midtrimester abortion by dilatation and evacuation using dilapan and digoxin. Paper presented at 13th Annual Meeting of the National Abortion Federation, San Francisco, April 4, 1989.

62. Wu, YT: Suction in artificial abortion: 300 cases, *Chin J Obstet Gynecol* 6:447, 1958.

Chapter 63

CERVICAL CERCLAGE

Donald R. Coustan

Cervical incompetence was described by Palmer and La-Comme[56] in 1948. The placement of a suture around the cervix, known as *cerclage,* was first popularized by Shirodkar[66] in 1955, when he described the use of fascia for this procedure. Numerous other procedures have been proposed and popularized during the past four decades, and virtually every obstetrician has a favorite approach. What is most striking is the relative dearth of data addressing the supposed condition for which this procedure is used, the *incompetent cervix.* This diagnosis is often applied but rarely proven. Although it has been estimated to complicate as many as 1% of all pregnancies,[50] its true prevalence is more likely to be in the range of 0.05 to 0.2%.[6,27,73] Textbooks of obstetrics define incompetent cervix as the functional inability to retain a pregnancy in utero until term. The "classic history" of painless dilation of the cervix eventuating in delivery between 16 and 28 weeks' gestation (or later) is obviously a retrospective diagnosis. Attempts to make the diagnosis prospectively, whether in the nonpregnant state by passage of a no. 8 Hegar dilator or no. 16 foley catheter, or in the pregnant woman by serial digital examination of the cervix, remain unproven. Floyd[23] performed serial vaginal examinations of 100 women whose pregnancies went to at least 36 weeks. By the sixth month of pregnancy, 15% of nulliparas were 1 cm dilated, as were 72% of parous women. In fact, 36% of parous individuals manifested cervical dilation of 2 cm or more. Similarly, Parikh and Mehta[57] found that 16% of nulliparas and 17% of parous women had an "open" cervix (dilation of at least one fingertip) at 21 to 28 weeks. Such women manifested a prematurity rate of 14%, not much different from the 11% among those with closed cervixes. Schaffner and Schanzer[62] examined 299 women at 28 to 32 weeks' gestation. At 28 weeks, the cervixes of 7% were dilated 2 to 3 cm at the internal os, and by 32 weeks 32% were dilated to this extent. Premature births occurred in 6.1% of the dilated

group and 6.9% of those with closed cervixes, despite the fact that no treatment was provided those with dilated cervixes. More recently, Bouyer et al[8] reported a townwide, population-based study in which women were examined at each prenatal visit. Among nulliparous women, 3% had an "open cervix" (at least one fingertip at the internal os) at 25 to 28 weeks, as did 6.5% at 29 to 31 weeks and 9.6% at 32 to 34 weeks. For parous women, the corresponding figures were 5.6%, 13.3%, and 14%. This variable (open cervix) carried with it a relative risk for preterm birth of 4.6 at 25 to 28 weeks in nulliparas and 3 in parous women. However, no mention is made of incompetent cervix or cerclage in the paper, and the open cervix was generally treated with increased rest. Thus in this study one cannot distinguish between cervical dilation and incompetent cervix as a risk factor for preterm labor.

The ideal way to test the hypothesis that incompetent cervix is an entity that is appropriately treated by cerclage would be a randomized trial of the procedure in patients deemed to have the condition by virtue of the "classical history." Most published studies compare pregnancy outcome among women undergoing cerclage with past pregnancy performance. Such studies are bound to demonstrate an apparent benefit for the procedure, since studies of subsequent pregnancies among women with one[58] or two[4] consecutive midtrimester losses demonstrate term birth rates of approximately 70%, even without intervention. Thus, any procedure applied to a group of women with previous midtrimester losses would be expected to have a 70% success rate even if the procedure were no better than a placebo. This lesson should have been learned from studies on the use of progestational agents to prevent spontaneous abortion[28,65] and from the diethylstilbestrol (DES) tragedy. If incompetent cervix is a distinct entity, correctable by cerclage, one would expect that patients with this condition undergoing the procedure would demonstrate better reproductive performance than patients without the condition, whose previous losses were caused by preterm labor. In fact, Barford and Rosen[5] found just the opposite. Two randomized trials of cerclage have been published.[37,60] Because of ethical concerns about the use of an untreated control group, neither study focused on patients with a classical history or signs of incompetent cervix. Instead, both studies were of patients at high or moderate risk for preterm delivery. In neither study did cerclage afford any benefit, and in both studies there was increased morbidity among patients receiving cerclage. Because patients with classical histories were not the subjects of the above investigations, the only conclusion that can be drawn is that pregnancies of women at high risk of preterm labor who do not have such classic incompetent cervix histories do not benefit from cerclage. This finding is particularly important in light of published recommendations for "aggressive" prophylactic use of this procedure to prevent pregnancy wastage.[16] In 1988 a preliminary report was published by the MRC/RCOG Working Party on Cervical Cerclage.[49] At the time of publication 905 pregnant women without classical histories but whose obstetricians were uncertain whether to recommend cerclage had been randomly allocated; approximately half received cervical cerclage and half did not. Those treated with cerclage manifested a slightly but significantly lower likelihood of delivery before 33 weeks than did the untreated pregnancies (13% versus 18%, p = 0.03) and a similar decrease in the likelihood of delivering a baby weighing less than 1500 grams (11% versus 16%). Because the difference was so small, the trial is continuing.

An understanding of the pathophysiology of incompetent cervix should form the basis for approaches to diagnosis and intervention strategies. The cervix is primarily composed of fibrous and connective tissue, with a small amount of smooth muscle. The smooth muscle is more abundant at the upper portion of the cervix, as the isthmus is approached. As the second trimester begins, the isthmus starts to unfold and the functional internal os moves downward. Before this time the uterus and cervix grow ahead of the enlarging conceptus, and the cervix is apparently not responsible for retaining the pregnancy.[17] Thus incompetent cervix is not believed to be responsible for pregnancy loss before 14 to 16 weeks' gestation. An understanding of the genesis of the incompetent cervix may well have to wait for elucidation of the biochemical changes that occur in the cervix during pregnancy, particularly as term approaches, a process usually referred to as "ripening." This poorly understood process, which transforms the cervix from a firm, unyielding structure to a buttery soft, easily negotiated portal for fetal egress, is almost certainly mediated by the hormonal changes of pregnancy. Possible candidates for this role include estrogens, prostaglandins, and relaxin. Another promising area of investigation is the chemical composition of the cervix. Leppert et al[40] have demonstrated decreased elastin content in cervical biopsies of women with classical incompetent cervix compared to normal pregnant and nonpregnant control women. Rech-

berger, Uldbjerg, and Oxlurd[59] found evidence of increased collagen turnover in cervical biopsies from presumed incompetent cervices compared to normal controls. Kiwi et al,[36] using a cervical balloon, found the "elastance" of the cervixes of nonpregnant women with clinical histories of incompetent cervix to be significantly lower than that of normal controls. Clinical applicability of this elastance test is not yet clear.

Studies of incompetent cervix are made difficult by the likelihood that both congenital and acquired forms exist. Trauma to the cervix, as may occur from forceful dilation, cone biopsy, or obstetric laceration, may be associated with this condition. There is also evidence that DES exposure in utero may lead to congenital predisposition toward this problem. Whether multiple causes may lead to a common problem, such as loss of elastin content in the cervix, remains to be established.

INDICATIONS FOR CERCLAGE

Despite the relatively nihilistic view of incompetent cervix that emerges from a review of the scientific literature, it remains true that cerclage is commonly performed in patients suspected of having this abnormality. The clinician must decide, on an individual basis, when to place a cerclage. Some guidelines may be useful in making such a decision. What follows is based upon my approach to this clinical problem, with reference to the pertinent literature where data are available.

The patient whose most recent previous pregnancy ended in painless dilation of the cervix, culminating in relatively painless and rapid labor in the midtrimester, presents little problem in decision making. Most clinicians would place a cerclage in the cervix of such a patient. It was previously the practice to wait until the first trimester had passed in order to lessen the chance of an operative procedure being followed by a spontaneous first trimester abortion unrelated to incompetent cervix. However, the identification of fetal heart motion by ultrasound allows earlier intervention, if desired, since the odds of miscarriage decrease markedly once fetal viability is documented.

The patient with a previous midtrimester or early third trimester delivery but without a classic history presents more of a problem. In patients at an advanced state of cervical dilation but with painful contractions during the midtrimester, there always remains the possibility that silent cervical dilation went undetected and that cervical stretching ultimately caused uterine contractions. Thus the typical clues to incompetent cervix may have been missed. Similarly, patients with preterm premature rupture of membranes and a dilated cervix may have experienced this problem because of cervical dilation, with exposure of the membranes to mechanical and bacteriologic stimuli leading to disruption of membrane integrity. Finally, it seems possible that preterm labor and delivery leading to forceful dilation of a cervix that may be "unripe" could cause cervical trauma. Thus, at least theoretically, such patients may be at risk for subsequent pregnancy loss related to incompetent cervix. The data cited in the first section of this chapter lend no support to the concept of "prophylactic" cervical cerclage in such cases. A reasonable approach, then, is to consider such pregnancies at risk for incompetent cervix. McDonald's early description of incompetent cervix[46] cited symptoms of vaginal discharge, lower abdominal discomfort, or the sensation of a lump in the vagina. Such complaints should always prompt a vaginal examination in a patient believed to be at risk. Cervical examinations performed at weekly intervals may allow the placement of a cerclage in a timely fashion once cervical softening and dilation, or effacement combined with palpable thinning of the lower uterine segment, occur. This approach leaves open the possibility that cervical change may occur and precipitate labor and delivery during the interval between examinations. On the other hand, the placement of a cerclage without clear-cut indications entails definite risk without definite benefit. Risks include those inherent in anesthesia, whether general or conduction. In addition, maternal sepsis[32] and even death[22] have been reported. Other risks include preterm labor, rupture of membranes, cervical injury, and cervical stenosis.[1]

As ultrasound equipment has advanced, yielding better and better resolution, there has been increasing interest in the use of this modality to visualize the lower uterine segment and internal cervical os, structures that are relatively inaccessible to the examining finger. Sarti et al[61] described a case of already diagnosed incompetent cervix, in which cerclage had been performed, in which ultrasound demonstrated a distended upper cervix that appeared closed when the urinary bladder was filled. Brook et al[10] reported that the internal os was significantly wider among patients scheduled for cerclage (2.57 ± .36 cm) than in normal controls (1.67 ± .23 cm). A number of subsequent investigators have reported ultrasonic evidence of incompetent cervix, including prolapse of the membranes into the upper portion of the cervix[70] and shortening of the cervix and a dilated endocervical canal.[34] Mahran[45] suggested that an internal os diameter of 15 mm or more during the first trimester or 20 mm or more during the second trimester was diagnostic for incompetent cervix. Varma, Patel, and Pillai[71] found that a "short cervix" (less than 2.5 cm) was not a particularly bad sign so long as the cervical canal was closed (less than 5 mm in width) and the width of the entire cervix at the level of the internal os was less than 3 cm. A canal width greater than 7 mm with herniation of the amniotic membrane containing fetal parts was considered an ominous sign. Measurement of cervical canal width was felt to be the most useful predictor of incompetent cervix. It seems eminently reasonable that ultrasound would be useful in making the diagnosis of incompetent cervix in individuals without a classic history, and this approach is gaining popularity. However, it must be borne in mind that no series has reported the function of this diagnostic tool in a blinded fashion. Ultrasonographic diagnosis of incompetent cervix leading to cerclage becomes a

self-fulfilling prophecy, and data are not available on the fate of such patients if left untreated. Furthermore, at least one case has been reported of an ultrasonographic examination showing a somewhat short but closed cervix followed by a vaginal exam 20 minutes later revealing 4 to 5 cm dilation.[74] Thus, not all cases of incompetent cervix can be detected with ultrasonography. Brown et al[11] published preliminary data suggesting that vaginal sonography may have advantages compared to more traditional transabdominal sonography with respect to cervical evaluation.

The indications for cerclage thus far described have been based upon previous pregnancy performance; the recommendation has been placement of a suture when the history is classic, and close observation in other cases. Digital and sonographic examinations may be helpful in determining which of the latter group of patients require intervention. However, another group of patients considered for cerclage by many clinicians includes women who have not experienced a reproductive loss as yet but whose histories contain certain risk factors believed to be associated with cervical incompetence. Whether cerclage should be performed prophylactically, to minimize the likelihood that cervical dilation will advance between examinations so as to preclude treatment, is controversial. Risk factors that have been cited in the literature include DES exposure in utero, previous cone biopsy of the cervix, previous voluntary interruption(s) of pregnancy, structural uterine abnormalities, placenta previa, and multiple gestation.

Exposure to DES in utero has been associated with reproductive wastage, particularly prematurity and midtrimester loss,[15] but not specifically with incompetent cervix except in the form of case reports or series.[26,68] In one recent case-control study,[69] DES-exposed gravidas were significantly more likely to have a cerclage than normal controls, but the diagnosis of incompetent cervix was not always clear. In a prospective but nonrandomized study, Ludmir et al[43] followed 63 DES-exposed patients using a standard protocol. Cerclage was placed prophylactically in 26 who had a previous midtrimester loss or hypoplastic cervix on examination. The other 37 patients were managed expectantly. Of the latter, 16 (44%) underwent emergency cerclage because of cervical change. All of the 5 perinatal deaths occurred in the 21 patients who received neither an elective nor an emergency cerclage. These patients also delivered significantly earlier than those who received cerclage. The authors concluded that strong consideration should be given to early cerclage placement in DES-exposed gravidas. Because of the nonrandomized nature of the study, confirming data would be helpful; none have been reported as yet.

A history of cervical cone biopsy is often considered a risk factor for cervical incompetence. It stands to reason that removal of a large portion of the cervix may weaken the structure, particularly if the internal cervical os is included in the biopsy. However, determination of the amount of risk associated with a particular individual's biopsy remains problematic. Lee[38] noted that 14% of 106 pregnancies following cone biopsy ended in midtrimester abortions or premature births. In a 1979 literature review, Weber and Obel[72] noted that when all series including 25 or more patients were combined, 7% of 577 pregnancies eventuated in premature delivery, with only 2 patients receiving cerclage. Because the various studies considered included patients with differing depths and widths of cone biopsy, it is still impossible to conclude that cone biopsy carries no risk for incompetent cervix. Leiman, Harrison, and Rubin[39] reviewed 88 pregnancies occurring after cone biopsy, dividing the cone biopsy procedures into large (maximum cone height more than 2 cm and/or cone volume more than 4 cc) and small cones. Large cones (by height) were performed in 23 patients and small cones in 65. Patients having large cones experienced a 52% rate of second trimester abortion or preterm delivery, while those with small cones experienced a 21% rate of these complications. Tests of statistical significance were not applied in this paper. Buller and Jones[12] found no effect of cone biopsy on second trimester abortion or prematurity rates, using the patients' pregnancy performance before conization as their own controls. Moinian and Andersch,[48] on the other hand, reported a seven-fold increase in second trimester abortion after conization, with 19% of patients ultimately receiving cerclage. The latter two studies did not report on the extent of the cone biopsy procedures, and this may be the critical issue. It appears most reasonable that patients with a previous cone biopsy and no intervening term pregnancies be managed expectantly with weekly or biweekly cervical examinations after the 16th week of pregnancy. Goldberg, Altaras, and Bloch[25] recently reported a procedure for combining cone biopsy during pregnancy with cervical cerclage.

It seems logical that cervical trauma caused by induced abortion might predispose to incompetent cervix in subsequent pregnancies. Bracken[9] reviewed the world's literature pertaining to perinatal complications in pregnancies subsequent to induced abortion. While some studies showed increased rates of second trimester spontaneous abortion compared to control pregnancies, others did not. No conclusion could be reached, although the authors suggested that abortion by dilation and curettage (D and C) may carry a higher risk for subsequent pregnancy loss than abortion by suction aspiration. Harlap et al[31] found a relative risk of 3.27 for midtrimester losses among nulliparous women who had induced abortion by D and C, a risk that disappeared after cervical dilation with laminaria was introduced. Levin et al[41] found a significantly increased likelihood (relative risk 4.7) of two or more previous induced abortions among women with pregnancy loss between 20 and 27 weeks compared to women with term pregnancies but no increased likelihood of having had only one previous induced abortion. In the latter series the method of abortion or degree of cervical dilation could not explain the subsequent losses. In another group of women, the same authors[63] confirmed no apparent increase in risk with one previous induced abortion. Unfortunately, none of the available studies addressed the issue of incompetent cervix. We are thus left with the possibility that multiple induced abortions may increase the risk of subsequent midtrimester pregnancy loss, and we can speculate that some of these losses might possibly be related to incompetent cervix. Clearly there is inadequate evidence to support prophylactic cerclage in such patients. Whether women with two or more previous induced abortions require frequent cervical exams remains to be elucidated.

Abramovici, Faktor, and Pascal[2] reported on 15 women with congenital uterine anomalies and previous reproductive losses who were treated with cerclage despite the absence of clinical or radiologic evidence of incompetent cervix. All of the patients delivered surviving infants, 13 of them at term. The authors concluded that the reproductive outcomes were so much better than in previous pregnancies that cerclage should be performed in such patients before surgical correction of the anomalies is attempted. Unfortunately, no control group was available for comparison, so we do not know how these 15 women would have done without the surgery. Cerclage cannot be recommended for such patients at the present time.

Arias[3] performed a randomized trial of McDonald cerclage in 25 patients with bleeding at 24 to 30 weeks and sonographic evidence of placenta previa. The 13 patients treated with cerclage had later deliveries (35 versus 32 weeks), larger birth weight (2709 versus 1812 g), and fewer neonatal complications than did the 12 patients not receiving a cerclage. Patients receiving cerclage also spent less time in hospital. While Arias concluded that his results support the use of cervical cerclage in patients with placenta previa, no confirmatory data have yet become available.

Multiple gestation represents a clinical situation in which preterm birth is an ever present risk. Although incompetent cervix has not been shown to occur with increased frequency in such pregnancies, it is not surprising that cerclage has been applied as a possible means of preventing prematurity. Zakut, Insler, and Serr[76] performed cerclage at 12 to 15 weeks' gestation on 20 women with multiple pregnancies induced by gonadotropin therapy. The pregnancy outcomes were compared with those of 20 other women with similar gonadotropin-induced multiple gestations, not treated with cerclage. Pregnancies treated with cerclage resulted in significantly more surviving offspring and significantly longer duration of gestation. Admirably, because therapy was not randomly allocated in the latter study, some of the same authors[19] later carried out a randomized trial of cerclage in 50 ovulation-induced twin pregnancies. The perinatal outcomes were remarkably similar, with 45% of sutured and 48% of nonsutured pregnancies ending in premature delivery and 18% and 15%, respectively, ending in neonatal death. These studies point out the tremendous importance of using appropriate control groups when studying clinical interventions. A recent study[18] found no difference in outcomes between twin pregnancies treated with cerclage and those treated with bedrest. Cerclage was associated with a significantly increased incidence of premature rupture of membranes, but perinatal outcomes were otherwise similar. The authors concluded that cerclage offered an improved quality of life over bedrest, but another conclusion would be that since the efficacy of bedrest in twin gestation remains unproven, neither therapy is superior. Currently available evidence does not support the routine use of cerclage to prevent prematurity in multiple gestations.

Contraindications to cerclage include active labor, active uterine bleeding, rupture of membranes, intra-amniotic infection, and the known presence of major congenital anomalies incompatible with life. The use of bedrest and/or vaginal pessaries has been advocated as an alternative to cerclage but has not gained widespread popularity.

In summary, then, cerclage appears to be an appropriate intervention when the history for incompetent cervix is classic (i.e., a previous pregnancy culminating in delivery during the second or early third trimester, in which painless cervical dilation was followed by relatively painless labor). Other situations, such as DES exposure, previous second or early third trimester birth without a classic history, multiple previous pregnancy terminations, or multiple gestations, merit frequent cervical examinations and perhaps ultrasound examinations, with cerclage reserved for those patients demonstrating cervical change.

PROCEDURES

The choice of one cerclage procedure over another has no clear scientific foundation. At present no randomized "head-to-head" comparison studies have been carried out. Outcomes of the two most common procedures, the Shirodkar and McDonald, appeared to be similar in one retrospective review of 251 cerclage operations.[30] Therefore, in this section I will describe the commonly performed procedures and recount the apparent advantages and disadvantages of each.

Shirodkar procedure

As originally described by Shirodkar,[66] this operation was performed as follows:

1. A strip of fascia lata ¼ inch wide and 4½ inches long, is removed from the outer side of the thigh, and each end of this strip is transfixed with a linen suture.
2. The cervix is pulled down, a transverse incision is made above the cervix as in anterior colporrhaphy, and the bladder is pushed well up above the internal os.
3. The cervix is then pulled forward, toward the symphysis pubis, and a vertical incision is made in the posterior vaginal wall, again at and above the internal os, going *only* through the vaginal wall.
4. Through the right and left corner of the anterior incision an aneurysm needle is passed between the cervix and the vaginal wall until its eye comes out of the posterior incision.
5. The linen attached to each end of the fascia is passed through the eye of the aneurysm needle, and the right end

of the fascia is pulled retrovaginally forward into the anterior incision. The same thing is done from the left side.
6. The two ends of the strip cross each other in front of the cervix and are tightened to close the internal os. The operator's left index finger in the internal os will indicate how much to pull on the strips. The assistant should be holding one end of the strip with an artery forceps.
7. The two ends are stitched together by a number of stitches that take a bite of the muscle fibers of the lowest part of the lower uterine segment, using a small curved needle and fine linen.
8. Extra portions of the fascia are cut out, and the anterior and posterior incisions are closed with chromic catgut No. 0.

Later refinements by Shirodkar[67] included switching from fascia lata to no. 2 Dacron suture and tying the suture posteriorly.

A number of other modifications to Shirodkar's original operation have been suggested. Fascia has been replaced by newer synthetic materials, most often a Mersilene band 5 mm in width or no. 2 Mersilene thread.[67] Druzin and Berkeley[20] suggested the use of a White tonsil forceps with medium curve to grasp the tissue between the anterior and posterior incisions and retract it laterally, allowing the use of an atraumatic Mayo needle swedged onto the Mersilene band (rather than the aneurysm needle previously recommended) to place the suture through the paracervical tissue on each side. Caspi et al[13] described a modification wherein a single transverse incision in the anterior fornix is used. A monofilament nylon suture 0.6 mm in diameter is passed on each side, under the mucosa at the level of the internal os, from the anterior incision to exit through the mucosa of the posterior cervix, and is then tied. The procedure was compared to the modified technique of Shirodkar[67] in a randomized fashion, the subjects being 90 patients with previous failed McDonald procedure or with cervical anatomy felt to be unfavorable for McDonald cerclage. Similar pregnancy outcomes were noted with the two procedures. The investigators believe that the newer modification has the advantages of simplicity, ease of removal, and lower incidence of severe vaginal discharge.

Advantages often cited for the Shirodkar procedure center around the fact that the anterior mucosal incision and reflection of the bladder upward allow the stitch to be placed high on the cervix, near the location of the internal os. In addition, most of the suture is buried under the mucosa. Disadvantages include occasional difficulty in removal of the suture at term, particularly if a Mersilene band is utilized. Although at one time many operators left the suture in place and performed cesarean section delivery, I favor removal of the stitch at term with vaginal delivery planned.

Following is a description of the Shirodkar procedure as I perform it:

1. Regional anesthesia is preferred, since patients

awakening from general anesthesia sometimes cough and retch, which may put particular strain on the cerclage and membranes. Nevertheless, either method of anesthesia is acceptable, and the choice should be made in a collaborative manner, with the patient, anesthesiologist, and obstetrician involved in the process.

2. The patient is placed in the lithotomy position in stirrups. Assuming that the procedure is being done prior to cervical dilation, the vagina is prepped with Betadine in the usual fashion. The bladder is not emptied unless it is overdistended; a semifilled bladder allows easier visualization of the cervicovesical reflection.

3. A long, weighted speculum is placed in the posterior vagina. The anterior and posterior lips of the cervix are grasped with ring forceps, or with tenacula if that is impossible. Care should be exercised not to lacerate the cervix if tenacula are used.

4. Because bleeding from the anterior mucosal incision may obscure the operator's view of the posterior cervix, the posterior mucosal incision is made first (Fig. 63-1). A 2-cm vertical incision is begun approximately 2.5 cm proximal to the external os and carried upward. The plane between the cervical mucosa and the cervical substance is entered using blunt dissection.

5. The cervicovesical reflection is identified by moving the cervix cephalad and caudad, allowing visualization of the slight ballooning of the bladder. The anterior mucosal incision, approximately 2 cm long, is made transversely at the reflection (Fig. 63-2). The appropriate tissue plane is identified by blunt dissection. The bladder is reflected superiorly bluntly, exposing the cervix as close to the level of the internal os as possible.

6. A large tonsil forceps with medium curve or a long curved Allis clamp is used to bring the mucosa and paracervical tissue laterally (Fig. 63-3, A and B). One blade of the clamp is inserted in the anterior incision and the other in the posterior incision on the left side of the cervix. As the clamp is closed, the tissues are drawn away from the substance of the cervix.

7. Although many obstetricians prefer a Mersilene strip, I have noted difficulty in the removal of such sutures once they have become scarred into the substance of the cervix. Therefore, I prefer to use a 0.6-mm monofilament nylon suture, swedged onto a medium-sized atraumatic curved needle. Because the suture will be tied posteriorly to prevent erosion of an anterior knot into the bladder, the first bite of tissue is taken from posterior to anterior (Fig. 63-

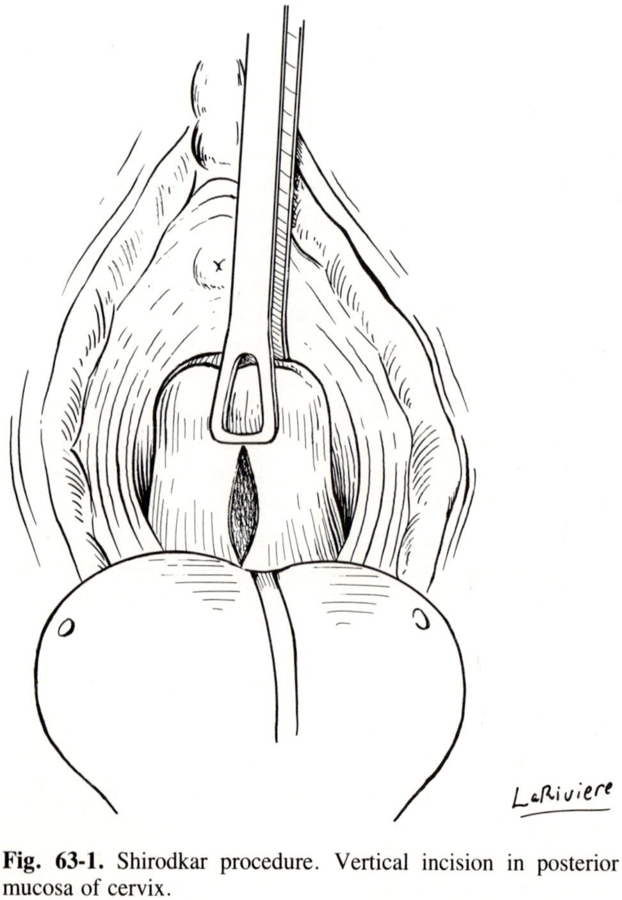

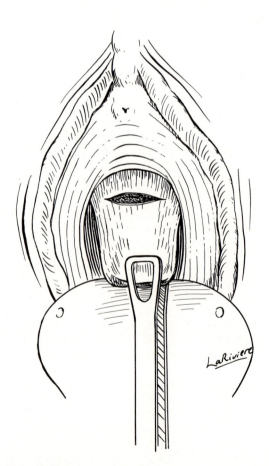

Fig. 63-1. Shirodkar procedure. Vertical incision in posterior mucosa of cervix.

Fig. 63-2. Shirodkar procedure. Transverse incision in anterior mucosa of cervix.

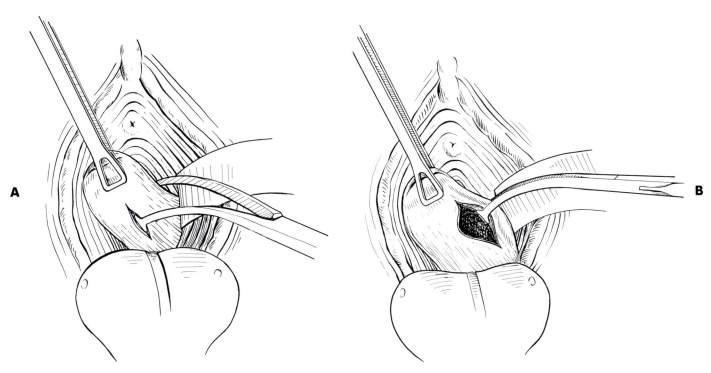

Fig. 63-3. Shirodkar procedure. long, curved Allis clamp encompassing tissue between anterior and posterior mucosal incisions on patient's left side. **A,** Jaws of clamp are open. **B,** Jaws of clamp have been closed, drawing paracervical tissues laterally.

4). The needle is grasped at about its midpoint in a long, preferably curved, needleholder. The needle tip is placed just beyond the tip of the clamp holding the paracervical tissue, with the needle's curvature going in a direction opposite to the curvature of the cervix. This orientation helps to avoid the needle tip's "wandering" into the endocervical canal. The needle is driven directly upward through the paracervical tissue, emerging in the anterior mucosal incision.

8. The above process is repeated on the right side of the cervix, except that the needle is driven from anterior to posterior, emerging in the posterior mucosal incision (Fig. 63-5).

9. The nylon suture is then anchored to the anterior cervical substance at the level of the internal os. Although a permanent silk suture is preferred by many for this step, I believe it is better to use an absorbable suture to avoid leaving a foreign body in the area after the pregnancy has been completed. Therefore, no. 0 chromic or no. 00 polyglycolic acid (or some similar substance) is used for this purpose (Fig. 63-6). It is assumed that by the time the absorbable suture has deteriorated, the nylon suture will have scarred in so that slippage will be unlikely.

10. The cerclage should now be tied. The assistant should insert a fingertip into the endocervical canal

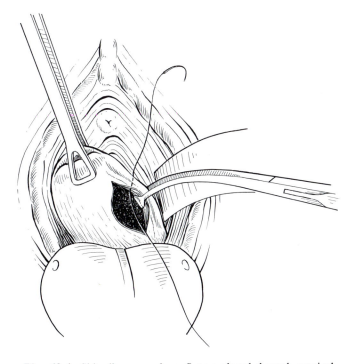

Fig. 63-4. Shirodkar procedure. Suture placed through cervical tissue on patient's left side, with needle inserted from posterior to anterior.

Fig. 63-5. Shirodkar procedure. Suture placed through cervical tissue on patient's right side, with needle inserted from anterior to posterior.

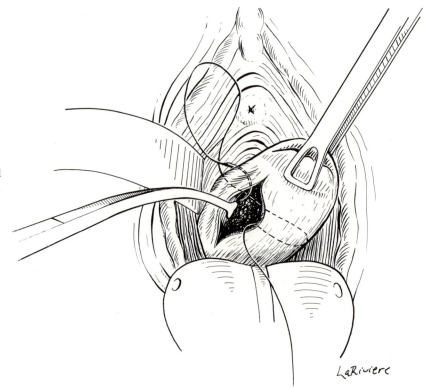

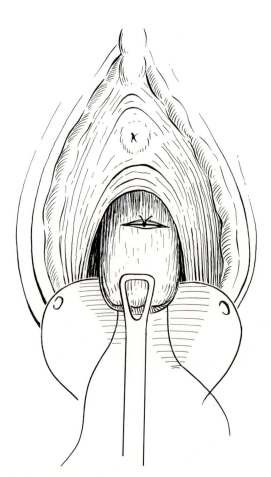

Fig. 63-6. Shirodkar procedure. Absorbable suture used to anchor cerclage stitch to cervical substance under anterior mucosal incision.

to the level of the internal os. A surgeon's knot is then tied, and the knot is snugged down as the assistant slowly withdraws the fingertip. The internal os should be very slightly open once the procedure is completed. Four or five more throws are taken in the knot. The long ends of the suture are then held in a small mosquito forceps.

11. The edges of the anterior mucosal incision are then approximated using a running, locking no. 00 chromic suture for hemostasis (Fig. 63-7).

12. The edges of the posterior incision can be approximated using interrupted no. 00 chromic sutures on each side of the emerging cerclage stitch.

13. The cerclage suture ends are then trimmed but left approximately 3 cm long (Fig. 63-8) to allow easy identification and manipulation when it is time to remove the suture.

14. The patient should be warned of the likelihood that pieces of absorbable suture material may be discharged from the vagina in 1 to 2 weeks after the procedure, and that these do not represent the cerclage coming out.

15. Once the patient is fully recovered from anesthesia she may be kept in the hospital for overnight observation of possible uterine activity and discharged the next morning.

Perioperative antibiotics and/or tocolysis are not employed routinely in my center when Shirodkar cerclage is performed prior to cervical effacement and/or dilation. Although Novy, Ducsay, and Stanczyk[54] identified increases

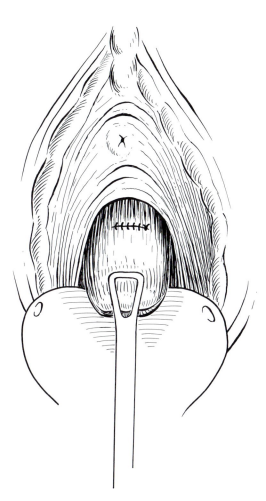

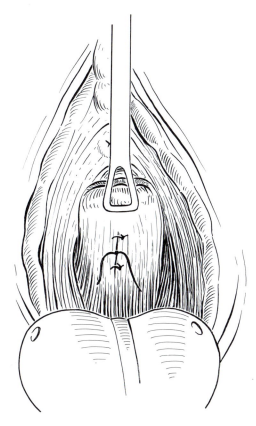

Fig. 63-8. Shirodkar procedure. Posterior view of completed cerclage.

Fig. 63-7. Shirodkar procedure. Anterior mucosal incision closed with running absorbable suture, burying cerclage stitch.

in circulating prostaglandin metabolite levels immediately after vaginal and abdominal cerclage procedures, these were generally transient and returned to baseline levels within 6 to 8 hours of the procedure. They were not associated with adverse outcomes unless the cervix was in an advanced state of dilation and effacement, the uterus was already irritable, or the membranes prolapsed or ruptured. The authors concluded that routine tocolysis was not indicated after nonemergency cerclage.

McDonald procedure

As originally described by McDonald,[46] who reported on 70 cases performed at an advanced state of dilation with a 43% success rate (surviving babies), this procedure was performed in the following manner:

The bladder having been emptied, the cervix is exposed and grasped at each quadrant by Allis' or Babcock forceps. If necessary the bulging bag of membranes is reduced by one or two dampened swabs held on sponge forceps. . . . A purse-string suture of no. 4 Mersilk on a Mayo needle is inserted around the exo-cervix as high as possible to approximate to the level of the internal os. This is at the junction of the rugose vagina and

smooth cervix. Five or six bites with the needle are made, with special attention to the stitches behind the cervix. These are difficult to insert and must be deep. If the ligature pulls out later, it is always from this portion, the silk remaining attached to the anterior lip. The stitch is pulled tight enough to close the internal os, the knot being made in front of the cervix and the ends left long enough to facilitate subsequent division.

McDonald[47] later reported an 80% success rate with his subsequent 25 procedures, an improvement that he attributed to prophylactic suturing at 14 weeks' gestation. He also switched from silk suture to no. 4 braided Mersilene suture material.

Advantages of the McDonald procedure may include its relative simplicity and bloodlessness (compared to the Shirodkar cerclage). Mucosal incisions are not required. Although some authorities recommend the Shirodkar procedure when the cervix is markedly effaced, I have found the McDonald procedure more practical under these difficult circumstances. Occasionally it is helpful to place a second McDonald suture above or below the first after the initial cerclage has initiated the reconstitution of the cervix. Disadvantages of the McDonald procedure include the fact that generally it is not placed as high on the cervix, and it is not anchored as well into the cervical substance as is the Shirodkar. Therefore, it may be more likely to pull through or slip (although controlled studies addressing this issue have not been reported).

Following is a description of the McDonald operation as I perform it:

1. Regional anesthesia is preferred, since patients awakening from general anesthesia sometimes cough and retch, which may put particular strain on the cerclage and membranes. Nevertheless, either method of anesthesia is acceptable, and the choice should be made in a collaborative manner, with the patient, anesthesiologist, and obstetrician involved in the process.

2. The patient is placed in the lithotomy position in stirrups. Assuming that the procedure is being done prior to cervical dilation, the vagina is prepped with Betadine in the usual fashion. If the cervix is already dilated the prep is applied to the vulva but not into the vaginal cavity itself.

3. A long, weighted speculum is placed in the posterior vagina. The anterior and posterior lips of the cervix are grasped with ring forceps, or with tenacula if that is impossible. Care should be exercised not to lacerate the cervix if tenacula are used.

4. A 0.6-mm monofilament nylon suture, swedged to a medium-sized curved atraumatic needle, is grasped at its midportion with a long, curved needleholder. The curvature of the needle is oriented opposite the curvature of the cervix. The first bite of tissue is taken as high on the cervix as possible by entering the needle into the submucosa of the posterior cervix at approximately the 6 o'clock position and bringing it out at approximately the 4 o'clock position (Fig. 63-9). The needle is reinserted into the cervical mucosa at the 2 o'clock position and emerges at the 12:30 position. It is reinserted at the 11:30 position and reemerges at the 10 o'clock position. It is finally reinserted at the 8 o'clock position and reemerges at the 6 o'clock position. Care must be taken to obtain adequate purchase of the cervical connective tissue but not to bury the needle too deeply in the cervix lest the endocervical canal be traversed. Such a "transcervical" suture might lead to sawing through of the membranes and is also bound to be less effective than the usual cerclage.

5. Once the needle has been removed from the end of the suture, the purse string can be drawn closed. First, a finger should be inserted into the endocervical canal to ascertain that the suture has not violated this space. Then the operator places a surgeon's knot into the stitch and cinches it down on the posterior aspect of the cervix (Fig. 63-10) as the assistant's finger is slowly withdrawn from the canal. A slight opening should remain at the internal os. Four or five more throws are placed into the knot, and the ends are trimmed to about 2 to 3 cm in length to allow easy identification and manipulation at the time removal is planned.

Abdominal cerclage

Some patients manifest severe cervical injuries, and others have apparent congenital absence of the portio vaginalis of the cervix, rendering Shirodkar or McDonald cerclage technically difficult or impossible. Benson and Durfee[7] described an abdominal approach to cerclage, a procedure that was applied to congenitally short or surgically amputated cervixes and those with marked scarring, deep notching, multiple defects, or penetrating lacerations of the fornixes. Novy[51] has popularized this procedure and added the indications of "wide or extensive cervical conization, cervico-vaginal fistulas following abortion, or a previously failed vaginal approach to cervical cerclage." In addition, Novy suggested using this procedure in pregnant patients with cervical effacement that precluded high placement of a vaginal cerclage. Although his first report described only 4 cases, Novy[52] later reported on 16 patients treated with transabdominal cerclage during a 14-year interval, including 22 pregnancies, 21 of which resulted in living children. Indications for the procedure in these patients included marked scarring after failed vaginal cerclage (N = 6), abnormally short or amputated cervix (N = 5), deep forniceal lacerations (N = 3), and marked cervical effacement with dilation less than 4 cm and intact membranes (N = 3). The last 3 patients are of great interest because the procedures were performed at 22 to 26 weeks and all 3 went to term. Mahran[44] reported 10 cases

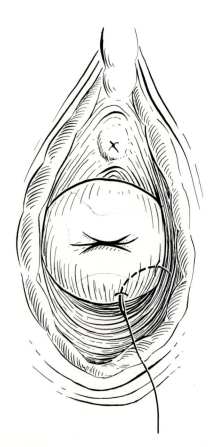

Fig. 63-9. McDonald procedure. First bite of cervical substance is taken from 6 o'clock to 4 o'clock position.

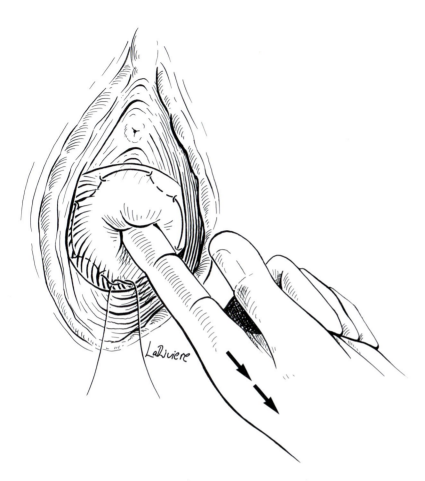

Fig. 63-10. McDonald procedure. Purse-string placement has been completed. The knot is tied posteriorly and snugged down as assistant withdraws finger from cervical canal.

of abdominal cerclage placed for very short or absent cervix with poor reproductive history, 7 of which resulted in perinatal survival. More recently, Herron and Parer[33] reported 9 abdominal cerclage procedures on 8 patients who had failed vaginal cerclage with deep traumatic defects (N = 6) or extremely short cervix (N = 2) and previous fetal salvage rate of only 5 of 25 pregnancies going beyond the first trimester. After cerclage, 13 pregnancies resulted in 11 births at 36 weeks or more and 2 fetal losses. Recently Novy[53] reported the results of an additional 20 abdominal cerclage procedures performed since 1982. The perinatal survival rate was 90%. Over the past 12 years, I have performed 10 abdominal cerclage procedures with 12 pregnancies, 11 of which resulted in surviving children. Indications for such a procedure are exceedingly rare; Novy[52] noted that in his center there was 1 abdominal cerclage for every 6 vaginal cerclage procedures, and it should be noted that his center presumably receives referrals specifically for this procedure. My own guidelines for patient selection include the following:

1. Previous failed vaginal cerclage with scarring or lacerations rendering vaginal cerclage technically very difficult
2. Absent or very hypoplastic cervix with history of pregnancy loss fitting classical description of incompetent cervix

Specifically, I have not placed an abdominal cerclage in a patient with a scarred or apparently absent cervix who has not had a previous typical pregnancy loss. A high proportion of such patients go through pregnancy successfully because, although the portio vaginalis of the cervix is apparently lacking, the internal os is presumably intact. Whether such patients can be diagnosed by ultrasound before their first pregnancy loss cannot be answered without controlled studies. Some have advocated this procedure when there is severe cervicitis, but this is controversial.

Advantages to abdominal cerclage include the obvious fact that it is performed in patients who cannot be treated successfully with vaginal cerclage. Clearly the cerclage can be placed higher on the cervix, at the level of the internal os, with the abdominal approach. Theoretically there should be a lower risk of infection since the procedure is done through the peritoneal cavity, a clean operative field. The main disadvantage of abdominal cerclage, and it is an important problem, is that the patient must undergo two laparotomies since most authors advocate delivery by cesarean section. An even greater problem is the pregnancy that eventuates in fetal death or preterm labor prior to viability after abdominal cerclage; here a laparotomy is usually necessary even though no living child will result. Novy[53] has reported 2 cases in which spontaneous abortions at 13 and 14 weeks were treated with D & E, with abdominal cerclage sutures left in place. Infection, hemorrhage, injury to intrabdominal structures, and disfigurement from the abdominal incision are all potential complications. Thus the procedure must be reserved for highly selected cases.

Following is my approach to abdominal cerclage, which is based upon Novy's descriptions[51-53]:

1. The procedure is planned for the end of the first trimester or the early second trimester, after fetal viability has been documented. It is important to wait until the highest risk of spontaneous first trimester abortion has passed, so that the necessary laparotomy is unlikely to be followed immediately by a second laparotomy.

2. An indwelling catheter is placed in the bladder. Although conduction anesthesia is my preference because of the decreased likelihood of postoperative retching, general anesthesia is also commonly employed. Both Pfannenstiel and vertical abdominal incisions have been advocated. Because of my experience with what seemed to be the excessive manipulation necessary to bring the gravid uterus up and into a Pfannenstiel incision in 2 cases, I strongly favor the vertical abdominal incision.

3. Once the peritoneal cavity is opened the bladder flap is incised transversely for approximately 5 cm at its reflection on the uterus, just above the level of the internal cervical os (Fig. 63-11). The bladder flap is advanced downward bluntly for only about 5 cm.

4. The uterine fundus is wrapped in a laparotomy pad moistened with warm saline, and the uterus is brought up into the abdominal incision, putting the cervix on some degree of traction. The uterine artery on one side of the cervix is palpated and then visualized, splitting into ascending and descending branches (Fig. 63-12). The relatively avascular space lateral to the cervix but medial to the branches of the uterine artery is identified. This space is then enlarged by the assistant, using lateral traction on the uterine vessels.

5. A 5-mm Mersilene tape swedged onto a needle is then placed through the avascular space from anterior to posterior.

6. If bleeding is encountered at this point, it is usually controlled by gentle pressure. On one occasion I found it necessary to use hemostatic clips for this purpose.

7. The same process is repeated on the other side of the uterus except that the needle carrying the Mersilene tape is now passed from posterior to anterior so that

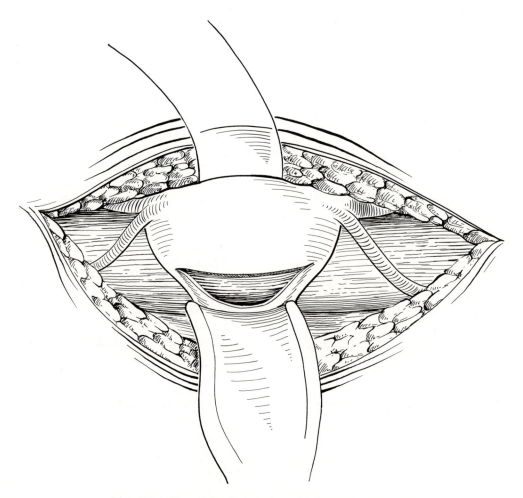

Fig. 63-11. Transabdominal cerclage: Bladder flap is created.

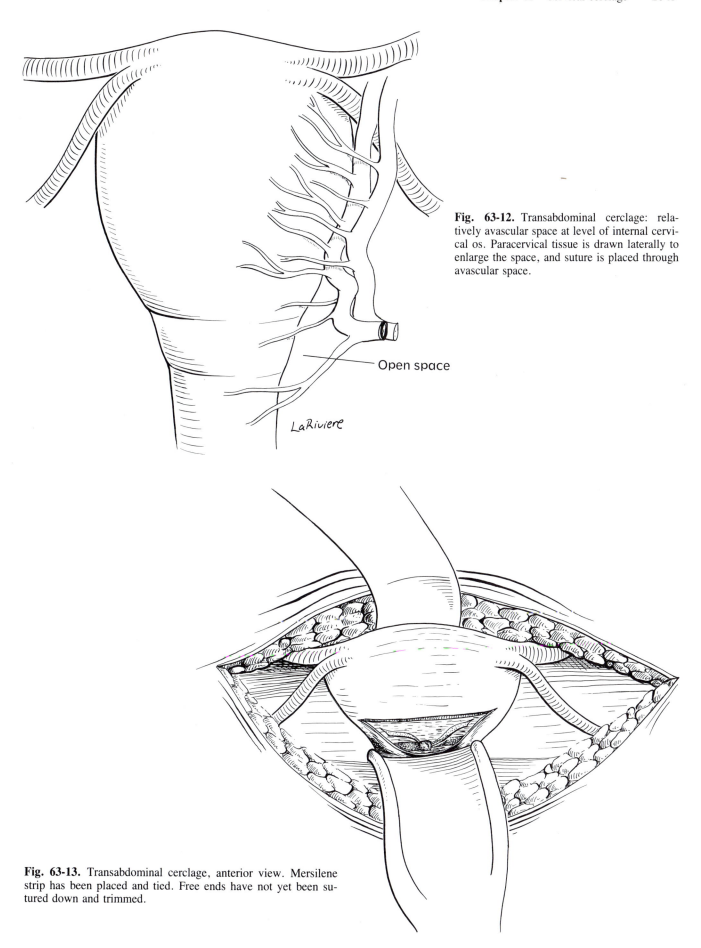

Fig. 63-12. Transabdominal cerclage: relatively avascular space at level of internal cervical os. Paracervical tissue is drawn laterally to enlarge the space, and suture is placed through avascular space.

Open space

LaRiviere

Fig. 63-13. Transabdominal cerclage, anterior view. Mersilene strip has been placed and tied. Free ends have not yet been sutured down and trimmed.

the knot can be placed anteriorly (Fig. 63-13). Although a posterior knot might enable the removal of the cerclage through a posterior colpotomy, the manipulations necessary to tie and secure the knot are much more difficult when attempted posterior to the gravid uterus.

8. Care must be taken to insure that the Mersilene tape is flat all the way around and not twisted. A square knot is placed anterior to the internal os, compressing the cervical tissue but not too tightly. The free ends of the tape are secured to the band by no. 3-0 silk sutures placed approximately 1 to 2 cm distal to the knot. The remaining free ends are then cut away (Fig. 63-14). The posterior portion of the band passes around the isthmus of the uterus at about the level of insertion of the uterosacral ligaments and is easily palpable and visible from behind as the uterus is drawn into the incision. Later it will become encased in scar tissue.

9. The bladder flap, peritoneal cavity, and abdominal incision are closed routinely.

Emergency cerclage

All three of the above procedures for cervical incompetence are best performed prior to cervical dilation and effacement. However, as noted in the section on indications, many patients do not have the classic history that indicates prophylactic cerclage in the late first or early second trimester. Such patients are managed expectantly, with cerclage reserved for those who manifest cervical change demonstrated clinically or by ultrasound. Therefore many cerclage procedures are performed emergently rather than prophylactically. At least two studies have reported a lower success rate (50% and 59%) with emergent cerclage than with prophylactic cerclage (86% and 81%), although in neither was the number of cases sufficient to reach statistical significance.[27,30] If emergent cerclage procedures truly have a lower success rate, the supposition is that the cervical incompetence advanced too far before intervention. However, an alternative explanation would be that some prophylactic procedures are done in patients who do not need them, and are thus bound to have favorable outcomes.

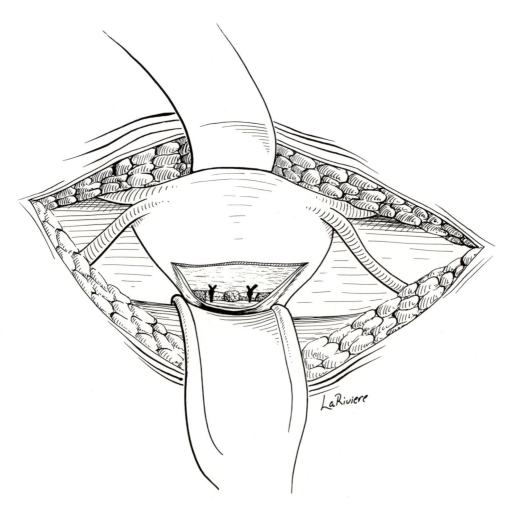

Fig. 63-14. Transabdominal cerclage, anterior view, just before closure of bladder flap and completion of procedure.

The most important step in performing emergency cerclage is making the diagnosis. Other causes of premature cervical dilation must be ruled out, specifically preterm labor. Thus external monitoring of uterine contractions should be performed. If regular uterine contractions are present, tocolysis should be considered. Abruptio placentae should be part of the differential diagnosis and is considered a relative contraindication to tocolysis and probably an absolute contraindication to cerclage. In the absence of evidence of abruption, tocolysis can be initiated. Only if uterine contractions can be successfully inhibited, and the clinician is convinced that preterm labor was the *result* of cervical dilation rather than the cause of it, should emergency cerclage be considered. Steps should be taken to rule out chorioamnionitis if contractions are present. Even in the absence of contractions, cervical cultures should be obtained to rule out specific organisms such as group B streptococci, although the cerclage procedure need not be delayed pending results.

The choice of procedure for emergency cerclage is not universally agreed upon. While the Shirodkar procedure unquestionably gains access to "higher territory," closer to the internal os, it may be particularly difficult to carry out successfully in a markedly effaced and dilated cervix. Novy[52] advocates the abdominal procedure in such cases. In our experience, the McDonald procedure has worked well, although we have not attempted an abdominal cerclage under conditions of cervical dilation and effacement. Schulman and Farmakides[64] recommend a modification of the McDonald procedure for patients with failed cerclage needing reoperation. Prolene suture, no. 0, is used, and multiple small bites are taken. Two circumferential sutures are placed and tied anteriorly. No comparative results are available.

Cerclage is clearly contraindicated in the presence of ruptured membranes. However, a number of investigators have published descriptions of approaches to the dilated cervix with bulging, unruptured membranes. In his original description of the procedure, McDonald[46] suggested using a moistened swab on a sponge forceps to reduce the bulging membranes. Goodlin[29] suggested transabdominal amniocentesis to reduce the tension in the amniotic cavity and allow retraction of "hourglassing" membranes. We have used this approach on occasion, with limited success. Olátunbosun and Dyck[55] recommended the placement of such patients in steep Trendelenberg position under general anesthesia and the use of 6 to 10 cervical stay sutures of no. 00 silk, then using traction on these sutures to cause the membranes to fall back into the uterine cavity before placing the cerclage. Recently Katz and Chez[35] suggested that filling the bladder by instilling 400 to 500 ml of normal saline may lead to a retraction of the amniotic sac into the uterine cavity, thus allowing cerclage.

Charles and Edwards[14] recommended the use of prophylactic antibiotics when emergency cerclage is performed. They found a 2.6-fold increase in chorioamnionitis when cerclage was performed after, compared to before, 18 weeks' gestation and a tripling in the likelihood of preterm PROM. It is our practice to prescribe a 3-day course of broad-spectrum antibiotics beginning just before emergency cerclage, although data are not available to allow a specific rational choice of type or duration of therapy.

Similarly, it has been our practice to use tocolysis with terbutaline subcutaneously (0.25 mg every 4 to 6 hours) for the first 24 hours in patients undergoing emergency cerclage with a dilated cervix, particularly if uterine irritability is present. No controlled trials are available to evaluate this practice.

Although maternal sepsis[21,32,42] and death[22] have been reported, particularly with ruptured membranes and a cerclage left in place, Yeast and Garite[75] reported on 32 patients managed expectantly with preterm PROM and cerclage in place. The cerclage was removed immediately in each case. The patients were compared to 32 matched controls with PROM but without cerclage in place. Latency periods and infectious complications were similar in both groups, suggesting that the presence of a preexisting cerclage in the face of preterm PROM is not a contraindication to expectant management so long as the cerclage is removed. The management of preterm PROM with an abdominal cerclage in place remains speculative. While I have not personally encountered this situation, my inclination would be to manage with non-intervention, since removal of the abdominal cerclage would involve a laparotomy, and the intraabdominal location of the suture should not predispose to infection with ruptured membranes.

FOLLOW-UP CARE

Patients who have undergone vaginal cerclage prophylactically are usually discharged from the hospital on the day of or the day after the procedure provided that their condition is stable. Patients who have undergone elective abdominal cerclage are kept in the hospital as for any laparotomy, 3 to 4 days if there are no complications. When cerclage has been performed emergently, for a dilated and/or effaced cervix, the patient may require a longer period of rest and observation, to detect preterm labor if it supervenes. Once discharged, patients with cerclage in place are usually asked to observe "pelvic precautions," avoiding coitus or the placement of any object in the vagina. Those who have had an elective procedure are allowed to resume other normal activities and are examined weekly to ascertain the integrity of the cerclage. Women whose cervixes were dilated and effaced, particularly if they were at an advanced state of dilation, are often asked to restrict their activities and may require bedrest at home. This advice is individualized. All patients with cerclage are instructed to report any signs of cervical change, including vaginal or back pressure, increased discharge, pelvic ache, or cramps.

The timing of cerclage removal has not been studied in a controlled manner. However, it seems reasonable that the cerclage be removed at such a time as the clinician would be willing to deliver the baby electively (i.e., at 38 weeks or beyond). Although some patients may ask that the cerclage be removed at an earlier point, for convenience, this approach could lead to early delivery with its attendant risks. On the other hand, it has been our practice to remove the cerclage in any patient with significant contractions at a gestational age when we would not ordinarily be willing to institute tocolysis (i.e., 36 weeks or beyond). The logic behind such a policy is that uterine contractions in the face of a sutured cervix could lead to rupture of the uterus or avulsion of the cervix. Patients should be prepared for the possibility that their pregnancies may extend post term despite the removal of the cerclage. Whether this phenomenon represents scarring of the cervix from the cerclage or mistaken diagnosis of incompetent cervix or neither remains unknown. When an abdominal cerclage has been placed we generally plan elective cesarean section at term. If labor supervenes the cesarean section can be performed on an emergency basis, or tocolysis utilized if the onset of labor is prior to term.

Finally, it is worth mentioning that the very name of the condition for which cerclage is prescribed is an unfortunate choice of words. In his essay "The Incompetent Cervix: Words That Can Hurt," Fox [24] notes that the definition of *incompetent* includes "lacking in qualities (as maturity, capacity, initiative, intelligence) necessary to effective independent action . . . one incapable of doing properly what is required." He concludes, "In light of these last meanings, it is easy to see how a mother grieving over the death of her premature infant might be additionally upset by being told by her physician that the premature birth resulted from her 'incompetent cervix.' " Fox cites several examples of patients reporting a tremendous sense of guilt and worthlessness because of this diagnosis and experiencing real relief when the nature of the condition was better explained to them. My own experience has been similar, and I support Fox's suggestion that the name be changed to some less judgmental term such as *premature cervical dilatation,* although the latter is not specific enough to convey the absence of labor or other causes.

REFERENCES

1. Aarnoudse JG, Huisjes HJ: Complications of cerclage, *Acta Obstet Gynecol Scand* 58:255, 1979.
2. Abramovici H, Faktor JH, Pascal B: Congenital uterine malformations as indication for cervical suture (cerclage) in habitual abortion and premature delivery, *Int J Fertil* 28:161, 1983.
3. Arias F: Cervical cerclage for the temporary treatment of patients with placenta previa, *Obstet Gynecol* 71:545, 1988.
4. Bakketeig L, Hoffman HJ, Harley EE: The tendency to repeat gestational age and birth weight in successive births, *Am J Obstet Gynecol* 135:1086, 1979.
5. Barford DA, Rosen MG: Cervical incompetence: diagnosis and outcome, *Obstet Gynecol* 64:159, 1984.
6. Bengtsson LP: Cervical insufficiency, *Acta Obstet Gynecol Scand* suppl 47:9, 1968.
7. Benson RC, Durfee R: Transabdominal cervicoisthmic cerclage during pregnancy for the treatment of cervical incompetence, *Obstet Gynecol* 25:145, 1965.
8. Bouyer J et al: Maturation signs of the cervix and prediction of preterm birth, *Obstet Gynecol* 68:209, 1986.
9. Bracken MB: Induced abortion as a risk factor for perinatal complications: a review, *Yale J Biol Med* 51:539, 1978.
10. Brook I et al: Ultrasonography in the diagnosis of cervical incompetence in pregnancy—a new diagnostic approach, *Br J Obstet Gynaecol* 88:640, 1981.
11. Brown JE et al: Transabdominal and transvaginal endosonography: evaluation of the cervix and lower uterine segment in pregnancy, *Am J Obstet Gynecol* 155:721, 1986.
12. Buller RE, Jones HW III: Pregnancy following cervical conization, *Am J Obstet Gynecol* 142:506, 1982.
13. Caspi E et al: Cervical internal os cerclage: description of a new technique and comparison with Shirodkar operation, *Am J Perinatol* 7:347, 1990.
14. Charles D, Edwards WR: Infectious complications of cervical cerclage, *Am J Obstet Gynecol* 141:1065, 1981.
15. Cousins L et al: Reproductive outcome of women exposed to diethylstilbestrol in utero, *Obstet Gynecol* 56:70, 1980.
16. Crombleholme WR et al: Cervical cerclage: an aggressive approach to threatened or recurrent pregnancy wastage, *Am J Obstet Gynecol* 146:168, 1983.
17. Danforth DN: The fibrous nature of the human cervix and its relation to the isthmic segment in the gravid and nongravid uteri, *Am J Obstet Gynecol* 53:541, 1947.
18. Del Valle G et al: Comparison between the use of prophylactic cerclage and bedrest in twin gestation, *Am J Obstet Gynecol* 164:408, 1991.
19. Dor J et al: Elective cervical suture of twin pregnancies diagnosed ultrasonically in the first trimester following induced ovulation, *Gynecol Obstet Invest* 13:55, 1982.
20. Druzin ML, Berkeley AS: A simplified approach to Shirodkar cerclage procedure, *Surg Gynecol Obstet* 162:375, 1986.
21. Dubouloz P, Maye D, Béguin F: Cerclage et infections: etude clinique et thérapeutique, *J Gynecol Obstet Biol Reprod* 9:671, 1980.
22. Dunn LJ, Robinson JC, Steer CM: Maternal death following suture of the incompetent cervix during pregnancy, *Am J Obstet Gynecol* 78:335, 1959.
23. Floyd WS: Cervical dilatation in the mid-trimester of pregnancy, *Obstet Gynecol* 18:380, 1961.
24. Fox HA: The incompetent cervix: words that can hurt, *Am J Obstet Gynecol* 147:462, 1983.
25. Goldberg GL, Altaras MM, Bloch B: Cone cerclage in pregnancy, *Obstet Gynecol* 77:315, 1991.
26. Goldstein DP: Incompetent cervix in offspring exposed to diethylstilbestrol in utero, *Obstet Gynecol* 52(suppl):73s, 1978.
27. Goldstein PJ, Wolff RJ: The incompetent cervix: a survey of survivors, *Obstet Gynecol* 23:752, 1964.
28. Goldzieher JW: Double-blind trial of a progestin in habitual abortion, *JAMA* 188:651, 1964.
29. Goodlin RC: Cervical incompetence, hourglass membranes, and amniocentesis, *Obstet Gynecol* 54:748, 1979.
30. Harger JH: Comparison of success and morbidity in cervical cerclage procedures, *Obstet Gynecol* 56:543, 1980.
31. Harlap S et al: Prospective study of spontaneous fetal losses after induced abortion, *N Engl J Med* 301:677, 1979.
32. Heinemann M, Tang C, Kramer EE: Placental bacteremia and maternal sepsis complicating Shirodkar procedure, *Am J Obstet Gynecol* 128:226, 1977.
33. Herron MA, Parer JT: Transabdominal cerclage for fetal wastage due to cervical incompetence, *Obstet Gynecol* 71:865, 1988.
34. Jackson G et al: Diagnostic ultrasound in the assessment of patients with incompetent cervix, *Br J Obstet Gynaecol* 91:232, 1984.
35. Katz M, Chez RA: Reducing prolapsed membranes, *Contemp Ob/Gyn* 35:48, 1990.
36. Kiwi R et al: Determination of the elastic properties of the cervix, *Obstet Gynecol* 71:568, 1988.
37. Lazar P et al: Multicentred controlled trial of cervical cerclage in

women at moderate risk of preterm delivery, *Br J Obstet Gynaecol* 91:731, 1984.

38. Lee NH: The effect of cone biopsy on subsequent pregnancy outcome, *Gynecol Oncol* 6:1, 1978.

39. Leiman G, Harrison NA, Rubin A: Pregnancy following conization of the cervix: complications related to cone size, *Am J Obstet Gynecol* 136:14, 1980.

40. Leppert PC et al: Decreased elastic fibers and desmosine content in incompetent cervix, *Am J Obstet Gynecol* 157:1134, 1987.

41. Levin AA et al: Association of induced abortion with subsequent pregnancy loss, *JAMA* 243:2495, 1980.

42. Lindberg BS: Maternal sepsis, uterine rupture and coagulopathy complicating cervical cerclage, *Acta Obstet Gynecol Scand* 58:317, 1979.

43. Ludmir J et al: Management of the diethylstilbestrol-exposed pregnant patient: a prospective study, *Am J Obstet Gynecol* 157:665, 1987.

44. Mahran M: Transabdominal cervical cerclage during pregnancy: a modified technique, *Obstet Gynecol* 52:502, 1978.

45. Mahran M: *The role of ultrasound in the diagnosis and management of the incompetent cervix.* In Kurjak A, editor: *Recent advances in ultrasound diagnosis,* vol 2, New York, 1980, Excerpta-Medica.

46. McDonald IA: Suture of the cervix for inevitable miscarriage, *J Obstet Gynaecol Br Emp* 64:346, 1957.

47. McDonald IA: Incompetent cervix as a cause of recurrent abortion, *J Obstet Gynaecol Br Commonw* 70:105, 1963.

48. Moinian M, Andersch B: Does cervical conization increase the risk of complications in subsequent pregnancies? *Acta Obstet Gynecol Scand* 61:101, 1982.

49. MRC/RCOG Working Party on Cervical Cerclage: Interim report of the Medical Research Council/Royal College of Obstetricians and Gynaecologists multicentre randomized trial of cervical cerclage, *Br J Obstet Gynaecol* 95:437, 1988.

50. Niebyl J: Detecting signs and symptoms of incompetent cervix, *Contemp Ob/Gyn* 28:37, 1990.

51. Novy MJ: Managing reproductive failure by transabdominal isthmic cerclage, *Contemp Ob/Gyn* 10:17, 1977.

52. Novy MJ: Transabdominal cervicoisthmic cerclage for the management of repetitive abortion and premature delivery, *Am J Obstet Gynecol* 143:44, 1982.

53. Novy MJ: Transabdominal cervicoisthmic cerclage: a reappraisal 25 years after its introduction, *Am J Obstet Gynecol* 164:1635, 1991.

54. Novy MJ, Ducsay CA, Stanczyk FZ: Plasma concentrations of prostaglandin F_{2a} and prostaglandin E_2 metabolites after transabdominal and transvaginal cervical cerclage, *Am J Obstet Gynecol* 156:1543, 1987.

55. Olátunbosun OA, Dyck F: Cervical cerclage operation for a dilated cervix, *Obstet Gynecol* 57:166, 1981.

56. Palmer R, LaComme M: Le beance de l'orifice interne, cause d'avortement s repitetion? Une observation de dechirure cervicoisthmique reparee chiurgicalement, avec gestation a term consecutive, *Gynecol Obstet* (Paris) 47:905, 1948.

57. Parikh MN, Mehta AC: Internal cervical os during the second half of pregnancy, *J Obstet Gynaecol Br Commw* 68:818, 1961.

58. Ratten GJ: Etiology of delivery during the second trimester and performance in subsequent pregnancies, *Med J Aust* 2:654, 1981.

59. Rechberger T, Uldbjerg N, Oxlund H: Connective tissue changes in the cervix during normal pregnancy and pregnancy complicated by cervical incompetence, *Obstet Gynecol* 71:563, 1988.

60. Rush RW et al: A randomized controlled trial of cervical cerclage in women at high risk of spontaneous preterm delivery, *Br J Obstet Gynaecol* 91:724, 1984.

61. Sarti DA et al: Ultrasonic visualization of a dilated cervix during pregnancy, *Radiology* 130:417, 1979.

62. Schaffner F, Schanzer SN: Cervical dilatation in the early third trimester, *Obstet Gynecol* 27:130, 1966.

63. Schoenbaum SC et al: Outcome of the delivery following an induced or spontaneous abortion, *Am J Obstet Gynecol* 136:19, 1980.

64. Schulman H, Farmakides G: Surgical approach to failed cervical cerclage, *J Reprod Med* 30:626, 1985.

65. Shearman RP, Garrett WJ: Double-blind study of effect of 17-hydroxyprogesterone caproate on abortion rate, *Brit Med J* 1:292, 1963.

66. Shirodkar VN: A new method of operative treatment for habitual abortions in the second trimester of pregnancy, *The Antiseptic* 52:299, 1955.

67. Shirodkar VN: Discussion following Barter RH et al: Further experience with the Shirodkar operation, *Am J Obstet Gynecol* 85:795, 1963.

68. Singer MS, Hochman M: Incompetent cervix in a hormone-exposed offspring, *Obstet Gynecol* 51:625, 1978.

69. Thorp JM Jr et al: Antepartum and intrapartum events in women exposed in utero to diethylstilbestrol, *Obstet Gynecol* 76:828, 1990.

70. Vaalamo P, Kivikoski A: The incompetent cervix during pregnancy diagnosed by ultrasound, *Acta Obstet Gynecol Scand* 62:19, 1983.

71. Varma TR, Patel RH, Pillai U: Ultrasonic assessment of cervix in "at risk" patients, *Acta Obstet Gynecol Scand* 65:147, 1986.

72. Weber T, Obel E: Pregnancy complications following conization of the uterine cervix, *Acta Obstet Gynecol Scand* 58:259, 1979.

73. Weingold AB, Palmer JI, Stone ML: Cervical incompetency: a therapeutic enigma, *Fertil Steril* 19:244, 1968.

74. Witter FR: Negative sonographic findings followed by rapid cervical dilatation due to cervical incompetence, *Obstet Gynecol* 64:136, 1984.

75. Yeast JD, Garite TR: The role of cervical cerclage in the management of preterm premature rupture of the membranes, *Am J Obstet Gynecol* 158:106, 1988.

76. Zakut H, Insler V, Serr DM: Elective cervical suture in preventing premature delivery in multiple pregnancies, *Isr J Med Sci* 13:488, 1977.

Chapter 64

EPISIOTOMY, REPAIR OF FRESH OBSTETRIC LACERATIONS, SYMPHYSIOTOMY

David H. Nichols

EPISIOTOMY

Although episiotomy was intended to prevent perineal tearing, providing the alternate of repair of a fresh surgical "incision" to that of the jagged edges of the perineal tear, there were large areas of interest in using episiotomy as a safe aid in shortening the second stage of labor. At the height of its popularity, this operation, often combined with "prophylactic" low forceps application, was practiced upon women of all ages in the Western world, and America in particular, and at a time when the relative inelasticity of tissues of the parturient now in her 30's was not as commonly encountered as it has become during the 80's and 90's.

The first truly significant, objectively documented study that correlated the management of labor and delivery with subsequent evidence of maternal soft tissue injuries was reported by Gainey in 1943. No equally significant study appeared in the U.S. literature until 1955, when Gainey reported the results of his comparison of specific, documented injuries in two series of 1000 patients each. Gainey had personally delivered and assessed the postpartum evidence of injury in each patient in both series. There was, however, an essential difference in the management of labor in patients in the two series. He had performed an episiotomy in the first group only when there was a maternal or fetal indication for it—either to avoid "impending" perineal laceration or to hasten delivery because of "fetal distress." In every instance in the second series, he had performed an episiotomy at the outlet station of the pre-

senting part, after which he had accomplished all deliveries by low or outlet forceps (except in 27 instances that required forceps rotation and 40 breech presentations in which the fetuses were delivered by "breech assists" with forceps to the aftercoming head). Gainey found that performing episiotomy and controlling the delivery of the fetal head by "outlet" or "prophylactic" forceps provided significant protection for the vagina, urogenital diaphragm, and perineum.

Almost any obstetric procedure that had become "routine" has lost much of its popularity, and episiotomy, as such, is no exception.

Although there is no clear-cut objective evidence that episiotomy significantly reduces the incidence of soft tissue damage requiring future reconstructive surgery, one is mindful of the large number of current parturients who have chosen to have their babies later in life, often starting their families after they have reached the age of 30. Because the "aging" tissues have apparently lost some of their elasticity, it appears that the obstetric incidence of significant vaginal and perineal tears and soft tissue damages is increased in this group, suggesting the long-range desirability of a more liberal application of timely episiotomy. Once performed, and anatomically repaired, the applicability of episiotomy with future deliveries for the same patient remains the same. This thinking presumes that the timeliness of the episiotomy was such that it was performed before the soft tissue damages had occurred, and occasionally this requires that it be done during the end of the second stage of labor but before crowning of the fetal head.

The duration of the second stage of labor to some extent determines the capability of the vaginal and perineal musculature to respond safely to stretching. If labor has been short or precipitate, such ability to stretch is usually compromised, suggesting further the desirability of timely episiotomy, and similarly the episiotomy may be "protective" in the case of a prolonged second stage of labor. Some indication of good elastic distensibility of the pelvic soft tissue may be inferred by observation of the extent and width of striae appearing on the patient's abdomen and breast. This was observed and reported by Magdi who coined the phrase "elastic index," as he suggested clinical relevance between many wide striae and decreased elasticity with increased likelihood of parturient tearing.

Gentle manual dilation of the perineum near the end of the second stage of labor, by well-lubricated downward and side-to-side pressure by the examiner's hand, has been described as an "ironing out" maneuver. It takes several minutes to accomplish, and one may start with the introduction of two fingerwidths, palm down, and gentle side-to-side pressure. A third (and then a fourth) finger is inserted when it can be accommodated, and the process is gently continued with emphasis on making posteriorly directed pressure.

Types of episiotomy

If one has decided to perform episiotomy, usually coincident with some lack of elasticity of the perineal tissues, the choice between a midline and mediolateral site for the episiotomy incision depends largely on the experience of the obstetrician or gynecologist. The obvious site of a previous episiotomy, the position of the baby's presenting part, the thickness or rigidity of the patient's perineum, and the obstetric perception of an impending severe laceration that risks fourth-degree extension, are all factors. Intentional midline episioproctotomy was recommended in the late 1960s, but, although the long-term results were most satisfactory and associated with a reduced incidence of subsequent rectocele and soft tissue damage, the increased amount of immediate postpartum pain and discomfort, especially in the current presence of almost mandatory reduction in length of hospital stay, has caused the procedure to be abandoned. Given a parturient patient who has had successful repair of a previous rectovaginal fistula, many obstetricians would opt for a subsequent *mediolateral* episiotomy, performed before crowning of the presenting fetal part. When a midline episiotomy or perineal tear threatens to interrupt the external sphincter or extend to become a fourth-degree perineal laceration, a deliberate and timely incision can be made at the base of the opened perineum off to one side (the "hockey stick" extension) directing the extension away from the rectal lumen.

There appears to be little indication for a bilateral mediolateral episiotomy.

Technique of repair

The technique of repair is as important as the choice of site for episiotomy. The goal is to put back together the soft tissues that had been incised, having arrested by ligation the free bleeding that was created. The anatomy of the undamaged perineum is shown in Fig. 64-1. Administration of a pudendal block is shown in Fig. 64-2. This approximation is far easier to do with a midline episiotomy repair (Figs. 64-3 through 64-9) than a mediolateral one because the incised tissues with the former are bilaterally symmetrical. With repair of a mediolateral episiotomy (Figs. 64-10 and 64-11) in contrast, the bulbocavernosus muscle often has been incised and the anterior extremity has retracted into the labia (Fig. 64-12). If such is the case, the retracted end should be deliberately sought and anchored to the perineum by a separate suture. The vaginal wall can be approximated by either running subcuticular stitching, using a small gauge (00 or 000) chromic or polyglycolic acid suture, or either running or interrupted through-and-through sutures. The subepithelial tissues are best approximated by buried interrupted stitches, and the perineal skin is closed by a running subcuticular suture or through-and-through, according to the operator's preference (Fig. 64-13). The pelvic muscles are displaced laterally after delivery (Fig. 64-14).

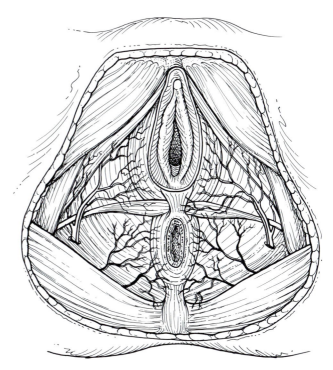

Fig. 64-1. The anatomy of the perineum after removal of the skin and subcutaneous tissue. The perineal body is the center of the hub of a wheel that includes the transverse perinei, the capsule of the external anal sphincter, and the bulbocavernosus muscles. The blood vessels enter from the side, and their branches may be cut by episiotomy at the five, six and seven o'clock positions. Mediolateral episiotomy transects the superficial muscles of the perineum, but the midline episiotomy does not.

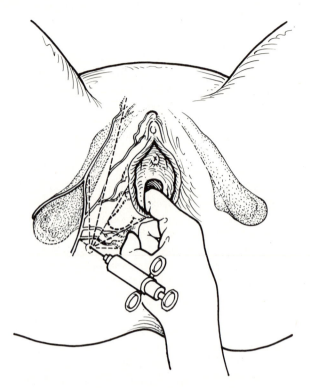

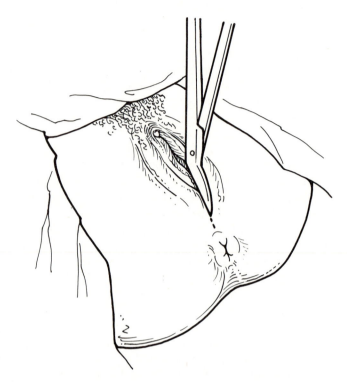

Fig. 64-2. The pudendal block. The pudendal nerve can be effectively blocked by a local anesthetic, effectively anesthetizing the perineum. The tip of the obstetrician's right index finger is placed overlying the right ischial spine. The pudendal nerve and artery are directly behind the spine. A pudendal block, to be effective, must be done on each side. The tip of a long needle attached to a syringe of local anesthetic is injected through the skin medial to the ischial tuberosity and headed toward the ischial spine, which is identified by palpation. Anesthetic material is injected into the tissues around the pudendal nerve, and additional anesthetic agent may be injected along the site of the dashed lines, as shown.

Fig. 64-3. A midline episiotomy is made through the anterior portion of the perineal body in the six o'clock position as shown.

After repair of an episiotomy, a rectal examination should be done, and, if a stitch in the rectum is discovered, it should be cut, usually on the rectal side, after which the ends fully withdraw and disappear into the deeper tissues. Cutting such a suture not only lessens the amount of postpartum pain and discomfort, but reduces the tendency for local necrosis at the suture site, lessening the chance of a postpartum rectovaginal fistula.

Aftercare

In many patients, the postpartum perineal pain may induce some degree of spasm of the levator ani muscle, inhibiting the spontaneous voiding process and making catheterization necessary. Should this become evident, the administration of an alpha-adrenergic blocking agent usually relaxes the "reflex" urethral spasm sufficiently to permit voiding, provided that the bladder has not become temporarily paralyzed by having become overdistended. An example of such a blocking agent (also useful for the same purpose after any procedure that by pain inhibits muscular

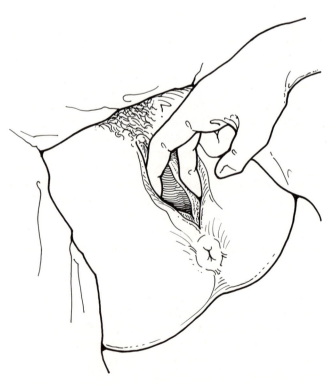

Fig. 64-4. The temporarily gaping introitus after midline episiotomy.

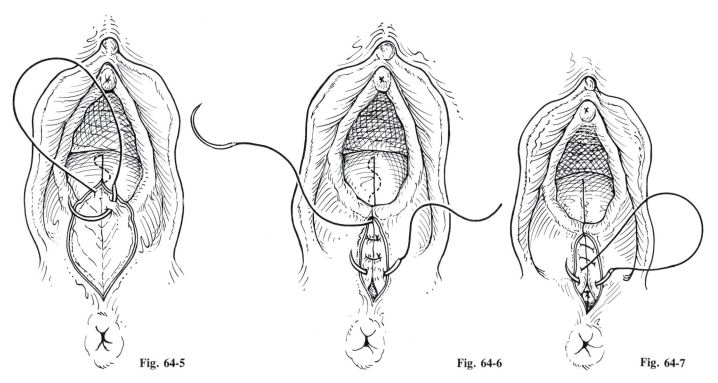

Fig. 64-5. **Fig. 64-6.** **Fig. 64-7.**

Fig. 64-5. Midline episiotomy is repaired by a running subcuticular suture beneath the vaginal incision and starting at its very top. This is carried down to the hymenal margin.

Fig. 64-6. Bisected portions of the perineal body are reunited by a series of interrupted sutures.

Fig. 64-7. If desired, the vaginal suture may be continued as a running layer to reunite the sides of the perineal body.

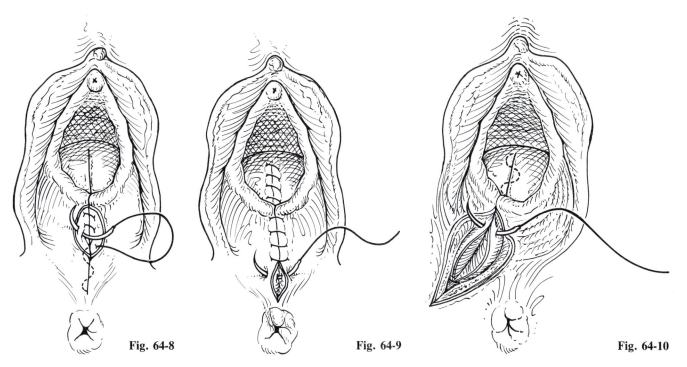

Fig. 64-8. **Fig. 64-9.** **Fig. 64-10.**

Fig. 64-8. When this has reached the bottom of the episiotomy, it is returned to the hymenal margin as a running subcuticular suture.

Fig. 64-9. Alternately, the skin of the vagina and other perineal body may be reunited by a series of interrupted sutures.

Fig. 64-10. Repair of a right mediolateral episiotomy. The vaginal portion of the incision is reunited by a running subcuticular suture placed according to the path indicated by the dashed line. The series of deep interrupted stitches reunite the deeper stitches of the perineal incision as shown.

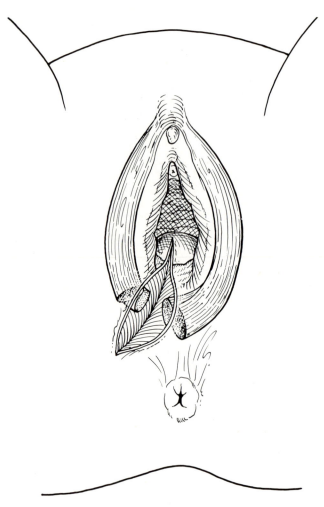

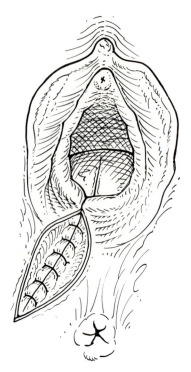

Fig. 64-12. When the deeper tissues have been reunited, as shown, the subcutaneous layer is closed by a running subcuticular suture.

Fig. 64-11. A special effort is made to find the retracted free end of the bulbocavernosus muscle and reattach it to the perineal body. The retracted ends of the cut muscle are shown. These must be reunited to the perineal body if an anatomic restoration is to be accomplished.

relaxation, i.e., hemorrhoidectomy, appendectomy, herniorrhaphy) is phenoxybenzamine (Dibenzyline), 10 mg dose, by mouth. Adequate postpartum analgesia inhibits perineal pain, often precluding the necessity for catheterization. Early ambulation also has a salutory effect in reestablishing voiding, because many women are unable to void when lying down, having conditioned themselves to this eventuality since their childhood toilet training. Application of ice packs to the perineum is comforting during the first 18 hours postpartum while the patient is hospitalized. Local applications of cotton balls saturated with witch hazel are soothing to the perineum.

The perineum should be inspected daily during hospitalization, usually with the patient in the lateral recumbent or Sims' position, and, if the perineum is unusually tender or inflamed, local heat is helpful after the first postpartum day. This may be in the form of a heat lamp or the heat from a blow-type hair dryer initially, because the skin incision does not become water-tight until after the second

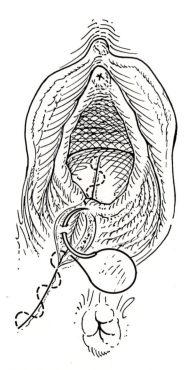

Fig. 64-13. When the deeper tissues have been reapproximated, the skin of the perineum is reapproximated by a running subcuticular suture placed as shown.

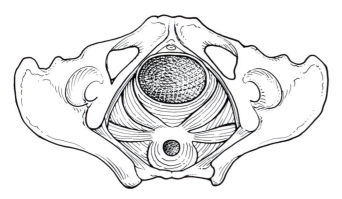

Fig. 64-14. The introitus and subcutaneous muscles at the time of vaginal delivery. Compare this with Fig. 64-1, and notice the lateral displacement of the muscles during obstetric delivery.

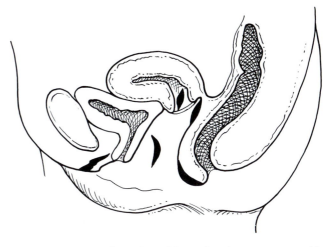

Fig. 64-15. The various sites of laceration that may occur with confinement are identified by the blackened areas. Note that laceration may occur in the cervix and lower uterine segment, the vault of the vagina, the perineum, the lateral wall of the vagina, and anterior to the urethra.

postpartum or postoperative day. After the second day, warm water sitz baths, two or three times a day, may be comforting.

Attention to bowel habit is important, because perineal pain may inhibit defecation, and it is important to inhibit the development of a fecal impaction. Stool softeners and gentle laxatives, often the use of a rectal laxative suppository (glycerin or Dulcolax), may be necessary.

Perineal infection, although rare, should be taken seriously, because the severe consequence of development of synergistic bacterial gangrene or even necrotizing fasciitis is possible. The latter may develop unexpectedly after discharge from the hospital so attention must be given to postpartum communication from the patient concerning her perineum.

Postpartum hematoma of the vulva and episiotomy site produces local disfiguration and pain. The site should be watched carefully, because the veins of the vulva have no valves, and continued bleeding can occur, distending all of the soft tissues and compartments of the pelvis. Progressive enlargement is evident, often with accompanying discoloration. Such sutures are taken out as might be removed to provide exposure and evacuation of clots, and the raw surfaces are inspected. Any bleeding vessels that can be identified are clamped and tied, and the hematoma cavity is packed, for which iodoform gauze is useful.

Should there be postpartum breakdown of an episiotomy, usually secondary to infection, débridement of necrotic tissues is done and the tissues should be given time for the necrosis to be discarded, edema to subside, and purulence to be replaced by granulation tissue before redébridement and rerepair, the latter using interrupted absorbable sutures. There may be no hurry for rerepair to be accomplished, because if the need for this becomes evident after discharge from the hospital, the new mother also requires time to arrange for the care of her newborn.

LACERATIONS OF THE PELVIS

The cervix and vagina should be inspected for the presence of lacerations (Fig. 64-15), which may be repaired

promptly, with adequate visualization provided by appropriate retractors, usually using interrupted sutures of absorbable material. Blood vessels that are found bleeding should, of course, be clamped and tied. Most lacerations should be repaired as soon after delivery as possible.

Degrees of tearing

A first-degree laceration of the perineum is one that extends through the vaginal and perineal skin and superficial tissues of the perineal body. Débridement is rarely necessary, and a single layer of interrupted sutures placed about 1 cm apart suffices in the majority of cases.

Second-degree perineal laceration, on the other hand, extends deeply into the soft tissues of the perineum, sometimes down to but not including the external anal sphincter, and generally involves disruption of some fibers of the transverse perineal muscles. A layer of buried interrupted sutures is placed, and a superficial layer of through-and-through absorbable interrupted stitches finishes the repair. Damage from unexposed stretching to the smooth and striated muscles and soft unexposed tissues of the perineum has already been done and will not likely be repaired or restored by repair at this time.

Third-degree laceration extends through the skin and tissues of the perineum and portions or all of the external anal sphincter. This should also be repaired by a series of interrupted sutures reuniting the sides of the perineal body, and each severed end of the external anal sphincter is identified and grasped by an Allis clamp or hemostat and brought together by two interrupted mattress sutures of long-lasting absorbable suture material such as Maxon or PDS, placed at right angles to one another (Fig. 64-16).

Although the patient may be on a regular house diet, special attention should be given to keeping the stool on the soft side, using stool softeners as necessary during the

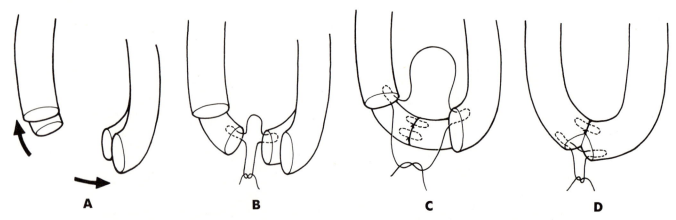

Fig. 64-16. The details of suture placement reuniting the severed ends of the perineal muscles are shown. **A,** The ends of the muscles tend to retract from the site of their incision, as indicated by the black arrows. **B,** The ends of the muscle are identified and reapproximated by a series of interrupted sutures, the deeper ones being placed first. **C,** When these have been tied, additional interrupted sutures are placed in the ends of the transected muscle in its more superficial portion. **D,** The appearance when these are tied.

first month postpartum, and restoration of bowel habits with regular movement is the immediate goal. Perineal resistive exercises of the Kegel type (15 squeezes of 3 seconds' duration six times a day) are useful for 3 months postpartum. Appropriate laxative stimulation, if necessary, helps avoid fecal impaction, and a mental or written note is appended to the patient's chart to consider strongly a mediolateral episiotomy with the next confinement.

Fourth-degree laceration, although occasionally unavoidable, is an obstetric tragedy and its' repair and the aftercare require the undivided attention of the patient's obstetrician. Laceration is more common in the presence of a relatively inelastic perineum, especially during a violent labor, that has compromised the ability of the perineal tissues to stretch slowly to accommodate the passage of the fetal presenting part.

A fourth-degree laceration may occur within a few seconds, usually followed by the explosive delivery of the fetus. The laceration does not undergo spontaneous restorative healing, leaving the patient with a strong likelihood of fecal incontinence. Most should be repaired immediately after delivery of the placenta and inspection of the birth canal.

Repair of fourth-degree laceration

Any necessary débridement should be accomplished, the injury site should be irrigated with sterile saline, and the necessary components for anatomic reconstruction should be identified and tagged if necessary. The full extent of the laceration in the anterior rectal wall is exposed (Figs. 64-17, 64-18) and approximated from side to side by submucosal running suture all the way down to the margin of the anal skin. A second layer of running suture will invert the first, taking some of the tension from the first layer closure, which may be helpful during the heal-

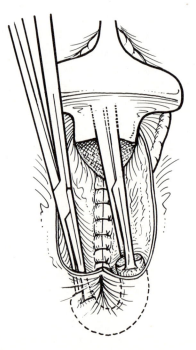

Fig. 64-17. Repair of a fourth-degree laceration. The torn edges of the rectal submucosa and muscularis are reunited by the series of interrupted sutures as shown, and the cut edges of the external anal sphincter are grasped with Allis clamps.

ing process. If not previously accomplished, the retracted ends of the external anal sphincter are grasped with Allis clamps, and mattress sutures of long-lasting absorbable polyglycolic acid type are placed, but not yet tied (Fig. 64-19). The vaginal wall is approximated from side to side by suture, and careful side-to-side placement of interrupted absorbable sutures begins the reconstruction of the perineal body and perineum. These stitches are carefully tied as

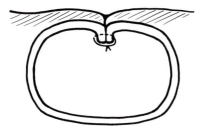

Fig. 64-18. When there is considerable bleeding from the rectal edges of the tear in the rectal mucosa, it may be controlled by a series of stitches that invert the mucosa into the rectal lumen. These stitches are tied so that the suture knot is on the interior surface of the rectum.

they are placed, with the tension sufficient to approximate the tissues, but not so tightly as to strangulate the tissues in which they have been placed. When all have been placed and tied, the sutures previously placed uniting the ends of the severed anal sphincter are tied, and the perineum and skin are closed, usually using interrupted absorbable sutures. Rectovaginal fistula after a fourth-degree laceration is highly litiginous! Fistula formation should be prevented by careful control of diet and resumption of good bowel habits postpartum and until the tissues have fully healed. A low-residue diet is initiated, and the patient is started on daily doses of stool softeners and bulk producers. Careful attention must be given to initiation of the first bowel movement, and, if this has not occurred after 48 hours postpartum, a mild laxative is given, such as milk of magnesia with cascara. After the first bowel movement, a regular diet may be initiated, although daily stool softeners and laxatives should be continued for a month until a history of regular daily bowel movements has been reported.

Immediately after the repair of even a routine episiotomy, rectal examination should be done to check for an unexpected hole between rectum and vagina above the site of the episiotomy repair, and, if one is found, it should, of course, be repaired at this time. If a stitch is found transgressing the rectum, it should be cut transrectally, to lessen the chance of rectovaginal fistula.

Failure to respect the tremendous intrarectal pressures that can be generated during forceful evacuation of the first large bolus of hard stool some 7 to 10 days after delivery and repair may compromise the integrity of the anterior rectal wall portion of the repair—with disruption of its cranial portion, through both rectal and vaginal wall, with the production of a rectovaginal fistula! The patient will date her incontinence of gas and feces to that first postpartum bowel movement. In general, I believe this unwelcome eventuality to be due to mismanagement of postpartum bowel habits more than to any technical imprecision in the repair of a fourth-degree laceration.

When breakdown of a fourth-degree laceration has been noted while the postpartum patient is still in the hospital, there is usually much coexistent edema, local infection,

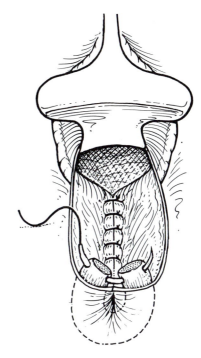

Fig. 64-19. The Allis clamps are replaced with transfixion ligatures reuniting the ends of the external anal sphincter.

pain, and some necrosis. Most obstetricians and gynecologists elect to recommend repair after some 3 months postpartum, when pain, infection, and edema have subsided, and provision has been made for the care of the newborn baby. These fistulas are repaired without the coincident performance of a complementary colostomy, using an appropriate repair as described in Chapter 29. Generally speaking, if the perineal repair and anal sphincter reunification have healed effectively, it is not essential to redivide the healed areas by recreation of a fourth-degree laceration for the repair, because on occasion the rerepair may break down with disruption of a previously healed strategic tissue. Should the patient request and be prepared for an "immediate" rerepair, this can be offered as a consideration, although she must understand that a small percentage do not heal properly and require another rerepair some months in the future. Should the patient be prepared to take her chances with "immediate rerepair," she should be placed immediately on a clear liquid diet, frequent sitz baths, and heat to the perineum, rinsing the area twice daily with 5% hydrogen peroxide solution, and experiencing gentle daily débridement of any necrotic tissue, until purulence, pain, and edema have subsided, and a preoperative mechanical and appropriate antibiotic bowel prep (NuLytely, Erythromycin-Neomycin, or Mefoxin) is given. Because healing of the uninfected tissues is incomplete, a fresh wound is recreated at surgery and repaired. Antibiotics and a clear liquid diet are continued postoperatively, along with abundant analgesia, local heat, and daily stool softeners such as Colace. Beginning the third postoperative day, a low-residue diet may be started, but the patient is not discharged until after the first bowel movement. The low-residue diet is continued for 3 weeks after discharge, with periodic phone calls from the office staff to the patient to solicit and answer any relevant questions.

Postpartum rectovaginal fistula

This fistula is more common in the patient over age 40, in whom tissue elasticity and distensibility are reduced, after breakdown of the repair of a fourth-degree laceration, or it may come from unrecognized buttonholing of the anterior rectal and posterior vaginal wall coincident with episiotomy. In this instance, incontinence of gas should be noted within the first 2 postpartum days. A postpartum rectovaginal fistula that does not make itself known for 7 to 14 days after delivery may be more likely caused by necrosis at the site of an episiotomy suture placed through the posterior vaginal wall and inadvertently through the anterior wall of the rectum. A digital examination of the rectum should always be done after episiotomy repair, so any such transgressing suture can be identified and promptly cut. Usually, if it is cut on the rectal side, it retracts promptly from the rectum and toward the vagina and out of harm's way.

Paravaginal hematomas

This may be found, usually unexpectedly, immediately after delivery and will be present as a discreet and spongy localized fullness in the region of the ischial spine. They are usually unilateral and may represent unexpected trauma to the pudendal blood vessels. Because of their arterial component and the lack of counterpressure on the cranial side of the hematoma, expansion within the vaginal and subvaginal tissues and more particularly into the retroperitoneal tissues of the pelvis is to be expected, which, if undetected, can give rise to a most disproportionate degree of pelvic pain. These hematomas can contain up to 1200 ml of blood clot. There is no place for expectant treatment of these hematomas. If they are detected immediately after delivery, the full thickness of the vaginal wall should be incised longitudinally, and the clot should be evacuated. If individual bleeding vessels are encountered, they should be clamped and the clamp should be replaced by a transfixion ligature. If they have retracted within the side wall of the pelvis and are not visible, the hematoma cavity should be tightly packed with gauze, preferably iodoform, which is shortened in 12 hours and generally removed in 24 hours. This compression effectively controls residual bleeding by counterpressure, and the wound and vaginal incision generally heal promptly and with no sequelae.

If the hematoma occurs on the side or at the site of an episiotomy, the stitches are removed, the clot is evacuated, and the episiotomy is rerepaired while using interrupted sutures. Postpartum purplish discoloration of the vulvar skin is to be expected, but the associated edema rapidly subsides. Supravaginal hematomas, although most uncommon, may be suspected by an unexplained rise in the pulse rate and coincident drop in blood pressure. One

can be confirmed by a falling hematocrit, and an ill-defined pelvic fullness, usually unilateral, may be perceived by manual examination. These should be watched carefully, and, if palpable suprapubically, the height should be marked on the patient's abdominal skin, so one can observe objectively whether an increase in size evolves. If it does not, expectant treatment may suffice, but, if the mass enlarges, laparotomy should be performed, the clot should be evacuated, and the area should be drained.

SYMPHYSIOTOMY

In usual North American practice situations, emergency symphysiotomy is not a substitute for cesarean section, but it is a welcome solution to obstructed labor in many parts of the world (underdeveloped regions including South America, Central Africa, Asia, and various parts of Australia and New Zealand) where facilities for emergency cesarean section are unavailable. Timely symphysiotomy may be not only life-saving for the fetus but may spare the mother the incalculable pain and suffering of massive disability, or of maternal death.

Although documentation of the operation is over 200 years old, it was reintroduced into obstetric technology by the South American, Zarate, who published a detailed experience and description of the operation in 1955. Important but somewhat sporadic contributions have been published in the international literature since then.

Indications for symphysiotomy

Indications for symphysiotomy are:

- A modest degree of fetal pelvic disproportion, with the membranes ruptured and the cervix fully dilated; progress of fetal descent has become arrested, either inlet midpelvic or, more rarely, outlet (in the latter circumstance, separation of the pubis does not ensure appreciable separation of bones at the outlet).
- Unexpected arrest of a non-hydrocephalic aftercoming head during breech delivery through a fully dilated cervix. Delivery of a living, undamaged fetus is otherwise improbable in a clinical setting in which emergency cesarean section is neither safe nor technically feasible.

Most of the patients will be primagravidas, although an occasional indication may be seen where the unmolded aftercoming head of a baby presenting by breech may become trapped within the bony pelvis and may be salvaged. If it is to be effective, symphysiotomy must be implemented without delay.

Technique for symphysiotomy

The operation is simple, although it requires technical precision. For a proper indication, it can be performed under local anesthesia in about 5 minutes. The technique is a modification from Zarate's description and is as follows:

The patient is in the lithotomy position her legs should be firmly held by two assistants (Fig. 64-20, *A* through *C*).

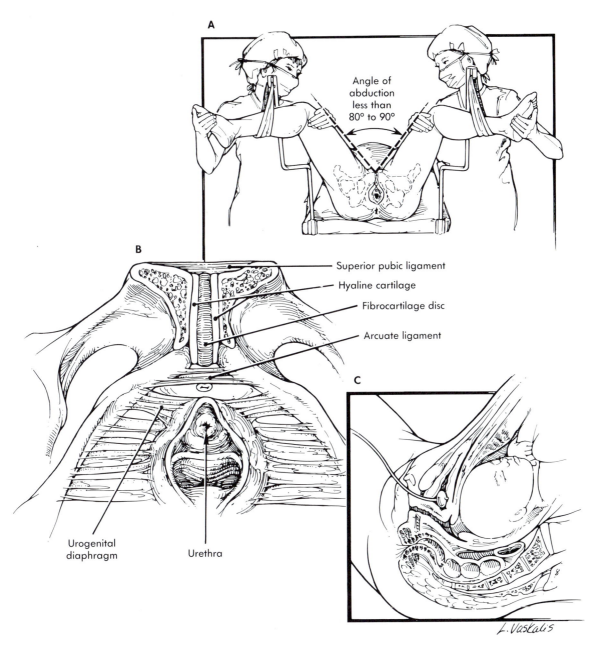

Fig. 64-20. Symphysiotomy. **A,** The patient's legs are supported. The angle of abduction must be between 80 and 90 degrees. **B,** Basic anatomy of the pubis symphysis. **C,** Sagittal section of the pelvis during labor. A catheter has been inserted into the bladder.

Continued.

A local anesthetic solution is infiltrated into the skin above the symphysis and then around the joint, and a transurethral catheter is passed and left in place.

The skin and tissues of the mons pubis are infiltrated, and the needle is directed into the joint of the symphysis pubis where more local anesthetic is injected. This step, as pointed out by Menticoglou, identifies the joint space and the needle can be left in situ as a guide wire if desired (Crichton and Seedat, 1963) (Fig. 64-20, *D* and *E*). The index and middle fingers of the left hand are introduced palm side up into the vagina. The index finger pushes the

catheter and urethra to one side, and the middle finger remains on the posterior aspect of the pubic joint to make sure the scalpel blade, when it is almost through the joint, does not penetrate too deeply. The scalpel (an old-type, one-piece scalpel without detachable blade, or a modern scalpel with a no. 20 blade) is used to make a short incision 0.5 cm above the upper edge of the pubis and directly toward the center of the joint.

The scalpel is held in the right hand, and the hypothenar eminence may rest on the pubic region to keep strict control over the movements of the knife. The scalpel is

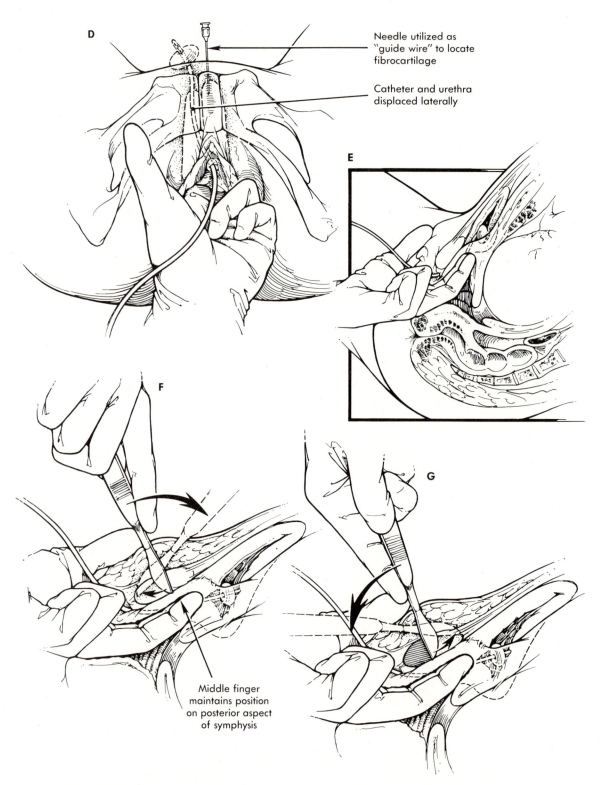

Needle utilized as
"guide wire" to locate
fibrocartilage

Catheter and urethra
displaced laterally

Middle finger
maintains position
on posterior aspect
of symphysis

Fig. 64-20, cont'd. D, An anesthetic has been injected, and the needle of the syringe is used as a guide wire to locate the pubic fibrocartilage. The fingers of the operator's left hand displace the catheter and urethra to one side. This is shown in sagittal drawing in **E. F,** A scalpel is held perpendicular to the skin, with the cutting edge toward the operator, and is directed posteriorly until it can be felt by the vaginal fingers. With a gentle rocking motion, as indicated by the arrows, the superior and anterior ligaments are divided down to the upper part of the arcuate ligament. The knife handle is lowered toward the maternal abdomen, and, using the upper part of the symphysis as a fulcrum, the knife cuts through the lower half of the symphysis. **G,** The knife is removed, turned 180 degrees, and reintroduced through the same stab incision, and the handle is lowered, cutting the upper half of the symphysis. The maximal separation of the pubis should not exceed 3.5 cm and is controlled by counterpressure by the leg holders.

grasped like a pencil, except that the ring and the little fingers are maximally flexed with their tips pressed against the palm of the hand and the scalpel is kept in a strict sagittal plane, resisting the natural tendency to give the hand the lateral inclination used for writing (Zarate, 1955).

This method is a subcutaneous partial symphysiotomy, which is simple, rapid, and associated with a minimum of complications.

The two vaginal fingers monitor the position of the scalpel blade to make sure it does not penetrate too deeply.

The knife is held perpendicular to the skin overlying the symphysis. The cutting edge of the blade faces the operator, and the knife enters 1 cm below the upper edge of the pubis. If the knife is placed perpendicularly and in the midline, it meets little resistance and only minimal force is needed to direct it posteriorly until the tip of the blade is felt by the vaginal fingers. If resistance is encountered, the blade has deviated laterally and is hitting the articular surface of one of the pubic bones; the blade is withdrawn a few millimeters, recentered and readvanced.

The knife is carried down to the center of the upper part of the joint in an almost vertical position (Fig. 64-20, *F*). With gentle rocking movements, the superior and anterior ligaments are divided with the joint down to and including the upper part of the arcuate ligament. When the scalpel tip is felt through the anterior vaginal wall (which must not be pierced), the knife handle is lowered toward the maternal abdomen and, using the upper part of the symphysis pubis as a fulcrum, the blade cuts through the lower half of the symphysis. The knife is removed, turned 180 degrees so that the cutting edge faces away from the operator, and reintroduced through the same stab incision in the skin. By lowering the handle toward the operator, the upper half of the symphysis will be divided (Fig. 64-20, *G*). The vaginal finger can identify any ligaments left to be divided. When the middle finger in the vagina can fit into the space created by the separation of the pubic bones, the symphysiotomy is complete. Alternately, the joint may be only partially divided, the posterior ligament and lower fibers of the arcuate ligament being left intact. These subsequently rupture either by gentle abduction of the legs by the assistants or as the presenting part descends with continuing labor. The separation of the pubis should not exceed 3.5 cm and is controlled by counterpressure by the leg holders. The skin is closed by one or two interrupted sutures, and any bleeding is controlled by external tamponade.

After the operation, delivery of the fetus is frequently spontaneous and rapid. Forceps should be avoided if possible, although use of the vacuum extractor during a uterine contraction can be recommended should further interference with the progress of labor be required. A generous episiotomy should be made in the primagravida, and when necessary in the multipara. Postpartum, a tight binder is applied around the pelvis at the level of the trochanters and a catheter is left in place for 4 or 5 days.

Postoperative care

Ambulation should be encouraged as soon as the patient wishes to get up, although she should be aided in walking for which she should use short, shuffling steps. The patient should be warned against undue exercise during at least 3 months postpartum.

Immediate complications from symphysiotomy are uncommon. Hemorrhage from the vascular bed over the pubis is sometimes profuse and is said to always stop as soon as the baby is born and may be controlled before delivery by firm pressure. Infection at the operative site may occur but may usually be prevented by appropriate antibiotics. Soft tissue injury is rare. The patient may sustain damage to the urethra, usually consequent to a technical error during the procedure, and, rarely, the patient may develop urinary stress incontinence.

The operation should not be undertaken before labor in the patient with obvious disproportion, nor early in labor, because the latter may be unnecessary if there is adequate molding of the head or occasionally the patient experiences spontaneous separation of the symphysis during labor.

The one exception to this rule is that, in cases of modest disproportion, the operation may be undertaken earlier in the second stage of labor in a patient with breech presentation, provided that the baby's buttocks have descended at least to the midcavity. If the baby is dead, it is better delivered by a destruction operation on the fetus; in the patient with a scar of a previous cesarean section, repeat cesarean section is by far the safest choice. Similarly, the head of a hydrocephalic infant is better delivered by compression of the skull (often by needling through the occipital foramen) than by symphysiotomy, unless the obstetrician wishes to perform cesarean section.

Long-term orthopedic disability is reported to be uncommon; occasional cases of spontaneous pubic separation are seen during antepartum care or in early labor in any large obstetric practice.

Complications of symphysiotomy

Recorded complications of symphysiotomy include:

1. Cystotomy or urethrotomy with or without formation of a subsequent vesicovaginal or urethrovaginal fistula
2. Urinary stress incontinence
3. Fever with abscess formation
4. Severe hemorrhage
5. Orthopedic disability when intrapartum pubic separation improperly exceeded 2.5 cm, thus subjecting the sacroiliac articulation to permanent and symptomatic damage from avulsion or overstretching.

Once performed, however, symphysiotomy is a logistic situation in which the patient will be likely to continue and to reproduce in the future. The accommodation of reseparation of the pubis during subsequent labor may occur "automatically," negating the requirements for cesarean section at a site where this operation is not available, or for repeat cesarean section if the patient's problem resulting from the initial disproportion had been solved previously by primary cesarean section.

SUGGESTED READINGS

Atlee HB: *The gist of obstetrics,* Springfield, IL, 1957, Charles C Thomas, p 164.

Buxton BH, Muram D: *Episiotomy.* In Sciarra J, editor: *Gynecology and obstetrics,* vol 2, Philadelphia, 1991, JB Lippincott, p 1.

Chrichton D, Seedat EK: The technique of symphysiotomy, *S Afr Med J* 37:227, 1963.

Cibils LA: Rupture of the symphysis pubis, *Obstet Gynecol* 38:407, 1971.

Combs CA, Robertson PA, Laros RJ: Risk factors for third-degree and fourth-degree perineal lacerations in forceps and vacuum deliveries, *Am J Obstet Gynecol* 63:100, 1990.

Cunningham CB, Pilkington JW: Complete perineotomy, *Am J Obstet Gynecol* 70:1225, 1955.

DeLee JB: The prophylactic forceps operation, *Am J Obstet Gynecol* 1:34, 1920.

Dewhurst J: *Integrated obstetrics and gynaecology for postgraduates,* ed 3, London, 1981, Blackwell, p 456.

Finn WF: The outcome of pregnancy following vaginal operations, *Am J Obstet Gynecol* 56:291, 1948.

Fleming AR: Complete perineotomy, *Obstet Gynecol* 16:172, 1960.

Gainey HL: Postpartum observation of pelvic tissue damage, *Am J Obstet Gynecol* 45:457, 1943.

Gainey HL: Postpartum observation of pelvic tissue damage: further studies, *Am J Obstet Gynecol* 70:800, 1955.

Gebbie D: Symphysiotomy, *Clin Obstet Gynecol* 9:663, 1982.

Gellman E, Cherry SH, Merkatz IR: *Complications of pregnancy: medical, surgical, gynecologic, psychosocial, and perinatal,* ed 4, Baltimore, 1991, Williams & Wilkins, p 1061.

Goodlin RC: On protection of the maternal perineum during birth, *Obstet Gynecol* 62:393, 1983.

Hartfield VJ: Subcutaneous symphysiotomy—time for a reappraisal? *Aust NZ J Obstet Gynaecol* 13:147, 1973.

Hartfield VJ: Symphysiotomy for shoulder dystocia (letter to the editor), *Am J Obstet Gynecol* 155:228, 1986.

Hauth JC et al: Early repair of an external sphincter ani muscle and rectal mucosal dehiscence, *Obstet Gynecol* 67:806, 1986.

Inmon WB: Mediolateral episiotomy, *South Med J* 53:257, 1960.

Magdi I: Obstetric Injuries of the perineum, *J Obstet Gynaecol Brit Emp* 49:687, 1942.

Menticoglou SM: Symphysiotomy for the trapped aftercoming parts of the breech: a review of the literature and a plea for its use, *Aust NZ J Obstet Gynaecol* 30:1, 1990.

Nichols DH, Randall CL: *Vaginal surgery,* ed 3, Baltimore, 1989, Williams & Wilkins, p 46.

Pritchard JA, MacDonald PC, Gant NF: *Williams obstetrics,* ed 17, Norwalk, CT, 1985, Appleton-Century-Crofts, p 348.

Quilligan EJ, Zuspan FP: *Douglas, Stromm, operative obstetrics,* ed 4, New York, 1982, Appleton-Century-Crofts, p 697.

Rageth JC, Buerklen A, Hirsch HA: Long-term sequelae of episiotomies, *Z Geburtshilfe Perinatol* 193:233, 1989.

Shiono P et al: Midline episiotomies: more harm than good? *Obstet Gynecol* 75:765, 1990.

Snyder RR, Hammond TR, Hankins GDV: Human papillomavirus associated with poor healing of episiotomy repairs, *Obstet Gynecol* 76:664, 1990.

van Roosmalen J: Safe motherhood: cesarean section or symphysiotomy? *Am J Obstet Gynecol* 163:1, 1990.

Willson JR: Prophylactic episiotomy to minimize soft tissue damage, *Infect in Surg* July: 399, 1987.

Yetman TJ, Nolan TE: Vaginal birth after cesarean section: a reappraisal of risk, *Am J Obstet Gynecol* 161:1119, 1989.

Zarate E: Sinfisiotomia subcutanea (Frank), *La Semana Medicale* (Buenos Aires) 23:379, 1916.

Zarate E: *Subcutaneous partial symphysiotomy* (English edition), Buenos Aires, 1955, TICA.

Chapter 65

SAFETY OF FORCEPS VAGINAL DELIVERY AND PRINCIPLES OF APPLICATION

Marshall W. Carpenter

Evidence of the use of obstetric forceps for the delivery of a living child dates to Avicenna (AD 980-1037).[25,37] The modern era of forceps design and application began with the development of the two-part forceps incorporating a cephalic curve by the Chamberlen family in the sixteenth century. By the mid-eighteenth century, use of forceps was commonplace. Over 600 modifications in design have been made since. The more notable design developments include interlocking handles,[13] incorporation of a pelvic curve,[26] a sliding lock in a forceps lacking a pelvic curve for cephalic rotation and correction of asynclitism,[23] and an asymmetric forceps for application in the anterioposterior diameter of the maternal pelvis in cases of arrest of descent in an occiput transverse position (deep transverse arrest).[2] The often colorful history of forceps development is described by Richardson et al,[35] Speert,[37] and Rovinsky.[36]

Before the period of modern obstetrical practice, the primary objective of operative obstetrics was the prevention of significant maternal morbidity and death. Obstetric forceps offered maternal salvage in arrested labor by the prevention of uterine rupture by either destructive delivery of the stillborn infant or, later, by manipulation of the usually live fetus, avoiding the morbidity attendant to the classical vertical cesarean section. The present rationale for the use of forceps in vaginal delivery is substantially different and should be understood in the context of modern operative obstetric care. This has been characterized over the past 40 years by the use of the low transverse uterine incision for abdominal delivery, the application of balanced regional and inhalational anesthesia, the availability of modern blood banking technique, antibiotic ther-

apy, and, finally, by the advent of the means of antepartum fetal surveillance. Consequently, the present rationale for the use of obstetric forceps balances the risk of morbidity from cesarean section and the perinatal risk from the possible attendant delay of delivery on the one hand and, on the other hand, the risk of maternal and perinatal injury that may be associated with their use.

The following examines prior investigations that have been influential and have allowed some insight into the principles of forceps delivery today. The reader is referred to the several excellent texts[9,28,32,33,36] that describe the technique of the application of various forceps, which is not addressed here.

MATERNAL MORBIDITY ASSOCIATED WITH FORCEPS DELIVERY

The use of obstetric forceps has always been recognized as bearing both maternal and fetal risks. The former include vaginal, bladder, urethral, cervical, perineal, and neural injury. The more serious of these attended high forceps application and application before full cervical dilatation, thereby justifying the proscription of both of these practices.

The risk of severe maternal trauma from low forceps delivery is negligible. Most morbidity is limited to perineal lacerations. These occur commonly with spontaneous vaginal delivery of large babies. Because large babies are over-represented among forceps deliveries, several authors have concluded that fetal size rather than the application of forceps determined the risk of perineal trauma. Nyirjesy et al, in an era when 40% of infants were delivered by low forceps, found no increase in the incidence of second- and third-degree perineal lacerations nor of cervical lacerations in women delivered by forceps after the head was visible at the introitus.[31]

Maternal morbidity from mid forceps delivery may be greater than that from outlet forceps or spontaneous vaginal delivery. The overall risk of maternal trauma from mid forceps delivery has been estimated to be between 6% and 40%.[22,38] In an analysis of 1000 consecutive mid forceps deliveries on an obstetric service with a 3.9% section rate and a 1.9% mid forceps rate, Cosgrove noted a 6% rate of third- and fourth-degree perineal lacerations, a 16% incidence of vaginal laceration, a 3% rate of cervical laceration (80% of which were associated with forceps rotation), and a 0.3% rate of bladder injury.[7] Dierker,[10] in an era when mid forceps had fallen to 0.8% of live births, compared rates of maternal trauma with indicated (fetal distress, arrest disorders, and so forth) mid forceps delivery with all other deliveries. Indicated mid forceps deliveries had a rate of cervical laceration three times (12%) and third-degree perineal laceration seven times (46%) that found among the other deliveries. Compared to Nyirjesy's data two decades earlier, there was a similar risk of cervical laceration but a tenfold higher third-degree laceration rate in this later study. Kirk found that maternal complications were not associated with mode of delivery, but had an association with fetal weight and pelvic capacity.[24]

Risks from mid forceps delivery should be contrasted with maternal risks derived from cesarean section. Both Evrard and Cunningham have documented an increased febrile morbidity of 11% to 51% associated with maternal cesarean section.[8,15] Evrard also documented a twenty-six-fold increase in maternal mortality associated with cesarean section.[14]

PERINATAL MORTALITY ASSOCIATED WITH MID FORCEPS

The consideration of the use of forceps requires the appraisal of short- and long-term fetal risks resulting from the use of forceps. Immediate fetal risks attributable to forceps use include facial bruising and lacerations, neural injury (particularly to the facial nerve), skull fracture, cephalohematoma, and intracranial hemorrhage. Neither serious maternal nor fetal injury has been associated with "low" forceps delivery.[17,30,31] Yet forceps application at a higher station than the perineum or their use in rotation of the fetal head has generated much controversy with respect to their causal relationship to injury to mother and child.

Initial studies in the 1950s and 1960s pointed to an increase in perinatal mortality associated with the use of mid forceps. Taylor concluded in 1953 that the morbidity resulting from mid forceps deliveries was so great (a perinatal mortality rate of 25% and additional perinatal morbidity of 30%) that they should be replaced, in most circumstances, by abdominal delivery.[39] However, this perspective was based on only 31 procedures performed over 8 years, without documentation of cases excluded from the report, without enumeration of the nature of the birth inju-

ries or the indications and clinical conditions of their use, and without provision of an appropriate control group. Cosgrove[7] noted that 93% of fetal deaths occurred when mid forceps were applied at 0 to +2 station. However, these authors also noted that a decreased overall perinatal mortality was associated with mid forceps delivery. Nyirjesy[31] showed no association between mid forceps delivery and perinatal mortality. Because perinatal mortality in later series is extremely small, the use of this outcome is no longer helpful in determining perinatal risk and the relative safety of mid forceps.

Uncontrolled studies

Most recent studies have focused on the risk of trauma to the fetus from mid forceps. Harkins noted a 6% morbidity including respiratory depression, cephalohematoma, sepsis, facial palsy, and feeding problems. Weinberg et al[41] examined 1150 mid forceps deliveries and described three cephalohematomas, two transient Erb's palsies, and two facial paralyses. Cooke[6] noted a high rate of fetal trauma in mid forceps deliveries, including cephalohematoma, facial palsy, Erb's palsy, and skull fracture. There were no controls in this study, however. Dunlop[12] examined perinatal outcome in 201 easy, 77 "moderate," and 24 difficult consecutive mid forceps deliveries as defined by the operator's report. He noted two babies with facial paralysis, a stillbirth due to cord prolapse, a neonatal death due to prematurity, and 13 babies with 5-minute Apgar scores less than 7.

Controlled studies

Hepner[19] found a similar rate of facial palsy in forceps compared with nonforceps vaginal delivery with a rate of 6.3% among 159 forceps deliveries versus 6.45% among 716 spontaneous vaginal deliveries. Cooke[6] found fetal morbidity in 14 of 71 mid forceps, 2 of 37 cesarean sections, and 3 of 15 vacuum deliveries performed in cases where there was greater than 2-hour second-stage labor. The morbidity in the first group included fetal asphyxia, laceration, cephalohematoma, meconium aspiration, and sepsis. However, a skull fracture and a cephalohematoma were found in the cesarean section group. The indications for delivery were not indicated in this investigation. However, 90% of the fetal morbidity was found in those mid forceps characterized as being difficult. Dudley[11] compared indicated with elective mid forceps deliveries and found depressed Apgar scores in 3 of 42 in the former group and in only 1 of 75 in the latter. Hughey[20] examined 458 mid forceps deliveries controlled with only 17 abdominal deliveries (selecting criteria not given) and found an "unfavorable fetal outcome" in 30% of the former and 0% of the latter deliveries.

Chiswick and James[5] used spontaneous vaginal deliveries as controls and found an increased perinatal mortality, increased fetal trauma, an increase in the delay in respirations, and abnormal neurologic behavior. However, when these authors controlled for the indication for mid forceps and excluded cases with fetal distress, only "abnormal neurological behavior" (defined as "apathy or irritability as determined by the resident physician") remained as an association with forceps delivery.

Dierker[10] examined 176 mid forceps deliveries performed in the course of 21,414 deliveries (0.8%). Mid forceps deliveries were compared to deliveries at cesarean section for the same indications. There was no difference in perinatal morbidity when dystocia was the indication for delivery. In fact, there was a higher rate of depressed 5-minute Apgar scores among infants delivered abdominally compared to those delivered by mid forceps. The incidence shoulder dystocia, seventh nerve and brachioplexus palsy, seizures, and central nervous system (CNS) hemorrhage was not higher in the mid forceps group compared to the other groups. This is an important study because it compares mid forceps delivery with cesarean section stratified by indication for operative delivery and avoids the comparison with spontaneous vaginal delivery, which, for reasons of pelvic dystocia or fetal distress, does not represent a comparable group. The study is also done during a period when fetal monitoring was routine. Therefore, it is more relevant to present practice than data derived from the pre-fetal monitoring era.

Gilstrap et al[18] examined the incidence of neonatal acidosis among 177 elective low forceps, 293 indicated low forceps and 234 indicated mid forceps deliveries and 303 spontaneous and 111 abdominal deliveries. No association of fetal acid–base status or trauma with mode of delivery was found except that cephalohematoma was more prevalent after spontaneous delivery. Traub et al[40] also compared neonatal outcome from successful Kielland rotation deliveries with those from cesarean sections in second-stage labor and failed Kielland applications. There were no differences in Apgar score, need for resuscitation, jaundice, and abnormal neurologic behavior.[40]

LONG-TERM PEDIATRIC MORBIDITY ASSOCIATED WITH MID FORCEPS DELIVERY

The effect of antecedent mid forceps delivery on late pediatric morbidity is difficult to identify because the relationship is confounded by the conditions and management of labor and delivery that may independently affect subsequent development. Additionally, factors that may affect immediate outcome independent of forceps use, such as fetal asphyxia, may significantly bias follow-up surveillance and the interpretation of later measures of neurologic, intellectual, and school performance. Earlier studies (summarized by Richardson et al[35]) offer a mixed verdict on the existence of an association of mid forceps delivery with subsequent neurodevelopmental impairment. These studies provided inadequate controls for the clinical conditions that resulted in mid forceps use, however.

Little contemporary data are available relating prospectively ascertained delivery events (including cord blood studies) to subsequent long-term morbidity with respect to mode of delivery. Studies, now approximately 15 years

old, are based on data from the National Collaborative Perinatal Project, which is based on 55,000 deliveries in 12 medical centers during the 1950s. Broman et al[4] analyzed development in 4-year-old offspring from the entire project and found that children delivered by mid forceps had an increased IQ compared to those delivered spontaneously. Birthweight was not controlled for in their analysis.

Friedman[17] examined data in 26,760 births from the National Collaborative Perinatal Project. Among 155 patients with labor "dystocia" weighing 2500 g or more, those delivered by mid forceps had lower IQs (99.8) than those delivered with low forceps (103) or born spontaneously (106). Missing from both studies were control groups of children born by cesarean section. In fact, in Friedman's study there was a similar decrease in IQ scores in each group if an arrest disorder was present as compared to prolonged latent phase or protraction disorders. This suggests that labor abnormalities or other clinical circumstances associated with the use of mid forceps may, independent of forceps use, result in neonatal morbidity.

Whether arrest disorders per se increase the risk for abnormal neonatal outcome has been controversial. Friedman[16] noted increased perinatal mortality and an increased risk of low Apgar scores with arrest disorders. Bottoms,[3] however, in an era characterized by the general availability of electronic fetal monitoring and scalp blood pH sampling, noted no increase in perinatal morbidity with arrest disorders irrespective of route of delivery. These data suggest that increased perinatal mortality or morbidity associated with arrest disorders may be found only in the group that has inadequate assessment of fetal respiratory status during labor.

It is also troublesome that in Friedman's study[17] the group that were delivered vaginally had a higher IQ than the project as a whole. Those in the experimental group had a lower IQ than the whole group who had mid forceps deliveries. Also, there was no control over gender, socio-economic status, and mother's education, all of which have been found to have an impact on IQ tests. McBride et al[27] compared 175 mid forceps with 188 low forceps to 101 elective cesarean sections and 207 spontaneous deliveries. These authors found that family background was a more powerful predictor of IQ than method of delivery. These data suggest that other factors than just mid forceps delivery per se have a powerful impact on IQ and other integrative neurologic test outcomes.

A follow-up study of all 62 males delivered by forceps and all 38 males delivered by vacuum extraction in a Norwegian hospital examined intelligence scores from military draft examinations at 18 years of age.[29] Those delivered by Kielland forceps had a higher mean intelligence score, whereas the vacuum group's score reflected the national average.

Probably the best lesson to be learned from these studies is that all the data sets lose their relevancy as the practice of perinatal care changes and improves. If the impact of changes in technology and care are substantial, it must be accounted for in contemporary data to examine the effects of therapeutic interventions, including forceps delivery.

INDICATIONS FOR MID OR LOW FORCEPS DELIVERY

Indications for mid or low forceps delivery are either fetal or maternal (see box at right). Operative vaginal delivery provides an advantage to the fetus if the mechanics of pelvic passage are improved by application of forceps or if the timing of delivery is thereby improved. Consequently, malposition of the fetal cranium with respect to the maternal pelvis (asynclitism, persistent occiput posterior, or deep transverse arrest identified during a prolonged second stage of labor) suggests forceps delivery. Some authors have opined that mechanical forces on the premature fetal brain are reduced if forceps are used during delivery of the fetal head, thereby reducing risk of intracranial injury. Also, hemorrhage from an acute abruptio placentae or vasa previa or signs of fetal asphyxia from a prolapsed umbilical cord or other causes in the context of second-stage labor may indicate immediate forceps delivery if this can be accomplished more rapidly than abdominal delivery. However, prolongation of second-stage labor per se is not a medical indication for forceps delivery. The ability to carry out fetal heart rate monitoring and fetal scalp blood pH measurement allows the identification of the fetus unable to tolerate labor. In labors, during which a healthy fetus is confirmed, either other indications may be found to justify forceps delivery, or appropriate decision making in the context of an elective forceps delivery should take place.

Maternal indications for operative vaginal delivery are several. Many maternal diseases provide absolute or relative contraindications to prolonged, intense effort, which characterizes second-stage labor. These include pulmonary insufficiency, cardiac lesions that result in a low, fixed cardiac output, and neuromuscular diseases such as myasthenia gravis. Maternal propulsive effort may be lacking or significantly diminished in paraplegia, neuromuscular diseases, with asthma or other pulmonary disease, or with dense regional anesthesia. If these deficits result in an arrest in second-stage labor, forceps delivery may be justified. Several maternal conditions may contradict prolonged periods of bearing down that reflexly occurs as the fetal head descends through the true pelvis. These include intracranial arteriovenous malformations, Marfan's syndrome with aortic dilatation, prior pneumothorax, and retinal detachment. Also, maternal obstetric sepsis, hemorrhage, deceminated intravascular coagulation, cardiac or pulmonary dysfunction or seizures may make forceps delivery preferable to waiting through a long second stage of labor.

THE CHANGING CLASSIFICATION OF FORCEPS DELIVERIES

Much of the controversy attending the issue of maternal and fetal safety of forceps deliveries has resulted from in-

---

> **Indications for forceps delivery**
>
> *Fetal indications*
>
> 1. Signs of fetal asphyxia or hemorrhage
> 2. Malposition of fetal head associated with prolongation of second stage of labor
> 3. Low fetal weight associated with prematurity
> 4. Prolapse of umbilical cord
>
> *Maternal indications*
>
> 1. Maternal cardiac, pulmonary, or neuromuscular disease contradicting prolonged second-stage labor
> 2. Failed maternal propulsive efforts associated with prolonged second-stage labor
> 3. Maternal conditions contradicting prolonged maternal propulsive efforts
> 4. Maternal sepsis, hemorrhage, disseminated intravascular coagulation (DIC), cardiopulmonary dysfunction, seizures

---

adequate definitions of the fetal station, position, and other conditions in which the deliveries were carried out, from small sample size, and from inadequate or inappropriate selection of control subjects. In part, as a response to the first source of confusion, recent reclassifications of types of forceps deliveries have been attempted. The American College of Obstetricians and Gynecologists (ACOG) Committee Opinion Number 71 is a recent attempt to create criteria for forceps application in cephalic presentations.[1] These new criteria (Table 65-1) have been chosen in response to the above investigations, which have suggested that station gained by the fetal skull and the degree to which rotation is required both influence the maternal and perinatal safety of the operation. These criteria should provide the basis for a more accurate comparison of the effect of various forceps applications on perinatal outcome.

CRITERIA FOR FORCEPS APPLICATION

An indication for forceps use is not an adequate justification for their application. Only when forceps can be applied and traction can be employed safely can their use be defended. In fact, conclusions about the safety of mid forceps use are limited primarily by the retrospective nature of most investigations. The result of the retrospective character of data retrieval in most studies is that neither the rationale for the choice of patient nor the conditions under which the forceps were applied can be adequately described or controlled for in analysis.

Consequently, much of the existing consensus about safety guidelines in the application is based on clinical experience and opinion rather than prospective controlled observational cohort studies or randomized trials in the present era. Nevertheless, there is fairly uniform agreement about the criteria for forceps application, which must be addressed before their use (see box at right). The operator or his or her assistant should be experienced and

Table 65-1. Changes in classification of forceps deliveries according to station and rotation

Type of procedure	1980 criteria*	1989 criteria†
Outlet	1. Not included in classification	1. Scalp visible at the introitus without separating labia 2. Fetal skull at pelvic floor 3. Sagittal suture within 45 degrees of anteroposterior position 4. Fetal head at or on perineum
Low	1. Fetal head at the perineal floor 2. Sagittal suture in the anteroposterior diameter	1. Leading point of fetal head ≥+2 station but not on pelvic floor 2. Group a: rotation ≤45 degrees Group b: rotation >45 degrees
Low mid forceps	1. Biparietal diameter at or below the ischial spines 2. Leading point of fetal head within finger breadth of perineum between contractions 3. Head fills hollow of sacrum	1. Not included in classification
Mid forceps	1. Lowermost part of fetal skull reaches or is below the ischial spines 2. Head fills hollow of sacrum	1. Station above +2 station 2. Head engaged
High	1. Leading point of fetal head above level of ischial spines	1. Not included in classification

*Pritchard-MacDonald: *Williams Obstetrics,* ed 16, Norwalk, Conn, 1980, Appleton-Century-Crofts.
†ACOG Committee Opinion: *Obstetric forceps,* no. 71, August 1989.

Criteria for forceps application in cephalic presentation

Appropriately experienced and skilled operator
Ruptured membranes
Fully dilated cervix
Empty bladder
Effective anesthesia
Pelvic architecture assessment
Estimated fetal weight less than 4000 to 4500 g
Engaged fetal head
Known fetal presentation
Known fetal cranial position

---

skilled in the use of the particular forceps employed. The membranes should be ruptured, the cervix fully dilated, and the bladder demonstrated to be empty by use of an urethral catheter. Appropriate local or regional anesthesia is required, but not for the application of forceps, which should, when properly used, provoke minimal discomfort. Rather, anesthesia allows the cooperation of the patient during forceps rotation and traction, thereby minimizing the risk of vaginal and perineal trauma. The pelvic architecture should be assessed by palpation before application for forceps. The fetal size estimate should be less than 4000 to 4500 g, although published opinion differs on this limit. The fetal presenting part and its position (occipital

position, asynclitism, deflexion, and so forth) should be known.

The fetal biparietal diameter should be engaged in the pelvic inlet. This is assessed, usually, by noting the descent of the leading point of the fetal head relative to the clinically determined midplane of the pelvis (defined by the two ischial spines and the inferior aspect of the symphysis pubis). Molding of the fetal cranium, especially in a persistent occiput posterior position may falsely suggest fetal cranial engagement. Generally, engagement of the fetal head can be confirmed in these cases by noting filling of the sacral hollow by the fetal cranium.

REFERENCES

1. ACOG Committee Opinion: *Obstetric forceps,* no. 71, August 1989.
2. Barton LG, Caldwell VOE, Studdifnd WE Sr: A new obstetric forceps, *Am J Obstet Gynecol* 15:16, 1928.
3. Bottoms SF, Hirsch VJ, Sokol RJ: Medical management of arrest disorders of labor: a current overview, *Am J Obstet Gynecol.* 156:935-939, 1987.
4. Broman SH, Nichols PL, Kennedy WA: *Preschool IQ: prenatal and early development correlates,* Hillsdale, NJ, 1975, Erlbaum Associates.
5. Chiswick ML, James DK: Kielland's forceps: association with neonatal morbidity and mortality, *Br Med J* 1:7, 1979.
6. Cooke WA: Evaluation of the mid-forceps delivery, *Am J Obstet Gynecol* 99:327, 1967.
7. Cosgrove RA, Weaver OS: An analysis of 1000 consecutive midforceps operations, *Am J Obstet Gynecol* 73:556, 1957.
8. Cunningham FG et al: Infectious morbidity following cesarean sections, *Obstet Gynecol* 52:656, 1978.
9. Dennen's forceps deliveries, ed 3, Philadelphia, 1989, FA Davis Co.

10. Dierker LJ et al: The midforceps: maternal and neonatal outcomes, *Am J Obstet Gynecol* 152:176-183, 1985.

11. Dudley AG, Markham SM, McNie TMG: Elective versus indicated midforceps delivery, *Obstet Gynecol* 37:19, 1971.

12. Dunlap DL: Midforceps operations at the University of Alberta Hospital (1965-1967), *Am J Obstet Gynecol* 103:471, 1969.

13. Duser: 1734.

14. Evrard FR, Gold EM: Cesarean section and maternal mortality in Rhode Island: incidence and risk factors, 1965-1975, *Obstet Gynecol* 50:133, 1977.

15. Evrard JR, Gold EM, Cahill T: Cesarean section—a contemporary assessment, *J Reprod Med* 24:147, 1980.

16. Friedman: *Clin Obstet Gynecol* 16:172, 1973.

17. Friedman EA, Sachtleben MR, Bresky PA: Dysfunctional labor XII. Long-term effects on infant, *Am J Obstet Gynecol* 127:779, 1977.

18. Gilstrap LC et al: Neonatal acidosis and method of delivery, *Obstet Gynecol* 63:681, 1984.

19. Hepner WR: Some observations on facial paresis in the newborn infant: etiology and incidence, *Pediatrics* 8:494, 1951.

20. Hughey MJ, McElin TW, Lussky R: Forceps operation in perspective. I. Midforceps rotation operations, *J Reprod Med* 20:253, 1978.

21. Kadar N: Do midforceps deliveries really impair subsequent intelligence quotient scores? *Am J Obstet Gynecol* 153:233-235, 1985.

22. Kane HF, Parker HP: An analysis of 569 forceps operations, *Am J Obstet Gynecol* 31:657, 1936.

23. Kielland: 1916.

24. Kirk RF, Keumholz BA, Callagan DA: The midforceps operation prognosis based on pelvic capacity and fetal weight, *Obstet Gynecol* 15:447, 1960.

25. Laufe LE: *Obstetric forceps,* New York, 1968, Hoeber Medical Division, Harper & Row.

26. Leviet: 1744.

27. Mcbride WG et al: Method of delivery and developmental outcome at five years of age, *Med J Aust* 1:301, 1979.

28. Myerscough PR: *Munro Kerr's operative obstetrics,* ed 10, 1982, Bailliere Tindall.

29. Nilsen ST: Boys born by forceps and vacuum extraction examined at 18 years of age, *Acta Obstet Gynecol Scand* 63:549-554, 1984.

30. Niswander KR, Gordon M: Safety of the low-forceps operation, *Am J Obstet Gynecol* 117:619, 1973.

31. Nyirjesy L, Pierce WF: Perinatal mortality and maternal morbidity in spontaneous and forceps vaginal deliveries. *Am J Obstet Gynecol* 89:568, 1964.

32. O'Grady P: *Modern instrumental delivery,* 1988, Williams & Wilkins.

33. Oxoron: *Human labor and birth,* ed 4, 1980, Appleton-Century-Crofts.

34. Pritchard-MacDonald: *Williams Obstetrics,* ed 16, 1980, Appleton-Century-Crofts.

35. Richardson DA, Evans MI, Cibils LA: Midforceps delivery: a critical review, *Am J Obstet Gynecol* 145:621, 1983.

36. Rovinsky JJ: *Forceps delivery.* In Iffy L, Lancet M, Kessler I, editors: *Operative perinatology invasive obstetric techniques,* New York, 1984, Macmillan.

37. Speert H: The obstetric forceps, *Clin Obstet Gynecol* 3:761, 1960.

38. Steer CM: Effect of type of delivery on future child bearing, *Am J Obstet Gynecol* 60:395, 1950.

39. Taylor ES: Can mid-forceps operations be eliminated? *Obstet Gynecol* 2:302, 1953.

40. Traub AI et al: A continuing use of Kielland's forceps? *Br J Obstet Gynaecol* 91:894, 1984.

41. Weinberg A: Present status of forceps operations, *Am J Surg* 83:143, 1952.

Chapter 66

ADVANCED ECTOPIC PREGNANCY

John R. Oliver
Richard H. Paul

Often, the terms *ectopic pregnancy* and *abdominal pregnancy* are used interchangeably. In this chapter, however, ectopic pregnancy is a general term used to encompass any pregnancy that develops after implantation of the blastocyst anywhere other than the endometrium lining the uterine cavity. On the other hand, abdominal pregnancy is a form of ectopic pregnancy, specifically, pregnancy that develops in any portion of the peritoneal cavity. Extrauterine is synonymous with ectopic.

In 1903, J. Whitridge Williams in the first edition of Williams' *Obstetrics*[38] wrote regarding ectopic pregnancy that, "the operation is still one of the most dangerous which the gynaecologist is called upon to perform." This statement is still true today. Many of the controversies with regard to the management of advanced ectopic pregnancies that existed in 1903 still exist today. Fortunately, this condition is very rare. The key to optimizing maternal morbidity and mortality is the early detection and treatment of all extrauterine gestations. With the advent of ultrasound and other methods of early pregnancy detection, the incidence of advanced ectopic pregnancies should decline. When an advanced ectopic pregnancy is encountered, the surgeon is faced with decisions regarding the timing of delivery and the management of the placenta, which may have a significant impact on both maternal and fetal outcomes.

Reported maternal mortality for ectopic pregnancies in 1886 was about 89%. By 1933, mortality had dropped to 32%. As blood transfusions became available, mortality continued to decrease and by 1948 was 15%. As antibiotics became available to treat the severe infections that occurred in these patients, mortality declined even further. By 1957, mortality for patients with abdominal pregnancies was 2%.[17]

There are six types of extrauterine pregnancy:

1. *Primary ovarian pregnancy:* The incidence of ovarian pregnancies has been reported to be about 1 per 6970 deliveries or 0.7 to 1.0 per 100 ectopic gestations.[28] Spiegelberg in 1878 defined ovarian pregnancies using four strict pathologic criteria that are still in use today: (1) The tube on the affected side must be intact, (2) the gestational site must occupy the normal position of the ovary, (3) the gestational site must be connected to the uterus by the ovarian ligament, and (4) histologically identified ovarian tissue must be identified in the sac wall.[2,13,28] Usually, ovarian pregnancies are identified in the first trimester.[20,39] King[20] described one study of ovarian pregnancy in which 60 cases were diagnosed in the first trimester, 11 cases in the second trimester, and 11 in the third trimester. Seven third-trimester fetuses were stillborn, and four were living (two with gross deformities).

2. *Primary abdominal pregnancy:* This type of ectopic pregnancy is very rare with only 24 cases of primary abdominal pregnancy reported in 1968.[12] Studdiford in 1942 gave a strict definition for primary abdominal pregnancy that is still used today: (1) Normal tubes and ovaries, (2) no evidence of uteroplacental fistula, and (3) the pregnancy is implanted only on the peritoneal surface and early enough in the gestation to eliminate the possibility of secondary implantation of a ruptured tubal gestation.[2,5,12,28] This third definition makes it impossible to distinguish advanced primary abdominal pregnancies from advanced secondary ectopic pregnancies because the placental implantation usually involves the uterus tubes and ovaries to some extent in both types of abdominal pregnancies. The majority of pri-

mary abdominal pregnancies are implanted in and around the cul-de-sac.[12,14] However, in a recent case at Los Angeles County-University of Southern California (USC) Medical Center, a primary abdominal pregnancy was implanted on the infundibulopelvic ligament about 6 cm above the ovary. This points out the need for careful, detailed abdominal exploration when performing laparoscopy or celiotomy on a patient for a suspected ectopic gestation, especially if the tubes appear to be normal. Perhaps the most unusual locations for implantation of a primary abdominal pregnancy are the liver and spleen. Six cases of splenic and four of hepatic pregnancies have been reported.*

3. *Secondary abdominal pregnancy:* This is the most common type of advanced ectopic pregnancy.[2,20,28] The gestation ruptures through the tube, aborts out of the end of the tube, or ruptures through a previous uterine scar retaining enough placental function to continue supporting the pregnancy. The reported incidence ranges from 1 per 782 deliveries[40] to 1 per 50,820 deliveries.[35] Recent reports have ranged from 1 per 7,095[10] deliveries to 1 per 10,200.[29] Approximately 1 in 70 ectopic pregnancies are abdominal, although this incidence may be higher in regions where early prenatal care is not obtained.[1,10] In advanced extrauterine pregnancies due to tubal rupture or abortion, the placenta usually involves portions of the uterus, tubes, ovaries, cul-de-sac, broad ligament, and other pelvic structures. In advanced extrauterine pregnancies due to rupture of a uterine scar, the placenta might remain completely inside the uterine cavity.[8]

4. *Primary tubal pregnancy:* Most tubal pregnancies rupture in the first trimester. However, King[20] reported five cases that had advanced to term. All of these were located in the interstitial portion of the tube. Interstitial pregnancies are often incorrectly called cornual pregnancies.

5. *Intraligamentous pregnancy:* This occurs when a tubal pregnancy ruptures into the broad ligament with the pregnancy growing between the anterior and posterior leaves of the broad ligament. The incidence is reported to range from 1 per 49,765 to 1 per 183,900 pregnancies.[2] As the pregnancy progresses, the placenta may erode and invade the sigmoid colon, rectum, vagina, bladder, and anterior abdominal wall. The placenta may form fistulous tracts with these structures. King[20] describes an example with the patient having passed per rectum what she thought was chicken bone. Careful examination reveale_ that this was a fetal femur. At surgery, the patient was found to have an intraligamentous pregnancy demise that had formed an amniocolic fistula.

6. *Rudimentary horn (cornual) pregnancy:* This type of pregnancy is very rare. The reported incidence is 1 per 100,000 pregnancies.[2] It occurs when the pregnancy

develops in the noncommunicating horn of a bicornuate uterus. For this to occur, the spermatozoa or the fertilized ovum must migrate transperitoneally. O'Leary[26] reported that only 11% of cornual pregnancies went to term, whereas 89% ruptured before term. Only seven surviving infants have been reported.[2] A recently managed pregnancy of this type at Los Angeles County-USC Medical Center occurred in the noncommunicating right horn with its tube and ovary located adjacent to the cecum. This case emphasizes the need for careful exploration when performing laparoscopy or exploratory celiotomy for a suspected ectopic gestation.

The risk for advanced extrauterine gestations depends on the type and site of implantation. Primary abdominal pregnancy is so rare that cases probably represent spontaneous incidents and no significant identifiable risk factors are present. Primary tubal pregnancies, secondary abdominal pregnancies, and intraligamentous pregnancies present similar historic risk factors. A history of salpingitis or prior tubal surgery is an identifiable risk factor.[5,8,10] Low gravidity as well as long-standing secondary infertility are additional risk factors. These women tend to be older, with an average age of about 30 years.* Primary ovarian pregnancy has risk factors similar to tubal pregnancies in general, except that women with ovarian pregnancies are less likely to have a history of infertility.[13] Obviously, for a rudimentary horn pregnancy to occur, a woman must have a bicornuate uterus with a noncommunicating horn.

It should be emphasized that hysterectomy does not preclude the occurrence of an extrauterine pregnancy. There have been ectopic pregnancies reported that have occurred years after hysterectomy.[23,25]

DIAGNOSIS

Much progress has been made in the diagnosis of extrauterine and abdominal pregnancies. The first report of an ectopic pregnancy was made by Albucasis (936-1013), a famous Arabic physician who lived in Cordova, Spain. One of his patients developed an abscess near the umbilicus and started to pass bones from the wound. Realizing that the abdomen does not contain bones, he explored the wound, removed many more bones, and made the diagnosis of ectopic pregnancy. The patient survived. Most ectopic pregnancies were diagnosed in this manner or at autopsy until the late nineteenth century when reports began to appear describing successful delivery of live fetuses with survival of the mother.[20] The most important contribution decreasing maternal morbidity and mortality from ectopic pregnancies was early diagnosis and treatment.[2,14] Patients with an ectopic pregnancy that can be treated in the first trimester or early second trimester should have morbidity and mortality similar to the more common tubal gestation.

Patient history

The history can be helpful in establishing the diagnosis of ectopic pregnancy. King[20] described five stages through which abdominal pregnancies pass:

1. The symptoms of early pregnancy. These are similar to the symptoms of a normal pregnancy (missed menses, morning sickness, breast tenderness, and so forth).
2. A phase of threatened or actual rupture.[2,5,11,20,40] King was able to obtain a history of onset of severe low abdominal pain in 6 of the 12 patients he reported. The onset of pain occurred between 6 and 16 weeks of gestation. The patient may have some vaginal bleeding at this time.[20] An excellent example of this stage was recently encountered at the Los Angeles County-USC Medical Center. The patient presented 9 weeks after her last normal menstrual period with symptoms of low abdominal pain and vaginal bleeding. She had developed sudden onset of lower abdominal pain 2 weeks earlier and was seen by a physician who told her she had an infection and prescribed antibiotics. She sought further treatment at our facility because her symptoms had not resolved. Her urine pregnancy test was positive, and ultrasonography revealed a fetus with cardiac motion in the left adnexa. At exploratory celiotomy, the patient was found to have a ruptured left fallopian tube with implantation of the gestational sac on the posterior leaf of the left broad ligament. A left salpingo-oophorectomy was performed, and the patient's postoperative course was uncomplicated. As exemplified by this case, morbidity and mortality can be minimized if operative intervention occurs during these first two phases.
3. Symptoms of continuation of the pregnancy. King[20] points out that most patients have sought treatment before this stage occurs. Delke et al[10] reported that 8 out of the 10 patients in their study had care before 16 weeks of gestation. Patients in this phase may complain of abdominal pain and painful fetal movements. They also frequently have nausea and vomiting that persist throughout pregnancy. The patient notes increasing abdominal size as expected with a normal intrauterine pregnancy. Patients with abdominal pregnancies do not experience Braxton Hicks contractions. They may complain that the fetus is unusually high in the abdomen.*
4. A history of false labor. King obtained this history in 6 of his 12 patients, with passage of a decidual cast in 5 of the 6. This false labor usually occurs near term, and fetal movements may decrease or cease.[3,7,11,20,40]
5. Later clinical manifestations. Should the fetus die, the patient has a decrease in abdominal size, but she may continue to have abdominal pain and gastrointestinal complaints (frequent bowel movements, tenesmus). Eventually, there is a return of menses, and the patient might conceive again.[7,20,40]

*References 2, 3, 7, 8, 11, 20, 28, 29, 40.

Physical examination

The physical examination can be helpful in making the diagnosis of ectopic pregnancy. It would seem that the fetal parts should be easily palpable in an abdominal pregnancy. This, however, is rarely the case. The presence of easily palpable fetal parts should raise one's suspicion about the possibility of an ectopic pregnancy, but the absence of this finding in no way excludes the diagnosis. If a mass is palpable separate from the uterus, ectopic pregnancy should be suspected. The fetus is often in an abnormal presentation. If fetal heart tones are auscultated, they may be unusually loud. If the patient has a fetal demise, the diagnosis of ectopic pregnancy should be considered. The cervix may be unusually high and displaced either laterally or anteriorly. It is usually closed and uneffaced. Historically, patients with intraligamentous pregnancies often form fistulous tracts with the rectum, vagina, bladder, or abdominal wall through which they pass the fetal bones and tissue.*

Diagnostic tests

Several tests can aid in the diagnosis of ectopic pregnancy. The patient usually has a positive urine or serum beta-human chorionic gonadotropin (HCG) unless the fetus has been dead for a long time. About 70% of the patients are anemic.[28] There has been a report of an ectopic pregnancy with maternal serum alpha-fetoprotein values in a range usually only seen with hepatomas and endodermal sinus tumors (greater than 20 multiples of the median). Future studies may reveal if this is a useful test.[36] Culdocentesis and paracentesis have been used to diagnose ectopic pregnancies. However, a negative test does not rule out the diagnosis.[15] Measuring the uterine depth with a sound should be avoided. If the diagnosis is incorrect, the membranes may be ruptured with potential harm of the fetus. A case has been reported in which the uterus was perforated into the sac of an abdominal pregnancy with the subsequent development of amnionitis in the pregnancy.[7] Failure of the cervix to dilate in response to oxytocin or prostaglandins is also suggestive of ectopic pregnancy.†

Historically, several radiographic tests have aided in the diagnosis of ectopic pregnancy. The simplest is the abdominal x-ray, which Hibbard[15] did not find to be very useful. However, Clark and Guy[8] recommended an anteroposterior view and an upright lateral view. The anteroposterior view might show the maternal bowel intimately associated with the fetus. The pathognomonic x-ray finding for ectopic pregnancy is presence of the fetal skull behind the anterior border of the maternal spine. Hysterosalpingography has been used to confirm the diagnosis of ectopic pregnancy. However, it should be used with great caution and is largely supplanted by ultrasonography.‡

Ultrasound is extremely valuable in diagnosing extrau-

*References 2, 3, 5, 7, 8, 10, 11, 15, 20, 28, 29, 40.
†References 2, 3, 5, 10, 11, 28, 29, 40.
‡References 3, 5, 7, 8, 10, 11, 20, 28, 29, 40.

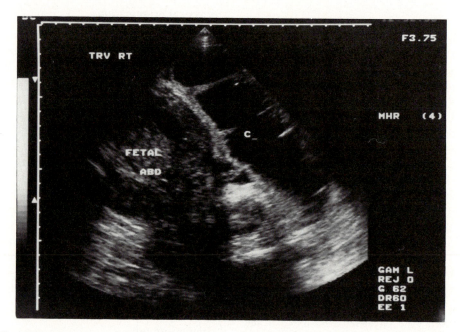

Fig. 66-1. Ultrasound of an abdominal pregnancy, which demonstrates the fetal abdomen in close proximity to the maternal colon *(C)* with no intervening uterus. (Courtesy Richard E. Frates, M.D.)

terine pregnancy, particularly early in the gestation. The diagnosis becomes more difficult as the pregnancy progresses. Delke et al[10] reported that of five patients with ectopic pregnancies undergoing ultrasound evaluation, two were misdiagnosed as having intrauterine pregnancies (at 28 weeks and 39 weeks). Important ultrasound findings include (1) a small uterus with minimal internal uterine echoes, (2) the fetal head and body located outside of the uterus, (3) an ectopic placenta, (4) the fetal body and maternal bladder not separated by uterine wall, and (5) the identification of fetal parts close to the maternal abdominal wall (Fig. 66-1).[2,28] Magnetic resonance imaging (MRI) may also prove to be of benefit in diagnosing ectopic pregnancy.[34]

Management

There has been much controversy with regard to the optimal management of ectopic pregnancies. First, there has been controversy regarding the timing of delivery. Should the patient have surgery as soon as the ectopic pregnancy is diagnosed, or should the delivery be delayed if the fetus is close to viability to improve its chances for survival? Additional controversy has focused on the management of the placenta. Should the placenta be removed or left in the abdomen at the time of surgery? If the placenta is left in the abdomen, should the patient in contemporary practice receive methotrexate to accelerate the resorption of the fetal placenta? These issues may be addressed by reviewing the history of advanced extrauterine pregnancies.

The first successful delivery of an ectopic pregnancy occurred in Sigerhausen, Switzerland, in 1500. Elizabeth

Nufer, whose husband Jacob was the local swine-gelder, had been in labor for several days. She was attended by 13 midwives and several lithotomists without success. In an act of desperation, her husband decided to deliver the baby abdominally. After receiving permission from the local magistrate, he placed his wife on a table and after one stroke with his knife delivered a healthy, crying infant. He closed the incision, and Elizabeth recovered. She subsequently had five intrauterine pregnancies including twins. The first reported successful delivery of an ectopic pregnancy in the United States was in 1759 by a surgeon in New York, Dr. John Bard.[20] Turnbul in London in 1791 was the first to recommend leaving the placenta in situ at the time of surgery for an abdominal pregnancy.[17]

In 1888, Dr. Lawson Tait published his *Lectures on Ectopic Pregnancy and Pelvic Hematocele,* which firmly established surgery as the treatment of choice for ectopic gestations. He was one of the first to recognize the management dilemma of the placenta in advanced ectopic pregnancy and described this as the "crux of the discussion." He left the placenta in situ in three and removed the placenta in two with all patients surviving.[20]

The surgical management of an advanced extrauterine gestation is determined somewhat by the type of gestation. Patients with a pregnancy in a rudimentary horn require resection of the horn along with the tube on that side. Obviously, if the fetus is potentially viable, it should be delivered before resection of the rudimentary horn. Otherwise, it may be left intact to prevent unnecessary blood loss. If the patient does not desire fertility and is hemodynamically stable, a total hysterectomy may be considered. These patients should have an intravenous pyelogram performed postoperatively because of the association of renal anomalies with this condition.[2,28]

Similar recommendations can be made for advanced interstitial pregnancies. If the fetus is viable, it should be removed through a large linear salpingostomy incision before performing the salpingectomy. Otherwise, the fetus and tube may be removed intact. In the patient who does not desire future fertility, a total abdominal hysterectomy with salpingo-oophorectomy of the involved side is probably the safest procedure. This might be best performed by first performing a salpingo-oophorectomy followed by hysterectomy with the interstitial pregnancy out of the way.

Ovarian pregnancies often are associated with hemoperitoneum at the time of diagnosis because of the vascularity of the ovary. Hallatt reported that 81% of the ovarian pregnancies in his series had more than 500 ml of hemoperitoneum at the time of surgery. Most cases, if diagnosed early, can be treated by performing ovarian wedge resection or ovarian cystectomy.[13] Williams et al[39] reported the delivery of a live infant from a term ovarian pregnancy.

Intraligamentous pregnancies are much more likely to progress to term than ovarian, or interstitial pregnancies. Paterson and Grant[27] reviewed 48 cases and found that there were 23 live births (with 6 subsequent neonatal deaths). It is unusual to have significant hemoperitoneum with an intraligamentous pregnancy because the pregnancy is confined between the leaves of the broad ligament. There are often adhesions between the omentum and bowel and the superior aspect of the gestational sac. The placenta is usually not a problem in intraligamentous pregnancies. It should be removed at the time of surgery.[2,28] Paterson and Grant[27] reported a single maternal death in their series of 48 cases. This occurred as a result of hemorrhage in a patient whose placenta was not removed. It should be remembered that intraligamentous pregnancies are the most likely to form fistulous tracts between the gestational sac and the rectum, vagina, bladder, or abdominal wall especially when the demise has been present for some time.[20] In such patients, Gastrografin enemas and cystograms before surgery may identify fistulous tracts to the bladder, rectum, or abdominal wall. These patients also benefit from bowel preparation with laxatives and antibiotics should rectal or sigmoid resection be necessary. Obviously, these recommendations apply only to the patient who is stable before surgery.

Of all advanced extrauterine pregnancies, the abdominal pregnancy is by far the most complex and challenging to manage. It is also the most controversial. The patient is at significant risk for developing massive hemorrhage at the time of surgery and is also at risk for developing hemoperitoneum before delivery. This raises an important management question: Should an abdominal pregnancy be delivered as soon as it is diagnosed, or should delivery be delayed to enhance fetal viability?

If the pregnancy is diagnosed in the first trimester or the early second trimester, surgery should be performed without delay. In more advanced abdominal gestations, with patient consent and willingness to spend the remainder of her pregnancy in the hospital, it is not unreasonable to delay delivery for several reasons: (1) The fetus may achieve relative maturity. (2) The patient can be delivered immediately should bleeding or deterioration occur. (3) There is no evidence that the risk of massive hemorrhage at the time of delivery is increased by expectant management. In patients who elect expectant management, one should obtain serial hemoglobin or hematocrit determinations. There must always be at least four units of blood typed and cross-matched. Symptoms of false labor should lead to delivery because false labor historically has often preceded fetal death. Fetal surveillance should be done twice weekly. Amniocentesis has unwittingly been performed in abdominal pregnancies, but the risk of rupture of the gestational sac contraindicates the use of this procedure. Ultrasound dating criteria for fetal maturity are likely to be of questionable value because the fetus' growth is probably retarded. Therefore, relative maturity has to be assessed, and the fetus is delivered as deemed maturationally appropriate.

In abdominal pregnancy with a fetal demise, there is also controversy about the timing of delivery. Waiting has been advocated because the placenta is easier to remove at the time of surgery and would less likely be associated with massive hemorrhage. It should be noted, however, that massive hemorrhage has been reported as long as 7 years after the demise occurred.[7,17] Therefore, delay is probably of little value in such patients. If delay is necessary for any reason, the patient must be observed in the hospital. Serial hematocrits must be performed, and blood must be immediately available.

In patients presenting initially in shock with evidence of massive hemoperitoneum, surgery must occur as soon as possible. In elective, planned procedures, the patient should have a bowel preparation with laxatives and antibiotics. Although bowel injury rarely occurs in patients with abdominal pregnancy, when it does, the results can be devastating.[15] All patients should have antibiotic prophylaxis and postoperative therapy because of the significant risk of infection, particularly when the placenta is not removed.

At the time of surgery, adhesions between the gestational sac omentum and abdominal wall are likely to be encountered.[20] Once the infant has been delivered, the surgeon is faced with the next management decision. Should the placenta be removed or left inside the abdomen at the time of delivery? Often, the placenta separates on its own after delivery of the fetus, thus answering the question for the surgeon. A surgeon who decides to remove the placenta should be prepared for massive hemorrhage. If possible, the blood supply to the placenta should be identified and ligated before removal of the placenta. The surgeon should not hesitate to perform salpingo-oophorectomy or even hysterectomy if this is necessary to control the bleeding, particularly if the patient does not desire future fertility. If the blood supply to the placenta involves a loop of bowel, the surgeon should be prepared to resect a portion of the bowel to control the bleeding. Control of bleeding from arteries and veins is vital; however, the surgeon should expect some continued arteriolar and capillary oozing from the placental bed. Many surgeons feel uncomfortable in closing the abdomen without achieving total hemostasis. However, strict hemostasis is often not possible in these patients. Application of coagulation-enhancing agents such as Gelfoam, Avitene, or Surgicell alone or in combination with gauze packing to tamponade the placental bed has been used to control the bleeding.[3,8,15,40] An umbrella packing brought out through the posterior cul-de-sac has not been reported but might be useful for controlling blood loss.

Sandberg and Pelligra[32] reported on the use of the medical antigravity suit or Medical Anti-Shock Trousers (MAST; David Clark Co., Inc., Worcester, Massachusetts) to control hemorrhage in three patients with abdominal pregnancies. Two of the patients underwent surgery at 30 weeks gestation, and the third patient underwent surgery at about 20 weeks gestation. In two of the patients, complete spontaneous separation of the placenta occurred at the time of surgery. One of the patients had partial separation of the placenta at the time of surgery. In all three patients, complete hemostasis was not possible at the time of surgery. These patients were placed in a MAST suit at a pressure of 20 to 30 mm Hg. All the patients showed a dramatic improvement in their hemodynamic status while the MAST suits were in place. Two of the patients remained intubated while the suits were inflated. One of the patients required reexploration to ligate a bleeding artery 2 days later. This emphasizes the importance of initial control of arterial bleeding at the time of surgery because the medical antigravity suit cannot effectively control arterial bleeding once the suit is deflated. Another patient required reexploration on the fourteenth day to remove the placental tissue that had been left behind at the initial surgery. Other complications encountered included adult respiratory distress in one patient, the formation blisters on the thighs of one patient, and the inadvertent ligation of a ureter at the initial surgery that resulted in a subsequent nephrectomy for a nonfunctioning kidney.

If after surgery the patient continues to demonstrate evidence of intraperitoneal bleeding, angiographic arterial embolization can be considered to control hemorrhage. Kivikoski et al[21] reported a case in which this was done with satisfactory results. If successful, this procedure may avoid a second celiotomy.

Our opinion supports initial placental removal at the time of surgery. Review of the literature clearly demonstrates that both maternal morbidity and mortality are reduced when the placenta is initially removed. Hibbard[15] reported 23 cases of abdominal pregnancy that occurred at Los Angeles County-USC Medical Center. The placenta was left in situ in four of these patients, all of whom de-

veloped subsequent significant infections. Only 2 of the remaining 19 patients in whom the placenta was removed developed infections. Furthermore, there was no evidence that leaving the placenta in situ reduced the need for blood replacement. The four patients in whom the placenta was left in situ received an average of 2835 ml (range of 2000 to 5000 ml) of blood. The remaining 19 patients in whom the placenta was removed received an average of 2132 ml (range of 500 to 5,000 ml) of blood. The one death occurred in a patient in whom the placenta had implanted into the wall of the rectosigmoid colon. The placenta spontaneously separated at the time of surgery and a 2-cm perforation of the rectosigmoid colon was identified and repaired. This patient died 4 days later from sepsis due to overwhelming fecal peritonitis despite antibiotic therapy.

Hreshchyshyn et al[17] reviewed the world literature and found 101 cases of abdominal pregnancy between 1950 and 1957. The placenta was completely removed in 65 patients and partially removed in another 7 patients. Only 17.5% of these patients required more than 20 days of hospitalization. In the remaining 29 patients, the placenta was left in situ, and 47.5% of these patients required hospitalization for more than 20 days. The majority of the patients in whom the placenta was left in situ had symptoms of abdominal pain, intermittent fever, and general malaise for months to years. These patients often required repeat celiotomies to remove the placenta because of hemorrhage, persistent pain, intermittent partial intestinal obstruction, and to drain abscesses. Two maternal deaths occurred in cases with the placenta left in situ. A higher mortality rate when the placenta was left in situ had previously been reported. Beacham et al[3] in their review of the literature and their personal experience at Charity Hospital in New Orleans found a higher maternal mortality when the placenta was left in situ. The usual causes of death in all patients with abdominal pregnancies include hemorrhage, sepsis, renal failure, and chronic blood loss.[5]

Although the literature and our opinion suggest initial removal, we cannot say that the placenta should never be left in situ. One can imagine a case of an unstable patient in whom the blood loss expected from attempted removal of the placenta would result in an exsanguination death on the operating table. Obviously, clinical judgment is required on the part of the surgeon to determine if the patient falls into this category. It should be noted, however, that when the placenta is left in situ it can spontaneously separate postoperatively, resulting in massive hemorrhage. We recommend that when the placenta is left in situ, the placenta should be drained of as much blood as possible and the umbilical cord should be cut at its insertion site into the placenta. Plans should be made to reoperate under stable conditions to remove the placenta to minimize the morbidity anticipated in these patients. Ultrasound and gallium scanning have been used to follow resorption of the placenta when it was left in the abdomen after celiotomy.[4,31,34]

In 1965, Hreshchyshyn et al[18] reported the first case in

which methotrexate was given to a patient in whom the placenta was left in situ after removal of a abdominal pregnancy. The goal was to promote destruction of the trophoblast resulting in a decrease in lifespan and vascularity for the placenta. The patient was followed with serial human chorionic gonadotropin (HCG) titers until they returned to a nonpregnant value. Four months later, the patient was reexplored, and the placenta was removed with minimal blood loss. Three more case reports followed involving four patients in whom the placenta was left in situ and methotrexate was given.[22,33,37] Methotrexate was given to one of these patients even though the HCG titers had returned to a nonpregnant value. It should be stressed that two of these patients were reexplored to remove the placenta; the two not reexplored had palpable masses at the time of examination 1 year after therapy. The value of methotrexate was questioned in one of the reports.[37]

Not all of the reports of methotrexate use have satisfactory outcomes. Rahman et al[29] in Saudi Arabia reported on ten cases of abdominal pregnancy. In three of the patients, the placenta was removed. The placenta was partially removed in one patient, and in six the placenta was left in situ. Five of the six were treated with methotrexate. Two of these patients died from sepsis. These authors rightfully questioned the efficacy of methotrexate. Methotrexate does cause myelosuppression and may pose unacceptable risks in patients prone to sepsis.

There is little information in the literature regarding fetal outcome. Perinatal mortality as high as 95% has been reported.[3] However, these rates can be deceiving because many times intervention occurred as soon as the diagnosis of abdominal pregnancy was made. This resulted in the delivery of many infants who subsequently died from the effects of preterm delivery. Survival as high as 50% to 70% is reported when only viable infants are considered. The most thorough discussion of fetal outcome is by Tan and Wee in Singapore. They evaluated eight cases of abdominal pregnancy that occurred between 1958 and 1968. Three of the fetuses were stillborn. Of the five living infants, one had microcephaly and died at 8 months of age. Three of the infants had deformities, which were felt to be pressure deformities resulting from oligohydramnios. These deformities included talipes equinovarus; webbing of the neck, elbows, and knees; torticollis; and facial asymmetry (Fig. 66-2). The incidence of such deformities has been reported to be about 20% to 40%.[28,29,35] All four of the surviving infants showed normal development.[35]

In cases of demise, the fetus is initially macerated like any other demise. It will gradually become mummified or develop into adipocere (degeneration into a greasy yellow substance). Fetuses retained in the abdomen for years become lithopedions (calcified). King[20] describes three types of lithopedions:

1. Lithotecnon (43%) is a calcified fetus only.
2. Lithokelyphopedion (31%) is a calcified fetus, membranes and placenta.
3. Lithokelyphos (26%) is calcification of the membranes only. The fetus becomes mummified or skeletonized.

In conclusion, the operation for abdominal pregnancies is "still one of the most dangerous which the gynaecologist is called upon to perform."[38] The key to preventing significant maternal morbidity and mortality is early diagnosis and treatment. Patients with advanced abdominal pregnancies may be closely monitored in the hospital until 36 to 38 weeks in an effort to optimize fetal outcome. At the time of surgery, every effort should be made to remove the placenta and control the arterial bleeding. Continued bleeding may respond to treatment with the MAST suit or angiographic embolization. If the placenta is initially left in situ, it should be removed after the patient becomes stable. There is minimal evidence to support actively the use of methotrexate in abdominal pregnancies. Living infants delivered near term can usually be expected to have normal development. There are no easy cookbook recipes for management of advanced extrauterine pregnancies. Sound clinical judgment must be applied to each case.

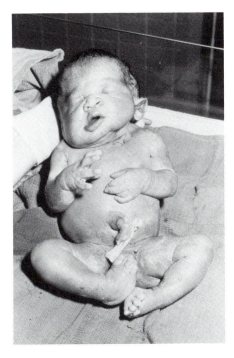

Fig. 66-2. Newborn infant of an advanced abdominal pregnancy. Notice the facial asymmetry and the limb deformities.

REFERENCES

1. Alto W: Is there a greater incidence of abdominal pregnancy in developing countries? Report of four cases, *Med J Aust* 151(7):412, 1989.
2. Bayless RB: Nontubal ectopic pregnancy, *Clin Obstet Gynecol* 30(1):81, 1968.
3. Beacham WD et al: Abdominal pregnancy at Charity Hospital in New Orleans, *Am J Obstet Gynecol* 84(10):1257, 1962.
4. Belfar HL, Kurtz AB, Wapner RJ: Long-term follow-up after removal of an abdominal pregnancy: Ultrasound evaluation of the involuting placenta, *J Ultrasound Med* 5(9):521, 1986.

5. Bendvold E, Raabe N: Abdominal pregnancy: A case report and brief review of the literature, *Acta Obstet Gynecol Scand* 62:377, 1983.

6. Caruso V, Hall WHJ: Primary abdominal pregnancy in the spleen: A case report, *Pathology* 16:93, 1984.

7. Charlewood GP, Culiner A: Advanced extrauterine pregnancy: Fifty two cases, *J Obstet Gynaecol Br Emp* 62:555, 1955.

8. Clark JFJ, Guy RS: Abdominal pregnancy, *Am J Obstet Gynecol* 96(4):511, 1966.

9. Cohen JM et al: Imaging of a viable full-term abdominal pregnancy, *AJR* 145:407, 1985.

10. Delke I, Veridiano NP, Tancer ML: Abdominal pregnancy: Review of current management an addition of 10 cases, *Obstet Gynecol* 60(2):200, 1982.

11. Foster HW, Moore DT: Abdominal pregnancy: Report of 12 cases, *Obstet Gynecol* 30(2):249, 1967.

12. Friedrich EG Jr, Rankin CA Jr: Primary pelvic peritoneal pregnancy, *Obstet Gynecol* 31(5):649, 1968.

13. Hallatt JG: Primary ovarian pregnancy: A report of 25 cases, *Am J Obstet Gynecol* 143:55, 1982.

14. Hallatt JG, Grove JA: Abdominal pregnancy: A study of twenty-one consecutive cases, *Am J Obstet Gynecol* 152(4):444, 1985.

15. Hibbard LT: The management of secondary abdominal pregnancy, *Am J Obstet Gynecol* 74(3):543, 1957.

16. Hietala SO, Andersson M, Emdin SO: Ectopic pregnancy in the liver: Report of a case and angiographic findings, *Acta Chir Scand* 149:633, 1983.

17. Hreshchyshyn MM, Bogen B, Loughran CH: What is the actual present-day management of the placenta in late abdominal pregnancy? Analysis of 101 cases, *Am J Obstet Gynecol* 81(2):302, 1961.

18. Hreshchyshyn MM, Naples JD, Randall CL: Amethopterin in abdominal pregnancy, *Am J Obstet Gynecol* 93(2);286, 1965.

19. Huber DE, Martin SD, Orlay G: A case report of splenic pregnancy, *Aust NZ J Surg* 54:81, 1984.

20. King G: Advanced extrauterine pregnancy, *Am J Obstet Gynecol* 67(4):712, 1954.

21. Kivikoski AI et al: Angiographic arterial embolization to control hemorrhage in abdominal pregnancy: A case report, *Obstet Gynecol* 71(3):456, 1988.

22. Lathrop JC, Bowles GE: Methotrexate in abdominal pregnancy: Report of a case, *Obstet Gynecol* 32(1):81, 1968.

23. Meizner I et al: Abdominal pregnancy following hysterectomy, *Isr J Med Sci* 19:283, 1983.

24. Mitchell RW, Teare AJ: Primary hepatic pregnancy: A case report and review, *S Afr Med J* 65:220, 1984.

25. Niebyl JR: Pregnancy following total hysterectomy, *Am J Obstet Gynecol* 119:512, 1974.

26. O'Leary IL, O'Leary JA: Rudimentary horn pregnancy, *Obstet Gynecol* 22:371, 1963.

27. Paterson WG, Grant KA: Advanced intraligamentous pregnancy: Report of a case, review of the literature and a discussion of the biological implications. *Obstet Gynecol Surv* 30:715, 1975.

28. Peterson HB: Extratubal pregnancies: Diagnosis and treatment, *J Reprod Med* 31(2):108, 1986.

29. Rahman MS et al: Advanced abdominal pregnancy—Observations in 10 cases, *Obstet Gynecol* 59(3):366, 1982.

30. Reddy KSP, Modgill VK: Intraperitoneal bleeding due to primary splenic pregnancy, *Br J Surg* 70:564, 1983.

31. Rettenmaier MA et al: The use of gallium scanning and determination of human chorionic gonadotropin to evaluate resorption of an abdominal placenta, *Am J Obstet Gynecol* 146(4):471, 1983.

32. Sandberg EC, Pelligra R: The medical antigravity suit for management of surgically uncontrollable bleeding associated with abdominal pregnancy, *Am J Obstet Gynecol* 146(5):519, 1983.

33. St. Clair JT, Wheeler DA, Fish SA: Methotrexate in abdominal pregnancy, *JAMA* 208(3):529, 1969.

34. Spanta R et al: Abdominal pregnancy: Magnetic resonance identification with ultrasonographic follow-up of placental involution, *Am J Obstet Gynecol* 157(4):887, 1987.

35. Tan KL, Wee JH: The paediatric aspects of advanced abdominal pregnancy, *J Obstet Gynecol Br Cwlth* 76:1021, 1969.

36. Tromans PM et al: Abdominal pregnancy associated with an extremely elevated serum alphafetoprotein: Case report, *Br J Obstet Gynaecol* 91:296, 1984.

37. Weinberg PC, Pauerstein CJ: Methotrexate and the abdominal placenta, *Obstet Gynecol* 33(6):837, 1969.

38. Williams JW: *Obstetrics*, Norwalk, 1903, Appleton.

39. Williams PC, Malvar PC, Kraft JR: Term ovarian pregnancy with delivery of a live female infant, *Am J Obstet Gynecol* 142:589, 1982.

40. Zuspan FP, Quilligan EJ, Rosenblum JM: Abdominal pregnancy, *Am J Obstet Gynecol* 74(2):259, 1957.

Chapter 67

CESAREAN SECTION

Raphael Durfee

Cesarean Section—"That smash and grab raid"!

LAWSON TAIT

Removal of a child from the body of its mother by an abdominal incision was the first incision of the abdominal wall in history; the only other so-called major surgery from prehistoric and ancient times was trepanation. Early abdominal deliveries were done for religious or mythologic reasons and almost invariably on dead or agonal women. It is possible that the concept of abdominal delivery was introduced by one or both of two means; one, the discovery of a live unborn fetus at the time of animal sacrifice; or, two, the deliberate or accidental evacuation of a human pregnant uterus by a sword of a conqueror. There are some factual records of cesarean section in legal documents, mythologic poems and prose, and written legends of several peoples.

The earliest record of performance of cesarean section in ancient times is from Sumer, where it was reported that the operation was performed on slaves in the second millennium BC. In a cuneiform written tablet, which was a legal document also from Sumer, there was reference to precedence of inheritance. This was to remain with the first child born by normal vaginal delivery rather than by abdominal means. A statement was made that "the child was pulled out," an inference that this was from the abdomen and not the pelvis. There is another illustration from Sumer of a seal on which there are depicted surgical instruments and a figure stated to be a person who delivered children. These artifacts establish the fact that the operation was done earlier than 2000 BC.

The use of cesarean was involved in innumerable problems not all medical. Laws were created to control its use, and medical discussions and confrontations have continued to the present day. The procedure developed very slowly and painfully, and it was not until the later part of the 1700s but especially in the 1800s that its use became accelerated because of the advances in anesthesia, hemostasis, antisepsis, and the application of uterine suture.

In the early to middle 1900s, the operation became acceptable and has been so ever since. The cesarean operation is so widely used today that it may well be a matter of abuse. Modern challenges to 24% to 26% cesarean section rates may bring about an effort to reduce this operative furor!

ORIGIN OF THE TERM: CESAREAN SECTION

"That operation is called Cesarean by which any way is opened for the child than that destined for it by nature" (L. Baudelocque, 1790). Vaginal cesarean was not a term preferred by Williams, who stated in 1903 that "vaginal hysterotomy" is correct. The term cesarean section should not be applied to a laparotomy for abdominal pregnancy. Confusion about this matter led to false reports of early successful cesarean operations. Many texts that deal with the cesarean section present misinformation about the origin of the term. Etymologists are fascinated with this term because it is a unique word formation. There is a persistent repetition of error by historians who have simply followed their predecessors' statements for information without the authenticity of such material. *Cesarean section* is a phrase that uses two words with similar meanings. This is defined as a pleonasm. The derivation of each of these words is complex because of the ancient historic references to the matter.

Pliny, who some refer to as a "lying historian," was in error when he stated that some of the Caesars, Julius in particular, were delivered by an abdominal incision. *"Caesar,"* derived from the Latin verb *caedo*—to cut. The name was assumed by several Roman emperors so that ultimately the word *Caesar* became a synonym for *imperator*—emperor. *Caesus*—cut, from the same Latin root, *caedo*—to cut, may have been the origin of the term *Caesar*. Festus stated that those persons delivered by abdominal incision were called *"caesones."* Isidorus of Seville firmly and erroneously established the relationship between the operation and the person Julius Caesar and referred to such persons as *"Caesares."* According to Pundel, Rousset, author of the first text on the subject, became confused with Pliny's Latin text; de Chauliac and Roesslin both perpetuated the story, and it has been repeated in print as late as March 1985. The myth was preserved through the Middle Ages in many manuscripts and in the 1300s in *The Faits des Romains* and only in the first printed version of *The Twelve Caesars* written in the second century AD by Suetonius and printed in 1506. This text includes a woodblock print that purports to be the first picturization of a cesarean section, but this is an error (Fig. 67-1).

More probable origins for this elusive pleonasm are derived from some form of Latin words meaning to cut or to kill. The Latin verb *caedo, caedere, cecidi, caesum* means to cut or to kill. An adverb from *caesium,* from *caedo,* means with cutting. There is no identifiable word *caesones* or *caesares* in Cassell's Latin Dictionary.

Another possibility is that the term arose from the *Lex Regia* or *Lex Caesara* (The King's Law), ascribed to Numa Pompilius in 716 BC.

There is also some confusion about the second part of the phrase, which probably arose from the verb *seco, secare, secui, sectum,* meaning to cut. The noun for this is *sectio* (f).

It is stated that Rousset used "section" in his first book but in the author's copy are the words "enfantement cesarien." Bauhin, about a year later, published Rousset's book, and in the index of that text are listed the following: *Caesarea sectio,* page 163; *Casaream sectione,* page 188; *Caesarei partus,* page 3; and *Partus Caesarei definito,* page 1. Guillemeau in 1598 used the phrase "cesarienne section" thus discrediting the point that this combination was first used by Raynaud in 1737 and as is indicated it was Bauhin who first used the combination.

Modern terminology is an Anglicized version of the French spelling *cesarienne;* thus we are provided with the words cesarean section, which eliminates the confusion over Caesar and this operation for all time.

CESAREAN SECTION FROM 2000 BC TO THE EIGHTEENTH CENTURY

There are few records of the cesarean operation from 120 AD to 1115. Gestein von Gerstadt was delivered by postmortem cesarean in 1115. The earliest confirmed delivery of a living child by the abdominal route was Gorgias of Leontine, Sicily, in 508 BC. Gebhardt, the Bishop of Constance, was delivered in 919 AD; Count Lingsow, known as Ingentius the Abbey of Saint Gall was delivered in 949. Both were postmortem deliveries of premature infants, and the children were placed in the abdomen of a newly killed pig because the pig fat stayed warm and moist for a longer time than any other animal. These served as excellent rural incubators.

de Castro reported the birth of Sancho Garcia or Mayer of Navarre who was delivered by a brave strong Spanish nobleman when Sancho's mother was killed by the Saracens; he saw the child's arm had protruded through the wound in the mother's abdomen, pulled it free, and it lived and breathed at once. The nobleman educated his little miracle who later became the King of Navarre in the twelfth century.

One of the more controversial royal deliveries concerned Edward VII, son of Henry VIII and Jane Seymour. Because of a failed labor, the king was questioned as to whether such an operation should be done because it was usually fatal. He presumably replied, "Proceed, for it is easier to find another wife than a son and heir." There were several songs and ballads about this sung in the pubs and ale houses in London in 1537, which mirrored popular opinion, but apparently was not true.

Cesarean for the live woman

The first unquestioned successful cesarean section for a live woman performed by a physician was by Trautmann and Seest in 1610 AD in Wittenberg. From this time the operation was used rarely, but, as time passed, its use increased in spite of high maternal mortality. Cesarean section for the live woman is truly an operation of the late 1800s and the twentieth century. When the first cesarean section was done for a live woman is unknown, unless the statement in the Sushruta Samhita is acceptable. The reference to cesarean section for women slaves in Sumer probably involved live women to ensure live children, otherwise why sacrifice the slave? Reference was made to Hua T'o, a great surgeon in the Han Dynasty in China, who purportedly performed cesarean section in 120 AD. This operation was mentioned again in the Tang Dynasty and was a postmortem procedure.

deLee wrote that in the Talmud, *Kareth Habetan* was the term used for midline delivery postmortem and *Jotze Dophan* was the term used for delivery through a flank incision for live women. In the Misnah of the Talmud, there are several references to cesarean section; the Talmud is not a medical manuscript but rather an interpretation of the rules and customs of human conduct. For many years, the records have been debated by scholarly rabbis, and it is apparent that the operation was performed on both live and dead women. For example, it is stated that a woman who delivered by cesarean section did not have to undergo the postpartum purification rites usually associated with vaginal delivery. These rites were very specific and strictly enforced. If the operation had not been done, there would have been no reason to include it in the Talmud. There are no other reports of the operation for a live woman that can be verified with certainty until about 1500 AD.

The cesarean birth of Julius Caesar caught the fancy of the miniature printers of the 1300s particularly in a text entitled *The Faits des Romains* where there is a print in an edition in the late 1200s of the birth of Caesar that because of the valid date establishes this as the first illustration of cesarean section in the literature. There were several other prints in later editions of *The Faits des Romains* in the 1300s.

In 1500, there was the famous case of the pig gelder, Nufer, who recorded that he performed a cesarean section for his wife who had an apparent unsolvable labor condition; she and the child survived. This documented operation is the first proven case known to have been successfully done for a live woman not by a physician.

van Roonhuyze, 1663, one of the more famous of the early surgeons who performed operations on women, produced a text that illustrated the technique of cesarean for live women. He illustrated a postmortem laparotomy for a ruptured uterus. Scultetus in 1666 published the first text on this matter in detail (Fig. 67-1), in which he described a cesarean for a live woman.

CLASSICAL, FUNDAL, CORPOREAL CESAREAN SECTION

In the eighteenth century, the cesarean operation had undergone many influences affecting its use. These varied from absolute forbiddance to use for religious purposes (e.g., baptism of the child as fostered by the strong Christian church). The majority of physicians involved in obstetric care were strongly opposed to the employment of cesarean except in the obviously moribund or recently expired woman. The few who advocated the use of cesarean when the mother was alive and in good condition were severely castigated by their peers but, nevertheless, persisted in their attitude. Of these pioneers, Levret and Baudelocque in France were the leading protagonists for cesarean and each realized that a contracted pelvis beyond a certain reasonable point indicated one of two possibilities for evacuation of the fetus; embryotomy with decapitation or cesarean section. Opinions concerning destruction of a living child in utero were as divided and as vehement as attitudes in contemporary times are about abortion. Severe

desperation brought about unusual solutions; one of the most unique was the operation of symphysiotomy proposed by Sigault in 1768. This procedure, which is still used in modern times in Third World countries, permitted an increase in size of the inner bony pelvis but was accompanied by several risks, one of the worst of which was the compromise in the ability of the patient to walk normally after delivery. There were decades of public and private discussions about these matters, especially in England. However, Hull was a strong advocate of cesarean in uterine rupture and even in cases of abdominal pregnancy if the child was alive. He received some support from Smellie, but, in general, the operation was not popular in England. One occurrence in the eighteenth century could have decreased the high mortality of the cesarean operation and that was the introduction of suture placement in the uterine wound by Lebas in 1769. Strangely, this concept was not used for nearly 70 years!

Most of the first cesarean sections in England and America were done by midwives, charlatans, or women themselves. Bennett presumably was the first to do cesarean section in the United States in 1794 in Virginia. King in 1975 disproved the Bennett priority very conclusively and stated unequivocally that the first cesarean section in the United States was done by Richmond in 1827 in Newton, Ohio. In the nineteenth century, obstetrics, gynecology, and general surgery all began to proliferate and prosper because of the solution to the three absolute requirements for successful surgery. These were and still remain: control of bleeding—hemostasis; control of pain—anesthesia; control of infection—asepsis.

In spite of the amazing difference produced by the three solutions to surgical problems, mortality for the cesarean operation was inordinately high. This was not due as much to the inherent possible fatality of the procedure as to the timing of the operation. The search continued for an im-

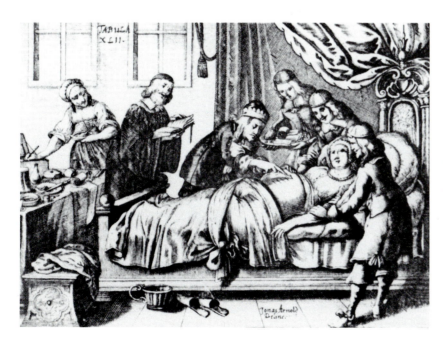

Fig. 67-1. Cesarean section for a live woman. (From *Armamentarium chirurgicum*, Frankfurt, 1666, J Scultetus. In Ricci V: *The development of gynecological surgery and instruments*, Philadelphia, 1949, Blakiston, Co.)

proved operation, and one of the first and most dramatic was the postdelivery hysterectomy created by Porro in 1876. The idea for such a procedure was originated by Porro's predecessors and actually a cesarean delivery was followed by a hysterectomy for hemorrhage from myomas by Storer in Boston in 1869. Unfortunately, Storer's patient died; otherwise, he would have had the famous name that accompanies cesarean hysterectomy. There were several additions to the Porro operation, but the fact that it was considered mutilating made its use as a routine procedure unacceptable to many operators. The last hysterectomy with abdominal exteriorization of the cervical stump after cesarean section was done by Davis in the 1920s in the United States. Modifications of abdominal and uterine incisions were abundant in these years; packs and drains both cervical and through the wounds were also numerous and not very successful. In 1817, Barlow was the second to suture the uterine wound in England. Very few followed this addition except in the United States where it was frequently successfully used. The next important contribution to the cesarean operation occurred in 1882.

Uterine suture was a very controversial matter in 1882 when two German surgeons, Kehrer and Sanger, introduced adequate and entirely useful methods for closure of the uterine wound. The Sanger operation closed the uterine fundus, and the Kehrer operation closed a transverse lower uterine segment. If Kehrer had been more aggressive in reporting his procedure, the lower uterine segment operation probably would have been used 40 years before it was recognized. Various modifications of the Sanger closure have been introduced to contemporary times. Management of the abdominal wound is another area in which many modifications have been introduced.

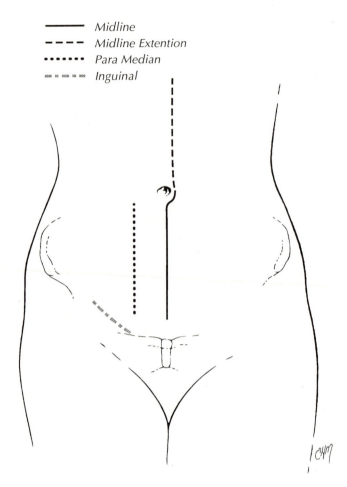

— Midline
--- Midline Extension
····· Para Median
⚬⚬ ⚬ ⚬⚬ ⚬ ⚬⚬ Inguinal

Fig. 67-2. Vertical and oblique abdominal incisions. Adapted from several illustrations.

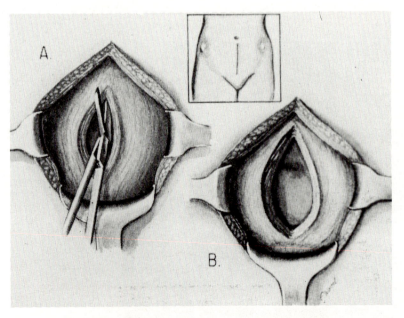

Fig. 67-3. Vertical uterine incision. (From Bonica J: *Principles and practice of obstetric analgesia and anesthesia,* vol. 2, Philadelphia, 1967, FA Davis.)

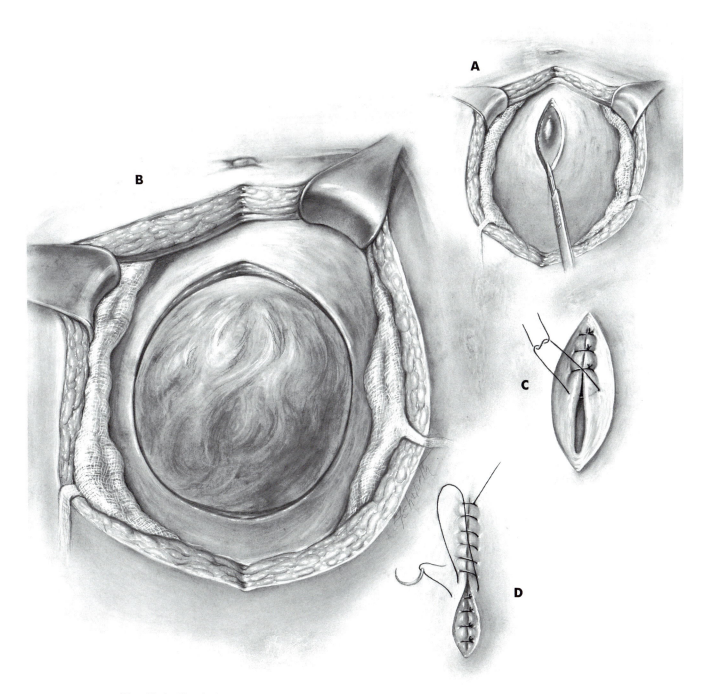

Fig. 67-4. Classical cesarean section: breech delivery. **A,** Vertical incision. **B,** Fetal head delivery. **C,** First layer closure. **D,** Second layer closure. (From Moir J: *Munro Kerr's operative obstetrics,* 6th ed., London, 1956, Bailliere, Tindall and Cox.)

Fundal cesarean has an important but limited use in modern obstetrics. Another procedure closely associated with an incision in the uterine fundus is one used in certain cases of indicated late abortion or early prematurity and is referred to as abdominal hysterotomy.

Another answer to the problem of the high mortality and morbidity of fundal cesarean was to pursue a method of entering the uterine cavity extraperitoneally. These are discussed in the section entitled "Extraperitoneal Cesarean Section." Still another solution was the use of an intraperitoneal lower uterine segment incision.

Fundal or classical technique

Fundal cesarean is performed usually with a vertical abdominal incision (Fig. 67-2). The peritoneum is opened vertically, and a vertical incision is made usually in the upper middle of the anterior uterine fundus. This is done with a scalpel and completed with a blunt-nosed scissors (Fig. 67-3). The delivery is accomplished with the placenta and membranes (Fig. 67-4), the uterine cavity is explored, and the wound is closed with either 00 chromic catgut or polyglycolic acid suture by the surgeon's choice. A running stitch or interrupted figure-of-eight sutures may be placed in the deep portion of the wound (Fig. 67-5). The endometrial layer should not be included in the suture and, if possible, a two-suture closure of the uterine wall is desirable if the tissues can be well approximated and hemostasis is complete. The serosa may be inverted or closed with a fine 5-0 or 6-0 suture to reduce the number of postoperative adhesions (Fig. 67-6).

Fundal cesarean is indicated in most premature births in which the fetus is at risk, all premature abnormal presentations especially breech, in cases of high anterior implantation of the placenta, term gestation transverse presentation with the back anterior or down, in many anomalies such as fused twins, in cases in which an anterior myoma blocks the low uterine segment, and in cases of extreme emergency when time is all important and the delivery must be accomplished as soon as possible. Fundal cesarean should probably be repeated if a second or more pregnancies ensue, but a low-segment operation has been suggested. Vaginal delivery in a subsequent pregnancy is a controversial point; if certain prerequisites are present, normal onset of labor may be carefully followed and, if the previous indication is absent, the presentation is vertex, and labor progress rapidly, then normal vaginal delivery can be accomplished. The risk of uterine rupture, however, is higher than with the low-segment operation, and many are of the opinion that labor should not be induced in these patients.

More blood may be lost with a fundal cesarean, hemostasis may be difficult, and the wound may be difficult to close (Fig. 67-7). Regional anesthesia probably cannot be

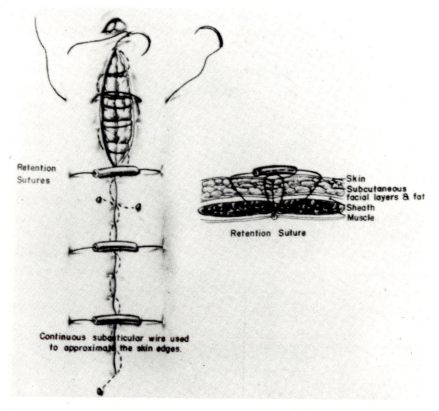

Fig. 67-5. Classical cesarean section: uterine incision closure with retention sutures. (From Riva H: *Transabdominal techniques in cesarean section: clinical obstetrics and gynecology,* vol. 2, New York, 1959, Harper.)

used, and the uterus should be eventrated postdelivery to facilitate wound closure.

Abdominal hysterotomy has a limited use, but it should be used in cases of indicated late abortion that cannot be delivered vaginally. The procedure is a miniclassical operation and is best conducted under general anesthesia. A vertical incision is usually made, but a high transverse in the interest of aesthetics can be done. The uterine incision is vertical but can be lower than for fundal cesarean. Management is much the same, but usually the patient can be dismissed early (Figs. 67-8 and 67-9).

LOW-SEGMENT CESAREAN SECTION

Not until 1805 was there any reference to a low uterine approach for delivery; deLee gives Osiander credit for being the originator of the low-segment cesarean. Osiander decided that there were many advantages to making an incision in the dependent portion of the uterus and performed such an operation, according to deLee, in 1915.

Kehrer outlined and illustrated the technique for low-segment cesarean section with a plan for closure of the uterine wound in 1882. Pfannenstiel failed in 1908 to perform an extraperitoneal dissection; he then cut the uterine

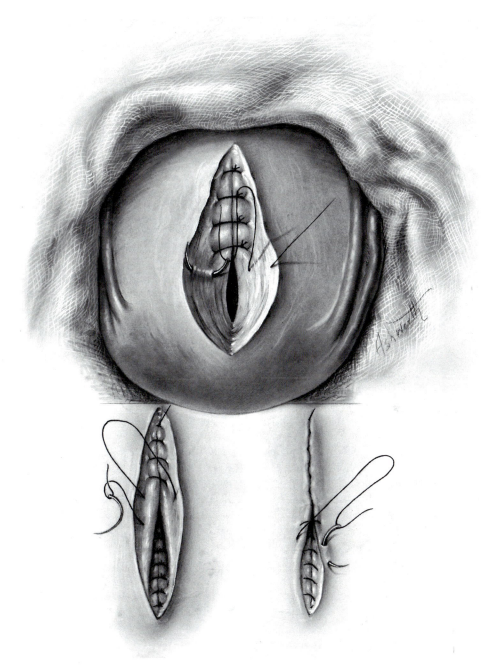

Fig. 67-6. Classical cesarean section: uterine incision closure. Three layers: interrupted; continuous; subserosal or through and through.

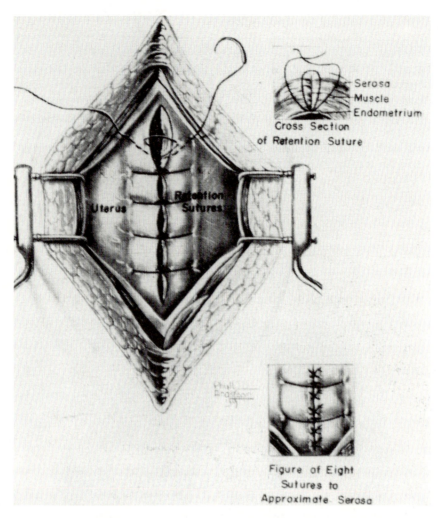

Fig. 67-7. Classical cesarean section: abdominal incision closure with retention sutures. (From Riva H: *Transabdominal techniques in cesarean section: clinical obstetrics and gynecology,* vol 2, New York, 1959, Harper.)

serosa as in hysterectomy, advanced the bladder downward, entered the low portion of the uterus, and successfully delivered a child. He resurrected the transperitoneal, easy low uterine segment cesarean section in this manner. By 1912, he reported 33 cases with only one maternal death! Opitz in 1911 used a vertical abdominal incision, dissected the uterine serosa, used a vertical low-segment incision, and closed the serosa carefully over the sutured uterine incision. Kronig, a year later, introduced another precursor to the modern operation: he raised the bladder serosa high over the tip of the closed vertical uterine incision, which theoretically sealed the uterine cavity completely. However, a failed procedure done in this manner that resulted in mortality from peritonitis induced Beck and deLee in 1919 to perform what came to be known as a "two-flap" closure for low-segment operations.

de Lee and Cornell reported 145 cases in 1922 with remarkable results. The procedure became popular in England where St. G. Wilson in 1931 proposed the use of a *transverse incision* in the low uterine wall and declared

that this brought about a return to a single-flap closure of the uterine wound and furthermore the entire incision was in the lowest part of the uterus or even in the dilated cervix. This was the first known transverse uterine incision since Kehrer. Wilson was supported in his contention by Kerr who curved the incision downward for some time but eventually curved it upward as did all his colleagues.

There are several small detailed modifications of this operation, but only one is of true importance. It is now recognized that peritoneal cuts or separations heal from inside the area, which eliminates the serosal closure after low-segment cesarean. This means that the bladder will not be used to cover the surgical area but will remain in its normal anatomical area. This should prevent dense adhesion formation between the bladder and the anterior uterine wall and help eliminate that problem at the time of hysterectomy at a later date.

Modern technique for this operation follows. Preoperative management of an elective low-segment operation is fairly simple.

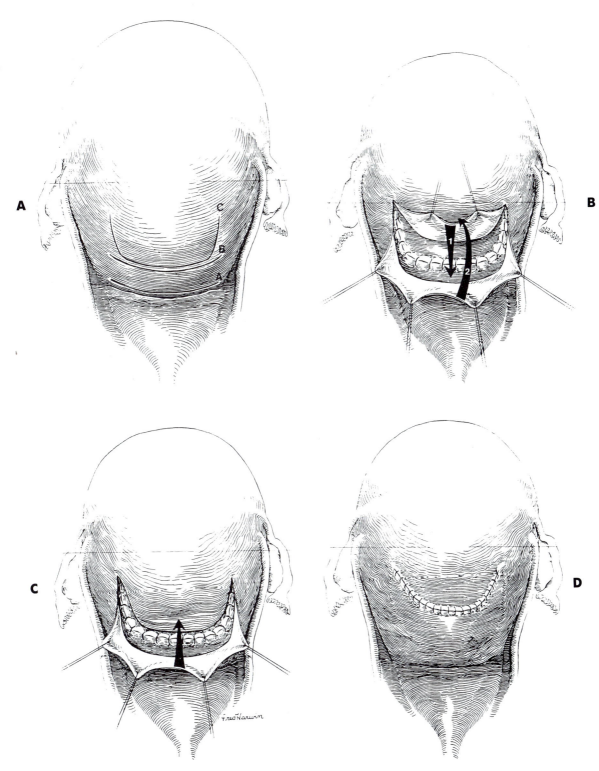

Fig. 67-8. "Low classical" cesarean. **A,** *a & b,* Two possible incisions are too low. *c,* In the lower third of uterine fundus, a modified Bailey incision. **B,** Fundal incision, serosal closure: *1,* upper serosal flap; *2,* lower serosal flap. **C,** Serosal flaps for suture. **D,** Serosal suture closure. (From Drufee R: *Low classical cesarean section OB-GYN survey,* vol 21, Baltimore, 1970, Williams & Wilkins.)

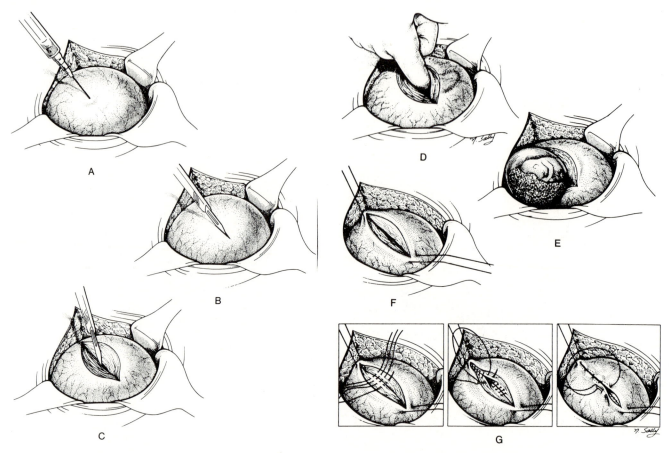

Fig. 67-9. Abdominal hysterotomy. **A,** Serosal injection. **B,** Initial incision. **C,** Second incision. **D,** Finger dissection of placenta. **E,** Evacuation of pregnancy. **F,** Traction sutures for closure. **G,** Three-step uterine incision closure. (From Quilligan and Zuspan: *Douglas-Stromme operative obstetrics,* Norwalk, Conn., 1982, Appleton, Century, Crofts.)

Cesarean section surgical technique

Low uterine segment (LUS) cesarean section is the most frequently used operation for abdominal delivery in contemporary obstetrics. The usual preoperative preparations are made with attention to any unusual details. The patient's position must not be supine and is best shifted approximately 15 degrees to the left; this is easily accomplished by the use of one or more towels under the buttocks on the opposite side. A catheter should be placed in the bladder, and the fluid should be emptied; the catheter is left in situ. Bath towels are frequently placed bilaterally along the lower body to absorb any overflow of amniotic fluid or blood. An adherent plastic drape is often used to help keep the operative field dry. When the peritoneum has been opened, large laparotomy sponges may be placed along the uterine adnexal gutters to prevent spill of uterine contents into the peritoneal cavity.

Transverse abdominal incisions began to be used in the early 1900s. Anatomical studies of the muscle orientation in the uterine body, the low uterine segment, and the cervix by Goerttler (Fig. 67-10) provided information for the

evolution of transverse incisions in the low uterine segment or the completely dilated cervix.

A high straight transverse abdominal incision was inherited from the past but was not adaptable to the LUS operation (Fig. 67-11). Bardenhaer in 1881 described a wide curved lower abdominal incision in which the rectus muscles were transected after ligation of the inferior hypogastric vessels to provide maximal exposure of the lower abdomen and pelvis. Maylard modified this extensive transverse incision by reduction of its length and also transected the rectus muscles. Pfannenstiel changed the location of the incision, slightly altered the curve, dissected the abdominal fascia from the anterior recti in both directions, retracted the muscles with Fritsch abdominal retractors, and did not transect the muscle. Cherney further modified these incisions by excision of the rectus muscles at the insertion of the conjoined tendon on the superior aspect of the pubic symphysis. Various incisions for the lower uterine area have been proposed (Fig. 67-12). Each of these was used for specific purposes and to adapt to different situations such as available space for delivery of the child,

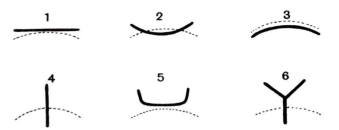

Fig. 67-12. Some incisions shown in relation to the uterovesical reflection of peritoneum. *1,* Doerfler; *2,* type used by many, including the author; *3,* Munro Kerr's incision; *4,* vertical incision; *5,* Bailey's "trapdoor" incision; *6,* Drüner's incision. (From Marshall CM: *Cesarean section: lower segment operation,* London, 1939, John Wright & Sons, Bristol & Simpkin Marshall.)

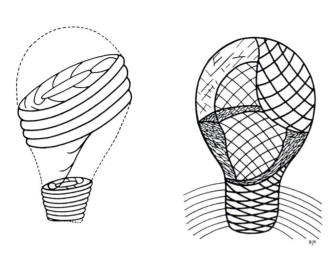

Fig. 67-10. Diagrammatic representation of muscle arrangement in the uterus and cervix. (From Goettler. In Marshall CM: *Cesarean section: lower segment operation,* London, 1939, John Wright & Sons, Bristol & Simpkin Marshall.)

· · · · · · *Straight*
※ ※ ※ ※ ※ *Bardenhauer*
⸺⸺⸺ *Pfannenstiel*
– – – – *Cherney*
· · · · · · · *Maylard*

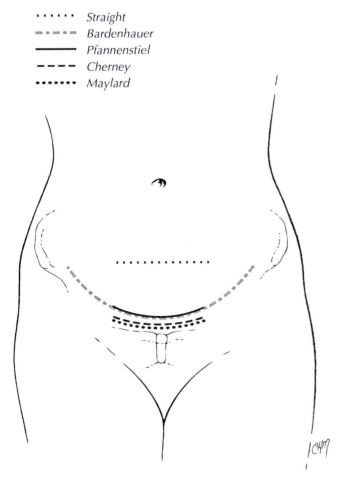

Fig. 67-11. Transverse abdominal incisions.

the presence of large aberrant vessels, and a large or several undiagnosed myomas. A scar from previous surgery, either abdominal or uterine, is almost always excised. Most transverse incisions are made when the fetal pole is vertical; vertical incisions are made for premature breech, in cases of unformed lower uterine segment or a contraction ring, and for hysterotomy (Fig. 67-13).

Care must be taken with use of a transverse incision not to extend the cut into the lateral uterine vessels. The incision can be made with a scalpel (Fig. 67-14) followed by bilateral extension with finger traction (Fig. 67-15). The incision can also be made with a blunt-nosed scissors, but one must be sure not to cut too far laterally. Figure-of-eight sutures can be placed at both ends of the incision, but it is easy to perforate a vessel with a needle. A clamp can be used bilaterally to limit the extent of the incision as well. If more space is needed, the incision can be converted into a partial vertical extension. It is better to convert the incision into a form of "trap door" with vertical extensions bilaterally (Fig. 67-16, *A*) or with a single laterally placed vertical J-shaped incision on one side or the other. A single central incision cephalad toward the fundus may be made (Fig. 67-16, *B*). This T-shaped incision does not heal as readily as the trap door or J type of extension because of the nature of the wound edges. A vertical incision or extension should not enter either the fundus or the vagina if at all possible. A fundal extension may compromise the possibility for vaginal delivery at a later date. An extremely rapid delivery can be accomplished with a good transverse incision and may readily avoid a fundal delivery. All areas of blood loss are clamped but not ligated until after the delivery just as in the case of a fundal incision made for the same reason, speed.

Regardless of the type of transverse low-segment incision that has been elected, it is ordinarily retrovesical. The vesical plica is dissected with the uterine and bladder serosa, and the bladder is directed downward. This is a simple but very important move and may only be complicated by dense adhesions between the posterior bladder wall and the anterior low uterine segment wall. These are usually from a previous cesarean. If this is exceptionally difficult, a layer of so-called uterine fascia may be available and the

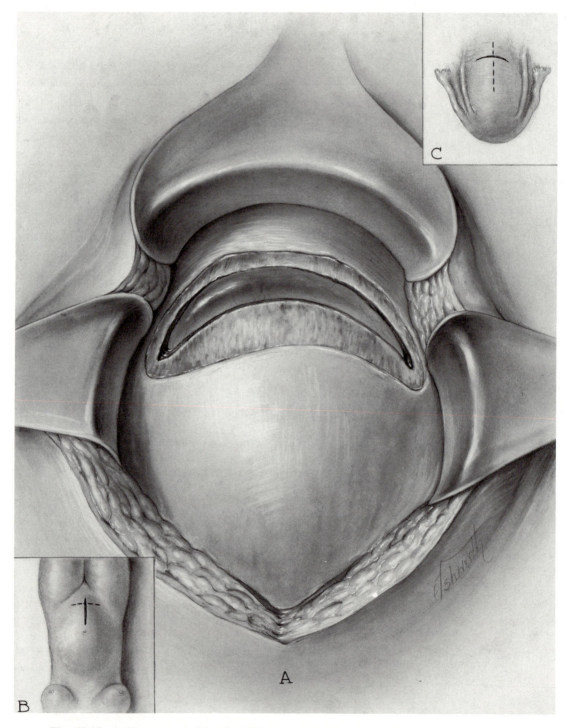

Fig. 67-13. A, Transverse incision for LUS cesarean section. **B,** Indicates vertical incision. **C,** Two abdominal incisions.

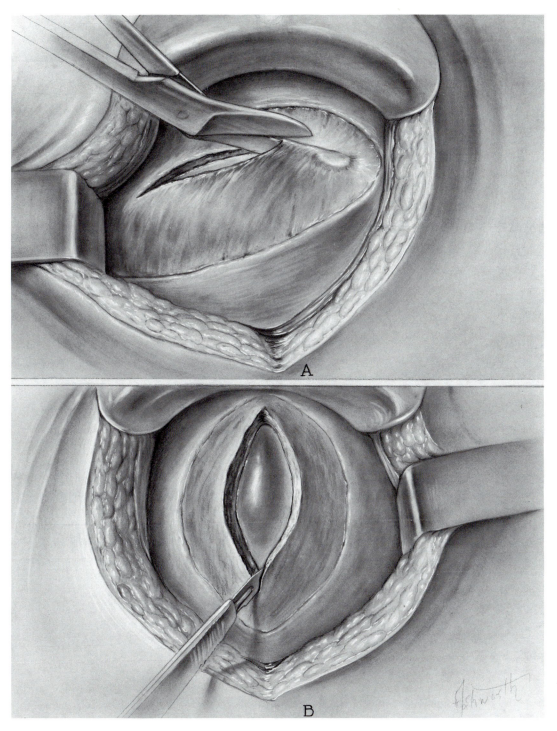

Fig. 67-14. LUS incision methods. **A,** Blunt scissors, transverse. **B,** Scalpel, vertical.

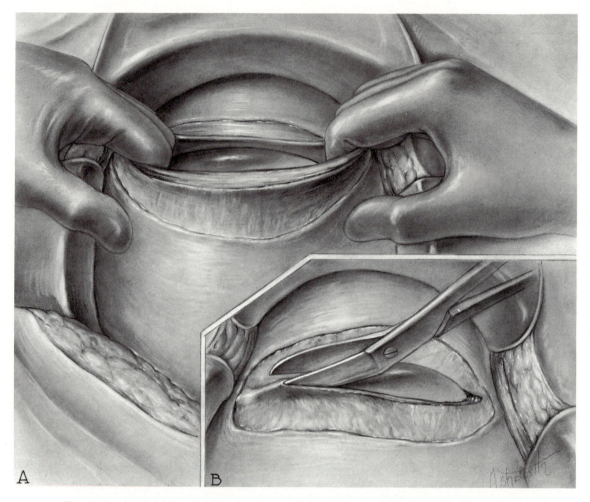

Fig. 67-15. LUS transverse incision extension. **A,** With finger traction. **B,** With blunt scissors.

dissection can be performed under this layer, which permits mobilization of the tissues. Care must be taken not to split or thin the bladder muscle and, of course, not to perforate the vesical mucosa. If this should occur, it should be repaired immediately if there is no reason for immediate delivery. Sharp dissection may be effective, but the curved portion of the scissors must face the uterine tissues.

When the uterine tissue is thin, incision of the fetus is possible and should be guarded against. If there is a considerable wide, thin scar, this can be excised at the time of uterine closure. The edges of the uterine wound can be held with any one of four or five kinds of clamps (Fig. 67-17), many of which have been made for this purpose. Ring clamps in the corners of the uterine wound may prevent blood loss. The membranes are ruptured if intact, and delivery is accomplished. The uterus may be eventrated at this point to make it easier to close the wound or massage the uterine body if it is not contracted from previous medication. The wound edges can be trimmed at this point, if, as noted above, there is excessive scar tissue or if there has been a silent rupture or division of the previous scar.

Delivery of a child from a uterine incision

Neurophysiologists are convinced that each human brain comes with a given number of nerve cells that are never replaced nor do they heal if injured. If these irreplaceable cells are damaged in a vulnerable portion of the brain, they are gone forever. Everyone who takes a child out of the uterus through an incision must remember that fact. If the performance of a cesarean operation is done to preserve the baby's brain as opposed to a traumatic vaginal delivery or because of an obstetric accident, the care with which the child's body and especially its brain are removed from the uterus must be absolute. There is no excuse for trauma to a child in cesarean section delivery—*none!* Methods for such delivery need to be reviewed and analyzed constantly to improve the results of cesarean delivery. If a child's brain, spine, clavicles, abdominal contents, or limbs are damaged by inept delivery through uterine and abdominal incisions, the operator is absolutely liable for the consequences.

There are several methods for cesarean delivery. It is common to place a finger in the child's mouth, turn the face into the wound (Fig. 67-18), and deliver the head by

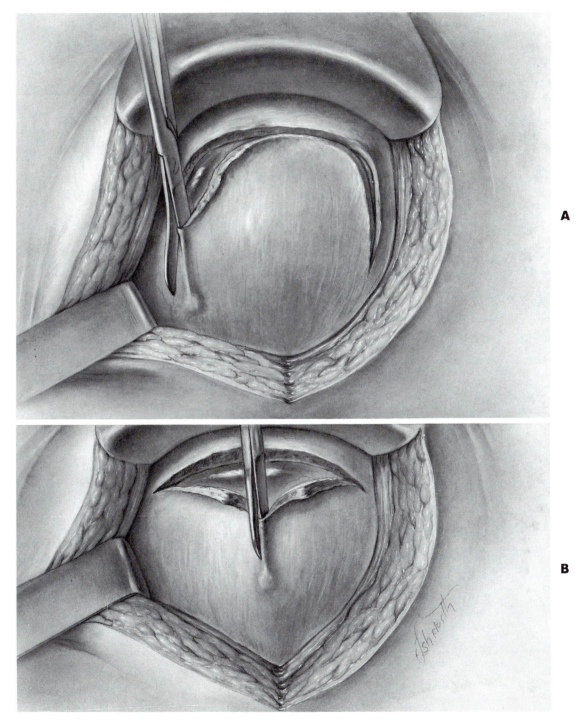

A

B

Fig. 67-16. LUS incision enlargement. **A,** Bailey type lateral incisions. **B,** Vertical or "T" extension.

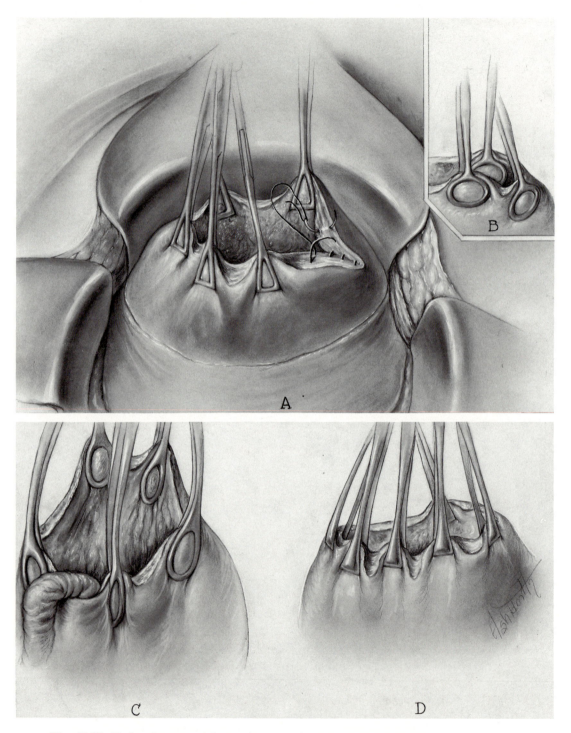

Fig. 67-17. Various instruments for traction on uterine wound edges for suture closure. **A,** Pennington clamps. **B,** Oval clamps. **C,** Long ring forceps. **D,** Long Allis forceps.

gentle flexion over the bottom of the wound. It is frequently helpful to pass two fingers of each hand bilaterally along the sides of the head (Fig. 67-19). A simple and safe method is to apply carefully a forceps that has been specially made for this purpose to the proper area of the fetal head (Fig. 67-20), then use gentle traction. If the fit of the instrument is too tight or the traction too difficult, the incisions should be enlarged as needed. Vacuum traction is a viable alternative to forceps. The head may be guided into the incision by a scalp forceps as suggested by Kustner. A vectis may be applied carefully using one blade of a small fenestrated forceps or a Murless type or Torpin blade. Oc-

casionally, bilateral gentle pressure from above on the mother's flanks may facilitate removal of the head, but it should *never* be done with the aftercoming head of a breech.

Delivery of a breech at cesarean requires equal or more skill than a vaginal delivery; this is even more important when dealing with a premature breech presentation. Both incisions may be made a little larger in the beginning when one knows that a breech is presenting; a vertical incision may be especially advantageous with a premature frank breech or a transverse presentation. Conversion of frank breech to a single footling requires intrauterine manipulation, which can frequently be easier than when attempted vaginally. All traction must be very gentle. There should be absolutely *no twisting of the spine at any time*. Each arm must be delivered without force, traction, or direct pressure. The aftercoming head must be managed under complete control; it is especially important not to allow a sudden expulsion of the head through the wound because such sudden decompression produces trauma to the base of the brain. Very careful use of small forceps with the aftercoming head may be most helpful but requires experience and skill. Pressure must *never* be put on the aftercoming

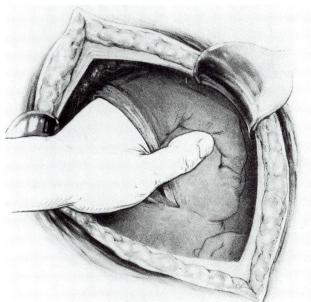

Fig. 67-18. Finger to mouth maneuver to change position of the fetal head. (From Doderlein A: *Doderlein-Kronig operative gynakologie,* Leipzig, 1924, Georg Thieme.)

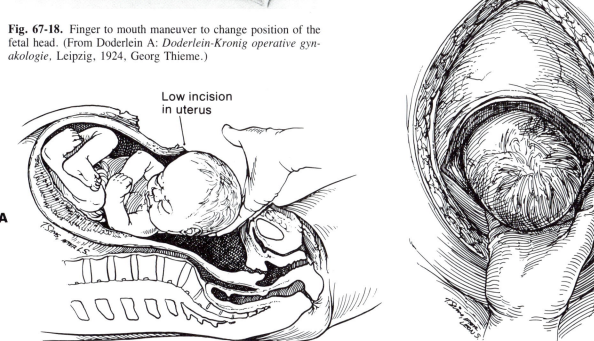

Fig. 67-19. Manual delivery of fetal head at LUS cesarean section. **A,** Lateral view. **B,** Anterior view. (From Pritchard J, MacDonald P, Gent N: *Williams' obstetrics,* ed 17, Norwalk, Conn., 1985, Appleton, Century, Crofts.)

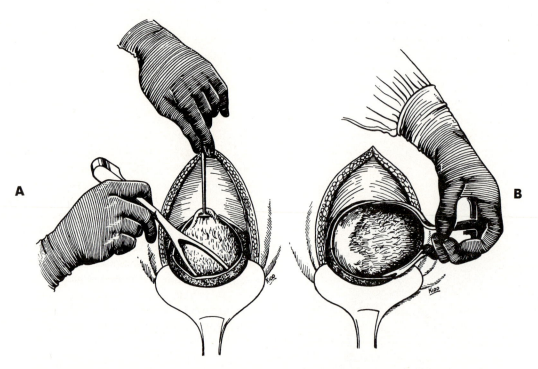

Fig. 67-20. Forceps delivery at LUS cesarean section. **A,** Scalp forceps and application of Obs forceps. single blade can be used as a vectis. **B,** Forceps application to transverse fetal head position. (From Marshall CM: *Cesarean section: lower segment operation,* London, 1939, John Wright & Sons, Bristol & Simpkin Marshall.)

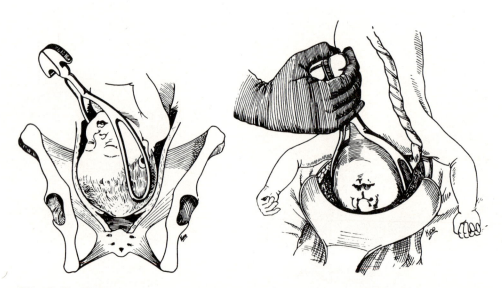

Fig. 67-21. Forceps application to impacted fetal head at LUS cesarean section. (From Marshall CM: *Cesarean section: lower segment operation,* London, 1939, John Wright & Sons, Bristol & Simpkin Marshall.)

head from above because of the danger of herniation of brain tissue through the foramen!

Delivery of an impacted presenting part may prove to be difficult and can damage the fetus. A molded, tightly impacted head deep in the pelvis, as seen after a long, difficult labor, sometimes requires vaginal assistance (Fig. 67-21). Two suggestions to solve the problem are: relief of the impaction before the cesarean, or simultaneous relief of the impaction from above and below at the time of the cesarean. Such manipulations must be unusually gentle because of the increased vulnerability of the fetal head and risk of trauma to the maternal soft tissues. Larger than usual incisions are mandatory in complicated cases. If transverse abdominal incisions are used, those designed by Bardenhauer, Maylard, or Cherney should be considered.

In cases of impacted shoulder and arm especially with the back down, a long vertical incision is the best to allow for unusual intrauterine manipulation. If the vertical abdominal incision is made long enough, total uterine eventration may be used to complete difficult intrauterine manipulation for delivery. Fortunately, these situations are extremely rare.

Another situation that may require vaginal assistance is the upward pressure against a fetal part to hold it out of the pelvis in a case of prolapsed umbilical cord. If the membranes have not been ruptured, this may not be as important.

After a child has been delivered, mucus and fluids are aspirated by a bulb syringe or a deLee trap, the cord is doubly clamped and divided on the mother's abdomen, and blood specimens are taken. If contamination is suspected, the cord can be divided 6 inches from the fetal abdomen before the child is passed to the receiving team; the placental side of the cord is left inside the uterus. This is a moot point in modern obstetrics because of the efficiency of antibiotics in cases of potential or actual infection. The infant's introduction to the mother is done when expedient, and when she is awake. Oxytocin has been given in the intravenous (IV) system by this time, and the placenta is delivered, not by traction on the cord but usually manually with gentleness. The uterine cavity is inspected to be sure all the placental tissues have been removed. At this time, any areas of blood loss are clamped. In cases in which the cervix is tightly closed, a long, curved forceps can be passed through the cervical canal to allow for drainage later; suggestions have been made that a small drain or wick be placed in this area to be removed vaginally 12 hours later. There is no longer any mention of the use of a de Lee shuttle for this purpose.

If cesarean section hysterectomy is contemplated in a grave emergency, the uterine vessels are bilaterally clamped, cut, and tied. The adnexal structures and ligaments are all clamped but not ligated, and the body of the uterus may be easily removed by extension of the transverse incision around posteriorly, which quickly removes the uterine tissue mass; this allows the operator to proceed with the removal of the cervix and ligation of the various pedicles with much more space and better visualization of the pelvis. This procedure is especially helpful if there has been massive hemorrhage or abruptio placenta, where speed in removal of the uterine body facilitates hemostasis. Identification of the ureters and bladder is much more accurate as is location of the cervix and vagina, which can be difficult if the cervix has been completely dilated for some time. Ligation of all the pedicles is also much more accurate and without pressure to hurry unnecessarily.

Suture of the uterine incision

Suture closure of the uterine incision is a matter of some controversy. Alternatives are as follows:

1. Close the angles of the wound bilaterally with a single figure-of-eight suture of 00 polyglycolic or 0 chromic catgut. Follow with interrupted sutures of either material to close the myometrial layer; avoid the endometrial cavity and use a minimal amount of suture material to accomplish the closure. Or follow with a continuous suture of either material, and avoid the endometrial cavity but not with a locked stitch unless there is unusual blood loss, as may be the case if there has been some form of placenta previa in which case, interrupted figure-of-eight sutures may produce the best hemostasis without as much potential for tissue necrosis as with locked stitch.
2. Close the entire incision with a continuous or locked stitch of either 00 polyglycolic material or 0 chromic catgut. Avoid the endometrial cavity and keep the suture placements even, with traction that is neither too tight nor too loose. Make only one needle placement each time.
3. A second closure of superficial uterine tissues, not the serosa, may be performed at this time. This may be more indicated in elective cesarean section in which there has been no dilation of the cervix than in cases in which the reverse is true, because in the latter the tissues may be very thin and a single closure will suffice. Hemostasis is one of the important points, and this may be accomplished with a single figure-of-eight suture as indicated.
4. No second closure is indicated if the first is properly done, with the exception of the rare figure-of-eight for bleeding.
5. The serosa may not be closed at all (Fig. 67-22).
6. The serosa may be sutured above the closed incision line with three interrupted sutures of 0000 polyglycolic or 000 chromic catgut. The intent of these alternative methods is to prevent the formation of an undue amount of scar formation between the bladder and the lower uterine segment, which might seriously compromise either vaginal or abdominal hysterectomy at a later date.
7. Close the serosa, avoid the bladder, and use a fine continous suture carefully applied to seal the uterine suture line to prevent drainage from the uterus into the perito-

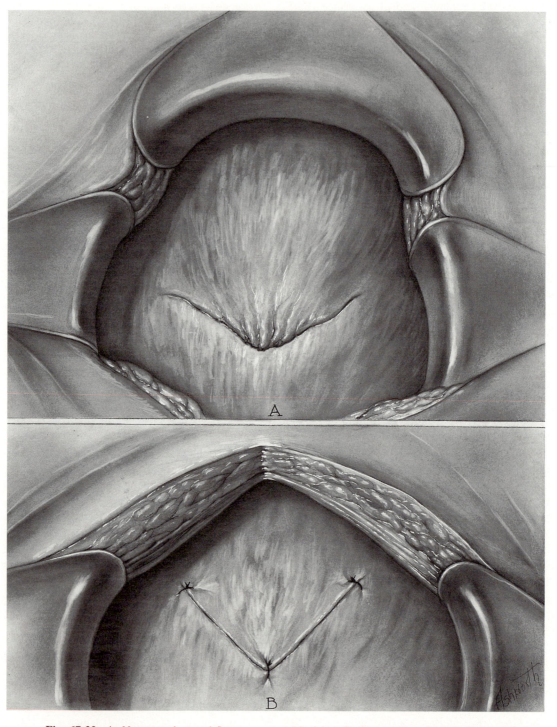

Fig. 67-22. A, Nonsutured serosal flap over sutured incision. **B,** Three-suture closure of serosa.

neal cavity; this is particularly true in cases of gross or potential severe intrauterine infection.

If eventrated, the uterus is returned to the pelvic cavity; the uterus should be kept moist at all times while it is external to the abdominal cavity.

Closure of the abdominal wound

The abdominal wound is closed by the operator's choice. Some do not close the parietal peritoneum. The fascia is closed with a continous suture of 00 polyglycolic material. The subcutaneous tissue may be closed with one or two interrupted sutures if the area is unusually thick; otherwise, the skin is closed with surgical clips or a fine subcuticular polyglycolic suture. Drains may be placed in the presence of obvious infection, and the wound is closed with interrupted sutures in the skin; in some rare cases, the abdominal wound may be left open down to the closed parietal peritoneum.

Results

This operation has been modified many times in small details, and these are merely a matter of choice. The basic procedure is as outlined. Low-segment cesarean is a very efficient successful procedure with minimal postoperative problems and can be repeated several times. Rupture of the scar is not common, and, when it occurs, there is usually no hemorrhage, frequently there is no pain. The size of the rupture may vary from 1 to 2 cm to the entire length, but rarely is the fetus found in the abdominal cavity. These weakened tissues have been dissected free at the ends of the operation, and freshened edges have been approximated with no repetition of the rupture at a later pregnancy. It is hoped that by avoidance of the use of suture to cover the area of the uterine incision with serosa that the scar formation between bladder and anterior uterine wall may not occur.

Postoperative management

Postoperative care after a simple, uncomplicated cesarean section is usually not difficult. The patient is taken to a postsurgical care unit where she is carefully monitored for at least 4 to 6 hours. Observation is made of fundal height, respiratory activity, blood pressure, and any possible evidence of hemorrhage. In modern obstetrics, pain control is frequently accomplished by repeated doses of the regional anesthetic that was used for the operation. Another method is the use of epidural or intrathecal Fentyl or another drug of choice. When this is no longer used, pain control is usually accomplished with parenteral opiates, which often are not needed, or by oral medications such as aspirin or acetaminophen and codeine or the synthetic codeines such as Percocet. Whenever possible, the doses should be minimal and frequent rather than large loaded doses. It should be kept in mind that lactation may prevent the use of these drugs for very long.

Modern operative technique saves blood and prevents

contamination of the peritoneal cavity by blood and amniotic fluid or meconium so that problems with nausea or bowel stasis are minimal. The bladder catheter is removed as soon as possible, and the patient is ambulated usually in 6 hours after she has left the postoperative unit. IV hydrations and supplemental glucose are administered until the patient takes solid food. She should be fed a diet as near to her usual normal intake as soon as possible. Such management with encouragement generally rehabilitates most normal women quickly. Bowel functions return rapidly, and convalescence can be carried out at home. Minor difficulties can be controlled with specific medication and treatment that varies to some extent by a physician's choice. A competent staff of nurses is invaluable in such cases, and the proper combination has the patient in a normal condition in a few days at the most. Management of the breast and lactation is especially dependent on knowledgeable nurses, and such help and encouragement are essential for an ideal nursing experience. Combined team effort returns the patient in good health and spirits to her home with minimal hospital stay, which is the goal of obstetrics today. This provides emotional and financial benefits.

EXTRAPERITONEAL CESAREAN SECTION

As the earliest of the concepts of low uterine segment operations were developed simultaneously, other ideas had evolved. These were more concerned with protection of the abdominal cavity from infection than the approach to the low segment of the cervix for delivery of the child. The information gained from these various dissections made the evolution and performance of true low-segment transperitoneal cesarean seem simple (Fig. 67-23). Throughout this time, extraperitoneal, peritoneal exclusion, uteroabdominal fistula, vaginal cesarean, and pseudoextraperitoneal operations were being introduced along with uterine eventrations that included a posterior fundal incision.

The true extraperitoneal operation involved dissections near the bladder in the adjacent tissues that admitted entrance to the dilated cervix or low uterine segment external to the peritoneal cavity (Fig. 67-24). There are two basic varieties: one is to dissect the vesical peritoneum from the anterior bladder wall and expose the low segment or dilated cervix to incisional entrance of sufficient size to permit delivery of a child; the other is to accomplish the same result by a lateral dissection of the vesical peritoneum and lateral exposure of the same anatomical area for the same purpose. At this point, it should be noted that the anatomy of the area inferior to the bladder and superior to the low uterine segment, dilated cervix and vagina, is distorted by the changes brought about by pregnancy and labor. Because most of these operations were performed at the end of a long and often complicated labor, some after attempted vaginal delivery, it was impossible to discern where the fully dilated and edematous cervix, vagina, and thin low uterine segment actually were, in relation to each other. This accounts for the discussions in regard to the

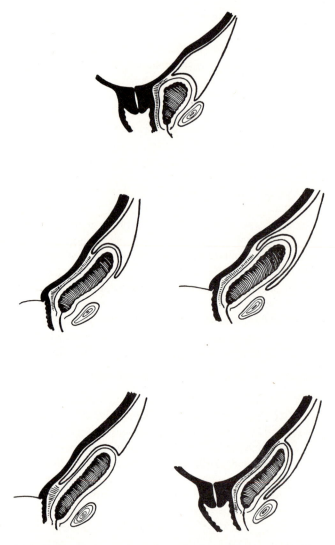

Fig. 67-23. Variations in peritoneal relationships to the bladder. (From Marshall CM: *Cesarean section: lower segment operation,* London, 1939, John Wright & Sons, Bristol & Simpkin Marshall.)

terminology of these operations, extraperitoneal or not: were these truly low-segment or cervical cesarean sections? The question is moot. As noted, the supravesical procedure was first conceived by Physick in 1824 in the United States (Fig. 67-25). A technique somewhat similar was proposed by Bell in 1837 in England, but was not quite as clearly defined. The extraperitoneal approach thus suggested was not accepted, and it was not until Skene and Thomas in 1874 and 1878 reviewed the operation of gastroelytrotomy, which was so named by Baudelocque in 1823. Thomas in 1870 described an operation much like that of Ritgen in which, after the proper dissection and manual dilation of the cervix, the cervix was brought through the vaginal incision and the child was delivered. This revived operation had a brief acceptance and then yielded to the other less exotic attempts at extraperitoneal cesarean. German and American surgeons were the most

active in the development of both supravesical and lateral approaches for delivery without peritoneal invasion.

In summary, the following are examples of these various methods:

1. *Gastroelytrotomy:* Begun by Ritgen, prompted by Baudelocque and Thomas.
2. *Extraperitoneal:* Retrovesical and paravesical techniques: paravesical dissection approaches the low uterine segment by lateral tissue manipulation, which extends behind the bladder and below the peritoneum, followed by lateral retraction of the bladder, which exposes the area of the anterior uterine wall for the incision for delivery. This was created by Latzko, who used one of Sellheim's several methods (Fig. 67-26). Since that time, 1908, Burns (1930), Norton (1935), and the author (1965) have simplified the dissection and allowed for increased space for delivery (Fig. 67-27). Doderlein in Europe used an inguinal incision.
3. *Retrovesical or supravesical dissection* originated with Physick in the United States and was securely established by Sellheim (Fig. 67-28). The operation was promoted by Waters, Leavitt, Cartwright, and Ricci. In this operation, the peritoneum is dissected from the anterior wall of the bladder through a T-shaped superficial incision, which permits it to be retracted inferiorly to expose the lower uterine segment for incision after the uterine peritoneal fold has been retracted anteriorly (Fig. 67-29). It has an advantage of increased space for delivery but has a high failure rate due to injury to the peritoneum. The anatomical relationships of these low operations are seen in Fig. 67-29, *A* (#3), *B* (#2), and *C* (#2).
4. *Peritoneal exclusion* was created by Frank in 1906. In this operation the parietal peritoneum was sutured to the upper visceral peritoneum, which closed off the peritoneal cavity (Fig. 67-30). There were several variations of this type of peritoneal suture placement, but, in reality, no sutured tissue was free from bacterial invasion and permeation. Peritoneal exclusion continued with many variations, which included ingenious methods using clamps, packing with various materials, and the use of a rubber dam.
5. *Uteroabdominal fistula formation* was first created by Pillore in France in 1845. He sutured the uterine incision edges to the abdominal incision, which allowed the uterine cavity to drain its contents exterior to the peritoneal cavity. This was followed by others, but it remained for Sellheim, who was disappointed by his previous three procedures, to establish this method.
6. *Pseudoextraperitoneal operations* have not been well accepted because they violate the principle of extraperitoneal surgery. It was first introduced by Aldridge in 1937 and performed in several different ways by others, which included the injection of methylene blue dye intraperitoneally to identify it for dissection.
7. Duhrssen and Solms in 1909 *combined vaginal cesar-*

Text continued on p. 1102.

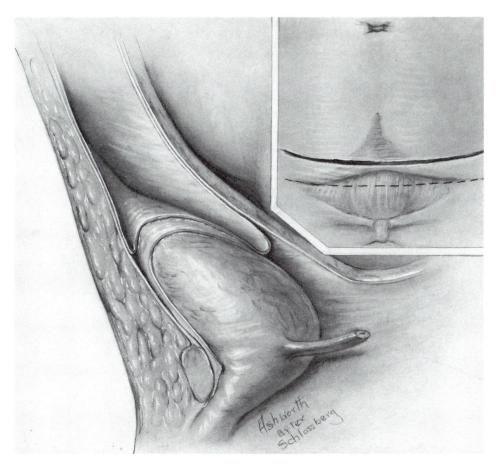

Fig. 67-24. Lateral anatomical view of anterior pelvic area. **A,** Peritoneum. **B,** Bladder. **C,** Perivesical "fascia." **D,** Anterior abdominal wall and incision relationship.

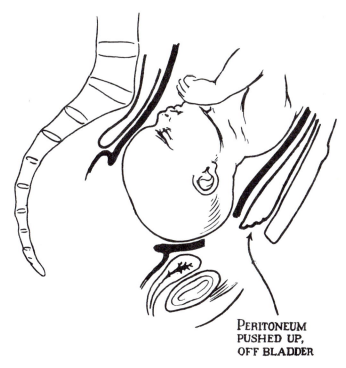

Fig. 67-25. Physicks' suprasymphysial supravesical approach to the LUS. (From DeLee J: Low or cervical cesarean section. *Am J Ob/Gyn* 10:610, 1925.)

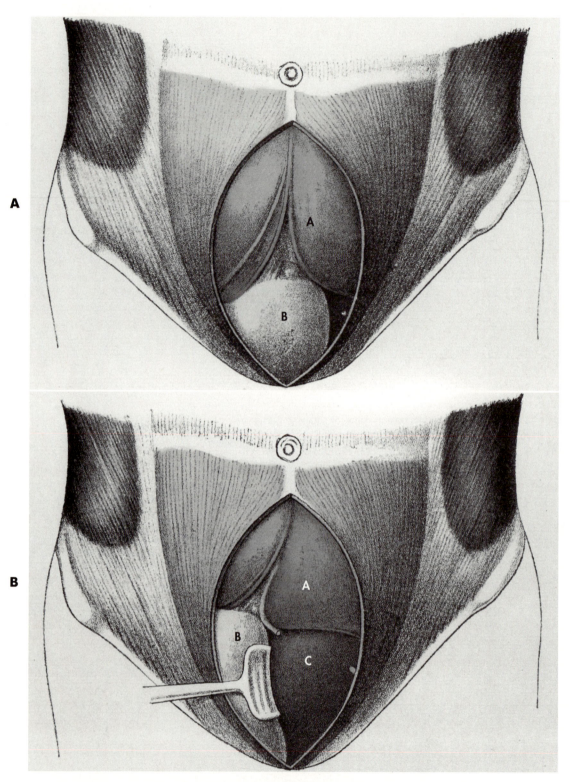

Fig. 67-26. Paravesical lateral cesarean section. **A,** Anatomical references. *A,* peritoneal folds; *B,* bladder. **B,** Uterine wall exposure. *A,* Peritoneum; *B,* bladder; *C,* uterine wall.

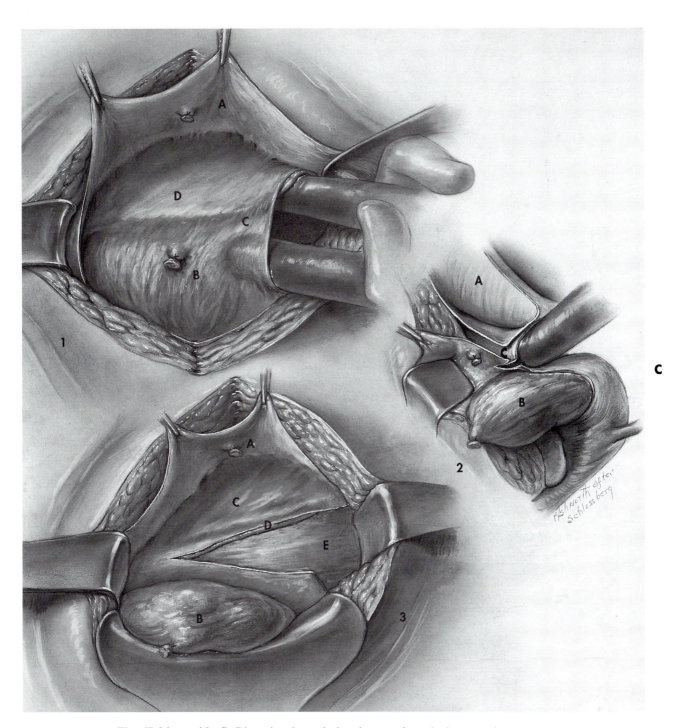

Fig. 67-26, cont'd. C, Dissecting the vesical peritoneum from the lower uterine segment.

Continued.

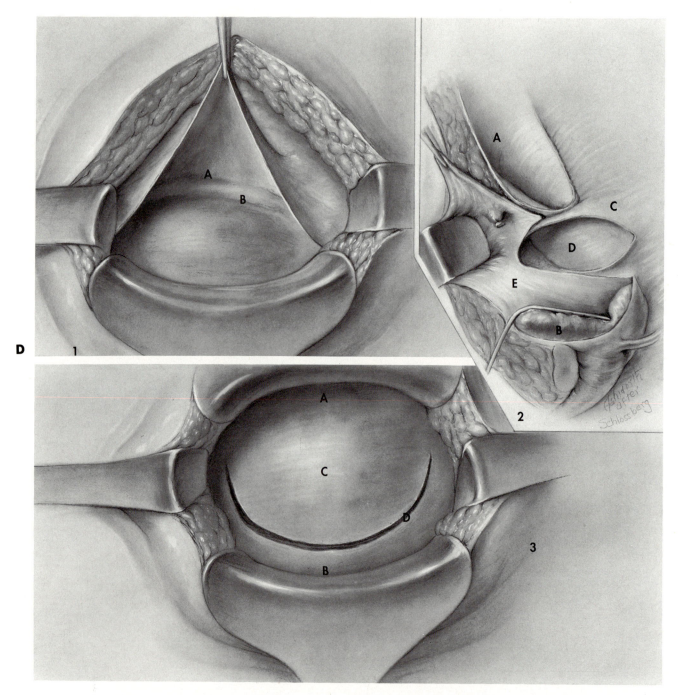

Fig. 67-26, cont'd. D, Extraperitoneal exposure of the lower uterine segment. (Adapted from Latzko W: *Wein Klin Wchnschr,* 22:477, 1909, and in Ricci J, Marr J: *Principles of extraperitoneal cesarean section,* Philadelphia, 1939, Blakiston Co.).

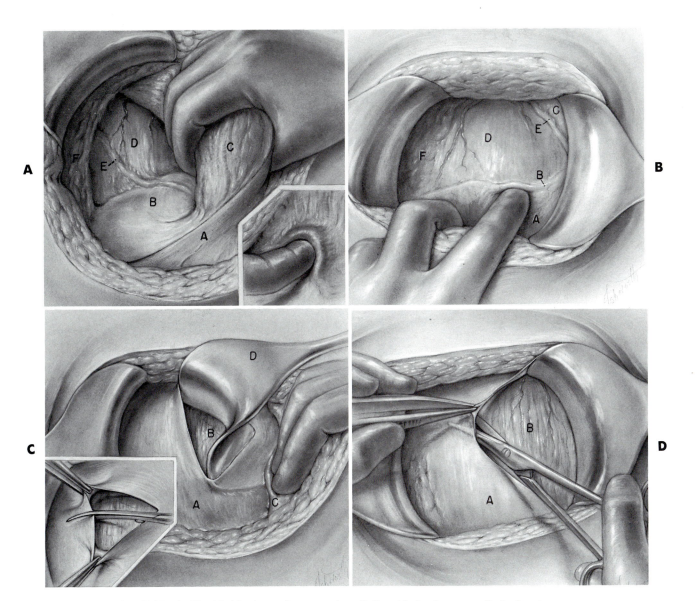

Fig. 67-27. A, The bladder is gently retracted medially with the fingers. *a,* Parietal peritoneum. *b,* Posterior peritoneal fold. *c,* Bladder. *d,* Lower uterine segment. *e,* Obliterated hypogastric artery. *f,* Fatty tissue and large vessels in the lateral pelvic space. *(Insert)* Method of dissecting with fingertip. **B,** Further progression in the blunt dissection of the area. *a,* Parietal peritoneum. *b,* Posterior peritoneal fold. *c,* Bladder retracted laterally. *d,* Lower uterine segment. *e,* Obliterated hypogastric artery. *f,* Fatty tissue and large vessels in the lateral pelvic space. **C,** *(Insert)* Method of extending the fascial incision. *(Main illustration)* Extension of the fascial dissection using the Fritsch retractor. Shows the next step in extension of the dissection enlarging the operative field. *a,* Superficial uterine fascia. *b,* Lower uterine segment. *c,* Edge of posterior peritoneal fold. *d,* Fritsch retractor. **D,** *a,* Superficial uterine fascia. *b,* Lower uterine segment. (From Durfee R: Elective extraperitoneal cesarean section, *SG & O,* 110:173, 1960.)

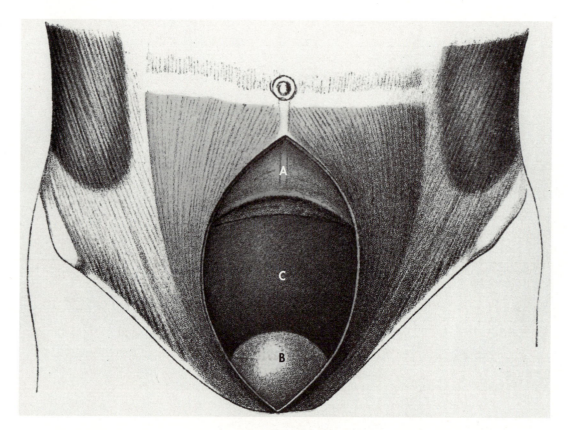

Fig. 67-28. Supravesical extraperitoneal cesarean section by Sellheim. *A,* Peritoneum. *B,* Bladder. *C,* LUS uterine wall. (Adapted from Latzko W: *Wein Klin Wchnschr,* 22:477, 1909, and in Ricci J: *Principles of extraperitoneal cesarean section,* Philadelphia, 1939, Blakiston Co.)

ean with a supra-Poupart's ligament approach. The abdominal operation was first done with exposure of the area, the vaginal incision was then performed, and the delivery was accomplished through the abdominal wound extraperitoneally.

All of the exotic procedures have yielded to either a paravesical or supravesical operation. When these operations are properly performed with care, skill, and knowledge of the anatomy of the area and the possible variations in the peritoneal folds, the procedure is successful.

INDICATIONS FOR CESAREAN SECTION

Primary indications for cesarean section were to remove a child from a dead woman perhaps to save it, but more so for satisfaction of rituals and religious reasons. With the appearance of Christianity, a child was removed for the purpose of baptism. Almost all of these were postmortem, but the use of cesarean for the dying produced more living children and led directly to the use of the operation in the living.

Rousset, in 1581, outlined the following indications for abdominal delivery: very large child, large twins, complications from myomas, fetal monstrosities, abnormal irreducible presentations, a contracted pelvis, a strictured uterus, a large vesicle stone, and an aged woman or one

too young. These are familiar and clearly were designed for cesarean for live women.

In spite of such a wide variety of indications, the high mortality associated with the operation reduced the indications for cesarean for the live woman to a totally contracted pelvis and nothing else. A very few intrepid operators used the operation for more than this single indication, but by 1747 Levret summed it all up into "an extreme contraction of the pelvis which caused the absolute impossibility for delivery through the natural passages." There were other conditions that had to be met. The child had to be alive and the pelvis so contracted that the obstetrician could not pass a hand through it to perform a version or embryotomy. Levret did not acknowledge blockage by fleshy tumors or the restraint caused by stenosis or constriction of the cervix or vagina because there were methods to circumvent these problems by less hazardous procedures than cesarean section. What these were is not clear. This opinion included placenta previa! By 1756, Crantz added the occasion of imminent uterine rupture as an indication. But neither this nor the presence of placenta previa was generally reason for performance of cesarean section.

The situation remained static until 1890 when Tait advocated the cesarean operation without question for hemor-

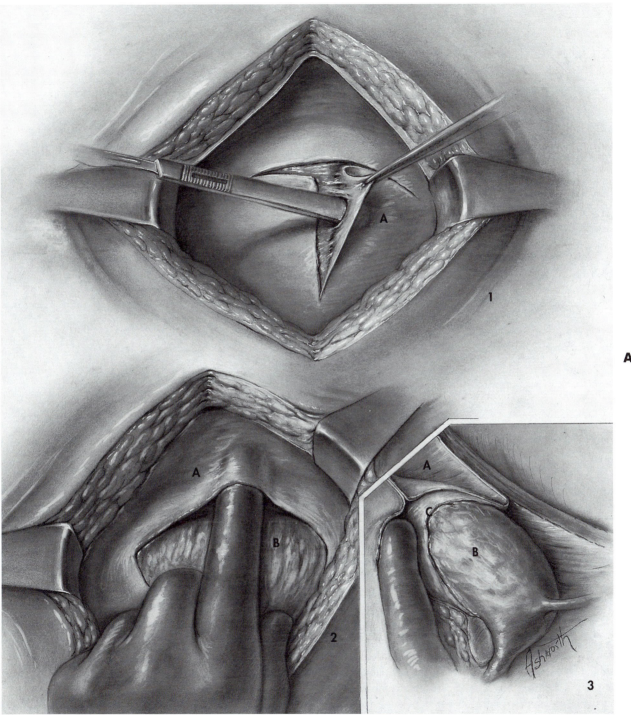

A

Fig. 67-29. Supravesical extraperitoneal cesarean section. **A,** *1A,* "T" incision over bladder; *2A,* paravesical "fascia"; *B,* bladder; *3A,* peritoneal cavity; *B,* bladder; *C,* paravesical "fascia."

Continued.

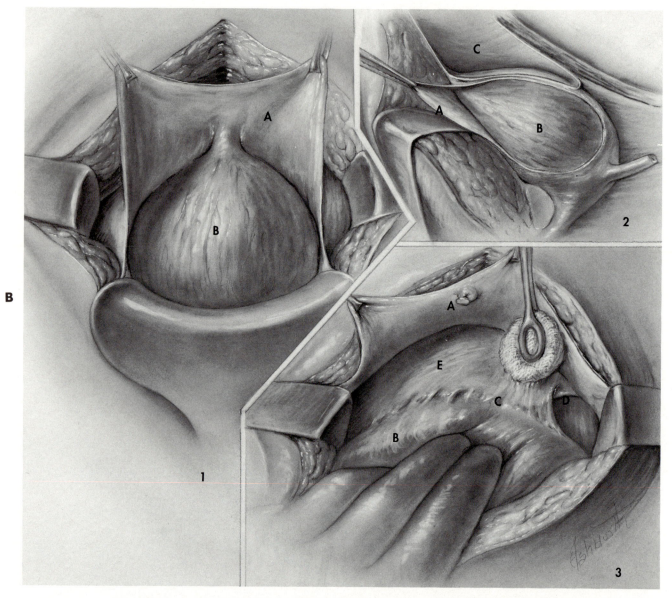

Fig. 67-29, cont'd. B, *1A,* Dissected superior paravesical "fascia"; *B,* bladder; *2A,* paravesical "fascia"; *B,* bladder; *C,* peritoneal cavity; *3A,* paravesical "fascia"; *B,* bladder; *C,* deep paravesical "fascia"; *D,* uterine wall; *E,* peritoneum.

rhage from placenta previa followed by hysterectomy; he did one of these in 1898 and succeeded in safe delivery of the mother, but the child died after 1 month, of pneumonia. In the United States in 1892, cesarean section for placenta previa was suggested by Ford; it was done by Hypes and Hulbert with no details. A badly overmanipulated patient was delivered by Sligh in 1892, but she was in such poor condition that she had no chance for survival. Bernays in the United States did the first successful operation in 1894, without hysterectomy; three other operations had been done in the United States before Tait's successful case. By 1901, Zinke advocated cesarean in cases of central placenta previa, with a closed cervix, in a primigravida not in labor, and

with hemorrhage not controlled by conservative methods. Kerr was opposed to this indication, but from 1902 to 1921 he changed his mind completely. In the next 50 years, the indication was more or less as it is today.

Another frequently fatal situation in obstetrics has been eclampsia. In 1788, Lauverjat suggested the use of cesarean for a convulsive woman; he did the operation four times in 1780. Each of these was postmortem and received a dead child each time. He stated that clearly the operation should be done while the mother was alive, because apparently the child would die before she did. In 1827, Richmond performed cesarean section for an eclamptic woman in the backwoods of the United States with success, Ben-

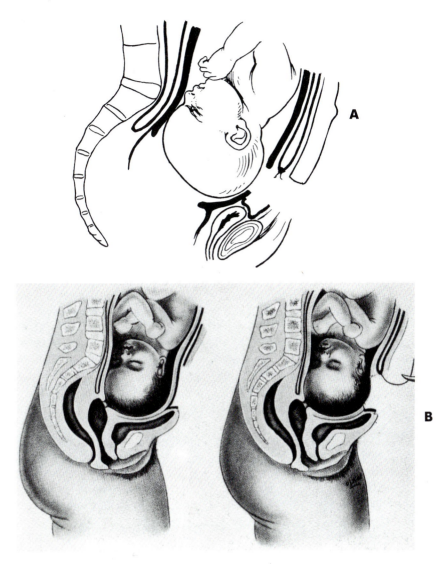

Fig. 67-30. Frank's peritoneal exclusion cesarean. (**A,** From de Lee: Low or cervical cesarean section. *Am J Ob/Gyn* 10:51, 1925. **B,** From Marshall JM: *Cesarean section: lower segment operation,* London, 1939, John Wright & Sons, Bristol & Simpkin Marshall.)

nett's wife also had toxemia. Pollack in 1904 reported that Van de Akker in 1875 was the first to perform the operation for eclampsia, but this is clearly not true. Foster reported a case in 1870, but it was Halbertsma in 1881 who established the real basis for cesarean in eclampsia. He repeated his opinion in 1889. There was much divided attitude about this practice, and, by 1937, it was agreed that a high percentage of the maternal deaths after cesarean section for this indication was because of absence of treatment, or the failure thereof, before surgery. Once again, the cesarean was an operation of last resort.

In the years that followed, cesarean section became safer with the recognition of the importance of "timing" of the application of the procedure in all indicated situations.

From 1940 to the present day, indications have been categorized by such definitions as "absolute" and "relative" for want of better terms. In some reports there are special divisions for fetal or maternal indications only. The following are some examples of the trends for the use of the operation.

"Absolute" indications in the era from 1940

1. A completely contracted pelvis
2. Central placenta previa with blood loss
3. Transverse presentation not amenable to version
4. Breech presentation in a primipara with borderline pelvis
5. Severe increasing toxemia with progression to eclampsia
6. Imminent uterine rupture
7. Premature separation of the placenta with severe abruption
8. Complete obstruction of the pelvis by nonremovable tumors or cysts
9. Prolapsed fetal cord without cervical dilatation above 3 cm

10. Severe threat to life or progressive maternal disease (e.g., severe uncontrollable diabetes, some cardiac diseases)
11. Previous pregnancy loss in labor or nonviable premature more than three times
12. Failed labor 18 to 24 hours in women over 40 or under 14 years of age
13. Moribund woman after pulmonary aspiration, with asphyxia; symptoms of amniotic fluid embolus; massive cardiovascular accident with coma
14. Invasive cervical carcinoma diagnosed at term
15. Paralytic poliomyelitis with paralysis to C-6 no longer an indication
16. Coma or brain death within range of fetal viability
17. Diagnosed uterine rupture, symptomatic with hemorrhage
18. Total soft tissue obstruction of the lower birth canal (e.g., nearly complete vaginal atresia, massive vulvar edema, or scar formation from trauma or severe genital burns)
19. Multiple pregnancy with unengaged fetal parts (e.g., triplets)
20. Massive fetal monstrosities not amenable to embryotomy

"Relative" indications from 1940

1. Cervical dystocia (i.e., failed dilation)
2. Failed onset of labor after attempted induction with ruptured membranes over 12 hours
3. Uterine atony in second stage of labor with high station of the presenting part, unengaged
4. Uterine contraction ring unresponsive to treatment
5. Failed forceps or vacuum extraction delivery
6. Premature separation of the placenta with severe abruption with failed response to conservative therapy
7. Unmanageable psychiatric disease (e.g., wild mania or sustained hysteria, not amenable to treatment). This may be questionable in contemporary obstetrics
8. Evidence of severe intrauterine infection and fetal distress with poor labor
9. Emergency development of extensive maternal disease (many examples)
10. Prolonged painful red degeneration of a large myoma
11. Abnormal fetal presentations in overdue elderly primipara with firm undilated cervix
12. Extensive pelvic plastic repair of extremely severe previous vaginal, cervical, or perineal trauma that included the rectum and/or bladder with fistula formation, successfully repaired
13. After extensive intraabdominal pelvic surgery, such as exenteration of extragenital organs
14. Moribund woman with severe chronic disease (e.g., carcinoma anywhere, advanced tuberculosis)
15. Highly valuable child with any complication
16. Failed test of labor
17. Prolapse of fetal arm or arm and leg

18. Obvious evidence of increased fetal distress diagnosed by electronic devices
19. Repeat cesarean section if original indication is still present
20. Any number of rare and exotic situations

Questionable indications from 1940

1. Patient and relatives request for cesarean section
2. Elective cesarean section to preserve tissues of the genital canal (e.g., Harris in Hollywood to preserve the sexual attractiveness of actresses)
3. Malingering hysteria and purported fear of labor and vaginal delivery
4. Herpes virus disease not active in the genital tract
5. Acquired immunodeficiency syndrome (AIDS)
6. "Once a cesarean always a cesarean"
7. To deliver a child on a special date (e.g., a relative's birthday, anniversary, or sibling's birthday, or by decision of an astrologist)
8. To guarantee a live child for royal succession or in some cases of involved inheritance
9. In nonpermanent cervical cerclage, with dilation
10. In cases of healed vesicovaginal fistula, in multipara with history of easy labor

Contraindications from 1940

1. Patient with a dead child and no other indication
2. Severe intrauterine infection, before antibiotic era, and now with severe maternal disseminated intravascular coagulation (DIC)
3. In a woman diagnosed with certainty dead more than 1 hour
4. Only for the purpose of baptism
5. Where any risk of cesarean section would be maternally fatal
6. Where there is no available anesthesia of any kind
7. For the purpose of sterilization only
8. In the presence of intraabdominal infection, nonobstetric

Contemporary fetal indications

1. Abnormal fetal heart rate pattern that persists and a fetal scalp pH of less than 7.2
2. Abnormal fetal heart rate with cardiac abnormalities
3. Low birthweight child with abnormal fetal heart rate or any other added problem, such as other than a normal vertex position, multiple gestation, long duration membrane rupture not responsive to amnioinfusion, any suspected evidence of even mild asphyxia
4. Abruptio placenta with live child and no maternal DIC
5. Placenta previa, central or with worrisome blood loss if near viability, failed conservative treatment with a hemorrhage will activate cesarean delivery
6. Active genital tract maternal herpes simplex virus
7. Idiopathic thrombocytopenic purpura (ITP) with low platelet count fetus
8. Hydrocephaly in certain cases

9. Highly valuable child
10. Prolapsed cord without labor, or prolapsed arm or arm and leg together

Contemporary maternal indications

1. Mechanical obstructions to the birth canal
2. Genital tract malignancy, cervical, vaginal carcinoma
3. Permanent cervical cerclage
4. Massive abruption of the placenta with imminent shock and potential interference with the blood clotting mechanism
5. Obstetric situations that require delivery not necessarily only for the fetus

Almost all the indications from the era of 1940 to 1975 with few exceptions, the term *absolute,* while not ideal, is no longer ruled out.

The extraperitoneal operation can be used in long, infected, debilitated cases in which prevention of gross contamination of the abdominal cavity may be the difference between life and death. It is acknowledged that it may not totally prevent peritonitis, but at least it prevents an overload of contaminated material. It can be done electively for purposes of instruction in a medical school environment.

The low-segment operation is the method of choice for most cases of cesarean section. Variations in techniques are essentially a matter of choice by the obstetrician.

The fundal operation is chosen for selected cases in which delivery through a low-segment incision would be compromised and especially in premature fetal malpresentations.

Abdominal hysterotomy is done in cases of indicated late abortion when labor induction is not feasible or possible.

Although vaginal hysterotomy is rarely used, it can be valuable in certain situations in which removal of a fetus is essential to save its life when it is not feasible to subject the patient to an abdominal operation.

COMPLICATIONS OF CESAREAN SECTION
Intraoperative complications

Uterine hemorrhage. Heavy sudden blood loss in the course of or at the start of the operation disturbs the surgeon-obstetrician and arises from several causes:

1. Uterine atony
2. Extension of incision into uterine vessels
3. Anterior implantation of the placenta or placenta previa
4. Premature placental separation with or without abruption
5. Myometrial damage from severe placental abruption
6. Incomplete removal of the placenta includes placental anomalies
7. Presence of myomata uteri
8. Suspected or unsuspected uterine rupture

9. Cervical or vaginal lacerations from attempts at vaginal delivery
10. Partial or complete placenta accreta
11. Failures of the blood clotting mechanism
12. Uterine trauma at the time of delivery of the fetus

Each of these problems is solved in a specific and individual manner. Uterine atony is solved by injection of oxytocic drugs, systemic and local; uterine massage and the use of hot packs; eventration and temporary or permanent occlusion of the uterine vessels; hysterectomy as a last resort. Uterine trauma, incision extension, and rupture are all managed by local hemostasis, the use of clamps and suture repair; vessel obstruction or hysterectomy may be necessary. Blood clotting problems are usually managed by the hematologist and anesthesiologist.

Placental abnormalities and hemorrhage. Position of the placenta in the uterus can cause any number of difficulties before, in the course of, and after delivery (Fig. 67-31). The posterior low level is an incursion into the pelvic space. The importance of recognition of this was emphasized by Stallworthy, who also strongly recommended detailed important care in such cases because the low level posterior placental position was exceedingly potentially dangerous. Not only can the placenta prematurely separate in this position, but the presence of the tissue mass prevents engagement of the fetal pole into the pelvic inlet. The latter may compromise management of placental separation blood loss. An anterior low-level placenta may cause similar problems but has the added disadvantage of impedance of a surgical approach through the anterior uterine wall at low-segment cesarean (Fig. 67-32). Management usually depends on the degree and frequency of blood loss, the position of the fetal pole at the onset of labor, and whether the presentation is vertex or breech. Encroachment of the placenta into the cervix with the subsequent interference with normal labor and delivery together with the increased incidence of hemorrhage is a frequent indication for cesarean. This is known as placenta previa. A central placenta previa almost always is an indication for operative delivery (Fig 67-31). A delivery through a LUS incision may require premature placental removal, incision of placental tissue, and penetration of the tissue mass to reach the fetal pole. Extensive hemorrhage can occur at this time. Rapid dissection, delivery, and immediate placental removal are mandatory (Fig. 67-33). In contemporary obstetrics, the diagnosis often can be made by ultrasound (US) examination.

When there is premature separation of the placenta, regardless of its position, which is known as abruption in certain circumstances, the operator must be prepared for unusual blood loss. Abruption is usually associated with a normally implanted placenta, and there may be several stages of severity (Fig. 67-34). In such cases, blood replacement is often necessary, hysterectomy may be required, the fetus may be compromised especially when premature, and the mother can be seriously involved.

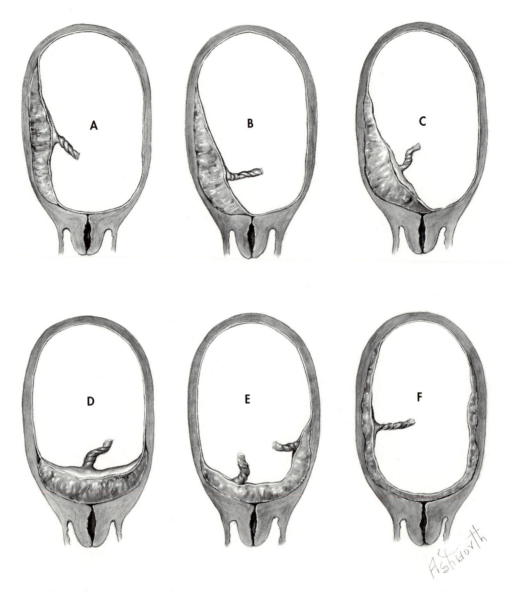

Fig. 67-31. Various placental positions. **A,** Low level. **B,** Marginal placenta previa. **C,** Partial placenta previa. **D,** Central placenta previa. **E,** Twin placenta previa. **F,** Placenta membranacea.

Whenever possible, all eventualities must be communicated to the patient and her relatives in detail before the operation. Massive intrusion of blood into the uterine wall may cause such trauma that the uterus cannot contract and a condition known as uteroplacental apoplexy (Couvelaire uterus) is observed. This often leads to the intense onset of shock, complicated by interference of the formation of normal blood clots and a condition known as disseminated intravascular coagulation (DIC), which may be a threat to the mother's life. Treatment involves the entire surgical team, which includes hematologists and laboratory personnel. If further surgery is necessary after the condition is brought under control, uterine or hypogastric artery ligation may be sufficient to stop the hemorrhage. If the uterus has been badly damaged, hysterectomy is indicated.

If the situation is not so severe, sustained external pres-

sure may control blood loss from the open placental bed after cesarean; if this does not suffice, sutures placed in the area may control blood loss. Intrauterine or intravenous medications may bring about sustained uterine contraction; hot packs may also be used.

If there should be a placenta accreta in association with placenta previa and blood loss persists after removal of all but the adherent portion, hysterectomy may be indicated (Fig. 67-35). Occasionally, if blood loss stops, the accreta may be left intact to be treated with methotrexate. This should begin immediately postoperatively. The patient should not nurse. She should be observed carefully with almost constant follow-up, and, if there are no complications, the methotrexate can be reversed as indicated. If one is fortunate, the placental tissue can be seen with a high-resolution US or magnetic resonance imaging (MRI), and,

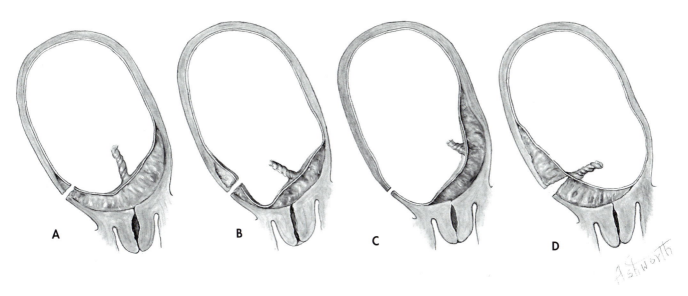

Fig. 67-32. Placental injury by an incision in the LUS wall. **A,** Placental edge entered. **B,** Placental lobe entered. **C,** Placenta missed. **D,** Center placenta entered.

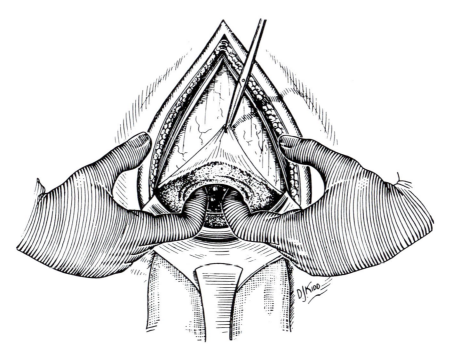

Fig. 67-33. Finger dissection of LUS cesarean section placenta previa. (From Marshall JM: *Cesarean section: lower segment operation,* London, 1939, John Wright & Sons, Bristol & Simpkin Marshall [from Geppert and Hauser].)

if it tends to disappear rapidly, the treatment may be successful. The progress can be followed with hormonal tests and charts of hormone concentration curve, as in the management of hydatid mole or choriocarcinoma. If hemorrhage or other complications such as infection, severe constant pain, or reaction to the chemotherapeutic agent become increased in severity, hysterectomy may have to be done. Actinomycin can be used, but its action is not reversible; sequential measureable titers are mandatory.

If a myoma that has undergone red degeneration is pedunculated, it may be removed without much difficulty. However, attempts to perform intramural myomectomy are not usually recommended because of excessive blood loss and additional creation of thinness of the uterine wall; there almost always is prolonged postoperative recovery. Use of the laser has future possibilities, and it remains to be seen if dissolution of myomatous tissue with the laser followed by polyglycolic suture closure of the wound will

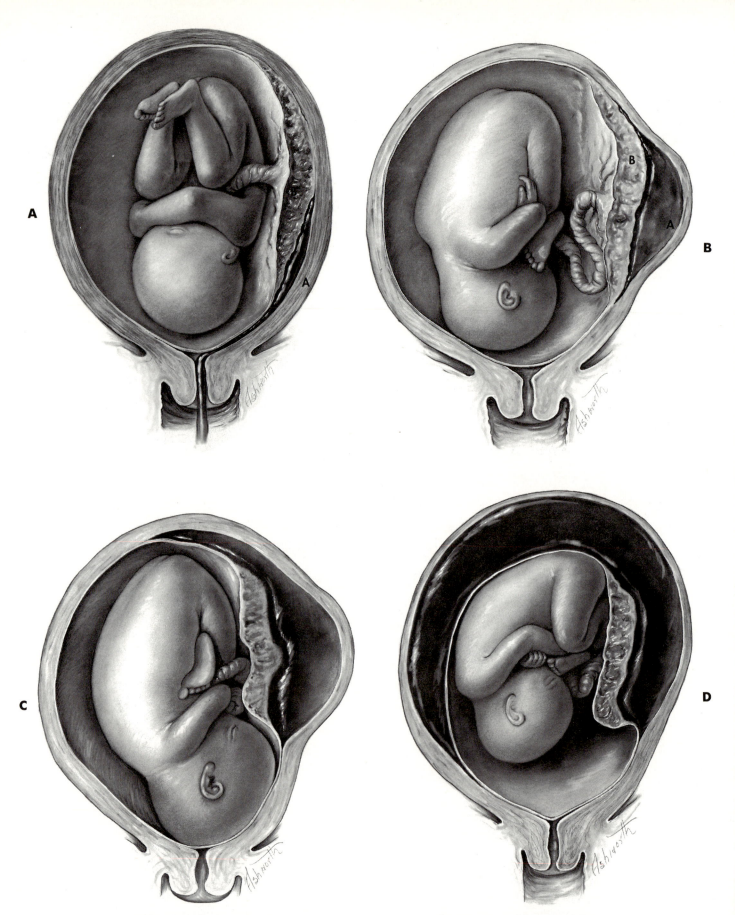

Fig. 67-34. Placental abruption. **A,** Early placental separation with blood loss. *A,* Area of minor separation; *B,* placenta. **B,** Early occult placenta separation. *A,* Blood clot; *B,* placenta. **C,** Moderately severe separation. *A,* Large blood clot; *B,* separated placenta. **D,** Total placental separation with uteroplacental apoplexy.

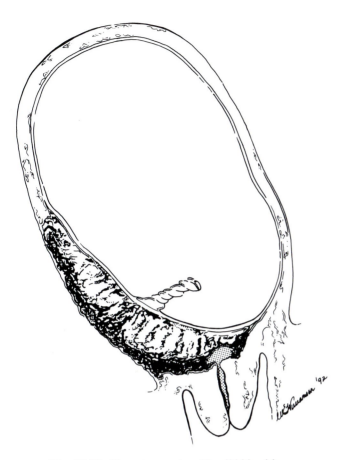

Fig. 67-35. Placenta accreta with mild blood loss.

permit myomectomy especially for control of blood loss at cesarean.

Urinary tract injury. Vesical laceration is easily repaired if recognized early in the operation; this can be done with a mucosal inversion suture in the bladder wall followed by a second layer for reinforcement. The bladder should be tested for integrity after closure and before suture closure of the abdominal cavity. It is more secure to use a serosal cover procedure over the uterine suture line and close the parietal peritoneum in such cases; drainage is arbitrary.

Ureteral avulsion, or partial or complete severance, is repairable usually with success if diagnosed at the time of the accident. Although all operators should know more than one method for ureteral anastomosis or repair, consultation with the specialized urologist is recommended, especially in the litiginous atmosphere of modern practice. Drainage is always provided, and wound closure is meticulous, *never by use of permanent sutures.*

Uterine infection. When the uterus is infected at the time of the cesarean, this is usually due to long and difficult labor, with extended time of membrane rupture and some trauma from attempted vaginal delivery. There is obvious endometritis and chorioamnionitis, which is treated during and after the operation with rigorous antibiotic ther-

apy. Minimal amounts of nonreactive absorbable suture material are used for closures, and, in such cases, the peritoneum is closed and the proper areas are drained; if the infection is extremely severe, the abdominal wound may be left open down to the peritoneal or fascial layer. Severe acute thrombophlebitis associated with extensive uterine infection is rarely seen in the United States but is seen in Third World countries. This requires intensive detailed complicated care and generally is not an intraoperative problem.

Gastrointestinal problems. Intraoperative problems with the bowel usually have to do with adhesions and possible bowel injuries associated with lysis of these tissues. This may occur with trauma associated with adhesion separation from previous surgery. Instant repair is indicated; if bowel resection is needed, this should be done by a general surgeon. As a rule, bowel surgery is contraindicated with cesarean section.

Lethal or near-lethal accidents. Amniotic fluid embolism, with a sudden pulmonary crisis, is usually a problem for anesthesia; minimal manipulatory termination of the cesarean is indicated (Fig. 67-36). Other severe accidents such as vascular or fatty pulmonary embolism, cardiac arrest, severe convulsions, or coma require the immediate attention of a team, which presumably is available in every modern operating suite. Attention to the child, if undelivered, is essential; hemostasis should be complete. Placental removal is best allowed to be spontaneous, and wound closures are delayed until the patient's condition permits such activity. The wounds should be closed routinely if the patient expires.

Postoperative complications

The majority of postoperative problems include postanesthesia complications, which are frequently pulmonary difficulties. Situations such as postspinal headache or paraesthesias related to conduction anesthesia are not ordinarily cared for exclusively by the obstetrician. The development of endometritis with or without peritonitis requires extensive supportive treatment and specific high-dose combinations of antibiotics. Ileus is not common in modern times, but, when it occurs, treatment should be IV hydration, no oral intake, careful and complete laboratory studies, and close observation. US or x-ray studies may reveal the severity of the problem and lead to more active treatment such as nasogastric suction or, in severe cases, the passage of a Miller-Abbott tube. Urinary tract infection is common postoperatively and is usually managed with post culture-specific antibiotics and hydration; failure to respond to usual treatment leads to suspicion of urinary tract injury. Wound infection that appears 2 or 3 days after cesarean may be from an unsuspected infected uterus before the operation or, more commonly, from a contaminant at the time of surgery. With the meticulous care with which surgery is done today, none of these should occur. Usually a break in technique is the responsible factor, and every effort should be made to prevent wound infection in other-

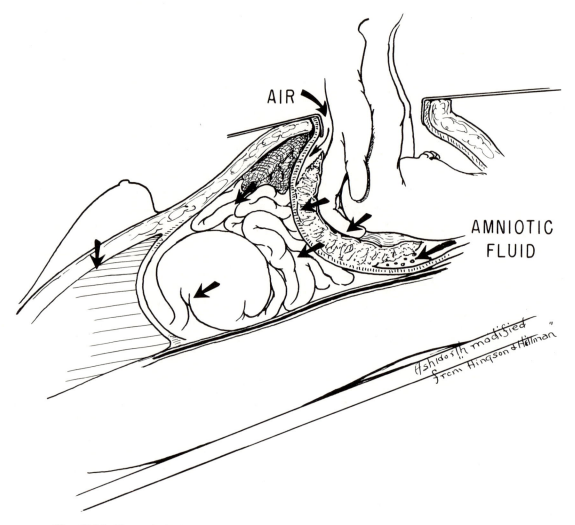

AIR

AMNIOTIC FLUID

Ashidosth modified from Hingson & Hellman

Fig. 67-36. Theoretical etiology of an amniotic fluid embolus or an air embolus at cesarean section.

wise clean cases. Details of the methods of performance of the operation must be reviewed and examined constantly. Wound infections are now related to a classification of the conditions of the genital tract at the time of surgery.

These vary from primary clean to totally infected. Some wounds may be predicted to break down with infection on this basis, and prophylactic antibiotics may be effective in the reduction of the severity and numbers of these. Drainage should be properly employed in wounds in which infection is probable. An infected wound should be treated by exposure to the fascia and the use of local, established methods for management. Wounds may be closed by first or second intention. In cases of dehiscence, the wound should be debrided if necessary, closed loosely with Smead-Jones or retention sutures, and managed with local methods. In cases in which there is bowel protrusion, closures should be accomplished in the operating room. Supportive measures of all kinds are available for use in these cases. "Necrotizing fasciitis" is the most formidable of wound problems and requires early diagnosis, extensive

debridement, several times, a combination of at least three antibiotics, and hyperbaric oxygen. Final treatment may require skin grafts.

Postsurgical convulsions in eclampsia are managed as aggressively as before surgery. Postsurgical hemorrhage may be due to uterine atony, incomplete placental removal or accreta, or blood loss from the wound. US frequently makes the diagnosis for a probable specific cause of the blood loss. Treatment includes exploration, as indicated, to produce hemostasis in the uterine wound.

CESAREAN SECTION ANESTHESIA

General inhalation anesthetics discovered in the early 1800s by Morton et al were introduced early by Simpson into use in conduct of labor and delivery. Ether, chloroform, and nitrous oxide were used until the early 1900s when cyclopropane and thiopentothal were added. Potential risks for both mother and child were recognized, so, when the regional anesthetic agents were devised, prompt use of them for cesarean section developed. All anesthetic

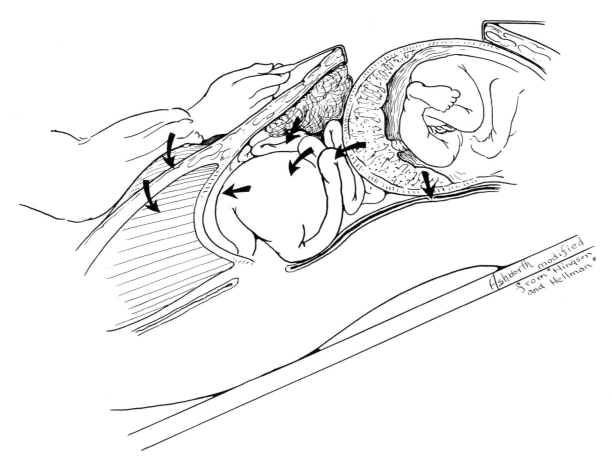

Fig. 67-37. Effect of pressure from several sources to produce hypotension with flat supine position at cesarean section.

agents virtually removed the agony of abdominal surgery and solved most of the problems of pain control with operative procedures. Most important was the recognition of the effect of these agents on the fetus as well as the mother. The adaption of anesthesia for cesarean section with this knowledge facilitated the rise of the anesthesia specialist, especially in obstetrics, such as Apgar.

Conduction anesthesia was used in cases in which the fetus or the mother was in a grave situation and in which a rapid delivery was mandatory. Induction with intravenous pentothal in small doses, the addition of nitrous oxide and oxygen followed by intravenous curare, and perhaps the addition of one of the halogenated agents as indicated is a method of choice for certain emergency cesarean sections. Regional anesthesia is more popular for most operations and frequently can be used both for a test of labor and the subsequent cesarean sections when necessary.

Regional anesthesia began with carefully administered and monitored intrathecal or spinal anesthesia for cesarean section. This was followed by caudal anesthesia, known as a "low-lying" epidural. Continuous caudal epidural was then developed with use of a catheter in the caudal space to replenish the anesthetic agent as needed; this could be successfully used for the conduct of labor and also for a cesarean section when necessary without the addition of

another medication. In contemporary obstetrics, this has been replaced with epidural anesthesia, which accomplishes a similar result and may be easier to administer with reduced risks.

Inhalation anesthesia must be monitored for the inherent risks of inhalation of gastric contents, anoxia, hypotension, and concentration of anesthetic agents in the fetus. Regional anesthesia must be monitored for inherent risks of hypotension, a possibly fatal elevation level, and postanesthesia complications such as headache, meningeal irritation, and other rare problems. Position of the patient for cesarean section is paramount to prevent compression of the great vessels and is prevented by turning the patient's body to the left approximately 15 to 20 degrees (Fig. 67-37). Intravenous lines are mandatory, and, in the case of conduction (inhalation) anesthesia, *so is tracheal intubation, the only sure method to prevent aspiration.*

Local infiltration anesthesia for cesarean section has specific indications. Certain points with its use must be considered. The patient should have a minimal nonthreatening amount of sedation—just enough to alleviate anxiety and fear. She should be verbally encouraged throughout the procedure with explanation as to what is going on and what to expect in the way of sensation from time to time. At best, the operation should be considered less

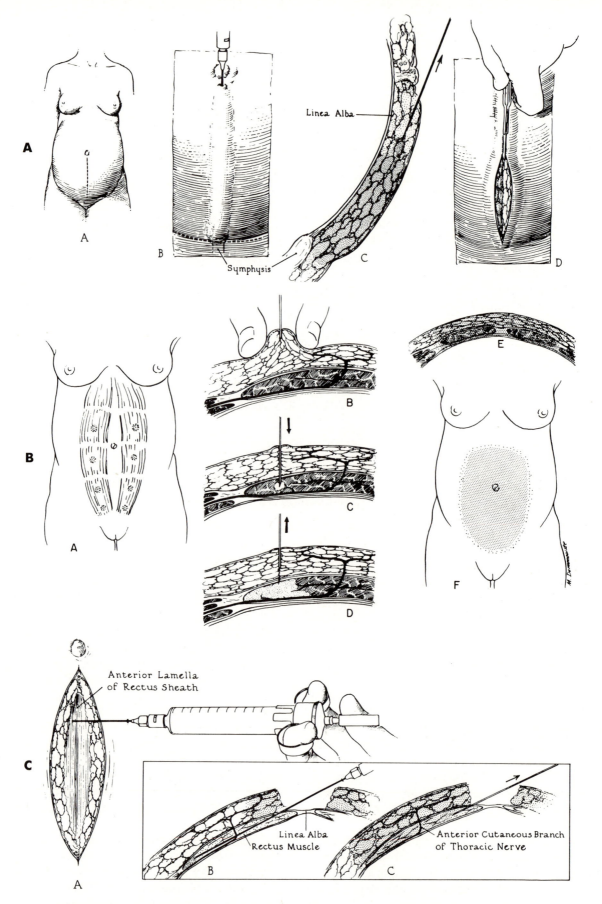

Fig. 67-38. Local anesthesia for cesarean section midline incision. **A,** *A,* Incision line; *B,* superficial injection; *C,* detailed illustration; *D,* superficial incision. **B,** *A,* Areas for injection; *B* through *E,* details of injection; *F,* area of anesthesia. **C,** Details of injection. **D,** *A,* Extended injection; *B,* detail; *C,* area of anesthesia.

painful than vaginal delivery without anesthesia. The choice of local anesthetic is arbitrary, but what must be always carefully considered, as with continuous epidural or spinal techniques, is the *quality and quantity* as well as low concentration of the agents used. The primary indications for local anesthesia are: (1) circumstances in which there is no anesthesiologist available or perhaps not even another physician obtainable; (2) cases in which endotracheal intubation is impossible and it is important to provide exceedingly light anesthesia with a high oxygen content combined with the use of local injection; (3) neuromuscular diseases such as myasthenia gravis in which muscular relaxation medications should be avoided; and (4) patients with failed regional attempts at spinal or epidural who wish to be awake (Fig. 67-38).

Special application of anesthesia is evident for patients who are high risk (e.g., patients with toxemia, eclampsia, chronic hypertension, any heart disease, hepatitis, diabetes, pulmonary disease, placental abruption, severe chronic or acute anemia).

Regional anesthesia for cesarean for breech delivery appears to be the method of choice. Because it has been observed that there can be some effect on the fetal brain by epidural or spinal anesthetics, these side actions are prevented as much as possible. Any deleterious effect from regional anesthesia is probably due to an unexplained overdose of the metabolites of the anesthetic agent, hypotension, or sedative drugs. Because the morbidity of breech delivery by cesarean section is not yet acceptable, this could be corrected by improved management of the delivery at the time of the operation. There is no question that the brain can be easily traumatized by a careless or unnecessarily difficult delivery of a breech through the ce-

sarean wounds. The same skill and art of obstetric management of these presentations must be used in these cases as much or more than in vaginal delivery. All of these factors are highly increased and magnified in the case of the premature breech. The outcome of vaginal delivery of a premature breech is also not acceptable, and, for many reasons, the usual performance of cesarean in these cases can be very different. Difference in placement and size of both incisions is essential, and the care with which anesthesia and manipulation at delivery are done is greatly intensified. Occasionally, a uterine muscle-relaxing agent will facilitate removal of the child, especially when there is an unformed low uterine segment.

Evaluation of the child at delivery

At delivery, the child has been very carefully monitored throughout labor or evaluated before an elective operation. Abdominal and scalp records have been taken, and blood studies have been done. Characteristic tracings are seen by monitor. At delivery, some idea of the child's condition exists. The Apgar score is taken immediately either before or after the cord is cut. An Apgar score reads:

Sign	0	1	2
Heart rate		Slow (below 100)	Over 100
Respiratory effort	Absent	Slow, irregular	Good, crying
Muscle tone	Absent	Some extremity flexion	Active motion
Reflex irritability	Flaccid	Grimace	Vigorous cry
Color	Blue or pale	Extremities blue Body pink	Completely pink

The original Apgar score used 0-3 for 0, 4-7 for 1, 8-10.

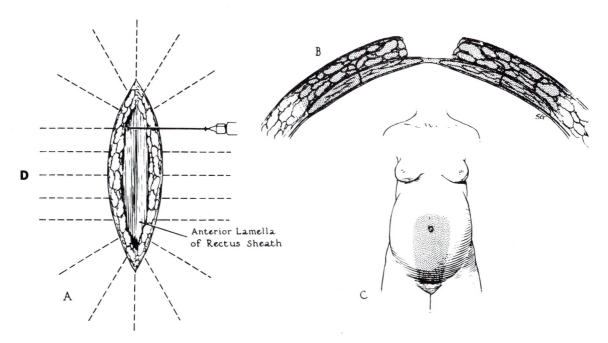

Anterior Lamella of Rectus Sheath

Fig. 67-38, cont'd. For legend see opposite page. (From Bonica J: *Principles and practice of obstetric analgesia and anesthesia,* Vol. 1, Philadelphia, 1967, FA Davis.)

There must be an integrated, close relationship between all members of the team that is prepared to care for the vulnerable child in many obstetric matters. This team includes the perinatologist, who is the keystone of modern obstetric practice. Unquestionably, the presence of a highly trained specialized anesthesiologist at all cases of cesarean section will reduce morbidity even more.

ADJUNCTIVE SURGERY WITH CESAREAN SECTION

Questions with regard to surgery other than the cesarean section arise with regard to appendectomy, herniorrhaphy, ovariectomy, myomectomy, gastrointestinal surgery, panniculectomy, correction of uterine anomalies, and tubal ligation. In general, each of these has a very specific indication; routine appendectomy at every operation is not recommended. Excision of ovarian cysts or paraovarian cysts is indicated if there are no complicating factors related to the primary operation. If the cesarean section has been elective without any complications, excision of pedunculated myomata may be performed without risk. Subserous myomata, unless they interfere with closure of the uterine wound, should not be removed. Uterine anomalies should not be repaired, with the exception of a small uterine horn or sacculation. Excision of a previous defective myometrial scar may be performed.

Tubal ligation must be done with attention to the increased vascularity of the mesosalpinx; the more simple procedures such as Pomeroy or Parkland are the most popular. The tube should be ligated with at least *1-0 and preferably #1 plain catgut;* this produces the greatest immediate local tissue reaction, which is desirable. The Uchida procedure is the most dependable with an almost nonexistent failure rate (when properly performed). On the other hand, if poorly performed, it requires more time and skill and can result in local bleeding or hematoma formation. Ampullary fimbriectomy such as the Kroner, with use of 1-0 plain catgut as a ligature, double tied is simple and effective; except in rare circumstances, an Irving procedure is not indicated at cesarean section. Because of the added time of operation and the increased blood loss, total hysterectomy at the time of cesarean section is not usually indicated for sterilization. Good postoperative recovery is directly related to operating time, low tissue trauma, minimal blood loss, and reduced size and amount of suture material.

Any severe gastrointestinal disease that includes the gallbladder should be dealt with by a consultant. Panniculectomy should not be done; repair of a symptomatic hernia, if small and simple, can be done at cesarean section. Umbilical hernia, which is common in pregnancy, can be repaired very easily. Superficial plastic surgery can be done currently with the cesarean under local anesthesia, but extensive tissue dissection and any surgery on the breasts should be avoided.

ELECTIVE CESAREAN SECTION AND POSTCESAREAN VAGINAL DELIVERY
Elective cesarean section

A repeated cesarean section is performed for conditions in which a trial of labor is not indicated. Some examples of this are: previous classical operation, poorly healed postcesarean section scar, the presence of the same indication for which the previous operation was done, evidence of imminent uterine rupture, fetal indications that preclude vaginal delivery at any time, and central placenta previa.

The single most important consideration in elective or repeated cesarean section is "timing." The maturity of the fetus must be established without any doubt. This is one of the most serious failures in the use of the elective operation and should be one that never occurs in modern obstetric practice. Fetal pulmonary maturity can be determined by several factors. Whenever possible, the determination of accurate gestational dates is essential. Reliable dates can be supported by records of ovulation when available. Early pregnancy tests done by the patient have become common and are reliable when positive on a given date in relation to the last menstrual period. Pelvic examination, accurate estimation of fundal height, determination of a fetal heart, and "quickening" all indicate accuracy of conception time. US determinations are more reliable to determine fetal age and size at various times in the pregnancy and are used with increased accuracy to judge overall fetal maturity. Invasive studies such as amniocentesis with determination of lecithin-sphingomyelin (L:S) ratio, while moderately risky, are nevertheless very valuable markers of lung maturity. It is obvious that careful prenatal care and exact records together with the information from fetal maturity determinations are absolutely necessary to establish both fetal whole body and lung maturity. It may be necessary to allow the patient to go into labor and then perform the operation with further estimation of fetal maturity whenever possible. Failure to be particularly precise about this matter may be disastrous, for RDS and HMD may produce a damaged child, which could have been avoided and will lead, if nothing else, to indefensible litigation.

Postcesarean vaginal delivery

Now that the "once a cesarean section always a cesarean section" theory has been put to rest, the practice to permit vaginal delivery after a previous cesarean section has reached a proportion of approximately 65%. This is true even after more than one previous cesarean section in the past 10 years. If the original indication is absent, previous postoperative course was uneventful, and there are no other contraindications, vaginal delivery after cesarean section has become very successful. Rupture of the uterine scar is relatively rare. The use of very dilute oxytoxic agents to enhance labor has been without event; vaginal delivery has progressed readily. If the patient has had a vaginal delivery either before or after a previous cesarean section, her chances of success are high. Prostaglandin gels have been used to ripen the cervix in several cases without noticeable deleterious effect. If there are suspicions that the scar may have ruptured, an immediate cesarean section can be performed. This means that vaginal delivery after cesarean section should be done in an adequate environment with a full backup of personnel available for major surgery.

CESAREAN SECTION ETHICAL AND LEGAL CONSIDERATIONS
Definitions

ethics right or wrong, good or bad, moral obligation (Webster Law); a rule of conduct imposed by authority (Oxford Dictionary)

life animate existence (Oxford Dictionary)

murder to kill a human being intentionally, unlawfully, with malice aforethought; to kill wickedly or inhumanely (Oxford Dictionary). To kill a person secretly as opposed to openly (old English law). To kill a person under circumstances defined by statute (Webster's Dictionary).

In the sense of ethics, a decision between two of its elements and the concept of moral obligation, a third element, is involved in questions of the correct use of the cesarean operation. In the earliest of times, moral obligation was the primary consideration in these decisions. In India, a child was removed postmortem by abdominal incision to provide it with a separate burial in the ground rather than by cremation with its mother. In Sumer, 2000 BC, female slaves were delivered by cesarean section, details unknown; legal preference for inheritance was given to the child born by "normal" means. According to the Talmud, a child was removed from an agonal woman in childbirth even on the occasion of the Sabbath. In 1751, when cesarean mortality was extremely high, Burton stated that to abandon an undeliverable live woman with a live child to certain death was unpardonable; because to neglect to save a person when one has the power to save her makes him an accessory to her death, and to decline the operation under the circumstances described above made him an accessory to the death of two persons.

Questions are raised by these historic references.

Questions

What was the justification of the separation of two persons at the time of death during childbirth?

Was there religious custom that required the establishment of independence for the child?

What was the importance that the identification of the unborn child be verified by release from the prison of its dead mother's body?

Whatever the reasons were for the separation of child and mother postmortem, the infant was removed by abdominal incision in most cases for many centuries without emphasis or reference to the principle of right or wrong.

The first legal reference to this practice is in the *Lex Regia* of Numa Pompilius 715 BC (see Chapter 1). The child should always be removed from a dead woman's body.

The strongest impact of thought on this matter was by the Christian church and the importance of the right of baptism. Before and all through the Middle Ages, there was movement of the nuns into midwifery; males were excluded even from the examination of a female except in rare instances of embryotomy by instrumentation. Questions arose in the minds of these midwives that concerned certain situations.

If there is no clear evidence of fetal movement, how can one be certain that a child is still alive after the death of its mother?

How can one be sure the mother is truly dead and the child is not alive?

How long after a mother's death can a child survive in utero?

Does baptism of a newly dead child entitle it to the proper quality of life after death?

If no knowledgeable person is present at a woman's death with a viable child in utero, can a "lay" person perform postmortem cesarean section?

Does any public or religious authority or relative have to give permission for postmortem operation in such cases?

What is the punishment for failure to rescue a live child postmortem?

Most of these questions, until very recently, have never been adequately answered and there are those who are still not sure of all the answers. One of the motivations to write about obstetric matters was ostensibly for the education of midwives; almost all the earliest obstetric texts were for this purpose. There was intense pressure to remove a child for baptism, if not to save its life, and this led to many strange practices including the pretense of life in a postmortem child so that it could be baptized and properly buried. It has been suggested that maternal death was even hurried to allow for abdominal delivery. In the 1500s, Estienne was the first to suggest cesarean section in the moribund woman. He depicted a certain area and kind of abdominal incision for this purpose. In the past, ethics, the law, and religious matters came into conflict, and Estienne's suggestion of the agonal cesarean, as it was referred to, helped solve some of this dilemma.

Even in contemporary times, "when does the soul enter the fetus?" is the most vexatious question. Is an unborn fetus a person? When does a fetus really become *viable* without life support in a highly technical neonatal intensive care nursery? Aside from this point in the decision for cesarean, consider the incredible impact of this matter in questions of abortion.

The matter of the soul was debated by literally thousands of religious people in the Western world and millions in the Eastern world and still is. For an historic landmark in the West, there is the philosophic attitude of Tertullian in 200 AD who was the greatest protagonist of the soul for many years. His opinion was that the fetus was a living organism from conception and did not acquire life at birth. He was convinced that the soul was in the fetus from the beginning and considered various obstetric procedures such as embryotomy on a living child. He referred to an instrument that caused a violent secret intrauterine death without the obvious dismemberment of embryotomy. This was a long, bronze, sharp, stylet, called a "foeticide," which was inserted into the fetal head in utero, which caused a fetal death. Later in this same reference, Tertullian referred to the use of an abdominal incision to deliver a child for preservation of its "soul." This adherence to the concept of the soul caused an ethical problem when embryotomy was considered because, if it was carried out with a live child, it can be judged as being murder.

Should a woman be sacrificed to preserve a child, if not for life, at least for baptism? An English translation of Trotula leaves little doubt how the midwives were advised: "When the woman is feeble and the chylde may naught comyn out, then it is better that the chylde be slayne than the moder of the chylde also dye." According to St. Paul (Rom. 3:8) no woman should be sacrificed for the purpose of saving the child: "Evil should not be done that good may come." In the 1500s, on the other hand, is the famous quote of Henry VIII regarding the fate of Jane Seymour: "Save the child by all means, for it is easier to get wives than male heirs." In 1513, Roesslin in his text on advice to midwives implied the presence of males at the time of cesarean section, even though one midwife in the 1300s had apparently performed seven successful operations.

At a meeting of the faculty of Doctors of Theology in France in 1733, four questions were asked for solution:

1. Can one use the cesarean operation to save a mother and child when there is a good prognosis to save one or the other by the procedure? The answer: One can use the operation when the best prognosis is good for both mother and child.

2. Can one prejudice a mother, to obtain a secure salvation for the child when her certain death will be caused by the operation? The answer: If the operation will cause certain death, one cannot use it as a remedy. There is more in the answer, but, in summary, it was said that God who gives us life, alone can dispose of it; one cannot do evil to do good; the mother's consent does not make the operation legal; she is not in a state to give away that which is not hers to give; one cannot compare the temporal life of the mother with the spiritual life of the child, because one compares the mother's homicide with the child's misfortune and this assures the homicide is a crime without excuse, whereas the child's misfortune, deplorable as it is, does not charge anyone.

3. When the loss of both mother and child is anticipated because of the circumstances that surround

them, can one be expected to use the cesarean section for the one who has the better chance of survival? The answer: In such a case, even if there is no certainty of success with the operation for either, it is permissible to use it. One can certainly use a doubtful cure in a hopeless disease. One would not use the operation, however, to accelerate a death to obtain a life.

4. Finally, if one can save only the mother or the child by the use of the operation, with good prognosis for the other, which of the two is preferable? The answer: In response to this, the Council regarded the respect for the question to a court of law, but there is always the requirement of mercy. If one does not abide by the law, one can sacrifice the child's life for that of the mother; but mercy demands that a mother may prefer the preservation of the child's rightful life. We have the right to preserve the life God has given us, and we are empowered to take away the refuge when to do so rejects that which needs it. (This is a rough translation from Pundel.)

In 1752, Fra Cangiamila in his text, "Embryologie Sacree," very strongly indicated the opinion of the Christian church about the absolute importance of salvation of the soul through baptism. There were implications of the tendency to favor the child in this writing, and he reported on more than 112 cases of postmortem cesarean section with successful infant baptism. This historic background provides consideration of some aspects of these heavy decisions in contemporary obstetrics. For example, from a legal point of view, a physician who dismembers a live child in utero because it cannot be delivered vaginally or another who performs a cesarean section for a live child with full knowledge that such an operation will kill the mother could be liable for a charge of murder. Murder charges have never been brought probably because of the involuntary nature of inescapable circumstances. However, if either child or mother or both die because of neglect, ignorance or failure to perform the duties of an obstetrician in accord with established minimum standards, or if the physician is under the influence of drugs or alcohol and is totally incompetent to accomplish *anything* properly, such a person may be liable for more than just malpractice.

In the 1700s, every possible solution was explored and Sigault, in 1768, proposed a method to increase the size of the internal bony pelvis by splitting the cartilage of the pubic symphysis. This procedure has many sequelae but is still used in some countries. For over 150 years, the discussions raged as to the ultimate anterior-posterior internal measurement that would not permit even an embryotomy. Several women were left to die with a partially dismembered dead fetus still in utero in the mistaken belief that such treatment did not constitute murder as much as the use of the cesarean operation. As of 1843, the cesarean was considered the most brutal operation in medicine, condemned by every principle of humanity, philosophy, and religion. No one understood that long difficult labors with ruptured membranes and multiple internal and external manipulations before performance of a cesarean *compromised the operation completely*. By 1865, Radford stated that no physician had cause to commit murder of the unborn and that the lack of reasonable estimate of the child's value had led to destruction of infants for which there was no compensation. Barnes, who greatly favored embryotomy, was of the opinion that physicians should not employ vengeance against the woman who could not deliver vaginally, by use of cesarean section as punishment. In 1880, Kinkead in Ireland remarked that a live unborn child has as much a right to life as the mother has to hers. At that time, the earlier philosophy was repeated that, in the end, the mother has the inalienable right of survival even if it means destruction of the child, because both she and the physician were answerable to God and the child was not. The impact of anesthesia, antisepsis, hemostasis, and suture of the uterine wound was immeasurable and between 1880 and 1940 cesarean section mortality was 5% or less. The operation became more improved as to "timing," and indications were observed early in labor or often even before.

Injudicious use of the operation arose with improvement, and this may be a problem in modern times. Two major problems still existed in the early twentieth century: the continued risk and presence of intraabdominal infection and uterine rupture with a subsequent pregnancy. This led to the dictum, "once a cesarean always a cesarean" and stimulated invention of the low uterine segment and extraperitoneal operations and caused investigation of certain indications. As the safety of the operation increased, these questions became more important from the standpoint of the ethical use of cesarean:

1. Should cesarean be performed when the child is dead?
2. Can the parents or relatives demand that the operation be done?
3. Should cesarean section be done without a medical indication, such as high social value of the child?
4. Is preservation of the soft tissue of the pelvis a reason for performance of the operation?
5. Are most abnormal fetal presentations always delivered by cesarean?
6. Should the operation ever be performed for gross fetal abnormalities?
7. What are the ethics of performance of a cesarean for a moribund woman?
8. Is a failed induction of labor with ruptured membranes after 48 hours an indication for the operation?
9. Are severe psychoses or unstable personalities contraindications for vaginal delivery?
10. Is an abnormal fear of labor or the loss of three premature infants compensated by elective cesarean?

All of these reasons have been used for performance of cesarean many times. The ethical considerations of these various problems are rarely discussed with the parents; some overly conservative obstetricians would not consider most of these at any time for cesarean section. The moral integrity of the obstetrician in attendance has been questioned on occasion, and absence of it may have been correct. The importance of truth as one sees it, with all the available information and perhaps the opinion of another, equally ethical physician, may solve some of these unacceptable practices. Instruction of the importance of absolute personal integrity in medicine has been considered since before the second millennium BC. In cases involving two or more lives, this integrity must be complete.

As this century moves on, lawsuits and open criticism in the media; ethical considerations by the public in other areas of reproductive medicine such as abortion, in vitro fertilization, surrogate parents, preservation of fertilized ova, use of fetal organs for transplantation, artificial insemination especially in parents of the same sex: and improvements in intrauterine surgery have all influenced the use of cesarean section in the United States.

Terms such as right to life, right for perfection, wrongful life, and maternal denial of the operation are now in the public eye almost on a daily basis. Consideration of court-ordered cesarean section regardless of the parent's wishes is a potential devastation in obstetric practice. Incursion of the law into medicine in obstetrics began, as has been seen, with the *Lex Regia* in 715 BC. This was preserved in the Justinian Code, and the principle was reviewed in 1139. Rules of conduct in relation to cesarean section were established in Europe in various countries. One of the most extensive was the decree in 1749 by Charles III of Spain made in Sicily, which empowered priests and other laypersons in the Catholic Church to perform postmortem cesarean in the absence of a physician. This decree was the basis for postmortem cesarean performed by Catholic priests in the early days of California and Mexico.

In France, postmortem cesarean was decided by the physician and the family; if the Catholic Church insisted on the operation, *it was never supported by the law*. In the early 1800s, there was punishment for burial of a woman with a viable child without an examination by an expert to decide to save the child.

In another country, cesarean operations could only be done by a specialist unless there was sudden death, in which case any physician could do it. Viability was set at 6 months' gestation. Postmortem cesarean had to be performed with the same care and diligence as if the woman was alive. Some of the laws in Europe were enacted as late as 1835. The multiplicity and sometimes discrepancy in these legal decrees indicated the confusion over the ethics of performance of cesarean section. The only law still known in the United States is a state law that requires the permission of a husband or near relative to allow a postmortem operation whenever possible.

In contemporary practice there are several items for consideration, for example, negligence, which is composed of duty, breach, causation, injury. It is the obligation of the obstetrician to use all knowledge, skill, care, and diligence in management of all decisions with regard to the kind of birth required for the best outcome. When is referral indicated? Should there always be a second opinion? Informed consent should always contain at least the reason for the operation, the risks, the potential complications, alternatives, consequences if not performed, and recuperation. Other matters are concerned with the timely cesarean, the failure to perform it at all or at the wrong time, failure to perform the operation properly, the problems of the broken instruments, presence of a foreign body in the uterus or peritoneal cavity, and the principle that the surgeon is still responsible for everything and everyone in the operating room.

Some situations must be considered in the use of the cesarean operation that might not be usually recognized: What is the legal status of a child who is killed in utero by a bullet, dies during intrauterine fetal surgery, dies because its mother is killed or injured either accidentally or maliciously, dies from prematurity because of elective cesarean, or dies from maternal drug overdosage or extreme alcoholism? These are mostly matters for attorneys, and, yet, this begins another dilemma: What are the mother's rights to permit or request a cesarean, and what are the child's rights for delivery by cesarean rather than by vaginal delivery no matter how difficult.

Cases have been filed in the courts in which the person who caused the violent death of the child either directly or indirectly is indicted for second-degree murder. Recent cases reported in the media with potential if not actual legal consequences are as follows:

1. A young woman was admitted in labor in an Emergency Room, with no prenatal care, in deep coma and knowledge that she had taken a recent heavy dose of crack cocaine. There was fetal tachycardia. She delivered a newly dead infant in 3 hours. The mother may be indicted for manslaughter or murder on the basis of violation of the fetal right to life.

2. A young woman, who was an intense chronic drug user throughout her pregnancy, delivered a newly stillborn child. She was not indicted because of very low mentality and an inability to recognize the gravity of her situation. She was recommended for custodial care.

3. A young male was arrested, indicted, and convicted of second-degree murder of an unborn child. He struck the automobile in which the mother was being driven while he was under the influence of drugs and alcohol. She suffered severe injuries and deep hemorrhagic shock, which led to the death of her 7-months' premature child delivered by emergency cesarean section. The defendant showed no remorse and was sentenced to a long prison term without parole. At issue were the rights of the unborn child and whether a 7-months' premature child could survive outside the mother's body.

4. A case is under consideration for indictment of a severely chronic alcoholic young woman, drunk throughout her pregnancy, who delivered a child so severely compromised by fetal alcohol syndrome that it could not survive. There are no extenuating circumstances.

5. There are two recent cases of trauma to an unborn infant by gunfire. One was a "drive-by shooting," which resulted in trauma to the abdomen and uterus and an injury to the fetal zygomatic arch and the external ear on the same side. The mother survived. The second was a gunshot trauma of the abdomen at the time of the recent Los Angeles riots. This random bullet lodged in the fetal arm, which prevented it from entrance to vital areas. Both of these involve questions of assault with a deadly weapon upon the unborn child.

The precedence for these cases is not strong, and it remains to be seen what the law will ultimately do with such conditions. It is the role of any physician who is involved in obstetrics to enter into discussion of all of these things, and it is also the role of obstetric organizations to impact as strongly as possible in the creation of solutions that are reasonable, moral, ethical, and correct for all concerned.

CONTEMPORARY CESAREAN SECTION

The primary concern with the use of cesarean delivery, aside from life itself, is the preservation of the fetal brain. Everyone who conceives is entitled to a perfect child regardless of any of the factors that mediate against this. This single element is probably the most important cause of the high cesarean rate in modern American obstetrics. Litigation involves the liability of the obstetrician in cases of the imperfect child and almost never its parents, especially the mother (see Chap. 10).

The human brain develops as the largest single organ in the embryo and at 38 to 40 weeks weighs an average of 350 g. It doubles in size by the sixth month of neonatal life, averaging about 700 g. It doubles again by 3 years of age. Preservation of this remarkable organ must begin early in prenatal life. During this time, critical influences that affect the brain occur. These may be beneficial under normal conditions but may produce devastation when adverse environmental factors are present. Toxic poisons can enter the fragile vulnerable brain cells as a result of almost all drugs ingested by the mother. The more toxic the drug, the greater is the damage. The effects of so-called benign medication or foods that may impair these cells are not reversible. Nerve cell damage is observed in cases of starvation or inadequate diet, irradiation, and trauma. Neurophysiologists state that millions of nerve cells never reproduce. They cannot repair themselves. They cannot be replaced. Once injured or killed, these cells are lost (see Chapter 6).

The effects of the conduct of prenatal care, no matter how exact and careful, may be negated by the rigors of labor, trauma of delivery, obstetric accident, uteroplacental insufficiency, or inherent genetic defects, among other things. Modern obstetric practice uses an incredible array of scientific devices and chemical materials to facilitate the care of the fetal brain before, during, and after labor and delivery. This includes the judicious use of cesarean section to respond to indicators of fetal trouble, failing labor, or maternal physiologic problems.

Knowledge of predictable difficulty in the obstetric situation is essential in the never-ending battle for preservation of the fetal brain. Information derived from US and numerous other testing methods may lead to cesarean section as the method of choice for delivery even without a test of labor or trial of induction of labor. This obviously is in the interest of preservation of the fetal brain. Obstetric accidents such as premature separation of the placenta, prolapse of the fetal cord, sudden or increased development of fetal distress, or uterine hemorrhage with central placental previa, for example, all indicate immediate surgical intervention, again, especially for preservation of the fetal brain. Some maternal illnesses may have a profound influence on developing brain cells, and the progression or intensification of such disease leads to the performance of elective cesarean, even premature, rather than induced premature labor. Otherwise, obstetric situations are obvious, such as failed labor, disproportion between the fetus and maternal pelvis, and several others, as indicators for avoidance of traumatic vaginal delivery by performance of cesarean.

Some of the effects of instrumental delivery on the fetal brain are incompletely known, and there are undoubtedly subtle effects on the fetal brain by these maneuvers that are as yet unknown, regardless of the skill and competence of the specialized obstetrician.

Ricci and Marr in 1942 stated: "Of what value is the adroit forceps (or vacuum extractor) delivery of a woman in prolonged labor if every muscle and every fiber is stretched and attenuated beyond resiliency, if the perineal body becomes relaxed, scarred and functionless, initiating a trial of distressing pelvic symptoms? Of what value is a type of delivery which (thus) destroys the natural tone of the vagina and starts the gradual descent of the cervix and fundus necessitating an eventual drastic repair." The author would add, perhaps of even greater importance, of what value are such deliveries and ill-timed interventions if there is permanent damage to the fragile cells of the infant brain, with the recollection that a high percentage of "nerve cells" never replace themselves; once damaged, forever damaged, they are not restored. The disastrous effects of asphyxia, internal cerebral blood loss either gross or microscopic, and laceration or distortion of brain tissues by trauma and edema set the stage for the tragedy of the kind of damage in which all variations of cerebral palsy are only partial results.

Cesarean section is, of course, no panacea against these damages to the fetus by any means, but, if its use is judicious as to "timing," true indication, and other factors, it is potentially a positive influence in the production of a healthy child. External elements such as prematurity, poor surgical ability, careless delivery of the child through abdominal or uterine incisions of improper size or placement, improper anesthesia producing anoxia or toxic effects, maternal hypotension, excessive blood loss before delivery all influence the success of cesarean delivery.

The inability to guarantee a perfect child by abdominal delivery is cause for careful deliberation with regard to frivolous or convenient use of the operation. One must be prepared to defend both sides of the case; the operation should have been done earlier, or electively, or later, or not at all!

The passage of time and the potential increase in knowledge and sophistication in the management of the reproductive process from start to finish, which includes cesarean section, should assist all physicians to reach a much higher success with the product "the perfect child."

SUGGESTED READINGS

1. Apgar V: Proposal for a new method of evaluation of the newborn, *Anesth Analg* 32:260, 1953.
2. Baas J: *Outlines of the history of medicine,* Huntington, NY, 1971, Robert E Kreiger (Translated by H Handerson; originally published in 1889).
3. Baudelocque J: *L'art des accouchements,* ed 3, Paris, 1796, Chez Mequignon.
4. Bauhin C: *Hysteromotokia by Francisco Rousset,* ed 1, Basle, Conrad Valdkirch, 1581 (Translated by C Bauhin).
5. Beck A: Low segment cesarean section, *Am J Obstet* 79:179, 1919.
6. Benirshke K: *Pathology of the placenta,* New York, 1991, Springer-Verlag.
7. Bhishagratna K: *The Sushruta Samhita Varanasi,* ed 2, India, 1963, Chowkhamba Sanskrit Series Office.
8. Blumenfeld-Kosinski R: *Not of woman born,* Ithaca, NY, 1990, Cornell University Press.
9. Boley J: Caesarean section, *Can Med Assoc J,* 32:557, 1935.
10. Bonica J: *Principles and practice of obstetrical analgesia and anesthesia,* Philadelphia, 1967, FA Davis.
11. Bumm E: *Geburtshulfe,* ed 17.
12. Burns H: The Latzko extraperitonial caesarean section, *Am J Obstet Gynecol* 19:759, 1930.
13. Cangiamila F: *Embryologica sacra,* Milan, 1751 (abridged into French, 1762, Chez Nyon).
14. Cartwright E: Retrovesical extraperitoneas cesarean section, *Am J Obstet Gynecol,* 39:423, 1940.
15. de Lee J: Newer methods of cesarean section, *JAMA* 73:91-95, 1919.
16. de Lee J: An illustrated history of the low or cervical cesarean sections, *Am J Obstet Gynecol* 10:503-520, 582-583, 1925.
17. Dionis M: *Cours d'operation de chirurgie,* Paris, 1740, Chez d'Henry.
18. Doderlein A: *Operative Gynakologie Doderlein-Kronig,* ed 5, Leipzig, 1924, Georg Thieme.
19. Duhrssen A: Vaginaler Kaiserschnitt bei Eklampsie, *Arch Gynakol* 39:235.

20. Durfee R: Extraperitoneal cesarean section, *Surg Gynecol Obstet* 1962.
21. Durfee R: "Low classical" cesarean section, *Ob-Gyn Survey* 27:624, 1972.
22. Estienne C: *La dissection de partis du corps,* Paris, 1546, Chez Simon de Colines.
23. Finan M et al: The "Allis" text for easy cesarean delivery, *Surg Gynecol Obstet (Int Abstr Surg Suppl)* 174:22, May 1992.
24. Kehrer F: Ueber ein modifiziertes Verfahren beim Kaiserschnitte, *Arch Gynakol* 19:177, 1882.
25. King A: The legacy of Jesse Bennet's cesarean section, *Bull Hist Med* 2:242-250, 1976.
26. Kinght A: Life and times of J Bennett, MD, *S Hist Mag* 2:1-13, 1892.
27. Latzko W: Extraperitonealer Kaiserschnitt, *Wien Klin Wchnschr* 22:477-482, 1909.
28. Marshall C: *Caesarean section lower segment operation,* Bristol, 1939, John Wright & Sons.
29. Maygrier J: *Midwifery Illustrated 1833 (Translated by A. Doane.)*
30. Mercurio S: *La comare o raccoglitrice,* ed 2, Venice, Italy, 1713, Domenico, Lovisa.
31. Norton J: Latzko extraperitoneal caesarean section, *Am J Ob/Gyn* 30:209, 1935.
32. Opitz E: Die Kaiserschnitt, *Zent f Gynak* 35:270, 1911.
33. Osiander F: *Handbuch der Entbindungkunst,* Tubingen, Ger, 1820.
34. Phelan J, Clark S: *Cesarean delivery,* New York, 1988, D Appleton.
35. Poidevin L: *Caesarean section scars,* Springfield, 1956, Charles C Thomas.
36. Porro E: Dell'amputazione utero-ovarica come complemento di taglio caesareo, *Annal univers di med e chirurg* 5:237, 1876.
37. Preuss J: *Biblical and talmudic medicine,* New York, 1978 Sanhedrin Press (Translated by F Rosner.)
38. Pundel G: *Histoire de l'operation cesarienne,* Brussels, 1969.
39. Ricci J, Marr J: *Principles of extraperitoneal caesarean section,* Philadelphia, 1942, The Blakiston Co.
40. Ricci J: *The development of gynecological surgery and instruments,* Philadelphia, 1949, The Blakiston Co.
41. Ricci J: *The geneology of gynecology,* Philadelphia, 1950, The Blakiston Co.
42. Roonhuyze H: *Heel-konstige aanmerkkingen betreffende de gebrekken der vrouwen,* Amsterdam, 1663, (translated into English London, 1676).
43. Rosslin E: *Rosengarten,* Munich, 1910, reprint G Klein & Carl Kuhn (originally published 1513).
44. Rueff J: *De conceptu et generatione hominis.*
45. Sanger M: Die kaiserschnitt, *Arch f Gynak* 19:370, 1882.
46. Scultetus J: *Armamentarium chirurgicum,* Frankfort, 1666.
47. Siebold EV: *Geschichte der geburtshulfe,* ed 2, Tubingen, 1901, Franz Pietzcker.
48. Suetonius C: *The historie of twelve caesars,* London, 1931, Frederick Etchells & Hugh Macdonald (Reprint by Oxford University Press; originally published in English 1606).
49. *Sushruta.* In *The Sushruta Samhita Varanasi,* ed 2, India, 1963, Chowkhamba Sanskrit Series Office.
50. Tertullian: In Ricci: *The geneology of gynecology,* Philadelphia, 1950, The Blakiston Co.
51. Waters E: Retrovesical extraperitoneal cesarean section, *Am J Ob/Gyn* 39:423, 1940.
52. Williams J: *Obstetrics,* ed 17, Baltimore, 1989, Williams & Wilkins.
53. Young J: *Caesarean section,* London, 1944, HK Lewis & Co.

DICTIONARIES

1. *Cassell's new latin dictionary,* New York, 1960, Funk & Wagnalls Co (Originally published in 1854).
2. *Cassell's new german dictionary,* New York, 1959 Funk & Wagnalls Co.
3. *Cassell's new french dictionary,* New York, Funk & Wagnalls Co.
4. Klein's Etymological Dictionary
5. Oxford Dictionary
6. Webster's Dictionary
7. The Holy Bible, King James version

Chapter 68

CESAREAN HYSTERECTOMY

David L. Barclay

EVOLUTION OF THE OPERATION

Cesarean hysterectomy evolved as a life-saving procedure to prevent death after cesarean section. When the uterus, with a gaping wound, was returned to the peritoneal cavity after cesarean section; maternal mortality approached 100% as a result of intraperitoneal hemorrhage and spillage of infected uterine contents. Animal experiments suggested that the uterus was not an essential organ, and it was thought that removal might reduce the prohibitive postoperative mortality. Porro, in 1876, reported the first successful hysterectomy at the time of cesarean section. However, within six years, Sanger introduced closure of the uterine incision with multiple sutures, which obviated the need for a hysterectomy. The Sanger operation became known as the conservative cesarean section and the Porro operation as the radical cesarean section. The Porro operation was reserved for the treatment of uncontrollable hemorrhage and uterine infection after cesarean section.

Interest in the operation as an elective procedure was rekindled with the advent of improved antimicrobial agents and relatively safe blood banking procedures in the 1940s. These developments expanded the indications for all elective operations, including cesarean hysterectomy. During the next two decades, reports from major clinics showed elective cesarean hysterectomy to be considered a suitable procedure for sterilization at the time of an obstetrically indicated cesarean section. In addition, total cesarean hysterectomy was recommended in place of the Porro procedure, which consisted of a subtotal hysterectomy and bilateral salpingo-oophorectomy. This enthusiasm began to wane in the latter part of the 1970s. By the 1980s, publications reflected an adverse attitude to the elective operation, and in many major centers the operation was reserved for emergency indications only.

Era of speculation: 1768-1868

Joseph Cavallini, in 1768, published his experience with experiments on dogs and sheep in which he removed the uterus at the time of delivery. His conclusions were as follows: "All which things having been duly weighed, I do not doubt that the uterus is not at all necessary to life; but whether it may be plucked out with impunity from the human body, we cannot be certain without a further series of experiments of this kind which perhaps a more fortunate generation will attain."[48]

In 1809 Dr. G. P. Michaelis of Marburg suggested that amputation of the uterus after removal of the fetus might make cesarean section a less dangerous operation. Although Dr. James Blundell confined himself to experiments on animals, in 1828 he suggested in his lectures on obstetrics at Guy's Hospital that he was inclined to believe that the dangers of the cesarean operation might be considerably diminished by removal of the uterus. He encouraged adoption of this change in the method of operating in successive lectures and editions of his book on obstetrics. Despite the great mortality accompanying cesarean section in Great Britain, no surgeon in that country ever tested the value of his suggestion. He died at the age of 87, in the year 1878, by which time other surgeons had proved his views to be correct. The history of cesarean section has been reviewed in great detail by Young.[48]

The first operations: 1868-1876

Horatio Robinson Storer performed the first cesarean hysterectomy on a woman.[43] Storer was a strong individualist who received his degree from the Harvard Medical School in 1853 and continued his training in Paris and London. In 1855 he entered general practice in Boston but soon broke with tradition and announced himself a specialist in the diseases of women. He became the first American physician to teach gynecology as a separate subject and was the first surgeon to wear rubber gloves while operating. His staunch independence resulted in his removal from the Harvard faculty in 1866, which was the year in which he performed the fourth successful abdominal hysterectomy in the United States.

Storer and his associate, Bixby, performed the first cesarean hysterectomy on July 21, 1868. Storer had seen the patient on July 16, 1868, and determined that vaginal delivery would be impossible, even with craniotomy, because of a large abdominal tumor obstructing the birth canal. The onset of labor occurred on July 18 and, despite active labor and rupture of the membranes, the presenting part could not enter the pelvis. Surgery was delayed until the morning of the 21st, when the operation was performed using chloroform anesthesia. A large uterine fibroid complicated the operation and caused extensive hemorrhage. The male child and placenta were badly decomposed, and hemorrhage was profuse. After cesarean section, a metallic cord was firmly tied around the lower uterine segment. The corpus and adnexa were excised and the cervical stump exteriorized. The patient succumbed to infection on the third postoperative day.

In contrast to Storer's unplanned emergency operation, Eduardo Porro of Pavia, Italy, carefully planned and exe-

cuted the 26-minute operation that he performed on May 21, 1876.[43] Prior to that operation, no woman had ever survived a cesarean section in Pavia. The patient was a 25-year-old primagravid dwarf who had a skeletal deformity complicated by rickets, resulting in absolute disproportion. Porro felt that a cesarean section was mandatory, discussed the matter with his colleagues, and planned the operation very carefully. The patient, Julia Cavallini, sought religious support and finally consented to the operation after 6 hours of labor. Essentially, a classical cesarean section was performed, after which there was profuse hemorrhage from the uterine incision. The corpus and adnexa were delivered through the incision, and a wire snare of Cintrat was placed around them and drawn tightly at the level of the internal os. The structures could then be excised and the cervical stump exteriorized through the lower pole of the incision. Peritoneal toilet was accomplished, and a large curved clamp was placed through the vagina and cul-de-sac into the peritoneal cavity for insertion of a large drainage tube. The uterine stump was incorporated into the lower angle of the wound and painted with an antiseptic. The snare was removed with the gangrenous portion of the uterine stump on the fourth postoperative day and the vaginal drain removed the following week. By definition, a Porro operation is a subtotal hysterectomy and bilateral salpingo-oophorectomy.

Porro assumed the Chair of Obstetrics at the university at Pavia in 1875 and remained until 1882, when he became head of the School of Obstetrics of Milan. In 1902 he wounded his hand during an operation on an infected patient and died from sepsis. His statue stands in the courtyard of the Women's Hospital at the University of Milan (Fig. 68-1).

There was serious question about the morality of the operation; he discussed the issue at great length with the bishop of Pavia, who sanctioned the hysterectomy as a procedure for saving the patient's life. Only with this backing could Porro present his operation to the Medical Congress of Turin. The keys to his success were planning of the operation prior to prolonged labor and rupture of the membranes, use of chloroform anesthesia, and adherence to Lister's principles of asepsis. The operation was accepted in European countries but was not favorably considered in Great Britain or the United States. At the Vienna Lying In Hospital during the previous 100 years, not a single woman had recovered after cesarean section. From 1787 until the first successful Porro operation in Paris in 1879, all cesarean section patients had died at the Maternity Hospital at Paris. Nevertheless, in 1879 Harris of the United States was not ready to accept the operation and called it an "unsexing and mutilating procedure."[48]

Evolution of operative technique

Modifications of the operative procedure began shortly after the report of Porro's operation. Muller, in 1878, delivered the uterus through the abdominal incision and constricted the lower uterine segment with an elastic tube, af-

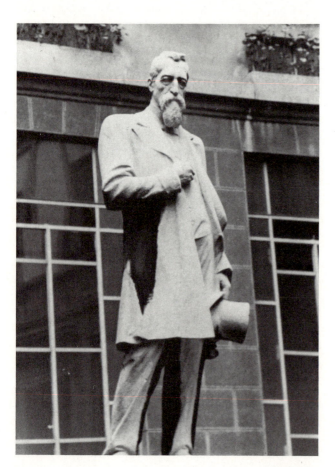

Fig. 68-1. Statue of Professor Eduardo Porro in the courtyard of the Instituto Obstetrico Ginecologico L. Mangiagalli Dell 'Universita' Di Milano. (Courtesy of Professor G.B. Candiani.)

ter which the uterus was incised, delivery effected, and the corpus amputated. The concept was that the peritoneal cavity would be protected from contamination.[19] However, the constrictor caused asphyxia of the child. The first Porro-type cesarean hysterectomy in the United States was performed in 1880 by Isaac Taylor of New York. The cervical stump was returned to the abdominal cavity after hemostasis had been secured, and no drains were employed. Unfortunately, the patient died of a pulmonary embolism on the 26th postoperative day. The first 50 cases of "cesarean ovarohysterectomy" from the world literature were reported by Harris[27] of Philadelphia in 1880; there were 29 maternal deaths and 7 fetal deaths; 23 of the operations had been performed in Italy and 11 in Australia. The first successful cesarean hysterectomy in the United States was performed using the Porro-Muller technique by Richardson in 1881. In that same year, Spencer Wells performed the first total cesarean hysterectomy for cancer of the cervix. Goodson performed the first in the United Kingdom in 1884, using a transverse incision that was extended laterally by traction; this was the first reference to the low segment operation. In addition, he summarized 134 Porro operations, indicating that return of the cervical stump to the peritoneal cavity was associated with a 77% mortality compared to a 53% mortality for exteriorization.[19] Von Waerz, in 1892, introduced specific vessel ligation and returned the cervix to the peritoneal cavity in uninfected patients; otherwise it was exteriorized. By 1901 the overall maternal mortality was 24.8% in the 1097 operations that had been reported.[19]

Only six years after the first successful Porro operation, Max Sanger, a German surgeon, introduced the use of a large number of sutures, deep and superficial, to secure perfect closure of the uterine wound and prevent spillage of blood and lochia into the peritoneal cavity. As noted above, this came to be called the conservative cesarean section, or Sanger operation, while the Porro operation was called the radical cesarean operation. Although Sanger was not the first to close the uterine incision, he described the procedure in detail. The conservative cesarean section became the procedure of choice, and cesarean hysterectomy in the United States was limited to emergency situations such as infection after prolonged labor and hemorrhage. Cesarean hysterectomy was replaced by the low cervical or extraperitoneal procedure for the treatment of intrauterine infection.[48] The Johns Hopkins experience was reported by J.W. Harris[26] in 1922: 64 of 223 cesarean sections were followed by a subtotal hysterectomy, with a maternal mortality of 4.68%. Interestingly, 8 operations were performed for sterilization. Sterilization was also listed as an indication for cesarean hysterectomy by Lash and Cummings[30] in 1935.

Evolution of indications

Until the early 1940s, little emphasis was placed on elective sterilization by hysterectomy at the time of cesarean section. At the University of Rochester in 1945, Wil-

son[47] reported that 8.7% of all cesarean sections included a hysterectomy; indications were hemorrhage, uterine pathology, intrapartum infection, and also sterilization. A review in 1947 indicated that in the United States about 2.54% of cesareans were terminated by hysterectomy, with a maternal mortality of 5.2% in contrast to 3.42% for cesarean birth. The results of elective operations were not analyzed separately from those of life-saving procedures.[41] The results of 153 cases of cesarean hysterectomy performed since 1931 were reported by Dieckman in 1948.[17] Again, some operations had been performed strictly for sterilization.

In the early 1940s, expansion of indications for all elective operations, including elective cesarean hysterectomy, was fostered by the increased availability of antimicrobial drugs and the introduction of blood banking procedures. Davis,[17] of Chicago, advocated total cesarean hysterectomy for elective sterilization, removal of the diseased uterus, or removal of the uterus no longer functionally useful for a woman near the climacteric. At the Chicago Lying In Hospital, from July 1, 1947, to April 1, 1951, 140 of 700 cesareans were terminated by hysterectomy. Dyer, Nix, and Weed,[21] in 1953, emphasized the fact that cesarean hysterectomy was the method of choice for surgical removal of a diseased uterus and reported 84 cases of total hysterectomy. They strongly advocated total cesarean hysterectomy, and they described the technique of passing a finger into the vagina through the cervical canal to identify the lower limits of the cervix. In 1951 it became the policy of the Tulane service, Charity Hospital, New Orleans, to perform a total operation. This decision was made after review of 3 patients who had died after a subtotal operation for a ruptured uterus that had extended into the cervix and vaginal fornix, resulting in postoperative hemorrhage.[3] Refinements of the operative technique of total hysterectomy were described by Bradbury[10] in 1955. A radical hysterectomy and pelvic lymphadenectomy for treatment of cancer of the cervix was reported by Brunchweig and Barber[12] in 1958. Cesarean hysterectomy was openly advocated as a sterilization procedure during the remainder of the 1950s.[4]

Cesarean hysterectomy, primarily for elective reasons, was further advocated in the 1960s, although most authors felt that a cesarean section should not be performed simply for the purpose of removing the uterus. In 1963 Pletsch and Sandberg[37] raised the question of whether or not cesarean hysterectomy should replace cesarean delivery and tubal ligation for sterilization. The "post-tubal ligation syndrome" was a concern to some, and Weed[46] questioned the fate of the postcesarean uterus. One half of the September 1969 issue of *Clinical Obstetrics and Gynecology* was devoted to articles on the subject.[44] From January 1, 1938, to September 1, 1959, 1000 cesarean hysterectomies had been performed at the Charity Hospital in New Orleans.[3] All operations were performed after 28-week gestation and following abdominal delivery. The operations were further classified as either elective or emergency procedures; the latter designation included only those operations performed to prevent exsanguination from profuse hemorrhage. If uterine rupture had occurred, the case was included as abdominal delivery and emergency hysterectomy. There were 800 elective and 200 emergency hysterectomies, which constituted 15.3% of all cesarean sections performed during that period of time.

During the 1970s, the incidence of cesarean hysterectomy decreased throughout the country, and although some private institutions retained enthusiasm for it, teaching services were losing interest. The first paper[9] appeared comparing the characteristics of elective cesarean hysterectomy with cesarean birth, with or without tubal ligation. Two papers[1,8] reported the use of primary cesarean hysterectomy to accomplish delivery and removal of the uterus for carcinoma in situ of the cervix. Three review articles were published during that decade.[4,28,32] Altogether, 866 cesarean hysterectomies performed between 1938 and 1967 were reported from the Tulane service, Charity Hospital in New Orleans.[4] The changing indications and modifications of the operative procedure over that 30-year period were reviewed with particular reference to discontinuance of the subtotal operation in 1951. Despite the continued popularity of the operation during that decade, notes of caution were voiced, particularly in a paper by Haynes and Martin.[28]

During the decade of the 1980s, publications emphasized the role of cesarean hysterectomy for management of uncontrolled hemorrhage and perhaps for the treatment of concurrent uterine pathology identified at the time of an obstetrically indicated cesarean section.[4] The latter was only a relative indication, depending upon the experience of the surgeon. A recent review[25] from Charity Hospital in New Orleans indicated that between 1984 and 1988 a total of 129 cesarean hysterectomies were performed after 4891 cesarean sections; 107 were classified as elective and 22 as emergency operations. In a recent update tape,[7] Clark, from the University of Southern California, indicated that at his institution a cesarean hysterectomy was performed in roughly one of 200 cesareans, primarily for control of hemorrhage. During this decade, concern was voiced about the adequacy of residency training for the young physician who might be confronted with the need to perform an emergency postpartum hysterectomy. In summary, outside of a few institutions, cesarean hysterectomy has again become a rather uncommon procedure.

CURRENT INDICATIONS FOR CESAREAN HYSTERECTOMY
Emergency hysterectomy

An emergency cesarean hysterectomy is by definition a life-saving procedure performed to control hemorrhage. The causes of postpartum hemorrhage fall into roughly four categories: uterine atony, placental disorders, ruptured uterus, and extension of the cesarean incision into the uterine vessels. In 1984 Clark et al[16] reported that 43% of emergency hysterectomies in their series were per-

formed for uterine atony. This is somewhat less than the 67% incidence reported by O'Leary and Steer.[32,33] In the Tulane series,[4] extending from 1938 to 1967, 31.6% of operations were performed for that indication. In the early years of that study, the Couvelaire uterus associated with abruptio placenta and a consumption coagulopathy was a common indication. Hysterectomy is, of course, an option of last resort and this is currently an infrequent indication. Clark et al[16] found that hysterectomy for atony had a statistically significant association with amnionitis, oxytocin augmentation of labor, cesarean section for labor arrest, preoperative magnesium sulfate infusion, and increased fetal weight. In 23% of their patients there was no identifiable risk factor causing the atony. A hysterectomy for uterine fibroids in a patient who has undergone an obstetrically indicated cesarean would be classified as elective. However, uterine fibroids may interfere with closure of the uterine incision and contractility of the corpus, causing hemorrhage.

Bleeding from the placental site usually involves the noncontractile lower uterine segment in a patient who has undergone a cesarean section for placenta previa. The lower segment is less resistant to penetration by the placenta, causing placenta accreta, increta, or percreta; the last may result in laceration of the uterine vessels when the placenta is removed. The placenta may penetrate through a previous low segment incision and into the base of the bladder. Placenta accreta in excess of that noted in the older literature is emerging as a major indication for hysterectomy, particularly in patients who have undergone a previous cesarean section.[40] The sharp rise in the cesarean section rate in this country during the past decade may account for this increase.

Uterine rupture is currently the third most common indication for emergency cesarean hysterectomy. In the older literature, separation of a low segment scar identified at the time of cesarean section was the prime indication for elective removal of the uterus. Even in the less muscular fibers of the lower uterine segment, it is not surprising that an incision in an involuting organ would not heal well. Separation of a low segment scar seldom results in either fetal loss or bleeding. On the other hand, frank rupture of a prior classical uterine incision is a catastrophic event, often resulting in expulsion of the fetus into the abdominal cavity and near inversion of the uterus. Spontaneous rupture of the unscarred uterus frequently results from extension of an old cervical laceration; therefore, total hysterectomy is mandatory, and an associated vaginal laceration, which could result in postoperative hemorrhage, must not be overlooked. Spontaneous rupture of an intact uterus is infrequent and can be associated with blunt trauma to the abdomen, which compresses the uterus against the sacral promontory, lacerating the posterior wall.[20]

Extension of a low transverse incision into the uterine vessels or the cervix and vagina is an uncommon occurrence. In patients of low parity, an extended incision can usually be repaired. Care must be taken to prevent damage to the ureter or bladder. Bleeding is not completely controlled by ligation of the anterior division of one or both hypogastric arteries, although pulse pressure in the uterine artery is decreased.[13,16,34] Ligation of the uterine artery at its origin is usually necessary and can be accomplished by developing the pararectal and paravesical spaces. The ureter is identified and the vessels secured with clips, but venous bleeding remains a problem because of the increased vascularity of the pelvis in pregnancy. Throughout the repair procedure, the ureters must be identified by palpation or visualized before placing ligatures or clips.[23]

Elective cesarean hysterectomy

Indications for elective cesarean hysterectomy fall into two categories: pathologic conditions in the pelvis and elective or medically indicated sterilization. These indications are relative, and the frequency with which the operation is performed depends upon the philosophy of the particular obstetrical unit. In some obstetric units, an elective cesarean hysterectomy has never been performed. Primary cesarean section to allow an associated hysterectomy may occasionally be performed for uterine pathology such as leiomyomata or carcinoma in situ of the cervix. Early invasive cancer of the cervix can be treated by a primary cesarean delivery and radical hysterectomy with pelvic lymphadenectomy.[12,42,45]

Since 1980 few publications have suggested elective cesarean hysterectomy as a means of sterilization. In 1980 Britton[11] reported 112 elective cesarean hysterectomies, of which 74 were planned and performed for sterilization; the remaining patients underwent hysterectomy for uterine or other gynecologic pathology or for medically indicated sterilization. Plauché, Gruich, and Bourgeois[35] in 1981, reported 108 cesarean hysterectomies performed in a private practice setting; 46.3% were for the purpose of sterilization. There is little current support for this method of sterilization without the presence of associated uterine or pelvic pathology. Although the failure rate of tubal ligation performed at the time of cesarean section is somewhat higher than that of an interval operation, it is considered to be the method of choice in conjunction with abdominal delivery. Although the fate of the postcesarean uterus has been questioned, it has been suggested that 25% of these patients will undergo a subsequent hysterectomy.[46] In general, interval hysterectomy is thought to present fewer complications.

Uterine pathology indicating a cesarean hysterectomy is usually listed as carcinoma in situ of the cervix, uterine fibroids, or severe intrauterine infection. The advent of improved antibiotic therapy has obviated the need for hysterectomy in cases of infection, although with advanced pelvic sepsis it is an important adjunctive form of therapy, particularly in diabetic and otherwise compromised patients.

Carcinoma in situ of the cervix can usually be accu-rately diagnosed during pregnancy by colposcopy. If invasive disease has been excluded, vaginal delivery is allowed and the cervix treated by an appropriate means after the postpartum period. However, some patients who would be candidates for hysterectomy may wish to proceed with completion of treatment at the time of delivery. In 1977, a satisfactory fetal and maternal outcome was reported for 32 patients treated by cesarean hysterectomy for carcinoma in situ of the cervix.[8] The operations were planned and performed before the onset of labor; therefore, adequate removal of the cervix was accomplished without difficulty.

Uterine leiomyomata are seldom an indication for cesarean delivery unless there is interference with the labor and delivery process. If an interval hysterectomy were planned for treatment of large uterine fibroids, hysterectomy after an obstetrically indicated cesarean section would be appropriate in the hands of an experienced surgeon. This approach appeals to patients and is cost-effective.

A controversial indication for elective cesarean hysterectomy is the "thin uterine scar."[4] Cesarean section scars may vary from thin, white, avascular scars to asymptomatic complete dehiscences. Most low-segment scars can be repaired, but a defective vertical scar extending into the corpus or a T incision may not heal well. Most surgeons would choose to perform a tubal ligation to prevent future pregnancies; however, in the past, hysterectomy was performed in hospitals where tubal ligation was prohibited.

Interval vaginal hysterectomy and repairs would be the treatment of choice for uterine prolapse and vaginal relaxation. If a cesarean hysterectomy is performed for this indication, the uterosacral ligaments should be plicated and a suprapubic urethrovesical suspension performed.[5,9]

If bilateral adnexal pathology is identified at the time of cesarean section, a hysterectomy is ordinarily performed also. Care must be taken not to misinterpret bilateral adnexal enlargement that is due to benign hyperactio luteinalis or luteoma of pregnancy.

Other reported indications for elective cesarean hysterectomy are dysfunctional uterine bleeding, adenomyosis, endometriosis, and other forms of pelvic pathology that would be infrequently identified at the time of cesarean section.

THE SURGICAL PROCEDURE

A cesarean hysterectomy is distinctly different from a hysterectomy in the nonpregnant patient. The tissues are soft and pliable, and the uterine and paravesical veins are markedly distended. Constant tension on the uterine corpus attenuates the very engorged uterine vessels and allows sharp dissection throughout.

Preparation for the operation is that usually undertaken for a patient undergoing an elective cesarean section. Vaginal cleansing has not been routinely carried out. The patient's blood is typed and screened so that blood will be available if needed. For a planned operation, autologous blood can be stored.[14] A short course of prophylactic antibiotics is prescribed and is the same as that used by the surgeon for cesarean delivery. Consent-to-sterilization forms are completed, and the patient is counseled in regard to the irreversibility of the infertility that is a secondary consequence of this operation.

Basic surgical principles that facilitate the operation are as follows:

1. The skin incision may be vertical or transverse.
2. Dissection of the vesicouterine space is carried out before incision of the uterus.
3. A vertical or transverse uterine incision in the lower segment can be used, although the vertical incision facilitates constant tension on the corpus.
4. The uterine corpus is placed on constant tension by the first assistant.
5. Sharp dissection allows the uterine vessels, particularly the veins, to be skeletonized.
6. Vascular pedicles are secured with clamps and cut but not ligated until the uterine vessels on both sides have been secured.
7. Low ligation of the uterine vascular pedicles requires that the ureters be identified by palpation.
8. Compression of the lower uterine segment between the thumb and forefinger allows one to "milk" the soft dilated cervix above the fingers and secure the vagina with angle clamps.

Either general or conduction anesthesia is used, whichever is ordinarily used for cesarean section.[15,29] A vertical or low transverse abdominal incision can be used. It is usually easier to develop the bladder flap over the present-ing part before the uterine cavity is opened; adhesions from a prior cesarean section require sharp dissection. Although the dilated veins over the bladder may appear formidable, sharp dissection and gentle blunt dissection can usually avoid entry into the venous channels.

After delivery of the newborn, the uterus is delivered from the abdominal cavity. The placenta is removed only if it separates easily; otherwise it is left in place. If the uterine incision tends to bleed, it can be secured with large sutures or simply clamped with small ring forceps. It is important to move quickly and secure vascular pedicles without delay. The corpus is placed on constant tension by the first assistant, which maintains anatomic relationships and decreases blood loss (Fig. 68-2). If the need for cesarean hysterectomy has been determined preoperatively, a vertical incision facilitates delivery of the newborn, and the first assistant's finger can be placed into the upper pole of the incision to maintain constant traction on the uterus throughout the procedure. A self-retaining retractor is placed and gauze sponges packed into the cul-de-sac.

If oophorectomy is not indicated, the operation is begun on one side by placing a clamp on the round ligament, which is cut, and the anterior leaf of the broad ligament is incised to join the bladder flap incision. The avascular space in the broad ligament is penetrated, and the utero-ovarian ligament and fallopian tube are doubly clamped and cut, with a third clamp securing the proximal pedicle to prevent back bleeding. With constant tension on the corpus, the broad ligament is incised sharply with the scissors and the uterine vessels skeletonized (Fig. 68-3). This dissection progresses so quickly and easily that the uterine

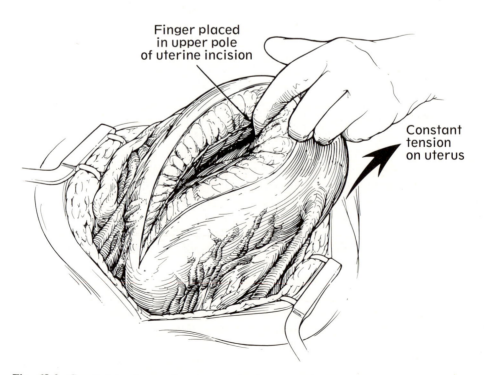

Finger placed
in upper pole
of uterine incision

Constant
tension
on uterus

Fig. 68-2. Constant tension on the uterus maintains anatomic relationships and attenuates the uterine vessels, which facilitates sharp dissection.

vessels may be skeletonized to the cardinal tunnel, jeopardizing the ureter. The clamp is placed on the uterine vessels quite low on the cervix. As a consequence, the vesicouterine space should be reinspected to be certain that the angle of the bladder has been adequately mobilized and perhaps elevated with a retractor. Since the tissues of the cardinal ligament are quite soft and pliable, the ureters can be readily rolled between the thumb and forefinger for precise identification before placing the clamp on the uterine vessels (Figs. 68-4 and 68-5).

After performing a similar dissection on the opposite side and clamping the uterine vessels, the major vascular pedicles have been secured. A proximal clamp is placed on the uterine vessels on either side to prevent back bleeding, after which the uterine vascular pedicles are cut and secured with a stick tie. The round ligament pedicle is secured in a similar manner. The uteroovarian pedicle, however, is quite large and requires a free tie followed by a stick tie. If the ties are placed too close to the ovary, there is a tendency for the suture to cut through the ovarian parenchyma, resulting in intraoperative or postoperative bleeding. As a consequence, about 6% to 10% of patients receive a unilateral salpingo-oophorectomy.[4,9] If the pedicle is entirely too large, the ovarian portion may be secured separately.

The need for additional pedicles can be determined by compressing the lower uterine segment between the thumb and forefinger. This assists in identification of the very soft cervix, which is difficult to define, particularly in the patient who has undergone much cervical dilatation and effacement. Compression of the lower segment tends to "milk" the uterine cervix upward for identification (Fig. 68-6). The adequacy of dissection of the bladder from the upper vagina is again assessed. An additional pedicle is usually required at the base of the cardinal ligament and may include the attenuated uterosacral ligament. The pedicle is grasped with a straight Kocher or Heaney clamp that is allowed to slide off the lateral portion of the cervix and grasp the base of the cardinal ligament. A knife is used to cut a wedge-shaped pedicle that is tied with a suture ligature, which may include and retie the adjacent uterine vascular pedicle. A retractor is placed beneath the bladder reflection to assure that space has been adequately developed, and the cervix is again identified by palpation. A curved Heaney clamp can then be placed on each angle of the vagina, the vagina incised, and the specimen removed. If there is uncertainty about the cervix, the anterior vaginal wall can be opened and the Heaney clamps then placed on each angle of the vagina before circumscribing the remainder of the vagina.

The mucosa of the cut edge of the vagina tends to retract; therefore, Kocher clamps are placed on the anterior and posterior vaginal walls. A figure-eight suture is placed at each angle of the vagina, making certain that the angle of the vaginal mucosa is included and secured to the base of the cardinal ligament. The remainder of the vaginal cuff is closed with figure-eight sutures. If the surgeon prefers to leave the vaginal cuff open, the entire edge can simply be

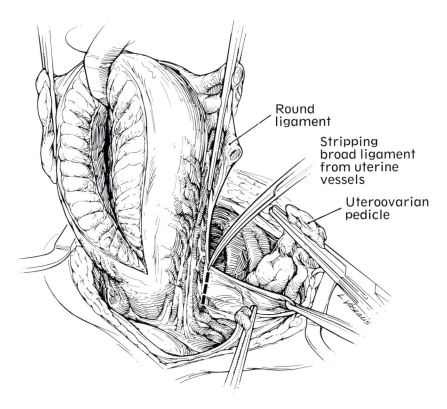

Round ligament

Stripping broad ligament from uterine vessels

Uteroovarian pedicle

Fig. 68-3. Vascular pedicles are clamped but not ligated until the uterine vessels are secured. Uterine vessels are skeletonized by sharp dissection.

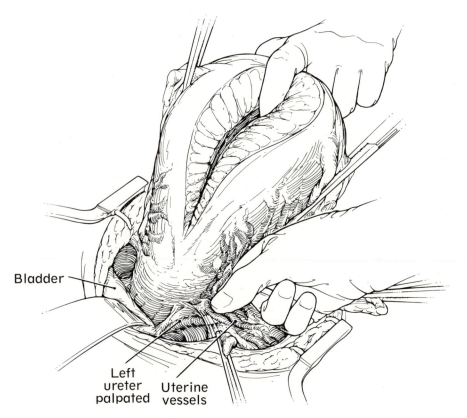

Fig. 68-4. Ureter is rolled between thumb and forefinger and bladder is retracted before uterine vessels are clamped.

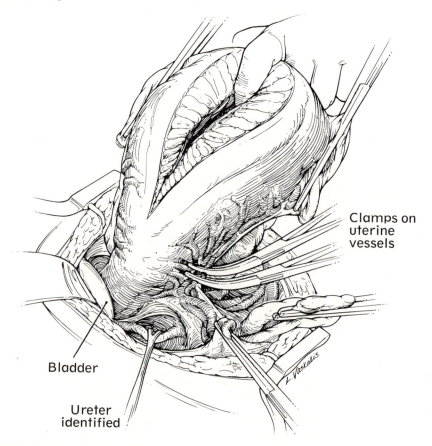

Fig. 68-5. Babcock clamp placed on distal ureter for demonstration purposes. Ureter and bladder are at risk when uterine vessels are clamped.

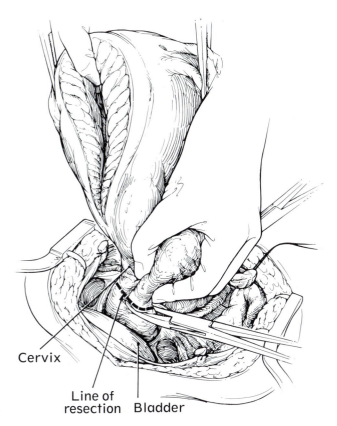

Fig. 68-6. With constant traction on uterus, upper vagina is compressed to "milk" the soft cervix above the fingers. A clamp can then be placed on each angle of the vagina.

run with a locking suture. (Within 24 to 48 hours postoperatively, the vaginal cuff that is left open is probably functionally closed, although it is easier to open if there is a pelvic hematoma.) The pelvis is thoroughly inspected and irrigated, and hemostasis is secured. The ovarian pedicle is secured to the adjacent round ligament and not attached to the vaginal cuff. A transvaginal T tube or extraperitoneal drain is used at the discretion of the surgeon. Ordinarily drainage is not necessary if prophylactic antibiotics are used. I do not reperitonealize the pelvis after any hysterectomy, although this is a debatable issue and the surgeon's choice.

The described surgical technique represents my own bias.[5] A low transverse uterine incision may decrease blood loss from the cesarean section, but constant tension on the corpus is easier with a vertical incision. There may be hesitancy in developing the vesicouterine space before incising the uterus for delivery, but the space is more easily and thoroughly developed over the presenting part, particularly if there have been prior cesarean sections and there is scar tissue in the space. If there is uncertainty about identification of the ureters by palpation, the uterine vessels can be taken at a higher level; however, this requires several pedicles along each side of the uterus, close to the cervix. The lower limits of the cervix can be identified by incising the cervix anteriorly or by entering the vagina posteriorly. This causes additional contamination of the operative field, however, and delineation of the cervix, if well effaced, may still be difficult. Extrusion of mucus from the cervical glands has been suggested by Plauché as a helpful indicator of the lower edge of the cervix.[7] Particularly with emergency cesarean hysterectomies, a variable number of patients reportedly have retained a remnant of cervix. Absorbable suture of polyglycolic and/or chromic catgut is used throughout the operation.

In an emergency situation, in the hands of a surgeon who has had little experience with the operation, subtotal hysterectomy is an acceptable alternative. However, one must be certain that a uterine tear has not extended into the cervix or fornix of the vagina, a problem not resolved by subtotal hysterectomy. After ligation of the uterine vessels, the corpus is amputated and the cervix simply closed.

OPERATIVE COMPLICATIONS

The surgical complications of cesarean hysterectomy are not unique to the operation, but their frequency of occurrence is greater. Operating time may be prolonged, and the frequency of blood transfusion and urinary tract injury is increased. In experienced hands, the average elective operation takes less than 90 minutes, which is approximately 30 minutes longer than a cesarean section, with or without tubal ligation.[9] Plauché et al[35] reported an average operating time of about 65 minutes for a series of elective operations that Plauché performed. The duration of emergency operations depends primarily on the amount of time spent attempting to stop bleeding before a decision is made to remove the uterus. Clark et al,[16] reporting on a series of emergency operations, noted an approximately 3-hour operating time.

The incidence and quantity of blood transfusion depend upon the indications for the operation, whether emergency or elective, the experience of the surgeon, and the extent of pelvic pathology. A hysterectomy performed after a cesarean for a bleeding complication, such as placenta previa, obviously increases the need for blood replacement. In my series,[9] approximately 20% of patients undergoing elective cesarean hysterectomy received a transfusion, but 4% of those undergoing cesarean delivery, with or without tubal ligation, were transfused. The mean preoperative hematocrit in patients undergoing cesarean hysterectomy was 35.6% ± 3.5%; 13 of the 47 transfused patients were admitted to the hospital with a hematocrit of 30% or less, and 1 had undergone a cesarean delivery for bleeding. Plauché, Gruich, and Bourgeois[35] reported that 11.8% of private patients undergoing an elective operation received a transfusion. Fluid administration during the operation can often maintain vital sign stability until equilibration in the recovery room necessitates transfusion. Pritchard et al[39] demonstrated that a gravida at term can lose 1 L of blood with little or no hemodilution in the postpartum period. It may be reasonable for the patient scheduled to undergo a planned elective cesarean hysterectomy to store a unit of her own blood several weeks preoperatively.[14] Some authors[24,34] have recommended ligation of the anterior division of the hypogastric artery prior to hysterectomy, but this has had little influence on the amount of blood loss or incidence of transfusion. Clark et al[16] have also found this to be true during emergency hysterectomy for hemorrhage. On the other hand, if a uterine vessel retracts into the cardinal ligament adjacent to the ureter or there is excessive bleeding for other reasons, one should open the pararectal and paravesical spaces and place a clip on the anterior division of the hypogastric artery and on the uterine artery at its origin. Pulse pressure in the uterine artery is decreased after ligation of the anterior division and may assist in defining the site of bleeding.[13] The importance of operative technique cannot be overemphasized: constant tissue tension, sharp dissection, and development of the vesicouterine space before delivery of the presenting part are imperative if one is to maintain control of the operation and minimize blood loss.

Bladder entry and ureteral injury are recognized complications of cesarean hysterectomy but also occur with cesarean section. In my series,[9] 4 of 390 patients undergoing repeat cesarean section without hysterectomy sustained bladder entry and repair with satisfactory healing; 4 of 242 patients undergoing an elective cesarean hysterectomy sustained bladder entry, all among the 114 patients undergoing a repeat cesarean birth. Eisenhop et al[23] reported 23 inadvertent bladder entries and 29 diagnostic cystotomies in a series of 5376 primary and 2151 repeat cesarean sections. The diagnostic cystotomies were performed to evaluate for ureteral injury. Bladder entry is ordinarily recognized, repaired, and heals uneventfully; most fistulas probably result from inadvertent inclusion of bladder wall during closure of the vaginal cuff or separation of bladder muscle such that the adjacent mucosa undergoes subsequent necrosis. Leakage of urine usually occurs within the first 10 days postoperatively. Some authors[31] have recommended that the bladder be partially distended with methylene blue or sterile milk before or after the hysterectomy to detect an unrecognized entry. A lacerated bladder wall is closed in two layers, using absorbable suture, and the catheter is left in place for approximately 7 to 10 days.

Ureteral injury is a greater risk during cesarean hysterectomy than during abdominal or vaginal hysterectomy in the nonpregnant patient. The ureter is most often injured with ligation of the uterine vessels. However, when salpingo-oophorectomy is performed, the ureter should be identified at the pelvic brim before securing the infundibulopelvic ligament. My technique of cesarean hysterectomy can be used only if the surgeon is confident that the course of the ureter can be identified by palpation. If there is a question of ureteral injury, one can open the bladder extraperitoneally, identify the ureteral orifice, and pass a retrograde ureteral catheter. Another alternative is to perform a linear ureterotomy at the pelvic brim and thread a ureteral catheter into the bladder. Partial severance of the ureter may be detected by injection of methylene blue into the ureteral lumen at the pelvic brim. In my series of 242 elective cesarean hysterectomies,[9] there was injury to 1 ureter,

which was recognized, repaired, and healed satisfactorily, and the hospital stay was not prolonged. In the Tulane series of 866 cesarean hysterectomies performed over a 30-year period,[4] there were 4 ureteral injuries, of which 3 were recognized, repaired, and healed satisfactorily and 1 was repaired during the postoperative period. Plauché, Gruich, and Bourgeois[35] reported no ureteral injuries in a series of 108 elective and emergency operations performed in a private hospital. Mickal and Plauché[31] reported 808 consecutive operations at the Charity Hospital in New Orleans; there were 30 bladder entries, 7 vesicovaginal fistulas, and 2 ureteral fistulas. It should be emphasized again that since dissection and skeletonization of the uterine vessels progress easily in pregnancy, there is a tendency to clamp the uterine vessels quite low. If one cannot be certain of the location of the ureter by palpation, the uterine vessels should be taken high but this means multiple pedicles on each side of the uterus.

It should be noted that Eisenhop et al[23] reported 7 patients who sustained ureteral injury among 7527 who underwent cesarean section: 5 of the ureteral ligations occurred during control of bleeding from extension of a uterine incision into the broad ligament; in 1 patient the uterine incision extended into the trigone of the bladder; in another patient the ureter was compromised during evacuation of a retroperitoneal hematoma. Because the ureters are always at risk during a pelvic operation, the importance of learning to visualize the ureter or define its course by palpation is obvious.

POSTOPERATIVE COMPLICATIONS

Febrile morbidity secondary to infection of the operative site and bleeding are the primary postoperative complications. In most studies the incidence of febrile morbidity is less after cesarean hysterectomy than following cesarean delivery. This is particularly true if there has been prolonged labor or evidence of intrauterine infection. In my series,[9] febrile morbidity after elective cesarean hysterectomy was 31% compared to 55% after cesarean and 34% after cesarean delivery and tubal ligation. The cesarean tubal ligation and cesarean hysterectomy patients, by and large, underwent a planned operation before the onset of labor. In addition, the study was made during an era when prophylactic antibiotics were not used. In a recent study, Gonsoulin et al[25] reported an 18.3% incidence of febrile morbidity after elective cesarean hysterectomy where prophylactic antibiotics were used. Although vaginal cuff infection is the most common source of febrile morbidity, urinary tract infection, pulmonary atelectasis, wound infection, thrombophlebitis, and breast inflammation must all be considered.

Postoperative ovarian abscess is a special cause of postoperative febrile morbidity after cesarean hysterectomy: 6 of 12 cases reviewed by me had occurred after cesarean hysterectomy. The latent period between the operation and acute symptoms was as long as 300 days. The ovary in pregnancy is particularly susceptible to infection. Sutures on the utero-ovarian ligament may cut through and fracture the ovarian cortex sufficiently to allow entry of organisms.

The incidence of postoperative bleeding after abdominal hysterectomy is approximately 0.7% and after a vaginal hysterectomy, approximately 2%, in the nonpregnant patient.[2,18,22,38] Postoperative bleeding, consisting of intra-abdominal or vaginal hemorrhage, expanding vaginal cuff or retroperitoneal hematoma or incisional bleeding that requires suturing, occurs after approximately 3% to 4% of elective cesarean hysterectomies.[4,7,9,31] Intraperitoneal hemorrhage necessitates secondary surgery in approximately 1% to 2% of patients. The site of bleeding is most often the utero-ovarian ligament, which may require unilateral salpingo-oophorectomy. Bleeding from the area of the vaginal cuff or uterine vessels is difficult to identify immediately. A pack can be placed in the pelvis and the retroperitoneal space entered for identification of the anterior division of the hypogastric and uterine arteries at the pelvic sidewall on either side, and the vessels can be secured with clips. The hypogastric venous system is markedly dilated during pregnancy, and care must be taken to avoid injury to those vessels. This approach ordinarily slows bleeding sufficiently to allow specific identification and ligation of bleeding points. Again, the ureter must be identified and protected. After a number of transfusions, a consumption coagulopathy is a consideration. Treatment of large vaginal or retroperitoneal hematomas must be individualized as one would after any type of hysterectomy. After an emergency operation for uterine rupture, care should be taken not to overlook an extension of the uterine tear into the vaginal fornix; this is particularly true if a subtotal operation has been performed.

Addition of hysterectomy to cesarean delivery should increase the average hospital stay by 1 day or less. Currently, that would mean approximately a 4-day postoperative hospital stay.[7,9]

One would expect a no greater postoperative death rate after cesarean hysterectomy than after an elective cesarean section alone or, for that matter, abdominal or vaginal hysterectomy in the nonpregnant patient. The indication for the operation, such as uterine rupture or severe intrauterine infection, is usually the determining factor in postoperative outcome.

SUMMARY

The evolution of the cesarean hysterectomy operation has been reviewed. The operation was devised to prevent death from hemorrhage and sepsis after cesarean section. Need for the operation was obviated by closure of the uterine incision, aseptic surgical techniques, and extraperitoneal cesarean section.

Performance of an emergency cesarean hysterectomy, defined as an operation to prevent death from hemorrhage, has not been questioned. Introduction of transfusion therapy and antibiotics in the 1940s expanded indications for all elective surgery, including elective cesarean hysterectomy. Until perhaps the mid 1970s, the elective operation, even for sterilization only, was advocated by many authors. That enthusiasm has now waned, and the question is whether or not enough operations are being performed to maintain surgical skills.

The surgical technique of cesarean hysterectomy is different from that of hysterectomy in the nonpregnant patient. Those differences must be recognized and taught, preferably during an elective operation. An emergency operation in untrained hands can be hazardous.

The complications of cesarean hysterectomy, primarily hemorrhage and urinary tract injury, are well recognized. Approximately 10% to 20% of patients undergoing an elective operation, particularly in an indigent population, require transfusion—often 1 U of packed red blood cells. The incidence of postoperative bleeding is approximately 4%, and 1% of patients require reoperation. Bladder entry occurs even during cesarean section, but if recognized, repair is usually successful. An occasional vesicovaginal fistula or ureteral injury occurs in association with cesarean hysterectomy. The incidence of these complications should be interpreted in the context of similar occurrences during or after abdominal or vaginal hysterectomy in nonpregnant patients.

Each surgeon, on the basis of surgical experience, must decide in conjunction with each patient whether or not elective hysterectomy at the time of cesarean section is in the patient's best interest.

REFERENCES

1. Abitbol MM, Benjamin F, Gastillo N: Cesarean hysterectomy in the treatment of carcinoma in situ of the cervix diagnosed during pregnancy, *Am J Obstet Gynecol* 117:909, 1973.
2. Amirikio H, Evans TN: Ten year review of hysterectomies: trends, indications and risks, *Am J Obstet Gynecol* 134:431, 1979.
3. Barclay DL: Cesarean hysterectomy at the Charity Hospital in New Orleans—1000 consecutive operations, *Clin Obstet Gynecol* 12:635, 1969.
4. Barclay DL: Cesarean hysterectomy—thirty years experience, *Obstet Gynecol* 35:120, 1970.
5. Barclay DL: Current ob/gyn techniques. Surgical Communications, Inc, vol 1, no 3, Ortho Pharmaceutical Corp., 1976.
6. Barclay DL: *Cesarean hysterectomy*. In Phelan JP, Clark SL, editors: *Cesarean delivery*, New York, 1988, Elsevier.
7. Barclay DL, Clark SL, Plauché WC: Cesarean hysterectomy, update tape, *Am College Obstet Gynecol*, vol 11, 1986.
8. Barclay DL, Frueh DM, Hawks BL: Carcinoma in situ of the cervix in pregnancy: treatment with primary cesarean hysterectomy, *Gynecol Oncol* 5:357, 1977.
9. Barclay DL et al: Elective cesarean hysterectomy: a 5 year comparison with cesarean section, *Am J Obstet Gynecol* 124:900, 1976.
10. Bradbury WC: Cesarean hysterectomy, *West J Surg* 63:232, 1955.
11. Britton JJ: Sterilization by cesarean hysterectomy, *Am J Obstet Gynecol* 173:887, 1980.
12. Brunschwig A, Barber HR: Cesarean section immediately followed by radical hysterectomy and pelvic node excision, *Am J Obstet Gynecol* 76:199, 1958.
13. Burchell CR: Physiology of internal iliac artery ligation, *J Obstet Gynecol Brit Cwlth* 75:642, 1968.
14. Chestnut DH: Autologous blood for elective cesarean hysterectomy, *Am J Obstet Gynecol* 150:796, 1984 (letter).
15. Chestnut DH, Redick LF: Continuous epidural anesthesia for elective cesarean hysterectomy, *South Med J* 78:1168, 1985.

16. Clark SL et al: Emergency hysterectomy for obstetric hemorrhage, *Obstet Gynecol* 64:376, 1984.

17. Davis ME: Complete cesarean hysterectomy: logical advance in modern obstetric surgery, *Am J Obstet Gynecol* 63:838, 1951.

18. Dicker RC et al: Complications of abdominal and vaginal hysterectomy among women of reproductive age in the United States, *Am J Obstet Gynecol* 144:841, 1982.

19. Durfee RB: Evolution of cesarean hysterectomy, *Clin Obstet Gynecol* 12:575, 1969.

20. Dyer I, Barclay DL: Accidental trauma complicating pregnancy and delivery, *Am J Obstet Gynecol* 83:907, 1962.

21. Dyer I, Nix FG, Weed JC: Total cesarean hysterectomy at cesarean section and in the immediate puerperal period, *Obstet Gynecol* 65:517, 1953.

22. Easterday CL, Grimes DA, Riggs JA: Hysterectomy in the United States, *Obstet Gynecol* 62:203, 1983.

23. Eisenhop SM et al: Urinary tract injury during cesarean section, *Obstet Gynecol* 60:591, 1982.

24. Evans S, McShane P: The efficacy of internal iliac artery ligation in obstetric hemorrhage, *Surg Gynecol Obstet* 160:250, 1985.

25. Gonsoulin et al: Elective versus emergency cesarean hysterectomy cases in a residency program setting: a review of 129 cases 1984-1988, *Am J Obstet Gynecol* 1992 (in press).

26. Harris JW: A study of the results obtained in sixty-four cesarean sections terminated by supravaginal hysterectomy, *Bull Johns Hopkins Hosp* 33:318, 1922.

27. Harris RP: Results of the first fifty cases of "caesarean ovaro-hysterectomy," 1869-1880, *Am J Med Sci* 80:129, 1880.

28. Haynes DM, Martin BJ Jr: Cesarean hysterectomy: a twenty-five year review, *Am J Obstet Gynecol* 134:393, 1979.

29. LaPlatney DR, O'Leary JA: Anesthetic considerations in cesarean hysterectomy, *Anesth-Analg (Cleveland)* 49:328, 1970.

30. Lash AF, Cummings WG: Porro cesarean section, *Am J Obstet Gynecol* 30:199, 1935.

31. Mickal A, Plauché WC: *Cesarean hysterectomy,* Mediguide to Ob/Gyn. Lawrence DellCorte Publications, Inc. Miles Pharmaceuticals vol 4, no 1, 1985.

32. O'Leary JA: Cesarean hysterectomy: a 15 year review, *J Reprod Med* 4:231, 1970.

33. O'Leary JA, Steer CE: A 10 year review of cesarean hysterectomy, *Am J Obstet Gynecol* 90:227, 1964.

34. Pelosi M, Langer A, Hung C: Prophylactic internal iliac artery ligation at cesarean hysterectomy, *Am J Obstet Gynecol* 121:394, 1975.

35. Plauché WC, Gruich FG, and Bourgeois MO: Hysterectomy at the time of cesarean section: analysis of 108 cases, *Obstet Gynecol* 58:459, 1981.

36. Plauché WC et al: Cesarean hysterectomy at Louisiana State University, 1975 through 1981, *South Med J* 76:1261, 1983.

37. Pletsch TD, Sandberg EC: Cesarean hysterectomy for sterilization, *Am J Obstet Gynecol* 85:254, 1963.

38. Pratt JH: Common complications of vaginal hysterectomy, *Clin Obstet Gynecol* 19:645, 1976.

39. Pritchard JA et al: Blood volume changes in pregnancy and the puerperium. II. Red blood cell loss and changes in apparent blood volume during and following vaginal delivery, cesarean section and cesarean section plus total hysterectomy, *Am J Obstet Gynecol* 84:1271, 1962.

40. Read JA et al: Placenta accreta: changing clinical aspects and outcome, *Obstet Gynecol* 56:31, 1980.

41. Reis RA, DeCosta EJ: Cesarean hysterectomy, *JAMA* 134:775, 1947.

42. Sall S, Rini S, Pineda A: Surgical management of invasive carcinoma of the cervix in pregnancy, *Obstet Gynecol* 118:1, 1974.

43. Speert H: Eduardo Porro and cesarean hysterectomy, *Surg Gynecol Obstet* 106:245, 1958.

44. Symposium: Cesarean hysterectomy, *Clin Obstet Gynecol* 12:652, 1969.

45. Thompson JD et al: The surgical management of invasive cancer of the cervix in pregnancy, *Am J Obstet Gynecol* 121:853, 1975.

46. Weed JC: The fate of the post cesarean uterus, *Obstet Gynecol* 14:780, 1960.

47. Wilson KM: The role of Porro cesarean section in modern obstetrics, *Am J Obstet Gynecol* 50:761, 1945.

48. Young JH: *Cesarean section: the history and development of the operation from earliest times,* London, 1944, Lewis & Co.

Chapter 69

RUPTURE OF THE UTERUS

Warren C. Plauché

Rupture of the uterus is encountered by the obstetrician-gynecologist in two principal contexts: obstetric and nonobstetric. Obstetric uterine ruptures may be sudden spontaneous events, separation of previous uterine scars, or tears at the time of traumatic deliveries. Nonobstetric uterine ruptures are likely to result from instrumental perforations, tumor infiltration, or infections.

The box below lists prominent causes of obstetric uterine rupture. The box below, right, lists common causes of nonobstetric uterine rupture. Whatever the cause, uterine

rupture requires prompt attention and considered decision making by the attending physician.

OBSTETRIC UTERINE RUPTURE

Rupture of the pregnant uterus can be among the most dramatic of surgical obstetric complications. Careful study of uterine rupture reveals that nearly half of the cases are not dramatic or life-threatening events.[49] Many separations of previous uterine scars, while technically classified as uterine ruptures, occur with few symptoms or signs. These

---

Obstetric uterine rupture—contributing causes

- I. Uterine scar dehiscence
- II. Trauma
  - A. Direct
    - Penetrating wounds
    - Intrauterine manipulations
    - Forceps application and rotation
    - Postpartum curettage
    - Manual placental extraction
    - External or internal version
  - B. Indirect
    - Blunt trauma—blows, seat belts
    - Manual fundal pressure
    - Extension of cervical tears
- III. Inappropriate use of oxytocics
- IV. Grandmultiparity
- V. Fetal problems
  - Macrosomia, malposition, anomalies, destructive procedures
- VI. Placenta percreta
- VII. Tumors
  - Trophoblastic disease, cervical carcinoma
- VIII. Extratubal ectopic gestations
  - Cornual, intramural, cervical, sacculation, rudimentary horn

---

Classification of nonobstetric uterine rupture

- I. Trauma
  - A. Instrumental perforation
    1. Dilatation and curettage—sharp or suction curettage
    2. Hysteroscopy
    3. Laparoscopy trocar
    4. Intrauterine contraceptive device placement or retrieval
  - B. Penetrating traumatic wounds
- II. Tumor invasion
  - A. Uterine malignancies
    1. Sarcoma
    2. Choriocarcinoma
    3. Epidermoid cervical carcinoma
    4. Adenocarcinoma
  - B. Metastatic disease
  - C. Radiation therapy
- III. Infections
  - A. Pyometra
  - B. Myometrial abcesses
  - C. *Clostridium, Bacteroides* infections
- IV. Surgical wound dehiscences
  - A. Hysterotomy
  - B. Myomectomy
  - C. Reunification of double uterus

separations are discovered incidentally at the time of repeat cesarean operations or uterine exploration after vaginal delivery.

Asymptomatic dehiscences should be considered separately from major life-threatening uterine ruptures. The obstetric literature contains many papers on uterine rupture that combine cases of all degrees of severity. The combined morbidity and outcome statistics and management suggestions do not relate well to individual cases.

Studies of uterine rupture from referral centers focus on catastrophic ruptures. Conclusions of such studies cannot be held to apply to minor uterine wound dehiscences.[49] Conversely, studies of minimal cesarean wound separations do not prepare physicians for the problems of massive uterine rupture.

Prevalence

Kieffer in 1964 reported 9300 cases of uterine rupture from a survey of a 30-year span of the world's English language literature.[27] Surveyed reports estimated the total incidence of rupture of the gravid uterus variously from a high of 1 in 800 deliveries to a low of 1 in 3000.

Eden et al reported 1 obstetric uterine rupture per 1424 deliveries among the Duke University Medical Center records of 53 years beginning in 1931.[15,16] Separate analysis of the last decade of the Duke experience showed a tenfold increase in the cesarean delivery rate but an incidence of only 1 rupture per 2251 deliveries.

By contrast, Van der Merwe and Ombelet, in South Africa, reported 89 uterine ruptures among 77,133 deliveries for an overall incidence of 1 per 866 deliveries.[67] More than half (53%) of these cases were ruptured previous section scars.

Shrinsky and Benson in 1978 reported a 25-year study in which 1 uterine rupture per 2695 deliveries occurred on their University of Oregon service.[61] Their survey of the world literature is difficult to interpret. Thirty-three papers between 1945 and 1975 showed a broad variation in the incidence of uterine rupture from 1 in 93 deliveries to 1 in 4900 deliveries.[61] Some papers reported only complete major ruptures; others included all uterine wound separations.

The author in 1984 reported an incidence of 1 in 2174 deliveries during the preceding decade of catastrophic, life-threatening uterine rupture on the Louisiana State University Charity Hospital service.[49] The mean incidence of complete rupture of the uterus from our English literature survey was 1 in 1148 deliveries.

A current best estimate of the probability of major catastrophic uterine rupture is 1 in 2200 deliveries. Scar dehiscences after previous uterine incisions occur 40 to 50 times more frequently, in 2% to 4% of cases.*

Causes

Dehiscence of previous scars. The principal cause of rupture of the pregnant uterus, responsible for 50% to 70%

*References 5, 28, 39, 40, 42, 51.

of all cases and 30% of catastrophic cases, is the previous uterine scar. The large majority of scars that result in uterine rupture are those from previous cesarean births.

Osmers et al reported necrosis of the lower uterine segment above previous uterine scars as the pathologic cause of scar fenestration in late pregnancy.[45] Histologic examination indicated that the rupture process developed in several stages, rather than as an acute event. A form of pressure necrosis was postulated.

Nielsen et al in 1989 reported the conclusions of a large prospective study from Sweden of the incidence of rupture and dehiscence of previous cesarean scars.[44] Uterine scar dehiscence was defined as separation of the scar without rupture of the chorioamniotic membranes. Uterine rupture implied open rupture into the peritoneal cavity of both the uterine wall and chorioamniotic membranes.

Nielsen's 10-year study followed 2036 women with previous cesarean delivery. Trial of labor was attempted in 1008 patients and was successful in 92.2%. Uterine scar dehiscence occurred in 4% of previous section cases, and uterine rupture occurred in 0.6%. Two of the ruptures occurred before labor, both in T incision scars. The true incidence of dehiscence in this study is uncertain because the authors did not examine the interior of the uterus after vaginal delivery in all cases.

Among the author's Louisiana State University series of 23 catastrophic uterine ruptures, fourteen (61.3%) patients had previous cesarean deliveries.[49] Trials of labor in 307 patients with previous cesarean scars of all types, including unknown scars, were examined by our University Medical Center affiliate in 1987. Two major uterine ruptures required emergency hysterectomies, and seven dehiscences of uterine scars required repair (2.9%).[71]

Yetman and Nolan reviewed vaginal birth after cesarean section (VBAC) at the Naval Hospital in Portsmouth, Virginia.[72] The scar separation rate in these 224 VBAC cases was 1.79%. Two of the four scar separations were catastrophic ruptures requiring hysterectomy to control hemorrhage.

One of the lowest incidences of rupture of previous cesarean scars is that reported by Meehan and Magani from University Hospital in Galway between 1972 and 1987.[38] This group found only six true scar ruptures (1 in 225, 0.44%) among 1350 VBAC patients.

Uterine scars from hysterotomies, myomectomies, perforations from sharp or suction curettage, and even laparoscopy trochar punctures have been related to uterine rupture.[19,37] Deaton et al reported a rare case of spontaneous uterine rupture in pregnancy after hysteroscopic lysis of intrauterine adhesions in a case of Asherman's syndrome.[11] These events make up less than 10% of the cases. The widely held belief that myometrial incisions that do not enter the endometrial cavity will not subsequently rupture is unsubstantiated.

Dunnihoo et al investigated the effect of closure method on uterine scar integrity in rabbits.[13] Two wounds were made in each uterine horn. Continuous everted, continuous inverted, interrupted everted, and interrupted inverted methods were used. No significant difference was found in the tensile strength of these scars after 28 to 30 days.

Endomyometritis was formerly thought to be an important factor in uterine rupture after previous cesarean birth. Close examination reveals an inconsistent relationship between postpartum infection and wound rupture. Post cesarean endomyometritis is not an absolute indicator of weak or defective wound healing.[58]

Jones and Mitler reported rupture of the uterus in a gravid bicornuate uterus infected with *Bacteroides* and *Clostridium* organisms.[25] Lindberg recorded a case of uterine rupture from a beta-hemolytic streptococcal infection after cervical circlage.[29]

Uteri involved in severe postpartum infections occasionally develop early postdelivery dehiscence of the cesarean wound. The infected dehiscence site is often localized by adherence of the wound site to the anterior abdominal wall. Omentum and bowel further seal off the infection. Little or no myometrium remains between the abdominal wall and the chorioamniotic sac at the time of a subsequent pregnancy. Trial of labor in such a situation risks uterine rupture. It is difficult for obstetricians to detect this type of abnormal wound healing. Indeed, it is not currently possible prospectively to evaluate the strength of any myometrial scar.

Trauma

Direct. Trauma is responsible for approximately 20% of obstetric uterine ruptures. Trauma may be related to direct obstetric maneuvers or indirect external forces. The majority of traumatic ruptures due to obstetric manipulations are associated with forceps deliveries. Reviews of uterine rupture from 1930 to 1970 usually cited Kielland forceps and rotation maneuvers as the most frequent forceps operations causing uterine rupture.[61] Forceps delivery also increases the number of extensions of cervical tears into the lower uterine segment.

Obstetric manipulations of the fetus contribute a small share of uterine injuries. Older studies found internal podalic version of transverse lies and breech extractions to be involved in 4% to 6% of uterine ruptures.[61] External version has only occasionally resulted in uterine rupture since the advent of effective tocolytic agents.

Indirect. Auto accidents, stab wounds, and gunshot wounds are the principal causes of uterine rupture from external trauma. These cases comprise no more than 10% of ruptures.[49,63] The English language obstetric literature contains only 22 cases of stab wounds of the pregnant uterus.[12] A small number of papers describe gunshot and other penetrating wounds of the pregnant uterus. Franger et al found only nine cases in the literature of self-inflicted gunshot wounds to the pregnant uterus.[17]

Motor vehicle and seat belt injuries to mothers and fetuses have been carefully studied.[14] These traumatic uterine ruptures are often severe and frequently involve injury to the bowel, bladder, spleen, kidney, liver, soft tissues, and pelvic bones.

Inappropriate use of oxytocics. Rupture of the gravid uterus was also historically related to oxytocin administration.[6] Present methods demand supervised administration of carefully measured, minute quantities of dilute oxytocin. Attendants immediately stop administration of the drug if hyperstimulation occurs. Uterine contractions can be monitored by internal pressure transducers so both timing and intensity of contractions are known. Under these circumstances, hyperstimulation of the uterus should be rare.

The availability of prostaglandins for uterine stimulation raises the question of safety of oxytocics once again. McCarthy and McQueen in 1980 reported uterine rupture complicating intraamniotic prostaglandin E_2 for second trimester abortion.[36] Valenzuela et al, Sawyer et al, and others have recorded cases of rupture of the uterus after intravaginal suppositories of prostaglandin E_2 were used to ripen the cervix at term.[56,66]

Prostaglandins are very powerful oxytocic agents. Their physiologic action closely resembles the normal process of labor. Their pharmacologic instability has made it difficult to develop a delivery system that approaches the safety of carefully metered intravenous oxytocin. Prostaglandins are not, at the time of this writing, approved by the Food and Drug Administration (FDA) for induction of labor or other use in late pregnancy.

Multiparity, fetal problems, and placenta percreta. Parity of five or more has been associated with rupture of the unscarred uterus.[49,61,67] Multiparity, oxytocin misuse, fetal macrosomia and excessive fundal pressure for delivery formerly contributed to obstetric uterine rupture in multiparas. These factors are rare in modern case collections. Unsuspected macrosomia, malpositions, anomalies, and cephalopelvic disproportion remain serious considerations as we enter an era of more universal trial of labor for patients with previous cesarean scars.

Spontaneous rupture of the intact pregnant uterus is usually unanticipated and dramatic.[46,64,69] Ruptures of the intact uterus comprised 38% of our Charity Hospital series of catastrophic ruptures and 70% of our literature survey of complete uterine rupture.[49]

Spontaneous obstetric uterine ruptures often defy explanation.[70] Liu et al found irreversible cell injury in fibers of the lower uterine segment in ruptures of the intact uterus during labor. They believed that severe, longstanding pressure of the fetal presentation during prolonged labor was the essential pathophysiologic change.[30] These findings do not explain spontaneous midpregnancy rupture of an apparently normal uterus.

Small subgroups in the spectrum of spontaneous uterine rupture relate to congenitally weak areas of the myometrial wall, fetal macrosomia, or hydramnios. Makar et al reported an unusual case of spontaneous perforation of the uterus after red degeneration of a myoma in a pregnant patient.[33] The uterus may be more prone to obstetric rupture in women who were exposed to diethylstilbesterol (DES) in utero.[3]

Rare instances of spontaneous uterine rupture are associated with placenta percreta or invasive moles in which the placental villi grow entirely through the uterine wall. Nagy reported such a case of major uterine rupture due to placenta percreta that resulted in fetal demise.[43]

Extratubal ectopic gestations. An important group of spontaneous rupture cases are related to abnormal pregnancy implantation sites. Nidation of the developing pregnancy normally takes place in the endometrial cavity. Occasionally, the ovum implants within the uterus but not in the normal uterine cavity. The result is cornual, intramural, or cervical pregnancy, or pregnancy in a uterine sacculation or in a rudimentary horn (Table 69-1). These rare ectopic gestations comprise 6% of ectopic pregnancies and a similarly small percentage of uterine ruptures.

Cornual pregnancy. Cornual and interstitial pregnancies comprise 4% to 5% of all ectopic gestations.[50] These are the most frequent of pregnancies within the uterine wall. Cornual pregnancies are nidations that take place in the thinned portion of the uterus near the ostia of the fallopian tubes. Interstitial pregnancies are tubal gestations in the portion of the fallopian tube that traverses the myometrial wall. Cornual and interstitial pregnancies are clinically indistinguishable. Pregnancies at these sites grow normally for several months then rupture through the cornual portion of the uterus with disastrous effect.

Previous tubal surgery is the factor most commonly associated with cornual pregnancy.[50,55,68] Cornual pregnancies give few warnings of their presence before catastrophic rupture in the middle trimester. The uterus may feel asymmetric in early pregnancy. The examiner often describes the possibility of a fundal leiomyoma. Ultrasound may show the gestational sac to be in an unusual location high in one corner of the endometrial cavity. The appearance mimics pregnancy in one horn of a bicornuate uterus. The examiner cannot distinguish the two without prior knowledge of the anatomy.

The true nature of the disorder becomes overt when the patient develops sudden severe pain, shock, and signs of intraperitoneal hemorrhage. An occasional case advances far into the third trimester without rupture.

The management of cornual pregnancy is surgical. In early unruptured cases, the cornu is resected around the implantation. The defect is closed in two or three layers as for a classical cesarean incision.

Surgical exploration of an advanced ruptured cornual pregnancy reveals one side of the upper uterus violently blown outward. The fetus is usually free in the abdominal cavity. The cavity in the uterus has a ragged wall of torn myometrium and placental tissue. Bleeding is brisk, and a large amount of blood collects in the pelvis and abdominal cavity. The Cell Saver filter system can be used to return some of the intraperitoneal blood to the vascular system by autotransfusion.

Surgical options include cornual suture reconstruction, cornual resection and repair, and hysterectomy. Hysterectomy is often necessary to gain control of blood loss and because of extensive damage to the uterus. Previous ectopic gestations have already threatened the health and lives of many of these patients.

It is often possible to perform a more conservative cornual repair. Every effort is made to repair the uterus when the patient has expressed a wish to become pregnant again. The edges of the rupture are debrided and the defect is closed with two or three layers of 0 chromic or 00 polyglycolic/polyglactan absorbable suture. Long-term follow-up of repaired cases are too few to predict accurately the course of later pregnancy.

Beckmann and Ron-El each reported cases of coexistent normal implantations and cornual gestations.[7,55] They resected the cornual gestations early in pregnancy. The normally implanted pregnancies continued until cesarean delivery near term without further complication.

Brandes et al reported successful treatment of a cornual pregnancy with systemic methotrexate.[8] The presumed diagnosis was gestational trophoblastic disease for which the patient received an 8-day course of methotrexate. A cornual gestation suspected on later hysterosalpingogram was confirmed by laparoscopy. The cornual pregnancy resolved without further surgery. The authors commented on the possible utility of this method when surgery is contraindicated or for patients who wish future pregnancies.

Methotrexate management of cornual pregnancy presumes reliable prerupture diagnosis, which is, unfortunately, quite unusual. Early, reliable detection of extratubal ectopic gestation would make nonsurgical management feasible.

Intramural pregnancy. Intramural pregnancies develop within the uterine wall. They must be separate from the uterine cavity and fallopian tube and surrounded by myometrium to support this diagnosis. There must be no congenital sacculation, diverticulum, or congenital anomaly of the uterus. We found only 19 reported cases in literature searches from 1924 to the present.

It is difficult to point out etiologic or clinical features of so rare a phenomenon. The most consistently reported associated pathologic finding is deficient decidua in the endometrial cavity. Previous uterine trauma or infection are consistent cohorts. The etiologic pattern resembles that of placenta accreta.

Table 69-1. Ectopic implantation sites within the uterine wall

Site	Percentage of all ectopic pregnancies (%)
Abnormal uterine implantations	4.9–5.6
Interstitial	(4.1)
Cornual	(0.3–0.7)
Cervical	(0.1–0.2)
Intramural	(0.3–0.5)
Sacculation	(0.1)
Rudimentary horn	(0.08)
Intraligamentous from uterine rupture	0.1–0.2

Intramural pregnancies give few signs before they rupture in the second trimester. The patient complains of severe pain in the lower abdomen and has signs of peritoneal irritation and hypovolemia. Intramural pregnancy is an operating table diagnosis in most cases.

Treatment of ruptured intramural pregnancy includes exploratory laparotomy and blood transfusion. Damage to the uterus is usually extensive enough to require hysterectomy. Hysterectomy in the presence of widespread trauma and hematoma formation is always challenging. Hemostasis and a clear operating field are difficult to obtain. The ureters and large pelvic vessels are at risk during dissection. Ligation of the internal iliac arteries or aortic compression can provide temporary hemostasis to allow the surgeon to identify anatomic landmarks.

Maternal and fetal morbidity and mortality with rupture of intramural pregnancies are similar to spontaneous rupture of normally implanted gestations.

Cervical pregnancies. Cervical pregnancy is a most unusual manifestation of ectopic gestation and a dangerous one. Studdiford defined cervical pregnancy as nidation and development of the fertilized ovum within the structure of the cervix, the uterine corpus remaining uninvolved.[62] Surgical pathologic specimens must show cervical glands adjacent to the placenta. The placenta must intimately attach to the cervix below the entrance of the uterine vessels. There must be no fetal elements in the corpus uteri.

Jauchler and Baker in 1970 found 37 reported cases in their broad search of the literature.[24] Twenty-two of these cases were unconfirmed by surgical pathologic specimens. Shinagawa and Nagayama reported an unusually large series of 19 cases of cervical pregnancy among several thousand therapeutic abortion cases from Japan.[60] Published studies variously estimate the incidence at 1 in 2400 to 1 in 18,000 pregnancies. It is difficult to determine the true incidence of so rare a condition.

Schneider proposed that slowing of ovum transit or acceleration of its implantation capability produces tubal or cornual gestations.[57] Similar logic indicates that speeding of ovum transit or delayed nidation occasionally produces cervical pregnancy.

Trauma or infectious injury to the endometrium play a role in development of cervical as well as other ectopic gestations. All but one of Shinagawa's 19 cases had previous elective abortions.[60] Each of the five cases in the report by Parente et al had previous curettages.[47] This group found that 25 of 31 cases of cervical pregnancy from the literature had previous uterine curettages.

Thomsen and Johansen in 1961 reported two patients with cervical pregnancy, both of whom had previous therapeutic abortions; one also had a previous cesarean delivery.[65] Four of the eight most recently reported cervical pregnancy cases had previous cesarean deliveries.[24,65]

Uterine scarring may speed the passage of the fertilized egg or delay its implantation. This usually results in undetected abortion. Cervical gestation occurs if the fertilized ovum implants in cervical glands.

There are two possible clinical courses for cervical pregnancies. They may grow and eventually rupture the cervix, or they may abort. The latter course is much more common. Advanced cervical pregnancy is very rare.

Cervical pregnancies mimic threatened abortions early in their course. The patient displays signs and positive tests for pregnancy. There is a varying period of amenorrhea, usually of 6 to 12 weeks. Vaginal bleeding without cramping pain brings the patient to the physician. The cervix is discolored and enlarged. The external os is usually open. It may be possible to palpate the uterus as a mass separate from and above the cervical mass.

Incomplete or inevitable abortion is the usual presumptive diagnosis. There is little indication of the extent of the problem until attempts at evacuation begin. Bleeding that does not respond to oxytocic agents quickly becomes profuse. Packing of the evacuated cavity may temporarily slow or stop the hemorrhage, but bleeding frequently recurs. New hemostatic materials such as Avitene or fibrin glue can be helpful in such situations. Transfemoral embolization of branches of the internal iliac arteries can also be attempted.

Hysterectomy is necessary when efforts at hemostasis fail to control bleeding. Enlargement of the cervix and pericervical hemorrhage distort anatomic relationships. Dissection must proceed with caution.

Pelosi described and illustrated an inventive cervicotomy approach to cervical pregnancy evacuation.[48] He ascribed the method to Dubrovici of Rumania. He placed hemostatic sutures at the 3 o'clock and 9 o'clock positions at the lateral edges of the cervix. Incision of the vaginal mucosa permitted reflection of the bladder from the cervix and isthmus. Anterior cervicotomy opened the cervical canal and permitted digital removal and curettage of the gestation. Sutures were used to close the cervical and vaginal incisions.

Our current management sequence for cervical pregnancy is transcervical evacuation, application of pressure by cervical packing with hemostatic agents and gauze. We perform embolization or hysterectomy if hemostasis is not secure.

Uterine sacculations. Uterine sacculation is a rare developmental defect in the muscle layers of the uterine wall that resembles a diverticulum of the bowel. Uterine sacculations most frequently occur on the posterior surface of the uterus. Nidation in these sites can enfold and grow as though within the uterine wall. The clinical presentation, signs, symptoms, and management of these cases are the same as intramural gestations. The one pregnancy in a sacculation that we managed carried to term and was discovered at the time of cesarean delivery for failure to progress. Uterine rupture in the middle or last trimester is the more common course.

Rudimentary horn pregnancies. Most rudimentary uterine horns do not communicate with the principal endometrial cavity. Pregnancy in these anomalous uterine horns is rare. Most cases end in uterine rupture or death and mummification of the fetus. Heinonen and Aro were able to find only five cases of pregnancy in a rudimentary horn in which both the mother and baby survived.[22] The clinical course closely resembles that of cornual gestations.

Morbidity and mortality

The threat of obstetric uterine rupture to mother and baby varies with the length of gestation at the time of rupture and with placental implantation in relation to the rupture site. Additional factors include the presence or absence of previous uterine scars, the extent of the rupture, and the inciting event, spontaneous or traumatic. The variables are so numerous that estimations of morbidity and mortality are best confined to specific types of uterine rupture.

Asymptomatic dehiscences of previous cesarean scars are the most frequent type of uterine rupture encountered in the practice of obstetrics and gynecology. All obstetric surgeons have encountered separations in thin, white, relatively avascular scars through which amniotic membranes are visible or extruded. Morbidity is minimal in most cases. Problems occur when placental implantation is directly beneath the dehiscence, when lateral extension lacerates the uterine vessels, or when membranes rupture, spilling uterine contents into the peritoneal cavity.

Rupture of a previous uterine scar usually results in less blood loss and threat to the life of the baby and mother than does rupture of the intact organ.[17] Our literature survey from 1978 to 1983 indicated a maternal mortality of 13.5% for 162 complete ruptures of the intact uterus. All patients survived the 38 complete ruptures of the scarred uterus. Fetal mortality was 76.1% in complete ruptures of the intact uterus, compared to 32.4% in complete ruptures of the scarred uterus.[49]

The review of Van der Merwe and Ombelet confirmed these findings.[67] Among 89 complete uterine ruptures, all maternal deaths occurred in ruptures of the intact uterus. Fetal mortality was 71% for complete ruptures of the intact uterus but only 36% in ruptures of the scarred uterus.[67]

Ruptures of the scarred uterus clearly present only a small threat to the life of the mother when operating facilities, surgical skills, and blood transfusions are readily available. Complete rupture of the scarred uterus threatens the life of a third of the babies despite dramatic improvement in neonatal intensive care.

Extensive ruptures of uterine scars before term occur most often in uteri that bear vertical scars extending into the fundal portion of the uterus. Classical incisions comprised 68% of the ruptures of vertical scars and 12% of all catastrophic ruptures in our published review.[49]

Separation of a classical scar opens a large portion of the anterior uterine wall. This disrupts large uterine vascular channels and is likely to expose a portion of the placental implantation site. Both of these factors provoke brisk bleeding. Rupture of classical scars is often a sudden dramatic event accompanied by intraperitoneal and vaginal bleeding, abdominal pain, and fetal distress or death.

Sixty percent of uterine scar disruptions occur in transverse scars.[39] Many intrapartal dehiscences of transverse cesarean scars are partial, small, and asymptomatic. Transverse scars are much less vascular and less likely to involve the placental implantation site than vertical scars. Therefore, the threat to mother and baby is much reduced unless there is extension into the uterine vascular bundle.

Traumatic injuries are among the most difficult cases of obstetric uterine rupture. Auto accidents, gunshot wounds, and stab wounds to the abdomen of pregnant patients carry high morbidity and mortality risk for the mother and especially for the fetus. Franger et al reported the perinatal mortality from gunshot wounds of the uterus at 47% to 71%.[17] Such cases are seldom simple and often require the skills of a multidisciplinary team of surgeons.

Spontaneous rupture of the intact pregnant uterus is another catastrophic although rare event that poses great risk to mother and baby. Spontaneous rupture of the intact uterus before term is much more devastating than most scar separations that occur during labor. Spontaneous uterine ruptures of normal implantations may occur at any time during pregnancy but are most common in the last trimester.

Spontaneous ruptures of aberrant implantations in the cornual portion of the uterus or in anomalous uterine horns usually occur in the middle trimester of gestation. Cervical pregnancies often perforate or hemorrhage in the first trimester. These ruptures may be life-threatening for the mother and are usually fatal to the fetus.

Diagnosis

Dehiscence of the central portion of previous transverse uterine scars usually occurs without many symptoms or signs. These ruptures are encountered as incidental findings at the time of repeat cesarean delivery or at the time of uterine exploration after delivery.

The box below outlines clinical features of diagnostic value in cases of overt uterine rupture. The classic signs are vaginal hemorrhage, shock, cessation of labor, and re-

---

> **Obstetric uterine rupture: Intrapartal diagnosis***
>
> Maternal anxiety, diaphoresis
> Vascular instability and shock
> Vaginal bleeding
> Fetal distress or demise
> Pain not associated with contractions
> Cessation of labor
> Recession of presenting part
> Easily palpable fetal parts through abdominal wall
> Point tenderness of uterus
> Ultrasound evidence of rupture or extrusion of uterine contents
> Decompression of intrauterine pressure catheter
> Signs of peritoneal irritation

*All diagnostic signs and symptoms may be present in varying degrees or may be entirely absent.

cession of the presenting part. This tetrad is easily recognized but seldom seen.

Absence of premonitory signs precludes intervention early in the disorder in most cases. There have been instances of fortuitous recognition of asymptomatic uterine dehiscence by ultrasound imaging.[2,45] Osmers et al recognized a 1.4% risk of asymptomatic fenestration after cesarean section with visualization of the lower uterus by ultrasound.[45] They admitted that prediction of uterine scar rupture was rarely possible.

There are other signs of early overt uterine rupture. Occasionally, fetal stress or distress is detected during electronic monitoring. The mother may complain of unusual suprapubic discomfort or tenderness. These signs appear immediately preceding or during the rupture event.

Loss of pressure in an intrauterine pressure transducer system occurs in some cases of uterine rupture. Loss of catheter pressure occurs in normal labor monitoring often enough to make it unreliable for the diagnosis of uterine rupture. Rodriguez et al reviewed 76 cases of uterine rupture of which 39 had intrauterine pressure catheters in place. Loss of catheter pressure was not observed in any of these patients.[54]

Interval hysterograms or ultrasound imaging before labor may identify distorted or thin uterine scars. An abnormal scar appearance does not always presage rupture, nor does visual perfection of a scar guarantee its tensile strength. There are, at present, no reliable signs, symptoms, or tests that allow the physician to predict which scars or uteri will remain intact or which will rupture.

Massive spontaneous or traumatic prepartal uterine ruptures are suspected from the patient's history plus signs of shock, vaginal bleeding, fetal death, or distress, and an acute abdominal emergency. Confirmation of diagnosis is by laparotomy.

Intrapartal ruptures of the uterus are usually found among cases of severe postpartum hemorrhage after difficult labor or instrumental delivery. Confirmation of the diagnosis in these cases depends on careful examination of the genital tract to rule out other causes of postpartum bleeding. Diagnosis of uterine rupture depends on detecting a rent in the wall of the uterus by manual exploration of the uterine cavity.

Postpartum manual exploration of the uterus. The dominant hand is carefully introduced into the uterus, and the endometrial cavity is palpated in a systematic fashion. The examiner should feel for a gap in the wall of the uterus. The lower uterine segment after vaginal delivery is thin and soft. This segment may be normal yet feel almost as though no uterine wall exists. It is very difficult to be certain of the presence or absence of a lower segment tear under these circumstances.

Anterior isthmic or upper cervical ruptures are identified when the fingers pass through a rent and are felt by the abdominal hand. The inside fingers feel as though they are just beneath the skin of the anterior abdominal wall in thin patients. Palpation of bowel or other organs is certain

confirmation of major rupture but is seldom detected in ruptures of the lower uterus. Posterior ruptures of the uterus are difficult to detect. Although not rare, they are often not considered by the examiner.

Massive bleeding often signals a lateral tear into the major uterine vessels. The lateral portion of the isthmus of the uterus and the upper cervix are assessed carefully. Incomplete ruptures are particularly difficult to detect. The fingers may enter a complete rupture and pass right into the broad ligament. The diagnosis is then sufficiently confirmed to warrant laparotomy.

Complete ruptures that extend into the anterior fundal portion of the uterus are easier to detect than lower segment ruptures. The uterine muscle at the junction of the upper cervix and myometrium normally forms a firm ring that can be palpated around its entire circumference. A gap in this ring signals a rupture of the uterus until proven otherwise. Complete ruptures allow the examining fingers to pass into the peritoneal cavity. Palpation of extrauterine organs may be possible. There can even be intrusion of bowel or omentum through the laceration into the uterine cavity. The diagnosis is then obvious, and immediate laparotomy is indicated.

The obstetrician is often uncertain about the assessment of uterine integrity after delivery, particularly when faced with an unexplained postpartum hemorrhage. The uterine cavity after normal delivery should be examined frequently to become accustomed to the feel of the normal organ. The fingers can then more reliably detect an abnormality.

Given a massive postpartum hemorrhage unresponsive to oxytocics with no other obvious cause, uterine rupture must be suspected. Laparotomy is the appropriate confirmatory step as soon as preparations are complete. Attempts should be made to stabilize the patient while operating facilities, anesthesia, and blood replacement are quickly prepared. The patient often cannot be stabilized in the presence of massive uterine rupture until bleeding is surgically secured.

Management

Asymptomatic uterine scar dehiscence. Uterine scars should be carefully evaluated after every subsequent delivery. The integrity of the previous scar determines current management and influences advice about future pregnancies.

Small, asymptomatic dehiscences encountered at the time of repeat cesarean operation are simply debrided and closed with the new cesarean incision.

The uterine cavity should be explored manually after each vaginal birth after cesarean (VBAC). If a small dehiscence is detected but is entirely asymptomatic and not bleeding, current management favors observation of the patient and spontaneous healing. Large separations combined with postpartum hemorrhage demand exploratory surgery. Many cases fall between these extremes and must be individually managed, usually by surgical repair.

What about further pregnancies and surgical sterilization after a uterine rupture? If the patient wants another pregnancy, we recommend repeat cesarean birth near term without labor. That operation usually includes surgical sterilization by tubal ligation or hysterectomy, depending on coexisting problems. If the patient is certain she wants no more pregnancies, peripartal hysterectomy at the time of uterine rupture is offered. Repair and tubal sterilization are suggested if the patient does not agree to hysterectomy.

Major, complete uterine rupture. Catastrophic obstetric uterine rupture is among the most dramatic and difficult of obstetric problems. Such uterine ruptures challenge the skills and ingenuity of the most meticulously trained obstetric surgical team. The box below outlines the limited choices available to an operator addressing the problem of major uterine rupture.

Uterine packing. Packing the uterus for postpartum hemorrhage was commonplace in the era preceding safe obstetric surgery. Packing a uterus when uterine rupture is diagnosed or suspected is only a stopgap measure, seldom a definitive treatment. Blood loss can be reduced while preparations are made for definitive surgical treatment. An incomplete laceration without major arterial bleeding may occasionally be controlled with a pack.

The obstetrician who chooses to use an intrauterine pack must introduce fold after fold of gauze packing into the uterine cavity.

The end of a Kerlix or other long gauze roll is grasped with curved uterine dressing forceps or a long Kelly clamp. The first segment of packing is placed into one cornu of the uterine cavity. The forceps are withdrawn. Another length of packing is grasped just outside the cervix and placed carefully into the opposite uterine cornu. Packing proceeds from one side to the other until the uterine cavity is filled with tightly packed folds of gauze. Oxytocics ensure tight application of the uterus around the pack. Broad-spectrum antibiotic coverage is wise after placement of a uterine pack.

Uterine packing has several possible complications, including perforation of the uterus and endomyometritis. Placing a uterine pack can extend a previous laceration of the uterus. Uterine packing requires repeated entries into the uterine cavity with an instrument that can perforate the uterus. Bacteria are introduced into the uterus with each transition of the cervix.

Obstetric uterine rupture: Management options

Uterine packing*
Debridement and repair
Peripartal hysterectomy
    Subtotal (supracervical)
    Complete
Internal iliac artery ligation*

*Auxiliary procedure, seldom definitive therapy.

Packing is most often temporary until more definitive surgery is performed. A pack occasionally yields total control of postpartum hemorrhage. The successful pack should be left in place no longer than 12 to 24 hours. It is then removed slowly and gently while oxytocics are administered to ensure tight uterine contraction. Only analgesia, not general anesthesia, is required for removal of a uterine pack.

Uterine packing and expectant management do not allow assessment of retroperitoneal or intraperitoneal bleeding. The extent of the injury to the uterus or other abdominal organs cannot be evaluated. Therefore, uterine packing is seldom the wisest management choice for uterine rupture in modern obstetrics.[64] Extensive ruptures of the uterus are better managed by exploratory surgery with either repair of the defect or removal of the uterus.

Repair or removal of uterus. Should we repair or remove the uterus that has sustained a complete rupture? The obstetric surgeon who is trained and capable of rapid, safe peripartal hysterectomy can choose to repair the rent in the uterus or to remove the uterus.

The uterus that has explosive damage and is beyond safe repair should be removed. Removal of the uterus may also be offered for less severe ruptures when multiparous patients with previous cesarean deliveries do not want more children. The presence of other gynecologic disorders such as uterine leiomyomata may influence this decision.

Repair rather than removal of the ruptured uterus has found favor in recent literature on this subject. Aguero and Kizer from Caracas reported suture repairs in 462 (67.5%) of 684 uterine ruptures and dehiscences.[4] Their survey of the literature revealed the prevalence of suture repair for uterine rupture to be 41.3%.

Sheth from Bombay reported a series of 110 uterine ruptures of which 66 (63%) were managed by suture repair.[59] Reyes-Ceja et al of Mexico reported 100 uterine ruptures of which 65% were managed by hysteroraphy rather than hysterectomy.[52] The above investigators all felt that, in their environments, repair was safer than hysterectomy.

Repair of major uterine ruptures is much like the layered closure of a classical cesarean incision. Principles include rapid control of blood loss, clear visualization of the extent of the injury, debridement, and accurate reapproximation of the uterine wall.

Control of bleeding at the site of rupture may entail uterine artery ligation, internal iliac artery ligation, or even transient compression of the aorta. The object is to stabilize the patient as quickly as possible and clear the operative field for the definitive repair or hysterectomy.

Once the decision is made to attempt repair of the uterus, the rupture site should be debrided of all necrotic or damaged tissues. The remaining wound is closed in layers with absorbable suture such as 0 chromic or 00 polyglycolic/polyglactin suture. Two or three layers of suture are usually required for secure closure of ruptures in the

Table 69-2. Pregnancies after suture repair of obstetric uterine rupture: Literature review: 1964-1989

	No.	Rate (%)
Patients	209	
Pregnancies	271	
Site of original scar		
Classical	96	48
Lower segment	34	16
Not recorded or no scar	73	36
Reruptures	25	11.9
Maternal deaths	2	0.9
Perinatal deaths	12*	5.9

*Abortions not included.

thick fundus of the uterus. The first layer of continuous suture is deep in the myometrium, inverting the endometrium into the uterine cavity. A second layer of continuous suture closes the middle third of the myometrium. A final layer neatly closes the serosa and subserosal layer of the myometrium.

Rerupture after repair. The fate of the repaired uterine rupture in subsequent pregnancy is becoming more clear as a body of literature builds on this subject. The Sheth study reported 21 pregnancies in 13 patients who had suture repairs of previous uterine ruptures. Of 17 pregnancies after repair of a lower segment rupture, repeat rupture occurred in only one. Three of four pregnancies after repair of a fundal rupture reruptured, and only one child survived.[59]

Reyes-Ceja's group recorded 22 pregnancies in 19 patients with previous uterine rupture.[52] It was the policy of these authors to deliver their patients by cesarean operation at 38 weeks gestation. Eight pregnancies culminated, however, in vaginal delivery. Only one repeat uterine rupture was encountered (4.5%). Pregnancy after repaired uterine rupture was felt to be appropriate by the Reyes-Ceja group. They suggested that there was international consensus that patients with pregnancies after repair of uterine rupture should have cesarean deliveries.

Ritchie in 1971 reported a personal series of 36 pregnancies in 28 patients after uterine rupture.[53] There were two reruptures of classical incision rupture repairs (5.5%). Ritchie's literature survey was divided into two eras. The classical cesarean era before 1932 revealed 86 pregnancies after uterine rupture with 52 (61%) repeat ruptures. The literature from 1932 to 1970 contained 253 pregnancies in 194 patients with previous uterine rupture. Rerupture occurred in 10% of cases and resulted in 2 maternal deaths (0.8%) and 11 perinatal deaths (5.9%). Ruptures of classical scars dominated these statistics and were responsible for the most severe cases. Table 69-2 summarizes pregnancy outcomes after uterine rupture repair collected from the recent literature.*

The body of recent literature indicates a modest risk of

*References 15, 18, 44, 51, 52, 53, 59, 67.

rerupture and a small risk of maternal death for patients with previous suture repair of uterine ruptures. Most of the risk of rerupture accrues to cases of repaired fundal rupture. Tubal sterilization with rupture repair or hysterectomy should be considered for patients who experience major fundal rupture unless the patient insists on future pregnancies. Repaired ruptures of the lower segment appear safer for another pregnancy.

Internal iliac (hypogastric) artery ligation. Ligation of the anterior division of the internal iliac (hypogastric) arteries can reduce blood flow to the site of a major uterine rupture and clear the operating field for safe dissection. Ligation must usually be performed on both sides because of extensive collateral circulation. Internal iliac ligation is an auxiliary operation to control blood loss and is not sufficient treatment for most cases of rupture of the gravid uterus. Transient aortic compression can be used when nothing else will stem the hemorrhagic tide.

The internal iliac arteries are approached on each side by opening the parietal peritoneum on the lateral pelvic wall from the insertion of the round ligament cephalad. There are more direct routes to these vessels, but the round ligament is always a safe place to begin this dissection, even with extensive pelvic contusions and hematomas.

The medial peritoneal edge of the above incision is reflected medially. The ureter is readily identified on the undersurface of this flap and will remain safe from injury during further dissection.

The common iliac artery is palpated at the pelvic brim and followed caudad to its bifurcation. The posterior branch is the internal iliac artery, which courses medial and deep to the external iliac vessels. The first branch of the internal iliac is usually the superior gluteal artery, which courses posterior and deep to the dissection. The intention is to ligate the internal iliac artery just distal to this first branch. Ligation above this branch can occasionally result in presacral necrosis.

A small right-angled clamp, such as a Munion clamp, is useful to dissect away carefully the connective tissue around the internal iliac artery. Care must be taken in the depths of this dissection to avoid injury to large veins nearby. The internal iliac vein lies immediately beneath and lateral to the internal iliac artery. The external iliac vein lies lateral and slightly posterior to the dissection.

The curved clamp is passed beneath the internal iliac artery from lateral to medial. The clamp is opened, and a double strand of permanent suture is placed within its jaws. The suture is drawn beneath the vessel and upward as a double strand. The sutures are tied as two separate vascular ties a few millimeters apart. The surgeon must check to be sure that pulsations are good in the external iliac or femoral artery distal to the field before tying these sutures. The vessel need not be divided. The peritoneum is closed with 00 chromic running suture or left open if rapid progression of the case is necessary.

Hysterectomy. Removal of the ruptured uterus is a proper choice when the uterus is damaged beyond safe repair or when other measures fail to stop the blood loss. Hysterectomy in these cases may be a life-saving procedure. The procedure for cesarean hysterectomy is discussed in detail in Chapter 68.

The entire abdomen is examined, and injuries to other organs are repaired. The bowel, bladder, ureters, and adnexal structures are at greatest risk. Organs as distant as the liver and spleen may be involved in blunt trauma cases or penetrating wounds to the pregnant abdomen.

The superiority of complete versus subtotal peripartal hysterectomy has been argued for years. A uterine rupture confined to the fundus of the uterus in an unstable patient can be addressed by subtotal (supracervical) hysterectomy. This operation is certainly faster and easier than complete hysterectomy. It is difficult to identify the lower extent of a uterine tear at the time of operation. If the rupture extends into the lower segment and cervix, subtotal hysterectomy will not suffice. Total hysterectomy is recommended whenever feasible.

NONOBSTETRIC UTERINE RUPTURE
Causes

Rupture of the nonpregnant uterus is a rare event whose causes are outlined in the box on p. 1135, right. The most common cause is instrumentation during gynecologic operative procedures.[31] Operative procedures for abortion are included in this discussion although abortions are clearly not "nonobstetric."

Trauma. Most surgical uterine ruptures are perforations during dilation and curettage (D and C). Perforations are reported to occur in 0.63% of gynecologic D and Cs and 0.2% of obstetric D and Cs.[21,31] Grimes felt that perforations were three to four times more common with sharp curettage than with suction curettage.[21] Mittal and Misra did not confirm this impression but reported a 0.4% incidence of uterine perforation with vacuum aspiration of first trimester pregnancies.[41]

Kaali et al found that only a small proportion (0.13%) of uterine perforations were recognized during the performance of first trimester abortions. When laparoscopy for sterilization followed the D and C, unrecognized perforation was noted in 1.98% of cases.[26] Multiparas appear to have three times greater risk of perforation at the time of obstetric D and C than primiparas. The Centers for Disease Control in 1988 reported that D and C for abortion resulted in a maternal death rate of 0.6 per 100,000 abortions.[21]

Uterine perforations occasionally occur at the time of hysteroscopy and hysteroscopic resection of uterine polyps, adhesions, leiomyomas, and congenital septae.

Introduction and removal of intrauterine contraceptive devices (IUDs) were responsible for a number of uterine perforations in the 1970s and 1980s. Abramovici et al reported a prevalence of perforation of 1 per 1000 IUD insertions.[1]

Small IUDs introduced with pointed carriers were particularly apt to cause uterine perforation. Perforation was more common with postpartum insertions. Abramovici et al reported nine perforations resulting from insertion of the Lippes loop and Cu-7 devices.[1] Perforation incidents related to IUDs became less common as the IUD became a less frequently used form of contraception.

Tumor invasion. Aggressive uterine tumors infiltrate and eventually penetrate the uterine wall. Uterine ruptures are most common with mixed mesodermal tumors, sarcomas, and choriocarcinomas.[32] Rupture is rarely associated with adenocarcinomas of the endometrium whose habit is polypoid growth. Cervical epidermoid malignancies perforate the uterus as they extend cephalad and lateral. Rupture of the uterus has also been reported to result from red degeneration of leiomyomas.[33]

Treatment of uterine tumors by radiation can result in uterine rupture by several mechanisms. Direct perforations may occur at the time of placement of intracavitary or intracervical radiation sources. Matsuyama et al found evidence of uterine perforation in 6 of 61 patients at the time of small source insertion for brachytherapy.[35] Makin and Hunter used computed tomography (CT) scans to identify perforations during afterloading intracavitary radiation treatment for carcinoma of the cervix. Three percent of the patients had unrecognized perforations.[34] Postradiation necrosis may result in uterine perforation and genital fistulas.

Infections. Virulent infections can cause necrosis and rupture of the uterine wall. The most dramatic examples are ruptures of pyometras. Rupture of the uterus from pyometra is a rare event usually associated with weakening of the uterine wall by tumors. Peritonitis and septic shock follow shortly after rupture of pyometra. The review of Hosking contains 12 cases of spontaneous uterine perforation of pyometras.[23] *Clostridium* and *Bacteroides* infections of the myometrial wall can also cause its disruption and rapidly spreading peritonitis.

Surgical wound dehiscence. Uterine rupture due to ischemic necrosis is occasionally seen at the site of uterine surgical wounds. Wound dehiscence from necrosis or infection is rare after gynecologic procedures. It is more common in cesarean operations performed after prolonged labor when genital tract bacteria have colonized the lower uterine segment.

Management

Most instrumental perforations of the uterus occur at the time of dilatation and curetage (D and C). The uterine sound or the endometrial sharp or suction curette can easily perforate the myometrial wall, particularly if some physiologic or disease process has weakened the wall. Important considerations when planning the management of D and C perforations include the size and depth of the injury, bleeding and hemodynamic stability of the patient, the indication for the procedure, and the need to complete the procedure.

The size and depth of the injury are very difficult to determine but are important to further management. Incomplete ruptures are often not recognized. Most D and C injuries are small perforations at the time of introduction of instruments into the uterine cavity. Extensive injuries occur when sweeps of the curette are taken after perforation has occurred.

Other pelvic organs can be injured at the time of uterine perforation or laceration. The author has managed a case in which the posterior wall of the uterus was lacerated along its entire length at the time of curettage for abortion. The anterior wall of the sigmoid colon also sustained a full-thickness 6-cm laceration.

The presence or absence of bleeding or hemodynamic instability influences management decisions. When perforation causes significant bleeding or when the injury seems to be large and injury to other organs is suspected, the procedure should be stopped, and the intraabdominal situation should be evaluated carefully. Laparoscopy is very useful to assess the extent of uterine injury, the presence of expanding hematomas, or injury to adjacent structures.[26]

Large injuries usually require laparotomy and suture repair for hemostasis and proper healing. Laparotomy should be performed if the surgeon cannot exclude injury to the bowel or other abdominal or pelvic organs or if expanding hematomas are detected. Perforations due to external penetrating trauma such as bullet wounds require laparotomy even though they may initially appear to be small and asymptomatic.[18,37]

Whether to continue curettage after perforation is detected depends on the indication for the procedure and the stage of the operation at the time of perforation. If it is necessary to continue curettage after perforation, it can safely be done under laparoscopic visualization. Direct visualization assures the surgeon of the size and location of the original injury and avoids extending the injury.

Small perforations that are not bleeding can usually be managed conservatively by observation of the patient for bleeding or signs of peritoneal irritation. Kaali et al managed 22 patients with perforations at the time of D and C for abortion in this way with no immediate or late complications.[26]

Small perforations that are bleeding can often be closed at laparotomy with one or two hemostatic stitches of 0 chromic or 00 polyglycolic suture material. Larger injuries to the uterine wall are closed in layers similar to the closure of a hysterotomy or cesarean section wound.

The entire abdomen and pelvis should be explored if laparotomy is undertaken. Any perforations or lacerations of bowel, bladder, or other organs must be closed. Any foreign bodies must be removed. The peritoneal cavity is cleansed and irrigated before closure of the abdominal wall.

SUMMARY

The spectrum of conditions relating to rupture of the uterus includes both obstetric and nonobstetric events. The recent literature relating to the causes, recognition, and management of uterine rupture is herein reviewed.

This chapter focused attention on obstetric spontaneous uterine rupture, postcesarean scar separation, and extratu-

bal ectopic gestations as they relate to rupture of the pregnant uterus. The clinical indications for repair or removal of the ruptured uterus and methods of hemostasis, including uterine packing and internal iliac artery ligation, were described.

Nonobstetric uterine rupture may be due to instrumental perforation, tumors, or infections. Management options for nonobstetric rupture were related to the acuity of the problem and the extent of the injury to the uterus.

All trained obstetrician-gynecologists should be prepared to manage the potentially life-threatening complication of rupture of the uterus.

REFERENCES

1. Abramovici H et al: Removal of completely perforating IUDs by explorative laparotomy, *Int J Fertil* 32:279, 1987.
2. Acton CM: The ultrasonic appearance of a ruptured uterus, *Austral Radiol* 22:254, 1978.
3. Adams DM, Druzin ML, Cderqvist LL: Intrapartum uterine rupture, *Obstet Gynecol* 73:471, 1989.
4. Aguero O, Kizer S: Suture of the uterine rupture, *Obstet Gynecol* 31:806, 1968.
5. American College of Obstetricians and Gynecologists: *Guidelines for vaginal delivery after a cesarean birth. Statements of the Committee on Obstetrics: Maternal and Fetal Medicine.* Washington, DC, 1982, 1984, 1988, 1989.
6. Awais GM, Lebherz TB: Ruptured uterus: a complication of oxytocin induction and high parity, *Obstet Gynecol* 36:465, 1970.
7. Beckmann CRB, Tomasi AM, Thomason JL: Combined interstitial and intrauterine pregnancy: cornual resection in early pregnancy and cesarean delivery at term, *Am J Obstet Gynecol* 149:83, 1984.
8. Brandes MC et al: Treatment of cornual pregnancy with methotrexate: case report, *Am J Obstet Gynecol* 155:655, 1986.
9. Champion PM, Tessitore NJL: Broad ligament pregnancy, *Am J Obstet Gynecol* 36:281, 1938.
10. Chestnut D et al: Peripartum hysterectomy, *Obstet Gynecol* 65:365, 1985.
11. Deaton JL, Maier D, Andreoli J Jr: Spontaneous uterine rupture during pregnancy after treatment of Asherman's syndrome, *Am J Obstet Gynecol* 160:1053, 1989.
12. Degefu S et al: Stab wound of the gravid uterus: a case report and literature update, *J LA State Med Soc* 140:39, 1988.
13. Dunnihoo DR et al: An evaluation of uterine scar integrity after cesarean section in rabbits, *Obstet Gynecol* 73:390, 1989.
14. Dyer I, Barclay DL: Accidental trauma complicating pregnancy, *Am J Obstet Gynecol* 83:907, 1962.
15. Eden RD, Parker RT, Gall SA: Rupture of the pregnant uterus: a 53-year review, *Obstet Gynecol* 68:671, 1986.
16. Eden TW, Lockyer C, editors: *Gynecology,* p 210, New York, 1928, Macmillan.
17. Franger AL, Buchsbaum HJ, Peaceman AM: Abdominal gunshot wounds in pregnancy, *Am J Obstet Gynecol* 160:1124, 1989.
18. Garnett JD: Uterine rupture during pregnancy: an analysis of 133 patients, *Obstet Gynecol* 23:898, 1964.
19. Golan A, Sanbank O, Tear AJ: Trauma in late pregnancy, *S Afr Med J* 547:161, 1980.
20. Graham AR: Trial of labor following previous cesarean section, *Am J Obstet Gynecol* 149:35, 1984.
21. Grimes D: *Surgical management of abortion.* In Thompson J and Rock J, editors: *Telinde's operative gynecology,* ed 7, J.B. Lippincott, Philadelphia p 339, 1992.
22. Heinonen PK, Aro P: Rupture of pregnant noncommunicating uterine horn with fetal salvage, *Eur J Obstet Gynecol Reprod Biol* 27:261, 1988.
23. Hosking SW: Spontaneous perforation of a pyometra presenting as generalized peritonitis, *Postgrad Med J* 61:645, 1985.

24. Jauchler GW, Baker RL: Cervical pregnancy: review of the literature and a case report, *Obstet Gynecol* 35:870, 1970.

25. Jones DE, Mitler LK: Rupture of a gravid bicornuate uterus in a primigravida associated with clostridial and *Bacteriodes* infection, *J Reprod Med* 21:185, 1978.

26. Kaali SG, Szigetvari IA, Bartfai GS: The frequency and management of uterine perforation during first-trimester abortions, *Am J Obstet Gynecol* 161:406, 1989.

27. Kieffer WS: Rupture of the uterus, *Am J Obstet Gynecol* 89:335, 1964.

28. Lavin J et al: Vaginal delivery in patients with a prior cesarean section, *Am J Obstet Gynecol* 59:135, 1982.

29. Lindberg BS: Maternal sepsis, uterine rupture and coagulopathy complicating cervical cerclage, *Acta Obstet Gynecol Scand* 58:317, 1979.

30. Liu A et al: Pathophysiologic mechanism of uterine rupture during labor, *Chinese Med J* 98(3):161, 1985.

31. Mackenzie IZ, Bibby JG: Critical assessment of dilatation and curettage in 1029 women, *Lancet* ii:566, 1978.

32. Maiman M et al: Uterine rupture secondary to a malignant mixed mesodermal (mullerian) tumor: a case report, *Gynecol Oncol* 30:137, 1988.

33. Makar AP et al: A case report of unusual complication of myomatous uterus in pregnancy: spontaneous perforation of myoma after red degeneration, *Europ J Obstet Gynecol Reprod Biol* 31:289, 1989.

34. Makin WP, Hunter RD: CT scanning in intracavitary therapy: Unexpected findings in "straightforward" insertions, *Radiother Oncol* 13:253, 1988.

35. Matsuyama T et al: Uterine perforation at the time of brachytherapy for the carcinoma of the uterine cervix, *Gynecol Oncol* 23:205, 1986.

36. McCarthy T, McQueen J: Uterine rupture as a complication of second trimester abortion using intraamniotic prostaglandin E₂ and augmentation with other oxytocic prostaglandins 19:869, 1980.

37. McNabey W, Smith EI: Penetrating wound of the gravid uterus, *J Trauma* 12:1024, 1972.

38. Meehan FP, Magani IM: True rupture of the cesarean section scar (a 15 year review, 1972-1987), *Br J Obstet Gynecol Reprod Biol* 30:129, 1989.

39. Meier P, Porreco R: Trial of labor following cesarean section: a two year experience, *Am J Obstet Gynecol* 144:671, 1982.

40. Merrill BS, Gibbs CE: Planned vaginal delivery following cesarean section, *Obstet Gynecol* 52:50, 1978.

41. Mittal S, Misra SL: Uterine perforation following medical termination of pregnancy by vacuum aspiration, *Int J Gynaec Obstet* 23:45, 1985.

42. Morrison J: Vaginal delivery after cesarean section, *Am J Obstet Gynecol* 146:262, 1983.

43. Nagy PS: Placenta percreta induced uterine rupture and resulted in intraabdominal abortion, *Am J Obstet Gynecol* 161:1185, 1989.

44. Nielsen TF, Ljungblad U, Hagberg H: Rupture and dehiscence of cesarean section scar during pregnancy and delivery, *Am J Obstet Gynecol* 160:569, 1989.

45. Osmers R et al: Sonographic detection of an asymptomatic rupture of the uterus due to necrosis during the third trimester, *Int J Gynecol Obstet* 26:279, 1988.

46. Palerme GR, Friedman EA: Rupture of the gravid uterus in the third trimester, *Am J Obstet Gynecol* 94:571, 1966.

47. Parente JT et al: Cervical pregnancy analysis: A review and report of 5 cases, *Obstet Gynecol* 62:79, 1983.

48. Pelosi MA: *Cervical pregnancy*. In Iffy L, Charles D, editors: *Operative perinatology*, New York, 1984, Macmillan.

49. Plauche' WC, Von Almen W, Muller R: Catastrophic uterine rupture, *Obstet Gynecol* 64:792, 1984.

50. Pritchard JA, MacDonald PC, Gant NF: *Ectopic pregnancy*. In *Williams obstetrics*, ed 17, Norwalk, CT, 1989, Appleton-Century-Crofts.

51. Pruett KM, Kirshon B, Cotton DB: Unknown uterine scar and trial of labor, *Am J Obstet Gynecol* 159:807, 1988.

52. Reyes-Ceja L et al: Pregnancy following previous uterine rupture. Study of 19 patients. *Obstet Gynecol* 34:387, 1969.

53. Ritchie EH: Pregnancy after rupture of the pregnant uterus, *J Obstet Gynecol Br Commwlth* 78:642, 1971.

54. Rodriguez MH et al: Uterine rupture: are intrauterine pressure catheters useful in the diagnosis? *Obstet Gynecol* 161:666, 1989.

55. Ron-El R et al: Term delivery following mid-trimester ruptured cornual pregnancy with combined intrauterine pregnancy. Case report, *Br J Obstet Gynaecol*, 95:619, 1987.

56. Sawyer MM et al: Third-trimester uterine rupture associated with vaginal prostaglandin E₂, *Am J Obstet Gynecol* 140:710, 1981.

57. Schneider P: Distal ectopic pregnancy, *Am J Surg* 12:526, 1946.

58. Schwartz OH, Paddock R, Bortnick AR: The cesarean scar, an experimental study, *Am J Obstet Gynecol* 25:962, 1938.

59. Sheth SS: Results of treatment of rupture of the uterus by suturing, *J Obstet Gynecol Br Commwlth* 75:55, 1968.

60. Shinagawa S, Nagayama M: Cervical pregnancy as a possible sequel of induced abortion. Report of 19 cases, *Am J Obstet Gynecol* 105:282, 1969.

61. Shrinsky DC, Benson RC: Rupture of the pregnant uterus: a review, *Obstet Gynecol Surv* 33:217, 1978.

62. Studdiford WE: Cervical pregnancy: a partial review of the literature and a report of two probable cases, *Am J Obstet Gynecol* 49:160, 1945.

63. Taylor HW, Slate WG: *Surgery and trauma during pregnancy*. In Iffy L, Charles J, editors: *Operative perinatology*, ed 1, New York, 1984, MacMillan.

64. Taylor PJ, Cumming DC: Spontaneous rupture of a primigravid uterus, *J Reprod Med* 22:168, 1979.

65. Thomsen M, Johansen F: Two cases of cervical pregnancy, *Acta Obstet Gynecol Scand* 40:99, 1961.

66. Valenzuela G et al: Uterine rupture at term with vaginal prostaglandin E₂, *Am J Obstet Gynecol* 138:1223, 1980.

67. Van der Merwe JV, Ombelet WUAM: Rupture of the uterus: A changing picture, *Arch Gynecol* 240:159, 1987.

68. Wechstein LN: Current perspectives on ectopic pregnancy, *Obstet Gynecol Surv* 40:259, 1985.

69. Weingold AB et al: Rupture of the gravid uterus, *Surg Gynecol Obstet* 21:1233, 1966.

70. Wolfe SA, Neigus I: Broad-ligament pregnancy with report of three early cases, *Am J Obstet Gynecol* 66:106, 1953.

71. Woodbridge A, Gonsoulin W: *Trial of labor after cesarean birth: the UMC Lafayette experience*. LSU resident research day presentation, New Orleans, Oct 1988.

72. Yetman TJ, Nolan TE: Vaginal birth after cesarean section: a reappraisal of risk, *Am J Obstet Gynecol* 161:1119, 1989.

Chapter 70

INVERSION OF THE UTERUS

David H. Nichols

DEFINITION AND TYPES

A turning inside-out, or inversion, of the uterus may be incomplete, in which only the uterine fundus is inverted to varying degrees, or complete, in which the entire endometrial cavity is everted.

Das' historic review[8] of uterine inversion notes that it was recorded as long ago as 2500 BC.

Degrees[33]

First-degree inversion of the uterus is incomplete, and the inverted cavity is said to extend to the cervix, but not beyond the cervical ring. Because at times it may be self-correcting, its frequency may be greater than reported.

Second-degree uterine inversion is the most common type reported. The inverted endometrial cavity extends through the cervical ring, but it does not descend as far as the patient's perineum.

Third degree, or complete, inversion extends to the perineum.

NONOBSTETRIC INVERSION OF THE UTERUS
Etiology and diagnosis

Downward traction to the uterine fundus from an attached pedunculated submucosal leiomyoma or other neoplasm, combined with longstanding myometrial contraction as an attempt by the uterus to rid itself of such a perceived "foreign body" may invert the uterine fundus along with the tumor. The lesion may be found on routine examination often in the presence of a chronic bloody discharge.[16]

Treatment

The condition should be treated initially by transvaginal amputation of the tumor, being careful that the surgery be extraperitoneal at this time, because the prolapsed lesion is usually infected. If subsequent hysterectomy is contem-plated, the uterus should be given several weeks for the infection to subside to lessen the risk of peritonitis.

Fundal inversion coincident with a prolapsed leiomyoma can be identified by careful bimanual pelvic or rectal examination whereby the gynecologist, while palpating the top of the uterine fundus, feels for the characteristic dimple in the fundus. Finding such a dimple forewarns of the possibility of unexpectedly transecting the inverted fundus along with removal of the prolapsed tumor and, by opening into the peritoneal cavity, risking peritonitis (Fig. 70-1).

When such a dimple has been identified, the stalk of the pedicle should be transected near its attachment to the prolapsed tumor. The base of the stalk may be ligated or cauterized for hemostasis, and the remaining stalk is permitted to retract within the uterine cavity. Freed of the tumor, the partially inverted uterine fundus usually reverts to normal over a period of a few weeks.

PUERPERAL UTERINE INVERSION
Etiology and diagnosis

Most of the uterine inversions that are encountered are accidents of labor and delivery. The frequency with which obstetric uterine inversion is encountered varies from 1:1000 to 1:6500 deliveries,[6,26,33,36] the different rates possibly reflecting the rate of detection and diagnosis.

Obstetric uterine inversion occurs unexpectedly during the third stage of labor, possibly when a portion of the uterine fundus becomes indented (as from traction to an unseparated placenta, or presence of a short umbilical cord), and the remaining muscle of the uterus contracts around the invaginated portion as it would around a foreign body[24,25] and, in attempting to expel it, turns itself inside-out.[20]

Puerperal inversion is most common among the primip-arous[2,3,30] and is seen more frequently among patients

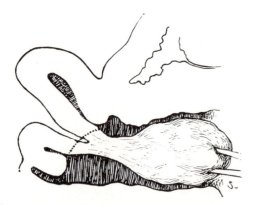

Fig. 70-1. One of the dangers of myomectomy in the presence of a partial uterine inversion is shown. If the pedicle stalk is divided at the site of the dotted line, the peritoneal cavity would be opened, risking peritonitis. (From Crossen HS, Crossen RJ: *Operative gynecology*, ed 6, St Louis, CV Mosby, 1948.)

who were receiving intravenous $MgSO_4$ for treatment of preeclampsia.[26,33,35]

In most instances, the condition occurs spontaneously without demonstrable obvious cause, although it is more common among nullipara, especially those with a previous first-trimester pregnancy loss.

Subsequent recurrence of inversion in the same patient has been reported.[38] Deep anesthesia causing uterine relaxation after delivery has been noted.[2,18,29] Plaut[34] cautions against membrane traction during delivery of the placenta as possibly etiologic, and Harris[5,17] recommends routine exploration of the uterine cavity after every delivery to detect early inversion and treat it immediately. An association with prolonged labor has been suggested.[39]

Careful management of the third stage of labor is the most important factor in preventing this serious complication.

Treatment

Acute inversion. Immediate recognition of the inversion with prompt reposit of the uterus may prevent the alarming hemorrhage and consequent shock associated with the condition.[28,30] Often, deep general anesthesia may be required, such as under the fluorinated hydrocarbon halothane (Fluothane) given in high concentration to provide rapid, maximal relaxation.[1,5]

Ninety percent of the reported deaths from postpartum uterine inversion occur within the first 2 hours after delivery[11] and are caused by hemorrhage or shock.[20]

Administration of an oxytocic to the patient with uterine inversion before it is reduced makes replacement of the fundus more difficult.[4]

When acute uterine inversion is first recognized, two large-bore intravenous lines carrying Ringer's lactate are immediately started[5,6] and immediate professional assistance including an anesthetist is requested. A transfusion of whole blood should be started, instilled under mechani-

cal pressure if necessary, as soon as the likely need has become evident. To lessen the size of the raw endouterine surface from which hemorrhage can arise, the operator may leave the unseparated placenta attached to the fundus until the latter has been replaced within the abdomen.[2,5,13,26]

Transvaginal treatment of acute inversion. The Johnson technique[23] of applying steady pressure to the periphery of the inverted fundus, usually posteriorly, is useful, especially if it can be performed before the myometrium becomes contracted. The entire hand of the operator is placed in the vagina, with the finger tips at the uterocervical junction and the fundus in the palm. Pressure is applied so the entire uterus is lifted out of the pelvis to the level of the umbilicus where countertraction of the uterine ligaments exerts pressure to widen the cervical ring pulling the fundus back through it.[20] If myometrial spasm and contraction rings impede the reinversion, tocolytics as well as deep general anesthesia may be helpful. $MgSO_4$ may be given intravenously, 1 g per minute for 4 minutes, to relax the uterus.[6,13] If this is not effective, 0.125 to 0.25 mg of terbutaline may be given intravenously.[27]

Before the hand is removed from the reposited uterus, the uterine fundus may be elevated against the anterior abdominal wall and an oxytocic or prostaglandin is injected through the abdominal wall directly into the uterus. The hand is withdrawn only when the uterus has contracted firmly.[5,6,36] If bleeding persists and examination has ruled out rupture or perforation of the uterus, an intrauterine packing may be inserted for 24 hours.[32]

If the above technique is not successful in repositing the uterus, the Jones' method[24,25] may be attempted. The gloved fingers are placed in the center of the inverted fundus while pressing slowly upward. Countertraction with ring forceps applied to the cervix may be helpful.[20]

One should use whichever method seems to be most effective in the individual case.

O'Sullivan[32] suggests another method whereby the obstetrician's hand replaces the inverted uterus within the vagina, and, with hand and wrist occluding the introitus, an intravenous infusion tube is passed into the posterior vaginal fornix and saline is run rapidly into the upper vagina, the hydraulic pressure so created reverts the uterus.[15] Unless the reposited uterus contracts firmly, it may reinvert,[21] requiring that it be watched carefully postpartum.

Unlike the reports of Kitchen[26] and of Donald,[9] Platt and Druzen's review[33] of their own cases did not support the view that prophylactic antibiotic use is indicated in patients with uterine inversion.

Transabdominal surgical approach. If the transvaginal methods of reposing the acutely inverted uterus fail, laparotomy should be considered.

The Huntington procedure[20,22] should be tried first, in which the abdominal peritoneal side of the uterus is grasped on both sides with Allis clamps about 2 cm below the ring and upward traction is applied. Additional forceps are placed below the original pair, successively picking up

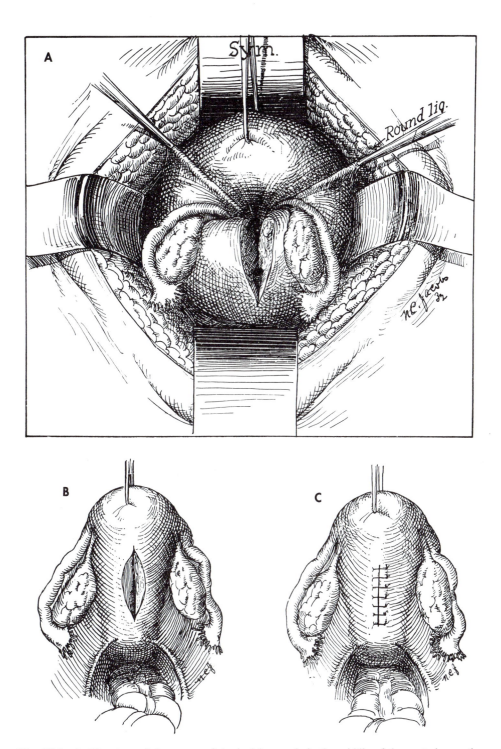

Fig. 70-2. A, The site and the extent of the incision made in the middle of the posterior portion of the constricting ring are shown. The inverted fundus can be replaced by pressure from below, through the vagina, or by traction from above, according to the method of Huntington and Irving. An incision of approximately 1 inch in length usually suffices, but, if necessary, this can be enlarged somewhat. The constricting ring should be incised as it lies, the incision will then be in the region of the lower uterine segment rather than in the upper portion, thus rendering the uterus safer for future childbearing. **B,** Diagrammatic illustration of the uterus after it has been replaced. The incision in the posterior wall will be closed by two layers of sutures: an intramuscular layer of interrupted sutures and a continuous seromuscular layer. (In the diagram, the incision is represented at a rather higher level than usual.) **C,** The uterine incision is closed. If there is any tendency toward backward displacement, some form of uterine suspension may be employed. (From Wilson K: Inversion of the uterus, *Am J Obstet Gynecol* 28:738, 1934.)

portions of the uterus until the inversion is completely reposited. Simultaneous transvaginal pressure by an assistant's hand in the patient's vagina may be helpful.

If success cannot be achieved by the Huntington maneuver, as might be noted when the inversion is of longer duration, the Haultain[19] procedure may be used.[10,19,20] In this transabdominal operation, a longitudinal incision is made in the posterior uterine wall over and through the contraction ring. A finger may be introduced through the uterine incision to a point below the inverted fundus, and reduction is effected by applying pressure with this finger against the fundus[7] or by simultaneous pressure from the fingers of an assistant, which are placed in the patient's vagina. The reposition completed, the uterine incision is repaired transabdominally by a series of interrupted stitches (Fig. 70-1).

Chronic uterine inversion. When a patient with an undetected uterine inversion has survived for months, a large degree of uterine involution will have taken place in the postpartum uterus, and the condition may be described as "chronic" inversion. When the condition is associated with a nonobstetric etiology, it may be present for years. The patient may describe a bloody vaginal discharge of long duration, and upon pelvic examination the presence of a dusky dark red mass protruding from the uterine cervix will be noted as well as the palpable dimple at the top of the shortened uterine fundus, perhaps best identified by bimanual palpation of the uterus during rectal examination.

Transvaginal surgery. A vaginal approach to reposition of the inverted fundus may be preferable for the chronic case because of better access to the operative site and the more limited intraperitoneal manipulation than would be necessary with the transabdominal operation.

In the older Küstner operation,[14,31] a transvaginal transverse colpotomy and incision of the full thickness of the cervix at the 6 o'clock position carried up through the posterior uterine wall are made (Fig. 70-2) and the inversion is reposited. The incision in the posterior uterine wall and cervix is repaired, as is the original transverse incision and colpotomy in the vagina. Disadvantages of the Küstner operation are that there is greater risk of pelvic adhesion formation to the recently sutured posterior uterine wall than there would be to a similar incision in the anterior wall, and the posterior uterine incision is not available for palpation during subsequent pregnancy, possibly masking a silent or impending uterine rupture.

These objections are overcome when the somewhat newer transvaginal Spinelli operation[7,12,31,37] is performed (Fig. 70-3). The anterior vaginal wall is made tense against the countertraction of a retractor and is incised transversely just above the anterior cervical lip. The bladder is dissected from the cervix and lower uterine segment. A midline incision is made through the cervix at the 12

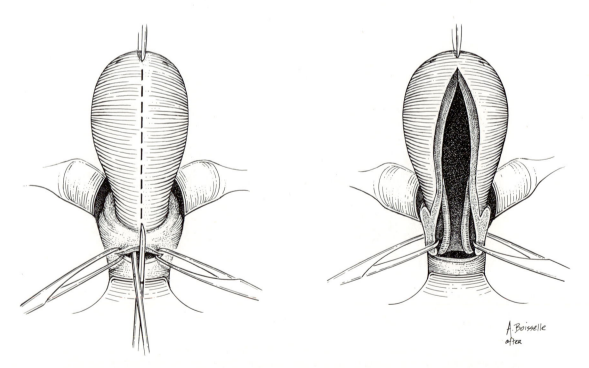

Fig. 70-3. The Küstner operation for chronic inversion of the uterus is shown. The posterior cul-de-sac has been opened, and the cervix and posterior wall of the uterus should be incised along the path of the broken line as shown in the drawing on the left. When this has been completed, as shown in the drawing to the right, thumb pressure along the sides of the uterus produce reversion, the wounds are closed with interrupted sutures, and the uterus is replaced in the pelvic cavity. The colpotomy is then closed. (From Nichols DH, Randall CL: *Vaginal surgery,* ed 3, Baltimore, Williams & Wilkins, 1989.)

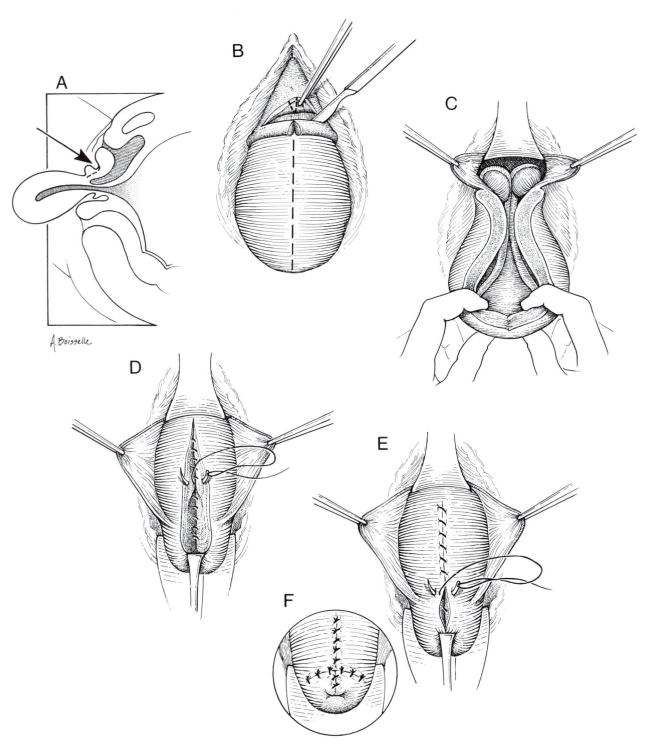

Fig. 70-4. The Spinelli operation for chronic inversion of the uterus is illustrated. The cervix is split in the midline and carefully separated from the bladder as shown by the dotted line in **A.** The anterior wall of the everted uterus is split along the path of the dotted line in **B. C,** By pressure with the operator's index fingers and thumbs, the uterus is turned outside-in. **D,** The myometrium is reapproximated by two layers of running PGA suture. **E,** The serosal surface is reapproximated by a single layer. **F,** The vaginal skin is reapproximated with interrupted sutures, as is the full thickness of the cervix. (From Nichols DH, Randall CL: *Vaginal surgery,* ed 3, Baltimore, Williams & Wilkins, 1989.)

o'clock position, completely dividing the constriction ring. The incision is carried in the midline to the uterine fundus. The uterus is reverted by hooking one's forefingers into the incision on the exposed endometrial surface and making counterpressure with the thumbs on its peritoneal side, forcing the fundus upward much in the manner that one would use to turn a cut tennis ball inside-out (Fig. 70-4, *A* through *C*). As much myometrium and endometrium as bulge into the uterine incision are trimmed as longitudinal wedges to permit coaption of all layers of myometrium and peritoneum without tension. The vertical incision in the cervix is closed by side-to-side interrupted sutures, and the transverse vaginal skin is approximated as shown (Fig. 70-4 *D* through *F*).

Future obstetric delivery, in most instances, should be by elective cesarean section 2 weeks before term in patients who have experienced such a hysterotomy.

Hysterectomy. Vaginal or abdominal hysterectomy may be advised for the patient in whom reinversion continues or in whom extensive tissue necrosis and infection are observed.

REFERENCES

1. Albright GA et al: *Anesthesia in obstetrics—maternal, fetal, and neonatal aspects,* ed 2, Boston, 1986, Butterworths.
2. Bell JE Jr, Wilson GF, Wilson LA: Puerperal inversion of the uterus, *Am J Obstet Gynecol* 66:767, 1953.
3. Bunke JW, Hofmeister FJ: Uterine inversion—obstetrical entity or oddity, *Am J Obstet Gynecol* 91:934, 1965.
4. Burrus JH, Lampley CG Jr: Acute puerperal inversion of the uterus, *NC Med J* 26:502, 1965.
5. Catanzarite VA, Grossman R: How to manage uterine inversion, *Contemp Ob/Gyn* 28:81, 1986.
6. Catanzarite VA et al: New approaches to the management of acute puerperal uterine inversion, *Obstet Gynecol* 68:75, 1986.
7. Crossen HS, Crossen RJ: *Operative gynecology,* ed 6, St Louis, Mosby–Year Book, 1948, p 424.
8. Das P: Inversion of the uterus, *Br J Obstet Gynaecol* 47:525, 1940.
9. Donald I: *Practical obstetric problems,* ed. 4, Philadelphia, 1969, JB Lippincott, p 609.
10. Easterday CL, Reid D: Inversion of puerperal uterus managed by Haultain technique, *Am J Obstet Gynecol* 78:1224, 1959.
11. Eastman NJ, Hellman LM: Williams' obstetrics, ed 13, New York, 1966, Appleton-Century-Crofts.
12. Greenhill JP: *Surgical gynecology,* ed 2, Chicago, 1957, Mosby–Year Book, p 198.
13. Grossman RA: Magnesium sulfate for uterine inversion, *J Reprod Med* 26:261, 1981.
14. Halban J: *Gynäkologische Operationslehre.* Wien, 1932, Urban and Schwarzenberg, p 196.
15. Halles RW: The use of intravaginal hydrolic pressure douches, *Am J Obstet Gynecol* 56:133, 1948.
16. Hanton EM, Kempers RD: Puerperal inversion of the uterus, *Postgrad Med* 36:541, 1964.
17. Harris BA: Acute puerperal inversion of the uterus, *Clin Obstet Gynecol* 27:134, 1984.
18. Harris RE, Dunnihoo DR: Inversion of the uterus in a patient under halothane anesthesia, *Obstet Gynecol* 27:655, 1966.
19. Haultain FWN: The treatment of chronic uterine inversion by abdominal hysterotomy, with a successful case, *Br Med J* 2:974, 1901.
20. Hess H: Uterine inversion, *Female Patient* 7:1, 1982.
21. Heyl PS, Stubblefield PG, Phillippee M: Recurrent inversion of the puerperal uterus managed with 15(S)-15-methyl prostaglandin F2-alpha and uterine packing, *Obstet Gynecol* 63:263, 1984.
22. Huntington JL: Acute inversion of the uterus, *Boston Med Surg J* 184:376, 1921.
23. Johnson AB: A new concept in the replacement of the inverted uterus and a report of nine cases, *Am J Obstet Gynecol* 57:557, 1949.
24. Jones WC: Inversion of the uterus with report of a case occurring during the puerperium and caused by a fibroid, *Surg Gynecol Obstet* 16:632, 1913.
25. Jones WC: Reports of two cases of postpartum inversion of the uterus with discussion of the pathogenesis of obstetrical inversion, *Am J Obstet* 69:982, 1914.
26. Kitchen D et al: Puerperal inversion of the uterus, *Am J Obstet Gynecol,* 123:51, 1975.
27. Kovacs VW, DeVore GR: Management of acute and subacute puerperal uterine inversion with terbutaline sulfate, *Am J Obstet Gynecol* 150:784, 1984.
28. Lee W et al: Acute inversion of the uterus, *Obstet Gynecol* 51:144, 1978.
29. Marcus MB, Brandt ML: Acute puerperal inversion of the uterus complicated by lower nephron nephrosis, *Obstet Gynecol* 9:725, 1957.
30. Mehra U, Ostapowicz F: Acute puerperal inversion of the uterus in a primipara, *Obstet Gynecol* 47:30, 1976.
31. Nichols DH, Randall CL: *Vaginal surgery,* ed 3, Baltimore, 1989, Williams & Wilkins, p 456.
32. O'Sullivan JV: Acute inversion of the uterus, *Br Med J* 2:282, 1945.
33. Platt LD, Druzin ML: Acute puerperal inversion of the uterus, *Am J Obstet Gynecol* 141:187, 1981.
34. Plaut GS: Chronic puerperal inversion of the uterus, *Postgrad Med J* 37:164, 1961.
35. Pritchard JA, MacDonald PC, Gant NF: *Williams Obstetrics,* ed 17, Norwalk, 1985, Appleton-Century-Crofts, p 715.
36. Shah-Hosseini R, Evrard JR: Puerperal uterine inversion, *Obstet Gynecol* 73:567, 1989.
37. Spinelli PC: Cura chirurgica conservative dell' inversione cronica dell' utero col processo kehrer, *Arch Ital Cinecol* 2:7, 1899.
38. Steffen E: Puerperal inversion of the uterus occurring in consecutive pregnancies in the same patient, *Am J Obstet Gynecol* 74:655, 1957.
39. Watson T, Besch N, Bowes WA Jr: Management of acute and subacute puerperal inversion of the uterus, *Obstet Gynecol* 55:12, 1980.

Chapter 71

SURGICAL THERAPY OF GESTATIONAL TROPHOBLASTIC DISEASE

John T. Soper
Charles B. Hammond

The term *gestational trophoblastic disease* (GTD) includes a wide range of clinically and histologically defined neoplasms derived from the human trophoblast, ranging from benign molar pregnancies with spontaneous resolution after evacuation to highly malignant gestational choriocarcinoma. Several factors have contributed to GTD becoming among the most curable forms of human solid tumors, including the widespread availability of sensitive and specific assays for human chorionic gonadotrophin (hGC), development of effective chemotherapy, integration of appropriate surgical intervention with chemotherapy, and individualization of chemotherapeutic regimens for patients with malignant GTD based on recognized risk factors. Although GTD afflicts young women during their prime reproductive years and can be a potentially devastating illness, the majority of women with malignant GTD can be cured using contemporary approaches to management.

The primary management of women with partial and complete hydatidiform mole is through surgical evacuation coupled with close monitoring of hCG levels. In patients who develop postmolar malignant GTD or gestational choriocarcinoma, chemotherapy has largely replaced surgery as the primary therapeutic modality. However, surgical procedures are often useful in the management of women with malignant GTD. Specific surgical techniques will not be reviewed in detail in this chapter, but the integration of surgery into the management of women with GTD will be presented.

HYDATIDIFORM MOLE

Two distinct entities of molar gestations, partial and complete moles, have recently been defined on the basis of cytogenetic, histopathologic, and clinical characteristics (Table 71-1). The majority of partial moles have a 69, XXX or 69, XXY karyotype derived from both maternal and paternal genome.[2,17,39-43] Often partial moles have clinical or histologic evidence of a fetus (e.g., amniotic membranes, fetal vessels with fetal red blood cells) and have irregular hydropic changes of chorionic villi with focal trophoblastic proliferation.[2,17,39-43] Because of the only modest increase in placental size and trophoblastic mass, the uterus is usually enlarged less than would be anticipated from the duration of gestation or is compatible with dates. Clinically and ultrasonographically, partial moles most often present as threatened or missed spontaneous abortions. Malignant sequelae, usually consisting of persistent (nonmetastatic) GTD, develop in less than 10% of patients after evacuation of partial hydatidiform moles.[2]

In contrast, complete hydatidiform moles have a 46, XX or 46, XY karyotype derived from the paternal genome.* Histologically these are characterized by absence of fetal development and diffuse, often massive hydropic degeneration of chorionic villi with diffuse trophoblastic proliferation.[39,40] The uterus is often enlarged more than would be expected based on gestational age. The clinical and ultrasonographic diagnosis is most often that of hyda-

*References 1, 4, 16, 18, 39, 40.

Table 71-1. Partial versus complete hydatidiform mole

	Partial mole	Complete mole
Cytogenetic analysis	69, XXX	46, XX
	Occasional 69, XXY	Occasional 46, XY
	Paternal + maternal origin	Paternal origin
Pathology features		
Fetus, amnion, fetal vessels	Frequent	Rare
Hydropic villi	Variable, irregular	Diffuse, often pronounced
Trophoblastic proliferation	Focal, slight to moderate	Variable, often pronounced
Clinical features		
Clinical/ultrasound diagnosis	Missed abortion	Molar pregnancy
Uterus large for dates	Rare	25% to 50%
Malignant sequelae	< 10%	10% to 30%

tidiform mole. In contrast to partial moles, patients with complete moles have approximately a 20% incidence of malignant sequelae after evacuation, with 10% to 20% of these having metastatic disease.[8,24,31]

Despite these differences, the management and surveillance of partial and complete molar gestations are similar. Once the diagnosis is suggested by clinical findings or ultrasound, the workup of a patient with a molar gestation involves screening for metastatic disease and stabilizing the patient for evacuation. The evaluation consists of a complete physical examination, baseline hCG level, chest x-ray, hematologic profile, renal and liver function tests, and thyroid function tests. If the uterus is larger than 14 to 16 weeks' size or the patient has pregnancy-induced hypertension, arterial blood gases should be obtained preoperatively because many of these patients develop respiratory insufficiency after evacuation. A baseline ultrasound should be obtained to screen for the presence of thecalutein cysts.

Evacuation of hydatidiform mole

Several techniques for evacuation of hydatidiform moles have been used in the past, including induction of labor with oxytocin or prostaglandins, hysterotomy, cervical dilatation with suction curettage (D and C), and hysterectomy. Of these, we recommend suction D and C or, if the patient desires sterilization, abdominal hysterectomy.

Suction curettage. The patient should be hemodynamically stable, with correction of preoperative anemia and stabilization of pregnancy-induced hypertension or systemic manifestations of hyperthyroidism, if these are present. If the uterus is more than 14 to 16 weeks' gestational size, a central line should be placed for intraoperative central venous pressure monitoring and rapid administration of fluids or blood products during the procedure. At least 2 U of blood and a laparotomy set should be available in the operating room.

We follow these steps for suction D and C of a hydatidiform mole:

1. The cervix is dilated gently with Pratt dilators.

2. The largest available suction canula (14 to 16 mm) is introduced through the cervix into the midendometrial cavity. Since the myometrium is often distended and soft, no attempt is made to sound the uterus to the fundus in order to avoid uterine perforation.

3. During suction curettage, one hand is placed on the fundus to assist in achieving uterine contraction through fundal massage and to sense involution of the uterus during evacuation of the uterine contents.

4. Suction is applied, and the canula is initially rotated to evacuate uterine contents. The majority of the hydatidiform mole will be removed using this maneuver without requiring vigorous curettage.

5. Pitocin in a concentration of 20 U/L is begun only after cervical dilatation has been completed and the suction curettage started to prevent contractions against an undilated cervix.

6. As the uterine fundus involutes with evacuation and uterine contraction, completion of evacuation of the uterine contents is performed using gentle curettage with the suction canula.

7. After evacuation of uterine contents with the suction canula, the endometrium is gently curetted using a large sharp curette to ensure complete evacuation. Also, this may yield the diagnosis of invasive mole (chorioadenoma destruens) if villi are seen invading the myometrium directly without intervening endometrium. The diagnosis of invasive mole is an indication for chemotherapy, but it is extremely difficult to make from the uterine curettings.

8. Pitocin infusion is continued for 12 to 24 hours following evacuation, until vaginal bleeding is minimal.

Hysterectomy. In women who desire sterilization, hysterectomy offers the advantages of simultaneous evacuation of hydatidiform mole and sterilization. Additionally, performance of hysterectomy decreases the risk of malignant sequelae to approximately 3.5% from the 20% anticipated for those treated with D and C.[8] However, since hysterectomy does not eliminate the potential for malignant sequelae, all women must be monitored for hCG levels after hysterectomy. We recommend a simple total abdominal hysterectomy as the procedure of choice in women with hydatidiform mole because of uterine enlargement and, rarely, adnexal or intraabdominal metastases. Most women with hydatidiform mole are younger than 40 years; therefore the adnexa should not be removed unless the patient is perimenopausal or there are obvious adnexal metastases. Theca-lutein cysts usually regress spontaneously following evacuation or hysterectomy and do not need to be drained or removed unless torsion or intraoperative rupture has occurred.

Other techniques of molar evacuation. Induction of labor with oxytocin or prostaglandins produces an increased risk of disseminating trophoblast through the systemic circulation caused by uterine contractions against an undilated cervix. Blood loss may be great, and evacuation is often incomplete, requiring suction D and C.[32] Hysterotomy is also associated with increased blood loss compared to suction D and C. The vertical uterine incision frequently results in a need for cesarean section to deliver subsequent pregnancies. This is an important consideration in the majority of these patients, who are in the prime reproductive age group. Additionally, Tow[46] found that evacuation of hydatidiform mole with hysterotomy resulted in a greater incidence of postmolar malignant sequelae than did suction D and C.

Complications associated with evacuation

Theca-lutein cysts. Clinically evident (larger than 5-cm) theca-lutein cysts are detectable in approximately one fourth of women with hydatidiform mole, with additional smaller cysts often detected by ultrasound alone.[8,26] Histologically and physiologically these are similar to conditions of iatrogenic ovarian hyperstimulation caused by exogenous gonadotrophin/hCG administration for ovulation induction. These cysts will usually spontaneously regress with evacuation of the hydatidiform mole and diminishing hCG levels. It is very rare for a patient to develop overt ovarian hyperstimulation with fluid retention and/or ascites. However, an occasional patient will develop ovarian torsion or rupture and bleeding of the cysts, requiring oophorectomy.[26]

Montz, Schlaerth, and Morrow[26] studied the natural history of theca-lutein cysts. They reported that the presence of these cysts was associated with both acute complications of molar evacuation and subsequent development of postmolar malignant GTD. Although cyst size did not affect the incidence of postmolar GTD, bilaterality or theca-lutein cysts associated with a complication of molar evacuation increased the risk of postmolar GTD to approximately 75%, with a risk of 52% for patients who had theca-lutein cysts but lacked bilaterality. In addition, 16% of the theca-lutein cysts developed 2 to 13 weeks after evacuation, and these were also associated with a 75% risk

of postmolar GTD. Others have documented an increased risk of postmolar GTD when theca-lutein cysts are associated with uterine enlargement greater than dates.[8,31]

Theca-lutein cysts usually regress spontaneously with diminishing hCG levels, but approximately 30% enlarge in response to the rising hCG levels associated with postmolar GTD.[46] Occasionally theca-lutein cysts persist for several months beyond hCG level remission.[46]

Respiratory distress syndrome. Many potential causes for respiratory distress exist during evacuation of molar gestation, including trophoblastic deportation, high-output congestive heart failure caused by anemia or hyperthyroidism, preeclampsia, and iatrogenic fluid overload. Pulmonary complications appear in approximately one quarter of all patients with uterine size more than 16 weeks' gestation.[47] In a small series of patients studied with invasive central monitoring during suction D and C, a transient impairment of left ventricular function was observed during general anesthesia.[7] This might contribute to the development of pulmonary edema in unmonitored patients given large volumes of crystalloid during the procedure. In general, pulmonary complications should be managed with ventilator support and central monitoring with a Swan-Ganz catheter to measure pulmonary wedge pressures and thus accurately determine fluid status and the need for blood products or diuresis. All patients should have a chest x-ray after evacuation of hydatidiform mole to rule out significant trophoblastic deportation or pulmonary edema.

Uterine perforation. Fortunately, uterine perforation rarely occurs as an acute complication during suction D and C for hydatidiform mole.[32] If perforation is recognized, the suction should be immediately discontinued and the rate of Pitocin infusion increased. Laparoscopy or laparotomy should be performed to assess the site of perforation. If hemostasis is adequate and there is no damage to the gastrointestinal organs, curettage can be completed under direct visualization.

Rarely, uterine perforation occurs during or after suction D and C in a focus of deep myometrial penetration by invasive mole. Surgical management should be individualized based on the site and extent of perforation. Although some patients require hysterectomy, anecdotal case reports have suggested that individual patients with invasive moles can be treated with segmental resection and repair of the affected myometrium.[4] Perforation occurs most frequently in the midline of the uterine fundus. The full-thickness myometrial incision usually requires cesarean section for delivery of subsequent pregnancies.

Management after molar evacuation

Monitoring of serial quantitative serum hCG levels is the only reliable means for detecting malignant sequelae of hydatidiform mole.[8,24,31] One of any number of sensitive assays employing polyclonal or monoclonal antibodies to either whole-molecule or total-beta hCG fragments can be used for monitoring. A baseline level should be obtained within 48 hours of evacuation and serial levels followed at 1-week intervals until normal hCG levels are attained. Levels should then be followed at 1- to 2-month intervals to ensure that spontaneous remission is sustained beyond 6 to 12 months. It is rare to observe reelevation of hCG caused by malignant GTD after more than 6 months of normal hCG levels without an intercurrent pregnancy. Physical examination and chest x-ray should be repeated every 2 to 4 weeks as long as the hCG level is more than 1000 ImU/ml. Patients who have not undergone hysterectomy should use active contraception until sustained regression has been documented. Usually oral contraceptives are recommended since these do not increase the risk of malignant sequelae.[4]

Malignant sequelae following evacuation of hydatidiform mole are diagnosed if the hCG levels rise acutely or if they plateau (±10%) over more than 2 to 3 weeks. Additionally, the histologic diagnosis of choriocarcinoma or invasive mole, or the appearance of metastatic disease, is an indication for chemotherapy.

Patients with malignant sequelae after hydatidiform moles frequently develop vaginal bleeding and uterine enlargement. The efficacy of a secondary D and C to remove additional trophoblastic tissue and allow spontaneous regression has never been prospectively evaluated. Schlaerth, Morrow, and Rodriguez[30] retrospectively reviewed their experience with secondary D and C among women with GTD. The majority exhibited either a transient decrease in hCG levels followed by a subsequent rise or no effect of curettage upon hCG levels. Only 20% entered spontaneous remission after secondary D and C. Others[11,19] have observed that secondary D and C affects management in only about 10% of patients. We have been reluctant to recommend an attempt at secondary therapeutic D and C unless there is marked hemorrhage, because of the documented lack of success, increased chance of uterine perforation or infection, and possible risk of delaying therapy, which might result in uterine perforation or metastases from clinically occult intrauterine or extrauterine foci of malignant GTD.

SURGICAL MANAGEMENT OF MALIGNANT GTD

The development of effective chemotherapy has diminished the role of surgery for therapy of women with malignant GTD. However, many procedures are useful adjuncts when integrated into the management of patients with malignant GTD. Primary or delayed hysterectomy may remove central disease, and removal of distant metastases may result in the cure of highly selected women with isolated foci of drug-resistant disease.[12] We perform extirpative procedures (e.g., hysterectomy) under coverage of chemotherapy, to minimize the possibility of metastasis induced by surgical manipulation of tissues. There does not appear to be an increase in morbidity using this combined modality approach.[12,20,21] In approximately 30% of patients with high-risk metastatic disease, one or more surgi-

cal procedures will be performed during therapy, either as a planned therapeutic maneuver or to treat complications of the disease, such as hemorrhage or abscess, and allow continuation of chemotherapy.[12] Finally, we have used indwelling double- or triple-lumen central catheters for prolonged venous access in most women with high-risk disease, who often require prolonged chemotherapy, blood product support, or total parenteral nutrition during therapy.

General management

Approximately half to two thirds of cases of malignant GTD follow molar pregnancies. Gestational choriocarcinomas derived from term pregnancies, spontaneous abortions, and tubal pregnancies account for the remainder. Although the diagnosis of malignant GTD after hydatidiform mole is usually made promptly, malignant GTD resulting from other pregnancies is often diagnosed later in the course of the disease, and patients are frequently seen first with nongynecologic signs and symptoms.[13,25] It should be stressed that any woman in the reproductive age group with abnormal uterine bleeding, or metastases to the lungs, central nervous system, liver, or other distant sites from an unknown primary site of malignancy, must have the diagnosis of GTD excluded with a screening test for hCG.

Usually, malignant GTD initially invades the myometrium and penetrates small uterine vessels. Venous metastasis then occurs, resulting in pulmonary and/or vaginal metastases. Usually, systemic hematogenous metastases occur only after pulmonary metastases have become established.[37] Occasionally, pulmonary metastases are not detected by conventional chest x-ray.[27] Therefore all women with malignant GTD should have a complete metastatic survey before initial therapy, consisting of chest x-ray or computed tomography (CT) scan and CT scans of the brain, abdomen, and pelvis. A pretherapy hCG level should be obtained in addition to complete blood count and renal and liver function tests.

Anatomic stage of malignant GTD is assigned by International Federation of Gynecology and Obstetrics (FIGO) criteria[28]:

Stage I	Confined to the uterine corpus
Stage II	Vaginal or pelvic metastases
Stage III	Pulmonary metastases
Stage IV	Other systemic metastases

However, initial therapy is assigned on the basis of the risk for failure of primary single-agent chemotherapy. Either the Hammond, Weed, and Currie[12] clinical classification (see box) or the World Health Organization (WHO) prognostic index score[50] (Table 71-2) are used to determine whether the patient has low-risk or high-risk disease. In general, single-agent regimens of methotrexate or dactinomycin are used to treat patients with nonmetastatic or low-risk metastatic GTD, while those with high-risk metastatic GTD should be treated initially with multiagent chemotherapy.[9,12,14,23,35] Triple therapy with methotrexate-dactinomycin-chlorambucil or cyclophosphamide (MAC)

Hammond clinical classification

I. Nonmetastatic GTD: no evidence of disease outside of uterus—not assigned to prognostic category

II. Metastatic GTD: any metastases

A. Good prognosis metastatic GTD

1. Short duration (< 4 months)
2. Low hCG level (< 40,000 mIu/mL serum B-hCG)
3. No metastases to brain or liver
4. No antecedent term pregnancy
5. No prior chemotherapy

B. Poor prognosis metastatic GTD: any high-risk factor

1. Long duration (> 4 months)
2. High pretreatment hCG level (> 40,000 mIu/ml serum B-hCG)
3. Brain or liver metastases
4. Antecedent term pregnancy
5. Prior chemotherapy

From Hammond CB, Weed JC, and Currie JL: The role of operation in the current therapy of gestational trophoblastic disease, *Am J Obstet Gynecol* 136:844, 1980.

is often used, but patients with high WHO prognostic index scores are probably best treated with etoposide-containing regimens, since their prognosis is very poor even when MAC chemotherapy is employed.[9] Table 71-3 displays clinical groupings, therapy, and expected outcome. In general, the majority of women with malignant GTD can be cured with available chemotherapeutic regimens.

Pretherapy D and C

The theoretical benefits of a pretherapy D and C before the first cycle of chemotherapy for malignant GTD include "debulking" of the intrauterine tumor and detection of histologic changes that might correlate with response to chemotherapy. Potential disadvantages include perforation and the introduction of infection during uterine manipulation. The efficacy of routine pretherapy D and C for the purpose of debulking intrauterine disease has never been tested prospectively. Berkowitz et al[3] evaluated their experience with routine pretherapy D and C in 37 patients with nonmetastatic postmolar GTD: 20 (54%) had no tissue detected by pretherapy D and C, and 19 of these developed sustained remission with limited chemotherapy. Patients having intrauterine disease with a worsened histology were at risk for failure of initial chemotherapy. None of their patients suffered uterine perforation or other complications. However, Schlaerth, Morrow, and Rodriguez[30] documented an 8.1% incidence of uterine perforation during D and C performed in this setting, and 2 of the 3 patients with perforation required hysterectomy. We prefer to reserve secondary D and C for patients who experience significant uterine bleeding during chemotherapy.

Hysterectomy

Before effective chemotherapy was widely available, Brewer, Smith, and Pratt[5] reported a 2-year survival rate of 40% for women with nonmetastatic choriocarcinoma and only 15% for those with metastatic choriocarcinoma who were treated with hysterectomy alone. Although chemotherapy has markedly improved the outlook of women with malignant GTD, both primary and delayed hysterectomy continues to play a role in the management of patients with malignant GTD. However, primary hysterectomy is not indicated for younger patients who wish to preserve childbearing capacity.

Among 194 women with nonmetastatic or good prognosis metastatic malignant GTD reported from our institution,[12] there was a 100% sustained remission rate whether patients were treated with chemotherapy alone or chemo-

Table 71-2. World Health Organization prognostic index score for GTD

| | Score* | | | |
Prognostic factors	0	1	2	4
Age (y)	≤ 39	> 39	—	—
Antecedent pregnancy	Hydatidiform mole	Abortion	Term	—
Interval+	< 4	4-6	7-12	>12
hCG (IU/l)	< 10^3	10^3-10^4	10^4-10^5	>10^5
ABO groups (female X male)	—	O X A / O X A	B / AB	—
Largest tumor, including uterine tumor	—	3-5 cm	> 5 cm	—
Site of metastases	—	Spleen, kidney	Gastrointestinal tract, liver	Brain
Number of metastases identified	—	1-4	4-8	> 8
Prior chemotherapy	—	—	Single drug	Two or more agents

*The total score for a patient is obtained by adding the individual scores for each prognostic factor. A total score of 0–4 = low risk, 5–7 = intermediate risk, > 8 = high risk.

†Months from antecedent pregnancy.

From World Health Organization Scientific Group: Gestational Trophoblastic Disease, Tech Rep Series 692, Geneva, 1983, World Health Organization.

Table 71-3. Management summary for GTD

Category*	Therapy	Survival (%)
Nonmetastatic GTD	Primary: methotrexate regimens Salvage: dactinomycin hysterectomy	> 99
Metastatic GTD, good prognosis (WHO PI ≤ 4)	Primary: methotrexate or dactinomycin Salvage: alternative single agent hysterectomy thoracotomy	> 99
Metastatic GTD, poor prognosis (WHO PI > 4)	Primary MAC or EMA-CO† Salvage: combination regimens individualized surgical resection(s)	60–85

*Hammond criteria[30]

†Selected patients may receive brain or liver radiation therapy.

WHO PI = World Health Organization prognostic index score; MAC = methotrexate-dactinomycin-chlorambucil/cytoxan; EMA-CO = alternating cycles of etoposide-methotrexate-dactinomycin/cyclophosphamide-vincristine.

therapy combined with hysterectomy. Of those who wished to retain fertility, 89% were able to, and many have had subsequent viable pregnancies. All 32 patients treated with primary hysterectomy and primary chemotherapy achieved sustained remission compared to 87% who achieved sustained remission using initial single-agent chemotherapy alone. However, for patients who underwent primary hysterectomy the total hospitalization times were shorter, total number of courses of chemotherapy lower, and total chemotherapy dosages lower. Therefore, primary hysterectomy is indicated for patients with nonmetastatic or good prognosis metastatic GTD who do not desire to preserve childbearing capacity.

Delayed hysterectomy may be considered for patients who fail to respond to initial chemotherapy. In our experience,[12] almost all patients with nonmetastatic and good prognosis metastatic GTD who were treated with delayed hysterectomy after the failure of primary single-agent chemotherapy achieved a sustained remission without requiring multiagent chemotherapy.

Primary or delayed hysterectomy may be considered in selected patients with poor prognosis metastatic GTD who have a small extrauterine tumor burden, but in general the procedure is not as beneficial as in those with more limited disease.[12] This reflects the relatively large amount of extrauterine disease present in many of these patients. Nevertheless, primary or delayed hysterectomy may be beneficial for selected patients in this disease category.

The majority of women undergoing hysterectomy for malignant GTD have been treated with total abdominal hysterectomy, with or without preservation of the adnexa. This allows visualization of intraabdominal organs to assess for extrauterine metastases, which are rarely encountered in patients with limited disease. However, we have occasionally performed vaginal hysterectomies in women with low risk nonmetastatic GTD who have a small uterus and desire primary hysterectomy as sterilization during

their initial course of chemotherapy. We have not encountered any significant complications using standard vaginal hysterectomy techniques.

Pulmonary resection

Thoracotomy with pulmonary wedge resection or partial lobectomy is the most frequently performed surgical procedure for extirpation of distant drug-resistant metastases of GTD. Pulmonary resection can be performed safely under the coverage of chemotherapy, but it is not necessary to resect pulmonary disease in the majority of patients. Although those with persistent pulmonary nodules on chest x-ray that persist during chemotherapy may be at increased risk for recurrent GTD, radiographic evidence of tumor regression may lag far behind the hCG level response.[22,49] Some patients have persistent pulmonary nodules that have gradually resolved over several months of follow-up after completion of chemotherapy. Therefore there is no justification for the indiscriminate resection of pulmonary metastases that persist on chest x-ray during chemotherapy with a satisfactory hCG level response or after induction of hCG level remission.

Resection of pulmonary nodules in highly selected women with drug-resistant disease may be successful in inducing remission.[10,33,34,45] Before performing thoracotomy, however, it is important to exclude the possibility of active disease elsewhere. We recommend rescreening these patients with CT evaluation of the brain, thorax, and abdomen and simultaneous cerebrospinal fluid and serum beta hCG levels to search for occult extrapulmonary metastases. If the patient has not undergone hysterectomy, active pelvic disease should also be excluded radiographically with angiography or magnetic resonance imaging (MRI).

Tomoda et al[45] reviewed indications for planned resection of pulmonary metastases of GTD. They proposed the following criteria for successful resection: (1) good surgical candidate, (2) primary malignancy controlled (uterus excised or no evidence of pelvic disease on angiographic studies), (3) no evidence of other metastases, (4) solitary pulmonary lesion, and (5) persistent hCG level of < 1000 ImU/ml. In their series, 14 (93%) of 15 patients who satisfied these criteria survived after pulmonary resection compared to none of the 4 patients who had one or more unfavorable clinical feature. Other investigators[10,33,34,45] have also reported that prompt hCG level remission after resection of an isolated pulmonary nodule predicts a favorable outcome.

Craniotomy

Central nervous system metastases are clinically or radiographically detected in 8% to 15% of women with metastatic GTD and are associated with a worse prognosis than lung or vaginal metastases.* These metastases are highly vascular and have a tendency for hemorrhage, often early in the course of therapy, when patients may develop acute neurologic deterioration. The major goals of therapy are early detection of brain metastases through complete radiographic evaluation of the patient before initiating chemotherapy, stabilization of neurologic status, and institution of appropriate therapy. Craniotomy to obtain tissue for the diagnosis of GTD is not indicated. Any women of reproductive age with brain metastases or cerebral hemorrhage of unexplained cause should be screened for GTD with an hCG level.[13,21] If the hCG level is elevated and pregnancy excluded, therapy can be instituted without a tissue diagnosis.

In the United States, whole brain irradiation has been used in an attempt to prevent hemorrhage from brain metastases.[12,14,35,38,48] In contrast, Rustin et al[29] recommend early craniotomy and intrathecal methotrexate in an attempt to eradicate brain lesions. Both approaches appear to be fairly successful, and in stark contrast to patients with brain metastases from other solid tumors, the majority of women who are seen with primary brain metastases of malignant GTD will survive.

Craniotomy for resection of drug-resistant lesions is justified only rarely and then only for carefully selected patients who do not have evidence of metastatic disease elsewhere. In general we reserve craniotomy for patients who require acute decompression of hemorrhagic lesions, to allow stabilization and institution of therapy.

Other extirpative procedures

Occasionally, surgical extirpation of disease involving other sites is beneficial in treating women during primary or salvage therapy of malignant GTD.[12] Vaginal metastases are highly vascular, originating via metastasis through the submucosal venous plexus,[37] and should not be resected or biopsied unless they represent the only site of drug-resistant disease. Rare patients are seen with intraabdominal metastasis or gastrointestinal involvement,

which will require resection of involved structures in an effort to stabilize the patient during therapy.[12] Additionally, a few patients with unilateral renal metastases and limited systemic disease burden have been successfully managed by integrating primary or salvage nephrectomy with chemotherapy.[36]

Central venous catheters

A surgical procedure that we frequently use in the management of patients with poor prognosis metastatic GTD is insertion of a tunneled Hickman-Broviac catheter for central venous access.[6,15,44] This provides reliable venous access in women who require long-term chemotherapy, nutritional support, and support with antibiotics or blood components. The catheter is inserted under fluoroscopic guidance and tunneled subcutaneously to reduce infectious complications. Multiple lumen catheters are preferentially inserted so that one lumen can be reserved for total parenteral nutrition. Each patient is instructed in the care of the catheter site, and the catheters are maintained by a special nursing team while in the hospital to reduce infectious complications. Despite the use of strict aseptic techniques, some catheter-related sepsis, skin infections, or thrombosis will occur, requiring removal of the catheter.[6,15,44] Nevertheless, these aid in the care of patients with high-risk disease.

SUMMARY

Although the development of effective chemotherapy has resulted in improved survival of patients with GTD, surgery remains an important part of the integrated management of these women. The coordination of chemotherapy, surgery, and radiation therapy requires the availability of sensitive hCG assays and physicians with experience in the treatment of these diseases. Patients undergoing intensive therapy for poor-prognosis GTD are best managed by physicians with experience in coordinating a multidisciplinary approach to the treatment of GTD.

REFERENCES

1. Bagshawe KD: Risk and prognostic factors in trophoblastic neoplasia, *Cancer* 38:1373, 1976.
2. Berkowitz RS, Goldstein DP, Bernstein MR: Natural history of partial molar pregnancy, *Obstet Gynecol* 66:677, 1983.
3. Berkowitz RS et al: Pretreatment curettage—a predictor of chemotherapy response in gestational trophoblastic neoplasia, *Gynecol Oncol* 10:39, 1980.
4. Berkowitz RS et al: Oral contraceptives and post-molar trophoblastic disease, *Obstet Gynecol* 58:474, 1981.
5. Brewer JI, Smith RT, Pratt GB: Choriocarcinoma: absolute survival rates of 122 patients treated by hysterectomy, *Am J Obstet Gynecol* 85:84, 1963.
6. Broviac JW, Cole JS, Scribner BH: A silicone rubber atrial catheter for prolonged parenteral alimentation, *Surg Gynecol Obstet* 136:602, 1972.
7. Cotton DB et al: Hemodynamic observations in evacuation of molar pregnancy, *Am J Obstet Gynecol* 138:6, 1980.
8. Curry SL et al: Hydatidiform mole: diagnosis, management and long-term follow up in 347 patients, *Obstet Gynecol* 45:1, 1975.
9. DuBeshter B et al: Metastatic gestational trophoblastic disease: expe-

*References 1, 9, 12, 14, 23, 29, 35, 38, 48.

rience at the New England Trophoblastic Disease Center, 1965–1985, *Obstet Gynecol* 69:390, 1987.

10. Edwards JL, Makey AR, Bagshawe KD: The role of thoracotomy in the management of pulmonary metastases of gestational choriocarcinoma, *Clin Oncol* 1:329, 1975.

11. Flam F, Lundstrom V: The value of endometrial curettage in the follow up of hydatidiform mole, *Acta Obstet Gynecol Scand* 67:649, 1988.

12. Hammond CB, Weed JC, Currie JL: The role of operation in the current therapy of gestational trophoblastic disease, *Am J Obstet Gynecol* 136:844, 1980.

13. Hammond CB et al: Diagnostic problems of choriocarcinoma and related trophoblastic neoplasms, *Obstet Gynecol* 29:224, 1967.

14. Hammond CB et al: Treatment of metastatic trophoblastic disease: good and poor prognosis, *Am J Obstet Gynecol* 115:451, 1973.

15. Hickman RO et al: A modified right atrial catheter for access to the venous system in marrow transplant recipients, *Surg Gynecol Obstet* 148:871, 1979.

16. Jacobs PA et al: Mechanism of origin of complete hydatidiform moles, *Nature* 286:714, 1980.

17. Jacobs PA et al: Human triploidy: relationship between paternal origin of the additional haploid complement and development of partial hydatidiform mole, *Ann Hum Genet* 46:223, 1982.

18. Kajii T et al: XX and XY complete moles: clinical and morphologic correlations, *Am J Obstet Gynecol* 150:57, 1984.

19. Lao TT, Lee FH, Yeung SS: Repeat curettage after evacuation of hydatidiform mole: an appraisal, *Acta Obstet Gynecol Scand* 66:305, 1987.

20. Lewis J Jr, Ketcham AS, Hertz R: Surgical intervention during chemotherapy of gestational trophoblastic neoplasms, *Cancer* 19:1517, 1966.

21. Lewis J Jr et al: The treatment of trophoblastic disease with the rationale for the use of adjunctive chemotherapy at the time of the indicated operation, *Am J Obstet Gynecol* 96:710, 1966.

22. Libshitz HI, Barber CE, Hammond CB: The pulmonary metastases of choriocarcinoma, *Obstet Gynecol* 49:412, 1977.

23. Lurain JR et al: Gestational trophoblastic disease: treatment results at the Brewer Trophoblastic Disease Center, *Obstet Gynecol* 60:354, 1982.

24. Lurain JR et al: Natural history of hydatidiform mole after primary evacuation, *Am J Obstet Gynecol* 145:591, 1983.

25. Magrath IT, Golding PR, Bagshawe KD: Medical presentation of choriocarcinoma, *Br Med J* 2:633, 1971.

26. Montz FJ, Schlaerth JB, Morrow CB: The natural history of theca lutein cysts, *Obstet Gynecol* 72:247, 1988.

27. Mutch DG et al: Role of computed axial tomography of the chest in staging patients with non-metastatic gestational trophoblastic disease, *Obstet Gynecol* 68:348, 1986.

28. Pettersson F et al, editors: *Annual report on the results of treatment in gynecologic cancer,* vol 19, Stockholm, 1985, International Federation of Gynecology and Obstetrics.

29. Rustin GJS et al: Weekly alternating etoposide, methotrexate and actinomycin/vincristine and cyclophosphamide chemotherapy for the treatment of CNS metastases of choriocarcinoma, *J Clin Oncol* 7:900, 1989.

30. Schlaerth JB, Morrow CP, Rodriguez M: Diagnostic and therapeutic curettage in gestational trophoblastic disease, *Am J Obstet Gynecol* 162:1465, 1990.

31. Schlaerth JB et al: Prognostic characteristics of serum human chorionic gonadotropin titer regression following molar pregnancy, *Obstet Gynecol* 58:478, 1981.

32. Schlaerth JB et al: Initial management of hydatidiform mole, *Am J Obstet Gynecol* 158:1299, 1988.

33. Shirley RL, Goldstein DP, Collins JJ Jr: The role of thoracotomy in management of patients with chest metastases from gestational trophoblastic disease, *J Thorac Cardiovasc Surg* 63:545, 1972.

34. Sink JD, Hammond CB, Young WG: Pulmonary resection in the management of metastases from choriocarcinoma, *J Thorac Cardiovasc Surg* 81:830, 1981.

35. Soper JT, Clarke-Pearson DL, Hammond CB: Metastatic gestational trophoblastic disease: prognostic factors in previously untreated patients, *Obstet Gynecol* 71:338, 1988.

36. Soper JT et al: Renal metastases of gestational trophoblastic disease: a report of eight cases, *Obstet Gynecol* 72:796, 1988.

37. Sung H et al: A staging system of gestational trophoblastic neoplasms based on the development of the disease, *Chin Med J* 97:557, 1984.

38. Surwit EA, Hammond CB: Treatment of metastatic trophoblastic disease with poor prognosis, *Obstet Gynecol* 55:565, 1980.

39. Szulman AE: Syndromes of hydatidiform moles: partial versus complete, *J Reprod Med* 29:788, 1984.

40. Szulman AE, Surti U: The syndromes of hydatidiform moles. I. Cytogenetics and morphologic correlations, *Am J Obstet Gynecol* 131:665, 1978.

41. Szulman AE, Surti U: The syndromes of hydatidiform moles. II. Morphologic evolution of the complete and partial mole, *Am J Obstet Gynecol* 132:20, 1978.

42. Szulman AE, Surti U: The clinicopathologic profile of the partial hydatidiform mole, *Obstet Gynecol* 59:597, 1982.

43. Szulman AE et al: Human triploidy: association with partial moles and non-molar conceptuses, *Hum Pathol* 12:1016, 1981.

44. Thomas HJ et al: Hickman-Broviac catheters, *Am J Surg* 140:791, 1980.

45. Tomoda Y et al: Surgical indications for resection in pulmonary metastases of choriocarcinoma, *Cancer* 46:2723, 1980.

46. Tow WSH: The place of hysterotomy in the treatment of hydatidiform mole, *Aust N Z J Obstet Gynaecol* 7:97, 1967.

47. Twiggs CB, Morrow CP, Schlaerth JB: Acute pulmonary complications of molar pregnancy, *Am J Obstet Gynecol* 135:189, 1979.

48. Weed JC, Hammond CB: Cerebral metastatic choriocarcinoma: intensive therapy and prognosis, *Obstet Gynecol* 55:89, 1980.

49. Wong LC, Ma HK: Persistent chest opacity in trophoblastic disease: is thoracotomy justified? *Aust N Z J Obstet Gynaecol* 23:237, 1983.

50. World Health Organization Scientific Group: *Gestational trophoblastic disease,* Tech Rep Series 692, Geneva, 1983, World Health Organization.

Part XI

GYNECOLOGIC SURGERY

Chapter 72

PENETRATING WOUNDS OF THE PREGNANT UTERUS AND FETUS*

Thomas L. Ball†
David H. Nichols

GENERAL CONSIDERATIONS

The presence of the pregnant uterus modifies the type of injury that is sustained from objects penetrating the abdominal wall and perineum. The pregnant uterus affords protection to the other viscera and displaces the abdominal and pelvic contents to somewhat different locations, depending on the duration of the pregnancy. Many pregnant women have been injured by bullets, shrapnel, and other objects capable of inflicting a penetrating wound during recent military conflicts, in which attacks on military targets in the vicinity of large cities were commonplace. It is expected that many more such accidents will happen in any future conflict, because it would not be possible, at least in the early stages of an attack, to single out pregnant women for evacuation. Other factors that increase the likelihood that these injuries will occur include the trend for women to remain actively employed during pregnancy, an increase in women undertaking jobs that are considered more hazardous, and the increase in violence in society in general.

ETIOLOGY AND PATHOLOGIC ANATOMY

In civilian accidents, the most common penetrating object is an accidentally discharged bullet. The accidents occurring during the bombing of large cities place secondary objects in motion by the explosion. The change in the position of the peritoneal reflections of the bladder, uterus,

*Modified from Ball TL: *Gynecologic surgery and urology*, ed 2, St. Louis, 1963, Mosby.
†Deceased.

and bowel in the various months of pregnancy is the most important factor in determining the type of injury. The protection given to other abdominal organs by the pregnant uterus and fetus varies with the duration of pregnancy, and organs that are ordinarily vulnerable to penetrating wounds of the abdomen are less so in the presence of a term pregnancy. Figure 72-1 shows some of the common wounds that may occur with the fetus at term. The bowel is crowded into the upper abdomen at this time, and a penetrating wound entering above the fundus might be expected to penetrate several loops of bowel. Perforations of the bowel, whether in the presence of a pregnancy or not, tend to occur in multiples of two. This fact should be remembered in exploring the abdomen after accidents, because fragments passing through a segment of bowel have a wound of entrance and a wound of exit. The fragment may pass through the bowel and the uterine wall to lodge in the placenta. This may cause a premature separation of the placenta, with concealed bleeding. The fragment may enter the uterus and cause a laceration of the cord, with death of the fetus. The deflection of fragments from bony structures within the pelvis, with the creation of secondary fragments of bone, causes many bizarre wounds. Wounds from missiles in which the entrance is in the perineum are less serious if they are below the levator muscle (Fig. 72-1). The possible course of these missiles is determined to decide whether supralevator or infralevator injuries or a combination of both has occurred. Lacerations of the cervix and vagina occur and may preclude vaginal delivery.

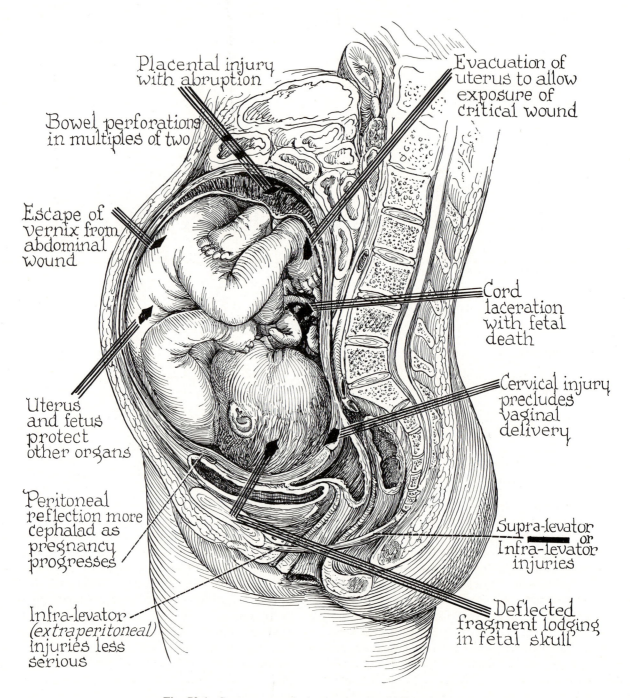

Placental injury
with abruption

Evacuation of
uterus to allow
exposure of
critical wound

Bowel perforations
in multiples of two

Escape of
vernix from
abdominal
wound

Cord
laceration
with fetal
death

Uterus
and fetus
protect
other organs

Cervical injury
precludes
vaginal
delivery

Peritoneal
reflection more
cephalad as
pregnancy
progresses

Supra-levator
or
Infra-levator
injuries

Infra-levator
(extraperitoneal)
injuries less
serious

Deflected
fragment lodging
in fetal skull

Fig. 72-1. Common wounds that may occur with fetus at term.

There is almost an unlimited combination of wounds that may occur in addition to those injuries sustained by the fetus. In assessing the probable damage, the surgeon constantly keeps in mind the change in the peritoneal reflection and the position of the fetus, placenta, and abdominal and pelvic viscera at the various weeks of pregnancy. Despite the apparent vulnerability of the fetus and pregnant mother to such penetrating wounds, the number of case reports is relatively small and the survival rate is reasonably good. There are no statistical studies available to suggest the number of casualties that may be anticipated among pregnant women during a mass attack. They have undoubtedly occurred in considerable numbers, but seldom, under wartime conditions, does the physician stop to analyze the individual factors resulting from the pregnancy that may have influenced the type of wounds observed.

SYMPTOMS AND DIAGNOSIS

The wounds of entrance and exit are noted on all parts of the chest, abdomen, and perineum. The wound of entrance is usually smaller than the wound of exit and may be further identified by threads of cloth or grease from the object along the edges of the entrance hole. Amniotic fluid, as well as vernix, may escape from the abdominal wound, and this confirms a perforation of the uterine wall. The passage of meconium in the abdominal wound suggests severe injury, with death of the fetus or severe injuries to the fetus. If x-ray facilities are available, the fetus and placental site are studied to locate objects or bullets that may have lodged in either the fetus or placenta. Fragments of shrapnel and other objects have been passed in the lochia after penetrating wounds of the pregnant uterus and subsequent delivery. Injuries to other organs in conjunction with the pregnant uterus may not show the characteristic signs and symptoms seen in the nonpregnant state due to their displacement and the added confusing factors resulting from injury to the pregnant uterus or fetus. Many injuries are not diagnosed until the uterus is emptied and an exploratory laparotomy is performed.

SURGICAL PRINCIPLES

The surgical principles in dealing with penetrating wounds during pregnancy are discussed under four headings: (1) abdominal injuries involving the pregnant uterus with the fetus alive and viable, (2) abdominal injury not affecting the pregnant uterus with the fetus alive and viable, (3) abdominal injuries that have a favorable prognosis but with a fetus that is premature or not viable, and (4) abdominal or perineal injuries with no involvement of the uterus itself in which labor is either in progress or imminent. There are many other possible situations, each of which must be evaluated individually. If the fetus is alive and viable, the abdominal injuries are repaired, usually after evacuation of the uterus by cesarean section. The obstetrician decides at this time whether a Porro section or a section hysterectomy should be done, depending on the extent of the damage to the uterus. The judgment of the obstetrician in this decision is the result of many years of experience and skill in determining the future capabilities of the uterus and the possible complications that would result from its retention. Injuries that do not affect the uterus, in which the fetus is alive and viable, are managed by evacuating the uterus to facilitate the repair of other organs. In exceptional cases the pregnant uterus is removed to manage wounds in the pelvis in which the presence of the recently evacuated uterus causes technical difficulties. The presence of a premature fetus and an abdominal injury with a favorable prognosis again requires the skill and judgment of the obstetrician to decide whether or not the pregnancy can be allowed to continue or whether the uterus must be evacuated and the fetus lost. Many factors enter into the final decision, but, if it appears that the patient is going into premature labor, the most conservative course is to evacuate the uterus at the time of abdominal surgery. If study of the abdominal wounds and uterus indicates that the prognosis is just as favorable with the uterus remaining, the uterus is left and measures are taken to prevent premature labor. Subsequently, the patient can be expected to deliver vaginally provided there are no injuries to

the perineum or vagina that would contraindicate this method of delivery. The problem of managing abdominal injuries while labor is in progress requires judgment as to the mode of delivery. Abdominal hemorrhage or perforation of the bowel or other vital organs cannot wait the termination of labor and a vaginal delivery. A cesarean section is done and uterine contractions are stopped by a general anesthetic, regardless of the cervical dilatation. If delivery is imminent, one might be faced with the problem of delivering the infant vaginally and immediately proceeding with a laparotomy for multiple abdominal injuries that may not have seriously affected the uterus.

PROGNOSIS

Some of the factors influencing the outcome of the patient with a perforating wound of the abdomen in the presence of a pregnant uterus are as follows: the greater the number of perforations and the greater the length of time between injury and treatment, the higher the mortality; the further the pregnancy is advanced, and therefore occupying more space, the greater is the chance of uterine injury. The contractility of the uterine musculature, however, permits severe lacerations without exsanguinating the patient. Experience in labor with a previously myomectomized uterus has taught us that the organ need seldom be sacrificed for any lacerations caused by perforating objects. The age of the patient is a consideration. Older gravidas do not tolerate abdominal wounds as well as younger patients because of arteriosclerotic changes in the vessel walls that prevent vasoconstriction. The location of wounds in the abdominal viscera is an important factor. A tear in the left colon, with the escape of formed fecal material, does not produce the dramatic symptoms of a lacerated stomach, with the escape of a large quantity of gastric contents. It likewise does not produce symptoms as soon as lesions of the small bowel, with pouring of liquid contents into the peritoneal cavity. Lack of symptoms due to the escape of formed fecal material may delay surgery, and time is a factor in the ultimate prognosis. In reviewing many of these injuries, one cannot help but be impressed with the remarkably safe locale the fetus occupies in utero, compared with the rest of us on the outside.

RUPTURE OF THE PREGNANT UTERUS BY EXTERNAL VIOLENCE

Rupture of the pregnant uterus by external violence, such as automobile accidents, falls, and crushing injuries from other accidents, is quite uncommon despite the large number of pregnant women exposed to these possibilities. Patients usually show a laceration or contusion of the abdominal wall. The signs of primary shock, loss of fetal heartbeat, and a tetanic contraction of the uterus indicate an intraabdominal and uterine catastrophe. Examination of the abdomen reveals the tender uterus and suggestive signs of intraabdominal hemorrhage. The pulse rate continues to rise, whereas the blood pressure falls, and immediate preparations must be made to combat shock and prepare the patient for operation. Treatment consists of a laparotomy, with the decision as to the preservation of the uterus being made by the obstetrician for each individual case. The fetus is frequently lost, and the placenta and fetus may be found free in the abdominal cavity. After expulsion of the fetus into the peritoneal cavity, the uterus contracts down around the point of rupture and serious hemorrhage is less likely to occur. The obstetrician decides whether the uterus can be preserved as a functional organ. If so, the rent in the uterus is repaired in layers, and systematic examination of all of the pelvic and abdominal viscera is done to exclude injury to any other organs. If not, immediate hysterectomy is performed.

BIBLIOGRAPHY

Armstrong CL, Andreson PS: Metallic intrauterine foreign body in term pregnancy, *Am J Obstet Gynecol* 78:442, 1959.

Beattie J, Daly R: Gunshot wound of the pregnant uterus, *Am J Obstet Gynecol* 80:772, 1960.

Belkap R: Gunshot wound of the pregnant uterus, *J Maine MA* 30:13, 1939.

Black B: Surgical treatment with recovery in a case of perineo-abdominal shotgun wounds from close range with multiple injuries to viscera, *Surg Clin North Am* 24:952, 1944.

Echerling B: Obstetrical approach to abdominal war wounds late in pregnancy, *J Obstet Gynaecol Br Emp* 57:747, 1950.

Elias M: Rupture of the pregnant uterus by external violence, *Lancet* 2:253, 1950.

Flamrich E: Gunshot wounds of the pregnant uterus, *Zentralbl Tynak* 65:25, 1941.

Fowler R: Gunshot wounds of the pregnant uterus, *New York J Med* 11:525, 1911.

Gourlay N: Accidental rupture of the female urethra, *J Obstet Gynaecol Br Emp* 67:991, 1960.

Helsper J: Nonperforating wounds of the abdomen, *Am J Surg* 90:580, 1955.

Holters O, Daversa B: Bullet wound of a gravid uterus with intestinal perforation, *Am J Obstet Gynecol* 56:985, 1948.

Jacobus W: Gunshot wound of the gravid uterus, *Am J Obstet Gynecol* 63:687, 1952.

Kobak A, Hurwitz C: Gunshot wounds of the pregnant uterus, *Obstet Gynecol* 4:383, 1954.

Motta M, Vianna G: Bullet wound in a pregnant uterus, *Rev de gynec e d'obst* 23:319, 1929.

Placintianu G, Turcanu G: Bullet wound in a pregnant uterus at term, *Spitalul* 48:224, 1928.

Souter RJ de N: Penetrating gunshot wound of a pregnant uterus, *Med J Aust* 2:111, 1947.

Zondek B: Shrapnel shot through the placenta, *Lancet* 1:674, 1947.

Chapter 73

ADDITIONAL INTERNATIONAL PERSPECTIVES

Lejla V. Adamyan

The elaboration of principally new methods of surgical intervention and the improvement of traditional techniques characterize the modern period of operative gynecology. A number of advances in the fields of polymeric chemistry and physics during the twentieth century have contributed to these developments in operative gynecology. Together, these developments have widened significantly the possibilities for surgical intervention in cases of varying etiology and severity, even making surgical treatment effective in some cases in which it had previously been considered inappropriate.

Among the most promising developments are (1) the use of biologic glues, such as fibrin glue; (2) the embolization of internal iliac arteries; (3) the use of preserved dura mater; (4) the use of laparoscopy in the treatment of, for example, congenital disorders, endometriosis, and postoperative rehabilitation; (5) cryotherapy and laser therapy in the surgical treatment of severe forms of endometriosis; and (6) colpopoiesis (formation of a new vagina) in patients with both vaginal and uterine aplasia.

BIOLOGIC GLUES

Despite the use of modern suturing instruments (e.g., electrical and laser devices) in reconstructive surgery, patients frequently develop adhesions and other complications postoperatively, partly because traditional methods of suturing wound edges may deform tissues, disturb the microcirculation, and cause local ischemia as a result of tension along the suture lines. Infections along puncture routes and local tissue reactions to suture materials may result in excessive adhesion formation and may lead to subsequent malfunction of the involved organ. Surgeons in many different countries have been seeking some means of nonsuture anastomosis and wound sealing that does not have such disadvantages.

Biologic glues may be used not only in reconstructive operations on the genital organs (e.g., reconstruction of the uterine tubes), but also for hemostasis (i.e., in the place of hermetic sutures) in patients with a high risk of hemorrhage or with abnormalities of coagulation. The medical glues used in gynecologic surgery are cyanoacrylate, sulfacrylate, and fibrin sealants. For the last 30 years, the use of cyanoacrylate sealants has been widespread in different fields of surgery all over the world. These sealants have a number of disadvantages, however. For example, they resolve slowly, and toxic decomposition products may have an adverse effect on tissue regeneration. Studies conducted to find ways to resolve these problems led to the development of biocompatible biologic glue.

The sealing and hemostatic properties of fibrinogen have attracted physicians' attention for several centuries; the use of blood preparations with such properties dates back to the end of the eighteenth century. In 1909, Bergel[5] reported the use of fibrin as a protective and curative preparation, and, in 1915 to 1916, Grey[10] and Harvey[11] reported using it to control hemorrhage from parenchymatous organs. Since highly purified blood plasma factors became commercially available, the problems of the use of blood products have been extensively studied in Western Europe, the United States, and the former Soviet Union.

Fibrin glue is a two-component sealant. The primary component is human fibrinogen produced by cryoprecipitation or lyophilization; this component contains factor XIII dissolved in aprotinin. The second component is an application solution that contains lyophilized thrombin and calcium salts.

Mechanism of fibrin glue action

In the end phase of the biologic process of blood coagulation, fibrinogen becomes unstable fibrin, which is then stabilized by the action of factor XII in the presence of calcium ions. Aprotinin prevents the lysis of the fibrin, resulting in the formation of a fibrin clot. The mechanism of fibrin glue action is similar. After the application of fibrin glue, numerous fibrin fibers attach themselves to the wound edges, sealing the edges and controlling diffuse bleeding from small vessels. The network of fibers provides sufficient tension strength and acts as a framework for the ingrowing fibroblasts from which connective tissue is formed, thus ensuring firm adherence of the wound edges.

In their experimental work, Hedelin and associates[12] implanted both Teflon cylinders that were empty and Teflon cylinders that were filled with 0.5% to 1% fibrin clots in the backs of rats. Microscopic and histologic examinations 1, 2, and 4 weeks after the implantation showed that all the cylinders were completely filled with granulation tissue. As early as 2 weeks after the implantation, however, granulation tissue with growing capillary buds had begun to replace the fibrin clots.

Applications of fibrin glue

Used as separate components, fibrin glues are sometimes applied with the help of the Duploject double syringe, which consists of a holder for two disposable syringes of equal volume operated simultaneously by pistons; in this case, volumes of the two components are mixed in the joining piece of the syringe clip. The fibrin glue components can also be applied in succession. When bleeding is diffuse, fibrin glue may be applied using a spray.

Surgeons in European countries such as Austria, Germany, Italy, and Great Britain generally use different modifications of commercial fibrin glue (e.g., Tissucol, Tissel, Beriplast, Sony-1, Sony-2), but those in the United States usually prefer fibrin glue made of fresh-frozen plasma obtained from a single donor or from the patient. Russian surgeons sometimes use fibrin glues that are commercially produced by the Tissucol and Beriplast companies, but may use a homemade fibrin glue.

Fibrin glue is appropriate for use in reconstructive operations on uterine tubes for infertility[2,3]; in wedge-shaped resection of ovaries, myomectomy, and metroplasty; in procedures to achieve hemostasis in the parametrium; in excisions for retrocervical endometriosis; and in a one-stage operation of colpopoiesis in which pelvic peritoneum is used.

Fibrin glue has been used successfully to treat premature rupture of the amniotic sac in the second trimester of pregnancy.[4,7-9,13,14] Fibrin glue injected into the cervical canal 3 to 4 cm above the internal cervical os and introduced from several syringes, in combination with tocolytic and antibiotic therapy, was effective for sealing the amniotic sac. Electron microscopy had shown that after the sac has been sealed, amniotic membrane regeneration was promoted at the site of the defect. Baumgarten believed that

fibrin sealing of the amniotic membranes, although safely attempted at an earlier stage of gestation, was most successful after the 32nd week. Fibrin glue has been shown to be advantageous for control of diffuse capillary bleeding when no specific bleeding source can be identified.[15] It has been used to close a small vesicovaginal fistula after the epithelial lining had been removed by a sharp curette.[16] Some authors believed that fibrin formed a scaffolding for migratory fibrinoblasts and promoted the ingrowth of capillaries.[6,12] The article by Adamyan, Myinbayev and Kulakov[1] reviewing the literature concerning the use of fibrin glue in obstetrics and gynecology is followed by an extensive and comprehensive bibliography.

Reconstructive surgery on uterine tubes. Fibrin glue may be used for implantation of uterine tubes into the uterus, isthmus-isthmus anastomosis, ampulla-ampulla anastomosis, and fimbrioplasty. In all these procedures, surgeons may use fibrin glue either to unite tissues without sutures or to stabilize suture lines.

In the implantation of tubes into the uterus after the primary procedures of the operation, fibrin glue can join the serous coat of the uterine tube and the serous coat of the uterus. In a tubal anastomosis that involves a silicon stent, the operator may use fibrin glue for a sutureless anastomosis of the tubes or in a combined technique of suture strengthening and tubal anastomosis. In fimbrioplasty, fibrin glue completely replaces suture materials.

Fibrin gluing for a tubal anastomosis requires

- Thrombin, two ampules, 800 units each
- Calcium chloride solution, 5.0 ml (40 mmol/L)
- Fibrinogen, 1 ampule (0.7 g of coagulating protein)
- Water for injection, 10 ml
- Two disposable syringes
- Four disposable needles

Each of the two ampules of thrombin is dissolved in 1.5 ml of calcium chloride. To ensure the complete dissolution of the thrombin, it is necessary to shake the ampules well. Then 0.7 g of lyophilized fibrinogen is dissolved in 10 ml of water for injection. Before the solution is made, the ampule must be shaken well to separate the powder from the wall; when the water has been added, the mixture should be shaken again. The components are applied to the tissue surface in the following sequence: thrombin, fibrinogen, thrombin, fibrinogen.

When the patient is under general anesthesia, the operator brings both uterine tubes out through the anterior abdominal wall incision and dissects them in the area of the occlusions. Then, to approximate the cut edges of the uterine horns, the operator inserts polyvinyl chloride plastic (PM-1/92) stents that are 1.33 to 2 mm in diameter and 22 cm in length. For a sutureless anastomosis, the operator places fibrin glue in the gap between the uterine tubes and presses the cut margins closely together for 2 to 3 minutes. Another application of fibrin glue over the serous coat increases the strength of the anastomosis. If a combined method is appropriate, two sutures, one in the area of attachment of the mesosalpinx and the other on the opposite side, may be placed, but not tied, before the first application of fibrin glue; the sutures are tied before the second application of fibrin glue.

Clinical data on more than 700 operations completed with the use of fibrin glue and more than 450 microsurgical procedures performed on the uterine tubes of infertile women indicate that this new biologic adhesive is a promising tool for gynecologic surgeons. Fibrin glue has been found to have several advantages, perhaps because it is made of natural blood components. It is absorbed within 10 to 15 days after the operation, never causes foreign body tissue reaction, and stimulates wound healing. In addition, fibrin glue reduces the number of postoperative adhesions, decreases the operating time required, and, as shown by the pregnancy rate among women who have undergone procedures in which fibrin glue was used, effectively maintains the anatomic patency and functional activity of the uterine tubes. Fibrin glue also contributes to hemostasis, controlling capillary oozing and making it possible to use fewer sutures. The clinical applications of fibrin glue for sutureless tissue connection are not widespread, however, because of the high cost of the commercial preparations.

Ovarian surgical procedures. In resection or biopsy of the ovaries, surgeons may use fibrin glue to achieve hemostasis or to seal the layer of the resected ovaries. The operative technique is rather simple in laparotomy. It is more difficult in laparoscopy, because the glue components undergo polymerization very rapidly and the application of fibrin glue through a laparoscope requires a long syringe and a large amount of glue. In the future, hemostasis by means of fibrin glue may become more important in laparoscopy, because surgeon-endoscopists are likely to be performing more and more procedures that require hemostasis in areas where the placement of sutures risks coagulation difficulties.

Myomectomy and metroplasty. During myomectomy and metroplasty, fibrin glue is useful for uniting the uterine serous coat without sutures, strengthening the suture lines, maintaining hemostasis, and creating a single suture-glue complex on the surface of the uterus. In the majority of cases, postoperative adhesions that lead to disorders of the female reproductive system complicate surgery for uterine myomata. These adhesions may be associated with ischemia of the uterine tissue caused by multiple sutures. A well-performed anastomosis with fibrin glue may prevent or reduce the number of serous sutures and, thus, eliminate ischemia. Furthermore, the application of additional fibrin glue on the uterine suture reduces the possibility of adhesion formation, provided polymerization has occurred.

The use of fibrin glue after the excision of the retrocervical endometrium or the rectouterine hollow enables a surgeon to stop bleeding without the use of dangerous sutures in the parametrium and the rectovaginal septum.

EMBOLIZATION OF INTERNAL ILIAC ARTERIES

The commonly used hemostatic techniques (e.g., ligation, electrocoagulation, excision of bleeding tissues, or even removal of the whole organ) involve an external approach to vessels. In the practice of medicine, however, situations sometimes arise in which the usual methods of hemostasis either are impossible or require difficult procedures that risk the life of the patient. A new approach to hemostasis in surgery—intravascular blockade of a bleeding vessel by means of artificial emboli made of hydrogel—is reducing the risks of surgery for patients in these situations.

In obstetrics and gynecology, embolization is indicated in cases of pelvic angiodysplasia and angioma in combination with any genital pathology that requires operative intervention, such as

- Uterine and adnexal tumors
- Congenital abnormalities
- Genital fistulas
- Large extraperitoneal tumors
- Pregnancy and labor associated with pronounced disorders of the pelvic vascular system
- Varicosity of pelvic veins
- Profuse coagulopathic postpartum uterine hemorrhage in association with disseminated intravascular coagulation (DIC) syndrome caused by blood diseases (e.g., Werlhof's disease, von Willebrand's disease)

Although extraperitoneal tumors make up only 0.03% to 0.3% of all growths, extraperitoneal tumors and pelvic hemangiomas are of particular concern, especially in women of reproductive age. The presence of these pathologic processes near the internal genitals, bladder and urinary canals, rectosigmoid part of the intestine, and iliac arteries (at the level or after their bifurcation) presents a high risk for hemorrhage both intraoperatively and postoperatively, and was once considered a contraindication for pregnancy and labor. Embolization of the internal iliac arteries decreases this risk.

The search for optimal occlusive materials has accompanied the resolution of the clinical problems that have arisen in the development of this technique. The main requirement is "medical cleanliness," the absence of low molecular weight additives that can have a negative effect on the patient. In addition, the material should be biocompatible; it should cause minimal inflammatory reaction and must cause no general toxic, carcinogenic, or allergic disturbances. Finally, it should be highly resistant to the influence of body substances.

Emboli made of hydrogel (poly-2-hydroxiethylmetankrilat), created in collaboration with coworkers of the Vishnevsky Institute of Surgery, the Institute of Macromolecular Chemistry, and the Institute of the Chemical Physics attached to the Russian Academy of Medical Science, appear to be the most promising. As a rule, the emboli are in the form of small balls that are 0.05 to 1.5 mm in diameter or cylinders that are 0.5 to 4 mm in diameter and vary in length. They have a spongelike structure; the pores make up approximately 50% to 60% of the volume and may be altered in form and diameter.

Mechanism of emboli action

When introduced into a vessel, an embolus swells and blocks the vessel. In spite of the pressure that it exerts on the vessel walls, the swollen embolus does not irritate or damage them. It induces hypercoagulation as early as the first day after its implantation into the vessel bed. The trigger factor for the hypercoagulation in the first hours after embolization appears to be the aggregation of thrombocytes, followed by the activation of other factors. Thrombus-forming factors are activated even in patients who have severe hypercoagulation disorders and whose hemorrhage may be life-threatening. With a reduction in anticoagulation parameters, hypercoagulation may last as long as 3 days; coagulation then decreases and becomes normal 10 to 15 days after embolization.

Simultaneously with hypercoagulation, blood proteins are absorbed along the surface of the embolus, strengthening the process of local thrombus formation. Later, connective tissue penetrates the pores of the embolus, making repatency of the vessel impossible and preventing hemorrhage.

Embolization procedures

Patients with angiodysplasias and extraperitoneal tumors need angiography to determine the peculiarities of vascularization of the tumor, as well as the diameter and topography of the vessels. The location of the tumor and its proximity to other organs and tissues determine the appropriate route of surgical access: laparotomy line, vaginal access, combined abdominovaginogenital access. The new generation of roentgenocontrast emboli has facilitated the medical procedure, because their movement is easier to monitor and control than was that of emboli used in the past. In addition, roentgenocontrast emboli with silver iodide are bactericidal, thus eliminating the risk of local tissue infection around them.

There are two methods of embolization: closed selective and open intraoperative. The two methods do not compete with each other and are sometimes used in the treatment of a single patient. The indication determines the method used.

Closed selective embolization is performed in a special operating room equipped with an electronic optical transformer that has a television device. In the first step of the procedure after the administration of local anesthesia, the operator inserts a catheter into the femoral artery. Then, the operator uses angiography to determine the character of the disorder, to identify the site of bleeding, and to control the position of the catheter in the vessel space. After introducing the emboli into the catheter lumen, the operator pushes them into the vessel until occlusion is complete. In general, 3 to 5 ml of saline and 30 to 40 emboli are required for one embolization. Control angiography follows the procedure so that the operator can determine precisely the locations and effect of the emboli.

In open, intraoperative embolization, which is useful for patients with angiodysplasias of the pelvis and extraperitoneal tumors, the operator introduces the emboli through a special syringe inserted into the great vessel exposed during the operative procedure.

Effectiveness of embolization

Nine patients with pelvic hemangiomas who underwent embolization of the internal iliac arteries up to their third or fourth branches for prophylaxis of hemorrhage in the period from 1 to 5 years before pregnancy were able to deliver infants successfully, although cesarean delivery was indicated. There was a significant decrease in the amount of hemangiomic tissue in the uterus, permitting preservation of the uterus in six patients; extravaginal extirpation of the uterus was necessary in only three patients. None of the patients experienced hemorrhage in the postoperative period.

Similarly, preliminary embolization, arteriography, and endovascular occlusion of the branches of the internal iliac artery with the help of hydrogelic emboli in four patients with extraperitoneal tumors permitted operative treatment for the tumors with minimum hemorrhage. Observations indicate that patients with extraperitoneal pelvic tumors can undergo surgery either in inpatient gynecologic facilities with the assistance of a general or vascular surgeon, or in general surgical facilities with the assistance of a gynecologist. When the extraperitoneal tumor is in the small pelvis (and has the form of sand glass) and has encroached on the perineal tissues, two surgical teams should be ready for two operative approaches: abdominovaginal or abdominoperineal.

These studies have proved the effectiveness of preoperative angiography with subsequent endovascular occlusion of major vessels in preventing intraoperative complications. Preoperative embolization of the internal iliac artery on the side affected by an extraperitoneal tumor or angiodysplasia not only ensures minimum hemorrhage, but also improves visualization and reduces trauma, which is especially important for surgery of the small pelvis. Embolization of the internal iliac arteries has also been shown to be extremely effective in arresting massive postnatal hemorrhage (2.5 L) in women with von Willebrand's disease when other methods of coagulation were unsuccessful.

USE OF PRESERVED DURA MATER

In a number of cases, surgical interventions fail to produce the desired results, especially reoperations associated with defects and scars in the tissue. Because the introduction of polymeric materials (e.g., lavsan and capron) has not always been successful in reconstructive and plastic operations in patients with uterine myoma and cervicovaginal, urogenital, and intestinovaginal fistulas, preserved tissues from the dura mater are being used to repair defects of the muscular tissue and to strengthen sutures placed during gynecologic operations.

Since World War II when surgeons first noted that dura mater is an effective barrier capable of preventing infections, neurosurgeons; abdominal, thoracic, cardiac, and vascular surgeons; traumatologists; otolaryngologists; ophthalmologists; and urologists have found transplants of these tissues to be useful in various types of operations. For example, it is possible to use such tissue to repair extensive defects of breast and abdomen, to close hermetically the stumps of bronchi, to recreate the cardiac valve apparatus, to block terminal defects of blood vessels, and to eliminate fistulas and defects of the digestive system.

The dura mater is preserved by freezing, lyophilization, or by chemical treatment with a mixture of 0.5% to 4% solution of formalin, 96% of glycerol, and 0.5% to 2% of ethylonoxide solution or b-propiolactone to retain its structural and functional features up to the moment of the operation. The many collagenic and elastic fibers that interlace in various directions give the dura mater its mechanical properties of strength, elasticity, and solidness. Because its cellular elements are limited in number, dura mater transplants have rather low immunologic activity and produce no clinical and morphologic signs of transplant rejection or sensitization of a recipient.

Personal experience with 63 patients indicates that dura mater transplants are appropriate for gynecologic reconstructive and plastic operations in patients with pronounced defects and scarring changes (e.g., defects of uterine development, uterine myomata, vaginal operations, uterine prolapse, or prolapse of the vaginal stump).

EARLY POSTOPERATIVE LAPAROSCOPY

The role of laparoscopy in gynecology in the past has been limited primarily to the diagnosis of disease in the internal reproductive organs. During recent years, surgeons have found laparoscopy to be a useful route for surgery, and in planning a postoperative rehabilitation program, in evaluating reparative regeneration processes after different surgical procedures, and in determining the prognosis for restoration of reproductive function after surgery. All these aspects are of the utmost importance in modern gynecologic surgery because of the increasing number of reconstructive procedures performed in an effort to establish or restore fertility in sterile women. In some myomectomies, repairs of incorrect uterine development, and partial resections of the uterine tubes, however, the results are still unsatisfactory.

Despite the recent large-scale introductions of microsurgery, areactive sutures, lasers, and the use of different dextrans in various surgical procedures, the incidence of adhesion development after gynecologic surgical procedures remains high. Laparoscopic reinspection by means of traditional techniques long after surgery is less effective, and due to dense adhesions can be dangerous. Only an early postoperative laparoscopy can provide the information required to correct any "fresh," reversible deviations that have followed surgery. Even if the surgery has been unsuccessful and the early laparoscopic inspection reveals the reocclusion of the uterine tubes or bowel adhesions, the surgeon can at least inform the patient of the prognosis at an early date.

After completing the initial laparotomy, the operator inserts two-channel silicon drainage tubes, 8 and 11 mm in diameter, through the counterapertures in the left and right hypogastric areas and fixes them to the skin of the front abdominal wall with capron sutures. The inner part of the drainage tubes is 5 cm long; the outer part is 10 to 15 cm long. The outer openings of the tubes are connected to hermetic and sterile devices for draining the wound secretions under negative pressure.

Laparoscopic inspection takes place on the fourth or fifth day after the reconstructive procedure. The operator first closes one of the tubes. The other tube, after being shortened and washed both inside and out, serves for the carbon dioxide pneumoperitoneum. As for the usual diagnostic laparoscopy, 1.5 to 2 L of gas are generally enough.

To begin the procedure, the operator inserts an optical system through the wide (11 mm) drain and a manipulator through the narrow drain. The operator examines the condition of the peritoneum of the small pelvis, the quantity and character of the exudate in the abdomen, and the condition of the tissues on which surgery was performed (e.g., the presence of hyperemia or edema, the status of sutures and adhesions). The patency of the tubes is tested by means of indigo-carmine hydrotubation. Fresh adhesions are separated, and hemostasis is achieved with bipolar coagulation of the blood vessels in the area. The abdomen is irrigated with isotonic saline solution, 0.01% chlorhexidine solution, or dextran.

After completing the laparoscopy, the operator removes the drains from the peritoneal cavity. There have been no reported complications associated with early postoperative laparoscopy.

SURGICAL TREATMENT OF ENDOMETRIOSIS

During the past few years, several researchers have been investigating the use of endoscopic surgery, electrocoagulation, cryodestruction, and carbon dioxide lasers in the treatment of endometriosis.

Changes were evident in all parts of the neuroendocrine system in the patients studied. For example, they experienced disorders in the cyclic increases and decreases in the level of gonadotropic and steroid hormones, as well as in the proportional relationships of these hormones; even so, the principal parameters of ovulation in the periovulatory period were normal. Also manifested were disorders of the estrogen and progesterone receptor systems in the endometrium. In fact, in patients with endometriotic foci the progesterone content in the peritoneal fluid decreased to half, with a high percentage of degenerative oocytes. There were clear irritative changes of diencephal activity, as shown by electroencephalography; some changes in the rate of metabolism, as shown by electronic paramagnetic resonance; and severe morphofunctional changes in the endometrium and in endometriotic foci, as shown by electron microscopy. Changes were greatest in patients with extended ovarian endometriosis.

To ensure the accuracy of diagnosis, serum levels of cancer antigen CA-125 were performed on 325 patients before and after surgery. In 92% of patients with endometriosis in stages II through IV or with recurring disease, the results of these tests were abnormal.

The patient's age, the site of the disease process, the stage of expansion, the desire for fertility, and the possibility of hormone therapy determined the extent of the operations.

Endometriotic ovarian cysts

If the patient with endometriosis had an ovarian cyst, removal of the cyst was the first step of treatment. In stages I and II, such cysts could be removed by means of laparoscopic electrocoagulation and laser techniques. Patients who had more severe forms of the disease, as the majority of the patients in this study did, generally required a laparotomy so that the surgeon could resect the ovaries up to the healthy tissues and clear the endometriotic foci by carbon dioxide laser. The use of the focused ray of the laser to remove the capsule of the endometriotic cyst or the use of the defocused ray in the field of cystic foci after the removal of the capsule not only facilitated the procedure, but also contributed to hemostasis, decreased the incidence of postoperative complications, and reduced the risk of recurrence of the endometriosis.

When the endometriotic ovarian cysts had initiated a reactive inflammation in the rectouterine pouch that obliterated the cul-de-sac or when adhesions of the intestine, urinary bladder, and appendix accompanied the cysts, the operator removed the appendix and dissected the adhesions.

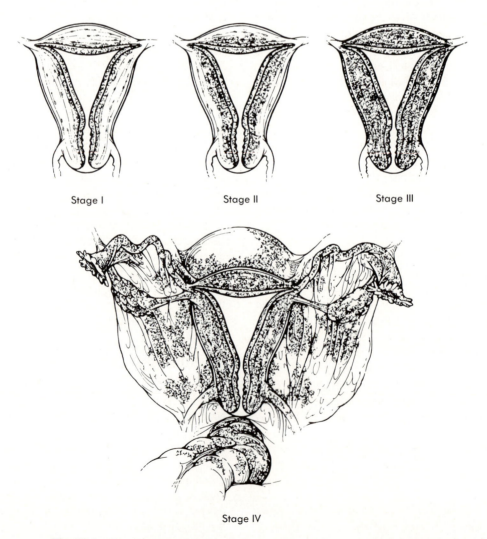

Stage I   Stage II   Stage III

Stage IV

Fig. 73-1. Classification of adenomyosis according to the extent of the disease.

Sometimes, technical hindrances made the operations extremely difficult.

Adenomyosis (internal uterine endometriosis)

Data obtained through ultrasound examination, hysterosalpingography, and hysteroscopy indicated the stage of adenomyosis among patients in the study group. The disease was classified according to the following stages (Fig. 73-1):

- Stage I: Involvement of up to one third of the myometrium
- Stage II: Involvement of tissues to the middle part of the muscular layer
- Stage III: Involvement of the entire uterine wall
- Stage IV: Involvement of tissues to the parietal peritoneum and surrounding organs

The first step in the treatment of adenomyosis was the administration of gestagens and antigonadotropins, 400 to 600 mg/day for 6 to 9 months. If the endometriosis involved the isthmus or penetrated the serous covering, however, this conservative treatment was not effective. The diffuse form of adenomyosis required hysterectomy, with or without adnexectomy.

For young infertile women with nodular adenomyosis, it was sometimes possible to perform a reconstructive operation on the uterus by resecting the myometrium and part of the endometrium with a carbon dioxide laser. The borders of the affected area in these instances were determined preoperatively and intraoperatively by means of contact ultrasonography and use of the radionuclide P-32 in the uterine tissue.

Retrocervical endometriosis

Like patients with adenomyosis, patients with retrocervical endometriosis in the study group were classified according to the extent of their disease (Fig. 73-2):

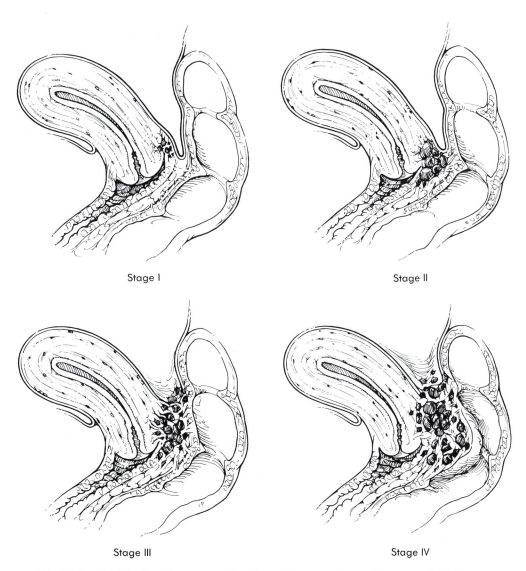

Stage I

Stage II

Stage III

Stage IV

Fig. 73-2. Classification of retrocervical endometriosis according to the extent of the disease.

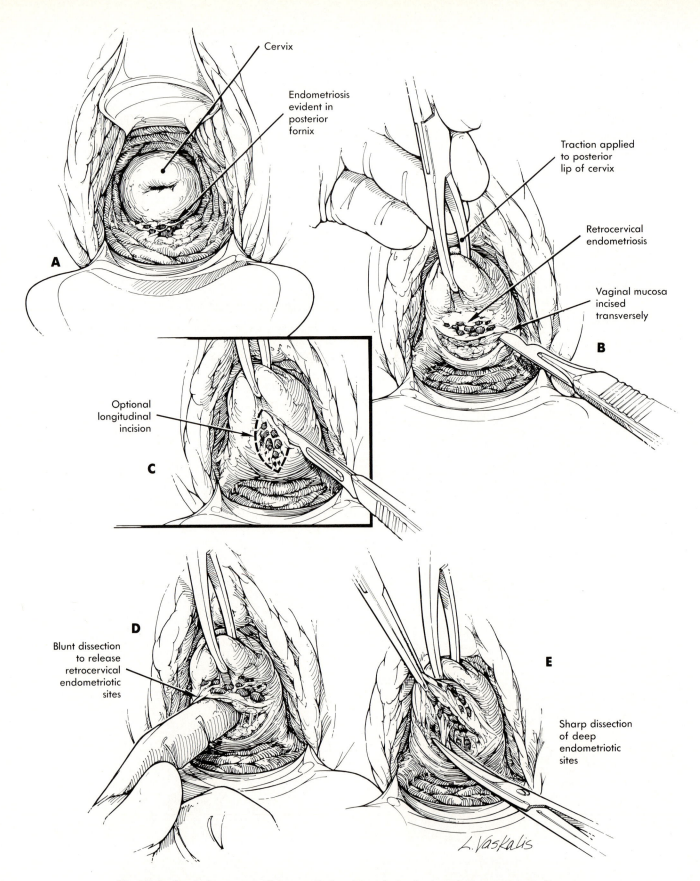

Fig. 73-3. Surgical treatment of retrocervical endometriosis. **A,** A vaginal speculum displays the areas of endometriosis visible in the posterior vaginal fornix. **B,** While upward traction is made to a tenaculum applied to the posterior lip of the cervix, a transverse incision is made through the full thickness of the vaginal wall. **C,** An alternate option is for longitudinal incision, depending on the configuration of the disease process. **D,** Blunt finger dissection may free the endometriotic foci. **E,** Sharp dissection with scissors or laser may be used if necessary.

Continued.

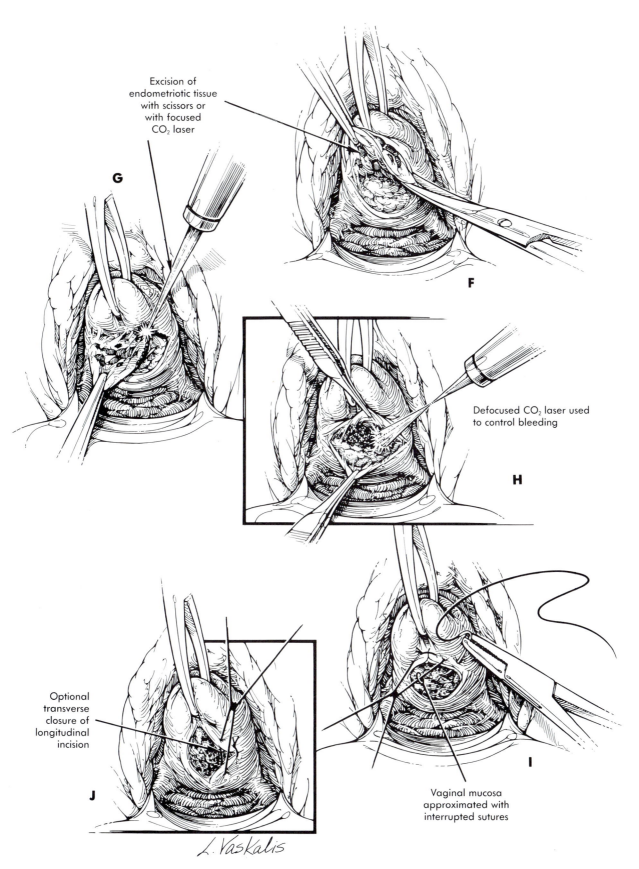

Fig. 73-3, cont'd. F, Excision of endometriotic tissue by sharp dissection. **G,** Alternatively, the tissues may be dissected by the focused beam of a CO_2 laser. **H,** Bleeding after excision of the endometriosis may be controlled by the defocused laser. **I,** The vaginal wall (mucosa) is closed transversely using interrupted absorbable sutures. **J,** Alternatively, the vaginal wall may be closed longitudinally.

Excision of endometriotic tissue with scissors or with focused CO_2 laser

Defocused CO_2 laser used to control bleeding

Optional transverse closure of longitudinal incision

Vaginal mucosa approximated with interrupted sutures

L. Vaskalis

- Stage I: Endometriotic lesions were confined to the rectovaginal cellular tissue in the area of the vaginal vault.
- Stage II: Endometriotic tissue had invaded the cervix and penetrated the vaginal wall, causing fibrosis and small cyst formation.
- Stage III: Lesions had spread into the sacrouterine ligaments and the rectal serosa.
- Stage IV: The rectal wall, rectosigmoid zone, and rectouterine peritoneum were completely involved, and the rectouterine pouch was totally obliterated.

The surgical methods used in the treatment of patients with retrocervical endometriosis included (1) the removal of foci by scalpel, (2) evaporation by carbon dioxide laser, (3) cryodestruction, and (4) electrocoagulation. In patients who underwent laser treatment, the focused ray was applied for tissue dissection and the evaporation of endometriotic foci; the defocused ray was applied for the additional treatment of the most severe cases of retrocervical endometriosis. The operator sometimes used a vaginal route, sometimes an abdominal route, and sometimes a combination of the two (i.e., laparoscopy and vaginal access).

Combined treatment procedure. The patient who is to undergo a combined treatment procedure for endometriosis is prepared for surgery as if the procedure were a bowel operation, and general anesthesia is administered. After performing laparoscopy and hysteroscopy according to routine procedures, the operator introduces the vaginal speculum and fixes the posterior lip of the cervix in a position as far as possible toward the front (Fig. 73-3, *A*). The operator incises the vaginal mucosa at the level of the posterior fornix either longitudinally or transversely, depending on the site of the endometriosis (Fig. 73-3, *B* and *C*). Grasping the lesion with bowel clamps, the operator removes the tissue from the vaginal side with a carbon dioxide laser focused ray (Fig. 73-3, *D* through *G*). If the removal of the endometriosis is successful, there is no need for a special culdotomy; however, use of the defocused carbon dioxide laser may be necessary to control bleeding from the site of the endometriosis (Fig. 73-3, *H*). The vaginal mucosa is then repaired with interrupted absorbable sutures (Fig. 73-3, *I* and *J*).

For patients with endometriosis at stage II or III, the operator uses a manipulator and a laparoscope to perform posterior colpotomy under direct vision and to remove as much endometriotic tissue as possible from the retrocervical cellular tissue (Fig. 73-4). To prevent a bowel injury, the operator controls the rectum by holding and moving the peritoneum with the manipulator. After a thorough inspection, the operator uses the focused ray of a carbon dioxide laser to dissect the endometriotic tissue from both the peritoneal side and the vaginal side.

If cryogenic equipment is available, it is advisable to perform a cryodestruction of the endometriotic lesions in the area of the sacrouterine ligament, a procedure that takes 3 minutes. The use of both the carbon dioxide laser and cryodestruction simplifies the technical performance of the operative procedures and reduces the frequency of complications and recurrences. Hormonal therapy with antigonadotropins, gestagens (e.g., gestrinone), and gonadotropin-releasing hormone agonists is often helpful; if hormonal therapy fails to produce any effect or if accompanying disease contraindicates a trial of hormonal therapy, hysterectomy is necessary.

The combined treatment is appropriate for young women who are infertile or dysmenorrheic and hope to preserve their reproductive function. Women who are 35 years of age or older and have completed their families generally undergo hysterectomy for retrocervical endometriosis. When the disease has reached stage IV, the combined approach to surgery is not always adequate because the entire pathologically altered area cannot be completely removed.

Surgery on adjacent organs. If the preliminary urologic and endoscopic examination reveals involvement of the adjacent organs (e.g., bladder and intestine) in the endometriosis, the gynecologic surgeon should consult a specialist in the involved area. The most serious operations are those in which the endometriosis has invaded the bladder walls and urinary tract. In these patients, the operator (1) reconstructs the urinary tract at the level of the endometriotic lesions, with dissection of the occlusion; (2) implants the distal part of the ureter into the bladder from one or two sides; and (3) performs a sigmocystoplasty.

Invasion of the walls of the bladder and the ureter, resulting in a scarring deformity; renal disorders of filtration secretion; hydroureters; and dilation of the urinary tract because of pronounced stenosis of distal parts due to endometriosis are indications for sigmocystoplasty. In this procedure, the operator resects the part of the bladder invaded by endometriosis, cuts a flap from the wall of the sigmoid colon to use in reconstructing the bladder wall, implants the distal parts of the ureter into the sigmoid colon, reconstructs the bladder, and creates a urinary sac from the wall of the sigmoid colon. This operation often has complications, but it is the procedure of choice if hormonal therapy has no effect or is contraindicated.

Postoperative treatment

Every patient who has undergone surgical treatment for endometriosis should have an individualized program of rehabilitation. The primary task of postoperative care is to prevent complications, reduce the risk of recurrence, and eliminate secondary functional disturbances such as neuroendocrine insufficiency or vascular dystonia.

In general, postoperative rehabilitation is a complex regimen that includes several types of care. For example, exercise therapy and the administration of antibiotics and

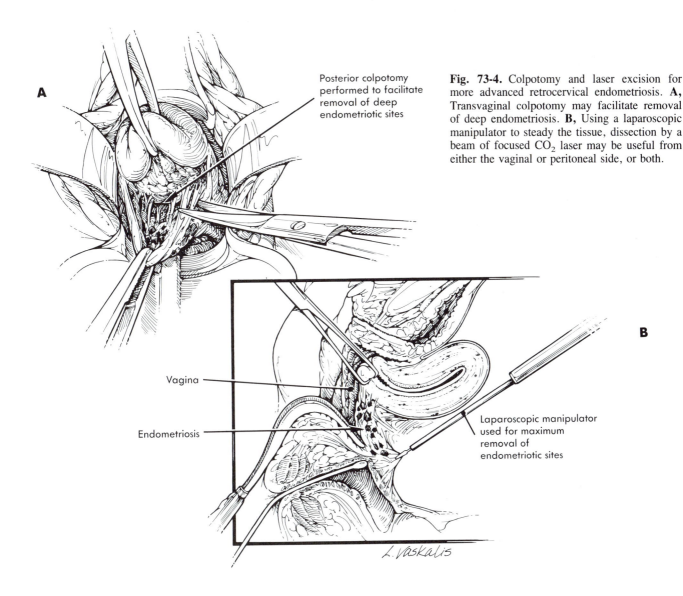

Posterior colpotomy performed to facilitate removal of deep endometriotic sites

Fig. 73-4. Colpotomy and laser excision for more advanced retrocervical endometriosis. **A,** Transvaginal colpotomy may facilitate removal of deep endometriosis. **B,** Using a laparoscopic manipulator to steady the tissue, dissection by a beam of focused CO_2 laser may be useful from either the vaginal or peritoneal side, or both.

Vagina

Endometriosis

Laparoscopic manipulator used for maximum removal of endometriotic sites

L. Vaskalis

anticoagulants are both normally part of the regimen. The application of a variable magnetic field during the first postoperative days not only has antiinflammatory, dehydratic, hypocoagulant, and analgesic effects, but also activates immunocompensatory mechanisms. Hyperbaric oxygenation is helpful in the prophylaxis and treatment of intestinal ileus after laparotomy, and it has a normalizing effect in tissues, organs, and systems. Hyperbaric oxygenation also stimulates the receptor systems of trigger organs.

Treatment with radon may be helpful for its anti-inflammatory effect, restoration of metabolic processes on the cellular level, regulation of the nervous system and ovarian function, and stimulation of compensatory-rehabilitative functions. Severe psychoemotional and neuroendocrine disorders are indications for iod-bromatherapy in the form of baths and vaginal irrigations. The therapeutic value of this therapy is in its sedative effect and in its positive influence on the glucocorticoid function of the adre-

nal cortex, thyroid gland function, and hypothalamo-hypophyseal ovarian system.

Hormonal therapy may be necessary to correct endocrine dysfunction. Data suggest that gestagens may prove useful in the treatment of patients with endometriosis because they suppress the gonadotropic function of the hypophysis, decrease the steroid production of the ovaries, and have a positive local effect on the level of receptors of the endometrium and endometriotic lesions. The rationale for the use of antigonadotropins in the treatment of severe endometriosis is based on the fact that danazol, an active steroid, suppresses the secretion of gonadotropins and induces atrophy and regression in the tissue of endometriotic heterotopies.

During the last 5 years, patients with endometriosis have been given agonists of hormone-releasing preparations (e.g., Baserelin) in a dose of 300 to 400 mg. The administration of such agonists produces a temporary medical oophorectomy and, as a result, leads to the atrophy and regression of endometriotic lesions. Research is now being conducted on treatment with the agonists of prostaglandins and immunomodulators.

The final results of treatment for endometriosis depend on the severity of the condition at diagnosis, the difficulty of operative intervention, the effect of rehabilitative and hormonal therapy, and the degree of disruption to the reproductive system before surgery. Dynamic supervision, including ultrasound examination (once in 3 months) and CA-125 tests (once in 3 months), is essential during the postoperative period.

COLPOPOIESIS IN VAGINAL AND UTERINE APLASIAS

Over the last century, gynecologic surgeons have tried a variety of methods to create an artificial vagina for patients with vaginal and uterine aplasias, but none has been completely satisfactory. In an effort to develop a simpler, more effective technique, surgeons have devised a one-stage colpopoiesis in which the pelvic peritoneum is used as a reconstructive material.

As in all methods of operative treatment for vaginal aplasia, the most important stage is the creation of the bed for the future vagina, because there is always a danger of wounding the bladder or rectum. The patient is placed on the table in the supine position with the legs wide apart. The patient's pelvis is placed so that the surgeon can manipulate the tissues with a vaginal retractor.

One-stage colpopoiesis of pelvic peritoneum

After the labia minora are spread wide apart, the operator makes a 3- to 4-cm incision in the vaginal orifice along the lower edge of the labia minor between the urethra and the rectum (Fig. 73-5, A and B). The operator dissects not only the epithelial coat, but also 1 to 1.5 cm of the deeper fascia (Fig. 73-5, C). When the fascial plate is open (Fig. 73-5, D), the operator inserts two fingers and moves them straight ahead as far as the peritoneum of the small pelvis, dividing the tissues between the bladder and the rectum (Fig. 73-5, E). (In another technique, the operator may insert a speculum deeper and deeper to separate these tissues.) The movement of the fingers (or the speculum) from side to side creates a rather wide canal in which the operator will subsequently place the transplant.

In some cases, the operator can separate the tissues between the bladder and the rectum rather easily; if the tissue must be dissected near the bladder or the rectum, however, there is a risk that the adjacent organ may be injured. Although this injury is the most frequently occurring complication of the procedure, its incidence is actually very low (approximately 1% in 500 patients). In the event of such an injury, the operator sutures the wound and continues the procedure. When pulled down later, the peritoneum will cover a wound in the rectum and facilitate healing. If the bladder is injured, a catheter should remain in the bladder for 5 to 7 days. After an injury to the rectum, the pa-

tient should be given antibiotic therapy, be placed on a liquid diet, and be followed as if she had undergone a rectovaginal fistula repair.

The dissection is continued until the pelvic peritoneum has been exposed and incised transversely (Fig. 73-5, F).

The pelvic peritoneum appears as a sagging, thin, pale yellow plate. The most difficult stage of the operation is the identification of the peritoneum. To make it easier, the operator may use one of the following procedures:

1. Injection of indigo-carmine solution into the bladder so that the bladder mucosa can be identified before it is inadvertently opened.
2. Puncture of the abdominal cavity through the vagina and aspiration of its contents. If the needle is placed into the abdominal cavity, light, amber peritoneal fluid is always seen.
3. Traction on the peritoneum applied with the manipulator of a laparoscope to avoid trauma to the adjacent organs.

The operator takes the peritoneum with long forceps, opens it, pulls it down (Fig. 73-5, G), and sutures it to the skin in the vaginal orifice (Fig. 73-5, H). Then, using the rudiment of the uterus, the operator forms a vaginal fornix from the side of the vagina by placing three or four catgut sutures with a small round needle. If there is no uterine rudiment, the operator sutures the peritoneum separately to the bladder walls, rectum, and back wall of the pelvis with separate catgut sutures (Fig. 73-5, I through K). If there are any difficulties in forming the vaginal tunnel, the operator should also use a laparoscope.

Laparoscopic colpopoiesis

A laparoscopic examination is helpful to determine the precise abnormality of genital development. In patients with vaginal and uterine aplasia, laparoscopy may reveal a muscular "embankment" positioned in the center of the small pelvis transversely between the bladder and the rectum (Fig. 73-6, A). The peritoneum of the small pelvis in this area has ample mobility. Generally, the most mobile part of the peritoneum is approximately 5 to 7 cm behind the muscular embankment.

The operator incises the perineum midway between the urethra and anus transversely. In general, the best place for this incision is the lower edge of the labia minora, where they meet the skin of the perineum. Using both blunt and sharp dissection to make a tunnel between the bladder wall and the rectum, the operator reaches the small pelvis peritoneum. The operator then uses a laparoscopic manipulator to move the peritoneum so that he or she can open it from the vaginal side, dissect it, and pull it to the dissected skin of the vagina (Fig. 73-6, B).

The peritoneum is fixed with separate catgut sutures to the perineal skin around the full circumference, and the vaginal fornix is created from the small pelvis peritoneum that covers the bladder and front wall of the rectum (Fig.

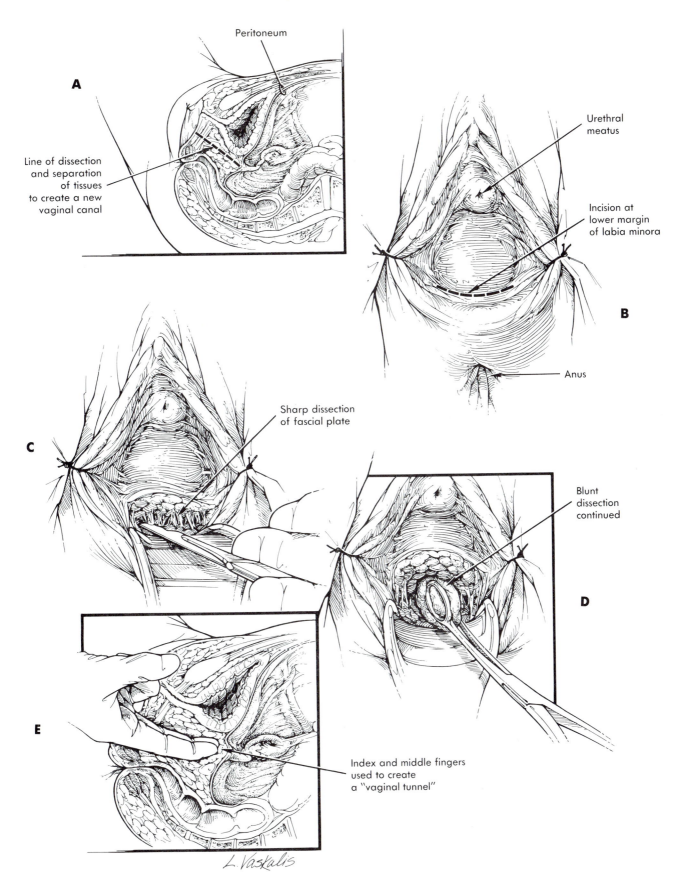

A

Peritoneum

Line of dissection
and separation
of tissues
to create a new
vaginal canal

Urethral
meatus

Incision at
lower margin
of labia minora

B

Anus

Sharp dissection
of fascial plate

C

Blunt
dissection
continued

D

E

Index and middle fingers
used to create
a "vaginal tunnel"

L. Vaskalis

Fig. 73-5. One-stage colpopoiesis using peritoneum to line the new vagina. **A,** Sagittal view of a patient with vaginal agenesis. The pathway of dissection to create a new vagina is shown by the broken line. **B,** A transverse incision between the lower edges of the labia minora is made at the site indicated by the broken line. **C,** Sharp dissection of the subepithelial fascial plate begins as shown. **D,** It is continued bluntly in a cranial direction. **E,** The tissues between bladder and rectum are divided by dissection using two fingers, palm side up.

Continued.

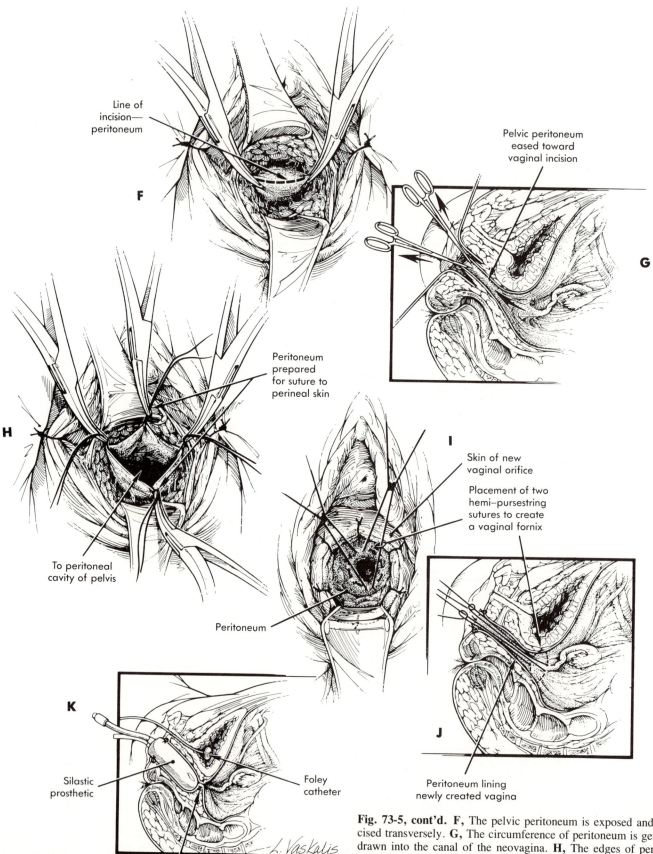

Line of incision— peritoneum

Pelvic peritoneum eased toward vaginal incision

F

G

Peritoneum prepared for suture to perineal skin

H

To peritoneal cavity of pelvis

Peritoneum

I

Skin of new vaginal orifice

Placement of two hemi-pursestring sutures to create a vaginal fornix

K

Silastic prosthetic

Foley catheter

J

Peritoneum lining newly created vagina

Vaginal fornix created

—L. Vaskalis

Fig. 73-5, cont'd. F, The pelvic peritoneum is exposed and incised transversely. **G,** The circumference of peritoneum is gently drawn into the canal of the neovagina. **H,** The edges of peritoneum are sewn to the skin of the vaginal orifice. **I,** The peritoneal cavity is closed by two hemi-pursestring sutures placed high in the neovagina. **J,** Closing of the peritoneal cavity is shown in sagittal drawing. **K,** A Foley catheter is inserted into the bladder, and a silicone prosthesis is inserted into the vagina.

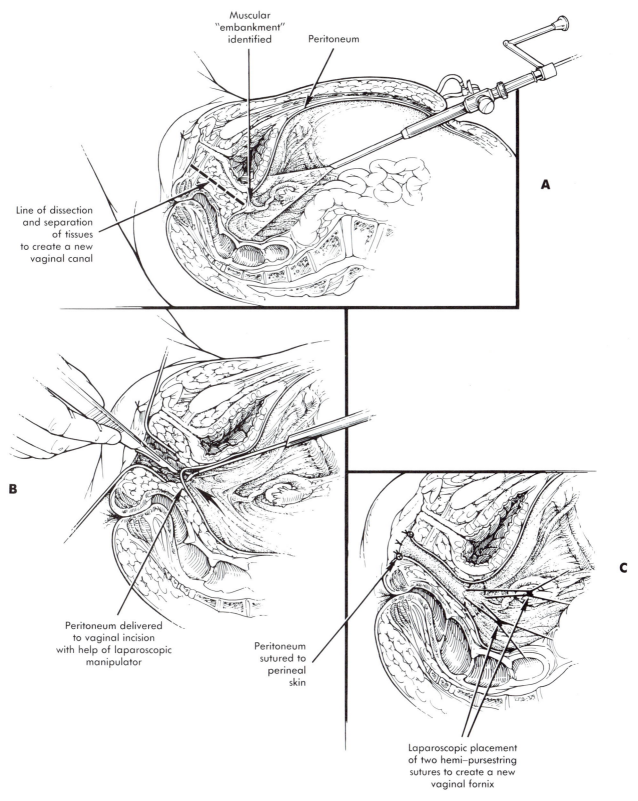

Muscular "embankment" identified

Peritoneum

A

Line of dissection and separation of tissues to create a new vaginal canal

B

Peritoneum delivered to vaginal incision with help of laparoscopic manipulator

Peritoneum sutured to perineal skin

C

Laparoscopic placement of two hemi-pursestring sutures to create a new vaginal fornix

Fig. 73-6. Laparoscopy-assisted colpopoiesis. **A,** Laparoscopic examination of the pelvis is performed. The site of transvaginal dissection for creation of a neovagina is shown by the dashed line. **B,** Using a laparoscopic probe or manipulator may help to deliver the peritoneum to the new tunnel. The peritoneum is opened transversely. **C,** The cut edges of peritoneum are sewn to the skin of the vaginal orifice, and the peritoneal cavity is closed by two hemi-pursestring sutures placed through the laparoscope.

73-6, *C*). The operator can perform the latter reconstructive procedure either from the peritoneal cavity, by using the laparoscope, or from the vaginal side. Separate purse-string sutures of absorbable material (e.g., Dexon, Vicryl) are placed longitudinally 10 to 12 cm from the vaginal orifice. In some cases, the operator creates the fornix center by connecting the muscular embankment to the bladder peritoneum.

Results of surgery

A one-stage colpopoiesis with the use of the pelvic peritoneum seldom takes more than 25 to 45 minutes, but it results in a new vagina, which, when lined up with growth of squamous epithelium from the orifice, is physiologically similar to a natural one. It has an acid pH, for example. Furthermore, after epithelialization, the new vagina has the same cyclic changes. Coitus is permissible 10 to 15 days after the surgery.

REFERENCES

1. Adamyan LV, Myinbayev OA, Kulakov VI: Use of fibrin glue in obstetrics and gynecology: a review of the literature, *Int J Fertil* 36:76, 1991.
2. Akuns KB: Nonsuture method of salpingo-salpingoanastomosis using fibrin tube, *Sovetskaya Med* 1:82, 1965.
3. Akuns KB: Salpingostomy using fibrin tube, *Akusherstvo Gynecol* 7:71, 1968.
4. Baumgarten K, Moser S: The technique of fibrin adhesion for premature rupture of the membranes during pregnancy, *J Perinat Med* 14(1):43, 1986.
5. Bergel S: Über Wirkungen des Fibrins, *Deutsch Med Wochenschr* 35:663, 1909.
6. Bruhn H et al: *Regulation der Fibroblastenproliferation durch Fibrinogen/Fibrin, Fironectin und Faktor XIII*. In Schimpf K, editor: *Fibrinogen, fibrin and fibrin glue*, Stuttgart, New York, 1980, FK Schattauer, p 217.
7. Genz HJ: Die Behandlung des vorzeitigen Blasensprungs durch Fibrinklebung, *Med Welt* 30(42):1557, 1979.
8. Genz HJ, Gerlach H, Metzger H: *Behandlung des vorzeitige Blasensprungs durch Fibrinklebung*. In Deutscher E, Zechner, editors: *Fibrinolyse, Thrombose, Hämostase*, Stuttgart, New York, 1980, p 698.
9. Genz HJ et al: *Antibiotikahaltiger Fibrinkleber zur Behandlung des vorzeitigen Blasensprungs in Perinatale Medizine*. In Dudenhausen JW, Saling E, editors: *Perinatale Medizine*, Band IX. Stuttgart, 1982, Tieme.
10. Grey EC: Fibrin as a hemostatic in cerebral surgery, *Surg Gynecol Obstet* 21:452, 1915.
11. Harvey SC: The use of fibrin paper and forms in surgery, *Boston Med Surg J* 174:6, 1916.
12. Hedelin H et al: Influence of fibrin clots on development of granulation tissue in preformed cavities, *Surg Gynecol Obstet* 154(3):1982.
13. Kulakov VI et al: The use of fibrin glue in gynecological reconstructive plastic operations, *Akusherstvo Gynecol* 1990.
14. Kurz CS, Huch A: Fibrin sealing: an advanced therapy in dealing with premature rupture of membranes, *J Perinat Med* 10:66, 1982.
15. Moront MG et al: The use of topical fibrin glue at cannulation sites in neonates, *Surg Gynecol Obstet* 166(4):358, 1988.
16. Petersson S et al: Fibrin occlusion of a vesicovaginal fistula, *Lancet* i(8122):933, 1979.

EPILOGUE

Because of a predictable constant increase in the cost of hospitalization and in the number of older women requiring surgical care for restoration of quality of life, the need for more sophisticated gynecologic surgery to be done safely will increase almost exponentially in the years ahead. These needs appear to be international in scope and demand, and to preserve their cost effectiveness will require progressively longer periods of surgical training and experience. In most instances this will require a constant refinement of available skill to include those not all equally well developed in the surgeons presently practicing and will embrace operative pelviscopy, transvaginal pelvic reconstruction of all types, and a full menu of transabdominal gynecology, gynecologic urology, and reconstruction of the dysfunctional sigmoid colon and rectum. In all probability a large volume of surgery will be done in the future by a smaller number of better surgeons—those who can operate consistently with the lowest complication rates and provide a minimal necessity for reoperation. Surgical mediocrity will not be excusable.

New combinations of operative procedures embracing the above will come into focus, and it is conceivable, for example, that the future operation of choice for invasive squamous cell carcinoma of the cervix might be laparoscopic pelvic lympadenectomy, followed by the Schaüta radical vaginal hysterectomy in appropriate cases in which the greatest diameter of the tumor is less than 4 cm. In selected cases this may provide for the safe removal of the largest amount of tissue in the shortest operating time.

It has been demonstrated that all variety of gynecologic surgery can be done through the laparoscope, but it must be proven that such laparoscopic surgery is not only better for the patient but is cost effective for society in general, and furthermore, that it can be taught effectively to willing gynecologic surgeons. Measurements of this efficacy must coincide with development and implementation of a credentialing process for such surgery that will safeguard the best interests of the patient. Further new techniques will evolve, and they must be adequately tested before they are made available widely. Since the needs of women are so similar in so many nations and cultures throughout the world, politically free cooperation between physicians and surgeons including the exchange of both teaching and learning personnel and implementation of ideas and significant concepts will speed this process immeasurably.

INDEX

The letter *f* following a page number indicates a figure; the letter *t* indicates a table.

A

Abbe-McIndoe-Read procedure, 798, 800*f*
Abbe-McIndoe vagina, 412-413*f*
  full or partial, 416-417
Abdominal bleeding, as gynecologic symptom, 102-103
Abdominal evisceration, 199-203, 201*f*, 202*f*
Abdominal hysterectomy, 11, 19-21, 226; *See also* Hysterectomy
  for benign disease, 19-20
  complications in, 297
  for endometrial cancer, 532-533
    additional procedures in, 534
    intrafascial technique for, 532
    and kind of hysterectomy, 533-534
    operating personnel in, 534-535
  indications for, 297
  infection from, 226
  for malignancy, 20
  support of vaginal vault at time of total, 537-538
  technical considerations, 515
    American technique, 515-517, 516*f*, 518*f*, 519*f*, 520*f*, 521, 522*f*
    Japanese technique, 521, 523*f*, 524-530*f*, 531*f*
    hospitalization following, 531
    psychological preparation of patient for, 531-532
  in Twentieth Century, 20-21
  versus vaginal hysterectomy, 297, 298*t*
Abdominal masses, as gynecologic symptom, 103
Abdominal myomectomy, 610-618*f*
Abdominal pain, as gynecologic symptom, 102
Abdominal pregnancy, 1067, 1071
Abortion, 1016*t*
  correlation with conization, 267-268
  first trimester
    complications of
      bladder injury, 1024
      bowel injury, 1023-1024
      hematometra, 1023
      hemorrhage, 1023
      perforation, 1023
      postabortal triad, 1023
    in reduction of multifetal pregnancies, 1022
    surgical techniques, 1016-1017
      medical abortion, 1021-1022
      minisuction, 1021, 1022*f*
      standard vacuum curettage, 1017*t*-1021*f*, 1018*f*
  induced, and incompetent cervix, 1034
  infection from, 226-227
  recurrent, as indication for hysteroscopy, 751
  second trimester
    choice of procedure, 1028
      fetal death in utero, 1028-1029
    complications
      disseminated intravascular coagulopathy (DIC), 1027
      failed abortion, 1027-1028*f*

labor induction methods
    dilatation and evacuation (D and E), 1025-1026*f*
    hypertonic saline, 1026
    intraamniotic urea, 1026-1027
    intrauterine prostaglandins, 1027
    oxytocin, 1027
    systemic prostaglandins, 1027
  suction curettage in, 258
  in third trimester, 1029
Abruption, as complication in cesarean section, 1107-1108, 1110*f*
Abruptio placentae, 1045
Abscess
  appendiceal, 922-924
  Bartholin's, 239
  diverticular, 924
  formation
    following vaginal hysterectomy, 226
    as postoperative complication, 136-137
  ovarian, 1132
  tuboovarian, 225, 636-638
Acquired immunodeficiency syndrome (AIDS)
  and blood exposure in operating room, 163
  and ethical considerations, 155
  risk in postoperative blood transfusion, 114
  risk in use of amnion, 414, 801, 802
  risk in use of cryoparticipate, 214
  and surgical glove perforation, 127
ACTH, and surgical stress, 82
Actinomycin
  for gestational trophoblastic neoplasms, 699
  for placental accreta, 1109
Adenocarcinoma, 928
Adenomyosis, 541, 1172*f*, 1173
Adenomyosis interna, and need for dilation and curettage, 257
Adhesions
  intrauterine
    hysteroscopy in, 755*ft*-756*t*
    labial, 797, 798
  laparoscopy for
    dense adhesions, 744
    filmy adhesions, 744*f*
    prevention of, 744
      needle and trocar insertion, 744
  small-intestine, 925, 927
Adjunctive surgery, with cesarean section, 1116
Adnexa, 541
Adnexal surgery for benign disease, 652
  choosing surgical approach, 653
    oophorectomy and oophorocystectomy, 654-656, 655*f*-657*f*, 658*f*, 659
    ovarian preservation at hysterectomy, 659
    parovarian cysts, 659
    tubal cysts, 659
    vascular surgical anatomy of adnexum, 653-654
  preoperative diagnosis and management, 652-653
Adnexectomy, 653, 654, 659
Afibrinogenemia, congenital, 210
Agenesis
  of breast, 981-983
  of vagina, 825
AIDS; *see* Acquired immunodeficiency syndrome (AIDS)

Alanine, 90
Alkeran, 697
Alkylating drugs, 697
Allis forceps, 829
Alpha-fetoprotein, 693
Ambulatory surgery
  of Bartholin's gland, 239
  biopsy of vulva, 239, 240*f*
  cervical intraepithelial neoplasia, 253, 256, 257
  dilation and curettage, 257-258, 259*f*, 260, 261*f*
  endometrial biopsy, 260, 262*f*
  excision of endometrial or endocervical polyp, 253, 254*f*, 255*f*
  excision of vaginal apex, 248, 250*f*, 251*f*, 252*f*, 253*f*
  lesions of urethra of the hymen, 242, 245*f*, 246*f*, 247*f*, 248
  obstructed vagina, 248
  vulvar vestibular syndrome, 242, 248
  Wolffian duct cyst, 253, 255*f*
American Association of Gynecologic Laparoscopists, 6
Amine test, 631
Amino acid metabolism, 94-95
Amniocentesis
  in abdominal pregnancy, 1071
  historical perspectives of, 1009
  risks of, 1010-1011
  technique of, 1010*f*
  in timing cesarean section, 1116
  utility of, 1009-1010
Amniotic fluid embolism, as complication in cesarean section, 1111, 1112*f*
Ampullary fembriectomy, 1116
Anal warts, laser vaporizations of, 281
Anastomosis
  cornual, 775-783*f*, 794
  end-to-end, 928, 929*f*
  results of, 746
  side-to-side, 928
  techniques of, 928-929, 930*f*-933*f*, 934*f*
  tubotubal, 783-788*f*
Anatomic stress urinary incontinence, 832
Anemia
  as complication following myomectomy, 620
  correction of, prior to myomectomy, 609-610
  as postoperative complication, 143
Anesthesia, 8-9
  for cesarean hysterectomy, 1128
  for cesarean section, 1112-1113*f*, 1114*f*, 1115*f*
  for dilation and evaluation, 1026
  for tubal patency restoration, 768
  for vesicovaginal fistula, 873
Anorectal prolapse, types and combinations of, 505
Anterior abdominal wall, anatomy of, 167, 168*f*, 169*f*, 170*f*, 171
Anterior colporrhaphy, 842
Anterior cystocele, 336*f*-337
Antibiotics
  for postoperative infection, 228, 232*t*-233
  prophylactic administration of, 112